MW00838000

Comprehensive Handbook of Pediatric Audiology

Second Edition

Comprehensive Handbook of Pediatric Audiology

Second Edition

Anne Marie Tharpe, PhD
Richard Seewald, PhD

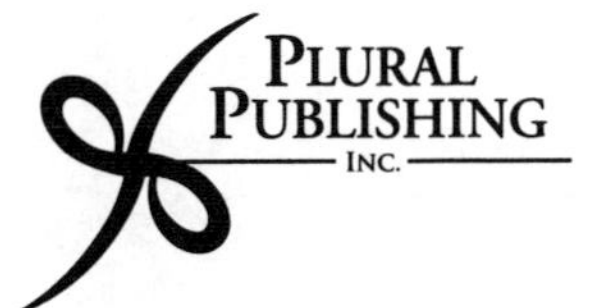

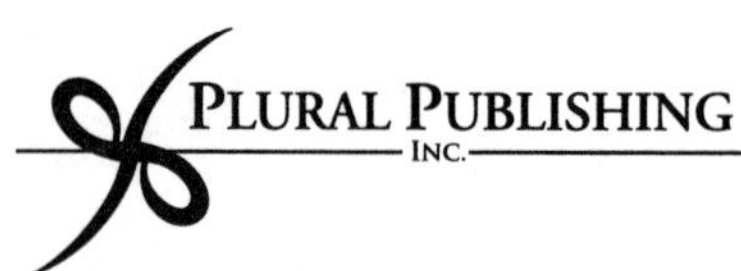

5521 Ruffin Road
San Diego, CA 92123

e-mail: info@pluralpublishing.com
Website: http://www.pluralpublishing.com

Typeset in 10/12 Palatino by Flanagan's Publishing Services, Inc.
Printed in the United States of America by McNaughton & Gunn, Inc.
20 19 18   2 3 4 5

Library of Congress Cataloging-in-Publication Data

Names: Tharpe, Anne Marie, editor. | Seewald, Richard C., editor.
Title: Comprehensive handbook of pediatric audiology / [edited by] Anne Marie Tharpe, Richard Seewald.
Description: Second edition. | San Diego, CA : Plural, [2017] | Includes bibliographical references and index.
Identifiers: LCCN 2015042632 | ISBN 9781597566155 (alk. paper) | ISBN 1597566152 (alk. paper)
Subjects: | MESH: Hearing Disorders. | Child. | Hearing Tests. | Hearing. | Infant.
Classification: LCC RF291.5.C45 | NLM WV 271 | DDC 618.92/09789—dc23
LC record available at http://lccn.loc.gov/2015042632

Contents

Foreword by Fred H. Bess, PhD ix
Acknowledgments xi
Contributors xiii

I Typical Auditory Development **1**

1 Hearing Development: Embryology of the Ear 3
Mark Hill

2 Biologic Development of the Auditory System From Periphery to Cortex 23
Robert V. Harrison

3 Infant Speech Perception 49
Derek M. Houston

4 Auditory Development in Children With Normal Hearing 67
Lynne A. Werner and Lori J. Leibold

II Etiology and Medical Considerations **87**

5 Descriptive Epidemiology of Childhood Hearing Impairment 89
Adrian Davis and Katrina A.S. Davis

6 Genetics of Childhood Hearing Loss 133
Linda J. Hood and Bronya J.B. Keats

7 Medical Considerations for Infants and Young Children With Hearing Loss: A Pediatrician's Perspective 149
Betty R. Vohr

8 Medical Considerations for Infants and Children With Hearing Loss: An Otologist's Perspective 163
Craig A. Buchman and Oliver F. Adunka

9 Current Issues in Preventable Hearing Loss 181
Andrea Hillock-Dunn and Christopher Spankovich

III Types of Hearing Loss in Children **205**

10 Conductive Hearing Loss in Children: Otitis Media With Effusion and Congenital Conditions 207
Lisa L. Hunter and Daniel I. Choo

11 Auditory Neuropathy Spectrum Disorder 227
Gary Rance and Arnold Starr

12 Management of Children With Auditory Neuropathy Spectrum Disorder (ANSD) 247
Patricia A. Roush

13 (Central) Auditory Processing Disorders in Children 269
Prudence Allen

14 Pseudohypacusis: False and Exaggerated Hearing Loss 295
James E. Peck

IV Early Identification of Hearing Loss **307**

15 Principles and Methods of Newborn Hearing Screening 309
Martyn Hyde

16 Newborn Hearing Screening Program Evaluation and Quality 349
Martyn Hyde

17 Screening for Hearing Loss and Middle Ear Disorders: Beyond the Newborn Period 383
Jackson Roush and Nicole E. Corbin

18 Newborn Hearing Screening Program Implementation: Early Hearing Detection and Intervention 413
Kathryn L. Beauchaine, Jeffrey K. Hoffman, and Diane L. Sabo

V Audiologic Assessment of Children **447**

19 Middle Ear Measurement 449
Lisa L. Hunter and Chelsea M. Blankenship

20 Otoacoustic Emissions in Infants and Children: An Updated Approach 475
Carolina Abdala, Margaret Winter, and Christopher A. Shera

21 Threshold Assessment in Infants Using the Frequency-Specific Auditory Brainstem Response and Auditory Steady-State Response 505
Susan A. Small and David R. Stapells

22 Electrophysiological Assessment of Hearing With Auditory Middle Latency and Auditory Late Responses — 551
James W. Hall III and Anuradha R. Bantwal

23 Behavioral Audiometry in Infants and Children — 591
Allan O. Diefendorf and Anne Marie Tharpe

24 Audiologic Considerations for Children With Complex Developmental Conditions — 609
Allan O. Diefendorf, Kathleen R. Corbin, Rebecca Trepcos-Klingler, and Amanda S. Weinzierl

VI Hearing Technologies — 629

25 Current Approaches to the Fitting of Amplification to Infants and Young Children — 631
Marlene P. Bagatto and Susan D. Scollie

26 Hearing Instrument Orientation for Children and Their Families — 659
Anne Marie Tharpe, Hollea A.M. Ryan, and Samantha J. Gustafson

27 Remote Microphone Systems and Communication Access for Children — 677
Jace Wolfe, Dawna Lewis, and Leisha R. Eiten

28 Measuring Outcomes of Infants and Children With Hearing Loss — 713
Teresa Y.C. Ching, Sanna Y.L. Hou, and Vicky W. Zhang

29 Cochlear Implants for Children: Promoting Auditory Development With Electrical Pulses — 739
Karen A. Gordon

30 Care of Children Who Use Cochlear Implants — 761
Marilyn Neault

31 Other Hearing Devices: Bone Conduction — 781
Bill Hodgetts

32 The Future of Auditory Implants — 793
René H. Gifford

VII Management of Childhood Hearing Loss — 813

33 History of the Management of Hearing Loss in Children — 815
Andrée Durieux-Smith and Elizabeth M. Fitzpatrick

34 Facilitating Communication in Infants and Toddlers With Hearing Loss — 829
Melody Harrison

35 Potential Meets Reality in Early Intervention for Children With Hearing Loss 849
Amy McConkey Robbins

36 Support for Adolescents With Hearing Loss 871
Kris English

37 Minimal Hearing Loss in Children 887
Heather Porter, Fred H. Bess, and Anne Marie Tharpe

38 Moderate to Profound Sensory/Neural Hearing Loss in Children 915
Karen C. Johnson, Amy S. Martinez, Laurie S. Eisenberg, and Dianne M. Hammes Ganguly

39 School-Age Children 941
Carolyne Edwards

40 Providing Services in Educational Contexts: Defining the Role of the Educational Audiologist 961
Patricia M. Chute and Mary Ellen Nevins

Index *973*

Foreword

It is difficult to pinpoint when the term *pediatric audiology* actually came into common usage. We can only assume that the concept of pediatric audiology began shortly after the development of the discipline of audiology during and following World War II. We do know that Canfield, an otolaryngologist from Yale University, made one of the earliest references to pediatric audiology in his seminal book *Audiology, The Science of Hearing* (1949). However, long before the 1940s, historical writings clearly show that early civilization experienced and appreciated the problems associated with deafness in childhood. Indeed, Greek and Latin writers referenced the plight of the deaf on several occasions in the Bible.

During the Renaissance through to the latter part of the 19th century, we read about teachers and priests who were dedicated to serving children with hearing loss. This was a period in deaf education sometimes referred to as "the age of teaching"; it was an era in which the oral method clashed with teachings that emphasized the use of signs and finger spelling. Such well-recognized teachers as Pedro Ponce de León and Juan Pablo Bonet of Spain, Samuel Heinicke of Germany, Abbe Charles Michel de l'Epee of France, and Thomas Braidwood of Scotland were early pioneers of methods and techniques for educating young deaf children. One well-known scholar who brought specific teaching methods and philosophies from Europe to America was Thomas Gallaudet. After studying with de L'Epee in Paris, Gallaudet returned to the United States and established the first school for deaf children in Hartford, Connecticut, in 1817. The school was called the American Asylum for the Education and Instruction of the Deaf and Dumb.

During the early 20th century, pediatric audiology was not yet a recognized specialty, but educational and health care professionals throughout the United States became involved by necessity in the identification, assessment, and management of very young children with hearing loss. Perhaps most notable was the work of Sir Alexander and Lady Irene Ewing who worked tirelessly to serve young children with hearing loss in Great Britain. As early as 1919, Irene Ewing opened a hearing clinic at Manchester University. The Ewings, more than anyone during this period, influenced professionals throughout the world on issues pertaining to the identification and management of childhood deafness. They introduced some of the fundamental concepts now associated with pediatric audiology: the benefits of early identification and intervention including hearing aids, the importance of parent-home training for the development of speech and language, and the effective approaches for testing young children with hearing loss. By most accounts, this was the beginning of pediatric audiology.

By the late 1950s and early 1960s, a small group of audiologists was beginning to focus its efforts on young children, and we began to hear the term *pediatric audiology* on a more frequent basis; soon thereafter, training programs started to offer specialty tracks in pediatric audiology. There were few books dedicated to young children with hearing loss. As there was no single text that met the specific needs of pediatric audiologists or university training programs, several resource books were considered essential reading. These books included *Educational Guidance and the Deaf Child* (Ewing, 1957), and *New Opportunities for Deaf Children* by Sir Alexander Ewing (1959); *Auditory Disorders in Children* by Myklebust (1954); *Deafness in Childhood* by McConnell and Ward (1967); and *Hearing and Deafness* by Davis and Silverman (1960).

Clinical protocols related to identification, assessment, and hearing aid fitting for very young children also was limited. Evidence-based procedures had not yet been developed, and clinicians working with children were forced to rely mostly on intuition and common sense for their clinical decision making—clinical practice was probably more art than science. As Liden and Harford (1985) observed, pediatric audiologists "waved their magic wand and sprinkled whiffle dust to make the child's invisible reactions visible" (p. 6). Importantly, robust clinical tools commonly used today, such as electroacoustic immittance measures, auditory brainstem responses, and otoacoustic emissions, were not yet available to pediatric audiologists for the identification, assessment, and management of children with hearing loss. Although the profession of audiology recognized the importance of early identification of hearing loss in children, the average age of identification in the United States was 3 to 4 years, and there was a significant lag between the age when a child was identified and the age when a child actually received a hearing aid. Hearing aids were large, unattractive, and produced a great deal of distortion. Receiver buttons were used to modify the electroacoustic responses of hearing aids, and Y-cords served to provide a child with bilateral amplification. Hearing aid fitting was accomplished using a comparative approach for aided sound-field behavioral thresholds. The hearing aid that provided the most threshold improvement with the least amount of irregularity across frequencies was thought to provide the best speech understanding and subsequently was the hearing aid of choice. Because it was difficult to obtain accurate thresholds on young children using behavioral methodology, the fitting strategy was an ongoing process sometimes taking more than a year to finalize.

The contents of this new edition (second) of *Comprehensive Handbook of Pediatric Audiology*, serve as a stunning reminder of how far we have come since those early years in our efforts to serve young children with hearing loss and their families. Indeed, one cannot help but be impressed with the many positive changes that have occurred since the first edition of this book. Today, better graduate education, advanced technology, and innovative clinical research have brought about significant improvements in early identification of hearing loss, audiological assessment, the selection and evaluation of amplification, and the management strategies used with young deaf children. We now have the ability to identify hearing loss in the vast majority of newborns, obtain reliable frequency-specific threshold information on infants and toddlers, and objectively fit young babies with digital hearing aids and other assistive devices. The advent of cochlear implantation has resulted in significant improvements in the speech, language, and listening skills of children with severe-to-profound bilateral sensorineural hearing loss. We also have witnessed improvements in technology and medical care that have brought about changes in the prevalence of causation and severity of hearing loss. The second edition of *Comprehensive Handbook of Pediatric Audiology* addresses all of the relevant issues impacting today's young children with hearing loss and their families. It is exciting to see in one volume comprehensive coverage of contemporary trends in pediatric audiology. No doubt, the information contained within this new edition will be of value to those who seek to better understand the perplexities of childhood deafness and motivate others to search for newer and better ways to serve young children with deafness.

A portion of the proceeds from this book will be dedicated to a student scholarship fund at Vanderbilt University named in memory of Judith S. Gravel, an outstanding alumna of Vanderbilt University and one of the true giants of pediatric audiology. In fact, it was Judy Gravel who originally envisioned the need for a book in audiology that focused on pediatric hearing loss. Her presence can be seen throughout the entirety of this book simply by reviewing the references at the end of each chapter that highlight her diversity of interest areas and contributions to the profession. Although Judy was taken from us at a young age, her life was filled with love, fun, and accomplishments that far exceeded her years. To be sure, we are all so very fortunate that she shared her many gifts with us.

—Fred H. Bess, PhD

References

Canfield, N. (1949). *Audiology: The science of hearing—A developing professional specialty*. Springfield, IL: Charles C. Thompson.

Davis, H., & Silverman, S. R. (1960). *Hearing and deafness*. New York, NY: Holt, Rinehart and Winston.

Ewing, A.W.G. (1957). *Educational guidance and the deaf child*. Manchester, UK: Manchester University Press.

Ewing, A.W.G. (1959). *New opportunities for deaf children*. Manchester, UK: Manchester University Press.

Liden, G., & Harford, E. R. (1985). The pediatric audiologist: From magician to clinician. *Ear and Hearing*, 6(1), 6–9.

McConnell, F., & Ward, P. H. (Eds.). (1967). *Deafness in childhood*. Nashville, TN: Vanderbilt University Press.

Myklebust, H. (1954). *Auditory disorders in children: A manual for differential diagnosis*. New York, NY: Grune and Stratton.

Acknowledgments

The concept and original outline for this book were developed at a meeting with Dr. Judith Gravel in July 2006. Judy was a big dreamer and saw a great need for a comprehensive text in the area of pediatric audiology. With a twinkle in her eye, she referred to this book as "the mothership." By the end of this meeting, the Table of Contents included chapters covering every conceivable topic related to the basic sciences, screening, assessment, and management associated with childhood hearing and hearing loss. It was her vision and passion that led to the development of this book. Two weeks following the July 2006 meeting with Judy, she was diagnosed with cancer. We lost Judy on December 31, 2008. Throughout her courageous battle with cancer, we asked Judy on numerous occasions if she wanted to continue the work on the book. Our queries were always greeted with silence. When Judy became silent the answer was always clear. To discontinue work on this project was never an option for Judy. We have done all that we could to ensure this book lives up to Judy's dream. We thank you, Judy.

It is possible that our work on this book had more missed deadlines than the book has pages. Nonetheless, throughout this journey we have always had the support, expertise, and patience of the exceptional group at Plural Publishing. Specifically, we would like to thank Angie Singh for her genuine encouragement and support from the very start. Throughout the process, Valerie Johns, Kalie Koscielak, and Nicole Bowman have always been there to nudge us along gently and to help us with even the smallest editorial detail. We cannot imagine having a more positive and informed group with whom to work.

We offer a special thank you to Samantha Gustafson. Her amazing organizational skills, and overall management of the editing process kept us on track for the last year and a half. We simply could not have done it without her! We are also grateful to Melanie Jordan who took on the tremendous task of verifying thousands of references for us. And, of course, we would like to thank the 68 authors who took time from their research, clinical, and administrative activities to share their knowledge, experiences, and wisdom with the readers of this volume.

Finally, we would like to thank our life partners Jim and Carol for their unqualified support of our work on this project—we promise to make up for lost time!

—Anne Marie Tharpe and Richard Seewald

Contributors

Carolina Abdala, PhD
Professor
Tina and Rick Caruso Department of Otolaryngology-Head and Neck Surgery
Keck School of Medicine
University of Southern California
Los Angeles, California
Chapter 20

Oliver F. Adunka, MD, FACS
Professor and Division Director
Department of Otolaryngology-Head and Neck Surgery
The Ohio State University Wexner Medical Center
Director, Pediatric Otology
Nationwide Children's Hospital
Columbus, Ohio
Chapter 8

Prudence Allen, PhD
Director
National Centre for Audiology
Associate Professor
School of Communication Sciences and Disorders
Faculty of Health Sciences
The University of Western Ontario
London, Ontario, Canada
Chapter 13

Marlene P. Bagatto, AuD, PhD
Adjunct Research Professor
National Centre for Audiology
Western University
London, Ontario, Canada
Chapter 25

Anuradha R. Bantwal, MSc (Audiology and Speech Rehabilitation)
Visiting Faculty
Ali Yavar Jung National Institute for the Hearing Handicapped
Audiologist and Speech-Language Pathologist
AURED—Aural Education for the Hearing Impaired
Mumbai, India
Chapter 22

Kathryn L. Beauchaine, MA, CCC-A
Audiology Coordinator, Hearing and Balance Center
Boys Town National Research Hospital
Omaha, Nebraska
Chapter 18

Fred H. Bess, PhD
Vickie and Thomas Flood Professor
Department of Hearing and Speech Sciences
Vanderbilt Bill Wilkerson Center
Vanderbilt University School of Medicine
Director
National Center for Childhood Deafness and Family Communication
Nashville, Tennessee
Chapter 37

Chelsea M. Blankenship, AuD
PhD Student
University of Cincinnati
Cincinnati, Ohio
Chapter 19

Craig A. Buchman, MD, FACS
Lindburg Professor and Chair
Department of Otolaryngology
Washington University School of Medicine
St. Louis, Missouri
Chapter 8

Teresa Y.C. Ching, PhD
Senior Research Scientist
Team Leader for Rehabilitation Procedures
National Acoustic Laboratories
Sydney, Australia
Chapter 28

Daniel I. Choo, MD, FACS, FAAP
Professor and Director
Division of Pediatric Otolaryngology Head and Neck Surgery
Cincinnati Children's Hospital Medical Center
Department of Otolaryngology Head and Neck Surgery
University of Cincinnati
Cincinnati, Ohio
Chapter 10

Patricia M. Chute, EdD, CCC-A
Dean
School of Health Professions
New York Institute of Technology
Health Policy Fellow
Old Westbury, New York
Chapter 40

Kathleen R. Corbin, MA, CCC-A
Audiologist
Riley Hospital for Children at Indiana University Health
Indianapolis, Indiana
Chapter 24

Nicole E. Corbin, AuD
Department of Allied Health Sciences
Division of Speech and Hearing Sciences
University of North Carolina School of Medicine
Chapel Hill, North Carolina
Chapter 17

Adrian Davis, OBE, FFPH, FSS, FRSA, PhD
Director
AD CAVE Solutions Ltd.
Honorary Professor of Hearing and Communication
University College London
London, United Kingdom
Chapter 5

Katrina A.S. Davis, MB, BChir, MRCPsych
Research Associate
Department of Psychological Medicine
Institute of Psychiatry, Psychology, and Neuroscience
King's College London
London, United Kingdom
Chapter 5

Allan O. Diefendorf, PhD
Professor Emeritus
Indiana University School of Medicine
Visiting Professor
Butler University
Indianapolis, Indiana
Chapters 23 and 24

Andrée Durieux-Smith, PhD, FCAHS
Professor Emeritus
Faculty of Health Sciences
University of Ottawa
Ottawa, Ontario, Canada
Chapter 33

Carolyne Edwards, MCISc, MBA
Director, Auditory Management Services
Executive Director and Senior Faculty
Gestalt Institute of Toronto
Toronto, Ontario, Canada
Chapter 39

Laurie S. Eisenberg, PhD
Professor of Research Otolaryngology
USC Caruso Family Center for Childhood Communication
Tina and Rick Caruso Department of Otolaryngology-Head and Neck Surgery
Keck School of Medicine
University of Southern California
Los Angeles, California
Chapter 38

Leisha R. Eiten, AuD, CCC-A
Clinical Coordinator

Boys Town National Research Hospital
Omaha, Nebraska
Chapter 27

Kris English, PhD
Professor and Interim School Director
School of Speech Pathology and Audiology
The University of Akron
Akron, Ohio
Chapter 36

Elizabeth M. Fitzpatrick, PhD
Associate Professor
Faculty of Health Sciences
University of Ottawa
Senior Scientist
Children's Hospital of Eastern Ontario Research Institute
Ottawa, Canada
Chapter 33

Dianne M. Hammes Ganguly, MA, CCC-SLP
Assistant Professor of Clinical Otolaryngology
USC Caruso Family Center for Childhood Communication
Tina and Rick Caruso Department of Otolaryngology-Head and Neck Surgery
Keck School of Medicine
University of Southern California
Los Angeles, California
Chapter 38

René H. Gifford, PhD
Associate Professor, Hearing and Speech Sciences
Director, Cochlear Implant Program
Associate Director, Implantable Hearing Technologies
Vanderbilt Bill Wilkerson Center
Nashville, Tennessee
Chapter 32

Karen A. Gordon, PhD, Reg. CASPLO, CCC-A
Bastable-Potts Health Clinician Scientist in Hearing Impairment
Archie's Cochlear Implant Laboratory, The Hospital for Sick Children
Associate Professor, Department of Otolaryngology-Head and Neck Surgery
University of Toronto
Toronto, Canada
Chapter 29

Samantha J. Gustafson, AuD
Department of Hearing and Speech Sciences
Vanderbilt Bill Wilkerson Center
Vanderbilt University School of Medicine
Nashville, Tennessee
Chapter 26

James W. Hall III, PhD
Professor
Osborne College of Audiology
Salus University
Elkins Park, PA
Professor
College of Communication Sciences and Disorders
University of Hawaii
Honolulu, HI
Extraordinary Professor
Department of Audiology and Speech Pathology
University of Pretoria
Pretoria, South Africa
Chapter 22

Melody Harrison, PhD, CCC-SLP
Professor
Division of Speech and Hearing Sciences
Department of Allied Health Sciences
University of North Carolina School of Medicine
Chapel Hill, North Carolina
Chapter 34

Robert V. Harrison, PhD, DSc
Professor and Director of Research
Department of Otolaryngology-Head and Neck Surgery
University of Toronto
Senior Scientist
Program in Neuroscience and Mental Health
The Hospital for Sick Children
Toronto, Canada
Chapter 2

Mark Hill, PhD
Head of Embryology
School of Medical Sciences, Medicine
UNSW Australia
Sydney, Australia
Chapter 1

Andrea Hillock-Dunn, AuD, PhD, CCC-A
Assistant Professor
Department of Hearing and Speech Sciences
Vanderbilt University
Associate Director
Division of Pediatric Audiology
Vanderbilt Bill Wilkerson Center
Nashville, Tennessee
Chapter 9

Bill Hodgetts, PhD
Associate Professor
University of Alberta
Program Director, Bone Conduction Amplification
Institute for Reconstructive Sciences in Medicine
Misericordia Hospital
Edmonton, Canada
Chapter 31

Jeffrey K. Hoffman, MS, CCC-A
Outreach Coordinator
Early Childhood Hearing Outreach (ECHO) Initiative
NCHAM—National Center for Hearing Assessment and Management
Utah State University
Logan, Utah
Chapter 18

Linda J. Hood, PhD
Professor
Department of Hearing and Speech Sciences
Associate Director for Research
National Center for Childhood Deafness
Vanderbilt Bill Wilkerson Center
Vanderbilt University
Nashville, TN
Honorary Professor
School of Health and Rehabilitation Sciences
University of Queensland
Brisbane, Australia
Chapter 6

Sanna Y.L. Hou
Paediatric Research Audiologist
National Acoustic Laboratories
Sydney, Australia
Chapter 28

Derek M. Houston, PhD
Associate Professor
Department of Otolaryngology-Head and Neck Surgery
The Ohio State University College of Medicine
Columbus, Ohio
Chapter 3

Lisa L. Hunter, PhD
Scientific Director, Audiology
Communication Sciences Research Center
Cincinnati Children's Hospital Medical Center
Professor
Otolaryngology and Communication Sciences and Disorders
University of Cincinnati
Cincinnati, Ohio
Chapters 10 and 19

Martyn Hyde, BSc, PhD
Professor
Department of Otolaryngology
University of Toronto
Consultant
British Columbia Early Hearing Program
Ontario Infant Hearing Program
Toronto, Canada
Chapters 15 and 16

Karen C. Johnson, PhD
USC Caruso Family Center for Childhood Communication

Tina and Rick Caruso Department of Otolaryngology-Head and Neck Surgery
Keck School of Medicine
University of Southern California
Los Angeles, California
Chapter 38

Bronya J.B. Keats, PhD
Professor and Head Emeritus
Department of Genetics
Louisiana State University Health Sciences Center
New Orleans, Louisiana
Chapter 6

Lori J. Leibold, PhD
Director, Center for Hearing Research
Boys Town National Research Hospital
Omaha, Nebraska
Chapter 4

Dawna Lewis, PhD
Director
Listening and Learning Laboratory
Boys Town National Research Hospital
Omaha, Nebraska
Chapter 27

Amy S. Martinez, MA
Assistant Professor of Clinical Otolaryngology
USC Caruso Family Center for Childhood Communication
Tina and Rick Caruso Department of Otolaryngology-Head and Neck Surgery
Keck School of Medicine
University of Southern California
Los Angeles, California
Chapter 38

Marilyn Neault, PhD
Director
Habilitative Audiology Program
Boston Children's Hospital
Assistant Professor of Otology and Laryngology
Harvard Medical School
Boston, Massachusetts
Chapter 30

Mary Ellen Nevins, EdD
Professor and Director of Auditory-Based Intervention
University of Arkansas for Medical Sciences
Little Rock, Arkansas
Chapter 40

James E. Peck, PhD
Associate Professor Emeritus
Division of Audiology
Department of Otolaryngology and Communicative Sciences
University of Mississippi Medical Center
Jackson, Mississippi
Chapter 14

Heather Porter, PhD, CCC-A
Postdoctoral Fellow
USC Caruso Family Center for Childhood Communication
Tina and Rick Caruso Department of Otolaryngology-Head and Neck Surgery
Keck School of Medicine
University of Southern California
Los Angeles, California
Chapter 37

Gary Rance, PhD, MSc, BEd, Dip Aud, MAudSA(cc)
Associate Professor
Department of Audiology and Speech Pathology
The University of Melbourne
Melbourne, Australia
Chapter 11

Amy McConkey Robbins, MS, CCC-SLP, LSLS Cert. AVT
Speech-Language Pathologist
Communication Consulting Services
Indianapolis, Indiana
Chapter 35

Jackson Roush, PhD
Professor and Director
Division of Speech and Hearing Sciences
Department of Allied Health Sciences
University of North Carolina School of Medicine
Chapel Hill, North Carolina
Chapter 17

Patricia A. Roush, AuD
Associate Professor
Department of Otolaryngology-Head and Neck Surgery
University of North Carolina at Chapel Hill
Director of Pediatric Audiology
University of North Carolina Hospitals
Chapel Hill, North Carolina
Chapter 12

Hollea A.M. Ryan, AuD, PhD
Assistant Professor
Samford University
Birmingham, Alabama
Chapter 26

Diane L. Sabo, PhD
Hearing Screening Program Manager
Audiology Systems, Inc.
Schaumburg, Illinois
Chapter 18

Susan D. Scollie, PhD
Associate Professor
School of Communication Sciences and Disorders
Principal Investigator
National Centre for Audiology
Faculty of Health Sciences
University of Western Ontario
London, Ontario, Canada
Chapter 25

Richard Seewald, PhD
Distinguished University Professor Emeritus
School of Communication Sciences and Disorders
National Centre for Audiology
Faculty of Health Sciences
University of Western Ontario
London, Ontario, Canada

Christopher A. Shera, PhD
Professor
Otology and Laryngology
Harvard Medical School
Boston, Massachusetts
Chapter 20

Susan A. Small, PhD
Hamber Professor of Clinical Audiology
School of Audiology and Speech Sciences
University of British Columbia
Vancouver, British Columbia, Canada
Chapter 21

Christopher Spankovich, AuD, PhD, MPH
Associate Professor
Department of Otolaryngology and Communicative Sciences
University of Mississippi Medical Center
Jackson, Mississippi
Chapter 9

David R. Stapells, PhD
Professor Emeritus
School of Audiology and Speech Sciences
University of British Columbia
Vancouver, British Columbia, Canada
Chapter 21

Arnold Starr, MD
Professor Emeritus
Department of Neurology and Neurobiology
University California at Irvine
Irvine, California
Chapter 11

Anne Marie Tharpe, PhD
Professor and Chair
Department of Hearing and Speech Sciences

Associate Director
Vanderbilt Bill Wilkerson Center
Vanderbilt University School of Medicine
Nashville, Tennessee
Chapters 23, 26, and 37

Rebecca Trepcos-Klingler, MA, CCC-A
Audiologist
Riley Hospital for Children at Indiana University Health
Indianapolis, Indiana
Chapter 24

Betty R. Vohr, MD
Professor of Pediatrics
Alpert Medical School of Brown University
Medical Director, Rhode Island Hearing Assessment Program
Director, Neonatal Follow-up
Women and Infants Hospital
Providence, Rhode Island
Chapter 7

Amanda S. Weinzierl, AuD, CCC-A
Audiologist
Riley Hospital for Children at Indiana University Health
Indianapolis, Indiana
Chapter 24

Lynne A. Werner, PhD
Professor
University of Washington
Seattle, Washington
Chapter 4

Margaret Winter, MS, CCC-A
Associate Professor of Clinical Otolaryngology
USC Caruso Family Center for Childhood Communication
University of Southern California
Los Angeles, California
Chapter 20

Jace Wolfe, PhD
Hearts for Hearing
Oklahoma City, Oklahoma
Chapter 27

Vicky W. Zhang, PhD
Paediatric Research Audiologist
National Acoustic Laboratories
Sydney, Australia
Chapter 28

This book is dedicated to our dear friend and colleague Judith S. Gravel, whose vision for this volume guided our every step. Judy was beautifully unique. She was a scholar, a scientist, a teacher, and a master clinician whose career exemplified the highest standards of professionalism and ethical conduct. Above all, she was a warm and caring person with a remarkable way of bringing out the best in everyone whose life she touched, including children whom she loved the most.

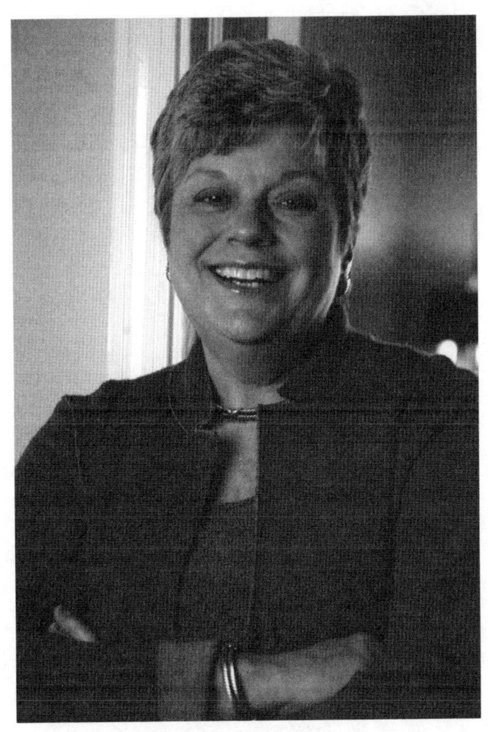

Dr. Judith S. Gravel
December 1948–December 2008

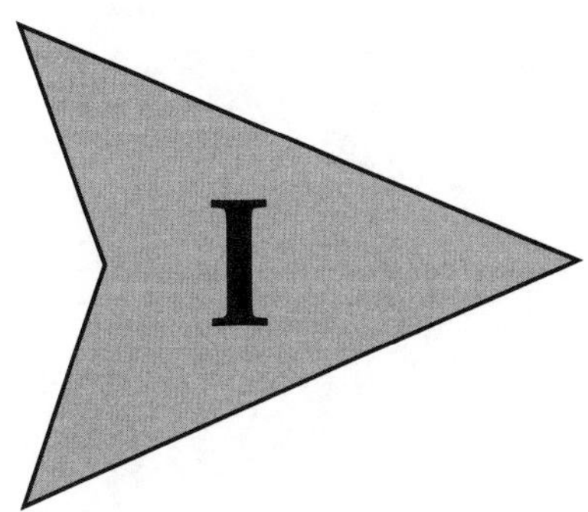

Typical Auditory Development

Hearing Development: Embryology of the Ear

Mark Hill

Developmental Origins

Human embryology at the turn of the last century identified selected aspects of ear structural development as part of the overall study of the development of the head and nervous system in studies by Thyng (1914). Studies of animal models played an important role in the early history of auditory embryology. For example, as early as 1911, Jenkinson examined the embryological development of the middle ear in mice. Studies of embryonic human external ears followed in the 1930s (Wood-Jones & Wen, 1934). The chicken model was also used around this time for studying the development of the central auditory pathway (Levi-Montalcini, 1949). In the 1940s and 1950s, research focused on the relationship between the human auditory system and the general embryonic stages of development (Streeter, 1942, 1948, 1951). It was not until the 1950s that hearing development research took off with many studies on embryological, anatomic, and neurologic development. Today, a search of the PubMed reference abstract database with "development of hearing" will return more than 10,000 studies. The current studies mainly utilize animal models and study the molecular mechanisms of development. In particular, genetic and teratological studies have and are identifying a growing number of specific genes and teratogens associated with auditory abnormal embryology. Our current understanding of developmental mechanisms and gene function has led to potential future treatment of genetic deafness through gene therapy (Askew et al., 2015).

This chapter introduces the embryology time course of the human ear as divided by the three anatomic divisions (Figure 1–1, external, middle, and inner). The description also draws on the many animal model studies that have helped us further understand human auditory development. Examples are given of embryologic studies currently unraveling the complex signaling pathways involved in development. Many of these pathways involve a regulated sequence of secreted growth factors, transcription factor "switches," gap junctions, and adhesive interactions choreographed into a back-and-forth signaling process between developing ear structures and surrounding tissues. Finally, a brief overview of critical periods of embryologic development in relationship to genetic and environment conditions is given. Note that neurologic and postnatal development is covered elsewhere in this text (see Chapters 2 and 4) and in recent reviews (Fritzsch, Knipper, & Friauf, 2015; Litovsky, 2015). Human embryology stages and the organ of audition and equilibrium are also described in the online resource Embryology (http://tiny.cc/Hearing_Development).

General Human Embryology

When staging human prenatal development, there is an important consideration and sometimes confusion when reading the literature. Embryologists consider fertilization to initiate development and all following staging commences from this point in time. Clinicians, other than with in vitro fertilization (IVF), cannot easily ascertain the time of fertilization. In this case, a far easier and more predictable timing is from when the mother is not pregnant, that is, the last menstrual period (LMP). Therefore, there is often approximately a 2-week difference, as fertilization occurs after ovulation at the midpoint of the menstrual cycle. For example,

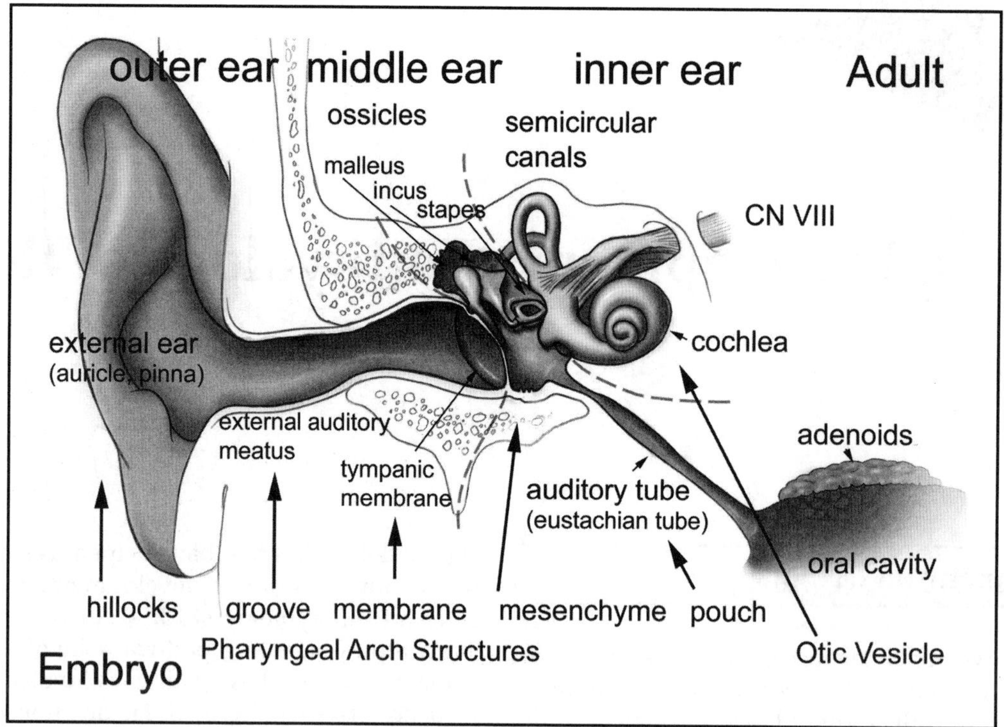

FIGURE 1–1. General anatomy of the adult ear and the equivalent embryonic structures from which each component is derived. The inner ear forms from the surface otic placode forming the otic vesicle (or otocyst), which contributes the membranous labyrinth and cranial ganglia. The middle and external ear form from components from pharyngeal Arch 1 and 2. (Image based on NIH imagebank and National Institute on Deafness and Other Communication Disorders [NIDCD].)

postfertilization Week 3 is clinically Week 5 LMP. All timings described in this current chapter refer to embryologic dates from fertilization.

In the first 3 weeks of development, the embryo forms initially as three main layers (trilaminar), or germ layers, from which all tissues of the embryo derive. These three layers are the ectoderm (forms all neural tissue and the surface epithelium); the mesoderm (forms most connective tissues of the body; muscle, bone, cartilage); the endoderm (forms the lining epithelium of the gastrointestinal, urogenital, and respiratory tract). Each of these layers begins as a simple circular disk of cells stacked like dinner plates. The three layers later will segment themselves into different regions, which contribute to specific tissues. Specialized senses such as hearing and vision will have contributions from all three of these embryonic germ layers during their complex developmental process.

In the fourth week of development, organogenesis begins throughout the embryo, which converts the trilaminar embryo into anatomically identifiable organs and tissues. In humans, the first 8 weeks of development are described as the embryonic period when organogenesis occurs. This is followed by the fetal period when continued growth and differentiation of mainly preexisting tissues and organs occurs. Classically, the embryonic period has been divided into 23 Carnegie stages, describing development as a series of observable changes in external appearance and features of the embryo. Stage 1 begins at fertilization, Stage 7 at implantation at the end of the first week, and Stage 23 the end of the embryonic period in the eighth week. The same classification can be applied to embryos of many different species, allowing direct developmental comparisons although over different time periods for each species stage. This classification has also been useful for studying the embryological development of human hearing and balance using a variety of animal models (mainly chicken, mouse, rat, and zebrafish), which will be referred to within this chapter.

Normal embryonic system development, including hearing, requires a combination of developmental signaling mechanisms. These mechanisms include short- and long-distance interactions by secretions (growth factors, hormones, and ionic changes), adhesive interactions (cell-cell, cell-extracellular matrix), and a subsequent cascade of transcription factors (DNA binding proteins). These transcription factors activate key genes required at specific developmental stages and eventually the adult pattern of gene expression in that cell or tissue.

Clinically, the embryonic period can also be seen to occupy most of the first trimester, and the fetal period occupies the second and third trimester of human development. This division of development is also an important consideration when we look at the critical periods of development that can be impacted by teratogens. This chapter includes brief coverage of some molecular regulatory mechanisms of normal development, as perturbations of these signaling pathways relate to abnormalities of hearing and balance. The following sections cover initially the early embryonic development of all three anatomic ear divisions, which are followed by later fetal development and detailed development of the cochlear and key auditory components.

Early Inner Ear

The earliest external feature of auditory development is the appearance on the ectoderm of the embryo surface in the head region of otic placodes (for a review, see Whitfield, 2015). These placodes form as a pair of the series of placodal regions that form initially at the edge of the neural plate. The otic placodes are two small circular regions of ectoderm on the lateral surface of the developing head and the first "visible" pair of sensory placodes that eventually will contribute to each sensory system (hearing, vision, smell, and taste). In other species, there can be additional sensory placodes that contribute to sensory systems not present in humans. The otic placode lies closely associated with, but separate from, the neural tube level that corresponds to the hindbrain region of the neural tube. This localization with the neural tube later can be further positioned as adjacent to rhombomere 5 and 6 segmental subdivisions of the hindbrain.

The otic placode is a single layer of ectodermal cells organized in a columnar epithelium, which differs in cell shape from the surrounding cuboidal epithelia that will contribute the epithelia of the skin. In the zebrafish model, a number of specific genes are involved in initial induction of the otic placode including both growth factors (FGF3 and FGF8) and transcription factors (dlx3b, dlx4b, and foxi1; Solomon, Kwak, & Fritz, 2004).

Proliferation of the otic placode cells leads to an inward folding, or invagination, giving the external appearance of a depression on the lateral sides of the early developing neck region. The epithelium is still a single layer of cells, which continues to invaginate until the edges of the disc of cells come into apposition on the embryo surface. In the mouse model, placodal invagination but not specification requires placodal expression of the transcription factor Sox9 (Barrionuevo et al., 2008).

Further invagination leads to the edges of the placode coming into close apposition and then fusing to form a hollow, fluid-filled sac; this structure is then renamed as the *otic vesicle* or *otocyst* (Figure 1–2). The otic vesicle is the primordium of all the inner ear structures, including the cochleovestibular neurons of the future cranial nerve eight (CN VIII). The otic vesicle is now lost from the embryo surface and sits embedded within the mesenchyme, embryonic connective tissue, behind the first and second pharyngeal arches. The otic vesicle is surrounded by a number of developmental structures including the fifth rhombomere (medially), the anterior cardinal vein (laterally), and developing cranial ganglia (rostro-caudally). These events of otic placode formation, invagination, and otic vesicle formation all occur within the third week of human development.

Otic Vesicle Development

The inner ear membranous labyrinth has two major linked components, the vestibular system (semicircular canals) and the auditory system (cochlea duct). Both are derived from the otic vesicle. This section will detail the early events of otic vesicle differentiation followed by specific notes on the later development of both systems.

By the fourth week, the otic vesicle is a spherical epithelial fluid-filled ball at the level of rhombomere 5 and 6 (Hatch, Noyes, Wang, Wright, & Mansour, 2007). During this week, neuroblasts delaminate to form the primordial of the vestibulocochlear (statoacoustic) ganglion, the vesicle elongates, and the walls also change in relative thickness. This initial elongated portion of the otic vesicle will form the endolymphatic sac.

The beginning of otic vesicle differentiation is the localized expression of transforming growth factor-β2 (Okano et al., 2005). The site (see Figure 1–2) of this expression in the otic wall locates cells that will delaminate and contribute to formation of the statoacoustic

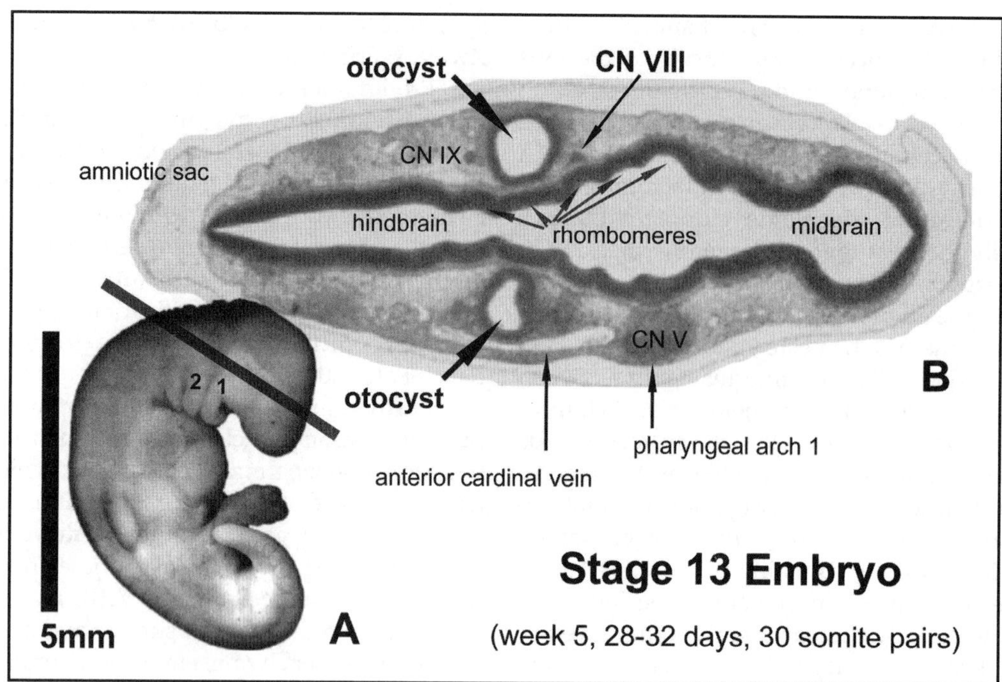

FIGURE 1–2. Stage 13 embryo (Week 5) showing otocyst that will form the inner ear. **A.** Ventrolateral view of the whole embryo with 5-mm scale bar. At this stage of development, no middle or external ear structures are apparent and will be derived later from pharyngeal arches 1 and 2 (*labeled*). **B.** The gray bar through the head indicates the plane of cross section, which is a cross section of the head showing the size and position of the otic vesicles. At this stage of development, the vesicles lie within the head mesenchyme behind pharyngeal Arch 1 and 2 and in close apposition to the developing hindbrain. Note the close position of the otic vesicle to the rhombomeres, hindbrain folds that represent the initial segmentation of the hindbrain. Also shown are developing cranial ganglia and blood vessel lying adjacent to the otic vesicles. The wall of the otic vesicle at this stage is a simple epithelium.

ganglion or cranial nerve CN VIII (Andermann, Ungos, & Raible, 2002; Represa, Moro, Gato, Pastor, & Barbosa, 1990). These cells remain adjacent to the otic vesicle residing in the surrounding cellular mesenchyme, a mixture of mesoderm and neural crest cells, the latter contributing to the ganglia (Bruska & Wozniak, 2000; Wikstrom & Anniko, 1987). Cells within the ganglia differentiate into both neural and supporting glial cells. The neural cells eventually develop a bipolar morphology, extending central processes toward the neural tube and peripherally into the sensory epithelium of the vestibular apparatus and cochlea. Ganglionic neuron processes extend centrally toward the neural tube region that will form the medial geniculate nuclei. Divisions of the cochlear ganglion (spiral) from the vestibular ganglion have been identified to occur in human embryos between Carnegie stages 18 and 19 (44 to 46 postovulatory days; Ulatowska-Blaszyk & Bruska, 1999). Growth of processes toward the sensory epithelia is potentially driven by chemoattractant and repulsion cues (for a review, see Fekete & Campero, 2007). The neurotrophin family and their high-affinity Trk receptors control innervation of the cochlea during embryonic development. Mouse models point to a role for both brain-derived neurotrophic factor (Bdnf) and neurotrophin 3 (Nt3; Schimmang et al., 2003).

In humans, the cochlea nerve fibers in the prosensory domain appear at Week 6 and commence synaptogenesis in Week 9 (Pechriggl et al., 2015). The ganglion neurons differentiate to form two distinct populations on the basis of their location within the ganglia and soma size, central Type I large and peripheral Type II small cells. Note that more Type II ganglion cells have been identified in neonates, within the middle and apical turns, than in adults (Chiong, Burgess, & Nadol, 1993). This suggests an ongoing postnatal differentiation within the ganglion. An earlier study identified the associated glial cells do not myelinate the ganglion fibers, either in the fetus or neonate, and only thin myelination was observed in the elderly (Arnold, 1987). A more recent study identified in the fetal period cochlear, Schwann cell myelination (24 weeks) distally, and a later glial myelination (26 weeks) proximally (Moore & Linthicum, 2001).

In the fourth week, the endolymphatic sac extends initially from the otic vesicle as a small diverticulum, with the main otic body forming the primordia of the utricle and the saccule (Figure 1–3). Regional differentiation of the utricle and saccule is regulated by the transcription factors Otx1 (Beisel, Wang-Lundberg, Maklad, & Fritzsch, 2005) and Pax5 (Kwak et al., 2006), both members of the homeobox gene family. The endolymphatic sac's mature function is both secretory and absorptive. The endolymphatic sac begins initially as an extending "single-lumen pouchlike structure," which in humans goes on to develop through the fetal period and into the first postnatal year into a series of tubular structures (Bagger-Sjoback, 1991; Ng, 2000; Ng & Linthicum, 1998). This mature tubular structure is not seen in other species (Ng & Linthicum, 1998).

The adult endolymphatic sac is filled with endolymphatic fluid with a unique composition of high potassium and low sodium ions (Grunder, Muller, & Ruppersberg, 2001). Both the vestibular and cochlear epithelial cells secrete endolymphatic fluid. It is not known in humans at what stage of development this ionic status is achieved. In the rat, adult sodium levels are seen in the first week after birth, while both potassium

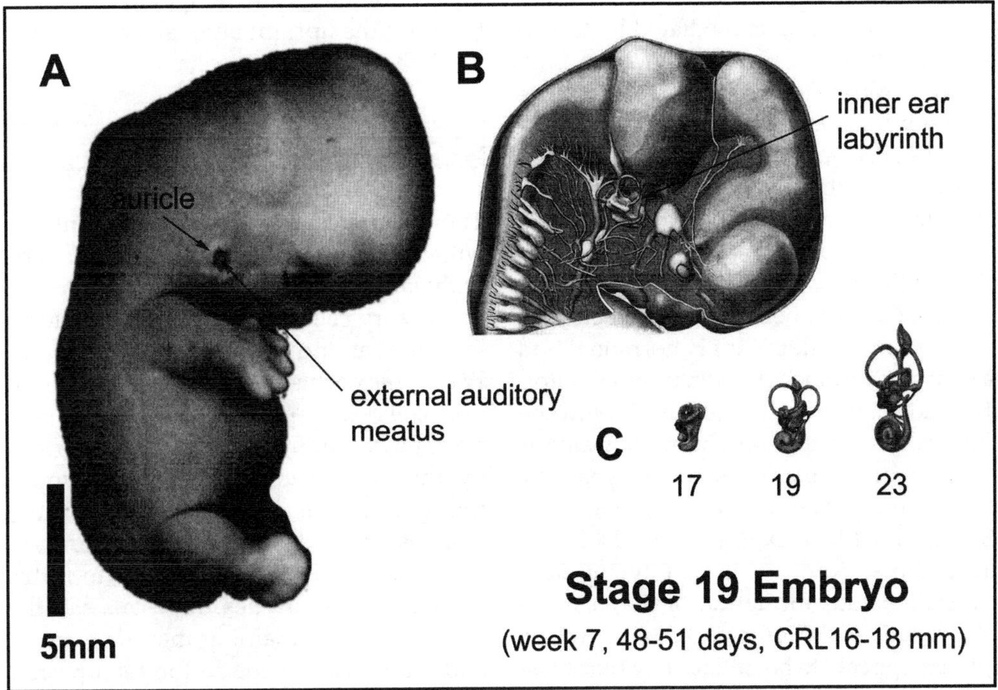

FIGURE 1–3. Stage 19 embryo (Week 7) showing the ear development features. **A.** Lateral view of the whole embryo with 5-mm scale bar. Note the pharyngeal arches have differentiated and are no longer visible on the surface. The external ear (auricle) has formed from hillocks on pharyngeal arch 1 and arch 2. Note the relative position of the ear just above the neck and at the level of the lower jaw. The external auditory meatus is enlarged and ends at a meatal plug. **B.** Historic image (Thyng, 1914) cutaway view of same stage embryo showing the position and appearance of the inner ear relative to the developing brain and other cranial ganglia. **C.** The relative size and shape of the inner ear labyrinth at Weeks 6, 7, and 8. By the end of the embryonic period (Week 8), the inner ear labyrinth approximates the shape of the adult structure.

and chloride levels are below the normal adult levels (Bosher & Warren, 1971). A similar postnatal increase in potassium ion levels occurs in the mouse (Anniko & Nordemar, 1980; Anniko & Wroblewski, 1981), and in chickens this rise occurs before hatching (Masetto, Zucca, Botta, & Valli, 2005).

The otic vesicle in the fifth week (at stage 16) extends a second process at the region where the saccule is forming and at the opposite pole from the developing endolymphatic sac (Yasuda, Yamada, Uwabe, Shiota, & Yasuda, 2007). This otic extension is the initial primordia of the cochlear duct and at this stage is a simple epithelial fluid-filled sac. Over the next 2 weeks (Week 5 to 7), from Stage 16 to 22, the cochlea not only elongates and rotates, it begins to differentiate the organ of Corti, but this will not fully form until well into the fetal period. The cochlear ganglion neurons grow into this developing structure and will contact developing hair cells within the organ of Corti. As in other developing neuronal systems, neuronal development and survival appear to be mediated by target-derived secreted growth factors, in this system both brain-derived neurotrophic factor (BDNF) and neurotrophin 3 (NT3; Bernd, Zhang, Yao, & Rozenberg, 1994; Camarero et al., 2001; Fekete & Campero, 2007; Fritzsch, Pirvola, & Ylikoski, 1999; Hossain, Brumwell, & Morest, 2002; Wei, Jin, Jarlebark, Scarfone, & Ulfendahl, 2007). Similarly, hair cell survival is also regulated by the growth BDNF and fibroblast growth factor-2 (FGF-2; Cristobal et al., 2002). The other regulatory factor for spiral ganglion neuron development is hormonal and related to fetal thyroid hormone (Rueda, Prieto, Cantos, Sala, & Merchan, 2003). Initial synaptogenesis between developing hair cells and the ganglionic neurons is directly onto neuronal cell bodies (somatic synapses) and only later do a network of dendritic spinous synapses form (Sobkowicz, Slapnick, & August, 2002).

It is during the seventh week of development that the otic vesicle begins formation of the vestibular semicircular canals (see Figure 1–3). Semicircular canal development appears to be initiated by fibroblast growth factor locally upregulating bone morphogenetic protein 2 (*BMP2*) expression (Chang, Brigande, Fekete, & Wu, 2004). A related *BMP4* (Omata et al., 2007) and neuronal calcium sensor 1 (*NCS1*; Blasiole et al., 2005) appear to also control early development of the semicircular canals. Three otic vesicle outpocketings from the utricular region indicate the location of the future semicircular canals. A recent study in human embryos (Yasuda et al., 2007) has established the morphogenesis time course of the three semicircular canals. At Stage 17, the anterior and posterior semicircular ducts begin to form. By Stage 18, the epithelia at the core of these outpocketings fuse, die by apoptosis, and are replaced by mesenchyme. By Stage 19, these canals have the structural "loop" appearance. The lateral semicircular canal appears slightly delayed but by Stage 19 has a similar morphology.

Chondrification of surrounding mesenchyme begins in the first week of fetal development (Week 9) forming the otic capsule (Figures 1–4 and 1–5). In the second trimester (Weeks 12 to 16), the cartilage adjacent to the membranous labyrinth breaks down forming the perilymphatic space in which the membranous labyrinth will now float. Ossification of the surrounding capsule, the bony labyrinth, occurs between Weeks 16 and 24 of fetal development. The bony labyrinth anatomically is within the petrous portion of the temporal bone and encloses all the inner ear structures. The human bony labyrinth is unique and differs from even those of other primates, in size, shape, and orientation. These differences are thought to derive from the cranial base and the upright bipedal locomotion in humans.

Cochlear Development

The otic vesicle pseudostratified epithelial cells differentiate through regulated signaling into four distinct pathways forming cochlear prosensory cells, vestibular prosensory cells, neurons in the auditory and vestibular ganglia, and nonsensory epithelia (Kelley, 2007). Within the cochlear duct, a chamber, sensory cells, support cells, and specialized extracellular matrices will eventually differentiate from this primordia formed by the otic vesicle. The mesenchyme surrounding the cochlear duct along its length vacuolates to form a series of fluid-filled spaces. These spaces coalesce either side of the cochlear duct to form two parallel perilymphatic cavities, the scala vestibuli and scala tympani. The remaining mesenchyme will chondrify and later ossify through the fetal period to form the bony labyrinth in which the membranous labyrinth resides. The adult cochlear size is achieved by 16 to 17 weeks gestation (see Figure 1–4).

The specialized auditory component within the cochlea is referred to as the organ of Corti, named after the Italian anatomist Marquis Alfonso Giacomo Gaspare Corti (1822–1876) who carried out microscopic analysis of human and other species cochleas. The most studied animal model of cochlea development is that of the mouse (then guinea pig and gerbil), with several knockouts mimicking human hearing loss and in

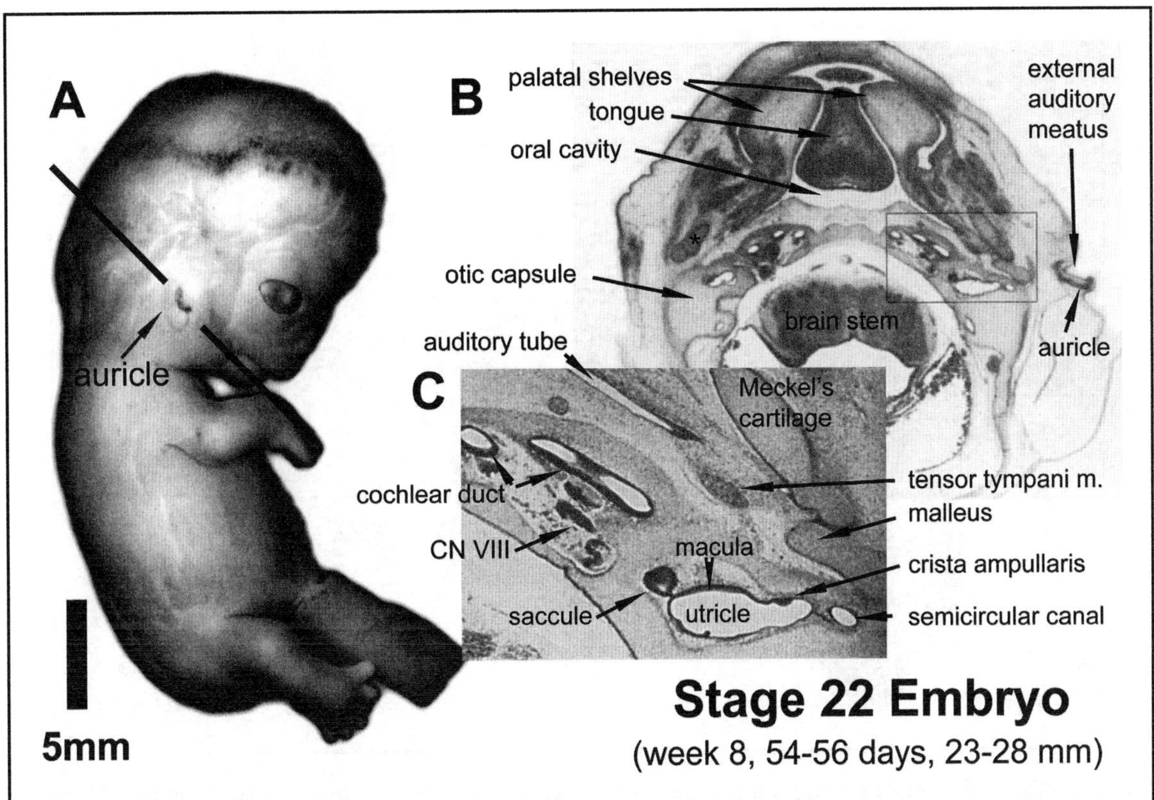

FIGURE 1–4. Stage 22 embryo (Week 8) showing the embryo near the end of the embryonic period. **A.** Lateral view of the whole embryo with 5-mm scale bar. Note the well-developed external ear with simplified adult structure and narrower meatal opening. The gray bar through the head indicates the plane of cross section for (**B**) and (**C**). **B.** Cross section of the head at the plane of the skull base and oral cavity to the top. The otic capsule is well formed by this stage containing all the membranous labyrinth structures. It is still a cartilaginous structure ventral to the brainstem and lying behind the oral cavity. The tongue occupies the floor of the oral cavity with the unfused palatal shelves lying lateral and the auditory tubes clearly shown on the posterior wall. The external ear is visible on the right-hand side of the head with a band of cartilage (dark stain) within the auricle. **C.** The gray box indicates detail of inner and middle ear development. The middle ear cavity has not yet formed, and the ossicles (malleus shown) are embedded in mesenchyme that is being lost. The tensor tympani muscle is differentiating in the adjacent mesenchyme. The inner ear membranous labyrinth has formed its adult external structure. The section through the turns of the cochlear duct shows the internal cochlea structure is still underdeveloped; in contrast, the balance region is more developed.

contrast to humans, where the onset of hearing occurs postnatally. The molecular differentiation of the individual cells that form the specialized organ of Corti has been recently reviewed (Kelley, 2007).

The first structure to form is Kollicker's organ, or greater epithelial ridge, a transient epithelial structure lying beneath the tectorial membrane from which some of the specialized cells of the organ of Corti are formed. The adjacent lesser epithelial ridge is separated initially by a notch from the greater epithelial ridge and will contribute the outer hair cells. Following generation of the hair and pillar cells, Kollicker's organ will then regress and generate the inner sulcus.

A study of the human developing cochlea (Figure 1–6) during the embryonic to early fetal period shows the sex-determining region Y (SRY)–related high mobility group (HMG)-box transcription factors (*SOX2* and *SOX9*) are key early markers of the proneural region of the duct epithelium (Locher et al., 2014). A detailed histological study has been made of the

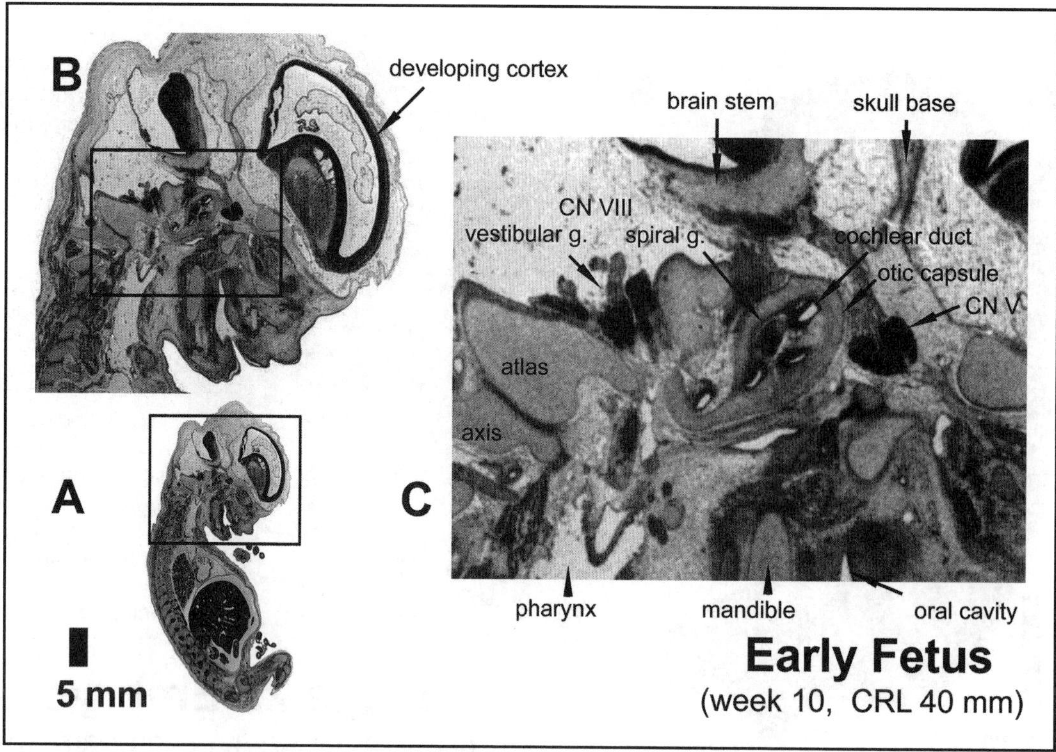

FIGURE 1–5. Fetal development (Week 10) showing the early fetal cochlea. **A.** Sagittal section through the whole fetus with 5-mm scale bar. **B.** The gray box indicates this region; enlarged view of head showing the anatomic position and size of the cochlea relative to the developing brain, mouth, and vertebral column. Note the large trigeminal ganglia (CN V) and relatively underdeveloped cortex above the basal ganglia. **C.** The gray box indicates this region; enlarged view of cochlea showing sections through turns of the cochlear duct in the otic capsule. The cranial ganglia CN VIII (vestibulocochlear nerve, auditory-vestibular nerve, or statoacoustic nerve) has clearly separated vestibular and cochlear divisions. Note the position of the oral cavity, mandible, and pharynx lying directly beneath the otic capsule.

human timeline of development of both the temporal bone and the organ of Corti (Bibas et al., 2008; see Table 1–1 and Figure 1–3). The recent morphological developmental timeline suggests that auditory function begins after the Week 20 (LMP) time point, later than the Week 14 time point suggested by other studies. Note that not only the cochlea, but also the cochlear nerve and central pathways need to develop for a functioning central neural pathway to occur (Sanchez Del Rey, Sanchez Fernandez, Martinez Ibarguen, & Santaolalla Montoya, 1995).

Audition through the fetal period is by bone conduction, not mediated by the middle ear. The bone conduction is initiated as sound-induced fluid vibration of the amniotic fluid, generating low-frequency vibrations within the developing skull and its contents (Sohmer, Perez, Sichel, Priner, & Freeman, 2001).

A key regulator in hair cell production is Math1, the homolog of the Drosophila proneural gene atonal, which regulates the total number of hair cells produced. This gene is in turn negatively regulated by the hairy and enhancer of split (HES) family of factors, which has been shown to be a general negative regulator of neurogenesis (Petrovic, Galvez, Neves, Abello, & Giraldez, 2015; Zheng, Shou, Guillemot, Kageyama, & Gao, 2000).

Another gene involved in early hair cell proliferation, but not differentiation, is the expression of the retinoblastoma protein pRb (Sage et al., 2006). Later differentiation of hair and support pillar cells appears to rely initially on a lateral inhibition process mediated through the Notch signaling pathway (Daudet, Ariza-McNaughton, & Lewis, 2007). Outer hair cell differentiation also requires further signaling by the

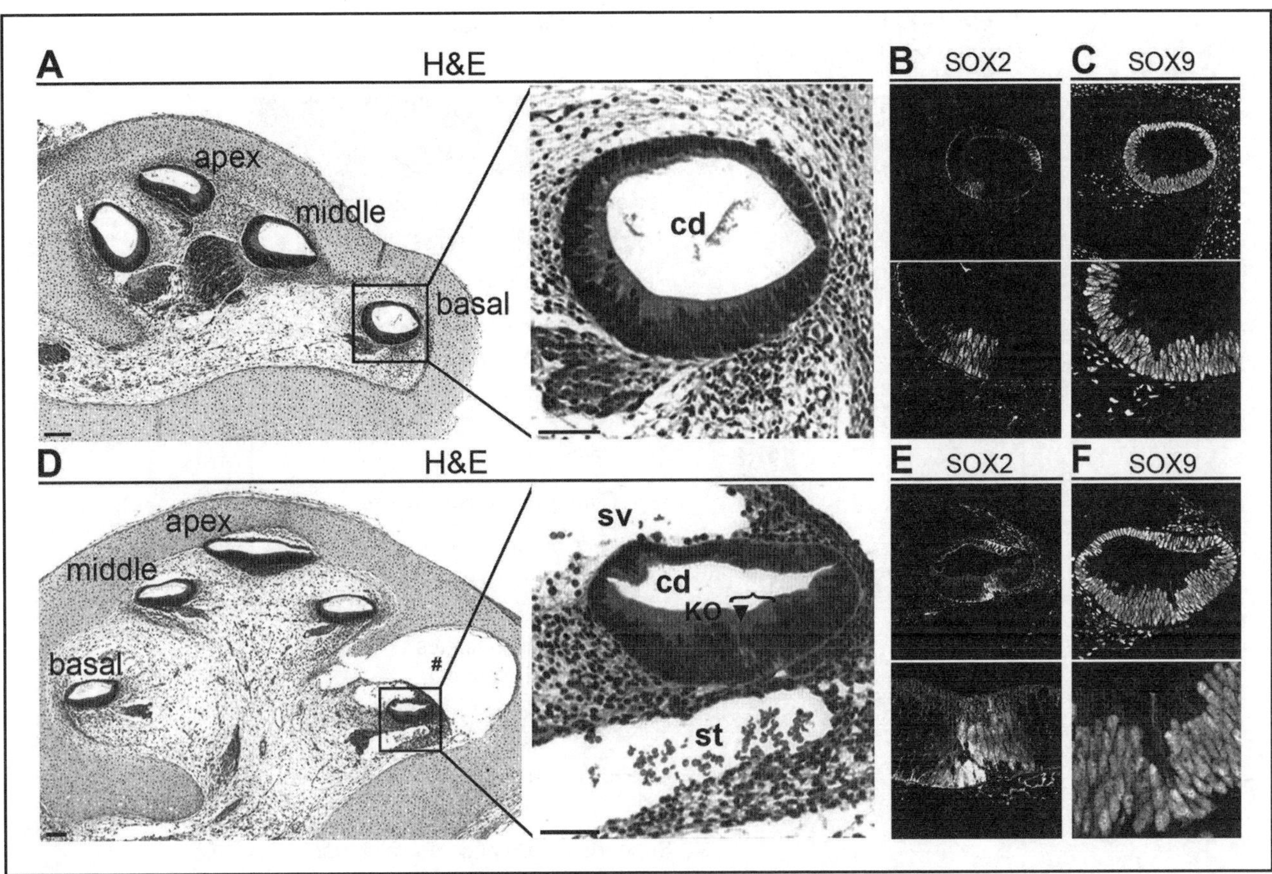

FIGURE 1–6. Late embryonic (Week 8, A) to early fetal (Week 10, D) human cochlea showing localized gene expression of the transcription factors Sry-Related Hmg-Box Gene 2 (SOX2; B and E) in the prosensory domain and SOX9 (C and F) in the basal turn of the cochlear duct epithelium and otic capsule. Mutations in both SOX2 (3q26.33; http://www.omim.org/entry/184429) and SOX9 (17q24.3; http://www.omim.org/entry/608160) have been associated with sensorineural hearing loss. (cd, cochlear duct; KO, Kölliker's organ; sv, scala vestibuli; st, scala tympani. Scale bars = 100 µm [all lower magnifications] or 50 µm [all higher magnifications]; Figure modified from Locher et al., 2014. With permission.)

Pou4f3 (Brn3.1, Brn3c) transcription factor activation of growth factor-independent 1 (Gfi1; Hertzano et al., 2004). Mouse Pou4f3 knockout, a model for human autosomal dominant nonsyndromic progressive hearing loss, shows a specific developmental degeneration of outer hair cells (Hertzano et al., 2004).

Later hair cell neural transmission occurs through voltage-gated calcium channels opening when mechanical stimulation depolarizes the hair cell membrane, and the resulting calcium influx triggers neurotransmitter release. In animal models, these channels are expressed very early in hair cell development and may have additional developmental functions within these cells (Hafidi & Dulon, 2004; Waka, Knipper, & Engel, 2003). Finally, fetal thyroid hormone contributes a hormonal role in the differentiation of hair cells and their subsequent innervation by spiral ganglion neurons (Rueda et al., 2003).

Much research has focused on the development of hair cells, but much less is known about the other main cochlear cell population with the same embryonic origin, the supporting cells. There are five distinct supporting cell types: Hensen's cells, Deiters' cells, pillar cells, inner phalangeal cells, and border cells. Developmentally, these supporting cells interact through signaling and by contact with hair cells to establish their mosaic pattern of distribution (for a review, see Wan, Corfas, & Stone, 2013). Postnatally, they may also provide protection (May et al., 2013) and be involved in recycling of damaged hair cells.

Table 1–1. Late Embryonic and Fetal Development of Both the Cochlea and Organ of Corti

LMP Week	*Postovulatory Week*	*Event*
10	8	Tectorial membrane primordium found throughout cochlea turns
14	12	Hair cells at the basal turn
		Oval space located between inner and outer hair cells in the basal turn
14–15	12–13	Hensen's cells present
17	15	Pillar cells present
		Spiral limbus increases in size
		Kollicker's organ
20	18	Tunnel of Corti opens
21–25	19–23	Tunnel of Corti continues to open upward from the base
25	23	Cochlea is adult size
26	24	Inner sulcus a single layer of flattened cells
		Supporting cells become columnar

Source: Data from A. G. Bibas et al. (2008), based on the study of 81 human fetal temporal bones.

The stria vascularis within the cochlea produces by ionic regulation endocochlear potential and contacts both perilymph and endolymph fluids (Johnson & Spoendlin, 1966; Nin et al., 2008). In humans, the earliest strial cell differentiation occurs during Week 9 (11 weeks LMP) as a ridge of epithelial cells on the lateral wall of the cochlear duct (Bibas, Liang, Michaels, & Wright, 2000). By Week 12 (14 weeks LMP), the three major strial cell types are present: marginal, intermediate, and basal cells (Lavigne-Rebillard & Bagger-Sjoback, 1992). The intermediate cells of the stria vascularis are neural crest–derived melanocytes, which are capable of continuous replication (Conlee, Gerity, & Bennett, 1994). By Week 19 (21 weeks LMP) the stria vascularis appears adult in structure but is not mature until the third trimester (Lavigne-Rebillard & Bagger-Sjoback, 1992). Atrophy occurs postnatally in the elderly of both the stria vascularis and spiral ganglion (Suzuki et al., 2006).

Vestibular Development

The short tube of the ductus reuniens connects the cochlear duct to the vestibular components of the membranous labyrinth (see Figure 1–4). The saccule and utricle are the two dilatations of the membranous labyrinth in the vestibule. The utricle is a connecting chamber that communicates with the semicircular canals. The saccule communicates with the utricle, and the two combine to form the endolymphatic duct, a sac that ends blindly in the temporal bone.

In the utricle and saccule are the maculae utriculi and maculae sacculi, respectively. These lie perpendicular to one another, and each consists of supporting (sustentacular) cells and hair cells. The hair cells have long cilia that are embedded in an otolithic membrane. The otolithic membrane contains otoliths, which are small crystalline bodies of calcium carbonate. Position changes of the head stimulate the otolithic membrane, and this stimulation is picked up by nerve endings between the hair cells. The maculae are concerned with the detection of linear movement of the head. The semicircular canals achieve adult size by 17 to 19 weeks gestation, with the lateral canal being the most slowly growing.

Early Middle Ear

Middle ear development begins closely associated with head formation and involves both the foregut tube (pharynx) and the pharyngeal arches. Pharyngeal arches form the main anatomical structures of the head and neck, including all components of the middle and outer ear.

Pharyngeal arches (branchial arches) are named by their location and shape, wrapping externally around the ventral surface of the pharynx and forming an "arch" shape. In humans, a series of five pharyngeal arches (1, 2, 3, 4, 6) form in sequence rostro-caudally (head to tail), Arch 5 apparently does not form, and Arches 4 and 6 soon fuse together. This leaves a series of four externally visible arches in the head region, with Arch 2 eventually growing over the inferior arches so that they are lost from the embryo surface.

Pharyngeal arches 1 and 2 are the main contributors to the middle and outer ear. Each of the arches has a similar overall structure with contributions from all three germ cell layers, but each arch will form different anatomical components of the head and neck. Each arch is covered with ectoderm (embryo surface) and lined with endoderm (pharynx) and separated from each other by a membrane formed by these two layers. The arches are composed of unsegmented head mesoderm, which is invaded by neural crest cells to form initially mesenchyme, a term used to describe an embryonic undifferentiated connective tissue. The mesenchyme differentiates to form the same series of components within each arch: a band of cartilage, an artery, and a vein. During later development these pharyngeal arch structures are extensively remodeled.

Middle Ear Auditory Ossicles

The three middle ear bones or auditory ossicles (malleus, incus, stapes) are formed from the cartilage template found within pharyngeal arches 1 and 2. These bones are commonly named the hammer (malleus), anvil (incus), and stirrup (stapes), and the cartilage bands are historically named after two German anatomists and are called Meckel's cartilage (first pharyngeal arch; named after Johann Friedrich Meckel, 1781–1833) and Reichert's cartilage (second pharyngeal arch; named after Karl Bogislaus Reichert, 1811–1883). There are several theories as to how each arch cartilage contributes individual components of the middle ear ossicles (Whyte et al., 2008; Whyte Orozco et al., 2003). Meckel's cartilage first appears histologically at Stage 16 (Orliaguet, Darcha, Dechelotte, & Vanneuville, 1994) and Reichert's cartilage slightly later.

The early stages of auditory ossicle development all occur within the solid mesenchyme of the pharyngeal arches until the eighth month of development, then within a fluid-filled space for the final month, and finally only postnatal in the neonate in the air-filled tympanic cavity. This transition in auditory ossicle environment means that the middle ear does not function correctly until after birth, and any prenatal conduction to the cochlea must be mediated through bone conduction. During development of the tympanic cavity, the auditory ossicles are held in their correct anatomic positions by supporting ligaments. Arch cartilages ossify by the process of endochondral ossification, where a preexisting cartilage template is first formed and later replaced by bone. Endochondral ossification is the main process of bone formation throughout the entire skeleton, except for the cranial vault and the clavicle that ossify by a process of intramembranous ossification.

Initially, the malleus and incus form as a single structure, and it is only later that they separate to form two separate bones. Ossification continues through the entire fetal period, and the newly formed bones also have a transient bone marrow cavity (Yokoyama, Iino, Kakizaki, & Murakami, 1999). The marrow cavity is still present at birth, in both the malleus and the incus, and with continued ossification is lost during the first 2 years after birth. Postnatally, first the malleus and then the incus lose their marrow spaces (Yokoyama et al., 1999).

Middle Ear Muscles

The middle ear also contains the two smallest muscles of the body, the stapedius and tensor tympani muscles, which both differentiate from arch mesenchyme (see Figure 1–5). These muscles form and differentiate in a similar fashion to other developing skeletal muscle. Initially, myoblasts proliferate under the influence of growth factors in the region of where the muscle will form. Myoblasts are the embryonic undifferentiated single cells of all skeletal muscles. The myoblasts' numbers reach a critical concentration, often depleting locally secreted growth factors, migrate, align, and commence to fuse plasma membranes. These fusion events form multinucleated myotubes, into which additional myoblasts continue to fuse at each end. The mechanisms regulating myoblast fusion are still being investigated (suggested signaling mechanisms include adhesion, immunoglobulin superfamily proteins, metalloproteases, potassium ion channels, and calcium). These myotubes that form are the second main stage of muscle cellular differentiation.

Depending on the size and structure of the muscle, a later second round of myoblast fusion events might occur around these early forming primary myotubes. The myotubes begin to upregulate and express the contractile proteins involved in forming the molecular contractile apparatus within muscle. The striated muscle contractile apparatus is called the sarcomere, which is the basic unit of contraction. The two major proteins are actin and myosin, which interact to shorten the single sarcomere, and the serial organization of thousands of sarcomeres within the muscle fiber leads to overall anatomical contraction. Sarcomeres initially form at the edge of developing myotubes and in many cases require innervation to complete their organization to form the mature muscle fiber. Innervation of muscle is therefore the final key to skeletal muscle differentiation, and functioning, denervated muscle will atrophy.

The type (isoform) of myosin and actin expressed by individual muscle fibers determines the contractile properties of the muscle fiber: slow (Type 1) or fast (Type 2A, 2X, 2B) twitch; oxidative (1, 2A), glycolytic (2B), or a mixture of both (2X) metabolisms. The adult muscle fiber isoform will then be regulated by the activity type of the innervating neuron. There is also some evidence to suggest a role for some hormonal regulation of muscle differentiation pattern. A single neuron will innervate a group of fibers all with the same contractile properties. The neuron together with the group of individual muscle fibers it innervates is called a motor unit.

Little is known about the developmental or adult muscle fiber types present in the human tensor tympani and stapedius muscles. In other skeletal muscles, the initial myotubes form as primary embryonic slow fibers being surrounded later by secondary fast fibers. Both primary and secondary fibers are then converted into their final adult fiber type by the innervating neuron. There is some fiber type analysis from animal model studies, including avian (Counter, Hellstrand, & Borg, 1987), rabbit (Vita, Muglia, Germana, Pennica, & Carfi, 1983), and cat (Lyon & Malmgren, 1982, 1988). The adult tensor tympani is classed as a mixed muscle containing slow (Type 1) and fast (Type 2A, and probably 2X) muscle fibers. The adult mammalian stapedius muscle contains mainly (77%) fast oxidative glycolytic-type muscle fibers and the avian muscle only contains fast fibers (Counter et al., 1987).

Both muscles carry out their contractile function postnatally. The tensor tympani's contraction pulls the malleus and tenses the tympanic membrane dampening auditory ossicle movement. The tensor tympani muscle cells arise from beside the auditory tube, the cartilaginous portion, and the muscle inserts into the malleus at the manubrium near the root. The tensor tympani will be innervated by cranial nerve five (CN V, trigeminal nerve). The second muscle, the stapedius muscle, will contract to pull the stapes and dampens auditory ossicle movement. This muscle is innervated by cranial nerve seven (CN VII, facial nerve). The main cranial nerve associated with hearing and balance is cranial nerve eight (CN VIII, vestibulocochlear nerve) or auditory-vestibular nerve or statoacoustic nerve. A brief summary of cranial nerve development is described later in this chapter and elsewhere (see Chapter 2).

Middle Ear Auditory Tube and Tympanic Cavity

The auditory tube, eustachian tube (named after Bartolomeo Eustachi, 1500–1574), otopharyngeal or pharyngotympanic tube develops from the first pharyngeal pouch and is lined with endoderm. This narrow cavity links the pharynx to the middle ear and is continuous with the tympanic cavity (see Figure 1–5). The auditory tube has two main functions: ventilation, to allow the equalization of pressure in the middle ear, and clearance, to allow the middle ear fluid continuously produced by the epithelial lining to drain from the middle ear.

In normal human development, the auditory tube has an almost straight posterolateral to anteromedial pathway. The main growth of the auditory tube occurs in extension and lumen of the cartilaginous portion in the fetal period between Weeks 16 and 28 (Swarts, Rood, & Doyle, 1986).

At birth, and in the young child, the tube is shorter (8–9 mm) compared to the adult length (17–18 mm), runs almost horizontal, and is narrower in diameter. Head growth in the child to adult size results in a longer, wider tube that runs at approximately 45 degrees to the horizontal. The auditory tube is also normally closed and is opened by muscles—in the infant this is only a single muscle, the tensor palati muscle. In the adult, the auditory tube is now opened by two separate muscles, the tensor palati and levator palati muscles.

The above developmental factors combine to contribute to the increased frequency of middle ear infections arising in the young child. The short length leads to easier transmission of infection from oral cavity to middle ear. The opening beside the adenoids and narrow lumen leads to easy blockage during infection and inflammation. Finally, the almost horizontal pathway leads to poor middle ear drainage.

The middle ear cavity or tympanic cavity is formed by an expansion of the pharynx. The initial early cavity lining is formed by the pharyngeal endoderm epithelium. The epithelium will then continue to expand, to eventually also line the entire mastoid antrum.

The adult middle ear, like the inner ear, eventually will lie within the petrous portion of temporal bone. Initially, both the middle and inner ear form within mesenchyme, embryonic connective tissue, forming the otic capsule, and this will also form the base of the skull. The mesenchyme differentiates first to form cartilage, forming a structure known as the chondrocranium. This initial cartilage is gradually replaced by bone forming at a number of sites within the cartilage, ossification centers. The initial bone that is formed also contains marrow spaces that disappear with ongoing ossification (Yokoyama et al., 1999). Between the weeks 16 and 24, centers of ossification appear in the remaining cartilage of the otic capsule, and these continue to ossify to eventually form mastoid process of temporal bone (Nemzek et al., 1996).

Early External Ear Development

The outer ear consists of the auricle (pinna), the external auditory meatus (ear canal), and the outer layer of the tympanic membrane. The first and second pharyngeal arches contribute the auricle, each contributing three auricular hillocks. Each of the auricular hillocks (small hills) is a mesenchymal swelling covered in ectoderm observable on the embryo surface and will contribute an individual anatomical component of the external ear (Figure 1–7). These hillocks are initially located low on the developing head, at the level of the neck, and both change their relative position with head growth and are extensively remodeled during the late embryonic period (Weeks 5–8). By the end of Week 8, the basic structure of the external auricle has been formed, but it still lies well below its final anatomical position. Some abnormalities of external ear structure and position are both indicators of developmental problems requiring further investigation; this is discussed later in the chapter. These abnormalities can relate to the development of hearing as well as to other internal systems that develop over a similar time course.

The external auditory meatus develops from the first pharyngeal cleft, which lies externally between the first two arches. It is the only cleft that will form a structure in the developing embryo. The embryonic canal is blocked by a temporary meatal plug, which forms at the end of the embryonic period and remains for a variable period through fetal development. The epithelial lining is derived from the ectoderm germ layer and also contributes the outer layer of the tympanic membrane. Failure of the meatal plug to degenerate can lead to deafness. A detailed time course of human meatal development has been previously described and published by Nishimura and Kumoi (1992).

Later in the fetal period toward the end of the second trimester, within the epithelium two types of associated glands differentiate, sebaceous and modified apocrine glands, which in the postnatal period begin to secrete cerumen, or ear wax (Wright, 1997). The cerumen is composed of exfoliated epithelial keratin and gland secretions also containing antimicrobial peptides (Supp, Karpinski, & Boyce, 2004). These glandular secretions are altered postnatally and mature at puberty (Wright, 1997).

After the embryonic period, both the auricle and external canal continue to grow through the fetal period and into the postnatal period, reaching their young adult size at about 9 years of age (Wright, 1997). The external ear then continues to grow in size slowly through the entire adult life.

The tympanic membrane or eardrum has contributions from all three germ layers. The external auditory meatus is lined with surface ectoderm, which is continuous with the outer tympanic membrane. The tympanic cavity forms from the pharynx and is lined with endoderm, which is continuous with the inner tympanic membrane. Lying between the two layers is a thin layer of mesenchymal connective tissue, the fibrous stratum.

Cranial Nerve Development

There are 12 pairs of cranial nerves numbered in rostrocaudal (head to tail) sequence and developing initially beside the neural tube at the level of the hindbrain. The cranial nerves are traditionally numbered by Roman

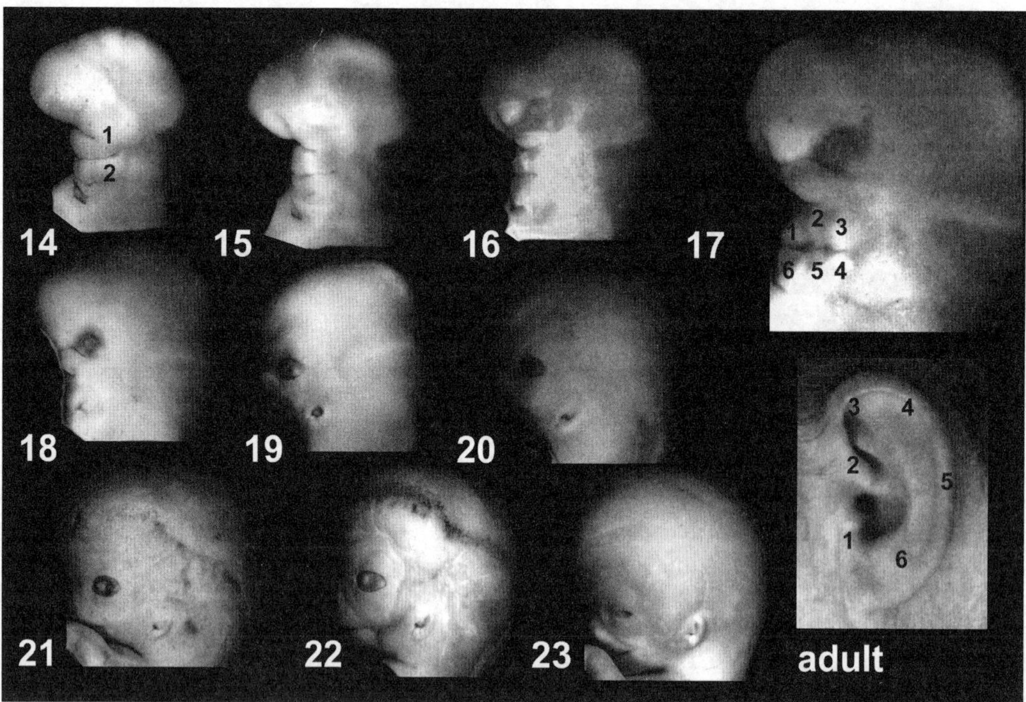

FIGURE 1–7. Embryonic development of the external ear from Stage 14 (Week 5) to Stage 23 (Week 8) compared to the adult ear. Lateral views of the heads are not shown to scale, and there is a fivefold increase in size between Stages 14 and 23. During Week 5 (Stage 14 to 15), pharyngeal arches 1 and 2 are visible separated by the first pharyngeal groove, which will form the external auditory meatus. In Week 6 (Stages 16 and 17), separate hillocks appear on the surfaces of pharyngeal arches 1 and 2, which will contribute the structure of the external ear. Stage 17 is enlarged to show the numbered hillocks, and equivalent regions are shown in the adult ear. Importantly, note the changing relative position of the external ear with head growth and development from below the lower jaw to between the level of the nose and eye by the end of the embryonic period. Embryo images are modified from the Kyoto collection, courtesy of Professor Kohei Shiota and Shigehito Yamada.

numerals as well as have names based on their adult function. As discussed previously, the middle ear muscles are supplied by motor divisions of different cranial nerves. The tensor tympani will be innervated by the mandibular division of the trigeminal nerve (CN V). The stapedius muscle is innervated by the tympanic branch of the facial nerve (CN VII), and the cochlea and vestibular apparatus are supplied by statoacoustic or vestibulocochlear ganglion (CN VIII). The neurons have a dependence during development for their survival on at least two known secreted growth factors, brain-derived neurotrophic factor (BDNF) and neurotrophin 3 (NT3). BNDF and NT-3 bind TrkB and TrkC receptors, respectively, on the surface of these neurons. The growth factors may also have differential functions in identifying either vestibular or cochlear targets within the inner ear (Tessarollo, Coppola, & Fritzsch, 2004).

Abnormalities

Human pregnancy and development are generally robust processes, and in dealing with abnormalities this can sometimes be forgotten. All abnormalities of human development can be grouped into three main categories: genetic, environmental, and unknown (undetermined). The complex origins of all components of hearing and the long time-course of development expose this system to a large number of different environmental effects. To further complicate diagnosis and prognosis, all the environmental factors below have different combinatorial effects, and exposure at different times of the pregnancy can also lead to entirely different developmental outcomes. The sensory systems too have the combined effects of abnormalities in both or either of the sensory components or structures (conductive) and the sensorineural pathway. This also may mean that an abnormality will occur in combinations of outer, middle, and inner ear structures. Two notable recent changes in our general understanding of human abnormalities include increasing incidence of fetal alcohol syndrome and the fetal origins hypothesis that states that prenatal developmental effects impact postnatally on lifelong health outcomes.

The external ear (auricle) is also an excellent indicator or marker for other, not as easily detectible, internal developmental abnormalities. The commonly detected abnormalities include sinuses, tags, and position on the head. In many cases, this is related to the development of the external ear and head overlapping with these internal systems, for example, the correlation of ear abnormalities with kidney developmental abnormalities. Another currently relevant correlation is a low or uneven ear/head position with the growing occurrence of fetal alcohol syndrome.

This chapter includes a brief overview and a few sample disorders of some hearing abnormalities, due to the large number of different genetic associations. More details are shown online at http://tiny.cc/Hearing_Abnormalities (Hill, 2015).

Genetic

In human development, the majority of major genetic abnormalities are thought to be lost in the first 2 weeks of development as the zygote, then morula and blastocyst fail to develop correctly and complete implantation. Genetic abnormalities can be further grouped into chromosomal aneuploidies (abnormal chromosome numbers, e.g., Down syndrome, trisomy 13), translocation of chromosomal segments, and, finally, single gene mutations. The single gene mutations can be of four main types: autosomal (non-sex chromosome) and X-linked, and in both cases can be a dominant (expressed) or a recessive (carrier) trait. These genetic mutations are now often well documented in terms of systematic effects. Single gene mutations are also defined by the gene location using the following combination of chromosome number (1 to 22, X or Y), letter (p or q, referring to the short or long "arm" of each chromosome), and number (variable referring to position with reference to banding pattern on folded chromosome). The gene location as yet also may not be exactly located or span two reference locations.

Online Mendelian Inheritance in Man (OMIM; http://omim.org) is a searchable compendium of human genes and genetic phenotypes, and it contains both reference links for this next section of notes and detailed clinical synopses. A search of OMIM with the term "hearing" results in more than 900 different entries, and nearly 400 entries have a clinical synopsis. Many of these genetic disorders that affect hearing are also part of multisystem genetic syndromes. The usefulness of the OMIM database is shown in the following example: Congenital autosomal dominant deafness (DFNA36, http://www.omim.org/entry/606705) is caused by mutations in the transmembrane channel–like gene 1 (TMC1, 9q21.13, http://www.omim.org/entry/606706). With this knowledge, a mouse model of deafness (*Beethoven*) that is a knockout of Tmc1 has been generated. Hearing in this deaf mouse model has recently been restored by gene therapy (Askew et al., 2015).

Environmental

The many different environmental effects, described as "teratogens," have been more typically described as "maternal effects." This term though is both outdated and stigmatizing to parents. Some environmental effects can be directly due to maternal behavior/lifestyle (e.g., diet, drugs, smoking, or alcohol) or a preexisting maternal condition (e.g., diabetes), often before pregnancy has been detected. However, there are many other developmental environmental effects that are not directly controlled by the mother. These include infections (bacterial, viral, parasites), hyperthermia, environmental contaminants (heavy metals, polychlorinated biphenyls), and radiation.

External Ear

Low or uneven set ears indicate a developmental abnormality of head growth and development and can be unique to the ear or relate to other conditions. Some of these external abnormalities are indicative of middle ear bone abnormalities: thickened lobes (abnormal incus and stapes), smaller "cup" ears with absent cartilage (Mennonite genetic kindred absence of incus and stapes), or absent superior crus (congenital ossicle fixation). Other non-hearing-associated abnormalities include Klippel-Feil syndrome, cardiac, and urogenital (kidney and gonad) abnormalities.

Anotia or absence of the ear is due to the pharyngeal arch hillocks failing to form and impacts also on the external auditory meatus and middle ear bones. This is sometimes grouped with microtia. Known genetic associations include mandibulofacial dysostosis, Treacher Collins syndrome (5q32-q33.1), hemifacial microsomia (14q32), and congenital aural atresia (18q22.3-q23).

Microtia or small ear has a cup ear or overfolded auricle and might have absence of the external auditory meatus. Genetically, there are nearly 40 different associations including syndromes, hearing and vision abnormalities, neurological abnormalities, clefting of the palate and face, and other musculoskeletal abnormalities. Environmentally, maternal drugs including thalidomide and retinoic acid have also caused microtia. This condition is repaired surgically using cartilage derived from the rib to reconstruct the external ear. Auriculocondylar syndrome (question mark ear) also can be repaired by this cartilage transfer operation; it is a rare syndrome with variable hearing loss and facial effects.

Auricular fistulas (an abnormal connection or passageway) and sinuses (cavities) are usually harmless. Preauricular sinus occurs in 0.25% births, is bilateral (hereditary) in 25% to 50% of cases, and unilateral (slightly more in the left). They are developmental and generally occur on the surface in the anterior margin of the ascending limb of the helix, and the duct runs inward to the perichondrium of the auricular cartilage and in some cases extends into the parotid gland. Some genetic associations vary from prevalent to rare syndromes and include hemifacial microsomia (914q32), Townes and Brocks syndrome (16q12.1), branchiooculofacial syndrome (96p24), and velocardiofacial syndrome (22q11.2). Sinuses postnatally are also common sites of infections.

Auricular appendages (tags) bilateral or unilateral (one or both ears) are quite common and often not associated with other developmental conditions other than those shown above. Stenosis (narrowing) of the external auditory meatus is uncommon and postnatally can be due to chronic otitis externa or acquired atresia. The condition can be treated surgically by meatoplasty (reconstructive surgery of the canal) alone, though acquired atresia requires removal of the soft tissue plug and a split skin graft.

The external ear can also be diagnostic for fetal alcohol syndrome (FAS), the most serious of the fetal alcohol spectrum disorders (FASDs). FASD is an umbrella term used to describe the range of effects that can occur in an individual whose mother drank alcohol during pregnancy, and is not intended as a clinical diagnosis. The effects can include physical, mental, behavioral, and learning disabilities with possible lifelong implications. There is also evidence that FAS is directly associated with delayed auditory function, sensorineural hearing loss, and intermittent conductive hearing loss due to recurrent serous otitis media (Church & Abel, 1998). Fetal alcohol effect (FAE) is the less obvious form and has the neurological effects without the external physiologic features. It presents as learning difficulties or delayed milestones. The infant with FAS will have lower or uneven external ear position. The auricle also may feature a curve at the top part of the ear, which is underdeveloped and folded over parallel to the curve beneath. This appearance is often described as a "railroad track" ear.

Middle Ear

There are many middle ear abnormalities that mainly affect the middle ear ossicle formation and can also incorporate effects on the facial nerve. The majority (90%) of infants with Trisomy 21 (Down syndrome) have hearing loss due to conduction abnormalities.

The absence of middle ear ossicles can be associated with a range of conditions and syndromes, including dwarfism and achondrogenesis. The most common bones to be absent are the incus and stapes. Fixation of the stapes by fibrous tissue can occur in association with cochlear abnormalities of oval window absence and in several syndromes including X-linked deafness 2 DFNX2 (Xq21.1), branchiootorenal syndrome (8q13.3; Senel et al., 2009), and Beckwith-Wiedemann syndrome (11p15.5, 11p15.5, 11p15.5, 5q35; Paulsen, 1973).

Persistent stapedial artery occurs in the fetus, as the stapedial artery initially lies between the foramen of the stapes and is lost before birth. If this regression fails, it can lead to a persistent stapedial artery that will affect conduction through the middle ear ossicle chain. This condition can be seen in hemifacial microsomia (14q32), a reasonably common sporadic and rare familial autosomal dominant abnormality of the first and second pharyngeal arch derivatives (Carvalho, Song, Vargervik, & Lalwani, 1999).

The middle ear cavity can be delayed in either formation or size, leading to variable conduction effects. This can be seen with oligohydramnios caused by renal agenesis, such as in branchiootorenal syndrome (8q13.3).

Inner Ear

Inner ear cochlear and semicircular canal abnormalities are generally due to many different genetic effects and are both conducting and sensorineural related. In addition to specific gene mutations, the trisomies (chromosomal aneuploidy) have inner ear abnormalities. Infants with Trisomy 21 (Down syndrome) can have a range of conduction defects, and more recently, inner ear defects have been reported (Blaser et al., 2006).

Infants with Trisomy 13 (Patau syndrome) can have an underdeveloped cochlear duct and saccule. Infants with Trisomy 18 (Edwards syndrome) lack spiral ganglia and have other middle ear abnormalities.

Michel aplasia is an extremely rare abnormality showing complete absence of the inner ear labyrinth. This loss of inner ear structures is similar to that seen in the autosomal recessive LAMM syndrome, which consists of labyrinthine aplasia, microtia, and microdontia. LAMM syndrome is caused by mutations in just the single gene encoding fibroblast growth factor 3 (11q13). FGF3 is a transmembrane receptor involved in developmental signaling including cell proliferation and vascular growth.

Pendred syndrome (7q31) is one of the most common (1% to 10% of hereditary deafness) inner ear deafness syndromes, autosomally recessive with abnormalities of the cochlea, enlarged vestibular aqueduct, sensorineural hearing loss, and diffuse thyroid enlargement (goiter; Phelps et al., 1998). The condition is caused by a mutation in the gene encoding an anion transporter (SLC26A4) protein called pendrin (Everett et al., 1997). More recently, a growing number of human genetic studies and animal model studies have identified gene mutations (OMIM 67 entries) that can impact on general cochlear and, specifically, hair cell development.

Several examples of prenatal infections that impact inner ear development are also mentioned. Rubella is the most well-known viral infection with severe impact on hearing through effects on cochlear duct and saccular development (Vermeif-Keers, 1975). In some countries with poor vaccination records, gestational rubella can be responsible for a significant proportion of reported deafness (Bento, Castilho, Sakae, Andrade, & Zugaib, 2005; Niedzielska, Katska, & Szymula, 2000). Other viral infections have also been shown to impact hearing: cytomegalovirus (CMV) inner ear vascular effects and herpes simplex 2 viremia can cause both hemorrhagic and necrotic lesions. Interestingly, the mouse model of CMV-related hearing loss suggests that the main effect is due to the inflammatory response rather than the direct effects of infection (Bradford et al., 2015). Toxoplasmosis infection caused by the protist *Toxoplasma gondii* being present in uncooked meat and contact with cat feces is rarely serious postnatally in children or adults. In contrast, a maternally derived infection of the fetus can lead to spontaneous abortion and a range of developmental effects including deafness (Brown, Chau, Atashband, Westerberg, & Kozak, 2009).

This chapter has provided a brief introduction to the normal and abnormal development of hearing and the related genetic and environmental effects. Other chapters in this textbook expand on the clinical aspects of these topics and additional disorders, as well as covering issues relating to neonatal hearing testing and diagnosis.

Acknowledgments. The author wishes to thank Judith Gravel, Richard Seewald, and Anne Marie Tharpe for the original chapter invitation. I thank again my wife Leighana for her support during preparation of this new edition of the chapter. I apologize to any of my colleagues whose work was not cited in this review because of length constraints.

References

Andermann, P., Ungos, J., & Raible, D. W. (2002). Neurogenin1 defines zebrafish cranial sensory ganglia precursors. *Developmental Biology, 251*(1), 45–58.

Anniko, M., & Nordemar, H. (1980). Embryogenesis of the inner ear. IV. Post-natal maturation of the secretory epithelia of the inner ear in correlation with the elemental composition in the endolymphatic space. *Archives of Oto-rhinolaryngology-Head and Neck Surgery, 229*(3–4), 281–288.

Anniko, M., & Wroblewski, R. (1981). Elemental composition of the developing inner ear. *Annals of Otolology, Rhinology & Laryngology, 90*(1 Pt. 1), 25–32.

Arnold, W. (1987). Myelination of the human spiral ganglion. *Acta Otolaryngologica, 104*(Suppl. 436), 76–84.

Askew, C., Rochat, C., Pan, B., Asai, Y., Ahmed, H., Child, E., . . . Holt, J. R. (2015). Tmc gene therapy restores auditory function in deaf mice. *Science Translational Medicine, 7*(295), 295ra108.

Bagger-Sjoback, D. (1991). Embryology of the human endolymphatic duct and sac. *Journal of Oto-Rhino-Laryngology and Its Related Specialties, 53*(2), 61–67.

Barrionuevo, F., Naumann, A., Bagheri-Fam, S., Speth, V., Taketo, M. M., Scherer, G., & Neubuser, A. (2008). Sox9 is required for invagination of the otic placode in mice. *Developmental Biology, 317*(1), 213–224.

Beisel, K. W., Wang-Lundberg, Y., Maklad, A., & Fritzsch, B. (2005). Development and evolution of the vestibular sensory apparatus of the mammalian ear. *Journal of Vestibular Research, 15*(5–6), 225–241.

Bento, R. F., Castilho, A. M., Sakae, F. A., Andrade, J. Q., & Zugaib, M. (2005). Auditory brainstem response and otoacoustic emission assessment of hearing-impaired children of mothers who contracted rubella during pregnancy. *Acta Otolaryngologica, 125*(5), 492–494.

Bernd, P., Zhang, D., Yao, L., & Rozenberg, I. (1994). The potential role of nerve growth factor, brain-derived neurotrophic factor and neurotrophin-3 in avian cochlear and vestibular ganglia development. *International Journal of Developmental Neuroscience, 12*(8), 709–723.

Bibas, A., Liang, J., Michaels, L., & Wright, A. (2000). The development of the stria vascularis in the human foetus. *Clinical Otolaryngology and Allied Sciences, 25*(2), 126–129.

Bibas, A. G., Xenellis, J., Michaels, L., Anagnostopoulou, S., Ferekidis, E., & Wright, A. (2008). Temporal bone study of development of the organ of Corti: Correlation between auditory function and anatomical structure. *Journal of Laryngology and Otology, 122*(4), 336–342.

Blaser, S., Propst, E. J., Martin, D., Feigenbaum, A., James, A. L., Shannon, P., & Papsin, B. C. (2006). Inner ear dysplasia is common in children with Down syndrome (trisomy 21). *Laryngoscope, 116*(12), 2113–2119.

Blasiole, B., Kabbani, N., Boehmler, W., Thisse, B., Thisse, C., Canfield, V., & Levenson, R. (2005). Neuronal calcium sensor-1 gene ncs-1a is essential for semicircular canal formation in zebrafish inner ear. *Journal of Neurobiology, 64*(3), 285–297.

Bosher, S. K., & Warren, R. L. (1971). A study of the electrochemistry and osmotic relationships of the cochlear fluids in the neonatal rat at the time of the development of the endocochlear potential. *Journal of Physiology, 212*(3), 739–761.

Bradford, R. D., Yoo, Y. G., Golemac, M., Pugel, E. P., Jonjic, S., & Britt, W. J. (2015). Murine CMV-induced hearing loss is associated with inner ear inflammation and loss of spiral ganglia neurons. *PLOS Pathogens, 11*(4), e1004774.

Brown, E. D., Chau, J. K., Atashband, S., Westerberg, B. D., & Kozak, F. K. (2009). A systematic review of neonatal toxoplasmosis exposure and sensorineural hearing loss. *International Journal of Pediatric Otorhinolaryngology, 73*(5), 707–711.

Bruska, M., & Wozniak, W. (2000). The origin of cells of the cochlear ganglion in early human embryos. *Folia Morphologica (Warsz), 59*(4), 233–238.

Camarero, G., Avendano, C., Fernandez-Moreno, C., Villar, A., Contreras, J., de Pablo, F., . . . Varela-Nieto, I. (2001). Delayed inner ear maturation and neuronal loss in postnatal Igf-1-deficient mice. *Journal of Neuroscience, 21*(19), 7630–7641.

Carvalho, G. J., Song, C. S., Vargervik, K., & Lalwani, A. K. (1999). Auditory and facial nerve dysfunction in patients with hemifacial microsomia. *Archives of Otolaryngology-Head and Neck Surgery, 125*(2), 209–212.

Chang, W., Brigande, J. V., Fekete, D. M., & Wu, D. K. (2004). The development of semicircular canals in the inner ear: Role of FGFs in sensory cristae. *Development, 131*(17), 4201–4211.

Chiong, C. M., Burgess, B. J., & Nadol, J. B., Jr. (1993). Postnatal maturation of human spiral ganglion cells: Light and electron microscopic observations. *Hearing Research, 67*(1–2), 211–219.

Church, M. W., & Abel, E. L. (1998). Fetal alcohol syndrome. Hearing, speech, language, and vestibular disorders. *Obstetrics and Gynecology Clinics of North America, 25*(1), 85–97.

Conlee, J. W., Gerity, L. C., & Bennett, M. L. (1994). Ongoing proliferation of melanocytes in the stria vascularis of adult guinea pigs. *Hearing Research, 79*(1–2), 115–122.

Counter, S. A., Hellstrand, E., & Borg, E. (1987). A histochemical characterization of muscle fiber types in the avian M. stapedius. *Comparative Biochemistry and Physiology A, 86*(1), 185–187.

Cristobal, R., Popper, P., Lopez, I., Micevych, P., De Vellis, J., & Honrubia, V. (2002). In vivo and in vitro localization of brain-derived neurotrophic factor, fibroblast growth factor-2 and their receptors in the bullfrog vestibular end organs. *Molecular Brain Research, 102*(1–2), 83–99.

Daudet, N., Ariza-McNaughton, L., & Lewis, J. (2007). Notch signalling is needed to maintain, but not to initiate, the formation of prosensory patches in the chick inner ear. *Development, 134*(12), 2369–2378.

Everett, L. A., Glaser, B., Beck, J. C., Idol, J. R., Buchs, A., Heyman, M., . . . Green, E. D. (1997). Pendred syndrome is caused by mutations in a putative sulphate transporter gene (PDS). *Nature Genetics, 17*(4), 411–422.

Fekete, D. M., & Campero, A. M. (2007). Axon guidance in the inner ear. *International Journal of Developmental Biology, 51*(6–7), 549–556.

Fritzsch, B., Knipper, M., & Friauf, E. (2015). Auditory system: Development, genetics, function, aging, and diseases. *Cell Tissue Research, 361*(1), 1–6.

Fritzsch, B., Pirvola, U., & Ylikoski, J. (1999). Making and breaking the innervation of the ear: Neurotrophic support during ear development and its clinical implications. *Cell Tissue Research, 295*(3), 369–382.

Grunder, S., Muller, A., & Ruppersberg, J. P. (2001). Developmental and cellular expression pattern of epithelial sodium channel alpha, beta and gamma subunits in the inner ear of the rat. *European Journal of Neuroscience, 13*(4), 641–648.

Hafidi, A., & Dulon, D. (2004). Developmental expression of Ca(v)1.3 (alpha1d) calcium channels in the mouse inner ear. *Brain Research Developmental Brain Research, 150*(2), 167–175.

Hatch, E. P., Noyes, C. A., Wang, X., Wright, T. J., & Mansour, S. L. (2007). Fgf3 is required for dorsal patterning and morphogenesis of the inner ear epithelium. *Development, 134*(20), 3615–3625.

Hertzano, R., Montcouquiol, M., Rashi-Elkeles, S., Elkon, R., Yucel, R., Frankel, W. N., . . . Avraham, K. B. (2004). Transcription profiling of inner ears from Pou4f3 (ddl/ddl) identifies Gfi1 as a target of the Pou4f3 deafness gene. *Human Molecular Genetics, 13*(18), 2143–2153.

Hill, M. A. (2015). *Embryology sensory—Hearing and balance development*. Retrieved August 1, 2015, from https://embryology.med.unsw.edu.au/embryology/index.php/Sensory_-_Hearing_and_Balance_Development

Hossain, W. A., Brumwell, C. L., & Morest, D. K. (2002). Sequential interactions of fibroblast growth factor-2, brain-derived neurotrophic factor, neurotrophin-3, and their receptors define critical periods in the development of cochlear ganglion cells. *Experimental Neurology, 175*(1), 138–151.

Jenkinson, J. W. (1911). The development of the ear-bones in the mouse. *Journal of Anatomy and Physiology,* 45(Pt. 4), 305–318.

Johnson, R. L., & Spoendlin, H. H. (1966). Structural evidence of secretion in the stria vascularis. *Annals of Otology, Rhinology & Laryngology, 75*(1), 127–138.

Kelley, M. W. (2007). Cellular commitment and differentiation in the organ of Corti. *International Journal of Developmental Biology, 51*(6–7), 571–583.

Kwak, S. J., Vemaraju, S., Moorman, S. J., Zeddies, D., Popper, A. N., & Riley, B. B. (2006). Zebrafish pax5 regulates development of the utricular macula and vestibular function. *Developmental Dynamics, 235*(11), 3026–3038.

Lavigne-Rebillard, M., & Bagger-Sjoback, D. (1992). Development of the human stria vascularis. *Hearing Research, 64*(1), 39–51.

Levi-Montalcini, R. (1949). The development to the acoustico-vestibular centers in the chick embryo in the absence of the afferent root fibers and of descending fiber tracts. *Journal of Comprehensive Neurology, 91*(2), 209–241.

Litovsky, R. (2015). Development of the auditory system. *Handbook of Clinical Neurology, 129*, 55–72.

Locher, H., de Groot, J. C., van Iperen, L., Huisman, M. A., Frijns, J. H., & Chuva de Sousa Lopes, S. M. (2014). Distribution and development of peripheral glial cells in the human fetal cochlea. *PLOS One, 9*(1), e88066.

Lyon, M. J., & Malmgren, L. T. (1982). A histochemical characterization of muscle fiber types in the middle ear muscles of the cat. 1. The stapedius muscle. *Acta Otolaryngologica, 94*(1–2), 99–109.

Lyon, M. J., & Malmgren, L. T. (1988). Muscle fiber types in the cat middle ear muscles. II. Tensor tympani. *Archives of Otolaryngology-Head and Neck Surgery, 114*(4), 404–409.

Masetto, S., Zucca, G., Botta, L., & Valli, P. (2005). Endolymphatic potassium of the chicken vestibule during embryonic development. *International Journal of Developmental Neuroscience, 23*(5), 439–448.

May, L. A., Kramarenko, II, Brandon, C. S., Voelkel-Johnson, C., Roy, S., Truong, K., . . . Cunningham, L. L. (2013). Inner ear supporting cells protect hair cells by secreting HSP70. *Journal of Clinical Investigation, 123*(8), 3577–3587.

Moore, J. K., & Linthicum, F. H., Jr. (2001). Myelination of the human auditory nerve: Different time courses for Schwann cell and glial myelin. *Annals of Otology, Rhinology & Laryngology, 110*(7 Pt. 1), 655–661.

Nemzek, W. R., Brodie, H. A., Chong, B. W., Babcook, C. J., Hecht, S. T., Salamat, S., . . . Seibert, J. A. (1996). Imaging findings of the developing temporal bone in fetal specimens. *American Journal of Neuroradiology, 17*(8), 1467–1477.

Ng, M. (2000). Postnasal maturation of the human endolymphatic sac. *Laryngoscope, 110*(9), 1452–1456.

Ng, M., & Linthicum, F. H. (1998). Morphology of the developing human endolymphatic sac. *Laryngoscope, 108*(2), 190–194.

Niedzielska, G., Katska, E., & Szymula, D. (2000). Hearing defects in children born of mothers suffering from rubella in the first trimester of pregnancy. *International Journal of Pediatric Otorhinolaryngology, 54*(1), 1–5.

Nin, F., Hibino, H., Doi, K., Suzuki, T., Hisa, Y., & Kurachi, Y. (2008). The endocochlear potential depends on two K+ diffusion potentials and an electrical barrier in the stria vascularis of the inner ear. *Proceedings of the National Academy of Sciences, USA, 105*(5), 1751–1756.

Nishimura, Y., & Kumoi, T. (1992). The embryologic development of the human external auditory meatus. Preliminary report. *Acta Otolaryngologica, 112*(3), 496–503.

Okano, J., Takigawa, T., Seki, K., Suzuki, S., Shiota, K., & Ishibashi, M. (2005). Transforming growth factor beta 2 promotes the formation of the mouse cochleovestibular ganglion in organ culture. *International Journal of Developmental Biology, 49*(1), 23–31.

Omata, Y., Nojima, Y., Nakayama, S., Okamoto, H., Nakamura, H., & Funahashi, J. (2007). Role of bone morphogenetic protein 4 in zebrafish semicircular canal development. *Developmental Growth and Differentiation, 49*(9), 711–719.

Orliaguet, T., Darcha, C., Dechelotte, P., & Vanneuville, G. (1994). Meckel's cartilage in the human embryo and fetus. *Anatomical Record, 238*(4), 491–497.

Paulsen, K. (1973). Otological features in exomphalos-macroglossia-gigantism syndrome (Wiedemann's syndrome). *Zeitschrift für Laryngologie, Rhinologie, Otologie und ihre Grenzgebiete, 52*(11), 793–798.

Pechriggl, E. J., Bitsche, M., Glueckert, R., Rask-Andersen, H., Blumer, M. J., Schrott-Fischer, A., & Fritsch, H. (2015). Development of the innervation of the human inner ear. *Developmental Neurobiology, 75*(7), 683–702.

Petrovic, J., Galvez, H., Neves, J., Abello, G., & Giraldez, F. (2015). Differential regulation of Hes/Hey genes during inner ear development. *Developmental Neurobiology, 75*(7), 703–720.

Phelps, P. D., Coffey, R. A., Trembath, R. C., Luxon, L. M., Grossman, A. B., Britton, K. E., . . . Reardon, W. (1998). Radiological malformations of the ear in Pendred syndrome. *Clinical Radiology, 53*(4), 268–273.

Represa, J. J., Moro, J. A., Gato, A., Pastor, F., & Barbosa, E. (1990). Patterns of epithelial cell death during early development of the human inner ear. *Annals of Otology, Rhinology & Laryngology, 99*(6 Pt. 1), 482–488.

Rueda, J., Prieto, J. J., Cantos, R., Sala, M. L., & Merchan, J. A. (2003). Hypothyroidism prevents developmental neuronal loss during auditory organ development. *Neuroscience Research, 45*(4), 401–408.

Sage, C., Huang, M., Vollrath, M. A., Brown, M. C., Hinds, P. W., Corey, D. P., . . . Chen, Z. Y. (2006). Essential role of retinoblastoma protein in mammalian hair cell development and hearing. *Proceedings of the National Academy of Sciences, USA, 103*(19), 7345–7350.

Sanchez Del Rey, A., Sanchez Fernandez, J. M., Martinez Ibarguen, A., & Santaolalla Montoya, F. (1995). Morphologic and morphometric study of human spiral ganglion development. *Acta Otolaryngologica, 115*(2), 211–217.

Schimmang, T., Tan, J., Muller, M., Zimmermann, U., Rohbock, K., Kopschall, I., . . . Knipper, M. (2003). Lack of Bdnf and TrkB signalling in the postnatal cochlea leads to a spatial reshaping of innervation along the tonotopic axis and hearing loss. *Development, 130*(19), 4741–4750.

Senel, E., Kocak, H., Akbiyik, F., Saylam, G., Gulleroglu, B. N., & Senel, S. (2009). From a branchial fistula to a branchiootorenal syndrome: A case report and review of the literature. *Journal of Pediatric Surgery, 44*(3), 623–625.

Sobkowicz, H. M., Slapnick, S. M., & August, B. K. (2002). Differentiation of spinous synapses in the mouse organ of corti. *Synapse, 45*(1), 10–24.

Sohmer, H., Perez, R., Sichel, J. Y., Priner, R., & Freeman, S. (2001). The pathway enabling external sounds to reach and excite the fetal inner ear. *Audiology and Neuro-Otology, 6*(3), 109–116.

Solomon, K. S., Kwak, S. J., & Fritz, A. (2004). Genetic interactions underlying otic placode induction and formation. *Developmental Dynamics, 230*(3), 419–433.

Streeter, G. L. (1942). Developmental horizons in human embryos: Description of age group XI, 13 to 20 somites and age group XII, 21 to 29 somites. *Contributions to Embryology, 30*, 211–245.

Streeter, G. L. (1948). Developmental horizons in human embryos: Description of age groups XV, XVI, XVII and XVIII, being the third issue of a survey of the Carnegie Collection. *Contributions to Embryology, 32*, 133–203.

Streeter, G. L. (1951). Developmental horizons in human embryos: Description of age groups XIX, XX, XXI, XXII XXIII, being the fifth issue of a survey of the Carnegie Collection. *Contributions to Embryology, 34*, 165–196.

Supp, D. M., Karpinski, A. C., & Boyce, S. T. (2004). Expression of human beta-defensins HBD-1, HBD-2, and HBD-3 in cultured keratinocytes and skin substitutes. *Burns, 30*(7), 643–648.

Suzuki, T., Nomoto, Y., Nakagawa, T., Kuwahata, N., Ogawa, H., Suzuki, Y., . . . Omori, K. (2006). Age-dependent degeneration of the stria vascularis in human cochleae. *Laryngoscope, 116*(10), 1846–1850.

Swarts, J. D., Rood, S. R., & Doyle, W. J. (1986). Fetal development of the auditory tube and paratubal musculature. *Cleft Palate Journal, 23*(4), 289–311.

Tessarollo, L., Coppola, V., & Fritzsch, B. (2004). NT-3 replacement with brain-derived neurotrophic factor redirects vestibular nerve fibers to the cochlea. *Journal of Neuroscience, 24*(10), 2575–2584.

Thyng, F. W. (1914). The anatomy of a 17.8 mm human embryo. *American Journal of Anatomy, 14*, 31–113.

Ulatowska-Blaszyk, K., & Bruska, M. (1999). The cochlear ganglion in human embryos of developmental stages 18 and 19. *Folia Morphohologica (Warsz), 58*(1), 29–35.

Vermeif-Keers, C. (1975). Primary congenital aphakia and the rubella syndrome. *Teratology, 11*(3), 257–265.

Vita, G., Muglia, U., Germana, G., Pennica, F., & Carfi, F. (1983). Histochemical characteristics of rabbit stapedius muscle. *Experimental Neurology, 81*(2), 511–516.

Waka, N., Knipper, M., & Engel, J. (2003). Localization of the calcium channel subunits Cav1.2 (alpha1C) and Cav2.3 (alpha1E) in the mouse organ of Corti. *Histology and Histopathology, 18*(4), 1115–1123.

Wan, G., Corfas, G., & Stone, J. S. (2013). Inner ear supporting cells: Rethinking the silent majority. *Seminars in Cell and Developmental Biology, 24*(5), 448–459.

Wei, D., Jin, Z., Jarlebark, L., Scarfone, E., & Ulfendahl, M. (2007). Survival, synaptogenesis, and regeneration of adult mouse spiral ganglion neurons in vitro. *Developmental Neurobiology, 67*(1), 108–122.

Whitfield, T. T. (2015). Development of the inner ear. *Current Opinions in Genetic Development, 32*, 112–118.

Whyte, J., Cisneros, A., Yus, C., Obon, J., Whyte, A., Serrano, P., . . . Vera, A. (2008). Development of the dynamic structure (force lines) of the middle ear ossicles in human foetuses. *Histology and Histopathology, 23*(9), 1049–1060.

Whyte Orozco, J., Cisneros Gimeno, A. I., Urieta Carpi, J. J., Yus Gotor, C., Ganet Sole, J., Torres del Puerto, A., & Sarrat Torreguitart, R. (2003). [Ontogenic peculiarities of the human tympanic ossicular chain]. *Acta Otorrinolaringologica Espanola, 54*(1), 1–10.

Wikstrom, S. O., & Anniko, M. (1987). Early development of the stato-acoustic and facial ganglia. *Acta Otolaryngologica, 104*(1–2), 166–174.

Wood-Jones, F., & Wen, I.C. (1934). The development of the external ear. *Journal of Anatomy*, 68(Pt 4), 525–533.

Wright, C. G. (1997). Development of the human external ear. *Journal of the American Academy of Audiology, 8*(6), 379–382.

Yasuda, M., Yamada, S., Uwabe, C., Shiota, K., & Yasuda, Y. (2007). Three-dimensional analysis of inner ear development in human embryos. *Anatomical Science International, 82*(3), 156–163.

Yokoyama, T., Iino, Y., Kakizaki, K., & Murakami, Y. (1999). Human temporal bone study on the postnatal ossification process of auditory ossicles. *Laryngoscope, 109*(6), 927–930.

Zheng, J. L., Shou, J., Guillemot, F., Kageyama, R., & Gao, W. Q. (2000). Hes1 is a negative regulator of inner ear hair cell differentiation. *Development, 127*(21), 4551–4560.

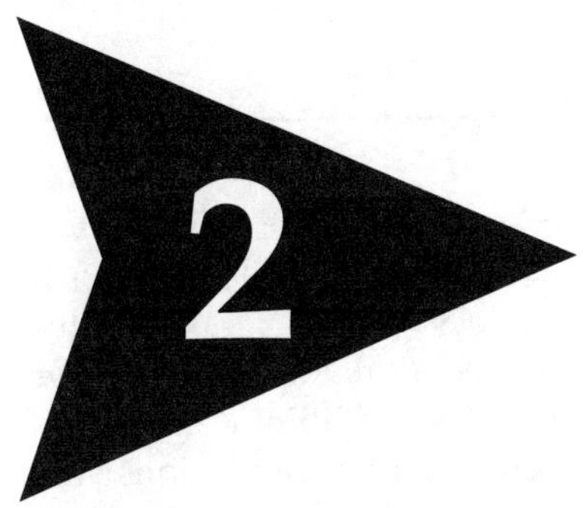

Biologic Development of the Auditory System From Periphery to Cortex

Robert V. Harrison

Introduction

At birth, the human cochlea is almost fully developed; however, the central auditory pathways are definitely not "ready to go." The system takes over a decade for its maturation and even beyond then, further development (plasticity and learning) in some auditory brain areas continues throughout life. In pediatric audiology, the important questions are not only about how hearing loss affects an infant's immediate communication skills, but also about the long-term impact of early impairment on the development of the auditory brain. Importantly, before we can optimize interventions for hearing loss in children, we must fully appreciate the developmental processes that the treatment or therapy will impact, and how we can take advantage of this development.

One obvious example of how we already capitalize on auditory development is the cochlear implantation of congenitally deaf infants. Our knowledge of age-related plasticity has prompted us to seek early detection of hearing loss through newborn hearing screening, and to provide an implant as early as possible. We now appreciate that the auditory system specifically develops to take advantage of the very limited sound information provided by an implant device. When young and plastic, the brain does a great job and eventually communication ability and language development in implanted children approaches normal.

This chapter provides an outline of important stages in the normal development of the auditory system, and also describes how hearing loss can influence such development. The coverage will deal with fundamental physiologic concepts rather than specific clinical issues, which are comprehensively covered in other sections of this handbook. The chapter describes some basic aspects of developmental plasticity in the auditory system and discusses associated concepts, such as age-related plasticity and "sensitive periods" during development. This introduction provides a useful background to later chapters in this handbook dealing with hearing loss and child development, and the early identification of hearing loss in childhood.

The Beginning and the End of Hearing Development

Perhaps the first task in considering the development of the auditory system is to define a starting point and to ask when we first hear. This question is more philosophical than biological, not least because it depends on what we mean by "hear." Does hearing start when cochlear hair cells can first be activated by acoustic signals? If we can detect that neurons in the auditory brainstem are excited by acoustic stimuli (e.g., with auditory brain stem response [ABR] tests), or if we can record middle latency responses from auditory cortex, does that imply "hearing," or do we require behavioral evidence? Even if there is a behavioral response such as a head orientation or an eye blink (startle) reflex, is this "hearing," or do we need proof of conscious perception of sound? Determination of when we first hear sound is not so simple, and when a question is posed such as, "Can my baby hear in utero?" the answer is not so easy.

At the other end of the developmental time continuum, we can ask when the development of the auditory system is complete. If we consider simple patterns of neural activity in primary auditory cortex, we might say at age 1 to 2 years in humans. If we think about more complex processing in core auditory areas, we can consider late puberty to be a significant endpoint. However, as we must all recognize, higher levels of cortex, including auditory memory, speech/language regions, and speech motor areas are always developing, always "plastic." If we consider that brain neuroplasticity is the norm, then the development of the auditory system never really ends. In between these not so easily defined endpoints, we do have a mainline auditory system development, which has been studied anatomically and physiologically in various animal models, and which in humans can be monitored by various test methods.

In the context of pediatric audiology, we obviously need to understand the system development and, most importantly, appreciate the concept of age-related plasticity in the auditory system. In other words, how does the plasticity (the ability of neural networks to remodel) of the developing auditory system reduce over time? Furthermore, we need to recognize that there might be sensitive (or critical) periods during development such that intervention strategies can be planned for maximal benefit. In this chapter, we first consider some important developmental epochs at the level of the inner ear, including when cochlear hair cells connect up with the brain, when other components of the organ of Corti (e.g., tectorial membrane) are ready to activate hair cells optimally and, thus, when environmental acoustic stimuli can effectively activate the cochlea. This is followed by a brief description of central auditory pathway development up to core auditory cortex based on both animal models and human data. Some of the work reviewed relates to normal auditory system maturation, and other studies show us the effects of hearing impairment on system development. A particular emphasis is on research that indicates how acoustically driven activity of the auditory system acts to guide its development. In the final section, clinical issues that relate to developmental plasticity are discussed.

The Early Growth of the Auditory Periphery

The sequence of embryologic development of the inner ear has been extensively studied in various animal models and is well described in Chapter 1 of this volume. In the human, when cochlear hair cells start to differentiate within the otocyst (about 2 months after conception), there is evidence of the formation of presynaptic structures (Pujol, 1986). Within a few weeks, the hair cells have formed synaptic connections with cochlear afferent neurons; however, hair cell function in terms of the transduction of mechanical stimuli lags behind. At that time, the stereocilia are still not fully developed, and the final maturation of the tectorial membrane is incomplete (Lim & Anniko, 1986).

Figure 2–1 provides a summary of the developmental timelines for the human cochlea from conception to the neonatal period. The lower captions note key features of anatomical growth; evidence of function is listed in the upper section. A very important stage in the functional development of the cochlea is tectorial membrane maturation. Figure 2–2 illustrates some salient features of tectorial membrane development. In humans, the inner (IHCs) and outer hair cells (OHCs) differentiate in the otocyst early on, around 8 to 10 weeks postconception. Both IHCs and OHCs are well differentiated and innervated long before the tectorial membrane has grown into position. Before this time, hair cells may transduce some mechanical signals, but the role of OHCs as a biomechanical amplifier, and the normal mode of stimulation of the IHCs (fluid streaming in the subtectorial space) is not possible. As a result, low threshold signal detection and cochlear frequency selectivity are likely not evident until late stages of gestation.

When an animal is born, the state of these important developmental stages differs considerably between species. Many altricious mammals are born in an immature state (e.g., mice and rats) and have a postnatal onset of hearing. On the other hand, the human is a relatively precocious species and has a well-developed cochlea at birth similar to, for example, the chinchilla (which makes the latter an appropriate animal model for studies related to human auditory development). To illustrate such species differences, Figure 2–3 shows the sensory epithelium of the mouse cochlea at birth compared with that of the chinchilla (that is similar to the human condition).

In the mouse (left-hand panel), note the excessive tissue on the surfaces of cells surrounding the hair cells. This is evidence of the subtectorial meshwork that, after birth, is still active in secreting and forming the tectorial membrane. At this stage, the normal deflection of OHC stereocilia by tectorial membrane or by fluid motion beneath it (to activate IHCs) is clearly not effective. Contrast this to the sensory epithelium of the newborn chinchilla (right panel) where the subtectorial

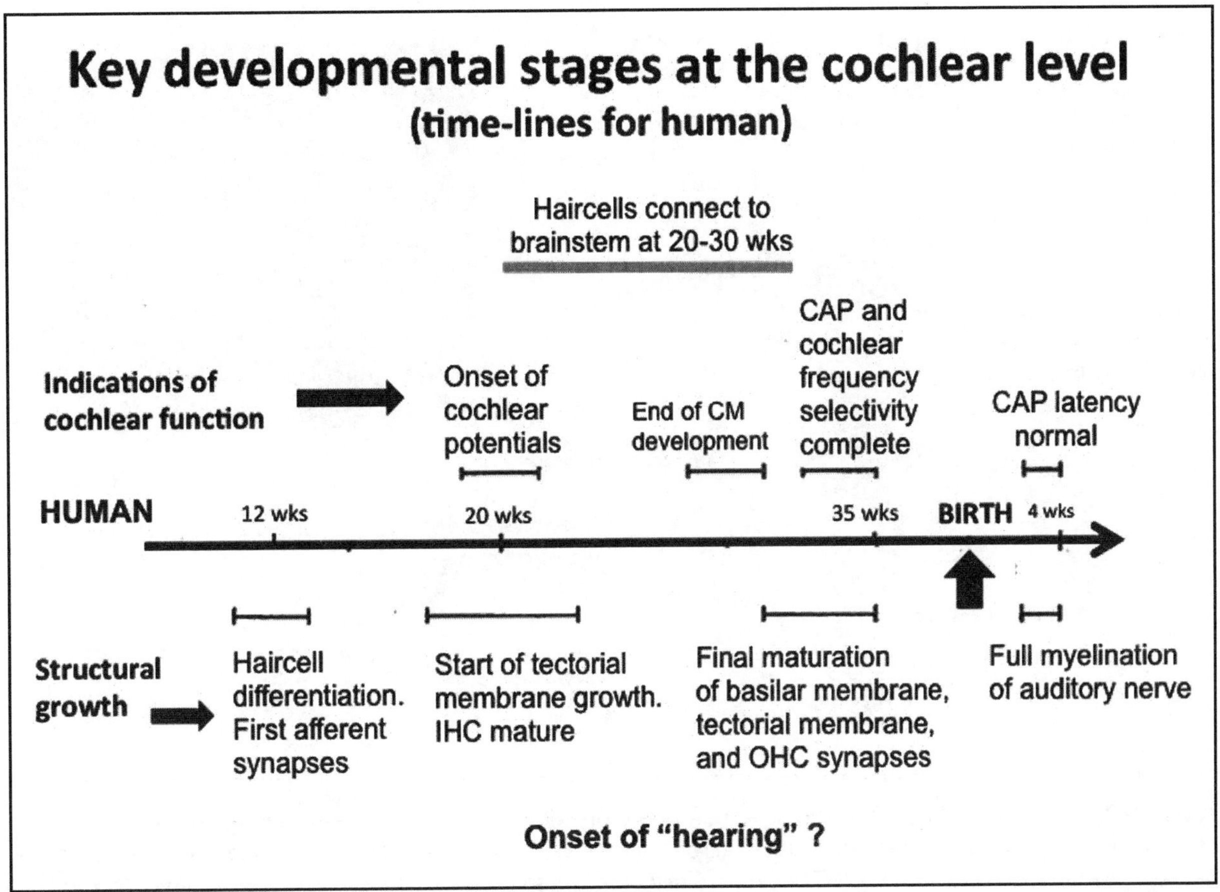

FIGURE 2–1. Key structural and functional stages in human cochlear development. (CM, cochlear microphonic; CAP cochlear action potential; IHC, inner hair cell; OHC, outer hair cell.)

space (i.e., surface of the reticular lamina) is clear. In this species, as with humans, the cochlea is fully functional at birth (Harrison, Cullen, Takeno, & Mount, 1996).

Connecting the Cochlea to the Brain

Not only does the human cochlea function well before birth, but cochlear afferent connections from hair cells to the cochlear nucleus of the brainstem are also well established. Essentially, the auditory nuclei of the brainstem and midbrain arise at about the same time as the inner ear formation. Some of the key aspects of connecting the cochlea to the auditory brain are summarized schematically in Figure 2–4. Immature neurons derived from the otocyst produce centrally directed processes that grow toward, and split to send branches to three brainstem (cochlear nucleus) areas. These are, or become, the anteroventral cochlear nucleus (AVCN), posteroventral-cochlear nucleus (PVCN), and dorsal cochlear nucleus (DCN). These neurons connect hair cells along the cochlear length with target cells in the cochlear nucleus in a topographic fashion, resulting in the systematic tonotopic mapping seen in the mature subject. Strictly speaking, the neural projections should be described as cochleotopic rather than tonotopic, but most often (but not always) the terms can be interchanged. This ordered "wiring pattern" occurs before the system has auditory input—that is, before there is acoustically activated neural activity. However, there may be a role for spontaneous (i.e., intrinsically arising) neural activity in these early developmental stages. In humans, most of the connections are complete at 20 to 30 weeks gestational age. When the neural connections have been established, the maintenance and survival of target cells in the cochlear nucleus depend on activity in the cochlear nerve whether intrinsic (spontaneous activity) or extrinsic (stimulus driven). For more comprehensive reviews, see Romand (1983) and Rubel, Parks, and Zirpel (2004).

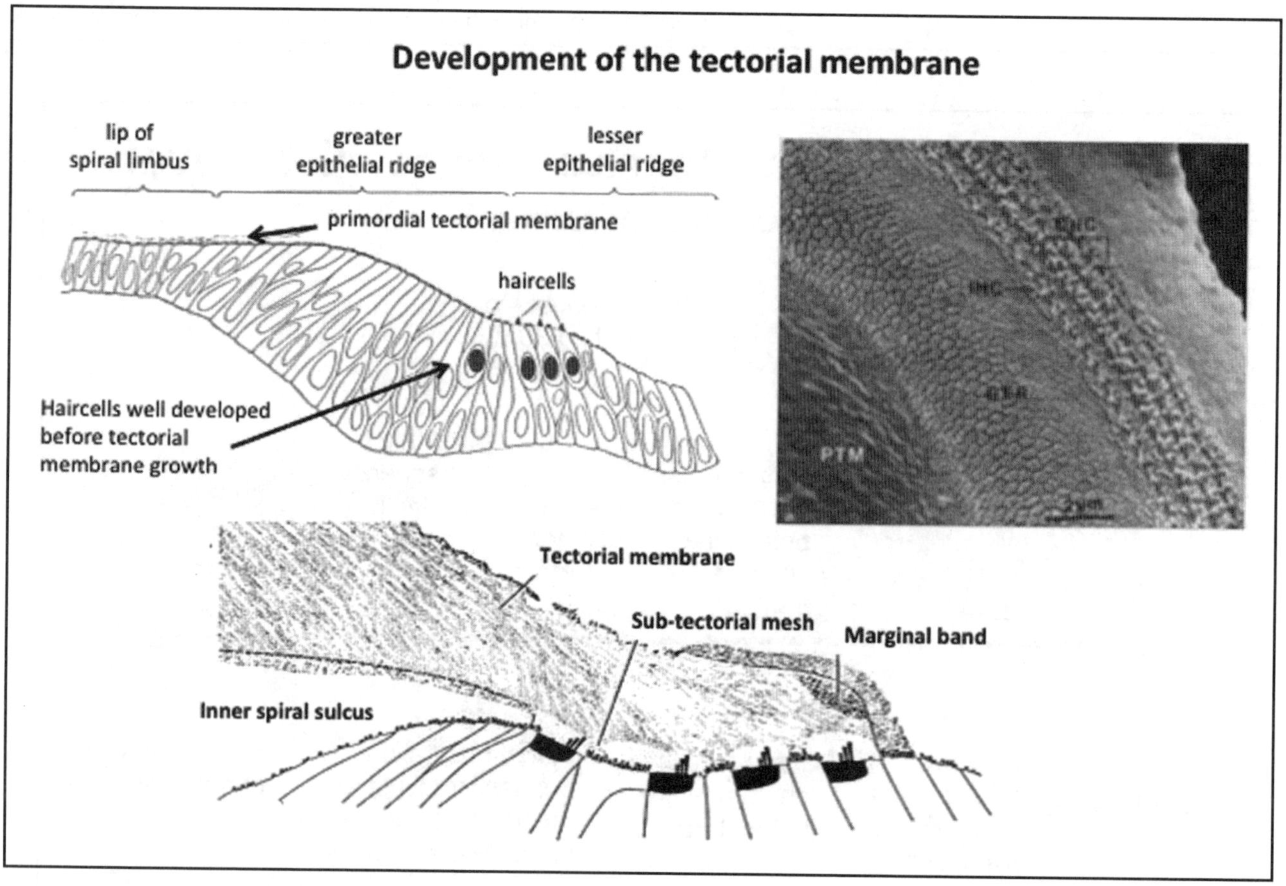

FIGURE 2–2. Some aspects of early tectorial membrane growth. *Upper left:* Cross-sectional view at initial stage of membrane production. *Upper right:* Scanning electron micrograph of immature sensory surface. *Lower panel:* Intermediate stage of membrane maturation. (PTM, primordial tectorial membrane; Adapted from data of Lim & Anniko, 1986.)

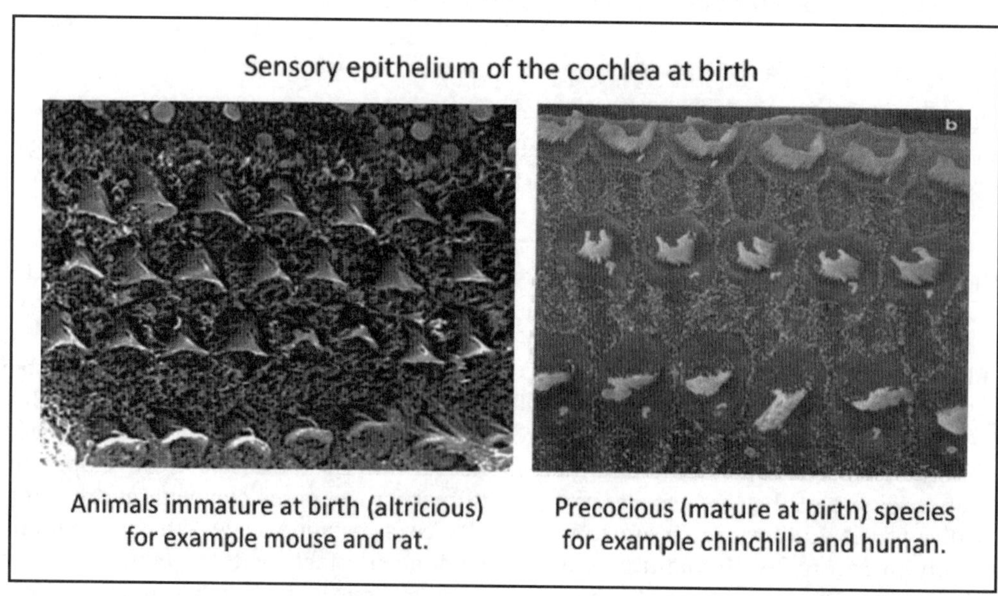

FIGURE 2–3. Scanning electron micrographs of the cochlear sensory epithelium at birth from an altricious species (mouse; *left panel*) compared with a precocious animal (chinchilla; *right panel*).

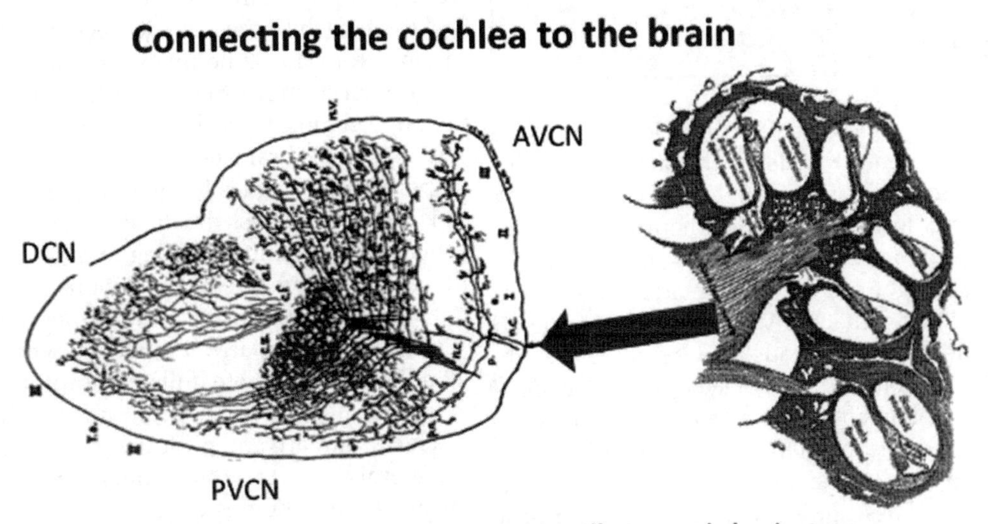

- Immature neurons in the otocyst grow centrally towards brainstem.
- They split (twice) to connect with target cells in AVCN, PVCN and DCN.
- Mid regions of the cochlea connect up first, apical and basal areas later.
- Initial projections/connections are cochleotopic.
- Initial wiring occurs before any sound driven auditory input.
- May be a role for intrinsic (spontaneous) activity.
- Connections in humans complete at 20-30 wks (10-20 wks before birth)

FIGURE 2–4. Some salient processes in the development of connections between the cochlea and auditory brainstem. (AVCN, anteroventral cochlear nucleus; PVCN, posteroventral cochlear nucleus; DCN, dorsal cochlear nucleus.)

When Do We First "Hear"?

In humans, anatomic connections of cochlea to brain are complete at 10 to 20 weeks before birth, and toward the end of that period there is some evidence of auditory function. For example, ABR waveforms can be measured in 15-week premature neonates (Graziani, Weitzman, & Velasco, 1968), and sound-evoked blink startle reflex (ultrasound imaging in utero) shows responses at 24 to 25 weeks gestational age (Birnholz & Benacerraf, 1983). As discussed earlier, tectorial membrane maturation is required for low threshold cochlear activation and also for cochlear frequency selectivity; thus, it is unlikely that these develop until 30 to 35 weeks of gestation. The sensory epithelium of mid-frequency regions of the cochlea is the first to develop and connect with the brainstem. The development of more apical and basal areas follows later such that even 6 months after birth, high- and low-frequency thresholds continue to improve (e.g., Olsho, 1986; Trehub, Schneider, & Endman, 1980).

It is clear that mid-frequency regions of the cochlea and neural connections through much of the auditory pathway can be activated during the third trimester. However, does this mean that the unborn baby can "hear" in the normal perceptual sense, and if so, what can he or she possibly hear? Clearly environmental sounds will be much attenuated by the completely fluid-filled system. Normal middle-ear impedance matching mechanism will not work, and the cochlea will be essentially stimulated by something similar to a bone conduction pathway. On the other hand, maternal sounds (e.g., mother's voice and heartbeat) will be somewhat effective as stimuli, as will acoustic signals directly applied to the body in the mode of a bone conduction hearing aid.

Central Auditory Pathway Development

During the same period that the cochlea is linking to the brainstem, more central nuclei in the superior olivary complex, auditory midbrain, and thalamus are forming and connecting. In these locations, neuron formation and migration, axon out-growth, and synaptic connections to other target cells are also made before there is any acoustic-driven activity, but there might be an important role for spontaneous activity in the system, especially for the consolidation of synapses. There does not appear to be any particular sequence of connectivity (e.g., from the peripheral to central), but rather there is overlapping development of connections, and both the ascending and descending neural pathways appear to be formed at the same time (Rubel et al., 2004). As is the case in the cochlear nucleus, more central connections are topographically organized so as to eventually achieve cochleotopic/tonotopic mapping throughout. This initial order clearly does not depend on stimulus-driven cochlear activity, because that is not yet present. Again, it is likely that intrinsically arising (spontaneous) neural activity has a significant role (Lippe, 1994). Later, it is clear that acoustically driven neural signals will act to consolidate synaptic connections and refine cochleotopic projections. There is good evidence (some of which is reviewed below) that abnormal patterns of activity at the cochlear nerve level during an early postnatal period can have significant influence on tonotopic organization in central auditory areas.

Developmental Plasticity of the Binaural Hearing System

The earliest studies of neuroplasticity in auditory system development were pioneering anatomic studies by Levi-Montalcini (1949) who demonstrated that unilateral otocyst removal (in chick embryo) resulted in abnormal central auditory neuron projections. Many other more recent studies in mammals have similarly shown that unilateral cochlear ablation results in the development of unusual innervation patterns in the brainstem (e.g., Hashisaki & Rubel, 1989; Kitzes, 1984; Moore, 1994; Moore & Kitzes, 1985; Parks & Jackson, 1986). Figure 2–5 illustrates some of the effects of neonatal cochlear ablation (in gerbil) on brainstem "wiring" (Kitzes, 1984, 1996). During normal development, target neurons of the medial and lateral nuclei of the superior olive and the medial nucleus of the trapezoid body receive input from both cochleas, but after cochlear ablation, each of these nuclei receive two inputs originating from the same unablated side. Such abnormal neural connections that result from neonatal cochlear ablation significantly change the response properties of neurons in the brainstem and midbrain. Although these experimental studies involve whole cochlear ablation, it is likely that a less drastic lesion, such as a profound unilateral congenital hearing loss, will similarly result in abnormal brainstem connections.

It might be supposed that there are few clinical situations in pediatric audiology where the extreme condition of complete unilateral profound hearing loss exists. However, consider an infant with a unilateral cochlear implant and profound hearing loss in the contralateral ear. In this case, from an early age of cochlear implantation, there is effectively a unilateral auditory input stimulating the development of the auditory brain. There are some parallels between an infant with one cochlear implant and an animal model where, during early development, only one cochlea is functional. Is it possible that some of the abnormal neural connections seen in animal models of unilateral cochlear ablation will arise in the unilaterally implanted infant?

We do have to consider, as previously noted above, the issue of precocious (well-developed at birth) versus altricious species. For any infant given a cochlear implant, the new electrically generated activity patterns will be imposed on an already well-formed central auditory system and thus might not produce the radically abnormal innervation patterns found in some of the animal models. But, if there has been no extrinsic input to an infant because of profound deafness, the central pathways may still be awaiting consolidation by stimulus-driven activity. If this comes from one (implanted) side only, the final innervation patterns could be significantly abnormal.

Perhaps more clinically relevant are studies in which the balance of input to the two ears has been less extensively altered, for example, by unilateral plugging (unilateral conductive hearing loss). Experimental manipulations like this have shown, in some animal models, to result in significant impairment in bilateral function. For example, experiments in the barn owl (Knudsen, 1984; Knudsen, Esterly, & Knudsen, 1984) and in the ferret (Moore, Hutchings, King, & Kowalchuk, 1989; Moore, King, McAlpine, Martin, & Hutchings, 1993; Moore et al., 1999) show that early disruption of bilateral input can result in significant impairment of sound localization ability. In humans, the most common condition in which there can be an unbalanced auditory input during early life is that resulting from chronic or recurring otitis media

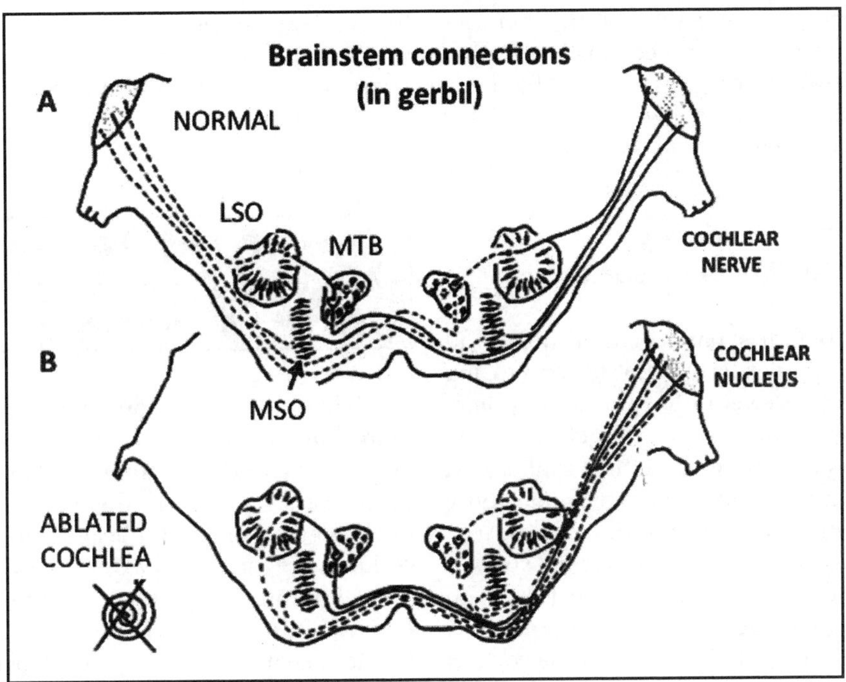

FIGURE 2–5. The effect of unilateral cochlear ablation on the development of neural pathways in the auditory brainstem (gerbil model; Adapted with permission from Kitzes, L. M. [1986]. The role of binaural innervations. In R. J. Ruben, T. R. Van der Water, and E. W. Rubel [Eds.], *The biology of change in otolaryngology* [p. 188]. The Netherlands: Elsevier Press. Copyright Elsevier 1986.)

in infants. There is some evidence that such a condition can result in impaired auditory function (e.g., Hogan & Moore, 2003) and perhaps delays in language development.

Another condition in which unbalanced auditory input could occur is when an infant with hearing loss in both ears is only provided with unilateral hearing aid amplification. Of course, our standard practice for infant aiding is bilateral amplification because of the improved threshold sensitivity, signal detection in noise, and sound localization. We could add a further benefit, that of providing a balanced binaural input during early system maturation.

In summary, we can think of the auditory system as being a fully integrated binaural system that requires, during development and perhaps later, a balanced input from both sides. Experimental or clinical situations when balanced input is not the case will potentially result in some degree of abnormal structure and function of brainstem and midbrain auditory centers. For readers interested in a more comprehensive review of the plasticity of binaural hearing, see Moore and King (2004).

Intrinsic Versus Extrinsic Influences During Development

Another important concept to consider in auditory system development is the issue of extrinsic versus intrinsic influence: *extrinsic* meaning acoustically driven neural activity from the periphery as opposed to *intrinsic* meaning signals such as local spontaneous discharge, activity from descending auditory pathways or, at the highest levels, intrinsic activity in corticocortical connections. Mention has already been made of the possible role of spontaneous neural activity in the formation or consolidation of synaptic connections in the auditory brainstem. In studies of the auditory brainstem, there is some evidence that spontaneous discharge in cochlear afferent neurons (preceding any acoustically driven neural activity) appears to have a role in establishing central connections (e.g., Lippe, 1994). Similarly, in the visual system, retinal level spontaneous activity appears to have a role in central visual system development (e.g., Cang et al., 2005; Meister, Wong, Baylor, & Schatz, 1991). At the level of cortex, other types of intrinsic signals have to be considered, not the least of which includes activity from other sensory systems, and reciprocal connections with other brain systems. Detailed coverage is not possible here, but for useful discussion see reviews by Pallas (2001) and Newton and Sur (2005).

The Development of Auditory Connections at the Level of Cortex

The number of potential synaptic connections and the corresponding complexity of auditory processing increase with ascending level in the auditory system. Up to the thalamic level, the system is largely activated by auditory signals originating from the periphery. At the cortical level, many more pathways of connectivity develop including projections to multimodal sensory cortex, speech areas, and nonsensory regions such as memory, motor, and arousal systems. Most of these connection pathways are reciprocal. Furthermore, it appears that system plasticity is greater at the cortical level (or at least maintained for longer) than in more peripheral auditory areas.

We can gain an impression about the remarkable degree of this cortical plasticity, especially during early development, from experiments in which the sensory inputs to the cortex are rewired, as well as in demonstrations of cross-modal plasticity. In one type of sensory rerouting experiment, visual neurons from the retina have been directed to the early developing medial geniculate nucleus of the (auditory) thalamus (Roe, Pallas, Kwon, & Sur, 1992; Sharma, Angelucci, & Sur, 2000). As a result, cells in the auditory cortex are driven by visual input and develop visual response characteristics normally associated with primary visual cortex (e.g., retinotopic organization and visual contour orientation selectivity). Such studies reveal how sensory areas that we normally assume to be "devoted" to one sense, can in fact take on a role for neural processing of a different sensory modality. We could say that the auditory cortex is not reserved for hearing. In experimental or natural circumstances when one modality of sensory input is absent, the cortical area normally associated with processing that sensory information becomes available to process some other sensory modality. For example, in congenitally blind humans, the visual areas are driven by somatosensory input (Sadato et al., 1996) and are also involved in auditory tasks (Kujala et al., 1997). Similarly, visual processing occurs in "auditory" cortical regions of congenitally deaf subjects (Neville, Schmidt, & Kutas, 1983). This extremely plastic reorganization ability in the cortex has some clinical implications. For example, if the auditory cortex of a congenitally deaf adult has been taken over for other functions, will there be adequate cortical space for processing if the subject is provided with a cochlear implant?

Evoked Potential Measures of Human Auditory System Development

Much has been learned about the maturational changes in the human auditory system by systematic studies of auditory evoked potentials as a function of age. Some of the classic studies in this regard have been carried out by Eggermont and colleagues in normal infants and children (Eggermont, 1985, 1988; Eggermont & Salamy, 1988; Ponton, Eggermont, Kwong, & Don, 2000; for review, see Ponton & Eggermont, 2007). Complementary to such monitoring in those with normal hearing are studies of auditory-evoked potentials elicited by electrical stimulation in subjects with cochlear implants (e.g., Gordon, Papsin, & Harrison, 2003; Ponton, Don, Eggermont, Waring, & Masuda, 1996; Ponton & Eggermont, 2001). Some of this work is reviewed later in this chapter (see also Chapter 27 on cochlear implants for children).

It is clear from these studies that at birth, ABR and middle latency responses from the thalamocortex can be detected, but all differ in amplitude and are longer in latency compared with the adult subject. During maturation, waveform peak latencies become reduced, with the earliest ABR waveform component from cochlear nerve having normal values within a few weeks of birth. Later components such as wave P5, originating from the auditory midbrain, continue to reduce in latency for a few years after birth. These ABR changes during development are illustrated in the left panel of Figure 2–6. On a longer time scale, auditory-evoked potentials originating at the cortical level continue to show developmental changes for many years, including increasing detectability, changes in amplitude, and a reduction in latency. These cortical potentials are finally "mature" (are adult-like in waveform morphology) in adolescent children. This is illustrated in Figure 2–6 (right-hand panel; Ponton & Eggermont, 2001). Note in particular the change, with increasing age, of the waveform shape from being one dominant positive peak in the two earliest age groups (5–7 years, 8–9 years), and thereafter the emergence of a second positive peak to the waveform.

These distinct changes clearly indicate that cortical maturational processes continue through adolescence.

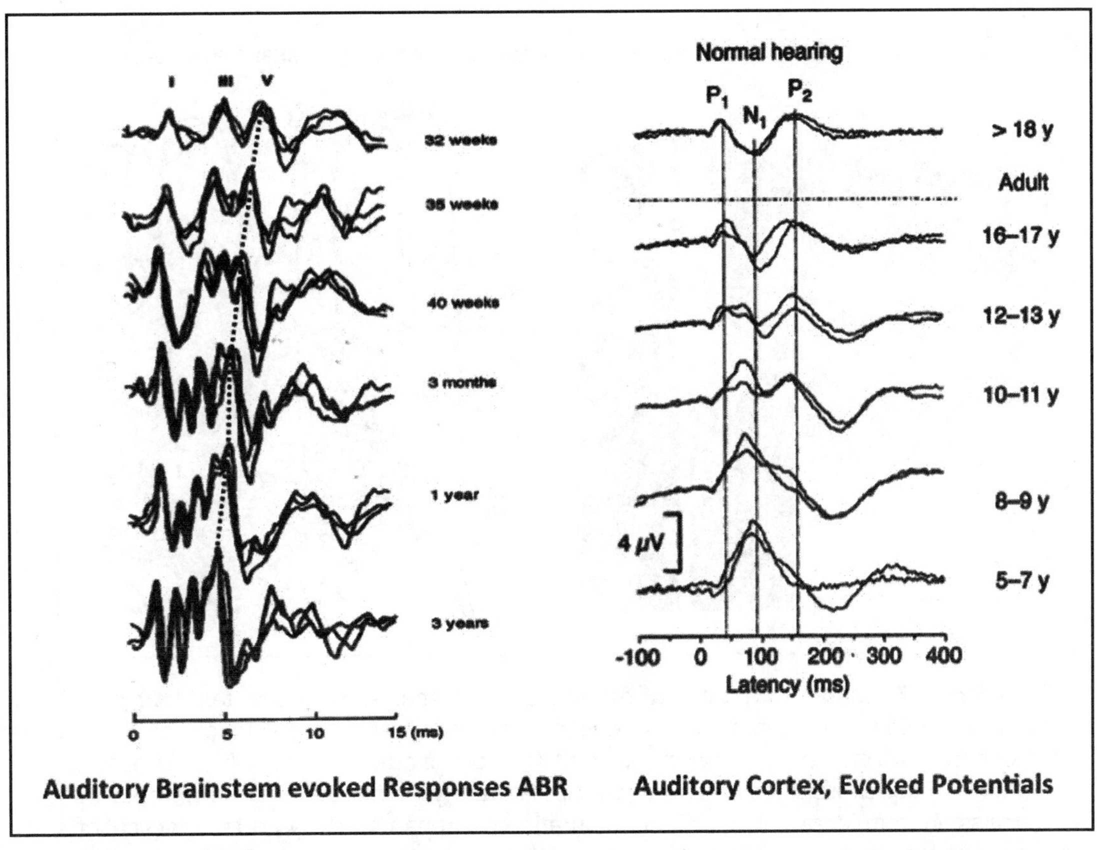

FIGURE 2–6. Auditory system maturation as measured with auditory-evoked potential recordings. *Left panel:* ABR waveforms in normal-hearing infants of various ages. *Right panel:* Evoked potential from auditory cortex in normal-hearing children and adults of various ages. (Adapted from C. W. Ponton & J. J. Eggermont, 2007.)

These cortical potential waveform changes approximate in time with neurofilament maturation in deeper cortical layers, as shown in human tissue studies by Moore (2002), and might be correlated in some way. Figure 2–7 illustrates the findings of the anatomical study by Moore (left panel). Note in particular the dense labeling in all cortical layers of the 11-year specimen compared with those from younger subjects. Thus, we have both functional and anatomical evidence of the relatively lengthy time course of human auditory cortex development.

Another perspective on the developmental progression within the auditory system is to note when different types of auditory-evoked potentials are fully mature (i.e., have adult-like characteristics). As a rule of thumb, cochlear action potentials are mature within weeks of birth, and the ABR is adult-like within 3 to 5 years. Potentials from the thalamocortical input pathways (i.e., middle latency response) and the later auditory-evoked cortical potentials are mature by about 14 years of age. Later auditory potentials originating in cortical areas beyond primary auditory cortex (e.g., P300) can take up to 20 years to show full maturity. These auditory-evoked response studies have provided a general picture of the developmental changes in the auditory pathways. Latency and amplitude characteristics of waveform peaks reflect the number and synchronicity of underlying neurons activated by acoustic stimuli.

In general, it can be concluded that throughout the system, with age, there is a decrease in neural transmission time, perhaps related to increased myelination of neurons or to increased efficacy of synaptic transmission. Increases in peak amplitudes of waveforms indicate increases in either number of neurons contributing, or more synchronized responses, or perhaps structural/orientation changes to auditory array pathways that create more effective dipole sources for scalp-recorded signals. More detailed information about system development is difficult to judge from

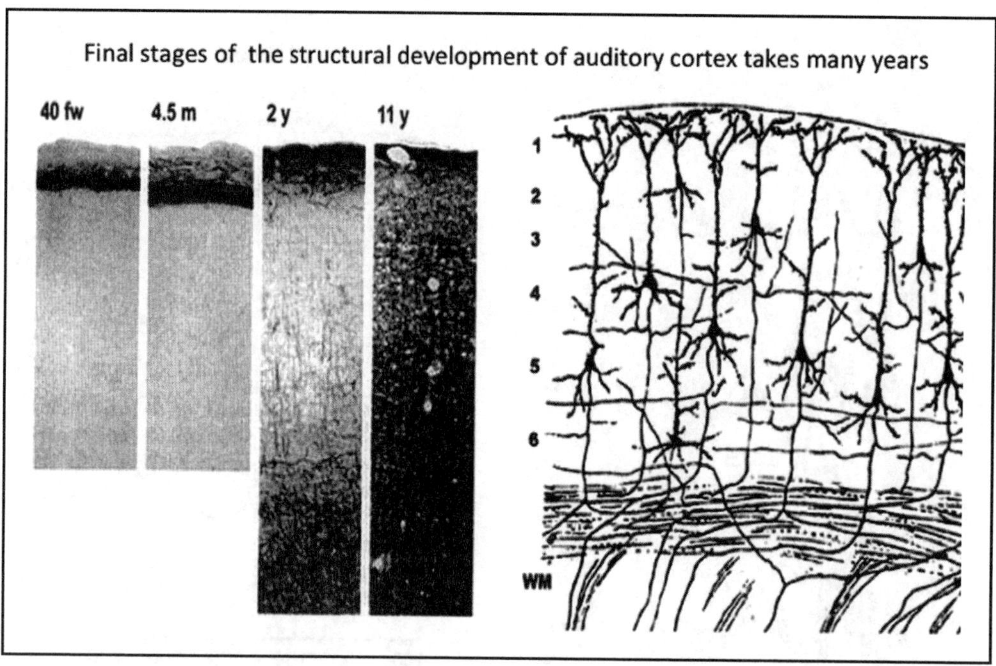

FIGURE 2–7. Long-term postnatal maturation of human auditory cortex. *Left panel:* Immunolabeled neurofilaments in a section of cortical tissue from subjects at 40 fetal weeks (fw), 4.5 months (m), 2 years (y), and 11 years of age. *Right panel:* Laminar organization of cortex from the classical work of Ramon y Cajal. (Left panel reprinted with permission from Moore, J. K. [2002]. Maturation of human auditory cortex: Implications for speech perception. *Annals of Otology, Rhinology, Laryngology, 189*[Suppl.], 7–10. Copyright Annals Publishing Company.)

such standard clinical electrophysiological studies, not least because scalp recorded signals can have complex waveforms that reflect not only the number and synchronicity of neurons firing, but also the (multiple) source distribution of contributing current sources. However, there have been many methodological refinements such as multichannel EEG recordings allowing dipole source analysis, and new technologies such as magnetoencephalography (MEG), and functional magnetic resonance imaging (fMRI). In the future, systematic investigations using such tools undoubtedly will provide us with much more detail about human auditory system development.

Experimental animal studies can provide some detail about developmental processes in the auditory cortex with age. Figure 2–8 illustrates the increasing complexity of processing in cortical neurons with development in a chinchilla model (Pienkowski & Harrison, 2005). At birth, most cortical neurons have a "simple response" to one sound frequency. This is illustrated in the central panels and shows the frequency-time response plot of a cortical cell in a 3-day-old (P3) animal. In contrast, the right-hand panels show a typical "complex response" from a neuron in the adult subject. The upper left histogram plots the increase during development of the proportion of cortical cells with a complex response. Thus, at postnatal day 3 (P3), 90% of cortical cells are of the simple type and only 10% have complex responses. In the adult, 40% of cells show a complex response. These complex cortical responses are in part the result of the development of local neural interactions between cells. It is perhaps relevant to think of the human anatomical data in Figure 2–7 (Moore, 2002) indicating the maturation of cortical interneurons during adolescence.

Evoked Potential Studies in Children With Cochlear Implants

In children with cochlear implants, measurement of evoked potentials provides a tool to study developmental plasticity that results from electrical activation of the cochlea (Eggermont, Ponton, Don, Waring,

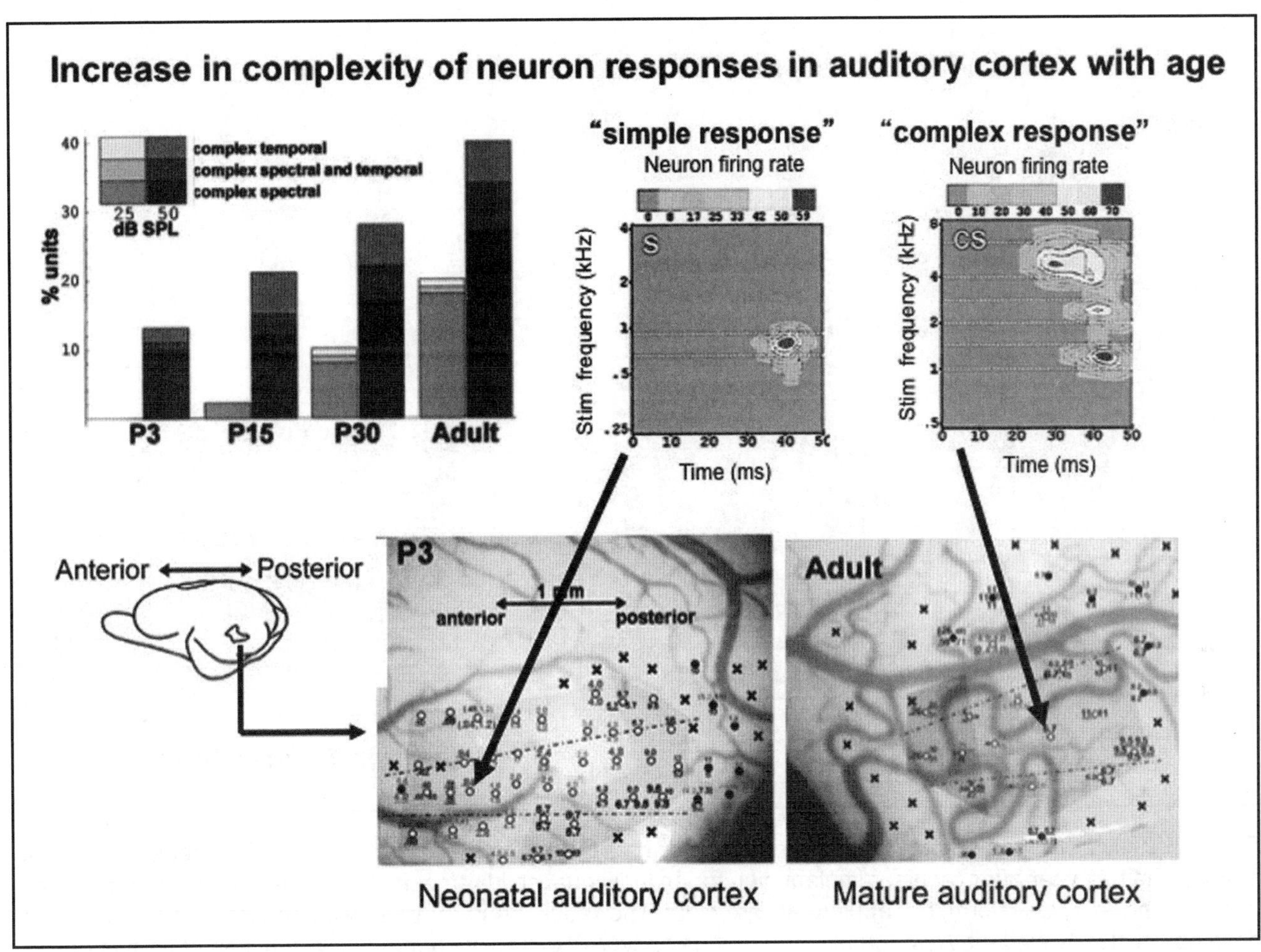

FIGURE 2–8. Increase in complexity of neuron responses in auditory cortex during development. The lower diagrams show cortical surface and neuron recoding sites for two example responses in a chinchilla model. In the upper central panel is a "simple response" from a cell in the neonatal (P3) animal. This spectro-temporal plot shows how the neuron simply responds to only a single sound frequency (0.8 kHz). In the right-hand panel, a "complex response" is shown in which the neuron responds to a number of different sound frequencies. This response complexity is typical in the adult subject. The upper left-hand plot shows the increase in the percentage of complex cell responses with developmental age. (Based on data from Pienkowski & Harrison, 2005.)

& Kwong, 1997; Gordon, Papsin, & Harrison, 2003, 2005, 2006, 2007; Ponton, Don, Eggermont, Waring, & Masuda, 1996). The following studies serve to illustrate some aspects of developmental plasticity as it relates to cochlear implantation.

The left panel of Figure 2–9 shows a series of electrically evoked ABR measures made at initial implant device turn-on, and then at time intervals up to 1 year after implantation (Gordon, Papsin, & Harrison, 2006). The electrical artifact from cochlear electrode stimulation obscures the earliest peaks of the ABR waveform, but waves eIII and eV are evident. As the auditory system of this child is electrically activated, we note the reduction in these peak latencies over time (highlighted by dashed line connecting eV peaks). In the pooled data of the right-hand graph, changes in ABR latency are plotted as a function of time. The solid line (lower curve) represents latencies in children with cochlear implants, and "time in sound" for them starts from initial stimulation with the cochlear implant device. The thinner-line upper plots represent data from normal-hearing children; here time in sound starts at birth. For all subjects, the time scale represents time exposed to sound. Note here that the trajectories of these functions, whether normal changes from birth or changes in implant patients from day of activation, are similar.

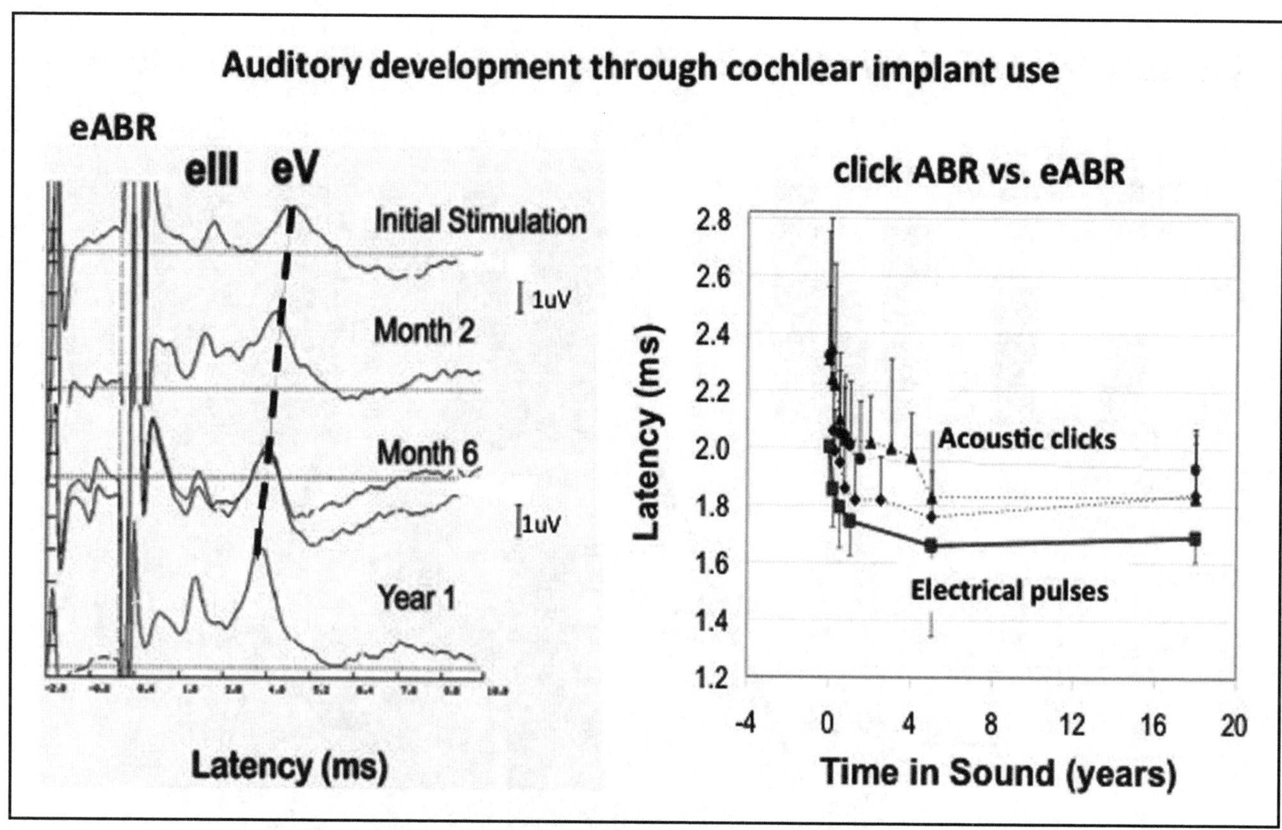

FIGURE 2–9. *Left panel:* Electrically evoked auditory brainstem evoked responses (eABRs) measured at time intervals up to 1 year after cochlear implantation for an individual child. An electrical artifact obscures the earliest peaks of the ABR waveform, but eIII and eV are clear. The reduction in eV peak latency as the auditory system develops is clearly evident. *Right panel:* Pooled data show ABR latency changes as a function of time in normal infants (click evoked ABR; time zero is birth). Solid data line shows eABR latency in children with cochlear implants; time zero is at initial stimulation with the device. (Figure modified from Gordon, Papsin, & Harrison, 2006.)

The only difference is the overall shorter latency of the electrically evoked responses. These data suggest that the electrical stimulation of the cochlea drives a developmental process similar to that initiated at hearing onset in the normal newborn infant. Importantly, this also suggests a cochlear implant device in a congenitally deaf infant has two roles: one is to provide hearing, the other is to promote development.

A second example of the use of evoked potentials to study neuroplasticity in children with cochlear implants relates to bilateral cochlear implantation. We previously discussed experimental animal studies in which one cochlea was ablated during early development and that resulted in the formation of abnormal "wiring" in the auditory brainstem. Such investigations strongly hint at the importance of having balanced, bilateral input to the auditory system for normal development. The experimental conditions in those studies are not dissimilar to those of a congenitally deaf infant with unilateral cochlear activation through a single cochlear implant. How abnormal is the development of auditory pathways under these circumstances? More importantly, if the child later receives another cochlear implant on the opposite side, can it effectively restore the balanced auditory system that is likely essential for binaural hearing?

Figure 2–10 shows a series of electrically evoked ABRs from two children. On the left, Child A had simultaneous bilateral cochlear implantation. Child B (right) had a 2-year delay between left and right ear implantation (Gordon, Valero, & Papsin, 2007; Papsin & Gordon, 2008). In the lower panels, for each subject, eABR waveforms evoked by separate stimulation of left and right ears are shown from initial stimulation

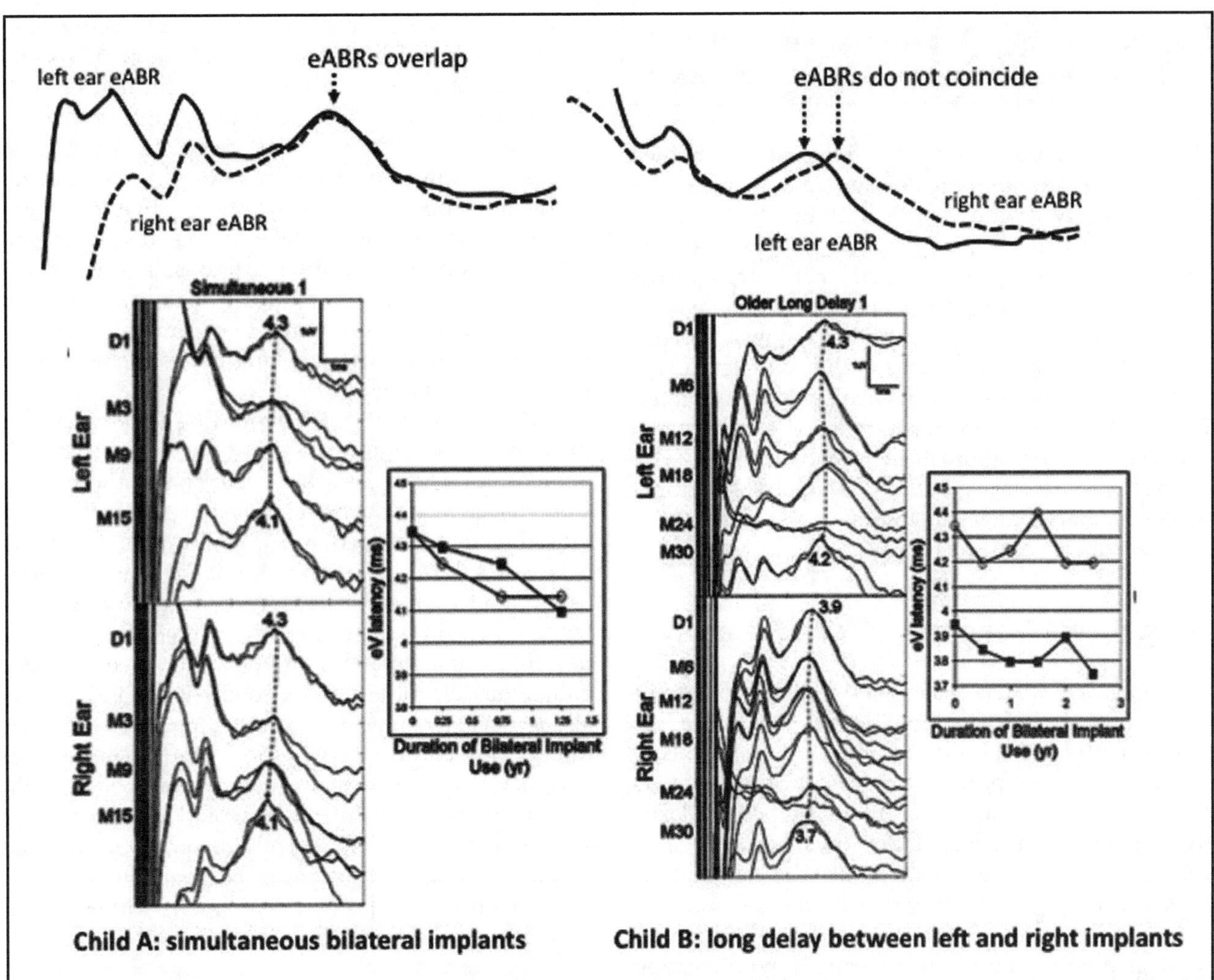

FIGURE 2–10. Electrically evoked auditory brainstem responses (eABRs) from two children measured at time of implant activation (D1) and at intervals indicated in months. Child A (*left panels*) had simultaneous bilateral cochlear implantation. Child B (*right panels*) had a 2-year delay between left and right ear implantation. For both children, eV latency is plotted as a function of duration of bilateral implant use. The upper waveforms are superimposed left ear and right ear evoked eABRs measured at time of device activation. For Child A, eABR waveforms from both sides overlap. For Child B, eABR waveforms do not superimpose, either initially or after many years of bilateral implant use. (Modified from Gordon, Valero, & Papsin, 2007.)

on day 1 (D1) and at intervals labeled in months (M3 to M30). For each ear, the eV latency measures are plotted as a function of duration of bilateral implant use. At the top of the figure, for each child, eABR waveforms measured from left and right ears on day 1 are superimposed. For the simultaneous bilateral implanted child, eABRs (note wave V) are coincident in time. For the nonsimultaneous bilaterally implanted child, the eABR waveforms do not superimpose, either initially or after many years of bilateral implant use. In order to achieve useful binaural hearing (including sound localization and improved speech signal-to-noise ratio), auditory signals from the two implanted ears should reach brainstem and midbrain areas at the same time. The take home message from this study is that if there is a long delay between the times of implantation of each ear, this timing coincidence will not occur, and true binaural hearing will not be achieved (Papsin & Gordon, 2008).

Development, Maintenance, and Plasticity of Tonotopic Projections

Patterns of neural activity generated at the cochlear level are influential in the development, maintenance, and plasticity of the central auditory brain. When abnormal cochlear activity patterns exist from an early age, tonotopic (cochleotopic) map reorganization occurs in core auditory cortex. In addition, there is significant reorganization to frequency maps at subcortical levels, for example, in the auditory thalamus and midbrain. In contrast, when cochlear activity pattern changes are induced in an adult model (e.g., by partial cochlear deafferentation), there is reorganization of frequency maps in cortex, but little evidence of midbrain tonotopic map change suggesting an age-related plasticity at subcortical levels in the auditory system.

What Do We Mean by the Term *Plasticity*?

The term *plasticity* has been used by authors to describe very different aspects of brain development or reorganization, and we should be careful to avoid making inappropriate comparisons of different types of plasticity. Consider some of the different types of plasticity that have been reported. One obvious classification relates to the research methods used to demonstrate plastic change. Plasticity has been demonstrated in anatomical studies (e.g., abnormal neural structures, new, or altered axonal pathways). Numerous types of functional studies have revealed plasticity including fMRI measures, evoked potential recordings, and physiological experiments at cellular, membrane, or ion channel levels. We also have a wide range of behavioral studies from standard audiologic tests through to detailed psychophysical studies that demonstrate plastic change.

Another important dimension of plasticity is its time course. Auditory system plasticity has been described over time spans from minutes and hours, through months and years. An example of rapid plasticity is the observation of auditory neuron receptive field alteration (both excitatory and inhibitory frequency tuning curves), which can occur within tens of minutes after induction of cochlear lesions, or partial deafferentation (e.g., Boettcher & Salvi, 1993; Wang, Salvi, & Powers, 1996). It is reasonable to suppose that short-term plastic change reflects relatively small-scale neural alterations, with subtle synaptic modifications to existing neural networks. More extensive auditory system reorganization appears to occur over a longer time course. This is clear from numerous electrophysiological studies showing a modification of central tonotopic mapping as a result of cochlear lesions or partial deafferentation. In these studies, the time course of plastic change appears to be completed over many weeks or months. In such cases, extensive reorganization is often observed, which suggests that long-term processes such as new axonal growth and synaptogenesis have occurred in addition to a consolidation of synaptic changes. To use a computer analogy, short-term plasticity might be considered to be software changes, whereas long-term changes might also include hardwiring modifications.

Most importantly, we should be very careful to distinguish the neural plasticity during early development, as opposed to that occurring in the mature subject. Age related or developmental plasticity relates most directly to this pediatric audiology handbook. As we discuss next in relation to tonotopic map reorganization after cochlear lesions, more extensive changes result when the system input is altered during early development compared to in the adult. In considering animal model studies of developmental plasticity, it is also important to note, as already emphasized, whether the species is altricious or precocious. The human peripheral auditory system is well developed at birth, and an animal model of choice would be a precocious species such as chinchilla. In other words, it may not be accurate to make cross-species comparisons between altricious mice and precocious humans without some developmental timeline correction factor.

Reorganization of Tonotopic Maps After Cochlear Lesions

Cochleotopic projections can be considered as a mainline organizational feature of the auditory system. Just as the sensory epithelium of the skin surface or the retina have orderly central projections, so too in the auditory system, the topographical order of ascending neurons is well maintained from the sensory epithelium of the cochlea up to cortex (e.g., Merzenich & Brugge, 1973; Reale & Imig, 1980). Strictly speaking, we should refer to this projection system as cochleotopic, in analogy with the similarly organized retinotopic visual system and the somatotopic pathways of the somatosensory system. The interchangeability of the terms *cochleotopic* and *tonotopic* is possible because of the place coding of sound frequency along the cochlear length. However, some caution is advised on the interchangeability of these terms when considering systems having pathologic cochleas. Under such conditions, considerable distortion of the normal place coding of sound frequency is possible. The term *tonotopic* becomes somewhat inappropriate when considering a cochlea electrically stimulated with an electrode array.

The tonotopic map in primary auditory cortex in an animal model can be determined by recording from cortical neurons at several sites (Figure 2–11). Each data point indicates the microelectrode recording site, and the sound frequency to which neuron(s) respond best (often called the characteristic frequency) is indicated in kilohertz (kHz). This cortical tonotopic map reflects a relatively direct organizational "point-to-point" neural projection system from the cochlear sensory epithelium to this orderly tonotopic map at the level of cortex. The isofrequency contours that are drawn through the cortical map are plotted at octave intervals and show that, normally, sound frequency octaves are relatively evenly represented in cortex.

Figure 2–12 shows the cortical tonotopic map in a cat treated at birth with amikacin, an aminoglycoside antibiotic that is ototoxic in high concentration. Such treatment results in bilateral cochlear hair cell degeneration, particularly in the cochlear base (high-frequency region). In this case, histological examination of the cochlea showed that the basal region was totally damaged with both IHCs and OHCs destroyed, but in more apical areas, above the 6- to 8-kHz region, a normal sensory epithelium was present. This is consistent

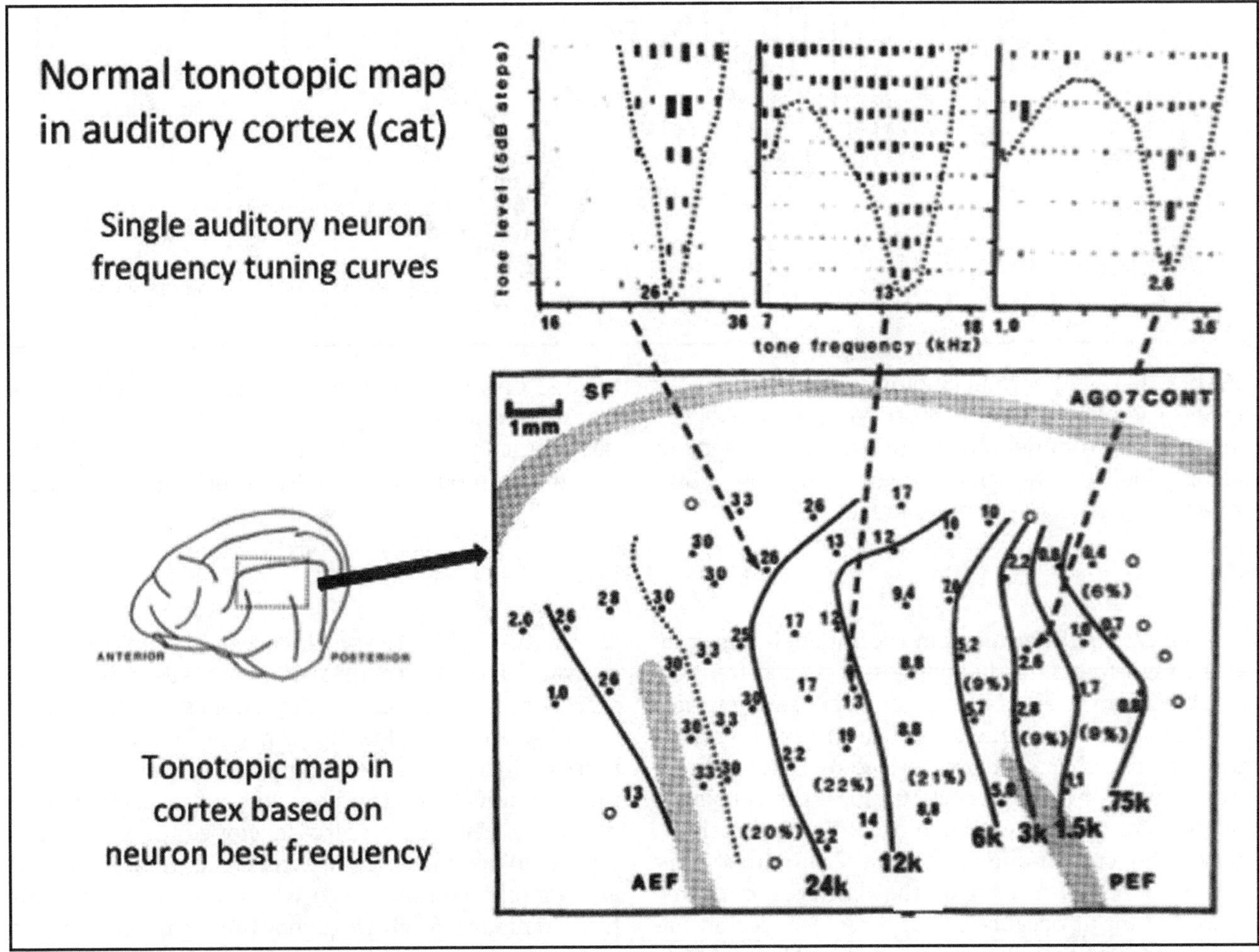

FIGURE 2–11. Cochleotopic or tonotopic map in normal cat auditory cortex as determined by single unit mapping (Harrison, Nagasawa, Smith, Stanton, & Mount, 1991). At each indicated electrode position, the frequency tuning of neural units is determined from receptive field raster plots as indicated in the three upper panels. The stimulus frequency that evokes a response at minimum threshold (characteristic frequency, CF) is indicated on the tonotopic map in kilohertz (kHz). Isofrequency contours shown are at octave intervals. (AEF, anterior ectosylvian fissure; PEF, posterior ectosylvian fissure; SF, sylvian fissure.)

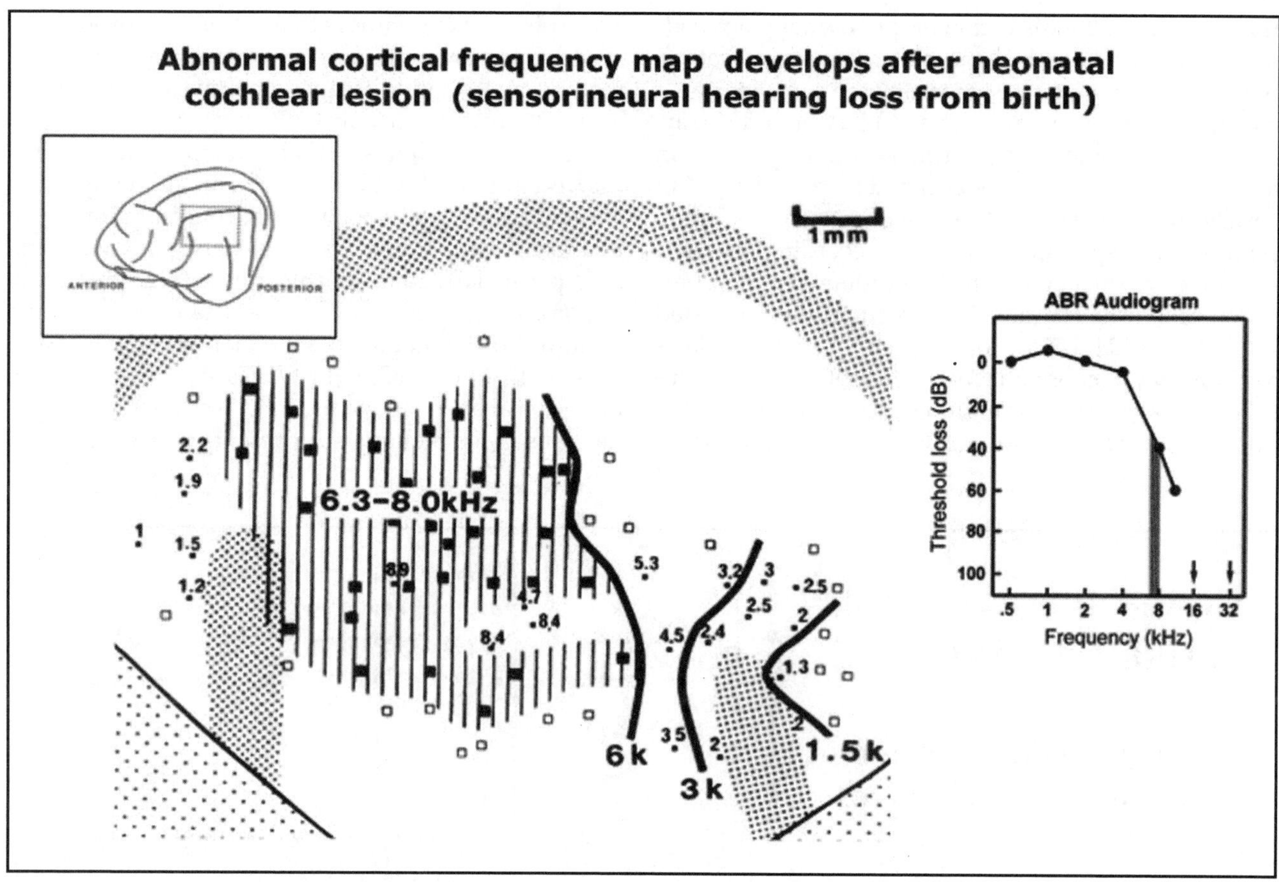

FIGURE 2–12. Abnormal tonotopic maps that developed after a basal cochlear lesion (amikacin treatment; cat model). The effect of the cochlear damage is reflected in the ABR-derived audiogram of the left panel. Tonotopic maps plotted from neuron characteristic frequency data; isofrequency contours are at octave intervals. Cross-hatching indicates regions in which all neurons have similar tuning properties. (Based on data from Harrison, Nagasawa, Smith, Stanton, & Mount, 1991.)

with the cat's ABR audiogram (right panel) that indicates a high-frequency hearing loss to sound frequencies above 6 to 8 kHz, but normal response thresholds to lower stimulus frequencies. The cortical tonotopic map for this subject is characterized by a normal representation of low frequencies, up to 6 kHz, consistent with a histologically normal middle-to-apical cochlear region and corresponding normal ABR thresholds. However, the cortical region that has been deprived of normal input because of basal cochlear lesion has developed such that all neurons are tuned to about 6 to 8 kHz (shown as the crosshatched area). The boundary region of the cochlear lesion (i.e., the 6–8 kHz region) is abnormally over-represented in terms of cortical space. This suggests that surviving hair cells near the lesion boundary eventually become connected with large numbers of cortical neurons (Harrison et al., 1991).

Figure 2–13 shows results from a subject where amikacin-induced cochlear damage was more extensive, with a severe basal lesion and also scattered hair cell loss up to apical, low-frequency cochlea areas. This is reflected in the ABR audiogram (right panel) that shows a gradually increasing auditory loss across all frequencies measured. This subject also developed a cortical tonotopic map in which there was a very large isofrequency area (shown crosshatched) where almost all neurons have common 6.6 kHz frequency tuning. In addition, the low-frequency region of the tonotopic map is severely distorted compared to normal (compare the irregular, closely-spaced isofrequency contours with those in the normal cat of Figure 2–11). It should be obvious, from studies such as these, that the cortical frequency map development is guided in large part by the pattern of neural excitation originating at the cochlear level.

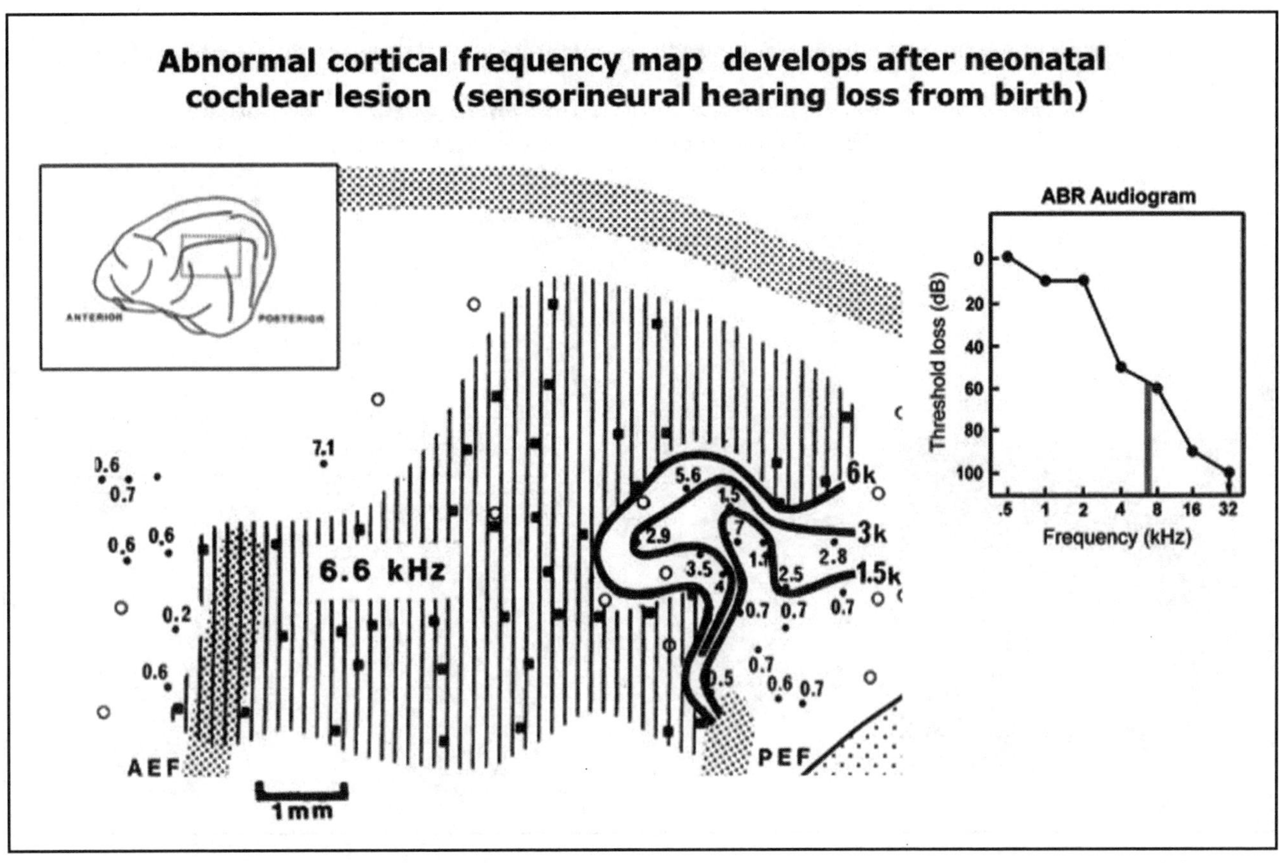

FIGURE 2–13. The cortical frequency map in a kitten reared with a high-frequency cochlear hearing loss from birth as indicated by the ABR audiogram in the right-hand panel (Harrison, Nagasawa, Smith, Stanton, & Mount, 1991). The crosshatched area shows a monotonic area in which all neurons are tuned to about 6.6 kHz. (AEF, anterior ectosylvian fissure; PEF, posterior ectosylvian fissure.)

The experimental results described above were from studies in which the cochlear lesions were induced in neonatal animals (Harrison et al., 1991). Qualitatively similar results are also found at the cortical level if the lesions are made in the adult animals. However, the spatial extent of such cortical map reorganization is much less extensive after cochlear damage in the mature subject compared with that resulting from neonatal lesions (Kakigi, Hirakawa, Harel, Mount, & Harrison, 2000; Rajan, Irvine, Wise, & Heil, 1993; Robertson & Irvine, 1989; Schwaber, Garraghty, & Kaas, 1993).

Tonotopic Map Reorganization at Subcortical Levels

Although many experiments show sensory map reorganization at the cortical level, it does not necessarily follow that the neural alterations are intrinsically cortical. Mapping changes can reflect (wholly or in part) rewiring at lower levels in the system. In the case of developmental plasticity of tonotopic maps in auditory cortex, this is the case. In cats with tonotopic map reorganization shown, for example, in Figures 2–12 and 2–13, neural tracer studies labeling input pathways show that the auditory thalamus has similarly reorganized tonotopic maps (Stanton & Harrison, 2000).

More direct evidence of subcortical frequency map reorganization after cochlear lesions in a developmental model can be observed at the level of the inferior colliculus (IC; Harrison, Ibrahim, & Mount, 1998). Plot A of Figure 2–14 shows, for a normal control animal (chinchilla), the characteristic frequency (CF)–based tonotopic map within the central nucleus of IC. The upper plot shows the tonotopic progression of neuron CF as the electrode penetrates IC in a dorsoventral direction, as illustrated in the lower diagrams. Panel B shows IC tonotopic organization after a basal

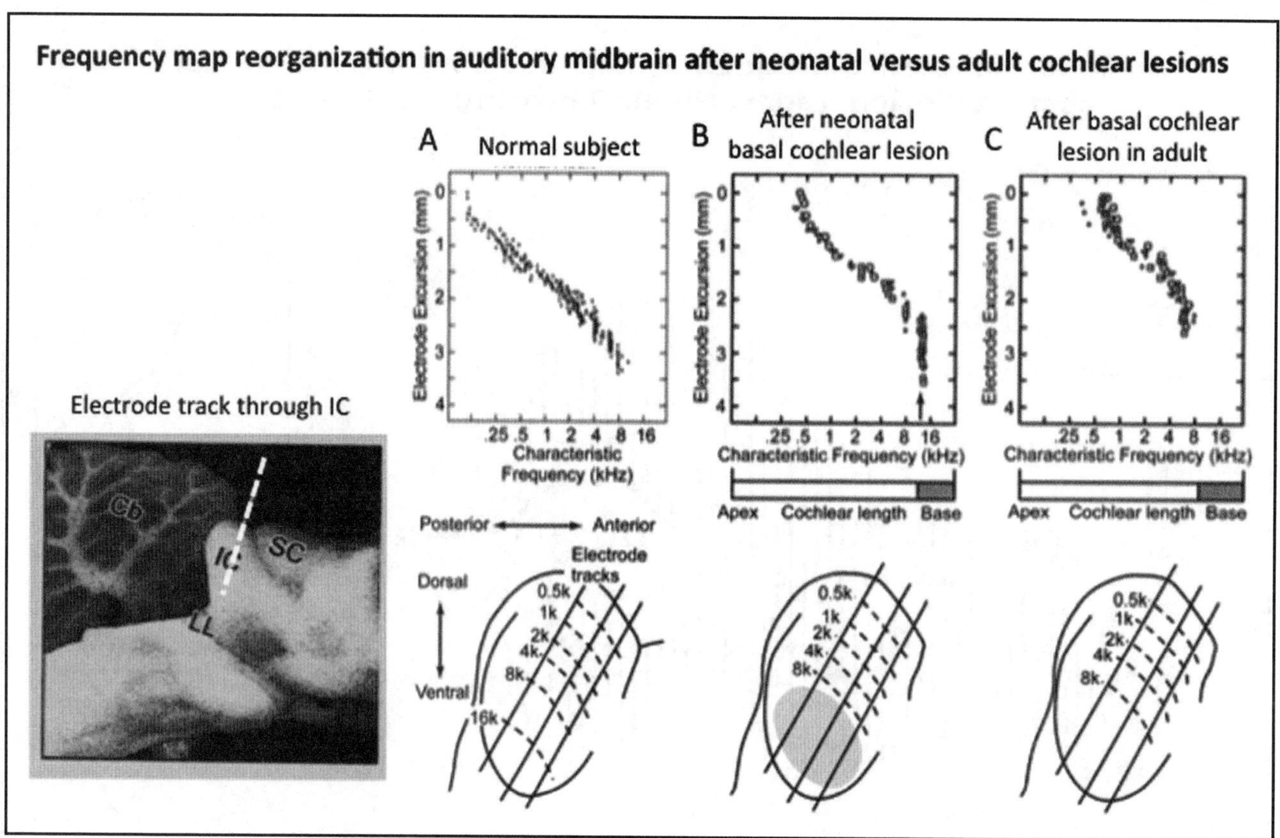

FIGURE 2–14. Tonotopic maps in the central nucleus of inferior colliculus (IC) of the chinchilla. All maps were derived from single neuron recordings in electrode tracks along the dorsoventral axis of IC as shown in the lower panels. The upper graphs plot neuron CF as a function of electrode excursion. The lower diagrams represent the tonotopic maps, with isofrequency contours indicated at octave intervals. Results from a normal animal are shown in *A*, compared with a subject (*B*) in which a basal cochlear lesion was made within days of birth (IC tonotopic map derived 4 months later). In the map (*lower right-hand plot*), the crosshatched area shows the ventral region of IC in which all neurons had a common CF. In plot *C*, a basal cochlear lesion was made in an adult animal, and the resulting IC frequency map is shown. There is little evidence of map reorganization. (Cb, cerebellum; IC, inferior colliculus; LL, lateral lemniscus; SC, superior colliculus. Based on data from Harrison, Ibrahim, & Mount, 1998.)

cochlear lesion made by amikacin drug treatment in a neonatal animal. The cochlear lesion is indicated on the horizontal bar plot. The graph of unit CF versus position within the dorsoventral IC axis clearly indicates that a large region of IC contains neurons tuned to about 10 kHz (arrow symbol). This region of over-representation of one frequency is analogous to the large monotonic regions found in cortical maps after neonatal cochlear lesions. Collectively, these data demonstrate that when cochlear lesions exist during an early developmental period, tonotopic map reorganization occurs not only in auditory cortex but also at subcortical levels. The studies discussed here demonstrate remapping at thalamic and midbrain levels, and it is likely that similar reorganization also exists at the brainstem level.

Can such subcortical reorganization occur in the mature animal after cochlear lesions? Some data suggest that at the level of IC, it does not. Thus, in Figure 2–14, Panel B illustrates the tonotopic map change in IC after a neonatal cochlear lesion, compared with a subject (Panel C) in which a similar lesion was made in a mature animal (based on data from Harrison, 2001). Note that there is no isofrequency region in IC, the de-afferented ventral area of IC being "silent" (no neurons respond to sound stimulation). At the level of the cochlear nucleus, there is also little evidence of tonotopic map reorganization resulting from cochlear lesions made in the mature subject (Kaltenbach, Meleca, & Falzarano, 1996; Rajan & Irvine, 1998). It appears that despite considerable plasticity at all levels of the auditory pathways during early development, plasticity is much reduced in the peripheral pathways as a subject matures.

Tonotopic Map Reorganization After Chronic Local Excitation of the Neonatal Cochlea

The studies outlined above have shown that drastic reductions in neural activity levels from cochlear lesions (partial cochlear de-afferentation) can modify the development of central tonotopic projections. What happens if instead of reducing activity we locally increase cochlear excitation?

In one such experiment (Stanton & Harrison, 1996), kittens were reared for many weeks after birth in an environment where an 8-kHz acoustic signal was constantly present, at a level of 55 to 60 dB SPL (measured level at ear canal). Being suprathreshold, the stimulus activated cochlear neurons across a 7- to 12-kHz range. The tonal stimulus was frequency modulated (±1 kHz; once per second) so as to avoid adaptation effects and possible cochlear hair cell trauma. Some months after this initial rearing period, cortical tonotopic maps were assessed as illustrated in Figure 2–15. Compared to a normal, age-matched control (upper-right panel), a kitten reared in the tonal environment (lower right) showed a significant increase in the cortical space devoted to the frequency region extending from 8 to

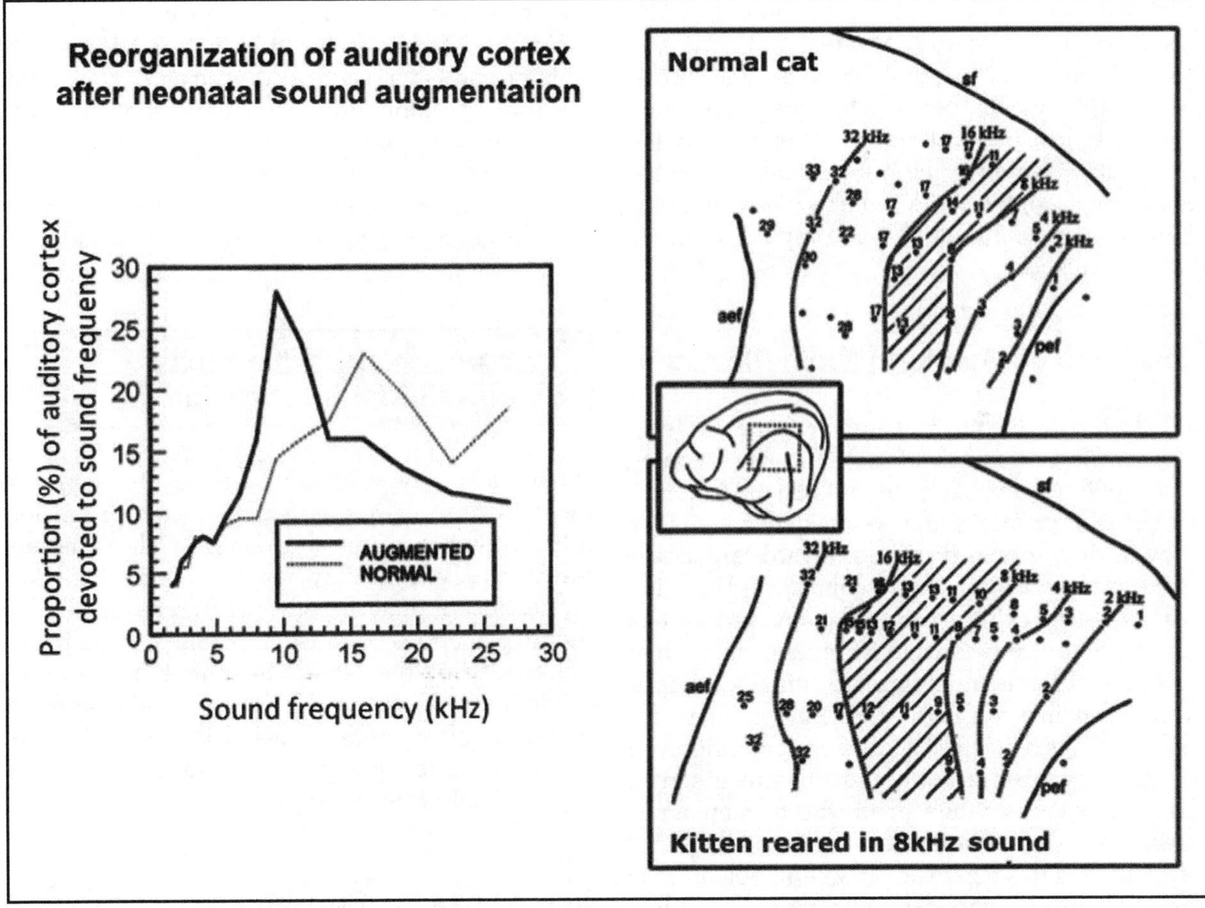

FIGURE 2–15. Tonotopic map in cat auditory cortex resulting from chronic local cochlear activation in the neonate. The upper right-hand frequency map is from a normal control cat. The lower plot is the cortical map in an animal reared postnatally for a month in an acoustic environment with a constant 8 kHz sound signal. Isofrequency contours are drawn at octave intervals. In both examples, the 8- to16-kHz octave interval is crosshatched to emphasize the main difference between the experimental and control subject. The left-hand plot shows pooled data from three experimental sound-reared (augmented) animals and three controls. The graph plots the proportion of auditory cortex representing sound stimulus frequencies. (sf, sylvian fissure; aef, anterior ectosylvian fissure; pef, posterior ectosylvian fissure. Based on data from Stanton & Harrison, 1996.)

12 kHz. Compare the crosshatched 8 to 16 kHz (one octave) frequency region in the experimental animal versus the control. The graph on the left plots pooled data from experimentally sound exposed kittens ($n = 3$) and age-matched controls ($n = 3$). It shows the proportion of auditory cortex devoted to different frequencies. It is supposed that the chronic increase in firing rate of neurons in the mid-frequency area of the cochlea level during an early postnatal period has resulted in an over-representation of those sound frequencies in auditory cortex. Note that for these experimental studies, the environmental tonal stimulus was passive and had no obvious behavioral significance for the animal. In experiments in the mature animal, such stimulus driven cortical reorganization appears only possible when the acoustic stimulus has behavioral significance (e.g., is part of an attention or conditioning task) or in experimental conditions involving forebrain (nucleus basalis) activation (Kilgard & Merzenich, 1998; Weinberger & Bakin, 1998). We could suppose that during an early developmental period when the whole auditory brain is plastic, any stimulus-driven activity has the potential to "remodel" the system. After this critical or sensitive period, the cortex remains plastic but only when the acoustic stimulus has some important significance to the subject.

Mechanisms of (Auditory) Brain Plasticity

Neural plasticity is the result of numerous mechanisms, some of which we understand in detail, some vaguely, and many of which are likely still unknown. The development of a functional neural system depends first on the growth of neuronal processes toward target cells and the establishment of synaptic linkages. These initial stages will provide a coarsely connected system that can be followed by anatomic refinements such as by "pruning" of unwanted or underutilized synaptic connections. For any individual synapse, there are many known mechanisms that can adjust its efficacy or "strength." A detailed review of synaptic strengthening mechanisms is beyond the scope of this text, but a few key principles should be mentioned. Two terms that are often cited in this regard are long-term potentiation (LTP) and Hebbian synaptic strengthening. The former refers to mechanisms in which synaptic transmission is improved after repeated stimulation. A number of pre- and postsynaptic factors have been identified that can achieve this result, including the well-known changes to the effectiveness of *N*-methyl-D-aspartate (NMDA) postsynaptic receptors (see review by Rauschecker, 1991).

Hebbian processes, originally postulated by Donald Hebb (1949), are those where synapses between cells are strengthened when pre- and postsynaptic cells are simultaneously active. The catch phrase here is "cells that fire together, wire together." Besides synapses, other neuronal structures can modify to improve signal transmission, for example, increased myelination of axons as well as other types of neuron-glia cell interactions. All of these known processes are likely in operation during the development of auditory pathways, particularly at early stages when the system is most plastic. In addition to synaptic strengthening, there are also mechanisms that will consolidate and maintain any "programmed" neural network.

As mentioned previously, during early development and in later maturation there are both intrinsic and extrinsic factors that play a role in guiding or driving the process. In this chapter, we have concentrated on the main extrinsic factor, that is, acoustically driven activity, and have seen that during early development this input certainly does drive the organization of the central auditory brain. To complete this chapter, let us take from this review of auditory system development (from cochlea to cortex) some important concepts that are relevant to clinical issues in pediatric audiology.

Auditory System Plasticity: Some Clinical Implications

What do our new insights about neural plasticity mean in practical terms for healthcare professionals dealing with hearing and deafness? In some areas, the new knowledge may have little immediate impact on healthcare practice, other than offering some further explanations of cause of certain symptoms (e.g., understanding the genesis of some types of tinnitus, or loudness perception disorders). In other areas, new scientific information particularly about age-related plasticity of the auditory system has already changed hearing healthcare and patient management.

Some Possible Consequences of Abnormal Auditory System Development

Experimental animal studies (as illustrated in Figures 2–12 and 2–13) clearly indicate that early sensorineural hearing loss will result in some organizational change at the cortical level. A common feature of reorganization is the development of isofrequency regions where certain sound frequencies (or, strictly speaking, cochlear positions) are over-represented. It is still unclear whether such changes have any functional significance. In other words, we do not know whether reorganization improves auditory processing within the range of the residual hearing. On the negative side, one might speculate that such isofrequency areas will contribute to perceptual problems such as loudness recruitment, and perhaps the generation of certain types of tinnitus. In the experimental animals depicted in Figures 2–12 and 2–13 with large monotonic regions in auditory cortex, certain acoustic stimulus frequencies will activate extensive areas of auditory cortex. Given that perceptual loudness is related to the number of neurons active, it is difficult to imagine that this degree of cortical activation will not result in a perceived abnormal increase in loudness (loudness recruitment).

In regard to tinnitus, a few speculative comments are worth making. First, certain types of tinnitus could arise from groups of auditory neurons that develop self-perpetuating activity. The brain is full of network connections that might allow, for example, local and reciprocal intracortical connections, or thalamocortical feedback loops. With our understanding that synaptic efficacy can be considerably increased by long-term potentiation and Hebbian mechanisms, it is easy to conceive of local circuits being reinforced to the point of "ringing" (i.e., having a positive feedback mode). For this and other reasons, the need for extensive and continuous inhibitory control within the brain is obvious. When there are extensive isofrequency areas in auditory cortex, with the potential for massive synchronous activity, it is possible that such inhibitory mechanisms cannot sufficiently suppress positive feedback processes that could lead to self-generated percepts of sound (i.e., tinnitus). An even simpler mechanism for tinnitus production is plausible. Suppose that the synchronous firing of these extensive isofrequency neural populations results in them all being connected together. This is quite feasible; remember Hebb's rule that "cells that fire together, wire together." If we assume that conscious perception has some basis in cortical neuronal activity, then perhaps even very low levels of activity in a vast, linked network of cells could give rise to a chronic sound sensation. For more useful review and discussion about tinnitus generation, see Eggermont (2007, 2008, 2012).

In light of experimental data on plasticity, one final comment about tinnitus is relevant. There is much discussion about the different types and origins of tinnitus. One distinction often made is between "central" and "peripheral" tinnitus. The studies on central auditory plasticity draw attention to the fact that a cochlear lesion can cause central reorganization. It is plausible that some traumatic event at the cochlear level, causing either reduced cochlear nerve activity levels (e.g., after hair cell loss) or much increased neural firing such as injury discharges from damaged or degenerating neurons, could promote central neural connection patterns, resulting in cortical over-representation (as in shown in the examples of this chapter). Thus, in many cases, a tinnitus sensation is caused by overactivity in central auditory neurons; however, this is linked with an initial, peripheral event (cochlear lesion). This notion complicates the distinction between a central versus peripheral origin of the tinnitus.

Early Hearing Loss Detection and Intervention

The take-home message from numerous clinical observations and experimental studies, some described in this text, is that early auditory system development is, in large part, dependent on the pattern of neural activity from the periphery. This means that a hearing loss during early development will significantly impact central auditory brain development. For normal central development, it is clear that there needs to be normal (or near normal) cochlear function during the time window when the system is most plastic and thus influenced by extrinsic signals. Perhaps there is a critical period during which cochlear function needs to be particularly intact. The concepts and concerns raised by developmental neural plasticity experiments (in all sensory systems) have heightened an appreciation about age-related plasticity and have been responsible for major initiatives for early detection and intervention in sensorineural hearing loss. This has, importantly, led to the implementation of universal infant hearing screening programs in many health care jurisdictions.

Most of the animal studies of plasticity that clearly show central structural and functional alterations involve extreme experimental manipulations, such as total cochlear ablation or partial deafferentation. However, it is logical to suppose that more subtle types of cochlear dysfunction will alter peripheral stimulation patterns and thus influence auditory system development. Thus, a mild sensorineural hearing loss, or a chronic conductive hearing loss (e.g., from repeated episodes of otitis media), particularly in the very young, might well alter normal central pathway development. Similarly, an asymmetric hearing loss, which might not be considered clinically significant, may also have an impact on binaural auditory system development.

One of the difficulties with testing or "proving" such hypotheses is that any abnormal auditory development will not be immediately apparent but show up much later in time. For example, neonatal hearing disorders that might lead to problems in language development will only become evident 3 or 4 years later when such development can be assessed. Research in this area can be problematic, especially to gather solid experimental evidence; for example in a prospective, randomized controlled study. Rather than dismissing or ignoring a potential hearing development problem for lack of real evidence, a good practical strategy is to assume the worst, and make every possible effort to normalize hearing during early postnatal years. Pediatric audiologists and other clinicians already take this approach, for example, by making the early detection of hearing problems a priority through neonatal or infant hearing screening programs. Equally important is the timely diagnostic follow-up from such screening and the early intervention with hearing aids, cochlear implants, and auditory habilitation training.

There are still many unanswered questions about age-related plasticity. Perhaps the most important are whether there are developmental time windows within which interventions will be most effective. In other words, are there critical periods not to be missed? Importantly, are there stages in development when the door has effectively closed for an intervention (hearing prosthesis or training therapy program)? When cochlear implants for children became widely available, an important question asked was whether, for congenitally deaf infants, there was a critical or sensitive period after which implantation was of limited benefit. The consensus from many studies was that there was always some benefit, no matter what the duration of deafness, but that children implanted before the age of about 6 years progressed significantly better in speech understanding tests and language development. Some results of one such study are shown in Figure 2–16 (Harrison, Gordon, & Mount, 2005). Children with severe-to-profound hearing loss from birth ($n = 82$) were tested with a battery of speech perception tests before and at

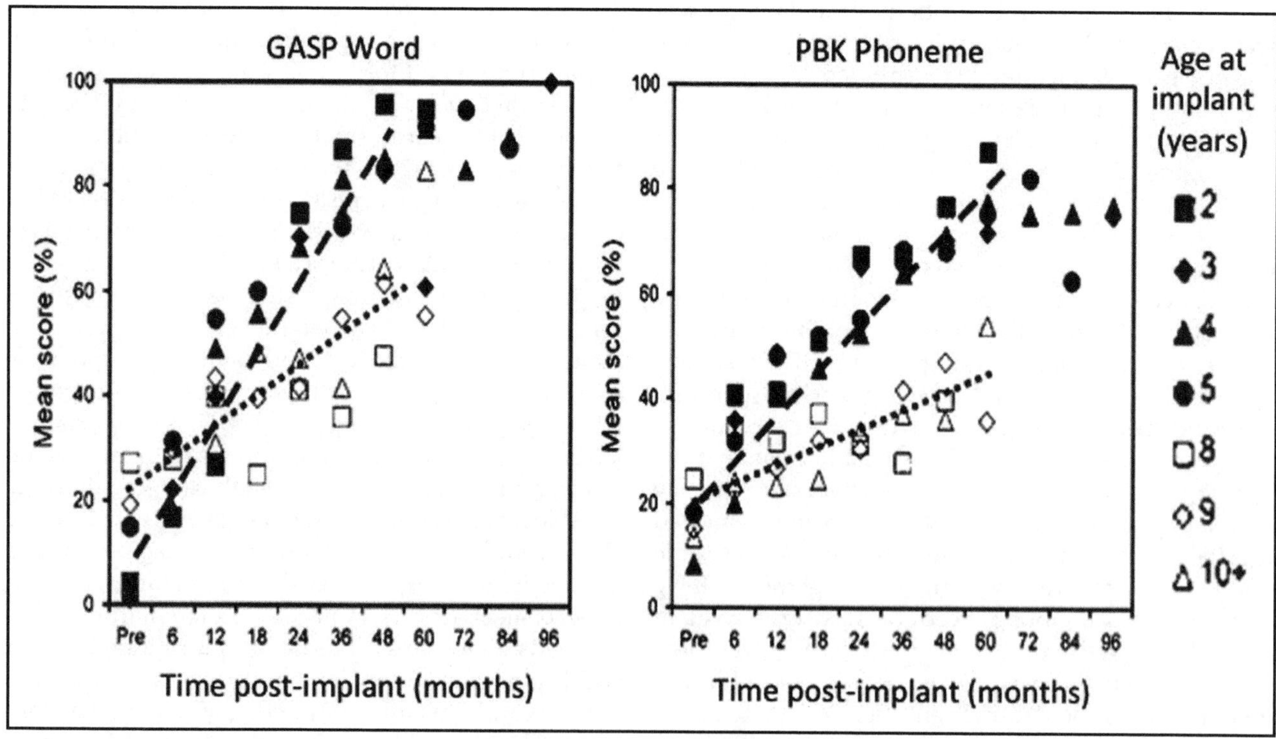

FIGURE 2–16. Development of speech perception in congenitally deaf children ($n = 82$) with cochlear implantation provided at different ages. Scores in GASP word test (*left panel*) and in the PBK phoneme test (*right panel*), preimplant (Pre) and at intervals up to 96 months postimplantation. Mean values are shown for each age-at-implant group, as indicated by the symbols (*key on far right*). Filled symbols and dashed lines represent results for children who were implanted before 6 years of age. The open symbols and dotted line show scores for later implanted children (Harrison, Gordon, & Mount, 2005).

regular intervals after receiving a cochlear implant. The children were grouped into subsets by age. In the figure, these age groups are coded with symbols shown in the key to the right of the data. Filled symbols (and the dashed line) represent children implanted before 6 years of age, and open symbols (and dotted line) show data from children implanted after 6 years of age. Note there is a categorical difference in the performance on these typical example tasks (GASP word and PBK phoneme tests) between children implanted before versus after age 6 years (Harrison et al., 2005).

Cochlear Implants in Children: Stimulating Central Auditory Development

The central auditory system development is significantly guided by cochlear activity patterns. It follows that a cochlear implant, or other hearing prosthesis provided to a young infant, will have a dual purpose. Not only does the device provide "hearing," but the augmented stimulation of the cochlear nerve will also have an influence on central auditory system development. Many questions arise from this notion. First, is a stimulation paradigm designed to provide good auditory input for hearing the most optimal for influencing developmental change? Perhaps we should design hearing prostheses that are constantly activating the system, even when not being used for "hearing." That way they can constantly provide stimulation to the developing auditory brain. Another issue relating to cochlear implants is that for the early implanted, congenitally deaf infant, it is likely that the pattern of stimulation from a specific cochlear implant device drives the development of an atypical central auditory system. If so, what does this mean for replacing devices or changing speech coding paradigms later in life, especially if a sensitive period of early development is passed and the system is less plastic?

A related issue concerns bilateral cochlear implantation. It can be argued that to most closely emulate natural auditory system development, we would like a balanced binaural activation implemented as early as possible. Hence, for the congenitally deaf infant, simultaneous binaural cochlear implantation should be (or become, resource permitting) the optimal intervention. However, what about the provision of a second implant in children already implanted in one ear? If we suppose that activity patterns from one cochlear implant have driven auditory system development in a particular way, can new contralateral activity integrate with the previously established monaural pathway? Is there an overall age-related plasticity during which conversion from monaural to binaural input is useful? Is there a delay of cochlear implantation of each ear beyond which the benefits of binaural hearing are not realized? These are important questions that are just being answered, and the research and discussion around Figure 2–10 in this chapter are providing a clearer understanding of these issues. Children with simultaneous binaural cochlear implants have auditory activity in the brainstem and midbrain that can integrate information from both ears. Children with many years of delay between implantation of each ear do not appear to have that capability and will likely not achieve the benefits of binaural hearing such as sound localization and improved speech understanding in noise (Gordon, Valero, & Papsin, 2007; Papsin & Gordon, 2008).

Some Final Thoughts

We now clearly understand that throughout life, the brain, including the auditory areas, maintains some plasticity and can be rewired, reprogrammed, and taught new tricks. In the adult, plasticity appears to be predominantly at the cortical level, and reprograming is mainly achieved through active attention to tasks and, sometimes difficult learning procedures. On the other hand, the developing brain is enormously plastic. Thus, in neonates and young infants, the developing central auditory system can be significantly influenced by patterns of auditory activity from the periphery. During early development, plasticity is not confined to auditory cortex, and all levels of the pathway from the brainstem up can be (re)organized by auditory input. In pediatric audiology, we must be aware of this plasticity during early years and work to take advantage of this sensitive period in early development. Interventions are more effective at age 6 months than at 6 years. We should also bear in mind that early interventions such as provision of hearing aids, cochlear implant devices, and auditory training therapies will be influential not just in helping a child to hear better in the short term, but also in guiding the long-term development of the auditory brain.

This chapter has provided only some key studies related to auditory development. Some of the references given are chapters in multiauthor texts dealing broadly with hearing development and plasticity, and generally those volumes provide more comprehensive coverage for those with further interest.

References

Birnholz, J. C., & Benacerraf, B. R. (1983). The development of human fetal hearing. *Science, 222*, 516–518.

Boettcher, F. A., & Salvi, R. J. (1993). Functional changes in the ventral cochlear nucleus following acute acoustic overstimulation. *Journal of the Acoustical Society of America, 94*, 2123–2134.

Cang, J., Rentería, R. C., Kaneko, M., Liu X., Copenhagen, D. R., & Stryker, M. P. (2005). Development of precise maps in visual cortex requires patterned spontaneous activity in the retina. *Neuron, 48*, 797–809.

Eggermont, J. J. (1985). Evoked potentials as indicators of auditory maturation. *Acta Otolaryngologica, 421*(Suppl), 41–47.

Eggermont, J. J. (1988). On the rate of maturation of sensory evoked potentials. *Electroencephalography and Clinical Neurophysiology, 70*, 293–305.

Eggermont, J. J. (2007). Pathophysiology of tinnitus. *Progress in Brain Research, 166*, 19–35.

Eggermont, J. J. (2008). Role of auditory cortex in noise- and drug-induced tinnitus. *American Journal of Audiology, 17*, 162–169.

Eggermont, J. J. (2012). *The neuroscience of tinnitus*. Oxford, UK: Oxford University Press.

Eggermont, J. J., Ponton, C. W., Don, M., Waring, M. D., & Kwong, B. (1997). Maturational delays in cortical evoked potentials in cochlear implant users. *Acta Otolaryngologica, 117*, 161–163.

Eggermont, J. J., & Salamy, A. (1988). A maturational time course for the ABR in preterm and full term infants. *Hearing Research, 33*, 37–47.

Gordon, K. A., Papsin, B. C., & Harrison, R. V. (2003). Activity-dependent developmental plasticity of the auditory brainstem in children who use cochlear implants. *Ear and Hearing, 24*, 485–500.

Gordon, K. A., Papsin, B. C., & Harrison, R. V. (2005). Effects of cochlear implant use on the electrically evoked middle latency response in children. *Hearing Research, 204*, 78–89.

Gordon, K. A., Papsin, B. C., & Harrison, R. V. (2006). An evoked potential study of the developmental time course of the auditory nerve and brainstem in children using cochlear implants. *Audiology and Neurootology, 11*, 7–23.

Gordon, K. A., Papsin, B. C., & Harrison, R. V. (2007). Auditory brainstem activity and development evoked by apical versus basal cochlear implant electrode stimulation in children. *Clinical Neurophysiology, 118*, 1671–1684.

Gordon, K. A., Valero, J., & Papsin, B. C. (2007). Auditory brainstem activity in children with 9–30 months of bilateral cochlear implant use. *Hearing Research, 233*, 97–107.

Graziani, L. J., Weitzman, E. D., & Velasco, M. S. (1968). Neurologic maturation and auditory evoked responses in low birth weight infants. *Pediatrics, 41*, 483–494.

Harrison, R. V. (2001). Age related tonotopic map plasticity in the central auditory pathways. *Scandinavian Audiology, 30*(Suppl. 53), 8–14.

Harrison, R. V., Cullen, J. R., Takeno, S., & Mount, R. J. (1996). The neonatal chinchilla cochlea: Morphological and functional study. *Scanning Microscopy, 10*, 889–894.

Harrison, R. V., Gordon, K. A., & Mount, R. J. (2005). Is there a critical period for cochlear implantation in congenitally deaf children? Analyses of hearing and speech perception performance after implantation. *Developmental Psychobiology, 46*, 252–261.

Harrison, R. V., Ibrahim, D., & Mount, R. J. (1998). Plasticity of tonotopic maps in auditory midbrain following partial cochlear damage in the developing chinchilla. *Experimental Brain Research, 123*, 449–460.

Harrison, R. V., Nagasawa, A., Smith, D. W., Stanton, S., & Mount, R. J. (1991). Reorganization of auditory cortex after neonatal high frequency cochlear hearing loss. *Hearing Research, 54*, 11–19.

Hashisaki, G. T., & Rubel, E. W. (1989). Effects of unilateral cochlea removal on anteroventral cochlear nucleus neurons in developing gerbils. *Journal of Comprehensive Neurology, 283*, 465–473.

Hebb, D. O. (1949). *The organization of behavior*. New York, NY: Wiley.

Hogan, S. C., & Moore, D. R. (2003). Impaired binaural hearing in children produced by a threshold level of middle ear disease. *Journal of the Association for Research in Otolaryngology, 4*, 123–129.

Kakigi, A., Hirakawa, H., Harel, N., Mount, R. J., & Harrison, R. V. (2000). Tonotopic mapping in auditory cortex of the adult chinchilla with amikacin-induced cochlear lesions. *Audiology, 39*, 53–160.

Kaltenbach, J. A., Meleca, R. J., & Falzarano, P. R. (1996). Alterations in the tonotopic map of cochlear nucleus following cochlear damage. In R. J. Salvi, D. Henderson, F. Fiorino, & V. Colletti (Eds.), *Auditory system plasticity and regeneration* (pp. 317–332). New York, NY: Thieme Medical.

Kilgard, M. P., & Merzenich, M. M. (1998). Cortical map reorganization enabled by nucleus basalis activity. *Science, 279*, 1714–1718.

Kitzes, L. M. (1984). Some physiological consequences of neonatal cochlear destruction in the inferior colliculus of the gerbil, *Meriones unguiculatus*. *Brain Research, 306*, 171–178.

Kitzes, L. M. (1986). The role of binaural innervation in the development of the auditory brainstem. In R. J. Ruben, T. R. Van De Water, & E. W. Rubel (Eds.), *The biology of change in otolaryngology* (pp. 185–199). Amsterdam, the Netherlands: Elsevier Science.

Kitzes, L. M. (1996). Anatomical and physiological changes in the brainstem induced by neonatal ablation of the cochlea. In R. J. Salvi, D. Henderson, F. Fiorino, & V. Colletti (Eds.), *Auditory system plasticity and regeneration*. New York, NY: Thieme Medical.

Knudsen, E. I. (1984). The role of auditory experience in the development and maintenance of sound localization. *Trends in Neuroscience, 7*, 326–330.

Knudsen, E. I., Esterly, S. D., & Knudsen, P. F. (1984). Monaural occlusion alters sounds localization during a sensitive period in the barn owl. *Journal of Neuroscience, 4*, 1001–1011.

Kujala, T., Alho, K., Huotilainen, M., Ilmoniemi, R. J., Lehtokoski, A., Leinonen, A., & Näätänen, R. (1997). Electrophysiological evidence or cross-modal plasticity in humans with early- and late-onset blindness. *Psychophysiology, 34*, 213–216.

Levi-Montalcini, R. (1949). Development of the acousticovestibular centers in the chick embryo in the absence of the afferent root fibres and of descending fiber tracts. *Journal of Comparative Neurology, 91*, 209–242.

Lim, D. J., & Anniko, M. (1986). Correlative development of sensory cells and overlying membrane of the inner ear: Micromechanical aspects. In R. J. Ruben, T. R. Van De Water, & E. W. Rubel (Eds.), *The biology of change in otolaryngology* (pp. 55–69). Amsterdam, the Netherlands: Elsevier Science.

Lippe, W. R. (1994). Rhythmic spontaneous activity in the developing avian auditory system. *Journal of Neuroscience, 14*, 1486–1495.

Meister, M., Wong, R. O., Baylor, D. A., & Schatz, C. J. (1991). Synchronous bursts of action potentials in ganglion cells of the developing mammalian retina. *Science, 252*, 939–943.

Merzenich, M. M., & Brugge, J. F. (1973). Representations of the cochlear partition on the superior temporal plane of the macaque monkey. *Brain Research, 50*, 275–296.

Moore, D. R. (1994). Auditory brainstem of the ferret: Long survival following cochlear removal progressively changes projections from the cochlear nucleus to the inferior colliculus. *Journal of Comparative Neurology, 339*, 301–310.

Moore, D. R., Hine, J. E., Jiang, Z. D., Matsuda, H., Parsons, C. H., & King, A. J. (1999). Conductive hearing loss produces a reversible binaural hearing impairment. *Journal of Neuroscience, 19*, 8704–8711.

Moore, D. R., Hutchings, M. E., King, A. J., & Kowalchuk, N. E. (1989). Auditory brainstem of the ferret: Some effects of rearing with a unilateral ear plug on the cochlea, cochlear nucleus, and projections to the inferior colliculus. *Journal of Neuroscience, 9*, 1213–1222.

Moore, D. R., & King, A. J. (2004). Plasticity of binaural systems. In R. R. Fay & A. N. Popper (Eds.), *Plasticity of the auditory system* (pp. 96–172). New York, NY: Springer Science.

Moore, D. R., King, A. J., McAlpine, D., Martin, R. L., & Hutchings, M. E. (1993). Functional consequences of neonatal unilateral cochlear removal. *Progress in Brain Research, 97*, 127–133.

Moore, D. R., & Kitzes, L. M. (1985). Projections from the cochlear nucleus to the inferior colliculus in normal and neonatally cochlea-ablated gerbils. *Journal of Comparative Neurology, 240*, 180–195.

Moore, J. K. (2002). Maturation of human auditory cortex: Implications for speech perception. *Annals of Otology, Rhinology & Laryngology, 189*(Suppl.), 7–10.

Neville, H. J., Schmidt, A., & Kutas, M. (1983). Altered visual-evoked potentials in congenitally deaf adults. *Brain Research, 266*, 127–132.

Newton, J. R., & Sur, M. (2005). Rewiring cortex: Functional plasticity of the auditory cortex during development. In J. Syka & M. M. Merzenich (Eds.), *Plasticity and signal representation in the auditory system* (pp. 127–137). New York, NY: Springer Science.

Olsho, L. W. (1986). Early development of human frequency resolution. In R. J. Ruben, T. R. Van De Water, & E. W. Rubel (Eds.), *The biology of change in otolaryngology* (pp. 71–90). Amsterdam, the Netherlands: Elsevier Science.

Pallas, S. L. (2001). Intrinsic and extrinsic factors that shape neocortical specification. *Trends in Neuroscience, 24*, 417–432.

Papsin, B. C., & Gordon, K. A. (2008). Bilateral cochlear implants should be standard for children with bilateral sensorineural deafness. *Current Opinion in Otolaryngology & Head and Neck Surgery, 16*, 69–74.

Parks, T. N., & Jackson, H. (1986). Early destruction of the ear induces formation of a new functional brainstem auditory pathway. In R. J. Ruben, T. R. Van De Water, & E. W. Rubel (Eds.), *The biology of change in otolaryngology* (pp. 225–234). Amsterdam, the Netherlands: Elsevier Science.

Pienkowski, M., & Harrison, R. V. (2005). Tone frequency maps and receptive fields in developing chinchilla auditory cortex. *Journal of Neurophysiology, 93*, 454–466.

Ponton, C. W., Don, M., Eggermont, J. J., Waring, M. D., & Masuda, A. (1996). Maturation of human cortical auditory function, difference between normal hearing and cochlear implanted children. *Ear and Hearing, 17*, 430–437.

Ponton, C. W., & Eggermont, J. J. (2001). Of kittens and kids: Altered cortical maturation following profound deafness and cochlear implant use. *Audiology and Neurootology, 6*, 363–380.

Ponton, C. W., & Eggermont, J. J. (2007). Electrophysiological measures of human auditory system maturation: Relationship with neuroanatomy and behavior. In R. F. Burkard, M. Don, & J. J. Eggermont (Eds.), *Auditory evoked potentials. Basic principles and clinical application* (pp. 385–402). Baltimore, MD: Lippincott Williams & Wilkins.

Ponton, C. W., Eggermont, J. J., Kwong, B., & Don, M. (2000). Maturation of human central auditory system activity: Evidence from multichannel evoked potentials. *Clinical Neurophysiology, 111*, 220–236.

Pujol, R. (1986). Synaptic plasticity in the developing cochlea. In R. J. Ruben, T. R. Van De Water, & E. W. Rubel (Eds.), *The biology of change in otolaryngology* (pp. 47–54). Amsterdam, the Netherlands: Elsevier Science.

Rajan, R., & Irvine, D. R. F. (1998). Absence of plasticity of the frequency map in dorsal cochlear nucleus of adult cats after unilateral partial cochlear lesions. *Journal of Comparative Neurology, 399*, 35–46.

Rajan, R., Irvine, D. R. F., Wise, L. Z., & Heil, P. (1993). Effect of unilateral partial cochlear lesions in adult cats on the representation of lesioned and unlesioned cochleas in primary auditory cortex. *Journal of Comparative Neurology, 338*, 17–49.

Rauschecker, J. P. (1991). Mechanisms of visual plasticity: Hebb synapses, NMDA receptors and beyond. *Physiological Reviews, 71*, 587–615.

Reale, R., & Imig, T. (1980). Tonotopic organization in auditory cortex of the cat. *Journal of Comparative Neurology, 338*, 265–291.

Robertson, D., & Irvine, D. R. F. (1989). Plasticity of frequency organization in auditory cortex of guinea pigs with partial unilateral deafness. *Journal of Comparative Neurology, 282,* 456–471.

Roe, A. W., Pallas, S. L., Kwon, Y. H., & Sur, M. (1992). Visual projections routed to the auditory pathway in ferrets: Receptive fields of visual neurons in primary auditory cortex. *Journal of Neuroscience, 12,* 3651–3664.

Romand, R. (1983). Development of the cochlea. In R. Romand (Ed.), *Development of the auditory and vestibular systems* (pp. 47–88). New York, NY: Academic Press.

Rubel, E. W., Parks, T. N., & Zirpel, L. (2004). Assembling, connecting and maintaining the cochlear nucleus. In R. R. Fay, & A. N. Popper (Eds.), *Plasticity of the auditory system* (pp. 8–48). Baltimore, MD: Springer Science.

Sadato, N., Pascual-Leone, A., Grafman, J., Ibañez, V., Deiber, M. P., Dold, G., & Hallett, M. (1996). Activation of the primary visual cortex by Braille reading in blind subjects. *Nature, 380,* 526–528.

Schwaber, M. K., Garraghty, P. E., & Kaas, J. H. (1993). Neuroplasticity of the adult primate auditory cortex following cochlear hearing loss. *American Journal of Otolaryngology, 14,* 252–258.

Sharma, J., Angelucci, A., & Sur, M. (2000). Induction of visual orientation modules in auditory cortex. *Nature, 404,* 841–847.

Stanton, S. G., & Harrison, R. V. (1996). Neonatal auditory augmentation modifies cochleotopic mapping in primary auditory cortex of the cat. *Auditory Neuroscience, 2,* 97–107.

Stanton, S. G., & Harrison, R. V. (2000). Projections from the medial geniculate body to primary auditory cortex in neonatally deafened cats. *Journal of Comparative Neurology, 426,* 117–129.

Trehub, S. E., Schneider, B. A., & Endman, M. (1980). Developmental changes in infants' sensitivity to octave-band noises. *Journal of Experimental Child Psychology, 29,* 283–293.

Wang, J., Salvi, R. J., & Powers, N. (1996). Plasticity of response properties of inferior colliculus neurons following acute cochlear damage. *Journal of Neurophysiology, 75,* 171–183.

Weinberger, N. M., & Bakin, J. S. (1998). Learning-induced physiological memory in adult primary auditory cortex: Receptive fields plasticity, model, and mechanisms. *Audiology and Neurootology, 3,* 145–167.

Infant Speech Perception

Derek M. Houston

Introduction

Speech perception can be described as a mode of hearing specialized for speech. When people engage in conversation, they do not hear simply the information conveyed in a waveform or a spectrogram. Instead, they perceive linguistic and indexical information that conveys words and sentences as well as identifying qualitative characteristics of the talkers. People are able to extract linguistic and indexical information from speech because of the specialized way the human hearing instrument is tuned. Accordingly, the study of infant speech perception is concerned with the tuning of that instrument during early development.

A complete understanding of how speech perception develops would require descriptions of the initial and end states of infants' speech perception and an explanation of how the change of state happens. The field of infant speech perception is not yet able to describe with certainty exactly what information infants perceive from speech at any stage of development or what drives speech perception to change with development and language experience. Nevertheless, developmental scientists have made a great deal of progress over the last 45 years toward these goals.

Early work in infant speech perception was strongly influenced by Noam Chomsky's theories, which were revolutionizing the field of linguistics at the time. Chomsky (1968, 1975) posited that language was not learnable from the input alone and required a specialized universal language acquisition device that was innately endowed to humans. Because of this prevailing view, most work focused on identifying speech perception skills that were thought to be innate and universal. Gradually, however, infant speech perception scientists have focused increasingly more on what infants are able to learn from the input, and mounting evidence suggests that general learning mechanisms might play a larger role in language acquisition than previously thought (Behme & Deacon, 2008).

This chapter reviews what is known about normal-hearing infants' initial preferences and sensitivities to both suprasegmental properties of speech (e.g., stress, intonation, rhythm) and fine-grained information contained in phonemes. I then discuss learning mechanisms that have been found to play a role in tuning infants' speech perception skills. Finally, we describe the speech perception skills that infants acquire as a result of these learning mechanisms, which put them in a position to build a vocabulary and acquire language.

Birth to Six Months: Initial Preferences and Sensitivities

The aim of this section is to describe infants' speech perception skills during the early postnatal period. However, this period might not reflect infants' initial state because fetuses are able to hear and learn in utero. Fetuses demonstrate consistent responses to auditory stimulation by 25 to 29 weeks gestational age (Birnholz & Benacerraf, 1983), which means that full-term newborns have more than 2 months of auditory experience. In utero experience can shape the initial postnatal state, and we consider its role in the initial postnatal state of speech perception.

The fetal hearing experience might affect some aspects of speech perception more than others. Studies of the in utero acoustic environment suggest that frequencies above 1000 Hz are attenuated 20 to 30 dB in transmission to fetuses (e.g., Lecanuet et al., 1998), suggesting that they have, at best, limited access to acoustic information important for discriminating segmental information, especially consonants. However, one recent study challenges this conclusion. Moon, Lagercrantz, and Kuhl (2013) investigated Swedish and American neonates' sucking responses to Swedish and English vowels. They found that neonates responded differentially to native and nonnative variants of vowels. Because most of the information that differentiates vowels is above 1000 Hz, the findings suggest usable access to frequencies up to 2600 Hz in utero (Huotilainen, 2013). Further research might reveal access to even higher frequencies. In the meantime, there is ample research suggesting that fetuses have access to the lower frequencies necessary for perception of suprasegmental aspects of speech. We review some of that research below.

Perception of Suprasegmental Information

Suprasegmental information, such as intonation and rhythm, transmits very well to fetuses. Several research teams have investigated how prenatal experience with suprasegmental information affects infants' early speech perception. One issue of interest is whether or not fetuses encode suprasegmental information into memory. If so, their in utero experience with speech might affect their initial postnatal speech processing and preferences.

Evidence of Early Encoding

There is evidence that fetuses not only have access to auditory information, they also encode speech information into memory—especially suprasegmental information. Both newborns and fetuses demonstrate the ability to discriminate their native language from a foreign language (Kisilevsky et al., 2009; Mehler et al., 1988; Moon, Cooper, & Fifer, 1993; Nazzi, Bertoncini, & Mehler, 1998) and their mother's voice from another woman's voice (DeCasper & Fifer, 1980; Kisilevsky et al., 2003). Both of these abilities presumably rely in large part on sensitivity to suprasegmental information.

To explore the possibility that suprasegmental properties encoded during the last trimester persist in memory, DeCasper and colleagues investigated newborns' and fetuses' memory of their mothers' speech. They instructed women to read a nursery rhyme three times a day, starting 6 weeks before their due date. Newborns showed a preference for the familiar nursery rhyme over a novel nursery rhyme (DeCasper & Spence, 1986). A follow-up investigation found that fetuses who were tested 2 weeks before birth showed differential heart rate responses for the familiar compared to a novel rhyme (DeCasper, Lecanuet, Busnel, Granier-Deferre, & Maugeais, 1994). Thus, 4 weeks of exposure for a few minutes a day is *sufficient* for fetuses to encode some properties of a nursery rhyme. However, it is unknown at this time how much exposure is *necessary* for fetuses to encode suprasegmental properties of their language, their mother's voice, or a nursery rhyme.

Recent studies have investigated how long representations of sounds persist in fetal memories. Granier-Deferre, Bassereau, Ribeiro, Jacquet, and Decasper (2011) found that fetuses exposed to a piano melody at 35 to 37 weeks gestation exhibited memory of the melody 6 weeks later. Krueger and Garvan (2014) found that 38-week fetuses demonstrated memory of a nursery rhyme to which they had been exposed regularly from 28 to 34 weeks gestation. Further research is needed to test the limits of fetal memory for speech and music.

Sensitivity to Rhythm and Intonation

The above findings suggest that infants are highly attuned to what they hear in utero. But what aspects of speech are they encoding? One possibility is that infants' ability to discriminate what they hear in utero from novel stimuli might reflect simple pattern-matching skills. However, their discrimination abilities might instead reflect a more general attunement to suprasegmental properties of speech. Nazzi, Bertoncini, and Mehler (1998) investigated this possibility by testing newborn infants' discrimination of languages to which they were not exposed to in utero. Specifically, they investigated the role of rhythm—the timing of syllables in a language—in infants' language discrimination. French newborns demonstrated discrimination of unfamiliar languages that were rhythmically dissimilar (English and Japanese) but not languages that were rhythmically similar (English and Dutch), suggesting they had a general sensitivity to rhythmic information in speech.

As discussed later in the chapter, infants' sensitivity to the rhythmic properties of speech appears to play an important role in their later speech segmentation skills—that is, their ability to locate word boundaries in the context of fluent speech. It is therefore tempting to assume that infants' ability to discriminate languages that are rhythmically different means that they are especially sensitive to rhythmic properties of speech. However, the rhythm of speech correlates strongly with its intonation, and it is not clear if infants rely mainly on rhythm or intonation to discriminate languages (Ramus, 2002). Whatever the case, infants' sensitivity to suprasegmental properties of speech seems to be general rather than limited to only the speech to which they were exposed in utero. In the next section, we discuss the role that infant sensitivity to suprasegmental properties might play in their processing of speech.

Effects of Rhythm and Intonation on Early Speech Processing: Preference for Infant-Directed Speech

Not only are infants able to discriminate suprasegmental properties, several investigations suggest that these properties play a role in infants' attention to speech and what information they extract. With respect to attention, adults speak differently to infants than they do to other adults or even older children, especially when they want to engage infants' attention. *Infant-directed speech* (IDS) and *adult-directed speech* (ADS) differ in their rhythmic and intonational properties. IDS is characterized as being slower (longer durations of syllables and pauses), higher pitched, and having greater pitch excursions than ADS. Infants demonstrate greater attention to IDS than to ADS, at least during the first 6 months of life (Cooper & Aslin, 1990; Fernald, 1985; Fernald & Kuhl, 1987; Werker & McLeod, 1989). After that, there is mixed evidence for greater attention to IDS than ADS up to 16 months of age (Hayashi, Tamekawa, & Kiritani, 2001; Newman & Hussain, 2006; Segal & Newman, 2015).

The advantage of IDS over ADS in capturing infants' attention does not appear to depend much, if at all, on infants' experience with IDS. Cooper and Aslin (1990) assessed attention to IDS and ADS in 2-day-olds and 1-month-olds and found that both groups of infants demonstrated longer looking times when presented with IDS than when presented with ADS. Given our previous discussion of fetal sensitivities to speech, we might speculate that in utero experience plays a role in infants' attention to IDS. However, fetuses are exposed to ADS more than to IDS (unless the pregnant mother speaks more to infants than to adults and older children); thus, it seems very unlikely that newborns' increased attention to IDS could be due to their exposure to speech (which is mainly ADS) during the fetal period.

If infants' attention to IDS is not due to experience, then it is likely something about the acoustic properties of IDS that draws infants' attention to it. To investigate the relative contributions of the pitch (as measured by F0), intensity, and duration characteristics of IDS on capturing infants' attention, Fernald and Kuhl (1987) presented infants with one of three types of IDS and ADS computer-synthesized speech. Each type of synthesized speech preserved one characteristic that differentiated IDS and ADS and equalized the other two characteristics; all speech types were devoid of any lexical information. The investigators found that 4-month-olds showed greater attention to the IDS only when the pitch was preserved, suggesting that the pitch characteristics of IDS are what captures infants' attention (Fernald & Kuhl, 1987). Follow-up studies suggested that the aspect of pitch most important for infants' preference for IDS is intonation rather than the mean pitch height (Fernald, 1993). However, more recently, Singh, Morgan, and Best (2002) found that 6-month-olds preferred speech that conveyed positive affect to speech that conveyed neutral affect, regardless of whether it was IDS or ADS. Moreover, infants showed no preference for IDS over ADS when they controlled for affect. In fact, infants preferred ADS to IDS when presented with positive-affect ADS and neutral-affect IDS. Also, infants responded more positively to IDS that expresses approval than IDS that expresses disapproval (Fernald, 1993). These findings suggest that infants prefer IDS because it generally conveys a positive affect, which is carried primarily through intonation (Fernald, 1989).

Taken together, research on young infants' sensitivity to suprasegmental information suggests that they are attuned to the rhythmic and intonational properties of speech at birth and even before. They prefer intonation that conveys emotional information. There is no strong evidence that infants have a similar kind of preference for a particular type of rhythm, but they are able to discriminate rhythmic differences at very young ages. It is not clear what drives infants to attend to rhythmic properties. It is possible that because intonation and rhythm are highly correlated, attention to intonation may contribute to sensitivity to rhythm. Infants' attention to rhythmic properties plays an important role in the development of more advanced speech perception skills, as we discuss later in this chapter. However, for now, we continue to focus on speech perception skills during early infancy. We now turn to their perceptual sensitivities to segmental information in speech.

Perception of Segmental Information

Segmental information refers to the acoustic properties of speech that differentiate phonemes. Given that much of the high-frequency acoustic information that distinguishes phonemes is not available to fetuses because of in utero filtering, we might expect young infants to be poor at discriminating phonemes. But despite the lack of experience with high-frequency segmental information in utero, newborns and young infants demonstrate sensitivities to fine-grained changes in segmental information.

Categorical Perception

The earliest infant speech perception research was motivated by findings that adults perceived some acoustic-phonetic dimensions categorically rather than continuously (Liberman, Harris, Hoffman, & Griffith, 1957). For example, *voice onset time* (VOT) is the time between the release of an articulation for a stop consonant (e.g., [p, b, t, d, k, g]) and the onset of voicing. Although VOT varies along a continuum, adults perceive VOT categorically (Liberman, Harris, Kinney, & Lane, 1961). In English, stop consonants with relatively short VOTs (0–20 msec) are perceived as *voiced* (e.g., [b, d, g]), and those with relatively long VOTs (>30 msec) are perceived as *voiceless* (e.g., [p, t, k]). They are considered to be perceived categorically because listeners are very poor at discriminating within-category changes in VOT (e.g., 0 and 20 msec VOTs or 40 and 60 msec VOTs) but can readily discriminate changes in VOT that cross VOT categories (e.g., 20 and 40 msec VOTs) even when the objective differences in VOT are identical. At issue in the late 1960s was whether or not categorical perception was due to innate auditory sensitivities or due to experience—learning the phonology of the ambient language.

To test whether or not infants were innately endowed with speech discrimination abilities that were attuned to language, Peter Eimas and his colleagues tested 1- and 4-month-old infants' ability to discriminate synthesized versions of [ba]-[pa] that varied along the VOT continuum. To test young infants, Eimas, Siqueland, Jusczyk, and Vigorito (1971) used the high-amplitude sucking (HAS) paradigm. In the HAS paradigm, infants suck on a non-nutritive pacifier that is connected to a computer that registers each suck. During the habituation phase, infants are presented with one stimulus each time they suck until their sucking rate decreases to a habituation criterion. They are then presented with a novel stimulus (experimental group) or the same stimulus (control group), and their sucking times are analyzed to determine if the presentation of the novel stimulus elicits an increase in sucking rate, suggesting infants can discriminate the two stimuli. Eimas and colleagues found that 1- and 4-month-old infants showed discrimination of the same VOTs as adults, suggesting that they also perceived VOT categorically. Numerous follow-up studies have shown that infants categorically discriminate voicing, place-of-articulation, and manner-of-articulation (e.g., Eimas, 1974, 1975; Eimas & Miller, 1980a, 1980b; Eimas et al., 1971), suggesting that infants are born with a perceptual system that is tuned to detect acoustic-phonetic properties important for identifying phonemes in many of the world's languages.

Some more recent work suggests that infants' discrimination of consonants is not as fixed or as strictly categorical as previously thought. Maye, Werker, and Gerken (2002) tested the effects of input on infants' discrimination of VOT contrasts. They familiarized infants with repetitions of eight unaspirated alveolar stops that varied in VOT from [da] to [ta]. One group of infants was presented with relatively more tokens from the middle of the VOT range (unimodal distribution), and the other group was presented with relatively more tokens from the two endpoints of the VOT range (bimodal distribution). They then tested infants' discrimination of [da] and [ta] and found that only the group familiarized with the bimodal distribution demonstrated discrimination.

Whereas Maye et al. (2002) found that infants can fail to discriminate across category boundaries under some stimulus conditions, McMurray and Aslin (2005) found that infants can discriminate VOTs within category boundaries under some testing conditions. They used a head-turn preference procedure (described in more detail later) to assess 8-month-olds' discrimination of prototypical and nonprototypical tokens of [ba] and [pa]. Unlike previous studies that used a habituation/dishabituation procedure, McMurray and Aslin (2005) found that infants could discriminate tokens that fell within phoneme categories. Taken together, these and a growing number of other findings (Burns, Yoshida, Hill, & Werker, 2007; Hoonhorst et al., 2009; Liu & Kager, 2015; Narayan, Werker, & Beddor, 2010; Sato, Sogabe, & Mazuka, 2010) suggest that although infants may have some initial auditory sensitivities to particular acoustic-phonetic cues, these sensitivities are not rigid and can be influenced by linguistic input.

Although the above work suggests that many consonant contrasts can be perceived categorically, investigations on the perception of vowels suggest that they are perceived more continuously. Unlike consonants, adults discriminate steady-state vowels in a continuous rather than a categorical manner (Fry, Abramson, Eimas, & Liberman, 1962; Pisoni, 1973; Stevens, Liberman, Studdert-Kennedy, & Ohman, 1969). Swoboda, Morse, and Leavitt (1976) discovered that 2-month-olds not only discriminated [i] and [ê] but also discriminated vowel sounds that fell within the same vowel category but differed with respect to formant frequencies, suggesting that, like adults, young infants also perceive vowels in a continuous manner.

Sensitivity to Phoneme Inventory

The above findings suggest that, like their ability to discriminate suprasegmental properties of speech, young infants are able to discriminate segmental properties after little to no experience with language. However, the above findings tell us very little about infants' ability to encode phonemes into long-term memory. Evidence that they can encode suprasegmental information into long-term memory comes from studies reviewed in the previous section in which infants respond differently to the familiar rhythmic and intonational characteristics of their mothers' speech than to the speech of another woman and to a familiar nursery rhyme than to an unfamiliar one. Responding to familiarity requires not only the ability to discriminate familiar and unfamiliar stimuli, but also the ability to associate a familiar sample of speech to representations of that speech stored in long-term memory. In contrast, a finding of discrimination where one stimulus is presented until habituation is reached and then a novel stimulus is presented requires infants to store speech information into memory for only a very brief period of time.

If infants are able to encode segmental information of the ambient language into their long-term memory as they do suprasegmental information, they should show similar attentional preferences for native segmental information as they do for native suprasegmental information. Jusczyk, Friederici, Wessels, Svenkerud, and Jusczyk (1993) tested this possibility by assessing 6- and 9-month-old English-learning infants' preferences for English words versus foreign words that differed from English words in phoneme inventories, rhythmic properties, or both. Infants demonstrated longer looking times for their native rhythm versus a foreign rhythm (low-pass filtered Norwegian) but not for their native phoneme inventory versus a language with a similar rhythm but dissimilar phoneme inventory (Dutch). Nine-month-olds, in contrast, showed preferences based on both rhythm and phoneme inventories, suggesting that familiarity with native segmental characteristics emerges later than familiarity with native suprasegmental characteristics.

Effects of Language Experience on Speech Discrimination

Many phonemes are common across most languages, and early work on speech discrimination in infants focused on their ability to discriminate those common phonemes. However, some phonemes are particular to one or just a few of the world's languages. For example, in Hindi there are two types of "d" sounds. One is similar to the English "d" ([d]—produced by the tongue releasing down from the teeth); the other—a *retroflex* "d" [ɖ]—is produced by pulling the tongue back from the teeth. Non-Hindi speakers have difficulty hearing the difference between these two "d" sounds. Werker and Tees (1984) wanted to know if infants could discriminate phonemic contrasts that occurred in some languages but were difficult for adults who did not speak those languages to discriminate. They tested three age groups (6–8 months, 8–10 months, and 10–12 months) from three language backgrounds (English, Hindi, and Nthlakapmx) on several consonant contrasts. Werker and Tees (1984) found that younger infants were able to discriminate all of the contrasts, but 10- to 12-month-olds could discriminate only those that were linguistically relevant in their native language, suggesting that consonant discrimination is affected by language input.

The effect of language input on speech discrimination has been investigated with vowels as well. Kuhl, Williams, Lacerda, Stevens, and Lindblom (1992) tested English-learning and Swedish-learning infants' discrimination of variants of the English vowel [i] and the Swedish vowel [y]. The two groups of infants showed different patterns of results, suggesting that language background affected their discrimination of the vowels. Specifically, when infants were presented with variants of [i], English-learning infants were less likely to discriminate two variants that were acoustically similar to the prototypical English [i] than two variants that were less similar to the prototype, even though the variants in each pair were equally similar to each other. Swedish-learning infants, by contrast, were just as likely to discriminate both pairs of the English [i] variants. When infants were presented with variants of the Swedish vowel [y], the group differences were reversed; only the Swedish-learning infants' discrimination was affected by similarity to the prototype. Kuhl (1991, 1993) described these findings as representing a "perceptual magnet effect" in which the distribution of vowel variants in the ambient language shapes infants' perceptual systems such that they perceive variants within a vowel category to be more like the prototype of that category. However, Polka and Bohn (1996) found no evidence of a perceptual magnet effect when they tested English-learning and German-learning infants' discrimination of the German and English contrasts. Instead, these findings and others suggest that vowels on the periphery of the F1/F2 acoustic space serve as universal perceptual attractors (Polka & Bohn, 2003, 2011).

These and similar findings (Best, McRoberts, & Sithole, 1988; Trehub, 1976; Tsushima et al., 1994; Werker & Lalonde, 1988) led to a *universalist* view of infant speech discrimination—that infants are born able to discriminate any phonemic contrast that could potentially be relevant to any of the world's languages; and then, with experience, infants lose the ability to discriminate contrasts that are not relevant for their language (e.g., Eimas, Miller, & Jusczyk, 1987; Werker & Pegg, 1992). However, since then, the picture of infants' speech discrimination abilities has become more complex. For example, some non-native phoneme contrasts fall into the same phoneme category in English (e.g., the Hindi [ɖ]), but many speech sounds (e.g., African clicks) do not fall into any phonemic category of English speakers. Best, McRoberts, Lafleur, and Silver-Isenstadt (1995) found that such contrasts remain easy to discriminate for English-speaking adults and older infants. These findings provide evidence against a strong universalist view that infants lose the ability to discriminate all sounds that are not linguistically relevant.

One limitation of a universalist view of speech discrimination is that it does not take into consideration subphonemic information that, although not relevant for distinguishing words, is relevant for other aspects of speech perception and language acquisition. Allophones (context-dependent variants of phonemes) specify details for how words are produced in the native language and can play a role in speech segmentation. For example, initial stops are aspirated in English but not in French—"port" is pronounced [pʰort] in English, but in French "porte" (door) is pronounced [port]. Stops are unaspirated in other positions in English (e.g., "sport"). To sound like a native English speaker, English-learning infants must encode allophonic information even though it does not differentiate words. Hohne and Jusczyk (1994) tested infants' discrimination of words and word pairs such as "nitrates" and "night rates." The same strings of phonemes comprise these sequences but differ with respect to some of the allophonic information: the "t" in "nitrates" is aspirated, released, and retroflexed; the "t" in "night rates" is unaspirated, unreleased, and not retroflexed. Also, the "r" is devoiced in "nitrates" but not in "night rates." Two-month-olds demonstrated discrimination of these allophones (Hohne & Jusczyk, 1994). Subsequent investigations of infants' use of allophonic information (discussed below) suggest that infants do not lose their ability to discriminate this fine-grained information.

Another challenge to a universalist view of speech discrimination is that some contrasts, rather than being discriminable universally during early infancy, require language experience before they can be discriminated. Lacerda (1993) found that Swedish-learning 6- to 12-month-olds could discriminate between [a] and [ʌ] but not between [a] and [ɑ], both of which are linguistically relevant in Swedish. Similarly, Lasky, Syrdal-Lasky, and Klein (1975) tested Spanish-learning 4.5- to 6-month-olds on three different VOT contrasts. They found that the Spanish-learning infants were able to discriminate a pair of speech sounds that was irrelevant for Spanish but relevant for English, but did not discriminate a contrast that is distinctive in Spanish. More recent work suggests that VOT boundaries shift to what is appropriate for the ambient language at around 8 to 10 months of age (Burns et al., 2007; Hoonhorst et al., 2009; Liu & Kager, 2015).

Other recent investigations have demonstrated that discrimination of some contrasts improves with language experience from infancy through adulthood (Narayan et al., 2010; Polka, Colantonio, & Sundara, 2001; Sato et al., 2010; Sundara, Polka, & Genesee, 2006; Tsao, Lui, & Kuhl, 2006). For example, English-learning infants and children improve in their ability to discriminate the [d]-[ð] contrast, whereas French-learning infants and children do not (Polka et al., 2001; Sundara et al., 2006). Taken together, the findings point to an early perceptual system that is able to discriminate most contrasts of the world's languages, and then through experience with language input, infants become more sensitive to sounds that are relevant for their language and less sensitive to contrasts that are not linguistically relevant.

Six Months to One Year: Demonstrations of Learning

Given that infants seem to learn something about the organization of sounds in their language by the second half of the first year of life, it is worth considering what kinds of learning mechanisms are required to allow this auditory-perceptual learning to occur. This section will describe some of the specific learning abilities of infants that might interact with their innate auditory and perceptual abilities to transition them from universal perceivers to having perceptual systems tuned to the native language.

Mechanisms of Learning in Infants

Several learning mechanisms contribute to the development of language-specific speech perception skills. These learning mechanisms include, but are not limited to, recognition memory, associative learning, and statistical learning. Each of these learning mechanisms has been studied extensively by developmental scientists, and a full review of them is beyond the scope of this chapter. Instead, we will briefly describe what these mechanisms are and provide some evidence that infants possess these learning mechanisms.

Recognition Memory

Recognition is a very basic form of learning. In order to recognize something, it must be encoded into memory. Visual recognition memory has been investigated much more than auditory recognition memory. One way developmental scientists have investigated visual recognition memory is by using habituation/dishabituation paradigms (Colombo, Shaddy, Richman, Maikranz, & Blaga, 2004; Fagan & McGrath, 1981; Rose & Feldman, 1997; Rose, Feldman, & Jankowski, 2001). Infants are presented with an object or photograph of a face repeatedly until they habituate to it (i.e., decrease their looking time). Then they are presented with both a novel and the habituated object. Longer looking to the novel than to the habituated object indicates recognition of the object the child has already seen. Recognition memory improves significantly during the first year of life (Rose et al., 2001) and correlates with later cognitive and language outcomes (Rose, Feldman, & Wallace, 1992; Rose, Feldman, Wallace, & McCarton, 1991), suggesting that it is an important skill for cognitive and language development.

Some examples of infants' recognition memory for speech have already been reviewed above. Preferences for native language and mother's voice suggest recognition. Work with older infants suggests that infants' representations of speech sounds become more generalizable with experience and development. For example, Houston and Jusczyk (2000) tested infants' ability to recognize familiarized words when presented with a different voice. They found that 10.5-month-olds but not 7.5-month-olds were able to recognize words across talkers of the opposite sex, suggesting that 7.5-month-olds encode talker-specific information in memory and that this affects how they recognize words (see also Houston, 1999; Houston & Jusczyk, 2003). These findings illustrate how the development of recognition memory skills is important for correctly identifying words as novel and old, which is an important skill for learning the meaning of words across different contexts. Later, we discuss some additional examples of how the development of recognition memory skills affects speech perception in infants.

Associative Learning

Associative learning is highly relevant to language acquisition; word learning is a sophisticated type of associative learning. But well before infants utter their first words, their associative learning skills develop in nonlinguistic domains. In the visual domain, early associative learning plays an important role in forming categories of objects. Younger and Cohen (1986) investigated 4-, 7-, and 10-month-olds' use of correlated attributes (e.g., long neck associated with large ears and short neck associated with small ears) to form categories of novel animal drawings. They found that normal-hearing 7-month-olds but not 4-month-olds could learn correlations among attributes when all attributes were perfectly correlated and that normal-hearing 10-month-olds but not 7-month-olds could learn correlations among attributes when some of the attributes were correlated and others were not. Similar studies have found that older infants can learn correlations among objects' parts and their motion trajectories (Rakison & Poulin-Dubois, 2002).

In the auditory domain, young infants can learn simple associations, such as the relationship between vocal affect and facial expressions (Kahana-Kalman & Walker-Andrews, 2001; Walker, 1982; Walker-Andrews, 1986). Older infants learn to associate complex strings of speech sounds (i.e., words) with objects, actions, attributes, and experiences. The development of associative learning skills plays important roles in various aspects of language acquisition, some of which will be discussed later.

Statistical Learning

Statistical learning is related to associative learning. But rather than learning that x is associated with y, statistical learning involves learning the probability of y given x. In the visual domain, infants' statistical learning skills have been investigated by assessing their ability to learn visual sequences. Young infants (3- to 4-month-olds) can learn simple two- and three-location spatiotemporal patterns (Clohessy, Posner, & Rothbart, 2001; Haith, Hazan, & Goodman, 1988; Wentworth, Haith, & Hood, 2002), whereas older infants are able to learn more complex spatiotemporal sequences (Clohessy et al., 2001; Kirkham, Slemmer, Richardson, & Johnson, 2007).

In a seminal study on auditory statistical learning, Saffran, Aslin and Newport (1996) tested 8-month-olds' ability to detect syllable sequences within a 2-minute continuous stream of synthetic consonant-vowel syllables. The speech stream consisted of four 3-syllable sequences with no pauses between sequences. Thus, the only way infants could learn the sequences was by encoding the transitional probabilities of the syllables. For example, if one of the four sequences was /da/ro/pi/, then the probability of /ro/ following /da/ and of /pi/ following /ro/ would both be 1.0. However, /pi/

would be followed by one of three syllables. Saffran et al. found that 8-month-olds showed a novelty preference for sequences that had lower transitional probabilities in the speech stream (e.g., /pi/go/) compared with sequences that had high transitional probabilities (e.g., /da/ro/). These findings and others suggest that infants are sensitive to the statistical properties of speech sounds in their language.

Motivation for Social Interaction and Exploration

Although children readily learn language, it does require some effort. Innate speech perception capacities and learning mechanisms do not by themselves explain language acquisition. Infants' motivations and intentions play an important role in language development (Bloom & Tinker, 2001). Infants are dependent on their caregivers for physical and emotional needs and are thus motivated to communicate with their caregivers (Locke, 1993). What infants attend to in speech depends on their needs, which change with development. At the beginning of life, infants might seek only social-emotional information from speech and might attend mainly to prosodic information. As infants become more sophisticated, they attend to other aspects of speech that are more relevant to language acquisition. Moreover, motivation to attend to one type of information (e.g., prosody for affect) might set the groundwork for acquiring knowledge useful for obtaining other types of information (e.g., word boundaries) that are useful for obtaining later goals (e.g., understanding what the caregiver is trying to communicate).

Infants' speech perception changes through the interaction of cognitive, social, and linguistic factors. With development, infants are motivated for increasingly more sophisticated communication. Attention to speech and increasingly sophisticated learning mechanisms result in infants forming mental representations that shape how speech is perceived. And, because the input to the learning mechanisms differs across languages, infants form language-specific representations that result in language-specific perception of speech.

Organizing the Suprasegmentals

We learned earlier that newborns are able to discriminate the rhythmic properties of languages when languages fall into different rhythmic classes. That initial sensitivity to rhythmic information forms the basis for the ability to detect rhythmic information that relates to linguistic units in speech, such as clauses, phrases, and words. Being able to detect these linguistic structures may play a role in infants' ability to develop a vocabulary and acquire a grammar.

Utterance-Level Prosody

Utterances tend to contain one or more clauses, and clauses contain one or more phrases. An implicit understanding of clausal and phrasal organization in speech is important for language comprehension and production. Clauses and phrases influence the prosody of speech. For example, pauses tend to occur more often at clause and phrase boundaries than within clauses or phrases. It is possible that perceiving grammatical units within utterances (e.g., clauses) might be a first step in acquiring a grammar.

Hirsh-Pasek et al. (1987) investigated infants' sensitivity to prosodic markings of clause boundaries in fluent speech. They presented 6- and 9-month-olds with passages of natural infant-directed speech in which 1-s pauses were inserted either between or within clauses. Both groups of infants looked longer when pauses were between clauses than when they were within clauses, suggesting that by 6 months of age, English-learning infants have become familiarized with the prosodic cohesiveness of clauses in English.

Infants' sensitivity to the prosody of syntactic structures appears also to play a role in recognizing familiar sequences of words in the context of fluent speech. Nazzi, Kemler Nelson, Jusczyk, and Jusczyk (2000) investigated this in English-learning infants. Six-month-olds were familiarized with sequences of words (e.g., rabbits eat leafy vegetables) and then were presented with passages in which the sequence of words occurred either within a clause (e.g., . . . rabbits eat leafy vegetables . . .), or between clauses (e.g., . . . rabbits eat. Leafy vegetables . . .). Infants demonstrated recognition of the words only when they occurred within clauses (see also Soderstrom, Seidl, Kemler Nelson, & Jusczyk, 2003). Six- and 9-month-old English-learning infants show similar encoding effects for the prosodic structure of phrases (Soderstrom, Kemler Nelson, & Jusczyk, 2005). More recent research suggests that boundary information also plays a role in the development of word segmentation skills (Johnson, Seidl, & Tyler, 2014).

There are several possible prosodic cues that can play a role in infants' perception of prosodic structure cohesiveness (e.g., pauses, lengthening of vowels before clause boundaries, intonation). English-learning infants appear to use multiple cues fairly equally at 4 months of age (Seidl & Cristiá, 2008) but then rely mainly on pitch cues by 6 months of age (Seidl, 2007). The cues that infants rely on also seem to be language dependent (Johnson & Seidl, 2008; Wellmann et al., 2012). Taken together, the studies of infants' sensitivity to prosodic structure suggest that infants might begin parsing speech into prosodic units at a very young age using multiple cues and then eventually learn to rely on particular cues. Statistical and associative learning are involved such that infants learn via statistical learning which prosodic boundary cues co-occur most often with other prosodic boundary cues and then associate those cues with clausal and phrasal boundaries.

Language discrimination studies provide additional evidence of infants' developing sensitivity to prosodic information. Recall that newborns are able to discriminate languages that differ rhythmically (Nazzi et al., 1998). Nazzi, Jusczyk, and Johnson (2000) found that by 5 months of age, English-learning infants can discriminate their native language (e.g., American English) from languages (e.g., Dutch) and dialects (e.g., British English) within their same rhythmic class but cannot discriminate two foreign languages (e.g., Dutch and German) from the same rhythmic class. The investigators concluded that because 5-month-olds do not show language discrimination based on segmental information in previous work (Jusczyk, Friederici, et al., 1993), their discrimination was most likely due to an increased sensitivity to prosodic information that allowed the infants to detect subtle differences in rhythmic properties between the languages and dialects.

The above findings suggest that infants develop increasing familiarity with the prosodic properties of speech, including prosodic cues to linguistic units. This development suggests that there are learning mechanisms that transform infants from having a universal sensitivity to prosodic information to having a perceptual system tuned to the prosodic properties of the ambient language. First, recognition memory is required to identify units of speech as having rhythmic structure consistent with being clauses or phrases. Second, statistical learning is required to learn that certain rhythmic units (e.g., clauses) tend to co-occur with pauses, but other rhythmic units (e.g., a sequence of words across a clause boundary) are not associated with a pause.

Word-Level Prosody

The research reviewed so far has informed us about infants' sensitivity to the organization of large prosodic units and intonational patterns, which might be an important first step in children's acquisition of syntax. But we have said very little so far about infants' sensitivity to smaller rhythmic units. Young infants are able to discriminate isolated words that differ in stress pattern (Jusczyk & Thompson, 1977) just as they are able to discriminate isolated words and syllables that differ by one phoneme (reviewed above). But to what extent are they sensitive to the rhythmic properties of words in the real world? In other words, do infants encode the rhythmic properties of words in the ambient language and build up implicit knowledge—via statistical learning—of the frequencies of different rhythmic patterns of words? Before we review the research that has addressed this question, we should first consider why sensitivity to the rhythmic properties of words might be important for speech comprehension. One important role for the rhythmic properties of words in speech comprehension is the role it plays in the process of segmenting words from the context of fluent speech (i.e., speech segmentation).

Speech segmentation is a major topic in speech science because natural speech does not contain obvious acoustic cues to word boundaries (Cole & Jakimik, 1980). We perceive word boundaries because we are able to segment continuous speech into words (listening to someone speak an unfamiliar language is an easy way to appreciate this fact). Although fluent speech does not reliably contain obvious word boundaries, people are, of course, able to segment fluent speech once they know a language. Knowing the words of a language is probably the most important factor for segmenting speech—recognizing a word informs the listener of the onset of the following word. But there are also acoustic cues that become useful for segmentation as listeners gain implicit knowledge of the language, including the rhythmic properties of words.

One model of speech segmentation that emphasizes the importance of word rhythm is Anne Cutler's metrical segmentation strategy (MSS) model. The MSS asserts that in some languages, including English, listeners are attuned to strong[1] syllables as the primary acoustic cue for speech segmentation. In languages like English, strong syllables can serve as cues for segmentation because of their distribution in the language. Cutler and Carter (1987) conducted a corpus investigation of English and found that approximately 90% of content words in English begin with a strong syllable.

[1]The term *strong syllable* is nearly synonymous with the term *stressed syllable*. A strong syllable is any syllable that has a fully realized (i.e., nonreduced) vowel. A stressed syllable is a syllable that is more perceptually salient than its neighboring syllables. To illustrate, take the spondee "mailman." Both syllables are strong because their vowels are fully realized. However, neither syllable has lexical stress because they have similar perceptual salience.

Thus, if listeners assumed that every strong syllable they heard marked the onset of a word, they would be correct most of the time. Cutler and colleagues tested this idea experimentally in a number of studies with adults and found that English speakers do indeed tend to perceive strong syllables as word onsets (Cutler & Butterfield, 1992; Cutler & Norris, 1988; McQueen, Norris, & Cutler, 1994).

As important a role that word rhythm might play in adults' ability to segment speech, it might play an even greater role in the development of speech segmentation during infancy. Unlike adults, infants do not have a developed lexicon to help them identify words in fluent speech. And although infants might learn some words from hearing them often in isolation (e.g., "hi," "daddy"), the vast majority of words are not uttered in isolation, even to infants. An analysis of speech to an infant over a 3-week period found that 90% to 95% of utterances contained more than one word (van de Weijer, 1998). Even when caregivers are instructed to teach words, they present the novel words in isolation only 20% of the time (Woodward & Aslin, 1990). Thus, being able to segment words from the context of fluent speech is an important skill for language acquisition.

Understanding the role word rhythm might play in infant speech segmentation returns us to the question of infants' sensitivity to the rhythmic properties of words. To address this question, Jusczyk, Cutler, and Redanz (1993) presented 6- and 9-month-old English-learning infants with lists of strong/weak words and lists of weak/strong words. They found that 9-month-olds oriented longer to the words that follow the predominant stress pattern of English (strong/weak), but 6-month-olds did not. Similarly, Echols, Crowhurst, and Childers (1997) presented infants with trisyllabic weak/strong/weak sequences that contained a pause either before or after the strong syllable. They found that 9-month-old English-learning infants preferred sequences with the pause before the strong syllable, which preserved the strong/weak structure. These findings suggest that over the course of at least 6 months of exposure to English, infants build up the implicit knowledge that strong/weak words are more common than weak/strong words. In other words, their statistical learning skills enable them to acquire sensitivity to the predominant stress pattern of words in their language.

Findings that English-learning infants become sensitive to the predominant stress pattern of words in their language led Peter Jusczyk and his colleagues to investigate the role of lexical stress in the development of speech segmentation skills. They did this by using a variant of the head-turn preference procedure (HPP) to directly assess infants' ability to detect different types of familiarized words in the context of fluent speech. In the HPP, infants are first familiarized with two words —one word per trial repeated up to 20 times. Then during a test phase, they are presented with four passages—two of which contain the familiarized words. Their attention to each passage is measured by the amount of time they orient to a light that is located in front of the loudspeaker presenting the passages and which blinks during the presentation of each passage. Seminal work using this methodology suggests that infants orient longer to the presentation of passages containing the familiarized words than to other passages when they are able to segment and recognize the familiarized words from the context of fluent speech (Jusczyk & Aslin, 1995). An alternative version of the HPP involves presenting two of the four passages during the familiarization period and then presenting the two familiarized words and two unfamiliar words during the test phase. These two variants of the HPP have been found to produce identical results (Jusczyk & Aslin, 1995; Jusczyk, Houston, & Newsome, 1999).

Using the HPP, Jusczyk, Houston, and Newsome (1999) assessed 7.5- and 10.5-month-old English-learning infants' ability to segment strong/weak and weak/strong words from fluent speech. They found that 7.5-month-olds were able to segment strong/weak but not weak/strong words from fluent speech. Instead, infants showed evidence of segmenting only the strong syllable of weak/strong words. When 7.5-month-olds were familiarized with just the strong syllable of weak/strong words (e.g., tar from guitar) they oriented longer to passages containing the corresponding weak/strong whole words (e.g., guitar). However, when they were familiarized with the whole words (e.g., guitar), they did not orient longer to the passages containing the familiarized words.[2] In other words, *tar* matched better to what 7.5-month-olds heard in passages containing *guitar* than did *guitar*. However, by 10.5 months of age, English-learning infants show the opposite pattern of results.

Jusczyk, Houston, and Newsome (1999) interpreted the findings with the strong/weak and weak/strong words as follows: English-learning infants begin segmenting words from fluent speech using a type of metrical segmentation strategy: They assume

[2]For both conditions, identical results were found when infants were tested with the passages-first variant of the HPP.

that strong syllables mark word onsets. When a strong syllable is followed by the same weak syllable consistently—as is the case when a strong/weak word occurs often in a passage—then infants will treat the strong/weak word as a cohesive unit. To test this interpretation, they created new passages for the weak/strong words in which each weak/strong word was consistently followed by the same function word (e.g., guitar is). Infants were presented with two of the passages and then tested on either the strong syllables of the target words or with strong/weak nonwords formed from the strong syllable of the weak/strong words and the following function word (e.g., tar-is). Unlike the previous experiment with weak/strong words, 7.5-month-olds did not demonstrate segmentation of the strong syllable from the weak/strong words in the passages. Instead, they demonstrated recognition of the strong/weak pseudowords (e.g., taris). These findings suggest that 7.5-month-old English-learning infants use a strong version of the MSS to segment words from fluent speech such that they segment strong/weak units even when they cross word boundaries.

Using a strong version of the MSS allows English-learning infants to segment most words from fluent speech correctly. However, as seen in the findings of Jusczyk et al. (1999), a strong version of MSS results in mis-segmenting words that do not follow the predominant stress pattern of English. Thus, if infants use a strong version of the MSS, they must eventually adopt a less strong version and incorporate other information in their segmentation strategy. To investigate the use of this strong version of the MSS in older infants, Jusczyk et al. (1999) also tested 10.5-month-olds with the passages in which the weak/strong target words were always followed by the same function word. Unlike 7.5-month-olds, 10.5-month-olds did not demonstrate recognition when presented with the pseudowords (e.g., taris). However, they did demonstrate recognition when presented with the weak/strong words (e.g., guitar) during testing, suggesting that 10.5-month-old English-learning infants correctly segment weak/strong words from fluent speech even when they are consistently followed by the same function word.

Taken together, the above findings and others (Houston, Jusczyk, Kuijpers, Coolen, & Cutler, 2000; Houston, Santelmann, & Jusczyk, 2004; Johnson & Jusczyk, 2001) suggest that infants use statistical learning to infer the rhythmic structure of words in their language, and then that learning influences their processing of fluent speech. The initial segmentation strategy that develops from acquiring knowledge about the rhythmic properties of words does not always result in correct segmentation, so infants must acquire knowledge about other segmentation cues. We discuss what some of those other cues are next.

Meaningful Segmental Information

We learned earlier that young infants demonstrate discrimination of phonetic segments even when the differences between those segments do not differentiate words in their language. We also learned that toward the end of the first year of life, infants lose the ability to discriminate some non-native contrasts. On the surface, it appears that infants become less sensitive to segmental information. However, investigations of infants' sensitivity to segmental properties in their language suggest that infants learn much about how phonetic segments are distributed and organized in the ambient language during the first year of life. This statistical learning about the distributional properties of segmental information, in turn, shapes more advanced speech perception processes, such as infants' perception of word boundaries in fluent speech (i.e., speech segmentation). The following sections review investigations of older infants' sensitivity to several types of segmental information and what role these acquired sensitivities play in segmenting words from fluent speech.

Phonotactic Probabilities

The term *phonotactics* refers to the ordering of segments in languages. Languages differ greatly with respect to what clusters of phonemes are permissible in various positions within and between words and syllables. In English syllables, for example, each consonant before a vowel must be more sonorous than the previous segment and less sonorous than the subsequent segment ([s] is an exception). Thus, the word *plan* is possible, but the word *lpan* is not in English. Moreover, the word *pkan* is not possible because [p] and [k] have equal sonority. In other languages, such as Polish, syllable-initial consonant clusters can contain two voiceless stops in a row. In addition to phonotactic rules, there are phonotactic probabilities. Phonotactic probabilities refer to the occurrence of segment pairs within and between words and syllables. For example, the pair [s]-[d] occurs more often between words than within words in English, whereas the pair [s]-[t] occurs more often within words than between words. Sensitivity to these kinds of phonotactic probabilities can provide information about likely word boundaries in fluent speech.

Infants appear to become sensitive to phonotactic rules and probabilities at around the same time they show sensitivity to the predominant stress pattern of words in their language. Jusczyk, Friederici, Wessels, Svenkerud, and Jusczyk (1993) tested English-learning and Dutch-learning infants with lists of words that were either phonotactically legal in English and not in Dutch or vice versa. Dutch- and English-learning 9-month-olds both oriented longer to lists of words that were legal in their native language. Six-month-olds showed no preferences. Similarly, Friederici and Wessels (1993) found that Dutch-learning 9-month-olds but not 6-month-olds attended longer to nonwords with phonotactically permissible word onsets and offsets than to nonwords with phonotactically impermissible onsets and offsets, even though the impermissible onsets were permissible as offsets and vice versa. Jusczyk, Luce, and Charles-Luce (1994) found that 9-month-old English-learning infants attended longer to lists of words with higher phonotactic probabilities than to lists of words with relatively lower phonotactic probabilities even though none of the words had any sequences that were phonotactically impermissible.

Like sensitivity to lexical stress, sensitivity to phonotactic probabilities appears to play a role in infants' segmentation abilities. Mattys and Jusczyk (2001) used the HPP to investigate 9-month-old English-learning infants' segmentation of words from fluent speech that had either easy or difficult phonotactic boundary information. Similar to Jusczyk, Houston, and Newsome (1999), infants were familiarized with two passages, each containing several instances of a target word. However, in this experiment, they manipulated the words that surrounded the target words such that they provided either good or poor phonotactic boundary information. Infants were able to segment the words from fluent speech only when the phonotactic boundary information for the target words was good at the onset, offset, or both. These findings suggest that by 9 months of age, English-learning infants acquire knowledge about the frequency of occurrence of phoneme sequences within words and can use this information to segment words from fluent speech.

Subphonemic Cues

So far, we have reviewed speech cues infants use for segmenting words from fluent speech that are at the clause, phrase, syllable, and phoneme levels of acoustic-phonetic information. As discussed earlier, infants appear to be sensitive not only to these levels of acoustic-phonetic information, but also to subphonemic information in speech (Hohne & Jusczyk, 1994; McMurray & Aslin, 2005). It is possible that subphonemic information may play a role in infant speech segmentation. Using the HPP, Jusczyk, Hohne, and Bauman (1999) investigated English-learning infants' sensitivity to allophonic information as a cue to word segmentation. Infants were familiarized with two-syllable items (e.g., nitrates) and tested for recognition of those sequences in fluent speech. Jusczyk et al. found that 10.5-month-olds but not 9-month-olds listened longer to the passages containing the exact match (e.g., nitrates) than to passages containing an allophonic variant (night rates) of the familiarized items, suggesting that only the older infants relied on allophonic information to segment words from fluent speech.

Subsequent investigations have provided additional evidence that infants are sensitive to subphonemic cues to word segmentation. By 8 months of age, English-learning infants' segmentation of three-word sequences is affected by whether they are produced as single words (e.g., catalog) versus three-word phrases (e.g., cat a log; Johnson, 2003; Johnson & Jusczyk, 2001). By 12 months of age, English-learning infants demonstrate sensitivity to subtle acoustic-phonetic word boundary information (e.g., [toga][lore] versus [toe][galore]) when segmenting strong/weak sequences (e.g., toga) from fluent speech (Johnson, 2008). Taken together, these studies suggest that a variety of subphonemic cues play a role in infants' speech segmentation, especially by the end of their first year of life.

Infants' sensitivity to segmental information as cues to word segmentation is acquired as a result of their experience to language and their developing learning mechanisms. Most of the segmental cues to segmentation discussed in this section are not universal across languages. So for these cues to be useful for segmentation, statistical and associative learning is necessary to learn which phoneme sequences and subphonemic variants are associated with word boundaries and which are not. However, in order to learn which segmental cues are associated with word boundaries, infants must be able to segment at least some words from fluent speech. As a solution to this apparent chicken-and-egg problem, Jusczyk (1997, 2002) posited that English-learning infants use a divide-and-conquer strategy: they first segment strong/weak units from fluent speech and then analyze the strong/weak units to discover other segmentation cues. This is a plausible strategy for English-learning infants to use because of the rhythmic properties of English words. Recent evidence suggests that in languages with different rhythmic properties, infants adopt other segmentation strategies (Nazzi, Iakimova, Bertoncini, Frédonie, & Alcantara, 2006).

Nonphonetically Based Segmentation Cues

Most work on infant speech segmentation has focused on the role that acoustic-phonetic properties play.

However, there are other types of information infants can exploit to segment words from fluent speech. Earlier we reviewed work by Saffran et al. (1996), which found that statistical learning skills enable 8-month-olds to compute transitional probabilities of syllables. For example, if an infant notices that occurrences of the syllable [ma] are usually followed by the syllable [mi] and that what precedes [ma] and what follows [mi] is highly variable, this statistical information might contribute to helping the infant segment [ma]-[mi] as a cohesive unit from fluent speech. And then if an infant is able to recognize a familiar word like "mommy" in an utterance, then that word can serve as a wedge to help segment the surrounding words. A recent investigation found just that. Bortfeld, Morgan, Golinkoff, and Rathbun (2005) tested 6-month-olds' segmentation of words from fluent speech that were preceded by words they already knew (e.g., "mommy"). In contrast to earlier studies showing that 6-month-olds could not segment words from fluent speech (Jusczyk & Aslin, 1995), Bortfeld et al. (2005) found that 6-month-olds could segment words from fluent speech, but only when preceded by a word they already knew. These findings suggest that word recognition plays an important role in segmenting novel words from fluent speech.

Conclusions

The field of infant speech perception has grown immensely over the last 40 years, and this review of the work is, as a consequence, very incomplete. Many of the most important studies in the field were left out. More thorough reviews of the field can be found elsewhere (Jusczyk, 1997; Saffran, Werker, & Werner, 2006). The purpose of this chapter is to provide some understanding of how our hearing instrument becomes tuned to process speech. We first reviewed some of what is known about infants' early speech perception abilities and then described some of the developments in speech perception during the second half of the first year of life that put infants in a position to segment words from fluent speech. Finally, I described some general learning mechanisms that play a role in the development of speech perception skills.

Gaining a better understanding of how cognitive mechanisms affect speech perception development in typically developing normal-hearing infants contributes to our general understanding of language development. This knowledge also might have clinical implications for infants and children with congenital hearing loss. With impoverished auditory input, general cognitive skills might be particularly important for hearing-impaired infants' ability to achieve successful language outcomes. Future work exploring the links between specific cognitive and speech perception skills in both normal-hearing and hearing-impaired infants could provide valuable information to clinicians, especially if methods of improving cognitive skills in infants can be developed. Moreover, comparing normal-hearing and hearing-impaired infants' speech perception skills can provide insight into the effects of early auditory experience on the development of early speech perception and language skills (Horn, Houston, & Miyamoto, 2007; Houston, Pisoni, Kirk, Ying, & Miyamoto, 2003; Houston, Ying, Pisoni, & Kirk, 2003).

Acknowledgments. Preparation of this chapter was facilitated by a Research Grant from NIDCD (DC006235) and support from the Philip F. Holton Fund. The author would like to thank Carissa Shafto for helpful comments on a previous version of this chapter.

References

Behme, C., & Deacon, S. H. (2008). Language learning in infancy: Does the empirical evidence support a domain specific language acquisition device? *Philosophical Psychology, 21*(5), 641–671.

Best, C. T., McRoberts, G. W., Lafleur, R., & Silver-Isenstadt, J. (1995). Divergent developmental patterns for infants' perception of two nonnative consonant contrasts. *Infant Behavior and Development, 18*, 339–350.

Best, C. T., McRoberts, G. W., & Sithole, N. M. (1988). Examination of the perceptual re-organization for speech contrasts: Zulu click discrimination by English-speaking adults and infants. *Journal of Experimental Psychology: Human Perception and Performance, 14*, 345–360.

Birnholz, J. C., & Benacerraf, B. B. (1983). The development of human fetal hearing. *Science, 222*, 516–518.

Bloom, L., & Tinker, E. (2001). The intentionality model and language acquisition: Engagement, effort, and the essential tension in development. *Monographs of the Society for Research in Child Development, 66*(4), 1–91.

Bortfeld, H., Morgan, J. L., Golinkoff, R. M., & Rathbun, K. (2005). Mommy and me: Familiar names help launch babies into speech-stream segmentation. *Psychological Science, 15*(4), 298–304.

Burns, T. C., Yoshida, K. A., Hill, K., & Werker, J. F. (2007). The development of phonetic representation in bilingual and monolingual infants. *Applied Psycholinguistics, 28*(3), 455–474.

Chomsky, N. (1968). *Language and mind.* New York, NY: Harcourt Brace.

Chomsky, N. (1975). *Reflections on language.* New York, NY: Pantheon Books.

Clohessy, A. B., Posner, M. I., & Rothbart, M. K. (2001). Development of the functional visual field. *Acta Psychologica, 106*(1–2), 51–68.

Cole, R. A., & Jakimik, J. (1980). A model of speech perception. In R. A. Cole (Ed.), *Perception and production of fluent speech* (pp. 133–163). Hillsdale, NJ: Erlbaum.

Colombo, J., Shaddy, D. J., Richman, W. A., Maikranz, J. M., & Blaga, O. M. (2004). The developmental course of habituation in infancy and preschool outcome. *Infancy, 5*(1), 1–38.

Cooper, R. P., & Aslin, R. N. (1990). Preference for infant-directed speech in the first month after birth. *Child Development, 61*, 1584–1595.

Cutler, A., & Butterfield, S. (1992). Rhythmic cues to speech segmentation: Evidence from juncture misperception. *Journal of Memory and Language, 31*(2), 218–236.

Cutler, A., & Carter, D. M. (1987). The predominance of strong initial syllables in the English vocabulary. *Computer Speech and Language, 2*, 133–142.

Cutler, A., & Norris, D. (1988). The role of strong syllables in segmentation for lexical access. *Journal of Experimental Psychology: Human Perception and Performance, 14*(1), 113–121.

DeCasper, A. J., & Fifer, W. P. (1980). Of human bonding: Newborns prefer their mothers' voices. *Science, 208*, 1174–1176.

DeCasper, A. J., Lecanuet, J. P., Busnel, M. C., Granier-Deferre, C., & Maugeais, R. (1994). Fetal reactions to recurrent maternal speech. *Infant Behavior and Development, 17*, 159–164.

DeCasper, A. J., & Spence, M. J. (1986). Prenatal maternal speech influences newborns' perception of speech sounds. *Infant Behavior and Development, 9*, 133–150.

Echols, C. H., Crowhurst, M. J., & Childers, J. (1997). Perception of rhythmic units in speech by infants and adults. *Journal of Memory and Language, 36*, 202–225.

Eimas, P. D. (1974). Auditory and linguistic processing of cues for place of articulation by infants. *Perception & Psychophysics, 16*, 513–521.

Eimas, P. D. (1975). Auditory and phonetic coding of the cues for speech: Discrimination of the [r-l] distinction by young infants. *Perception and Psychophysics, 18*, 341–347.

Eimas, P. D., & Miller, J. L. (1980a). Contextual effects in infant speech perception. *Science, 209*, 1140–1141.

Eimas, P. D., & Miller, J. L. (1980b). Discrimination of the information for manner of articulation. *Infant Behavior and Development, 3*, 367–375.

Eimas, P. D., Miller, J. L., & Jusczyk, P. W. (1987). On infant speech perception and the acquisition of language. In H. Stevan (Ed.), *Categorical perception: The groundwork of cognition* (pp. 161–195). New York, NY: Cambridge University Press.

Eimas, P. D., Siqueland, E. R., Jusczyk, P., & Vigorito, J. (1971). Speech perception in infants. *Science, 171*(968), 303–306.

Fagan, J. F., & McGrath, S. K. (1981). Infant recognition memory and later intelligence. *Intelligence, 5*, 121–130.

Fernald, A. (1985). Four-month-old infants prefer to listen to motherese. *Infant Behavior and Development, 8*, 181–195.

Fernald, A. (1989). Intonation and communicative intent in mothers' speech to infants: Is the melody the message? *Child Development, 60*, 1497–1510.

Fernald, A. (1993). Approval and disapproval: Infant responsiveness to vocal affect in familiar and unfamiliar languages. *Child Development, 64*(3), 657–674.

Fernald, A., & Kuhl, P. K. (1987). Acoustic determinants of infant preference for Motherese speech. *Infant Behavior and Development, 10*, 279–293.

Friederici, A. D., & Wessels, J. M. I. (1993). Phonotactic knowledge and its use in infant speech perception. *Perception and Psychophysics, 54*, 287–295.

Fry, D. B., Abramson, A. S., Eimas, P. D., & Liberman, A. M. (1962). The identification and discrimination of synthetic vowels. *Language and Speech, 5*, 171–189.

Granier-Deferre, C., Bassereau, S., Ribeiro, A., Jacquet, A. Y., & Decasper, A. J. (2011). A melodic contour repeatedly experienced by human near-term fetuses elicits a profound cardiac reaction one month after birth. *PloS One, 6*(2), e17304.

Haith, M. M., Hazan, C., & Goodman, G. S. (1988). Expectation and anticipation of dynamic visual events by 3.5-month-old babies. *Child Development, 59*, 467–479.

Hayashi, A., Tamekawa, Y., & Kiritani, S. (2001). Developmental change in auditory preferences for speech stimuli in Japanese infants. *Journal of Speech, Language, and Hearing Research, 44*(6), 1189. doi:10.1044/1092-4388

Hirsh-Pasek, K., Kemler Nelson, D. G., Jusczyk, P. W., Cassidy, K. W., Druss, B., & Kennedy, L. (1987). Clauses are perceptual units for young infants. *Cognition, 26*(3), 269–286.

Hohne, E. A., & Jusczyk, P. W. (1994). Two-month-old infants' sensitivity to allophonic differences. *Perception and Psychophysics, 56*(6), 613–623.

Hoonhorst, I., Colin, C., Markessis, E., Radeau, M., Deltenre, P., & Serniclaes, W. (2009). French native speakers in the making: From language-general to language-specific voicing boundaries. *Journal of Experimental Child Psychology, 104*(4), 353–366. doi:10.1016/j.jecp.2009.07.005

Horn, D. L., Houston, D. M., & Miyamoto, R. T. (2007). Speech discrimination skills in deaf infants before and after cochlear implantation. *Audiological Medicine, 5*, 232–241.

Houston, D. M. (1999). *The role of talker variability in infant word representations* (Doctoral dissertation). Johns Hopkins University, Baltimore, MD.

Houston, D. M., & Jusczyk, P. W. (2000). The role of talker-specific information in word segmentation by infants. *Journal of Experimental Psychology: Human Perception and Performance, 26*(5), 1570–1582.

Houston, D. M., & Jusczyk, P. W. (2003). Infants' long-term memory for the sound patterns of words and voices. *Journal of Experimental Psychology: Human Perception and Performance, 29*(6), 1143–1154.

Houston, D. M., Jusczyk, P. W., Kuijpers, C., Coolen, R., & Cutler, A. (2000). Cross-language word segmentation by 9-month-olds. *Psychonomic Bulletin & Review, 7*, 504–509.

Houston, D. M., Pisoni, D. B., Kirk, K. I., Ying, E., & Miyamoto, R. T. (2003). Speech perception skills of deaf infants following cochlear implantation: A first report. *International Journal of Pediatric Otorhinolaryngology, 67*, 479–495.

Houston, D. M., Santelmann, L., & Jusczyk, P. W. (2004). English-learning infants' segmentation of trisyllabic words from fluent speech. *Language and Cognitive Processes, 19*(1), 97–136.

Houston, D. M., Ying, E., Pisoni, D. B., & Kirk, K. I. (2003). Development of pre word-learning skills in infants with cochlear implants. *Volta Review, 103*(Monograph 4), 303–326.

Huotilainen, M. (2013). A new dimension on foetal language learning. *Acta Paediatrica (Oslo, Norway, 102*(2), 102–103.

Johnson, E. K. (2003). *Word segmentation during infancy: The role of subphonemic cues to word boundaries* (Doctoral dissertation). Johns Hopkins University, Baltimore, MD.

Johnson, E. K. (2008). Infants' use of prosodically conditioned acoustic-phonetic cues to extract words from speech. *Journal of Acoustical Society of America, 123*(6), EL144–148.

Johnson, E. K., & Jusczyk, P. W. (2001). Word segmentation by 8-month-olds: When speech cues count more than statistics. *Journal of Memory and Language, 44*, 548–567.

Johnson, E. K., & Seidl, A. (2008). Clause segmentation by 6-month-old infants: A cross-linguistic perspective. *Infancy, 13*(5), 440–455.

Johnson, E. K., Seidl, A., & Tyler, M. D. (2014). The edge factor in early word segmentation: Utterance-level prosody enables word form extraction by 6-month-olds. *PloS One, 9*(1), e83546.

Jusczyk, P. W. (1997). *The discovery of spoken language.* Cambridge, MA: MIT Press.

Jusczyk, P. W. (2002). How infants adapt speech-processing capacities to native-language structure. *Current Directions in Psychological Science, 11*(1), 18.

Jusczyk, P. W., & Aslin, R. N. (1995). Infants' detection of the sound patterns of words in fluent speech. *Cognitive Psychology, 29*(1), 1–23.

Jusczyk, P. W., Cutler, A., & Redanz, N. J. (1993). Infants' preference for the predominant stress patterns of English words. *Child Development, 64*(3), 675–687.

Jusczyk, P. W., Friederici, A. D., Wessels, J., Svenkerud, V. Y., & Jusczyk, A. M. (1993). Infants' sensitivity to the sound patterns of native language words. *Journal of Memory and Language, 32*, 402–420.

Jusczyk, P. W., Hohne, E. A., & Bauman, A. (1999). Infants' sensitivity to allophonic cues for word segmentation. *Perception and Psychophysics, 61*, 1465–1476.

Jusczyk, P. W., Houston, D. M., & Newsome, M. (1999). The beginnings of word segmentation in English-learning infants. *Cognitive Psychology, 39*, 159–207.

Jusczyk, P. W., Luce, P. A., & Charles-Luce, J. (1994). Infants' sensitivity to phonotactic patterns in the native language. *Journal of Memory and Language, 33*(5), 630–645.

Jusczyk, P. W., & Thompson, E. (1977). Perception of a phonetic contrast in multisyllabic utterances by 2-month-old infants. *Perception and Psychophysics, 23*(2), 105–109.

Kahana-Kalman, R., & Walker-Andrews, A. S. (2001). The role of person familiarity in young infants' perception of emotional expressions. *Child Development, 72*(2), 352–369.

Kirkham, N. Z., Slemmer, J. A., Richardson, D. C., & Johnson, S. P. (2007). Location, location, location: Development of spatiotemporal sequence learning in infancy. *Child Development, 78*(5), 1559–1571.

Kisilevsky, B. S., Hains, S. M., Brown, C. A., Lee, C. T., Cowperthwaite, B., Stutzman, S. S., . . . Wang, Z. (2009). Fetal sensitivity to properties of maternal speech and language. *Infant Behavior and Development, 32*(1), 59–71.

Kisilevsky, B. S., Hains, S. M., Lee, K., Xie, X., Huang, H., Ye, H. H., . . . Wang, Z. (2003). Effects of experience on fetal voice recognition. *Psychological Science, 14*(3), 220–224.

Krueger, C., & Garvan, C. (2014). Emergence and retention of learning in early fetal development. *Infant Behavior & Development, 37*(2), 162–173.

Kuhl, P. K. (1991). Human adults and human infants show a "perceptual magnet effect" for the prototypes of speech categories, monkeys do not. *Perception and Psychophysics, 50*, 93–107.

Kuhl, P. K. (1993). Innate predispositions and the effects of experience in speech perception: The native language magnet theory. In B. de Boysson-Bardies, S. de Schonen, P. Jusczyk, P. McNeilage, & J. Morton (Eds.), *Developmental neurocognition: Speech and face processing in the first year of life* (pp. 259–274). Dordrecht, the Netherlands: Kluwer.

Kuhl, P. K., Williams, K. A., Lacerda, F., Stevens, K. N., & Lindblom, B. (1992). Linguistic experiences alter phonetic perception in infants by 6 months of age. *Science, 255*, 606–608.

Lacerda, F. (1993). Sonority contrasts dominate young infants' vowel perception. In *PERILUS XVII* (pp. 55–63). Stockholm University, Sweden.

Lasky, R. E., Syrdal-Lasky, A., & Klein, R. E. (1975). VOT discrimination by four to six and a half month old infants from Spanish environments. *Journal of Experimental Child Psychology, 20*, 215–225.

Lecanuet, J. P., Gautheron, B., Locatelli, A., Schaal, B., Jacquet, A. Y., & Busnel, M. C. (1998). What sounds reach fetuses: Biological and nonbiological modeling of the transmission of pure tones. *Developmental Psychobiology, 33*(3), 203–219.

Liberman, A. M., Harris, K. S., Hoffman, H. S., & Griffith, B. C. (1957). The discrimination of speech sounds within and across phoneme boundaries. *Journal of Experimental Psychology, 54*, 358–368.

Liberman, A. M., Harris, K. S., Kinney, J. A., & Lane, H. L. (1961). The discrimination of relative-onset time of the components of certain speech and non-speech patterns. *Journal of Experimental Psychology, 61*, 379–388.

Liu, L., & Kager, R. (2015). Bilingual exposure influences infant VOT perception. *Infant Behavior & Development, 38*, 27–36. doi:10.1016/j.infbeh.2014.12.004

Locke, J. L. (1993). *The child's path to spoken language.* Cambridge, MA: Harvard University Press.

Mattys, S. L., & Jusczyk, P. W. (2001). Phonotactic cues for segmentation of fluent speech by infants. *Cognition, 78*(2), 91–121.

Maye, J., Werker, J. F., & Gerken, L. (2002). Infant sensitivity to distributional information can affect phonetic discrimination. *Cognition, 82*, B101–B111.

McMurray, B., & Aslin, R. N. (2005). Infants are sensitive to within-category variation in speech perception. *Cognition, 95*(2), B15–B26.

McQueen, J. M., Norris, D., & Cutler, A. (1994). Competition in spoken word recognition: Spotting words in other

words. *Journal of Experimental Psychology: Learning, Memory, and Cognition, 20*(3), 621–638.
Mehler, J., Jusczyk, P., Lambertz, G., Halsted, N., Bertoncini, J., & Amiel-Tison, C. (1988). A precursor of language acquisition in young infants. *Cognition, 29*(2), 143–178.
Moon, C., Cooper, R. P., & Fifer, W. P. (1993). Two-day old infants prefer their native language. *Infant Behavior and Development, 16*, 495–500.
Moon, C., Lagercrantz, H., & Kuhl, P. K. (2013). Language experienced in utero affects vowel perception after birth: A two-country study. *Acta Paediatrica, 102*(2), 156–160.
Narayan, C. R., Werker, J. F., & Beddor, P. S. (2010). The interaction between acoustic salience and language experience in developmental speech perception: Evidence from nasal place discrimination. *Developmental Science, 13*(3), 407–420.
Nazzi, T., Bertoncini, J., & Mehler, J. (1998). Language discrimination by newborns: Toward an understanding of the role of rhythm. *Journal of Experimental Psychology: Human Perception and Performance, 24*(3), 756–766.
Nazzi, T., Iakimova, G., Bertoncini, J., Frédonie, S., & Alcantara, C. (2006). Early segmentation of fluent speech by infants acquiring French: Emerging evidence for crosslinguistic differences. *Journal of Memory and Language, 54*, 283–299.
Nazzi, T., Jusczyk, P. W., & Johnson, E. K. (2000). Language discrimination by English-learning 5-month-olds: Effects of rhythm and familiarity. *Journal of Memory and Language, 43*(1), 1–19.
Nazzi, T., Kemler Nelson, D. G. K., Jusczyk, P. W., & Jusczyk, A. M. (2000). Six-month-olds detection of clauses embedded in continuous speech: Effects of prosodic well-formedness. *Infancy, 1*(1), 123–147.
Newman, R. S., & Hussain, I. (2006). Changes in preference for infant-directed speech in low and moderate noise by 4.5-to 13-month-olds. *Infancy*, 10(1), 61–76.
Pisoni, D. B. (1973). Auditory and phonetic memory codes in the discrimination of consonants and vowels. *Perception and Psychophysics, 13*, 253–260.
Polka, L., & Bohn, O. S. (1996). A cross-language comparison of vowel perception in English-learning and German-learning infants. *Journal of the Acoustical Society of America, 100*(1), 577–592.
Polka, L., & Bohn, O. S. (2003). Asymmetries in vowel perception. *Speech Communication, 41*(1), 221–231.
Polka, L., & Bohn, O. (2011). Natural referent vowel (NRV) framework: An emerging view of early phonetic development. *Journal of Phonetics, 39*(4), 467–478.
Polka, L., Colantonio, C., & Sundara, M. (2001). A cross-language comparison of /d/-/ð/ perception: Evidence for a new developmental pattern. *Journal of the Acoustical Society of America, 109*(5), 2190–2201.
Rakison, D. H., & Poulin-Dubois, D. (2002). You go this way and I'll go that way: Developmental changes in infants' detection of correlations among static and dynamic features in motion events. *Child Development, 73*(3), 682–699.
Ramus, F. (2002). Language discrimination by newborns: Teasing apart phonotactic, rhythmic, and intonational cues. *Annual Review of Language Acquisition, 2*, 85–115.
Rose, S. A., & Feldman, J. F. (1997). Memory and speed: Their role in the relation of infant information processing to later IQ. *Child Development, 68*(4), 630–641.
Rose, S. A., Feldman, J. F., & Jankowski, J. J. (2001). Visual short-term memory in the first year of life: Capacity and recency effects. *Developmental Psychology, 37*(4), 539–549.
Rose, S. A., Feldman, J. F., & Wallace, I. F. (1992). Infant information processing in relation to six-year cognitive outcomes. *Child Development, 63*, 1126–1141.
Rose, S. A., Feldman, J. F., Wallace, I. F., & McCarton, C. (1991). Information processing at 1 year: Relation to birth status and developmental outcome during the first 5 years. *Developmental Psychology, 27*(5), 723–737.
Saffran, J. R., Aslin, R. N., & Newport, E. L. (1996). Statistical learning by 8-month-old infants. *Science, 274*, 1926–1928.
Saffran, J. R., Werker, J., & Werner, L. (2006). The infant's auditory world: Hearing, speech and the beginnings of language. In R. Siegler & D. Kuhn (Eds.), *Handbook of child development* (pp. 58–108). New York, NY: Wiley.
Sato, Y., Sogabe, Y., & Mazuka, R. (2010). Discrimination of phonemic vowel length by japanese infants. *Developmental Psychology, 46*(1), 106–119.
Segal, J., & Newman, R. S. (2015). Infant preferences for structural and prosodic properties of infant-directed speech in the second year of life. *Infancy, 20(3)*, 339–351.
Seidl, A. (2007). Infants' use and weighting of prosodic cues in clause segmentation. *Journal of Memory and Language, 57*(1), 24–48.
Seidl, A., & Cristià, A. (2008). Developmental changes in the weighting of prosodic cues. *Developmental Science, 11*(4), 596–606.
Singh, L., Morgan, J. L., & Best, C. T. (2002). Infants listening preferences: Baby talk or happy talk? *Infancy, 3*(3), 365–394.
Soderstrom, M., Nelson, D. G. K., & Jusczyk, P. W. (2005). Six-month-olds recognize clauses embedded in different passages of fluent speech. *Infant Behavior and Development, 28*(1), 87–94.
Soderstrom, M., Seidl, A., Kemler Nelson, D. G., & Jusczyk, P. W. (2003). The prosodic bootstrapping of phrases: Evidence from prelinguistic infants. *Journal of Memory and Language, 49*(2), 249–267.
Stevens, K. N., Liberman, A. M., Studdert-Kennedy, M. G., & Ohman, S. E. G. (1969). Cross-language study of vowel perception. *Language and Speech, 12*, 1–23.
Sundara, M., Polka, L., & Genesee, F. (2006). Language-experience facilitates discrimination of /d-th/ in monolingual and bilingual acquisition of English. *Cognition, 100*(2), 369–388.
Swoboda, P., Morse, P. A., & Leavitt, L. A. (1976). Continuous vowel discrimination in normal and at-risk infants. *Child Development, 47*, 459–465.
Trehub, S. E. (1976). The discrimination of foreign speech contrasts by infants and adults. *Child Development, 47*, 466–472.
Tsao, F. M., Liu, H. M., & Kuhl, P. K. (2006). Perception of native and non-native affricate-fricative contrasts: Cross-

language tests on adults and infants. *Journal of the Acoustical Society of America*, *120*(4), 2285–2294.

Tsushima, T., Takizawa, O., Sasaki, M., Siraki, S., Nishi, K., Kohno, M., . . . Best, C. (1994, September). *Discrimination of English /r-l/ and /w-y/ by Japanese infants at 6–12 months: Language specific developmental changes in speech perception abilities.* In The 3rd International Conference on Spoken Language Processing (pp. 57–61), Yokohama, Japan..

van de Weijer, J. (1998). *Language input for word discovery.* Nijmegen, the Netherlands: Kluwer.

Walker, A. S. (1982). Intermodal perception of expressive behaviors by human infants. *Journal of Experimental Child Psychology*, *33*(3), 514–535.

Walker-Andrews, A. S. (1986). Intermodal perception of expressive behaviors: Relation of eye and voice. *Developmental Psychology*, *22*(3), 373–377.

Wellmann, C., Holzgrefe, J., Truckenbrodt, H., Wartenburger, I., & Höhle, B. (2012). How each prosodic boundary cue matters: Evidence from German infants. *Frontiers in Psychology*, *3*, 580.

Wentworth, N., Haith, M. M., & Hood, R. (2002). Spatiotemporal regularity and interevent contingencies as information for infants' visual expectations. *Infancy*, *3*(3), 303–321.

Werker, J. F., & Lalonde, C. E. (1988). Cross-Language speech perception: Initial capabilities and developmental change. *Developmental Psychology*, *24*, 672–683.

Werker, J. F., & McLeod, P. J. (1989). Infant preference for both male and female infant-directed talk: A developmental study of attentional and affective responsiveness. *Canadian Journal of Psychology*, *43*, 230–246.

Werker, J. F., & Pegg, J. E. (1992). Infant speech perception and phonological acquisition. In C. A. Ferguson, L. Menn, & C. Stoel-Gammon (Eds.), *Phonological development: Models, research, implications* (pp. 285–311). Timonium, MD: York Press.

Werker, J. F., & Tees, R. C. (1984). Cross-Language speech perception: Evidence for perceptual reorganization during the first year of life. *Infant Behavior and Development*, *7*, 49–63.

Woodward, J. Z., & Aslin, R. N. (1990). *Segmentation cues in maternal speech to infants.* Paper presented at the seventh biennial meeting of the international conference on infant studies. Montreal, Quebec, Canada.

Younger, B. A., & Cohen, L. B. (1986). Developmental change in infants' perception of correlations among attributes. *Child Development*, *57*(3), 803–815.

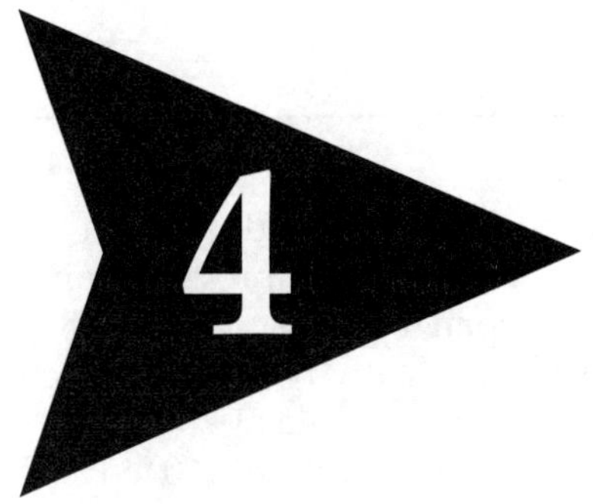

Auditory Development in Children With Normal Hearing

Lynne A. Werner and Lori J. Leibold

Why Study Auditory Development?

One of the first things that students learn when they begin to study pediatric audiology is that infants come into the world ready to learn about sound. Students are often surprised to learn that hearing, although functional, is still immature in infancy and that it continues to develop into adolescence. This may seem particularly perplexing once it is realized that the cochlea of a newborn infant responds much like that of an adult. If the inner ear is mature, why does hearing continue to develop?

Because most people with hearing loss have otherwise normally functioning brains connected to their disordered ears, it is easy to forget that without that mature brain function, hearing could be difficult or even impossible. In fact, it appears that much of what develops about hearing during infancy and childhood resides not in the peripheral auditory system, but in the nervous system. Infants and children learn about sound, what is important in sound, and what is less important, as well as what sounds mean. What infants and children learn about sound eventually makes them rapid and efficient processors of sound, but it takes a long time to learn all the details of complex sounds such as speech.

Obviously, experience with sound is critical to auditory development. Infants and children with hearing loss must pass through the same stages of auditory development as infants and children with normal hearing, but their ability to learn about sound is likely to be limited by their hearing impairment. Very little is known about auditory development in children with hearing loss. However, by carefully documenting how hearing develops in children with normal hearing, we can develop hypotheses about what specific types of auditory experience are important to development. Moreover, understanding the typical developmental time course allows us to predict how a hearing loss, amplification, or electric stimulation would change auditory development. The studies reviewed in this chapter used behavioral responses to assess a broad range of auditory abilities, from detecting tones in quiet to detecting speech in a background of competing speech. In the study of auditory development, as in audiology, behavior is considered the "gold standard" of hearing. The studies of infants generally use a conditioned-response procedure to assess hearing; infants are rewarded by interesting sounds or interesting sights for responding to the test sounds. Visual reinforcement audiometry (VRA) is a clinical example of this type of procedure. The studies of children generally use the same sort of procedure to test children as one would use to test adults; children are asked to push a button to indicate when they hear the test sound. A detailed account of these methods and their limitations can be found in Werner and Rubel (1992) and in Werner and Marean (1995).

Development of Sound Detection: Absolute Sensitivity

Age-Related Changes

Absolute auditory sensitivity refers to the ability to detect a sound in quiet. In the audiology clinic, the typical measure of absolute sensitivity is the pure-tone audiogram. Several laboratories studying auditory development have consistently and reliably observed systematic age-related changes in absolute sensitivity (e.g., Olsho, Koch, Carter, Halpin, & Spetner, 1988; Tharpe & Ashmead, 2001; Trehub, Schneider, & Endman, 1980; reviewed by Werner, 2007). Although the most substantial of these changes occur during infancy (e.g., Tharpe & Ashmead, 2001), progressive improvements in sound detection have been observed until approximately 10 years of age (e.g., Trehub, Schneider, Morrongiello, & Thorpe, 1988).

Figure 4–1 shows the estimated audibility curve, the function that relates absolute sensitivity to acoustic frequency, at 1 month, 3 months, 6 months, 4 years, 10 years, and for adults, using data published by Werner and Marean (1996). The sounds used in the studies summarized in Figure 4–1 were pure tones or noise bands. It is clear from Figure 4–1 that developmental improvements in absolute sensitivity are not uniform across frequency. The most rapid changes in absolute thresholds occur in early infancy at high frequencies. In contrast, low-frequency thresholds mature more gradually. Whereas the average threshold in quiet at 4000 Hz improves by about 20 dB between 1 and 3 months of age, the average threshold at 500 Hz improves by only 10 dB across the same age span (e.g., Olsho et al., 1988). Note that although absolute sensitivity does not reach adult levels until about 10 years of age at all frequencies, absolute auditory thresholds are within 10 to 15 dB of adults' thresholds by about 6 months of age (e.g., Trehub et al., 1988). Thus, 6-month-old infants generally can respond within audiometrically normal limits by the time that VRA becomes clinically feasible (reviewed by Gravel & Hood, 1998). It should be noted that infants' absolute threshold is even closer to adults' absolute threshold for a broadband noise (Werner & Boike, 2001).

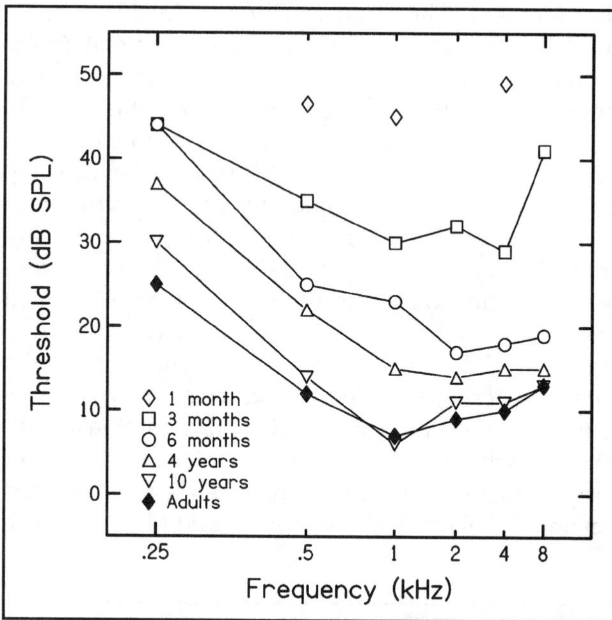

FIGURE 4–1. The audibility curve at different ages. Notice that absolute thresholds are rather high in the first months after birth. High-frequency thresholds improve the most in the first 6 postnatal months, so that high-frequency thresholds reach adult values before low-frequency thresholds. Low-frequency thresholds continue to improve into childhood.

Sources of Age-Related Change

The development of the conductive apparatus appears to be an important contributor to age-related changes in the shape of the audibility curve (e.g., Keefe, Bulen, Arehart, & Burns, 1993; Keefe, Burns, Bulen, & Campbell, 1994). Anatomic changes in the ear canal and middle ear system have been documented during infancy and childhood, including a lengthening of the ear canal (e.g., Keefe et al., 1993), an increase in the volume of the middle ear cavities (e.g., Eby & Nadol, 1986), and changes in the density and orientation of surrounding tissues (e.g., Ikui, Sando, & Fujita, 1997; Ruah, Schachern, Zelterman, Paparella, & Yoon, 1991). As a consequence of these anatomic changes, the conduction of sound energy through the conductive apparatus becomes progressively more efficient with increasing age during infancy (Keefe et al., 1993, 1994; reviewed by Keefe & Levi, 1996), and is not adultlike until 11 years of age (Okabe, Sachiko, Hareo, Tanetoshi, & Hiroaki, 1988). Consistent with developmental changes in absolute sensitivity (e.g., Olsho, Koch, Carter, Halpin, et al., 1988; Tharpe & Ashmead, 2001; Trehub et al., 1980), however, the largest improvements in conductive efficiency occur during the first 6 months of life (Keefe et al., 1993, 1994). For example, the amount of sound energy transmitted through the middle ear is approximately 20 dB less for a 1-month-old infant than for an adult at high frequencies, but improves to within 10 dB compared to an adult by 6 months of age (Keefe et al., 1994). Of particular relevance to pediatric audiologists is the fact that improvements in middle ear efficiency directly influence behavioral thresholds. For example, Werner and Holmer (2002) demonstrated that improvements in middle ear conductance between 3 months of age and adulthood can account for approximately 8 dB of the improvement in behavioral threshold estimates.

Converging evidence indicates that neither the rapid improvements in absolute auditory sensitivity occurring in early infancy nor the later progressive improvements occurring into childhood can be accounted for by maturation of the inner ear. The inner ear starts to function in utero by at least 22 weeks gestational age (e.g., Birnholz & Benacerraf, 1983; Pujol, Lavigne-Rebillard, & Uziel, 1991). In addition, anatomic, histologic, and physiologic data indicate mature cochlear function at term birth (e.g., Bargones & Burns, 1988; Lavigne-Rebillard & Pujol, 1987, 1988).

One physiologic method that has often been used to study cochlear function during infancy is the measurement of otoacoustic emissions (OAEs), sounds that are generated by the cochlea in response to stimulation. OAEs can be measured in the ear canal and provide a noninvasive indicator of normal cochlear function. Abdala, Oba, and Ramanathan (2008) reported that OAE amplitude increased with age at some frequencies in preterm infants, and that the amplitude of OAEs was higher in term infants than in adults, particularly at certain frequencies. The amplitude of OAEs, however, did not change between birth and 6 months postnatal age in full-term infants, an age range over which absolute thresholds change considerably. It appears that most of the reported age-related differences in OAE level reflect infants' immature conductive transmission (Abdala & Keefe, 2006; Keefe & Abdala, 2007).

Inefficient neural transmission through the auditory pathways in the brainstem also appears to play a role in the development of absolute sensitivity during early infancy (e.g., Gorga, Kaminski, Beauchaine, Jesteadt, & Neely, 1989; Ponton, Moore, & Eggermont, 1996; Werner, Folsom, & Mancl, 1994). Moreover, this inefficient neural transmission is related to absolute sensitivity prior to 6 months of age. Werner et al. (1994) demonstrated that auditory brainstem response (ABR) Wave I to V interwave latency predicts high-frequency behavioral thresholds for 3-month-olds, but not for 6-month-olds. One explanation for this result is that improvements in synaptic efficiency in the auditory brainstem occur between 3 and 6 months of age.

Conductive and brainstem immaturities do not account for all of the behavioral threshold immaturities that have been observed. In fact, by 7 months of age only a relatively small effect of conductive immaturity appears to remain (e.g., Keefe et al., 1994).

It has been suggested that infants and young children perform more poorly than adults on behavioral measures because they are inattentive or "off-task" on a certain proportion of trials. However, models of inattention account for only a small portion (2–3 dB) of the observed threshold immaturity (e.g., Viemeister & Schlauch, 1992; Wightman & Allen, 1992). Rather, it appears that some of the developmental changes in absolute sensitivity are the result of immature processing efficiency. Processing efficiency is a central phenomenon that is influenced by attention, motivation, memory, and selective attention (e.g., Bargones & Werner, 1994; Bargones, Werner, & Marean, 1995; Werner & Boike, 2001). For example, it has been suggested that infants and young children listen less selectively than adults. Whereas adults listen selectively for an expected signal in a detection task (e.g., Dai, Scharf, & Buus, 1991), infants monitor a broad range of frequencies during detection (Bargones & Werner, 1994). This inability to direct attention to the appropriate frequency appears to account for a substantial part of early behavioral threshold immaturity (e.g., Werner & Boike, 2001). It also explains why infants' absolute thresholds are more like those of adults for broadband than for narrowband sounds (e.g., Werner & Boike, 2001).

Development of the Basic Representations of Sound

Acousticians describe sound in two ways—in the time domain and in the frequency domain. The time domain representation of sound is pressure as a function of time and is often referred to as the time waveform. The frequency domain representation of sound has two components: the amplitude of sound as a function of frequency, called the *amplitude spectrum*, and the phase of sound as a function of frequency, called the *phase spectrum*. These representations of sound are illustrated in Figure 4–2. The peripheral auditory system also represents sound in the time domain (the "temporal" representation) and in the frequency domain (the "spectral" representation), although neither representation is complete and distortion free. These neural representations of sound are also shown in Figure 4–2. It is useful to think about hearing and hearing development in terms of the auditory system's representation of the time waveform and the amplitude spectrum.

Development of the Spectral Representation of Sound

A simple way to test a listener's representation of the amplitude spectrum is to measure a threshold for a tone or a narrow band of noise in broadband noise.

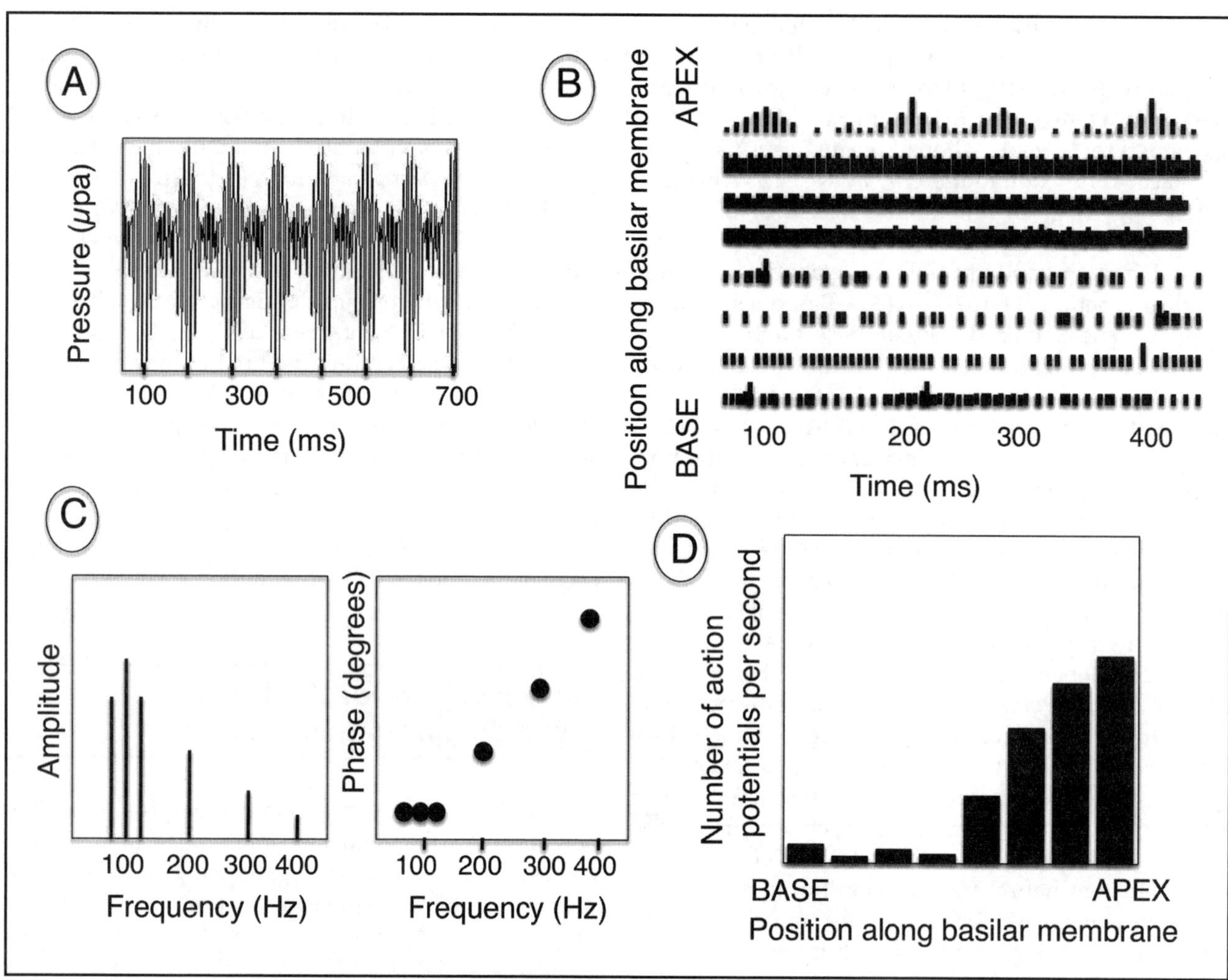

FIGURE 4–2. A comparison of acoustic and neural representations of sound. Sounds can be described in terms of their waveform, pressure as a function of time (**A**). An equivalent representation is the frequency domain representation (**C**). The sound is described in terms of its amplitude spectrum—amplitude as a function of frequency—and its phase spectrum—starting phase as a function of frequency. The auditory nerve carries two similar representations of sound. Neurons from each position along the basilar membrane respond in synchrony with the waveform of sound in each frequency band (**B**). Each bar represents the number of action potentials produced in a group of neurons at a particular position along the basilar membrane at each point in time. A taller bar indicates a larger number of action potentials. The neurons near the apex of the basilar membrane respond more when the amplitude of the waveform is high and less when the amplitude of the waveform is low. The other neural representation of sound is similar to the amplitude spectrum (**D**). Neurons from each position along the basilar membrane respond to a limited range of frequencies. Neurons respond more when the amplitude of sound within their frequency range is high and less when the amplitude of sound in their frequency range is low. Notice that there is some spontaneous activity in the basal (high-frequency) neurons even though there is no high-frequency energy in the sound (**B** and **D**). The phase spectrum of sound is not represented directly in the auditory nerve.

Schneider, Trehub, Morongiello, and Thorpe (1989) measured thresholds for a noise band masked by a broadband noise in listeners ranging from 6 months, through childhood, to adulthood. A summary of their results is shown in Figure 4–3. At 6 months, the masked threshold is about 15 dB higher than in adulthood. This difference grows progressively smaller as children grow older. Schneider et al. (1989) report that by

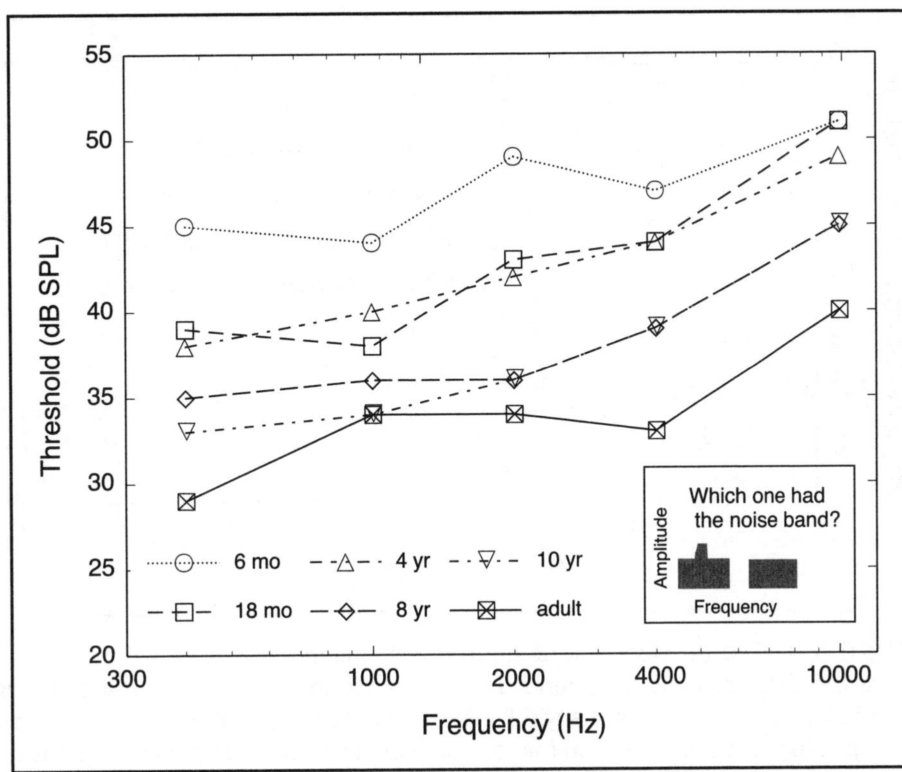

FIGURE 4–3. Threshold for an octave band of noise masked by a broadband noise, as a function of the center frequency of the noise band, for listeners of various ages, as reported by Schneider et al. (1989). Notice that masked threshold improves progressively with age up to about 10 years of age in this study. The masked threshold matures at about the same rate at all frequencies.

8 years, the masked threshold is only a little worse than that seen in adults. By some other reports, 6-year-olds are adultlike in threshold for a tone in noise (e.g., Hall & Grose, 1991).

Age-Related Changes

The amplitude spectrum plots amplitude, or intensity, as a function of frequency. Thus, to represent the amplitude spectrum, the auditory system must represent both the frequency and the intensity of sound. Consequently, maturation of the representation of frequency or intensity could be responsible for maturation of the spectral representation of sound. The precision of the representation of frequency, also known as frequency resolution, has been studied in infants and children using several different masking procedures (Hall & Grose, 1991; Olsho, 1985; Schneider, Morrongiello, & Trehub, 1990; Spetner & Olsho, 1990). Spetner and Olsho (1990), for example, tested frequency resolution in 3- and 6-month-old infants at 500, 1000, and 4000 Hz. They found that 6-month-olds were like adults in frequency resolution at all frequencies. Three-month-olds also had mature frequency resolution at 500 and 1000 Hz but had poorer frequency resolution than adults and older infants at 4000 Hz. Mature frequency resolution has also been reported in preschool children (e.g., Hall & Grose, 1991).

Maturation of the representation of intensity has been studied in two ways. One is intensity discrimination, in which the listener is asked to detect an intensity change in a sound or to choose the more intense of two sounds. The result is expressed as the change in intensity, expressed in decibels (dB), that a listener can just discriminate, the intensity difference limen (DL). Several studies have examined the development of intensity discrimination in infants and children; the results of these studies are summarized in Figure 4–4. The performance of 6-month-olds in these studies can be quite variable; in some studies infants could only discriminate a 12 dB change in intensity, and in others

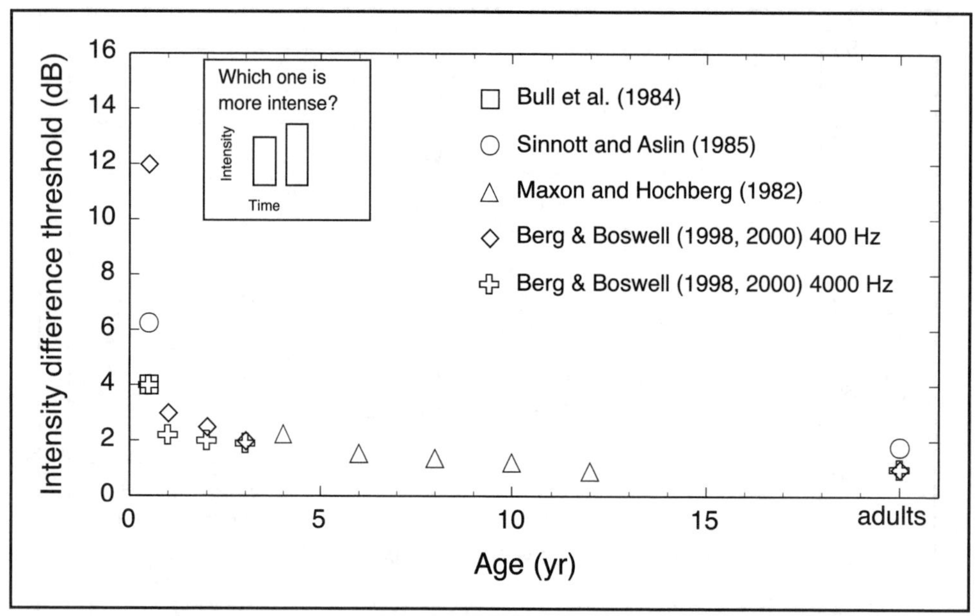

FIGURE 4–4. The development of intensity discrimination. The listener's task is to respond to the more intense sound. The difference in intensity that a listener can just discriminate gets smaller as the listener gets older, up to about 5 years of age, although even preschool children can discriminate fairly small changes in intensity.

they could discriminate a 4 dB change in intensity. Infants discriminate the smallest intensity changes for broadband sounds and at high frequencies (Berg & Boswell, 1998; Bull, Eilers, & Oller, 1984). At 12 months and beyond, however, intensity discrimination is consistently fairly good, and the intensity DL decreases from about 3 dB at 12 months to 1 to 2 dB at 6 years.

Another way to assess the representation of intensity in the auditory system is to ask the listener to report the loudness of a sound. It is not easy to get an infant to report how loud a sound is, but Leibold and Werner (2002) used the time it took infants to respond to a sound as an indication of loudness. Loudness had been shown in several studies to be related to reaction time in adults; adults respond faster when a sound is louder (e.g., Humes & Ahlstrom, 1984). Leibold and Werner found that infants also responded faster to more intense sounds, but infants' reaction time changed much more for a given change in intensity than did adults' reaction time. Thus, it is possible that loudness increases more with an increase in intensity for infants than for adults. By the time a child is 5 years old, it is possible to get the child to draw a line or provide a numerical estimate to express how loud something sounds to them. A 5-year-old's performance on these tests is comparable to that of an adult (e.g., Collins & Gescheider, 1989).

Thus, it appears that frequency resolution is immature at birth, at least at high frequencies, but matures during early infancy. The representation of intensity might still be rather immature in infants, but it matures quickly throughout the preschool period. The spectral representation of sound, then, is fairly precise in later infancy and probably adultlike by the time children begin kindergarten.

Sources of Age-Related Change

Postnatal maturation of the cochlea is probably not involved in the early development of the representation of the amplitude spectrum. As noted above, OAEs provide a noninvasive method for studying cochlear function, even in infants. OAEs for newborns increase in amplitude as the intensity of sound is increased in a similar way as OAEs for adults (Abdala, 2000). An OAE at a specific frequency can be suppressed, or masked, by sounds over about the same range of freqeuncies in newborns' and adults' ears (Abdala, Keefe, & Oba, 2007). Although some subtle differences between infant and adult cochlear responses have been reported (e.g., Dhar & Abdala, 2007; Moleti et al., 2008), at least some of these differences are actually due to middle ear immaturity (Abdala et al., 2007; Keefe & Abdala, 2007). In general, then, these results suggest that both frequency and intensity are represented in a mature way by the newborn's cochlea.

Immature frequency resolution before 6 months of age is apparently due to neural immaturity; frequency resolution measured in the cochlea is mature in newborns (e.g., Abdala & Sininger, 1996), but frequency resolution in the brainstem is immature in young infants as indicated by ABR (Abdala & Folsom, 1995; Folsom & Wynne, 1987). However, ABR results also indicate that frequency resolution is adultlike by 6 months of age (Abdala & Folsom, 1995; Folsom & Wynne, 1987). During the months after birth, it is likely that the connections between neurons in the auditory system are refined with exposure to sound (e.g., Sanes & Constantine-Paton, 1985). The refinement is reflected in maturation of frequency resolution.

However, there is little evidence that primary neural maturation contributes to age-related improvements in intensity resolution. The ABR increases in amplitude and decreases in latency as the intensity of the evoking sound is increased. If auditory neurons were not representing intensity accurately, we would expect to find that greater increases in intensity might be required to produce a certain amplitude or latency change for infants than for adults. Although ABR amplitude and latencies change as infants grow older, the effect of changing sound intensity is the same for infants as it is for adults (Gorga et al., 1989).

A small contributor to infants' immature tone-in-noise detection thresholds is their inability to stay on task during testing, as noted previously. A more important contributor is the way that infants listen to complex sounds. To detect a tone in noise at a low intensity, a listener must focus on the frequencies close to that of the tone. Adult listeners do this so well that they do not even hear tones that are presented at frequencies far from those of a target tone (e.g., Schlauch & Hafter, 1991). However, infants appear to listen broadly over a wide frequency range even when it would be beneficial to listen selectively (e.g., Bargones & Werner, 1994). It is not clear when children are able to listen as selectively as do adults (Leibold & Neff, 2007). Listening broadly over frequency is likely to be informative when infants and children are just learning about sounds in their environment. However, the disadvantage of broad listening is that competing sounds and noise are more detrimental to hearing for young listeners.

Development of the Temporal Representation of Sound

The auditory system's representation of the time waveform, or temporal characteristics, of sound provides information that the spectral representation cannot. For example, listeners can discriminate smaller changes in the frequency of a sound using its temporal, rather than spectral, representation (Moore, 1973). Furthermore, some slow changes in a sound over time, such as those that indicate prosody and intonation of speech, are carried by the temporal representation of sound (Rosen, 1989).

Pitch Perception

Age-Related Changes

Pitch is the perceptual dimension along which sounds are arranged from "high" to "low." In general, pitch varies with the frequency of a sound. Olsho, Koch, and Halpin (1987) reported that 3-month-old infants were poorer than adults at discriminating changes in the frequency of pure tones, particularly high-frequency (4000 Hz) tones. In contrast, 6- and 12-month-old infants could discriminate changes in the frequency of a pure tone as well as adults at 4000 Hz, but they were poorer than adults at discriminating changes in frequency and not much better than 3-month-olds at lower frequencies. Studies of preschool and school-age children indicated that low-frequency pure-tone discrimination continues to improve into the school years, but that high-frequency discrimination is quite good, even in 3-year-olds, as would be predicted from the infant studies (Hill, Hogben, & Bishop, 2005; Maxon & Hochberg, 1982). These age-related changes in pure-tone frequency discrimination are summarized in Figure 4–5.

Real-world sounds are rarely pure tones. Complex sounds that have distinct pitch consist of a fundamental frequency plus a set of harmonic frequencies. The pitch of such sounds corresponds to the pitch associated with the fundamental frequency, but if the fundamental frequency is filtered out, the remaining harmonics are still perceived as having the pitch of the fundamental. Thus, it is clear that complex pitch involves integrating information across frequency. Moreover, the perception of complex pitch depends on the temporal representation of sound. The development of complex pitch perception has not been well studied. Clarkson and her colleagues (Clarkson & Clifton, 1985, 1995; Clarkson, Martin, & Miciek, 1996; Clarkson & Rogers, 1995; Montgomery & Clarkson, 1997) have demonstrated that 7-month-old infants hear complex pitch much like adults (Figure 4–6), although there are circumstances in which infants of this age do not hear less salient pitches. Although neonates have been shown to discriminate large changes in the pitch of complex tones (Jeffrey & Cohen, 1971), there is no evidence that infants are extracting complex pitch from

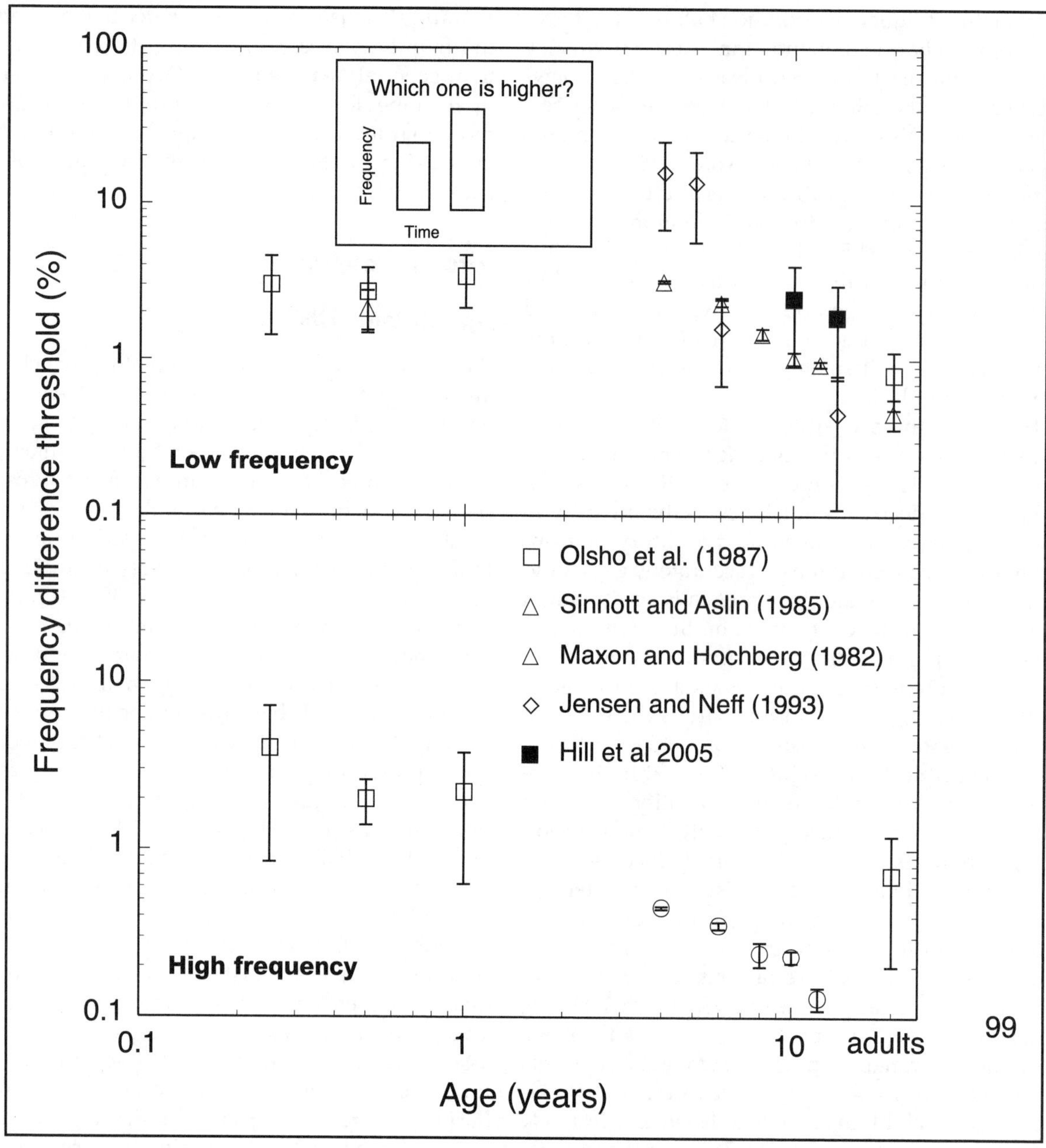

FIGURE 4–5. The development of frequency discrimination. The listener's task is to respond to the higher frequency tone. The difference in frequency that a listener can just discriminate gets smaller as the listener gets older, and for low-frequency tones this improvement continues into the school years. For high-frequency tones, 6- and 12-month-old infants are not very different from adults; notice that the error bars around the data points for these infants and all of the child groups overlap with the error bars around the adult data point. High-frequency pure-tone discrimination appears to mature earlier than low-frequency discrimination.

such sounds. By one report, 4-month-olds hear complex pitch poorly, and 2-month-olds not at all (Clarkson, Montgomery, Miciek, & Larson, 1998). It is not clear when children are able to hear complex pitch in all of the conditions in which adults hear it, although 5-year-old children have been shown to hear some subtle pitches like adults (Edwards, Giaschi, Low, & Edgell, 2005; Koelsch et al., 2003).

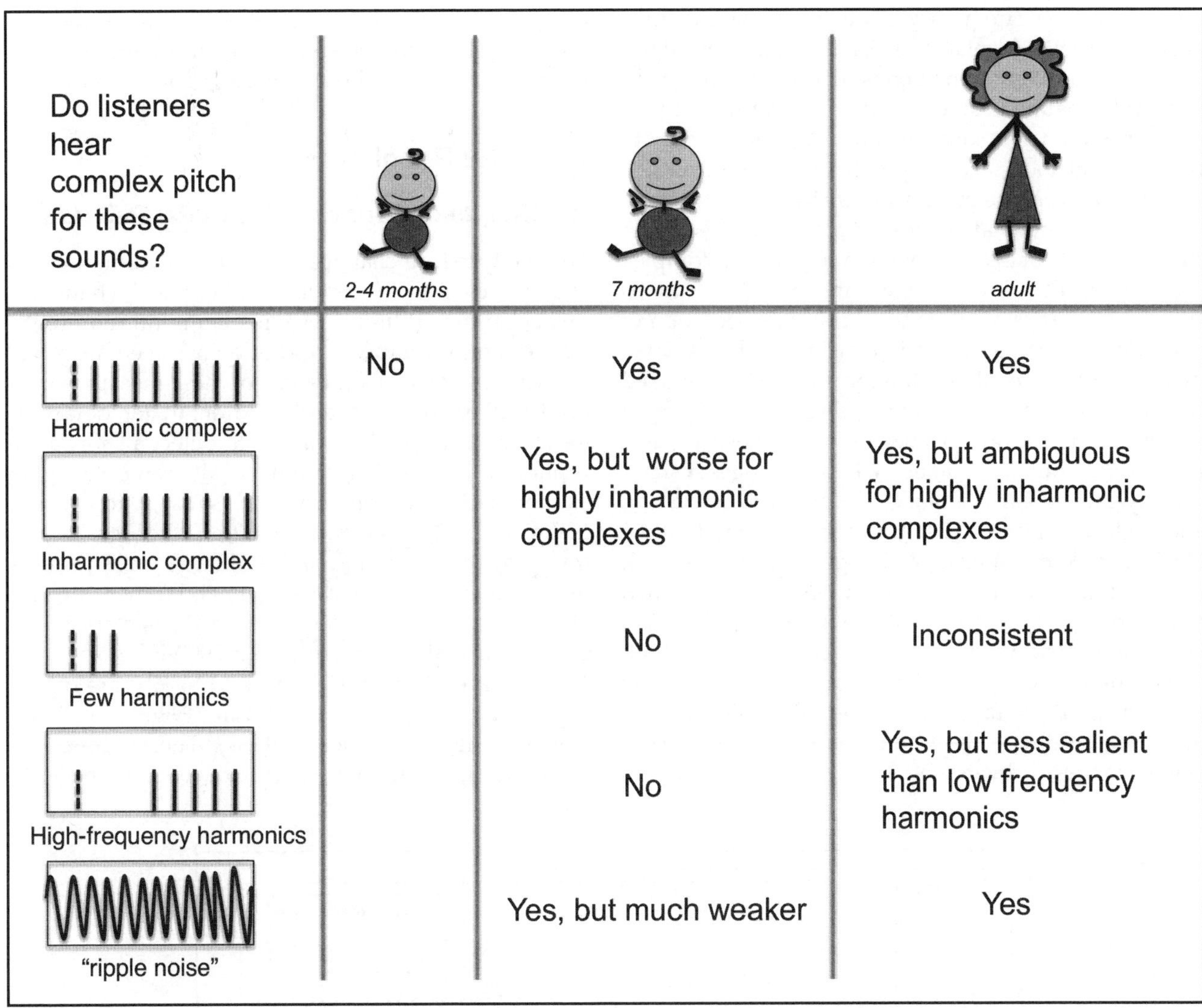

FIGURE 4–6. The development of complex pitch perception. Adults hear complex pitch in all of the sounds whose amplitude spectra are shown in the left-hand column. In each amplitude spectrum, the fundamental frequency of the complex is shown as a dashed line but is not physically present in the sound. Two-month-old infants do not appear to hear complex pitch, and 4-month-olds hear it poorly. Seven-month-olds and adults hear complex pitch in many of the same sounds, but when the pitch is weak for adults, the pitch is much weaker or absent for 7-month-olds.

Sources of Age-Related Change

Although pitch perception clearly involves the neural representation of the time waveform of sound, the so-called temporal representation, the neural representation of the amplitude spectrum, must also be involved. For example, people can discriminate changes in the frequency of pure tones at high frequencies, and the auditory system does not represent high-frequency information temporally (Pickles, 2008). Thus, that 3-month-old infants have particular difficulty discriminating between high-frequency tones is consistent with their immature high-frequency resolution, as described in the previous section of this chapter (Spetner & Olsho, 1990). Similarly, that 6-month-old infants can discriminate high-frequency tones as well as adults is consistent with their mature high-frequency resolution. Because low-frequency pure-tone discrimination is likely based on the temporal representation of sound, that even 12-month-old infants are immature at low-frequency pure-tone discrimination may mean that infants do not have precise temporal information. However, some evoked potential findings suggest that at least at low levels in the auditory system, the temporal representation of frequency is much like that in adults even in 1-month-old infants (Levi, Folsom, & Dobie, 1995).

The neural representation of both spectral and temporal information is involved in the perception of simple (pure-tone) and complex pitch. As described, both the temporal and spectral representations of sound sent to the brain from the ear are mature by 1 month of age. Thus, it is somewhat surprising that infants younger than 7 months of age do not seem to perceive complex pitch like adults. However, there are several indications that central processing of the neural representation of sound does not mature until later in childhood. First, evidence indicates that although the cortical-evoked response to changes in complex pitch are seen even in 2-month-olds, the organization of the response—which parts of the brain respond and when—changes systematically during early infancy (He, Hotson, & Trainor, 2007). He and Trainor (2009), moreover, found that the cortical-evoked response to changes in complex pitch occurred in 4-month-olds, but not 2-month-olds, when the fundamental was missing from the complex. Second, training seems to improve performance in both pure-tone frequency discrimination, especially at low frequencies (Buss, Taylor, & Leibold, 2014; Olsho, Koch, & Carter, 1988) and discrimination of subtle complex pitch changes (Edwards et al., 2005). Thus, it may be that infants and children have the neural representations they need to perceive pitch, but it takes time for them to learn to use those representations effectively.

Temporal Resolution

Age-Related Changes in Temporal Resolution

The ability to hear changes in a sound over time is called *temporal resolution*. Information about such changes is carried in the auditory system's temporal representation of sound. Temporal resolution has been measured in a variety of ways, and some of these measures have been applied to infants and children. In gap detection, for example, a listener is asked to detect a short interruption in an ongoing sound. Adults can detect gaps as short as 3 ms in some conditions (e.g., Eddins, Hall, & Grose, 1992). Infants, even 12-month-olds, in contrast, do not detect gaps shorter than about 30 ms (Trehub, Schneider, & Henderson, 1995; Werner, Marean, Halpin, Spetner, & Gillenwater, 1992). By preschool, the gap detection threshold in a 2000-Hz noise band has improved to about 12 ms, and by 6 years of age, gap detection appears to be mature (Wightman, Allen, Dolan, Kistler, & Jamieson, 1989). These age-related changes in gap detection are illustrated in Figure 4–7.

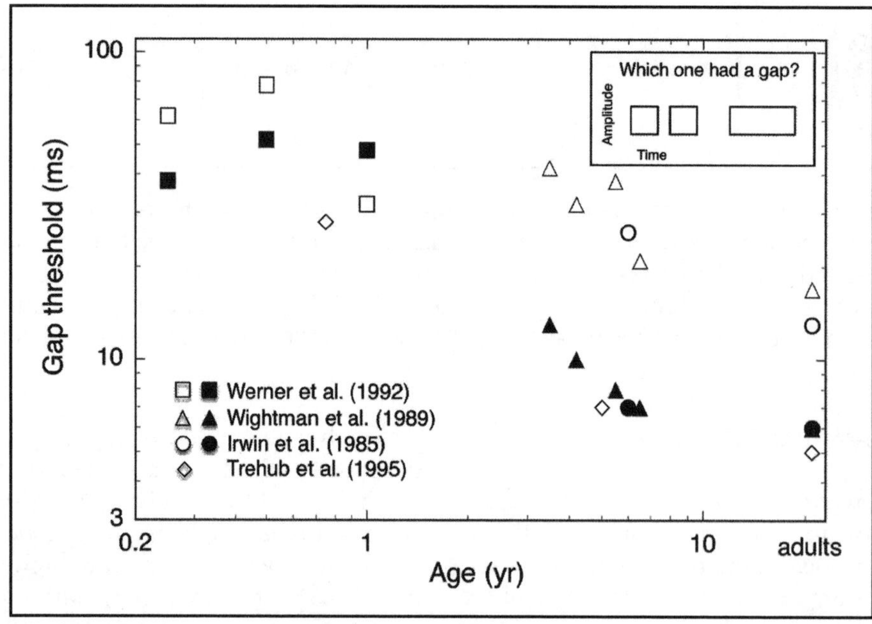

FIGURE 4–7. The development of gap detection. The listener's task is to respond when a very short interruption in an ongoing sound occurs. The unfilled symbols are gap thresholds for low-frequency sounds, and the filled symbols are gap thresholds for high-frequency sounds. Gap thresholds for both low- and high-frequency sounds improve with age, but high-frequency gap thresholds approach adult values at younger ages than low-frequency gap thresholds.

An issue with gap detection is that it depends not only on the auditory system's ability to follow a rapid change in sound, but also on the ability to represent a change in intensity. As noted above, the ability to represent a change in intensity may be immature in infants, so it is difficult to interpret the finding of poor gap detection performance. Another measure of temporal resolution is the temporal modulation transfer function (TMTF), which shows the amount of amplitude modulation required to detect modulation at different modulation rates (Viemeister, 1979). When the modulation rate is slow, the auditory system should have no trouble following the modulation, so the amount of modulation needed to hear the change will only depend on the system's ability to represent a change in intensity. However, as the modulation rate increases, the auditory system's ability to follow rapid changes begins to deteriorate. This will be reflected in an increase in the amount of modulation required for modulation detection (Figure 4–8). Thus, the modulation rate at which the amount of modulation required for detection starts to increase is a measure of temporal resolution, independent of intensity resolution. The TMTF of 4-year-old children has been shown to parallel that of adults (see Figure 4–8), indicating mature temporal resolution (Hall & Grose, 1994). However, recall that gap detection is immature at this age. There are few published data on infants' TMTF, although the data that are available suggest no obvious immaturity in this measure (Werner, 1996).

Sources of Age-Related Change

Electrophysiologic data on temporal resolution are consistent with the idea that temporal resolution is an early maturing ability. For example, auditory brainstem responses to the onset of sound following a temporal gap are similar to those of adults at 3 months of age (Werner, Folsom, Mancl, & Syapin, 2001). Furthermore, an evoked potential evoked by amplitude-modulated

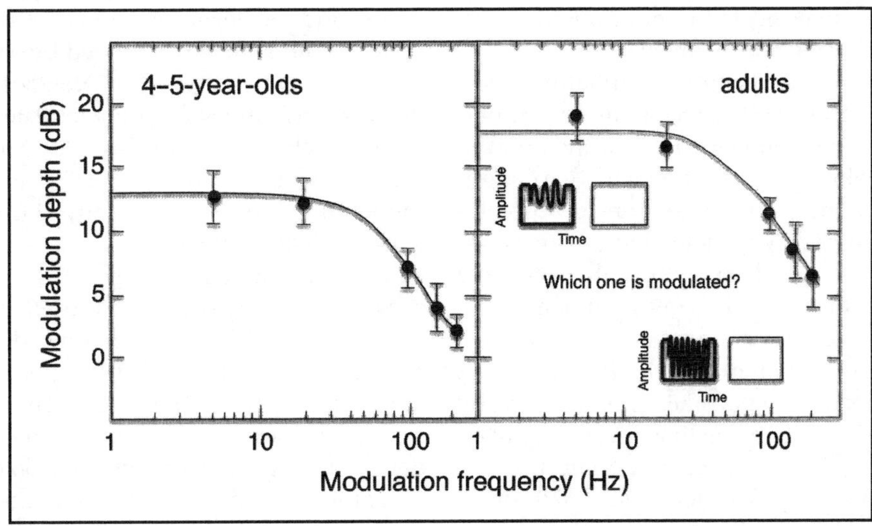

FIGURE 4–8. Temporal modulation transfer functions for 4- to 5-year-old children (*left panel*) and for adults (*right panel*), as reported by Hall and Grose (1994). The listener's task is to respond when the amplitude of a sound changes over time—that is, when the sound is amplitude modulated. In some conditions, the sound's amplitude changes slowly (*inset at top left of right panel*); in other cases, the sound's amplitude changes rapidly (*inset at bottom right of right panel*). How rapidly the sound is changing is the "modulation frequency" on the *x*-axis. The more rapid the modulation, the bigger, or "deeper," the modulation has to be for the listener to detect it. Notice that in the inset with the slowly changing sound, the modulation is not as deep as in the inset with the rapidly changing sound. The modulation depth, on the *y*-axis, can be thought of as how far down the amplitude has to go for the listener to detect the change. A value of 0 would mean that the amplitude has to go all the way off, whereas a value of 15 would mean that the amplitude only has to go down some of the way. Each data point plots the depth of modulation required to just detect modulation at a certain modulation frequency; the curves were fit to the data points. This shows that 4- to 5-year-olds generally need deeper modulation than adults do to detect modulation. Children's modulation threshold gets worse as the modulation frequency increases, however, just as that of adults. The curves are offset along the *y*-axis, but they are parallel to each other. This suggests that children's temporal resolution is similar to that of adults.

tones is similar in 1-month-olds and adults (Levi et al., 1995). Cortical potentials evoked by gaps in sound appear to be adultlike by 6 months of age, and although younger infants demonstrate a cortical response to gaps in sound, the morphology of the response is quite different from that seen in older infants (Trainor et al., 2003). Thus, it is possible that cortical development leads to early changes in temporal resolution, although there is no evidence that behavioral measures of temporal resolution change early in infancy. In sum, the available physiological evidence suggests that changes in a sound over time are accurately represented in the auditory system of infants and children.

If an infant's auditory system can represent temporal modulation in sound, why is an infant's gap detection performance so poor? One possibility is that immature gap detection reflects immature intensity resolution rather than immature temporal resolution. As noted above, infants are not as good as adults at discriminating a change in intensity, and loudness growth may be immature in infants. Although there are few electrophysiologic findings consistent with primary immaturity of the representation of intensity in the infant auditory system, this possibility cannot be dismissed.

Another possible explanation is immature selective attention. A listener will detect a gap in a sound most effectively if attention is focused on the point in time—a precise point in time—at which a gap might occur. If infants cannot direct attention to a precise point in time, then their gap detection performance would be poor compared to temporally selective adults. This could also explain why infants are particularly poor at detecting very short duration sounds. Werner, Parrish, and Holmer (2009) have examined infants' ability to focus on a particular point in time by comparing infants' detection of a tone that occurs at an expected time, compared to tones that occur at unexpected times. Interestingly, Werner et al. (2009) found that, like adults, infants detected tones at expected times better than they detected tones at unexpected times, indicating that they were listening selectively at the expected time. This finding argues against the idea that immature gap detection results from a failure to listen selectively in time, although it is not possible to determine whether infants' temporal attention is as precise as adults' attention from the results of Werner et al. (2009).

Spatial Hearing

From a developmental perspective, one of the more interesting aspects of hearing is spatial hearing. People are able to localize sound sources in space by using differences in the intensity and timing of sounds at the two ears and by reference to the shape of a sound's amplitude spectrum after it has passed through the external ear. All three of these acoustic cues to a sound source's location depend on the size of the head and the pinnas. Thus, as a child's head and ears grow, the acoustic cues associated with a particular location in space will change. Moreover, a small head and ears will provide a smaller cue than a large head and ears. Thus, infants and children are not only at an acoustic disadvantage when it comes to spatial hearing, but their brains must deal with a continually changing set of acoustic cues.

Age-Related Changes

Given the age-related differences in the acoustics that result from the growth of the head and ears, it will come as no surprise that infants and young children are not as good as adults at identifying the spatial location of a sound. For example, an adult will be able to tell that a sound source has moved by as little as 1° to the left or right (Blauert, 1983). Newborn infants can tell that a sound comes from the left or right (Field, Muir, Pilon, Sinclair, & Dodwell, 1980), but a sound source must move by as much as 27° before a 1-month-old can tell that the sound has moved (Morrongiello, Fenwick, & Chance, 1990). An 18-month-old can tell when a sound has moved left or right by 5°, and a 5-year-old can localize many sounds in the left-right dimension as well as adults (Litovsky & Ashmead, 1997). These age-related changes in the accuracy of sound localization are summarized in Figure 4–9. The ability to localize a sound in elevation—up or down—follows a similar developmental course (Morrongiello & Rocca, 1987).

However, in most studies of the development of sound localization, testing is conducted in a space in which reverberation is minimized. This is important, because in many situations, the sound reaches the ears directly from the source, followed by reverberations of the sound ("echoes") from walls and obstacles at other locations. To solve this problem, the auditory system bases its estimate of a sound's location primarily on the first sound that arrives at the ears. This is known as the precedence effect. Newborn infants do not demonstrate the precedence effect; they seem to hear both the direct sound and its echoes. However, by the time infants are 4 or 5 months old, they respond as if the first sound they hear gives the location of a sound source (see Figure 4–9; Clifton, Morrongiello, & Dowd, 1984). At the same time, infants and even 5-year-old children do not localize sound sources as accurately when there

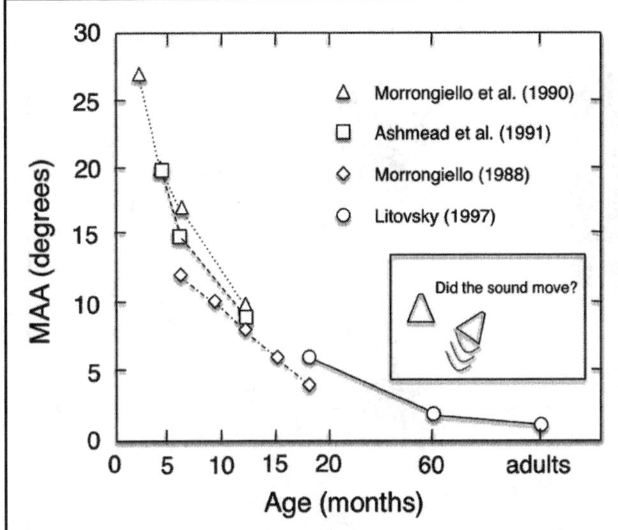

FIGURE 4–9. The development of the precision of sound localization in the left-right dimension. The listener's task is to respond when the location from which the sound is coming changes. The minimum audible angle (MAA) is the change in position, expressed in degrees of arc, which the listener can just detect. The MAA improves dramatically throughout infancy and reaches adult values around 5 years of age.

is reverberation, suggesting that the precedence effect is still immature at school age (Litovsky, 1997).

Sources of Age-Related Change

There are several possible explanations for infants' and young children's poor sound localization. These are illustrated in Figure 4–9.

As noted above, infants and young children may have difficulty localizing sounds because their small head and ears provide them with less acoustic information about a sound source's location. The data indicate that although the acoustics limit a young child's sound localization, they are not the only limitation. Clifton, Gwiazda, Bauer, Clarkson, and Held (1988) measured the distance between the ears in infants of different ages and calculated what the maximum acoustic differences between the ears would be at each age. What they found was that although the acoustic differences were smaller in younger infants, the differences were not small enough to account for the imprecise sound localization seen in infants.

To use the acoustic information about a sound's location, the ears must accurately represent the frequency, intensity, and timing of the sound, and the brain must be able to calculate the differences between the ears and to extract the shape of a sound's amplitude spectrum. As described above, the representation of sound reaching the brain from the ear is mature rather early in life. However, Ashmead, Davis, Whalen, and Odom (1991) found that infants were less accurate than adults at estimating differences in the arrival times of sounds at the two ears. This would suggest that the auditory system's ability to calculate differences between the ears is not yet mature in infancy. However, Ashmead et al. (1991) also showed that infant's poor arrival-time calculations were not poor enough to account for their imprecise sound localization.

Finally, to be able to figure out where a sound is coming from, the brain must "translate" an acoustic pattern into a particular spatial location. Although the development of this map of auditory space has not been studied in humans, it is known to depend on experience with sound in other species (Gray, 1992; Knudsen, 1985). Furthermore, people who are deprived of input to one ear for a time during development and then later have hearing in that ear restored, have a normal ability to discriminate the acoustic cues that specify a sound's location but are unable to say where a sound is coming from (Wilmington, Gray, & Jahrsdorfer, 1994). Thus, the development of sound localization may also depend on the formation of a map of auditory space.

Hearing in Complex Sound Environments

Natural environments contain multiple sources of competing sounds. Each source produces acoustic waveforms that vary in frequency and amplitude across time. In order to make sense of the overlapping mixture of sounds that reach the ears, listeners must determine which components were produced by the same source. This process is often referred to as sound source segregation (Bregman, 1990).

The developing child must learn speech and language in complex sound environments. For example, children are expected to follow directions spoken by their teacher in the classroom, despite hearing the voices of classmates and rumblings of cars driving on a nearby road (Figure 4–10). We do not yet know how children develop the ability to separate and select the most important sounds while ignoring sounds that are unrelated. Emerging data suggest, however, that the complex sound environments typical of everyday life pose considerable difficulty for infants and young children. Research conducted over the past 30 years has consistently shown that preschoolers and school-aged

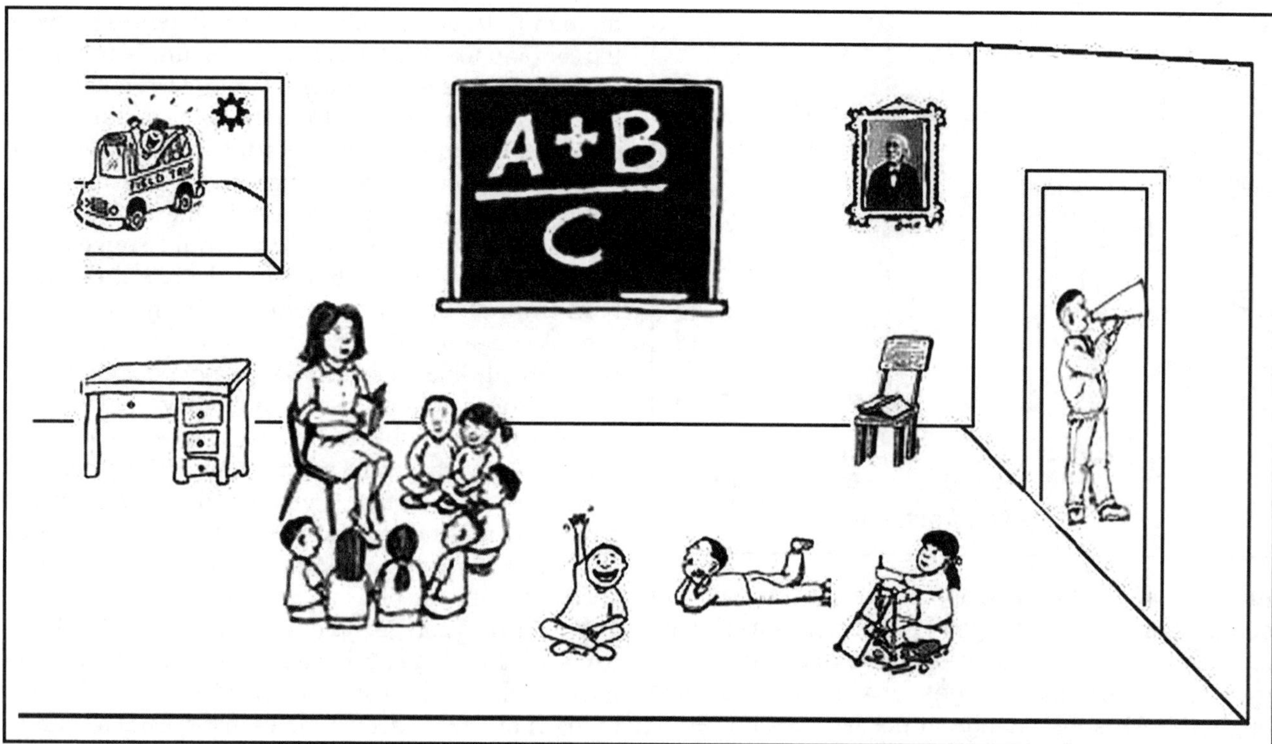

FIGURE 4–10. The problem of sound source segregation in the classroom. Children are asked to listen to one sound source—the teacher—in the presence of many other sound sources—other children's voices inside and outside the classroom, a school bus engine, clanking toys. The characteristics of sound that a listener might use to separate the sounds include differences in the fundamental frequency of the teacher and child voices, differences in the spatial location of the teacher and other sound sources, and differences in the pattern of sound over time.

children require a higher signal-to-noise ratio (SNR) compared to adults to achieve similar levels of performance on speech recognition tests in the presence of noise or speech maskers (e.g., Elliott et al., 1979; Nittrouer & Boothroyd, 1990; Wightman & Kistler, 2005). Similar to the studies of preschoolers and older children, Newman and Jusczyk (1996) found that infants could recognize their name embedded in a background of competing speech but needed a higher SNR to do so, relative to adults.

The increased susceptibility to interference from competing sounds observed during infancy and childhood appears to be different from the masking described in previous sections of this chapter (reviewed by Werner & Leibold, 2004). For example, Hall, Grose, Buss, and Dev (2002) demonstrated that child-adult differences in spondee word recognition were more pronounced for a two-talker competing sound than for a speech-shaped noise. These two distracting noises overlapped with the target words to the same extent in frequency and in time, and yet children had relatively greater difficulty hearing the target words when the distracter was speech. The pronounced developmental effects observed with increasing acoustic complexity might reflect immaturity in how children perceptually segregate the target sound from the competing background sounds.

Age-Related Change

Sound source segregation is often examined in adults by assessing auditory stream segregation (Bregman, 1990). Auditory streams can be thought of as sounds coming from different sources. People divide incoming sound complexes into separate auditory streams on the basis of acoustic similarities between frequency components. For example, components that come on and go off together will be heard as coming from the same source, but components with very different frequencies will be heard as coming from different sources (reviewed by Darwin & Carlyon, 1995; Yost, 1997). In a typical auditory streaming task, several components are presented, and one or more acoustic cues are manipulated. Listeners are asked to report whether they heard a single auditory stream or two distinct streams.

Studies of auditory streaming in infants indicate that auditory streaming processes are functional at birth (Demany, 1982; Fassbender, 1993; McAdams & Bertoncini, 1997; Winkler et al., 2003). Moreover, infants appear to be able to use several of the same acoustic cues used by adults to separate streams, including frequency proximity (Demany, 1982; Fassbender, 1993), intensity similarity (Fassbender, 1993), spectral similarity (Fassbender, 1993), timbre (McAdams & Bertoncini, 1997), and spatial location (McAdams & Bertoncini, 1997). However, larger acoustic differences in these potential cues were used for testing infants than for testing adults. In addition, only indirect measures of auditory streaming were used in the infant studies, because infants cannot be asked to say "one stream" or "two streams." Thus, it is as yet undetermined whether auditory streaming processes are fully adultlike during infancy or are functional, but immature.

Few studies have examined the auditory streaming abilities of preschoolers and school-aged children. However, in a recent study, Sussman, Wong, Horvath, Winkler, and Wang (2007) compared auditory streaming in children (5–11 years) and adults as a function of frequency proximity. Listeners heard a sequence of pure tones that differed in frequency. The frequency separation of the alternating pure tones was varied, and listeners were asked if they heard one or two auditory streams. A larger frequency separation was needed for children compared to adults before they would indicate that two streams were presented. Sussman et al. (2007) suggested that auditory stream segregation is functional early in life but matures with increasing age and experience throughout childhood.

Another promising approach to the study of sound source segregation during infancy and childhood is to examine whether acoustic cues shown to promote sound source segregation in adults provide infants and children with a release from "informational masking" (e.g., Kidd, Mason, Deliwala, Woods, & Colburn, 1994; Neff & Green, 1987; Watson, Wroton, Kelly, & Benbassat, 1975). Informational masking generally refers to masking that occurs even though the spectral and temporal representations of the sound provide enough detail to allow the listener to separate the target sound from the competing sound. For example, in an early study of informational masking, Neff and Green (1987) asked listeners to detect a 1000-Hz pure tone presented simultaneously with a multitonal masker. The individual frequency components of the multitonal masker were varied randomly on each presentation. For many adults, the introduction of variation in the masker had a large and detrimental effect on detection of the 1000-Hz tone even though the masker components were very different in frequency from the 1000-Hz tone.

Interestingly, manipulations of the acoustic properties of sound that promote sound source segregation, including spatial separation, asynchronous temporal onsets, and dissimilar temporal modulations, reduce informational masking for most adults who are susceptible to the effect (e.g., Arbogast, Mason, & Kidd, 2002; Durlach et al., 2003; Kidd et al., 1994; Neff, 1995; Oh & Lutfi, 1998). This suggests that informational masking could result from poor sound source segregation.

Researchers interested in auditory development have started to examine whether the acoustic cues that reduce informational masking in adults provide infants and children with a release from informational masking (e.g., Hall, Buss, & Grose, 2005; Leibold & Werner, 2006; Wightman, Callahan, Lutfi, Kistler, & Oh, 2003; Wightman & Kistler, 2005). The results of these initial studies indicate that children benefit from some, but not all, of the cues that improve adults' performance. Whereas the introduction of temporal asynchrony between a pure-tone signal and a multitonal masker improves thresholds for children and adults by a similar amount (Hall et al., 2005; Leibold & Neff, 2007), presenting the signal and masker to opposite headphones results in a large masking release for adults but does not benefit children (Hall et al., 2005; Wightman et al., 2003). For example, Wightman et al. (2003) measured detection thresholds for a 1000-Hz tone in the presence of a random-frequency, multitonal masker. Informational masking was observed for children and adults. However, masking was substantially reduced or eliminated in adults when signal and masker were presented to opposite ears. In contrast, improvement was significantly less for children in that condition.

Sources of Age-Related Change

The basic representation of sound provided to the brain of a typically developing 6-month-old appears to be adequate to support sound source segregation. Nonetheless, it is clear that the ability to separate target sounds embedded in competing background sounds is not mature until well into childhood. The sources of children's prolonged difficulties in complex sound environments are not well understood but appear to reflect maturation of higher-level neural structures and nonsensory or "central" auditory processes, such as sound source segregation. Understanding how infants and children perform sound source segregation is critical to understanding how children acquire speech and language in complex natural environments.

An important unresolved question for researchers and audiologists is to understand the influence of listening experience on the development of hearing in complex sound environments. Children become more efficient and flexible listeners as they learn about the important features of sound across different talkers and listening environments, but it is unclear how and when this process unfolds. Moreover, this development might well be prolonged or altered by hearing loss if access to sound is delayed or compromised.

Summary, Conclusions, and Principles of Development

Human auditory development begins before birth and continues into adolescence. The basic auditory capacities, the spectral and temporal representations of sound, are not completely mature at birth but are apparently adultlike by about 6 months of age. However, the ability to use the information that the ear provides the brain develops over a much longer time course. Infants and children progressively learn to separate a target sound from irrelevant sounds. As children grow older, they become sensitive to aspects of sounds that they previously appeared not to notice. Finally, children are able to choose the most informative aspects of sound to be efficient information processors. In addition, the abilities to break a sound down into separate sources and to match a pattern of sound to a particular location in space take time to develop. Although these abilities are present in rudimentary form in early infancy, they do not function effectively in the most complex listening conditions until adolescence.

References

Abdala, C. (2000). Distortion product otoacoustic emission (2f1-f2) amplitude growth in human adults and neonates. *Journal of the Acoustical Society of America, 107*, 446–456.

Abdala, C., & Folsom, R. C. (1995). The development of frequency resolution in humans as revealed by the auditory brain-stem response recorded with notched-noise masking. *Journal of the Acoustical Society of America, 98*, 921–930.

Abdala, C., & Keefe, D. H. (2006). Effects of middle-ear immaturity on distortion product otoacoustic emission suppression tuning in infant ears. *Journal of the Acoustical Society of America, 120*, 3832–3842.

Abdala, C., Keefe, D. H., & Oba, S. I. (2007). Distortion product otoacoustic emission suppression tuning and acoustic admittance in human infants: Birth through 6 months. *Journal of the Acoustical Society of America, 121*, 3617–3627.

Abdala, C., Oba, S., & Ramanathan, R. (2008). Changes in the DP-gram during the preterm and early postnatal period. *Ear and Hearing, 29*, 512–523.

Abdala, C., & Sininger, Y. S. (1996). The development of cochlear frequency resolution in the human auditory system. *Ear and Hearing, 17*, 374–385.

Arbogast, T. L., Mason, C. R., & Kidd, G. (2002). The effect of spatial separation on informational and energetic masking of speech. *Journal of the Acoustical Society of America, 112*, 2086–2098.

Ashmead, D. H., Davis, D., Whalen, T., & Odom, R. (1991). Sound localization and sensitivity to interaural time differences in human infants. *Child Development, 62*, 1211–1226.

Bargones, J. Y., & Burns, E. M. (1988). Suppression tuning curves for spontaneous otoacoustic emissions in infants and adults. *Journal of the Acoustical Society of America, 83*(5), 1809–1816.

Bargones, J. Y., & Werner, L. A. (1994). Adults listen selectively; infants do not. *Psychological Science, 5*, 170–174.

Bargones, J. Y., Werner, L. A., & Marean, G. C. (1995). Infant psychometric functions for detection: Mechanisms of immature sensitivity. *Journal of the Acoustical Society of America, 98*, 99–111.

Berg, K. M., & Boswell, A. E. (1998). Infants' detection of increments in lowand high-frequency noise. *Perception and Psychophysics, 60*, 1044–1051.

Berg, K. M., & Boswell, A. E. (2000). Noise increment detection in children 1 to 3 years of age. *Perception and Psychophysics, 62*(4), 868–873

Birnholz, J. C., & Benacerraf, B. R. (1983). The development of fetal hearing. *Science, 222*, 516–518.

Blauert, J. (1983). *Spatial hearing: The psychophysics of human sound localization* (J. S. Allen, Trans.). Cambridge, MA: MIT Press.

Bregman, A. S. (1990). *Auditory scene analysis: The perceptual organization of sound*. Cambridge, MA: MIT Press.

Bull, D., Eilers, R. E., & Oller, D. K. (1984). Infants' discrimination of intensity variation in multitsyllabic stimuli. *Journal of the Acoustical Society of America, 76*, 13–17.

Buss, E., Taylor, C. N., & Leibold, L. J. (2014). Factors affecting sensitivity to frequency change in school-age children and adults. *Journal of Speech, Language, and Hearing Research, 57*, 1972–1982.

Clarkson, M. G., & Clifton, R. K. (1985). Infant pitch perception: Evidence for responding to pitch categories and the missing fundamental. *Journal of the Acoustical Society of America, 77*, 1521–1528.

Clarkson, M. G., & Clifton, R. K. (1995). Infants' pitch perception: Inharmonic tonal complexes. *Journal of the Acoustical Society of America, 98*(3), 1372–1379.

Clarkson, M. G., Martin, R., & Miciek, S. (1996). Infants' perception of pitch: Number of harmonics. *Infant Behavior and Development, 19*, 191–197.

Clarkson, M. G., Montgomery, C. R., Miciek, S. G., & Larson, M. E. (1998). Perception of the pitch of the missing fundamental by 4-month-old infants. *Infant Behavior and Development, 21*, 343.

Clarkson, M. G., & Rogers, E. C. (1995). Infants require low-frequency energy to hear the pitch of the missing fundamental. *Journal of the Acoustical Society of America, 98*(1), 148–154.

Clifton, R. K., Gwiazda, J., Bauer, J., Clarkson, M., & Held, R. (1988). Growth in head size during infancy: Implications for sound localization. *Developmental Psychology, 24*, 477–483.

Clifton, R. K., Morrongiello, B. A., & Dowd, J. M. (1984). A developmental look at an auditory illusion: The precedence effect. *Developmental Psychobiology, 17*(5), 519–536.

Collins, A. A., & Gescheider, G. A. (1989). The measurement of loudness in individual children and adults by absolute magnitude estimation and cross-modality matching. *Journal of the Acoustical Society of America, 85*, 2012–2021.

Dai, H., Scharf, B., & Buus, S. (1991). Effective attenuation of signals in noise under focused attention. *Journal of the Acoustical Society of America, 89*(6), 2837–2842.

Darwin, C. J., & Carlyon, R. P. (1995). Auditory grouping. In B. C. J. Moore (Ed.), *Hearing* (pp. 387–424). New York, NY: Academic Press.

Demany, L. (1982). Auditory stream segregation in infancy. *Infant Behavior and Development, 5*, 261–276.

Dhar, S., & Abdala, C. (2007). A comparative study of distortion product-otoacoustic-emission fine structure in human newborns and adults with normal hearing. *Journal of the Acoustical Society of America, 122*, 2191–2202.

Durlach, N. I., Mason, C. R., Shinn-Cunningham, B. G., Arbogast, T. L., Colburn, H. S., & Kidd, G. (2003). Informational masking: Counteracting the effects of stimulus uncertainty by decreasing target-masker similarity. *Journal of the Acoustical Society of America, 114*, 368–379.

Eby, T. L., & Nadol, J. B., Jr. (1986). Postnatal growth of the human temporal bone. Implications for cochlear implants in children. *Annals of Otology, Rhinology, and Laryngology, 85*, 356–364.

Eddins, D. A., Hall, J. W., & Grose, J. H. (1992). The detection of temporal gaps as a function of frequency region and absolute noise bandwidth. *Journal of the Acoustical Society of America, 91*, 1069–1077.

Edwards, V. T., Giaschi, D. E., Low, P., & Edgell, D. (2005). Sensory and nonsensory influences on children's performance of dichotic pitch perception tasks. *Journal of the Acoustical Society of America, 117*, 3157–3164.

Elliott, L. L., Connors, S., Kille, E., Levin, S., Ball, K., & Katz, D. (1979). Children's understanding of monosyllabic nouns in quiet and noise. *Journal of the Acoustical Society of America, 66*, 12–21.

Fassbender, C. (1993). *Auditory grouping and segregation processes in infancy*. Norderstedt, Germany: Kaste Verlag.

Field, T. J., Muir, D., Pilon, R., Sinclair, M., & Dodwell, P. (1980). Infants' orientation to lateral sounds from birth to three months. *Child Development, 51*, 295–298.

Folsom, R. C., & Wynne, M. K. (1987). Auditory brain stem responses from human adults and infants: Wave V tuning curves. *Journal of the Acoustical Society of America, 81*, 412–417.

Gorga, M. P., Kaminski, J. R., Beauchaine, K. L., Jesteadt, W., & Neely, S. T. (1989). Auditory brainstem responses from children three months to three years of age: Normal patterns of response II. *Journal of Speech and Hearing Research, 32*, 281–288.

Gravel, J. S., & Hood, L. J. (1998). Pediatric audiological assessment. In F. Musiek & W. Rintelmann (Eds.), *Contemporary perspectives in hearing assessment* (pp. 305–326). Needham Heights, MA: Allyn & Bacon.

Gray, L. (1992). Interactions between sensory and nonsensory factors in the responses of newborn birds to sound. In L. A. Werner & E. W. Rubel (Eds.), *Developmental psychoacoustics* (pp. 89–112). Washington, DC: American Psychological Association.

Hall, J. W., Buss, E., & Grose, J. H. (2005). Informational masking release in children and adults. *Journal of the Acoustical Society of America, 118*, 1605–1613.

Hall, J. W., & Grose, J. H. (1991). Notched-noise measures of frequency selectivity in adults and children using fixed-masker-level and fixed-signal-level presentation. *Journal of Speech and Hearing Research, 34*, 651–660.

Hall, J. W., & Grose, J. H. (1994). Development of temporal resolution in children as measured by the temporal modulation transfer-function. *Journal of the Acoustical Society of America, 96*, 150–154.

Hall, J. W., Grose, J. H., Buss, E., & Dev, M. B. (2002). Spondee recognition in a two-talker masker and a speech-shaped noise masker in adults and children. *Ear and Hearing, 23*, 159–165.

He, C., Hotson, L., & Trainor, L. J. (2007). Mismatch responses to pitch changes in early infancy. *Journal of Cognitive Neuroscience, 19*, 878–892.

He, C., & Trainor, L. J. (2009). Finding the pitch of the missing fundamental in infants. *Journal of Neuroscience, 29*, 7718–7722.

Hill, P. R., Hogben, J. H., & Bishop, D. M. V. (2005). Auditory frequency discrimination in children with specific language impairment: A longitudinal study. *Journal of Speech Language and Hearing Research, 48*, 1136–1146.

Humes, L. E., & Ahlstrom, J. B. (1984). Relation between reaction time and loudness. *Journal of Speech and Hearing Research, 27*, 306–310.

Ikui, A., Sando, I., & Fujita, S. (1997). Postnatal change in angle between the tympanic annulus and surrounding structures: Computer-aided three-dimensional reconstruction study. *Annals of Otology, Rhinology, and Laryngology, 106*, 33–36.

Irwin, R. J., Ball, A. K. R., Kay, N., Stillman, J. A., & Rosser, J. (1985). The development of auditory temporal acuity in children. *Child Development, 56*, 614–620.

Jeffrey, W. E., & Cohen, L. B. (1971). Habituation in the human infant. In H. Reese (Ed.), *Advances in infancy research* (Vol. 6, pp. 63–99). New York, NY: Academic Press.

Jensen, J. K., & Neff, D. L. (1993). Development of basic auditory discrimination in preschool children. *Psychological Science, 4*(2), 104–107.

Keefe, D. H., & Abdala, C. (2007). Theory of forward and reverse middle-ear transmission applied to otoacoustic emissions in infant and adult ears. *Journal of the Acoustical Society of America, 121*, 978–993.

Keefe, D. H., Bulen, J. C., Arehart, K. H., & Burns, E. M. (1993). Ear-canal impedance and reflection coefficient in human infants and adults. *Journal of the Acoustical Society of America, 94*, 2617–2638.

Keefe, D. H., Burns, E. M., Bulen, J. C., & Campbell, S. L. (1994). Pressure transfer function from the diffuse field to the human infant ear canal. *Journal of the Acoustical Society of America, 95*, 355–371.

Keefe, D. H., & Levi, E. (1996). Maturation of the middle and external ears: Acoustic power-based responses and reflectance tympanometry. *Ear and Hearing, 17*, 361–373.

Kidd, G., Mason, C. R., Deliwala, P. S., Woods, W. S., & Colburn, H. S. (1994). Reducing informational masking by sound segregation. *Journal of the Acoustical Society of America, 95*, 3475–3480.

Knudsen, E. I. (1985). Experience alters the spatial tuning of auditory units in the optic tectum during a sensitive period in the barn owl. *Journal of Neuroscience, 5*, 3094–3109.

Koelsch, S., Grossmann, T., Gunter, T. C., Hahne, A., Schroger, E., & Friederici, A. D. (2003). Children processing music: Electric brain responses reveal musical competence and gender differences. *Journal of Cognitive Neuroscience, 15*, 683–693.

Lavigne-Rebillard, M., & Pujol, R. (1987). Surface aspects of the developing human organ of Corti. *Acta Otolaryngologica, 436*, 43–50.

Lavigne-Rebillard, M., & Pujol, R. (1988). Hair cell innervation in the fetal human cochlea. *Acta Otolaryngologica (Stockh.), 105*, 398–402.

Leibold, L., & Neff, D. L. (2007). Effects of masker-spectral variability and masker fringes in children and adults. *Journal of the Acoustical Society of America, 121*, 3666–3676.

Leibold, L., & Werner, W. A. (2002). Relationship between intensity and reaction time in normal hearing infants and adults. *Ear and Hearing, 23*, 92–97.

Leibold, L. J., & Werner, L. A. (2006). Effect of masker-frequency variability on the detection performance of infants and adults. *Journal of the Acoustical Society of America, 119*, 3960–3970.

Levi, E. C., Folsom, R. C., & Dobie, R. A. (1995). Coherence analysis of envelope-following responses (EFRs) and frequency-following responses (FFRs) in infants and adults. *Hearing Research, 89*, 21–27.

Litovsky, R. Y. (1997). Developmental changes in the precedence effect: Estimates of minimum audible angle. *Journal of the Acoustical Society of America, 102*(3), 1739–1745.

Litovsky, R. Y., & Ashmead, D. H. (1997). Development of binaural and spatial hearing in infants and children. In R. H. Gilkey & T. R. Anderson (Eds.), *Binaural and spatial hearing in real and virtual environments* (pp. 571–592). Mahwah, NJ: Lawrence Erlbaum Associates.

Maxon, A. B., & Hochberg, I. (1982). Development of psychoacoustic behavior: Sensitivity and discrimination. *Ear and Hearing, 3*(6), 301–308.

McAdams, S., & Bertoncini, J. (1997). Organization and discrimination of repeating sound sequences by newborn infants. *Journal of the Acoustical Society of America, 102*, 2945–2953.

Moleti, A., Sisto, R., Paglialonga, A., Sibella, F., Anteunis, L., Parazzini, M., & Tognola, G. (2008). Transient evoked otoacoustic emission latency and estimates of cochlear tuning in preterm neonates. *Journal of the Acoustical Society of America, 124*, 2984–2994.

Montgomery, C. R., & Clarkson, M. G. (1997). Infants' pitch perception: Masking by low- and high-frequency noises. *Journal of the Acoustical Society of America, 102*, 3665–3672.

Moore, B. C. J. (1973). Frequency difference limens for short-duration tones. *Journal of the Acoustical Society of America, 54*, 610–619.

Morrongiello, B. A. (1988). Infants' localization of sounds along two spatial dimensions: Horizontal and vertical axes. *Infant Behavior and Development, 11*, 127–143.

Morrongiello, B. A., Fenwick, K., & Chance, G. (1990). Sound localization acuity in very young infants: An observer-based testing procedure. *Developmental Psychology, 26*, 75–84.

Morrongiello, B. A., & Rocca, P. T. (1987). Infants' localization of sounds in the median sagittal plane: Effects of signal frequency. *Journal of the Acoustical Society of America, 82*, 900–905.

Neff, D. L. (1995). Signal properties that reduce masking by simultaneous, random-frequency maskers. *Journal of the Acoustical Society of America, 98*, 1909–1920.

Neff, D. L., & Green, D. M. (1987). Masking produced by spectral uncertainty with multicomponent maskers. *Perception and Psychophysics, 41*(5), 409–415.

Newman, R. S., & Jusczyk, P. W. (1996). The cocktail party effect in infants. *Perception and Psychophysics, 58*(8), 1145–1156.

Nittrouer, S., & Boothroyd, A. (1990). Context effects in phoneme and word recognition by young children and older adults. *Journal of the Acoustical Society of America, 87*, 2705–2715.

Oh, E. L., & Lutfi, R. A. (1998). Nonmonotonicity of informational masking. *Journal of the Acoustical Society of America, 104*, 3489–3499.

Okabe, K., Sachiko, T., Hareo, H., Tanetoshi, M., & Hiroaki, F. (1988). Acoustic impedance measurement on normal ears of children. *Journal of the Acoustical Society of Japan, 9*, 287–294.

Olsho, L. W. (1985). Infant auditory perception: Tonal masking. *Infant Behavior and Development, 8*(4), 371–384.

Olsho, L. W., Koch, E. G., & Carter, E. A. (1988). Nonsensory factors in infant frequency discrimination. *Infant Behavior and Development, 11*, 205–222.

Olsho, L. W., Koch, E. G., Carter, E. A., Halpin, C. F., & Spetner, N. B. (1988). Pure-tone sensitivity of human infants. *Journal of the Acoustical Society of America, 84*, 1316–1324.

Olsho, L. W., Koch, E. G., & Halpin, C. F. (1987). Level and age effects in infant frequency discrimination. *Journal of the Acoustical Society of America, 82*, 454–464.

Pickles, J. O. (2008). *An introduction to the physiology of hearing* (3rd ed.). Bingley, UK: Emerald Press.

Ponton, C. W., Moore, J. K., & Eggermont, J. J. (1996). Auditory brain stem response generation by parallel pathways: Differential maturation of axonal conduction time and synaptic transmission. *Ear and Hearing, 17*, 402–410.

Pujol, R., Lavigne-Rebillard, M., & Uziel, A. (1991). Development of the human cochlea. *Acta Otolaryngologica, 482*(Suppl.), 7–12.

Rosen, S. (1989). Temporal information in speech and its relevance for cochlear implants. In B. Fraypse & N. Cothard (Eds.), *Cochlear implants: Acquisitions and controversies* (pp. 3–26). Toulouse, France: Impasse La Caussade.

Ruah, C. B., Schachern, P. A., Zelterman, D., Paparella, M. M., & Yoon T. H. (1991). Age-related morphological changes in the human tympanic membrane. A light and electron microscopy study. *Archives of Otolaryngology-Head & Neck Surgery, 117*, 627–634.

Sanes, D. H., & Constantine-Paton, M. (1985). The sharpening of frequency tuning curves requires patterned activity during development in the mouse, *Mus musculus*. *Journal of Neuroscience, 5*, 1152–1166.

Schlauch, R. S., & Hafter, E. R. (1991). Listening bandwidths and frequency uncertainty in pure-tone signal detection. *Journal of the Acoustical Society of America, 90*, 1332–1339.

Schneider, B. A., Morrongiello, B. A., & Trehub, S. E. (1990). The size of the critical band in infants, children, and adults. *Journal of Experimental Psychology: Human Perception and Performance, 16*, 642–652.

Schneider, B. A., Trehub, S. E., Morrongiello, B. A., & Thorpe, L. A. (1989). Developmental changes in masked thresholds. *Journal of the Acoustical Society of America, 86*, 1733–1742.

Sinnott, J. M., & Aslin, R. N. (1985). Frequency and intensity discrimination in human infants and adults. *Journal of the Acoustical Society of America, 78*, 1986–1992.

Spetner, N. B., & Olsho, L. W. (1990). Auditory frequency resolution in human infancy. *Child Development, 61*, 632–652.

Sussman, E., Wong, R., Horvath, J., Winkler, I., & Wang, W. (2007). The development of the perceptual organization of sound by frequency separation in 5- to 11-year-old children. *Hearing Research, 225*, 117–127.

Tharpe, A. M., & Ashmead, D. H. (2001). A longitudinal investigation of infant auditory sensitivity. *American Journal of Audiology, 10*, 104–112.

Trainor, L., McFadden, M., Hodgson, L., Darragh, L., Barlow, J., Matsos, L., & Sonnadara, R. (2003). Changes in auditory cortex and the development of mismatch negativity between 2 and 6 months of age. *International Journal of Psychophysiology, 51*, 5–15.

Trehub, S. E., Schneider, B. A., & Endman, M. (1980). Developmental changes in infants' sensitivity to octave-band noises. *Journal of Experimental Child Psychology, 29*, 282–293.

Trehub, S. E., Schneider, B. A., & Henderson, J. (1995). Gap detection in infants, children and adults. *Journal of the Acoustical Society of America, 98*, 2532–2541.

Trehub, S. E., Schneider, B. A., Morrongiello, B. A., & Thorpe, L. A. (1988). Auditory sensitivity in school-age children. *Journal of Experimental Child Psychology, 46*, 273–285.

Viemeister, N. F. (1979). Temporal modulation transfer functions based upon modulation thresholds. *Journal of the Acoustical Society of America, 66*, 1364–1380.

Viemeister, N. F., & Schlauch, R. S. (1992). Issues in infant psychoacoustics. In L. A. Werner & E. W. Rubel (Eds.), *Developmental psychoacoustics* (pp. 191–210). Washington, DC: American Psychological Association.

Watson, C. S., Wroton, H. W., Kelly, W. J., & Benbassat, C. A. (1975). Factors in the discrimination of tonal patterns. I. Component frequency, temporal position, and silent intervals. *Journal of the Acoustical Society of America, 57*, 1175–1185.

Werner, L. A. (1996). The development of auditory behavior (or what the anatomists and physiologists have to explain). *Ear and Hearing, 17*, 438–446.

Werner, L. A. (2007). Issues in human auditory development. *Journal of Communication Disorders, 40*, 275–283.

Werner, L. A., & Boike, K. (2001). Infants' sensitivity to broadband noise. *Journal of the Acoustical Society of America, 109*, 2101–2111.

Werner, L. A., Folsom, R. C., & Mancl, L. R. (1994). The relationship between auditory brainstem response latencies and behavioral thresholds in normal hearing infants and adults. *Hearing Research, 77*, 88–98.

Werner, L. A., Folsom, R. C., Mancl, L. R., & Syapin, C. (2001). Human auditory brainstem response to temporal gaps in noise. *Journal of Speech, Language, and Hearing Research, 44*, 737–750.

Werner, L. A., & Holmer, N. M. (2002). *Infant hearing thresholds measured in the ear canal*. Paper presented at The American Auditory Society conference, Scottsdale, AZ.

Werner, L. A., & Leibold, L. J. (2004). Ecological developmental psychoacoustics. In J. Neuhoff (Ed.), *Ecological psychoacoustics* (pp. 192–219). San Diego, CA: Elsevier.

Werner, L. A., & Marean, G. C. (1995). *Human auditory development*. Boulder, CO: Westview Press.

Werner, L. A., & Marean, G. C. (1996). Methods for estimating infant thresholds. *Journal of the Acoustical Society of America, 90*, 1867–1875.

Werner, L. A., Marean, G. C., Halpin, C. F., Spetner, N. B., & Gillenwater, J. M. (1992). Infant auditory temporal acuity: Gap detection. *Child Development, 63*, 260–272.

Werner, L. A., Parrish, H. K., & Holmer, N. M. (2009). Effects of temporal uncertainty and temporal expectancy on infants' auditory sensitivity. *Journal of the Acoustical Society of America, 125*, 1040–1049.

Werner, L. A., & Rubel, E. W. (Eds.). (1992). *Developmental psychoacoustics*. Washington, DC: American Psychological Association.

Wightman, F., & Allen, P. (1992). Individual differences in auditory capability among preschool children. In L. A.

Werner & E. W. Rubel (Eds.), *Developmental psychoacoustics* (pp. 113–133). Washington, DC: American Psychological Association.

Wightman, F. L., Allen, P., Dolan, T., Kistler, D., & Jamieson, D. (1989). Temporal resolution in children. *Child Development, 60*, 611–624.

Wightman, F. L., Callahan, M. R., Lutfi, R. A., Kistler, D. J., & Oh, E. (2003). Children's detection of pure-tone signals: Informational masking with contralateral mask-ers. *Journal of the Acoustical Society of America, 113*, 3297–3305.

Wightman, F. L., & Kistler, D. J. (2005). Informational masking of speech in children: Effects of ipsilateral and contralateral distracters. *Journal of the Acoustical Society of America, 118*, 3164–3176.

Wilmington, D., Gray, L., & Jahrsdorfer, R. (1994). Binaural processing after corrected congenital unilateral conductive hearing loss. *Hearing Research, 74*, 99–114.

Winkler, I., Kushnerenko, E., Horvath, J., Ceponiene, R., Fellman, V., Huotilainen, M., . . . Sussman, E. (2003). Newborn infants can organize the auditory world. *Proceedings of the National Academy of Sciences of the United States of America, 100*, 11812–11815.

Yost, W. A. (1997). The cocktail party problem: Forty years later. In R. A. Gilkey & T. R. Anderson (Eds.), *Binaural and spatial hearing in real and virtual environments* (pp. 329–347). Hillsdale, NJ: Erlbaum.

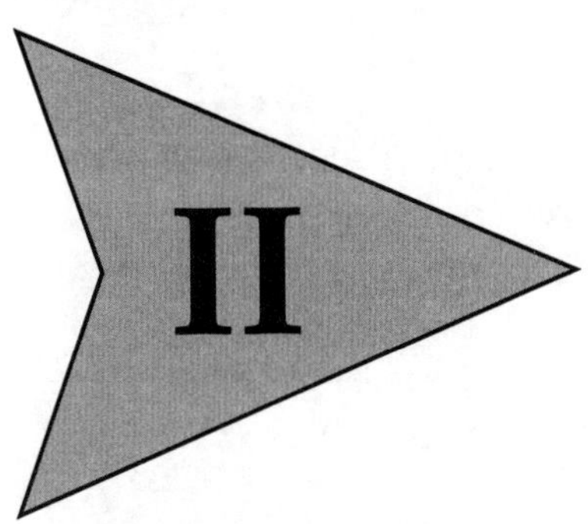

Etiology and Medical Considerations

Descriptive Epidemiology of Childhood Hearing Impairment

Adrian Davis and Katrina A.S. Davis

Introduction

The impact of hearing impairment on a newborn or developing child can be wide ranging and major. Not only does hearing impairment impact on method and quality of communication, but research also indicates potential difficulties in learning and education (Fitzpatrick, 2015; Stacey, Fortnum, Barton, & Summerfield, 2006), a risk of mental illness (Hindley, Hill, McGuigan, & Kitson, 1994; Theunissen et al., 2014), and restricted employment opportunities (Punch, Creed, & Hyde, 2005). As no child exists in isolation, an impairment also affects the family and systems supporting the child and family, whether they be statutory services or informal social networks (Hintermair, 2000). By nature of the depth of its impact for the individual, family, and local community, childhood deafness and hearing impairment represent an important public health issue.

Major epidemiologic influences on the prioritization for commissioning services are

1. the number of children living with deafness or hearing impairment (both recognized and yet to receive a diagnosis);
2. the degree and type of impairment and age of onset;
3. the predominant etiology of deafness; and
4. the potential costs and effectiveness of service provision, in both the prevention and amelioration of the limitations on the deaf by society (handicap).

However, the allocation of public resources to deafness and hearing impairment will depend not only on "need," but also on how this argument is presented. For example, is the argument made by public opinion and lobbying by patient advocacy groups and associations (National Deaf Children's Society, 2014; Society for Sound Hearing, 2015); how well is it received into local, national, and international politics; and what are the constraints, such as financial limitations?

Definitions

The two terms *prevalence* and *deafness* give potential for confusion. The term *prevalence* is used here to refer to the number of people in a defined population with a stated characteristic at a particular time, for example, the number of people who report a hearing problem in 2016. Sometimes, the prevalence is stated as a percentage of the population. A term related to prevalence is *incidence*, which is defined as the number of new cases in a defined population with a stated characteristic over a particular time period; for example, the number of people with a new hearing problem arising between January 1, 2016, and December 31, 2016. The term *deafness* has many dimensions, some of which have unwanted connotations. From a practical point of view, it is often difficult to decide how and where to draw the line between who is deaf and who is not, particularly when carrying out a survey to determine prevalence. To overcome this terminological problem, in the rest of this chapter the more easily quantifiable term *childhood hearing impairment* is used. Example definitions based on those used in the World Health Organization Global Burden of Disease project (WHO-GBD; Stevens et al.,

2012) are shown in Table 5–1, but the exact definition used in published work has varied between countries and study groups.

We refer to congenital hearing impairment, meaning that which is present and detectable using appropriate tests at or very soon after birth—the converse being postnatal hearing impairment. Where children experience temporary hearing impairment, such as otitis media with effusion (OME or "glue ear"), the individual consequences are not as severe as permanent childhood hearing impairment (PCHI), but the greater numbers of children with OME mean that temporary hearing loss does have considerable impact on services (Hoffman et al., 2013). Both congenital and acquired hearing impairments can be progressive in severity over time. The severity of hearing impairment is typically categorized as slight, mild, moderate, severe, and profound based on hearing thresholds, with thresholds taken from the better ear to describe bilateral hearing impairment or the worse ear when considering unilateral hearing impairment. Also, sometimes distinction is made between mechanisms or type of hearing impair-

Table 5–1. Proposed Definitions of Hearing Impairment

Pathology
Sensorineural: related to disease/deformity of the inner ear/cochlear nerve with an air-bone gap less than 15 dB HL averaged over 0.5, 1, and 2 kHz • *Sensory:* a subdivision of sensorineural related to disease or deformity in the cochlea • *Neural:* a subdivision of sensorineural related to a disease or deformity in the cochlear nerve • *Central:* sensorineural hearing loss related to a disease or deformity of the central nervous system beyond the cochlear nerve
Conductive: related to disease or deformity of the outer/middle ears. Audiometrically, there are normal bone conduction thresholds (less than 20 dB) and an air-bone gap greater than 15 dB averaged over 0.5, 1, and 2 kHz
Mixed: related to combined involvement of the outer/middle ears and the inner ear/cochlear nerve. Audiometrically greater than 20 dB HL in the bone conduction threshold together with greater than or equal to 15 dB air-bone gap averaged over 0.5, 1, and 2 kHz
Severity
Average hearing level: the level of the thresholds (in dB HL) measured in the better-hearing ear at 0.5, 1, 2, and 4 kHz.
Mild: average hearing level 20–34 dB
Moderate: average hearing level 35–49 dB
Moderately Severe: average hearing level 50–64 dB
Severe: average hearing level 65–79 dB
Profound: average hearing level >80 dB
Symmetry
Unilateral: one ear only has either a greater than 20 dB hearing impairment through 0.5, 1, and 2 kHz or one frequency exceeding 50 dB, with the other ear normal
Bilateral: greater than 20 dB hearing impairment through 0.5, 1, and 2 kHz or one frequency exceeding 50 dB in both ears
Asymmetric: greater than 10 dB difference between the ears in at least two frequencies, with the pure-tone average in the better ear exceeding 20 dB

ment in terms of sensory, neural, conductive, or mixed. WHO-GBD defines a bilateral deficit with better ear average thresholds 35 dB hearing level (HL) or greater as having the potential to benefit greatly from intervention, while acknowledging that mild and unilateral hearing loss also cause disability.

Prevalence

Estimates for the prevalence of childhood hearing impairment worldwide have been hindered by variations in how cases are defined and found between studies seeking to answer this question. The prevalence of hearing impairment as an indicator of population need for hearing services should not be estimated by clinical performance indicators such as the number of cochlear implants or hearing aids fitted each year, as the hidden nature of hearing impairment can lead to substantial unmet need. Instead, we have typically had to rely on cross-sectional epidemiological studies of retrospective ascertainment. One of the largest such studies, aimed at a calculation of prevalence of PCHI across the whole of the United Kingdom, was carried out by Fortnum and colleagues in the 1990s (Fortnum, Marshall, & Summerfield, 2002; Fortnum, Summerfield, Marshall, Davis, & Bamford, 2001). They approached both health and education professionals responsible for children with hearing impairment around the country, requesting details on every child with PCHI under their care. Professionals replied with over 26,000 sets of details. This allowed them to estimate the prevalence of moderate or greater PCHI in the United Kingdom was between one and two per 1,000 children. The inclusion of such large numbers in the study allowed a breakdown into subgroups, demonstrating the variability of prevalence across age and severity. This study and other "notification" studies have the weakness in that they include only those already identified, tending to underestimate the younger and milder cases, as well as the hard-to-reach populations such as the very poor and ethnic minorities.

An alternative is a cross-sectional survey, actively seeking children with a hearing impairment. These are not practical where impairment is at the levels found above, but come into their own when looking at milder impairment. Also in the 1990s, the Third U.S. National Health and Nutritional Examination Survey (NHANES III; Niskar et al., 1998) screened 6,497 children and found a detectable hearing loss in 14.9%, mostly unilateral and slight in severity. They found a small number of children with bilateral hearing loss of mild or greater severity, which they estimated had a point prevalence of between two and seven per 1,000 (>25 dB HL, better ear average of 0.5, 1, and 2 kHz) but could not say how likely this was to be a permanent or progressive impairment as opposed to a temporary one.

Although not an epidemiological study as such, results from the implementation of universal newborn hearing screening (UNHS) programs now have results from millions of babies, and provide a yield of hearing impairment detected per 1,000 babies screened. Depending on (a) the coverage (percentage of babies screened out of the total babies born), (b) the sensitivity of the test, and (c) the numbers of families returning for diagnostic assessment, the prevalence of congenital hearing impairment can be determined with increasing confidence. Prevalence estimates based on UNHS are in effect based on retrospective ascertainment, having the same limitations as other notification studies for milder cases and those not receiving health care.

English UNHS Data

We have reviewed the data from the first 7 years of the national universal newborn hearing screening program in the NHS in England (Wood, Sutton, & Davis, 2015). Over the 7 years from April 2006 until April 2013, the program achieved almost 97% coverage with 4.6 million babies screened. Among the babies referred from the screen, 93% received follow-up. A confirmed permanent bilateral hearing loss of moderate or greater severity was found in 5,463 cases over the course of follow-up. This leads to a rate of PCHI of 1.19 (95% 1.16–1.22) per 1,000 babies screened (≥40 dB HL better ear average [BEA] 0.5, 1, 2, and 4 kHz). A further 3,315 babies were found to have unilateral hearing loss. Although the bilateral hearing loss was many times more common for babies from neonatal intensive care units (NICUs) over their well peers (6.5 versus 0.86 per 1,000), most cases did not come from the NICUs, with well babies accounting for over 65% of cases found.

The information technology (IT) system that supports UNHS in England allows clinicians to record permanent hearing loss identified in a child that was covered by the UNHS program, whether or not the screen helped identify the child as needing audiology assessment. Analysis of the routes to identification can help identify subgroups that need more attention. For example, in Figure 5–1, we can see that a significant proportion (11%) of the people eventually diagnosed with hearing loss had initially passed the screen. At time of diagnosis of these children who had originally passed the screen, clinicians were asked to judge whether the

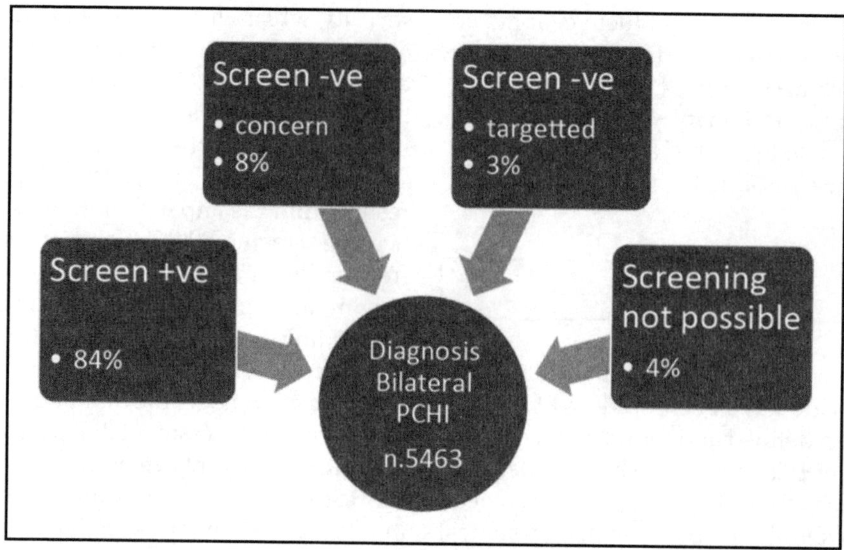

FIGURE 5–1. Routes to identification of a bilateral PCHI in children aged 1 to 7 years who were screened in the English universal newborn hearing screening program. (PCHI, permanent children hearing impairment; −ve, negative; +ve, positive.)

loss was likely to have been (a) present at birth but not picked up, (b) late-onset hearing loss, or (c) acquired postnatally; they split 25% present at birth (true-false negatives), 50% late-onset, and 25% acquired, of which over half were due to meningitis.

Severity

As the severity of a hearing impairment will affect its impact on a child and family and be an indicator of the extra help needed, studies that have been large enough stratify into severity bands. In the English UNHS data, of those who received evaluations, 54% had moderate, 27% severe, and 18% profound hearing loss. Figure 5–2 compares these results to UNHS data collated by the Centers for Disease Control (CDC) from the states across America for 2006 (CDC, 2008), the results of Polish UNHS program (Szyfter, Wrobel, Szyfter-Harris, & Greczka, 2013), and the large notification study in the United Kingdom (Fortnum et al., 2002). Data from CDC (2008) also include newborns diagnosed with mild bilateral hearing impairment, not shown in Figure 5–2. If they are included, they make up 23% of the total. However, UNHS programs are not particularly sensitive to mild hearing impairments—their aim is to catch potentially disabling losses prelingually—so these data are less robust.

The decision to concentrate screening on moderate and greater hearing impairment rather than increase sensitivity for mild cases is partly because it is much less clear what the needs are, both in terms of numbers of children with mild PCHI or impact on a child's development (Bamford, Uus, & Davis, 2005; Khairi Md Daud, Noor, Rahman, Sidek, & Mohamad, 2009; Wake et al., 2006). In terms of slight sensorineural hearing loss (SNHL), NHANES III (Niskar et al., 1998) found 16 per 1,000 cases of bilateral high-frequency loss, which they suggest is sensorineural, in their sample of 6- to 19-year-olds, whereas Wake et al. (2006) found less than half this rate in a sample of Australian school children aged 7 and 11 years (6.2 per 1,000). For mild SNHL, another study from the United States (Bess, Dodd-Murphy, & Parker, 1998) found 10 per 1,000 in a sample aged 9 to 15 years, whereas in the United Kingdom, a study of a group of 11-year-olds found 4 per 1,000 (Hall, Midgley, Steer, & Humphriss, 2011) and Wake et al. found 2.6 per 1,000. It is not clear to what extent the differences are due to methodology (such as the level of background noise during testing), the age of the children, or other demographics. The value of research in this area lies in identifying risk factors for hearing loss generally (for possible primary prevention), and factors associated with further deterioration of hearing and handicap from hearing loss (for possible secondary and tertiary prevention). In the developing world, mild hearing loss is many times more common

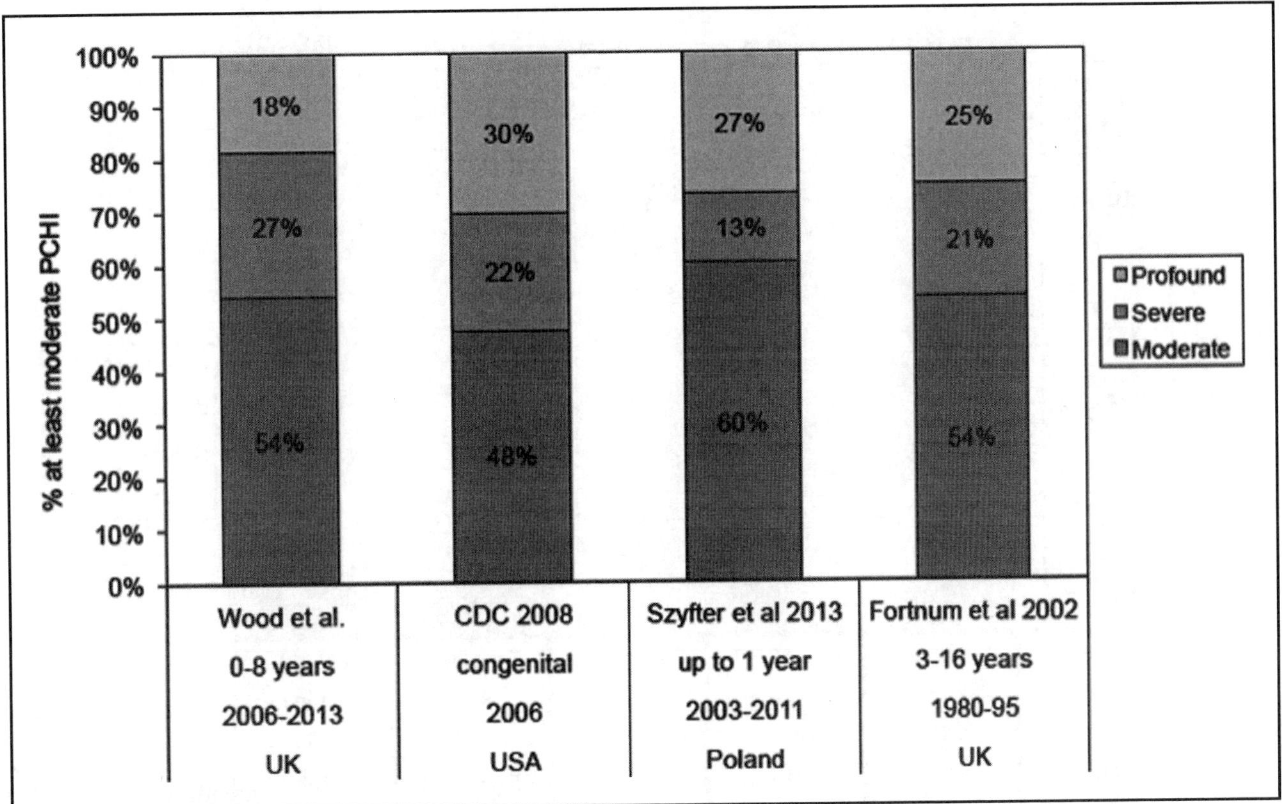

FIGURE 5–2. The severity distribution of permanent children hearing impairment (PCHI; moderate and greater) as reported in these populations.

(Khairi Md Daud et al., 2009), and a large proportion is related to active ear disease (such as chronic supporative otitis media), where identification for intervention might be warranted.

Site of Impairment

Some studies have published the distribution of the nature or "site" of the impairment—conductive in the outer or middle ear, or sensorineural (SNHL) in the inner ear and beyond. A subcategory of SNHL comprising neural and central hearing impairment, now known as auditory neuropathy spectrum disorder (ANSD), deserves special consideration in services with regard to newborn hearing screening. ANSD appears to be related to widespread neurological insult, especially hyperbilirubinemia, and associated with other abnormal findings (El-Badry, Hamdy, Sobhy, & Gamal, 2014; Kirkim, Serbetcioglu, Erdag, & Ceryan, 2008; Madden, Rutter, Hilbert, Greinwald, & Choo, 2002), but also occurs in apparently low-risk infants (Korver, van Zanten, Meuwese-Jongejeugd, van Straaten, & Oudesluys-Murphy, 2012). An infant with ANSD has a functioning inner ear, and thus may have normal otoacoustic emission (OAE) at birth, but further testing would reveal no, or abnormal, auditory brainstem response (ABR; Korver et al., 2012; Madden et al., 2002). ANSD will not be picked up by newborn hearing screening protocols that discharge all babies who pass OAE testing. The decision whether this protocol should be changed depends on (a) the prevalence of the disorder in the population and subgroups; and (b) the prognosis and management of children with ANSD.

Figure 5–3 shows six sets of results: two from UNHS data (CDC, 2008; Wood et al., 2015) and four specifically looking for ANSD (Foerst et al., 2006; Lotfi & Mehrkian, 2007; Sanyelbhaa Talaat, Kabel, Samy, & Elbadry, 2009; Tang, McPherson, Yuen, Wong, & Lee, 2004). The number of cases recorded in England is significantly higher than that recorded by the CDC ($p < 0.05$) but in line with other young cohorts in Figure 5–3. There is the suggestion that there is a change in hearing as the cohort ages, which could represent spontaneous improvement, show deterioration in the cochlear

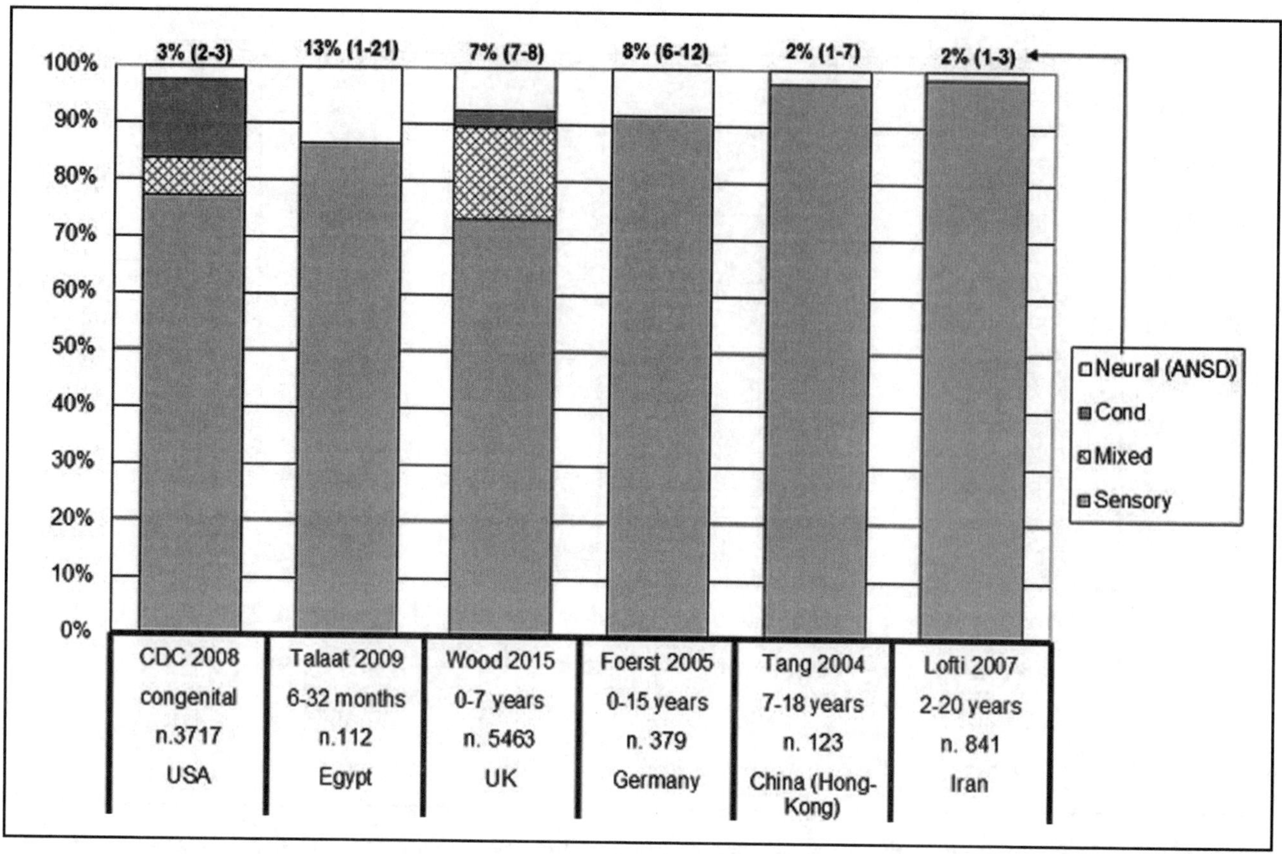

FIGURE 5–3. Site of hearing impairment in large surveys ordered by upper age bound: sensory, conductive, mixed, and auditory neuropathy spectrum disorder (ANSD), with proportion attributed to ANSD highlighted above (with 95% confidence intervals).

in some children with ANSD (hence a shift from ANSD to apparent SNHL), or be an artifact of some kind. Some studies have shown that up to one half of cases of auditory neuropathy are not picked up by newborn screening (Rodriguez Dominguez, Cubillana Herrero, Canizares Gallardo, & Perez Aguilera, 2007), which suggests that the results taken from UNHS could be under-representating the true prevalence. The English UNHS program screens NICU babies with OAE and ABR as first-line, but well babies with OAE alone. Of the 420 cases of ANSD in the follow-up data, only 6% had received a false-negative result at the original screening (compared to 11% for non-ANSD cases). There had been no false negatives from the NICU (accounting for 73% of the cases) but over 25% false negatives from the well babies.

The level of permanent conductive hearing loss seems greater in the U.S. cases. However, given that the size of conductive plus mixed conductive-sensory is approximately equal, it seems likely this is an issue of definition rather than true difference. It would be reasonable to presume that middle-ear problems contribute to the hearing loss of about 20% of all cases in both countries.

Variations in Prevalence

Age

True prevalence of PCHI is likely to vary across a population, but the prevalence in research studies varies for a variety of reasons, so it can be difficult to pick apart what variables in the population have what effect. One question that has been difficult to answer has been *when* children with PCHI develop hearing loss—at birth, as babies, or later? The answer to this will help plan screening and other services. The cross-sectional study by Fortnum and colleagues (Fortnum et al., 2001, 2002) found that the observed prevalence of moderate to profound PCHI increased from 1.1 per 1,000 at age 3 years, reaching a plateau at age 9 years with 2.1 per 1,000, implying that either children continued to develop PCHI well into their school years or were only finally recognized after they had started school.

A number of studies looking longitudinally have now been performed based around cohorts who received screening as newborns. Watkin and colleagues in the United Kingdom (Watkin & Baldwin, 2012) reported on the 6-year-old children known to the department with PCHI. Sixty-four had been identified by neonatal screen (1.79 per 1,000) and 46 had not, mostly mild and unilateral cases, making prevalence 3.09 per 1,000. Nine of those found after the screen had moderate or worse bilateral hearing loss (20% of all cases of moderate or worse hearing loss), and all had risk factors: five had meningitis, four a specific syndrome. In Austria, a group (Weichbold, Nekahm-Heis, & Welzl-Mueller, 2006a, 2006b) found postnatal loss making up around a quarter of known PCHI in their area by age 9 years. Of 23 postnatal cases they found, 18 had one of nine risk factors. In the Ostfold region of Norway (Nelson, Andersen, & Anderssen, 2015), a slightly different story was presented, in that, although similar numbers of babies with apparently normal screening tests developed hearing loss, only half had risk factors.

In Queensland, Australia, they looked at children who had any risk factors and found that 2.6% went on to develop postnatal PCHI (Beswick, Driscoll, Kei, Khan, & Glennon, 2013). In the Hubei Province of China, they looked only at children who had no risk factors and who had passed UNHS, finding that nearly 1 in 1,000 developed PCHI (with many more having potentially reversible conductive hearing loss), of which around a third was moderate or worse bilaterally (Chen, Fu, Luo, Zhang, & Yang, 2013).

The last two studies were involved in actively finding new cases, but most other studies are dependent on notification from services after a diagnosis has been made. Diagnosis might be delayed in cases where the impairment is not recognized or prioritized due to social and geographical barriers (Bush et al., 2014; Lai, Serraglio, & Martin, 2014), or where a child has complex needs arising from birth defects (Chapman et al., 2011).

Current evidence suggests that the apparent rise in prevalence with age is made up of

- children who acquire their impairment during childhood (e.g., meningitis in the Waltham Forest study);
- children whose cause of their hearing impairment is present at birth but manifest it later (e.g., craniofacial abnormalities in the Queensland study);
- children who have the confirmation of their hearing impairment delayed because of
  - screening methods that miss auditory neuropathy syndrome disorder (ANSD), mild bilateral and unilateral impairments (all factors in Waltham Forest), and other system delays; and
  - losses that are progressive or fluctuating (such as the conductive losses seen in Hubei).

English UNHS Data and Age

The UNHS program in England aims to complete assessment of 80% of babies identified by newborn screening within 6 months' gestational age, and assessment of 98% of babies by 12 months, so any diagnosis made after this could be thought of as delayed for one reason or another. Looking at the later diagnoses, it is necessary to adjust for the fact that the cohorts range from 1 to 7 years of age. After doing this, we find that 70% of all eventual diagnoses were made by 12 months, as shown in Figure 5–4. However, we are aware that clinicians did not always enter PCHI diagnosis for older children into the UNHS IT system, which could lead to underestimation of the number of diagnoses eventually made. From the figures we have, we arrive at a conservative projected 789 cases diagnosed between the ages of 1 and 7 years. Cases diagnosed later are not necessarily later onset—in fact, 48% of cases were thought to be congenital onset, with only 9% thought to be acquired, the rest were late-onset of congenital susceptibility, as shown in Figure 5–5.

Using UNHS data, we can estimate that the number of children diagnosed with bilateral disabling PCHI by age 7 years is in excess of 1.4 per 1,000, most of whom screened positive at birth (85%) and were diagnosed by 12 months of age (70%). In 7 years, just under 1,000 had their hearing loss "missed" by UNHS and picked up later (14%), while around 1,000 likely acquired a hearing loss after UNHS occurred (15%). Comparing this with the Austrian and Norwegian studies (Nelson et al., 2015; Weichbold, Nekahm-Heis, & Welzl-Mueller, 2006a, 2006b), it seems likely that services can expect that, in addition to the number of babies identified by UNHS, another 25% to 50% will become known later on, some of whom are predictable (e.g., babies who missed follow-up from failed screening, have craniofacial anomalies or survived meningitis) and many of whom are not. Although children seem at greater risk of developing hearing loss early on, congenital and other losses can also start or deteriorate later.

Aside from using data from the health services, one way to estimate the magnitude of need is enquiring in the education system. The British Association of Teachers of the Deaf carry out a survey of its members every year to see how many children in their area have been identified as potentially needing extra help due to hearing problems (Consortium for Research in Deaf Education, 2014). The teachers of the deaf identified

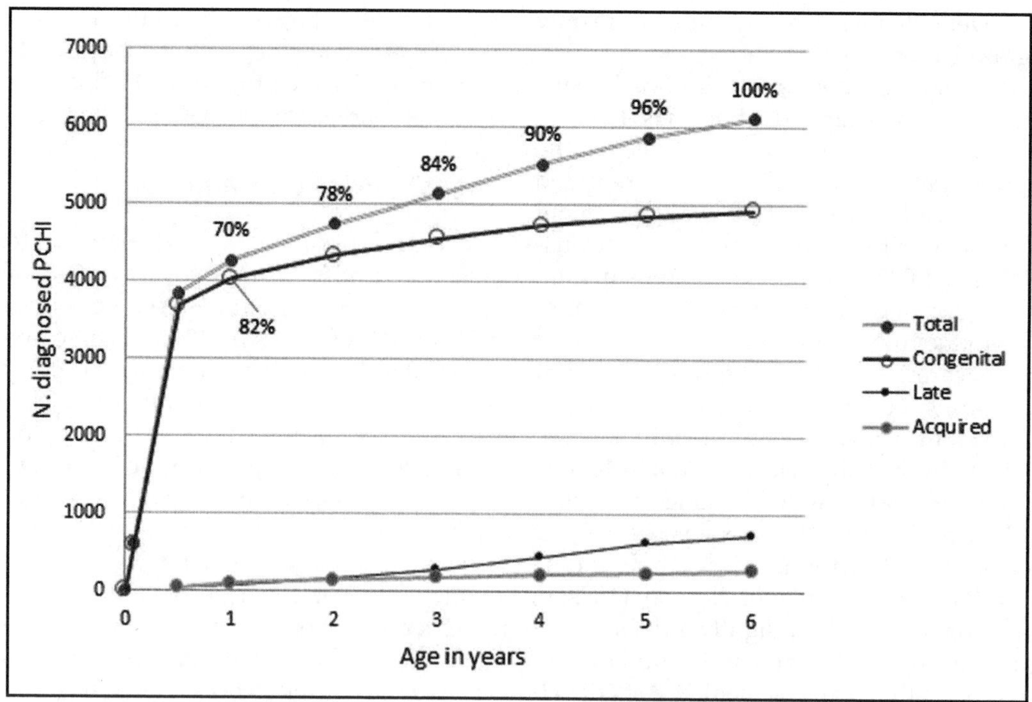

FIGURE 5–4. Age of diagnosis of PCHI in English screening cohort, numbers of children, and percentage of projected total by age 6 years. Estimation of timing of onset (congenital, hearing loss present soon after birth; late, cause of hearing loss presumed present at birth but hearing loss came later; acquired, cause of hearing loss came after birth) given by clinician on diagnosis. (PCHI, permanent children hearing impairment.)

40,614 such children in England. This equates to 3.6 per 1,000 children, well in excess of the numbers provided by the UNHS program. This fits with what we know from the Waltham Forest study where, once mild and unilateral losses were taken into account, the screen had identified only half of all cases of PCHI that were apparent by school age (Watkin & Baldwin, 2012). There will be a further contribution from persistent conductive loss such as otitis media with effusion (S.A. Wood, personal communication, 2015). For those not picked up at UNHS, the most important source for referral was parental suspicion (Bamford et al., 2007). Therefore, vigilance and attention to parental concern, for instance where this can be incorporated into systematic school screening, are essential throughout childhood so that children with mild, fluctuating, deteriorating, or unilateral hearing loss are identified to maximize their potential for learning speech and education.

Sex Ratio

Boys make up a slight, but significant, majority of the cases from large research studies of PCHI around the world, with a relative risk around 1.1 (see, for example, Fortnum et al., 2002). Because most unmanipulated populations have an approximately even split of male and female babies, this excess is due either to a higher prevalence or better detection. The consensus is that PCHI is more prevalent in boys. For poorly understood reasons, male babies have a higher incidence of perinatal problems and a higher prevalence of many congenital abnormalities (Di Renzo, Rosati, Sarti, Cruciani, & Cutuli, 2007; Kraemer, 2000), both of which correlate with hearing problems. They also are known to have more middle ear disease (Bennett & Haggard, 1998).

Country

Findings from the study in the Trent region of the United Kingdom (Fortnum & Davis, 1997) can be compared with studies done around the same time with similar methods and the same definitions of hearing impairment. For example, preliminary data were compared with data from Denmark (Davis & Parving, 1994) showing similar rates of PCHI, approximately 90% of which was presumed congenital. However, this head-

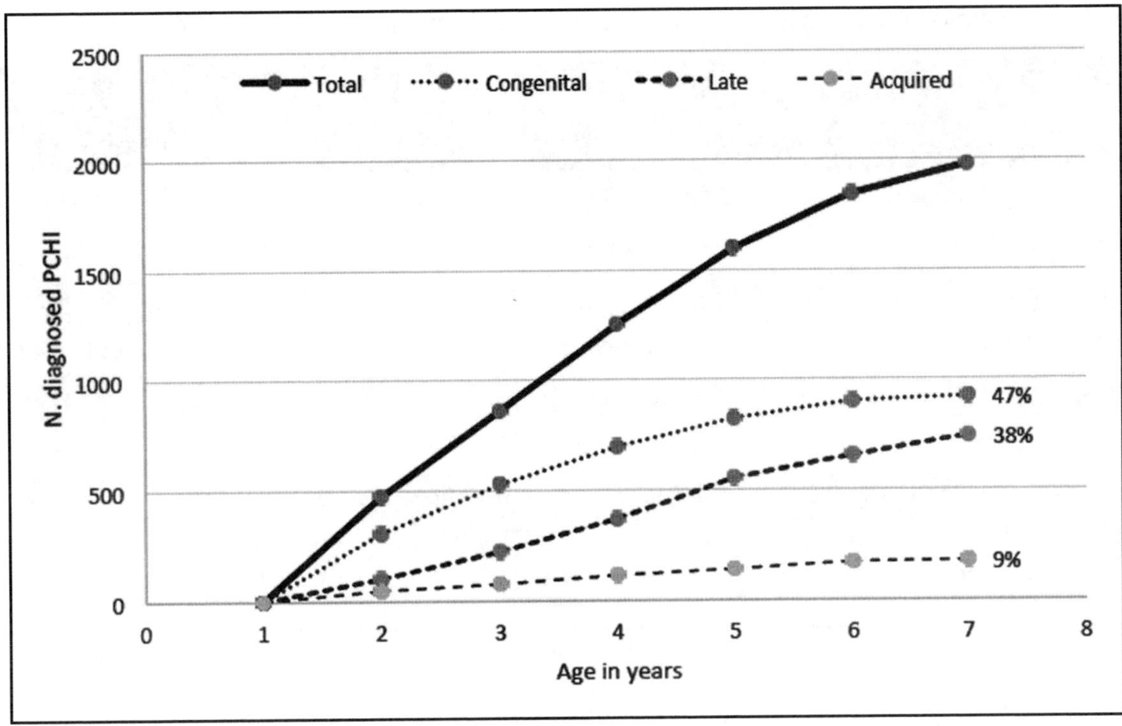

FIGURE 5–5. Projection of age of diagnosis for PCHI diagnosed after 1 year of age based on partial sample. Estimation of timing of onset (congenital, hearing loss present soon after birth; late, cause of hearing loss presumed present at birth but hearing loss came later; acquired, cause of hearing loss came after birth; PCHI, permanent children hearing impairment.)

line figure disguised some more subtle differences, including significantly more severely and profoundly hearing-impaired children in Denmark with higher levels of family history and lower levels of NICU admission than in England. Data used in comparative studies are shown in Table 5–2 (Baker, Crockett, Uus, Bamford, & Marteau, 2007; Maki-Torkko, Lindholm, Vayrynen, Leisti, & Sorri, 1998; Parving & Stephens, 1997; Uus & Davis, 2000). These results can also be compared against those from Atlanta, Georgia (Drews, Yeargin-Allsopp, Murphy, & Decoufle, 1994), although the study is less similar in design and definition. This demonstrates the differences in prevalence vary even between similar countries, and the differences between disparate countries are likely to be even greater.

Thus, data extrapolated from studies such as the Trent study might not be appropriate to plan services in less-developed countries. To overcome this bias, The World Health Organization (WHO) encourages countries to conduct random sample, population-based prevalence and etiology surveys of hearing impairment in children (WHO, 2015). Importantly, it publishes a protocol for good practice and enables studies to be more comparable. The survey protocol includes the identification of conductive and potentially reversible middle ear disease. This is appropriate in developing countries where the presence of middle ear disease is highly correlated with a long-term hearing loss and is in itself a major public health problem (Alberti, 1999; WHO, 2012; WHO & Acuin, 2004). These surveys and others were examined by the WHO Global Burden of Disease group, who built them into a model to make predictions about the prevalence of hearing loss broadly everywhere (Stevens et al., 2013). They estimate that in children aged 5 to 14 years, disabling hearing loss affects 1.4%, that is, 14 per 1,000, well in excess of any of the estimates from Table 5–2. This is because higher prevalence of hearing impairment was found to be positively associated with lower-income countries. To illustrate the point, Table 5–3 compares the rates of hearing loss at school age for a wider set of countries. The study from London, United Kingdom, was not a survey (Watkin & Baldwin, 2011), but it provides an accurate point of reference for five school surveys or screening pilots. Urban parts of Poland (Gierek, Gwozdz-Jezierska,

Table 5–2. Comparative Data Regarding Prevalence of PCHI From Europe and United States

Cohort	*Reference*	*Moderate or Greater*	*Profound *PTA > 90 dB; †PTA ≥ 95 dB*
Wales, United Kingdom (1975–1980)	Parving & Stephens, 1997	NR	0.41* (0.31–0.53)
Denmark (1975–1980)	Parving & Stephens, 1997	NR	0.45* (0.31–0.64)
Trent area, United Kingdom (1985–1990)	Fortnum & Davis, 1997	1.33 (1.22–1.45)	0.24† (0.20–0.30)
Denmark (1982–1988)	Davis & Parving, 1994	1.45 (1.25–1.68)	0.54† (0.42–0.69)
Oulu Area, Finland (1973–1992)	Maki-Torkko et al., 1998	1.19 (1.05–1.35)	0.36† (0.29–0.46)
Estonia (1985–1990)	Uus & Davis, 2000	1.72 (1.51–1.94)	NR
Glasgow, United Kingdom (1985–1994)	MacAndie, Kubba, & McFarlane, 2003	1.23 (1.03–1.46)	NR
Atlanta, Georgia, United States (1985–1987)	Drews et al., 1994	1.1 (0.9–1.4)	0.5* (0.4–0.7)

Note. Estimated prevalence per 1,000 live births (estimated 95% confidence intervals calculated for this table). *NR* = not reported.

Table 5–3. Estimated Prevalence of Bilateral Hearing Impairment in School-Aged Children Based on Survey Results

Study	*Screened*	*Bilateral SNHL Greater or Above Prevalence per 1,000 Children*	*Bilateral SNHL Severe or Profound Prevalence per 1,000 Children*
Waltham Forest, London, UK* Watkin & Baldwin, 2011	n. 100,096 5–6 years	1.5 (1.3–1.8)	0.3 @ 95 dB
Upper Silesia, Poland Gierek et al., 2009	n. 8,885 6–10 years	2.5 (1.6–3.7)	NR
Hubei Province, China Fu et al., 2010	n. 504,348 school children	1.6 (1.5–1.7)	0.8 @ 90 dB
Manicaland, Zimbabwe Westerberg et al., 2005	n. 5,528 4–18 years	6.2 (4.4–8.6)	2.7 @ 70 dB
Ilam, Ilam Province, Iran Sarafraz & Ahmadi, 2009	n. 785 6–7 years	15 (8.8–27)	NR
Rural Thailand and Bangkok Prasansuk, 2000	n. 12,395 6–15 years	35 (31–38)	0 @ 80 dB

Note. Estimated 95% confidence intervals calculated for this table. *Watkin & Baldwin (2011) is a notification study, not a survey. *NR* = not reported.

Markowski, & Witkowska, 2009) and China (Fu, Chen, Dong, & Zhang, 2010) are less developed than London, and the prevalence (after excluding solely conductive losses) is found to be raised. Iran (Sarafraz & Ahmadi, 2009), Zimbabwe (Westerberg et al., 2005), and Thailand (Prasansuk, 2000) are further removed and have many times the burden of PCHI. It should be noted that these surveys will underestimate numbers of children with severe hearing or other disabilities, as they are unlikely to attend these mainstream schools. However, it remains an efficient way to get a lower bound for estimates of prevalence and pick up reversible hearing loss for treatment. In Zimbabwe, Westerberg's team asked children if they knew anyone who did not attend school because they could not hear, and got three names. If those children had been attending, they would have made up 0.5 in 1,000.

Communities

The same factors that result in differences between countries will also influence communities within countries. There is some evidence to show that lower socioeconomic groups in developed countries have higher rates of hearing impairment. The U.S. Third National Health and Safety Examination Survey, NHANES III, found an overall prevalence of high-frequency hearing impairment (pure-tone average [PTA] across 3, 4, and 6 kHz ≥ 16 dB HL) in 6- to 19-year-olds was 127 per 1,000 and did not differ significantly across racial groups, but ranged from 79 (95% CI 51–107) in the highest income bracket to 163 (95% CI 136–189) in the lowest (Niskar et al., 1998). A different study in the United States asking parents about chronic disabilities in their children found reports of hearing impairment were not connected to poverty per se, but prevalence was increased in single-parent households (Kitsantas, Kornides, Cantiello, & Wu, 2013). The nationwide notification study in the United Kingdom (Fortnum et al., 2002) examined the rates geographically and found that the less affluent the area, the higher was the rate of PCHI. A separate study in Glasgow, United Kingdom, around the same time (Kubba, MacAndie, Ritchie, & MacFarlane, 2004) used a more sensitive measure of deprivation and confirmed the finding. They found that as well as the higher rate of perinatal problems, the more deprived groups had more cases of familial PCHI, suggesting that although deprivation might increase the risk of PCHI, having hearing impairment (or having PCHI in a family) might also predispose to deprivation. The WHO (2005) describes poverty and chronic disease as "interconnected in a vicious cycle." Poor people have a greater exposure to risks and decreased access to health services, predisposing them to disease and complications such as sensory impairment. People with disabilities such as sensory impairment have increased healthcare costs and reductions in income, pushing them into poverty. This cycle can be envisaged in individuals, families, whole communities, and even countries.

In developing countries, studies have also found a connection between increasing prevalence of hearing loss and poorer economic status (Tucci, Merson, & Wilson, 2010). For example, in poor, low-resource areas, the balance between elective or emergency caesarean section is different, and predisposes to perinatal complications and subsequent hearing loss (Olusanya & Solanke, 2009). Such explanations go some way to understanding why the prevalence of hearing impairment varies between urban and rural areas; although as for many things, this is rarely straightforward. For example, consider Tanzania where two studies (Bastos, Mallya, Ingvarsson, Reimer, & Andreasson, 1995; Minja & Machemba, 1996) found significantly higher prevalence rates of both ear disease and sensorineural hearing loss in rural areas, and previously undetected severe loss was only present in rural areas. However, high-frequency loss was more common in urban children (Bastos et al., 1995). Conversely, in Poland (a high-development country), a survey found conductive loss was more common in urban areas, and sensorineural hearing loss was more common in rural areas (Gierek et al., 2009). In Australia, it has been noted that Indigenous Australians have more middle ear pathology right from birth (Aithal, Aithal, Kei, & Driscoll, 2012), whereas children from an Asian background have more sensorineural loss (Wake et al., 2006).

The large numbers in the English UNHS data set can allow us to look at communities that we think might be disadvantaged. The program aims to record the ethnicity of babies and children diagnosed with PCHI. Table 5–4 compares this against birth registration data to show the prevalence for each ethnic group. There is a striking excess of hearing loss among the Asian group (mainly from the Indian subcontinent). The finding that children living in Britain with an Asian ethnic background are at particularly high risk for hearing impairment—and in particular, those with heritage in Pakistan or Bangladesh—has been made previously (Bajaj et al., 2009; Morton, Sharma, Nicholson, Broderick, & Poyser, 2002; Yoong, Feltbower, Spencer, & McKinney, 2005) as well as within Pakistan itself (Sajjad, Khattak, Bunn, & Mackenzie, 2008). There is no single explanation as to this phenomenon. The Asian group has proportionately more congenital seemingly

Table 5–4. Approximate Yield by Ethnic Group

**% of stated*	*Ethnicity of Births Registered (2007)**	*Relative Burden PCHI (2006–2013)**	*Estimated Prevalence (CI 95%)*	*Relative Risk (to White British)*
White British	69%	60%	1.03 (0.99–1.07)	1
Other	12%	11%	1.15 (1.05–1.26)	1.12
Black	7%	6%	0.99 (0.87–1.12)	0.96
Asian	11%	22%	2.44 (2.28–2.62)	2.38
–Asian Pakistani	4%	12%	3.27	3.18
–Asian Indian	3%	5%	1.76	1.72
–Asian Other	2%	2%	1.50	1.46
–Asian Bangladeshi	2%	3%	2.35	2.29
–Mixed White-Asian	1%	1%	1.22	1.19
Unstated	9%	29%		

Note. Asian, mainly from Indian subcontinent, with Chinese and Arab backgrounds included in "Other." Those with ethnicity unstated are excluded.

genetic causes, and consanguinity may play an important part, but an excess is also seen in unrelated parents of Asian backgrounds and in babies with mixed race where one parent is Asian (compared to those with other mixed parentage, who seem to have a slightly lower than average risk).

When looking at the efficacy of the newborn screen, there is evidence of disadvantage to people from Black backgrounds. As shown in Figure 5–6, babies from a Black background with PCHI seem more likely not to receive a timely diagnosis. On average, 18% of diagnoses are made over the age of 1 year, but for children from Black backgrounds, this rises to 29%. For presumed congenital losses, the figures were 20% versus 11%. There are a number of possible explanatory factors, such as perinatal illness, NICU stays, or the presence of auditory neuropathy syndrome disorder. But one suggestion is that people of Black ethnicity —or the areas in which they live—are not reached as well as others by the follow-up process, which deserves investigation. It is of relevance that an Australian study showed that ethnic-minority family status affects the time it takes to access early intervention for hearing loss (Lai et al., 2014), although not as much as geographical proximity. If the screen has a low efficacy for any group, there is the potential of underestimating the prevalence and need in that group, and so it is pertinent to notice that children of Black backgrounds had the lowest yield from the screen (although not significant).

Prevalence by UNHS

For an overview of congenital hearing impairment, the results of pilot studies of UNHS could be useful. Unfortunately, the structure and quality of the programs and reporting/publishing of results have shown great variety. Many study reports do not say what threshold they were using to define a "case," and where they have done so, the variation between them is such that an objective comparison is impossible. However, the volume and breadth of results between 2005 and 2015, which include studies from all eight WHO regions, deserves to be examined. We have calculated yields for moderate bilateral hearing impairment, corrected for under-ascertainment (treating all referred as though they have the same risk of having PCHI as those who returned for follow-up) from the following:

- High Income, Western Europe: Two national programs, seven multisite or regional programs, and six single-site programs (Adelola, Papanikolaou, Gormley, Lang, & Keogh, 2010; Attias et al., 2006; De Capua et al., 2007; Ghirri et al., 2011; Gilbey, Kraus,

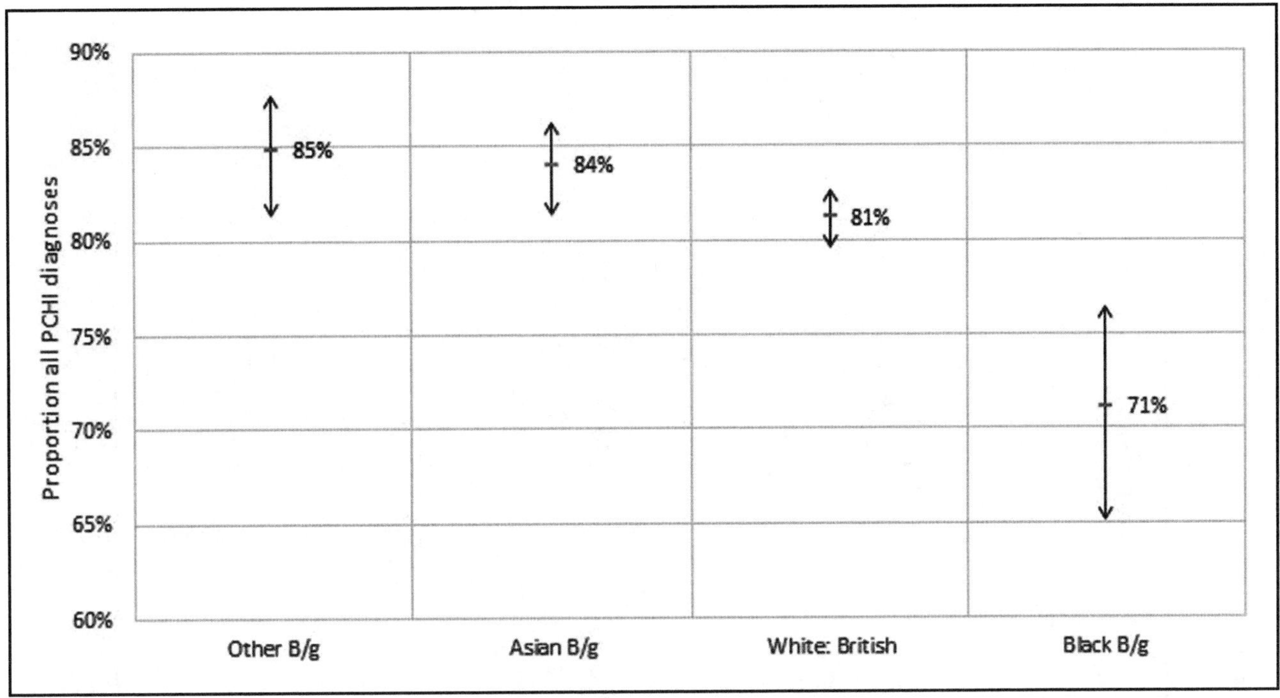

FIGURE 5–6. Proportion of diagnoses of PCHI diagnosed before 12 months by broad ethnic group over 7 years postuniversal newborn screening monitoring in England (with 95% confidence intervals). 29% with ethnicity not stated omitted. (PCHI, permanent children hearing impairment.)

Ghanayim, Sharabi-Nov, & Bretler, 2013; Gonzalez de Aledo Linos, Bonilla Miera, Morales Angulo, Gomez Da Casa, & Barrasa Benito, 2005; Korres et al., 2008; Langagne, Leveque, Schmidt, & Chays, 2010; Nelson et al., 2015; O'Connor, O'Sullivan, Behan, Norman, & Murphy, 2013; Rodriguez Dominguez, et al., 2007; Rohlfs et al., 2010; Schmidt, Leveque, Danvin, Leroux, & Chays, 2007; Uilenburg, Kauffman-de Boer, van der Ploeg, Oudesluys-Murphy, & Verkerk, 2009; Wood et al., 2015);

- Central/Eastern Europe and Central Asia, Central Europe: Two national programs (Jakubikova, Kabatova, Pavlovcinova, & Profant, 2009; Szyfter et al., 2013);
- Asia Pacific, Southeast Asia: Three single-site programs and a pilot study (Abdullah et al., 2006; Ahmad, Mohamad, Mansor, Daud, & Sidek, 2011; Mukari, Tan, & Abdullah, 2006; Tungvachirakul et al., 2011);
- East Asia, China, and Hong Kong: Two region programs, a single site and a pilot study (Huang et al., 2009; Huang et al., 2013; Lam, 2006; Nie et al., 2007);
- South Asia, India: Two single-site programs (Augustine et al., 2014; Rai & Thakur, 2013);
- Latin America and Carribean, Central Latin America: Single-site program (Yee-Arellano, Leal-Garza, & Pauli-Muller, 2006); and Tropical Latin America: Two single-site programs (Nivoloni Kde et al., 2010; Oliveira, Rodrigues, Aurelio, & Silva, 2013);
- Middle East and North Africa: One regional study and two single-site programs (Attias et al., 2006; Habib & Abdelgaffar, 2005; Özbay et al., 2014);
- Sub-Saharan Africa, West Africa: Two single-site programs (Olusanya, Wirz, & Luxon, 2008a).

Our interpretation of the results is plotted in Figure 5–7 against the Human Development Index for the country where the program was based. Human Development Index (HDI) is a measure created by the United Nations Development Program that combines life expectancy, years of schooling, and gross national income per capita (UN Development Programme, 2014). Figure 5–7 shows the large spread of yields, tending to be higher where development levels are lower and where there were many high-risk babies in the study. The HDI alone (as a power regression) explains around 18% of the variance for the majority of studies, but over 50% if the high-risk outliers are included. As study size increases, the results become both lower and

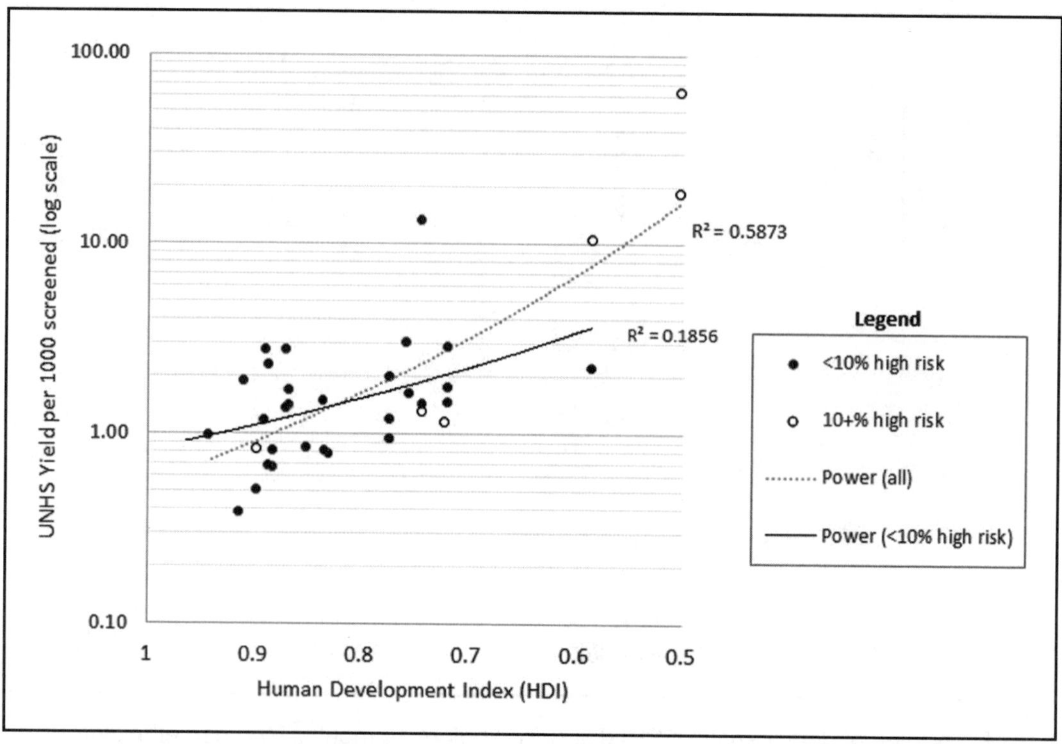

FIGURE 5–7. Worldwide universal newborn hearing screening yields by Human Development Index (HDI), with each point a published study listed in the text. The relationship between low development levels and high levels of congenital hearing loss shown by trend lines, with and without the highlighted studies with exceptional rates of high-risk babies.

more consistent. This could represent publication bias, inflating the prevalence, but these large studies tend to be in high-development areas, so this remains unclear.

There are a number of countries with nationwide access to universal newborn hearing screening for whom there have been published results, meaning we can make fairly reliable predictions from which related countries/programs can learn. Table 5–5 displays a selection of published results from Western Europe (O'Connor et al., 2013; Wood et al., 2015), Central Europe (Jakubikova et al., 2009; Szyfter et al., 2013), the United States (Centers for Disease Control and Prevention, 2015), Asia Pacific (Low, Pang, Ho, Lim, & Joseph, 2005), and the Middle East (Firoozbakht et al., 2014), along with a study on screening in two areas of China (Huang et al., 2009, 2013).The numbers screened and diagnosed with permanent hearing loss are directly compared, and also predicted numbers of babies per year (based on U.S. Government statistics for birth rate). The upper bound of this estimate is following adjustment for under-ascertainment, as above, where follow-up proportion has been given, or from the upper 95% confidence interval if not. The lower bound is from the 95% confidence interval. A uniform definition for hearing loss was needed to compare across studies, and permanent hearing loss of any cause with an average threshold of 40dB HL or greater in the better ear is used as a cutoff and described as "disabling" hearing loss. This was either taken directly from the study or extrapolated from other studies with similar procedures.

It can be seen in Table 5–5 that the programs screen at different levels and have different efficiency with follow-up. The low rate of follow-up in the United States leaves them with a low per 1,000 figure, and a wide uncertainty on numbers. The Polish uncertainty range appears low because there were no data on completeness of follow-up. Despite the differences in programs, the data point toward a significantly higher proportion of newborns having hearing loss in Singapore and China (or at least the parts of China where the screening was carried out) compared to the United Kingdom and United States.

Most infants with "disabling" hearing loss will need specialist intervention, so looking at this number will help with planning capacity for audiology services, teachers, amplification, and other support.

Table 5–5. Results From Seven National Universal Newborn Hearing Screening Programs and a Chinese Multiregion Program

First Author, Date	*Country*	*Number Screened*	*Threshold for Failed Screen (dB HL)*	*Follow-Up Rate*	*Diagnosed HL*	*Per 1,000*	*Disabling HL per 1,000*	*Birth Rate per 1,000*	*Births a Year*	*(Estimated) Children Born with PCHI/Year*	*(Estimated) Children Born With Disabling PCHI/Year*
Jakubikova (2009)	Slovakia	58,000	30		71	1.2	0.3	10.01	54,490	51–82	14–23
O'Connor (2013)	Ireland	11,738	40		15	1.3	0.5	15.18	73,361	46–141	19–56
Low (2005)	Singapore	36,095	40	84%	120	3.3	2.1	8.10	45,095	123–179	79–115
Szyfter (2013)	Poland	3,322,349	25		9,872	3.0	0.8	9.77	374,643	1,135–1,091	299–311
Wood (2015)	United Kingdom	4,591,350	40	93%	5,463	1.2	0.8	12.22	778,939	902–997	581–641
Firoozbakht (2014)	Iran	3,350,995	30	73%	9,741	2.9	0.9	18.23	1,473,726	4,199–5,842	1,260–1,752
CDC (2015)	United States	3,714,115	30	52%	5,088	1.4	0.4	13.42	4,279,532	5,702–11,327	1,710–3,398
Huang (2009)	China	28,428		64%	94	3.3	1.4	12.17	16,498,779	43,544–85,242	18,530–36,273

Note. Results from seven national universal newborn hearing screening programs and a Chinese multiregion program, highlighting the burden of congenital-onset hearing loss at levels considered disabling (>40 dB HL BEA). Where figures for disabling loss were not published, they have been estimated by extrapolating from studies using similar stated diagnostic thresholds; birth rates and population numbers from U.S. government statistics. Upper bound corrected for under-ascertainment where follow-up data are given. Range is otherwise 95% confidence interval around the estimate.

The United Kingdom needs to plan to help upward of 600 babies a year, Iran needs to plan for at least 1,200 babies, and Slovakia might see less than 20. The European countries provided breakdowns into severe and profound levels. Profound hearing loss occurred in 0.16 to 0.31 per 1,000 cases screened, and a country the size of the United Kingdom can expect to see 158 to 181 babies with profound PCHI a year found by UNHS and potentially benefitting from cochlear implantation. At the same ratio, China could expect to see 10,000 children needing implants per year, which is as many times the number of implantations carried out at any age in the whole of 1995 to 2012 (Liang & Mason, 2013).

Risk Factors

A widely used list of risk factors comes from the Joint Committee on Infant Hearing (Joint Committee on Infant Hearing, 2007), summarized in Table 5–6. The identification of some risk factors has come from understanding the etiology of PCHI, conversely, the etiology has sometimes been worked out after observational studies showed something as a risk factor. The study of the epidemiology of PCHI in the Trent region among children born from 1985 to 1993 (Fortnum & Davis, 1997) found that the majority of children with congenital PCHI of moderate or greater severity had one or more of just three risk factors: 29% had a stay in NICU ≥ 48 hours; 30% had a family history of PCHI; 12% had a craniofacial abnormality (CFA). By using these risk factors, they estimate a targeted newborn hearing screening program could detect 59% of congenital PCHI. Many places have used targeted screening as an efficient stepping stone toward universal screening (Rai & Thakur, 2013).

Even in places where universal screening is established, knowledge of risk factors helps to identify those for whom there is a risk of hearing impairment beyond the neonatal period, indicating the need for further observation of children as they develop. In studies of children who developed hearing loss postnatally, the vast majority have at least one of the Joint Committee on Infant Hearing risk factors (American Academy of Pediatrics, 2007), although the vast majority of children with a risk factor do not go on to develop PCHI (Beswick et al., 2013; Watkin & Baldwin, 2012; Weichbold et al., 2006a, 2006b). A recent review by the English UNHS group (Wood, Davis, & Sutton, 2013) found that 3% of children who passed UNHS had one or more known risk factors and were invited for targeted

Table 5–6. Risk Indicators Associated With Permanent Congenital, Delayed-Onset, or Progressive Hearing Loss in Childhood (Joint Committee on Infant Hearing, 2007)

Family history of permanent childhood hearing loss
In utero infections, such as CMV, herpes, rubella, syphilis, and toxoplasmosis
Neonatal intensive care of more than 5 days Extracorporeal membrane oxygenation Assisted ventilation Exposure to ototoxic medications (Gentamicin, Tobramycin, Furosemide, etc.) Hyperbilirubinemia that requires exchange transfusion
Craniofacial abnormalities, including those that involve the pinna, ear canal, ear tags, ear pits, and temporal bone abnormalities
Diagnosis of a syndrome associated with hearing loss, or physical findings suggestive of such a syndrome, such as neurofibromatosis, osteoporosis, or a white forelock
Neurodegenerative disorders
Culture-positive postnatal infections associated with sensorineural hearing loss, including bacterial and viral (especially herpes and varicella [chickenpox] viruses) meningitis
Head trauma, especially basal skull/temporal bone fracture that requires hospitalization
Chemotherapy

clinical follow-up assessment. This follow-up program aimed to identify children with bilateral moderate or greater hearing loss. They invited 70,000 families to follow-up, of which only 55% attended, from which 8,000 children were found to have nonpermanent, unilateral, or mild hearing loss, but only 73 were found to have more severe disorders. This gives an observed prevalence in this group of only 1.49 by the time they were discharged from surveillance—screening 670 children for every one found. Not all risk factors are equal: they found around one child for every 200 children screened had a congenital syndrome associated with hearing loss or craniofacial abnormalities (including Down syndrome). In future, of children who pass the newborn screening, only those with those syndromes or a congenital infection will be invited for targeted follow-up, cutting the proportion that are recalled from 3% to 0.25%. A study from Queensland Australia, mentioned previously, found the most important risk factors in their area were family history and craniofacial abnormalities (Beswick et al., 2013). All teams involved in UNHS protocols are encouraged to look at their own findings to optimize their knowledge and use of local risk factors.

Perinatal Risk Factors

A history of significant perinatal problems appears prominently in studies of risk factors for PCHI. A paper from the Metropolitan Atlanta Developmental Disability Surveillance Program (Van Naarden & Decoufle, 1999) concentrates on PCHI among children who were of low and very low birth weight (LBW < 2500 g but ≥ 1500 g, and VLBW < 1500 g) surviving to at least age 3 years. Of children born at normal birth weight, 0.37 per 1,000 had PCHI at age 3 years. Those children born with LBW had around 3.5 times this prevalence, and those VLBW were 14 times more likely to have PCHI (5.1 per 1,000). The babies included in the Atlanta Surveillance study were born in the 1980s, and since then developments in neonatal intensive care have meant that younger and smaller babies can be helped to survive. These babies might have increased rates of neurodevelopmental and sensory problems, although studies have been inconclusive, and it may be fair to say that although numbers with severe disability are increased, so are the proportion of NICU graduates surviving without any disability (Moore et al., 2012; Wilson-Costello, Friedman, Minich, Fanaroff, & Hack, 2005). Regarding hearing in particular, recent studies continue to show that very small babies treated in a modern NICU have risk of hearing loss an order of magnitude or more greater than their peers. For example, the rates of moderate or greater bilateral PCHI by age 3 years for these babies include

- ELBW (extremely low birth weight < 1000 g), Hong Kong born 2001 to 2002 (High Risk Follow-up Working Group, 2008)—40 per 1,000;
- ELBW, Canada born 1999 to 2006 (Synnes, Anson, Baum, & Usher, 2012)—87 per 1,000; and
- Born under 27 weeks gestation in the United Kingdom in 2007 (Moore et al., 2012)—53 per 1,000.

In the developing world, adverse perinatal conditions are also a prominent risk factor for developing PCHI. In Nigeria, parent-reported "difficult delivery" was associated with attending a deaf school in inner-city Lagos, with odds ratio 20.5 (Olusanya & Okolo, 2006). In Mexico City, a medical records re-view showed that 56% of children with prelingual SNHL had an "abnormal delivery" (Penazola-Lopez, Castillo-Maya, Garcia-Pedroza, & Sanchez-Lopez, 2004), and 11% were born weighing <1,500 g. As part of a study of UNHS in Nigeria, risk factors were investigated in babies who had been born outside of a hospital (Olusanya, Wirz, & Luxon, 2008b); the finding of PCHI was associated particularly with no skilled attendant at the birth (corrected odds ratio 4.2), and severe neonatal jaundice (corrected odds ratio 19). The sheer prevalence of unattended births in many developing countries, and other risk factors such as family history of hearing loss, mean that Joint Committee on Infant Hearing (JCIH) guidelines are helpful but need to be supplemented with local investigation (Botelho et al., 2010; Kanji & Khoza-Shangase, 2012; Olusanya, Okhakhu, & Somefun, 2011; Rai & Thakur, 2013).

Consanguinity as Risk Factor

Consanguinity is noted as a risk factor in a number of studies in the developing world and minority communities in developed countries. Results from some observational studies are shown in Table 5–7 (Al Khabori, 2004; Bener, Eihakeem, & Abdulhadi, 2005; Sajjad et al., 2008; Zakzouk, 2002). Although there is good reason to think consanguinity causes higher prevalence of hearing impairment, because of its link with disadvantage it is not easy to assess its true effects (Bajaj et al., 2009; Saggar & Bittles, 2008). The above-mentioned study in Lagos, Nigeria (Olusanya & Okolo, 2006), found that consanguinity had as big an effect on the risk of hearing impairment as did a family history of deafness (odds risk of 6.7 for consanguineous parents and 6.3 for family

Table 5–7. Rates of First-Cousin Marriage in Parents of Children With and Without PCHI

Country (Reference)	Method of Collecting Cases	Rate Consanguinity in Cases (%)	Method of Calculating Background Rate	Background Rate (%)
Saudi Arabia (Zakzouk, 2002a)	Cross-sectional hearing screening	30	Children passing screening	19
Qatar (Bener et al., 2005)	UNHS pilot	61	Children passing UNHS	25
Oman (Al Khabori, 2004)	Etiology investigation of known cases	70	Contemporary study (Rajab & Patton, 2000)	24
Pakistan (Sajjad, 2008)	Deaf school	86	Hearing children at immunization clinic	60

history). Some authors point out that consanguinity is a preventable risk factor that would be possible to reduce, but to do so would be no straightforward matter (WHO, 2006a).

Other Conditions

Risk factors are not independent—for example, a baby with craniofacial anomolies or prenatal infection is more likely to need NICU—but it is still found that the more risk factors, the more likely a baby is to have a hearing impairment (Bielecki, Horbulewicz, & Wolan, 2011; Martines et al., 2012; Turner, Lee, Boppana, Carlo, & Randolph, 2014). Risk factors are also not specific to hearing—many of them also predict other childhood disabilities (Moore et al., 2012; Synnes et al., 2012). That is, the Trent Study found that 40% of children with PCHI had at least one other congenital or neurodevelopmental problem or disabilitiy (Fortnum & Davis, 1997). This is important in two ways: children with disabilities have a greater potential complexity of need for identification and rehabilitation, and congenital/developmental problems bring children into contact with the health services. Therefore, there is both the need and the opportunity for active case finding (Bamford et al., 2007; Chapman et al., 2011). It is also worth bearing in mind that many chronic childhood illnesses appear to have a detrimental effect on children's hearing, including type 1 diabetes (Botelho, Carvalho, & Silva, 2014; Lin, Lin, Weng, & Chou, 2012) and HIV (Christopher, Edward, Sabrina, & Agnes, 2013; Torre et al., 2012). Greater complexity brings with it special challenges in management and rehabilitation, and services need to be prepared to address this in up to half of cases (Häkli, Luotonen, Bloigu, Majamaa, & Sorri, 2014; National Deaf Children's Society, 2014).

Major Etiologic Factors From a Worldwide Perspective

We have categorized the etiology of hearing impairment as arising genetically or being acquired pre-, peri-, or postnatally for a selection of recent etiologic studies in Table 5–8 and the accompanying Figure 5–8. The studies include children drawn from countries with a range of development levels. The studies from Western Europe (Deben, Janssens de Varebeke, Cox, & Van de Heyning, 2003; Elziere, Roman, Nicollas, & Triglia, 2012; Siem et al., 2010; Watkin & Baldwin, 2010), the United States (Wiley, Arjmand, Jareenmeinzen, & Dixon, 2011), Greece (Bajaj et al., 2009), and Saudi Arabia (Zakzouk & Al-Anazy, 2002) represent very highly developed nations. Oman (Al Khabori, 2004), Turkey (Ozturk et al., 2005), Brazil (de Nobrega, Weckx, & Juliano, 2005), and China (Fu et al., 2010) represent high human development nations. A study from Morocco (Aasham, Khandekar, Khabori, & Helmi, 2004) is the only one from a medium development country. Studies from Cameroon and Nigeria represent low development nations (Dunmade, Segun-Busari, Olajide, & Ologe, 2007; Lasisi, Ayodele, & Ijaduola, 2006; Wonkam et al., 2013). In collecting the data together, there is likely to be some overlap between categories because of the complicated nature of congenital disorders and differing definitions in different studies. We have not

Table 5–8. Selection of Etiological Reports for PCHI (bilateral, except where marked*), with Timing for the Insult Causing PCHI Categorized for This Table, by Country Where Study Took Place

First Author, Year	Siem, 2010; Watkins, 2010; Deben, 2003; Elziere, 2012	Wiley, 2011	Riga, 2005	Zakzouk, 2002	Al Khabori, 2004	Ozturk, 2005	de Nobrega, 2005	*Fu, 2010	Ridal, 2014	Wonkham, 2013	Lasisi, 2006	Dunmade, 2007
Location	Western Europe (amalgamated)	United States	Greece	Saudi Arabia	Oman	Turkey	Brazil	China	Morocco	Cameroon	Nigeria	Nigeria
Severity (thresholds dB HL average)	Various	>25 dB	Aids fitted	>76 dB	>60 dB	Deaf School	Any PCHI	>25 dB WE	Severe+	Severe+	Any SNHL	>71 dB
N	663	198	94	302	1400	840	442	813	250	582	103	115
Prenatal	**43%**	**48%**	**51%**	**64%**	**46%**	**52%**	**26%**	**29%**	**40%**	**15%**	**31%**	**3%**
Genetic	29%	28%	47%	52%	45%	51%	11%	6%	35%	15%	25%	0%
Nonsyndromic	*23%*	*21%*	*36%*	*47%*	*42%*	*35%*	*11%*	*6%*	*32%*	*13%*	*ns*	
Syndromic	*6%*	*7%*	*11%*	*5%*	*3%*	*16%*	*0%*	*0%*	*4%*	*2%*	*ns*	
Acquired	5%	ns	4%	9%	ns	1%	15%	ns	ns	ns	ns	1%
Rubella	*1%*	*ns*	*1%*	*3%*	*1%*	*0.6%*	*15%*	*ns*	*ns*	*1%*	*ns*	*1%*
Other	*4%*	*ns*	*3%*	*5%*	*ns*	*0.4%*	*ns*	*ns*	*ns*	*ns*	*ns*	
Unspecified	9%	20%	0%	3%	ns	ns	ns	ns	4%	ns	6%	3%
Perinatal	**13%**	**ns**	**31%**	**14%**	**12%**	**1%**	**13%**	**15%**	**8%**	**5%**	**14%**	**8%**
Postnatal	**8%**	**12%**	**3%**	**10%**	**8%**	**13%**	**12%**	**54%**	**19%**	**47%**	**53%**	**54%**
Systemic infection	*6%*	*4%*	*2%*	*10%*	*1%*	*12%*	*12%*	*0%*	*16%*	*41%*	*32%*	*32%*
Toxic	*1%*					*0%*		*31%*	*2%*	*6%*	*13%*	*3%*
Trauma	*0.5%*					*0%*			*1%*	*0%*	*1%*	
Ear/mastoid disease						*1%*		*1%*			*5%*	
Other	*0.5%*	*8%*	*1%*		*7%*	*0%*		*22%*		*ns*	*3%*	*18%*
Missing	**36%**	**40%**	**15%**	**12%**	**34%**	**12%**	**28%**	**3%**	**34%**	**33%**	**2%**	**35%**

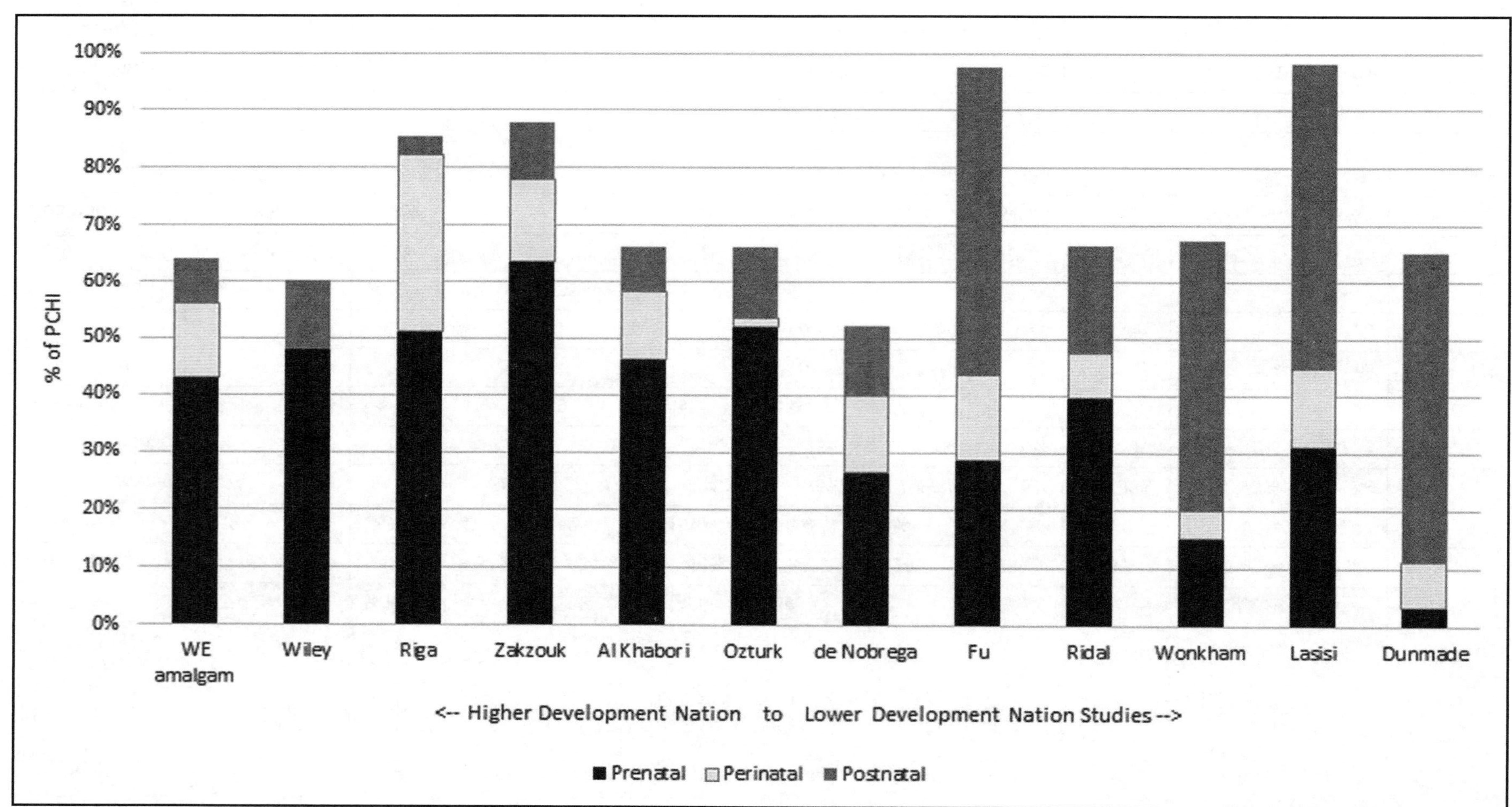

FIGURE 5–8. Studies from Table 5–8 with proportion of cases of PCHI thought to be due to pre-, peri-, and postnatal causes. Remainder is unknown timing (height is not related to prevalence; PCHI, permanent children hearing impairment.)

included craniofacial abnormality as an etiological category but, rather, as a risk factor or marker of some genetic, acquired, or multifactorial pathology (Tapadia, Cordero, & Helms, 2005). It can be seen that the size, age, and impairment level of the samples are all different, and this too will make comparison between studies difficult. But, it is possible to suggest some patterns. Most prominent is that the postnatally acquired proportion appears higher in lower development countries.

The proportion of hearing loss attributed to postnatal causes (both infectious and other) is plotted against the HDI for the country of study in Figure 5–9. This shows a moderate correlation between lower HDI and higher postnatal acquisition. This is both for infectious causes and others, although the latter observation is heavily influenced by one Chinese study. Along geographic lines there is also the hint that Africa might have a higher rate of infectious diseases, that the Middle East might have a higher genetic load, and that there is a higher relative contribution of perinatal causes in the other high-income countries, as shown in Figure 5–10, although caution should be taken not to draw conclusions due to the differing methodologies of the studies.

Unfortunately, it is common for a large percentage of cases to have unknown etiology. Collectively, the studies in Table 5–8 allocated 30% of cases of PCHI to unknown origin. The studies from Fu et al. in China and Lasisi et al. in Nigeria have a remarkably small proportion of unknown hearing loss, which probably represent how ubiquitous the proposed explanatory factors are (mainly ototoxic medication in China and systemic infection in Nigeria) making the suggestion of idiopathic deafness on an individual scale untenable. Where a greater proportion of children have known causes for their hearing loss, the larger proportion appears to be attributed to genetic causes, for example, between the Lasisi and Dunmade studies in Nigeria (although note different definitions of cases). In the Trent study, 41% of children did not have a known

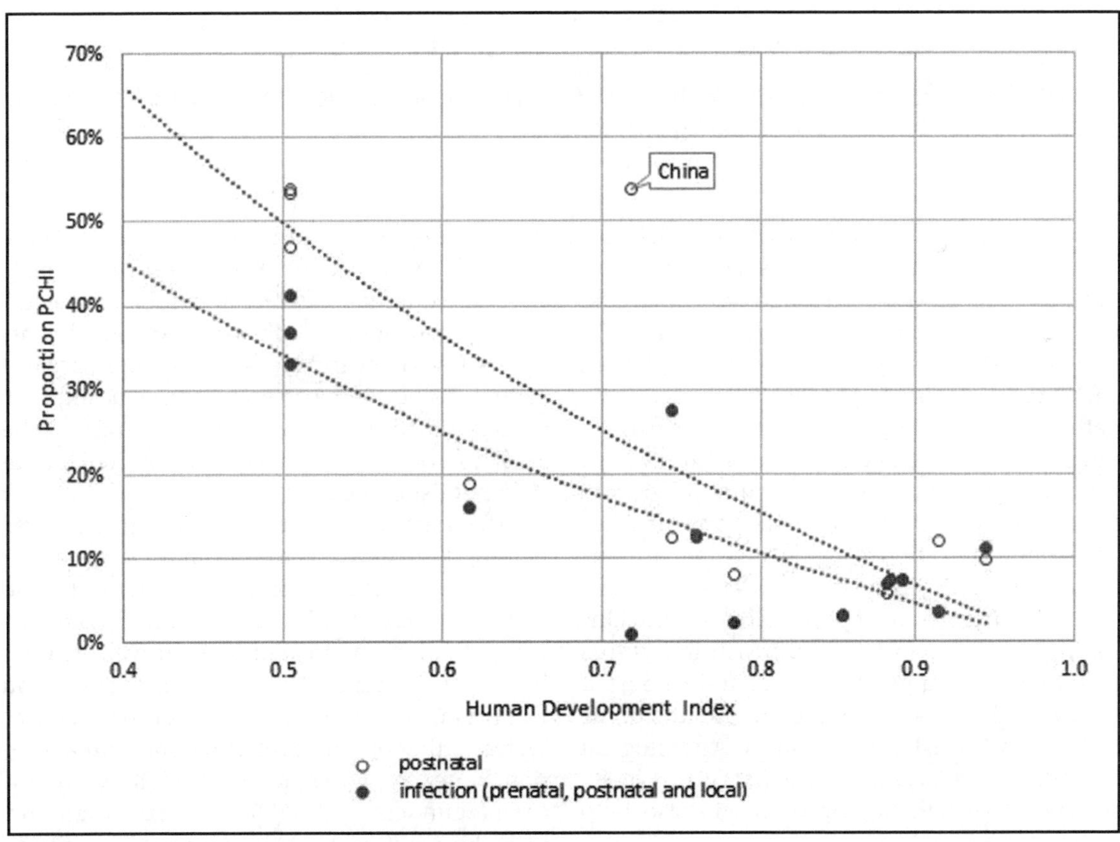

FIGURE 5–9. A regression of the results of the studies in Table 5–8. Proportion of cases of PCHI caused by postnatal insult (*open circle*) and infection (*closed circle*). Human Development Index (HDI) shows postnatally acquired proportion decreases with development level of country ($r^2 = 0.7$). China highlighted as significant outlier. (PCHI, permanent children hearing impairment.)

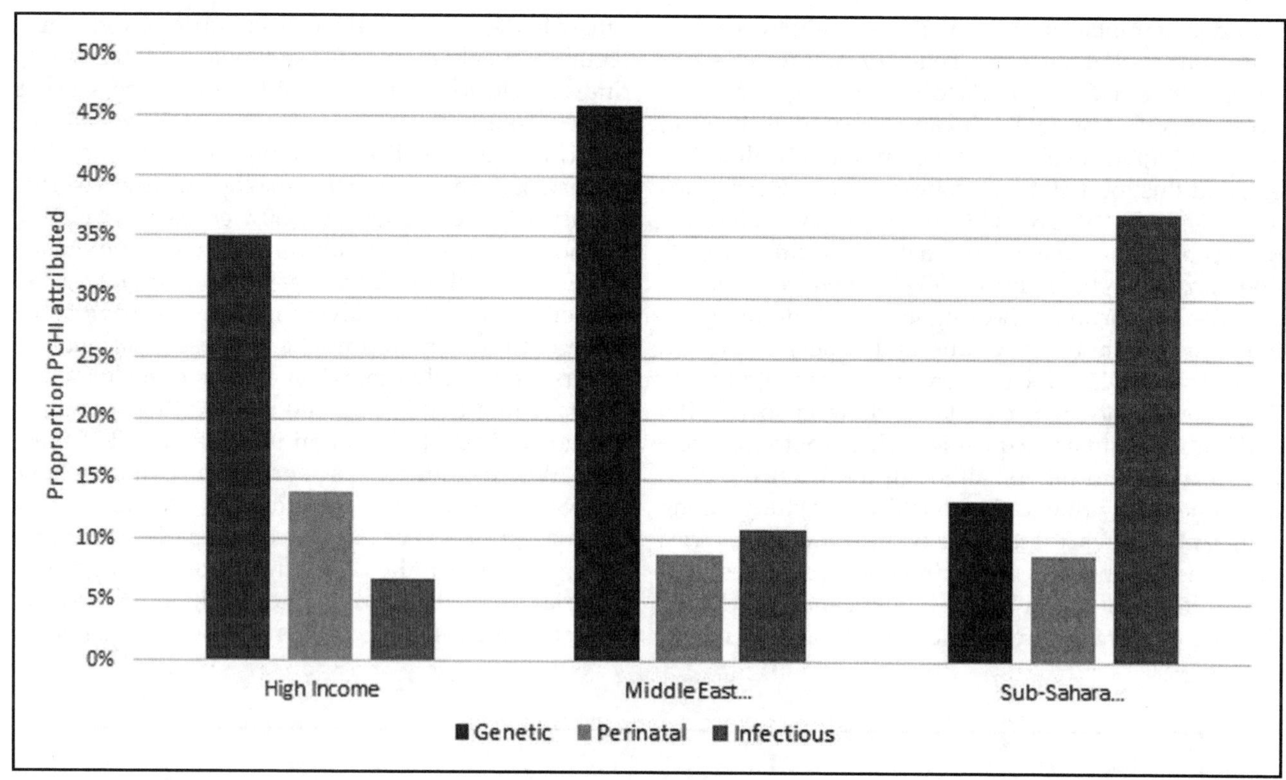

FIGURE 5–10. Three etiologies of PCHI in three WHO regions, using studies from Table 5–8 excluding China and Brazil. (PCHI, permanent children hearing impairment.)

etiology at identification. Nevertheless, it was possible to impute etiology from other data such as medical notes and this reduced the percentage of people who had no etiological information to approximately 25%. Taking this one step further, another study (Parker, Fortnum, Young, Davis, & Mueller, 2000) reported investigating 82 children from the Trent study using a questionnaire, home visit, and genetic test. They found eight children had a genetic syndrome not previously assigned, and seven additional cases had the most common genetic mutation causing hearing impairment in the United Kingdom, GJB2 35delG. There are a number of guidelines now available for clinicians investigating the cause of hearing loss in individual children, for example, a good practice guideline used for the Newborn Hearing Screening Programme in the United Kingdom (British Association of Audiological Physicians/British Association of Paediatricians, 2008), and this type of systematic approach will also help in research.

The presence of one possible etiology does not exclude another. For example, it is increasingly recognized that some mutations do not cause permanent hearing loss but lower the threshold for environmental insults pre-, peri-, and postnatally (Brent, 2004; Dyer, Strasnick, & Jacobson, 1998; Steel, 1998). Such mutations include the A1555G mitochondrial gene mutation, which might not affect a child's hearing at all, but predisposes to hearing loss, which might occur dramatically if a single dose of aminoglycoside antibiotic such as gentamicin is taken (Bitner-Glindzicz & Rahman, 2007; Kokotas, Petersen, & Willems, 2007). Causes can be synergistic, such as the compounded effect of a conductive hearing loss in children with a sensorineural hearing loss, which is too commonly missed (Ahmed, Kolo, Abah, & Oladigbolu, 2012; Oghan, Harputluoglu, Ozturk, Guclu, & Mayda, 2008) and something that can potentially be treated to improve functionality of hearing. Sometimes the number of potential causes for PCHI is increased due to the high prevalence of risk factors either on the level of the individual or population. For example, a study of PCHI in Nicaraguan children (Saunders et al., 2007) showed a high prevalence of PCHI (~180 per 1,000), with the majority (51%) of cases presenting with more than one potential etiology. Family history was present in 38%, prenatal infection found in over 30%, neonatal breathing problems in 28%, and aminoglycoside antibiotic use in 30%.

Changes Over Time

A school for deaf children in Copenhagen was used to study the causes of hearing loss in children attending in 1993 to 1994 (Parving & Hauch, 1994), and the results compared to cases evaluated 10 and 40 years previously in the same institution. They found that the frequency of congenital inherited hearing impairment increased steadily with time, whereas prenatal infections increased until the 1980s, then fell. There might also have been an increase in perinatal causes of PCHI and an increased complexity of the disabilities of these children (Admiraal & Huygen, 2000; Synnes et al., 2012). The changes in the developed world over the last few decades have shown the success of primary prevention. Measles, mumps, rubella, and meningitis are all implicated in PCHI and all have been the subject of immunization programs. Secondary prevention has also helped, with better nutrition and treatment leading to better outcomes from infections such as measles and meningitis. In contrast, comparing the etiology of sensorineural PCHI in Egypt between the 1970s and 1990s (Tantawy, Sobhy, Al-Farargy, & Shafik, 1998) and Nigeria between 1980 and 2000 (Dunmade et al., 2007) showed no significant change in infectious causes.

The rise of inherited PCHI in developed countries is not just in the proportion of genetic cases but in the actual numbers. In some cases, this reflects better survival of babies with life-threatening syndromes; in others, it is due to the increase in prevalence of particular mutations. It has been suggested that the frequency of PCHI caused by the connexin genes, *GJB2* and *GJB6*, might have doubled in the last 200 years due to the establishment of a Deaf community leading to healthier hearing-impaired adults (Tekin, 2009; Nance & Kearsey, 2004), thus decreasing the genetic selection for the unmutated forms of the connexin genes.

Genetic Hearing Impairment

It is thought that around half of all cases of PCHI have a genetic cause (Morton & Nance, 2006; Reardon, 1992) and the pattern shown in Figure 5–10 would seem to agree with this, at least in developed countries. Despite significant advances in the understanding of the molecular basis of hearing loss, identifying the precise genetic cause in an individual remains difficult. Hearing loss could result from a mutation in an estimated 300 to 500 genes, of which 120 have been identified so far. The majority of these genes are located on the autosomal chromosomes, up to 20% on the X-chromosome, and up to 20% in the maternally inherited mitochondrial DNA.

Genetic disorders were thought to be syndromic or nonsyndromic, and recessive or dominant, but increasing knowledge about the human genome and genetic epidemiology has shown that these distinctions are not as simple in reality. Phenotype-genotype relationships do not strictly follow Mendelian patterns (McHugh & Friedman, 2006; Wang et al., 2011), such that mutations in the same gene can have different effects in different racial groups, families, or individuals, probably due to gene-gene interactions and gene-environment interactions. Having acknowledged its limitations, the old nomenclature is sufficient for most clinical and epidemiologic purposes and will be used here.

Syndromic

Approximately 30% of genetic hearing impairment occurs as one of a number of developmental abnormalities—a syndrome (Häkli et al., 2014; Morton & Nance, 2006; Silan et al., 2004). Over 400 syndromes featuring PCHI have been described and many of the genetic abnormalities responsible identified. Syndromal hearing impairment can be sensorineural, conductive, or mixed. Many involve abnormalities of the temporal bone that can be seen on computed tomography (CT) scan (McClay et al., 2002; Reardon, 1992). The presence of a genetic syndrome in children with PCHI should not be overlooked as it can be important in determining prognosis and intervention measures, as well as for estimating the recurrence risks in the family (Mueller, 1996; Parker, Fortnum, Young, & Davis, 1999), but this is probably underestimated due to nonrecognition, as found in the follow-up to the Trent study (Parker et al., 2000).

Chromosomal syndromes, including Down and Turner syndromes, lead to increased risk of hearing impairment. Autosomal dominant disorders tend to be caused by genes with a developmental role, leading to abnormalities or symptoms detectable at birth. Autosomal recessive disorders, such as Usher and Pendred, tend to be caused by genes with metabolic roles leading to progressive symptoms. X-linked syndromes, such as Alport syndrome, affect males predominantly because they have only one X chromosome. Mitochondrial syndromes are inherited from the mother and are heterogeneous in expression (Hultcrantz, 2003; Keats, 2002; Kokotas et al., 2007; Park, Wilson, Stevens, Harward, & Hohler, 2012; Tapadia et al., 2005). The single-gene syndrome most commonly identified in people with PCHI is Waardenburg; Pendred syndrome is more common but has more variable hearing impairment (Morton

& Nance, 2006; Morzaria, Westerberg, & Kozak, 2004; Silan et al., 2004).

Nonsyndromic

Nonsyndromic genetic PCHI presentation is inherited in an autosomal recessive pattern in around 70% of cases (Morton & Nance, 2006; Petersen & Willems, 2006; Tekin, 2009). One gene whose mutations seem particularly important is *GJB2*—identified in 1997. This gene codes for a protein called connexin 26, a gap junction protein regulating the passage of ions in and out of human cells (OMIM, 2015; Ouyang et al., 2009). This is the most common gene to be found affected in studies in most of the world (Ouyang et al., 2009). In North America, Western Europe, and into the Middle East, the most common mutation is 35delG (Bonyadi, Fotouhi, & Esmaeili, 2014; Tekin et al., 2001), but in the Far East it is 235delC (Hayashi et al., 2011; Jiang et al., 2014). Whereas in Sub-Saharan Africa, the same genes are rarely found (Bosch et al., 2014; Javidnia et al., 2014; Kabahuma et al., 2011). Those found with the same allele or genotype can be affected differently (Beck et al., 2014); for instance, the *V37I* is a benign mutation in Western countries but appears to cause PCHI in Malaysia (Ruszymah et al., 2005).

Mitochondrial genes differ from nuclear genes in two major ways that affect inheritance. First, as mitochondria for an embryo are from the oocyte, all mitochondrial genes come from the mother alone. Second, there are multiple copies of mitochondrial DNA (mDNA) in each mitochondrion, and therefore, expression of a disease-causing gene is not inevitable, such that the clinical phenotype is much more variable than in autosomal mutations. The most common mutation causing PCHI worldwide is A1555G, which renders carriers susceptible to dramatic, profound deafness following standard doses of aminoglycoside antibiotics, discussed below (see Toxicity).

Testing for Genetic Disorders

As technology becomes available to analyze the genome for particular mutations rapidly, it is possible to use this technology (a) for research into genetic epidemiology of congenital hearing loss, (b) to provide more accurate diagnoses, and (c) for screening (Linden Phillips et al., 2013; Nivoloni Kde et al., 2010; Wang et al., 2011). Proponents of genetic screening (i.e., testing people without obvious hearing loss for genetic mutations associated with hearing loss) argue that it can highlight: (a) those children with genetic disorders who, through delayed-onset or other factors, are missed by UNHS; (b) those at risk of developing hearing loss due to environmental insult, which can then be avoided; and (c) carriers (who might also be more vulnerable themselves). Given the ethical, scientific, and clinical problems of predicting future outcomes on an individual scale (Brown & Rehm, 2001; Smith, 2001), it remains to be seen when or whether such genetic screening will become widespread.

Prenatal Infections

Maternal health affects a developing fetus, and especially when she has in infection that can pass to the fetus (Baecher-Lind, Miller, & Wilcox, 2010). The best known of these infections are known by the acronym TORCH—toxoplasma, rubella, cytomegalovirus, and herpes simplex—although there are many that are included as "O" for "Others," including syphilis, HIV, and viral hepatitis. The two individual infections that are noteworthy for the burden of hearing loss attributed to them are rubella and cytomegalovirus (Cohen, Durstenfeld, & Roehm, 2014), but infectious diseases are among etiologies that change the fastest, and epidemiologists, clinicians, and others must always be alert for emerging threats.

Rubella

If a mother is infected with rubella during the first 2 months of pregnancy there is a 90% chance of miscarriage or transmission to the fetus (Lambert, Strebel, Orenstein, Icenogle, & Poland, 2015). Congenital rubella syndrome (CRS) affects the eyes, ears, heart, and brain of the developing child. Hearing impairment is the most common permanent manifestation. During the 1970s to 1980s, congenital rubella was the most common reported cause of sensorineural hearing impairment in childhood, accounting for 16% to 22% of cases of hearing impairment in babies in Europe (Parving & Hauch, 1994). A single outbreak in the United States in 1964 to 1965 led to over 8,000 children being born with PCHI, with 3,500 having involvement of sight (Lambert et al., 2015). Where there is no vaccine, there are outbreaks seasonally, with large epidemics every 3 to 8 years, as herd immunity wanes among young children. A vaccination has the potential to eradicate rubella and thus end congenital rubella syndrome. As of 2000, the majority of the countries in the world provide a rubella vaccine (68% in 2012), giving a coverage of approximately 43% of the world's population. There is large regional variation, with The World Health Organization (WHO) American and European regions achieving 93% coverage. Endemic rubella is now gone from American regions. Yet in the African region, only 7% of countries vaccinated against rubella in 2012, which leaves endemic and epidemic rubella untouched. WHO urges combination of rubella vaccine with measles vaccine (2011a). At the 2011 level of vaccination in Africa, the WHO model predicts an incidence of CRS at 0.1 to 0.2 per 1,000 births annually, and 0.8 to 4 per 1,000 births during epidemics, which means a predicted 22,000 (95% CI 6,127–51,472) children with CRS born in Africa. A further 46,000 (95% CI 1,016–168,910) will be born each year in South-East Asia with CRS unless vaccination improves.

Cytomegalovirus (CMV)

CMV is a common chronic asymptomatic infection in adults, but when it infects the developing fetus and child, it gives rise to congenital CMV (cCMV), which can lead to perinatal and developmental abnormalities. Estimates vary as to the exact numbers of cCMV, but it appears to be the most common intrauterine infection in the developed world, and a major cause of congenitally acquired PCHI (Cannon, Griffiths, Aston, & Rawlinson, 2014; Cohen et al., 2014; Roizen, 2003). A review of studies on the epidemiology of cCMV (Goderis et al., 2014) reported the observed prevalence of cCMV to be 5.8 per 1,000 (range 3–22); around 10% is symptomatic at birth. Of those who have any symptoms at birth, there is high mortality, and half will develop a neurological or sensory disability—one third will experience hearing loss (mainly bilateral). Those asymptomatic at birth have a 1 in 10 risk of developing PCHI in the following years (often unilateral). As well as having delayed onset in some cases, there were also cases of progressive and fluctuating loss, all of which would be easy to miss until a child's development had been affected. CMV infection does not appear prominently in most studies of etiology because CMV infection can be otherwise silent (Townsend, Peckham, & Tookey, 2011). Where there has been positive case finding, for example, looking for CMV in stored dried heel-spot blood sample, the review suggests cCMV is involved in 10% to 20% of cases of PCHI (Goderis et al., 2014). cCMV is more likely to be found as the etiology where there is delayed onset or progressive, higher severity and/or unilateral hearing loss, and comorbid neurodevelopmental delay (Avettand-Fenoel et al., 2013; Barbi et al., 2003; Misono et al., 2011).

cCMV can be treated using IV antiviral treatment, which has been shown experimentally to prevent and treat some hearing loss for some babies, but treatment needs to start before the baby is a month old to be effective (Kimberlin et al., 2003). Because cCMV is often asymptomatic and easily confused with other causes of neonatal morbidity, in order to identify children early enough to benefit potentially from treatment, screening newborn babies for CMV might be a good solution. One proposed model is to offer saliva-based CMV screening where a baby has failed the screen for UNHS, as this can then be available around the same time as the audiology assessment, so that decisions can be made on treatment with both pieces of information, before 30 days after birth (Williams, Kadambari, et al., 2014). An evaluation by another team makes an argument for universal cCMV screening, saying it has the potential to benefit several thousand babies every year in the United States alone through improved use of pharmaceutical and nonpharmaceutical interventions (Cannon et al., 2014). Their numbers show that the number of children with disabilities among apparently asymptomatic children is much larger than from symptomatic, due to larger numbers. Their projected numbers are shown in Figure 5–11.

Maternal Drug Exposure

Drugs including streptomycin and quinine can destroy neural elements of the inner ear when the auditory system is developing, around 6 to 7 weeks postconception (Dyer et al., 1998). There are probably gene-environment/gene-toxin interactions involved in making particular drugs teratogenic in some mothers and pregnancies (Brent, 2004), such that it can be difficult to be definitive in identifying a drug as responsible for any individual case of PCHI, and difficult to advise mothers which medications are safe during pregnancy. Heavy alcohol intake during pregnancy has long been associated with poor outcomes including hearing loss, and maternal cigarette smoking is now also implicated in hearing impairment at birth (Durante, Ibidi, Lotufo, & Carvallo, 2011; Warren & Foudin, 2001). And, though this will not happen in every case, it is not possible to predict who is at risk, so women planning to become pregnant should be made aware of this.

Perinatal Factors

Neonates admitted to NICU for any reason have a risk of developing PCHI many times higher than those who have not (Davis & Wood, 1992), and even if not hearing impaired, have worse high-frequency hearing thresholds on average than children without perinatal complications (Razi & Das, 1994). There are many

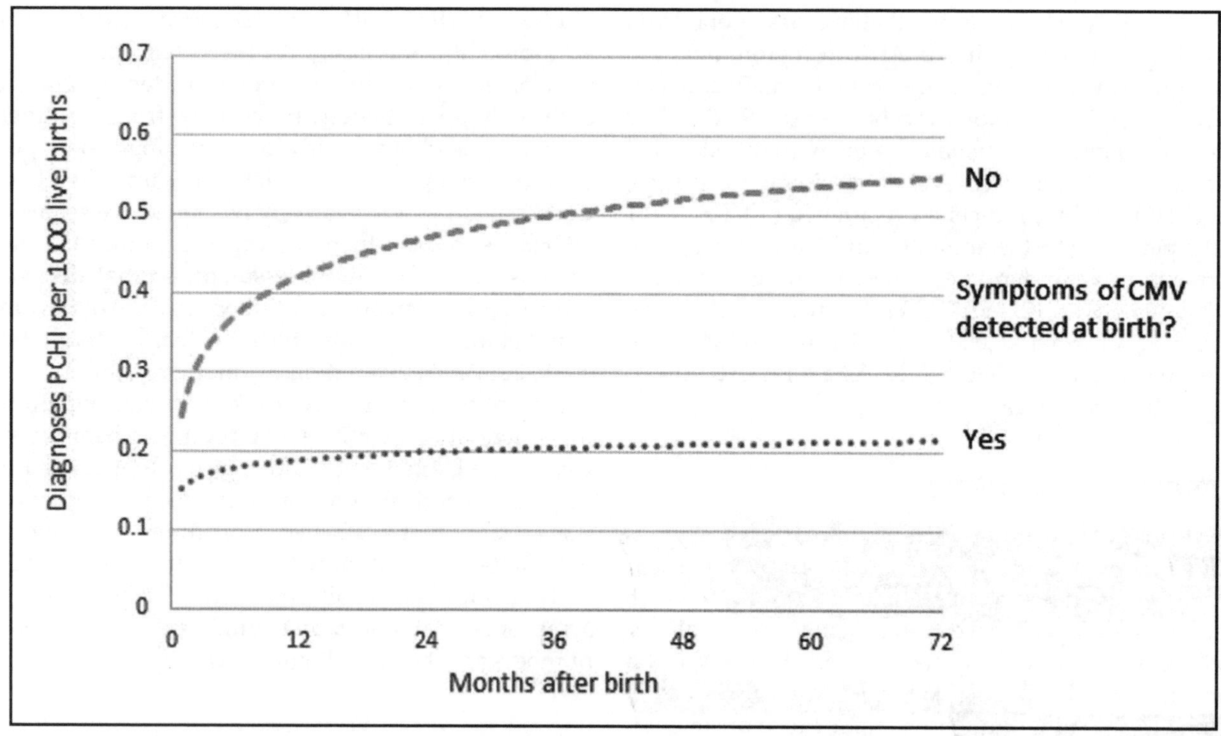

FIGURE 5–11. Estimated prevalence of cCMV-associated hearing loss in the population, numbers taken from Cannon et al., 2014. Of all babies who test positive for CMV, only 10% had symptoms of cCMV detected in the neonatal period. Higher rates of hearing loss in symptomatic, but higher numbers of asymptomatic babies makes mildly increased risk significant. (cCMV, congenital cytomegalovirus; PCHI, permanent children hearing impairment.)

factors that seem to predispose to PCHI in these babies, and they probably interact, such that in any one infant it would be almost impossible to pick one cause (Dennett et al., 2014; Martines, Martines, Mucia, Sciacca, & Salvago, 2013; Zimmerman & Lahav, 2013). Along with perinatal problems being a cause of congenital disease such as PCHI, prenatally determined congenital abnormalities can in turn lead to perinatal difficulties (Newton, 2001), making a causal link between any of these factors and hearing loss even more difficult to demonstrate.

A notable factor in the etiology of hearing loss for babies with perinatal illness is hyperbilirubinemia (a state of the waste product bilirubin building up in the circulation; a state also called *jaundice* or, when affecting the central nervous system, *kernicterus*). This is in the JCIH list of risk factors, but only where severe enough to need transfusion. It is also prominent in literature in the developing world (Olusanya, 2013). A review demonstrated that there is a dose-response relationship, with greater hearing abnormality following higher bilirubin levels and less hearing loss where the hyperbilirubinemia was successfully treated (Akinpelu, Waissbluth, & Daniel, 2013).

Postnatal Infections

Local

When discussing permanent hearing impairment, infection usually refers to systemic and neurological infections. But local infection, such as chronic suppurative otitis media (CSOM) and otitis media with effusion, needs inclusion, as it not only is a major cause of temporary hearing impairment, but it can cause persistent hearing problems, may delay the detection of permanent hearing impairment, and also has the potential to lead to permanent impairment (Czechowicz et al., 2010; Davidson, Hyde, & Alberti, 1989; Hoffman et al., 2013; Minja & Machemba, 1996). In the United Kingdom, school-entry screening finds that around 2.6% of 5-year-olds have temporary conductive hearing impairment, most likely to be OME (Fonseca, Forsyth,

& Neary, 2005). Five years is the peak age of presentation of OME in the United Kingdom (Bamford et al., 2007). Comparisons of point prevalence for conductive hearing loss from screening studies around the world show the following:

- India, 10.9% of 284 individuals ages 6 to 10 years (Jacob, Rupa, Job, & Joseph, 1997), 8.7% of 855 individuals aged 5 years (after wax removal; Rao, Subramanyam, Nair, & Rajashekhar, 2002);
- Turkey, 8.7% of 1,740 primary school children (Gultekin, Develioglu, Yener, Ozdemir, & Külekçi, 2010);
- Nigeria, 5.0% of 359 individuals from ages 4 to 10 years (Olusanya, Okolo, & Ijaduola, 2000);
- Swaziland, 3.3% of 2,480 individuals ages 5 to 15 years (Swart, Lemmer, Parbhoo, & Prescott, 1995);
- Peru (deprived area), 4.8% of 335 individuals aged 6 to 19 years (Czechowicz et al., 2010); and
- Malaysia, 2.1% of 234 individuals aged 11years (13% if hearing levels of 20–29 dB are included; Khairi Md Daud et al., 2009).

Long-term complications of local infection are more common in developing countries (Akinpelu & Amusa, 2007; Davidson et al., 1989), and the WHO estimates that over 90% of the burden of chronic ear infections is borne by countries in South-East Asia, Western Pacific, and African regions, along with ethnic minorities in the Pacific Rim (WHO & Acuin, 2004). But it should be remembered that repeated otitis media can lead to some degree of permanent hearing impairment even where health and health services are more robust (Jensen, Koch, & Homoe, 2013; Yehudai, Most, & Luntz, 2015; Yiengprugsawan, Hogan, & Strazdins, 2013). The WHO and its partners recognize that because a significant burden of persistent and permanent hearing impairment in the developing world is potentially due to reversible local ear disease, there is a need to educate and encourage community health teams to make managing common ear problems a priority (Ricard et al., 2004; Society for Sound Hearing, 2015; WHO, 2012). The WHO produces training resources under the heading "Primary ear and hearing care" (WHO, 2006b).

Systemic

Reports over a wide range of time and place have indicated that bacterial meningitis is one of the most common causes of acquired permanent childhood hearing impairment. In the English UNHS data, it was responsible for around 50% of the postnatally acquired documented cases. The systematic review by Morzaria found meningitis caused 44% (CI 95% 16–76) of postnatal cases and 3% (CI 95% 2.7–3.3) of all cases studied before 1990, and 31% (CI 95% 10–64)/2.6% (CI 95% 1.8–3.6), respectively, afterward (2004). Bacterial meningitis can be caused by a variety of pathogens, most commonly *Haemophilus influenzae* type b (Hib), *Streptococcus pneumoniae* (pneumococcus), and *Neisseria meningitidis* (meningococcus). For children who survive meningitis, sequelae can be severe, and disabling sensorineural hearing impairment, often profound, is one of the most common (Bedford et al., 2001). The incidence of post-meningitis hearing impairment in the literature varies greatly depending on population characteristics, illness variables, and definition of hearing impairment (Grimwood et al., 1995; Jusot, Tohon, Yazi, & Collard, 2013; Karanja, Oburra, Masinde, & Wamalwa, 2014; Koomen et al., 2003; Stein-Zamir et al., 2014; Wellman, Sommer, & McKenna, 2003; Worsoe, Caye-Thomasen, Brandt, Thomsen, & Ostergaard, 2010). For non-neonatal bacterial meningitis, it appears that around one in ten will suffer permanent disabling hearing impairment. Some risk factors for permanent and disabling hearing loss in children have been described:

1. Population level: High prevalence (e.g., living in the "meningitis belt" of Sahelian countries [Jusot et al., 2013]) and environmental factors such as overcrowding (WHO, 2013), and possibly some ethnicities have higher risk of meningitis and/or complications (D'Angio et al., 1995; O'Connor, Perry, & Lannigan, 2009);
2. Patient factors: Young age, which is more likely in high prevalence areas (Roine et al., 2014; WHO, 2013), comorbidity such as HIV (WHO, 2013; Worsoe et al., 2010), although a further study refutes this on a very high background rate of 66% hearing loss (Molyneux et al., 2003);
3. Illness factors: Acute neurological complications include convulsions (Grimwood et al., 1995; Kutz, Simon, Chennupati, Giannoni, & Manolidis, 2006; Roine et al., 2014), duration of symptoms before treatment (Koomen et al., 2003; Smith et al., 1988), and pneumococcus infection (Adachi, Ito, & Sakata; Koomen et al., 2003; Kutz et al., 2006; Wellman et al., 2003; Woolley et al., 1999).

Some meningitis strains are becoming resistant to penicillin-based antibiotics. This translates to a greater use of aminoglycosides as first line, and another reason why meningitis is a public health priority for which vaccines have been sought (Millar, 2011; WHO, 2013).

A vaccine against Hib was introduced in the United States in 1985 and is credited with a fall in the incidence of meningitis and subsequently reduced incidence of acquired hearing impairment (Wellman et al., 2003; Woolley et al., 1999; WHO, 2013). Pneumococcal meningitis has still been prevalent and is more likely to cause hearing loss (see above). An effective childhood vaccination became available in 2000 (the conjugate vaccine), and this too has shown to have protective effects for the individual and population in the United States (WHO, 2003). It also helps somewhat to protect against complications from *S. pneumoniae* otitis media (Lieu et al., 2000; WHO, 2003). Experience of the addition of a serogroup C *N. meningitidis*, "menC," vaccine to childhood immunization schedules in many developed countries has been positive, but outbreaks of other serotypes have led to a desire to widen this coverage, especially to add menB vaccination (Christensen, Trotter, Hickman, & Edmunds, 2014; Pace & Pollard, 2007). A breakthrough for the worldwide burden of disease due to meningitis is a vaccination for the meningococcal bacteria most often seen in the "meningitis belt"—the A serogroup of *N. meningitidis*, menA—which was introduced to 17 of the 26 high-risk countries between 2010 and 2015. Although vaccination programs are a start, adequate surveillance is necessary to use the different vaccines to their best effects (Vella & Pace, 2015), and there is further innovation needed to create vaccines with immunogenicity for wider ranges of serotypes and antibiotics to cover resistant disease (Braine, 2011; Ladhani & Ramsay, 2015).

An episode of measles has a much lower probability of causing permanent hearing loss (SNHL) than meningitis. But, overall risk from measles is high due to the much greater incidence of the infection. Measles is a viral illness, which, in past time, most children would catch between 6 months and 2 years of age (Cohen et al., 2014). Complications occur in around 30% cases, and include mouth ulcers, pneumonia, otitis media, and encephalitis. In developed countries, around 10% will need to be admitted to hospital, but in parts of the world where children are already malnourished, around 10% will die. In the Global Burden of Disease 1996, 5% of all deaths under 5 years were due to measles, and measles is also thought to be responsible for about 5% of PCHI (Cohen et al., 2014; Dunmade et al., 2007). Hearing impairment can occur through complication of otitis media, or as part of neural damage during encephalopathy, and can also possibly trigger otosclerosis (Cohen et al., 2014). The burden of measles has come down dramatically with WHO and others promoting a proven immunization strategy. But such strategies need continued vigilance. European countries were well on the way to eliminating measles in 2009 (as the Americas have done), when an epidemic swept into Western Europe putting over 7,000 people in hospital in 2009 to 2011, and killing nine, including seven children in France, because there had been a suboptimal rate of vaccination a few years previously (WHO, 2011b). However, the biggest burden of disease in 2011 came from the South-East Asia Region where they experience an incidence of around 25 per million population every year, which is around 35,000 people. There are no statistics on how many people are disabled by these preventable endemic and epidemic infections.

The mumps virus is related to measles, and can also cause sensorineural hearing loss, although unlike with measles, this is commonly unilateral (Cohen et al., 2014). Studies from Finland (Vartiainen & Karjalainen, 1998) and Sweden (Darin & Hanner, 1997) suggest great success in reducing mumps-related hearing loss, with no cases of mumps-induced hearing loss after a vaccine was introduced (although falling prior).

In countries without vaccination, the incidence of hearing loss due to preventable systemic infection remains high. In Nigeria, a survey of etiology in teaching hospitals showed that out of 115 cases of PCHI, those thought to be due to infection with measles numbered 16, meningitis 10, mumps 8, malaria 3, and "febrile illness" 21—together accounting for 50% of all cases (Dunmade et al., 2007). Note that it would be almost unheard of in the United Kingdom to have PCHI attributed to a "febrile illness" or even febrile convulsions, which is also often seen in studies from developing countries. A proportion of these may be misattribution of hearing loss from a less obvious cause. But the poor infrastructure that leads to late presentation of childhood illness, poor diagnostic facilities, and subsequent blind treatment that has probably contributed to any acquisition, also means it is impossible to tell if these children acquired PCHI through ototoxic drugs, through gross brain damage from a prolonged seizure or sepsis, or (most probably) postmeningitis.

Toxicity

Children can be given a number of ototoxic treatments, the most relevant being aminoglycoside antibiotics, such as gentamicin used in acute febrile infections and streptomycin used for tuberculosis. They cause renal toxicity and ototoxicity in almost everyone who receives a sufficiently high dose (Freeland, Jones, & Mohammed, 2010; Ruhl, Cable, & Martell, 2014), but some people have an inherited predisposition that means that even a single dose could result in permanent hearing loss (Bitner-Glindzicz et al., 2009; Fosso, Li, & Garneau-Tsodikova, 2014). A Japanese study of 459 unrelated individuals of all ages with SNHL found the A155G mitochondrial mutation in 5%, but in the 43 with potential aminoglycoside-induced hearing loss 46% had the mutation (Usami et al., 2000). The interaction between high numbers of mutations in mitochondrial DNA within a population and antibiotic requirements has led to some areas with particularly high rates (Fu et al., 2010; Liu et al., 2008; Malik, Pieter, Sudoyo, Kadir, & Marzuki, 2003; Ouyang et al., 2009; Tucci et al., 2010). Precautionary testing for special care babies and others at high risk of needing potent antibiotics has been tried (Bardien et al., 2009). Further studies on the prevalence of A155G are needed, and in the meantime, aminoglycosides should be used with caution, especially among those with family history of hearing loss (Maria Bitner-Glindzicz et al., 2009). In some parts of the world, the use of quinine-based drugs for malaria (McPherson & Swart, 1997) and in others cisplatin-based drugs for cancer contributes (Qaddoumi et al., 2012; Whelan et al., 2011) to acquired PCHI.

On a population level, there is evidence that some environmental pollutants might cause widespread reductions in hearing thresholds. These include passive cigarette smoke (Talaat, Metwaly, Khafagy, & Abdelraouf, 2014), lead (Abdel Rasoul, Al-Batanony, Mahrous, Abo-Salem, & Gabr, 2012; Shargorodsky, Curhan, Henderson, Eavey, & Curhan, 2011), and certain pesticides (Van Kerschaver, Boudewyns, Declau, Van de Heyning, & Wuyts, 2013).

Trauma and Noise

Head trauma, especially when involving pediatric temporal bone fracture, can cause dramatic hearing loss (Dunklebarger et al., 2014). Blast explosions can cause acoustic trauma due to dramatic damage to the structures of the ear (Mrena, Paakkonen, Back, Pirvola, & Ylikoski, 2004). Most worrying from a public health point of view though, is the trauma the delicate organ of Corti suffers from the cumulative effects of loud sounds over prolonged periods, termed *noise-induced hearing loss* (Burns & Robinson, 1970; Marlenga et al., 2012; WHO-PDH, 1997). Whereas exposure to loud sounds has traditionally been as military or occupation-related noise (that is, an unwanted sound), much of the exposure for the pediatric population comes from recreational sources, such as music played in clubs and regular attendance of major events, or through personal music players (Godlee, 1992). Concern over the rapid increase in use of personal music players led to the commissioning of a report by the European Commission Scientific Committee on Emerging and Newly Identified Health Risks (SCENIHR, 2008). This report found conflicting evidence on the risks of NIHL in children who listen to loud music, but cross-sectional studies have continued to show the possibility of a link (Henderson, Testa, & Hartnick, 2011; Williams, Carter, & Seeto, 2014; Xu et al., 2011). There seem to be environmental and genetic factors leading to susceptibility to the detrimental effects of noise in adults, and presumably children as well (Ecob et al., 2008; Henderson, Subramaniam, & Boettcher, 1993).

Global Burden of PCHI

In this chapter, we have seen that there are a number of aspects to the burden of disease from hearing impairment. First, there are the numbers who have hearing impairment from pre- and perinatal factors. These numbers appear to be related to human development, as shown in Figure 5–7, partly through known risk factors, but are also elevated in some ethnic backgrounds. A number of studies have found that around 70% to 80% of this PCHI can be detected by UNHS, while most of the rest develops before school entry and may well interfere with language acquisition.

Second, there are those who acquire hearing impairment postnatally. We know the proportion of postnatal to congenital is greatly elevated in poor countries, as shown by Figure 5–8. Generalizing about the five WHO country groups from Figures 5–9 and 5–10, and adding these two elements, shows the massive inequality of burden shown in Figure 5–12.

The last factor is the disability that every child with PCHI faces, which may vary. For example, the disability experienced by children varies by the availability of early detection and intervention, the educational and family support offered, the stigma hearing loss carries in their community, and any other disabilities they may have (Tucci et al., 2010).

It can be seen that the burden of permanent childhood hearing impairment follows poor health in a number of ways. Before birth, maternal poor health can give rise to prematurity and growth restriction, which are linked with hearing loss as well as other poor developmental outcomes (Kubba et al., 2004; MacDorman, Matthews, Mohangoo, & Zeitlin, 2014). Exposure to cigarette smoke (Durante et al., 2011), alcohol (Warren & Foudin, 2001) and infections in the womb (Cohen et al., 2014; Torre et al., 2012) are also detrimental in their own right. Lack of a skilled person attending birth has many poor outcomes, again including hearing problems (Olusanya, Wirz, & Luxon, 2008b). Jaundice, which

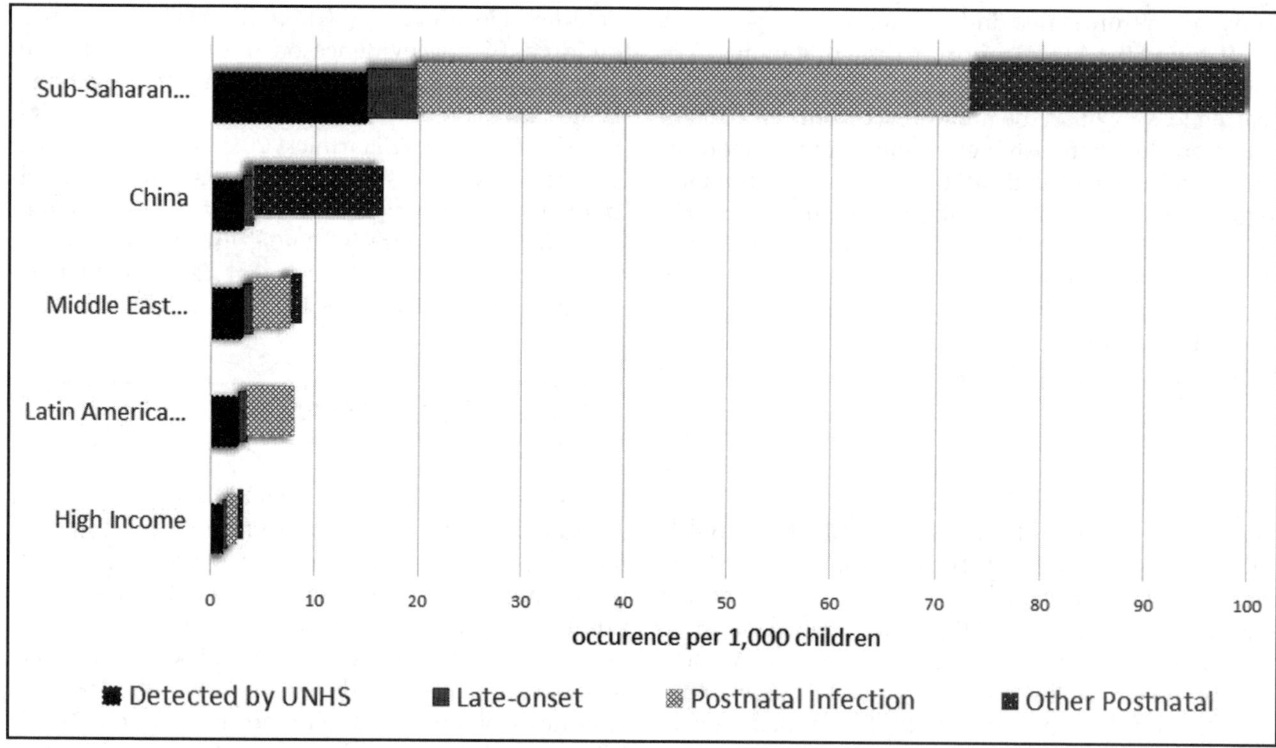

FIGURE 5–12. The burden of congenital and postnatally acquired PCHI, modeled using projected yield from universal newborn hearing screening from Figure 5–9 with late-onset correction, and the relative proportions from the studies in Table 5–8. An illustrative model of the burden of hearing impairment varying over region. (PCHI, permanent children hearing impairment.)

can be idiopathic but more commonly follows prematurity and congenital or neonatal infection, is toxic anywhere in the world; but, if there are no facilities to offer phototherapy and transfusion, the outcomes are more likely to be hearing loss and developmental delay (Olusanya, 2013).

Childhood infections such as measles are mostly harmless and preventable, but in children who already have malnutrition and dehydration, the outcomes are inevitably worse (Cohen et al., 2014). Other diseases such as meningitis are gradually being eliminated from the richer areas of the world but continue to rage elsewhere (Vella & Pace, 2015). And, because febrile illnesses are deadly, they are being treated in a blind manner with potent but toxic antibiotics (Tucci et al., 2010). Those who have the bad luck of genes that predispose them to hearing loss will come out the worst (Bitner-Glindzicz & Rahman, 2007). Chronic illnesses can damage the sensory and neural structures of hearing (Botelho et al., 2014; Naderpour, Mortazavi, Jabbari-Moghaddam, & Sharifi-Movaghar, 2011), while illnesses that damage the immune system, like certain cancers, HIV, and tuberculosis, predispose to virulent middle ear disease, and the drugs given to treat disease can again damage hearing (Olusanya, Neumann, & Saunders, 2014). Poverty can also follow chronic diseases and disabilities, especially when there is a lack of educational and employment opportunities (Olusanya et al., 2014; WHO, 2005). Poverty leads to overcrowding, predisposing to febrile illness and middle ear disease (Taha et al., 2010), that again lead to hearing loss and time away from school and work. In these circumstances, people rely on their families for survival, and there can be few opportunities to leave the village or family structure, leading to limited marital/reproductive choice, and the propagation of recessive disease genes (Saggar & Bittles, 2008).

Such a hypothesis should lead to some hope that in societies where health opportunities are low and hearing loss prevalence is high, improving health, in almost any way, can improve hearing. Antenatal, perinatal, and neonatal care—including advice to stop smoking, appropriate antiretrovirals, skilled attendant at births, better infection control in neonates, and phototherapy in rural clinics—would all help. Vaccination, promoting nutrition, and prompt treatment of dehydration would all help. Better access to diagnostics for febrile illness would help better target treatment to reduce complications and reserve ototoxic antibiotics to cases where they are needed. Encouraging better self-management of chronic illness might lead to reduced complications. Educational opportunities, even mandatory education (where there are appropriate opportunities), for the disabled as well as their well peers, can help break the cycle of inequality faced by those with hearing loss (Olusanya et al., 2014). Schemes to move families out of the subsistence trap and improve housing and social mobility will also help indirectly. Promotion of ear health is a specific intervention that promises to help those most at risk (WHO, 2012).

Early detection of hearing loss and specific rehabilitation such as hearing aids, cochlear implants, and teachers of the deaf are worthwhile goals in many places but are economically completely unattainable for many poor countries, partly because of the massive prevalence (Olusanya et al., 2014). Here, the aim should be primary prevention, with improved maternal and infant health and awareness-raising until prevalence has fallen.

Summary

In this chapter, we have looked at the epidemiology of childhood deafness and hearing impairment, particularly PCHI, as relevant to audiology service planning, clinical work, and research. Estimates of the prevalence of PCHI vary depending on definitions and population. In most moderate- to high-income (Westernized) countries, the true prevalence of bilateral PCHI of at least moderate severity that is detectable very soon after birth is probably 1.2 to 1.7 per 1,000 live births, of which around 20% to 30% will be profound hearing impairment. Around half as many again will be born with unilateral hearing loss. Many more will have milder hearing losses. The number of observed cases rises with age until around age 6 years, and this is due to a combination of acquired causes (mainly meningitis), delayed manifestation of hearing loss of pre- and perinatal cause, and delayed detection of congenital PCHI. Universal newborn hearing screening (UNHS) implementation has and will continue to cut the number of cases of moderate or greater hearing impairment that have a delayed diagnosis.

Comparing different populations shows that there are differences in the epidemiology in terms of overall prevalence, spread of severity, and etiology. Risk factors are the same across all populations, the main being family history, perinatal problems, and other congenital abnormality (especially craniofacial). Consanguinity, nonimmunization, lack of access to quality health care, and poverty probably also predispose to PCHI. Etiology is changing in developed countries, with infectious causes falling, and genetic and perinatal causes rising, while overall prevalence has stayed much the same. Genetic causes account for approaching half of cases in most high-income countries, but might be more in the Middle East and South Asia, probably related to consanguinity. The increase in recreational noise exposure does not seem to have had an effect on childhood hearing but may have the potential to accelerate age-related hearing loss that will affect these children as adults in decades to come. In developing countries, acquired causes such as systemic infection, otitis media, and ototoxicity still predominate.

How does our knowledge of the epidemiology of PCHI and the performance of current screening programs influence our understanding of the services that are needed? First, it shows the huge importance of immunization and other steps to prevent PCHI, both in reducing prevalence and freeing up resources to offer a better service to those that remain. Second, it shows there are different types of PCHI, so everyone referred after screening needs to have their needs assessed by well-networked high-quality diagnostic and treatment services. Parents and guardians are as important as ever in identifying problems and advocating (or delaying) contact with professionals, so they need to be educated, have access to appropriate information on service performance, and be involved where possible. Last, different countries, areas, and local communities will have different patterns of PCHI and different priorities, such that it is important for local professionals to agree on services specification, building on national and regional frameworks, to match the relevant epidemiology to the services needed to reduce burden for the children, families, and communities in their area.

References

Aasham, T., Khandekar, R., Khabori, M., & Helmi, S. A. (2004). Cost-effectiveness of audiometric screening of first-year preparatory pupils in Dhofar Region, Oman. *East Mediterranean Health Journal*, *10*(3), 303–308.

Abdel Rasoul, G. M., Al-Batanony, M. A., Mahrous, O. A., Abo-Salem, M. E., & Gabr, H. M. (2012). Environmental lead exposure among primary school children in Shebin El-Kom District, Menoufiya Governorate, Egypt. *The International Journal of Occupational and Environmental Medicine, 3*(4), 186–194.

Abdullah, A., Hazim, M. Y., Almyzan, A., Jamilah, A. G., Roslin, S., Ann, M. T., . . . Boo, N. Y. (2006). Newborn hearing screening: Experience in a Malaysian hospital. *Singapore Medical Journal, 47*(1), 60–64.

Adachi, N., Ito, K., & Sakata, H. (2010). Risk factors for hearing loss after pediatric meningitis in Japan. *Annals of Otology, Rhinology and Laryngology, 119*(5), 294–296.

Adelola, O. A., Papanikolaou, V., Gormley, P., Lang, J., & Keogh, I. J. (2010). Newborn hearing screening: A regional example for national care. *Irish Medical Journal, 103*(5), 146–149.

Admiraal, R. J., & Huygen, P. L. (2000). Changes in the etiology of hearing impairment in deaf-blind pupils and deaf infant pupils at an institute for the deaf. *International Journal of Pediatric Otorhinolaryngology, 55*(2), 133–142. doi:S0165-5876(00)00395-5 [pii]

Ahmad, A., Mohamad, I., Mansor, S., Daud, M. K., & Sidek, D. (2011). Outcome of a newborn hearing screening program in a tertiary hospital in Malaysia: The first five years. *Annals of Saudi Medicine, 31*(1), 24–28. doi:10.4103/0256-4947.75774

Ahmed, A. O., Kolo, E. S., Abah, E. R., & Oladigbolu, K. K. (2012). An appraisal of common otologic disorders as seen in a deaf population in North-Western Nigeria. *Annals of African Medicine, 11*(3), 153–156. doi:10.4103/1596-3519.96875

Aithal, S., Aithal, V., Kei, J., & Driscoll, C. (2012). Conductive hearing loss and middle ear pathology in young infants referred through a newborn universal hearing screening program in Australia [Research Support, Non-U.S. Gov't]. *Journal of the American Academy of Audiology, 23*(9), 673–685. doi:10.3766/jaaa.23.9.2

Akinpelu, O., & Amusa, Y. (2007). Otological diseases in Nigerian children. *Internet Journal of Otorhinolaryngology, 7*(1).

Akinpelu, O. V., Waissbluth, S., & Daniel, S. J. (2013). Auditory risk of hyperbilirubinemia in term newborns: A systematic review. [Review]. *International Journal of Pediatric Otorhinolaryngology, 77*(6), 898–905. doi:10.1016/j.ijporl.2013.03.029

Al Khabori, M. (2004). Causes of severe to profound deafness in Omani pediatric population. *International Journal of Pediatric Otorhinolaryngology, 68*(10), 1307–1313. doi:10.1016/j.ijporl.2004.05.002 S0165-5876(04)00154-5 [pii]

Alberti, P. W. (1999). Pediatric ear, nose and throat services' demands and resources: A global perspective. *International Journal of Pediatric Otorhinolaryngology, 49*(Suppl. 1), S1–S9.

Attias, J., Al-Masri, M., Abukader, L., Cohen, G., Merlov, P., Pratt, H., . . . Noyek, A. (2006). The prevalence of congenital and early-onset hearing loss in Jordanian and Israeli infants. *International Journal of Audiology, 45*(9), 528–536. doi:T403312W7U410632 [pii] 10.1080/14992020600810039

Augustine, A. M., Jana, A. K., Kuruvilla, K. A., Danda, S., Lepcha, A., Ebenezer, J., . . . Balraj, A. (2014). Neonatal hearing screening—Experience from a tertiary care hospital in southern India. [Research Support, Non-U.S. Gov't]. *Indian Pediatrics, 51*(3), 179–183.

Avettand-Fenoel, V., Marlin, S., Vauloup-Fellous, C., Loundon, N., Francois, M., Couloigner, V., . . . Leruez-Ville, M. (2013). Congenital cytomegalovirus is the second most frequent cause of bilateral hearing loss in young French children. [Research Support, Non-U.S. Gov't]. *Journal of Pediatrics, 162*(3), 593–599. doi:10.1016/j.jpeds.2012.08.009

Baecher-Lind, L. E., Miller, W. C., & Wilcox, A. J. (2010). Infectious disease and reproductive health: A Review. *Obstetrical & Gynecological Survey, 65*(1), 53–65. doi:10.1097/OGX.0b013e3181c9e7a1

Bajaj, Y., Sirimanna, T., Albert, D. M., Qadir, P., Jenkins, L., Cortina-Borja, M., & Bitner-Glindzicz, M. (2009). Causes of deafness in British Bangladeshi children: A prevalence twice that of the UK population cannot be accounted for by consanguinity alone. *Clinical Otolaryngology, 34*(2), 113–119. doi:COA1888 [pii]10.1111/j.1749-4486.2009.01888.x

Baker, H., Crockett, R., Uus, K., Bamford, J., & Marteau, T. (2007). Why don't health professionals check patient understanding? A questionnaire-based study. *Psychology Health and Medicine, 12*(3), 380–385. doi:778838613 [pii] 10.1080/13548500601133466

Bamford, J., Fortnum, H., Bristow, K., Smith, J., Vamvakas, G., Davies, L., . . . Hind, S. (2007). Current practice, accuracy, effectiveness and cost-effectiveness of the school entry hearing screen. *Health Technology Assessment, 11*(32), 1–168, iii–iv. doi:03/05/01 [pii]

Bamford, J., Uus, K., & Davis, A. (2005). Screening for hearing loss in childhood: Issues, evidence and current approaches in the UK. *Journal of Medical Screening, 12*(3), 119–124. doi:10.1258/0969141054855256

Barbi, M., Binda, S., Caroppo, S., Ambrosetti, U., Corbetta, C., & Sergi, P. (2003). A wider role for congenital cytomegalovirus infection in sensorineural hearing loss. *Pediatric Infectious Disease Journal, 22*(1), 39–42. doi:10.1097/01.inf.0000047673.38917.e4

Bardien, S., Human, H., Harris, T., Hefke, G., Veikondis, R., Schaaf, H. S., . . . de Jong, G. (2009). A rapid method for detection of five known mutations associated with aminoglycoside-induced deafness. *BMC Medical Genetics, 10*(2), 1471–2350.

Bastos, I., Mallya, J., Ingvarsson, L., Reimer, A., & Andreasson, L. (1995). Middle ear disease and hearing impairment in northern Tanzania. A prevalence study of schoolchildren in the Moshi and Monduli districts. *International Journal of Pediatric Otorhinolaryngology, 32*(1), 1–12. doi:016558769401904C [pii]

Beck, C., Pérez-Álvarez, J., Sigruener, A., Haubner, F., Seidler, T., Aslanidis, C., . . . Schmitz, G. (2014). Identification and genotype/phenotype correlation of mutations in a large German cohort with hearing loss. *European Archives of Oto-Rhino-Laryngology*, 1–12. doi:10.1007/s00405-014-3157-5

Bedford, H., de Louvois, J., Halket, S., Peckham, C., Hurley, R., & Harvey, D. (2001). Meningitis in infancy in England and Wales: Follow up at age 5 years. *BMJ, 323*(7312), 533–536.

Bener, A., Eihakeem, A. A., & Abdulhadi, K. (2005). Is there any association between consanguinity and hearing loss? *International Journal of Pediatric Otorhinolaryngology, 69*(3), 327–333. doi:S0165-5876(04)00334-9 [pii]10.1016/j.ijporl.2004.10.004

Bennett, K., & Haggard, M. (1998). Accumulation of factors influencing children's middle ear disease: Risk factor modelling on a large population cohort. *Journal of Epidemiology and Community Health, 52*(12), 786–793. doi:10.1136/jech.52.12.786

Bess, F. H., Dodd-Murphy, J., & Parker, R. A. (1998). Children with minimal sensorineural hearing loss: Prevalence, educational performance, and functional status. *Ear and Hearing, 19*(5), 339–354.

Beswick, R., Driscoll, C., Kei, J., Khan, A., & Glennon, S. (2013). Which risk factors predict postnatal hearing loss in children? *Journal of the American Academy of Audiology, 24*(3), 205–213. doi:10.3766/jaaa.24.3.6

Bielecki, I., Horbulewicz, A., & Wolan, T. (2011). Risk factors associated with hearing loss in infants: An analysis of 5282 referred neonates. *International Journal of Pediatric Otorhinolaryngology, 75*(7), 925–930. doi:http://dx.doi.org/10.1016/j.ijporl.2011.04.007

Bitner-Glindzicz, M., Pembrey, M., Duncan, A., Heron, J., Ring, S. M., Hall, A., & Rahman, S. (2009). Prevalence of mitochondrial 1555A->G mutation in European children. *New England Journal of Medicine, 360*(6), 640–642. doi:10.1056/NEJMc0806396

Bitner-Glindzicz, M., & Rahman, S. (2007). Ototoxicity caused by aminoglycosides. *BMJ, 335*(7624), 784–785. doi:335/7624/784 [pii]10.1136/bmj.39301.680266.AE

Bonyadi, M. J., Fotouhi, N., & Esmaeili, M. (2014). Spectrum and frequency of *GJB2* mutations causing deafness in the northwest of Iran. [Research Support, Non-U.S. Gov't]. *International Journal of Pediatric Otorhinolaryngology, 78*(4), 637–640. doi:10.1016/j.ijporl.2014.01.022

Bosch, J., Lebeko, K., Nziale, J. J., Dandara, C., Makubalo, N., & Wonkam, A. (2014). In search of genetic markers for nonsyndromic deafness in Africa: A study in Cameroonians and Black South Africans with the GJB6 and GJA1 candidate genes. [Research Support, Non-U.S. Gov't]. *Omics: Journal of Integrative Biology, 18*(7), 481–485. doi:10.1089/omi.2013.0166

Botelho, C. T., Carvalho, S. A., & Silva, I. N. (2014). Increased prevalence of early cochlear damage in young patients with type 1 diabetes detected by distortion product otoacoustic emissions. [Comparative Study Research Support, Non-U.S. Gov't]. *International Journal of Audiology, 53*(6), 402–408. doi:10.3109/14992027.2013.879341

Botelho, M. S., Silva, V. B., Arruda Lda, S., Kuniyoshi, I. C., Oliveira, L. L., & Oliveira, A. S. (2010). Newborn hearing screening in the Limiar Clinic in Porto Velho-Rondonia. *Brazilian Journal of Otorhinolaryngology, 76*(5), 605–610.

Braine, T. (2011). Race against time to develop new antibiotics. *Bulletin of the World Health Organization,* 89, 88–89. doi:10.2471/BLT.11.030211

Brent, R. L. (2004). Environmental causes of human congenital malformations: The pediatrician's role in dealing with these complex clinical problems caused by a multiplicity of environmental and genetic factors. *Pediatrics, 113* (4 Suppl), 957–968.

British Association of Audiological Physicians/British Association of Paediatricians in Audiology. (2008). *Guidelines for investigating infants with congenital hearing loss identified through the newborn hearing screening,* produced by the British Association of Audiovestibular Physicians and British Association of Pediatricians in Audiology. Retrieved from http://baap.org.uk/Resources/Documents,Guidelines ClinicalStandards.aspx

Brown, K. K., & Rehm, H. L. (2001). *Molecular diagnosis of hearing loss current protocols in human genetics.* New York, NY: Wiley.

Burns, W., & Robinson, D. W. (1970). An investigation of the effects of occupational noise on hearing. In: Sensorineural hearing loss. In G. E. W. Wonstenholme & J. Knight (Eds.), *Ciba Foundation Symposium* (pp. 177–192). New York, NY: Wiley.

Bush, M. L., Osetinsky, M., Shinn, J. B., Gal, T. J., Ding, X., Fardo, D. W., & Schoenberg, N. (2014). Assessment of Appalachian region pediatric hearing healthcare disparities and delays. [Research Support, N.I.H., Extramural]. *Laryngoscope, 124*(7), 1713–1717. doi:10.1002/lary.24588

Cannon, M. J., Griffiths, P. D., Aston, V., & Rawlinson, W. D. (2014). Universal newborn screening for congenital CMV infection: What is the evidence of potential benefit? *Reviews in Medical Virology,* 24(5), 291–230. doi:10.1002/rmv.1790

Centers for Disease Control and Prevention (CDC; 2008). Annual EHDI data. Early Hearing Detection & Intervention (EHDI) Program (September 29, 2008).

Centers for Disease Control and Prevention (CDC; 2015). 2013 annual data. Early Hearing Detection and Intervention (EHDI). Hearing Loss in Children. Retrieved from http://www.cdc.gov/ncbddd/hearingloss/ehdi-data2013.html

Chapman, D. A., Stampfel, C. C., Bodurtha, J. N., Dodson, K. M., Pandya, A., Lynch, K. B., & Kirby, R. S. (2011). Impact of co-occurring birth defects on the timing of newborn hearing screening and diagnosis. [Research Support, Non-U.S. Gov't Research Support, U.S. Gov't, P.H.S.] *American Journal of Audiology, 20*(2), 132–139. doi:10.1044/1059-0889(2011/10-0049

Chen, G., Fu, S., Luo, S., Zhang, W., & Yang, G. (2013). Screening of delayed-onset hearing loss in preschool children in the mid-south of China. *International Journal of Audiology, 52*(8), 568–571. doi:10.3109/14992027.2013.796408

Christensen, H., Trotter, C. L., Hickman, M., & Edmunds, W. J. (2014). Re-evaluating cost effectiveness of universal meningitis vaccination (Bexsero) in England: Modelling study. *BMJ, 349*(g5725), 1–18. doi:10.1136/bmj.g5725

Christopher, N., Edward, T., Sabrina, B. K., & Agnes, N. (2013). The prevalence of hearing impairment in the 6 months–5 years HIV/AIDS-positive patients attending pediatric infectious disease clinic at Mulago Hospital. *International Journal of Pediatric Otorhinolaryngology, 77*(2), 262–265. doi:10.1016/j.ijporl.2012.11.013

Cohen, B. E., Durstenfeld, A., & Roehm, P. C. (2014). Viral causes of hearing loss: A review for hearing health professionals. *Trends in Hearing, 18*, 1–17. doi:10.1177/2331216514541361

Consortium for Research in Deaf Education, C. (2014). *CRIDE report on 2014 survey on educational provision for deaf children: The British Association of Teachers of the Deaf, BATOD.* London, UK: National Deaf Children's Society.

Czechowicz, J. A., Messner, A. H., Alarcon-Matutti, E., Alarcon, J., Quinones-Calderon, G., Montano, S., & Zunt, J. R. (2010). Hearing impairment and poverty: The epidemiology of ear disease in Peruvian schoolchildren. *Otolaryngology-Head and Neck Surgery, 142*(2), 272–277. doi:S0194-5998(09)01660-X [pii]10.1016/j.otohns.2009.10.040

D'Angio, C. T., Froehlke, R. G., Plank, G. A., Meehan, D. J., Aguilar, C. M., Lande, M. B., & Hugar, L. (1995). Long-term outcome of *Haemophilus influenzae* meningitis in Navajo Indian children. *Archives of Pediatric Adolescent Medicine, 149*(9), 1001–1008.

Darin, N., & Hanner, P. (1997). Changes in prevalence, aetiology, age at detection, and associated disabilities in preschool children with hearing impairment born in Göteborg. *Developmental Medicine & Child Neurology, 39*(12), 797–802. doi:10.1111/j.1469-8749.1997.tb07545.x

Davidson, J., Hyde, M. L., & Alberti, P. W. (1989). Epidemiologic patterns in childhood hearing loss: A review. *International Journal of Pediatric Otorhinolaryngology, 17*(3), 239–266.

Davis, A., & Parving, A. (1994). Towards appropriate epidemiological data on childhood hearing disability: A comparative European study of birth cohorts 1982–88. *International Journal of Audiological Medicine, 3*(1), 35.

Davis, A., & Wood, S. (1992). The epidemiology of childhood hearing impairment: Factor relevant to planning of services. *British Journal of Audiology, 26*(2), 77–90.

De Capua, B., Costantini, D., Martufi, C., Latini, G., Gentile, M., & De Felice, C. (2007). Universal neonatal hearing screening: The Siena (Italy) experience on 19,700 newborns. *Early Human Development, 83*(9), 601–606. doi:S0378-3782(07)00002-3 [pii]10.1016/j.earlhumdev.2007.01.001

de Nobrega, M., Weckx, L. L., & Juliano, Y. (2005). Study of the hearing loss in children and adolescents, comparing the periods of 1990–1994 and 1994–2000. *International Journal of Pediatric Otorhinolaryngology, 69*(6), 829–838. doi:S0165-5876(05)00058-3 [pii]10.1016/j.ijporl.2005.01.019

Deben, K., Janssens de Varebeke, S., Cox, T., & Van de Heyning, P. (2003). Epidemiology of hearing impairment at three Flemish Institutes for Deaf and Speech Defective Children. *International Journal of Pediatric Otorhinolaryngology, 67*(9), 969–975. doi:S0165587603001861 [pii]

Deklerck, A. N., Acke, F. R., Janssens, S., & De Leenheer, E. M. R. (2015). Etiological approach in patients with unidentified hearing loss. *International Journal of Pediatric Otorhinolaryngology, 79*(2), 216–222. http://dx.doi.org/10.1016/j.ijporl.2014.12.012

Dennett, K. V., Fligor, B. J., Tracy, S., Wilson, J. M., Zurakowski, D., & Chen, C. (2014). Sensorineural hearing loss in congenital diaphragmatic hernia survivors is associated with postnatal management and not defect size. [Research Support, Non-U.S. Gov't]. *Journal of Pediatric Surgery, 49*(6), 895–899. doi:10.1016/j.jpedsurg.2014.01.049

Di Renzo, G., Rosati, A., Sarti, R., Cruciani, L., & Cutuli, A. (2007). Does fetal sex affect pregnancy outcome? *Gender Medicine, 4*(1), 19–30. doi:10.1016/S1550-8579(07)80004-0

Drews, C. D., Yeargin-Allsopp, M., Murphy, C. C., & Decoufle, P. (1994). Hearing impairment among 10-year-old children: Metropolitan Atlanta, 1985 through 1987. *American Journal of Public Health, 84*(7), 1164–1166.

Dunklebarger, J., Branstetter, B. T., Lincoln, A., Sippey, M., Cohen, M., Gaines, B., & Chi, D. (2014). Pediatric temporal bone fractures: Current trends and comparison of classification schemes. [Comparative study]. *Laryngoscope, 124*(3), 781–784. doi:10.1002/lary.21891

Dunmade, A. D., Segun-Busari, S., Olajide, T. G., & Ologe, F. E. (2007). Profound bilateral sensorineural hearing loss in Nigerian children: Any shift in etiology? *Journal of Deaf Studies and Deaf Education, 12*(1), 112–118. doi:enl019 [pii]10.1093/deafed/enl019

Durante, A. S., Ibidi, S. M., Lotufo, J. P., & Carvallo, R. M. (2011). Maternal smoking during pregnancy: Impact on otoacoustic emissions in neonates. [Research Support, Non-U.S. Gov't]. *International Journal of Pediatric Otorhinolaryngology, 75*(9), 1093–1098. doi:10.1016/j.ijporl.2011.05.023

Dyer, J. J., Strasnick, B., & Jacobson, J. T. (1998). Teratogenic hearing loss: A clinical perspective. *American Journal of Otology, 19*(5), 671–678.

Ecob, R., Sutton, G., Rudnicka, A., Smith, P., Power, C., Strachan, D., & Davis, A. (2008). Is the relation of social class to change in hearing threshold levels from childhood to middle age explained by noise, smoking, and drinking behavior? *International Journal of Audiology, 47*(3), 100–108. doi:791033452 [pii]10.1080/14992020701647942

El-Badry, M. M., Hamdy, N. A., Sobhy, S., & Gamal, R. (2014). Epileptiform electroencephalogram abnormality in children with congenital sensorineural hearing loss. *International Journal of Pediatric Otorhinolaryngology, 78*(4), 623–630. doi:10.1016/j.ijporl.2014.01.018

Elziere, M., Roman, S., Nicollas, R., & Triglia, J. M. (2012). Value of systematic aetiological investigation in children with sensorineural hearing loss. *European Annals of Otorhinolaryngology, Head and Neck Diseases, 129*(4), 185–189. doi:http://dx.doi.org/10.1016/j.anorl.2011.05.009

Firoozbakht, M., Mahmoudian, S., Alaeddini, F., Esmaeilzadeh, M., Rafiei, M., Firouzbakht, A., . . . Farhadi, M. (2014). Community-based newborn hearing screening programmed for early detection of permanent hearing loss in Iran: An eight-year cross-sectional study from 2005 to 2012. [Research Support, Non-U.S. Gov't]. *Journal of Medical Screening, 21*(1), 10–17. doi:10.1177/0969141314522992

Fitzpatrick, E. (2015). Neurocognitive development in congenitally deaf children. [Research Support, Non-U.S. Gov't Review]. *Handbook of Clinical Neurology, 129*, 335–356. doi:10.1016/B978-0-444-62630-1.00019-6

Foerst, A., Beutner, D., Lang-Roth, R., Huttenbrink, K.-B., von Wedel, H., & Walger, M. (2006). Prevalence of auditory neuropathy/synaptopathy in a population of children with profound hearing loss. *International Journal of Pediatric Otorhinolaryngology, 70*(8), 1415–1422.

Fonseca, S., Forsyth, H., & Neary, W. (2005). School hearing screening programmed in the UK: Practice and performance. *Archives of Disease in Childhood, 90*(2), 154–156. doi:90/2/154 [pii]10.1136/adc.2003.046979

Fortnum, H., & Davis, A. (1997). Epidemiology of permanent childhood hearing impairment in Trent Region, 1985–1993. *British Journal of Audiology, 31*(6), 409–446.

Fortnum, H. M., Marshall, D. H., & Summerfield, A. Q. (2002). Epidemiology of the UK population of hearing-impaired children, including characteristics of those with and without cochlear implants—Audiology, aetiology, comorbidity and affluence. *International Journal of Audiology, 41*(3), 170–179.

Fortnum, H. M., Summerfield, A. Q., Marshall, D. H., Davis, A. C., & Bamford, J. M. (2001). Prevalence of permanent childhood hearing impairment in the United Kingdom and implications for universal neonatal hearing screening: Questionnaire based ascertainment study. *BMJ, 323*(7312), 536–540.

Fosso, M. Y., Li, Y., & Garneau-Tsodikova, S. (2014). New trends in the use of aminoglycosides. [10.1039/C4MD00163J]. *Medicinal Chemical Communications, 5*(8), 1075–1091. doi:10.1039/c4md00163j

Freeland, A., Jones, J., & Mohammed, N. K. (2010). Sensorineural deafness in Tanzanian children—Is ototoxicity a significant cause? A pilot study. *International Journal of Pediatric Otorhinolaryngology, 74*(5), 516–519. doi:S0165-5876(10)00058-3 [pii]10.1016/j.ijporl.2010.02.010

Fu, S., Chen, G., Dong, J., & Zhang, L. (2010). Prevalence and etiology of hearing loss in primary and middle school students in the Hubei Province of China. [Research Support, Non-U.S. Gov't]. *Audiology & Neuro-Otology, 15*(6), 394–398. doi:10.1159/000307346

Ghirri, P., Liumbruno, A., Lunardi, S., Forli, F., Boldrini, A., Baggiani, A., & Berrettini, S. (2011). Universal neonatal audiological screening: Experience of the University Hospital of Pisa. *Italian Journal of Pediatrics, 37*, 16. doi:10.1186/1824-7288-37-16

Gierek, T., Gwozdz-Jezierska, M., Markowski, J., & Witkowska, M. (2009). The assessment of hearing organ of school children in Upper Silesia region. *International Journal of Pediatric Otorhinolaryngology, 73*(12), 1644–1649. doi:S0165-5876(09)00425-X [pii]10.1016/j.ijporl.2009.08.009

Gilbey, P., Kraus, C., Ghanayim, R., Sharabi-Nov, A., & Bretler, S. (2013). Universal newborn hearing screening in Zefat, Israel: The first two years. *International Journal of Pediatric Otorhinolaryngology, 77*(1), 97–100. http://dx.doi.org/10.1016/j.ijporl.2012.10.004

Goderis, J., De Leenheer, E., Smets, K., Van Hoecke, H., Keymeulen, A., & Dhooge, I. (2014). Hearing loss and congenital CMV infection: A systematic review. *Pediatrics, 134*(5), 972–982. doi:10.1542/peds.2014-1173

Godlee, F. (1992). Noise: Breaking the silence. *BMJ, 304*(6819), 110–113.

Gonzalez de Aledo Linos, A., Bonilla Miera, C., Morales Angulo, C., Gomez Da Casa, F., & Barrasa Benito, J. (2005). [Universal newborn hearing screening in Cantabria (Spain): results of the first two years]. *An Pediatr (Barc), 62*(2), 135–140. doi:13071310 [pii]

Grimwood, K., Anderson, V. A., Bond, L., Catroppa, C., Hore, R. L., Keir, E. H., . . . Roberton, D. M. (1995). Adverse outcomes of bacterial meningitis in school-age survivors. *Pediatrics, 95*(5), 646–656.

Gultekin, E., Develioglu, Ö. N., Yener, M., Ozdemir, I., & Külekçi, M. (2010). Prevalence and risk factors for persistent otitis media with effusion in primary school children in Istanbul, Turkey. *Auris Nasus Larynx, 37*(2), 145–149. doi:10.1016/j.anl.2009.05.002

Habib, H. S., & Abdelgaffar, H. (2005). Neonatal hearing screening with transient evoked otoacoustic emissions in Western Saudi Arabia. *International Journal of Pediatric Otorhinolaryngology, 69*(6), 839–842. doi:S0165-5876(05)00059-5 [pii]10.1016/j.ijporl.2005.01.018

Häkli, S., Luotonen, M., Bloigu, R., Majamaa, K., & Sorri, M. (2014). Childhood hearing impairment in northern Finland, etiology and additional disabilities. *International Journal of Pediatric Otorhinolaryngology, 78*(11), 1852–1856. http://dx.doi.org/10.1016/j.ijporl.2014.08.007

Hall, A. J., Midgley, E., Steer, C., & Humphriss, R. (2011). Prevalence and risk factors for mild and high-frequency bilateral sensorineural hearing loss at age 11 years old: A UK prospective cohort study. [Research Support, Non-U.S. Gov't]. *International Journal of Audiology, 50*(11), 809–814. doi:10.3109/14992027.2011.599869

Hayashi, C., Funayama, M., Li, Y., Kamiya, K., Kawano, A., Suzuki, M., . . . Ikeda, K. (2011). Prevalence of *GJB2* causing recessive profound non-syndromic deafness in Japanese children. [Comparative study]. *International Journal of Pediatric Otorhinolaryngology, 75*(2), 211–214. doi:10.1016/j.ijporl.2010.11.001

Henderson, D., Subramaniam, M., & Boettcher, F. A. (1993). Individual susceptibility to noise-induced hearing loss: An old topic revisited. *Ear and Hearing, 14*(3), 152–168.

Henderson, E., Testa, M. A., & Hartnick, C. (2011). Prevalence of noise-induced hearing-threshold shifts and hearing loss among US youths. *Pediatrics, 127*(1), e39–46. doi:10.1542/peds.2010-0926

High Risk Follow-up Working Group, K. R. (2008). Neurodevelopmental outcomes of extreme-low-birth-weight infants born between 2001 and 2002. *Hong Kong Medical Journal, 14*(1), 21–28.

Hindley, P. A., Hill, P. D., McGuigan, S., & Kitson, N. (1994). Psychiatric disorder in deaf and hearing impaired children and young people: A prevalence study. *Journal of Child Psychology and Psychiatry, 35*(5), 917–934.

Hintermair, M. (2000). Hearing impairment, social networks, and coping: The need for families with hearing-impaired children to relate to other parents and to hearing-impaired adults. *American Annals of the Deaf, 145*(1), 41–53.

Hoffman, H. J., Daly, K. A., Bainbridge, K. E., Casselbrant, M. L., Homoe, P., Kvestad, E., . . . Vernacchio, L. (2013). Advances in otitis media. Panel 1: Epidemiology, natural history, and risk factors. *Otolaryngology-Head and Neck Surgery, 148*(4 Suppl.), E1–E25.

Huang, H. M., Chiang, S. H., Shiau, Y. S., Yeh, W. Y., Ho, H. C., Wang, L., . . . Hsiao, K. J. (2013). The universal newborn hearing screening program of Taipei City. [Multicenter Study Research Support, Non-U.S. Gov't]. *International Journal of Pediatric Otorhinolaryngology, 77*(10), 1734–1737. doi:10.1016/j.ijporl.2013.08.004

Huang, L., Cai, Z., Zhang, H., Peng, S., Wu, D., Wang, L., . . . Han, D. (2009). [Study on multi-area universal newborn hearing screening in countryside of China]. *Lin Chung Er Bi Yan Hou Tou Jing Wai Ke Za Zhi, 23*(16), 737–742.

Hultcrantz, M. (2003). Ear and hearing problems in Turner's syndrome. *Acta Oto-laryngologica, 123*(2), 253–257.

Jacob, A., Rupa, V., Job, A., & Joseph, A. (1997). Hearing impairment and otitis media in a rural primary school in south India. *International Journal of Pediatric Otorhinolaryngology, 39*(2), 133–138. doi:S0165587696014796 [pii]

Jakubikova, J., Kabatova, Z., Pavlovcinova, G., & Profant, M. (2009). Newborn hearing screening and strategy for early detection of hearing loss in infants. *International Journal of Pediatric Otorhinolaryngology, 73*(4), 607–612. doi:S0165-5876(08)00596-X [pii]10.1016/j.ijporl.2008.12.006

Javidnia, H., Carson, N., Awubwa, M., Byaruhanga, R., Mack, D., & Vaccani, J. P. (2014). Connexin gene mutations among Ugandan patients with nonsyndromic sensorineural hearing loss. [Observational Study Research Support, Non-U.S. Gov't]. *Laryngoscope, 124*(9), E373–E376. doi:10.1002/lary.24697

Jensen, R. G., Koch, A., & Homoe, P. (2013). The risk of hearing loss in a population with a high prevalence of chronic suppurative otitis media. [Research Support, Non-U.S. Gov't]. *International Journal of Pediatric Otorhinolaryngology, 77*(9), 1530–1535. doi:10.1016/j.ijporl.2013.06.025

Jiang, H., Chen, J., Shan, X. J., Li, Y., He, J. G., & Yang, B. B. (2014). Prevalence and range of GJB2 and SLC26A4 mutations in patients with autosomal recessive nonsyndromic hearing loss. [Research Support, Non-U.S. Gov't]. *Molecular Medicine Reports, 10*(1), 379–386. doi:10.3892/mmr.2014.2148

Joint Committee on Infant Hearing (JCIH; 2007). Year 2007 Position Statement: Principles and guidelines for early hearing detection and intervention programs. *Pediatrics, 120*(4), 898–921. doi:10.1542/peds.2007-2333

Jusot, J. F., Tohon, Z., Yazi, A. A., & Collard, J. M. (2013). Significant sequelae after bacterial meningitis in Niger: A cohort study. [Research Support, Non-U.S. Gov't]. *BMC Infectious Diseases, 13*, 228. doi:10.1186/1471-2334-13-228

Kabahuma, R. I., Ouyang, X., Du, L. L., Yan, D., Hutchin, T., Ramsay, M., . . . Liu, X. Z. (2011). Absence of *GJB2* gene mutations, the *GJB6* deletion (GJB6-D13S1830) and four common mitochondrial mutations in nonsyndromic genetic hearing loss in a South African population. [Comparative Study Research Support, N.I.H., Extramural Research Support, Non-U.S. Gov't]. *International Journal of Pediatric Otorhinolaryngology, 75*(5), 611–617. doi:10.1016/j.ijporl.2011.01.029

Kanji, A., & Khoza-Shangase, K. (2012). The occurrence of high-risk factors for hearing loss in very-low-birth-weight neonates: A retrospective exploratory study of targeted hearing screening. *South African Journal of Communication Disorders. Die Suid-Afrikaanse tydskrif vir Kommunikasieafwykings, 59*, 3–7.

Karanja, B. W., Oburra, H. O., Masinde, P., & Wamalwa, D. (2014). Prevalence of hearing loss in children following bacterial meningitis in a tertiary referral hospital. *BMC Research Notes, 7*, 138. doi:10.1186/1756-0500-7-138

Keats, B. J. (2002). Genes and syndromic hearing loss. *Journal of Communication Disorders, 35*(4), 355–366.

Khairi Md Daud, M., Noor, R. M., Rahman, N. A., Sidek, D. S., & Mohamad, A. (2009). The effect of mild hearing loss on academic performance in primary school children. *International Journal of Pediatric Otorhinolaryngology, 74*(1), 67–70. doi:S0165-5876(09)00543-6 [pii]10.1016/j.ijporl.2009.10.013

Kimberlin, D. W., Lin, C. Y., Sanchez, P. J., Demmler, G. J., Dankner, W., Shelton, M., . . . Whitley, R. J. (2003). Effect of ganciclovir therapy on hearing in symptomatic congenital cytomegalovirus disease involving the central nervous system: A randomized, controlled trial. *Journal of Pediatrics, 143*(1), 16–25. doi:S0022347603001926 [pii]

Kirkim, G., Serbetcioglu, B., Erdag, T. K., & Ceryan, K. (2008). The frequency of auditory neuropathy detected by universal newborn hearing screening program. *International Journal of Pediatric Otorhinolaryngology, 72*(10), 1461–1469. doi:S0165-5876(08)00265-6 [pii]10.1016/j.ijporl.2008.06.010

Kitsantas, P., Kornides, M. L., Cantiello, J., & Wu, H. (2013). Chronic physical health conditions among children of different racial/ethnic backgrounds. [Research Support, N.I.H., Extramural]. *Public Health, 127*(6), 546–553. doi:10.1016/j.puhe.2013.02.006

Kokotas, H., Petersen, M. B., & Willems, P. J. (2007). Mitochondrial deafness. *Clinical Genetics, 71*(5), 379–391. doi:CGE800 [pii]10.1111/j.1399-0004.2007.00800.x

Koomen, I., Grobbee, D. E., Roord, J. J., Donders, R., Jennekens-Schinkel, A., & van Furth, A. M. (2003). Hearing loss at school age in survivors of bacterial meningitis: Assessment, incidence, and prediction. *Pediatrics, 112*(5), 1049–1053. doi:10.1542/peds.112.5.1049

Korres, S., Nikolopoulos, T. P., Peraki, E. E., Tsiakou, M., Karakitsou, M., Apostolopoulos, N., . . . Ferekidis, E. (2008). Outcomes and efficacy of newborn hearing screening: Strengths and weaknesses (success or failure?). *Laryngoscope, 118*(7), 1253–1256. doi:10.1097/MLG.0b013e31816d726c

Korver, A. M., van Zanten, G. A., Meuwese-Jongejeugd, A., van Straaten, H. L., & Oudesluys-Murphy, A. M. (2012). Auditory neuropathy in a low-risk population: A review of the literature. [Review]. *International Journal of Pediatric Otorhinolaryngology, 76*(12), 1708–1711. doi:10.1016/j.ijporl.2012.08.009

Kraemer, S. (2000). The fragile male. *British Medical Journal, 321*(7276), 1609–1612. doi:10.1136/bmj.321.7276.1609

Kubba, H., MacAndie, C., Ritchie, K., & MacFarlane, M. (2004). Is deafness a disease of poverty? The association between socio-economic deprivation and congenital hearing impairment. *International Journal of Audiology, 43*(3), 123–125.

Kutz, J. W., Simon, L. M., Chennupati, S. K., Giannoni, C. M., & Manolidis, S. (2006). Clinical predictors for hearing loss in children with bacterial meningitis. *Archives of Otolaryngology-Head and Neck Surgery, 132*(9), 941–945. doi:132/9/941 [pii]10.1001/archotol.132.9.941

Ladhani, S. N., & Ramsay, M. E. (2015). The story of Sisyphus: Why we need a universal pneumococcal vaccine to replace current conjugate vaccines. *Clinical Infectious Diseases, 61*(5), 776–778. doi:10.1093/cid/civ371

Lai, F. Y., Serraglio, C., & Martin, J. A. (2014). Examining potential barriers to early intervention access in Australian hearing impaired children. *International Journal of Pediatric Otorhinolaryngology, 78*(3), 507–512. doi:10.1016/j.ijporl.2013.12.032.

Lam, B. C. (2006). Newborn hearing screening in Hong Kong. *Hong Kong Medical Journal, 12*(3), 212–218.

Lambert, N., Strebel, P., Orenstein, W., Icenogle, J., & Poland, G. A. (2015). Rubella. *Lancet, 385*(9984), 2297–2307. http://dx.doi.org/10.1016/S0140-6736(14)60539-0

Langagne, T., Leveque, M., Schmidt, P., & Chays, A. (2010). Universal newborn hearing screening in the Champagne-Ardenne region: A 4-year follow-up after early diagnosis of hearing impairment. *International Journal of Pediatric Otorhinolaryngology, 74*(10), 1164–1170. doi:S0165-5876(10)00307-1 [pii]10.1016/j.ijporl.2010.07.005

Lasisi, O. A., Ayodele, J. K., & Ijaduola, G. T. A. (2006). Challenges in management of childhood sensorineural hearing loss in sub-Saharan Africa, Nigeria. *International Journal of Pediatric Otorhinolaryngology, 70*(4), 625–629. http://dx.doi.org/10.1016/j.ijporl.2005.08.009

Liang, Q., & Mason, B. (2013). Enter the dragon—China's journey to the hearing world. *Cochlear Implants International, 14*(Suppl. 1), S26–31. doi:10.1179/1467010013Z.0000000008010.1179/1467010013Z.000000000109

Lieu, T. A., Ray, G. T., Black, S. B., Butler, J. C., Klein, J. O., Breiman, R. F., . . . Shinefield, H. R. (2000). Projected cost-effectiveness of pneumococcal conjugate vaccination of healthy infants and young children. *Journal of the American Medical Association, 283*(11), 1460–1468. doi:jsc90347 [pii]

Lin, S. W., Lin, Y. S., Weng, S. F., & Chou, C. W. (2012). Risk of developing sudden sensorineural hearing loss in diabetic patients: A population-based cohort study. [Research Support, Non-U.S. Gov't]. *Otology & Neurotology, 33*(9), 1482–1488. doi:10.1097/MAO.0b013e318271397a

Linden Phillips, L., Bitner-Glindzicz, M., Lench, N., Steel, K. P., Langford, C., Dawson, S. J., . . . Packer, C. (2013). The future role of genetic screening to detect newborns at risk of childhood-onset hearing loss. [Research Support, Non-U.S. Gov't Review]. *International Journal of Audiology, 52*(2), 124–133. doi:10.3109/14992027.2012.733424

Liu, X. Z., Angeli, S., Ouyang, X. M., Liu, W., Ke, X. M., Liu, Y. H., . . . Yan, D. (2008). Audiological and genetic features of the mtDNA mutations. *Acta Otolaryngologica, 128*(7), 732–738. doi:788637768 [pii]10.1080/00016480701719011

Lotfi, Y., & Mehrkian, S. (2007). The prevalence of auditory neuropathy in students with hearing impairment in Tehran, Iran. *Archives of Iranian Medicine, 10*(2), 233–235. doi:0018 [pii]07102/AIM.0018

Low, W. K., Pang, K. Y., Ho, L. Y., Lim, S. B., & Joseph, R. (2005). Universal newborn hearing screening in Singapore: The need, implementation and challenges. *Annals Academy of Medicine Singapore, 34*(4), 301–306.

MacAndie, C., Kubba, H., & McFarlane, M. (2003). Epidemiology of permanent childhood hearing loss in Glasgow, 1985–1994. *Scottish Medical Journal, 48*(4), 117–119.

MacDorman, M. F., Matthews, T. J., Mohangoo, A. D., & Zeitlin, J. (2014). International comparisons of infant mortality and related factors: United States and Europe, 2010. In N. V. S. System (Ed.), *National Vital Statistics reports* (Vol. 63). Washington, DC: National Center for Health Statistics.

Madden, C., Rutter, M., Hilbert, L., Greinwald, J. H., Jr, & Choo, D. I. (2002). Clinical and audiological features in auditory neuropathy. *Archives of Otolaryngology-Head and Neck Surgery, 128*(9), 1026–1030. doi:10.1001/archotol.128.9.1026

Maki-Torkko, E. M., Lindholm, P. K., Vayrynen, M. R., Leisti, J. T., & Sorri, M. J. (1998). Epidemiology of moderate to profound childhood hearing impairments in northern Finland. Any changes in ten years? *Scandinavian Audiology, 27*(2), 95–103.

Malik, S. G., Pieter, N., Sudoyo, H., Kadir, A., & Marzuki, S. (2003). Prevalence of the mitochondrial DNA A1555G mutation in sensorineural deafness patients in island Southeast Asia. *Journal of Human Genetics, 48*(9), 480–483. doi:10.1007/s10038-003-0056-9

Marlenga, B., Berg, R. L., Linneman, J. G., Wood, D. J., Kirkhorn, S. R., & Pickett, W. (2012). Determinants of early-stage hearing loss among a cohort of young workers with 16-year follow-up. [Randomized Controlled Trial Research Support, U.S. Gov't, P.H.S.]. *Occupational and Environmental Medicine, 69*(7), 479–484. doi:10.1136/oemed-2011-100464

Martines, F., Martines, E., Mucia, M., Sciacca, V., & Salvago, P. (2013). Prelingual sensorineural hearing loss and infants at risk: Western Sicily report. *International Journal of Pediatric Otorhinolaryngology, 77*(4), 513–518. doi:10.1016/j.ijporl.2012.12.023

Martines, F., Salvago, P., Bentivegna, D., Bartolone, A., Dispenza, F., & Martines, E. (2012). Audiologic profile of infants at risk: Experience of a Western Sicily tertiary care centre. [Comparative study]. *International Journal of Pediatric Otorhinolaryngology, 76*(9), 1285–1291. doi:10.1016/j.ijporl.2012.05.020

McClay, J. E., Tandy, R., Grundfast, K., Choi, S., Vezina, G., Zalzal, G., & Willner, A. (2002). Major and minor temporal bone abnormalities in children with and without congenital sensorineural hearing loss. *Archives of Otolaryngology-Head and Neck Surgery, 128*(6), 664–671. doi:ooa00188 [pii]

McHugh, R. K., & Friedman, R. A. (2006). Genetics of hearing loss: Allelism and modifier genes produce a phenotypic continuum. *Anatomical Record Part A: Discoveries in Molecular,*

Cellular, and Evolutionary Biology, 288(4), 370–381. doi:10.1002/ar.a.20297

McPherson, B., & Swart, S. M. (1997). Childhood hearing loss in sub-Saharan Africa: A review and recommendations. *International Journal of Pediatric Otorhinolaryngology, 40*(1), 1–18. doi:http://dx.doi.org/10.1016/S0165-5876(97)01508-5

Millar, M. (2011). Can antibiotic use be both just and sustainable… or only more or less so? *Journal of Medical Ethics, 37*(3), 153–157. doi:10.1136/jme.2010.038042

Minja, B. M., & Machemba, A. (1996). Prevalence of otitis media, hearing impairment and cerumen impaction among school children in rural and urban Dar es Salaam, Tanzania. *International Journal of Pediatric Otorhinolaryngology, 37*(1), 29–34. doi:0165587696013638 [pii]

Misono, S., Sie, K. C., Weiss, N. S., Huang, M. L., Boeckh, M., Norton, S. J., & Yueh, B. (2011). Congenital cytomegalovirus infection in pediatric hearing loss. [Comparative Study Research Support, N.I.H., Extramural]. *Archives of Otolaryngology-Head and Neck Surgery, 137*(1), 47–53. doi:10.1001/archoto.2010.235

Molyneux, E. M., Tembo, M., Kayira, K., Bwanaisa, L., Mweneychanya, J., Njobvu, A., . . . Molyneux, M. E. (2003). The effect of HIV infection on paediatric bacterial meningitis in Blantyre, Malawi. *Archives of Disease in Childhood, 88*(12), 1112–1118. doi:10.1136/adc.88.12.1112

Moore, T., Hennessy, E. M., Myles, J., Johnson, S. J., Draper, E. S., Costeloe, K. L., & Marlow, N. (2012). Neurological and developmental outcome in extremely preterm children born in England in 1995 and 2006: The EPICure studies. [Comparative Study Research Support, Non-U.S. Gov't]. *BMJ, 345*, e7961. doi:10.1136/bmj.e7961

Morton, C. C., & Nance, W. E. (2006). Newborn hearing screening—A silent revolution. *New England Journal of Medicine, 354*(20), 2151–2164. doi:354/20/2151 [pii]10.1056/NEJMra050700

Morton, R., Sharma, V., Nicholson, J., Broderick, M., & Poyser, J. (2002). Disability in children from different ethnic populations. *Child Care Health and Development, 28*(1), 87–93. doi:245 [pii]

Morzaria, S., Westerberg, B. D., & Kozak, F. K. (2004). Systematic review of the etiology of bilateral sensorineural hearing loss in children. *International Journal of Pediatric Otorhinolaryngology, 68*(9), 1193–1198. doi:10.1016/j.ijporl.2004.04.013S0165587604001417 [pii]

Mrena, R., Paakkonen, R., Back, L., Pirvola, U., & Ylikoski, J. (2004). Otologic consequences of blast exposure: A Finnish case study of a shopping mall bomb explosion. *Acta Oto-laryngologica, 124*(8), 946–952. doi:000G27GDHBD8CBNX [pii]10.1080/00016480310017045

Mueller, R. (1996). Genetic counseling for hearing impairment. In A. Martini, A. Read, & D. Stephens (Eds.), *Genetics and hearing impairment* (pp. 255–264). London, UK: Whurr.

Mukari, S. Z., Tan, K. Y., & Abdullah, A. (2006). A pilot project on hospital-based universal newborn hearing screening: Lessons learned. *International Journal of Pediatric Otorhinolaryngology, 70*(5), 843–851. doi:S0165-5876(05)00453-2 [pii]10.1016/j.ijporl.2005.09.018

Naderpour, M., Mortazavi, F., Jabbari-Moghaddam, Y., & Sharifi-Movaghar, M. H. (2011). Auditory brain stem response and otoacoustic emission results in children with end-stage renal disease. [Comparative study]. *International Journal of Pediatric Otorhinolaryngology, 75*(5), 704–707. doi:10.1016/j.ijporl.2011.02.020

Nance, W. E., & Kearsey, M. J. (2004). Relevance of connexin deafness (DFNB1) to human evolution. *American Journal of Human Genetics, 74*(6), 1081-1087. doi:10.1086/420979S0002-9297(07)62835-3 [pii]

National Deaf Children's Society. (2014). Working together for deaf children. In NDCS (Ed.), *Impact Report 2013–2014*. Retrieved from http://www.ndcs.org.uk/about_us/impact_report_accounts/impact_report.html

Nelson, S., Andersen, R., & Anderssen, S. H. (2015). Hearing loss in children in Ostfold county 2000–9. *Tidsskrift for den Norske laegeforening: Tidsskrift for praktisk medicin, ny raekke, 135*(2), 132–136. doi:10.4045/tidsskr.13.0556

Newton, V. (2001). Adverse perinatal conditions and the inner ear. *Seminars in Neonatology, 6*(6), 543–551. doi:10.1053/siny.2001.0076 S1084-2756(01)90076-4 [pii]

Nie, W. Y., Wu, H. R., Qi, Y. S., Lin, Q., Zhang, M., Hou, Q., . . . Zhang, W. H. (2007). [Simultaneous screening program for newborns hearing and ocular diseases]. *Zhonghua Er Bi Yan Hou Tou Jing Wai Ke Za Zhi, 42*(2), 115–120.

Niskar, A. S., Kieszak, S. M., Holmes, A., Esteban, E., Rubin, C., & Brody, D. J. (1998). Prevalence of hearing loss among children 6 to 19 years of age: The Third National Health and Nutrition Examination Survey. *JAMA, 279*(14), 1071–1075. doi:joc72028 [pii]

Nivoloni Kde, A., da Silva-Costa, S. M., Pomilio, M. C., Pereira, T., Lopes Kde, C., de Moraes, V. C., . . . Sartorato, E. L. (2010). Newborn hearing screening and genetic testing in 8974 Brazilian neonates. [Research Support, Non-U.S. Gov't]. *International Journal of Pediatric Otorhinolaryngology, 74*(8), 926–929. doi:10.1016/j.ijporl.2010.05.015

O'Connor, A., O'Sullivan, P. G., Behan, L., Norman, G., & Murphy, B. (2013). Initial results from the newborn hearing screening programme in Ireland. *Irish Journal of Medical Science, 182*(4), 551–556. doi:10.1007/s11845-013-0924-z

O'Connor, T. E., Perry, C. F., & Lannigan, F. J. (2009). Complications of otitis media in Indigenous and non-Indigenous children. *Medical Journal of Australia, 191*(9 Suppl.), S60–S64. doi:oco10500_fm [pii]

Oghan, F., Harputluoglu, U., Ozturk, O., Guclu, E., & Mayda, A. (2008). Does the prevalence of otolaryngological diseases in deaf children differ from children without hearing impairment? *European Archives of Otorhinolaryngology, 265*(2), 223–226. doi:10.1007/s00405-007-0426-6

Oliveira, J. S., Rodrigues, L. B., Aurelio, F. S., & Silva, V. B. (2013). Risk factors and prevalence of newborn hearing loss in a private health care system of Porto Velho, Northern Brazil. *Revista paulista de pediatria: Orgao oficial da Sociedade de Pediatria de Sao Paulo, 31*(3), 299–305. doi:10.1590/S0103-05822013000300005

Olusanya, B. O. (2013). Letter: Investigating the burden of hyperbilirubinemia in resource-constrained settings. *Inter-*

national Journal of Pediatric Otorhinolaryngology, 77(9), 1626–1627. doi:http://dx.doi.org/10.1016/j.ijporl.2013.07.009

Olusanya, B. O., Neumann, K. J., & Saunders, J. E. (2014). The global burden of disabling hearing impairment: A call to action. *Bulletin of the World Health Organization*, 92, 367–373. doi:http://dx.doi.org/10.2471/BLT.13.128728

Olusanya, B. O., Okhakhu, A. L., & Somefun, A. O. (2011). Implementing the new WHO guidelines for the early detection of sensorineural hearing loss in newborns and infants in Nigeria. [Duplicate publication]. *Nigerian Quarterly Journal of Hospital Medicine, 21*(4), 324–326.

Olusanya, B. O., & Okolo, A. A. (2006). Adverse perinatal conditions in hearing-impaired children in a developing country. *Paediatric and Perinatal Epidemiology, 20*(5), 366–371. doi:PPE733 [pii]10.1111/j.1365-3016.2006.00733.x

Olusanya, B. O., Okolo, A. A., & Ijaduola, G. T. (2000). The hearing profile of Nigerian school children. *International Journal of Pediatric Otorhinolaryngology, 55*(3), 173–179. doi:S0165587600003931 [pii]

Olusanya, B. O., & Solanke, O. A. (2009). Maternal and neonatal factors associated with mode of delivery under a universal newborn hearing screening programme in Lagos, Nigeria. [Research Support, Non-U.S. Gov't]. *BMC Pregnancy and Childbirth, 9*, 41. doi:10.1186/1471-2393-9-41

Olusanya, B. O., Wirz, S. L., & Luxon, L. M. (2008a). Community-based infant hearing screening for early detection of permanent hearing loss in Lagos, Nigeria: A cross-sectional study. *Bulletin of the World Health Organization*, 86, 956–963. doi:10.2471/BLT.07.050005

Olusanya, B. O., Wirz, S. L., & Luxon, L. M. (2008b). Non-hospital delivery and permanent congenital and early-onset hearing loss in a developing country. *BJOG, 115*(11), 1419–1427. doi:BJO1871 [pii]10.1111/j.1471-0528.2008.01871.x

OMIM 121011. (2015, May). *Gap Junction Protein, Beta-2; GJB2.* Online Mendelian Inheritance in Man. Retrieved January 6, 2015, from http://www.omim.org/entry/121011

Ouyang, X. M., Yan, D., Yuan, H. J., Pu, D., Du, L. L., Han, D. Y., & Liu, X. Z. (2009). The genetic bases for non-syndromic hearing loss among Chinese. *Journal of Human Genetics, 54*(3), 131–140.

Özbay, İ., Kucur, C., Oğhan, F., Aksoy, S., Erdoğan, O., & Karakuş, Y. T. (2014). Newborn hearing screening results in an inner part of Aegean region. *Journal of Medical Updates, 4*(3).

Ozturk, O., Silan, F., Oghan, F., Egeli, E., Belli, S., Tokmak, A., . . . Zafer, C. (2005). Evaluation of deaf children in a large series in Turkey. *International Journal of Pediatric Otorhinolaryngology, 69*(3), 367–373. doi:S0165-5876(04)00365-9 [pii]10.1016/j.ijporl.2004.11.001

Pace, D., & Pollard, A. J. (2007). Meningococcal A, C, Y and W-135 polysaccharide-protein conjugate vaccines. *Archives of Disease in Childhood, 92*(10), 909–915. doi:10.1136/adc.2006.111500

Park, A. H., Wilson, M. A., Stevens, P. T., Harward, R., & Hohler, N. (2012). Identification of hearing loss in pediatric patients with Down syndrome. [Comparative Study Multicenter Study]. *Otolaryngology-Head and Neck Surgery, 146*(1), 135–140. doi:10.1177/0194599811425156

Parker, M. J., Fortnum, H., Young, I. D., & Davis, A. C. (1999). Variations in genetic assessment and recurrence risks quoted for childhood deafness: A survey of clinical geneticists. *Journal of Medical Genetics, 36*(2), 125–130.

Parker, M. J., Fortnum, H. M., Young, I. D., Davis, A. C., & Mueller, R. F. (2000). Population-based genetic study of childhood hearing impairment in the Trent Region of the United Kingdom. *Audiology, 39*(4), 226–231.

Parving, A., & Hauch, A. M. (1994). The causes of profound hearing impairment in a school for the deaf—A longitudinal study. *British Journal of Audiology, 28*(2), 63–69.

Parving, A., & Stephens, D. (1997). Profound permanent hearing impairment in childhood: Causative factors in two European countries. *Acta Otolaryngologica, 117*(2), 158–160.

Penazola-Lopez, Y. R., Castillo-Maya, G., Garcia-Pedroza, F., & Sanchez-Lopez, H. (2004). [Hypoacusis-deafness related to perinatal adverse conditions. According to the register available in a specialized unit of Ciudad de Mexico. Analysis according to birth weight]. *Acta Otorrinolaringologica Espanola, 55*(6), 252–259.

Petersen, M. B., & Willems, P. J. (2006). Non-syndromic, autosomal-recessive deafness. *Clinical Genetics, 69*(5), 371–392. doi:CGE613 [pii]10.1111/j.1399-0004.2006.00613.x

Prasansuk, S. (2000). Incidence/prevalence of sensorineural hearing impairment in Thailand and Southeast Asia. *Audiology, 39*(4), 207–211.

Punch, R., Creed, P. A., & Hyde, M. (2005). Predicting career development in hard-of-hearing adolescents in Australia. *Journal of Deaf Studies and Deaf Education, 10*(2), 146–160. doi:10/2/146 [pii]10.1093/deafed/eni015

Qaddoumi, I., Bass, J. K., Wu, J., Billups, C. A., Wozniak, A. W., Merchant, T. E., . . . Rodriguez-Galindo, C. (2012). Carboplatin-associated ototoxicity in children with retinoblastoma. [Research Support, N.I.H., Extramural Research Support, Non-U.S. Gov't]. *Journal of Clinical Oncology: Official Journal of the American Society of Clinical Oncology, 30*(10), 1034–1041. doi:10.1200/JCO.2011.36.9744

Rai, N., & Thakur, N. (2013). Universal screening of newborns to detect hearing impairment—Is it necessary? [Comparative study]. *International Journal of Pediatric Otorhinolaryngology, 77*(6), 1036–1041. doi:10.1016/j.ijporl.2013.04.006

Rao, R. S., Subramanyam, M. A., Nair, N. S., & Rajashekhar, B. (2002). Hearing impairment and ear diseases among children of school entry age in rural South India. *International Journal of Pediatric Otorhinolaryngology, 64*(2), 105–110. doi:S0165587602000320 [pii]

Razi, M. S., & Das, V. K. (1994). Effects of adverse perinatal events on hearing. *International Journal of Pediatric Otorhinolaryngology, 30*(1), 29–40.

Reardon, W. (1992). Genetic deafness. *Journal of Medical Genetics, 29*(8), 521–526.

Ricard, P., Santana-Hernandez, D., Smith, A., MacKenzie, I., Newton, V. E., Ratnesar, P., & Sirimanna, T. (2004). *Community Ear and Hearing Health Journal.* International Centre for Evidence in Disability. Retrieved from http://disabilitycentre.lshtm.ac.uk/key-publications/cehh-journal/

Rodriguez Dominguez, F. J., Cubillana Herrero, J. D., Canizares Gallardo, N., & Perez Aguilera, R. (2007). [Prevalence of auditory neuropathy: Prospective study in a tertiary-care center]. *Acta Otorrinolaringologica Espanola, 58*(6), 239–245. doi:13107617 [pii]

Rohlfs, A.-K., Wiesner, T., Drews, H., Müller, F., Breitfuß, A., Schiller, R., & Hess, M. (2010). Interdisciplinary approach to design, performance, and quality management in a multicenter newborn hearing screening project. *European Journal of Pediatrics, 169*(11), 1353–1360. doi:10.1007/s00431-010-1228-1

Roine, I., Pelkonen, T., Cruzeiro, M. L., Kataja, M., Aarnisalo, A., Peltola, H., & Pitkaranta, A. (2014). Fluctuation in hearing thresholds during recovery from childhood bacterial meningitis. [Research Support, Non-U.S. Gov't]. *Pediatric Infectious Disease Journal, 33*(3), 253–257. doi:10.1097/INF.0000000000000218

Roizen, N. J. (2003). Nongenetic causes of hearing loss. *Mental Retardation and Developmental Disabilities Research Review, 9*(2), 120–127. doi:10.1002/mrdd.10068

Ruhl, D. S., Cable, B. B., & Martell, D. W. (2014). Medication associated with hearing loss: 25 years of medical malpractice cases in the United States. *Otolaryngology-Head and Neck Surgery, 151*(3), 431–437. doi:10.1177/0194599814536850

Ruszymah, B. H., Wahida, I. F., Zakinah, Y., Zahari, Z., Norazlinda, M. D., Saim, L., & Aminuddin, B. S. (2005). Congenital deafness: High prevalence of a V37I mutation in the GJB2 gene among deaf school children in Alor Setar. *Medical Journal of Malaysia, 60*(3), 269–274.

Saggar, A. K., & Bittles, A. H. (2008). Consanguinity and child health. *Paediatric and Child Health, 18*(5), 244–249. doi:10.1016/j.paed.2008.02.008

Sajjad, M., Khattak, A. A., Bunn, J. E., & Mackenzie, I. (2008). Causes of childhood deafness in Pukhtoonkhwa Province of Pakistan and the role of consanguinity. *Journal of Laryngology and Otology, 122*(10), 1057–1063.

Sanyelbhaa Talaat, H., Kabel, A. H., Samy, H., & Elbadry, M. (2009). Prevalence of auditory neuropathy (AN) among infants and young children with severe to profound hearing loss. *International Journal of Pediatric Otorhinolaryngology, 73*(7), 937–939. doi:S0165-5876(09)00129-3 [pii]10.1016/j.ijporl.2009.03.009

Sarafraz, M., & Ahmadi, K. (2009). A practical screening model for hearing loss in Iranian school-aged children. *World Journal of Pediatrics, 5*(1), 46–50. doi:10.1007/s12519-009-0008-3

Saunders, J. E., Vaz, S., Greinwald, J. H., Lai, J., Morin, L., & Mojica, K. (2007). Prevalence and etiology of hearing loss in rural Nicaraguan children. *Laryngoscope, 117*(3), 387–398. doi:10.1097/MLG.0b013e31802e372600005537-200703000-00001 [pii]

SCENIHR. (2008). Potential health risks of exposure to noise from personal music players and mobile phones including a music playing function [Preliminary report]. K. Rydzynski & T. Jung (Eds.), *Brussels: European Commission, Scientific Committee on Emerging and Newly Identified Health Risks.* Retrieved September 10, 2015, from http://ec.europa.eu/health/archive/ph_risk/committees/04_scenihr/docs/scenihr_o_018.pdf

Schmidt, P., Leveque, M., Danvin, J. B., Leroux, B., & Chays, A. (2007). [Systematic hearing screening for newborns in the Champagne-Ardennes region: 32,500 births in 2 years of experience]. *Ann Otolaryngol Chir Cervicofac, 124*(4), 157–165. doi:S0003-438X(07)00009-6 [pii]10.1016/j.aorl.2006.10.004

Shargorodsky, J., Curhan, S. G., Henderson, E., Eavey, R., & Curhan, G. C. (2011). Heavy metals exposure and hearing loss in US adolescents. [Research Support, Non-U.S. Gov't]. *Archives of Otolaryngology-Head and Neck Surgery, 137*(12), 1183–1189. doi:10.1001/archoto.2011.202

Siem, G., Fagerheim, T., Jonsrud, C., Laurent, C., Teig, E., Harris, S., . . . Heimdal, K. (2010). Causes of hearing impairment in the Norwegian paediatric cochlear implant program. *International Journal of Audiology, 49*(8), 596–605. doi:10.3109/14992021003743269

Silan, F., Demirci, L., Egeli, A., Egeli, E., Onder, H. I., Ozturk, O., & Unal, Z. S. (2004). Syndromic etiology in children at schools for the deaf in Turkey. *International Journal of Pediatric Otorhinolaryngology, 68*(11), 1399–1406. doi:S0165-5876(04)00178-8 [pii]10.1016/j.ijporl.2004.05.007

Smith, A. W., Bradley, A. K., Wall, R. A., McPherson, B., Secka, A., Dunn, D. T., & Greenwood, B. M. (1988). Sequelae of epidemic meningococcal meningitis in Africa. *Transactions of the Royal Society of Tropical Medicine and Hygiene, 82*(2), 312–320.

Smith, R. H. (2001). Mutation screening for deafness: More than simply another diagnostic test. *Archives of Otolaryngology-Head and Neck Surgery, 127*(8), 941–942. doi:10.1001/archotol.127.8.941

Society for Sound Hearing. (2015). Awareness material. Retrieved June 1, 2015, from http://www.soundhearing2030.org/awareness

Stacey, P. C., Fortnum, H. M., Barton, G. R., & Summerfield, A. Q. (2006). Hearing-impaired children in the United Kingdom, I: Auditory performance, communication skills, educational achievements, quality of life, and cochlear implantation. *Ear and Hearing, 27*(2), 161–186. doi:10.1097/01.aud.0000202353.37567.b400003446-200604000-00007 [pii]

Steel, K. P. (1998). Progress in progressive hearing loss. *Science, 279*(5358), 1870–1871.

Stein-Zamir, C., Shoob, H., Sokolov, I., Kunbar, A., Abramson, N., & Zimmerman, D. (2014). The clinical features and long-term sequelae of invasive meningococcal disease in children. *Pediatric Infectious Disease Journal, 33*(7), 777–779. doi:10.1097/INF.0000000000000282

Stevens, G., Flaxman, S., Brunskill, E., Mascarenhas, M., Mathers, C. D., & Finucane, M. (2013). Global and regional hearing impairment prevalence: An analysis of 42 studies in 29 countries. [Research Support, Non-U.S. Gov't]. *European Journal of Public Health, 23*(1), 146–152. doi:10.1093/eurpub/ckr176

Stevens, G. A., Flaxman, S. M., Mascarenhas, M., Davis, K., Brunskill, E., Davis, A., . . . Mathers, C. D. (2012). Global and regional hearing impairment prevalence. In P. Alberti, V. Newton, & A. Smith (Eds.), *Prevention of hearing loss* (pp. 21–50). London, UK: Nova Science.

Swart, S. M., Lemmer, R., Parbhoo, J. N., & Prescott, C. A. (1995). A survey of ear and hearing disorders amongst a representative sample of grade 1 schoolchildren in Swaziland. *International Journal of Pediatric Otorhinolaryngology, 32*(1), 23–34. doi:016558769401109B [pii]

Synnes, A. R., Anson, S., Baum, J., & Usher, L. (2012). Incidence and pattern of hearing impairment in children with </= 800 g birthweight in British Columbia, Canada. [Research Support, Non-U.S. Gov't]. *Acta Paediatrica, 101*(2), e48–54. doi:10.1111/j.1651-2227.2011.02437.x

Szyfter, W., Wrobel, M. J., Szyfter-Harris, J., & Greczka, G. (2013). Hearing impairment in Polish infants. [Letter]. *Epidemiology, 24*(2), 333. doi:10.1097/EDE.0b013e31827b23a3

Taha, A. A., Pratt, S. R., Farahat, T. M., Abdel-Rasoul, G. M., Albtanony, M. A., Elrashiedy, A. L., . . . Zein, A. (2010). Prevalence and risk factors of hearing impairment among primary-school children in Shebin El-kom District, Egypt. *American Journal of Audiology, 19*(1), 46–60. doi:19/1/46 [pii]10.1044/1059-0889(2010/09-0030)

Talaat, H. S., Metwaly, M. A., Khafagy, A. H., & Abdelraouf, H. R. (2014). Dose passive smoking induce sensorineural hearing loss in children? *International Journal of Pediatric Otorhinolaryngology, 78*(1), 46–49. doi:10.1016/j.ijporl.2013.10.016

Tang, T. P., McPherson, B., Yuen, K. C., Wong, L. L., & Lee, J. S. (2004). Auditory neuropathy/auditory dys-synchrony in school children with hearing loss: Frequency of occurrence. *International Journal of Pediatric Otorhinolaryngology, 68*(2), 175–183. doi:S0165587603003768 [pii]

Tantawy, A. Z., Sobhy, O., Al-Farargy, M., & Shafik, M. (1998). Studying the etiology of deafness in the "deaf" schools of Alexandria. *Journal of Egyptian Public Health Association, 73*(1–2), 125–136.

Tapadia, M. D., Cordero, D. R., & Helms, J. A. (2005). It's all in your head: New insights into craniofacial development and deformation. *Journal of Anatomy, 207*(5), 461–477. doi:JOA484 [pii]10.1111/j.1469-7580.2005.00484.x

Tekin, M. (2009). Review Synthetic Report: Genomic architecture of deafness in Turkey reflects its rich past. *International Journal of Modern Anthropology, 1*(2), 39–51.

Tekin, M., Akar, N., Cin, S., Blanton, S. H., Xia, X. J., Liu, X. Z., . . . Pandya, A. (2001). Connexin 26 (GJB2) mutations in the Turkish population: Implications for the origin and high frequency of the 35delG mutation in Caucasians. *Human Genetics, 108*(5), 385–389.

Theunissen, S. C., Rieffe, C., Netten, A. P., Briaire, J. J., Soede, W., Schoones, J. W., & Frijns, J. H. (2014). Psychopathology and its risk and protective factors in hearing-impaired children and adolescents: A systematic review. [Research Support, Non-U.S. Gov't Review]. *JAMA Pediatrics, 168*(2), 170–177. doi:10.1001/jamapediatrics.2013.3974

Torre, P., 3rd, Zeldow, B., Hoffman, H. J., Buchanan, A., Siberry, G. K., Rice, M., . . . Williams, P. L. (2012). Hearing loss in perinatally HIV-infected and HIV-exposed but uninfected children and adolescents. [Research Support, N.I.H., Extramural Research Support, Non-U.S. Gov't]. *Pediatric Infectious Disease Journal, 31*(8), 835–841. doi:10.1097/INF.0b013e31825b9524

Townsend, C. L., Peckham, C. S., & Tookey, P. A. (2011). Surveillance of congenital cytomegalovirus in the UK and Ireland. *Archives of Disease in Childhood-Fetal and Neonatal Edition, 96*(6), F398–F403. doi:10.1136/adc.2010.199901

Tucci, D. L., Merson, M. H., & Wilson, B. S. (2010). A summary of the literature on global hearing impairment: Current status and priorities for action. *Otology & Neurotology, 31*(1), 31–41.

Tungvachirakul, V., Boonmee, S., Nualmoosik, T., Kamjohnjiraphun, J., Siripala, W., Sanghirun, W., . . . Potaporn, M. (2011). Newborn hearing screening at Rajavithi Hospital, Thailand: Hearing loss in infants not admitting in intensive care unit. [Evaluation Studies Research Support, Non-U.S. Gov't]. *Journal of the Medical Association of Thailand-Chotmaihet thangphaet, 94*(Suppl. 2), S108–S112.

Turner, K. M., Lee, H. C., Boppana, S. B., Carlo, W. A., & Randolph, D. A. (2014). Incidence and impact of CMV infection in very low birth weight infants. [Research Support, N.I.H., Extramural]. *Pediatrics, 133*(3), e609–e615. doi:10.1542/peds.2013-2217

Uilenburg, N., Kauffman-de Boer, M., van der Ploeg, K., Oudesluys-Murphy, A. M., & Verkerk, P. (2009). An implementation study of neonatal hearing screening in the Netherlands. *International Journal of Audiology, 48*(3), 108–116.

United Nations Development Programme. (2014). Sustaining human progress: Reducing vulnerability and building resilience. In UNDP (Ed.), *Human Development Reports New York: United Nations.* Retrieved from http://hdr.undp.org.

Usami, S.-i., Abe, S., Akita, J., Namba, A., Shinkawa, H., Ishii, M., . . . Komune, S. (2000). Prevalence of mitochondrial gene mutations among hearing impaired patients. *Journal of Medical Genetics, 37*(1), 38–40. doi:10.1136/jmg.37.1.38

Uus, K., & Davis, A. C. (2000). Epidemiology of permanent childhood hearing impairment in Estonia, 1985–1990. *Audiology, 39*(4), 192–197.

Van Kerschaver, E., Boudewyns, A. N., Declau, F., Van de Heyning, P. H., & Wuyts, F. L. (2013). Socio-demographic determinants of hearing impairment studied in 103,835 term babies. *European Journal of Public Health, 23*(1), 55–60. doi:10.1093/eurpub/cks010

Van Naarden, K., & Decoufle, P. (1999). Relative and attributable risks for moderate to profound bilateral sensorineural hearing impairment associated with lower birth weight in children 3 to 10 years old. *Pediatrics, 104*(4), 905–910. doi:10.1542/peds.104.4.905

Vartiainen, E., & Karjalainen, S. (1998). Prevalence and etiology of unilateral sensorineural hearing impairment in a Finnish childhood population. *International Journal of Pediatric Otorhinolaryngology, 43*(3), 253–259. doi:S0165587 69800010X [pii]

Vella, M., & Pace, D. (2015). Glycoconjugate vaccines: An update. *Expert Opinion on Biological Therapy, 15*(4), 529–546. doi:10.1517/14712598.2015.993375

Wake, M., Tobin, S., Cone-Wesson, B., Dahl, H. H., Gillam, L., McCormick, L., . . . Williams, J. (2006). Slight/mild sensorineural hearing loss in children. *Pediatrics, 118*(5), 1842–1851. doi:118/5/1842 [pii]10.1542/peds.2005-3168

Wang, Q. J., Zhao, Y. L., Rao, S. Q., Guo, Y. F., He, Y., Lan, L., . . . Shen, Y. (2011). Newborn hearing concurrent gene screening can improve care for hearing loss: A study on 14,913 Chinese newborns. [Research Support, Non-U.S. Gov't]. *International Journal of Pediatric Otorhinolaryngology, 75*(4), 535–542. doi:10.1016/j.ijporl.2011.01.016

Warren, K. R., & Foudin, L. L. (2001). Alcohol-related birth defects—The past, present, and future. *Alcohol Research and Health, 25*(3), 153–158.

Watkin, P. M., & Baldwin, M. (2011). Identifying deafness in early childhood: Requirements after the newborn hearing screen. *Archives of Disease in Childhood, 96*(1), 62–66. doi:10.1136/adc.2010.185819

Watkin, P., & Baldwin, M. (2012). The longitudinal follow up of a universal neonatal hearing screen: The implications for confirming deafness in childhood. [Comparative study]. *International Journal of Audiology, 51*(7), 519–528. doi:10.3109/14992027.2012.673237

Weichbold, V., Nekahm-Heis, D., & Welzl-Mueller, K. (2006a). Ten-year outcome of newborn hearing screening in Austria. *International Journal of Pediatric Otorhinolaryngoogyl, 70*(2), 235–240. doi:S0165-5876(05)00289-2 [pii]10.1016/j.ijporl.2005.06.006

Weichbold, V., Nekahm-Heis, D., & Welzl-Mueller, K. (2006b). Universal newborn hearing screening and postnatal hearing loss. *Pediatrics, 117*(4), e631–e636. doi:10.1542/peds.2005-1455

Wellman, M. B., Sommer, D. D., & McKenna, J. (2003). Sensorineural hearing loss in postmeningitic children. *Otology and Neurotology, 24*(6), 907–912.

Westerberg, B. D., Skowronski, D. M., Stewart, I. F., Stewart, L., Bernauer, M., & Mudarikwa, L. (2005). Prevalence of hearing loss in primary school children in Zimbabwe. *International Journal of Pediatric Otorhinolaryngology, 69*(4), 517–525.

Whelan, K., Stratton, K., Kawashima, T., Leisenring, W., Hayashi, S., Waterbor, J., . . . Mertens, A. C. (2011). Auditory complications in childhood cancer survivors: A report from the childhood cancer survivor study. [Comparative Study Multicenter Study Research Support, N.I.H., Extramural Research Support, Non-U.S. Gov't]. *Pediatric Blood and Cancer, 57*(1), 126–134. doi:10.1002/pbc.23025

Wiley, S., Arjmand, E., Jareenmeinzen, D., & Dixon, M. (2011). Findings from multidisciplinary evaluation of children with permanent hearing loss. *International Journal of Pediatric Otorhinolaryngology, 75*(8), 1040–1044. doi:S0165-5876(11)00269-2 [pii]10.1016/j.ijporl.2011.05.019

Williams, E. J., Kadambari, S., Berrington, J. E., Luck, S., Atkinson, C., Walter, S., . . . Davis, A. (2014). Feasibility and acceptability of targeted screening for congenital CMV-related hearing loss. *Archives of Disease in Childhood-Fetal and Neonatal Edition, 99*(3), 230–236..

Williams, W., Carter, L., & Seeto, M. (2014). Hearing threshold levels for a population of 11 to 35 year old Australian females and males. [Clinical Trial Research Support, Non-U.S. Gov't Validation Studies]. *International Journal of Audiology, 53*(5), 289–293. doi:10.3109/14992027.2013.873957

Wilson-Costello, D., Friedman, H., Minich, N., Fanaroff, A. A., & Hack, M. (2005). Improved survival rates with increased neurodevelopmental disability for extremely low birth weight infants in the 1990s. *Pediatrics, 115*(4), 997–1003. doi:115/4/997 [pii]10.1542/peds.2004-0221

Wonkam, A., Noubiap, J. J., Djomou, F., Fieggen, K., Njock, R., & Toure, G. B. (2013). Aetiology of childhood hearing loss in Cameroon (sub-Saharan Africa). *European Journal of Medical Genetics, 56*(1), 20–25. doi:10.1016/j.ejmg.2012.09.010

Wood, S. A., Davis, A. C., & Sutton, G. J. (2013). Effectiveness of targeted surveillance to identify moderate to profound permanent childhood hearing impairment in babies with risk factors who pass newborn screening. *International Journal of Audiology, 52*(6), 394–399. doi:10.3109/14992027.2013.769067

Wood, S. A., Sutton, G., & Davis, A. C. (2015). Performance and characteristics of the Newborn Hearing Screening Programme in England: The first seven years. *International Journal of Audiology, 54*(6), 353–358. doi:10.3109/14992027.2014.989548

Woolley, A. L., Kirk, K. A., Neumann, A. M., Jr., McWilliams, S. M., Murray, J., Freind, D., & Wiatrak, B. J. (1999). Risk factors for hearing loss from meningitis in children: The Children's Hospital experience. *Archives of Otolaryngology-Head and Neck Surgery, 125*(5), 509–514.

World Health Organization. (2003). Pneumococcal vaccination position paper. *Weekly Epidemiological Record, 78*(14), 110–119. Retrieved from http://www.who.int/wer

World Health Organization. (2005). *WHO global report. Preventing chronic disease: A vital investment.* Retrieved from http://www.who.int/chp/chronic_disease_report/contents/en/index.html

World Health Organization. (2006a). *Medical genetic services in developing countries: The ethical, legal and social implications of genetic testing and screening.* Retrieved from http://www.who.int/genomics/publications/GTS-MedicalGeneticServices-oct06.pdf

World Health Organization. (2006b). *Primary ear and hearing care [Training resource]: WHO—prevention of blindness and deafness.* Retrieved from http://www.who.int/pbd/deafness/activities/hearing_care/en/

World Health Organization. (2011a). Rubella vaccines: WHO position paper. *Weekly Epidemiological Record, 86*(29), 301–316. Retrieved from http://www.who.int/wer

World Health Organization. (2011b). Increased transmision and outbreaks of measles, European Region, 2011. *Weekly Epidemiological Record, 86*(49), 557–564. Retrieved from http://www.who.int/wer

World Health Organization. (2012). *Promoting ear and hearing care through community-based rehabilitation (CBR).* Retrieved from http://www.who.int/pbd/deafness

World Health Organization. (2013). *Haemophilus influenzae* type b (Hib) vaccination position paper. *Weekly Epidemiological Record, 88*(39), 413–428. Retrieved from http://www.who.int/wer

World Health Organization. (2015). *Prevention of blindness and deafness (PBD)—Epidemiology and economic analysis.* Retrieved September 10, 2015, from http://www.who.int/pbd/deafness/activities/epidemiology_economic_analysis

World Health Organization, & Acuin, J. (2004). Chronic suppurative otitis media: Burden of illness and management options. *Child and Adolescent Health and Development & Prevention of Blindness and Deafness.* Geneva, Switzerland: WHO. Retrieved from http://whqlibdoc.who.int/Publications/2004/9241591587.pdf

World Health Organization-PDH. (1997). Prevention of noise-induced hearing loss—Report of an informal consultation. Strategies for prevention of deafness and hearing impairment. Retrieved March 20, 2009, from http://www.who.int/pbd/deafness/en/noise.pdf

Worsoe, L., Caye-Thomasen, P., Brandt, C. T., Thomsen, J., & Ostergaard, C. (2010). Factors associated with the occurrence of hearing loss after pneumococcal meningitis. [Research Support, Non-U.S. Gov't]. *Clinical Infectious Diseases, 51*(8), 917–924. doi:10.1086/656409

Xu, Z., Li, Z., Chen, Y., He, Y., Chunyu, X., Wang, F., . . . Qiu, J. (2011). [Hearing the impact of MP3 on a survey of middle school students]. *Lin Chung Er Bi Yan Hou Tou Jing Wai Ke Za Zhi, 25*(4), 151–153.

Yee-Arellano, H. M., Leal-Garza, F., & Pauli-Muller, K. (2006). Universal newborn hearing screening in Mexico: Results of the first 2 years. *International Journal of Pediatric Otorhinolaryngology, 70*(11), 1863–1870. doi:S0165-5876(06)00206-0 [pii]10.1016/j.ijporl.2006.06.008

Yehudai, N., Most, T., & Luntz, M. (2015). Risk factors for sensorineural hearing loss in pediatric chronic otitis media. *International Journal of Pediatric Otorhinolaryngology, 79*(1), 26–30. doi:http://dx.doi.org/10.1016/j.ijporl.2014.10.025

Yiengprugsawan, V., Hogan, A., & Strazdins, L. (2013). Longitudinal analysis of ear infection and hearing impairment: Findings from 6-year prospective cohorts of Australian children. [Research Support, Non-U.S. Gov't]. *BMC Pediatrics, 13*, 28. doi:10.1186/1471-2431-13-28

Yoong, S. Y., Feltbower, R., Spencer, N., & McKinney, P. A. (2005). Families affected by deafness: Hospital services uptake in a multiethnic population. *Archives of Disease in Childhood, 90*(5), 454–459. doi:90/5/454 [pii]10.1136/adc.2003.046631

Zakzouk, S. (2002). Consanguinity and hearing impairment in developing countries: A custom to be discouraged. *Journal of Laryngology and Otology, 116*(10), 811–816. doi:10.1258/00222150260293628

Zakzouk, S. M., & Al-Anazy, F. (2002). Sensorineural hearing impaired children with unknown causes: A comprehensive etiological study. *International Journal of Pediatric Otorhinolaryngology, 64*(1), 17–21. doi:S0165587602000290 [pii]

Zimmerman, E., & Lahav, A. (2013). Ototoxicity in preterm infants: Effects of genetics, aminoglycosides, and loud environmental noise. *Journal of Perinatology, 33*(1), 3–8.

6

Genetics of Childhood Hearing Loss

Linda J. Hood and Bronya J.B. Keats

Introduction and Overview

Epidemiologic and Demographic Aspects of Genetic Hearing Loss

Congenital hearing loss occurs in approximately 1 to 2 of 1,000 births, and genetic factors account for at least 60% of childhood hearing loss. Genetic hearing loss is usually classified according to the presence (syndromic) or absence (nonsyndromic) of other clinical anomalies and the pattern of inheritance (autosomal, X-linked, dominant, recessive, mitochondrial). Over the past 20 years, more than 120 genes related to hearing loss have been described, and the causal mutations in patients can often be identified through genetic testing. Most cases (>70%) of childhood hearing loss are nonsyndromic with an autosomal recessive pattern of inheritance, and mutations in the *GJB2* gene that encodes the protein connexin 26 underlie as many as 50% of these cases in some populations.

A genetic etiology should be considered for every patient with a hearing problem. Even if a possible environmental cause is reported, a genetic cause cannot be ruled out. Conversely, if no obvious environmental insult or other cause can be determined, then the cause is most likely genetic. Also, it is important to realize that a family history of hearing loss is not necessary for the cause of a hearing loss to be related to a genetic source. For example, a child with autosomal recessive hearing loss is often the only affected person in the family (see below). Not all inherited hearing loss is present at birth; hereditary loss can also have later onset. This will be further discussed in the context of identification of hearing loss.

The Partnership of Geneticists and Audiologists

Accumulating knowledge about genetic causes of hearing loss and the steady increase in the sophistication of both auditory and genetic testing that is available provides options and opportunities for patients and their families to interact with professionals representing multiple disciplines. Audiologists and geneticists provide complementary roles in the process of identification and diagnosis of hearing loss, and partnerships can greatly enhance precise diagnosis, appropriate management of children with hearing loss, and the overall patient and family experience. With the wealth of information (and sometimes mis-information) available via the Internet, families often come to appointments with questions that different specialists are best prepared to address. Having readily available referral sources—in audiology for the geneticist and in genetics for the audiologist—can facilitate an efficient pathway through the diagnostic and management process.

Patterns of Inheritance

The human genome consists of 24 different types of chromosomes designated 1 to 22 (autosomes), X and Y (sex chromosomes). An offspring inherits one set of chromosomes from each parent, giving a total of 46 chromosomes (22 autosomal pairs plus XX or XY) in the nucleus of a cell. The major component of each of these chromosomes is a single molecule of deoxyribonucleic acid (DNA), which has a double helical structure, and is composed of a sugar-phosphate backbone and four bases called adenine (A), guanine (G), thymine (T), and cytosine (C). The double helix is formed through the pairing of A with T, and C with G, and the bases are held together by hydrogen bonds. Thus, knowing the sequence of bases on one DNA strand automatically gives the sequence on the other strand. This precise pairing means that DNA can replicate by separation of the two strands followed by each strand serving as a template for a new complementary strand.

Chromosomes can be differentiated from one another by size, centromere location, and the pattern of dark and light bands that is observed when various staining techniques are used. The arms on either side of the centromere (the area of constriction that demarcates the two arms) are designated "p" and "q" for the shorter and longer arm, respectively. The bands are numbered from the centromere outward to the end of the arm (known as the telomere) and have been subdivided numerous times as new banding methods were introduced. One of the uses of the banding is to give the approximate location of a gene (a sequence of bases coding for a specific protein). For example, a gene in the band numbered 2p11 is close to the centromere on the p arm of chromosome 2, while a gene in the band numbered 13q34 is toward the telomere on the q arm of chromosome 13.

Individuals inherit pairs of chromosomes and, therefore, pairs of genes, which are known as the individual's genotype. Occasionally one or both copies of a gene may contain a mutation that prevents formation of the normal form of the protein encoded by that gene. When this happens, the individual may have a clinically abnormal phenotype, such as hearing loss. If there is a family history of hearing loss, then this information can be used to construct a pedigree and determine if it is consistent with autosomal or X-linked inheritance, which may be further categorized as dominant or recessive.

The pattern of inheritance of hearing loss is probably autosomal dominant if some of the individuals in each generation have hearing loss, and both males and females are affected (Figure 6–1). The affected individuals usually have one normal (N) and one abnormal (D) copy of the gene related to the hearing loss, meaning that each offspring of an affected individual has a 50% chance of inheriting the abnormal copy. Examples of dominantly inherited syndromes are branchiootorenal (BOR), Waardenburg, and Treacher-Collins. If all individuals who inherit the abnormal gene exhibit features of the disease, penetrance is said to be complete. However, with some disorders, individuals who must have the abnormal gene (because, for example, they have an affected parent and an affected child) show no phenotypic signs. In this case, penetrance is said to be incomplete, perhaps due to the effect of other genetic factors or possibly environmental factors.

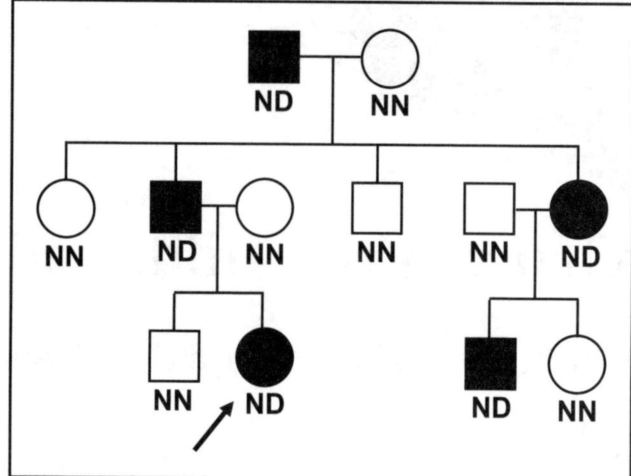

FIGURE 6–1. Three-generation pedigree depicting an autosomal dominant inheritance pattern.

The mode of inheritance is autosomal recessive if the hearing loss is found only in individuals who have two copies of the abnormal gene (genotype DD). If both parents are carriers of an abnormal (D) copy (that is, both have the genotype ND), their child might inherit two copies of D, one from each parent (Figure 6–2). In this situation, the child displays hearing loss, but neither parent is affected. The probability that a child of two carrier parents will be affected is one quarter. Note that family history is often negative with a recessive disorder because an abnormal form of the gene might be passed on from one (unaffected) carrier to the next for many generations before two individuals who are both carriers have an affected child. Examples of recessively inherited syndromes are Jervell and Lange-Nielsen, Pendred, Usher, and Wolfram.

Males have both an X and a Y chromosome; females have two X chromosomes. For X-linked inheritance, father-to-son transmission is not possible because a son must receive his X chromosome from his mother. For an X-linked recessive disorder, affected individuals are usually male because they have only one X chromosome. However, if the father is affected and the mother is a carrier, then both daughters and sons have a 50% chance of being affected. In contrast, all the daughters of affected fathers are affected for an X-linked dominant disorder with complete penetrance, and each child (whether male or female) of an affected female has a 50% chance of being affected (assuming the mother has the ND genotype and the father is unaffected). Alport

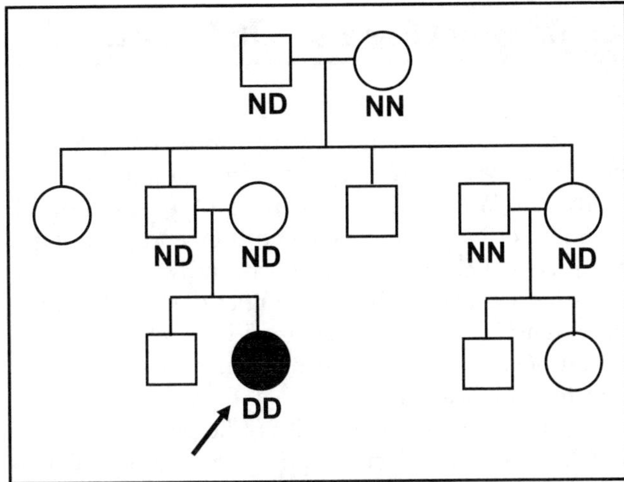

FIGURE 6–2. Three-generation pedigree depicting an autosomal recessive inheritance pattern.

is an example of a syndrome for which the pattern of inheritance is usually X-linked.

Mitochondria are small organelles that are located within the cytoplasm of a cell. A process called *oxidative phosphorylation* (OXPHOS) takes place in the mitochondria and is responsible for energy (ATP) production in the cell. Mitochondria are maternally inherited, and they have their own DNA (mtDNA). Thus, the expected family history for a disorder caused by a mtDNA mutation is that all children of an affected mother are affected, whereas children of an affected father are never affected. However, each mitochondrion has multiple copies of mtDNA, and each cell contains several hundred mitochondria. This means that cells may contain both mutant and normal copies of mtDNA, a condition known as *heteroplasmy* (as opposed to *homoplasmy* meaning that all the copies are the same). Children of an affected mother might inherit different percentages of mutant and normal mtDNA, which means that some might have more severe symptoms than others. If there are enough normal copies to provide the energy requirements of the cell, then normal function will be retained. But different cell types have differing energy requirements, so the effect of the mutant copies can vary from one organ to another. The organs with the most demand for energy are the skeletal muscle, heart, and brain. Thus, the typical symptoms found in mitochondrial disorders are muscle weakness, nervous system disorders, visual problems, hearing loss, and dementia.

Genetic hearing loss is not always the result of a mutation in a single gene. It might be one of multiple clinical findings associated with a chromosomal anomaly. For example, all or a large segment of a chromosome can be deleted, duplicated, or inverted, or one part of one chromosome might be attached to part of another chromosome, an event known as *translocation*. Children with Down syndrome usually have an extra copy of chromosome 21 (trisomy 21) giving them 47 chromosomes altogether, while those with Turner syndrome have 45 chromosomes because they have only one X chromosome and no Y. Hearing loss, particularly conductive hearing loss related to middle-ear anomalies, is often found in persons with Down syndrome.

In other situations, a mutation in a single gene can contribute to the hearing loss, but additional genetic or environmental factors might be required for the hearing loss to be present. This type of hearing loss is usually familial, but the pattern of inheritance is unclear; it is called *multifactorial inheritance*. Also, in taking a family history and interpreting a pedigree, it is very important to remember that hearing loss is relatively common, and the etiology might not be the same for all affected members of a family.

Genes associated with hearing loss have been localized to all chromosomes, including the X and Y chromosomes. Genetic loci (locations on chromosomes) associated with autosomal dominant forms of hearing loss are conventionally denoted as DFNA followed by a number that was assigned when the locus was mapped to a chromosome (e.g., DFNA1, DFNA2). Similar nomenclature is used for other forms: DFNB(number) for recessive hearing loss, DFNX (number) for X-linked hearing loss, DFNY(number) for Y-linked hearing loss, and a locus for a gene that modifies the hearing loss phenotype associated with another gene is given the label DFNM(number). An excellent source of up-to-date information that includes a listing of current loci associated with various forms of hearing loss can be found at the Hereditary Hearing Loss Homepage (http://hereditaryhearingloss.org) that was created and is maintained by Drs. Guy Van Camp and Richard J.H. Smith.

Nonsyndromic Hearing Loss

Genes associated with auditory function code for proteins that contribute to the development of the auditory system and underlie the many functions of specific structures of the external ear, middle ear, cochlea, vestibular system, and neural pathways. A mutation in any of these genes can lead to an abnormal protein and result in hearing loss. Additionally, within the same gene, there are often many different mutations that can cause hearing loss.

A high percentage of nonsyndromic hearing loss is associated with mutations in a gene named *GJB2*, which was the first identified form of autosomal recessive deafness, DFNB1 (Kelsell et al., 1997). *GJB2* maps to the chromosome position 13q11.12 and codes for the production of the protein connexin 26 (Cx26). Cx26 is one of a family of gap junction proteins that facilitate exchange of electrolytes, metabolites, and so on, between cells. In the inner ear, Cx26 is widely expressed in the cochlea, in supporting cells, and stria vascularis, and is thought to be important in endolymph equilibrium and maintaining high potassium levels in the scala media.

More than 80 mutations in *GJB2* have been reported, but certain mutations account for many cases of hearing loss. The most common mutations are 35delG, predominant in populations of European descent, 167delT found primarily in Ashkenazi Jewish persons, and 235delC in persons of Asian descent. Mutations in *GJB2* are usually associated with recessive hearing loss, but some mutations have been reported that result in dominant hearing loss (DFNA3) and also Vohwinkel's syndrome (sensorineural hearing loss and keratoderma). A significant number of children with recessive hearing loss have one *GJB2* mutation together with a deletion on the other copy of chromosome 13 involving a gene, *GJB6*, which is in very close proximity to *GJB2* and codes for another gap junction protein, connexin 30. Thus, evaluation of *GJB6* is often recommended following testing for *GJB2* mutations, if results of *GJB2* testing alone are not definitive.

Some gene mutations are associated with more severe hearing losses than others, though this is not a clear-cut rule, and sometimes individuals with the same mutations have different degrees of hearing loss. The lack of consistency might be due to influences of other genes. A general observation of the relationship between gene mutations and characteristics of a hearing loss is that mutations having more severe effects on production of the protein tend to be associated with more severe hearing losses. For example, the 35delG mutation in the *GJB2* gene is a deletion of a G at position 35 of the DNA coding sequence. Gene sequences are read in sets of three bases (codons), which specify the addition of a particular amino acid to the protein (or a stop). Presence of the 35delG mutation creates a premature stop codon, which instructs the process of protein creation to stop, resulting in a drastically truncated protein.

Genotype-Phenotype Relationships

The accumulation of increasingly more patients with hearing losses related to specific gene mutations allows study of relationships between genotype, an individual's underlying genetic constitution, and phenotype, the physical characteristics of an individual. Understanding genotype-phenotype relationships has been particularly possible for hearing losses related to *GJB2* mutations, given the high incidence of carriers and affected individuals.

One of the earliest studies of hearing loss related to *GJB2* mutations focused on two mutations, 35delG and 167delT, commonly found in populations of European descent and Ashkenazi Jewish persons, respectively. Severity of hearing loss in the 46 subjects studied ranged from mild to profound for homozygous 35delG mutations and from moderate to profound for those with homozygous 167delT and compound heterozygous (35delG/167delT) mutations (Cohn et al., 1999).

Subsequent studies have underscored the variation in hearing phenotype, even within specific genotypes, though clear trends have emerged as studies of larger numbers of patients became possible. In a large multicenter study, Snoeckx et al. (2005) performed a cross-sectional analysis of *GJB2* genotype and audiometric data from 1,531 persons from 16 different countries with autosomal recessive nonsyndromic hearing loss. A total of 153 different genotypes were found and were divided into three groups: homozygous truncating (T/T, n = 56), homozygous nontruncating (NT/NT, n = 30), and compound heterozygous truncating/nontruncating (T/NT, n = 67). The degree of hearing impairment associated with homozygous truncating mutations was significantly more severe than that associated with homozygous nontruncating mutations ($P < .0001$). The hearing loss associated with 48 different genotypes was less severe than that of 35delG homozygotes. Mild-to-moderate hearing impairment was found with several common mutations.

The homozygous 35delG genotype is characterized by severe-to-profound deafness in 82% to 90% of patients with this genotype (Azaiez, Van Camp, & Smith, 2006). When a 35delG mutation occurs in conjunction with another *GJB2* mutation, particularly a nontruncating mutation (T/NT), then the number of persons with severe-to-profound deafness is reduced. In contrast, when one *GJB2* truncating mutation occurs in conjunction with a *GJB6* deletion, the result is severe-to-profound deafness that is typically more severe than in 35delG homozygotes.

Discovery of these relationships between hearing phenotype and genotype has been possible in the case of *GJB2* because of the high incidence of this form of hearing loss in many populations. There is a need to develop large databases of pediatric (and adult) information with detailed auditory and genetic information to allow study of rare diseases and forms of hearing loss. The AudGenDB Project (http://audgendb.chop.edu) is one example of a project focused on compiling large amounts of auditory, medical, and genetic data that can be used in an open-access format to learn about characteristics of many forms of hearing loss.

The focus of the discussion thus far has been recessive hearing loss and mutations in *GJB2*; however, mutations in many other genes also are associated with recessive and dominant forms of nonsyndromic hearing loss. Adding to the complexity is the fact that mutations in the same gene may be associated with dominant or recessive hearing loss and both nonsyndromic and syndromic deafness. Thus, the same gene can be associated with different phenotypes and different patterns of inheritance, which underscores the importance of obtaining thorough history, observational, and evaluation information from all patients and their families.

Syndromes Associated With Hearing Loss

Syndromic hearing loss is often classified by association with other system disorders (Konigsmark & Gorlin, 1976; Toriello, Reardon, & Gorlin, 2004), and genes have been identified for many syndromes that involve hearing loss. Some of the common syndromes that include hearing loss are shown in Table 6–1, along with the other systems involved.

Syndromes involving hearing loss probably share molecular mechanisms that are abnormal in both the ear and the other affected organ systems. Understanding the molecular defect in one system should help in understanding processes underlying abnormal function in other systems impacted by genetic changes. However, in some cases, it is possible that the underlying causes do not share a common genetic source in the two systems, which would confound analysis and understanding of the apparent syndrome.

The following sections provide brief summaries of phenotype and genotype information related to some of the more common syndromes that involve hearing loss (presented in alphabetical order). The text

Table 6–1. Classification of Syndromic Forms of Hearing Loss by Association With Other System Disorders

System	Syndrome
Eye disorders	Usher
Endocrine disorders	Pendred Wolfram
Cardiac disorders	Jervell and Lange-Nielsen
Pigmentary disorders	Waardenburg
Renal disorders	Alport Branchial-oto-renal (BOR)
Musculoskeletal disorders	Stickler

Hereditary Hearing Loss and Its Syndromes (Toriello et al., 2004) is recommended for more detailed information about these and many other syndromes involving the auditory system. This text, an updated edition of the classic text from Gorlin, Toriello, and Cohen (1995), provides comprehensive information about characteristics, including visual depictions, and test results associated with syndromes involving hearing loss. Up-to-date information about the most common syndromes involving hearing loss is also available on the Hereditary Hearing Loss home page noted previously. For comprehensive information, the reader is referred to the website Online Mendelian Inheritance in Man (OMIM). OMIM provides an extensive online catalog of human genes and genetic disorders that is intended for use primarily by physicians and other professionals concerned with genetic disorders, by genetics researchers, and by advanced students in science and medicine.

Alport Syndrome

Alport syndrome is characterized by progressive loss of kidney function, sensorineural hearing loss, and sometimes visual defects. The incidence of Alport syndrome is approximately 1 in 50,000 live births. The most common inheritance pattern is X-linked, but it can also be autosomal recessive and autosomal dominant. The hearing loss is sensorineural in nature with higher frequencies affected to a greater degree, and onset is more often seen in older children and adolescents, though onset can be congenital. Autosomal dominant cases more often display a milder degree of hearing loss.

Visual defects involve ocular lesions and maculopathy. Alport is the second most common inherited cause of kidney failure and approximately 0.2% of adults and 3% of children in the United States with end-stage renal disease have been diagnosed with Alport syndrome.

Most cases of Alport syndrome are caused by mutations in the *COL4A5* gene on the q arm of the X chromosome (Xq22.3; Barker et al., 1990). Carrier females can show signs of the disease, but they are much less severely affected than males. The autosomal forms are associated with mutations in *COL4A3* and *COL4A4*, both located at 2q36.3 (Mochizuki et al., 1994). Recently, sequencing of these three genes in 87 Italian families that included members with a clinical diagnosis of Alport syndrome, identified mutations in 48 (55%) of the families. The results suggested a distribution of 65% X-linked, 31% autosomal dominant, and 4% autosomal recessive (Fallerini et al., 2014). The *COL4A3*, *COL4A4*, and *COL4A5* genes code for different chains of type IV collagen, which are major components of the structural matrix for the glomerular basement membrane in the kidney, the basilar membrane, spiral ligament, and stria vascularis in the inner ear, and in the eye.

Branchiootorenal (BOR) Syndrome

Branchiootorenal (BOR) syndrome has an incidence of about 1 in 40,000 and may account for about 2% of profound deafness. The branchial component of the syndrome name relates to anomalies involving the branchial arches in the structural development of the ear, and is present in about 50% of patients. Features of BOR include pre-auricular pits, branchial fistulae or cysts, and malformations of the external ear and middle ear. Patients with BOR syndrome have renal abnormalities that are a product of deformities in function and structure, varying in degree and effect on one or both kidneys.

Hearing loss associated with BOR is typically mixed but can be sensorineural or conductive. Onset of hearing loss ranges from birth to early adulthood with progression of hearing loss noted in about 30% of patients.

The pattern of inheritance is autosomal dominant with highly variable expression. The three identified genes related to BOR, *EYA1*, *SIX5*, and *SIX1*, on chromosomes 8q13.3, 19q13.32, and 14q23.1, respectively, are heavily involved in embryonic development, which is consistent with branchial arch abnormalities. Approximately 40% of patients have mutations in *EYA1*, and more than 80 different mutations have been reported (Abdelhak et al., 1997). The percentage with mutations in *SIX5* and *SIX1* is much smaller; additionally, for many affected individuals, mutations are not found in any of these three genes, so more remain to be identified.

Diagnosis of BOR, without positive family history, is based on the presence of either three or more major criteria or two major and two minor criteria. Major criteria are branchial arch abnormalities, pre-auricular pits, auricular deformity, deafness, and renal anomalies. Minor criteria include external auditory canal, middle ear, or inner ear anomalies, pre-auricular tags, and facial or palate abnormalities. There also is a variation of BOR that exists without evidence of renal dysfunction, which is known as branchio-otic syndrome (Kochhar et al., 2007).

CHARGE Syndrome

CHARGE syndrome stands for *c*oloboma, *h*eart defect, *a*tresia choane (also known as choanal atresia), *r*etarded growth and development, *g*enital abnormality, and *e*ar abnormality. Estimates of occurrence range from approximately 1 in 8,500 to 10,000 births. Characteristics vary among individuals. Many individuals have a hole in one of the structures of one or both eyes (coloboma), which forms during early development and may or may not affect vision. One or both nasal passages may be narrowed (choanal stenosis) or blocked (choanal atresia). Abnormal function of cranial nerves can result in swallowing problems, facial palsy/paralysis, diminished sense of smell, and mild-to-profound hearing loss. Nearly all individuals with CHARGE syndrome present with auricular deformities that are often asymmetric.

Mutations in the *CHD7* gene located at 8q12.1-q12.2 are responsible for about two thirds of cases with CHARGE syndrome (Zentner, Layman, Martin, & Schacheri, 2010). The protein encoded by the *CHD7* gene is a transcriptional regulator involved in chromatin remodeling. Mutations in *CHD7* result in production of abnormal protein that disrupts chromatin remodeling and neural crest gene expression, and are a likely cause of severe embryonic malformations seen on ultrasound (Sanlaville et al., 2006).

Jervell and Lange-Nielsen Syndrome

Jervell and Lange-Nielsen syndrome (JLNS) is a rare autosomal recessive disorder associated with congenital, bilateral sensorineural profound hearing loss and cardiac arrhythmia. The occurrence of JLNS is about 3 to 5 in 1,000,000 live births, though the prevalence varies among different world populations. About 1 in 100 infants identified with profound sensorineural hearing loss may have this recessively inherited syndrome. The importance of identifying this syndrome is highlighted by the characteristics of cardiac abnormalities, fainting spells, and sudden death. The cardiac abnormality is a long QT interval (the time period between two waves in the electrocardiogram), and when identified, cardiac problems can be managed, making the diagnosis a critical component of the workup of an infant or child identified with congenital sensorineural hearing loss. The importance of early diagnosis of this syndrome also supports the value of newborn hearing screening programs.

Mutations in two genes, *KCNQ1* and *KCNE1* on chromosomes 11p15 and 21q22, respectively, are associated with JLNS (Neyroud et al., 1997; Splawski et al., 1997). These genes code for proteins that are involved in the formation and function of potassium channels that regulate the flow of ions across cell membranes needed for normal function in the heart and inner ear (Schwartz et al., 2006). Approximately 90% of affected individuals have mutations in both copies of *KCNQ1*; the remaining 10% have mutations in both copies of *KCNE1*. Clinical manifestation of JLNS can be similar to other disorders, making comparison important in differential diagnosis. For example, Romano-Ward syndrome is a type of the more commonly occurring long QT syndrome that displays cardiac characteristics but not hearing loss.

MELAS and MERRF

MELAS is the acronym for mitochondrial encephalomyopathy, lactic acidosis, stroke-like episodes, and sensorineural hearing loss. Hearing loss is typically sensorineural in nature and severe. Characteristics of patients with MELAS are headaches, stroke-like episodes that can result in hemiparesis, seizures, growth deficiency, and lactic acidosis. Onset is typically in the first or second decade. Related pathology involves ragged-red fibers and other mitochondrial abnormalities observed in muscle.

MERRF denotes mitochondrial encephalomyopathy, myoclonus epilepsy, ragged-red fibers, and sensorineural hearing loss. MERRF is separated from other mitochondrial encephalomyopathies by the presence of myoclonic epilepsy. Onset occurs in the first decade or into adulthood, and the early symptoms can include myoclonic jerks and ataxia. Hearing loss is typically sensorineural but may also be neural in nature. Patients with MERRF/MELAS overlap syndrome experience symptoms of both disorders with variability among patients in severity and progression.

Several mutations in mtDNA are associated with MELAS and MERRF. These mutations are usually heteroplasmic and result in systemic neuromuscular dysfunction. The most common MELAS mutation, A3243G in the *MT-TL1* gene, has also been found in individuals with other clinical presentations, for example, sensorineural hearing loss and diabetes mellitus. The A8344G mutation in the *MT-TK* gene is the most common in patients with MERRF.

Pendred Syndrome

Pendred syndrome is one of the more common syndromes involving hearing loss with an incidence of 1 in 7,500. Other clinical findings in Pendred syndrome are goiter (enlarged thyroid) and enlarged vestibular aqueduct (EVA). Although goiter is the hallmark of the syndrome, it often does not present until patients are in young adulthood. Among patients with hearing loss and EVA, 86% were found to have a mutation in the *SLC26A4* gene (Reardon, Omahoney, Trembath, Jan, & Phelps, 2000). The pattern of inheritance is autosomal recessive, and hearing loss is characterized as profound, typically congenital, and sensorineural. This syndrome is thought to account for approximately 5% to 10% of children with severe or profound hearing loss, making it one of the most common forms of hearing loss.

Mutations in the *SLC26A4* gene explain about 50% of cases of Pendred syndrome (Everett et al., 1997). Located on chromosome 7q22.3, *SLC26A4* encodes a protein called pendrin that functions as a chloride and iodide transporter. Although more than 170 mutations have been reported, three mutations are found in about 55% of patients. Thus, genetic testing can initially be targeted to these three mutations. Another gene, *FOXI1*, on chromosome 5q35.1, codes for a protein that is involved in the regulation of *SLC26A4*, and mutations in *FOXI1* have been found in a small percentage of the Pendred patients who are heterozygous for a *SLC26A4* mutation, suggesting digenic inheritance (Yang et al., 2007). It should be noted that some mutations in *SLC26A4* are associated with nonsyndromic autosomal recessive hearing loss (DFNB4).

Stickler Syndrome

Stickler syndrome is one of the most common autosomal dominant disorders involving connective tissue. Collagen is a major structural component of cartilaginous tissues and is important for normal inner ear function due to its prevalence in structural components, including the tectorial membrane and supporting structures in the cochlea. Incidence among neonates is estimated to be about 1 in 7,500 to 9,000. Characteristics include midfacial hypoplasia and a flattened nasal bridge that give the appearance of a flattened facial profile, particularly in childhood, an abnormally small lower jaw, hearing loss, myopia, retinal detachment, joint hypermobility, and premature osteoarthritis. There are several subtypes that are differentiated based on inheritance pattern, different genotypes, and variable phenotypic characteristics. The most common type of hearing loss is sensorineural, mild-to-moderate sloping high-frequency hearing loss (Acke, Dhooge, Malfait, & De Leenheer, 2012). Mixed and conductive hearing losses can also occur, particularly in children and in patients with palatal defects as cleft palate occurs in some cases. Tympanometry might show hypermobile tympanic membranes.

Mutations in three collagen genes (*COL2A1*, *COL11A1*, and *COL11A2* on chromosomes 12q13.1, 1p21.1, and 6p21.3, respectively) are associated with autosomal dominant Stickler syndrome, subtyped as Types I, II, and III. Type I makes up about 75% of all Stickler patients. If ocular anomalies are present, the mutation is likely to be in *COL2A1* or *COL11A1*; if the patient has craniofacial and joint abnormalities but no ocular findings, then genetic testing would usually begin with *COL11A2*. Mutations in *COL11A2* have also been found in individuals with nonsyndromic hearing loss (DFNA13). Stickler Types IV and V are two rare autosomal recessive forms of the syndrome that are associated with homozygous mutations in *COL9A1* (6q13) and *COL9A2* (1p34.2), respectively.

Treacher Collins Syndrome

Treacher Collins syndrome is an autosomal dominant disorder that occurs in about 1 in 10,000 to 50,000 births. It is characterized by considerable phenotypic variability, and, unlike usual autosomal dominant inheritance, family history might be negative due to failure to recognize the disorder in a parent, incomplete penetrance, variable expressivity, or a new (de novo) mutation. Patients with Treacher Collins syndrome have congenital craniofacial abnormalities where bones of the head and face are underdeveloped or abnormally developed, such as an undersized jaw, undeveloped mandible, or cleft palate. Auditory characteristics typically relate to abnormalities of the external and middle ear, while inner ear structures are generally normal.

Mutations in the *TCOF1* gene that encodes a protein known as Treacle cause the majority of cases of Treacher Collins syndrome. This gene is located on chromosome 5q32 and more than 100 mutations have been described, most of which result in a premature stop codon. Approximately 60% of cases are due to new mutations, while in about 40% one of the parents has a mutation; however, because of incomplete penetrance or mild expression of the phenotype, the family members in previous generations with the mutation may not have been diagnosed. Recently, mutations in the genes *POLR1C* (6q21.1) and *POLR1D* (13q12.2) have been identified in individuals with Treacher Collins syndrome (Dauwerse et al., 2011). Treacher Collins syndrome can be linked to a lack of neural crest cells during embryologic development resulting in malformations of the maxillary and mandibular processes.

Usher Syndrome

Usher syndrome is characterized by hearing loss, retinitis pigmentosa (RP), a vision condition that involves progressive narrowing of the visual fields, and vestibular disorders. It is the most frequent cause of deafness accompanied by blindness in developed countries, accounting for greater than 50% of the deaf-blind population, about 18% of individuals with retinitis pigmentosa, and 3% to 6% of persons with congenital deafness. The inheritance pattern for Usher syndrome is autosomal recessive, and it is classified into three subtypes based on clinical findings related to degree of hearing loss, vestibular responses, and age at onset of RP. Profound congenital hearing loss, early onset of RP (in the first decade of life), and absent vestibular responses are found in patients with Type I Usher syndrome. Patients with Type II also have congenital hearing loss though more moderate in degree, later onset of RP, and vestibular responses are typically present. Type III has more variable characteristics including progressive hearing loss. Some forms of Usher syndrome are associated with certain populations, such as Usher Type IC, which is predominantly found in the Louisiana Acadian population (Keats, Nouri, Pelias, Deininger, & Litt, 1994). Confirmation of Usher syndrome is difficult at birth, and infants may be misdiagnosed with nonsyndromic congenital hearing loss until later determination of vision loss.

Eleven different genes that are associated with Usher syndrome have been identified so far, with others yet to be identified. Mutations in *MYO7A* (11q13.5), *USH1C* (11p15.1), *CDH23* (10q22.1), *PCDH15* (10q21.1), *SANS* (17q25.1), and *CIB2* (15q25.1) cause subtypes of Usher Type I. An added complication is that mutations in the first four of these genes have also been associated with nonsyndromic hearing loss. However, targeted genetic testing for a specific mutation in *USH1C* or *PCDH15* is likely to be successful for Usher I patients of Acadian or Ashkenazi Jewish ancestry, respectively. Testing for these mutations in Acadian and Ashkenazi Jewish infants with profound hearing loss might enable Usher I to be diagnosed well before the onset of RP.

Mutations in *USH2A* on chromosome 1q41 are responsible for 80% of Usher Type II; two other genes, *GPR98* (5q14.3) and *WHRN* (9q32) are associated with about 15% and 5%, respectively. Ebermann et al. (2010) suggested the possibility of digenic inheritance of Usher Type II involving mutations in *GPR98* and *PDZD7* (10q24.31). In addition to causing Usher II, *USH2A* mutations have also been found in 12% of patients with autosomal recessive RP. *WHRN* (*DFNB31*) mutations were first found in individuals with autosomal recessive nonsyndromic hearing loss (Mburu et al., 2003). Two Usher Type III genes, *CLRN1* (3q25.1) and *HARS* (5q31.3) have been identified; *CLRN1* mutations are relatively common in Finland.

The proteins encoded by the Usher I and II genes have been shown to interact with one another to form a large network that is necessary for normal function of the hair cells and stereocilia. A mutation in any one of these genes can disrupt the network.

Waardenburg Syndrome

Waardenburg syndrome is characterized by pigmentary abnormalities of the hair (white forelock), iris (heterochromia irides—different colored eyes), and skin. Another characteristic is wide-set eyes (dystopia canthorum). Hearing loss is sensorineural and has variable presentation, ranging from no hearing loss to profound unilateral or bilateral sensorineural hearing loss, and is progressive in some types. Clinical classifications of Waardenburg involve several subtypes dependent on presence or absence of various phenotype characteristics. In particular, dystopia canthorum is present in Type I and absent in Type II. Estimates of the prevalence of Waardenburg syndrome range from 1 in 20,000 to 1 in 40,000.

The inheritance pattern for Waardenburg syndrome is usually autosomal dominant with variable expression. However, Type IV, which is a combination of Type II and Hirschsprung disease, has an autosomal recessive pattern of inheritance. Six different genes are associated with Waardenburg syndrome (WS), and there are probably at least two more. Mutations in the *PAX3* gene on chromosome 2q36.1 are found in patients with both Type I and Type III (Type I plus upper limb abnormalities), while Type II is associated with mutations in *MITF* (3p14-p13) and *SNAI2* (8q11.21), as well as deletion of *SOX10* (22q13.1). The autosomal recessive form, Type IV, is caused by mutations in both copies of three genes: *EDNRB* (13q22.3), *EDN3* (20q13.32), and *SOX10*.

Symptoms of WS are differentiated into major and minor criteria. To make a diagnosis, a patient must have either two major criteria or one major and two minor criteria. Major criteria include congenital sensorineural, white forelock, iris pigmentation, dystopia canthorum, and affected first-degree relative. Minor criteria are abnormal skin pigmentation, medial eyebrow flare, high nasal root, hypoplastic nasal alae, and premature gray hair.

Wolfram Syndrome

Wolfram syndrome involves diabetes insipidus, diabetes mellitus, optic atrophy, and sensorineural deafness and is also referred to as DIDMOAD (diabetes insipidus, diabetes mellitus, optic atrophy, deafness). The rate of occurrence is between 1 in 150 and 1 in 175 of patients with juvenile diabetes (Gunn et al., 1976). Individuals can be small in stature and underweight. Onset of bilateral progressive loss of visual acuity leading to blindness occurs most frequently in the first decade of life. Hearing losses associated with Wolfram syndrome are bilateral and progressive, leading most often to moderate to severe sensorineural losses with poorer hearing in the higher frequencies.

Wolfram syndrome has an autosomal recessive pattern of inheritance and is caused by mutations in the *WFS1* gene on chromosome 4p16.1, which encodes a protein known as wolframin. Over 70 different mutations associated with Wolfram syndrome have been reported. Mutations in this gene are also associated with autosomal dominant low-frequency nonsyndromic hearing loss (DFNA6/14/38). A second type of Wolfram syndrome in which affected individuals also have defective platelet aggregation resulting in gastrointestinal ulceration and bleeding results from mutations in the *CISD2* gene on chromosome 4q24.

Aminoglycoside-Induced Deafness

Some individuals are at increased risk of deafness as a result of sensitivity to administration of low levels of aminoglycosides due to the presence of a mutation, A1555G, in the *MT-RNR1* gene of their maternally transmitted mtDNA (Prezant et al., 1993). This mutation is usually homoplasmic in affected individuals, and exposure to aminoglycosides such as streptomycin and gentamicin is not always a prerequisite for deafness. It is the most common mtDNA mutation associated with deafness and probably explains up to 1% of hearing loss in Caucasians; higher prevalences have been reported in Asian and Spanish patients.

Auditory Neuropathy/Dys-synchrony

Patients ranging in age from infants to adults are identified with auditory neuropathy/dys-synchrony (AN/AD; Berlin, Hood, & Rose, 2001; Starr, Picton, Sininger, Hood, & Berlin, 1996), which is also referred to as auditory neuropathy spectrum disorder (ANSD). AN/AD is characterized by the presence of responses associated with functional active cochlear processes related to outer hair cells and cochlear mechanics in the form of otoacoustic emissions or cochlear microphonics. Peripheral neural function at the level of the eighth nerve/brainstem is poor as characterized by absent or highly abnormal auditory brainstem responses (Berlin et al., 1998) and absent or abnormal middle ear muscle and medial olivocochlear reflexes (Berlin et al., 2005; Hood, Berlin, Bordelon, & Rose, 2003). Most patients with AN/AD show bilateral symptoms, though function can be asymmetric between ears, and cases of unilateral AN/AD have been documented (Berlin et al., 2010). Speech recognition is quite variable though generally much poorer than expected, particularly in noise. Some patients with AN/AD demonstrate timing problems (Zeng, Oba, Garde, Sininger, & Starr, 1999), which are suggestive of a disturbance in neural synchrony.

The mechanisms underlying AN/AD presently are unclear, and it is most likely that several mechanisms and etiologies exist. The mechanical transduction or other functional characteristics of the inner hair cells can be abnormal, the synaptic juncture between the inner hair cells and the cochlear branch of the vestibulocochlear (eighth) nerve might be affected, or the axons or cell bodies of the eighth nerve itself can be involved. Some patients, both children and adults, have no known etiology and no other identified neurological abnormalities. In other patients, the auditory findings can be associated with other peripheral neuropathies such as hereditary motor sensory neuropathy (Charcot-Marie-Tooth disease). Infants with neonatal abnormalities, including exchange transfusion, prematurity, and anoxia, have been reported with AN/AD (e.g., Deltenre, Mansbach, Bozet, Clercx, & Hecox, 1997).

Autosomal dominant, autosomal recessive, X-linked, and mitochondrial inheritance have all been reported for both syndromic and nonsyndromic AN/AD. Patients with syndromic AN/AD are often first diagnosed with peripheral neuropathy followed by the auditory neuropathy several years later, though this is not always the case. Mutations in HMSN genes such as *MPZ* are likely causes, particularly if the pattern of inheritance is autosomal dominant (Starr et al., 2003). Another gene that is highly expressed in nerves, *NDRG1*, was found to be associated with an autosomal recessive syndromic ANSD in the gypsy population (Kalaydjieva et al., 2000). Also, patients with X-linked recessive Mohr-Tranebjaerg syndrome have auditory neuropathy as do some patients with the mitochondrial disorder, Leber's hereditary optic neuropathy.

The majority of cases of nonsyndromic AN/AD are autosomal recessive, and the pure-tone loss can be severe to profound from infancy. Mutations in the gene *OTOF* (chromosome 2p23.3) that encodes a protein known as otoferlin are associated with recessive nonsyndromic AN (AUNB1). Varga et al. (2003) defined a group of patients with what they termed "nonsyndromic recessive auditory neuropathy," where patients displayed the classic features of AN/AD, and they found linkage to the *OTOF* gene. Some patients with *OTOF* mutations display a temperature-sensitive form of AN/AD (Marlin et al., 2010; Varga et al., 2006).

A nonsyndromic autosomal dominant form of AN (coded as AUNA1) is associated with the *DIAPH3* gene (13q21.2; Kim et al., 2004; Schoen et al., 2010). This dominant form of AN was identified in a multigenerational family of European descent with an average age of onset of hearing loss at 18 years.

Evaluation of Individuals With Hereditary Hearing Loss

Audiologists and geneticists are important partners in the evaluation and management of hereditary hearing loss. Thorough knowledge of a patient's family, medical, and other history is critical in accurately characterizing a hearing loss and understanding the etiology. Knowing whether other members of the immediate or extended family have a hearing loss or other medical or physical characteristics in common helps in determining whether a condition might be inherited and in discerning the pattern of inheritance. This information is helpful in guiding geneticists, audiologists, and physicians toward appropriate recommendations for genetic testing and can be invaluable in counseling patients and their families.

Determining whether a hearing loss might be genetic involves obtaining a family history and constructing a pedigree to follow the inheritance of a trait. A family pedigree includes information about the patient, parents, grandparents, siblings, aunts, and uncles, and may extend to many generations and extended family members. Pedigrees utilize standardized symbols and include information about key disorders or conditions, as well as ethnicity information. A graphic record of family health history through a pedigree can provide a clearer picture than a simple case history by establishing the lineage of possible inherited conditions and patterns of transmission of familial disorders. Obtaining a pedigree also provides professionals with an opportunity to establish rapport with a patient and his or her family. Construction of a family pedigree requires care in obtaining personal and family information as some instances might involve discussion of sensitive issues. Examples of family and health information to include in a pedigree are shown in Table 6–2.

Recording physical characteristics of a patient is another important part of the evaluation process. A dysmorphic evaluation includes examination of such factors as facial symmetry, the shape and size of the skull, ocular region, nose and midface, oral region and jaw, and external ears. Further evaluation involves the neck, chest, abdomen, limbs, skin, and hair. Medical follow-up testing can include an electrocardiogram (e.g., to evaluate the QT interval that is affected in Jervell and Lange-Nielsen syndrome), ophthalmological evaluation, imaging, and so on, depending on the results of previous evaluations.

Table 6–2. Family and Health Information to Include in a Pedigree

Gender
Birth date/Age
Age of death
Cause of death
Pregnancy
Pregnancy complications (e.g., miscarriage, stillbirth, pregnancy termination)
Relevant health information
Known medical problems
Ethnic background
Consanguinity
Date pedigree was drawn
Name of person who provided the data

There are some additional factors in a family history that increase suspicion of an inherited trait. These factors can include another family member with a chromosome abnormality or genetic disorder, a family history of a genetic disorder, and couples who have had more than two miscarriages. Individuals of almost every ethnic group have increased risks for particular genetic conditions.

Audiologists have many tools available to them for the evaluation of hearing sensitivity and auditory function at suprathreshold levels. Pure-tone audiograms provide information about the degree, configuration, and symmetry of a hearing loss and comparison of air and bone conduction thresholds, along with middle-ear measures, can help in defining the type of hearing loss as conductive, sensorineural, or mixed. In infants, auditory brainstem response (ABR) and auditory steady-state response (ASSR) methods can provide accurate estimates of threshold information via air and bone conduction.

It is fortunate that audiologists have many more sensitive methods available to characterize hearing loss beyond basic threshold measures. These tools serve two important purposes. First, methods such as OAE and middle-ear muscle reflexes provide valuable diagnostic information that allows accurate differentiation among hearing losses. For example, changes in OAEs have been demonstrated in persons with Waardenburg syndrome before changes in pure-tone thresholds are observed (Liu & Newton, 1997). Also, as we strive to better understand the relationships between genotype and phenotype, the more information that audiologists can obtain about auditory function, then the better geneticists can use this information to understand the role of various genes and functions of the proteins they encode.

Genetics and Newborn Hearing Screening

Molecular genetic testing has an important role in newborn hearing screening and diagnostic follow-up of identified hearing losses. When a hearing loss is identified, the inclusion of molecular genetic testing as part of the evaluation process can contribute to establishing the etiology of the hearing loss and can be informative in planning management. For example, identifying

Jervell and Lange-Nielsen syndrome in infants identified with hearing loss has obvious value in facilitating intervention prior to a potentially tragic outcome.

According to Nance (2007), four tests in the newborn period could detect the major causes of deafness. These include testing for (a) mutations in the connexin 26 (*GJB2*) gene and the connexin 30 (*GJB6*) gene; (b) the mtDNA A1555G mutation that increases susceptibility to aminoglycoside induced deafness; (c) *SLC26A4* mutations that are associated with Pendred syndrome and DFNB4, as well as an increased risk of nonsyndromic EVA in carriers; and (d) cytomegalovirus (CMV). Congenital CMV infection is a nongenetic cause for deafness at birth and in early childhood. Nance suggests that infants at risk could easily be detected by molecular testing of newborn blood spots for these traits.

Establishing the etiology of an identified hearing loss not only provides answers for parents, but also can be helpful in planning management appropriate to the characteristics of a particular genetic form. Furthermore, there are many questions related to hearing loss where genetic testing will likely have a future important role. For example, as knowledge increases related to the genetics of later onset hearing loss, then screening for genes related to these disorders in infants could avoid delays in identification.

Management of Patients and Families: A Team Approach

Partnering with geneticists and genetic counselors provides an important resource to audiologists, families, and all members of the health care team. Genetic and hereditary issues are not simple; questions and issues raised by genetic testing can challenge family and other personal relationships. The genetic counseling process integrates (a) collection and interpretation of family and medical histories to assess the chance of disease occurrence or recurrence; (b) education about inheritance, testing, management, prevention, resources, and research; and (c) counseling to promote informed choices and adaptation to the risk or condition. The website of the National Society of Genetic Counselors provides information that can be used in locating a genetic counselor (http://www.nsgc.org).

Conclusion

The availability of genetics information clearly advances the ability to understand and focus appropriate management on individuals with hearing loss. Although genetic evaluation provides great benefit, there is also potential for harm in revealing information about individuals and families that they may not wish to know. Thus, it is important to understand the ramifications of obtaining and sharing information about an individual's genetic makeup. The need to understand the ethical, legal, and social issues was recognized early on in the development and work of the Human Genome Project. Efforts have focused on deciding how genetic information should be used in relation to the privacy of genetic information, safe and effective introduction of genetic information in the clinical setting, and fairness in the use of genetic information. Additional work is directed toward preparing health professionals and society to use information effectively through professional and public education.

Sources of Information Related to Genetics and Hereditary Hearing Loss

"Genomics and Its Impact on Science and Society: The Human Genome Project and Beyond"

A primer on genetics from the U.S. Department of Energy, created in conjunction with the Human Genome Project, briefly covers basic genetics principles, an overview of the Human Genome Project, some facts about the human genome, medicine and the new genetics, and other benefits of genetic research.

http://web.ornl.gov/sci/techresources/Human_Genome/publicat/primer2001/index.shtml)

Online Mendelian Inheritance in Man (OMIM)

OMIM is a comprehensive, authoritative compendium of human genes and genetic phenotypes that is freely available and updated daily. Information is provided on clinical presentation, phenotypic characteristics, identified causative genes, and relevant references. OMIM is authored and edited at the McKusick-Nathans Institute of Genetic Medicine, Johns Hopkins University School of Medicine, under the direction of Dr. Ada Hamosh. Its official home is http://omim.org

http://www.ncbi.nlm.nih.gov/omim

Hereditary Hearing Loss Homepage

The Hereditary Hearing Loss Homepage aims to give an up-to-date overview of the genetics of hereditary hearing impairment for researchers and clinicians working in the field. The site lists data and links for all known gene localizations and identifications for monogenetic nonsyndromic hearing impairment. The most frequent monogenetic forms of syndromic hearing impairment are covered. The Hereditary Hearing Loss Homepage is maintained by Dr. Guy Van Camp, University of Antwerp, and Dr. Richard Smith, University of Iowa.

http://hereditaryhearingloss.org

Connexin-Deafness Homepage

This website maintains information specifically related to connexin and deafness, a mutations database, and references. Editors include Dr. Xavier Estivill and Dr. Paolo Gasparini.

http://davinci.crg.es/deafness/

"Understanding the Genetics of Deafness: A Guide for Patients and Families"

This is an information booklet for parents and patients from the Harvard Medical School Center for Hereditary Deafness.

http://hearing.harvard.edu/info/GeneticDeafnessBookletV2.pdf

A Parent's Guide to Genetics and Hearing Loss

This is an information booklet from the Centers for Disease Control and Prevention that addresses many of the questions that families have about the causes of hearing loss, including genetic causes.

http://www.cdc.gov/ncbddd/hearingloss/freematerials/parentsguide508.pdf

Gene Reviews

GeneReviews are expert-authored, peer-reviewed disease descriptions presented in a standardized format and focused on clinically relevant and medically actionable information on the diagnosis, management, and genetic counseling of patients and families with specific inherited conditions.

http://www.ncbi.nlm.nih.gov/books/NBK1116/

GeneTests

GeneTests is a medical genetics information resource developed for physicians, genetic counselors, and other healthcare providers and researchers. Two main components are a directory of over 600 international laboratories offering molecular genetic testing, biochemical genetic testing, and cytogenetic testing for more than 3,000 inherited disorders, and a directory of over 1,000 international genetics clinics providing diagnosis and genetic counseling services to patients and their families with known or suspected inherited disorders.

https://www.genetests.org

References

Abdelhak, S., Kalatzis, V., Heilig, R., Compain, S., Samson, D., Vincent, C., . . . Petit, C. (1997). A human homologue of the Drosophila eyes absent gene underlies branchio-oto-renal (BOR) syndrome and identifies a novel gene family. *Nature Genetics, 15,* 157–164.

Acke, F. R., Dhooge, I. J., Malfait, F., & De Leenheer, E. M. (2012). Hearing impairment in Stickler syndrome: A systematic review. *Orphanet Journal of Rare Disease, 7,* 84–93.

Azaiez, H., Van Camp, G., & Smith, R. J. H. (2006). Connexins and deafness: From molecules to disease. *Seminars in Hearing, 27,* 148–159.

Barker, D. F., Hostikka, S. L., Zhou, J., Chow, L. T., Oliphant, A. R., Gerken, S. C., . . . Tryggbason, K. (1990). Identification of mutations in the COL4A5 collagen gene in Alport Syndrome. *Science, 248,* 1224–1227.

Berlin, C. I., Bordelon, J., St. John, P., Wilensky, D., Hurley, A., Kluka, E., & Hood, L. J. (1998). Reversing click polarity may uncover auditory neuropathy in infants. *Ear and Hearing, 19,* 37–47.

Berlin, C. I., Hood, L. J., Morlet, T., Wilensky, D., Li, L., Rose-Mattingly, K., . . . Frisch, S. A. (2010). Multi-site diagnosis and management of 260 patients with auditory neuropathy/dys-synchrony (Auditory Neuropathy Spectrum Disorder). *International Journal of Audiology, 49,* 30–43.

Berlin, C. I., Hood, L. J., Morlet, T., Wilensky, D., St. John, P., Montgomery, E., & Thibodeaux, M. (2005). Absent or elevated middle ear muscle reflexes in the presence of normal otoacoustic emissions: A universal finding in 136 cases of auditory neuropathy/dys-synchrony. *Journal of the American Academy of Audiology. 16,* 546–553.

Berlin, C., Hood, L., & Rose, K. (2001). On renaming auditory neuropathy as auditory dys-synchrony: Implications for a clearer understanding of the underlying mechanisms and management options. *Audiology Today, 13,* 15–17.

Cohn, E. S., Kelley, P. M., Fowler, T. W., Gorga, M. P., Lefkowitz, D. M., Kuehn, H. J., . . . Kimberling, W. J. (1999). Clinical studies of families with hearing loss attributable to mutations in the connexin 26 gene (GJB2/DFNB1). *Pediatrics, 103,* 546–550.

Dauwerse, J. G., Dixon, J., Seland, S., Ruivenkamp, C. A. L., van Haeringen, A., Hoefsloot, L. H., . . . Wieczorek, D. (2011). Mutations in genes encoding subunits of RNA polymerases I and III cause Treacher Collins syndrome. *Nature Genetics, 43,* 20–22.

Deltenre, P., Mansbach, A. L., Bozet, C., Clercx, A., & Hecox, K. E. (1997). Auditory neuropathy: A report on three cases with early onsets and major neonatal illnesses. *Electroencephalography and Clinical Neurophysiology, 104,* 17–22.

Ebermann, I., Phillips, J., Liebau, M., Koenekoop, R., Schermer, B., Lopez, I., . . . Bolz, H. (2010). PDZD7 is a modifier of retinal disease and a contributor to digenic Usher syndrome. *Journal of Clinical Investigation, 120,* 1812–1823.

Everett, L., Glaser, B., Beck, J., Idol, J., Buchs, A., Heyman, M., . . . Green, E. (1997). Pendred syndrome is caused by mutations in a putative sulphate transporter gene (PDS). *Nature Genetics, 17,* 411–422.

Fallerini, C., Dosa, L., Tita, R., Del Prete, D., Feriozzi, S., Gai, G., . . . Ariani, F. (2014). Unbiased next generation sequencing analysis confirms the existence of autosomal dominant Alport syndrome in a relevant fraction of cases. *Clinical Genetics, 86,* 252–257.

Gorlin, R. J., Toriello, H. V., & Cohen, M. M. Jr. (1995). *Hereditary hearing loss and its syndromes.* Oxford, UK: Oxford University Press.

Gunn, T., Bortolussi, R., Little, J. M., Andermann, F., Fraser, F. C., & Belmonte, M. M. (1976). Juvenile diabetes mellitus, optic atrophy, sensory nerve deafness, and diabetes insipidus—A syndrome. *Journal of Pediatrics, 89,* 565–570.

Hood, L. J., Berlin, C. I., Bordelon, J., & Rose, K. (2003). Patients with auditory neuropathy/dys-synchrony lack efferent suppression of transient evoked otoacoustic emissions. *Journal of the American Academy of Audiology, 14,* 302–313.

Kalaydjieva, L., Gresham, D., Gooding, R., Heather, L., Baas, F., de Jonge, R., . . . Thomas, P. K. (2000). N-myc downstream-regulated gene 1 is mutated in hereditary motor and sensory neuropathy-Lom. *American Journal of Human Genetics, 67,* 47–58.

Keats, B. J. B., Nouri, N., Pelias, M. Z., Deininger, P. L., & Litt, M. (1994). Tightly linked flanking microsatellite markers for the Usher syndrome type I locus on the short arm of chromosome 11. *American Journal of Human Genetics, 54,* 681–686.

Kelsell, D. P., Dunlop, J., Stevens, H. P., Lench, N. J., Liang, J. N., Parry, G., . . . Leigh, I. M. (1997). Connexin 26 mutations in hereditary nonsyndromic sensorineural deafness. *Nature, 387,* 80–83.

Kim, T. B., Isaacson, B., Sivakumaran, T. A., Starr, A., Keats, B. J. B., & Lesperance, M. M. (2004). A gene responsible for autosomal dominant auditory neuropathy (AUNA1) maps to 13q14-21. *Journal of Medical Genetics, 41,* 872–876.

Kochhar, A., Fischer, S. M., Kimberling, W. J., & Smith, R. J. H. (2007). Branchio-oto-renal syndrome. *American Journal of Medical Genetics Part A, 143A,* 1671–1678.

Konigsmark, B. W., & Gorlin, R. J. (1976). *Genetic and metabolic deafness.* Philadelphia, PA: W.B. Saunders.

Liu, X. Z., & Newton, V. E. (1997). Distortion product emissions in normal-hearing and low-frequency hearing loss carriers of genes for Waardenburg's syndrome. *Annals of Otology Rhinology, and Laryngology, 106,* 220–225.

Marlin, S., Feldman, D., Nguyen, Y., Rouillon, I., Loundon, N., Jonard, L., . . . Denoyelle, F. (2010). Temperature-sensitive auditory neuropathy associated with an otoferlin mutation: Deafening fever! *Biochemical and Biophysical Research Communications, 394,* 737–742.

Mburu, P., Mustapha, M., Varela, A., Weil, D., El-Amraoui, A., Holme, R. H., . . . Brown, S. D. (2003). Defects in whirlin, a PDZ domain molecule involved in stereocilia elongation, cause deafness in the whirler mouse and families with DFNB31. *Nature Genetics, 34,* 421–428.

Mochizuki, T., Lemmink, H. H., Mariyama, M., Antignac, C., Gubler, M. C., Pirson, Y., . . . Reeders, S. T. (1994). Identification of mutations in the alpha 3(IV) and alpha 4(IV) collagen genes in autosomal recessive Alport syndrome. *Nature Genetics, 8,* 77–82.

Nance, W. (2007). How can newborn hearing screening be improved? *Audiology Today, 19,* 14–19.

Neyroud, N., Tesson, F., Denjoy, I., Leibovici, M., Donger, C., Barhanin, J., . . . Guicheney, P. (1997). A novel mutation in the potassium channel gene *KVLQT1* causes the Jervell and Lange-Nielsen cardioauditory syndrome. *Nature Genetics, 15,* 186–189.

Prezant, T. R., Agapian, J. V., Bohlman, M. C., Bu, X., Oztas, S., Qiu, W. Q., . . . Fischel-Ghodsian, N. (1993). Mitochondrial ribosomal RNA mutation associated with both antibiotic-induced and non-syndromic deafness. *Nature Genetics, 4,* 289–294.

Reardon, W., Omahoney, C. F., Trembath, R., Jan, H., & Phelps, P. D. (2000). Enlarged vestibular aqueduct: A radiological marker of Pendred syndrome, and mutation of the PDS gene. *Quarterly Journal of Medicine, 93,* 99–104.

Sanlaville, D., Etchevers, H. C., Gonzales, M., Martinovic, J., Clement-Ziza, M., Delezoide, A. L., . . . Attie-Bitach, T. (2006). Phenotypic spectrum of CHARGE syndrome in fetuses with CHD7 truncating mutations correlates with expression during human development. *Journal of Medical Genetics, 43,* 211–217.

Schoen, C. J., Emery, S. B., Thorne, M. C., Ammana, H. R., Sliwerska, E., Arnett, J., . . . Lesperance, M. M. (2010). Increased activity of diaphanous homolog 3 (DIAPH3)/diaphanous causes hearing defects in human with auditory neuropathy and in Drosophila. *Proceedings of the National Academy of Sciences USA, 107,* 13396–13401.

Schwartz, P. J., Spazzolini, C., Crotti, L., Bathen, J., Amlie, J. P., Timothy, K., . . . Denjoy, I. (2006). The Jervell and Lange-

Nielsen syndrome: Natural history, molecular basis, and clinical outcome. *Circulation, 113*, 783–790.

Snoeckx, R. L., Huygen, P. L. M., Feldmann, D., Marlin, S., Denoyelle, F., Waligora, J., . . . Van Camp, G. (2005). *GJB2* mutations and degree of hearing loss: A multicenter study. *American Journal of Human Genetics, 77*, 945–957.

Splawski, I., Timothy, K. W., Vincent, G. M., Atkinson, D. L., & Keating, M. T. (1997). Molecular basis of the long-QT syndrome associated with deafness. *New England Journal of Medicine, 336*, 1562–1567.

Starr, A., Michalewski, H. J., Zeng, F.-G., Fujikawa-Brooks, S., Linthicum, F., Kim. C. S., . . . Keats, B. J. B. (2003). Pathology and physiology of auditory neuropathy with a novel mutation in the *MPZ* gene (Tyr145Ser). *Brain, 126*, 1604–1619.

Starr, A., Picton, T. W., Sininger, Y., Hood, L. J., & Berlin, C. I. (1996). Auditory neuropathy. *Brain, 119*, 741–753.

Toriello, H. V., Reardon, W., & Gorlin, R. J. (2004). *Hereditary hearing loss and its syndromes* (2nd ed.). Oxford, UK: Oxford University Press.

Varga, R., Avenarius, M. R., Kelley, P. M., Keats, B. J., Berlin, C. I., Hood, L. J., . . . Kimberling, W. J. (2006). OTOF mutations revealed by genetic analysis of hearing loss families including a potential temperature sensitive auditory neuropathy allele. *Journal of Medical Genetics, 43*, 576–581.

Varga, R., Kelley, P. M., Keats, B. J., Starr, A., Leal, S. M., Cohn, E., & Kimberling, W. J. (2003). Non-syndromic recessive auditory neuropathy is the result of mutations in the otoferlin (OTOF) gene. *Journal of Medical Genetics, 40*, 45–50.

Yang, T., Vidarsson, H., Rodrigo-Blomqvist, S., Rosengren, S., Enerback, S., & Smith, R. J. H. (2007). Transcriptional control of SLC26A4 is involved in Pendred syndrome and non-syndromic enlargement of vestibular aqueduct (DFNB4). *American Journal of Human Genetics, 80*, 1055–1063.

Zeng, F.-G., Oba, S., Garde, S., Sininger, Y., & Starr, A. (1999). Temporal and speech processing deficits in auditory neuropathy. *Neuroreport, 10*, 3429-3435.

Zentner, G. E., Layman, W. S., Martin, D. M., & Scacheri, P. C. (2010). Molecular and phenotypic aspects of CHD7 mutation in CHARGE syndrome. *American Journal of Medical Genetics Part A, 152A*, 674–686.

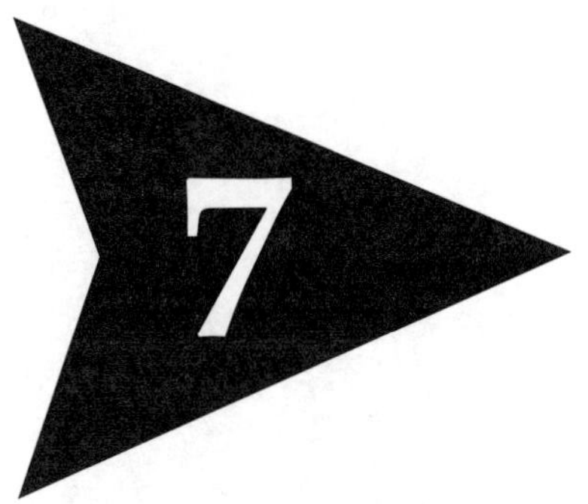

Medical Considerations for Infants and Young Children With Hearing Loss: A Pediatrician's Perspective

Betty R. Vohr

What Is the Medical Home?

The infant's pediatrician or primary health care provider is responsible for monitoring the general health, development, and well-being of the infant beginning in the newborn nursery. In 1999, the American Academy of Pediatrics (AAP) proposed the concept of a medical home for all children with special health care needs (2002). The medical home provides health care that is accessible, family centered, continuous, comprehensive, coordinated, compassionate, and culturally competent (AAP, 2002, 2010). The following sections describe the components of care required for infants and young children with permanent hearing loss, and the proposed role of the primary care provider and the medical home in coordinating and facilitating optimal care.

To maximize the outcome for infants with all degrees of congenital hearing loss, the hearing of all infants should be screened no later than 1 month of age. Every infant who does not pass the newborn screen should have a comprehensive audiologic diagnostic evaluation no later than 3 months of age, and infants with confirmed hearing loss should receive appropriate early intervention service by 6 months of age (AAP, 2007a). Figure 7–1 shows the algorithm developed to guide the pediatrician or primary health care provider in the management of infants relative to hearing screening, diagnosis, and intervention. The primary care physician's proposed role in this process is reviewed (AAP, 2010).

The Medical Home and Newborn Hearing Screening

The Joint Committee on Infant Hearing (JCIH) recommends as a benchmark that 4% or less of infants fail the newborn hearing screen (AAP, 2007a). The rate is usually higher for the neonatal intensive care unit (NICU) than for the well-baby nursery because of the risk factors for hearing loss associated with NICU care. Therefore, based on this benchmark, 40 of every 1,000 infants screened may fail the newborn screen. As the rate of congenital hearing loss is 2 per 1,000, there are approximately 38 infants with a false-positive screen. A false screen could be secondary to transient fluid in the middle ear, debris in the ear canal, upper airway congestion, excessive infant noise, background noise, or electrical noise. Because the cause of a fail is uncertain and might represent a true fail, it is important that the family return with the infant for the follow-up rescreen or diagnostic evaluation. Many states in the United States are currently achieving a 2% fail rate, which significantly reduces the false-positive rate.

It is currently recommended that families receive the results of the screen at the time of discharge from the birthing hospital and that physicians have access to the information, so that they can encourage the family to return for follow-up. Physicians must therefore be aware of the causes of a hearing screen fail and the types of permanent congenital hearing loss including sensorineural, permanent conductive, and neural/auditory neuropathy.

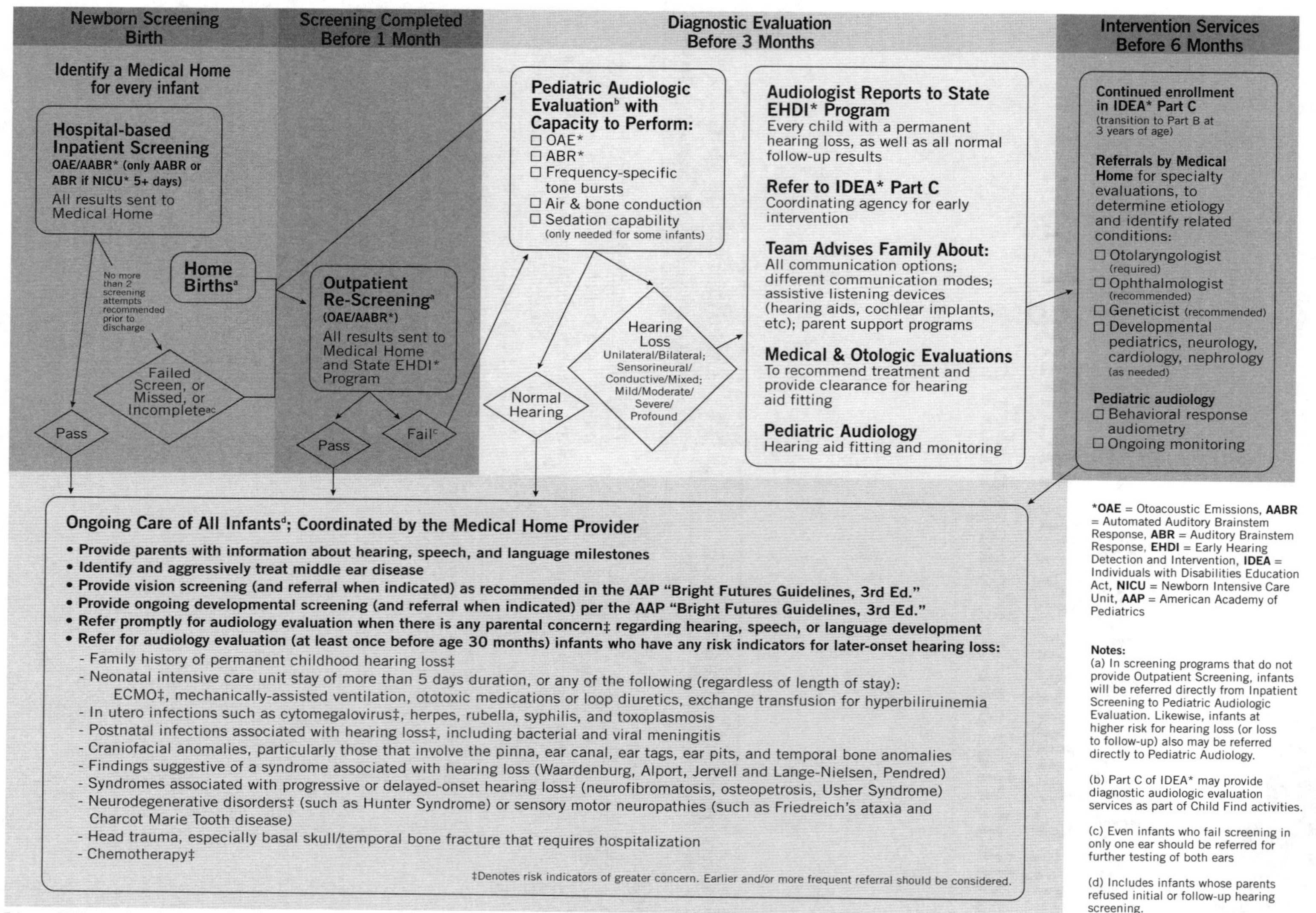

Figure 7–1. Universal newborn hearing screening, diagnosis, and intervention: guidelines for pediatric medical home providers (2010). Reprinted with permission from the American Academy of Pediatrics.

The Medical Home and Risk Factors for Neonatal and Late-Onset Hearing Loss

It is recommended that a history of risk factors be obtained or reviewed with the family at several time points: prior to delivery, during hospitalization, at discharge, and after discharge. The pediatrician or primary health care provider might meet with the family prior to delivery to obtain a detailed family history of risk factors that includes neonatal or late-onset hearing loss, syndromes, or disorders associated with hearing loss. If this is not possible, a meeting with the parents should take place prior to hospital discharge. The pediatrician or primary health care physician needs to review every infant's medical record or discharge summary for the medical history and the presence of risk factors. Some risk factors are associated with hearing loss at birth, and some require monitoring for delayed-onset or progressive hearing loss prior to discharge from the birthing hospital. The JCIH published an updated list of risk factors for hearing loss in 2007 that we will now review (AAP, 2007a).

Risk Factor 1

The first two recommendations depend on communication with the family. A family history of permanent childhood onset hearing loss, genetic disorders, or syndromes associated with hearing loss (Cone-Wesson et al., 2000; Morton & Nance, 2006) are important predictors of both neonatal and late-onset hearing loss. Studies have shown that at least 50% of congenital hearing loss is hereditary (Brookhouser, Worthington, & Kelly, 1994; Nance, 2003). It is recommended that a genetic consultation be offered to all families with a strong history of hearing loss or a newly identified infant with hearing loss. If appropriate, the evaluation should include genetic testing for nonsyndromic gene mutations such as *GJB2* (connexin-26) and syndromes commonly associated with early onset childhood sensorineural hearing loss (Denoyelle et al., 1999; Nance, 2003; Nance & Kearsey, 2004; Santos et al., 2005).

Risk Factor 2

Caregiver concern regarding hearing, speech, language, or developmental delay in the first 2 to 3 years of life is associated with an increased risk of late-onset hearing loss (Roizen, 1999). This is important, and professionals should not be complacent because of a passed newborn screen. The rate of permanent hearing loss in newborns is 2 to 3 per 1,000, and this rate increases up to 7 per 1,000 at school age (Bess, Dodd-Murphy, & Parker, 1998; Johnson et al., 2005). In a recent report, the prevalence of some degree of hearing loss by school age was 3.65/1,000 compared to a neonatal yield of 1.79/1,000 (Watkin & Baldwin, 2012).

Risk Factor 3

Recommendation 3 concerns infants admitted to the NICU. A new risk factor discussed in JCIH 2007 (AAP, 2007a) is for infants requiring neonatal intensive care or special care for greater than 5 days. This recommendation was added based on reports from the National Perinatal Research Center (NPIC) Quality Analytic Services. NPIC data indicated that approximately 25% of NICU and Level 2 infants (i.e., those who are premature or ill) have low-risk diagnoses, such as transient respiratory distress, temperature instability, or negative sepsis workup and are discharged by 5 days of age. As specific risk factors are often difficult for paraprofessional screeners to identify in the medical record, establishing a more general time criterion (>5 days in the NICU) was felt to be easier for universal implementation (AAP, 2007a). The initial wording of Risk Factor 3 resulted in some confusion, and it was subsequently reworded and a clarification was added to the JCIH website (http://jcih.org/posstatemts.htm) as follows:

> All infants with or without risk factors requiring neonatal intensive care for greater than 5 days, including any of the following: extracorporeal membrane oxygenation (ECMO), assisted ventilation, exposure to ototoxic medications (gentamycin and tobramycin) or loop diuretics (furosemide/lasix) are considered at increased risk of hearing loss. In addition, regardless of length of stay: hyperbilirubinemia requiring exchange transfusion.

Risk Factor 4

Risk Factor 4 is *in utero* infections, such as cytomegalovirus (CMV), herpes, rubella, syphilis, and toxoplasmosis (Fligor et al., 2005; Madden et al., 2005; Nance, Lim, & Dodson, 2006; Rivera et al., 2002). Screening for these infections is not routine and is implemented if there is maternal history or the infant presents with signs or symptoms suggestive of disease. Workup is indicated for infants with a history or clinical signs of intrauterine infection. CMV remains the most common infectious cause of early or delayed onset hearing loss (Fowler et al., 1997). Studies indicate that CMV polymerase chain reaction (PCR) of liquid or dried saliva yield 97% sensitivity and 99. 9% specificity, respectively, when compared to culture (Boppana et al., 2010; Ross et al., 2014). The finding of CMV in saliva does not confirm the presence and timing of active infection in infants as the virus has recently been recovered from the breast milk of seropositive mothers in the early weeks following birth (Josephson et al., 2014). Urine culture or PCR can be used to confirm infection in these children (Nozawa et al., 2007). Treatment of CMV-infected newborns with 6 weeks of parenteral ganciclovir therapy (6 mg/kg/dose, administered intravenously every 12 hours) was shown to protect against hearing deterioration and decreased the risk of developmental delays. Unfortunately, two systematic reviews of ganciclovir use identified significant toxicities and limited evidence for consistent benefit (Hamilton et al., 2014; Smets et al., 2006). Treatment of a small cohort of 23 symptomatic infants with intravenous ganciclovir for 6 weeks followed by oral ganciclovir for 12 months resulted in better auditory outcomes for infants with the extended treatment (Amir, Wolf, & Levy, 2010). A randomized trial that compared 6 months of therapy with valganciclovir with 6 weeks of therapy in neonates with symptomatic CMV disease reported that treatment for 6 months appeared to improve hearing and developmental outcomes modestly in the long term but not in the short term (Kimberlin et al., 2015). Side effects of episodes of Grade 3–4 neutropenia occurred in 21% of the 6-month group and 27% in the 6-week group. Discussion of risks and benefits of treatment with family and an infectious disease consult are indicated.

In addition, efforts at prevention of CMV have been attempted. A review of 24 studies reported that prevention of maternal infection using hygiene and behavioral interventions reduced maternal seroconversion rates during pregnancy, and treatment of maternal CMV infection with hyperimmune globulin (HIG) showed some evidence for efficacy in prevention of fetal infection and fetal/neonatal morbidity (Hamilton et al., 2014). However, more robust clinical evidence is required before HIG therapy can be routinely recommended. In addition, there is a need for a CMV vaccine.

Risk Factors 5 to 8

Risk Factors 5 to 8 are all associated with congenital abnormalities or syndromes. Risk Factor 5 is defined as craniofacial anomalies, including those involving the pinna, ear canal, ear tags, ear pits, and temporal bone anomalies (Cone-Wesson et al., 2000). These defects are common in both the well-baby nursery and the NICU. Risk Factor 6 includes physical findings, such as a white forelock, which are associated with a syndrome known to include sensorineural or permanent conductive hearing loss. Risk factor 6 also includes atresias (Cone-Wesson et al., 2000). Risk Factor 7 includes syndromes associated with hearing loss or progressive- or late-onset hearing loss, such as neurofibromatosis, osteopetrosis, and Usher's syndrome (Roizen, 2003). Other frequently identified syndromes include Waardenburg, Alport, Pendred, and Jervell and Lange-Nielson (Nance, 2003; Roizen, 2003). Risk Factor 8 consists of neurodegenerative disorders, such as Hunter syndrome, or sensory motor neuropathies such as Friedreich's ataxia and Charcot-Marie-Tooth disease (Roizen, 2003). Consultations with otolaryngology and genetics are indicated if a syndrome associated with hearing loss is suspected. In addition, the hearing of these children needs to be monitored longitudinally by a pediatric audiologist.

Risk Factor 9

Culture-positive postnatal infections associated with sensorineural hearing loss including confirmed bacterial and viral (especially herpes viruses and varicella) meningitis are important risk factors for hearing loss. Consultation with otolaryngology and audiology is indicated (Arditi et al., 1998; Biernath et al., 2006; Roizen, 2003).

Risk Factors 10 and 11

Risk Factors 10 and 11 are essentially postdischarge risk factors. Serious head trauma, especially basal skull or temporal bone fractures requiring hospitalization, is a risk factor for hearing loss in childhood (Lew et al., 2004; Vartialnen, Karjalainen, & Karja, 1985; Zimmerman, Ganzel, Windmill, Nazar, & Phillips, 1993). Although rare in the pediatric population, chemotherapy for children with leukemia or cancer remains a risk factor (Bertolini et al., 2004).

The Medical Home and Continued Surveillance

Children with a documented risk factor for hearing loss require close surveillance of hearing skills and language development and follow-up with audiology. For children with risk factors, the timing of hearing reevaluations by an audiologist should be individualized depending on the likelihood of a subsequent delayed-onset hearing loss. JCIH (AAP, 2007a) currently recommends that infants who pass the neonatal screening but have a risk factor should have at least one diagnostic audiology assessment by 24 to 30 months of age. Early and more frequent assessment may be indicated for CMV infection, syndromes associated with progressive hearing loss, neurodegenerative disorders, trauma, or culture-positive postnatal infections associated with sensorineural hearing loss. Also children who have received ECMO or chemotherapy and children for whom there is caregiver concern or a family history of hearing loss should have more immediate and more frequent assessments as clinically indicated (Fligor et al., 2005; Fowler et al., 1992; Madden et al., 2005; Rivera et al., 2002).

Medical Home: The Medical Workup and Care Coordination

The primary care physician assumes responsibility for coordinating comprehensive health care and working as a team member with the family, all key professionals, and others identified by the family as members of the team (AAP, 2007b). These efforts are initiated to ensure that no child is lost to follow-up, that all assessments occur in a timely fashion, and that all appropriate and individualized services are provided (Figure 7–2).

Aside from the partnership of the family with the primary provider, other team members include the hospital hearing screening staff, audiologist, otolaryngologist, geneticist, speech-language pathologist, and specialized early intervention providers. Additional team members might include an ophthalmologist, developmental pediatrician, deaf services, the deaf community, interpreter services, parent support groups, and third-party payers. There is a sequence of events that occurs and not all members of the team may be active at any one time. Participation depends on the needs and wishes of the family.

Management of the Child Who Fails the Screen

The first step is for the hospital screening staff to share the results of the screen with the primary physician and family. The physician proceeds to discuss the results with the family either before discharge from the birthing hospital or at the time of the first office visit, and to encourage the family to return for a rescreen or diagnostic evaluation. The physician then checks with the family at each subsequent office visit to determine if the rescreen has been completed, to facilitate the visit if it has not occurred, and to discuss the results with the family once the rescreen is completed.

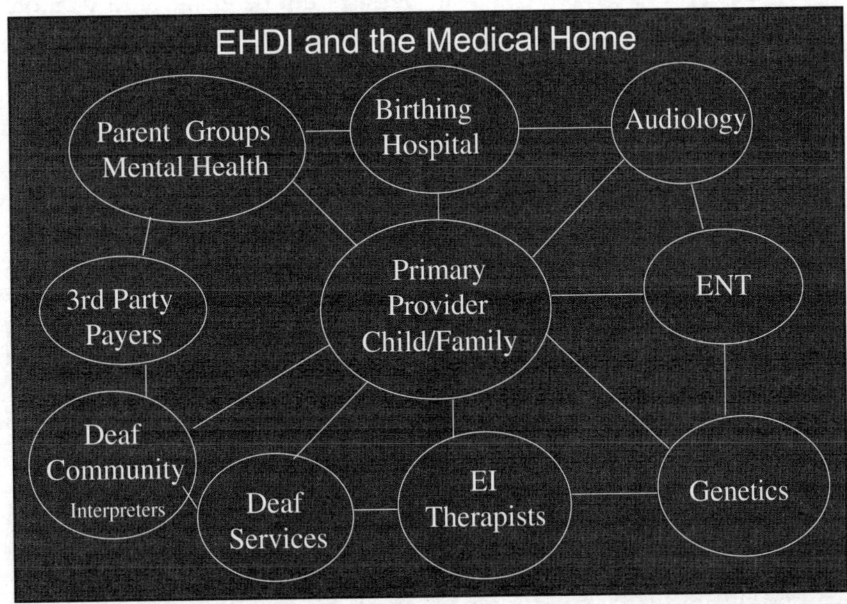

Figure 7–2. Potential members of the medical home team for the child and family. (ENT, ear, nose, and throat physician; EI, early interventionist.)

Management of the Child Who Passes the Screen or Rescreen

For the child who passes the screen or rescreen, the physician discusses the results with the family, shares that the screen pass does not mean that a subsequent hearing loss might not be identified, and informs the family that the child's hearing skills and development will be monitored. If the child has a risk factor for hearing loss, the primary care physician informs the family that a diagnostic audiologic evaluation will be completed at least once by 24 to 30 months of age. The referral for audiologic evaluation should be immediate if concerns arise regarding hearing skills or development.

In addition, the primary care physician is responsible for ongoing surveillance of parent concerns about language and hearing, auditory skills, and developmental milestones of all infants and children regardless of risk status, as outlined in the pediatric periodicity schedule published by the AAP (2000). This management approach permits the detection of children with either missed neonatal hearing loss or delayed-onset hearing loss and minimizes the risk of delayed diagnosis and intervention.

Management of the Child Who Fails the Rescreen and Is Referred for an Audiologic Diagnostic Evaluation

The physician ensures that the family takes the child for a diagnostic audiologic assessment to a center that has audiologists skilled in pediatric assessments as soon as possible. It is anticipated that the audiologist will call the pediatrician, discuss the findings, and send the test results for the child who does not pass. A complete report of the diagnostic assessment is sent to the primary care physician for all children evaluated whether they pass or fail. The pediatrician will then have a better understanding of the type and severity of hearing loss in order to support the recommendations of the audiologist and initiate the medical workup.

Management of the Child With a Failed Audiology Diagnostic Test

The pediatrician should schedule a meeting with the family as soon as possible to discuss the diagnosis, provide information, describe the next steps to be taken, and to be supportive of the family during a period of time in which they might experience significant stress. The benefits of active family participation in early intervention services and early amplification should be emphasized with the family (Yoshinaga-Itano, 2014). Communities might have a spectrum of pediatric diagnostic services and specialized early intervention programs. Families should be informed of programs appropriate for their infant. Many early hearing detection and intervention (EHDI) programs have developed guidebooks that are given to the family at the time of diagnosis that describe the available services. The primary care physician should also be aware of community resources and support the family choice of early intervention program and mode of communication.

Some components of the coordination can be implemented by different team members (see Figure 7–2). It is therefore important for the team members to communicate all interactions with the family and any actions taken with other team members. It is recommended that the audiologist facilitate a referral within 48 hours to the indicated specialized early intervention services chosen by the family. During the postdiagnosis appointment with the family, the physician reviews the family history again and reexamines the child for evidence of any craniofacial abnormalities or syndromes associated with hearing loss. It is important to emphasize to the family that their baby is still the same lovely baby, that the hearing loss was identified early, and that their baby will benefit from early intervention services and amplification (Yoshinaga-Itano, 2014).

The primary care physician must partner with the otolaryngologist. Every infant with confirmed hearing loss should be evaluated by an otolaryngologist with knowledge of pediatric hearing loss. Otolaryngologists who are skilled in childhood hearing loss will conduct a workup to determine the etiology of hearing loss and identify related risk indicators for hearing loss, including syndromes involving the head and neck. The otolaryngologist conducts a comprehensive assessment and provides recommendations and information to the family, audiologist, and primary health care provider on candidacy for amplification, assistive devices and surgical intervention, including reconstruction, bone-anchored hearing aids, and cochlear implantation.

Additional referrals can be made at that time for a developmental assessment, a genetics consultation, or other indicated specialist. The primary health care physician partners with other specialists to facilitate coordinated care for the infant and family. Because 30% to 40% of children with confirmed hearing loss will demonstrate developmental delays, comorbidities, or other disabilities, the primary care physician should closely monitor developmental milestones and initiate referrals related to suspected disabilities (AAP, 2006; Karchmer & Allen, 1999). The medical home algorithm for management of infants with either suspected or proven permanent hearing loss is seen in Figure 7–1 (AAP, 2010). Many families desire contact with another parent of a young child with a similar degree of hearing loss. Organizations such as Hands and Voices (http://www.handsandvoices.org) are excellent in facilitating a family meeting. Middle ear status should be monitored because the presence of middle ear effusion can further compromise hearing.

The Academy of Pediatrics has realized the importance of just-in-time responses of physicians to a new diagnosis. In addition to assuming responsibility to ensure that the audiologic assessment is conducted on infants who do not pass screening, the physician must initiate referrals for medical specialty evaluations necessary to determine the etiology of the hearing loss. Because of the association of hearing loss with other disabilities, including vision impairments, and the importance of vision for children with hearing loss, it is recommended that each child with a permanent hearing loss have at least one examination to assess visual acuity by an ophthalmologist experienced in evaluating infants.

It is estimated that at least 50% of congenital hearing loss is hereditary, and nearly 400 syndromes and 125 genes associated with hearing loss have already been identified (Huang, Zdanski, & Castillo, 2012; Mehra, Eavey, & Keamy, 2009; Nance, 2003). The geneticist will review the family history for specific genetic disorders or syndromes, examine the child, and complete genetic testing for syndromes or gene mutations for nondysmorphic hearing such as *GJB2* (connexin-26; Santos et al., 2005). Because of the prevalence of hereditary hearing loss, all families of children with confirmed hearing loss should be offered a genetics evaluation and counseling. This evaluation can provide families with information on etiology, prognosis, associated disorders, and the likelihood of hearing loss in future offspring.

The Medical Home and Surveillance

New recommendations for ongoing surveillance in the medical home for all infants with and without risk factors for hearing loss were published in JCIH (2007). Regular surveillance of developmental milestones, auditory skills, parental concerns, and middle ear status should be performed in the medical home, consistent with the AAP pediatric periodicity schedule (AAP, 2006; Geoffrey et al., 2014). In addition, all infants should have an objective standardized screening of global development with a validated assessment tool at 9, 18, and 24 to 30 months of age or at any time if the health care professional or family has concern (AAP, 2007a). Infants who do not pass the speech-language portion of a medical home global screening or for whom there is a concern regarding hearing or language should be referred for speech-language evaluation and audiology assessment.

The Medical Home and Middle Ear Disease

Middle Ear Effusion (OME)

The Agency for Healthcare Research and Quality clinical practice guidelines on otitis media with effusion (OME) were updated in 2004 to include all children 2 months to 12 years of age, including children with craniofacial abnormalities, neurologic abnormalities, and sensory deficits (AAP, 2004). The recommendations are based on the review of evidence and the collaborative efforts of the AAP, the American Academy of Family Medicine, and the American Academy of Otolaryngology, Head and Neck Surgery. OME is highly prevalent among young children, and approximately 90% of children have an episode of OME before starting school (Tos, 1984). OME is defined as the presence of middle ear fluid without signs or symptoms of acute ear infection. Recommendations related to diagnosis include (a) pneumatic otoscopy as the primary method to diagnose OME, and (b) physicians' documentation of laterality, duration of effusion, and severity of symptoms. Although 40% to 50% of children are asymptomatic (AAP, 2004; Lieberthal et al., 2013; Rosenfeld & Kay, 2003), children can have associated hearing loss, balance problems (Golz, Angel-Yeger, & Parush, 1998), or delayed speech or language. Children identified by the primary provider with persistent OME should be referred for consultation to an otolaryngologist. Children who become candidates for surgical intervention with tympanostomy include those with OME of greater than 3 to 4 months' duration with associated persistent hearing loss, recurrent or persistent OME in children at risk, and OME with associated structural injury to the tympanic membrane or middle ear. Tympanostomy is beneficial and has been shown to be associated with decreases in middle ear effusion and improved hearing (Rosenfeld et al., 2013).

Clinical practice guidelines for tympanostomy tubes in children were reported in 2013 (Rosenfeld et al., 2013). The group provided the following options: (a) clinicians may perform tympanostomy tube insertion in children with unilateral or bilateral OME for 3 months or longer (chronic OME) and symptoms that are likely attributable to OME including, but not limited to, vestibular problems, poor school performance, behavioral problems, ear discomfort, or reduced quality of life; and (b) clinicians may perform tympanostomy tube insertion in at-risk children with unilateral or bilateral OME that is unlikely to resolve quickly as reflected by a Type B (flat) tympanogram or persistence of effusion for 3 months or longer (chronic OME).

An important recommendation concerns children with OME who are at risk of speech, language, or learning problems, and includes children with permanent hearing loss (Table 7–1). Medical management of children in these categories of risk may be expanded as needed to include hearing testing, speech and language evaluations, amplification or amplification adjustment, and tympanostomy tubes.

The management approach for children without risk factors, in contrast, is based on the fact that most OME is self-limited (Lieberthal et al., 2013; Rosenfeld & Kay, 2003), and 75% to 90% spontaneously resolve in 3 months. Therefore, a 3-month period of observation is recommended. Evidence again suggests that no benefit is derived from the use of antihistamines or decongestants (AAP, 2004; Rosenfeld et al., 2013). In addition, no long-term benefits were identified for antimicrobial therapy or oral steroids. Children with persistent OME who are not at developmental risk are reexamined at 3- to 6-month intervals until either the OME resolves or a problem requiring intervention is identified.

Hearing testing is recommended for persistent OME when the child is considered at risk. Initial hearing screening is not appropriate in the primary care setting for children less than 4 years of age and should be completed at the birthing center. Hearing screenings with earphones can be performed in a primary setting if equipment and space are available for the child 4 years or older. Children under 4 years need to be referred to an audiologist. Children who fail the diagnostic hearing assessment at 20 dB HL or more need to be referred for language testing, and subsequently any child with a language delay needs to be referred for intervention services. Examples of language tests/screens that can be used in the primary care setting include the Early Language Milestone Scale (Coplan, 1993), the MacArthur Communicative Development Inventory (Fenson, 1993), the Language Development Survey (Rescoria, 1989), and Ages and Stages (Bricker & Squires, 1999).

Acute Otitis Media

Recommendations for acute otitis media management for children 2 months to 12 years by the Agency for Health Care Research and Quality are reviewed (AAP, 2004). Acute otitis media continues to be the most common infection diagnosed in children in the United States. The definition of acute otitis media depends on the following characteristics: (a) a history of acute onset of signs and symptoms, (b) the presence of middle ear effusion, and (c) signs and symptoms of inflammation

Table 7–1. Risk Factors for Developmental Difficulties

Risk Factors
Permanent hearing loss independent of OME
Suspected or diagnosed speech and language delay or disorder
Autism-spectrum disorder and other pervasive developmental disorders
Syndromes (e.g., Down) or craniofacial disorders with high prevalence of cognitive, speech, and language delays
Blindness or uncorrectable visual impairment
Cleft palate with or without visual impairment
Developmental delay

Note. Presented are sensory, physical, cognitive, or behavioral factors that place children who have OME at an increased risk for developmental difficulties (delay or disorder).

of the middle ear. The primary care physician must visualize the tympanic membrane for signs of middle ear effusion and inflammation to make the diagnosis. This is often challenging in uncooperative small infants and children with partially blocked ear canals or narrow ear canals.

Treatment includes pain management (acetaminophen or ibuprofen) as needed, and for children under 6 months of age, antibacterial treatment. For children older than 6 months, depending on severity of the illness, the options are antibacterial treatment or observation. Amoxicillin is currently the initial drug of choice. The recommendation of treatment for children with underlying permanent hearing loss and children at risk of language delays is antibacterial management.

The Medical Home and Children With Cochlear Implants

When cochlear implants first became available to children, the minimum age at implant was 2 years. Eligible children had to have bilateral, profound hearing loss. However, studies began to demonstrate that young congenitally deaf children with cochlear implants could learn to communicate orally. In addition, children with multiple disabilities could benefit from cochlear implants and develop auditory skills. As a result of these findings, candidacy criteria for pediatric cochlear implantation currently is 18 months or older for children with severe-to-profound bilateral sensorineural hearing loss, and 12 to 18 months for children with profound hearing loss. In cases of deafness due to meningitis, implants may be placed early in the first year of life. A lack of benefit in the development of auditory skills with amplification needs to be demonstrated. Children up to 7 years of age appear to derive the greatest benefit (Sharma, Dorman, & Kral, 2005).

Pediatricians need to be aware of key management criteria for children with cochlear implants. The child will need the services of an audiologist skilled in fitting hearing aids and providing implant services including programming of the speech processer. The team at the implant center should include a skilled pediatric otolaryngologist and pediatric anesthesiologist. Finally, it is important that appropriate speech and language therapy services be provided to facilitate and optimize oral communication skills.

According to the U.S. Food and Drug Administration (FDA), 38,000 children in the United States had received cochlear implants at the end of 2012 (FDA, 2015). Children with cochlear implants are at increased risk for bacterial meningitis compared to children in the general U.S. population (Bluestone, 2003; Reefhuis et al., 2003). Because of this risk, it is recommended that physicians monitor all patients with cochlear implants for meningitis and middle ear infections, but particularly children whose implants have a positioner (Biernath et al., 2006). *Streptococcus pneumoniae* is the most common pathogen causing bacterial meningitis in cochlear implant recipients of all ages (Manruqie, Cervera-Paz, Huarte, & Molina, 2004; Uchanski & Geers, 2003). Children less than 24 months of age with cochlear implants should receive PCV7, as recommended, and children ages 24 to 59 months with cochlear implants who have not received PCV7 should be vaccinated according to the high-risk schedule. The Centers for Disease Control and Prevention (CDC) recommends that children with implants also receive age-appropriate *Haemophilus influenzae* Type b (Hib) vaccines (CDC, Advisory Committee on Immunization, 2003).

Medical Home Stress and Impact on the Family

The Hearing Screen

Physicians need to be aware of the fact that parents perceive varying degrees of stress when they are informed that their infant has failed a newborn hearing screen. Although the possible cause could be either a false positive or a true fail, most parents will have some increase in worry until their infant is rescreened. NICU infants have higher false-positive rates and higher fail rates than well-baby nursery infants. In one study of well-baby nursery infants, parents reported increased "worry" at 2 to 8 weeks of age when they returned for the rescreen (Vohr, Letourneau, & McDermott, 2001). Mothers who were more informed about hearing screening experienced decreased worry. Physicians who understand the screening process can support the family whose infant fails the screen, encourage the family to return for the rescreen, and follow up with the family about the rescreen results. Stuart and colleagues (Stuart, Moretz, & Yang, 2000) administered the Parenting Stress Inventory at 1 month after discharge and found no differences in stress reported by mothers of infants who passed the screen and mothers of infants referred for further testing. This suggests that the stress and worry of a false positive is of short duration. Another study revealed that mothers of infants with a false-positive screen result did not report increased levels of stress or impact at 12 to 16, or 18 to 24 months, and that older maternal age (perhaps more parenting and screening experience) and greater family resources were protective against persistent stress, whereas NICU stay contributed to prolonged stress (Vohr et al., 2008).

The Audiology Diagnostic Fail

It has been proposed that there is a continuum of increasing stress for families whose infants are identified with hearing loss that increases as they progress through the hearing screen fail, rescreen fail, diagnostic fail, and intervention process (Kurtzer-White & Luterman, 2003). Abdala de Uzcategui and Yoshinaga-Itano (1997) conducted a study in which they sent mail interviews to families who had been referred for audiologic testing. Mothers reported feeling depressed, frustrated, and angry. Support and reassurance by the primary physician during this time is essential.

Parent perception of stress at the time of diagnosis varies significantly among parents. Parents who are culturally Deaf may have anticipated the diagnosis and be totally accepting. Hearing parents of children diagnosed with a hearing loss perceive greater stress that is, in part, related to the fear of disability (Abdala de Uzcategu & Yoshinaga-Itano, 1997; Barringer & Mauk, 1997; Brand & Coetzer, 1994; Clemens, Davis, & Bailey, 2000; Meadow-Orlans, 1990, 1995, 2001; Vohr et al., 2001; Weichbold & Welzl-Mueller, 2001). Approximately 95% of children with congenital hearing loss are born to hearing parents. Hearing parents might not know someone with a significant hearing loss and might feel isolated. Meadow-Orlans (1995) reported that mothers of infants who were deaf or hard of hearing perceived greater life stress (similar to that experienced with divorce, death in the family, moving, financial problems) than parents of hearing children. More recent studies have found similar parenting stress scores on the Parenting Stress Inventory for mothers of infants with hearing loss and mothers of hearing infants (Meadow-Orlans, 1995). Prompt sharing of results with the family and physician and referral to early intervention by the audiologist on the day of diagnosis might facilitate the provision of needed information and support to parents to mediate stress. Both younger maternal age and lower level of maternal education have been associated with greater perception of maternal stress associated with hearing loss (Meadow-Orlans, 1990).

Impact on the family is a measure of how the child's condition (hearing loss) produces change in the family. Categories of impact include financial impact, family burden, caretaker burden, and disruption of planning. In one study (Vohr et al., 2008), mothers of infants who did not pass the newborn hearing screening and were diagnosed with hearing loss reported significantly greater financial impact at 12 to 16 months of age and greater financial and caretaker burden at 18 to 24 months of age compared to mothers of infants who passed the screening process. This impact reflects "daily life" costs associated with hearing loss including amplification, speech and language therapy, and transportation for visits to specialists. If physicians become aware of financial difficulties experienced by the family, the Early Intervention case manager should be alerted to assist and empower the family to identify resources such as a hearing aid loaner program, respite care, and eligibility for financial assistance programs.

Calderon and Greenberg (1999) reported that social support was an important predictor of maternal adjustment for hearing mothers of children who are deaf or hard of hearing at school age. The physician can play an important role by informing and facilitating referral of the family to parent support groups such as Hands and Voices and Family Voices. As half of the children identified with congenital hearing loss are NICU graduates and approximately 40% of children with permanent hearing loss have other disabilities, these children might require the resources of a number of different medical and educational disciplines, adding to both the financial and emotional burden (Karchmer & Allen, 1999; Mitchell, 2004). As physicians become more informed about the needs of infants with hearing loss and their families, and community resources needed, they can become more effective members of the child/family EHDI team.

References

Abdala de Uzcategu, C., & Yoshinaga-Itano, C. (1997). Parents' reactions to newborn hearing screening. *Audiology Today*, *9*(1), 24–25.

American Academy of Pediatrics. (2000). Committee on Practice and Ambulatory Medicine. Recommendations for preventive pediatric health care. *Pediatrics*, *105*, 645–646.

American Academy of Pediatrics. (2002). Policy statement: The medical home. Medical Home Initiatives for Children With Special Needs Project Advisory Committee. *Pediatrics*, *110*(1), 184–186.

American Academy of Pediatrics. (2004). American Academy of Family Physicians, American Academy of Otolaryngology-Head and Neck Surgery, and American Academy of Pediatrics Subcommittee on Otitis Media With Effusion. Otitis media with effusion. *Pediatrics, 113*(5), 1412–1429.

American Academy of Pediatrics. (2006). Policy statement: Identifying infants and young children with developmental disorders in the medical home: An algorithm for developmental surveillance and screening. *Pediatrics, 118*(1), 405–420.

American Academy of Pediatrics. (2007a). Position statement: Principles and guidelines for early hearing detection and intervention programs. Joint Committee on Infant Hearing. *Pediatrics, 120*(4), 898–921.

American Academy of Pediatrics. (2007b). *Universal newborn hearing screening, diagnosis, and intervention: Guidelines for pediatric medical home providers.* Retrieved from http://www.medicalhomeinfo.org/screening/Screen%20Materials/Algorithm.pdf

American Academy of Pediatrics. (2010). T*ask Force on Improving the Effectiveness of Newborn Hearing Screening, Diagnosis, and Intervention. Universal newborn hearing screening, diagnosis, and intervention: Guidelines for pediatric medical home providers.* Elk Grove Village, IL: Author. Retrieved from http://www.medicalhomeinfo.org/downloads/pdfs/Algorithm1_2010.pdf

Amir, J., Wolf, D. G., & Levy, I. (2010). Treatment of symptomatic congenital cytomegalovirus infection with intravenous ganciclovir followed by long-term oral valganciclovir. *European Journal of Pediatrics, 169*(9), 1061–1067. doi:10.1007/s00431-010-1176-9

Arditi, M., Mason, E. O., Jr., Bradley, J. S., Tan, T. Q., Barson, W. J., Schutze, G. E., . . . Kaplan, S. L. (1998). Three-year multicenter surveillance of pneumococcal meningitis in children: Clinical characteristics, and outcome related to penicillin susceptibility and dexamethasone use. *Pediatrics, 102*(5), 1087–1097.

Barringer, D., & Mauk, G. (1997). Survey of parents' perspectives regarding hospital-based newborn hearing screening. *Audiology Today, 1*, 18–19.

Bertolini, P., Lassalle, M., Mercier, G., Raquin, M. A., Izzi, G., Corradini, N., & Hartmann, O. (2004). Platinum compound-related ototoxicity in children: Long-term follow-up reveals continuous worsening of hearing loss. *Journal of Pediatric Hematology Oncology, 26*, 649–655.

Bess, F. H., Dodd-Murphy, J., & Parker, R. A. (1998). Children with minimal sensorineural hearing loss: Prevalence, educational performance, and functional status. *Ear and Hearing, 19*(5), 339–353.

Biernath, K. R., Reefhuis, J., Whitney, C. G., Mann, E. A., Costa, P., Eichwald, J., & Boyle, C. (2006). Bacterial meningitis among children with cochlear implants beyond 24 months after implantation. *Pediatrics, 117*(2), 284–289.

Bluestone, C. D. (2003). Cochlear implants and meningitis: Update and recommendations for prevention. *Pediatric Infectious Disease Journal, 22*(5), 477–478. doi:10.1097/01.inf.0000068212.52052.53

Boppana, S. B., Ross, S. A., Novak, Z., Shimamura, M., Tolan, R. W., Jr., Palmer, A. L., . . . Fowler, K. B. (2010). Dried blood spot real-time polymerase chain reaction assays to screen newborns for congenital cytomegalovirus infection. *JAMA, 303*(14), 1375–1382. doi:10.1001/jama.2010.423303/14/1375 [pii]

Brand, H. J., & Coetzer, M. A. (1994). Parental response to their child's hearing impairment. *Psychological Reports, 75*(3 Pt 1), 1363–1368.

Bricker, D., & Squires, J. (1999). *Ages and Stages questionnaires: A parent-completed, child-monitoring system.* Baltimore, MD: Brookes.

Brookhouser, P. E., Worthington, D. W., & Kelly, W. J. (1994). Fluctuating and/or progressive sensorineural hearing loss in children. *Laryngoscope, 104*(8 Pt. 1), 958–964.

Calderon, R., & Greenberg, M. T. (1999). Stress and coping in hearing mothers of children with hearing loss: Factors affecting mother and child adjustment. *American Annals of the Deaf, 144*(1), 7–18.

Centers for Disease Control and Prevention. Advisory Committee on Immunization. (2003). Pneumococcal vaccination for cochlear implant candidates and recipients: Updated recommendations of the Advisory Committee on Immunization Practices. *MMWR Morbidity and Mortality Weekly Report, 52*(31), 739–740.

Clemens, C. J., Davis, S. A., & Bailey, A. R. (2000). The false-positive in universal newborn hearing screening. *Pediatrics, 106*(1), E7.

Cone-Wesson, B., Vohr, B. R., Sininger, Y. S., Widen, J. E., Folsom, R. C., Gorga, M. P., & Norton, S. J. (2000). Identification of neonatal hearing impairment: Infants with hearing loss. *Ear and Hearing, 21*(5), 488–507.

Coplan, J. (1993). *Early Language Milestone scale* (2nd ed.). Austin, TX: Pro-Ed.

Denoyelle, F., Marlin, S., Weil, D., Moatti, L., Chauvin, P., Garabedian, E. N., & Petit, C. (1999). Clinical features of the prevalent form of childhood deafness, DFNB1, due to a connexin-26 gene defect: Implications for genetic counselling. *Lancet, 353*(9161), 1298–1303.

Fenson, L., Dale, P. S., Resnick, J. S., Thal, D., Bates, E., Hartung, J. P., . . . Reilly, J. S. (1993). *The MacArthur Communicative Development Inventories: User's guide and technical manual.* San Diego, CA: Singular.

Fligor, B. J., Neault, M. W., Mullen, C. H., Feldman, H. A., & Jones, D. T. (2005). Factors associated with sensorineural hearing loss among survivors of extracorporeal membrane oxygenation therapy. *Pediatrics, 115*(6), 1519–1528.

Fowler, K., Stagno, S., Pass, R., Britt, W., Boll, T., & Alford, C. (1992). The outcome of congenital cytomegalovirus infection in relation to maternal antibody status. *New England Journal of Medicine, 326*(10), 663–667.

Fowler, K. B., McCollister, F. P., Dahle, A. J., Boppana, S., Britt, W. J., & Pass, R. F. (1997). Progressive and fluctuating sensorineural hearing loss in children with asymptomatic congenital cytomegalovirus infection. *Journal of Pediatrics, 130*(4), 624–630.

Geoffrey, R. S., Cynthia, B., Graham, A. B., 3rd, Brown, O. W., Hardin, A., Lessin, H. R., . . . Bright Futures Periodicity Schedule, W. (2014). 2014 recommendations for pediatric preventive health care. *Pediatrics, 133*(3), 568–570. doi:10.1542/peds.2013-4096

Golz, A., Angel-Yeger, B., & Parush, S. (1998). Evaluation of balance disturbances in children with middle ear effusion. *International Journal of Pediatric Otorhinolaryngology, 43*(1), 21–26.

Hamilton, S. T., van Zuylen, W., Shand, A., Scott, G. M., Naing, Z., Hall, B., . . . Rawlinson, W. D. (2014). Prevention of congenital cytomegalovirus complications by maternal and neonatal treatments: A systematic review. *Reviews in Medical Virology, 24*(6), 420–433. doi:10.1002/rmv.1814

Huang, B. Y., Zdanski, C., & Castillo, M. (2012). Pediatric sensorineural hearing loss, part 2: Syndromic and acquired causes. *AJNR American Journal of Neuroradiology, 33*(3), 399–406. doi:10.3174/ajnr.A2499

Johnson, J. L., White, K. R., Widen, J. E., Gravel, J. S., James, M., Kennalley, T., . . . Holstrum, J. (2005). A multicenter evaluation of how many infants with permanent hearing loss pass a two-stage otoacoustic emissions/automated auditory brainstem response newborn hearing screening protocol. *Pediatrics, 116*(3), 663–672.

Josephson, C. D., Caliendo, A. M., Easley, K. A., Knezevic, A., Shenvi, N., Hinkes, M. T., . . . Roback, J. D. (2014). Blood transfusion and breast milk transmission of cytomegalovirus in very low-birth-weight infants: A prospective cohort study. *JAMA Pediatrics, 168*(11), 1054–1062. doi:10.1001/jamapediatrics.2014.1360

Karchmer, M. A., & Allen, T. E. (1999). The functional assessment of deaf and hard of hearing students. *American Annals of the Deaf, 144*(2), 68–77.

Kimberlin, D. W., Jester, P. M., Sanchez, P. J., Ahmed, A., Arav-Boger, R., Michaels, M. G., . . . Infectious Diseases Collaborative Antiviral Study Group. (2015). Valganciclovir for symptomatic congenital cytomegalovirus disease. *New England Journal of Medicine, 372*(10), 933–943. doi:10.1056/NEJMoa1404599

Kurtzer-White, E., & Luterman, D. (2003). Families and children with hearing loss: Grief and coping. *Mental Retardation and Developmental Disabilities Research Reviews, 9*(4), 232–235.

Lew, H. L., Lee, E. H., Miyoshi, Y., Chang, D. G., Date, E. S., & Jerger, J. F. (2004). Brainstem auditory-evoked potentials as an objective tool for evaluating hearing dysfunction in traumatic brain injury. *American Journal of Physical Medicine Rehabilitation, 83*(3), 210–215.

Lieberthal, A. S., Carroll, A. E., Chonmaitree, T., Ganiats, T. G., Hoberman, A., Jackson, M. A., . . . Tunkel, D. E. (2013). The diagnosis and management of acute otitis media. *Pediatrics, 131*, e964. doi:10.1542/peds.2012-3488

Madden, C., Wiley, S., Schleiss, M., Benton, C., Meinzen-Derr, J., Greinwald, J., & Choo, D. (2005). Audiometric, clinical and educational outcomes in a pediatric symptomatic congenital cytomegalovirus (CMV) population with sensorineural hearing loss. *International Journal of Pediatric Otorhinolaryngology, 69*(9), 1191–1198.

Manruqie, M., Cervera-Paz, F., Huarte, A., & Molina, M. (2004). Advantages of cochlear implantation in prelingual deaf children before 2 years of age when compared with later implantation. *Laryngoscope, 114*(8), 1462–1469.

Meadow-Orlans, K. P. (1990). The impact of childhood hearing loss on the family. In D. F. Moores & K. P. Meadow-Orlans (Eds.), *Educational and developmental aspects of deafness* (pp. 11–23). Washington, DC: Gallaudet University Press.

Meadow-Orlans, K. P. (1995). Sources of stress for mothers and fathers of deaf and hard of hearing infants. *American Annals of the Deaf, 140*(4), 352–357.

Meadow-Orlans, K. P. (2001). Effects of mother and infant hearing status on interactions at twelve and eighteen months. *Journal of Deaf Studies and Deaf Education, 2*, 26–36.

Mehra, S., Eavey, R. D., & Keamy, D. G., Jr. (2009). The epidemiology of hearing impairment in the United States: Newborns, children, and adolescents. *Otolaryngology-Head and Neck Surgery, 140*(4), 461–472. doi:10.1016/j.otohns.2008.12.022

Mitchell, R. E. (2004). National profile of deaf and hard of hearing students in special education from weighted survey results. *American Annals of the Deaf, 149*(4), 336–349.

Morton, C. C., & Nance, W. E. (2006). Newborn hearing screening—A silent revolution. *New England Journal of Medicine, 354*(20), 2151–2164.

Nance, W. E. (2003). The genetics of deafness. *Mental Retardation and Developmental Disabilities Research Reviews, 9*(2), 109–119.

Nance, W. E., & Kearsey, M. J. (2004). Relevance of connexin deafness (DFNB1) to human evolution. *American Journal of Human Genetics, 74*(6), 1081–1087.

Nance, W. E., Lim, B. G., & Dodson, K. M. (2006). Importance of congenital cytomegalovirus infections as a cause for pre-lingual hearing loss. *Journal of Clinical Virology, 35*(2), 221–225.

Nozawa, N., Koyano, S., Yamamoto, Y., Inami, Y., Kurane, I., & Inoue, N. (2007). Real-time PCR assay using specimens on filter disks as a template for detection of cytomegalovirus in urine. *Journal of Clinical Microbiology, 45*(4), 1305–1307. doi:10.1128/JCM.02502-06

Reefhuis, J., Honein, M. A., Whitney, C. G., Chamany, S., Mann, E. A., Biernath, K. R., . . . Boyle, C. (2003). Risk of bacterial meningitis in children with cochlear implants. *New England Journal of Medicine, 349*(5), 435–445. doi:10.1056/NEJMoa031101349/5/435 [pii]

Rescoria, L. (1989). The Language Development Survey: A screening tool for delayed language in toddlers. *Journal of Speech and Hearing Disorders, 54*, 587–599.

Rivera, L., Boppana, S., Fowler, K. B., Britt, W. J., Stagno, S., & Pass, R. (2002). Predictors of hearing loss in children with symptomatic congenital cytomegalovirus infection. *Pediatrics, 110*(4), 762–767.

Roizen, N. J. (1999). Etiology of hearing loss in children. Nongenetic causes. *Pediatric Clinics of North America, 46*(1), 49–64.

Roizen, N. J. (2003). Nongenetic causes of hearing loss. *Mental Retardation and Developmental Disabilities Research Reviews, 9*(2), 120–127.

Rosenfeld, R. M., & Kay, D. (2003). Natural history of untreated otitis media. *Laryngoscope, 113*(10), 1645–1657.

Rosenfeld, R. M., Schwartz, S. R., Pynnonen, M. A., Tunkel, D. E., Hussey, H. M., Fichera, J. S., . . . Schellhase, K. G. (2013). Clinical practice guideline: Tympanostomy tubes in children. *Otolaryngology-Head and Neck Surgery, 149*(1 Suppl), S1–35. doi:10.1177/0194599813487302

Ross, S. A., Ahmed, A., Palmer, A. L., Michaels, M. G., Sanchez, P. J., Bernstein, D. I., . . . National Institute on Deafness and Other Communication Disorders CHIMES Study. (2014). Detection of congenital cytomegalovirus infection by real-time polymerase chain reaction analysis of saliva or urine specimens. *Journal of Infectious Diseases, 210*(9), 1415–1418. doi:10.1093/infdis/jiu263

Santos, R. L., Aulchenko, Y. S., Huygen, P. L., van der Donk, K. P., de Wijs, I. J., Kemperman, M. H., . . . Cremers, C. W. (2005). Hearing impairment in Dutch patients with connexin 26 (GJB2) and connexin 30 (GJB6) mutations. *International Journal of Pediatric Otorhinolaryngology, 69*(2), 165–174.

Sharma, A., Dorman, M. F., & Kral, A. (2005). The influence of a sensitive period on central auditory development in children with unilateral and bilateral cochlear implants. *Hearing Research, 203*(1–2), 134–143.

Smets, K., De Coen, K., Dhooge, I., Standaert, L., Laroche, S., Mahieu, L., . . . Boudewyns, A. (2006). Selecting neonates with congenital cytomegalovirus infection for ganciclovir therapy. *European Journal of Pediatrics, 165*(12), 885–890. doi:10.1007/s00431-006-0192-2

Stuart, A., Moretz, M., & Yang, E. Y. K. (2000). An investigation of maternal stress after neonatal hearing screening. *American Journal of Audiology, 9*, 135–141.

Tos, M. (1984). Epidemiology and natural history of secretory otitis. *American Journal of Otology, 5*(6), 459–462.

Uchanski, R., & Geers, A. (2003). Acoustic characteristics of the speech of young cochlear implant users: A comparison with normal-hearing age-mates. *Ear and Hearing, 24*(1 Suppl.), 90S–105S.

U.S. Food and Drug Administration (FDA; 2015). *Premarket to postmarket shift in clinical data requirements for cochlear implant device approvals in pediatric patients.* Retrieved from http://www.fda.gov/downloads/AdvisoryCommittees/CommitteesMeetingMaterials/MedicalDevices/MedicalDevicesAdvisoryCommittee/EarNoseandThroatDevicesPanel/UCM443996.pdf

Vartialnen, E., Karjalainen, S., & Karja, J. (1985). Auditory disorders following head injury in children. *Acta Oto-Laryngologica, 99*, 529–536.

Vohr, B. R., Jodoin-Krauzyk, J., Tucker, R., Johnson, M. J., Topol, D., & Ahlgren, M. (2008). Results of newborn screening for hearing loss: Effects on the family in the first 2 years of life. *Archives of Pediatrics and Adolescent Medicine, 162*(3), 205–211.

Vohr, B. R., Letourneau, K. S., & McDermott, C. (2001). Maternal worry about neonatal hearing screening. *Journal of Perinatology, 21*(1), 15–20.

Watkin, P., & Baldwin, M. (2012). The longitudinal follow-up of a universal neonatal hearing screen: The implications for confirming deafness in childhood. *International Journal of Audiology, 51*(7), 519–528. doi:10.3109/14992027.2012.673237

Weichbold, V., & Welzl-Mueller, K. (2001). Maternal concern about positive test results in universal newborn hearing screening. *Pediatrics, 108*(5), 1111–1116.

Yoshinaga-Itano, C. (2014). Principles and guidelines for early intervention after confirmation that a child is deaf or hard of hearing. *Journal of Deaf Studies and Deaf Education, 19*(2), 143–175. doi:10.1093/deafed/ent043

Zimmerman, W. D., Ganzel, T. M., Windmill, I. M., Nazar, G. B., & Phillips, M. (1993). Peripheral hearing loss following head trauma in children. *Laryngoscope, 103*, 87–91.

Medical Considerations for Infants and Children With Hearing Loss: An Otologist's Perspective

Craig A. Buchman and Oliver F. Adunka

Background and Protocol

Hearing loss is common among newborn infants with an incidence of 3 to 4 per 1,000 live births. Approximately 25% of these children have a severe-to-profound hearing loss, and the remaining are affected to a lesser degree. There also is a group of children who have passed their newborn hearing screen only to later be identified as having a progressive hearing disorder. Untreated hearing loss reduces sound and environmental awareness. This can result in delayed speech and language acquisition and impaired communication abilities. These individuals frequently attain lower levels of educational achievement than the normal hearing population, thereby adversely affecting employment opportunities and quality of life.

In the United States, universal newborn hearing screening has been mandated by law for all children in most states. Since the initiation of newborn infant hearing screening, a number of specialized programs have evolved to evaluate systematically and habilitate these children and provide a variety of resources for families. Many of these systems and processes have followed the recommendations of the 2007 Joint Committee on Infant Hearing (JCIH) statement that has been detailed elsewhere (American Academy of Pediatrics and Joint Committee on Infant Hearing, 2007). Despite these efforts, late-onset hearing loss might not be identified by newborn screening protocols. Risk factors for identifying late-onset hearing loss have also been developed (Joint Committee on Infant Hearing et al., 2013).

Following a failure result on the newborn infant hearing screen, a multidisciplinary approach and standardized protocols are needed to evaluate and treat these children. The multidisciplinary endeavor requires input from a diverse group of professionals with expertise in a variety of hearing-related disciplines. These areas are broadly depicted in Figure 8–1. It is common that certain disciplines might predominate during one phase of the process, while others frequently become more active later. Close cooperation through mutual respect for one another's skills and opinions forms the backbone for successful collaboration for the child's and family's benefit.

In an effort to create a timely diagnosis and early intervention, we have created a timeline for the events of the first year of life (Figure 8–2). Although not set in

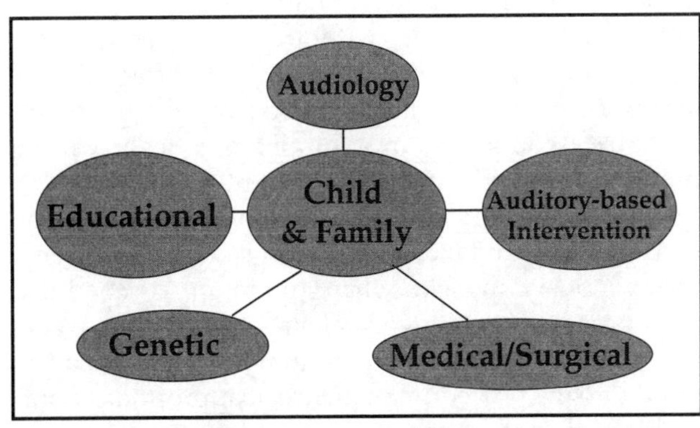

FIGURE 8–1. The Hearing Loss Team.

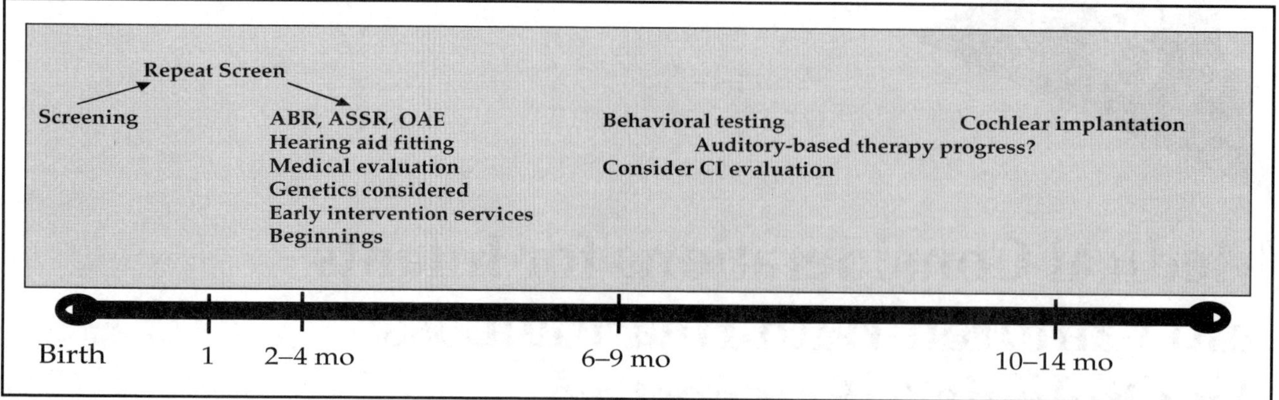

FIGURE 8–2. Timeline for diagnostic and therapeutic interventions for infants who fail a newborn infant screen.

stone, we believe this serves as a rough guide for the events of the first year of life as it relates to hearing loss and its management. The cornerstone goals of the first year are

1. *identification* of hearing loss and establishment of precise auditory thresholds;
2. *diagnosis* of the etiology for the hearing loss;
3. *intervention* through provision of appropriate treatment and technologies; and
4. *education* by providing information for families to help make decisions.

A comprehensive diagnostic hearing evaluation is the first required assessment following a confirmed "fail" or "refer" indication by the newborn infant hearing screening. At our center, this evaluation is carried out by a group of highly experienced audiologists with expertise in pediatric hearing testing. The initial follow-up testing for each child occurs under one of three environments: natural sleep, conscious sedation, or general anesthesia. Infants younger than about 3 months of age are tested in natural sleep, if possible. Babies older than this, without other medical contraindications, are sedated for testing. After medical clearance by a physician, a nurse from the hospital's pediatric sedation team administers a sedative and remains at bedside to monitor the entire session. Sedation can be accomplished with chloral hydrate delivered orally or midazolam (or other sedative) delivered intravenously. In cases where the infant is scheduled for a procedure under general anesthesia (e.g., surgery or imaging), the evoked potential testing is incorporated into the procedure sequence, if appropriate. Some children are not deemed candidates for safe, monitored conscious sedation, and so testing is carried out under the supervision of an anesthesiologist (i.e., general anesthesia). The duration of the test is usually dictated by the test environment, ranging from about 30 minutes in the operating room to over an hour under conscious sedation.

The importance of proper auditory brainstem response (ABR) testing cannot be overemphasized. Specifically, four frequencies (500, 1000, 2000, 4000 Hz) and clicks should be tested for each ear including bone conduction and a test run with a disconnected sound tube (to exclude electrical artifacts). Importantly, no single test modality is sufficient for precisely identifying the degree of hearing impairment in a baby (American Academy of Pediatrics and Joint Committee on Infant Hearing, 2007). Rather, a test battery is needed that can include a variety of measures such as ABR, auditory steady-state responses (ASSRs), otoacoustic emissions (OAEs), and tympanometry (immittance). Although reasonably accurate, each of these testing procedures has a variety of potential shortcomings. It is paramount that the individual administering the protocol be able to recognize and interpret the various test results within the context of these shortcomings (American Academy of Pediatrics and Joint Committee on Infant Hearing, 2007).

ABR, OAEs, and tympanometry form the backbone of the diagnostic testing protocol at our institution for infants who fail newborn screening. Our protocols have been detailed previously (Buchman et al., 2006; Hang et al., 2015). ASSR has also been used at our institution, although we have found such testing adds very little diagnostic information beyond conventional ABR. In a manner similar to ABR, ASSR can over- or underestimate the degree of hearing loss with overestimation being more common (Ahn, Lee, Kim, Yoon & Chung, 2007; Gorga et al., 2006; Stapells, Herdman,

Small, Dimitrijevic, & Hatton, 2005). ASSR is notably less accurate in patients with lesser degrees of hearing loss and is unable to identify those ears with the auditory neuropathy phenotype (Stapells et al., 2005; Tlumak, Rubinstein & Durrant, 2007). In subjects with profound hearing loss, ASSR can produce artifactual responses that are recorded as auditory thresholds when, in fact, they are produced by nonauditory centers (Gorga et al., 2004; Small & Stapells, 2004). Thus, it is critical that clinicians understand that these electrophysiological modalities are useful for estimating thresholds for the purposes of amplification fitting in children. However, they are not precise enough for making decisions regarding surgical intervention when destruction of the underlying residual hearing might occur as a sequelae of that intervention.

The otologist's role in caring for the hearing impaired child is to

1. *diagnose* hearing loss by identifying
   a. etiology and severity,
   b. specific anatomical relationships to functional findings,
   c. associated problems, and
   d. referrals to related professionals;
2. *treat* hearing loss by providing medical and surgical interventions;
3. *refer* for amplification and speech therapy;
4. *prevent* further hearing loss and other related complications through education of parents, children, and other health care providers; and
5. *communicate* with professionals on the hearing loss team.

The otologist's role usually commences once a hearing disorder has been identified. One exception might be the child who requires diagnostic audiology but is unable to be tested under natural sleep (compliance or advanced age) or sedation because of associated medical conditions, or when it is apparent that middle ear effusions need to be addressed in order to garner accurate test results. These children are taken to the operating room for general anesthesia. In this setting, the ears are examined using the operating microscope, and a determination regarding middle ear status is made. When a middle ear effusion is present, we prefer to place tympanostomy tubes, and the audiological testing protocol is subsequently carried out. Ear canal bleeding must be avoided as this might negatively impact testing results. Placement of otic drops is deferred until after the auditory testing has been concluded. If a hearing impairment has been identified, ear canal impressions for future hearing aid molds are typically taken during the same setting for convenience. Findings are subsequently entered into the newborn infant hearing screening database.

Following the initial audiological assessment, we have found that a search for a hearing loss etiology and associated medical conditions is critical and frequently impacts the treatment paradigm. Referrals are also made to the state early intervention services program at this juncture. *Early intervention services* refers to a variety of public state agencies working together to provide services for children with special needs age birth to 3 years. Early intervention services typically fund assistive technologies, and a speech and language pathologist becomes involved in the child's care plan. There are a growing number of speech-language pathologists who are trained and certified in the methods of auditory verbal therapy (AVT). Emerging evidence suggests that in the setting of an adequate auditory signal (either through amplification or a cochlear implant), auditory-based intervention provides for better acquisition of spoken language in hearing-impaired children than communication modes that include sign language (JCIH, 2013; Moog & Geers, 2003). However, the choice of communication strategy is certainly a very personal one for families of children who are hearing impaired. Every effort should be made to provide detailed information for families so that an informed decision can be made at this juncture.

Medical Diagnostic Evaluation

The medical evaluation focuses on trying to identify an etiology for the hearing loss and associated problems that might negatively impact communication or other health issues. Implicit is the fact that a detailed understanding of the causes of hearing loss in children is needed to identify the salient issues in a particular patient. An excellent review of the potential etiologies of hearing loss has been previously published (Morton & Nance, 2006). In addition to searching for the etiology of hearing loss, careful evaluation must identify disorders in vision, craniofacial malformations, and primary speech and auditory processing disorders to allow a comprehensive approach to the communication needs of a child and the family. Referrals among a variety of medical professionals are often needed.

Currently, available data estimate the incidence of hearing loss at birth to be 186 per 100,000, while the prevalence is roughly 270 per 100,000 at 4 years of age (Morton & Nance, 2006). Genetic factors appear to play a greater role than acquired causes at birth, while acquired cases become more prevalent later in life. There are more than 300 distinct hearing loss syndromes that have been identified by their association with other clinical features. Syndromic forms of hearing loss are less common, accounting for only 10% to 20% of new cases. However, a thorough understanding of these syndromes allows for relatively simple and rapid identification of the genetics and associated comorbidities that might affect a particular child. Nonsyndromic (55%) and acquired (35%) forms of hearing loss are responsible for most of the newly identified cases emerging from the newborn hearing screening process, and the etiologies can be somewhat more difficult or even impossible to identify (Morton & Nance, 2006). For all types of hearing impairment in children, evaluation by a geneticist with expertise in pediatric hearing loss can provide additional information for families.

A careful history, physical examination, and selective use of imaging studies and laboratory testing can identify the etiology of a child's hearing loss in many cases. In addition to knowing the details of the newborn infant screening and diagnostic auditory testing, the *medical history* should be thorough in the areas of pregnancy and complications, past medical/surgical history, and family history. Some of the details that should be extracted include the following:

1. Did the pregnancy progress to full term? Were there associated complications such as eclampsia, fetal distress, oligo- or polyhydramnios, bleeding, Rh incompatibility, premature rupture of membranes, or preterm labor?
2. Was there perinatal infection such as toxoplasmosis, herpes simplex, rubella, syphilis, or cytomegalovirus infection, Group B streptococcus, or other infection (TORCHeS)?
3. Was antibiotic treatment required? If yes, were aminoglycosides used?
4. Was perinatal hypoxia or meconium aspiration evident at the time of delivery?
5. Did the child spend time in the neonatal intensive care unit (NICU)? If so,
   a. What was the birth weight? (Below 1,500 grams?)
   b. Was the child on a ventilator? What duration?
   c. Were high oxygen concentrations needed?
   d. Were there blood transfusions?
   e. Was there intracranial hemorrhage?
   f. Was there necrotizing enterocolitis? This might be associated with the use of aminoglycoside antibiotics.
   g. Was there retinopathy of prematurity?
   h. Were there heart defects? If so, what type?
6. Was the child jaundiced? If so, how high was the bilirubin concentration, for what duration, and how was it treated?
7. Did the child have meningitis? Bacterial? If so, what organisms were present?
8. Did the infant require any surgeries?
9. What other medical disorders does the child have?
10. Are there difficulties with vision, feeding, or other bodily functions?
11. In addition to the usual medical history regarding medicines, allergies, and past surgeries, it is important to assess other family members with hearing disorders or disorders related to hearing loss. Attempts should be made to uncover both first- and second-degree relatives who have or have had hearing loss.

The *physical examination* is focused on trying to identify syndromic features, associated ear-specific disorders, and anatomic situations that would adversely affect communication. Although a detailed listing of these issues is beyond the scope of this manuscript, some specifics that are sought in the physical examination might include the following:

1. General appearance traits such as wide-set eyes, pigmentary changes such as heterochromic irides, and a white forelock of hair are consistent with Waardenburg syndrome.
2. Cervical fistulas and pits with ear deformities suggest branchiootorenal (BOR) syndrome.
3. Cleft lip/palate, down-slanting eyes, coloboma, low-set small external ears, and mandible and maxillary hypoplasia are seen in association with a conductive type of hearing loss that would possibly indicate Treacher Collins syndrome.
4. Palatal and lip clefts are seen in association with choanal atresia, external ear deformity, and facial paralysis that might raise the suspicion for CHARGE association or similar syndromes.
5. Microcephaly might be seen in association with perinatal cytomegalovirus (CMV) or rubella infection or other events such as birth asphyxia or brain underdevelopment.
6. The general neurologic status of the child should be assessed. Although this might not provide direct evidence for the etiology of the hearing loss, global neurological and cognitive impairment might clearly influence the effectiveness of a variety of interventions.
7. Otitis externa and otitis media should be assessed in all cases, as these can adversely affect precise

hearing loss assessment and the institution of amplification.

Radiographic Imaging

Radiological imaging is a critical aspect of the assessment of every child with newly identified hearing loss. In our program, imaging is recommended immediately after the diagnosis of hearing loss has been established by electrophysiological measures. Early anatomical assessment of the temporal bones; auditory, vestibular, and facial nerves; as well as brain might

1. further characterize the hearing loss *etiology;*
2. identify anatomical markers for hearing loss *progression;*
3. predict *poor prognosis* from interventions such as amplification and cochlear implantation; and
4. *identify lesions of the central nervous system that require medical/surgical intervention* for the overall health of the patient.

Classical studies of temporal bone and ear morphology have been carried out using histological/pathological techniques in a variety of conditions (Schuknecht, 1993). Thus, the structural characteristics of many of the hearing loss syndromes have been described and can broadly be classified into those with or without radiographically detectable abnormalities. Patients with isolated inner ear cellular or membranous labyrinthine disorders are not identifiable based on current imaging resolution. Conversely, labyrinthine malformations of the external, middle, and inner ears and internal auditory canal are clearly detectable using currently available imaging. Structural anomalies of the nerves of the internal auditory canal and brain are also resolvable in some cases. In general, high-resolution computed tomography (HRCT) is well suited for assessing the osseous structures (external auditory canal and middle ear), while magnetic resonance imaging (MRI) provides excellent soft tissue detail for looking at the cranial nerves and brain. The inner ear is well visualized using either MRI or HRCT. HRCT shows the osseous labyrinthine shell well, and MRI shows the fluids within the inner ear that conform to the otic capsule outline. The protocols that we use for these studies have been described previously (Adunka et al., 2006; Adunka, Jewells, & Buchman, 2007; Buchman et al., 2006).

There currently remains some debate regarding which of the various imaging modalities is most appropriate for assessing children with hearing loss (Adunka et al., 2006, 2007; Buchman et al., 2006; Parry, Booth & Roland, 2005; Trimble, Blaser, James, & Papsin, 2007). This controversy stems mostly from otologists' and radiologists' familiarity in interpreting HRCT for inner ear morphological changes. For cases of aural atresia and other conductive hearing losses, HRCT remains superior to MRI for assessing bony detail. Conversely, we prefer MRI rather than HRCT in all children with newly identified sensorineural hearing loss because it allows direct imaging of the cochlear nerves and brain. The consequences of missing either isolated cochlear nerve deficiency or unsuspected retrocochlear/brain pathology could be profound and might ultimately result in inappropriate treatment of the child. For example, cochlear implantation in an ear without a cochlear nerve or in an ear affected by a tumor could be devastating for the child and family. In cases of sensorineural hearing loss, we use supplementary HRCT only in cases where (a) semicircular canal defects are identified so that the anatomy of the facial nerve is determined, (b) inner ear obstruction is evident on MRI to determine further if the lesion is osseous or fibrous (postmeningitis), (c) the internal auditory canal is narrow to determine patency of the bony cochlear nerve canal, and (d) temporal bone pathology has been identified, such as in cases of tumors (Adunka et al., 2006, 2007; Buchman et al., 2006).

Inner ear malformations that are detectable on imaging studies are common in children with sensorineural hearing loss. Some studies have estimated that 20% to 30% of children with sensorineural hearing loss have some morphological abnormality of their inner ear (Coticchia, Gokhale, Waltonen, & Sumer, 2006). They can be conveniently divided into abnormalities of the cochlear and vestibular apparatus or abnormalities of the neural structures. Cochlear abnormalities can take the form of aplasia (absence or Michel aplasia; Figure 8–3), hypoplasia (small cochlea; Figure 8–4), or dysplasia. Cochlear dysplasias are usually characterized as an incomplete partitioning as in the classical Mondini malformation (Figure 8–5) or modiolar deficiency, as in X-linked stapes gusher syndrome (Figure 8–6). Vestibular morphological variants can also have aplasia, hypoplasia, or dysplasia and can affect the semicircular canals, otolithic organs, and the vestibular aqueduct. Vestibular aplasia is shown in Figure 8–7.

Children with inner ear or neural malformations might have no identifiable clinical syndrome. For instance, absent semicircular canals (see Figure 8–7) with or without cochlear hypoplasia and cochlear nerve deficiency are very common in children with CHARGE

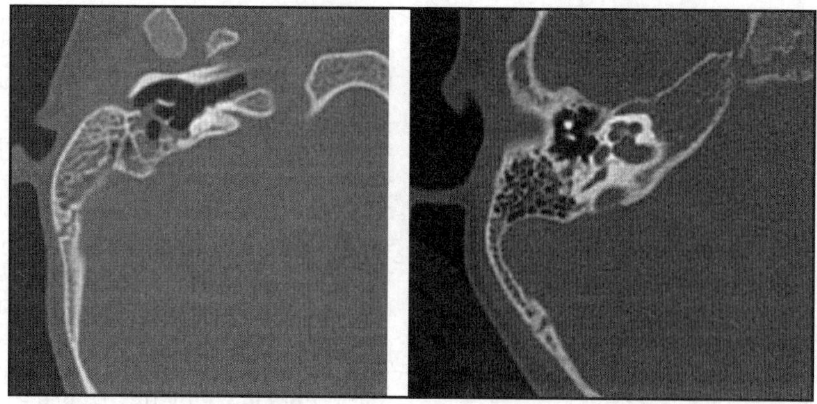

FIGURE 8–3. Michel aplasia (inner ear aplasia) on the left and normal inner ear right.

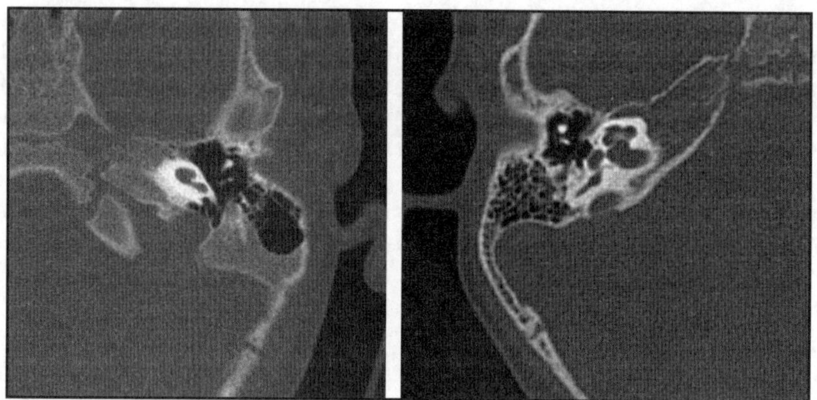

FIGURE 8–4. Cochlear hypoplasia (small cochlea) on left as compared to normal on right.

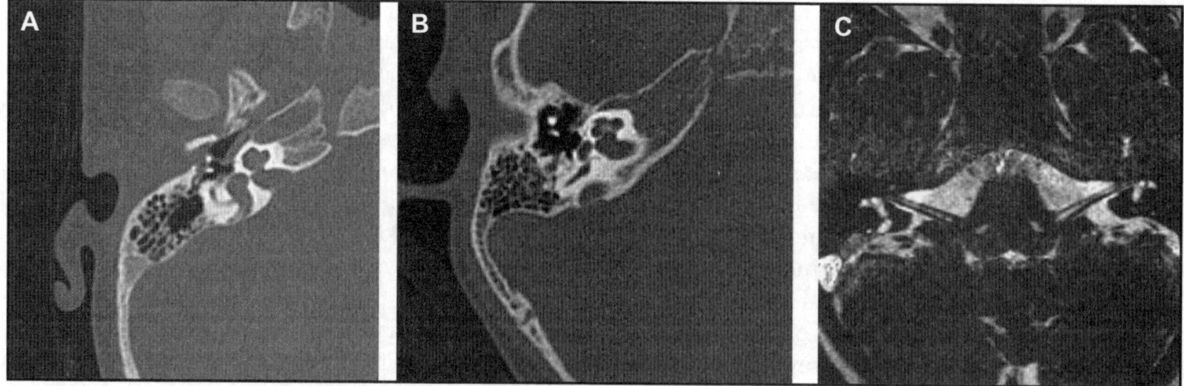

FIGURE 8–5. Mondini malformation (cochlear dysplasia, large vestibule, small horizontal canal, and enlarged vestibular aqueduct) as seen on HRCT (**A**) and MRI (**C**). A normal HRCT is shown in **B** for comparison.

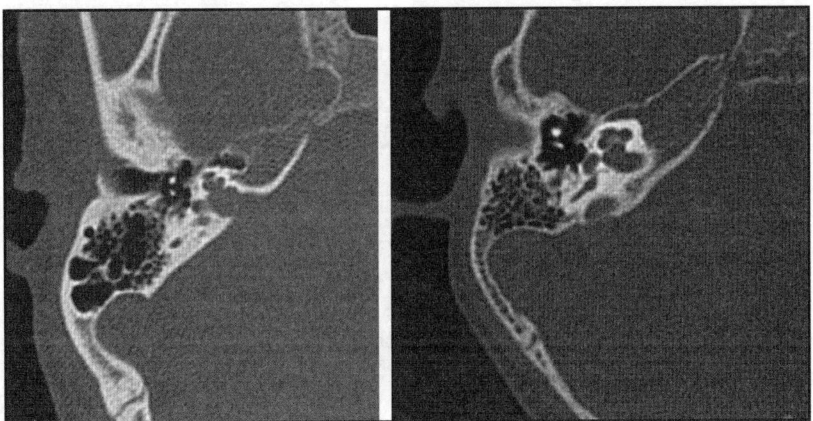

FIGURE 8–6. Cochlear dysplasia (modiolus deficiency) on the left from X-linked stapes gusher syndrome compared to normal right.

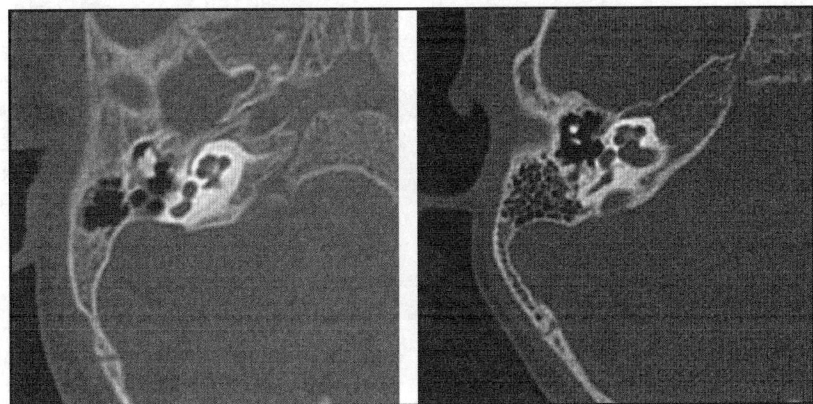

FIGURE 8–7. Vestibular aplasia (*left*) and normal inner ear (*right*).

association, VATER (vertebrae, anus, trachea, esophagus, and renal) or VACTERL (additional cardiac and limb conditions) syndrome or association, as well as branchiootorenal syndrome (BOR). An enlarged vestibular aqueduct (and endolymphatic duct) when seen in isolation or in association with an incompletely partitioned cochlea (Mondini's deformity; see Figure 8–5) might indicate that Pendred's syndrome is present. Children with Waardenburg's syndrome might also have inner ear malformations along the Mondini spectrum of findings. A bulbous or dilated internal auditory canal that widely communicates with a deficient cochlear modiolus is suggestive of the X-linked stapes gusher syndrome (see Figure 8–6; Morton & Nance, 2006).

Children with hearing loss can also have a variety of congenital and acquired changes to the central nervous system that are evident on imaging. Dandy-Walker syndrome is a congenital, developmental abnormality involving the cerebellum and posterior cranial fossa. The key features of this syndrome are enlargement of the fourth ventricle, a partial or complete absence of the cerebellar vermis, and cyst formation near the base of the skull. An increase in the size of the fluid spaces surrounding the brain as well as an increase in pressure might also be present (Parisi & Dobyns, 2003). Congenital CMV might result in microcephaly or cerebral calcifications and gliosis, which can be prominent in the temporal lobes. However, imaging findings can be difficult to distinguish from other viral infections of the central nervous system (Baskin & Hedlund, 2007). Meningitis from a variety of organisms can acutely result in varying degrees of brain edema, infarction, hydrocephalus, subdural pathology, and brain abscess that commonly leads to gliosis (Jan et al.,

2003). Inner ear involvement by inflammation and infection can result in labyrinthine obstruction from fibrosis and ultimate neo-ossification (Young, Hughes, Byrd, & Darling, 2000). Children with neurofibromatosis Type II can have bilateral acoustic neuromas that can present very early in life as well. In children born prematurely, radiographic sequelae from intraventricular hemorrhages and hydrocephalus can occur. Moreover, children with kernicterus and associated ANSD resulting from hyperbilirubinemia frequently have changes in the basal ganglia secondary to bilirubin staining (Katar, Akay, Taskesen, & Devecioglu, 2008).

In addition to changes in the brain, anatomical deficiency of the cochlear nerve can be identified on MRI (Adunka et al., 2006, 2007; Buchman et al., 2006). Although this disorder was originally described in children with inner ear malformations and very narrow internal auditory canals on HRCT, it has more recently been identified in children with normal inner ears and internal auditory canals. Moreover, it has been associated with a variety of syndromes such as CHARGE and VATER and can present in ears with electrophysiological evidence of ANSD on ABR testing. Figure 8–8 shows such an example (Adunka et al., 2006, 2007; Buchman et al., 2006).

Laboratory Assessment

Laboratory assessment is dictated, in part, by the patient's presenting situation. For children who have failed a newborn screening test and have undergone confirmatory testing that documents a sensorineural hearing loss, testing might include

1. electrocardiogram (EKG) to rule out Jervell and Lange-Nielsen syndrome;
2. Guthrie card polymerase chain reaction test (PCR) to rule out CMV infection;
3. connexin 26 and 30 mutation testing;
4. venereal disease research laboratory test (VDRL; syphilis);
5. erythrocyte sedimentation rate (ESR), complete blood count (CBC);
6. rheumatoid factor (RF), antinuclear cytoplasmic antibody (ANCA), antinuclear antibody (ANA), anticardiolipin antibody;
7. renal ultrasound to rule out BOR and urinalysis to rule out Alport's;
8. eye examination/electroretinography to rule out Usher; and
9. comprehensive molecular genetic testing (Alford et al., 2014).

In general, an EKG, CMV assessment, and connexin testing are offered to all families, and an eye examination with an ophthalmologist should be considered. Although the Jervell and Lange-Nielsen syndrome is exceedingly rare, a properly performed EKG can identify some cases. As there are treatments for this disorder that can be lifesaving, this simple and cheap test appears justified for all children with sensorineural hearing loss (Morton & Nance, 2006). For Usher's syndrome, the hearing loss usually presents prior to the onset of visual changes making detection in infancy difficult without an electroretinography (ERG). The VDRL is offered to families of children who have been adopted, where the background of the parents might be unknown or when a concern regarding syphilis exists. Tests listed in Items 5 and 6 (above) are considered in older children or adults with progressive hearing loss when autoimmune disorders might occur. Finally, the renal ultrasound is used in children with the clinical stigma of BOR where pits, ear tags, and microtia/atresia exist. Routine screening for Alport's is not currently carried out because the proteinuria/hematuria is usually later in onset (Morton & Nance, 2006). Today, there are resources available to do more thorough evaluation of the genetic etiology of hearing loss. When children have been tested as above with negative results, more detailed testing can be offered (Alford et al., 2014).

Protocol Variation: Auditory Neuropathy (AN) or Auditory Neuropathy Spectrum Disorder (ANSD)

ANSD is a clinical syndrome characterized by the presence of OAEs and cochlear microphonics (CM) suggesting present hair cell function in conjunction with absent or grossly abnormal ABRs (Starr, Picton, Sininger, Hood, & Berlin, 1996). ANSD is thought to account for up to 10% of newly diagnosed cases of hearing loss in children (Madden, Rutter, Hilbert, Greinwald, & Choo, 2002). Less than 10% of ANSD cases are thought to involve only one ear. With bilateral presentation, patients exhibit a wide range of auditory capabilities. Hearing thresholds for pure-tone detection can range from normal to profound levels (Madden et al., 2002; Rance, Cone-Wesson, Wunderlich, & Dowell, 2002). Recent studies in older children and adults suggest that these patients' perceptual abilities can be severely impaired for both pitch discrimination in the low frequencies as well as temporal processing tasks

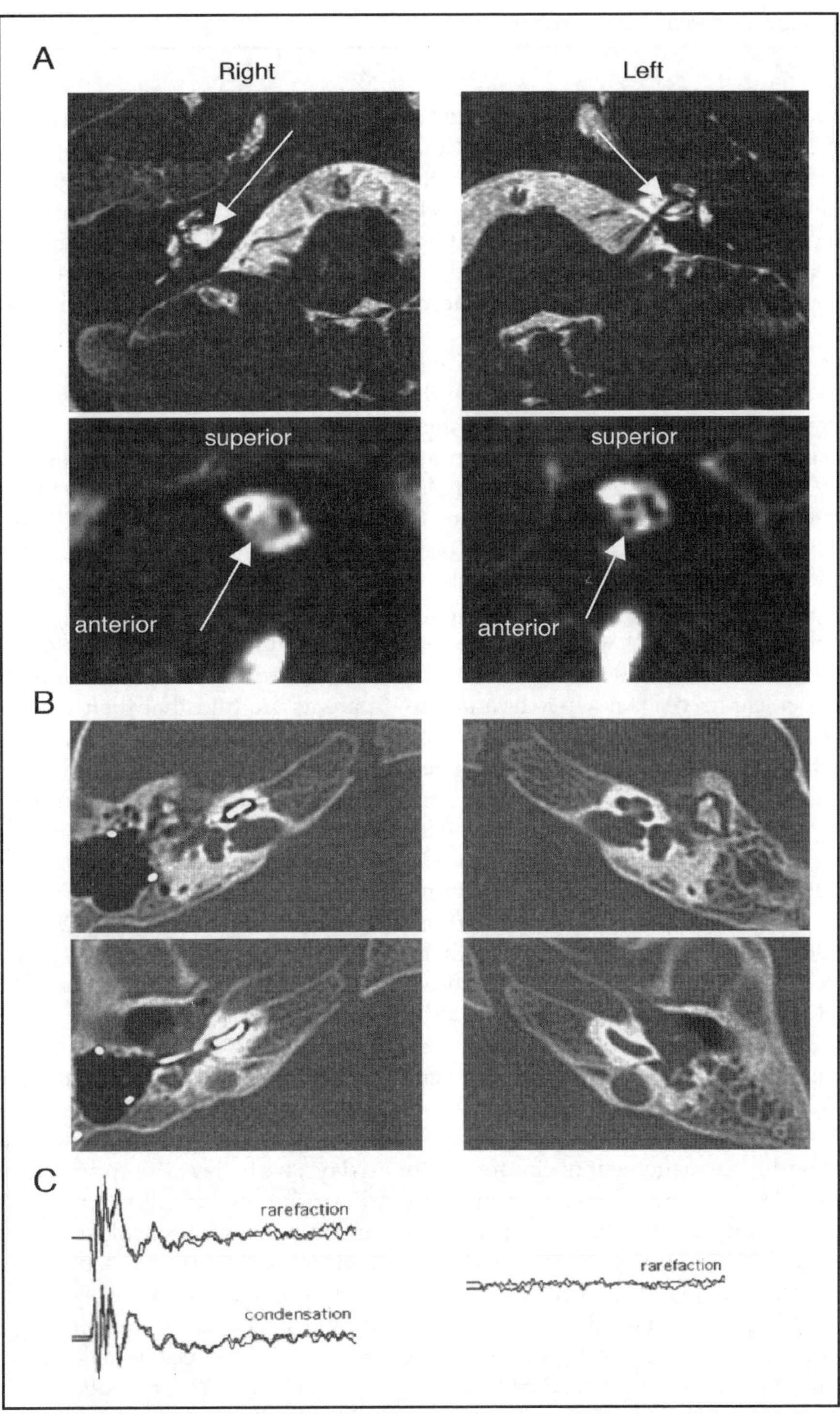

FIGURE 8–8. Cochlear nerve deficiency (right ear) in a child who experienced sudden hearing loss. **A.** MRI shows axial and parasagittal reconstructed images in a plane perpendicular to the IAC. In the left ear, four nerves (superior and inferior vestibular, facial and cochlear) are well visualized. In the right ear, the cochlear nerve is absent. The arrow points to the normal cochlear nerve on the left and the region of the absent cochlear nerve on the right. **B.** HRCT shows normal inner ear morphology and a satisfactorily placed cochlear implant in the ear without a cochlear nerve. **C.** The ABR shows a distinct cochlear microphonic in the right ear and no response in the ear with a normal nerve. The cochlear implant in the right ear provided limited perceptual abilities, and left cochlear implantation resulted in normal, open-set speech perception.

(Rance, McKay & Grayden, 2004; Zeng, Kong, Michalewski, & Starr, 2005). It has been hypothesized that lesions in the inner hair cells, the synapse between the inner hair cell and the auditory nerve, and the auditory nerve itself might account for the clinical findings (Berlin, Hood, Morlet, Rose, & Brashears, 2003a; Berlin, Morlet, & Hood, 2003b; Fuchs, Glowatzki, & Moser, 2003; Starr et al., 1996).

The etiology of ANSD appears to be multifactorial. Rather than a single lesion, it is plausible that the ANSD phenotype can result from a variety of lesions throughout the auditory pathway. Mutations in a number of genes (*MPZ, NDRG1, PMP22, OTOF, AUNA1*) have now been characterized in hereditary cases of ANSD (Varga et al., 2006). Associations have also been made between infectious (measles, mumps), metabolic (diabetes, hyperbilirubinemia, hypoxia), and neoplastic processes (acoustic neuroma), as well as prematurity (Rance et al., 1999; Starr et al., 2001). In most children with ANSD, the cochlear nerve is known to be anatomically present because residual hearing abilities exist. Many of these affected individuals have varying levels of pure-tone thresholds with disproportionately poor speech perception abilities. Because some children with ANSD who have received cochlear implants have had robust electrically evoked intracochlear compound action potentials (ECAPs) and good performance (Buss et al., 2002; Madden et al., 2002; Mason, De Michele, Stevens, Ruth, & Hashisaki, 2003), the abnormal hearing that some of these children have is thought to be due to disordered signal transduction at the inner hair cells, hair cell-dendrite synapse, or the cochlear neurons (e.g., ANSD; Berlin et al., 2003a, 2003b; Fuchs et al., 2003; Starr et al., 1996).

Opinions regarding management of children with ANSD vary widely. When hearing loss has been documented, conservative amplification has been proposed (Rance et al., 2002). On the contrary, other investigators believe that the distorted speech perception abilities resulting from ANSD preclude effective use of amplification (Berlin et al., 2003a). Regarding the utility of cochlear implantation in children with ANSD, limited data have demonstrated efficacy in many cases, implying that electrical stimulation might restore neural synchrony in some of these patients (Buss et al., 2002; Madden et al., 2002; Mason et al., 2003; Peterson et al., 2003; Sininger & Trautwein, 2002).

While at the University of North Carolina at Chapel Hill, we established a prospective, institutional review board (IRB)–approved protocol 5 years ago to study the clinical characteristics and outcomes of children with newly identified ANSD. The protocol was based on the premise that children with ANSD can have a diversity of clinical characteristics and auditory abilities, suggesting that some might benefit from certain interventions though others might not. We believed that some children with ANSD might have severely distorted perceptual abilities, as described above, while others might not. Thus, we chose to approach children with ANSD individually, assessing their perceptual abilities with and without amplification prior to considering cochlear implantation. Although this assessment and management paradigm sounds remarkably similar to that previously described for children without ANSD, some modifications were made in an attempt to understand better each child's perceptual abilities prior to instituting amplification or cochlear implantation. This management paradigm has been discussed in previous publications (Zdanski, Buchman, Roush, Teagle, & Brown, 2006).

In our program, when a child is identified with the electrophysiological characteristics of ANSD, the parents are told that their child has clear evidence of an auditory disorder. We also tell them that we cannot predict their child's auditory thresholds or speech perceptual abilities, and thus a period of careful observation ensues until an age when auditory thresholds can be determined. With highly experienced audiologists, thresholds are usually attainable using visual reinforcement audiometry (VRA) around 7 to 9 months corrected age. Should VRA demonstrate a significant hearing loss, a trial of amplification is instituted, based on real ear measures and prescriptive hearing aid targets. Should amplification prove fruitless in the setting of ongoing diagnostic and therapeutic speech and language therapy, cochlear implantation is then considered. Although this protocol does result in minor delays, we believe the approach is justified, so that children who can benefit from amplification are identified and inappropriate cochlear implantation is avoided. In children with multiple handicaps, VRA can frequently be impossible to obtain. For these children and their families, as well as the clinicians who care for them, rehabilitative decision making can be very difficult.

We are currently following approximately over 300 children with ANSD, all of whom had diagnostic electrophysiological testing carried out at our institution similar to that described previously. What is clear from looking at this group of children is that ANSD is a very heterogeneous group of disorders that presents with a common electrophysiological profile. Some children are profoundly affected by global and progressive neurological disease, and others are otherwise completely normal. Some children have a genetic form that is similar among affected siblings, and others have an association with prematurity, a stay in the

NICU, hyperbilirubinemia, and so on. When behavioral audiometry becomes possible, some children have near-normal pure-tone thresholds, while others have a profound hearing loss. Following determination of pure-tone thresholds, some children benefit from appropriately fitted amplification similar to those children with "typical sensorineural hearing loss," and others go on to cochlear implantation. Most of the children who have gone on to cochlear implantation have had severe-to-profound hearing loss and have met criteria for implantation based on conventional parameters. Very few children with ANSD and less than severe-to-profound hearing loss have received implants at our institution. Of this very select group of children with substantial residual hearing and ANSD, decision making on their behalf was very challenging for both the families and clinicians. In general, cochlear implantation has been very successful for most children with ANSD, although exceptions do exist. One group of children who provided significant insight into this disorder was those with anatomical cochlear nerve deficiency as detailed above (Buchman et al., 2006).

Medical Management of Hearing Loss in Children

The medical intervention for children with hearing loss depends on the type of hearing loss (conductive, sensorineural, mixed) and the functional-anatomical (or pathological) correlations that exist. Moreover, the desires and wishes of the family and child (in older children) are paramount. Patients and families not committed or interested in auditory-oral communication are by no means coerced into hearing restorative interventions unless medical necessity dictates such treatment. The details of every medical intervention for every type of hearing loss are beyond the scope of this work, but some generalizations can be made that might act as a rough guide for families and professionals.

Behavioral Audiometry

In our program, behavioral audiometric testing continues to form the backbone for decision making when medical/surgical intervention is being contemplated for a child. The shortcomings of both ABR and ASSR have been detailed previously. In short, these tests are clearly useful for estimating initial thresholds for the purposes of fitting amplification. Moreover, recent data from Hang et al. (2015) support the use of the "no-response ABR" in the decision-making process for children. Specifically, a "no-response" result on multiple frequency ABR in young children always resulted in progression to cochlear implantation in this study. Based on these results, we have adopted an approach that fast tracks such children to cochlear implantation following behavioral confirmation rather than spending long periods of time in hearing aid trials or repeated behavioral testing.

Hearing Restorative Medical Interventions

Hearing restorative medical interventions can be broadly classified into those that are disease specific or those that are not disease specific. Some examples of interventions that are not disease specific include referral for hearing aid evaluation and fitting or surgical placement of hearing devices such as cochlear implants, bone conduction devices, or auditory brainstem implants.

Cochlear Implants

Cochlear implants are reserved for those children with severe-to-profound sensorineural hearing loss (>90 dB) in the presence of anatomically intact cochleae and cochlear nerves. These children should also be enrolled in educational programs committed to an auditory-oral approach and demonstrate limited progress with speech and language development while using appropriately fitted amplification (http://www.nidcd.nih.gov/health/hearing/coch.asp). As the hearing loss is severe to profound, high-gain amplification is required, and these devices must be fitted using real ear measurements and according to prescribed hearing aid targets. In addition to the auditory and speech criteria listed above, participation in such a program requires significant commitment by the family members. In the best scenario, children are identified following birth by a newborn infant hearing screening program. Following verification in the first month of life, the diagnosis is confirmed by way of electrophysiological testing methods described above, and the trial of amplification is instituted. At the same time, the child is followed by a trained speech-language pathologist with experience in auditory-oral approaches. By 6 to 9 months of age, behavioral audiometry confirms the degree of hearing loss, and the therapist can provide feedback regarding auditory awareness and the development of the earliest vocalizations such as canonical babbling. When progress is evident, continued observation and therapy occur. Conversely, when the child is making limited progress, cochlear implantation is considered with the goal of getting the device implanted around the end of the first year of life (see Figure 8–2). Factors that might delay cochlear implantation beyond the first year of life include (a) delayed or inaccurate diagnosis, (b) delayed, underfitted, or nonused prescribed amplification, (c) lack of or inappropriate participation in a speech/language therapy trial, (d) medical comorbidities that delay diagnosis or preclude surgical intervention, (e) severe motor or cognitive developmental delays that hinder accurate auditory assessment, (f) diagnosis of ANSD, and (g) lack of commitment by the family. Later ages at implantation are also expected in children with progressive hearing loss, because these children achieve the severe-to-profound benchmark later in life and usually have better speech and language development because of their residual hearing.

Cochlear implant surgery takes roughly 90 min to 2 hr to perform at our institution. Following placement, intraoperative electrical telemetry is used to interrogate the device for integrity and to roughly estimate a starting point for programming in the postoperative period. Although complications are possible, they remain very unusual (Francis et al., 2008). Most children are implanted on an outpatient basis with anesthesia provided by a pediatric anesthesiologist. The children wear a head bandage for 3 to 5 days and return for a check approximately 1 week postoperatively. The device is usually activated 3 to 4 weeks postoperatively.

Outcomes following cochlear implantation in children are truly remarkable. Most children demonstrate significant closed-set speech perception ability with the benefit of visual cues after 1 year of usage. Open-set speech perception skills without the benefit of visual cues are usually evident after 2 to 3 years of device experience. Figure 8–9 demonstrates the results of speech perception testing using the phonetically balanced kindergarten (PBK; Haskins, 1949) word test for a group of 315 prelinguistic children implanted in our program as a function of years of implant usage and age at implantation. It is evident from the graph that earlier implantation is better for developing this skill.

Are bilateral cochlear implants better than unilateral implants in children? Recent evidence suggests that binaural implantation in postlinguistically deafened adults provides significant improvements for hearing in noise and sound localization abilities (Buss et al., 2008; Grantham, Ashmead, Ricketts, Labadie, &

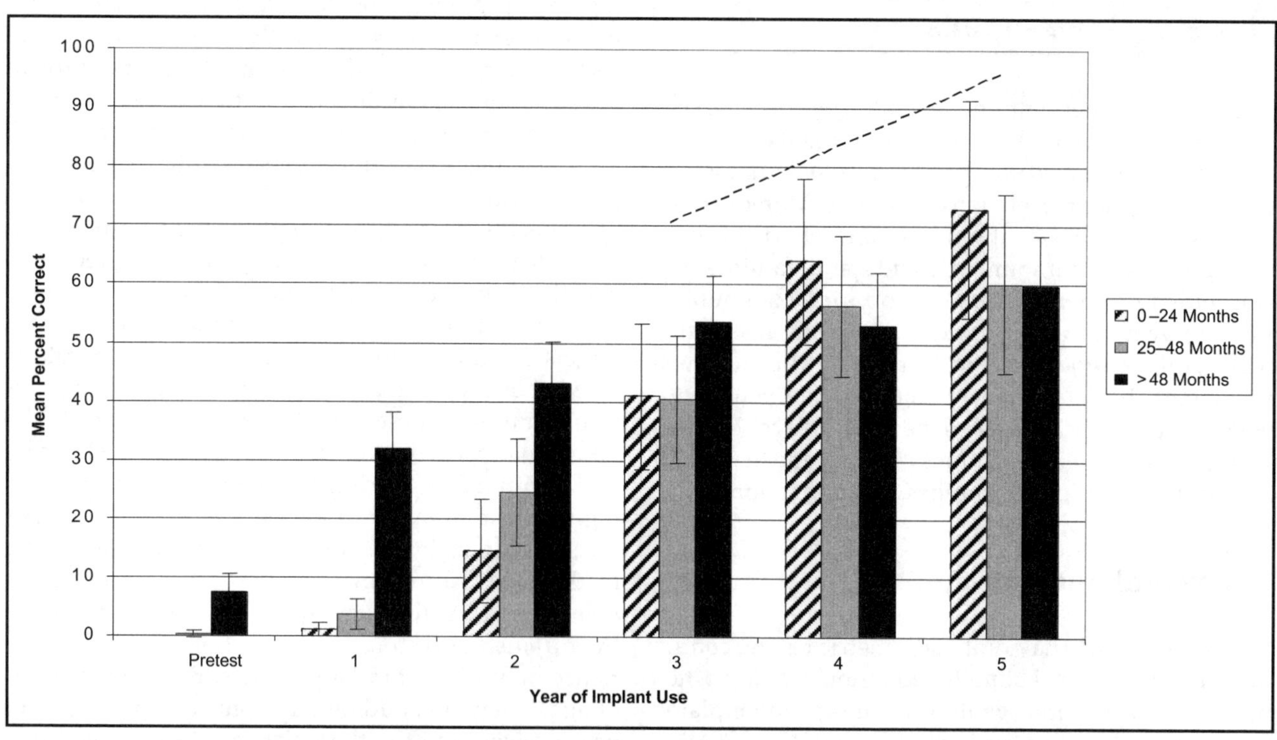

FIGURE 8–9. Phonetically balanced kindergarten (PBK) word scores as a function of duration of implant usage by age at implantation for 315 children with prelinguistic hearing loss. The dashed line indicates the scores for a group of children with normal hearing. In general, children implanted earlier ultimately achieve better scores at an earlier age than those children implanted later in life.

Haynes, 2007). In children, the data are only recently starting to emerge, but similar conclusions seem evident (Litovsky et al., 2006; Peters, Litovsky, Parkinson, & Lake, 2007). Only further research will determine whether there is a critical time window for developing these binaural skills in prelinguistic infants. Whether binaural implants will allow children to develop speech and language faster and to a higher level remains the critical unanswered question. What is clear regarding binaural implantation is that having a second device provides a backup should there be trouble with the equipment in one ear. Should the device problems require surgery, having the backup or second side device will prevent unwanted time "off the air."

Recent evidence suggests that children with sensorineural hearing loss with or without cochlear implants are at a higher risk for developing bacterial meningitis than the population in general (Biernath et al., 2006; Parner et al., 2007). It does appear from these data that cochlear implants impart an additional risk for contracting meningitis beyond that of having hearing loss alone. Although the factors responsible for this increased risk have not been completely elucidated, one particular model of cochlear implant device that used a separate electrode positioner was implicated as predisposing to meningitis at a much greater rate than other models. This model has been removed from the market. The findings of these studies also prompted the U.S. Food and Drug Administration (FDA) and the Centers for Disease Control and Prevention (CDC) to recommend routine vaccinations against the common bacteria implicated for cases of meningitis for all cochlear implantees. Thus, *Streptococcus pneumoniae* (i.e., pneumococcus) and *Haemophilus influenzae* Type B vaccinations are indicated for all children with cochlear implants. The pneumococcal vaccines include the heptavalent conjugate vaccine (Prevnar, Wyeth, Madison, New Jersey) for children less than age 2 years and the 23-valent polysaccharide vaccine (Pneumovax, Merck & Co, Whitehouse Station, New Jersey) after age 2 years and again 5 years later (before age 10 years). The precise recommendations of the CDC and FDA vaccine programs are available on the World Wide Web (http://www.cdc.gov/vaccines/vpd-vac/mening/cochlear/dis-cochlear-gen.htm). Currently, this vaccination is required prior to cochlear implantation in all children and adults in our program.

Implantable Bone Conduction Devices

Implantable bone conduction devices are used in children when significant conductive or mixed hearing loss exists and direct reconstruction of the hearing apparatus is either not feasible or not desired. This is relatively common in children with unilateral or poorly developed aural atresia. The current U.S. FDA-approved system for this application is the bone-anchored hearing appliance (BAHA; Cochlear Ltd. Macquarie University, NSW, Australia; Ponto, Oticon Medical, Askim, Sweden; Sophono, Boulder, Colorado). It is based on the concept of implanting an osseointegrated fixture into the skull to provide direct access to bone conduction of sound limiting the detrimental effects of soft tissue attenuation by the scalp. Low-gain amplification via osteo-oscillation is highly effective and very well tolerated. Implicit in the placement of such an implant is the need for a direct osseous connection; either via a percutaneous abutment or via an implantable magnetic system. With the percutaneous solutions, skin tolerance issues can be significant. Moreover, the skull of young children can be very thin precluding effective osseointegration. The BAHA is approved for use in children after age 5 years and is possible when skull thickness is sufficient (>3–4 mm). A preoperative CT scan can be useful in assessing skull thickness. The operation takes approximately 1 hour to perform and is usually outpatient surgery, although in children the operation is frequently performed in two stages. The device must heal for roughly 3 months prior to activation. It can be expected to provide auditory detection in the range of the bone conduction thresholds present on preoperative audiometric testing. The binaural benefits are only now becoming evident in congenitally affected patients (Kunst et al., 2008).

Auditory Brainstem Implants (ABIs)

Auditory brainstem implants (ABIs) are currently only approved for usage in the United States for children with cochlear nerve deficiency resulting from neurofibromatosis Type II. Although the initial results of ABIs in children without NF2 are interesting, further data regarding the risks and potential benefits are needed (Colletti, 2007). Currently, trials are ongoing in North Carolina, New York, Massachusetts, and California.

Ear Disease Management

Certain ear diseases that result in hearing loss can or must be addressed by way of disease-specific treatment of the underlying disorder. Examples of these disorders include otitis externa and otitis media, congenital ossicular malformations and atresia, sensorineural hearing losses resulting from inflammatory conditions, and tumors of the temporal bone and brain.

Otitis Externa

Otitis externa is defined as inflammation of the external auditory canal and commonly results from bacterial or fungal infection. The hallmark signs and symptoms of this disorder are pain with auricular motion, minimal discharge, and conductive hearing loss when canal swelling is substantial. These findings should prompt a visit to a physician with experience treating ear disorders. Otitis externa might follow ear canal trauma or contamination, such as that which occurs from swimming pools or bathtubs. In some instances, a poorly fitted hearing aid mold might cause pressure on the ear canal skin, thereby predisposing to infection. Treatment requires removal of the offending agent (foreign body or hearing aid ear mold) when present and application of an otic drop preparation containing either an acidifying or antimicrobial agent. When skin infection occurs outside of the ear canal, involving the pinna or surrounding soft tissues, an oral antimicrobial agent is also indicated. Patients with an immunocompromised state need to be treated particularly aggressively to prevent systemic infection and complications. Prevention in recurrent cases can usually be accomplished through careful cleaning and drying of hearing aid molds, removal of ear canal wax buildup, and prophylactic usage of drying agents (e.g., 50:50 mix of white vinegar and isopropyl alcohol) when the tympanic membrane is known to be intact (Buchman & Wambach, 2002).

Otitis Media

Otitis media is a primary inflammation of the middle ear space and commonly results from a bacterial or viral infection. Otitis media represents the most common ailment following the common cold for which a child will visit the doctor's office with a peak occurrence between the ages of 6 months and 2 years. Otitis media is commonly associated with episodes of upper respiratory tract infection and, thus, day care is a significant risk factor (Buchman & Das, 2003). The signs and symptoms of otitis media include some degree of conductive hearing loss with or without associated ear pain, fever, nausea, irritability, cold symptoms, and ear drainage if the tympanic membrane has ruptured. During episodes, fluid is evident behind the intact tympanic membrane and signs of inflammation might be present. Although the natural resolution rate is high, treatment is instituted to resolve pain more quickly, clear middle ear fluid, and prevent complications that at times can be severe and life threatening. Treatment of acute otitis media requires an oral antimicrobial agent and analgesics with follow-up to ensure the clearance of middle ear fluid. In otherwise uncomplicated cases, persistent middle ear fluid can take more than 3 months to resolve. Thus, associated conductive hearing loss should be expected. Tympanostomy tubes are considered for middle ear ventilation and drainage in an effort to decrease or eliminate the duration and severity of otitis media episodes, as well as to treat fluid- related hearing loss. Tympanostomy tubes are not routinely indicated for otherwise healthy children unless middle ear fluid persists for a prolonged period (>3–4 months) and is associated with significant hearing loss (>30 dB) or when the severity of otitis media episodes are severe and disabling. However, when children have other associated communication disorders such as permanent hearing loss, developmental delays in speech and language, craniofacial disorders, immune system disorders, or anatomical changes in the tympanic membrane that can predispose to complications, tube placement is considered earlier (Paradise & Bluestone, 2005).

Congenital Conductive Hearing Loss

Congenital conductive hearing loss can occur as a result of an isolated ossicular malformation or when external auditory canal atresia is present. For children with an isolated conductive loss with otherwise normal ear findings, stapes fixation represents the most common form of the disorder. Management of these children as infants is similar to those children with sensorineural hearing loss. That is, thresholds are determined, and amplification is fitted as early as possible. When an ear canal lumen is not present bilaterally, a bone conduction hearing aid is applied to take advantage of the excellent speech discrimination abilities that these children usually have. When the child is older, reconstructive surgical options versus BAHA can be considered.

For a child with a congenital conductive hearing loss, a nonspecific approach to the restoration of audition in the affected ear includes implantation of the BAHA device as described above (Kunst et al., 2008). For some families and children, the necessity for a percutaneous connector is unacceptable. Some payors will also not support this intervention because the price is considered prohibitive.

Another option for children with congenital conductive hearing loss is direct, surgical reconstruction. For the ear with an intact external auditory canal, this can be accomplished either through the canal or from a postauricular approach. When stapes fixation is identified, a stapedectomy or stapedotomy is possible with excellent hearing results anticipated. When the malleus or incus is involved, hearing outcomes might be slightly worse. Prior to considering middle ear exploration for congenital conductive hearing loss, preoperative imaging is needed to rule out an inner ear malformation that might predispose to intraoperative cerebrospinal fluid leakage and further hearing loss. This surgery is probably best carried out when the child is very cooperative and can understand the risks associated with such a surgery. This usually occurs around the age of 8 years or older (Welling, Merrell, Merz, & Dodson, 2003).

Reconstruction can also be considered for children with external auditory canal atresia. Indications for this procedure might include (a) bilateral involvement, (b) the presence of a developmental temporal bone cholesteatoma in the affected ear, or (c) when observation or the BAHA is unacceptable to the family for the previously mentioned reasons. This procedure is major otological surgery and requires a very cooperative patient in the postoperative period. The operation can take more than 4 hr and requires, in addition to an ear incision, a split thickness skin graft harvested from a site other than the head or neck (such as the leg or arm). Atresiaplasty is usually carried out after the time when the associated microtia surgery has been performed. Thus, most children undergo this surgery after the age of 7 or 8 years.

The results of atresiaplasty are quite variable and are dependent on the operating surgeon's experience, the healing of the patient, and the patient's anatomy. In general, roughly 75% of patients achieve a postoperative air-bone gap of less than 30 dB. In those with a patent ear canal that is dry, a conventional hearing aid is also possible, thereby obviating the need for a bone conductor (McKinnon & Jahrsdoerfer, 2002).

Inner Ear Malformations

Inner ear malformations are present in 20% to 30% of children with congenital sensorineural hearing loss. These children can present in a variety of ways. Although most will fail a newborn screen, some might not. Children with these anomalies clearly have a higher incidence of progressive hearing loss. It has been posited that sudden drops in hearing might be related to minor degrees of head trauma in these children. Many of these children will ultimately go on to cochlear implantation, which has a number of special considerations in this population (Buchman et al., 2004).

Although there is currently no available method to repair developmental anomalies of the inner ear, a few facts are important for managing these children. First, it important for families to recognize that progressive hearing loss is common in these children. Moreover, children with inner ear malformations are at a higher risk for developing meningitis than children without malformations. Families need to be educated regarding the signs and symptoms of meningitis and about aggressive treatment of otitis media. In this regard, these children should also be considered for preventive vaccination similar to children with cochlear implants. Finally, because of the association of sudden hearing changes and head trauma in these children, families are cautioned regarding their participation in contact sports and activities.

Acknowledgments. We would like to thank those individuals that work with me on a daily basis, to provide care for the hearing-impaired children we are so privileged to serve. Their efforts are no less than spectacular.

References

Adunka, O. F., Jewells, V., & Buchman, C. A. (2007). Value of computed tomography in the evaluation of children with cochlear nerve deficiency. *Otology and Neurotology, 28*(5), 597–604.

Adunka, O. F., Roush, P. A., Teagle, H. F., Brown, C. J., Zdanski, C. J., Jewells, V., & Buchman, C. A. (2006). Internal auditory canal morphology in children with cochlear nerve deficiency. *Otology and Neurotology, 27*(6), 793–801.

Ahn, J. H., Lee, H. S., Kim, Y. J., Yoon, T. H., & Chung, J. W. (2007). Comparing pure-tone audiometry and auditory steady state response for the measurement of hearing loss. *Otolaryngology-Head and Neck Surgery, 136*(6), 966–971.

Alford, R. L., Arnos, K. S., Fox, M., Lin, J. W., Palmer, C. G., Pandya, A., . . . Yoshinaga-Itano, C. (2014). ACMG Working Group on Update of Genetics Evaluation Guidelines for the Etiologic Diagnosis of Congenital Hearing Loss; Professional Practice and Guidelines Committee. American College of Medical Genetics and Genomics guideline for the clinical evaluation and etiologic diagnosis of hearing loss. *Genetic Medicine, 16*(4), 347–355.

American Academy of Pediatrics and Joint Committee on Infant Hearing. (2007). Year 2007 position statement: Principles and guidelines for early hearing detection and intervention programs. *Pediatrics, 120*(4), 898–921.

Baskin, H. J., & Hedlund, G. (2007). Neuroimaging of herpesvirus infections in children. *Pediatric Radiology, 37*(10), 949–963.

Berlin, C. I., Hood, L., Morlet, T., Rose, K., & Brashears, S. (2003a). Auditory neuropathy/dys-synchrony: Diagnosis and management. *Mental Retardation and Developmental Disability Research and Reviews, 9*(4), 225–231.

Berlin, C. I., Morlet, T., & Hood, L. J. (2003b). Auditory neuropathy/dyssynchrony: Its diagnosis and management. *Pediatric Clinics of North America, 50*(2), 331–340.

Biernath, K. R., Reefhuis, J., Whitney, C. G., Mann, E. A., Costa, P., Eichwald, J., & Boyle, C. (2006). Bacterial meningitis among children with cochlear implants beyond 24 months after implantation. *Pediatrics, 117*(2), 284–289.

Buchman, C. A., Copeland, B. J., Yu, K. K., Brown, C. J., Carrasco, V. N., & Pillsbury H. C. III. (2004). Cochlear implantation in children with congenital inner ear malformations. *Laryngoscope, 114*(2), 309–316.

Buchman, C. A., & Das, S. (2003). Prevention of acute otitis media during the common cold. In C. Alper, C. Bluestone, M. Casselbrant, J. Dohar, & E. Mandel (Eds.), *Advanced therapy of otitis media* (pp. 152–157). Hamilton, Ontario, Canada: B.C. Decker.

Buchman, C. A., Roush, P. A., Teagle, H. F., Brown, C. J., Zdanski, C. J., & Grose, J. H. (2006). Auditory neuropathy characteristics in children with cochlear nerve deficiency. *Ear and Hearing, 27*(4), 399–408.

Buchman, C. A., & Wambach, B. A. (2002). Otitis externa. In R. E. Rakel & E. T. Bope (Eds.), *Conn's current therapy* (pp. 114–117). Philadelphia, PA: W.B. Saunders.

Buss, E., Labadie, R., Brown, C., Gross, A., Grose, J., & Pillsbury, H. (2002). Outcome of cochlear implantation in pediatric auditory neuropathy. *Otology and Neurotology, 23*, 328–332.

Buss, E., Pillsbury, H. C., Buchman, C. A., Pillsbury, C. H., Clark, M. S., Haynes, D. S., . . . Barco, A. L. (2008). Multicenter U.S. bilateral MED-EL cochlear implantation study: Speech perception over the first year of use. *Ear and Hearing, 29*(1), 20–32.

Colletti, L. (2007). Beneficial auditory and cognitive effects of auditory brainstem implantation in children. *Acta Otolaryngologica, 127*(9), 943–946.

Coticchia, J. M., Gokhale, A., Waltonen, J., & Sumer, B. (2006). Characteristics of sensorineural hearing loss in children with inner ear anomalies. *American Journal of Otolaryngology, 27*(1), 33–38.

Francis, H. W., Buchman, C. A., Visaya, J. M., Wang, N. Y., Zwolan, T. A., Fink, N. E., . . . The CDaCI Investigative Team. (2008). Surgical factors in pediatric cochlear implantation and their early effects on electrode activation and functional outcomes. *Otology and Neurotology, 29*(4), 502–508.

Fuchs, P. A., Glowatzki, E., & Moser, T. (2003). The afferent synapse of cochlear hair cells. *Current Opinion in Neurobiology, 13*(4), 452–458.

Gorga, M. P., Johnson, T. A., Kaminski, J. R., Beauchaine, K. L., Garner, C. A., & Neely, S. T. (2006). Using a combination of click- and tone burst-evoked auditory brain stem response measurements to estimate pure-tone thresholds. *Ear and Hearing, 27*(1), 60–74.

Gorga, M. P., Neely, S. T., Hoover, B. M., Dierking, D. M., Beauchaine, K. L., & Manning, C. (2004). Determining the upper limits of stimulation for auditory steady-state response measurements. *Ear and Hearing, 25*(3), 302–307.

Grantham, D. W., Ashmead, D. H., Ricketts, T. A., Labadie, R. F., & Haynes, D. S. (2007). Horizontal-plane localization of noise and speech signals by postlingually deafened adults fitted with bilateral cochlear implants. *Ear and Hearing, 28*(4), 524–541.

Hang, A. X., Roush, P. A., Teagle, H. F., Zdanski, C., Pillsbury, H. C., Adunka, O. F., & Buchman, C. A. (2015). Is "no response" on diagnostic auditory brainstem response testing an indication for cochlear implantation in children? *Ear and Hearing, 36*(1), 8–13.

Haskins, H. (1949). *A phonetically balanced test of speech discrimination for children* (Unpublished master's thesis). Northwestern University: Evanston, IL.

Jan, W., Zimmerman, R. A., Bilaniuk, L. T., Hunter, J. V., Simon, E. M., & Haselgrove, J. (2003). Diffusion-weighted imaging in acute bacterial meningitis in infancy. *Neuroradiology, 45*(9), 634–639.

Joint Committee on Infant Hearing of the American Academy of Pediatrics, Muse, C., Harrison, J., Yoshinaga-Itano, C., Grimes, A., Brookhouser, P. E., . . . Martin, B. (2013). Supplement to the JCIH 2007 position statement: Principles and guidelines for early intervention after confirmation that a child is deaf or hard of hearing. *Pediatrics, 131*(4), e1324–e1349.

Katar, S., Akay, H. O., Taskesen, M., & Devecioglu, C. (2008). Clinical and cranial magnetic resonance imaging (MRI) findings of 21 patients with serious hyperbilirubinemia. *Journal of Child Neurology, 23*(4), 415–417.

Kunst, S. J., Leijendeckers, J. M., Mylanus, E. A., Hol, M. K., Snik, A. F., & Cremers, C. W. (2008). Bone-anchored hearing aid system application for unilateral congenital conductive hearing impairment: Audiometric results. *Otology and Neurotology, 29*(1), 2–7.

Litovsky, R. Y., Johnstone, P. M., Godar, S., Agrawal, S., Parkinson, A., Peters, R., & Lake, J. (2006). Bilateral cochlear implants in children: Localization acuity measured with minimum audible angle. *Ear and Hearing, 27*(1), 43–59.

Madden, C., Rutter, M., Hilbert, L., Greinwald, J. H. Jr., & Choo, D. I. (2002). Clinical and audiological features in auditory neuropathy. *Archives of Otolaryngology-Head and Neck Surgery, 128*(9), 1026–1030.

Mason, J. C., De Michele, A., Stevens, C., Ruth, R. A., & Hashisaki, G. T. (2003). Cochlear implantation in patients with auditory neuropathy of varied etiologies. *Laryngoscope, 113*(1), 45–49.

McKinnon, B. J., & Jahrsdoerfer, R. A. (2002). Congenital auricular atresia: Update on options for intervention and timing of repair. *Otolaryngologic Clinics of North America, 35*(4), 877–890.

Moog, J. S., & Geers, A. E. (2003). Epilogue: Major findings, conclusions and implications for deaf education. *Ear and Hearing, 24*(1 Suppl), 121S–125S.

Morton, C. C., & Nance, W. E. (2006). Newborn hearing screening—A silent revolution. *New England Journal of Medicine, 354*(20), 2151–2164.

Paradise, J. L., & Bluestone, C. D. (2005). Consultation with the specialist: Tympanostomy tubes: A contemporary guide to judicious use. *Pediatric Reviews, 26*(2), 61–66.

Parisi, M. A., & Dobyns, W. B. (2003). Human malformations of the midbrain and hindbrain: Review and proposed classification scheme. *Molecular Genetics and Metabolism, 80*(1–2), 36–53.

Parner, E. T., Reefhuis, J., Schendel, D., Thomsen, J. L., Ovesen, T., & Thorsen, P. (2007). Hearing loss diagnosis followed by meningitis in Danish children, 1995–2004. *Otolaryngology-Head and Neck Surgery, 136*(3), 428–433.

Parry, D. A., Booth, T., & Roland, P. S. (2005). Advantages of magnetic resonance imaging over computed tomography in preoperative evaluation of pediatric cochlear implant candidates. *Otology and Neurotology, 26*(5), 976–982.

Peters, B. R., Litovsky, R., Parkinson, A., & Lake, J. (2007). Importance of age and postimplantation experience on speech perception measures in children with sequential bilateral cochlear implants. *Otology and Neurotology, 28*(5), 649–657.

Peterson, A., Shallop, J., Driscoll, C., Breneman, A., Babb, J., Stoeckel, R., & Fabry, L. (2003). Outcomes of cochlear implantation in children with auditory neuropathy. *Journal of the American Academy of Audiology, 14*(4), 188–201.

Rance, G., Beer, D., Cone-Wesson, B., Shepard, R. K., Dowell, R. C., King, A. M., . . . Clark, G. M. (1999). Clinical findings for a group of infants and young children with auditory neuropathy. *Ear and Hearing, 20*(3), 238–263.

Rance, G., Cone-Wesson, B., Wunderlich, J., & Dowell, R. (2002). Speech perception and cortical event related potentials in children with auditory neuropathy. *Ear and Hearing, 23*(3), 239–253.

Rance, G., McKay, C., & Grayden, D. (2004). Perceptual characterization of children with auditory neuropathy. *Ear and Hearing, 25*(1), 34–46.

Schuknecht, H. F. (1993). *Pathology of the ear* (2nd ed.). Philadelphia, PA: Lea and Febiger.

Sininger, Y. S., & Trautwein, P. (2002). Electrical stimulation of the auditory nerve via cochlear implants in patients with auditory neuropathy. *Annals of Otology, Rhinology, and Laryngology, 189*, 29–31.

Small, S. A., & Stapells, D. R. (2004). Artifactual responses when recording auditory steady-state responses. *Ear and Hearing, 25*(6), 611–623.

Stapells, D. R., Herdman, A., Small, S. A., Dimitrijevic, A., & Hatton, J. (2005). Current status of the auditory steady-state responses for estimating an infant's audiogram. In R. C. Seewald & J. Bamford (Eds.), *A sound foundation through early amplification 2004: Proceedings of the third international conference* (pp. 43–59). Stäfa, Switzerland: Phonak AG.

Starr, A., Picton, T., Sininger, Y., Hood, L., & Berlin, C. (1996). Auditory neuropathy. *Brain, 119*, 741–753.

Starr, A., Sininger, Y., Nguyen, T., Michalewski, H. J., Oba, S., & Abdala, C. (2001). Cochlear receptor (microphonic and summating potentials, otoacoustic emissions) and auditory pathway (auditory brainstem potentials) activity in auditory neuropathy. *Ear and Hearing, 22*(2), 91–99.

Tlumak, A. I., Rubinstein, E., & Durrant, J. D. (2007). Meta-analysis of variables that affect accuracy of threshold estimation via measurement of the auditory steady-state response (ASSR). *International Journal of Audiology, 46*(11), 692–710.

Trimble, K., Blaser, S., James, A. L., & Papsin, B. C. (2007). Computed tomography and/or magnetic resonance imaging before pediatric cochlear implantation? Developing an investigative strategy. *Otology and Neurotology, 28*(3), 317–324.

Varga, R., Avenarius, M. R., Kelley, P. M., Keats, B. J., Berlin, C. I., Hood, L. J., . . . Kimberling, W. J. (2006). OTOF mutations revealed by genetic analysis of hearing loss families including a potential temperature sensitive auditory neuropathy allele. *Journal of Medical Genetics, 43*(7), 576–581.

Welling, D. B., Merrell, J. A., Merz, M., & Dodson, E. E. (2003). Predictive factors in pediatric stapedectomy. *Laryngoscope, 113*(9), 1515–1519.

Young, N. M., Hughes, C. A., Byrd, S. E., & Darling, C. (2000). Postmeningitic ossification in pediatric cochlear implantation. *Otolaryngology-Head and Neck Surgery, 122*(2), 183–188.

Zdanski, C. J., Buchman, C. A., Roush, P. A., Teagle, H. F. B., & Brown, C. J. (2006). Cochlear implantation in children with auditory neuropathy. *Perspectives on Hearing and Hearing Disorders in Childhood, 16*(1), 12–20.

Zeng, F. G., Kong, Y. Y., Michalewski, H. J., & Starr, A. (2005). Perceptual consequences of disrupted auditory nerve activity. *Journal of Neurophysiology, 93*(6), 3050–3063.

Current Issues in Preventable Hearing Loss

Andrea Hillock-Dunn and Christopher Spankovich

Introduction

Sensorineural hearing loss affects an estimated 1.8% of newborns and 3.5% of adolescents (Morton & Nance, 2006). It is well known that congenital and early onset hearing loss have significant and far-reaching consequences on receptive and expressive speech and language ability, learning, and health and wellness. Children with hearing loss are more likely to exhibit communication challenges, poor academic attainment, and social-emotional or self-esteem challenges. Although 50% or more of prelingual hearing loss is attributed to genetics (often unidentified nonsyndromic causes), 25% to 50% of early onset hearing loss is associated with environmental factors or unknown etiology (Morton, 1991; Smith, Bale, & White, 2005). A growing number of variables associated with acquired hearing loss have been identified, and the relationship of pre-, peri-, and postnatal factors and hearing outcomes are reviewed.

Prenatal to Perinatal Period

Disease and Infection and Hearing Loss

The Joint Committee on Infant Hearing (JCIH) position statement and supplement specifies risk factors for neonatal, congenital and delayed-onset hearing loss, and provides guidelines for diagnostic, rehabilitative, and early-intervention initiatives (2007, 2013); a full description of JCIH risk factors can be found in Chapter 7. Included among the risk indicators outlined by JCIH is diagnosis of pre- or postnatal virus or infection known to impact hearing. Although the association between maternal infection and fetal hearing damage is well established, fluctuation in the incidence of exposure has changed the global landscape of congenital, acquired hearing loss.

The term *TORCH* refers to a group of infections including toxoplasmosis, other (syphilis, varicella-zoster, parvovirus), rubella, cytomegalovirus (CMV), and herpes virus, which increase the risk of adverse health effects including hearing loss (JCIH, 2007). Two of these infections, rubella and CMV, remain relevant in the United States and abroad and will be explored.

Rubella

The last 40 years have seen a national and global decline in maternal rubella following licensure of a live vaccine in 1969 in the United States (Preblud, Serdula, Frank, & Hinman, 1980). Reported cases of rubella dropped from an estimated 12.5 million between 1964 and 1965 to a median of 11 cases annually from the mid-to-late 2000s (Centers for Disease Control and Prevention [CDC], 2015; Papania et al., 2014). Similarly, diagnoses of congenital rubella syndrome (CRS) decreased from roughly 20,000 to fewer than five infants annually over the same time span (CDC, 2015; Papania et al., 2014). Although rubella has been virtually eradicated in most industrialized nations, maternal rubella infection persists in some areas of the world. In 2002, only 48% of developing countries reported vaccine use, up from 28% in 1996 (Robertson, Featherstone, Gacic-Dobo, & Hersh, 2003). Furthermore, despite vaccination efforts, recent rubella epidemics (2012– 2013) have occurred in countries such as Poland and Japan, where most affected individuals reportedly had negative or unknown vaccination histories (CDC, 2013). Recent global estimates indicate that over 100,000 babies are born with CRS annually (Robertson et al., 2003). Sensorineural hearing loss remains the most common sequela of fetal rubella exposure, affecting more than half of children (e.g., Dammeyer, 2010). Higher rates of fetal infection are reported with earlier (first trimester) exposure (Webster, 1998).

Although rubella may manifest as a mild rash and fever in mothers, CRS produces more serious and enduring symptoms including congenital heart defect, deafness, and blindness. Sensorineural hearing loss in children with CRS typically develops in the first year of life and is commonly bilateral ranging from mild to profound. It is thought to arise from rubella-mediated cell death in the organ of Corti and stria vascularis as well as alterations in the endolymphatic fluid of the cochlea (Lee & Bowden, 2000; Webster, 1998).

Cytomegalovirus

Following the global decline in maternal rubella and CRS, congenital CMV supplanted rubella as the leading nongenetic cause of congenital hearing loss in the United States and other developed countries (Manicklal, Emery, Lazzarotto, Boppana, & Gupta, 2013). Seroprevalence rates vary globally, with higher infection rates reported in less developed countries (e.g., Cannon, 2009). In industrialized nations like the United States, approximately half of women of childbearing age show evidence of prior CMV infection as evidenced by the presence of CMV antibodies in the bloodstream (CDC, 2010). Predisposing factors for prior infection include sex (female predominance), ethnicity, household education level, and socioeconomic status (SES; e.g., Bate, Dollard, & Cannon, 2010; Colugnati, Staras, Dollard, & Cannon, 2007; Hyde, Schmid, & Cannon, 2010). Non-white women with lower SES and education levels, in crowded living conditions, and caring for young children (birth to 3 years) have higher seroprevalence and subconversion rates (Hyde et al., 2010).

One to 4% of women develop primary (first) CMV infection during pregnancy, resulting in fetal infection in roughly one third of cases (CDC, 2010). Conversely, the rate of fetal transmission (1.4%) is markedly lower in seropositive mothers with viral reactivation (CDC, 2010). CMV might go undetected or produce mild flu-like symptoms resembling mononucleosis in healthy mothers but have significant, lasting consequences on fetuses infected prenatally. In the United States, congenital CMV occurs in an estimated 0.6% to 1% of total live births, with symptoms displaying in 5% to 20% of cases (Cannon, 2009; CDC, 2010; Demmler, 1991; Fowler et al., 1997; Kenneson & Cannon, 2007; Madden et al., 2005). Manifestations of prenatal CMV infection can include intrauterine growth restriction, hearing or vision loss, seizures, microcephaly, and neurodevelopmental delays (Cannon, 2009; CDC, 2010). Sensorineural hearing loss can occur with symptomatic and asymptomatic CMV, but higher hearing loss prevalence is reported in symptomatic (35%–40%) versus asymptomatic (9%–11%) cases (e.g., Dollard, Grosse, & Ross, 2007; Fowler & Boppana, 2006; Fowler et al., 1997; Grosse, Ross, & Dollard, 2008). Congenital CMV infection can be identified through urine or saliva screenings performed before 2 to 3 weeks of life, but such screenings are not routinely performed in apparently healthy infants. Hence, it has been speculated that undiagnosed congenital (asymptomatic) CMV accounts for a portion of idiopathic early onset hearing loss (e.g., Fowler et al., 1997; Grosse et al., 2008).

Hearing loss presentation is variable but often severe-to-profound (Fowler & Boppana, 2006; Goderis et al., 2014; Madden et al., 2005). It is more commonly unilateral in asymptomatic patients, bilateral in symptomatic cases, and can fluctuate or progress (Fowler & Boppana, 2006; Fowler et al., 1997; Madden et al., 2005). Delayed-onset hearing loss has also been documented, resulting in a mean age at time of hearing loss identification of over 2 years (range = 1–5 years of age; Fowler et al., 1997). Given the risk for later-developing loss, audiologic monitoring is recommended for babies with known congenital CMV, regardless of newborn hearing screening result (Fowler et al., 1997; for a more in-depth description of CMV epidemiology, see reviews by Kenneson and Cannon [2007] and Manicklal et al. [2013]).

Like rubella, the mechanisms underlying CMV-related hearing damage are not completely understood, but it is speculated that damage is due to the direct action of the virus or the body's immune response to the virus. Temporal bone studies have identified the presence of viral antigens in various cochlear structures and inflammation and swelling of the cochlea and spiral ganglion cells, but the mechanism for hearing loss progression or delayed-onset loss remains nebulous (review by Cohen, Durstenfeld, & Roehm, 2014). Currently, experimental drug treatment studies are underway, which suggest that antivirals (e.g., ganciclovir) reduce viral shedding time in asymptomatic infants. However, as yet it is unclear whether faster shedding results in greater hearing preservation. For a more complete list of viral causes of hearing loss, hearing loss presentation, and so on, see Cohen et al. (2014).

Rubella and CMV can be passed between individuals through blood and bodily fluids including secretions or droplets from the nose or throat, urine, and breast milk. CMV can also be spread through semen or vaginal fluid. Fetal infection can arise from the transfer of infected blood via the placenta or from maternal to fetal blood or fluid exchange during the birth process. Although transmission can occur any time during pregnancy, the risk of miscarriage, rubella-associated birth defects, and symptomatic, congenital CMV is greatest for first-trimester exposure (Andrade et al., 2006); perinatal or early postnatal infections generally produce only mild, recoverable symptoms.

Vaccination programs have virtually eliminated rubella in the United States, but maternal rubella infection persists in less-developed nations. Currently, there is no CMV vaccine. Good hygiene practices such as frequent and diligent hand washing might reduce virus transmission, and continued research on antiviral therapy could further decrease the incidence of hearing loss and other symptoms from congenital infection (Kimberlin et al., 2003; Stowell et al., 2014).

Drugs and Hearing Loss

Research on fetal outcomes following gestational exposure to illicit, recreational, and prescribed drugs is limited, and conclusions regarding drug safety are generally tenuous. Methodological factors (e.g., small sample sizes, retrospective design) challenge studies and person-specific factors such as dosing, polysubstance use, medical conditions, access to health care, and so on, can modulate drug effects and limit conclusions. Drug use is generally not advised during pregnancy, except in cases of medical necessity. The U.S. Food and Drug Administration (FDA) has developed definitions and drug classifications to try to assign drug-related risk based on animal and human research. The safest drugs, Category A, do not pose any risk to the fetus based on human research, whereas Category X drugs have a proven risk to the fetus that outweighs possible benefit(s). Intermediary drug categories show evidence of possible fetal health risks such as hearing loss. Health effects have also been associated with exposure to some teratogenic chemicals such as polychlorinated biphenyls (PCBs), although drug labeling and category assignment might not be required for some pollutants.

Drugs and chemicals can reach the developing fetus through the placenta and might impact the fetus directly or indirectly by impairing maternal health, uterine status, or placental functioning. The placenta provides a blood and nutrient exchange between mother and baby, facilitates waste removal, and provides a protective barrier by reducing the passage of foreign agents from maternal blood into the fetal circulatory system. However, the protective function is imperfect as nearly all drugs achieve varying amounts of passive transplacental diffusion and some display active transport (Syme, Paxton, & Keelan, 2004). Variables influencing drug transfer include the degree of binding to plasma proteins, placenta metabolism, and features of the compound. Lipid-soluble, uncharged agents with lower molecular weights can cross more easily, resulting in greater fetal exposure. Gestational age at time of drug administration can also modulate fetal drug effects. Drug sensitivity varies during the course of auditory system development and with emerging hepatic and renal function, which affect the efficiency with which drugs are filtered and excreted by the fetus.

Prenatal drug exposure has been associated with both mild and more marked fetal health effects including intrauterine growth restriction, prematurity, neurological deficits, and hearing loss. Although the literature on fetal drug and chemical exposure is scant and many studies suffer from methodological limitations (e.g., retrospective, underpowered), various drugs and chemicals have been implicated as increasing hearing loss risk or causing alterations in auditory system functioning following fetal exposure.

Recreational and Social Drugs

A recent U.S. survey reported past-month illicit drug use in 5% of pregnant respondents ages 15 to 44 years (Aldworth, 2009), but studies have shown that prevalence estimates might be conservative due to underreporting (e.g., Ostrea, Brady, Gause, Raymundo, & Stevens, 1992). For example, in a study of newborns delivered in a high-risk, urban area, positive meconium drug screens indicative of cocaine, morphine, and cannabinoid exposure were identified in 88% of babies despite admitted drug use by only 11% of mothers (Ostrea et al., 1992). Reports across studies vary, but older, single, females with lower SES, receiving little prenatal care typically exhibit higher rates of prenatal drug use than the general population (e.g., Aldworth, 2009; Day, Cottreau, & Richardson, 1993; Ostrea et al., 1992). Ethnic and geographical trends in women of childbearing age suggest increased drug use in Native American/Alaska Native and bi- or multiracial individuals compared to other ethnic groups and women living in large, urban environments versus more rural settings (Aldworth, 2009). Recreational and social drug use during pregnancy may be related to depression among other factors (Hanna, Faden, & Dufour, 1994).

Heroin and Cocaine

Both opiates (e.g., heroin, methadone) and psychostimulants (e.g., cocaine) can impact fetal health and development, and presentation is variable. In humans, prenatal opiate exposure has been associated with intrauterine growth restriction (IUGR), low birth weight, neonatal abstinence syndrome, seizures, and developmental delays (e.g., language, motor, cognition; Bandstra, Morrow, Mansoor, & Accornero, 2010; Beckwith & Burke, 2015; Bunikowski et al., 1998; Naeye, Blanc, Leblanc, & Khatamee, 1973). Elevated risk of fetal growth restriction, neurologic events, and developmental challenges (e.g., language, attention, learning) have also been linked to prenatal cocaine use (e.g., Chasnoff, Burns, Schnoll, & Burns, 1985; Eyler, Behnke, Conlon, Woods, & Wobie, 1998; Singer et al., 2002; Zuckerman et al., 1989).

In addition, altered auditory system functioning has been reported in newborns with histories of prenatal drug exposure, but study findings vary. For example, Grimmer, Bührer, Aust, and Obladen (1999) observed no difference in auditory brainstem response (ABR) thresholds of infants with and without prenatal heroin exposure, but others noted prolonged wave V latency and I-V interpeak latencies in gestationally exposed newborns (Trammer, Aust, Köster, & Obladen, 1992). Aberrant ABR findings suggestive of central system effects have also been observed with prenatal cocaine exposure (Church, Crossland, Holmes, Overbeck, & Tilak, 1998; Cone-Wesson, 2005; Shih, Cone-Wesson, & Reddix, 1988). Cocaine-exposed rat pups showed delayed ABR maturation (Church et al., 1998), and prenatally cocaine-exposed babies had prolonged peak and interpeak latencies for later ABR components (III, V) indicating abnormality at or above the cochlear nucleus (Cone-Wesson, 2005; Shih et al., 1988). Although latency changes have also been reported in babies with IUGR and low birth weight without drug exposure histories (Salamy, 1984), prolongations are reportedly greater in those exposed to cocaine in utero (Cone-Wesson & Spingarn, 1993). The behavioral byproducts of latency alterations are currently unknown, but their association with delayed language function has been speculated (e.g., Cone-Wesson, 2005; Cone-Wesson, Kurtzberg, & Vaughan Jr, 1987).

Alcohol and Tobacco

Prenatal alcohol and tobacco use also has potential consequences on fetal health and hearing and is relatively common. In the National Survey of Drug Use and Health, 11% of pregnant respondents reported alcohol use (Aldworth, 2009). Consumption was characterized as binge (5+ drinks at same occasion) or heavy drinking (binge drinking >5 times in 30 days) by nearly half of women, and 6% of pregnant alcohol consumers reported first-trimester binge drinking. Factors associated with higher prenatal alcohol exposure risk and fetal alcohol spectrum disorder (FASD) include advanced maternal age, history of binge drinking, low SES, poor mental health (e.g., low self-esteem, depression), and alcohol abuse by a family member. Prevalence rates for fetal alcohol spectrum disorder vary, but a conservative estimate is 0.5 to 2 births per 1,000 in the United States (May & Gossage, 2001).

FAS sequelae include dysmorphic facial features (e.g., short palpebral fissures, cleft lip and/or palate), growth retardation, and central nervous system effects (e.g., cognitive and learning impairment, behavioral disorders). Facial malformations resulting from disrupted neural folding have implications for conductive hearing loss, and peripheral and central system effects have been speculated based on observations of cell death in the otic placode, vestibulocochlear ganglia, and brain malformations in ethanol-exposed mouse embryos (Du & Hamre, 2001; Goodlett & Horn, 2001; Kotch & Sulik, 1992). In vivo studies also suggest increased hearing loss risk following prenatal ethanol exposure. Church (1987) reported elevated ABR thresholds in 19% of alcohol-exposed rat pups, and prolonged ABR latencies reflecting delayed auditory maturation. However, consistent associations between prenatal alcohol exposure and hearing loss have not been reported in humans (e.g., Cohen-Kerem, Bar-Oz, Nulman, Papaioannou, & Koren, 2007; Cone-Wesson, 2005). But, prevalence of conductive hearing loss is quite high, and is likely associated with otitis media and eustachian tube dysfunction as is common in other children with craniofacial anomalies like cleft palate (Church, 1987).

Prenatal cigarette smoking is also surprisingly prevalent, and research suggests potential audiological symptoms in children with prenatal exposure. In a recent U.S. survey on drug use and health, over 16% of pregnant respondents reported past-month cigarette use (Aldworth, 2009). Many noxious compounds from cigarettes (e.g., nicotine, carbon monoxide) that are associated with adverse fetal health effects can be found in the fetal compartment (placenta and amniotic fluid; Behnke et al., 2013). These toxins are believed to cause hypoxia and vasoconstriction of placenta and umbilical vesicles, thus reducing fetal nutrient supply. Prenatal smoking reportedly increases risk of placental abruption, fetal distress, preterm birth, poor birth weight, sudden infant death syndrome (SIDs), and later developmental, behavioral, and health concerns or conditions (e.g., asthma; Cnattingius, 2004; Gilliland, Li, & Peters, 2001; Salihu & Wilson, 2007; Weitzman, Gortmaker, & Sobol, 1992). Cochlear structures such as the outer hair cells are particularly vulnerable to oxygen deprivation, and recent studies have reported reductions in the amplitude of transient-evoked otoacoustic emission (TEOAE) responses of newborns with a history of prenatal smoke exposure (Durante, Ibidi, Lotufo, & Carvallo, 2011; Korres et al., 2007). The association between TEOAE reductions and measures of hearing sensitivity remains to be fully elucidated, but a National Health and Nutrition study involving family interview and audiologic data collection in nearly 1,000 adolescents reported minor decrements in hearing sensitivity in children with a history of prenatal smoke exposure relative to unexposed controls (Weitzman, Govil, Liu, & Lalwani, 2013). Thresholds of adolescents with prenatal exposure were approximately 3 to 4 dB higher at 2000 and 6000 Hz for the poorer ear and at 6000 Hz for averaged ears. A higher rate of unilateral low-frequency sensorineural hearing loss was also reported in exposed versus unexposed groups (Weitzman et al., 2013). In addition to implications of modest ototoxic effects from maternal smoking, increased risk of middle ear dysfunction and ear infections has also been reported (e.g., Stathis, O'Callaghan, Najman, Anderson, & Bor, 1999).

Prescribed Drugs—Aminoglycosides

Despite medical recommendations discouraging use of medically unnecessary drugs during pregnancy, in the United States and elsewhere, there is a surprisingly high rate of prescribed prenatal (nonvitamin) drugs, including some known to cause possible fetal harm (e.g., Lacroix, Damase-Michel, Lapeyre-Mestre, & Montastruc, 2000; Malm, Martikainen, Klaukka, & Neuvonen, 2004; Olesen et al., 1999; Ostrea et al., 1992; Piper, Baum, & Kennedy, 1987). It is reported that more than half of women take a minimum of one prescription or nonprescription (over-the-counter) drug during pregnancy (Mitchell et al., 2011; Rubin, Ferencz, & Loffredo,1993). Trends from a longitudinal study of 30,000 mothers suggest a marked rise in maternal prescription and nonprescription drug use over the last 30 years, and a doubling in the rate of first trimester drug use (Mitchell et al., 2011).

Prenatal aminoglycoside use is of particular interest given the known potential ototoxic effects of these antibiotics. Such drugs (e.g., kanamycin, streptomycin, amikacin, gentamicin) are prescribed during pregnancy for the treatment of conditions such as kidney infections, chorioamnionitis, and tuberculosis (e.g., Kirkwood, Harris, Timar, & Koren, 2007; Niebyl, 2003). They destroy or slow the growth of gram-negative, aerobic bacteria by disrupting bacterial protein synthesis, and can cause auditory system damage. In animal studies, ototoxic effects appear to be associated with the timing of drug administration and are most conspicuous in the base of the cochlea (e.g., Dumas & Charachon, 1982; Onejeme & Khan, 1984; Uziel, Romand, & Marot, 1979). Uziel and colleagues (1979) reported decreased cochlear microphonic and compound action potential amplitudes (consistent with flat, sloping or high-frequency hearing loss) in newborn guinea pigs receiving in utero kanamycin exposure around the onset of auditory functioning (Uziel et al., 1979). Associations between the timing of kanamycin administration and auditory system vulnerability have also been reported by others. Inner ear dissection in rats exposed to kanamycin during (but not before or after) the period of cochlear development, beginning at 9 postnatal days versus prenatally in humans, revealed hair cell loss in the basal part of the cochlea and subtler cellular abnormalities more apically (Onejeme & Khan, 1984). Drug dosing is also a mitigating factor, and although human research on auditory outcomes following prenatal exposure is limited, older studies have suggested that in utero exposure following prolonged or high-dose kanamycin treatment can increase hearing loss risk in children (Jones, 1973; Nishimura & Tanimura, 1976).

Prenatal streptomycin administration has also been cautioned, although the science in humans is sparse. Small studies completed 50 years ago reported hearing loss and abnormal vestibular findings in a significant proportion of children with extended prenatal streptomycin exposure for the treatment of maternal tuberculosis, but confounding factors were present (Conway, 1965; Robinson & Cambon, 1964). More contemporary studies find a much lower rate of hearing loss in children with gestational streptomycin exposure (Donald, Doherty, & Van Zyl, 1991; Donald & Sellars, 1981). For example, Donald and colleagues reported one case of unilateral sensorineural hearing loss in a group of 30 children with first-trimester exposure (1991). Furthermore, epidemiological research shows no increase in birth defects with prenatal streptomycin administration (Czeizel, Rockenbauer, Olsen, & Sørensen, 2000). Nonetheless, additional research might help clarify possible risk(s) of exposure and the influence of relevant variables (e.g., timing and dosing) on fetal hearing outcomes.

Overall, studies suggest that prenatal kanamycin or streptomycin exposure might slightly increase risk of congenital hearing loss. Gentamicin, on the other hand, has generally been regarded as less ototoxic and remains preferred for the treatment of maternal infection. A recent study of 39 babies exposed to at least one dose of gentamicin at 28 weeks gestation (average) reported that all babies passed their initial newborn hearing screening or rescreening by otoacoustic emission (OAE) or automated auditory brainstem response

(AABR) testing (Kirkwood et al., 2007). Similar findings were reported in babies whose mothers were treated with gentamicin for chorioamnionitis prior to delivery. All 38 babies passed on initial screening or rescreening (Locksmith, Chin, Vu, Shattuck, & Hankins, 2005). However, the ability of screening tools to detect certain configurations of hearing loss and delayed-onset damage (potentially manifesting days to weeks after aminoglycoside exposure) is limited, rendering conclusions regarding fetal ototoxicity tenuous. Further diagnostic and behavioral testing in children with prenatal aminoglycoside exposure stands to improve our understanding of the risks of aminoglycoside exposure.

Gene-Drug Interaction: MT-RNR1 and Aminoglycoside-Induced Hearing Loss

As noted previously, the literature describing congenital hearing loss risk in humans following prenatal aminoglycoside exposure is limited. However, there is a rapidly growing body of research describing adverse hearing outcomes in children and adults with a genetic mutation that increases susceptibility to aminoglycoside-induced ototoxicity. And, whereas prenatal aminoglycoside prescription is relatively rare, perinatal aminoglycoside administration (hours to days after birth) is common, such as for the prophylactic treatment of suspected neonatal sepsis (e.g., Clark, Bloom, Spitzer, & Gerstmann, 2006; Grohskopf et al., 2005).

Mitochondrial mutations are estimated to account for roughly 1% of nonsyndromic, prelingual hearing loss (Morton, 2002), and gene-environment interactions have been shown to predispose some mutation carriers to developing sensorineural hearing loss following aminoglycoside exposure. The first of these mitochondrially encoded 12S RNA (MT-RNR1) gene mutations associated with aminoglycoside vulnerability (A1555G) was discovered in 1993 (Prezant et al., 1993). Since then, a growing literature has amassed documenting the mutation in families and sporadically in individuals (e.g., Estivill et al., 1998; Fischel-Ghodsian et al., 1997; Kupka et al., 2002; Li et al., 2004; Lu et al., 2010; Pandya et al., 1997). Other mitochondrial variants have also been identified as predisposing carriers to ototoxic drug effects (e.g., C1494T, G7444A), but the A1555G ribosomal RNA (rRNA) mutation remains the most frequently reported and studied (e.g., Leveque et al., 2007; Lu et al., 2010; Wei et al., 2013; Yuan et al., 2005).

Prevalence reports vary globally, suggesting differences in the A1555G mutation frequency across ethnicity. In Caucasian individuals with nonsyndromic hearing loss from the United States and Europe, genetic screenings uncovered a mutation frequency of 0.2% to 4% (Berrettini et al., 2008; Ealy, Lynch, Meyer, & Smith, 2011; Konings et al., 2008). Higher mutation rates have been reported in hearing-impaired individuals of Asian descent (3%–9%), which are further increased in studies including subjects with known aminoglycoside exposure (Li et al., 2005; Lu et al., 2010; Malik, Pieter, Sudoyo, Kadir, & Marzuki, 2003; Oshima, Kudo, & Ikeda, 2001; Wu, Chiu, Chen, & Hsu, 2007). However, differences in prescription practices could contribute to disparities in mutation frequency. Aminoglycosides are more readily administered in Asia compared to the United States, and aminoglycoside-induced hearing loss might therefore comprise a larger segment of the pediatric hearing-impaired population.

In two recent studies involving hearing and genetic screenings in Chinese and American babies, a similar prevalence of common mitochondrial mutations was seen (2%) and frequency of the A1555G variant (0.2%) was reported in newborns (Ealy et al., 2011; Zhang et al., 2013). Mutation frequencies also did not differ between babies in neonatal intensive care units (NICUs) versus general well-baby populations. All mutation carriers reportedly passed their hearing screening within 1 to 3 days after birth (Zhang et al., 2013), or before NICU discharge (10 days to 1 year following gentamicin treatment; Ealy et al., 2011). However, the sensitivity of screenings might be limited due to their inability to detect some types of hearing loss (e.g., configured and minimal/mild loss) and delayed ototoxic effects.

The aminoglycoside susceptibility affecting hearing in some MT-RNR1 carriers arises from a mutation at the A site of the 12S region of rRNA resulting in a base pair change (e.g., Prezant et al., 1993; Zhao et al., 2004). The change causes mitochondrial ribosomes to resemble bacteria to which aminoglycosides readily bind, leading to mitochondrial destruction in cochlear cells and ultimately hearing loss and vestibular problems (e.g., Guan, 2011; Prezant et al., 1993; Zhao et al., 2004). The damage preferentially affects cochlear and vestibular organs because aminoglycosides are harbored in high levels in cochlear fluid (Henley & Schacht, 1988). Although quickly excreted by the filtration action of the kidneys, thereby limiting tissue and organ damage (Edson & Terrell, 1999), due to their affinity for perilymphatic fluid aminoglycocides can persist and accumulate in the cochlea even after no longer being detected in the blood (Stupp, Rauch, Sous, Brun, & Lagler, 1967; Vrabec, Cody, & Ulrich, 1965). Hence, fetal serum levels (blood) might underestimate aminoglycoside concentration in cochlear fluid.

The time course for manifestation and stabilization of hearing loss in individuals with MT-RNR1 mutations is unclear, but considerable variability has been reported ranging from days to months or even years following aminoglycoside administration (e.g., Casano et al., 1999; Lu et al., 2010). Knowledge of the complex effects of drug type, dose, and treatment length is also limited, but even a single therapeutic dose has reportedly triggered mild hearing loss, and it is speculated that age and dose influence audiologic outcome (Yuan et al., 2005). Earlier age of exposure and higher cumulative dose(s) have been associated with more profound hearing loss (Guan, 2011; Yuan et al., 2005).

Although aminoglycoside exposure has been associated with hearing loss in mutation carriers, incomplete penetrance and phenotypic variation is reported as well as speculation that modifier genes or factors might influence hearing loss presentation (e.g., age of hearing loss onset, severity, progression; Guan, 2011). Audiometric presentation is variable, but many affected patients display sloping configurations (~75%), followed by flat (10%–15%), U-shaped, and rising patterns (Lu et al., 2010; Yuan et al., 2005). Hearing loss is commonly bilateral and in the severe-to-profound range, although milder losses and even normal hearing have been reported less frequently (Lu et al., 2010; Yelverton et al., 2013; Yuan et al., 2005). Some studies have also documented progressive hearing loss in mutation carriers without aminoglycoside exposure (e.g., Estivill et al., 1998; Guan, 2011; Lu et al., 2010), but others show no hearing loss penetrance in unexposed carriers (Wei et al., 2013). The potential influence of methodological confounds (i.e., reliance on accurate patient recall of drug history) cannot be ruled out, so further research is needed to develop a consensus on the likelihood of spontaneous hearing loss presentation in mutation carriers.

Although hearing loss predisposition is maternally inherited in MT-RNR1 carriers and therefore irreversible, eliminating aminoglycoside exposure could minimize or prevent hearing loss onset or progression. As noted earlier, aminoglycoside prescriptions are relatively conservative in the United States compared to other regions such as Asia, but an exception is in NICUs where the vast majority of babies receive one or more doses of these drugs (Clark et al., 2006). Genetic screening and consideration of case history information can limit or prevent aminoglycoside administration and hearing loss in presymptomatic carriers. One study reported that more than half of mutation carriers noted a positive family history of aminoglycoside-associated hearing loss illustrating the potential for patient interview and genetic counseling to prevent hearing loss (Fischel-Ghodsian et al., 1997). The American College of Medical Genetics has also recommended MT-RNR1 mutation screenings in patients with existing hearing loss and previous aminoglycoside exposure so that future drug treatment(s) might be altered to reduce further ototoxic effects in carriers (2002). Global initiatives focused on vaccination and infection control also remain critical because decreases in the prevalence of infection and disease will decrease the need for aminoglycoside administration and potentially the rate of acquired hearing loss in children with MT-RNR1 mutations.

Environmental Toxins

Use of prescribed or nonprescribed drugs can introduce fetal health risks that can be avoided or minimized through careful prescription practices or abstinence. Contrastingly, circulating environmental toxins can cause adverse fetal effects such as hearing loss from unknown exposure. For example, pregnant women living near hazardous waste facilities are more susceptible to air-borne polychlorinated biphenyl (PCB) exposure, or exposure from consumption of contaminated well water or fish (U.S. Environmental Protection Agency [EPA], 2015).

Polychlorinated biphenyls (PCBs) are synthetic chemicals manufactured in the United States between 1929 and 1979 for various applications and products. PCB use was voluntarily restricted to include only closed systems (e.g., transformers, capacitors, miscellaneous electrical equipment) around 1971 and ultimately banned shortly thereafter (1979) based on health concerns (e.g., cancer, reproductive, endocrine, and immune system effects, etc.). However, due to the stability of PCBs, the potential teratogenic effects of exposure remain relevant. Careful disposal is essential to prevent air and water contamination and subsequent exposure, especially in individuals residing near hazardous waste facilities (EPA, 2015). Although human studies have not directly studied prenatal PCB exposure, in utero exposure to Aroclor (a brand name for PCB) caused developmental disruptions in thyroid functioning resulting in postnatal hearing loss in Long Evans rat pups (Crofton & Rice, 1999; Goldey & Crofton, 1998). Exposed pups showed elevated acoustic startle response thresholds relative to control rats, and postnatal hormone replacement therapy mitigated auditory system effects, decreasing startle response amplitude (Goldey & Crofton, 1998). Findings suggest that drug treatment can potentially reverse ototoxic effects and restore hearing function.

Fetal hearing and global health hazards arise from a variety of known (e.g., prescription drugs) and unknown causes (e.g., chemical inhalation). Continued regulations regarding safe disposal of teratogenic agents such as PCBs can limit covert exposure, and careful prescription practices might minimize fetal drug effects. Furthermore, support programs might reduce fetal exposure to recreational or illicit drugs and chemicals and improve developmental outcomes through patient education regarding prenatal exposure risks, improved access to prenatal care, and cessation support or addiction treatment for women with drug dependence.

Noise and Hearing Loss

U.S. federal agencies provide recommendations and industry standards aimed at reducing hearing loss risk in noise-exposed workers such as through use of hearing protection and the establishment of noise dose limits (National Institute for Occupational Safety and Health [NIOSH], 1998; Occupational Safety and Health Administration [OSHA], 1997). However, sound abatement strategies and engineering controls (e.g., head worn earmuffs) developed to minimize noise hazard for workers may not be adequate for ensuring fetal hearing protection.

Over the last three decades, there has been an apparent change in the composition of the U.S. labor force (Bureau of Labor Statistics, 2012). Between 1972 and 2012, there was a nearly 15% rise in women in the workforce as well as an increase in the number of pregnant women working. In the mid-2000s over 50% of women continued working up until 1 month before their due date compared to 15% of women three decades before (Laughlin, 2011). Older mothers were more likely to work longer (U.S. Census Bureau, 2011). In the most recent survey from the U.S. Bureau of Labor Statistics (2014), it was reported that women comprised 47% of the workforce and nearly half of them were of childbearing age (16–44 years). Of those, roughly 10% were in industries that might increase risk of noise overexposure for mother and baby (e.g., manufacturing, transportation and utilities, construction, etc.).

Cochlear and auditory nerve cells become functional around 20 to 25 weeks gestation, and human babies can sense and respond to auditory stimulation at or beyond the end of the second trimester. For example, behavioral responses to vibroacoustic stimulation (e.g., blink-startle) can be consistently observed during ultrasound after 28 weeks gestation (Birnholz & Benacerraf, 1983). Evoked potential recordings indicate that early responses appear immature and sensitivity continues to improve with further system development throughout the third trimester and during the postnatal period (Lary, Briassoulis, de Vries, Dubowitz, & Dubowitz, 1985; Sininger, Abdala, & Cone-Wesson, 1997). However, speech, noise, and music can be readily detected in utero.

Sound passes easily into the uterine space, and comparison of broadband noise recordings made inside and outside pregnant ewes suggest that the abdomen acts much like a low-pass filter (Gerhardt, Abrams, & Oliver, 1990). There is a negligible decrease (<5 dB) or possible enhancement of frequencies below 250 Hz, a roughly 10 to 20 dB reduction in mid frequencies (250–1000 Hz), and 20 to 30 dB attenuation of high frequencies (>1000 Hz; e.g., Gerhardt et al., 1990; Peters, Gerhardt, Abrams, & Longmate, 1993; Vince, Armitage, Baldwin, Toner, & Moore, 1982; Vince, Billing, Baldwin, Toner, & Weller, 1985). Studies have further shown that fetal auditory stimulation primarily occurs through bone conduction as with underwater hearing in humans (Gerhardt, Huang, Arrington, Meixner, & Antonelli, 1996).

Despite elevated fetal hearing thresholds and signal attenuation or shaping by the abdomen, uterus, and amniotic fluid, there is the potential for hazardous levels of noise to reach the fetal head and ear. Animal studies have reported measurable changes in the bone-conduction ABRs of fetal sheep exposed to intense prolonged noise (120 dB SPL, 16 hr) played from loudspeakers placed near the pregnant ewe's flanks (Gerhardt, Pierson, Huang, Abrams, & Rarey, 1999; Huang, Gerhardt, Abrams, & Antonelli, 1997). Latency and amplitude increases were largest after exposure but remained significant after a recovery period of 2 to 3 weeks. ABR effects were generally most pronounced for lower-frequency tone-bursts, and histological analysis in animals with repeated prenatal broadband noise exposure localized hair cell damage to the apical and middle cochlear turns (Gerhardt et al., 1999). Overall, findings suggest that intense air-conducted signals can pass into the intrauterine space potentially damaging fetal hearing, and low-frequency hearing might be more vulnerable due to the relative ease with which those signals are transmitted.

Despite compelling animal research, evidence of fetal noise-induced hearing loss in humans is relatively weak. Occupational noise hazards have been associated with increased risks for gestational hypertension, preterm birth, and low birth weight (e.g., Dzhambov, Dimitrova, & Dimitrakova, 2014; Nurminen & Kurppa, 1989; Ristovska, Laszlo, & Hansell, 2014), but few studies have linked fetal noise exposure to adverse hearing outcomes in childhood. What limited research is available is somewhat conflicting. In a retrospective study by Lalande and colleagues (1986), an association between prenatal noise exposure and childhood sensorineural hearing loss was identified in 4- to 10-year-olds whose mothers worked in 65 to 95 dBA-8h noise for a minimum of 1 month during pregnancy. The proportion of children with elevated, poorer ear 4000 Hz thresholds was reportedly three to four times greater if mothers were exposed to higher ($L_{Aeq,9m}$ 85–95 dB) versus lower ($L_{Aeq,9m}$ 65–85 dB) noise doses during pregnancy. However, in a more recent study with greater methodological control, no difference in distortion product otoacoustic emission (DPOAE) amplitudes was reported between infants (birth to 6 months) with history of fetal noise exposure and a matched control group (Rocha et al., 2007). The exposure group was composed of babies whose mothers worked full time (8 hr/day, 5 days/week) in a nuts processing plant (80–90 dB A) for 8 to 9 months during pregnancy. Although DPOAE measures offer an objective, frequency-specific index of outer hair cell functioning suggesting no group difference, a caveat is that they are less sensitive to minimal or mild hearing loss and their relationship to hearing thresholds remains to be fully elucidated.

Observing safe noise limits during the perinatal period and thereafter is clearly warranted, and the potential dangers of auditory overexposure have been recognized. In addition to increased risk of sensorineural hearing loss, excessive noise can induce adverse physiologic changes such as increased heart rate, respiratory rate, and decreased O_2 saturation, especially in preterm infants (e.g., Brown, 2009; Wachman & Lahav, 2011). The American Academy of Pediatrics and others maintain that NICUs should not exceed levels of 45 to 50 dBA hourly and 65 to 70 dBA peak (American Academy of Pediatrics, 1997; Graven, 2000), but levels are frequently higher (especially within incubators). In U.S. and Canadian NICUs, equalized noise levels between 55 and 62 dBA and peak levels in excess of 120 dB have been reported (Darcy, Hancock, & Ware, 2008; Kent, Tan, Clarke, & Bardell, 2002; Krueger, Wall, Parker, & Nealis, 2005). Some respiratory and life support systems might further increase noise exposure risks in newborns (Bess et al., 1979; Surenthiran et al., 2003). Mean noise levels recorded from the postnasal space of preterm infants receiving continuous positive airways pressure (CPAP) were 102 dB at some frequencies, with higher levels observed with increasing flow rate (Surenthiran et al., 2003). The interactive effect of noise and aminoglycoside exposure, especially in infants with mitochondrial DNA mutations has also been speculated, and strategies for minimizing NICU noise have been extended (see review by Zimmerman & Lahav, 2013). Noise abatement techniques including use of silent alarms, acoustic damping material, and provider education might reduce perinatal noise exposure in NICUs (e.g., Milette, 2010; Zahr & de Traversay, 1994). Such initiatives have the potential to improve health and development and prevent or minimize acquired noise-induced hearing loss in newborns (e.g., Blackburn, 1998; Bremmer, Byers, & Kiehl, 2003; Brown, 2009; Zahr & de Traversay, 1994; Zimmerman & Lahav, 2013).

Postnatal Period

In the latter section of this chapter, prevention of postnatal acquired hearing loss will be discussed. It is defined herein as hearing loss occurring after the newborn period and, therefore, not identified by universal newborn hearing screening (UNHS). Determinants of hearing loss in children include nonmodifiable, possibly modifiable, and modifiable risk factors. Table 9–1 provides examples of determinants proposed for acquired hearing loss in pediatric populations. A preexisting hereditary form of hearing loss can be progressive in nature and thus go undetected by UNHS. Though technically the hearing loss in this example occurs postnatally, the outcome might be inevitable (at least not modifiable with today's technology) or be dependent on an additional risk factor. For example, the mitochondrial mutation of the 12S ribosomal RNA gene has been implicated as a predisposing factor in aminoglycoside ototoxicity (Bacino et al., 1995; Fischel-Ghodsian et al., 1997). Understanding genetic contributions to acquired hearing loss is critical and might lead to eventual treatments to prevent or reduce risk for hearing loss.

Table 9–1. Determinants Proposed for Acquired Hearing Loss in Pediatric Populations

Modifiable	*Nonmodifiable*
Noise and hearing protection use	Genetics
Diet	Sex
Lifestyle (exercise)	Race/ethnicity
Other environmental (e.g., chemicals, smoking/second-hand smoke)	Age
Possibly Modifiable	
Health, disease, medications	
Socioeconomic status/education, parental health	

The usual and customary view of acquired hearing loss is related to disease, drugs, noise, lifestyle, and other environmental factors. Currently, we cannot change an individual's genetics, we cannot change our age, and we cannot change our race/ethnicity. Though these factors might play a role in susceptibility to acquired hearing loss, there is little we can currently do to modify these factors for the purpose of prevention.

Disease/Infection and Hearing Loss

By far the most common disease/infection process contributing to hearing loss in children is otitis externa (OE) and otitis media (OM; Rovers et al., 2004). OE is inflammation of the external auditory canal most often caused by a bacterial infection and associated with warm water exposure. The most common pathogens are *Pseudomonas aeruginosa* and *Staphylococcus aureus*. Fungal involvement is uncommon in primary acute OE but may be more common in chronic OE or after treatment of acute OE with topical, or less often systemic, antibiotics. Topical antimicrobials are the primary method of treatment (Rosenfeld et al., 2014). OM represents a set of clinically defined phenotypes including acute OM, recurrent OM, chronic suppurative OM, OM with effusion, and chronic OM. The most common pathway for OM development is an upper respiratory infection that leads to suppuration of the middle ear with bacteria (most commonly, depending on region, *Streptococcus pneumoniae*, *Haemophilus influenzae*, and *Moraxella catarrhalis*; Bhutta, 2014). A more horizontal orientation and shorter length of the eustachian tube are associated with increased prevalence of OM in children (Dinc et al., 2015). It is estimated that there are an annual 2.4 million visits for OE and six million visits for OM in pediatric populations (Centers for Disease Control and Prevention [CDC], 2011; Marom et al., 2014). OM is the most common disease seen in pediatric populations with 80% of children estimated to experience at least one episode by 3 years of age (Teele et al., 1989). The hearing loss related to OE and OM is often conductive and transient in nature, but might still have a potential impact on speech-language development and academic performance (Roberts et al., 2004; Winskel, 2006). Chronic suppurative OM increases risk for some level of permanent loss (Jensen et al., 2013); however, studies with acute OM populations show minimal risk for permanent hearing damage (Boudewyns et al., 2011). An infection might also be secondary to other disorders that can contribute to hearing loss, such as craniofacial malformations (Phua et al., 2009).

Other conditions such as cholesteatomas (congenital and acquired) and tumors/lesions of the internal auditory canal, cerebellopontine angle, and brainstem can also present in pediatric populations. Cholesteatomas are noncancerous cystic lesions derived from an abnormal growth of keratinizing squamous epithelium in the temporal bone. Congenital cholesteatomas form prior to birth, while the acquired variant is related to retraction of the tympanic membrane due to chronic middle ear disease (i.e., chronic OM). Cholesteatomas are relatively rare (0.00003% incidence) but are often difficult to treat. Pediatric cholesteatomas are more infectious, aggressive, proliferative, and have less favorable prognoses compared to adult types (Kuo et al., 2015). Improved prevention of OM might lead to reduced incidence of acquired cholesteatomas in pediatric populations (Morita et al., 2015).

A significant amount of research has examined ways to reduce risk for OE and OM. Recommendations from experts to prevent OE include drying or ears thoroughly after water exposure, using swim plugs, and not inserting any foreign objects in the ear canal. Proper levels of chlorine and pH levels in swimming pools can also reduce risk (CDC, 2011). Prevention of OM is also a major public health concern related to cost, antibiotic utilization, and risk for permanent hearing loss. Current recommendations for treatment of OM include an observational approach with application of antibiotics limited to children with bilateral acute OM or with both OM and drainage (Venekamp et al., 2015). Significant decrease in rates of OM in the United States has been associated with advent of the 13-pneumococcal conjugate vaccine (PCV-13; Marom et al., 2014). However, other studies suggest no benefit from vaccination against pneumococci (El-Makhzangy et al., 2012). Other risk factors include day care entry before 2 years of age (increased risk), breastfeeding for 6 months (decreased risk), exposure to smoking or second-hand smoke (increased risk), use of pacifiers (increased risk), and poor nutrition (increased risk; Gisselsson-Solen et al., 2015). Tympanostomy tubes and adenoidectomy may shorten duration and reduce risk for further problems (Giebink, 2000).

Trauma

Trauma with and without temporal bone fracture and development of perilymphatic fistulas have also been reported in children (Huang et al., 2013). The most common cause of injury related to temporal bone fracture in children is motor vehicle accidents, followed by falls (Peerhentupa et al., 2010). Particular care should be taken in cases of preexisting enlarged vestibular aqueduct (EVA) and susceptibility to minor head injury, barotrauma, and noise. Noordman et al. (2015) found that 34% of patients with EVA experience significant hearing loss with minor head injuries. The risk for hearing loss was greater in patients with EVA who experienced previous spontaneous fluctuations in hearing not related to trauma.

Prevention of head injuries and barotrauma can reduce risk for trauma-related hearing loss. Early identification of predisposing factors such as EVA can help to mitigate hearing loss, particularly if preexisting hearing fluctuations are noted. Recommendations include limiting participation in contact sports, no scuba diving, and use of helmets (Noordman et al., 2015).

Drugs and Hearing Loss

The most common ototoxic medications used in children are aminoglycosides and platinum-based neoplastics. However, other drugs with ototoxic properties to consider include salicylate, loop diuretics, and quinine, although their effects can often be transient. Aminoglycosides are antibiotics that therapeutically target prokaryotic cells and exert their effect through inhibition of protein synthesis. We have previously discussed the mitochondrial 12S ribosomal RNA gene 1555G mutation associated with increased sensitivity to aminoglycoside drugs. Neoplastic drugs like cisplatin and carboplatin work by blocking transcription factors, thereby preventing both transcription and translation. This action in turn can send out DNA damage signals to trigger apoptosis (Schacht, Talaska, & Rybak, 2012). The hearing loss associated with aminoglycosides and platinum neoplastics is generally bilateral and begins at high frequencies (greater than 8 kHz), extending to lower frequencies with prolonged treatment.

The application of aminoglycosides in children includes treatment for sepsis and lung infections (Ibrahim et al., 2011) seen predominantly in the cystic fibrosis population. However, the reported risk for ototoxicity with aminoglycosides (El-Barbary et al., 2015; Mulheran et al., 2001) is relatively low compared to cisplatin. Platinum-based neoplastics are commonly used in treatment of osteosarcoma, neuroblastoma, hepatoblastoma, and germ cell tumors in children.

There is considerable variation in ototoxicity among and within both aminoglycosides and platinum-based neoplastics. For aminoglycosides, systematic neomycin is considered the most ototoxic (and why use is limited to topical administration), and for platinum neoplastics, cisplatin is considered the most ototoxic (Kotecha & Richardson, 1994; Schacht et al., 2012). The incidence of hearing loss related to aminoglycosides is variable with some suggesting 20% disturbance and other studies that include the testing of frequencies above 8 kHz showing 47% of patients with evidence of hearing loss. For platinum-based neoplastics, the reported incidence of hearing loss with carboplatin (second-generation platinum agent with less toxicity) is approximately 20% at high cumulative doses and up to 100% with high doses of cisplatin. However, there is great variation based on age, dose, and frequency of cisplatin treatment schedules, grading scales, and criteria for hearing loss (Bass & Bhagat, 2014; Langer et al., 2013). Younger children and higher cumulative doses ($\geq$400 mg/m^2) are associated with greater incidence of hearing loss (Coradini et al., 2007). Application of cranial radiation therapy for head-neck cancers can increase risk; however, limited data are available in pediatric populations (Bhandare et al., 2010).

Two primary areas of interest in ototoxicity monitoring are identification of early changes in auditory function (i.e., ototoxicity monitoring) and prevention of ototoxicity. Ototoxicity monitoring has focused primarily on application of extended high-frequency (EHF) audiometry (i.e., >8 kHz), use of OAEs, and grading scales. Numerous studies support EHF audiometry and OAEs for early identification of ototoxic pathology (Bhagat et al., 2010; Cooper et al., 2011; Knight et al., 2007; Stavroulaki et al., 1999; Yu et al., 2014). However, the benefit of earlier identification is limited by our current ability to intervene and prevent ototoxicity; therefore, current monitoring protocols have focused on changes in the 2 to 8 kHz region to manage loss as it begins to infringe upon speech frequencies. The testing approach is dependent on chronological and developmental age of the patient. See Bass and Baghat (2014) for a review and current recommendations for pediatric ototoxicity monitoring clinical protocols.

Numerous ototoxicity criteria or grading systems have been developed, which classify hearing loss differently, contributing to the large variance in incidence of ototoxicity seen across studies (see review by Langer et al., 2013). In 2010 recommendations made at the 42nd Congress of the International Society of Pediatric Oncology (SIOP) meeting were considered for development of a new scale called the SIOP Boston Ototoxicity Scale. The scale uses Grades 0 to 4 based on audiometric thresholds, with increase in grade indicating greater ototoxicity (Brock et al., 2012).

Prevention strategies involve alternative drugs, alternative dosing schedules, and adjunctive therapies; each of these has its limitations. Alternative drugs might not be as efficient or effective and development can be timely and expensive. Dosing schedules might be less efficient or effective and therefore not possible. Finally, adjunctive therapies or cotherapies might reduce the antitumor efficacy or antibacterial properties of these drugs that are treating potentially life-threatening pathologies.

Apramycin represents a potential alternative drug with reduced ototoxic effects. This naturally occurring aminoglycoside is widely used in veterinarian medicine and has excellent antimycobacterial activity. A designer aminoglycoside based on a modified biosynthetic precursor of gentamicin, called sisomicin, showed negligible ototoxicity of in vitro cochlear tissue (Steyger, 2015). Alternative dosing schedules might also influence susceptibility to hearing loss. Rademaker-Lakhai et al. (2006) demonstrated that doses below 60 mg/m^2 of cisplatin reduce risk for hearing loss. In addition, patients who received cisplatin treatment once a week for 6 weeks had lower risk of hearing loss than patients who received higher doses once every 2 weeks for 4 weeks.

The greatest focus of research to date is development of adjunctive prevention-based therapies. Numerous drugs have been studied, including alpha-lipoic acid (Rybak et al., 1999), sodium thiosulfate (Neuwelt et al., 1996), salicylate (Li et al., 2002), ebselen (Lynch et al., 2005), D-methionine (Campbell et al., 1996), amifostine (Church et al., 1995), ACEMg (Le Prell et al., 2014), *N*-acetylcysteine (Dickey et al., 2004), sound-conditioning (Roy et al., 2013), and thermal treatment (Spankovich et al., 2014). In addition, alternative delivery methods such as intratympanic injection with hydrogels (Engleder et al., 2014), intracochlear perfusion (Pararas et al., 2012), and diffusion of drugs across the tympanic membrane (Otonomy) are being explored to improve targeted protection and limit systemic effects that might alter antitumor efficacy. Another concern with patients on ototoxic drugs is increased risk for noise-induced hearing loss (NIHL; Peleva et al., 2014). Appropriate counseling on hearing conservation and reducing other environmental risk factors (e.g., chemicals, smoking, other ototoxic medications) is recommended.

Noise and Hearing Loss

Noise can damage the auditory system through direct mechanical trauma and metabolic changes that activate numerous cell death pathways (for review, see Le Prell et al., 2007). Historically, the effects of noise on hearing have been primarily focused on adult populations and occupational sources of noise. There is now a growing concern regarding risk for NIHL among children and contributions of nonoccupational sources of exposure. Niskar et al. (2001) provided one of the first estimates of prevalence of NIHL among children 6 to 19 years of age. The data came from the National Health and Nutrition Examination Survey (NHANES) III conducted from 1988 to 1994. The group defined NIHL as meeting criteria consistent with a "notch" configuration (i.e., at least 15 dB HL higher [poorer] at 3, 4, or 6 kHz than values at 0.5 and 1k Hz, and threshold at 8 kHz had to be at least 10 dB lower [better] than the maximum notch threshold). Tympanometry compliance measures were conducted to adjust for middle ear pathology. The overall prevalence of NIHL in one or both ears was 12.5%. This represented approximately 5.2 million children in the United States at that time. There were also noted sex and age effects, where males (14.8%) had significantly higher prevalence of NIHL than females (10.1%), and children aged 12 to 19 years (15.5%) had significantly greater prevalence of NIHL than younger children aged 6 to 11 years (8.5%).

More recently, Shargorodsky et al. (2010) received significant press with a study comparing NHANES data from 1988 to 1994 to data from 2005 to 2006 time periods. They reported a higher prevalence of hearing loss, here defined as pure-tone average (PTA; 3, 4, 6, and 8 kHz or 0.5, 1, and 2 kHz) greater than 15 dB HL, in the 2005 to 2006 time period (19.5%) compared to the 1988 to 1994 time period (14.9%). Though the authors discuss noise as a potential variable, they did not see a difference in prevalence of notched configurations. In addition, there was no adjustment or consideration for middle ear pathology. Henderson et al. (2011) investigated the prevalence of NIHL in the same dataset (NHANES) and time periods (i.e., 1988–1994 compared to 2005–2006) as Shargorodsky et al. (2010). Criteria for NIHL and hearing loss was identical to Niskar et al. (2001; that is, did not include 8 kHz) and influence of middle ear pathology was adjusted in the model. Overall, no significant increase in NIHL or high- or low-frequency hearing loss was found between survey periods. However, a significant increase in the prevalence of NIHL was found in stratified analyses in females. Despite no increase in overall prevalence of NIHL, there was a significant increase in reports of listening to music through headphones in the past 24 hr from 19.8% to 34.8% (note: the iPod was released in October 2001 with the one millionth unit sold by June 2003; iPod dominated over 70% of the personal listening device [PLD] market share during the 2005–2006 time period [Marsal, 2006]). Collectively, these studies suggest that NIHL remains a significant problem in youth populations, and females are now approaching males in prevalence of NIHL. It also points out a significant increase in use of music with headphones; however, there was not a significant relationship between use of headphones and likelihood of NIHL.

Personal Listening Devices

In recent years, there has been significant interest in the implications of PLDs and risk for NIHL. The output level of PLDs including portable compact disc players, MP3 players, and iPods has been reported as high as 139 dB (A) free field equivalent depending on type of headphone and PLD (Fligor & Cox, 2004; Kumar et al., 2009; Portnuff et al., 2011).

The levels that can be reached with a PLD pose a potential risk for NIHL. Portnuff et al. (2011) investigated use of PLD listening habits in adolescents aged 13 to 17 years of age. A small percentage of teenagers (14%) reported behavior that might increase risk for hearing loss. Measured listening levels, called chosen listening levels (CLL), were on average 74.1 dBA which is below risk levels. In addition, the median listening duration was 2 hr/day. The average CLL was higher in conditions where background noise was introduced, but below 85 dBA for all conditions suggesting the majority of youth use PLD at safe levels and durations. Similar findings have been reported in adolescents 10 to 17 years of age (Keith et al., 2011). However, other studies suggest that adolescents report playing their music at maximum levels and though aware of the risk, express low personal vulnerability (Vogel et al., 2008). In addition, slightly older populations (i.e., young adults) have shown risky listening behaviors, particularly in areas with high environmental noise (Levey et al., 2011, 2013; Fligor et al., 2014).

Counseling and education are needed to improve listening behaviors, particularly in high-level, high-duration users. Experts recommend use of sound limiters on devices, limitations to duration of listening based on level (e.g., 80–90 rule, listen to PLD with earbuds at 80% of maximum level for no greater than 90 minutes at a time), and noise-canceling/noise-isolating head/earphones that can reduce environmental noise.

Occupational Noise

Occupational noise in children might seem to be a minor issue today. However, many first jobs for adolescents and teenagers can include lawn care, construction, and other jobs involving use of heavy machinery and equipment that can pose a risk for hearing loss. Farm youth represent a unique population where children are exempt from child labor age restrictions. Youth of any age can be employed at any time, in any occupation in agriculture on a farm owned or operated by their caregiver (U.S. Department of Labor, 2007). A study in farm youth working on Vermont dairy farms found the average age youth started working was 8.4 years and during the summer months worked an average of 41.3 hr/week. Two of the ten children monitored exceeded the Occupational Safety and Health Administration's (OSHA) action level for noise exposure with noise doses of 206% and 127%. Noise sources included tractors, all-terrain vehicles, and chain saws, among others (Lander et al., 2007). In comparison to NHANES national representative data, youth working on Ohio farms had a higher prevalence of hearing loss and nearly twice the prevalence of notched audiograms (Renick et al., 2009). Marlenga et al. (2012) followed a cohort of young workers (mean age at inception 14.5 years) for 16 years as part of a hearing conservation intervention for high school students. The majority worked at some point in agricultural settings. However, other common sources of noise included recreational noise, occupational noise, and chemicals known or suspected to have ototoxic effects or implicated in increasing risk for NIHL. Over the 16-year period, 42.8% of males and 27.7% of females had decreases to hearing acuity greater than 15 dB at higher frequencies (maximum change at 3, 4, or 6 kHz). The risk factor analysis was limited to males in the study because of the small female sample size. The findings showed increased risk with occupational, recreational, as well as chemical exposures. The use of hearing protection devices (HPDs) appeared to mitigate the majority of these effects. However, use of HPDs among adolescents in farm environments was rare and sporadic (Reed et al., 2006).

Nonoccupational Noise Exposure

The majority of noise exposure associated with children is nonoccupational in nature. Noise exposure sources with potential risk for NIHL include, but are not limited to, toys, power tools, motorized vehicles (e.g., boats, jet ski, motorcycle), music (e.g., played and listened in home, car, concert/club venues, school or garage band, and via PLDs), movie theaters, use of firearms and firecrackers, sporting events, and others (Axelsson et al., 1985; Harrison, 2008; Hellstrom et al., 1992; Jokitulppo et al., 1997).

An early concern is application of sleep machines that commonly use white noise and environmental sounds with the goal to increase uninterrupted sleep.

One potential risk is the level and duration these sounds are played. A recent study found that many of these devices can reach levels greater than 85 dB SPL (A), which if played for 8 hr would exceed occupational noise limits for an 8-hr period (Hugh et al., 2014). A second concern is effects of broadband noise on development. Chang and Merzenich (2003) showed that rat pups exposed to continuous moderate levels of noise delayed the emergence of adult-like topographic representational order and refinement of response selectivity in the primary auditory cortex; similar effects were seen in shorter-term daily noise (10 hr) consistent with durations of sleep in infants and toddlers. There is limited evidence in humans to demonstrate delay in speech and language with use of sleep machines. A greater concern might be level and duration of noise. Parents should use caution in setting levels of these devices particularly when used for extended durations.

Loud toys are another risk factor for NIHL in children. There are no specific guidelines for safe limits of exposure to noisy toys. Federal regulations specify continuous sound produced by toys close to the ear should not exceed 65 dBA, and all other toys shall not exceed 85 dBA. Numerous papers have stressed the potential risk with sound levels produced by some toys (e.g., Axelsson et al., 1985; Hellstrom et al., 1992). The Sight and Hearing Association (SHA) selects a sample of toys each year that produce questionable noise levels. The noise levels are measured and published on the SHA website (http://sightandhearing.org) in advance of holiday shopping. Often covering the toy's speaker with tape or nontoxic glue is recommended to attenuate sound level (Weinreich et al., 2013); however, despite alterations, some toys might still produce potentially dangerous levels.

Another specific noise source of concern in youth is the use of firearms in hunting and target shooting. There are an estimated 1.6 million hunters in the United States between the ages of 6 and 15 years (U.S. Fish and Wildlife Service, 2006). A recent survey of youth shooting habits found that 78% began shooting before the age of 10 years. The majority reported they did not utilize hearing protection devices (HPD), and 10% reported constant tinnitus (Stewart et al., 2014).

The use of HPDs in children has received limited attention. A study by Chermak and Peters-McCarthy (1991) found that only 5.5% of children reported ever using HPDs while engaged in noisy actives. Numerous studies have examined knowledge and attitudes toward noise and barriers to HPD use and hearing conservation practices in young adult and adolescent populations (Crandell et al., 2004; Rawool et al., 2008; Widen et al., 2009). In brief, the findings indicated the majority of participants were aware that excessive noise can cause hearing damage (75%–95%), most did not believe they would lose hearing until an older age (76%), many thought hearing loss could be "fixed" with hearing aids (44%, it cannot), most never wore HPDs (72%–100%), participants with previous experience of hearing loss or tinnitus were more likely to wear HPDs, and a majority of participants would wear HPDs (85%) if provided free in a high-noise environment.

Prevention

To address the need for increased hearing conservation practices in young populations, educational programs and Web-based resources have been developed. For example, Dangerous Decibels is a public health partnership with the goal of reducing the incidence of NIHL and tinnitus. The program is founded in principles of health behavior theories including the transtheoretical model, the theory of planned behavior and reasoned action, the health belief model, and the social cognitive theory toward the goal of promoting healthy hearing behavior. The program has been demonstrated to improve knowledge, attitudes, and intended behaviors regarding sound exposure and use of hearing protection (Dell & Holmes, 2012; Griest et al., 2007), but follow-up has not addressed actual use of HPD, only intended behavior. Martin et al. (2013) evaluated and compared the effectiveness of NIHL prevention intervention in 1120 fourth-grade students. The intervention included (a) a classroom presentation by older-peer educators, (b) a classroom presentation by a health care professional, (c) exploration of a museum exhibition, and (d) exploration of an Internet-based virtual museum. The outcome examined the knowledge, attitudes, and intended behaviors in the students regarding healthy hearing behavior and use of HPDs. The classroom-based interventions were found to have the greatest impact. However, all intervention forms were recommended. Other programs include Cheers for Ears (Taljaard et al., 2013), Noisy Planet (NIDCD, http://www.noisyplanetnidcd.nih.gov /Pages/Default.aspx), Turn it to the Left (AAA, http://www.turnittotheleft.org), and Listen to your Buds (ASHA, http://www.asha.org/buds/).

The solution to reducing NIHL in children is to reduce the level and duration of exposure. However, many children and parents might be unaware of the long-term consequences of exposure to noise or lack knowledge or efficacy to prevent hearing loss. NIHL can be insidious, accumulating over time, with many not taking precautionary measures until already experiencing signs of damage (Rawool et al., 2008). A single exposure to loud sound can cause some aural fullness (i.e., plugged sensation) or even some ringing in the ears (i.e., tinnitus), but in most cases these symptoms subside shortly after the exposure. Those exposed might be under the impression that the resolved symptoms indicate that there was no damage or minimize perceived threat and susceptibility (Crandell et al., 2004; Newsom et al., 2012). Though the affects from a single exposure might indeed be limited, even a single noise exposure with recovered temporary effects can lead to later effects (Kujawa & Liberman, 2006).

The prevention of NIHL in children is dependent on (a) knowledge of noise risks and limitations to correct damage (relationship between noise intensity and duration), and (b) knowledge of the availability and types of HPDs for appropriate fit and application to different noise scenarios. Teenagers attending a concert might be less likely to use standard foam earplugs with high noise reduction ratings due to diminished fidelity and sound quality. However, they may be more likely to use musician ear plugs that have a lower attenuation rating, but still afford protection without sacrificing fidelity. Programs targeted at variable ages and populations (parents and children) are needed to increase awareness and encourage healthy hearing behaviors. Virtual experiences by application of filters and stimuli simulating tinnitus might allow children and parents to experience the effects of hearing loss and tinnitus in a safe manner to increase understanding of potential effects of noise. Furthermore, ensuring safe permissible noise levels at day cares and other venues (i.e., passive forms of prevention that do not require individual behavior change), supervising children's device usage, implementing level limiters, and enforcement of HPD use are encouraged. Other prevention strategies for NIHL exist including pharmacological approaches with agents similar to those being applied for ototoxic drugs (e.g. ACEMg, D-MET, ebselen, NAC, etc.)

The most common etiology of sensorineural hearing loss is unknown (Morzaria et al., 2004). Unknown should not be confused with idiopathic sudden sensorineural hearing loss. Numerous factors have been discussed that increase risk for hearing loss in pediatric populations. Vasconcellos et al. (2014) identified factors including birth weight, nutritional deficiencies, blood lead levels, and socioeconomic status. Understanding the risk factors is critical in targeting screening and preventive programs. Initiatives aimed at improving the health of babies and children through improved postnatal care (e.g., nutrition, vaccination, and so on), hearing conservation (e.g., reducing noise or smoke exposure), and alternative or preventative drug approaches can decrease risk for acquired hearing loss in children.

Summary

There are many sources of acquired preventable hearing loss arising from both pre- and postnatal exposure. Some are attributed to potentially unavoidable circumstances or events such as unforeseen injuries or trauma, or necessary interventions including therapeutic aminoglycoside treatment for disease. However, in other cases, hearing preservation might be achieved through proactive management of potentially harmful exposure (e.g., vaccination programs to prevent contraction of maternal disease, limiting noise exposure). Continued research and education surrounding safe listening practices and the factors potentially affecting hearing and the overall health and wellness of pregnant mothers and children is critical in reducing or preventing onset or progression of acquired hearing loss in youth.

References

Aldworth, J. (2009). *Results from the 2007 national survey on drug use and health: National findings*. Rockville, MD: Office of Applied Studies, NSDUH Series H-34, DHSS Publication No. SMA 08-4343.

American Academy of Audiology. *Turn it to the left*. Retrieved July 1, 2015, from http://www.turnittotheleft.org

American Academy of Pediatrics. (1997). Noise: A hazard for the fetus and newborn (RE9728). *Pediatrics, 100*(4), 1–10.

American College of Medical Genetics (ACMG; 2002). Genetics evaluation guidelines for the etiologic diagnosis of congenital hearing loss. *Genetics in Medicine, 4*(3), 162.

Andrade, J. Q., Bunduki, V., Curti, S. P., Figueiredo, C. A., de Oliveira, M. I., & Zugaib, M. (2006). Rubella in pregnancy: Intrauterine transmission and perinatal outcome during a Brazilian epidemic. *Journal of Clinical Virology, 35*(3), 285–291. doi:10.1016/j.jcv.2005.09.007

Axelsson, A., & Jerson, T. (1985). Listen to your buds; Noisy toys: a possible source of sensorineural hearing loss. *American Speech-Language Hearing Association, Pediatrics, 76*(4), 574–578.

Bacino, C. A., Prezant, T. R., Bu, X., Fournier, P., & Fischel-Ghodsian, N. (1995). Susceptibility mutations in the mitochondrial small ribosomal RNA gene in aminoglycoside induced deafness. *Pharmacogenetic, 5*(3), 165–172.

Bandstra, E. S., Morrow, C. E., Mansoor, E., & Accornero, V. H. (2010). Prenatal drug exposure: Infant and toddler outcomes. *Journal of Addictive Diseases, 29*(2), 245–258.

Bass, J. K., & Bhagat, S. P. (2014). Challenges in ototoxicity monitoring in the pediatric oncology population. *Journal of the American Academy of Audiology, 25*(8), 760–774.

Bate, S. L., Dollard, S. C., & Cannon, M. J. (2010). Cytomegalovirus seroprevalence in the United States: The national health and nutrition examination surveys, 1988–2004. *Clinical Infectious Diseases, 50*(11), 1439–1447. doi:10.1086/652438

Beckwith, A. M., & Burke, S. A. (2015). Identification of early developmental deficits in infants with prenatal heroin, methadone, and other opioid exposure. *Clinical Pediatriacs (Phila), 54*(4), 328–335. doi:10.1177/0009922814549545

Behnke, M., Smith, V. C., Levy, S., Ammerman, S. D., Gonzalez, P. K., Ryan, S. A., . . . Carlo, W. A. (2013). Prenatal substance abuse: Short-and long-term effects on the exposed fetus. *Pediatrics, 131*(3), e1009–e1024.

Berrettini, S., Forli, F., Passetti, S., Rocchi, A., Pollina, L., Cecchetti, D., . . . Siciliano, G. (2008). Mitochondrial non-syndromic sensorineural hearing loss: A clinical, audiological and pathological study from Italy, and revision of the literature. *Bioscience Reports, 28*, 49–59.

Bhagat, S. P., Bass, J. K., White, S. T., Qaddoumi I., Wilson, M. W., Wu, J., & Rodriguez-Galindo, C. (2010). Monitoring carboplatin ototoxicity with distortion-product otoacoustic emissions in children with retinoblastoma. *International Journal of Pediatric Otorhinolaryngology, 74*(10), 1156–1163.

Bhandare, N., Jackson, A., Eisbruch, A., Pan, C. C., Flickinger, J. C., Antonelli, P., & Mendenhall, W. M. (2010). Radiation therapy and hearing loss. *International Journal of Radiation Oncology, Biology and Physics, 76*(3), S50–S57.

Bhutta, M. F. (2014). Epidemiology and pathogenesis of otitis media: Construction of a phenotype landscape, *Audiology and Neurotology, 19*(3), 10–23.

Birnholz, J., & Benacerraf, B. (1983). The development of human fetal hearing. *Science, 222*(4623), 516–518. doi:10.1126/science.6623091

Blackburn, S. (1998). Environmental impact of the NICU on developmental outcomes. *Journal of Pediatric Nursing, 13*(5), 279–289.

Boudewyns, A., Declau, F., Van den Ende, J., Van Kerschaver, E., Dirckx, S., Hofkens-Van den Brandt, A., & Van de Heyning P. (2011). Otitis media with effusion: An underestimated cause of hearing loss in infants. *Otology and Neurotology, 32*(5), 799–804.

Bremmer, P., Byers, J. F., & Kiehl, E. (2003). Noise and the premature infant: Physiological effects and practice implications. *Journal of Obstetric, Gynecologic, & Neonatal Nursing, 32*(4), 447–454. doi:10.1177/0884217503255009

Brock, P. R., Knight, K. R., Freyer, D. R., Campbell, K. C., Steyger, P. S., Blakley, B. W. . . . Neuwelt, E. A. (2012). Platinum-induced ototoxicity in children: A consensus review on mechanisms, predisposition, and protection, including a new International Society of Pediatric Oncology Boston ototoxicity scale. *Journal of Clinical Oncology, 30*(19), 2408–2417.

Brown, G. (2009). NICU noise and the preterm infant. *Neonatal Network, 28*(3), 165–173.

Bunikowski, R., Grimmer, I., Heiser, A., Metze, B., Schafer, A., & Obladen, M. (1998). Neurodevelopmental outcome after prenatal exposure to opiates. *European Journal of Pediatrics, 157*(9), 724–730.

Campbell, K. C., Rybak, L. P., Meech, R. P., & Hughes, L. (1996). D-methionine provides excellent protection from cisplatin ototoxicity in the rat. *Hearing Research, 102*, 90–98.

Cannon, M. J. (2009). Congenital cytomegalovirus (CMV) epidemiology and awareness. *Journal of Clinical Virology, 46*(Suppl. 4), S6–S10. doi:10.1016/j.jcv.2009.09.002

Casano, R. A., Johnson, D. F., Bykhovskaya, Y., Torricelli, F., Bigozzi, M., & Fischel-Ghodsian, N. (1999). Inherited susceptibility to aminoglycoside ototoxicity: Genetic heterogeneity and clinical implications. *American Journal of Otolaryngology, 20*(3), 151–156.

Centers for Disease Control and Prevention. (2010). *Cytomegalovirus (CMV) and congenital CMV infection.* Retrieved from http://www.cdc.gov/cmv/congenital-infection.html

Centers for Disease Control and Prevention. (2011). Estimated burden of acute otitis externa—United States, 2003–2007. *Morbidity and Mortality Weekly Report (MMWR), 60*(19), 605–609. Retrieved from http://www.cdc.gov/mmwr/preview/mmwrhtml/mm6019a2.htm

Centers for Disease Control and Prevention. (2013). Nationwide rubella epidemic—Japan, 2013. *Morbidity and Mortality Weekly Report (MMWR), 62*(23), 457–462. Retrieved from http://www.cdc.gov/mmwr/preview/mmwrhtml/mm6223a1.htm

Centers for Disease Control and Prevention. (2015). Epidemiology and prevention of vaccine-preventable diseases. *The Pink Book* (13th ed.). Retrieved from http://www.cdc.gov/vaccines/pubs/pinkbook/downloads/rubella.pdf

Chang, E. F., & Merzenich, M. M. (2003). Environmental noise retards auditory cortical development. *Science, 300*(5618), 498–502.

Chasnoff, I. J., Burns, W. J., Schnoll, S. H., & Burns, K. A. (1985). Cocaine use in pregnancy. *New England Journal of Medicine*, 313(11), 666–669. doi:10.1056/NEJM198509123131105

Chermak, G. D., & Peters-McCarthy, E. (1991). The effectiveness of an eduational hearing conservation program for elementary school children. *Language, Speech, and Hearing Services in Schools, 22*, 308–312.

Church, M. (1987). Chronic in utero alcohol exposure affects auditory function in rats and in humans. *Alcohol, 4*(4), 231–239.

Church, M. W., Crossland, W. J., Holmes, P. A., Overbeck, G. W., & Tilak, J. P. (1998). Effects of prenatal cocaine on hearing, vision, growth, and behavior. *Annals of the New York Academy of Sciences, 846*(1), 12–28.

Church, M. W., Kaltenbach, J. A., Blakley, B. W., & Burgio, D. L. (1995). The comparative effects of sodium thiosulfate, diethyldithiocarbamate, fosfomycin, and WR-2721 on ameliorating cisplatin-induced ototoxicity. *Hearing Research, 86*, 195–203.

Clark, R. H., Bloom, B. T., Spitzer, A. R., & Gerstmann, D. R. (2006). Reported medication use in the neonatal intensive care unit: Data from a large national data set. *Pediatrics, 117*(6), 1979–1987. doi:10.1542/peds.2005-1707

Cnattingius, S. (2004). The epidemiology of smoking during pregnancy: Smoking prevalence, maternal characteristics, and pregnancy outcomes. *Nicotine & Tobacco Research, 6* (Suppl. 2), S125–S140. doi:10.1080/14622200410001669187

Cohen, B. E., Durstenfeld, A., & Roehm, P. C. (2014). Viral causes of hearing loss: A review for hearing health professionals. *Trends in Hearing, 18*. doi:10.1177/2331216514541361

Cohen-Kerem, R., Bar-Oz, B., Nulman, I., Papaioannou, V. A., & Koren, G. (2007). Hearing in children with fetal alcohol spectrum disorder (FASD). *Canadian Journal of Clinical Pharmacology, 14*(3), 307–312.

Colugnati, F. A., Staras, S. A., Dollard, S. C., & Cannon, M. J. (2007). Incidence of cytomegalovirus infection among the general population and pregnant women in the United States. *BMC Infectious Diseases, 7*, 71. doi:10.1186/1471-2334-7-71

Cone-Wesson, B. (2005). Prenatal alcohol and cocaine exposure: Influences on cognition, speech, language, and hearing. *Journal of Communication Disorders, 38*(4), 279–302.

Cone-Wesson, B., Kurtzberg, D., & Vaughan Jr, H. G. (1987). Electrophysiologic assessment of auditory pathways in high risk infants. *International Journal of Pediatric Otorhinolaryngology, 14*(2–3), 203–214. http://dx.doi.org/10.1016/0165-5876(87)90032-2

Cone-Wesson, B., & Spingarn, A. (1993). Effects of maternal cocaine abuse on neonatal auditory brainstem responses. *American Journal of Audiology, 2*(3), 48–54.

Conway, N. (1965). Streptomycin in pregnancy: Effect on the foetal ear. *BMJ, 2*(5456), 260–263.

Cooper, A. C., Commer, A. R., Finkelstein, M., Lipnik, P. G., Tollefson, L. M., Wilcox, R. A., & Hoff, D. S. (2011). Otoacoustic emissions screen results in critically ill neonates who received gentamicin in the first week of life. *Pharmacotherapy, 32*(7), 649–657.

Coradini, P. P., Cigana, L., Selistre, S. G., Rosito, L. S., & Brunetto, A. L. (2007). Ototoxicity from cisplatin therapy in childhood cancer. *Journal of Pediatric Hematology Oncology, 29*(6), 60–67.

Crandell, C., Mills, T. L., & Gauthier, R. (2004). Knoweldge, behaviors, and attitudes about hearing loss and hearing protection among racial/ethnically diverse young adults. *Journal of the National Medical Association, 96*(2), 176–186.

Crofton, K. M., & Rice, D. C. (1999). Low-frequency hearing loss following perinatal exposure to 3, 3′, 4, 4′, 5-pentachlorobiphenyl (PCB 126) in rats. *Neurotoxicology and Teratology, 21*(3), 299–301.

Czeizel, A. E., Rockenbauer, M., Olsen, J., & Sørensen, H. T. (2000). A teratological study of aminoglycoside antibiotic treatment during pregnancy. *Scandinavian Journal of Infectious Diseases, 32*(3), 309–313. doi:10.1080/00365540050165974

Dammeyer, J. (2010). Congenital rubella syndrome and delayed manifestations. *International Journal of Pediatric Otorhinolaryngology, 74*(9), 1067–1070. http://dx.doi.org/10.1016/j.ijporl.2010.06.007

Darcy, A. E., Hancock, L. E., & Ware, E. J. (2008). A descriptive study of noise in the neonatal intensive care unit ambient levels and perceptions of contributing factors. *Advances in Neonatal Care, 8*(3), 165–175. doi:10.1097/01.ANC.0000324341.24841.6e

Day, N. L., Cottreau, C. M., & Richardson, G. A. (1993). The epidemiology of alcohol, marijuana, and cocaine use among women of childbearing age and pregnant women. *Clinical Obstetrics and Gynecology, 36*(2), 232–245.

Dell, S. M., & Holmes, A. E. (2012). The effect of a hearing conservation program on adolescents' attitudes towards noise. *Noise and Health, 14*(56), 39–44.

Demmler, G. J. (1991). Infectious Diseases Society of America and Centers for Disease Control: Summary of a workshop on surveillance for congenital cytomegalovirus disease. *Review of Infectious Diseases, 13*(2), 315–329.

Dickey, D. T., Muldoon, L. L., Kraemer, D. F., & Neuwelt, E. A. (2004). Protection against cisplatin-induced ototoxicity by N-acetylcysteine in a rat model. *Hearing Research, 193*, 25–30.

Dinc, A. E, Damar, M., Ugur, M. B., Oz, I. I., Elicora, S. S., Biskin, S., & Tutar, H. (2015). Do the angle and the length of the eustachian tube influence the development of chronic otitis media? *Laryngoscope, 125*(9), 2187–2192.

Dollard, S. C., Grosse, S. D., & Ross, D. S. (2007). New estimates of the prevalence of neurological and sensory sequelae and mortality associated with congenital cytomegalovirus infection. *Reviews in Medical Virology, 17*(5), 355–363. doi:10.1002/rmv.544

Donald, P., Doherty, E., & Van Zyl, F. (1991). Hearing loss in the child following streptomycin administration during pregnancy. *Central African Journal of Medicine, 37*(8), 268.

Donald, P., & Sellars, S. (1981). Streptomycin ototoxicity in the unborn. *SA Medical Journal, 22*, 316–318.

Du, X., & Hamre, K. M. (2001). Increased cell death in the developing vestibulocochlear ganglion complex of the mouse after prenatal ethanol exposure. *Teratology, 64*(6), 301–310. doi:10.1002/tera.1085

Dumas, G., & Charachon, R. (1982). Ototoxicity of kanamycin in developing guinea pigs. *Acta Otolaryngologica, 94*(1–6), 203–212.

Durante, A. S., Ibidi, S. M., Lotufo, J. P., & Carvallo, R. M. (2011). Maternal smoking during pregnancy: Impact on otoacoustic emissions in neonates. *International Journal of Pediatric Otorhinolaryngology, 75*(9), 1093–1098. doi:10.1016/j.ijporl.2011.05.023

Dzhambov, A. M., Dimitrova, D. D., & Dimitrakova, E. D. (2014). Noise exposure during pregnancy, birth outcomes and fetal development: Meta-analyses using quality effects model. *Folia Medica (Plovdiv), 56*(3), 204–214.

Ealy, M., Lynch, K. A., Meyer, N. C., & Smith, R. J. H. (2011). The prevalence of mitochondrial mutations associated with aminoglycoside-induced sensorineural hearing loss in an NICU population. *Laryngoscope, 121*(6), 1184–1186. doi:10.1002/lary.21778

Edson, R. S., & Terrell, C. L. (1999). The aminoglycosides. *Mayo Clinic Proceedings, 74*(5), 519–528. http://dx.doi.org/10.4065/74.5.519

El-Barbary, M. N., Ismail, R. I., & Ibrahim, A. A. (2015). Gentamicin extended interval regimen and ototoxicity in neonates. *International Journal of Pediatric Otorhinolaryngology, 79*(8), 1294–1298.

El-Makhzangy, A. M., Ismail, N. M., Galal, S. B., Sobhy, T. S., & Hegazy, A. A. (2012). Can vaccination against pneumococci prevent otitis media with effusion? *European Archives of Otorhinolaryngology, 269*(9), 2021–2026.

Engleder, E., Honeder, C., Klobasa, J., Wirth, M., Arnoldner, C., & Gabor, F. (2014). Preclinical evaluation of thermoreversible triamcinolone acetonide hydrogels for drug delivery to the inner ear. *International Journal of Pharmaceutics, 471*, 297–302.

Estivill, X., Govea, N., Barcelo, E., Badenas, C., Romero, E., Moral, L., . . . Torroni, A. (1998). Familial progressive sensorineural deafness is mainly due to the mtDNA A1555G mutation and is enhanced by treatment of aminoglycosides. *American Journal of Human Genetics, 62*(1), 27–35.

Eyler, F. D., Behnke, M., Conlon, M., Woods, N. S., & Wobie, K. (1998). Birth outcome from a prospective, matched study of prenatal crack/cocaine use: I. Interactive and dose effects on health and growth. *Pediatrics, 101*(2), 229–236.

Fischel-Ghodsian, N., Prezant, T. R., Chaltraw, W. E., Wendt, K. A., Nelson, R. A., Arnos, K. S., & Falk, R. E. (1997). Mitochondrial gene mutation is a significant predisposing factor in aminoglycoside ototoxicity. *American Journal of Otolaryngology, 18*(3), 173–178.

Fligor, B. J., & Cox, L. C. (2004). Output levels of commercially available portable compact disc players and the potential risk to hearing, *Ear and Hearing, 25*(6), 513–527.

Fligor, B. J., Levey, S., & Levey, T. (2014). Cultural and demographic factors influencing noise exposure estimates from use of portable listening devices in an urban environment. *Journal of Speech Language and Hearing Research, 57*(4), 1535–1547.

Fowler, K. B., & Boppana, S. B. (2006). Congenital cytomegalovirus (CMV) infection and hearing deficit. *Journal of Clinical Virology, 35*(2), 226–231. doi:10.1016/j.jcv.2005.09.016

Fowler, K. B., McCollister, F. P., Dahle, A. J., Boppana, S., Britt, W. J., & Pass, R. F. (1997). Progressive and fluctuating sensorineural hearing loss in children with asymptomatic congenital cytomegalovirus infection. *Journal of Pediatrics, 130*(4), 624–630.

Gerhardt, K. J., Abrams, R. M., & Oliver, C. C. (1990). Sound environment of the fetal sheep. *American Journal of Obstetrics and Gynecology, 162*(1), 282–287.

Gerhardt, K. J., Huang, X., Arrington, K. E., Meixner, K., & Antonelli, P. J. (1996). Fetal sheep in utero hear through bone conduction. *American Journal of Otolaryngology, 17*(6), 374–379.

Gerhardt, K. J., Pierson, L. L., Huang, X., Abrams, R. M., & Rarey, K. E. (1999). Effects of intense noise exposure on fetal sheep auditory brain stem response and inner ear histology. *Ear and Hearing, 20*(1), 21–32.

Giebink, G. S. (2000). Otitis media prevention: Non-vaccine prophylaxis. *Vaccine, 19*, S129–S133.

Gilliland, F. D., Li, Y.-F., & Peters, J. M. (2001). Effects of maternal smoking during pregnancy and environmental tobacco smoke on asthma and wheezing in children. *American Journal of Respiratory and Critical Care Medicine, 163*(2), 429–436.

Gisselsson-Solen, M. (2015). Acute otitis media in children—Current treatment and prevention. *Current Infectious Disease Reports, 17*(5), 476.

Goderis, J., De Leenheer, E., Smets, K., Van Hoecke, H., Keymeulen, A., & Dhooge, I. (2014). Hearing loss and congenital CMV infection: A systematic review. *Pediatrics, 134*(5), 972–982.

Goldey, E. S., & Crofton, K. M. (1998). Thyroxine replacement attenuates hypothyroxinemia, hearing loss, and motor deficits following developmental exposure to Aroclor 1254 in rats. *Toxicological Sciences, 45*(1), 94–105.

Goodlett, C. R., & Horn, K. H. (2001). Mechanisms of alcohol-induced damage to the developing nervous system. *Alcohol Research and Health, 25*(3), 175–184.

Graven, S. N. (2000). Sound and the developing infant in the NICU: Conclusions and recommendations for care. *Journal of Perinatology, 20*(8 Pt 2), S88–S93.

Griest, S. E., Folmer, R. L., & Martin, W. H. (2007). Effectiveness of "Dangerous Decibels" a school-based hearing loss prevention program. *American Journal of Audiology, 16*(2), S165–S181.

Grimmer, I., Bührer, C., Aust, G., & Obladen, M. (1999). Hearing in newborn infants of opiate-addicted mothers. *European Journal of Pediatrics, 158*(8), 653–657. doi:10.1007/s004310051170

Grohskopf, L. A., Huskins, W. C., Sinkowitz-Cochran, R. L., Levine, G. L., Goldmann, D. A., Jarvis, W. R., & Network, t. P. P. (2005). Use of antimicrobial agents in United States neonatal and pediatric intensive care patients. *Pediatric Infectious Disease Journal, 24*(9), 766–773. doi:10.1097/01.inf.0000178064.55193.1c

Grosse, S. D., Ross, D. S., & Dollard, S. C. (2008). Congenital cytomegalovirus (CMV) infection as a cause of permanent bilateral hearing loss: A quantitative assessment. *Journal of Clinical Virology, 41*(2), 57–62. doi:10.1016/j.jcv.2007.09.004

Guan, M. X. (2011). Mitochondrial 12S rRNA mutations associated with aminoglycoside ototoxicity. *Mitochondrion, 11*(2), 237–245. http://dx.doi.org/10.1016/j.mito.2010.10.006

Hanna, E. Z., Faden, V. B., & Dufour, M. C. (1994). The motivational correlates of drinking, smoking, and illicit drug use during pregnancy. *Journal of Substance Abuse, 6*(2), 155–167. http://dx.doi.org/10.1016/S0899-3289(94)90181-3

Harrison, R. V. (2008). Noise-induced hearing loss in children: A less than silent environmental danger. *Paediatrics and Child Health, 13*(5), 377–382.

Hellstrom, P. A., Dengerink, H. A., & Axelsson, A. (1992). Noise levels from toys and recreational articles for children and teenagers. *British Journal of Audiology, 26*(5), 267–270.

Henderson, E., Testa, M. A., & Hartnick, C. (2011). Prevalence of noise-induced hearing threshold shifts and hearing loss among US youths. *Pediatrics, 127*, 39–46.

Henley, C. M., & Schacht, J. (1988). Pharmacokinetics of aminoglycoside antibiotics in blood, inner-ear fluids and tissues and their relationship to ototoxicity. *International Journal of Audiology, 27*(3), 137–146. doi:10.3109/00206098809081584

Huang, N. C., & Sataloff, R. T. (2011). Autoimmune inner ear disease in children. *Otology and Neurotology, 32*(2), 213–216.

Huang, X., Gerhardt, K. J., Abrams, R. M., & Antonelli, P. J. (1997). Temporary threshold shifts induced by low-pass and high-pass filtered noises in fetal sheep in utero. *Hearing Research, 113*(1–2), 173–181. http://dx.doi.org/10.1016/S0378-5955(97)00139-1

Huang, X., Xu, J., Xu, M., Zhou, L. F., Zang, R., Lang, L., . . . Zhang, Z. (2013). Clinical features of intracranial vestibular schwannomas. *Oncology Letters, 5*(1), 57–62.

Hugh, S. C., Wolter, N. E., Propst, E. J., Gordon, K. A., Cushing, S. L., & Paspsin, B. C. (2014). Infant sleep machines and hazardous sound pressure levels. *Pediatrics 133*(4), 677–681.

Hyde, T. B., Schmid, D. S., & Cannon, M. J. (2010). Cytomegalovirus seroconversion rates and risk factors: Implications for congenital CMV. *Reviews in Medical Virology, 20*(5), 311–326. doi:10.1002/rmv.659

Ibrahim, H. M., Kamel, T. B., Abdel-Salam, N. M., & Abu-Ata, S. R. (2011). Study of auditory function in children with chronic lung diseases. *International Journal of Pediatric Otorhinolaryngology, 75*(1), 39–42.

Jensen, R. G., Koch, A., & Homoe P. (2013). The risk of hearing loss in a population with a high prevalence of chronic suppurative otitis media. *International Journal of Pediatric Otorhinolaryngology, 77*(9), 1530–1535.

Joint Commission on Infant Hearing (JCIH; 2007). Year 2007 position statement: Principles and guidelines for early hearing detection and intervention programs. *Pediatrics, 120*(4), 898–921. doi:10.1542/peds.2007-2333

Joint Commission on Infant Hearing (JCIH; 2013). Supplement to the JCIH 2007 position statement: Principles and guidelines for early intervention after confirmation that a child is deaf or hard of hearing. *Pediatrics, 131*(4), e1324–e1349. doi:10.1542/peds.2013-0008

Jokitulppo, J. S., Bjork, E. A.,& Akaan-Penttila, E. (1997). Estimated leisure noise exposure and hearing symptoms in Finnish teenagers. *Scandinavian Audiology, 26*(4), 257–262.

Jones, H. C. (1973). Intrauterine ototoxicity. A case report and review of literature. *Journal of the National Medical Association, 65*(3), 201.

Keith, S. E., Michaud, D. S., Feder, K., Haider, I., Marro, L., Thompson, E., & Marcoux, A. M. (2011). MP3 player listening sound pressure levels among 10 to 17 year old students. *Journal of the Acoustical Society of America, 130*(5), 2756–2764.

Kenneson, A., & Cannon, M. J. (2007). Review and meta-analysis of the epidemiology of congenital cytomegalovirus (CMV) infection. *Reviews in Medical Virology, 17*(4), 253–276. doi:10.1002/rmv.535

Kent, W., Tan, A., Clarke, M. C., & Bardell, T. (2002). Excessive noise levels in the neonatal ICU: Potential effects on auditory system development. *Journal of Otolaryngology, 31*(6), 355–360.

Kimberlin, D. W., Lin, C.-Y., Sánchez, P. J., Demmler, G. J., Dankner, W., Shelton, M., . . . Whitley, R. J. (2003). Effect of ganciclovir therapy on hearing in symptomatic congenital cytomegalovirus disease involving the central nervous system: A randomized, controlled trial. *Journal of Pediatrics, 143*(1), 16–25. http://dx.doi.org/10.1016/S0022-3476(03)00192-6

Kirkwood, A., Harris, C., Timar, N., & Koren, G. (2007). Is gentamicin ototoxic to the fetus? *Journal of Obstetrics and Gynaecology Canada, 29*(2), 140–145.

Knight, K. R., Kraemer, D. F., Winter, C., & Neuwelt, E. A. (2007). Early changes in auditory function as a result of platinum chemotherapy: Use of extended high-frequency audiometry and evoked distortion produce otoacoustic emissions. *Journal of Clinical Oncology, 25*(10), 1190–1195.

Konings, A., Van Camp, G., Goethals, A., Van Eyken, E., Vandevelde, A., Azza, J. B., . . . Van Laer, L. (2008). Mutation analysis of mitochondrial DNA 12SrRNA and tRNASer (UCN) genes in non-syndromic hearing loss patients. *Mitochondrion, 8*(5), 377–382.

Korres, S., Riga, M., Balatsouras, D., Papadakis, C., Kanellos, P., & Ferekidis, E. (2007). Influence of smoking on developing cochlea. Does smoking during pregnancy affect the amplitudes of transient evoked otoacoustic emissions in newborns? *International Journal of Pediatric Otorhinolaryngology, 71*(5), 781–786. doi:10.1016/j.ijporl.2007.01.015

Kotch, L. E., & Sulik, K. K. (1992). Experimental fetal alcohol syndrome: Proposed pathogenic basis for a variety of associated facial and brain anomalies. *American Journal of Medical Genetics, 44*(2), 168–176. doi:10.1002/ajmg.1320440210

Kotecha, B., & Richardson, G. P. (1994). Ototoxicity in vitro: Effects of neomycin, gentamicin, dihydrostreptomycin, amikacin, spectinomycin, neamine, spermine and poly-L-lysine. *Hearing Research*, 73(2), 173–184.

Krueger, C., Wall, S., Parker, L., & Nealis, R. (2005). Elevated sound levels within a busy NICU. *Neonatal Network, 24*(6), 33–37. doi:10.1891/0730-0832.24.6.33

Kujawa, S. G., & Liberman, M. C. (2006). Acceleration of age-related hearing loss by early noise exposure: Evidence of a misspent youth. *Journal of Neuroscience, 26*(7), 2115–2123.

Kumar, A., Mathew, K., Alexander, S. A., & Kiran, C. (2009). Output sound pressure levels of personal music systems and their effect on hearing. *Noise Health, 11*(44), 132–140.

Kuo, C. L., Shiao, A. S., Yung, M., Sakagami, M., Sudhoff, H., Wang, C. H., Hsu, C. H., & Lien, C. F. (2015). Updates and knowledge gaps in cholesteatoma research. *BioMed Research International*, 2015, article ID 854024.

Kupka, S., Tóth, T., Wróbel, M., Zeißler, U., Szyfter, W., Szyfter, K., . . . Pfister, M. (2002). Mutation A1555G in the 12S rRNA gene and its epidemiological importance in German, Hungarian, and Polish patients. *Human Mutation, 19*(3), 308–309. doi:10.1002/humu.9017

Lacroix, I., Damase-Michel, C., Lapeyre-Mestre, M., & Montastruc, J. L. (2000). Prescription of drugs during pregnancy in France. *The Lancet, 356*(9243), 1735–1736. http://dx.doi.org/10.1016/S0140-6736(00)03209-8

Lander, L. I., Rudnick, S. N., & Perry, M. J. (2007). Assessing noise exposure in farm youths. *Journal of Agromedicine 12*(2), 25–32.

Langer, T., Zehnoff-Dinnesen, A., Radtke, S., Meitert, J., & Zolk, O. (2013). Understanding platinum-induced ototoxicity. *Trends in Pharmacological Sciences, 34*(8), 458–469.

Lary, S., Briassoulis, G., de Vries, L., Dubowitz, L. M. S., & Dubowitz, V. i. (1985). Hearing threshold in preterm and term infants by auditory brainstem response. *Journal of Pediatrics, 107*(4), 593–599. http://dx.doi.org/10.1016/S0022-3476(85)80030-5

Laughlin, L. (2011). *U.S. Census Bureau. Maternity leave and employment patterns of first-time mothers: 1961–2008.* Retrieved from https://www.census.gov/prod/2011pubs/p70-128.pdf

Le Prell, C. G., Hughes, L. F., & Miller, J. M. (2007). Free radical scavengers vitamins A, C, and E plus magnesium reduce noise trauma. *Free Radical Biology and Medicine, 42*(9), 1454–1463.

Le Prell, C. G., Ojano-Dirain, C., Rudnick, E. W., Nelson, M. A., DeRemer, S. J., Prieskorn, D. M., & Miller, J. M. (2014). Assessment of nutrient supplement to reduce gentamicin-induced ototoxicity. *Journal of the Assocication for Research in Otolaryngology, 15*(3), 375–393.

Lee, J. Y., & Bowden, D. S. (2000). Rubella virus replication and links to teratogenicity. *Clinical Microbiology Reviews, 13*(4), 571–587.

Leveque, M., Marlin, S., Jonard, L., Procaccio, V., Reynier, P., Amati-Bonneau, P., . . . Denoyelle, F. (2007). Whole mitochondrial genome screening in maternally inherited non-syndromic hearing impairment using a microarray resequencing mitochondrial DNA chip. *European Journal of Human Genetics, 15*(11), 1145–1155.

Levey, S., Fligor, B. J., Cutler, C., & Harushimana, I. (2013). Portable music player users: Cultural differences and potential dangers. *Noise Health, 15*(66), 296–300.

Levey, S., Levey, T., & Fligor, B. J. (2011). Noise exposure estimates of urban MP3 player users. *Journal of Speech, Language, and Hearing Research, 54*(1), 263–277.

Li, G., Sha, S. H., Zotova, E., Arezzo, J., Van De Water, T., & Schacht, J. (2002). Salicylate protects hearing and kidney function from cisplatin toxicity without compromising its oncolytic action. *Laboratory Investigation, 82*, 585–596.

Li, R., Xing, G., Yan, M., Cao, X., Liu, X. Z., Bu, X., & Guan, M. X. (2004). Cosegregation of C-insertion at position 961 with the A1555G mutation of the mitochondrial 12S rRNA gene in a large Chinese family with maternally inherited hearing loss. *American Journal of Medical Genetics Part A, 124*(2), 113–117.

Li, Z., Li, R., Chen, J., Liao, Z., Zhu, Y., Qian, Y., . . . Guan, M.-X. (2005). Mutational analysis of the mitochondrial 12S rRNA gene in Chinese pediatric subjects with aminoglycoside-induced and non-syndromic hearing loss. *Human Genetics, 117*(1), 9–15. doi:10.1007/s00439-005-1276-1

Locksmith, G. J., Chin, A., Vu, T., Shattuck, K. E., & Hankins, G. D. (2005). High compared with standard gentamicin dosing for chorioamnionitis: A comparison of maternal and fetal serum drug levels. *Obstetrics and Gynecology, 105*(3), 473–479.

Lu, J., Li, Z., Zhu, Y., Yang, A., Li, R., Zheng, J., . . . Guan, M. X. (2010). Mitochondrial 12S rRNA variants in 1642 Han Chinese pediatric subjects with aminoglycoside-induced and nonsyndromic hearing loss. *Mitochondrion, 10*(4), 380–390. doi:10.1016/j.mito.2010.01.007

Lynch, E. D., Gu, R., Pierce, C., & Kil, J. (2005). Reduction of acute cisplatin ototoxicity and nephrotoxicity in rats by oral administration of allopurinol and ebselen. *Hearing Research, 201*, 81–89.

Madden, C., Wiley, S., Schleiss, M., Benton, C., Meinzen-Derr, J., Greinwald, J., & Choo, D. (2005). Audiometric, clinical and educational outcomes in a pediatric symptomatic congenital cytomegalovirus (CMV) population with sensorineural hearing loss. *International Journal of Pediatric Otorhinolaryngology, 69*(9), 1191–1198. doi:10.1016/j.ijporl.2005.03.011

Mahboubi, H., Oliaei, S., Kiumehr, S., Dwabe, S., & Djalilian, H. R. (2013). The prevalence and characteristics of tinnitus in the youth population of the United States. *Laryngoscope, 123*(8), 2001–2008.

Malik, S., Pieter, N., Sudoyo, H., Kadir, A., & Marzuki, S. (2003). Prevalence of the mitochondrial DNA A1555G mutation in sensorineural deafness patients in island Southeast Asia. *Journal of Human Genetics, 48*(9), 480–483. doi:10.1007/s10038-003-0056-9

Malm, H., Martikainen, J., Klaukka, T., & Neuvonen, P. (2004). Prescription of hazardous drugs during pregnancy. *Drug Safety, 27*(12), 899–908. doi:10.2165/00002018-200427120-00006

Manicklal, S., Emery, V. C., Lazzarotto, T., Boppana, S. B., & Gupta, R. K. (2013). The "silent" global burden of congenital cytomegalovirus. *Clinical Microbiology Reviews, 26*(1), 86–102. doi:10.1128/CMR.00062-12

Marlenga, B., Berg, R. L., Linneman, J. G., Wood, D. J., Kirkhorn, S. R., & Pickett, W. (2012). Determinants of early-stage hearing loss among a cohort of young workers with 16-year follow-up. *Occupational and Environmental Medicine, 69*(7), 479–484.

Marom, T., Tan, A., Wilkinson, G. S., Pierson, K. S., Freeman, J. L., & Chonmaitree, T. (2014). Trends in otitis media-related health care use in the United States, 2001–2011. *JAMA Pediatrics, 168*(1), 68–75.

Marsal, K. (2006). iPod how big can it get? *Appleinsider*, May 24.

Martin, W. H., Griest, S. E., Sobel, J. L., & Howarth, L. C. (2013). Randomized trial of four noise-induced hearing loss and tinnitus prevention interventions for children. *International Journal of Audiology, 52*, S41–S49.

May, P. A., & Gossage, J. P. (2001). Estimating the prevalence of fetal alcohol syndrome: A summary. *Alcohol Research and Health, 25*(3), 159–167.

Milette, I. (2010). Decreasing noise level in our NICU: The impact of a noise awareness educational program. *Advances in Neonatal Care, 10*(6), 343–351. doi:10.1097/ANC.0b013e3181fc8108

Mitchell, A. A., Gilboa, S. M., Werler, M. M., Kelley, K. E., Louik, C., & Hernández-Díaz, S. (2011). Medication use during pregnancy, with particular focus on prescription drugs: 1976–2008. *American Journal of Obstetrics and Gynecology, 205*(1), 51.e51–51.e58. http://dx.doi.org/10.1016/j.ajog.2011.02.029

Morita, Y., Yamamoto, Y., Oshima, S., Takahashi, K., & Takahashi, S. (2015). Pediatric middle ear cholesteatoma: The comparative study of congenital cholesteatoma and acquired cholsteatoma. *European Archives of Otorhinolaryngology*. PMID: 26044405

Morton, C. C. (2002). Genetics, genomics and gene discovery in the auditory system. *Human Molecular Genetics, 11*(10), 1229–1240. doi:10.1093/hmg/11.10.1229

Morton, C. C., & Nance, W. E. (2006). Newborn hearing screening—A silent revolution. *New England Journal of Medicine, 354*(20), 2151–2164.

Morton, N. E. (1991). Genetic epidemiology of hearing impairment. *Annals of the New York Academy of Sciences, 630*, 16–31.

Morzaria, S., Weterberg, B. D., & Kozak, F. K. (2004). Systematic review of the etiology of bilateral sensorineural hearing loss in children. *International Journal of Pediatric Otorhinolaryngoogyl, 68*(9), 1193–1198.

Mulerhan, M., Degg, C., Burr, S., Morgan, D. W., & Stableforth, D. E. (2001). Occurrence and risk of cochleotoxicity in cystic fibrosis patients receiving repeated high-dose aminoglycoside therapy. *Antimicrobial Agents and Chemotherapy, 45*(9), 2502–2509.

Naeye, R. L., Blanc, W., Leblanc, W., & Khatamee, M. A. (1973). Fetal complications of maternal heroin addiction: Abnormal growth, infections, and episodes of stress. *Journal of Pediatrics, 83*(6), 1055–1061.

National Institute of Deafness and other Communication Disorders. Retrieved July 1, 2015, from http://www.noisy planetnidcd.nih.gov

National Institute for Occupational Safety and Health. (1998). *Criteria for a recommended standard: Occupational noise exposure. Revised criteria.* Retrieved from http://www.cdc.gov/98-126.html

Neuwelt, E. A., Brummett, R. E., Remsen, L. G., Kroll, R. A., Pagel, M. A., McCormick, C. I., . . . Muldoon, L. L. (1996). In vitro and animal studies of sodium thiosulfate as a potential chemoprotectant against carboplatin-induced ototoxicity. *Cancer, 56*, 706–709.

Newsom, J. T., Huguet, N., McCarthy, M. J., Ramage-Morin, P., Kaplan, M. S., Bernier, J., McFarland, B. H., & Oderkirk, J. (2012). Health behavior change following chronic illness in middle and later life. *Journal of Gerontology, 67B*(3), 279–288.

Niebyl, J. R. (2003). Antibiotics and other anti-infective agents in pregnancy and lactation. *American Journal of Perinatology, 20*(8), 405–414. doi:10.1055/s-2003-45391

Nishimura, H., & Tanimura, T. (1976). *Clinical aspects of the teratogenicity of drugs.* Ann Arbor, MI: University of Michigan.

Niskar, A. S., Kieszak, S. M., Holmes, A. E., Esteban, E., Rubin, C. & Brody, D. J. (2001). Estimated prevalence of noise-induced hearing threshold shifts among children 6 to 19 years of age: The Third National Health and Nutrition Examination Survey, 1988–1994, United States. *Pediatrics, 108*, 40–43.

Noordman, B. J., van Beeck Calkoen, E., Witte, B., Goverts, T., Hensen, E., & Merkus, P. (2015). Prognostic factors for sudden drops in hearing level after minor head injury in patients with enlarged vestibular aqueduct: A meta-analysis. *Otology and Neurotology, 36*(1), 4–11.

Nurminen, T., & Kurppa, K. (1989). Occupational noise exposure and course of pregnancy. *Scandinavian Journal of Work, Environment and Health, 15*(2), 117–124.

Occupational Safety and Health Administration. (1997). *OSHA Technical Manual (OTM).* Retrieved from https://www.osha.gov/dts/osta/otm/new_noise/#standards

Olesen, C., Hald Steffensen, F., Lauge Nielsen, G., Jong-van den Berg, L., Olsen, J., & Toft Sørensen, H. (1999). Drug use in first pregnancy and lactation: A population-based survey among Danish women. *European Journal of Clinical Pharmacology, 55*(2), 139–144. doi:10.1007/s00228005 0608

Onejeme, A. U., & Khan, K. M. (1984). Morphologic study of effects of kanamycin on the developing cochlea of the rat. *Teratology, 29*(1), 57–71.

Oshima, T., Kudo, T., & Ikeda, K. (2001). Point mutation of the mitochondrial genome in Japanese deaf-mutism. *ORL, 63*(6), 329–332.

Ostrea, E. M., Brady, M., Gause, S., Raymundo, A. L., & Stevens, M. (1992). Drug screening of newborns by meconium analysis: A large-scale, prospective, epidemiologic study. *Pediatrics, 89*(1), 107–113.

Pandya, A., Xia, X., Radnaabazar, J., Batsuuri, J., Dangaansuren, B., Fischel-Ghodsian, N., & Nance, W. (1997). Mutation in the mitochondrial 12S rRNA gene in two families from Mongolia with matrilineal aminoglycoside ototoxicity. *Journal of Medical Genetics, 34*(2), 169–172.

Papania, M. J., Wallace, G. S., Rota, P. A., Icenogle, J.P., Fiebelkorn, A.P., Armstrong, G.L., . . . Seward, J. (2014). Elimination of endemic measles, rubella, and congenital rubella syndrome from the Western hemisphere: The US experience. *JAMA Pediatrics, 168*(2), 148–155. doi:10.1001/jama pediatrics.2013.4342

Pararas, E. E., Borkholder, D. A., & Borenstein, J. T. (2012). Microsystems technologies for drug delivery to the inner ear. *Advanced Drug Delivery Reviews, 64*(14), 1650–1660.

Peleva, R., Aloy, E., Carret, A. S., & Daniel, S. J. (2014). Hearing loss in a pediatric patient following cisplatin chemotherapy and subsequent exposure to excessive noise. *International Journal of Pediatric Otorhinolaryngology 78*(12), 2301–2304.

Perheentupa, U., Kinnunen, I., Grenman, R., Aitasalo, K., & Maktie, A.A. (2010). Management and outcome of pediatric skull base fractures. *International Journal of Pediatric Otorhinolaryngology 74*(11), 1245–1250.

Peters, A. J., Gerhardt, K. J., Abrams, R. M., & Longmate, J. A. (1993). Three-dimensional intraabdominal sound pressures in sheep produced by airborne stimuli. *American Journal of Obstetrics and Gynecology, 169*(5), 1304–1315.

Phua, Y. S., Salkeld, L. J., & de Chalain, T. M. (2009). Middle ear disease in children with cleft palate: Protocols for management. *International Journal of Pediatric Otorhinolaryngology, 73*(2), 307–313.

Piper, J. M., Baum, C., & Kennedy, D. L. (1987). Prescription drug use before and during pregnancy in a Medicaid population. *American Journal of Obstetrics and Gynecology, 157*(1), 148–156. http://dx.doi.org/10.1016/S0002-9378(87)80368-X

Portnuff, C. D., Fligor, B. J., & Arehart, K. H. (2011). Teenage use of portable listening devices: A hazard to hearing? *Journal of the American Academcy of Audiology, 22*(10), 663–677.

Preblud, S. R., Serdula, M. K., Frank, J. A., Jr., & Hinman, A. R. (1980). From the Centers for Disease Control. Current status of rubella in the United States, 1969–1979. *Journal of Infectious Diseases,* 142(5), 776–779.

Prezant, T. R., Agapian, J. V., Bohlman, M. C., Bu, X. D., Oztas, S., Qiu, W. Q., . . . Fischelghodsian, N. (1993). Mitochondrial ribosomal-RNA mutation associated with both antibiotic-induced and non-syndromic deafness. *Nature Genetics, 4*(3), 289–294. doi:10.1038/Ng0793-289

Rademaker-Lakhai, J. M., Crul, M., Zuur, L., Baas, P., Beijnen, J. H., Simis, Y. J., …Schellens, J. H. (2006). Relationship between cisplatin administration and development of ototoxicity. *Journal of Clinical Oncology, 24*(6), 918–924.

Rawool, V. W., & Colligon-Wayne, L. A. (2008). Auditory lifestyles and beliefs to hearing loss among college students in the USA. *Noise Health, 10*(38), 1–10.

Reed, D. B., Browning, S. R., Westneat, S. C., & Kidd, P. S. (2006). Personal protective equipment use and safety behaviors among farm adolescents: Gender differences and predictors of work practices. *Journal of Rural Health, 22*(4), 314–320.

Renick, K. M., Crawford, J. M., & Wilkins, J. R. 3rd. (2009). Hearing loss among Ohio farm youth: A comparison to a national sample. *American Journal of Industrial Medicine, 52*(3), 233–239.

Ristovska, G., Laszlo, H. E., & Hansell, A. L. (2014). Reproductive outcomes associated with noise exposure—A systematic review of the literature. *International Journal of Environmental Research and Public Health, 11*(8), 7931–7952. doi:10.3390/ijerph110807931

Roberts, J. E., Rosenfeld, R. M., & Zeisel, S. A. (2004). Otitis media and speech and language: A meta-analysis of prospective studies. *Pediatrics, 113*(3), 238–248.

Robertson, S. E., Featherstone, D. A., Gacic-Dobo, M., & Hersh, B. S. (2003). Rubella and congenital rubella syndrome: Global update. *Revista Panamericana de Salud Pública, 14,* 306–315.

Robinson, G. C., & Cambon, K. G. (1964). Hearing loss in infants of tuberculous mothers treated with streptomycin during pregnancy. *New England Journal of Medicine, 271,* 949–951.

Rocha, E. B., Azevedo, M. F. d., & Ximenes Filho, J. A. (2007). Estudo da audição de crianças de gestantes expostas ao ruído ocupacional: Avaliação por emissões otoacústicas—produto de distorção. *Revista Brasileira de Otorrinolaringologia, 73,* 359–369.

Rosenfeld, R. M., Schwartz, S. R., Cannon, C. R., Roland, P. S., Simon, G. R., Kumar, K. A., . . . Robertson, P. J. (2014). Clincal practice guideline: Acute otitis externa executive summary. *Otolaryngology-Head and Neck Surgery, 150*(2), 161–168.

Rovers, M. M., & Zielhuis, G. A. (2004). Otitis media meta-analysis, *Pediatrics, 114*(2), 508–509.

Roy, S., Ryals, M. M., Van den Bruele, A. B., Fitzgerald, T. S., & Cunningham L. L. (2013). Sound preconditioning therapy inhibits ototoxic hearing loss in mice. *Journal of Clinical Investigation, 123*(11), 4945–4949.

Rubin, J. D., Ferencz, C., & Loffredo, C. (1993). Use of prescription and non-prescription drugs in pregnancy. *Journal of Clinical Epidemiology, 46*(6), 581–589. http://dx.doi.org/10.1016/0895-4356(93)90132-K

Rybak, L. P., Husain, K., Whitworth, C. & Somani, S. M. (1999). Dose dependent protection by lipoic acid against cisplatin induced ototoxicity in rats: Antioxidant defense system. *Toxicological Sciences, 47,* 195–202.

Salamy, A. (1984). Maturation of the auditory brainstem response from birth through early childhood. *Journal of Clinical Neurophysiology, 1*(3), 293–329.

Salihu, H. M., & Wilson, R. E. (2007). Epidemiology of prenatal smoking and perinatal outcomes. *Early Human Development, 83*(11), 713–720.

Schacht, J., Talaska, A. E., & Rybak, L. P. (2012). Cisplatin and aminoglycoside antibiotics: Hearing loss and its prevention. *Anatomical Record, 295*(11), 1837–1850.

Shargorodsky, J., Curhan, S. G., Curhan, G. C., & Eavey, R. (2010). Change in prevalence of hearing loss in US adolescents. *JAMA,304*(7), 772–778.

Shih, L., Cone-Wesson, B., & Reddix, B. (1988). Effects of maternal cocaine abuse on the neonatal auditory system. *International Journal of Pediatric Otorhinolaryngology, 15*(3), 245–251. http://dx.doi.org/10.1016/0165-5876(88)90079-1

Singer, L. T., Arendt, R., Minnes, S., Farkas, K., Salvatore, A., Kirchner, H.L., & Kleigman, R. (2002). Cognitive and motor outcomes of cocaine-exposed infants. *JAMA, 287*(15), 1952–1960. doi:10.1001/jama.287.15.1952

Sininger, Y. S., Abdala, C., & Cone-Wesson, B. (1997). Auditory threshold sensitivity of the human neonate as measured by the auditory brainstem response. *Hearing Research, 104*(1–2), 27–38. http://dx.doi.org/10.1016/S0378-5955(96)00178-5

Smith, R. J. H., Bale Jr, J. F., & White, K. R. (2005). Sensorineural hearing loss in children. *The Lancet, 365*(9462), 879–890. http://dx.doi.org/10.1016/S0140-6736(05)71047-3

Spankovich, C., Lobarinas, E., & Le Prell, C. G. (2014). Diametric effect of "localized" thermal exposure on cisplatin induced ototoxicity. *ARO Abstracts, 37,* 26.

Stathis, S. L., O'Callaghan, M., Najman, J. M., Anderson, M. J., & Bor, W. (1999). Maternal cigarette smoking during pregnancy is an independent predictor for symptoms of middle ear disease at five years' postdelivery. *Pediatrics, 104*(2), e16.

Stavroulaki, P., Apostolopoulos, N., Dinopoulou, D., Vossinakis, I., Tsakanikos, M., & Douniadakis, D. (1999). Otoacoustic emissions—An approach for monitoring aminoglycoside induced ototoxicity in children. *International Journal of Pediatric Otorhinolaryngology, 50*(3), 177–184.

Stewart, M., Meinke, D. K., Snyders, J. K., & Howerton, K. (2014). Shooting habits of youth recreational firearm users. *International Journal of Audiology, 53*(2), S26–S34.

Steyger, P. S. (2015). Novel aminoglycoside antibiotics show reduced ototoxicity risk. *Hearing Journal, 68*(4), 32–35.

Stowell, J. D., Forlin-Passoni, D., Radford, K., Bate, S. L., Dollard, S. C., Bialek, S. R., . . . Schmid, D. S. (2014). Cytomegalovirus survival and transferability and the effectiveness of common hand-washing agents against cytomegalovirus on live human hands. *Applied and Environmental Microbiology, 80*(2), 455–461. doi:10.1128/aem.03262-13

Stupp, H., Rauch, S., Sous, H., Brun, J., & Lagler, F. (1967). Kanamycin dosage and levels in ear and other organs. *Archives of Otolaryngology, 86*(5), 515–521.

Surenthiran, S. S., Wilbraham, K., May, J., Chant, T., Emmerson, A. J. B., & Newton, V. E. (2003). Noise levels within the ear and post-nasal space in neonates in intensive care. *Archives of Disease in Childhood-Fetal and Neonatal Edition, 88*(4), F315–F318. doi:10.1136/fn.88.4.F315

Syme, M. R., Paxton, J. W., & Keelan, J. A. (2004). Drug transfer and metabolism by the human placenta. *Clinical Pharmacokinetics, 43*(8), 487–514. doi:10.2165/00003088-200443080-00001

Taljaard, D. S., Leishman, N. F., & Eikelboom, R. H. (2013). Personal lisenting devices and the prevention of noise induced hearing loss in children: The Cheers for Ears Pilot Program. *Noise Health, 15*(65), 261–268.

Teele, D. W., Lein, J. O., & Rosner, B. (1989). Epidemiology of otitis media during the first seven years of life in children in greater Boston: A prospective cohort study. *Journal of Infectious Diseases, 160*(1), 83–94.

Trammer, R. M., Aust, G., Köster, K., & Obladen, M. (1992). Narcotic and nicotine effects on the neonatal auditory system. *Acta Paediatrica, 81*(12), 962–965.

U.S. Bureau of Labor Statistics. (2012). *Current Population Survey (CPS)/Graph by the Women's Bureau. U.S. Department of Labor—Quarter 4 data.* Retrieved from http://www.dol.gov/wb/stats/facts_over_time.htm

U.S. Bureau of Labor Statistics. (2014). *Survey and Employment Projections Program/Graph by the Women's Bureau, U.S. Department of Labor.* Retrieved from http://www.dol.gov/wb/stats/latest_annual_data.htm

U.S. Census Bureau. (2011). *Half of first-time mothers receive paid leave.* Retrieved from https://www.census.gov/sipp/source.html.

U.S. Department of Labor. (2007). Child labor requirements in agricultural occupations under the Fair Labor Standards Act, *Bulletin 102*.

U.S. Environmental Protection Agency. (2015). *Polychlorinated biphenyls (PCBs).* Retrieved from http://www.epa.gov/wastes/hazard/tsd/pcbs/about.htm

U.S. Fish & Wildlife Service. (2006). *National survey of fishing, hunting, and wildlife-associated recreation.* Retrieved from http://wsfrprograms.fws.gov/Subpages/NationalSurvey/National_Survey.htm

Uziel, A., Romand, R., & Marot, M. (1979). Electrophysiological study of the ototoxicity of kanamycin during development in guinea pigs. *Hearing Research, 1*(3), 203–211.

Vasconcellos, A. P., Kyle, M. E., Gilani, S., & Shin, J. J. (2014). Personally modifiable risk factors assocaited with pediatric hearing loss: A systematic review. *Otolaryngology-Head and Neck Surgery, 151*(1), 14–28.

Venekamp, R. P., Sanders, S. L., Glasziou, P. P., Del Mar, C. B., & Rovers, M. M. (2015). Antibiotics for acute otitis media in children. *Cochrane Database of Systematic Reviews*. doi:10.1002/14651858.CD000219.pub3

Vince, M., Billing, A., Baldwin, B., Toner, J., & Weller, C. (1985). Maternal vocalisations and other sounds in the fetal lamb's sound environment. *Early Human Development, 11*(2), 179–190.

Vince, M. A., Armitage, S. E., Baldwin, B., Toner, J., & Moore, B. C. (1982). The sound environment of the foetal sheep. *Behaviour, 81*(2), 296–315.

Vogel, I., Brug, J., Hosli, E. J., van der Ploeg, C. P., & Raat, H. (2008). MP3 players and hearing loss: Adolescent's perceptions of loud music and hearing conservation. *Journal of Pediatrics, 152*(3), 400–404.

Vrabec, D. P., Cody, D., & Ulrich, J. A. (1965). A study of the relative concentrations of antibiotics in the blood, spinal fluid, and perilymph in animals. *Annals of Otology, Rhinology, and Laryngology, 74*(3), 689–705.

Wachman, E. M., & Lahav, A. (2011). The effects of noise on preterm infants in the NICU. *Archives of Disease in Childhood-Fetal and Neonatal Edition, 96*(4), F305–F309.

Webster, W. S. (1998). Teratogen update: Congenital rubella. *Teratology, 58*(1), 13–23.

Wei, Q., Xu, D., Chen, Z., Li, H., Lu, Y., Liu, C., . . . Cao, X. (2013). Maternally transmitted aminoglycoside-induced and non-syndromic hearing loss caused by the 1494C > T mutation in the mitochondrial 12S rRNA gene in two Chinese families. *International Journal of Audiology, 52*(2), 98–103. doi:10.3109/14992027.2012.743046

Weinreich, H. M., Jabbour, N., Levine, S., & Yueh, B. (2013). Limiting hazardous noise exposure from noisy toys: Simple, sticky solutions. *Laryngoscope, 123*(9), 2240–2244.

Weitzman, M., Gortmaker, S., & Sobol, A. (1992). Maternal smoking and behavior problems of children. *Pediatrics, 90*(3), 342–349.

Weitzman, M., Govil, N., Liu, Y., & Lalwani, A. K. (2013). Maternal prenatal smoking and hearing loss among adolescents. *JAMA Otolaryngology-Head & Neck Surgery, 139*(7), 669–677. doi:10.1001/jamaoto.2013.3294

Werler, M. M., Mitchell, A. A., Hernandez-Diaz, S., & Honein, M. A. (2005). Use of over-the-counter medications during pregnancy. *American Journal of Obstetrics and Gynecology, 193*(3), 771–777. http://dx.doi.org/10.1016/j.ajog.2005.02.100

Widen, S. E., Holmes, A. E., Johnson, T., Bohlin, M., & Erlandsson, S. I. (2009). Hearing, use of hearing protection, and attitudes towards noise among young American adults. *International Journal of Audiology, 48*, 537–545.

Winskel, H. (2006). The effects of an early history of otitis media on children's language and literacy skill development. *British Journal of Educational Psychology, 76*(4), 727–744.

Wu, C. C., Chiu, Y. H., Chen, P. J., & Hsu, C. J. (2007). Prevalence and clinical features of the mitochondrial m.1555A>G mutation in Taiwanese patients with idiopathic sensorineural hearing loss and association of haplogroup F with low penetrance in three families. *Ear and Hearing, 28*(3), 332–342. doi:10.1097/AUD.0b013e318047941e

Yelverton, J. C., Arnos, K., Xia, X.-J., Nance, W. E., Pandya, A., & Dodson, K. M. (2013). The clinical and audiologic features of hearing loss due to mitochondrial mutations. *Otolaryngology-Head and Neck Surgery, 148*(6), 1017–1022. doi:10.1177/0194599813482705

Yu, K. K., Choi, C. H., An, Y. H., Kwak, M. Y., Gong, S. J., Yoon, S. W., & Shin, H. J. (2014). Comparison of the effectiveness of monitoring cisplatin-induced ototoxicity with extended high frequency pure-tone audiometry or distortion product otoacoustic emission. *Korean Journal of Audiology, 18*(2), 58–68.

Yuan, H., Qian, Y., Xu, Y., Cao, J., Bai, L., Shen, W., . . . Mo, J. Q. (2005). Cosegregation of the G7444A mutation in the mitochondrial COI/tRNASer (UCN) genes with the 12S rRNA A1555G mutation in a Chinese family with aminoglycoside-induced and nonsyndromic hearing loss. *American Journal of Medical Genetics Part A, 138*(2), 133–140.

Zahr, L. K., & de Traversay, J. (1994). Premature infant responses to noise reduction by earmuffs: Effects on behavioral and physiologic measures. *Journal of Perinatology, 15*(6), 448–455.

Zhang, J., Wang, P., Han, B., Ding, Y., Pan, L., Zou, J., . . . Wang, Q. (2013). Newborn hearing concurrent genetic screening for hearing impairment—A clinical practice in 58,397 neonates in Tianjin, China. *International Journal of Pediatric Otorhinolaryngology, 77*(12), 1929–1935. doi:10.1016/j.ijporl.2013.08.038

Zhao, H., Li, R., Wang, Q., Yan, Q., Deng, J.-H., Han, D., . . . Guan, M.X. (2004). Maternally inherited aminoglycoside-induced and nonsyndromic deafness is associated with the novel C1494T mutation in the mitochondrial 12S rRNA gene in a large Chinese family. *American Journal of Human Genetics, 74*(1), 139–152. http://dx.doi.org/10.1086/381133

Zimmerman, E., & Lahav, A. (2013). Ototoxicity in preterm infants: Effects of genetics, aminoglycosides, and loud environmental noise. *Journal of Perinatology, 33*(1), 3–8.

Zuckerman, B., Frank, D. A., Hingson, R., Amaro, H., Levenson, S. M., Kayne, H., . . . Fried, L. E. (1989). Effects of maternal marijuana and cocaine use on fetal growth. *New England Journal of Medicine, 320*(12), 762–768.

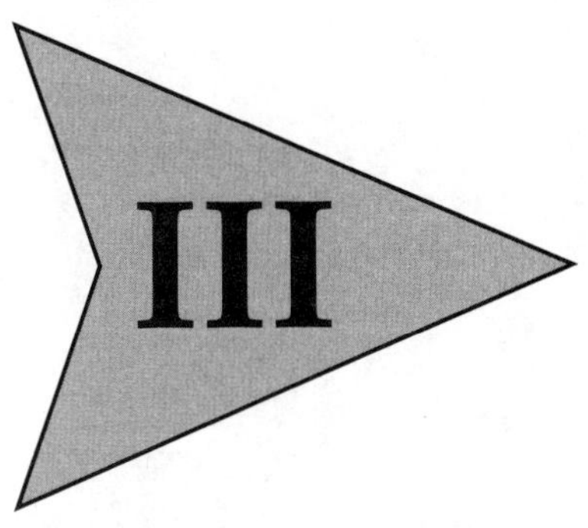

Types of Hearing Loss in Children

Conductive Hearing Loss in Children: Otitis Media With Effusion and Congenital Conditions

Lisa L. Hunter and Daniel I. Choo

Introduction

Conductive hearing loss in all its various forms presents as the most common clinical scenario faced on a daily basis by pediatric audiologists, from the newborn period through to adolescence. Conductive hearing loss (CHL) is defined as interference of the mechanical reception of sound by the cochlea resulting from loss of impedance matching by the middle ear. The presence of CHL is defined from a behavioral audiogram as significantly better bone conduction compared to air conduction, or air-bone gaps. Most audiologists clinically define "significant" air-bone gap as 10 dB at two or more frequencies, or 15 dB at one frequency. A finding of CHL on audiometry is supported by abnormal acoustic immittance, acoustic reflexes, otoacoustic emissions (OAEs), and threshold, bone-conduction auditory brainstem responses (ABR). Figure 10–1 illustrates a bilateral CHL of moderate degree in a young child with Down syndrome and otitis media with effusion (OME), along with associated test results. Preoperatively, hearing was affected in both ears across frequencies important for speech reception. Postoperatively, hearing levels were significantly improved but still poorer than in a child without a history of chronic OME.

Although behavioral audiometry is the gold standard for diagnosis of CHL, physiologic tests provide an important cross-reference to audiometry. In infants less than 9 months of age, the audiologist must rely solely on these physiologic tests to detect CHL. Infants who can perform visual reinforcement audiometry can usually also respond to bone-conduction speech and pure tones. To determine ear-specific air-bone gap, masking must be used, and in infants, they can often learn to ignore the masking noise without any special instruction, if reinforcement is provided for the speech and pure tones.

A wide range of pathologies involving the external, the middle and, rarely, the inner ear can exhibit CHL. The most common and treatable reasons for CHL are cerumen impaction and middle ear effusion. Because these are also the most easily observed with otoscopy, it is vital for audiologists to always perform otoscopy and to be comfortable with normal ear canal appearance and tympanic membrane landmarks.

In the case of an infant presenting for the first time to the audiology clinic, usually on referral from a newborn screening program, it is important to distinguish between transient and persistent forms of conductive or mixed hearing loss, distinct from sensorineural hearing loss. Congenital, persistent CHL also presents a classic genetic quest to distinguish between syndromic and nonsyndromic forms of the disorder. A carefully considered stepwise protocol of diagnostic tests with adequate levels of clinical evidence, as detailed in other chapters within this handbook, can assist audiologists in making the determination about type, degree, and configuration of the hearing loss as early as possible. Coupled with case history information and interdisciplinary consultation by otology, audiology, radiology, pediatrics, neurology, genetics, and orthopedics, as indicated, determination of etiology can be made at an early age. In the case of children beyond the first

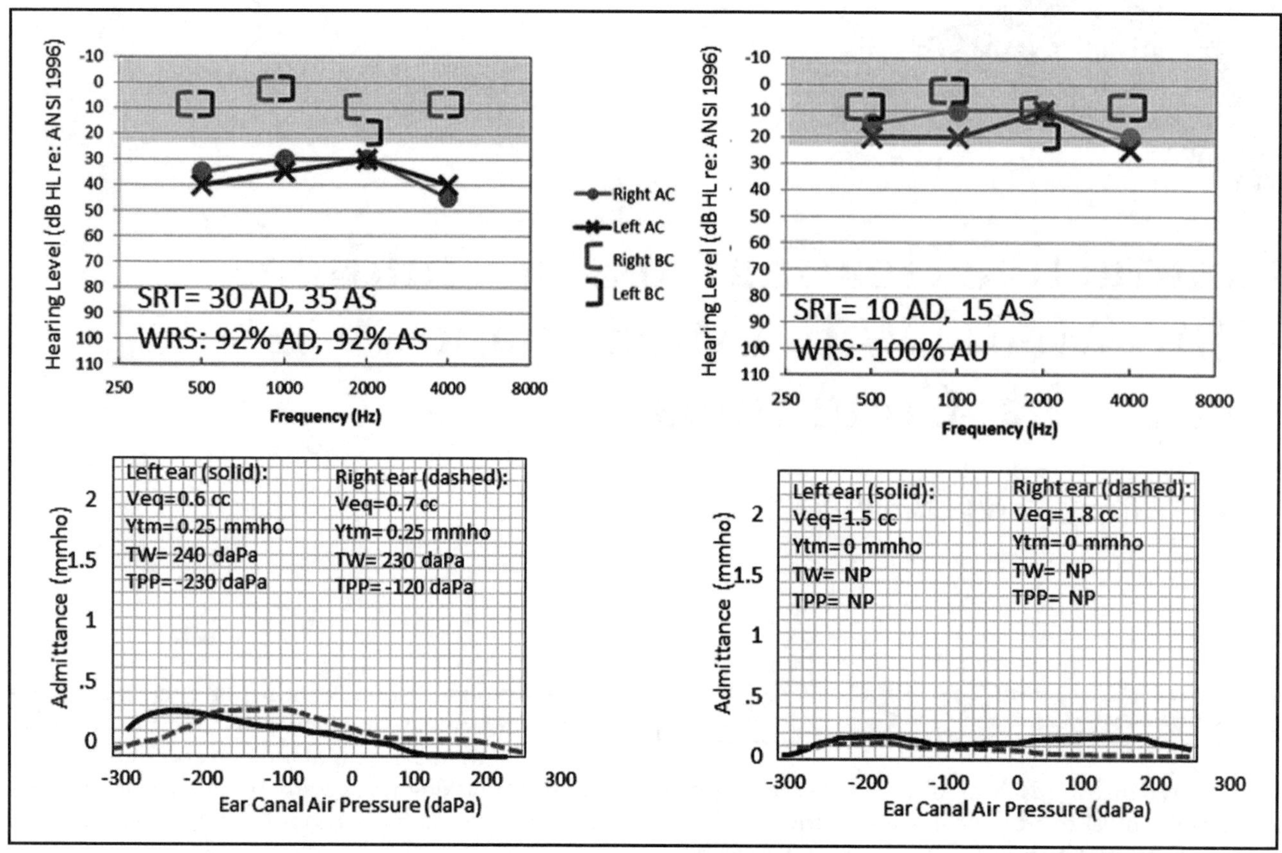

FIGURE 10–1. Bilateral conductive hearing loss due to otitis media with effusion. Preoperative (*left panel*) and post-ventilation tube insertion (*right panel*) hearing levels in a child with Down syndrome, tested using conditioned play audiometry. Specific factors such as craniofacial anomalies necessitate more frequent hearing testing and intervention, including surgery or coexisting medical problems. Behavioral audiologic testing method based on developmental age. (SRT, speech reception threshold; WRS, word recognition score; AS, left ear; AD, right ear; AU, both ears.)

6 months of age whose newborn screening was passed, the question of whether conductive loss is congenital or acquired is generally more clear, and the ubiquitous nature of otitis media with effusion means that most infants and children will present with transient as opposed to persistent CHL. In this chapter, we discuss various types of congenital and acquired CHL and the underlying epidemiologic, etiologic, diagnostic, and referral implications, taking an international perspective where supportive literature is available.

Recommendations of the Joint Committee on Infant Hearing for Middle Ear Conditions

The Joint Committee on Infant Hearing (JCIH) 2007 Position Statement identifies craniofacial anomalies as a risk factor for persistent congenital, delayed onset, or progressive hearing loss in childhood, including anomalies of the pinna, ear canal, ear tags, ear pits, and temporal bone anomalies. The JCIH recommends that a complete head and neck examination for craniofacial anomalies should document defects of the auricles, patency of the external ear canals, and status of the eardrum and middle ear structures. Atypical findings on eye examination, including irises of two different colors or abnormal positioning of the eyes, might signal stigmata of a syndrome that includes hearing loss. Congenital persistent CHL might be associated with craniofacial anomalies that are seen in disorders such as Down syndrome, Crouzon disease, Klippel Feil syndrome, and Goldenhar syndrome. The assessment of infants with these congenital anomalies should be coordinated with a team, including otolaryngology, clinical genetics, and others depending on the specific syndrome.

For all children, the JCIH recommends surveillance of middle ear status using pneumatic otoscopy and tympanometry at all well-child visits and referral of children with persistent middle ear effusion lasting for 3 months or longer for otologic evaluation. As noted by the JCIH, with regard to universal newborn hearing screening, both OAE and ABR screening technologies can be used to detect sensory (cochlear) hearing loss; however, both technologies might also be affected by outer or middle ear dysfunction. Consequently, transient conditions of the outer and middle ear might result in a "failed" screening result in the presence of normal cochlear and neural function.

Middle Ear Assessment in the Newborn

ABRs and OAEs, the primary procedures used in universal newborn hearing screening (UNHS) programs, are sensitive to the condition of the middle ear. For example, Hall, Smith, and Popelka (2004) found that CHL can persist for several weeks after birth. Stuart, Yang, and Green (1994) reported elevated (>10 dB) air-conducted ABR thresholds in neonates during the initial 48 hr after birth, whereas bone conducted ABR thresholds changed by less than 1 dB. Doyle, Burggraaff, Fujikawa, Jim, and MacArthur (1997) reported that newborn hearing screening pass rates in ears with occluding vernix were 66% for ABR, but only 38% for OAEs. Transient middle ear conditions might contribute to a "failed" result regardless of the presence of normal cochlear function due to decreased forward transmission of the stimulus and reverse transmission of the OAE signal through the middle ear.

Assessment of middle ear function is not currently part of UNHS protocols for well babies and graduates of neonatal intensive care units (NICUs) for several reasons (JCIH, 2007). First, pneumatic otoscopy and bone-conducted ABR are impractical in a UNHS protocol due to the use of ancillary screening personnel rather than audiologists or otologists. Tympanometry using a low-frequency probe tone is insensitive to middle ear dysfunction in newborns (Hunter & Margolis, 1992; Paradise, Smith, & Bluestone 1976; Sprague, Wiley, & Goldstein, 1985). Anatomical differences in infant ears, such as more compliant ear-canal walls (Holte, Margolis, & Cavanaugh, 1991), smaller ear canals, and middle ear spaces, and a more horizontal orientation of the tympanic membranes with respect to the axis of the ear canal contribute to developmental differences in tympanometry (Ikui, Sando, & Fujita, 1997; Ruah, Schachern, Zelterman, Paparella, & Yoon, 1991; Saunders, Kaltenback, & Relkin, 1983).

As discussed in Chapter 18, tympanometry using high probe-tone frequencies (up to 1 kHz) is currently recommended for diagnostic testing (after failed screening) by JCIH guidelines. Tympanometry using a 1-kHz probe tone is more sensitive to changes in middle ear status in infants younger than 4 months old compared to 0.226-kHz tympanometry (Alaerts, Lutz, & Woulters, 2007; Calandruccio, Fitzgerald, & Prieve 2006). Margolis, Bass-Ringdahl, Hanks, Holte, and Zapala (2003) reported that 1-kHz tympanometry is 91% specific in predicting distortion product OAE passes, but only 50% sensitive for distortion product OAE fails. Kei and colleagues (2003) reported 1-kHz tympanograms in 106 infants (1–6 days old) who passed a click-evoked OAE hearing screening. Single-peaked tympanograms were present in 92.3% of their sample. Baldwin (2006) reported sensitivity of 0.99 and specificity of 0.89 for 1-kHz tympanometry for infants with a mean age of 10 weeks but findings might not apply to neonates, as the youngest infant was 2 weeks old. Ambient-pressure energy reflectance and other acoustic transfer functions have been reported in children, infants, and neonates. Wideband acoustic immittance, a new test to assess middle ear status, is sensitive to middle ear disorders including otitis media with effusion, otosclerosis, ossicular discontinuity, and perforation of the tympanic membrane. Because wideband acoustic immittance can assess middle ear function in young infants, it could potentially be a useful tool in UNHS and early hearing detection and intervention (EHDI) programs.

Due to the use of ancillary screening personnel in many settings, a physiologic middle ear test such as wideband acoustic immittance that does not rely on subjective interpretation could improve UNHS programs. A need exists to understand whether infants who fail UNHS have sensorineural (SNHL) or CHL associated with middle ear dysfunction. The development of cost-effective tools to separate CHL from SNHL will allow UNHS systems to categorize type of hearing loss accurately, so that appropriate intervention can be initiated as soon as possible after birth.

Assessment of Children With Craniofacial Anomalies

Children with craniofacial anomalies who are at highest risk for chronic OME and CHL present special challenges for pediatric audiologists and craniofacial teams. As highlighted in the clinical practice guideline for otitis media with effusion by Rosenfeld et al. (in preparation), children at risk for speech or language delays would likely be further affected by hearing problems from OME, even though definitive studies are lacking. Children with craniofacial anomalies have a higher prevalence of chronic OME, hearing loss (conductive and sensorineural), and speech or language delays than children without these anomalies. In the United States, approximately 3% of babies are born with some type of birth defect, including craniofacial anomalies, Down syndrome (1.4 per 1,000), or cleft palate (1 per 1,000; Centers for Disease Control and Prevention [CDC], 2006). Often, these children have an associated problem of OME (JCIH, 2007). These children are more difficult to test if intellectual disability is present, and they typically require more frequent visits and routine use of physiologic measures, including ABR with sedation in order to determine hearing levels with certainty.

Congenital Aural Atresia and Microtia

It is important for audiologists to inspect a child's pinna for size, shape, landmarks, and position on the head. Each of the features can be related to hearing function and to the presence of certain congenital anomalies or syndromes. Figure 10–2 illustrates normal ear landmarks. The ear should be positioned approximately at the level of the horizontal line shown in Figure 10–2A. The ear should be rotated about 20 degrees posteriorly. Low-set ears are positioned lower than the horizontal line (Figure 10–2B), and often the ear is rotated posteriorly 30 degrees or more. This reflects an arrest in development, because the pinna rotates anteriorly and superiorly during fetal development.

The mildest and most common anomalies are ear tags, in which rudimentary soft tissue is present in front of the ear, and pits, which can be shallow or deep, and can be associated with branchial clefts. Low-set ears are commonly seen in a number of craniofacial syndromes. Congenital aural microtia and atresia are serious and complex birth malformations in which the auricle, the external auditory canal (EAC), the ossicles, and sometimes the cochlea or vestibule fail to develop completely. Microtia refers to underdevelopment of the auricle ("micro" means small and "otia" means ear), and can range from a normally shaped but smaller pinna to complete absence of the pinna with rudimentary soft tissue ear tags. Classification of microtia severity into three subtypes was originally proposed by Marx (1926). Examples of the three subtypes are shown in Figure 10–3, which illustrates anomalies of the EAC and pinna varying from normal, to a narrowed canal, to complete atresia or absence of the canal. Severity of EAC stenosis has been described by Schuknecht (1989) and Jahrsdoerfer, Yeakley, Aguilar, Cole, and Gray (1992). In Grade I microtia, the pinna is smaller than normal but the external canal is patent, and all of the normal ear structures are present. In Grade II, the external ear is malformed, the external canal is present but stenotic, and the middle ear space is small and the ossicles are malformed or fused. Grade III, the most severe, involves severe malformation or absence of the pinna, absence or complete stenosis of the external canal, and

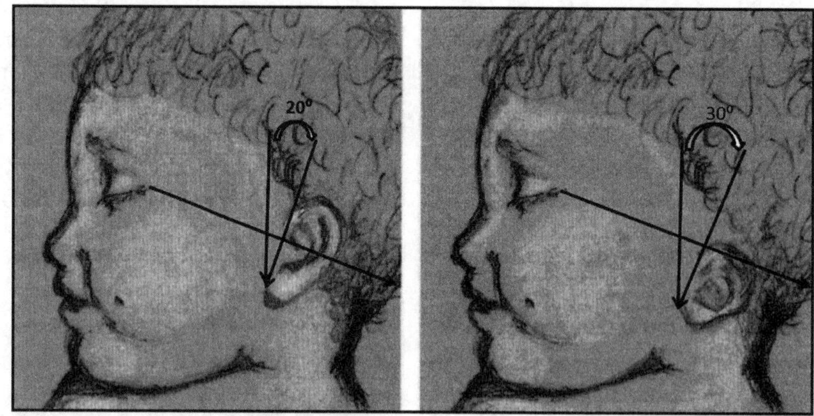

FIGURE 10–2. Facial structures in relation to the auricle. The ear should be positioned approximately at the level of the horizontal line from the outer canthus of the eye to the inion at the base of the skull as shown in **A**. The ear should be rotated about 20 degrees posteriorly. Low-set ears are positioned lower than the horizontal line as shown in **B**, and often the ear is rotated posteriorly 30 degrees or more.

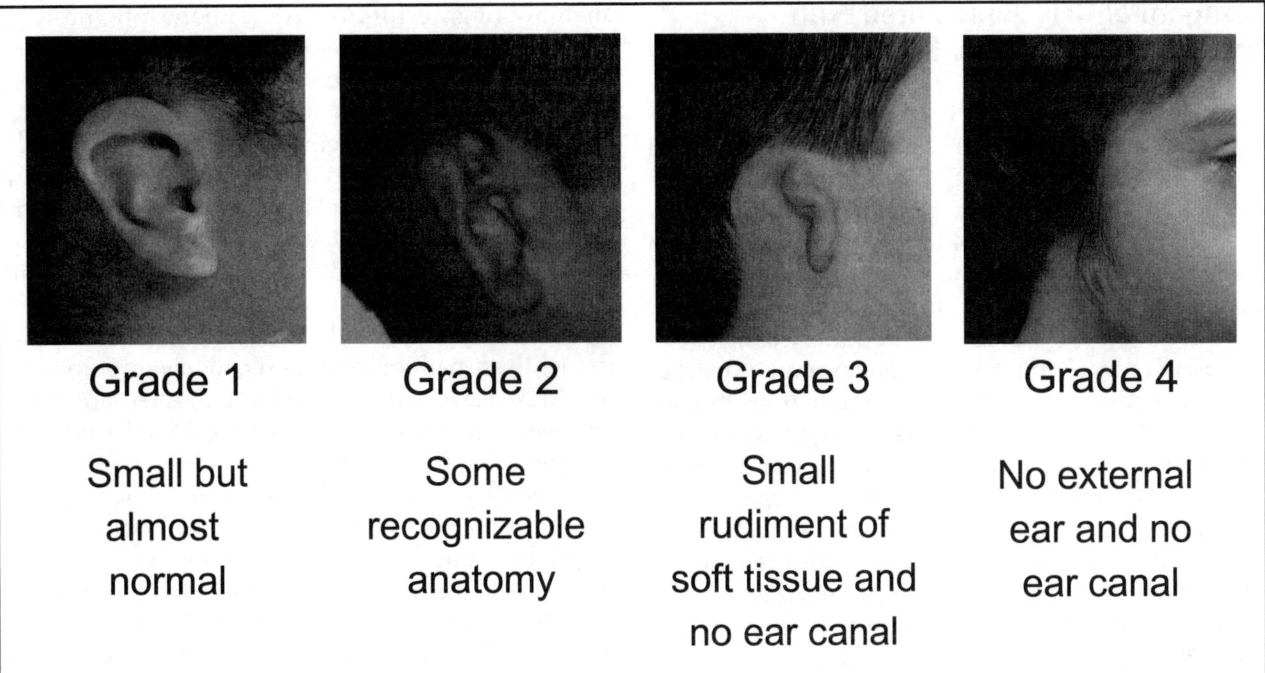

FIGURE 10–3. Classification of microtia severity into four subtypes originally described by Jahrsdoerfer et al. (1992). Microtia refers to the spectrum of deformities of the external ear and is typically categorized into four different grades. Grade 1 is a slightly smaller ear with the majority of the structure still present. Grade 2 has a little more deficiency of the ear structure. Grade 3 is absence of an external ear, with a peanut-like vestige, for lack of a better term. Grade 4, also known as anotia, is the total absence of the external ear. (Photo used with permission of Sheryl Lewin, M.D.)

absence or near absence of the middle ear space and ossicles. Atresia or stenosis of the external auditory canal is more common in microtia but also occurs frequently in cases of persistent CHL without microtia. Anomalies of the middle ear structures also occur frequently with microtia, and include stapes deformity, absence of the oval and round windows, facial nerve absence or anomalous development, poor pneumatization of the middle ear cells and space, and fusion of the malleus and incus into a columella-type structure. The incidence of inner ear abnormalities associated with microtia is estimated to be between 10% and 47% (Swartz & Faerber, 1985).

The era of high-resolution computerized tomography (CT) scanning has provided much greater detail regarding multiple anomalies, which are more common in children with syndromic forms of CHL than the general population (Tekes et al., 2013). The principle that "better developed outer ears go with better developed middle ears" has been demonstrated with high-resolution CT scanning (Ishimoto, Ito, & Yamasobo, 2005). As expected, this adage also holds true for hearing—better developed pinnae and ear canals correlate with better hearing function. A single genetic cause for microtia has not been identified, but there is evidence that it is associated with multifactorial genetic risk coupled with prenatal or intrauterine factors. The familial recurrence risk is estimated to be 5.7% (Takahashi & Maeda, 1982), but increases to 25% when all branchial arch abnormalities are considered (Tanzer, 1971). Known risk factors include rubella and maternal use of teratogenic drugs, including thalidomide, accutane, retinoic acid, and clomid. Although the overall incidence of microtia is estimated at 1 in 6,000 births, the risk appears to be greater in Japanese populations (1:4,000), and in Native American populations (1:2,000), especially in Navajos (1:1,000; Grabb, 1965). Unilateral microtia is thought to be a mild variant of hemifacial microsomia, which is the underdevelopment of half of the face. Microtia occurs in males twice as often as in females and occurs unilaterally in 70% to 90% of cases (Jafek, Nager, Strife, & Gayler, 1975; Schuknecht, 1989). Interestingly, microtia occurs in the right ear 55% to 65% of the time, possibly due to blood flow and growth signaling asymmetries (McKenzie & Craig, 1955; Poswillo, 1973).

Congenital CHL Associated With External Ear Malformations

In general, the degree of CHL corresponds to the severity (Grades I–IV; Jahrsdoerfer et al., 1992) of external and middle ear microtia. SNHL is more common in Grade III–IV microtia and is due to cochlear malformations. Approximately 40 hereditary hearing loss syndromes associated with external ear malformations and CHL have been identified (Allanson, 2004). In many of these syndromes, the auditory ossicles can be absent or malformed as well. For example, Treacher Collins syndrome includes malformation or absence of the malleus, incus and stapes, mastoid, absence of the external auditory canal, and occasional complete absence of the middle ear and epitympanic space. Bilateral hearing loss occurs in approximately half of the cases, and the degree of CHL corresponds to the degree of external ear stenosis (Pron, Galloway, Armstrong, & Posnick, 1993). Most of the known syndromes associated with external and middle ear malformations have been described in only sporadic cases or in a few families, and most are of autosomal recessive inheritance, sometimes associated with consanguinity (parents who are close relatives). Table 10–1 details the most common syndromes associated with external ear malformations, known hearing loss characteristics, and other associated congenital malformations.

Treatment for Aural Atresia

Congenital aural atresia is usually associated with moderate-to-severe CHL. Correction by conventional hearing devices is usually not possible because of the absence of an external auditory canal or pinna malformations. The options in treatment for congenital atresia include a bone-conduction hearing aid or CROS hearing aid, a bone-anchored hearing aid (BAHA) system, or atresiaplasty to create an ear canal/middle ear.

In the clinical evaluation of children with congenital atresia of the ear canal, CT scanning of the temporal bone provides clinicians with an excellent anatomical assessment of the middle and inner ears that then facilitates decision making. Those children with well-developed middle and inner ear anatomy (Figure 10–4A) are good candidates for aural atresia repair (opening and grafting of an ear canal, creation of a tympanic membrane, mobilization of the ossicular chain) with excellent chances of hearing improvement. Conversely, those children whose CT scans demonstrate poorly developed inner and middle ear anatomy (Figure 10–4B) have a poorer prognosis for hearing improvement following atresia repair surgery. In these instances, use of a bone-conduction hearing aid is typically recommended as the safer and more effective hearing management option.

A significant additional consideration in aural atresia management is the facial nerve. In children with congenital aural atresia, the atypical course of the facial nerve through the middle ear and mastoid compartments puts it at elevated risk for injury during atresia surgery. In cases where the nerve is aberrant and lying in the direct path of surgical repair, common practice would be to avoid surgery and pursue alternative hearing management options in order to avoid a potential iatrogenic facial nerve paralysis.

Decision making in the management of congenital aural atresia continues to be challenging from many perspectives. From a medical and audiologic perspective, the desire to restore normal native hearing without the need for a hearing appliance of any kind is balanced by the intrinsic difficulty of obtaining excellent hearing results with aural atresia surgery. The outstanding hearing outcomes offered by bone-conduction hearing aids/bone-anchored hearing aids is balanced by the need to use and maintain the hearing aid and the fairly common local infections/irritations associated with abutments required for percutaneous bone-anchored hearing aids. In this era of optimizing cost-effective hearing management strategies, it is unclear if higher up-front costs of aural atresia surgery or lifelong use of a bone-anchored hearing aid (with concomitant hearing aid replacements, batteries, and fitting costs) provide the better cost-effective option. An external bone-conduction device can be used on a headband during the first years of life, with good functional results. In a study of 12 children with atresia, Verhagen et al. (2008) reported they had an average air conduction pure-tone average (PTA) of 60 dB and achieved a gain of 33 dB (+/– or ±6 dB) with a bone-conduction device with a headband.

There are few evidence-based studies published to assist parents, otologists, and audiologists in objectively making treatment choices based on outcome data. An evidence-based review compared results of atresiaplasty with BAHA (Riemer et al., 2008). Included in this review, De Alarcon and Choo (2007) published an expert opinion on the current controversies in the treatment of aural atresia, citing studies that have shown positive outcomes for good surgical candidates. Candidacy was determined by using the Jahrsdoerfer scale (Jahrsdoerfer et al., 1992), along with high-resolution CT (HRCT), to predict the outcome from atresiaplasty.

Table 10–1. Syndromes Associated With External Ear Anomalies and Congenital Conductive Hearing Loss

Syndrome, Incidence, Genetics	*Ear Malformations*	*Hearing Loss Characteristics*	*Other Associated Malformations*
Treacher Collins syndrome (mandibulofacial dysostosis) Incidence 1:50,000 (Jahrsdoerfer & Jacobson, 1995). Autosomal dominant inheritance with variable expressivity; new mutations in 60% associated with paternal age	Agenesis or hypoplasia of the mastoid and antrum; external ear canal atresia or stenosis; middle ear agenesis, agenesis or malformation of the malleus, incus, stapes and oval window; cochlea and vestibular organs usually normal but may also be malformed	Bilateral conductive hearing loss (55%); generally moderate to severe and associated with degree of external canal malformation	Hypoplastic midface, coloboma of lower eyelid (75%), choanal atresia (few reports), macrostomia (cleft palate (35%)
Goldenhar syndrome (oculo-auriculo-vertebral spectrum or hemofacial microsomia) Incidence 1:3,500 to 1:5,600 (Bayraktar et al., 2005) Mostly sporadic but autosomal dominant inheritance in 1% to 2%	Usually unilateral; malformation varies from anotia to malformed auricular tissue displaced anterior/inferior to a mildly dysmorphic auricle; preauricular tags common; occasional isolated microtia	Conductive and sensorineural hearing loss (50%) due to diverse anomalies of external and middle ear; including ossicular hypoplasia, patulous eustachian tube, skull base abnormalities	Mild to marked facial asymmetry (65%), cleft lip/palate (7%–15%), eye anomalies (especially epibulbar dermoids, unilateral colobomas); facial nerve weakness, cranial nerve involvement, intracranial brain malformations, developmental delay, heart anomalies, renal, gastrointestinal and musculoskeletal anomalies
Branchiootorenal (BOR) syndrome or ear-pit hearing loss syndrome Incidence 1:40,000 (Fraser, Sproule, & Halal,1980) Autosomal dominant with variable expressivity; linkage to chromosome 8q	External ear anomalies (30%–60%), ranging from severe microtia to minor pinna anomalies (cup shaped, lopped, or hypoplastic); stenosis, malformation or upward slanting of ear canal; pre-auricular ear pits (70%–80%)	Hearing loss reported in 75%, including conductive (30%), sensorineural (20%), and mixed types (50%)	Long narrow face shape, facial nerve paralysis (10%), branchial cyst/fistulas (60%), structural renal anomalies (75%), functional renal anomalies (33%), ossicular malformations, congenital cholesteatoma, cochlear malformations including Mondini dysplasia
CHARGE Association (**C**oloboma, **H**eart defects, **A**tresia of choanae, **R**etarded growth and development, **G**enital hypoplasia, **E**ar anomalies and deafness) Heterogeneous, 6% recurrence risk; may be dominant in some cases	Characteristic short, wide pinna missing features such as tragus, helix; prominent anthelix and triangular concha; small or absent earlobes; ear canal stenosis and atresia rare	Hearing loss in 85%, ranging from mild to profound sensorineural or mixed hearing loss due to ossicular and cochlear anomalies, distinctive wedge-shaped hearing loss due to middle ear disease and sensorineural loss	Choanal atresia (blockage of the nasal passage), congenital heart disease (60%–70%), developmental, renal abnormalities (15%), tracheoesophageal problems, minor skeletal defects
Congenital aural atresia Incidence 1–5:10,000 Sporadic, no known inheritance patterns (Lambert, 2001)	Congenital atresia without other anomalies; microtia or anotia in 95% of cases; male:female ratio is 2:1, right ears affected more often (65%); more common in Native Americans (1:2,000)	Conductive hearing loss, generally moderate to severe depending on degree of stenosis and ossicular/middle ear abnormalities	No other associated anomalies

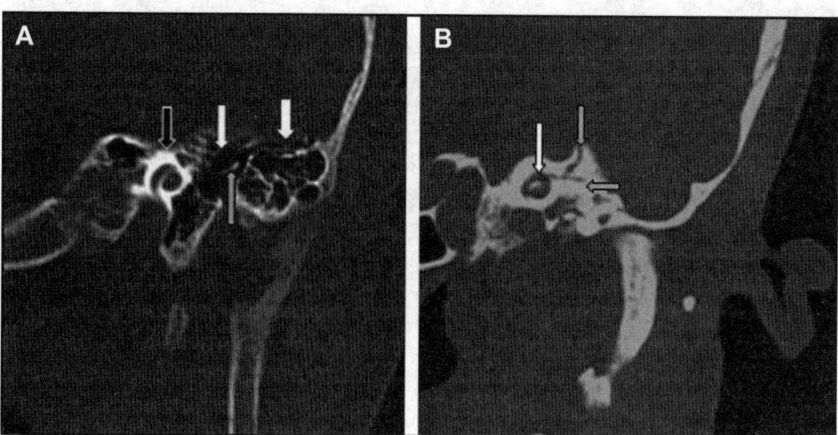

FIGURE 10–4. A. CT bone-window image of a left congenital aural atresia. The mastoid and middle ear are well aerated (*white arrows*) and sufficiently developed to allow surgical access to the middle ear ossicles (*gray arrow*). This type of anatomy offers a good prognosis for surgical reconstruction with good hearing results. Black arrow identifies the cochlea. **B.** In contrast to **A**, **B** depicts a very poorly developed temporal bone that would indicate that this patient is a poor candidate for surgical atresia repair. The mastoid and middle ear spaces are almost nonexistent, and the inner ear anatomy is also hypoplastic (poorly developed). The arrows indicate a hypoplastic cochlea (*white arrow*) and semicircular canals (*gray arrows*).

Patel and Shelton (2007) investigated 64 atresiaplasty cases and showed that stable short-term hearing results occurred after 32 surgeries and stable long-term hearing results occurred after 48 procedures. A retrospective study by Evans and Kazahaya (2007) compared both the outcomes and the costs of external auditory canal external auditory canal reconstruction and the BAHA system. Twenty-nine pediatric patients underwent external auditory canal reconstruction, and six pediatric patients underwent BAHA system surgery. BAHA system patients had more positive hearing outcomes (average hearing gain of 31.8 dB versus 17.3 dB for external auditory reconstruction), lower costs ($826 per dB hearing gain versus $2,910 per dB for external auditory canal reconstruction), and 93% of patients receiving external auditory canal reconstruction required some form of amplification postoperatively.

There are other articles in the otology literature that report the results of experienced surgeons who demonstrate improved hearing postoperatively for atresiaplasty, but the definitions of success vary considerably. Reducing the air-bone gap by 20 to 30 dB while showing improvement over preoperative hearing levels generally failed to improve hearing to the level of normal (Chang, Choi, & Hur, 2006; De La Cruz & Teufert, 2003; Digoy & Cueva, 2007; Evans & Kazahaya, 2007; Lambert, 1998; Patel & Shelton, 2007). Success is defined in these studies by improved hearing and stable hearing levels, rather than complete resolution of the air-bone gap, or speech reception thresholds (SRT) and pure-tone averages that fall within the normal range.

Studies of the BAHA system in achieving hearing outcomes within the normal range are also very few. Yellon (2007) reported on 13 children, 11 of whom had no complications and were using their devices. The mean postoperative SRT was 18.5 dB hearing level (HL) with a range of 14–25 dB. Evans and Kazahaya (2007) reported on six children who received surgery to implant the BAHA system, but audiometric postoperative data were only available on three of those children. The observed average gain was 31.8 dB HL, with an average SRT of 17.5 dB HL. There clearly is a need for studies with greater numbers of subjects that compare hearing outcomes from the use of an osseointegrated BAHA system and atresiaplasty. More recently, the new transcutaneous semi-implantable bone-conduction device that was developed in Germany in 2006 by Siegert et al. (2007) has been shown to produce an average of 43 dB HL PTA gain (33 dB HL SRT gain) in pediatric patients, with good parental satisfaction and fewer complications than the percutaneous BAHA device (Denoyelle et al., 2013).

Down Syndrome

Down syndrome, also known as trisomy 21, is a genetic disorder caused by an extra 21st chromosome (full or partial) and occurs with an incidence of 1/670 to 770 children born in the United States (Parker et al., 2010). Down syndrome is the most common chromosome disorder, and there are more than 400,000 people living with Down syndrome in the United States. OME is almost universal in children with Down syndrome, begins at a younger age, and persists to older ages than in typical children. Children with Down syndrome have a high incidence of conductive, mixed, and sensorineural hearing loss and are lost to follow-up at a higher rate than typically developing children (Park, Wilson, Stevens, Harward, & Hobler, 2012; Raut et al., 2011). Accordingly, the American Academy of Pediatrics (2001) has recommended that objective testing for hearing loss in children with Down syndrome should be done at birth to 3 months, and surveillance should continue during childhood.

Down syndrome has a distinct phenotype of facial dysmorphism, small stature, cardiac abnormalities, upper airway obstruction, obstructive sleep apnea, poor immune function, and subglottic stenosis. Ear, nose, and throat problems include stenotic ear canals and eustachian tube dysfunction, resulting in the development of ear infections and middle ear effusions.

Developmental and speech-language delay is associated with Down syndrome, affecting multiple areas that are important in assessment of hearing function, including nonverbal cognition, language learning, and social behavior. In addition, specific difficulties with speech and intelligibility, which are exacerbated by hearing loss, are associated with Down syndrome over and above the cognitive delay. The associated cognitive problems in children with Down syndrome make behavioral assessment problematic. Available studies in populations such as Down syndrome have found a 38% to 78% incidence of hearing loss, but if treated aggressively, hearing levels improve to the normal range for 86% to 98% (Paulsen, Weaver, & Macarthur, 2014; Shott, Joseph, & Heithaus, 2001). In a study of infants born with Down syndrome who were screened at birth and followed in a Down syndrome clinic, Raut et al. (2011) report that 82% of infants with Down syndrome had newborn hearing screening and hearing loss was diagnosed at a mean of 6.6 ± 3.3 months. The majority of these hearing losses (86%) were conductive, and were mild-moderate in more than half (57%). One third of those who were followed had normal hearing after treatment at 1 year of age. However, one third did not complete their audiological assessment. Hearing assessment is a lower priority for many parents of infants with Down syndrome during the first year of life compared to the overwhelming priorities of their other health care problems. Another recent study of NBHS and audiologic follow-up reported incidence of 38% with CHL due to otitis media, 6% with SNHL, and 3% with mixed HL (Park et al., 2012). In a population-based study in Norway (Austeng, Akre, & Falkenberge, 2013), 35% of children with Down syndrome at age 8 years had hearing levels worse than 25 dB HL in the better ear, with a higher incidence of SNHL (18%) compared to CHL (16%) and mixed HL (6%). Overall, OME is an ongoing problem in Down syndrome, and the majority of patients will require two or more sets of tubes during their childhood to achieve and maintain normal hearing (Paulson et al., 2014).

Cleft Lip and Palate (CLP)

Cleft lip and palate (CLP) is a congenital orofacial anomaly that occurs due to incomplete closure of the lip and palate during fetal development. CLP can be unilateral or bilateral and is one of the most common congenital anomalies affecting 1:500 live births worldwide. CLP affects hearing within the first 6 months of life due to eustachian tube dysfunction. Although middle ear effusion is common in healthy infants, it is nearly universal in infants with cleft lip and palate, which often persists into school age (Flynn, Moller, Jonsson, & Lohmander, 2009; Shah, 2004). Prior to surgery for palate closure, 92% to 99% of infants with cleft palate have OME due to eustachian tube dysfunction (Dhillon, 1988; Paradise & Bluestone, 1974; Schönweiler et al., 1999). Children with cleft palate have poor eustachian tube function due to a number of possible abnormalities (e.g., eustachian tube obstruction, narrow opening, and abnormal muscular control). Abnormal tubal function can persist even after palate repair.

CLP is also a common characteristic in many craniofacial conditions, including fetal alcohol, velocardiofacial, DiGeorge, CHARGE, and Down syndromes. These syndromes predispose affected children to recurrent ear infections and persistent middle ear effusion. A recent study of two groups of children (22 children with unilateral CLP, and 20 children without CLP) followed prospectively and longitudinally from 1 to 5 years of age was reported by Flynn et al. (2009). Assessments included otomicroscopy, tympanometry, and hearing assessment. Overall the children with unilateral CLP demonstrated a much higher prevalence of OME (75%) than children without CLP (19%).

A questionnaire sent to parents of children in a cleft palate registry in Ireland revealed that rates of middle ear disease were similar in children with isolated cleft palate and combined cleft lip and palate with considerably lower rates observed in children with cleft lip only (Sheahan, Miller, Sheahan, Earley, & Blayney, 2003). Rates of otitis media history, tube treatment, and current hearing loss were highest in 10- to 12-year-olds (65%, 83%, and 46%, respectively). OM onset typically was in the first year of life. Hearing was significantly poorer among those who had multiple tube surgeries, no doubt a marker for ongoing and recurrent middle ear disease.

Hearing loss due to OME has been found to be substantial in a study of 40 infants who range from 0 to 3 months old with cleft palate (Andrews, Chorbachi, Sirimanna, Sommerlad, & Hartley, 2004). In that study, thresholds measured with ABRs averaged 49 and 53 dB HL in the right and left ears, respectively. The conductive component was approximately 25 dB HL, and 83% of the infants with cleft palate had flat high-frequency tympanograms, consistent with middle ear effusion. Thus, it appears that middle ear effusion and CHL occur at an extremely high rate in children with cleft palate.

Acute Otitis Media and Otitis Media With Effusion

Acute otitis media (AOM) has a rapid onset, characteristic symptoms, and is of short duration. Otitis media with effusion (OME) is middle-ear fluid that remains after the acute infection is gone, or it can arise without signs or symptoms of acute infection. OME can produce CHL of 20 dB HL or greater in approximately 50% of cases (Hunter, Margolis, & Giebink, 1994; Sabo, Paradise, Kurs-Lasky, & Smith, 2003). Sabo et al. (2003) studied over 1,000 children with OME who were evaluated at least monthly with otoscopy and had hearing evaluations after 8 weeks of continuous middle ear effusion, as well as a sample of children without MEE. In this study, hearing threshold levels were 10 to 15 dB higher in the presence of bilateral MEE than in children without OME.

As shown in Figure 10–5, a wide range of hearing levels and hearing configurations exist in OME, which often is not recognized as it usually is characterized as mild, flat hearing loss (Margolis, Hunter, Rykken, & Giebink, 1993).

Incidence and prevalence rates are useful in reporting and following changes in the impact of AOM and OME in the pediatric population. The two rates provide different information. Prevalence conveys information about OME burden in a population at a given point in time and depends on both disease development and duration. Incidence measures new episodes of AOM/OME—that is, the probability of OM-free individuals developing OM over a specified time period.

Incidence and prevalence of AOM and OME vary widely around the globe. Variation in these two measures are likely related to (a) demographic characteristics of the group studied (e.g., age, race, ethnicity,

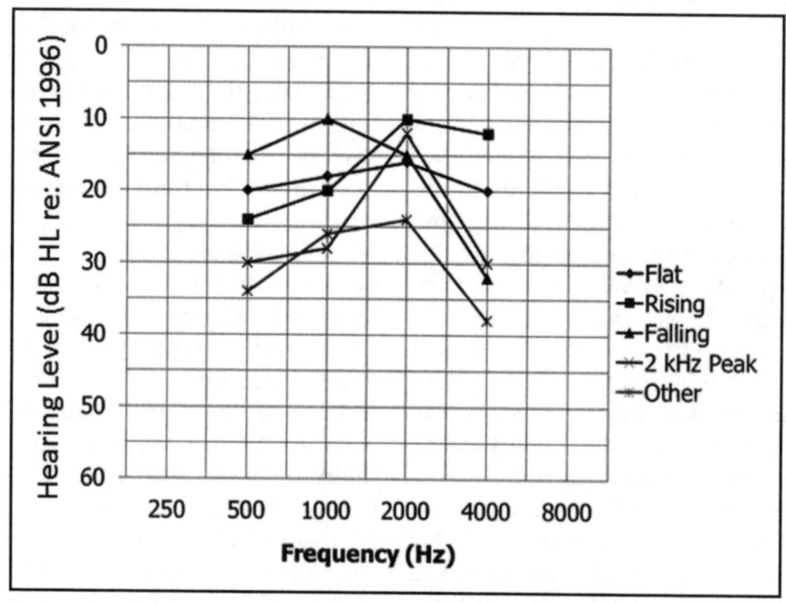

FIGURE 10–5. Average hearing levels in children with chronic otitis media with effusion classified into five distinct configurations.

socioeconomic status); (b) frequency and type of ascertainment (e.g., physician exam versus parent or self-report); and (c) the criteria used to diagnosis these two conditions. Population-based studies provide better estimates than convenience samples (such as daycare centers and schools), because they represent the broader community. Some of these studies have included hearing as a study factor in participants. There are several sources of incidence data. Information from over 8,000 parents of preschoolers collected in National Health and Nutrition Examination Survey (NHANES) III showed a nonsignificant 3% increase in reported rates of OM between 1988 and 1994 (Auringer, Lanphear, Kalkwarf, & Mansour, 2003). Significant increases of 5% in OM onset by 12 months and 6% in recurrent OM were also demonstrated. Children from low-income families and those with less-educated parents showed the greatest increase in these two measures. The Early Childhood Longitudinal Study Birth Cohort included over 8,000 children representative of 2001 U.S. births. Based on parent report of physician diagnosis, OM incidence was 39% by 9 months and 62% by 2 years of age (Hoffman, Park, Losonczy, & Chiu, 2007).

Since the licensure and routine use of the 7-valent pneumococcal conjugate vaccine (PCV-7) in 2000, important trends have emerged; overall OM incidence and prevalence rates have declined, particularly among young children (Grijalva et al., 2006; Zhou, Shefer, Kong, & Nuorti, 2008). Parent-reported recurrent OM incidence among children younger than 18 years also declined from 335 in 1,000 in 1997 to 214 in 1,000 in 2004 (U.S. Department of Health and Human Services [USDHHS], 2008). Similarly, physician office visits with an OM diagnosis declined from 118 to 78 per 100 children younger than 3 years old from 1997 to 2005, a 34% decrease (USDHHS, 2008).

International OM Rates

In the Netherlands, a retrospective cohort study of children younger than 13 years used data from the University Medical Center Utrecht Primary Care Network collected in 1995 to 2003 (Plasschaert, Rovers, Schilder, Verheij, & Hak, 2006). Among those under 2 years of age, AOM and OME incidence increased by 46% and 66%, respectively, whereas antibiotic prescription rates for AOM and OME increased by 45% and 25%. The contrast of declining rates in the United States and increasing rates in the Netherlands is most likely due to the later introduction of universal pneumococcal conjugate vaccination in the Netherlands in 2006 (Van Deursen et al., 2012). A database of over 2 million patients of 291 general practitioners in the United Kingdom was used to evaluate middle ear disease workload between 1991 and 2001 (Williamson, Benge, Mullee, & Little, 2006). AOM visits for 2- to 10-year-olds decreased from 105.3 to 34.7 per 1,000 over this period, whereas chronic OME visits were relatively stable (15.2 to 16.7 per 1,000 each year). In a study of Chinese kindergartners 3- to 6-year-olds (n = 3,013), the overall prevalence of OM diagnosed by a senior otolaryngologist using pneumatic otoscopy and tympanometry was 9.8%, with rates that were higher in 3- to 5-year-olds (11%–12%) and lower in 6-year-olds (6%; Chen, Lin, Hwang, & Ku, 2003). Longitudinal data on early AOM in the Oslo Birth Cohort revealed a 5% incidence before 6 months of age, and 28% incidence by 12 months (Bentdal, Karevold, Nafstad, & Kvaerner, 2007). Thirteen percent of 10-year-olds were reported to have AOM in the previous 12 months (Karevold, Kvestad, Nafstad, & Kvaerner, 2006). In Denmark, cumulative incidence of OM has not changed in recent years, despite less treatment with antibiotics (Todberg et al., 2014). The cumulative incidence of OM at 7 years was 60%; 16% had their first OM episode between 0 and 6 months of age, 44% between 7 and 18 months, and 40% between 19 months and 7 years. Four or more OM episodes before 7 years were reported by 40%. Thus, OM is a prevalent feature of childhood throughout the world, and while vaccination appears to have had some effect on AOM in countries that introduced universal vaccination in infancy, chronic OME does not appear to have declined overall and is still a significant health burden worldwide.

High-Risk Populations

Indigenous populations continue to suffer a considerable OM burden, but not all studies have evaluated hearing. A systematic review of population-based studies of OM incidence and prevalence in 250,000 children under 18 years old (Gunasekera, Hayson, Morris, & Craig, 2007) showed that OM prevalence in native populations is the highest of any group, such as in Alaskan Inuit and Australian aboriginals. Hearing impairment was present in 33% of Australian aboriginal children (Thorne, 2003) and 19% of Inuit children (Ayukawa, Lejeune, & Proulx, 2004). American Indian children in Minnesota had early OM onset, as 63% had OM and 30% failed OAE by 6 months of age (Daly, Pirie, Rhodes, Hunter, & Davey, 2007; Hunter, Davey, Kohtz, & Daly, 2007). In a Canadian indigenous population, children under 2 years old had 2.3 outpatient AOM visits per year (Dallaire, Dewailly, Vezina, Bruneau, & Ayotte, 2006). Among Australian aboriginal children, 41% had OME, 33% had AOM, and 40%

had tympanic membrane perforations by 18 months (Morris et al., 2005). Lehmann and colleagues (2008) reported that OM was detected in 55% of examinations in Aboriginal children and 26% of examinations in non-Aboriginal children; peak prevalence was 72% at age 5 to 9 months in Aboriginal children, and 40% at 10 to 14 months in non-Aboriginal children. Moderate-to-severe hearing loss was present in 32% of 47 Aboriginal children and 7% of 120 non-Aboriginal children aged 12 months or more. In another study of 280 western Australian children followed from birth to age 2 years, 74% of Aboriginal children and 45% of non-Aboriginal children had OM (Jacoby et al., 2008). In New Zealand Pacific Islander 2-year-olds (n = 1,001) who participated in a screening program, 75% failed the initial tympanometry screening. Of the 502 who attended the second screening at home or clinic, 51% failed. Of those failing two or three screens, 73% and 82% were determined to have OME or AOM (Paterson et al., 2006). Other countries that have high rates of poverty are also at high risk for chronic OM and hearing loss. For example, 2.5% of Nigerian children have chronic suppurative OM (Amusa, Ijadunola, & Onayade, 2005), and 47% of those cases have hearing loss (Lasisi et al., 2007a). Bottle feeding as well as poverty-related indices (lower socioeconomic status, crowding, malnutrition) are associated with chronic OM (Lasisi, Sulaiman, & Afolabi, 2007b). In Mozambique, overcrowding, exposure to tobacco and wood smoke, and a short duration of breastfeeding increased the risk of OM (da Costa, Navarro, Neves, & Martin, 2004). Chronic suppurative OM was experienced by 12% of children in Bangladesh (Biswas, Joarder, & Siddiquee, 2005). Factors that appear to contribute to higher rates of AOM, OME, and chronic OM among these high-risk populations include poverty, overcrowding, greater rates of smoking, or cooking smoke in the home. A lack of protective factors, such as breastfeeding, vaccinations, access to preventative care, high-quality daycare, clean water, and hygiene practices also play a role.

Effects of Genes and Environment on AOM/OME

Environmental and intrinsic factors each contribute to making infancy the period of greatest OM susceptibility. OM pathogens in the nose and throat have ready access to the middle ear via the shallow angle of the infant eustachian tube, relative to adults. The infant's immune system lacks the ability to mount an effective antibody response to infections that are commonly acquired in group child care or at home with siblings. Researchers have explored genes related to functions and processes that might be involved in early OM in infancy. A 5-year follow-up of the Pittsburgh twin and triplet cohort (Casselbrant et al., 2004) reported that heritability of total time with OME by age 5 years was 72%. Heritability refers to the proportion of variation in time with OME that can be attributed to genetic factors. Children undergoing tube surgery for chronic or recurrent OM and control children without OM histories had mucin 2 expression six times greater than control levels (Ubell, Kerschner, Wackym, & Burrows, 2008). Mucin 2 is a mucus-forming protein active in the middle ear and gut that plays a major role in chronic middle ear effusion, which often results in CHL. A Norwegian study of 4,247 twin pairs reported that genes involved in OM risk do not vary by gender (Kvestad et al., 2004).

Environmental and Other Risk Factors

Pacifier use, in a study of 495 children less than 4 years of age, was related to recurrent OM, but not to AOM (Rovers et al., 2008). A National Institute of Child Health and Human Development (NICHD) study was conducted among more than 11,000 children who entered daycare after 3 years of age. Those in settings with over six children had a 50% higher rate of OM from 3 to 4.5 years of age, and earlier daycare entry was not protective against OM (NICHD and Early Child Care Network, 2003). A 2003 study of more than 3,000 infants reported that supine sleeping decreased risk of OM by 30% to 40% by age 6 months compared to prone sleeping (Hunt et al., 2003). Jacoby's study of western Australian children reported that those exposed to tobacco smoke (64%) were 3.5 times more likely to have OM than those not exposed (Jacoby et al., 2008). Although 40% of non-Aboriginal children were exposed to tobacco smoke, this exposure did not significantly increase OM risk. Non-Aboriginal children were twice as likely to be diagnosed with OM if there were other children in the home, while very few Aboriginal children were in daycare and daycare did not increase their risk of OM. Among 6- to 12-year-olds identified with OME in a Greek screening program, exposure to tobacco smoke did not increase risk of OME (Xenellis et al., 2005). Earlier extrusion of ventilation tubes was reported in children whose parents smoked compared to children of nonsmokers (Praveen & Terry, 2005). A novel study in Germany and the Netherlands reported a slight but significant increase in OM by age 2 years in children with higher exposure to traffic-related pollutants identified by home address (Brauer et al., 2006). In a study of Pacific Islander children, predictive factors for OME included child care for 20 hr/week or more (Odds Ratio [OR] = 5.21) and a variety of respiratory and airway conditions in the prior year including draining ears (OR 2.10), more than five cough or cold illnesses (OR 1.91), frequent snoring (OR 2.60), and home treatment for breathing symptoms (OR 2.61; Paterson et al., 2007).

Researchers in Pennsylvania and Virginia studied middle ear effusion in 148 1- to 8-year-olds during the North American respiratory disease season (Mandel, Doyle, Winther, & Alper, 2008). Parents recorded information on onset and duration of respiratory illnesses throughout the study, and validated otoscopists performed ear exams weekly. Overall incidence of new OM episodes was about one per 100 child-days. Factors significantly related to respiratory disease (including OM) burden were young age, history of frequent colds, and parent occupation. Forty percent of OM episodes resolved within 1 week, and 75% to 90% by 1 month, whereas daily prevalence of OM ranged from 20% to 35% with peak prevalence in March. Analyses of National Health and Nutrition Examination Survey (NHANES) data collected in 1988 to 1994 revealed that shorter exclusive breastfeeding (<6 months) increased the risk of recurrent OM among children younger than 2 years about twofold, whereas exposure to both pre- and postnatal passive smoke increased ROM risk about 50% (Chandy, Howard, & Auringer, 2006). Clinicians should counsel families about these risk factors, and encourage mothers to breastfeed as long as possible; place infants on their back to sleep; advise parents not to smoke; avoid large group child care, if possible; and wash their hands as well as children's hands before eating, after diaper changing, toilet use, and coughing or sneezing.

Immunocompromise

Maternal antibodies are transferred in utero during pregnancy and to the infant at delivery (Englund, 2007), but maternal antibodies do not persist for very long. Infants do not begin to produce their own antibodies until 6 to 12 months of age (Glezen, 2003). Thus, otitis media incidence is high in the first year of life as a result of low levels of passive antibodies, coupled with the infant's exposure to pathogens carried by siblings and children in daycare. Besides low levels of antibodies or low antibody levels that affect all infants in early life, infants and children can have specific immunodeficiencies that increase the risk of OM and associated hearing loss. Primary specific immunodeficiency, the most common immune abnormality, results in defective antibody production, making individuals susceptible to respiratory diseases, including acute OM (Rynnel-Dagöö, 2004). Hereditary and congenital conditions that affect the immune system (e.g., Down syndrome, Turner syndrome) can also result in recurrent OM (Rynnel-Dagöö, 2004).

Children requiring organ or bone marrow transplants become immunocompromised as a result of treatments to reduce the likelihood of graft rejection. Other chronic conditions (e.g., diabetes, cancer) can increase the likelihood of immunodeficiency. A chart review of infectious diseases in 92 pediatric patients with primary immunodeficiencies revealed that 24% of those with antibody deficiency had OM, compared to 9% to 14% of those with cellular deficiency, combined deficiency, or phagocyte defect (Chang, Yang, & Chiang, 2006).

Treatment of OME and AOM

Guidelines for treatment of AOM and OME draw on the expertise of the Agency for Healthcare Research and Quality (AHRQ). These guidelines use common resources for literature review and incorporate similar criteria for recommendations. Recognizing that inappropriate diagnosis, treatment, and management of AOM and OME can prolong disease course and attendant CHL, primary care and specialist physician groups published evidence-based clinical practice guidelines for both OME in 2004, which was updated in 2016 by the American Academy of Otolaryngology (Rosenfeld et al., in preparation). Using levels of recommendation from "strongly recommended" to "not recommended," the OME panel graded the quality of evidence from published research ranging from A (randomized controlled trials) to D (expert opinion, case reports). The panel recommended identifying children at risk for speech, language, and learning problems for prompt assessment and early hearing evaluation. Watchful waiting for 3 months is recommended for the low-risk child with OME because of the likelihood of resolution in the majority of children. A child would be considered low risk unless he or she has one or more of the following: persistent hearing loss, suspected or diagnosed speech and language delay, autism spectrum disorder, other developmental disorders, Down syndrome, craniofacial anomalies associated with cognitive or speech and language delay, visual impairment, cleft palate, or developmental delay. The guidelines advocate hearing testing for children who have OME for 3 months or longer, are at high risk, or have language delay or speech problems. Surgically placed ventilation tubes are recommended unless findings indicate that additional procedures (e.g., adenoidectomy with or without tonsillectomy) are needed. The panel discourages population-based screening programs for OME among low-risk children, and routine treatment of OME with antihistamines, decongestants, antibiotics, and corticosteroids. The guidelines made no recommendations about complementary medicine or allergy management as OME treatment based on a lack of scientific evidence.

Guidelines for AOM (American Academy of Pediatrics and American Academy of Family Physicians, 2004) focus on diagnosis and initial treatment based on age and severity. The guideline advocates judicious use of antibiotics because inappropriate use results in high rates of resistance and multiple-resistant organisms, leading to the societal expense of developing and marketing new antimicrobials. The guidelines provide a detailed description of recommended diagnostic criteria for AOM: acute onset of signs and symptoms, presence of middle ear fluid, and symptoms of middle ear inflammation. Diagnosis in young children can be uncertain because middle ear fluid cannot be accurately ascertained (e.g., cerumen in the canal, narrow canal, lack of a proper seal for pneumatic otoscopy and tympanometry). Other recommendations include assessment and treatment of pain, observation as an option to treatment for uncomplicated AOM taking into account age, severity of illness, ability to follow-up, and diagnostic certainty. Antibacterial therapy was recommended for infants younger than 6 months, and for those 6 months or older to 2 years with severe illness and certain diagnosis. In this age group, if illness is not severe and diagnosis is uncertain, "watchful waiting" is an option. Children 2 years or older should be observed and receive pain medication if needed, but antibiotics should not be given unless OM is severe. Another recommendation is to prevent AOM by reducing risk factors. Complementary or alternative medicines were not recommended for AOM treatment because of inadequate data on effectiveness. Guidelines stress that observation is appropriate only when follow-up is possible and treatment can be provided if the illness worsens. A Cochrane Systematic Review of randomized controlled trials of ventilation tube placement for OME studied effects on hearing and a variety of other outcomes (e.g., quality of life, preventing adverse developmental outcomes; Lous et al., 2005). These authors concluded that the duration of effusion was reduced by 32% and hearing level was improved by 9 dB after 6 months and 6 dB by 12 months. No effect of tubes on speech and language was detected.

Chronic Middle Ear Disease and Conductive Hearing Loss

Whether due to chronic infections of the middle ear and mastoid or cholesteatoma-related middle ear problems, chronic ear disease is commonly associated with conductive hearing loss. The hearing loss can be attributed to chronic fluid involving the middle ear space, perforations of the tympanic membrane, erosion of the ossicles, or sclerotic fixation of the ossicular chain as a result of repetitive bouts of inflammation and scarring. The clinical and surgical management of chronic ear disease is typically guided by two objectives: (a) obtaining a dry and safe ear (free of infection or cholesteatoma), and (b) maintaining or establishing a good hearing ear. Unfortunately, these two goals often result in contradictory management strategies. For example, in the setting of cholesteatoma, aggressive surgical removal is the mainstay of treatment. This has classically involved removing any involved ossicles and removing the posterior external auditory canal (i.e., a canal wall down mastoidectomy or modified radical mastoidectomy) to obtain the widest exposure and most complete eradication of cholesteatoma from the middle ear and mastoid compartments. However, removing ossicles and altering the ear canal and tympanic membrane anatomy understandably have negative consequences for hearing. However, if more conservative surgical measures are taken to clean cholesteatoma or infection from the ear, there is the potential to leave residual disease in the ear that will then necessitate additional surgery down the road. Taken together, the management of chronic ear disease in patients is frequently associated with conductive hearing losses that requires either surgical repair or hearing aid intervention.

Reconstruction of the Tympanic Membrane

Myingoplasty specifically refers to surgical repair of the tympanic membrane. This can often be performed using simple materials in a transcanal procedure (e.g., paper patch or fat graft myringoplasty). This procedure is restricted to the tympanic membrane itself and does not involve the middle ear space proper. In contrast, a tympanoplasty routinely involves repair of a tympanic membrane defect but also entails cleaning out of the middle ear space (of cholesteatoma, infection, adhesions, etc.). Tympanoplasties can be performed either through the ear canal (transcanal) or through a postauricular incision. In tympanoplasty, temporalis fascia (harvested from an incision behind the ear) or tragal perichondrium are commonly used to repair the tympanic membrane. Tympanoplasty technique can also be further subclassified as either underlay/medial graft (graft placed medial to the tympanic membrane) or overlay/lateral graft (graft placed laterally on the tympanic membrane surface). Surgical results are largely dependent on the nature of the chronic ear disease more than on the surgical approach or repair technique. In general terms, closure of tympanic membrane defects via tympanoplasty is associated with a greater than 90% success rate.

Reconstruction of the Ossicular Chain

Over several decades, a variety of techniques have evolved for surgical reconstruction of ossicular chain defects. Depending on the ossicular problem as well as the surgeon preference, defects of the malleus, incus, and stapes can be reconstructed/replaced using autologous bone (e.g., incus interposition) or alternatively, using artificial ossicles (made out of hydroxyapatite, titanium, or a variety of other materials). When using autologous reconstruction, the most common scenario is one in which the incus is partially eroded and no longer in contact with the malleus or stapes. By first removing and then resculpting the incus, the reshaped incus can then be interposed between the malleus and stapes to reestablish continuity of the ossicular chain.

Alternatively, when a normal stapes is in place (regardless of the condition of the malleus and incus), a partial ossicular reconstruction prosthesis (PORP) can be seated on top of the stapes capitulum and either connected to the manubrium of the malleus or brought directly to the undersurface of the tympanic membrane in order to reestablish a sound conduction mechanism. In contrast, in many cases, the stapes superstructure is absent and only a footplate remains in the oval window. In this setting, a total ossicular reconstruction prosthesis (TORP) is needed to build a functional middle ear system. Both PORPs and TORPs are available in a variety of commercially available designs in several different biocompatible materials.

Hearing results from ossicular reconstruction are determined by several factors. The most significant factor is likely the overall health of the ear. Even when an "ideal" ossicular reconstruction is performed, an ear that is prone to recurrent infections or recurrent cholesteatoma will likely have poor long-term hearing outcomes. Particularly challenging are those ears with very poor eustachian tube dysfunction and chronically retracting tympanic membrane because of negative middle ear pressures. Under such clinical conditions, even the best of tympanic membrane and ossicular reconstructions will be susceptible to recurrent conductive hearing losses. In other scenarios, patients with healthy middle ear status and an intact stapes have an excellent hearing prognosis almost irrespective of the method of ossicular reconstruction performed. The stapes, in general, remains a key factor when discussing good hearing outcomes following chronic ear surgery. The stability of the ossicular reconstruction and the mechanical-acoustic advantages offered by an intact stapes likely explain the better hearing results.

Case Study

A 9-year-old girl presents with a history of recurrent cholesteatoma despite having undergone two prior ear surgeries. Her exam shows cholesteatoma debris in the ear canal and a thickened opaque tympanic membrane. Computed tomography (CT) scans demonstrate opacification of the middle ear and mastoid consistent with exam findings. Routine audiologic testing showed a moderate conductive hearing loss. Given the recurrent nature of the ear disease despite prior surgical treatment, the decision was made to perform a canal wall down mastoidectomy with an ossicular reconstruction.

Findings at the time of surgery showed extensive recurrent cholesteatomas that were eradicated with only the manubrium of the malleus and the stapes footplate remaining of the ossicular chain. After removing the posterior external auditory canal wall, a hydroxyapatite TORP was positioned directly on the stapes footplate and brought to the undersurface of the neotympanic membrane. In Figure 10–6A, a partially eroded incus has been reshaped into an autologous bony cap that has been seated on top of the stapes capitulum with the tympanic membrane then resting directly on top of the sculpted incus (arrows). Figure

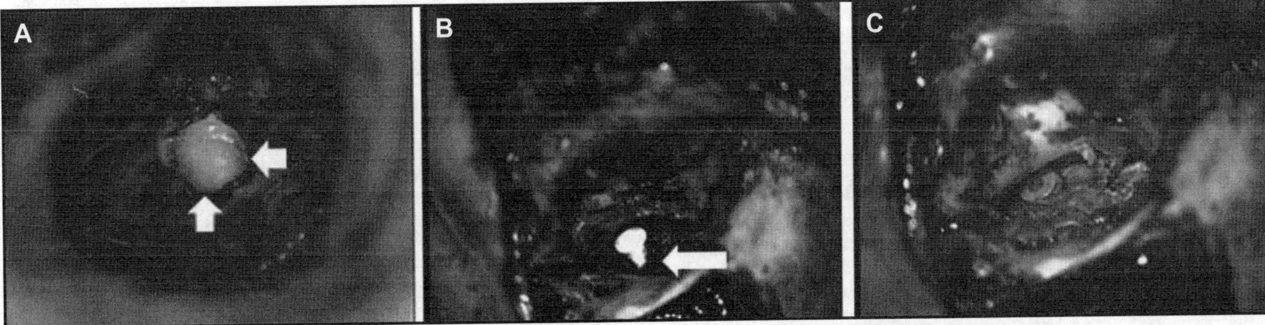

FIGURE 10–6. A. Incus interposition. **B.** Partial ossicular reconstruction (PORP). **C.** Tympanic membrane after PORP.

10–6B demonstrates partial ossicular reconstruction prosthesis (PORP) that is positioned directly on the stapes (arrow). The tympanic membrane has been lifted up and reflected forward to allow access to the middle ear space. Figure 10–6C shows the same ear as in Figure 10–3B with the tympanic membrane now laid back into its normal position. Note the ventilation tube in the tympanic membrane. Postoperative audiologic testing demonstrated a mild conductive hearing loss with an SRT of 25 dB and word recognition score of 100%. She was very successfully fit with a hearing aid for this ear 3 months postoperatively with excellent benefit.

Summary

It is vitally important for pediatric audiologists to be well acquainted with these various causes of CHL in infants and children, and to understand the best clinical practices for assessment and intervention for these children. Often, it seems that CHL is disregarded or downplayed as it is nearly a universal occurrence at some point in all children due to otitis media. Understanding the special issues related to assessment of the neonatal ear allows us to be more accurate in diagnoses of CHL, be it temporary or persistent. Knowledge of craniofacial characteristics of which to be alert during ear examinations and history can assist audiologists in making appropriate referrals to other medical professionals such as otology, genetics, and developmental pediatrics to assess the child for the presence of a syndrome. Finally, understanding the complexity of risk factors associated with recurrent and chronic otitis media can assist the audiologist in counseling parents on ways to reduce or prevent otitis media.

References

Alaerts, J., Lutz, H., & Woulters, J. (2007). Evaluation of middle ear function in young children: Clinical guidelines for the use of 226 and 1,000-Hz tympanometry. *Otology and Neurotology, 28*, 727–732.

Allanson, J. (2004). Genetic hearing loss associated with external ear abnormalities. In H. V. Toriello, W. Reardon, & R. J. Gorlin (Eds.), *Hereditary hearing loss and its syndromes* (Chapter 6). New York, NY: Oxford University Press.

American Academy of Pediatrics and American Academy of Family Physicians. (2004). Clinical practice guideline: Diagnosis and management of acute otitis media. *Pediatrics, 113*, 1451–1465.

American Academy of Pediatrics Committee on Genetics. (2001). Health supervision for children with Down syndrome. *Pediatrics, 107*, 442–449.

Amusa, Y. B., Ijadunola, I. K., & Onayade, O. O. (2005). Epidemiology of otitis media in a local tropical African population. *West African Journal of Medicine, 24*, 227–230.

Andrews, P. J., Chorbachi, R., Sirimanna, T., Sommerlad, B., & Hartley, B. E. J. (2004). Evaluation of hearing thresholds in 3 month-old children with a cleft palate: The basis for a selective policy for ventilation tube insertion at the time of palate repair. *Clinics in Otolaryngology, 29*, 10–17.

Auringer, P., Lanphear, B. P., Kalkwarf, H. J., & Mansour, M. E. (2003). Trends in otitis media among children in the United States. *Pediatrics, 112*, 514–520.

Austeng, M. E., Akre, H., & Falkenberge, E. (2013). Hearing level in children with Down syndrome at the age of eight. *Research in Developmental Disabilities, 34*, 2251–2256.

Ayukawa, H., Lejeune, P., & Proulx, J. F. (2004). Hearing screening outcomes in Inuit children in Nunavik, Quebec, Canada. *International Journal of Circumpolar Health, 63*(Suppl. 2), 309–311.

Baldwin, M. (2006). Choice of probe tone and classification of trace patterns in tympanometry undertaken in early infancy. *International Journal of Audiology, 45*, 417–427.

Bayraktar, S., Bayraktar, S. T., Ataoglu, E., Ayaz, A., & Elevli, M. (2005). Goldenhar's syndrome associated with multiple congenital abnormalities. *Journal of Tropical Pediatrics, 51*, 377–379.

Bentdal, Y., Karevold, A., Nafstad, P., & Kvaerner, K. J. (2007). Early acute otitis media. Predictor for AOM and respiratory infections in childhood? *International Journal of Pediatric Otorhinolaryngology, 71*, 1251–1259.

Biswas, A. C., Joarder, A. H., & Siddiquee, B. H. (2005). Prevalence of CSOM among rural school going children. *Mymensingh Medical Journal, 14*, 152–155.

Brauer, M., Gehring, U., Brunekreef, B., de Jongste, J., Gerritsen, J., Rovers, M., . . . Heinrich, J. (2006). Traffic-related air pollution and otitis media. *Environmental Health Perspectives, 114*, 1414–1418.

Calandruccio, L., Fitzgerald, T. S., & Prieve, B. A. (2006). Normative multifrequency tympanometry in infants and toddlers. *Journal of the American Academy of Audiology, 17*, 470–480.

Casselbrant, M. L., Mandel, E. M., Rockette, H. E., KursLasky, M., Fall, P. A., & Bluestone, C. D. (2004). The genetic component of middle ear disease in the first 5 years of life. *Archives of Otolaryngology-Head and Neck Surgery, 130*, 273–278.

Centers for Disease Control (CDC; 2006). Improved national prevalence estimates for 18 selected major birth defects—United States, 1999–2001. *Morbidity and Mortality Weekly Report, 54*, 1301–1305.

Chandy, C. J., Howard, C. R., & Auringer, P. (2006). Full breastfeeding duration and associated decrease in respiratory tract infection in US children. *Pediatrics, 117*, 425–432.

Chang, S. H., Yang, Y. H., & Chiang, B. L. (2006). Infectious pathogens in pediatric patients with primary immunodeficiencies. *Journal of Microbiology, Immunology and Infection, 39*, 503–515.

Chang, S. O., Choi, B. Y., & Hur, D. G. (2006). Analysis of the long-term hearing results after the surgical repair of aural atresia. *Laryngoscope, 166*(10), 1835–1841.

Chen, C. H., Lin, C. J., Hwang, Y. H., & Ku, C. J. (2003). Epidemiology of otitis media in Chinese children. *Clinics in Otolaryngology, 28*, 442–445.

Christensen, L. (2014, July). Understanding atresia, microtia, and the Baha system. *AudiologyOnline*, Article 12793. Retrieved June 25, 2015, from http://www.audiologyonline.com

da Costa, J. L., Navarro, A., Neves, J. B., & Martin, M. (2004). Household wood and charcoal smoke increases risk of otitis media in childhood in Maputo. *International Journal of Epidemiology, 33*, 573–578.

Dallaire, F., Dewailly, E., Vezina, C., Bruneau, S., & Ayotte, P. (2006). Portrait of outpatient visits and hospitalizations for acute infections in Nunavik preschool children. *Canadian Journal of Public Health, 97*, 362–368.

Daly, K. A., Pirie, P. L., Rhodes, K. L., Hunter, L. L., & Davey, C. S. (2007). Early otitis media among Minnesota American Indians: The little ears study. *American Journal of Public Health, 97*, 317–322.

De Alarcon, A., & Choo, D. I. (2007). Controversies in aural atresia repair. *Current Opinions in Otolaryngology and Head and Neck Surgery, 15*, 310–314.

De La Cruz, A., & Teufert, K. B. (2003). Congenital aural atresia surgery: Long-term results. *Otolaryngology-Head and Neck Surgery, 129*(1), 121–127.

Denoyelle F., Leboulanger N., Coudert C., Mazzaschi, O., Loundon, N., Vicaut, E., . . . Garabedian, E-N. (2013). New closed skin bone-anchored implant: Preliminary results in 6 children with ear atresia. *Otology and Neurotology, 34*, 275–281.

Dhillon, R. S. (1988). The middle ear in cleft palate children pre and post palatal closure. *Journal of the Royal Society of Medicine, 81*, 710–713.

Digoy, G. P., & Cueva, R. A. (2007). Congenital aural atresia: Review of short and long-term surgical results. *Otology and Neurotology, 28*, 54–60.

Doyle, K. J., Burggraaff, B., Fujikawa, S., Jim, J., & MacArthur, C. J. (1997). Neonatal hearing screening with otoscopy, auditory brain stem response, and otoacoustic emissions. *Otolaryngology-Head and Neck Surgery, 116*, 597–603.

Englund, J. A. (2007). The influence of maternal immunization on infant immune responses. *Journal of Comparative Pathology, 137*, S16–S19.

Evans, A. E., & Kazahaya, K. (2007). Canal atresia: Surgery or implantable hearing devices? The expert's question is revisited. *International Journal of Pediatric Otorhinolaryngology, 71*, 367–374.

Flynn, T., Moller, C., Jonsson, R., & Lohmander, A. (2009). The high prevalence of otitis media with effusion in children with cleft lip and palate as compared to children without clefts. *International Journal of Pediatric Otorhinolaryngology, 73*(10), 1441–1446.

Fraser, F. C., Sproule, J. R., & Halal, F. (1980). Frequency of the branchio-oto-renal (BOR) syndrome in children with profound hearing loss. *American Journal of Medical Genetics, 7*, 341–349.

Glezen, W. P. (2003). Effect of maternal antibodies on the infant immune response. *Vaccine, 28*, 3389–3392.

Grabb, W. (1965). The first and second bronchial arch syndrome. *Plastic and Reconstructive Surgery, 36*, 485.

Grijalva, C. G., Poehling, K. A., Nuorti, J. P., Zhu, Y., Martin, S. W., Edwards, K. M., & Griffin, M. R. (2006). National impact of universal childhood immunization with pneumococcal conjugate vaccine on outpatient medical care visits in the United States. *Pediatrics, 118*, 865–873.

Gunasekera, H., Hayson, L., Morris, P., & Craig, J. (2007). *The global burden of childhood otitis media and hearing impairment (HI): A systemic review*. Paper presented at the ninth International Symposium on Recent Advances in Otitis Media. St. Petersburg Beach, FL.

Hall, J. W., III., Smith, S. D., & Popelka, G. R. (2004). Newborn hearing screening with combined otoacoustic emissions and auditory brainstem responses. *Journal of the American Academy of Audiology, 15*, 414–425.

Hoffman, H. J., Park, J., Losonczy, K. G., & Chiu, M. S. (2007). *Risk factors, treatments, and other conditions associated with frequent ear infections in US children through 2 years of age: The Early Childhood Longitudinal Study Birth Cohort (ECLS-B)*. Paper presented at the ninth International Symposium on Recent Advances in Otitis Media. St. Petersburg Beach, FL.

Holte, L., Margolis, R. H., & Cavanaugh, R. M. (1991). Developmental changes in multifrequency tympanograms. *Audiology, 30*, 1–24.

Hunt, C. E., Lesko, S. M., Vezina, R. M., McCoy, R., Corwin, M. J., & Mandell, F. (2003). Infant sleep position and associated health outcomes. *Archives of Pediatric Adolescent Medicine, 157*, 469–474.

Hunter, L. L., Davey, C. S., Kohtz, A., & Daly, K. A. (2007). Hearing screening and middle ear measures in American Indian infants and toddlers. *International Journal of Pediatric Otorhinolaryngology, 71*, 1429–1438.

Hunter, L. L., & Margolis, R. H. (1992). Multifrequency tympanometry, current clinical application. *American Journal of Audiology, 1*, 33–43.

Hunter, L. L., Margolis, R. H., & Giebink, G. S. (1994). Identification of hearing loss in otitis media. *Annals of Otology, Rhinology, Laryngology, 163*(103, Suppl.), 59–61.

Ikui, A., Sando, I., & Fujita, S. (1997). Postnatal change in angle between the tympanic annulus and surrounding structures: Computer-aided three-dimensional reconstruction study. *Annals of Otolaryngology, Rhinology and Laryngology, 106*, 33–36.

Ishimoto, S., Ito, K., Yamasoba, T., Kondo, K., Karino, S., Takegoshi, H., & Kaga, K. (2005). Correlation between microtia and temporal bone malformation evaluated using grading systems. *Archives of Otolaryngology-Head and Neck Surgery, 131*, 326–329.

Jacoby, P. A., Coates, H. L., Arumgaswamy, A., Elsbury, D., Stokes, A., Monck, R., . . . Lehman, D. (2008). The effect of passive smoking on the risk of otitis media in Aboriginal and non-Aboriginal children in the Kalgoorlie-Boulder region of Western Australia. *Medical Journal of Australia, 188*, 599–603.

Jafek, B. W., Nager, G. T., Strife, J., & Gayler, R. W. (1975). Congenital aural atresia: An analysis of 311 cases. *Transactions of the Section Otolaryngology of the American Academy of Opthamology and Otolaryngology, 80*, 588–595.

Jahrsdoerfer, R. A., & Jacobson, J. T. (1995). Treacher Collins syndrome: Otologic and auditory management. *Journal of the American Academy of Audiology, 6*, 93–102.

Jahrsdoerfer, R. A., Yeakley, J. W., Aguilar, E. A., Cole, R. R., & Gray, L. C. (1992). Grading system for the selection of patients with congenital aural atresia. *American Journal of Otology, 13*, 6–12.

Joint Committee on Infant Hearing (JCIH; 2007). Year 2007 position statement: Principles and guidelines for early hearing detection and intervention programs. *Pediatrics, 120*, 898–921.

Karevold, G., Kvestad, E., Nafstad, P., & Kvaerner, K. J. (2006). Respiratory infections in schoolchildren: Co-morbidity and risk factors. *Archives of Diseases in Childhood, 91*, 391–395.

Kei, J., Allison-Levick, J., Dockray, J., Harrys, R., Kirkegard, C., Wong, J., . . . Tudehope, D. (2003). High-frequency (1000-Hz) tympanometry in normal neonates. *Journal of the American Academy of Audiology, 14*, 20–28.

Kvestad, E., Kvaerner, K. J., Roysamb, E., Tambs, K., Harris, J. R., & Magnus, P. (2004). Otitis media: Genetic factors and sex differences. *Twin Research, 7*, 239–244.

Lambert, P. R. (1998). Congenital aural atresia: Stability of surgical results. *Laryngoscope, 108*(12), 1801–1805.

Lambert, P. R. (2001). Congenital aural atresia. In B. J. Bailey, (Ed.), *Head and neck surgery: Otolaryngology* (pp. 1745–1757). Philadelphia, PA: Lippincott Williams and Wilkins.

Lasisi, A. O., Olaniyan, F. A., Muibi, S. A., Azeez, I. A., Abulwasiu, K. G., Lasisi, T. J., . . . Olayemi, O. (2007a). Clinical and demographic risk factors associated with chronic suppurative otitis media. *International Journal of Pediatric Otorhinolaryngology, 71*, 1549–1554.

Lasisi, A. O., Sulaiman, O. A., & Afolabi, O. A. (2007b). Socioeconomic status and hearing loss in chronic suppurative otitis media in Nigeria. *Annals of Tropical Paediatrics, 27*, 21–26.

Lehmann, D., Weeks, S., Jacoby, P., Elsbury, D., Finucane, J., Stokes, A., . . . Kalgoorlie Otitis Media Research Project Team. (2008). Absent otoacoustic emissions predict otitis media in young Aboriginal children: A birth cohort study in Aboriginal and non-Aboriginal children in an arid zone of Western Australia. *BMC Pediatrics, 8*, 32.

Lous, J., Burton, M. J., Felding, J. U., Ovesen, T., Rovers, M. M., & Williamson, I. (2005). Grommets (ventilation tubes) for hearing loss associated with otitis media with effusion in children. *Cochrane Database of Systematic Reviews*, Issue 1, Art. No. CD001801.

Mandel, E. M., Doyle, W. J., Winther, B., & Alper, C. (2008). The incidence, prevalence and burden of OM in unselected children aged 1–8 year followed by weekly otoscopy through the "common cold" season. *International Journal of Pediatric Otorhinolaryngology, 72*, 491–499.

Margolis, R. H., Bass-Ringdahl, S., Hanks, W. D., Holte, L., & Zapala, D. A. (2003). Tympanometry in newborn infants—1 kHz norms. *Journal of the American Academy of Audiology, 14*, 383–392.

Margolis, R. H., Hunter, L. L., Rykken, J. R., & Giebink, G. S. (1993). Effects of otitis media on extended high frequency hearing in children. *Annals of Otology, Rhinology, Laryngology, 102*, 1–5.

Marx, H. (1926). Die missbildungen des ohres. In F. Henke, & O. Lubarsh (Eds.), *Handbuch der spez path anatomie histology* (pp. 620–625). Berlin, Germany: Springer.

McKenzie, J., & Craig, J. (1955). Mandibulo-facial dysotosis (Treacher-Collins syndrome). *Archives of Diseases in Childhood, 30*, 391.

Morris, P. S., Leach, A. J., Silberberg, P., Mellon, G., Wilson, C., Hamilton, E., & Beissbarth, J. (2005). Otitis media in young Aboriginal children from remote communities in Northern and Central Australia: A cross-sectional survey. *BMC Pediatrics, 5*, 27.

NICHD and Early Child Care Network. (2003). Child care and communicable illness in children aged 37 to 54 months. *Archives of Pediatrics and Adolescent Medicine, 157*, 196–200.

Paradise, J. L., & Bluestone, C. D. (1974). Early treatment of the universal otitis media of infants with cleft palate. *Pediatrics, 53*, 48–54.

Paradise, J. L., Smith, C. G., & Bluestone, C. D. (1976). Tympanometric detection of middle ear effusion in infants and young children. *Pediatrics, 58*, 198–210.

Park, A. H., Wilson, M. A., Stevens, P. T., Harward, R., & Hohler, N. (2012). Identification of hearing loss in pediatric patients with Down syndrome. *Otolaryngology-Head and Neck Surgery, 146*, 135–140.

Parker, S. E., Mai, C. T., Canfield, M. A., Rickard, R., Wang, Y., Meyer, R. E., & Coreea, A. (2010). Updated national birth prevalence estimates for selected birth defects in the United States 2004–2006. *Birth Defects Research. Part A: Clinical and Molecular Teratology, 88*, 1008–1016.

Patel, N., & Shelton, C. (2007). The surgical learning curve in aural atresia surgery. *Laryngoscope, 117*(1), 67–73.

Paterson, J. E., Carter, S., Wallace, J., Ahmad, Z., Garett, N., & Silva, P. A. (2006). Pacific Island family study: The prevalence of chronic middle ear disease in 2-year-old Pacific Island children living in New Zealand. *International Journal of Pediatric Otorhinolaryngology, 70*, 1771–1778.

Paterson, J. E., Carter, S., Wallace, J., Ahmad, Z., Garett, N., & Silva, P. A. (2007). Pacific Island Families Study: Risk factors associated with otitis media with effusions among Pacific 2-year-old children. *International Journal of Pediatric Otorhinolaryngology, 71*, 1047–1054.

Paulson, L. M., Weaver, T. S., & Macarthur, C. J. (2014). Outcomes of tympanostomy tube placement in children with Down syndrome—A retrospective review. *International Journal of Pediatric Otorhinolaryngology, 78*, 223–226.

Plasschaert, A. I., Rovers, M. M., Schilder, A. G., Verheij, T. J., & Hak, E. (2006). Trends in doctor consultations, antibiotic prescription, and specialist referrals for otitis media in children: 1995–2003. *Pediatrics, 17,* 1879–1886.

Poswillo, D. E. (1973). The pathogenesis of first and second branchial arch syndrome. *Oral Surgery, 35,* 302.

Praveen, C. V., & Terry, R. M. (2005). Does passive smoking affect the outcome of grommet insertion in children? *Journal of Laryngology and Otology, 119,* 448–454.

Pron, G., Galloway, C., Armstrong, D., & Posnick, J. (1993). Ear malformation and hearing loss in patients with Treacher Collins syndrome. *Cleft Palate Craniofacial Journal, 30,* 97–103.

Raut, P., Sriram, B., Yeoh, A., Hee, K. Y., Lim, S. B., & Daniel, M. L. (2011). High prevalence of hearing loss in Down syndrome at first year of life. *Annals of the Academy of Medicine Singapore, 40,* 493–498.

Riemer, G., Castiglione, M., Ferrall-Pack, A., Staudigel, H., Summers, L., & Choo, D. (2008). *Best evidence statement on aural atresia.* Cincinnati Children's Hospital Medical Center unpublished evidence statement.

Rosenfeld, R. M., Shin, J. J, Schwartz, S. R., Coggins, R., Gagnon, L., Hackell, J. M., . . . Corrigan, M. D. (in preparation). *Clinical practice guideline: Otitis media with effusion (Update). Otolaryngology-Head and Neck Surgery.*

Rovers, M. M., Numans, M. E., Langenback, E., Grobee, D. E., Verheij, T. J., & Schilder, A. G. (2008). Is pacifier use a risk factor for acute otitis media? A dynamic cohort study. *Family Practice, 25,* 233–236.

Ruah, C. B., Schachern, P. A., Zelterman, D., Paparella, M. M., & Yoon, T. H. (1991). Age-related morphologic changes in the human tympanic membrane. A light and electron microscopic study. *Archives of Otolaryngology-Head and Neck Surgery, 117,* 627–634.

Rynnel-Dagöö, B. (2004): Acute otitis media and otitis media with effusion in the immunocompromised child. In C. Alper, C. Bluestone, M. Casselbrant, J. Dohar, & E. Mandel (Eds.), *Advanced therapy of otitis media* (pp. 462–464). Hamilton, Ontario, Canada: Decker.

Sabo, D. L., Paradise, J. L., Kurs-Lasky, M., & Smith, C. G. (2003). Hearing levels in infants and young children in relation to testing technique, age group, and the presence or absence of middle-ear effusion. *Ear and Hearing, 24,* 38–47.

Saunders, J. C., Kaltenback, J. A., & Relkin, E. M. (1983). The structural and functional development of the outer and middle ear. In R. Romand & M. R. Romand (Eds.), *Development of auditory and vestibular systems* (pp. 3–25). New York, NY: Academic Press.

Schönweiler, R., Lisson, J. A., Schönweiler, B., Eckardt, A., Ptok, M., Tränkmann, J., & Hausamen, J. E. (1999). A retrospective study of hearing, speech and language function in children with clefts following palatoplasty and veloplasty procedures at 18–24 months of age. *International Journal of Pediatrics in Otorhinolaryngology, 50,* 205–217.

Schuknecht, H. F. (1989). Congenital aural atresia. *Laryngoscope, 99,* 908–917.

Shah, U. K. (2004). Otitis media with effusion in craniofacial syndromes. In C. M. Alper, C. D. Bluestone, M. L. Casselbrant, J. E. Dohar, & E. M. Mandel, (Eds.), *Advanced therapy of otitis media* (pp. 468–473). Hamilton, Ontario, Canada: Decker.

Sheahan, P., Miller, I., Sheahan, J. N., Earley, M. J., & Blayney, A. W. (2003). Incidence and outcome of middle ear disease in cleft lip and palate. *International Journal of Pediatric Otorhinolaryngology, 67,* 785–793.

Shott, S. R., Joseph, A., & Heithaus, D. (2001). Hearing loss in children with Down syndrome. *International Journal of Pediatric Otorhinolaryngology, 61,* 199–205.

Siegert, R., Mattheis, S., & Kasic, J. (2007). Fully implantable hearing aids in patients with congenital auricular atresia. *Laryngoscope, 117,* 336–340.

Sprague, B. H., Wiley, T. L., & Goldstein, R. (1985). Tympanometric and acoustic-reflex studies in neonates. *Journal of Speech Hearing Research, 28,* 265–272.

Stuart, A., Yang, E. Y., & Green, W. B. (1994). Neonatal auditory brain-stem response thresholds to air and bone-conducted clicks. *Journal of the American Academy of Audiology, 5,* 163–172.

Swartz, J. D., & Faerber, E. N. (1985). Congenital malformations of the external and middle ear: High-resolution CT findings of surgical import. *American Journal of Roentgenology, 144,* 501–506.

Takahashi, H., & Maeda, K. (1982). Survey of familial occurrence in 171 microtia cases. *Japanese Journal Plastic Surgery, 15,* 310.

Tanzer, R. (1971). Total reconstruction of the auricle. The evolution of a plan of treatment. *Plastic and Reconstructive Surgery, 47,* 523.

Tekes, A., Ishman, S. L., Baugher, K. M., Brown, D. J., Lin, S. Y., Tunkel, D. E., . . . Huisman, T. A. (2013). Does microtia predict severity of temporal bone CT abnormalities in children with persistent conductive hearing loss? *Journal of Neuroradiology, 40,* 192–197.

Thorne, J. A. (2003). Middle ear problems in Aboriginal school children cause developmental and educational concerns. *Contemporary Nurse, 16,* 145–150.

Todberg, T., Koch, A., Andersson, M., Olsen, S. F., Lous, J., & Homøe, P. (2014). Incidence of otitis media in a contemporary Danish National Birth Cohort. *PLoS One, 29,* 9.

Ubell, M. L., Kerschner, J. E., Wackym, P. A., & Burrows, A. (2008). MUC2 expression in human middle ear epithelium of patients with otitis media. *Archives of Otolaryngology-Head and Neck Surgery, 134,* 39–41.

U.S. Department of Health and Human Services (DHHS; 2008). Vision and hearing. In *Healthy people 2010 midcourse review* (pp. 28–25). Washington, DC: U.S. Government Printing Office, December 2006.

Van Deursen, A. M., Verheij, T. J., Rovers, M. M., Veenhoven, R. H., Groenwold, R. H., Bonten, M. J., & Sanders, E. A. (2012). Trends in primary-care consultations, comorbidities, and antibiotic prescriptions for respiratory infections in The Netherlands before implementation of pneumococcal vaccines for infants. *Epidemiology and Infection, 140,* 823–834.

Verhagen, C. V., Hol, M. K., Coppens-Schellekens, W., Snik, A. F., & Cremers, C. W. (2008). The BAHA softband. A new treatment for young children with bilateral congenital aural atresia. *International Journal of Pediatric Otorhinolaryngology, 72*, 1455–1459.

Wiertsema, S. P., Herpers, B. L., Veenhoven, R. H., Salimans, M. M., Ruven, H. J., & Sanders, E. A. (2006). Functional polymorphisms in the mannan-binding lectin 2 gene: Effect on MBL levels and otitis media. *Journal of Allergy and Clinical Immunology, 117*, 1344–1350.

Williamson, I., Benge, S., Mullee, M., & Little, P. (2006). Consultations for middle ear disease, antibiotic prescribing and risk factors for reattendance: A case-linked cohort study. *British Journal of Genetic Practice, 56*, 170–175.

Xenellis, J., Paschalidis, J., Georgalas, C., Davilis, D., Tzagaroulakis, A., & Ferekidis, E. (2005). Factors influencing the presence of otitis media with effusion 16 months after initial diagnosis in a cohort of school-age children in rural Greece: A prospective study. *International Journal of Pediatric Otorhinolaryngology, 69*, 1641–1647.

Yellon, R. F. (2007). Bone anchored hearing aid in children —Prevention of complications. *Pediatric Otorhinolaryngology, 71*, 823–826.

Zhou, F., Shefer, A., Kong, Y., & Nuorti, J. P. (2008). Trends in acute otitis media-related health care utilization by privately insured young children in the US, 1997–2004. *Pediatrics, 121*, 253–260.

Auditory Neuropathy Spectrum Disorder

Gary Rance and Arnold Starr

Introduction

The recent development of objective measures of function of cochlear receptor elements (inner and outer hair cells), auditory nerve, and auditory brainstem pathways now allow the opportunity to define the site(s) of disorder at the levels responsible for "sensorineural" hearing loss. Disordered auditory nerve function affects the processing of auditory temporal cues and interferes with language comprehension, localization of sound sources, and binaural perceptions (Rance et al., 2012a; Zeng, Kong, Michaelewski, & Starr, 2005). Attention to clinical features such as age of onset, associated medical findings, imaging results, and family history are essential for defining the likely sites of the disorder as being "pre-neural" (affecting receptor elements and the formation or release of neural transmitters) and "neural" (affecting the function of auditory nerve and its brainstem connections). The nosology of the disorder includes "auditory neuropathy" (Starr, Picton, Sininger, Hood, & Berlin, 1996), "auditory neuropathy/dys-synchrony" (Berlin, Hood, & Rose, 2001), "auditory synaptopathy" (Moser et al., 2006), and "presynaptic and postsynaptic nerve disorder" (Starr, Sininger, & Pratt, 2000). The development of these descriptors reflects the fact that multiple pathological mechanisms may produce a common pattern of physiologic results. For example, the phenotype may result from specific loss of cochlear inner hair cells (Amatuzzi, Liberman, & Northrop, 2001), disordered release of neurotransmitter by inner hair cell ribbon synapses (Wynne et al., 2013), deafferentation accompanying loss of auditory nerve fibres (Starr et al., 2003), neural dys-synchrony or conduction block as a result of demyelination of nerve fibres (Rance et al., 2012a), and auditory nerve hypoplasia (Buchman et al., 2006). As a result, the term *auditory neuropathy spectrum disorder (ANSD)* has been developed to acknowledge this heterogeneity (Guidelines Development Conference, 2008). Differentiating the site(s) affected in an individual is an area of considerable research interest and remains a clinical challenge. What is clear is that the perceptual effects of this form of auditory disorder in both children and adults are quite different from those typically seen with sensory (cochlear) hearing loss. As up to 10% of children with permanent hearing deficit show evidence of ANSD, every pediatric audiologist must be able to identify the typical result pattern and have some insight into the disorder's particular management challenges. This chapter will address each of these issues as well as providing a neurological overview of auditory inner hair cell, auditory nerve, and auditory central pathway disorders.

Identification of ANSD

The clinical findings that suggest the presence of disrupted auditory nerve activity are the demonstration of cochlear (outer hair cell) integrity by cochlear microphonic or otoacoustic emission recordings, in conjunction with absence or marked abnormally of the auditory brainstem response (ABR). The demonstration of impaired auditory temporal perceptions independent of audibility changes is also a cardinal feature of the disorder but is not possible to demonstrate in newborns or infants using standard clinical techniques.

Auditory Brainstem Response

The ABR arises from neural activity occurring in the 10 to 15 ms immediately following an abrupt auditory stimulus (see Chapter 21 of this volume by Small and Stapells for details). In ears with significant peripheral (middle ear or cochlear) hearing loss, the threshold for ABR detection can be elevated or the response absent because the stimuli cannot be provided at a level sufficient to elicit recordable potentials in the auditory brainstem. In contrast, subjects with ANSD show absent or severely distorted ABRs at maximum presentation levels, not because the stimuli are insufficient to generate a response, but because the neural activities of auditory nerve and brainstem pathways are disrupted. Establishing ABR abnormality in such cases is relatively straightforward when the brainstem potentials are "absent" (or at least unrecordable). A present but "severely disrupted" response is more problematic, particularly when assessing premature infants who commonly display abnormal ABRs (with prolonged latency, reduced amplitude, etc.) as a result of incomplete myelination of auditory nerve and brainstem structures (Starr, Amlie, Martin, & Sanders, 1977). A commonly used definition (Sininger & Oba, 2001) for ABR abnormality consistent with ANSD is that the ABR be of low amplitude, prolonged latency, and only discernable to high-level stimuli (≥70 dB nHL). Some of the mechanisms by which the ABR can be disrupted in ANSD are described in the following sections.

Tests of Cochlear (Outer Hair Cell) Function

Evoked Otoacoustic Emissions (EOAE)

An otoacoustic emission is a release of sound energy produced within the cochlea that can be recorded in the ear canal (Kemp, 1978). This signal is thought to be the by-product of the mechanical activity of the outer hair cells (see Chapter 20 by Abdala, Winter, and Shera for details). EOAEs, in providing an indirect measure of this process, offer a means of distinguishing between sensory cell loss and ANSD. Ears with absent or significantly elevated ABRs due to sensory hearing loss typically show audiometric thresholds in the severe-to-profound range. Cochlear insult sufficient to produce a hearing loss of this degree typically disrupts the active mechanisms that produce the OAE resulting in nonresponse (Collet, Levy, & Veuillet, 1993; Lonsbury-Martin, Harris, Stagner, & Hawkins, 1990). EOAE presence in conjunction with significant ABR disruption therefore suggests ANSD rather than sensory-type hearing loss.

Cochlear Microphonic (CM)

The cochlear microphonic is a receptor potential produced by the polarization and depolarization of cochlear hair cells. The response is pre-neural and appears as an alternating current (AC) potential that provides a bioelectric analogue of the stimulus (Dallos & Cheatham, 1976). The potential is therefore unlike those produced by neural activity (such as the ABR), showing a direct phase relationship to the acoustic wave form. This relationship can be seen in Figure 11–5 where the CM reverses polarity as the stimuli are changed from rarefaction to compression clicks.

When recorded from extra-tympanic sites (such as the scalp), the CM is dominated by the activity of the outer hair cells because their numbers are thrice that of inner hair cells (Dallos, 1973; Norton, Ferguson, & Mascher, 1989). As such, this potential can be used in conjunction with the ABR to identify ANSD. As discussed previously, sensory hearing loss severe enough to prevent an ABR would be expected to affect cochlear OHC function. Hence, ANSD is indicated when the CM is present but the ABR disrupted. The reader is referred to Berlin et al. (1998), Rance et al. (1999), and Starr et al. (1991) for description of clinical CM recording procedures.

Possible Mechanisms Producing the ANSD Result Pattern

The absence of ABRs in subjects who can clearly "hear" the stimuli was disturbing when the phenomenon was first noticed in the 1970s and 1980s. A number of investigators described the paradox (Davis & Hirsh, 1979; Hildesheimer, Muchnik, & Rubinstein, 1985; Kraus, Ozdamar, Stein, & Reed, 1984) but could not realize the mechanisms. One of the authors (AS) saw such a child in 1989 and defined that in spite of the absence of ABRs, the cochlear microphonic receptor potentials were present. Just before publication (Starr et al., 1991), OAEs were demonstrated to be present.

A physiological model for this phenomenon is that auditory nerve input is not temporally precise to the repeated stimuli causing the averaged ABR to be absent or severely distorted, even though "hearing" the signals might not be affected. The distortion of the temporal processes is reflected in the inability to use temporal cues normally for life's daily perceptions.

The peripheral auditory system encodes temporal cues both at onset and during the stimulus, the latter particularly for low frequencies. The nerve and brainstem tracts discharge at a preferential phase of the low-frequency tones and produce a potential at the frequency of the tone recordable by scalp electrodes. These potentials are known as frequency following responses (FFRs) and are absent in ANSD. A second mechanism that would disrupt ABRs and auditory temporal perceptions would be a loss of the magnitude of the afferent input. This might result in cases with significantly reduced cochlear inner hair cell population, abnormal neurotransmitter release, abnormal synaptic function, or abnormal nerve fibers. Deafferentation can be actual loss of fibers or functional loss due to failure to activate the fibers.

Temporal bone analyses in patients with different etiologies of ANSD have been published. They have all shown loss of nerve fibers, abnormal myelin formation in some of the remaining nerve fibers, and preserved inner and outer hair cells. There is need for defining temporal bone studies in patients or animal models of inner hair cell disorders accompanying, for example, otoferlin gene mutations that affect neurotransmitter release by inner hair cells. We do not expect that the inner hair cells are lost or have abnormal potentials in this condition. Rather, the defect in neurotransmitter release will likely lead to atrophy and morphological changes of the nerve terminals (i.e., a trans-synaptic degeneration).

The definition of physiological processes responsible for the clinical picture of ANSD are difficult to address using auditory brainstem potential measures as these responses are typically absent and when present consist of a wave V generated by brainstem auditory structures. The registration of cochlear potentials from an electrode passed through the tympanic membrane and placed directly on the bony promontory or round window of the cochlea can reveal neural and cochlear receptor potentials not apparent in the ABR. Both children (McMahon, Patuzzi, Gibson, & Sanli, 2008) and adults (Santarelli, Starr, Michalewski, & Arslan, 2008; Santarelli et al., 2011, 2015) have been studied using these electrocochleographic methods (ECochG). Receptor summating potentials generated primarily by inner hair cells and cochlear microphonics generated primarily by outer hair cells appear normal. In contrast, auditory nerve compound action potentials (CAPs) are absent or present with low amplitudes consistent with disordered function of auditory nerve. Abnormally prolonged neural negative potentials are also evident in many patients with ANSD. This negative potential has been suggested to reflect activity of auditory nerve terminal dendrites accompanying abnormal generation of CAPs and abnormal synaptic function (transmitter release, transmitter binding) between inner hair cells and auditory nerve.

Medical Aspects of ANSD

ANSD is most common in the newborn population, particularly in premature babies and those who have medical illness. The major risk factors for ANSD include hyperbilirubinemia, hypoxia and accompanying metabolic acidosis, and exposure to antibiotics that are toxic to hair cells. For a review see Starr and Rance (2015).

Genetic causes of ANSD acting at the inner hair cells and their synapses with the auditory nerve include mutations of connexin 26 and of otoferlin and are expressed early in infancy (Santarelli, 2010). A variant of otoferlin mutation can be accompanied by a temperature-sensitive deafness (Starr et al., 1998) that is readily treated with acetaminophen that reduces body temperature.

Congenital disorders such as atresia of the auditory nerve can produce the picture of ANSD, and the diagnosis will be established with high-definition magnetic resonance imaging (MRI; Buchman et al., 2006). When should an MRI be done? We suggest that for all infants, correct diagnosis is important for parents and should be separated from therapeutic considerations such as decisions on cochlear implantation.

The etiologies described below occur as part of a general medical disorder, and these patients need to be evaluated by appropriate specialists such as neurologists, paediatricians, radiologists, and otologists. Infectious diseases due to bacterial involvement most commonly affect cochlear functions by involvement of both the auditory nerve and the arterial blood vessels supplying the cochlea. When the nerve is primarily affected, the clinical picture is of ANSD. If the arterial supply is not affected, ABR Wave I and CM and OAEs can be defined. When the arterial supply is compromised, both neural and cochlear receptor elements will be disrupted.

Infectious disorders due to viral involvement can have sequelae of hearing impairment due to auditory nerve involvement. Mumps and measles appear to have this association. The auditory nerve involvement in such cases can be unilateral.

Tumors of the brainstem and auditory vestibular nerve schwannomas can affect auditory nerve function by compression and, if the blood supply is not compromised, the ABR will be abnormal (absent or delayed components after a normal Wave I with preserved CMs and OAEs). Brain imaging and clinical examination will reveal such tumors, and clinical neurological examination will define disorders of cranial nerves such as III, IV, and VI controlling eye movements, VII controlling facial movements, and V controlling facial sensations. Neoplasms such as brainstem schwannomas are relatively slow growing and most common in middle-aged or elderly adult patients. However, recent work has shown that tumors (producing the ANSD result pattern) can present in newborns (Laury, Casey, McKay, & Germiller, 2009).

Genetic disorders affecting the auditory nerve as part of more general peripheral and cranial nerve involvement are common. The age of onset is typically after 8 years and can include mitochondrial disorders due to both the nuclear genes such as Friedreich ataxia (Cacace & Pinheiro, 2011; Rance et al., 2008), and dominant optic atrophy (OPA1 gene mutation; Santarelli et al., 2015), and other multisensory genetic disorders such as Leber's hereditary optic neuropathy (Rance et al., 2012c). In many of these generalized neuropathic conditions, deficits in auditory function present before symptoms in other sensory or motor systems (Starr et al., 1996).

Immune disorders can be accompanied by deafness typical of ANSD. For instance, deafness is reported in Guillain-Barré syndrome, an immune disorder affecting the proximal nerve roots and the proximal portions of the auditory nerve. Patients might be deaf and paralyzed and yet the prognosis for recovery is typically excellent though lengthy in time.

In summary, ANSD is a medical disorder affecting the output of the cochleae and their connections in the brainstem. Patients must be evaluated by a clinician skilled in neurology to define the site of affection. The audiologist can be suspicious of central auditory nerve problems when they detect either an absent or severely distorted ABR or a waveform complex associated with normal latency Wave I. Wave I is generated by the auditory nerve close to the cochlea and Wave II by the auditory nerve close to the brainstem. Waves III, IV, and V are generated by central auditory brainstem structures in the regions of cochlear nucleus (Wave III) and superior olive and lateral lemniscus (Waves IV and V).

Screening for ANSD

As discussed in the previous section, adult- and early childhood–onset forms of ANSD can be associated with progressive sensory motor neuropathies. However, the majority of pediatric ANSD cases do involve congenital or perinatal presentation (Sininger & Oba, 2001; Starr et al., 2000) and most diagnoses are made following infant hearing screening. This raises questions concerning the ways in which universal screening procedures should be configured to best capture affected babies. Clearly, programs employing only the OAE technique will miss a high proportion of ANSD cases as most affected infants show normal emissions.[1] For this reason, the Joint Committee on Infant Hearing (JCIH, 2007) has recommended that ABR be used as the screening measure, at least for babies housed in the neonatal intensive care unit (NICU), arguing that most affected children suffer a rocky neonatal course and hence are graduates of the special care nursery (Rance et al., 1999; Sininger & Oba, 2001).

OAE screening in the well-baby population might be less of an issue as the incidence of ANSD in this group is much lower. Furthermore, most babies who have a normal neonatal course and yet still suffer ANSD will have a genetic cause, so it should be possible to identify those in need of ABR screening on the basis of family history (hearing loss and sensory neuropathy). For screening programs employing OAE assessment, Berlin et al. (2005) have also suggested that middle ear muscle reflex (MEMR) testing can identify children in need of referral for ABR assessment (see later section in this chapter for details).

Prevalence

The prevalence of ANSD in adult and well-baby populations is yet to be determined. Data describing the proportion of affected children in high-risk populations are also sketchy, and estimates range from 0.23% to 9.63% (Table 11–1). The high variability reflects some methodological differences between studies and raises some important issues regarding the criteria for diagnosis of ANSD in early infancy. In particular, the age at which evoked potential assessments are carried out

[1]A number of studies have in fact indicated that in a high proportion (30%–50%) of ANSD cases, the OAE can disappear over time (Rance et al., 1999; Starr et al., 2000). Most reports of OAE deterioration have, however, occurred in the postneonatal period.

Table 11–1. Prevalence of Auditory Neuropathy Spectrum Disorder in "At-Risk" Infant Populations

Study	*Population*	*Number of Subjects*	*Number of ANSD Subjects*	*Percentage of Total (%)*
Stein et al. (1996)	Special care nursery	100	4	4.00
Psarommatis et al. (1997)	Intensive care unit	102	2	1.96
Rance et al. (1999)	"At-risk" infants	5,199	12	0.23
Berg et al. (2005)	Intensive care unit	1,194	115	9.63
Psarommatis et al. (2006)	Intensive care unit	1,150	25	2.17

also will affect the ANSD diagnosis rate in high-risk babies. Rance et al. (1999), for example, only included children who showed no ABR on repeated measures through the first year of life. Psarommatis et al. (2006) in contrast, considered that ≈1/50 of their ICU babies fit the ANSD pattern when assessed in the neonatal period, but subsequently found that in more than half of their ANSD cohort (12/20 cases), the ABR abnormalities had "resolved" when testing was repeated at 4 to 6 months of age.[2]

The proportion of children with permanent hearing disability showing the ANSD result pattern has been considered in a number of studies. Estimates vary (again probably reflecting methodological differences), but it appears that one in every 10 to 20 children with educationally significant hearing impairment will show evidence of normal cochlear (OHC) function and auditory pathway disorder (see Table 11–2 for details). It is likely that undiagnosed ANSD has always accounted for a proportion of permanent hearing loss. The high prevalence rates in recent studies (and anecdotal reports from neonatal screening programs) might, however, reflect an increase in the condition due to decreased mortality rates in very premature/low birth weight babies and the relatively high incidence of neurological consequences in those who survive (Rance et al., 1999).

Management (at Diagnosis)

Medical/Developmental Workup

All of the recommendations for initial management of children with sensorineural-type hearing loss by the Joint Committee on Infant Hearing (2007) are appropriate for babies with ANSD. These assessments include

1. pediatric and developmental evaluation and history,
2. otologic evaluation with imaging of the cochlear and auditory nerves (CT/MRI) and vestibular assessment,
3. medical genetics evaluation,
4. ophthalmologic assessment, and
5. communication development assessment and ongoing monitoring.

In addition, referral for neurological evaluation to assess peripheral and cranial nerve function is warranted in children with the ANSD result pattern.

Audiologic Follow-Up

As described in a previous section, diagnosing a baby with ANSD is relatively straightforward. Determining the child's auditory capacity in the infant period is rather more of a challenge.

One of the particular difficulties associated with early management of ANSD children relates to the inability of brainstem-evoked potential measures to predict the behavioral audiogram. Recent work (He, Teagle, Roush, Grose, & Buchman, 2013) has suggested that cortical auditory-evoked potential (CAEP) thresholds might predict hearing levels, but further investigation is required to confirm the efficacy of this technique.

Although sound audibility in children with ANSD does not predict the degree of functional disability (to the extent that peripheral hearing loss does), access to sound, in particular speech at conversational levels, still forms the basis of early intervention strategies (such as

[2]These authors recommend that diagnosis of ANSD be delayed in NICU graduates until 3 to 6 months corrected age.

Table 11–2. Prevalence of ANSD in Children With Permanent Hearing Loss

Study	*Population*	*Number of Cases Permanent Hearing Loss*	*Number of ANSD Cases*	*Percentage of Total (%)*
Kraus et al. (1984)	HI children	48	7	14.58
Park & Lee (1998)	HI children	139	7	5.04
Vohr, Carty, Moore, & Letourneau (1998)	Universal Screening	111	2	1.80
Rance et al. (1999)	"at-risk" infants	109	12	11.01
Berlin, Hood, & Morlet (2000)	HI children	1000	87	8.70
Cone-Wesson et al. (2000)	Universal Screening	56	3	5.36
Lee, McPherson, Yuen, & Wong (2001)	HI children	67	2	2.98
Madden, Rutter, Hilbert, Greinwald, & Choo (2002)	HI children	428	22	5.14
Tang et al. (2004)	HI children	56	1	1.78
Rance et al. (2005)	"at-risk" infants	290	19	6.55

Note. HI = hearing impaired.

hearing aid fitting). In listeners with ANSD who have complete ABR absence, behavioral hearing thresholds can vary from normal to profound levels (Rance et al., 1999). Children with present but abnormal ABR, tend to present with lesser degrees of loss, but in this group, ABR thresholds still show no relation to hearing level.

Auditory steady-state response (ASSR) thresholds also show no correlation with sound detection in listeners with ANSD. When stimuli modulated at high rates (70–100 Hz) are employed, responses can be obtained, suggesting that the ASSR requires a low degree of neural synchrony in the auditory brainstem (Rance et al., 1999). However, high-level signals (≥80 dB HL) are typically required to elicit the potential even in children who show subsequently normal behavioral audiograms (Attias, Buller, Rubel, & Raveh, 2006; Rance & Briggs, 2002; Rance, Dowell, Rickards, Beer, & Clark, 1998). The possibility of using lower modulation rates (e.g., 40 Hz) to elicit ASSRs from the auditory cortex in children with ANSD is yet to be fully explored.

Establishing sound detection levels in infants with ANSD requires careful evaluation of auditory behavior. Conditioned audiometric techniques (visual reinforcement audiometry or conditioned orientation audiometry) can be used in developmentally normal children from 6 months of age onward. In younger or delayed children, some information can be obtained using behavioral observation audiometry (BOA) techniques. To date, there have been few published findings describing BOA results in ANSD populations, but data from our laboratory suggest that minimum response levels obtained at younger than 6 months of age to speech and noisemaker stimuli can at least differentiate between those cases with normal, and those with elevated sound detection levels. Parental observation beyond the clinic including formal assessment tools (questionnaires) can also inform this process.

A number of recent reports have demonstrated that some children presenting with the ANSD result pattern in infancy can show "recovery" of the ABR and improvement in hearing thresholds (Attias & Raveh, 2007; Madden et al., 2002; Psarommatis et al., 2006; Stein et al., 1996). In most cases, this improvement has involved children with either hyperbilirubinemia or very low birth weight, and has occurred in the first year of life. These findings highlight a need for repeat ABR assessment and careful audiometric monitoring of infants with ANSD, particularly those who are NICU graduates. Long-term monitoring of children who have shown recovery is also warranted as it is not yet certain that restored neural synchrony in the auditory brainstem guarantees normal auditory perception in these cases.

The proportion of ANSD youngsters demonstrating ABR recovery is yet to be determined. In our laboratory, and the Australia-wide population, the proportion of babies showing improvement is relatively small. In fact, less than 5% of cases with the ANSD pattern in the neonatal period have shown ABR improvement on repeat assessment over the first 2 years of life. Establishing the likelihood of ABR development and its time course are clearly important clinical questions, potentially impacting upon infant assessment protocols (e.g., at what age should screening occur for high-risk populations? for how long should ABR status be monitored?), and both short- and long-term management decisions (e.g., when should amplification be provided or cochlear implantation considered?).

Audiologic Clinical Profile

Sound Detection Thresholds

Although some children show audiograms within the normal audiometric range (Berlin, Morlet, & Hood, 2003; Rance et al., 1999), most (>90%) present with impaired sound detection. Behavioral hearing thresholds range from normal to profound levels and are typically the same in both ears. Unilateral ANSD is most commonly associated with auditory nerve hypoplasia (cochlear nerve deficiency [CND]; Buchman et al., 2006). Average hearing levels in ears with CND are usually in the profound to total loss range. In radiologically normal children, they are evenly distributed across the audiometric spectrum (Madden et al., 2002; Rance et al., 1999; Sininger & Oba, 2001; Starr et al., 2000).

Audiograms with a low-frequency (reverse slope) configuration are common. Approximately 30% to 40% of reported ANSD children have shown poorest detection for stimuli in the 250 Hz to 500 Hz range. In contrast, the high-frequency configuration typical of sensory hearing loss only occurs in ≈10% of cases (Madden et al., 2002; Rance et al., 1999; Sininger & Oba, 2001; Vinay & Moore, 2007). This might reflect that low frequencies are encoded by both a place and temporal code, whereas high frequencies are encoded only by cochlear place of activation.

Fluctuation in sound detection has been a consistently reported feature of ANSD. Day-to-day variations in audiometric threshold (without directional trend) of 20 dB or more have been reported in some cases (Rance et al., 1999; Sininger & Oba, 2001). Occasionally, these fluctuations can be related to clinical changes in the subjects. Gorga, Stelmachowicz, Barlow, and Brookhouser (1995) and Starr et al. (1998), for example, have described a temperature-sensitive form of neuropathy (due to mutation of the otoferlin gene) where core body temperature increases of as little as 1° can result in dramatic auditory-evoked potential changes and temporary drops in both sound detection and speech understanding. However, in most ANSD cases, the cause of hearing level fluctuation is unknown.

Middle Ear Muscle Reflex

The middle ear muscle reflex (MEMR) is one of the two efferent reflexes modulated by the inner hair cells, eighth nerve, and auditory brainstem pathways and is consistently abnormal in cases of ANSD regardless of the subject's behavioral hearing levels[3] (Berlin et al., 2005; Sininger & Oba, 2001; Starr et al., 1996). In the most comprehensive study of the MEMR in ANSD patients, Berlin et al. (2005) found that the reflex was absent at all test frequencies and in all test conditions (ipsilateral/contralateral) in 88.3% of cases and that none of the 128 subjects showed a normal response pattern. As such, these authors recommend that tympanometry and MEMR testing be used as a triage procedure for all audiology patients and that MEMR testing be carried out to identify ANSD infants in screening programs that use only OAEs.

Cortical Auditory-Evoked Potentials

Despite the absence or severe disruption of ABRs in ears with ANSD, potentials from the auditory cortex including the middle latency response (Kraus et al.,1984; Starr et al., 1996), the cortical auditory-evoked potentials (Kraus et al., 2000; Kumar & Vanaja, 2008; Michalewski, Starr, Nguyen, Kong, & Zeng, 2005; Rance, Cone-Wesson, Wunderlich, & Dowell, 2002; Starr et al., 1996), mismatch negativity (Cone-Wesson, Rance, & Wunderlich, 2003), and the P300 cognitive potential (Starr et al., 1996) are recordable in some affected adults and children. That these potentials can be observed on occasion might reflect the fact that they are less dependent on synchronous neural firing than the ABR (Rance et al., 2005) and as such, might offer a broad measure of the degree of neural disruption in the central auditory

[3]The other is the medial olivocochlear reflex, which is responsible for suppression of the OAE by ipsilateral or contralateral masking and which is also absent in ears with ANSD (Hood, Berlin, Bordelon, & Rose, 2003).

pathways. Rance et al. (2002), for example, recorded obligatory cortical potentials (P_1-N_1-P_2) in a group of school-aged children with ANSD and found a high correlation between auditory processing ability (open-set speech understanding) and the presence or absence of the response. Furthermore, an acoustic change complex can also be elicited by stimulus changes (such as temporal gaps, intensity changes, and frequency variation) in a prolonged sound and difference limen are broadly consistent with those obtained behaviorally (Dimitrijevic et al., 2011; Michalewski, Starr, Zeng, & Dimitrijevic, 2009). As such, they offer the possibility of objective evaluation of auditory capacity (and potential for acoustic amplification benefit) in patients too young or unable to provide volitional responses (He et al., 2015). Another recent approach has been to measure the degree of cortical-level dys-synchrony using "time-frequency analysis," which measures phase locking of cortical oscillations to auditory stimuli (Nash-Kille & Sharma, 2014). Preliminary results indicate that children with ANSD show less cortical synchrony than controls with normal hearing and sensory loss, and refinement of the technique might allow estimation of auditory capacity in affected individuals.

Basic Auditory Processing

Disruption of the neural representation of sound in listeners with ANSD can result in severe perceptual deficits. Psychophysical studies exploring the ways in which this disruption affects basic auditory processing have revealed that the disorder produces a pattern of effects consistent with the physiologic profile of disruption. For example, frequency resolution (the capacity to separate or "resolve" frequency components in a complex signal) and intensity discrimination (the ability to identify level differences) are largely dependent on cochlear-level processing and are usually unaffected (Kraus et al., 2000; Rance, McKay, & Grayden, 2004; Rance et al., 2010a, 2012a; Zeng et al., 2005). In contrast, distortion of neural firing patterns in ANSD results in impaired temporal resolution (the ability to perceive signal changes over time) and disruption of the timing-based aspects of frequency discrimination (Rance et al., 2004, 2010a, 2012a; Starr et al., 1991; Zeng et al., 2005). Temporal resolution deficits most obviously affect the ability to identify brief gaps in continuous stimuli and to track rapid signal envelope changes in a complex signal (Figure 11–1).

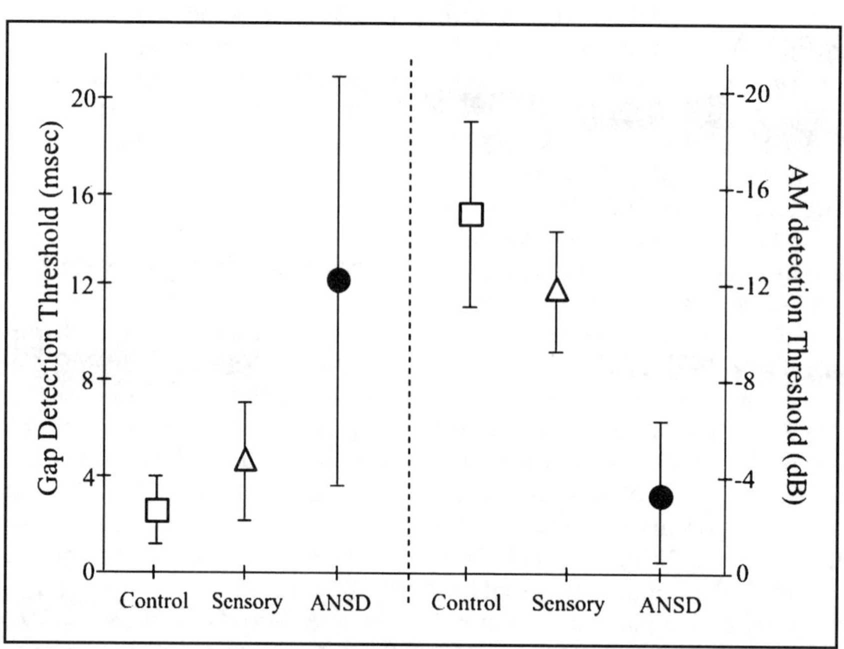

FIGURE 11–1. Auditory temporal processing in individuals with cochlear-sensory hearing loss and listeners with ANSD. Based on data presented in Starr et al. (1996, 2013); Zeng et al. (1999); Rance et al. (2004, 2010a, 2012a, 2012c); Dimitrijevic et al. (2011); and Wynne et al. (2013). Subjects with ANSD showed poorer gap detection ($P < .01$) and poorer AM detection (150 Hz) threshold than controls ($P < .001$). (ANSD, auditory neuropathy spectrum disorder; AM, amplitude modulation.)

Degree of temporal deficit varies across individuals, but processing deficits have been associated with each of the pathophysiologic mechanisms known to produce ANSD. For de-afferentiating disorders, thresholds of neuronal activation might be normal, but the nerve's capacity to convey timing cues in a complex signal might be limited, as the accurate representation of envelope patterns requires contributions from multiple neurons. Similarly, disorders affecting the synchrony of neural firing will affect the representation of timing information as temporal variations in the neural code distort the representation of signals carried by multiple neurons (Glowatzki, Grant, & Fuchs, 2008; Waxman, 1977).

In addition to suffering monaural temporal processing deficits, listeners with ANSD also show an impaired capacity to integrate binaural difference cues. The most obvious functional consequence of this deficit is a marked impairment in the ability to judge sound location. When sounds emanate from any direction other than directly in front of or behind the listener, the signal reaching each ear is subtly different. For example, an interaural level difference of up to 15 dB might be created by the head blocking the signal to the farther ear. In addition, interaural timing differences are produced by the unequal distance traveled to each ear. These difference cues, which may be as little at 50 μsec, are initially processed in the superior olivary complex of the brainstem where inputs from the left and right auditory nerves converge and are compared (Riedel & Kollmeier, 2002). In ANSD listeners, localization based on interaural level differences is typically unimpaired, but the temporally distorted inputs from the left and right auditory nerves cannot be effectively integrated. As a result, where normal listeners can identify sound direction changes of <3°, individuals with ANSD are typically unaware of direction changes up to 90° (Starr et al., 1991; Zeng et al., 2005).

Functional Hearing

Speech perception difficulty, and its consequent effects on communication, is an important clinical feature of ANSD. Figure 11–2 shows hearing quality-of-life questionnaire results for a group of school-aged children with normal sound detection and reveals considerably

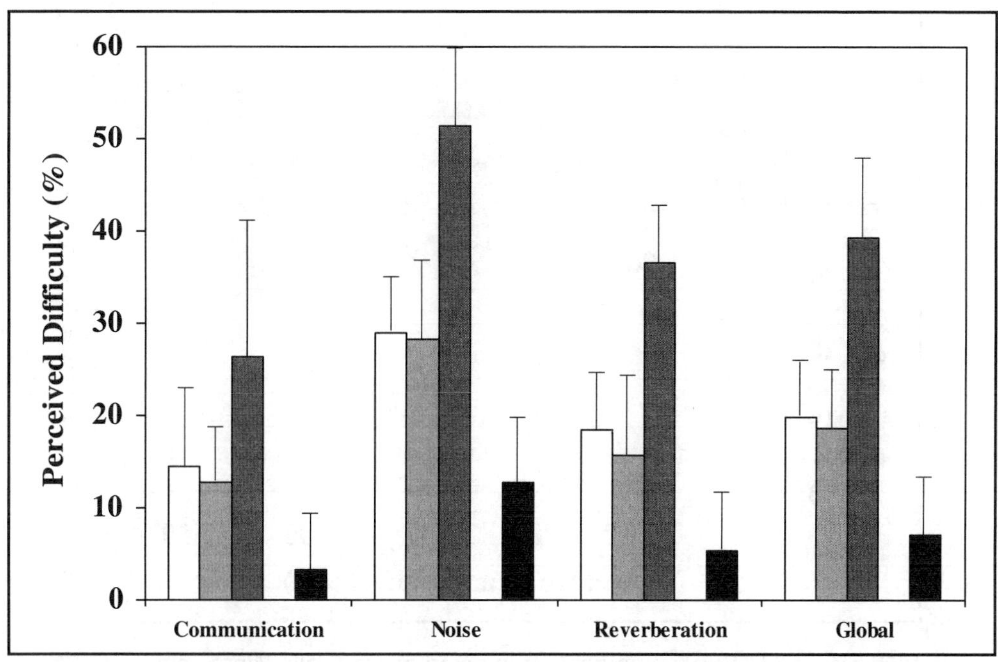

FIGURE 11–2. Hearing quality of life survey results (Abbreviated Profile of Hearing Aid Benefit [APHAB]) for school-aged children with perinatal ANSD (white bars; Rance et al., 2014), with Charcot-Marie-Tooth disease (type 1; light grey bars; Rance et al., 2012a) and with Friedreich ataxia (dark grey bars; Rance et al., 2010a). Each of these listeners with ANSD had normal or near–normal sound detection thresholds. The black bars show the findings for control subjects with normal sound detection. "Perceived Difficulty" is the proportion of everyday situations in which the participant suffers a significant listening/communication difficulty. (ANSD, auditory neuropathy spectrum disorder.)

higher degrees of everyday listening and communication difficulty than reported by matched controls.

Speech understanding difficulties are a consistently reported feature of ANSD. Almost all affected adults have shown perceptual deficits greater than predicted from their audiogram (Rance et al., 2008; Starr et al., 1996, 2000; Zeng, Oba, & Starr, 2001). Results in children have been more variable. At best, young ANSD listeners show speech perception test results comparable to their peers with sensory-type hearing loss. At worst, they show no functional hearing at all despite (in many cases) enjoying complete access to the normal speech spectrum. Figure 11–3 shows this broad spread of perceptual performance (for listening in quiet conditions) and reflects the lack of relationship between speech understanding and sound detection in children with ANSD. This mismatch between audibility and speech understanding suggests that distortion of supra-threshold cues is a major limiting factor in many cases. In fact, degree of temporal processing deficit is highly correlated with speech perception ability (Rance et al., 2004, 2010a, 2012a; Zeng et al., 2005). This relationship is reflected in Figure 11–3 where individuals with abnormal temporal processing typically show negligible (<25%), open-set speech perception, whereas those with normal temporal resolution demonstrate relatively normal speech scores.

The accurate resolution of timing cues is a prerequisite for speech perception. Discrimination of phonemes (individual speech sounds) in running speech, or even in single words requires that the listener not only identify the spectral shape of individual phonemes, but be able to continuously update this perception to track to flow of speech sounds. Brief temporal changes in the signal, such as silent period between a consonant burst and a following vowel (voice-onset-time) or the duration of a vowel, are often the only cues that differentiate speech sounds, and listeners with AN have particular difficulty identifying these acoustic markers (Rance et al., 2008, 2010a).

Speech Processing in Noise

Children with ANSD experience greater difficulties in background noise than individuals with normal audi-

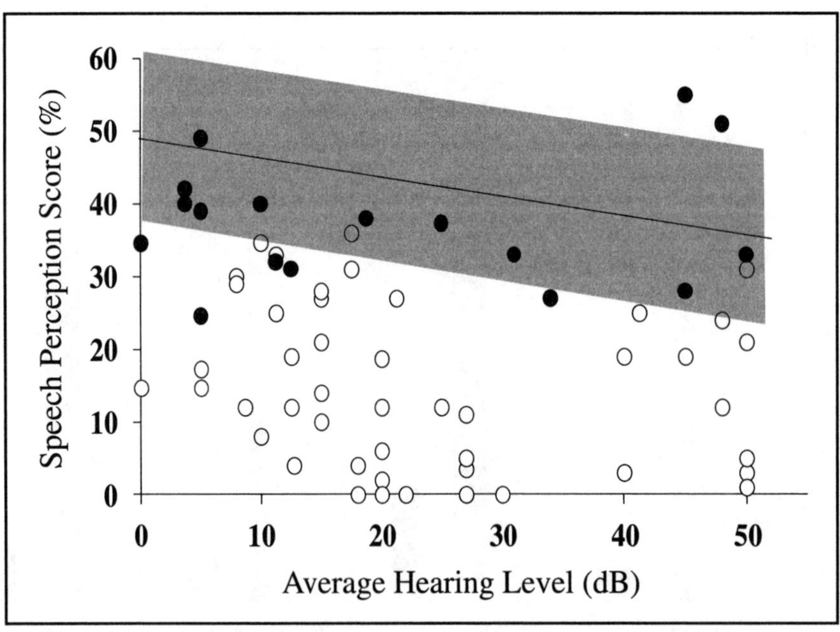

FIGURE 11–3. Speech perception in noise score (CNC-Word Test [0 dB SNR]) plotted as a function of hearing level for ANSD subjects presented in Rance et al. (2004, 2010a, 2012a, 2012b, 2012c, 2014). Filled circles represent individuals with normal auditory temporal resolution (amplitude modulation detection [150 Hz] task), and open circles represent participants with abnormal temporal resolution (>2 SD poorer than age-corrected norms). The shaded area shows the normal speech perception performance range for listeners with sensory hearing loss.

tory function and people with sensory hearing loss (Rance et al., 2007, 2008; Zeng et al., 2005; Figure 11–4).

Three possible explanations for this phenomenon are impaired gap listening, increased adaptation, and disrupted spatial listening.

Gap Listening

Psychophysical studies have shown exaggerated masking effects for tonal stimuli presented immediately before or immediately after a burst of noise (Zeng et al., 2005). As such, it appears that ANSD listeners are less able to separate sounds occurring successively. In everyday listening, where levels of background noise fluctuate, this temporal processing disorder may impair the listener's ability to use brief gaps in the noise to access the speech signal and optimize perception (Alcántara, Weisblatt, Moore, & Bolton, 2004).

Adaptation

Marked adaptation of signal loudness during constant stimulation has been reported for some forms of ANSD (Santarelli et al., 2008; Wynne et al., 2013). In affected listeners, the presence of continuous background noise could result in both an increase in activation threshold and an increase in the degree of neural dys-synchrony.

Spatial Listening

In everyday circumstances, auditory signals emanate from different directions, and sound localization cues can be used to separate a signal of interest from the background noise (Micheyl et al., 2007). ANSD disrupts the ability to focus on a particular signal based on its location, and consequently, an affected listener might require a relatively high signal-to-noise ratio (SNR) to understand speech in noise (Rance et al., 2012b). Spatial processing ability varies (in concert with temporal resolution), but overall, listeners with ANSD obtain approximately 5 dB less benefit from the separation of sound sources than controls. This degree of deficit is considerable, and for children with ANSD, developmentally significant. Signal-to-noise deficits of this order have been shown to reduce memory, motivation, and reading ability (Hetu, Truchon-Gagnon, & Bilodeau, 1990) and negatively impact overall academic achievement (Shield & Dockrell, 2008).

In summary, disruption of neural activity in the auditory pathways of children with ANSD can significantly affect the processing of timing cues. The severity of this temporal disruption is highly correlated with the overall level of functional disability (Rance et al., 2004; Zeng et al., 2005). However, the degree of temporal disruption is not consistent across subjects. As such,

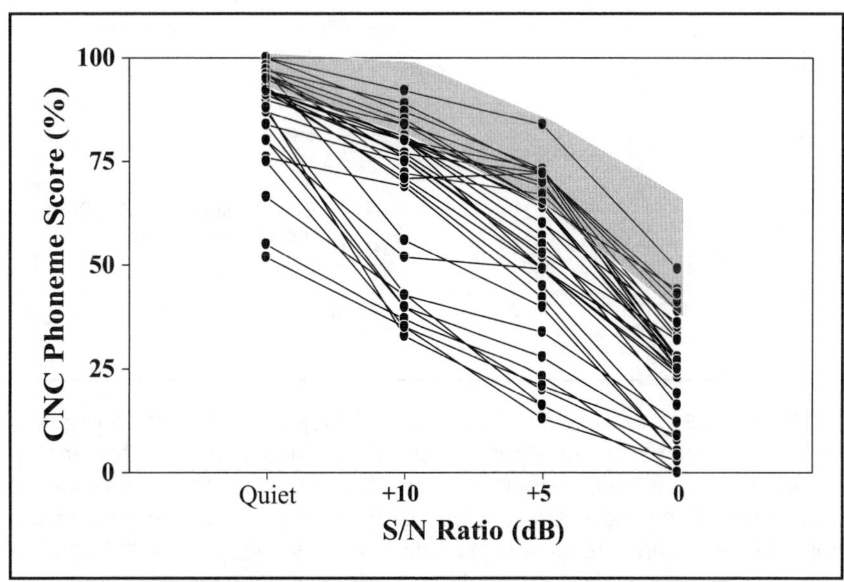

FIGURE 11–4. Open set speech perception scores for ANSD children with four-frequency average hearing thresholds <30 dB HL. Shown are scores for CNC-words presented in quiet and at +10 dB, +5 dB, and 0 dB signal-to-noise ratios. The shaded area represents the 95% performance range for age-matched controls.

the ability to quantify temporal processing in youngsters with ANSD offers a key to predicting their long-term capacity to use auditory cues.

Case Study (Auditory Processing)

Subject A was born at 32 weeks postconceptual age weighing 2.25 kg. Despite his prematurity, the infant presented with no neonatal risk factors for permanent hearing loss apart from hyperbilirubinemia (peak serum bilirubin level: 400 µmol/L) for which he received blood transfusion.

Click-ABR assessment was carried out at 1 month (corrected) age. Findings for the right ear showing a repeatable CM but absent ABR at maximum presentation levels are shown in Figure 11–5. Identical results were obtained for the left ear.[4] Transient otoacoustic emissions were present bilaterally. On the basis of these findings, Subject A was referred for medical (pediatric, neurologic, otologic) workup and was enrolled for early intervention support. Audiologic monitoring over the next 8 months showed consistent behavioral responses to speech and noisemaker stimuli at levels within the normal developmental range. As such, amplification was not recommended. Subsequent conditioned audiometric testing showed sound detection within normal limits for the left ear, and mild low-frequency threshold elevation in the right ear (Figure 11–6).

Subject A's speech, language, and general developmental progress were monitored and were considered normal at primary school entry (5 years of age). At this point he underwent a detailed speech perception and psychophysical assessment to evaluate his auditory processing ability. Figure 11–7 shows gap detection thresholds for Subject A and for a control cohort of children of equivalent age (5 to 7 years). In the left ear, his gap threshold was mildly elevated, suggesting only slightly impaired temporal resolution on this side.

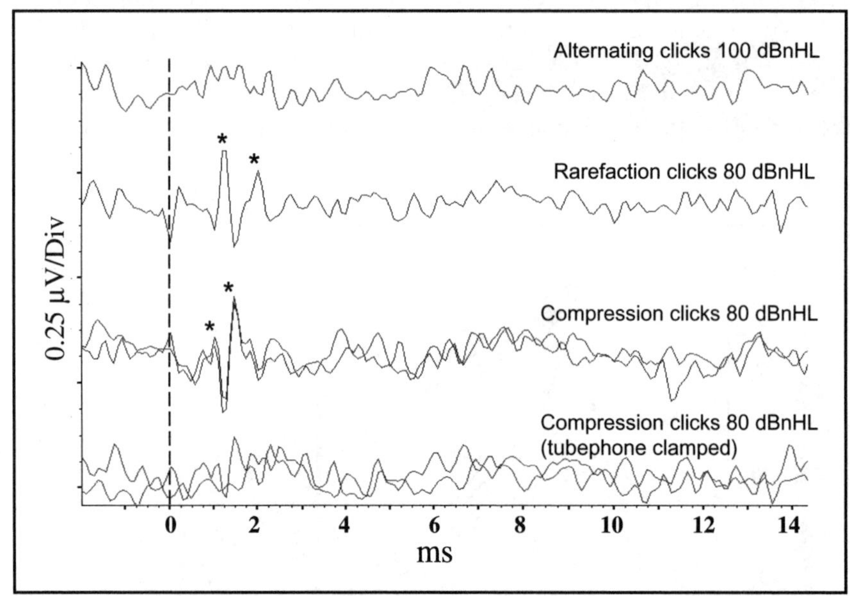

FIGURE 11–5. Averaged EEG tracings for Subject A. The dotted line represents the point of stimulus generation (at the transducer). The top tracing shows no recordable potentials to alternating acoustic clicks presented at 100 dB nHL. The middle tracings show cochlear microphonic responses but absent ABRs to unipolar stimuli at 80 dB nHL. Asterisks denote the positive peaks in the CM waveform. The bottom tracings were obtained to compression clicks presented with the tubephone clamped (no stimulus trials).

[4]Absent ABRs were also obtained on repeat assessment at 6 months, 12 months, and 5 years of age.

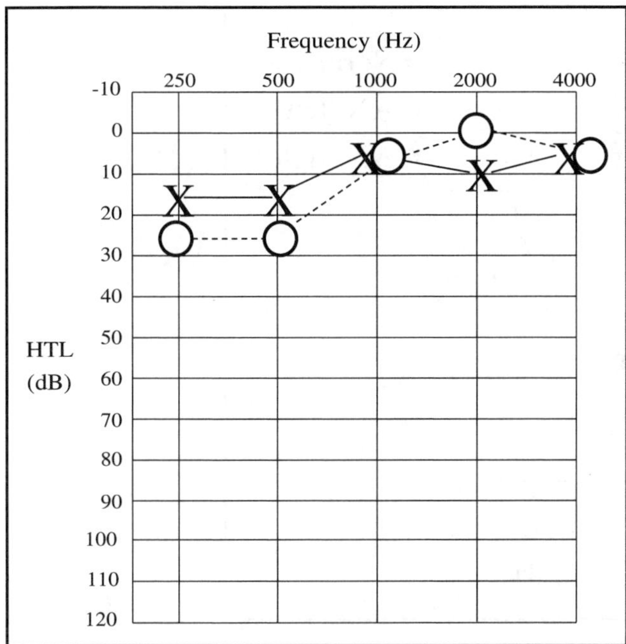

FIGURE 11–6. Conditioned audiometric thresholds for Subject A obtained at 8 months of age. Open circles represent hearing levels for the right ear, and X's show findings for the left ear.

However, temporal processing for stimuli presented to the right ear was significantly affected. This pattern was repeated on AM detection testing (Figure 11–8) where Subject A's ability to detect rapid amplitude changes in stimuli presented to the left ear was only mildly impaired, but results for the right ear were grossly abnormal.

Open-set speech perception results for Subject A reflected his temporal processing limitations. Figure 11–9 shows CNC-phoneme scores in four listening conditions. Speech understanding in quiet (+20 dB SNR) was relatively normal in both ears, but the introduction of background noise resulted in greater than typical deterioration in performance particularly in the psychophysically poorer (right) ear. These speech-in-noise difficulties were subsequently reflected in Subject A's school progress where both he and his teacher reported significant communication problems in the classroom. As such, he was fit with an FM listening device. He subsequently became a consistent device user and enjoyed significant benefit in the classroom (and in other challenging listening environments). Open-set speech perception testing in noise (+3 dB SNR) at age 6 years, 2 months revealed a CNC phoneme score of 25% in the unaided condition, improving to 98% in the aided.

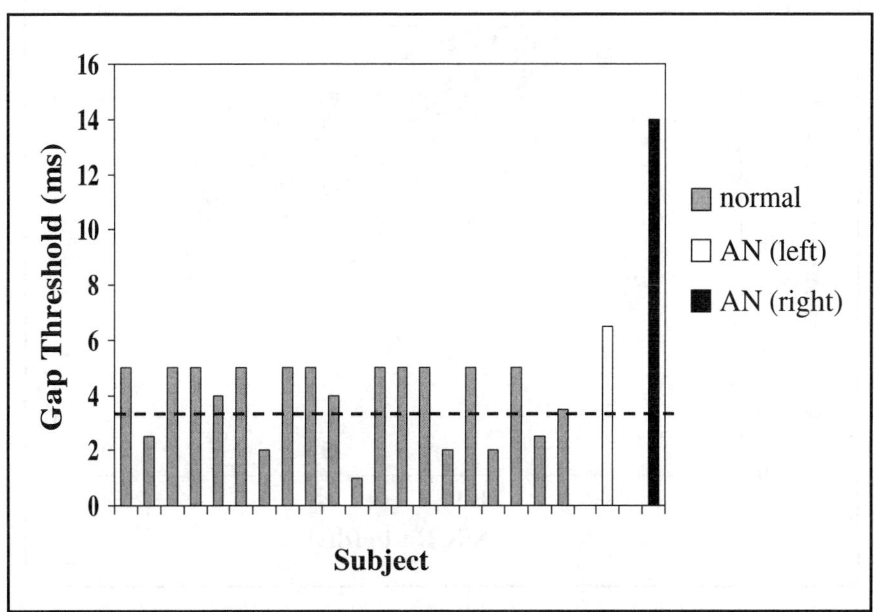

FIGURE 11–7. Threshold levels for gap detection in white noise presented at 70 dB SPL. Results for Subject A are represented by the white (left ear) and black (right ear) columns. The dashed line represents the mean detection threshold for a control group of school-aged children (5 to 7 years).

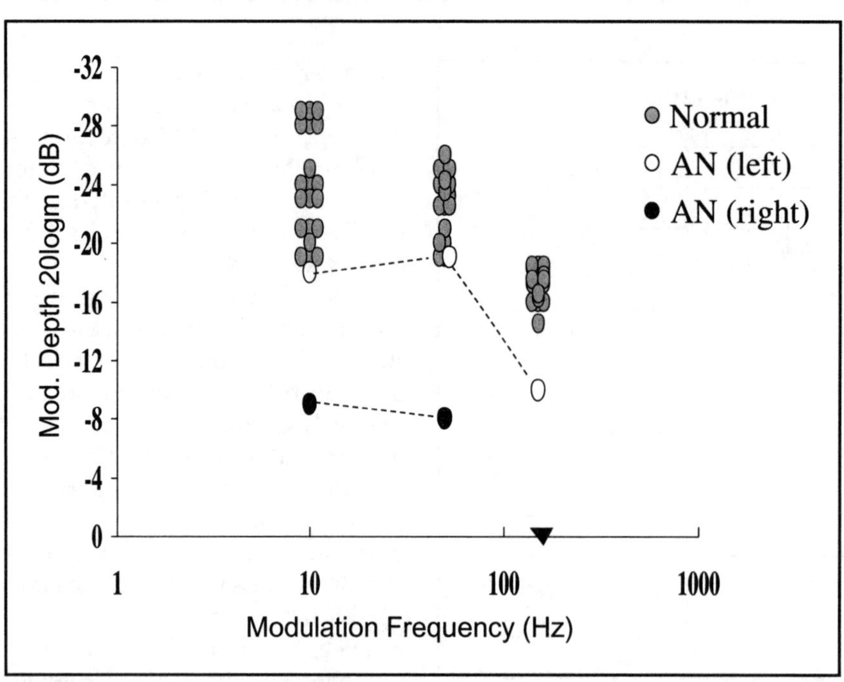

FIGURE 11–8. Amplitude modulation detection thresholds for white noise stimuli modulated at 10 Hz, 50 Hz, and 150 Hz. Findings for Subject A are represented by the white and black circles. Results for a control group of school-aged children are shown in gray (Rance et al., 2004).

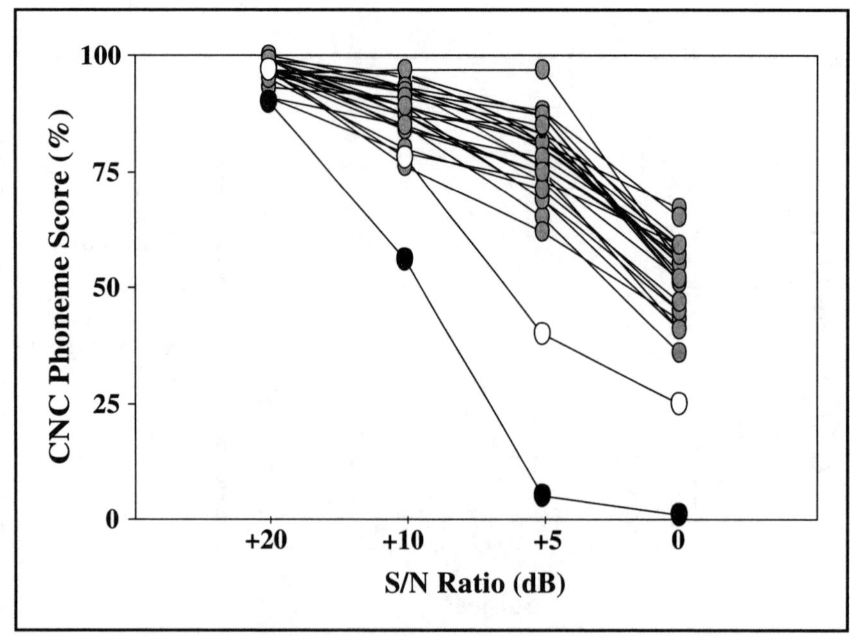

FIGURE 11–9. CNC-phoneme scores plotted as a function of listening condition. Results for Subject A are represented by the white and black circles. Findings for a control group of school-aged children are shown in gray (Rance et al., 2007).

Similarly, a 6-week device trial (as per Rance, Corben, Du Bourg, King, & Delatycki, 2010b) revealed clear differences in communication and listening ability with Abbreviated Profile of Hearing Aid Benefit (APHAB) global scores decreasing from 32% in the unaided, to normal levels (5%) in the FM-aided condition.

Case Summary

Findings for Subject A highlight the fact that it is possible for a child to have normal speech/language development, reasonably normal auditory temporal processing, and normal speech perception (at least in quiet) despite the absence of a recordable ABR. Comparing result patterns for the two ears also demonstrates the relationship between basic auditory processing abilities (measured psychophysically) and functional disability.

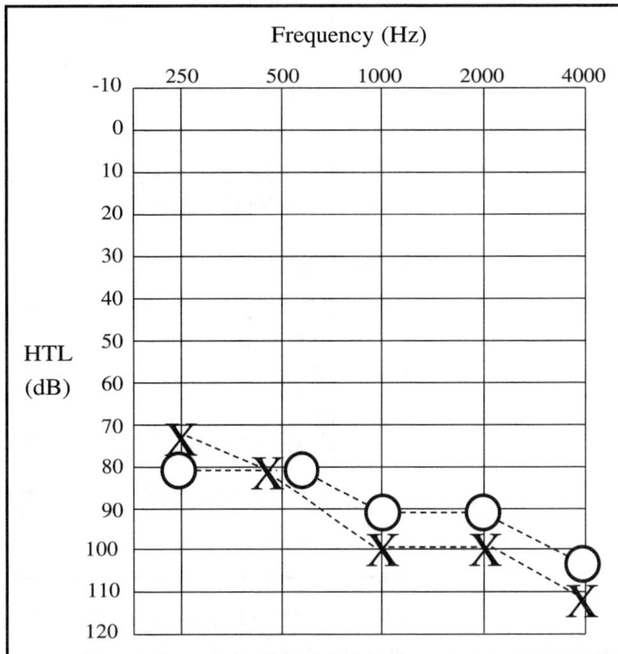

FIGURE 11–10. Conditioned audiometric thresholds for Subject B obtained at 8 months of age. Open circles represent hearing levels for the right ear, and X's show findings for the left ear.

Case Study (Management)

Child B suffered birth asphyxia when born at 38 weeks postconceptual age. Apart from severe oxygen deprivation, she presented with no risk factors for permanent hearing loss. Neonatal OAE screening showed normal responses bilaterally. However, severe-to-profound hearing loss was identified when she was reviewed at 9 months of age after her parents expressed concerns about her lack of auditory responsiveness (Figure 11–10). When transient OAE assessment again showed robust responses, she was referred for ABR assessment that showed the ANSD result pattern (Figure 11–11A).

Child B also underwent cortical auditory-evoked potential (CAEP) testing (Figure 11–12). Results of this assessment indicated that both speech and tonal stimuli could elicit electrical responses of normal latency and morphology at the level of the auditory cortex, if presented at high enough levels (100 dB sound pressure level [SPL]).

After an initial trial with low-gain hearing aids, which elicited no consistent response to sound, Child B was amplified to the degree of her hearing loss (NAL prescribed levels). She subsequently showed a capacity to use the amplified signal. Functional survey data (Meaningful Auditory Information Scale [MAIS-IT]) were used to track her auditory progress from 15 months of age when she began to show increased vocalization rates when aided, through to 2½ years of age, at which point she had developed an expressive vocabulary of ≈45 words. However, speech perception testing (at 3½ years) did highlight Child B's auditory limitations. Open-set word (Phonetically Balanced Kindergarten lists [PBK]) assessment showed perceptual levels below those expected for the typical young implantee (left ear aided, 34%; right ear aided, 40%; binaural aided, 40%). As such, it was recommended that she receive a cochlear implant in the left ear.

Child B was implanted with the CI-24 device at 4 years of age. Intraoperative EABR testing showed repeatable potentials to electrical pulses presented at typical current levels. This result suggested the presence of synchronized neural firing in the auditory brainstem (see Figure 11–11B).

Postoperatively, Child B has performed well with her cochlear implant.[5] At 14 years of age she scores at close to 100% on open-set speech perception tests in quiet, and in background noise understands more than the average implantee. Receptive and expressive language measures show only mild delay, and she has been successfully integrated into her local school.

[5]She originally wore the implant and hearing aid in concert but rejected the aid after 6 months of CI use.

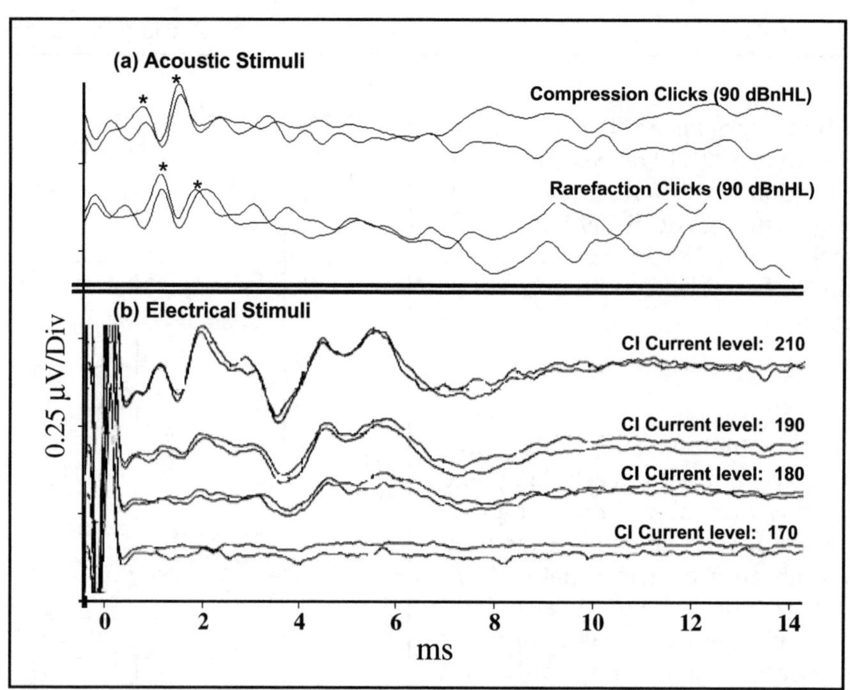

FIGURE 11–11. Averaged EEG tracings for Subject B. Section (a) shows potentials elicited by acoustic click stimuli at 90 dB nHL. Cochlear microphonic responses (*represented by the asterisks*) are present, but brainstem potentials are absent. Section (b) shows repeatable ABRs to electrical (cochlear implant generated) stimuli.

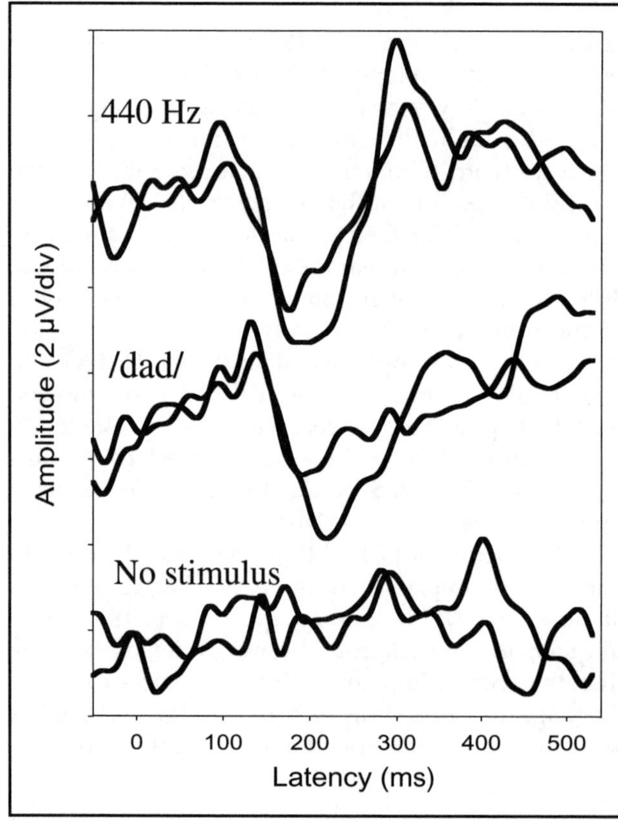

FIGURE 11–12. Cortical auditory-evoked potential (CAEP) responses for Subject B to 440 Hz tones (*top tracings*) and synthetic speech stimuli - /dad/ (*middle tracings*) presented at 100 dB SPL.

Case Summary

Clearly Child B has had a successful outcome with her CI and, as such, resembles most of the reported patients with ANSD who have followed this management path. She did receive her device relatively late (4 years), and we might expect an even better outcome had she been implanted earlier (although she did show good progress with amplification). Child B was in fact identified reasonably early in our series (early 1990s) and if seen now would probably be implanted younger (based on her limited access to the amplified speech spectrum). However, the question does remain, in children (like Child B) who show some ability to use their residual hearing, how do we determine whether amplification of implantation offers the best perceptual outcome?

Summary

A constant theme running through this chapter (and the literature on children with ANSD) is that sound audibility and auditory "perception" are not the same thing. If our experience with ANSD hearing loss has taught us anything, it is that auditory results, as measured by behavioral sound detection or electrophysiologic potentials, do not necessarily reflect function. Children with ANSD present with a common pattern of electrophysiologic and electroacoustic results, but their auditory capacity varies enormously. Developing methods that can quantify this capacity, predict long-term outcomes, and inform the management process remains a significant challenge for the future.

References

Alcántara, J. I., Weisblatt, E. J. L., Moore, B. C. J., & Bolton, P. F. (2004). Speech-in-noise perception in high-functioning individuals with autism or Asperger's syndrome. *Journal of Child Psychology and Psychiatry, 45*, 1107–1114.

Amatuzzi, M., Liberman, M. C., & Northrop, C. (2001). Selective inner hair cell loss in prematurity: A temporal bone study of infants from a neonatal intensive care unit. *Journal of the Association for Research in Otolaryngology, 12*(5), 595–604.

Attias, J., Buller, N., Rubel, Y., & Raveh, E. (2006). Multiple auditory steady-state responses in children and adults with normal hearing, sensorineural hearing loss or auditory neuropathy. *Annals of Otology, Rhinology, and Laryngology, 115*(4), 268–276.

Attias, J., & Raveh, H. (2007). Transient deafness in young cochlear implant candidates. *Audiology and Neurotology, 12*, 325–333.

Berlin, C. I., Bordelon, J., St.John, P., Wilenski, D., Hurley, A., Kluka, E., & Hood, L. J. (1998). Reversing click polarity may uncover auditory neuropathy in infants. *Ear and Hearing, 19*, 37–47.

Berlin, C. I., Hood, L. J., & Morlet, T. (2000). The search for auditory neuropathy patients and connexin 26 patients in schools for the deaf. *ARO Abstract, 23*, 23–24.

Berlin, C. I., Hood, L. J., Morlet, T., Wilenski, D., St. John, P., Montgomery, E., & Thibadaux, M. (2005). Absent or elevated middle ear muscle reflexes in the presence of normal otoacoustic emissions: A universal finding in 136 cases of auditory neuropathy/dys-synchrony. *Journal of the American Academy of Audiology, 16*, 546–553.

Berlin, C. I., Hood, L. J., & Rose, K. (2001). On renaming auditory neuropathy as auditory dys-synchrony. *Audiology Today, 13*, 15–17.

Berlin, C. I., Morlet, T., & Hood, L. J. (2003). Auditory neuropathy/dys-synhcrony: Its diagnosis and management. *Pediatric Clinics of North America, 50*, 331–340.

Buchman, C. A., Roush, P. A., Teagle, H. F. B., Brown, C., Zdanski, C. J., & Grose, J. H. (2006). Auditory neuropathy characteristics in children with cochlear nerve deficiency. *Ear and Hearing, 27*, 399–408.

Cacace, A. T., & Pinheiro, J. M. (2011). The mitochondrial connection in auditory neuropathy. *Audiology and Neurotology, 16*(6), 398–413.

Collet, L., Levy, V., & Veuillet, E. (1993). Click-evoked otoacoustic emissions and hearing threshold in sensorineural hearing loss. *Ear and Hearing, 14*(2), 141–143.

Cone-Wesson, B., Rance, G., & Wunderlich, J. L. (2003). Mismatch negativity in children with auditory neuropathy and sensorineural hearing loss. *Association of Research in Otolaryngology Abstract, 26*, 191.

Cone-Wesson, B., Vohr, B. R., Sininger, Y. S., Widen, J. E., Folsom, R. C., Gorga, M. P. & Norton, S. J. (2000). Identification of neonatal hearing impairment: Infants with hearing loss. *Ear and Hearing, 21*, 488–507.

Dallos, P. (1973). *The auditory periphery: Biophysics and physiology*. New York, NY: Academic Press.

Dallos, P., & Cheatham, M. A. (1976). Production of cochlear potentials by inner and outer hair cells. *Journal of the Acoustical Society of America, 60*, 510–512.

Davis, H., & Hirsh, S. K. (1979). The audiometric utility of the brain stem response to low frequency sounds. *Audiology, 15*, 181–195.

Dimitrijevic, A., Starr, A. M., Bhatt, S., Michalewski, H. J., Zeng, F. G., & Pratt, H. (2011). Auditory cortical N100 in pre- and post-synaptic auditory neuropathy to frequency or intensity changes of continuous tones. *Clinical Neurophysiology, 122*(3), 594–604.

Glowatzki, E., Grant, L., & Fuchs, P. (2008). Hair cell afferent synapses. *Current Opinion in Neurobiology, 18*(4), 389–395.

Gorga, M. P., Stelmachowicz, P. G., Barlow, S. M., & Brookhouser, P. E. (1995). Case of recurrent, sudden sensorineural hearing loss in a child. *Journal of the American Academy of Audiology, 6*, 163–172.

Guidelines Development Conference on the Identification and Management of Infants with Auditory Neuropathy. (2008). Retrieved from http://www.childrenscolorado.org/health-professionals/clinical-resources/auditory-neuropathy-spectrum-disorder-guidelines

He, S., Grose, J. H., Teagle, H. F., Woodard, J., Park, L. R., Hatch, D. R., . . . Buchman, C. A. (2015). Acoustically evoked auditory change complex in children with auditory neuropathy spectrum disorder: A potential objective tool for identifying cochlear implant candidates. *Ear and Hearing, 36*(3), 289–301.

He, S., Teagle, H. F., Roush, P., Grose, J. H., & Buchman, C. A. (2013). Objective hearing threshold estimation in children with auditory neuropathy spectrum disorder. *Laryngoscope, 123*(11), 2859–2861.

Hetu, R., Truchon-Gagnon, C., & Bilodeau, S. A. (1990). Problems of noise in school settings: A review of literature and the results of an exploratory study. *American Journal of Speech-Language Pathology, 14*, 31–38.

Hildesheimer, M., Muchnik, C., & Rubinstein, M. (1985). Problems in interpretation of brainstem-evoked response audiometry. *Audiology, 24*(5), 374–379.

Hood, L. J., Berlin, C. I., Bordelon, J., & Rose, K. (2003). Patients with auditory neuropathy/dys-synchrony lack efferent suppression of transient evoked otoacoustic emissions. *Journal of the American Academy of Audiology, 14*, 302–313.

Joint Committee on Infant Hearing (JCIH; 2007). Position statement: Principles and guidelines for early hearing detection and intervention programs. *Journal of Pediatrics, 120*, 898–921.

Kemp, D. T. (1978). Stimulated acoustic emission from the human auditory system. *Journal of Acoustical Society of America, 64*, 1386–1391.

Kraus, N., Bradlow, A. R., Cheatham, J., Cunningham, C. D., King, D. B., Koch, T. G., . . . Wright, B. A. (2000). Consequences of neural asynchrony: A case of auditory neuropathy. *Journal of the Association for Research in Otolaryngology, 1*(1), 33–45.

Kraus, N. A., Ozdamar, O., Stein, L., & Reed, N. (1984). Absent auditory brainstem response: Peripheral hearing loss or brainstem dysfunction? *Laryngoscope, 94*, 400–406.

Kumar, V., & Vanaja, C. S. (2008). Speech identification and cortical potentials in individuals with auditory neuropathy. *Behavioral and Brain Functions, 4*, 15.

Laury, A. M., Casey, S., McKay, S., & Germiller, J. A. (2009). Etiology of unilateral neural hearing loss in children. *International Journal of Pediatric Otorhinolaryngology, 73*(3), 417–427.

Lee, J. S. M., McPherson, B., Yuen, K. C. P., & Wong, L. L. N. (2001). Screening for auditory neuropathy in a school for hearing impaired children. *International Journal of Pediatric Otorhinolaryngology, 61*, 39–46.

Lonsbury-Martin, B. L., Harris, F. P., Stagner, B. B., & Hawkins, M. D. (1990). Distortion product emissions in humans: I. Basic properties in normally hearing subjects. *Annals of Otology, Rhinology, and Laryngology, 147*, 3–14.

Madden, C., Rutter, M., Hilbert, L., Greinwald, J., & Choo, D. (2002). Clinical and audiological features in auditory neuropathy. *Archives of Otolaryngology-Head and Neck Surgery, 128*, 1026–1030.

McMahon, C. M., Patuzzi, R. B., Gibson, W. B., & Sanli, H. (2008). Frequency-specific electrocochleography indicates that presynaptic and postsynaptic mechanisms of auditory neuropathy exist. *Ear and Hearing, 29*, 314–325.

Michalewski, H. J., Starr, A., Nguyen, T. T., Kong, Y-Y. & Zeng, F-G. (2005). Auditory temporal processes in normal-hearing individuals and in patients with auditory neuropathy. *Clinical Neurophysiology, 116*, 669–680.

Michalewski, H. J., Starr, A., Zeng, F. G., & Dimitrijevic, A. (2009). N100 cortical potentials accompanying disrupted auditory nerve activity in auditory neuropathy (AN): Effects of signal intensity and continuous noise. *Clinical Neurophysiology, 120*(7), 1352–1363.

Micheyl, C., Carlyon, R. P., Gutschalk, A., Melcher, J. R., Oxenham, A. J., Rauschecker, J. P., . . . Courtenay Wilson, E. (2007). The role of auditory cortex in the formation of auditory streams. *Hearing Research, 229*(1–2), 116–131.

Moser, T., Strenzke, N., Meyer, A., Lesinski-Shiedat, A., Lenarz, T., Beutner, D., . . . & Strutz, J. (2006). Diagnosis and therapy of auditory synaptopathy/neuropathy. *HNO, 54*(11), 833–839.

Nash-Kille, A., & Sharma, A. (2014). Inter-trial coherence as a marker of cortical phase synchrony in children with sensorineural hearing loss and auditory neuropathy spectrum disorder fitted with hearing aids and cochlear implants. *Clinical Neurophysiology, 125*(7), 1459–1470.

Norton, S. J., Ferguson, R., & Mascher, K. (1989). Evoked otoacoustic emissions and extratympanic cochlear microphonics recorded from human ears. *Abstracts of the twelfth midwinter research meeting of the Association for Research in Otolaryngology, 227*(A).

Park, M. S., & Lee, J. H. (1998). Diagnostic potential of distortion product otoacoustic emissions in severe or profound sensorineural hearing loss. *Acta Otolaryngologica* (Stockh), *118*, 496–500.

Psarommatis, I. M., Tsakanikos, M. D., Kontorgianni, A. D., Ntouniadakis, D. E., & Apostolopoulos, N. K. (1997). Profound hearing loss and presence of click-evoked otoacoustic emissions in the neonate: A report of two cases. *International Journal of Pediatric Otorhinolaryngology, 39*, 237–243.

Psarommatis, I. M., Riga, M., Douros, K., Koltsidopolous, P., Douniadakis, D., Kapetanakis, I., & Apostolopolous, N. (2006). Transient infantile auditory neuropathy and its clinical implications. *International Journal of Pediatric Otorhinolaryngology, 70*, 1629–1637.

Rance, G., Barker, E., Mok, M., Dowell, R., Rincon, A., & Garratt, R. (2007). Speech perception in noise for children with auditory neuropathy/dys-synchrony type hearing loss. *Ear and Hearing, 28*(3), 351–360.

Rance, G., Beer, D. E., Cone-Wesson, B., Shepherd, R. K., Dowell, R. C., King, A. K., . . . Clark, G. M. (1999). Clinical findings for a group of infants and young children with auditory neuropathy. *Ear and Hearing*, *20*, 238–252.

Rance, G., & Briggs, R. J. S. (2002). Assessment of hearing level in infants with significant hearing loss: The Melbourne experience with steady-state evoked potential threshold testing. *Annals of Otology, Rhinology, and Laryngology*, *111*(5), 22–28.

Rance, G., Corben, L., Barker, E., Carew, P., Chisari, D., Rogers, M., . . . Delatycki, M. (2010a). Auditory perception in individuals with Friedreich ataxia. *Audiology and Neurotology*, *15*, 229–240.

Rance, G., Cone-Wesson, B., Wunderlich, J., & Dowell, R. C. (2002). Speech perception and cortical event related potentials in children with auditory neuropathy. *Ear and Hearing*, *23*, 239–253.

Rance, G., Corben, L. A., Du Bourg, E., King, A., & Delatycki, M. B. (2010b). Successful treatment of auditory perceptual disorder in individuals with Friedreich ataxia. *Neuroscience*, *171*(2), 552–555.

Rance, G., Dowell, R. C., Rickards, F. W., Beer, D. E., & Clark, G. M. (1998). Steady-state evoked potential and behavioural hearing thresholds in a group of children with absent click-evoked auditory brainstem response. *Ear and Hearing*, *19*, 48–61.

Rance, G., Fava, R., Baldock, H., Chong, A., Barker, E., Corben, L., & Delatycki, M. (2008). Speech perception ability in individuals with Friedeich ataxia. *Brain*, *131*, 2002–2012.

Rance, G., Kearns, L. S., Tan, J., Gravina, A., Rosenfeld, L., Henley, L., . . . Mackey, D. A. (2012c). Auditory function in individuals within Leber's hereditary optic neuropathy pedigrees. *Journal of Neurology*, *259*(3), 542–550.

Rance, G., McKay, C., & Grayden, D. (2004). Perceptual characterisation of children with auditory neuropathy. *Ear and Hearing*, *25*, 34–46.

Rance, G., Roper, R., Symonds, L., Moody, L. J., Poulis, C., Dourlay, M., & Kelly, T. (2005). Hearing threshold estimation in infants using auditory steady state responses. *Journal of the American Academy of Audiology*, *16*, 293–302.

Rance, G., Ryan, M. M., Bayliss, K., Gill, K., O'Sullivan, C., & Whitechurch, M. (2012a). Auditory function in children with Charcot-Marie-Tooth disease. *Brain*, *135*, 1412–1422.

Rance, G., Ryan, M. M., Carew, P., Corben, L. A., Yiu, E., Tan, J., & Delatycki, M. B. (2012b). Binaural speech processing in individuals with auditory neuropathy. *Neuroscience*, *226*, 227–235.

Riedel, H., & Kollmeier, B. (2002). Auditory brain stem responses evoked by lateralized clicks: Is lateralization extracted from the human brain stem? *Hearing Research*, *163*, 12–26.

Santarelli, R. (2010). Information from cochlear potentials and genetic mutations helps localize the lesion site in auditory neuropathy. *Genome Medicine*, *2*(12), 91.

Santarelli, R., Rossi, R., Scimemi, P., Cama, E., Valentino, M. L., La Morgia, C., . . . Carelli, V. (2015). OPA1-related auditory neuropathy: Site of lesion and outcome of cochlear implantation. *Brain*, *138*(Pt 3), 563–576.

Santarelli, R., Starr, A., del Castillo, I., Huang, T., Scimemi, P., Cama, E., . . . Arslan, E. (2011). Presynaptic and postsynaptic mechanisms underlying auditory neuropathy in patients with mutations in the OTOF or OPA1 gene. *Audiological Medicine*, *9*(2), 59–66.

Santarelli, R., Starr, A., Michalewski, H. J., & Arslan, E. (2008). Neural and receptor cochlear potentials obtained by transtympanic electrocochleography in auditory neuropathy. *Clinical Neurophysiology*, *119*(5), 1028–1041.

Shield, B. M., & Dockrell, J. E. (2008). The effects of environmental and classroom noise on the academic attainments of primary school children. *Journal of the Acoustical Society of America*, *123*(1), 133–144.

Sininger, Y. S., & Oba, S. (2001). Patients with auditory neuropathy: Who are they and what can they hear? In Y. S. Sininger & A. Starr (Eds.), *Auditory neuropathy* (pp. 15–36). San Diego, CA: Singular.

Starr, A., Amlie, R. N., Martin, W. H., & Sanders, S. (1977). Development of auditory function in newborn infants revealed by auditory brainstem potentials. *Pediatrics*, *60*(6), 831–840.

Starr, A., McPherson, D., Patterson, J., Don, M., Luxford, W., Shannon, R., . . . Waring, M. (1991). Absence of both auditory evoked potentials and auditory percepts dependent on timing cues. *Brain*, *114*, 1157–1180.

Starr, A., Michalewski, H. J., Zeng, F. G., Fujikawa-Brooks, S., Linthicum, F., Kim, C. S., . . . Keats, B. (2003). Pathology and physiology of auditory neuropathy with a novel mutation in the MPZ gene (Tyr145→ Ser). *Brain*, *126*(7), 1604–1619.

Starr, A., Picton, T. W., Sininger, Y. S., Hood, L. J., & Berlin, C. I. (1996). Auditory neuropathy. *Brain*, *119*(3), 741–753.

Starr, A., & Rance, G. (2015). Auditory neuropathy. In M. J. Aminoff, F. Bolller, & D. F. Swaab (Eds.), *Handbook of clinical neurology* (pp. 495–508). Waltham, MA: Elsevier.

Starr, A., Sininger, Y. S., & Pratt, H. (2000). The varieties of auditory neuropathy. *Journal of Basic and Clinical Physiology and Pharmacology*, *11*(3), 215–230.

Starr, A., Sininger, Y. S., Winter, M., Derebery, M. J., Oba, S., & Michalewski, H. J. (1998). Transient deafness due to temperature-sensitive auditory neuropathy. *Ear and Hearing*, *19*, 169–179.

Stein, L., Tremblay, K., Pasternak, J., Banerjee, S., Lindermann, K., & Kraus, N. (1996). Brainstem abnormalities in neonates with normal otoacoustic emissions. *Ear and Hearing*, *17*(2), 197–213.

Tang, T. P. Y., McPherson, B., Yuen, K. C. P., Wong, L. L. N., & Lee, J. S. M. (2004). Auditory neuropathy/auditory dyssynchrony in school children with hearing loss: frequency of occurance. *International Journal of Pediatric Otorhinolaryngolology*, *68*, 175–183.

Vinay, & Moore, B. C. J. (2007). Ten(HL)-test results and psychophysical tuning curves for subjects with auditory neuropathy. *International Journal of Audiology*, *46*(1), 39–46.

Vohr, B. R., Carty, L. M., Moore, P. E., & Letourneau, K. (1998). The Rhode Island hearing assessment program: experience with statewide hearing screening (1993–1996). *Journal of Pediatrics*, *133*(3), 353–357.

Waxman, S. G. (1977). Conduction in myelinated, unmyelinated, and demyelinated fibers. *Archives of Neurology*, *34*(10), 585–589.

Wynne, D. P., Zeng, F. G., Bhatt, S., Michalewski, H. J., Dimitrijevic, A., & Starr, A. (2013). Loudness adaptation accompanying ribbon synapse and auditory nerve disorders. *Brain*, *136*(5), 1626–1638.

Zeng, F.-G., Kong, Y.,-Y., Michaelewski, H. J., & Starr, A. (2005). Perceptual consequences of disrupted auditory nerve activity. *Journal of Neurophysiology*, *93*, 3050–3063.

Zeng, F.-G., Oba, S., & Starr, A. (2001). Supra threshold processing deficits due to desynchronous neural activities in auditory neuropathy. In D. J. Breebaart, A. J. M. Houstma, A. Kohlrausch, V. F. Prijs, & R. Schoonhoven (Eds.), *Physiological and psychophysical bases of auditory function* (pp. 365–372). Maastricht, Netherlands: Shaker.

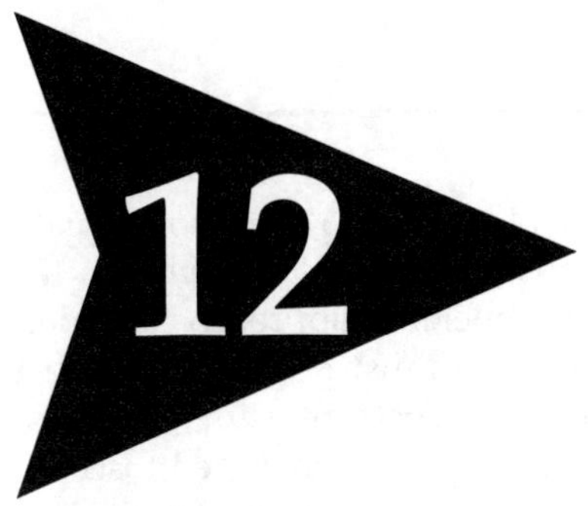

Management of Children With Auditory Neuropathy Spectrum Disorder (ANSD)

Patricia A. Roush

Introduction

In 1991, Arnold Starr and colleagues described an 11-year-old child with the paradoxical findings of absent auditory brainstem responses in the presence of normal cochlear microphonics (CMs) and otoacoustic emissions (OAEs). The child demonstrated severely impaired speech understanding despite a mild loss of hearing sensitivity. Further evaluation showed impaired temporal processing as exhibited by abnormal findings on a battery of psychophysical tests that included gap detection and binaural masking level differences. In 1996, Starr and colleagues reported on a group of 10 children and adults with similar findings (Starr, Picton, Sininger, Hood, & Berlin, 1996). Although the patients presented with no apparent neurologic involvement when their hearing impairments were first identified, eight of the ten showed later evidence of other peripheral neuropathies. Starr and colleagues coined the term *auditory neuropathy* (AN) to describe patients whose hearing impairment was attributed to "neuropathy of the auditory nerve."

Since the initial report by Starr and colleagues, it has become clear that individuals diagnosed with AN are a heterogeneous group even though they might exhibit common audiologic findings. Some individuals who exhibit the AN pattern might have a congenital form of the disorder resulting from a genetic mutation or pre- or perinatal causes, whereas others might have a later-onset form of the disorder associated with other peripheral neuropathies. Speculation regarding the underlying mechanisms of AN includes selective inner hair cell loss, a synaptic or myelinization disorder, or an auditory nerve disorder with other peripheral neuropathies (Starr, Sininger, & Pratt, 2000). Over the past decade, as universal newborn hearing screening has expanded and as audiologists have become more familiar with AN and its diagnosis, a growing number of infants and young children have been identified with this disorder. Characteristics of AN have been reported in children with histories of low birth weight, prematurity, neonatal insult, hyperbilirubinemia, perinatal asphyxia, artificial ventilation, and various infectious processes (Dowley et al., 2009; Mason, De Michele, Stevens, Ruth, & Hashisaki, 2003; Xoinis, Weirather, Mavoori, Shaha, & Iwamoto, 2007). Genetic abnormalities have also been identified, including those associated with the genes *OTOF*, *PMP22*, *MPZ*, and *NDRG1* (Kovach et al., 1999; Starr et al., 2003; Varga et al., 2006; Yasunaga et al., 1999). In 2006, Buchman and colleagues described a group of children who presented with physiologic test results typical of AN who subsequently were diagnosed by magnetic resonance imaging (MRI) as having cochlear nerve deficiency—that is, absent or small cochlear nerves.

Auditory neuropathy was initially thought to be rare; however, current estimates of prevalence range from 7% to 10% of children with permanent hearing loss (Madden, Rutter, Hilbert, Greinwald, & Choo, 2002; Rance, 2005). Considerable controversy exists regarding almost every aspect of the disorder including its etiology, site of lesion, treatment, and even the terminology used to describe it. In an effort to provide recommendations to clinicians working with these children, a panel was convened in June 2008 at an international conference in Como, Italy. The panel was charged with developing guidelines for identification and management of infants with AN (Guidelines Development Conference on the Identification and Management of Infants with Auditory Neuropathy, 2008). After extensive review and discussion, the term *auditory neuropathy spectrum disorder* (ANSD) was adopted as a way of describing the heterogeneous and multifaceted nature of the disorder.[1] Even so, current terminology remains inadequate because the level of dysfunction for many of the children with this condition might be central to the auditory nerve (Rapin & Gravel, 2003, 2006).

Further examination of this disorder, including information about etiology, possible mechanisms, and clinical characteristics, is provided in Chapter 11 by Rance and Starr in this volume. The present chapter addresses clinical management guidelines for pediatric audiologists and other professionals who work with these children.

Audiologic Evaluation

The Joint Committee on Infant Hearing (JCIH; American Academy of Pediatrics, 2007) recommends that a comprehensive audiological evaluation be performed for all infants referred from newborn screening by audiologists experienced in pediatric assessment. The recommended test battery includes physiologic measures and, when developmentally appropriate, behavioral measures. The goal of the diagnostic assessment is to determine the type of hearing loss and to estimate hearing sensitivity across a range of frequencies for each ear. The same comprehensive approach is needed to identify ANSD, and care must be taken to select and apply an appropriate electrophysiological test protocol. The initial battery should include otoscopic examination, immittance measures, auditory brainstem response (ABR) testing, and assessment of OAEs. When developmentally feasible, behavioral audiometry and speech perception measures should be included.

Diagnostic Criteria

In ANSD there is evidence of outer hair cell function while afferent neural conduction in the auditory pathway is disordered. Typical audiologic findings include absent or markedly abnormal ABR in combination with present cochlear microphonics (CM) and otoacoustic emissions (Figure 12–1).

Some earlier definitions of auditory neuropathy included present OAEs as a requirement for diagnosis. However, it is now recognized that OAEs might be present initially and disappear over time (Deltenre et al., 1999; Rance et al., 1999; Starr et al., 2001), and many infants with the disorder have present CM with absent emissions at the time of diagnosis, even when middle ear status is normal. Furthermore, both OAEs and CM provide evidence of outer hair cell function, albeit by different mechanisms. Thus, more recent

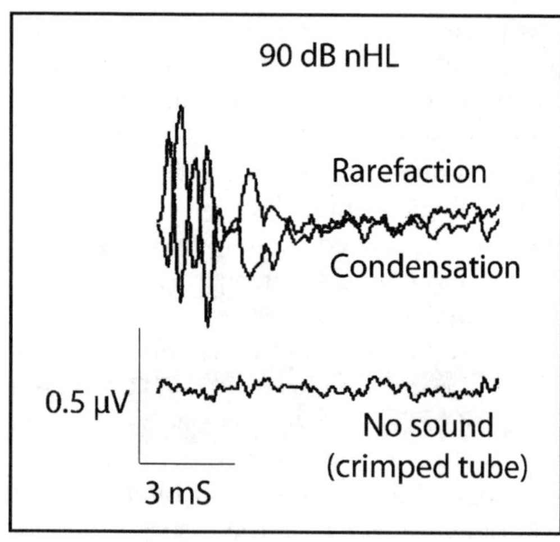

A

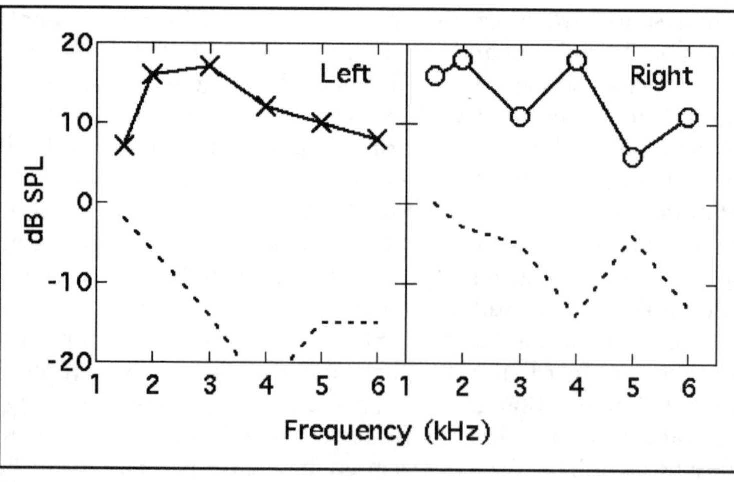

B

FIGURE 12–1. ABR (**A**) and OAE (**B**) test results for a child with auditory neuropathy spectrum disorder.

[1]The term *auditory neuropathy spectrum disorder* was suggested by Judith Gravel who noted the varied etiologies, presentations, and outcomes for children with similar electrophysiologic test findings.

descriptions of ANSD include either present OAEs or a present CM in combination with markedly abnormal or absent ABR.

Physiologic Measures

When diagnostic ABR testing using either click or tone burst stimuli shows no evidence of a neural response at high levels of stimulation, the clinician must determine if a CM is present. To accomplish this, ABR testing should be performed with insert earphones and high-intensity click stimuli (80–90 dB nHL) with separate response averages obtained for both *rarefaction* and *condensation* click polarities (Berlin et al., 1998; Starr et al., 2001). The CM occurs in the first few milliseconds of the response and, unlike neural responses, will show a reversal of the waveform when the stimulus polarity is inverted. If testing is limited to the evaluation of click stimuli with *alternating* polarity, the CM will not be evident because of cancellation and this might result in an incorrect diagnosis of profound sensory hearing loss in a child who actually has ANSD. To eliminate the possibility of incorrectly identifying stimulus artifact as the CM, a "sound interrupted/control run" should be completed by clamping or disconnecting the sound tube from the transducer while the stimulus is on, thereby preventing sound from entering the ear canal. This "sound interrupted/control run" should be completed without altering the spatial relationship between the transducer and the electrodes/leads (Rance et al., 1999). If the response observed remains without the stimulus entering the ear canal, the recorded response is a stimulus artifact rather than a cochlear microphonic. Insert earphones are required instead of standard headphones because inserts introduce a delay between the electrical signal at the transducer and the acoustic signal in the ear canal, further eliminating the possibility of electromagnetic stimulus artifact being incorrectly identified as the CM. Figure 12–2 shows an example of stimulus artifact *incorrectly* identified as CM.

As in all diagnostic ABR procedures, it is important to optimize recording conditions and to complete the testing with the infant sleeping quietly in either natural or sedated sleep. If an infant tested in natural sleep is too active for accurate, artifact-free assessment, it is better to reschedule the procedure and complete a sedated test than to risk an incorrect diagnosis due to poor recording conditions.

Both the amplitude and the latency of the CM vary in ANSD, so clinicians need to be familiar with the full range of possible test results (Starr et al., 2001). The characteristic pattern associated with the diagnosis of ANSD includes a "flat" ABR with no evidence of a neural response but with a present CM (see Figure 12–1). However, it is also possible to have a present CM in combination with markedly abnormal ABR morphology, as shown in Figure 12–3. In this case, early waveforms are absent, but a wave V is present and can be tracked down to lower intensity levels. In many cases like the one illustrated here, the wave V latency does not increase as intensity decreases as is typically expected.

With abnormal patterns like these, caution must be exercised in using the ABR to estimate behavioral thresholds because the minimal response levels obtained from the ABR might not correlate with the child's behavioral thresholds. Once the ANSD pattern has been identified, it is no longer possible to use the ABR to estimate the infant's behavioral thresholds, even when there is evidence of distal waveforms. At the time of this writing, controversy exists regarding whether these patients should be diagnosed as having

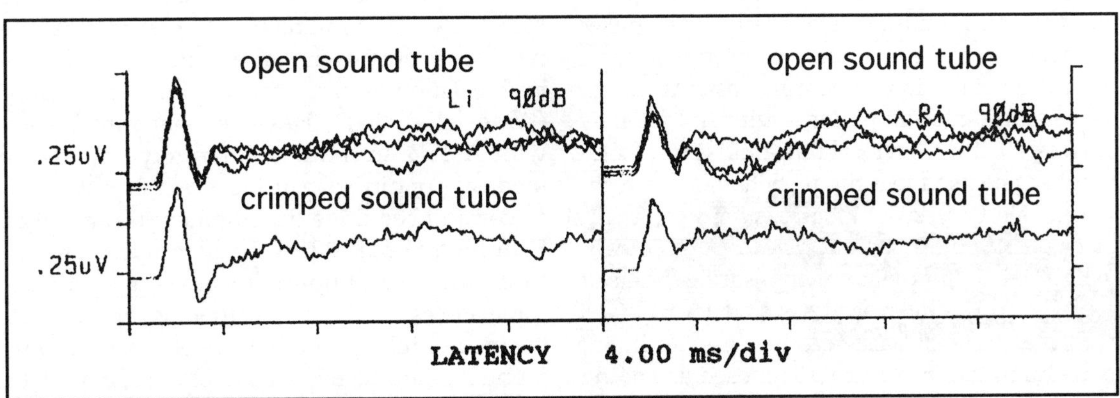

FIGURE 12–2. Example of stimulus artifact that might be misinterpreted as cochlear microphonic.

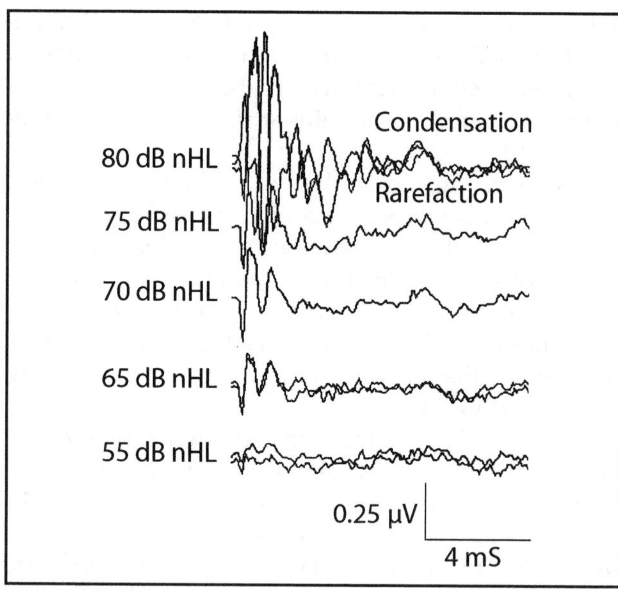

FIGURE 12–3. Abnormal auditory brainstem response showing cochlear microphonic with presence of distal waveforms.

ANSD. However, this electrophysiologic pattern is clearly abnormal, and these children should be closely monitored until behavioral audiograms are obtained and functional auditory abilities can be determined.

Caution is also needed when interpreting abnormal ABR findings obtained in infants prior to 34 to 36 weeks gestation as maturation of the auditory pathway might be incomplete. Furthermore, because cases of transient ANSD have been reported when the initial ABR was obtained in the first few months of life, the ABR should be repeated at a later point in time to confirm the diagnosis (Madden et al., 2002; Psarommatis et al., 2006; Raveh, Buller, Badrana, & Attias, 2007). This is especially important if there is a history of prematurity or hyperbilirubinemia (Xoinis et al., 2007).

In some clinics, auditory steady-state responses (ASSR) are used as the primary electrophysiologic measure in the evaluation of hearing loss. Although ASSRs can be measured in patients with ANSD, they do not correlate with behavioral thresholds and, therefore, should not be used to estimate behavioral thresholds (Rance et al., 1999, 2005). In cases where the ASSR is absent or when an infant is at risk for ANSD, ABR testing should be completed using single polarity click stimuli at a high intensity level to determine if a cochlear microphonic is present; otherwise, an infant with ANSD might be incorrectly diagnosed as having a profound sensory hearing loss. Other electrophysiologic measures such as cortical-evoked potentials and electrocochleography have also been explored in children with auditory neuropathy in an effort to determine the site of lesion (Rea & Gibson, 2003; Santarelli, Starr, Michalewski, & Arslan, 2008), to predict outcomes following treatment with amplification or cochlear implantation (He et al., 2015; Narne & Vanaja, 2008; Rance, Cone-Wesson, Wunderlich, & Dowell, 2002), and to attempt to estimate behavioral thresholds in children with ANSD who are young or difficult to test (He, Teagle, Roush, Grose, & Buchman, 2013; Pearce, Golding, & Dillon, 2007). These procedures, although still under investigation, hold promise for the future and warrant continued research.

Acoustic immittance measures (tympanometry and acoustic reflex testing) are also included in the comprehensive evaluation of ANSD. Middle ear muscle reflexes (MEMRs; both ipsilateral and contralateral) are usually absent or elevated in cases of ANSD (Berlin et al., 2005). For infants under 6 months of age, it is important to include a high-frequency (e.g., 1000 Hz) probe tone frequency (Margolis, Bass-Ringdahl, Hanks, Holte, & Zapala, 2003).

Behavioral Audiometry

Physiologic measures such as ABR and ASSR are not true tests of hearing in the perceptual sense, yet for many years these tests have enabled pediatric audiologists to make predictions regarding behavioral hearing thresholds. It is important to emphasize that in children with ANSD, thresholds cannot be predicted using ABR or ASSR. Thus, accurate behavioral audiometric procedures must be completed as soon as the child is developmentally capable of providing reliable responses. Behavioral audiometry using a conditioned response procedure such as visual reinforcement audiometry (VRA) can be initiated at a developmental level of 6 to 7 months. Using insert earphones attached to either foam tips or the infant's custom earmolds, it is often possible to obtain ear and frequency-specific measures by 7 to 9 months of age for typically developing infants (Widen et al., 2000). However, many infants identified with ANSD are born prematurely or have complex medical conditions putting them at risk for delayed motor and cognitive development (Teagle et al., 2010, Humphriss et al., 2013). These children are less likely to perform conditioned response procedures at the same age as healthy, typically developing infants, and testing at multiple intervals over a period of weeks or months might be required to obtain a complete audiogram. Furthermore, some infants with complex medical conditions or developmental delays might never be able to perform behavioral audiometry well enough to provide reliable estimates of hearing thresholds. In these cases behavioral observation audiometry (BOA) might be used; however, it is important to recognize the inter- and intrasubject variability inherent in this procedure (Widen, 1993, see also Chapter 23 by Diefendorf and Tharpe in this volume) and the limitations of BOA for purposes of hearing aid fitting. In cases where it is unlikely the infant will perform VRA reliably in a reasonable time frame for decisions regarding intervention, cortical-evoked potentials might be a useful supplement to behavioral audiometry for determining the child's auditory capacity (He et al., 2013; Pearce et al., 2007; Wunderlich & Cone-Wesson, 2006).

Medical Assessment

A comprehensive examination by an otolaryngologist is recommended for all children suspected of having ANSD. The otolaryngologist will obtain a medical history, perform a head and neck examination, and order laboratory studies as needed to determine the etiology of the hearing loss or to identify coexisting conditions. Radiologic assessment using MRI is essential in ANSD as the auditory neuropathy phenotype is often present in children who have cochlear nerve deficiency (Buchman et al., 2006). Furthermore, children with ANSD also have a higher incidence of other abnormal MRI findings. In a group of 118 children with ANSD who had imaging studies at the University of North Carolina, nearly 65% had at least one abnormal finding on MRI (Roche et al., 2010). The abnormalities identified in addition to cochlear nerve deficiency included prominent temporal horns; abnormalities of the brainstem, cerebellum, midbrain, or cerebrum; cerebrospinal fluid (CSF) and ventricular abnormalities; white matter changes; Dandy Walker malformation; and Arnold Chiari Type I malformation. In contrast, only approximately 30% of children with non-ANSD hearing loss have been reported to have abnormal MRI findings (Mafong, Shin, & Lalwani, 2002; Simons, Mandell, & Arjmand, 2006).

Other medical consultations include evaluation by an ophthalmologist to assess visual acuity and to rule out concomitant visual disorders, and referral for medical genetics to determine if there is a genetic basis for the disorder. Although not routinely recommended for children with sensory hearing loss, referral to a pediatric neurologist is recommended for children diagnosed with ANSD as some might have neurologic disease or other conditions requiring medical treatment. It is important to inform the child's primary care physician of the ANSD diagnosis and related findings, and to provide information regarding the auditory disorder and how it will be treated.

Evidence to Guide Management Decisions

Studies of children with ANSD show considerable variability in auditory capacity. Among the clinical characteristics reported are pure-tone thresholds that range from normal to profound; disproportionately poor speech recognition abilities for the degree of hearing loss; difficulty hearing in noise; and impaired temporal processing (Rance et al., 2002; Rance, McKay, & Grayden, 2004; Starr et al., 1996; Zeng & Liu, 2006; Zeng, Oba, Garde, Sininger, & Starr, 1999). It is important to recognize that the characteristics of ANSD vary, and not every individual diagnosed with the condition will present with the same symptoms or level of severity. Some children with ANSD have disproportionately poor speech recognition ability for their degree of hearing loss, whereas others perform at a level similar to peers with non-ANSD hearing loss. For example, Rance and colleagues (2002) in Australia compared unaided and aided speech perception abilities for a group of 15 children with ANSD to a group with typical sensory hearing loss matched for age and hearing level. Their results showed that approximately 50% of the children with ANSD had speech recognition scores that were similar to the children with sensory hearing loss; the other 50% showed essentially no open-set speech perception ability. Similarly, although it has been reported that children with ANSD have particular difficulty hearing in the presence of background noise (Gravel & Stapells, 1993; Kraus et al., 2000), a study by Rance and colleagues (2007) showed that children with typical sensorineural hearing loss and those with ANSD had more difficulty in noise than children with normal hearing. However, the effects were not consistent across subjects, and some children with ANSD showed relatively good speech perception abilities even at low signal-to-noise ratios.

Following the initial report by Starr and colleagues (1991) describing patients with what appeared to be a "neural" hearing loss, several journal articles and book chapters have included recommendations for clinical management. Recommendations included low-gain hearing aids or FM systems; low-gain hearing aids in one ear only; or the avoidance of hearing aid use altogether (Berlin, 1996, 1999; Berlin, Morlet, & Hood,

2003). Furthermore, because early reports described what appeared to be pathology of the auditory nerve, it was initially thought that cochlear implantation would not be beneficial (Cone-Wesson, Rance, & Sininger, 2001; Miyamoto, Kirk, Renshaw, & Hussain, 1999). Over time, as more young children diagnosed with ANSD have been evaluated, investigators have shown that both hearing aid use and cochlear implantation can be of benefit to some children with ANSD (Breneman, Gifford & Dejong, 2012; Buss et al., 2002; Ching et al., 2013; Rance et al., 1999, 2002; Rance & Barker, 2008; Rance, Barker, Sarant, & Ching, 2007; Teagle et al., 2010; Walker, McCreery, Spratford, & Roush, in press). The clinician's challenge is to determine, as soon as possible, whether or not hearing technology is needed and, if so, which technology will provide the most benefit for a particular child. Further research is needed to guide the clinician in predicting, at an early age, the technology and communication strategies that will be most beneficial for each child.

Hearing Aids and FM Systems

Currently available clinical tests provide limited information regarding site of lesion and, in many cases, it is difficult to predict whether a given child will benefit from amplification. In cases where there is residual hearing, and once reliable threshold estimates have been obtained, a trial period with amplification using an evidence-based hearing aid fitting protocol should be completed (e.g., American Academy of Audiology Clinical Practice Guidelines: Pediatric Amplification, 2013; Ontario Infant Hearing Program Protocol for the Provision of Amplification [Bagatto & Scollie, 2014]). This recommendation was also endorsed by the panel convened for the Guidelines Development Conference on the Identification and Management of Infants with Auditory Neuropathy (2008) in Como, Italy.

Established protocols for children include real ear measures or simulated real ear measures based on real-ear-to-coupler differences (RECDs) and use of a prescriptive hearing aid fitting method (e.g., Desired Sensation Level or National Acoustics Laboratory approaches), to ensure that speech at conversational levels is audible and comfortable. When managing amplification in these children, the clinician must keep in mind that ANSD is thought to cause a disruption in temporal rather than spectral processing (Rance et al., 2004; Zeng et al., 1999). As such, improving the audibility of the signal might not be sufficient to allow some children to make adequate progress with spoken language. Studies also have shown that in children with ANSD, it is possible to have varying degrees of temporal disruption (Rance et al., 2004). Thus, one might expect better performance with acoustic amplification in individuals who have milder forms of the disorder, although at the present time there is limited peer-reviewed literature regarding the benefits of amplification in children with ANSD (Roush, Frymark, Venediktov, & Wang, 2011).

Finally, considering the likelihood of difficulty hearing in the presence of background noise, use of a personal FM system by parents and other caregivers might be beneficial. As with children who have non-ANSD hearing loss, the use of an FM system in the classroom is especially important to reduce problems related to distance, reverberation, and background noise.

Evaluating Outcomes

Once hearing aids have been provided, it is important to evaluate the child's speech perception ability. Although evaluation of speech perception abilities in young children is challenging, a battery of age-appropriate tests, such as those used by cochlear implant teams, allows pediatric audiologists to evaluate a child's unaided and aided performance. Parent questionnaires such as the Infant-Toddler Meaningful Auditory Integration Scale (IT-MAIS; Zimmerman-Phillips, Osberger, & Robbins, 1997) and LittlEARS (Tsiakpini et al., 2004) and informal tests such as identification of body parts, as well as closed-set speech perception tests such as the Early Speech Perception test (ESP; Moog & Geers, 2003) might be useful in assessing progress when children are too young for open-set testing. Once the child is able to perform open-set speech recognition testing, measures such as the Multisyllabic Lexical Neighborhood Test (MLNT; Kirk, Pisoni, & Osberger, 1995) and the Lexical Neighborhood Test (LNT; Kirk, Pisoni, Sommers, Young, & Evanson, 1995) might be used. These tests use vocabulary in the lexicon of children under 5 years of age. For a review of speech recognition testing in children less than 3 years of age, see Eisenberg, Johnson, and Martinez (2005).

When children reach 5 years of age, the Phonetically Balanced Kindergarten (PBK) words (Haskins, 1949) can be used. It is important to use recorded speech materials whenever possible. In addition to evaluation of speech perception abilities, the child's speech and language development must be evaluated carefully to monitor communication milestones. As with young children who have sensory hearing loss, pediatric audiologists are advised to partner with speech-language pathologists and early intervention specialists. Experienced clinicians who know what to expect from children with varying degrees of sensory loss are essential to the process of monitoring communication development. Changes to an intervention strategy might be needed based on a child's progress and the preferences of the family.

Considerations for Cochlear Implantation

Children diagnosed with ANSD who exhibit severe-to-profound detection levels with stable thresholds over a period of several months, and whose families desire a spoken language approach, often are good candidates for cochlear implantation. For children without additional disabilities, decisions regarding cochlear implantation usually are uncomplicated once MRI has confirmed auditory nerve sufficiency (Buchman et al., 2006). Because of reports describing spontaneous improvement in auditory function in a subset of children with the ANSD phenotype, the guidelines developed at the Lake Como Conference recommend postponement of cochlear implantation until auditory test results (ABR and behavioral audiometry) are stable and demonstrate unequivocal evidence of permanent ANSD.

Decisions regarding the advisability of cochlear implantation for children with lesser degrees of hearing sensitivity loss are more challenging due to the range of functional abilities seen in this population and the difficulty determining the degree of impairment in very young children with ANSD. Because the behavioral pure-tone audiogram is of limited prognostic value in the prediction of aided benefit in children with ANSD, cochlear implantation should be considered even if audiometric thresholds are better than what typically would be considered when progress with conventional amplification is inadequate. For children with ANSD who have substantial residual hearing, an adequate trial with consistent use of amplification, appropriate early intervention services, and comprehensive evaluation by a team of professionals experienced in the evaluation and management of young children with hearing loss, are all prerequisites to cochlear implantation. For any child with a hearing disorder, a variety of factors might influence developmental outcomes. These factors include age at diagnosis and hearing aid fitting, consistency of hearing aid use, quality and intensity of early intervention, degree of parental involvement, and presence of additional developmental and medical conditions. The amount of time needed to determine benefit from hearing aid use will vary depending on each of these factors. Rather than identify an arbitrary time period for determining whether the child is receiving sufficient benefit from amplification, it is the role of pediatric audiologists, in partnership with the family and other team members, to identify the possible influence of each factor and its impact on developmental outcomes. Optimal management requires careful observation and a comprehensive team approach.

In the United States, candidacy for cochlear implantation is based on criteria developed by the U.S. Food and Drug Administration (FDA) using information obtained during clinical trials; the criteria specified on the device labeling vary by manufacturer. At the time of this writing, children between 12 and 18 to 24 months can be considered for cochlear implantation if they have a profound, bilateral sensorineural hearing loss. Children older than 18 months with severe-to-profound hearing loss can be considered for cochlear implantation if there is a failure to meet auditory milestones or if performance in the best-aided condition is less than 20% to 30% for MLNT or LNT at 70 dB SPL. The criteria for one manufacturer state that in children older than age 4 years, cochlear implantation can be considered if the score is less than 12% on PBK words or 30% on open-set sentences presented at 70 dB SPL. Although no specific FDA guidelines for cochlear implant candidacy currently exist for children with ANSD, professionals attempting to determine cochlear implant candidacy for children with ANSD who have less than a profound hearing loss should consider these general guidelines.

Counseling Families

Professionals who work with families of infants and young children with newly diagnosed hearing loss understand the critical role of counseling in helping a family understand the nature of a child's hearing loss and the implications of the diagnosis. Families need assistance with the emotional aspects of the new diagnosis and information they will need to make the best decisions for their child. This is a challenging process for the family and for the clinician. Families receiving a diagnosis of ANSD face additional challenges due to the uncertainties inherent at the time of the diagnosis and the complexities associated with management decisions for their child. When delivering a diagnosis of ANSD, it is important to share information based on the best available scientific evidence while providing the family with hope. For the young infant diagnosed with ANSD through electrophysiologic testing, the audiologist knows little more at the time of diagnosis than that the infant has an electrophysiologic pattern that is abnormal. Considering the heterogeneous nature of the disorder and range of functional outcomes, it makes little sense to make definitive predictions to the family regarding expected auditory behaviors until additional diagnostic information has been obtained.

For an infant only a few weeks of age, it might be appropriate simply to advise the family that the results of the ABR are not normal and that testing should be repeated in a few weeks. If the infant returns for a repeat study that yields similar results, additional information regarding ANSD should be provided to the family. For some families this might include showing them the ABR waveforms and contrasting them with expected results for children with non-ANSD hearing loss, as well as for a child with normal hearing sensitivity. Other families will prefer a more basic explanation. It is important for families to understand that an MRI will be needed to rule out cochlear nerve deficiency. Once cochlear nerve status has been determined, families will benefit from knowing the heterogeneous nature of ANSD and the variable outcomes associated with the disorder. It is important for families to understand that, unlike with non-ANSD hearing loss, the ABR does not assist in predicting the degree of hearing loss or in establishing thresholds for purposes of hearing aid fitting.

It is helpful for families to have a timeline for management during the first year including the need for medical evaluations, enrollment in intervention, and behavioral audiometry to establish thresholds beginning at 6 to 7 months of age. Families will need to understand that decisions regarding amplification might need to be deferred until behavioral audiometric thresholds can be established.

If a child is determined to be a good candidate for amplification, the family must understand the importance of full-time hearing aid use and the need to monitor communication milestones. Cochlear implantation can be discussed as one of several interventions that might be considered, but it should be explained that decisions regarding implantation need to be deferred until behavioral thresholds are established and benefit from hearing aid use has been determined. As discussed earlier, decisions regarding continuation of hearing aid use versus cochlear implantation must be made on an individual basis and determined by the needs of the child and the preferences of the family. Further research is needed to understand ANSD, its diagnosis, and its optimal management, but families should leave the clinic knowing that much can be done to facilitate their child's acquisition of functional communication ability.

Case Studies

As discussed above, the electrophysiologic test results that are characteristic of ANSD show a wide range of functional outcomes. The following case illustrations demonstrate the variable results obtained from children who exhibit the audiologic profile of ANSD. Key points are made to highlight the different habilitative recommendations made and outcomes obtained for each case.

Case 1

This child was born at 25 weeks gestation, with a history of hyperbilirubinemia that required an exchange transfusion. He was ventilated for 6 weeks and was on oxygen for 3 months. He did not pass his newborn hearing screen with automated ABR and was referred for diagnostic ABR testing. Following the ABR testing with tone bursts and clicks, the parents were told that the infant had a profound hearing loss, and he was fitted with high-gain hearing aids. The father had a job transfer and the family moved into our state. They were told that another ABR would be needed prior to acceptance into our program. On the day of the sedated ABR evaluation, the family reported that in spite of the diagnosis of profound hearing loss, they observed the baby respond to a variety of sounds at home and had even observed him startle to a loud sound.

Subsequent ABR testing showed an absent ABR with only a large CM present consistent with a diagnosis of ANSD. Otoacoustic emissions were absent bilaterally (Figure 12–4).

The diagnosis was explained to the family, and it was recommended that they discontinue use of the high-gain hearing aids until behavioral audiometry could be completed. The child was enrolled in an early intervention program, and the family was informed of various communication options. They chose spoken language as their initial communication approach and were assigned an auditory verbal therapist who provided weekly visits to the family's home. The child was seen by an otolaryngologist who recommended an MRI. The MRI showed normal inner ear anatomy with

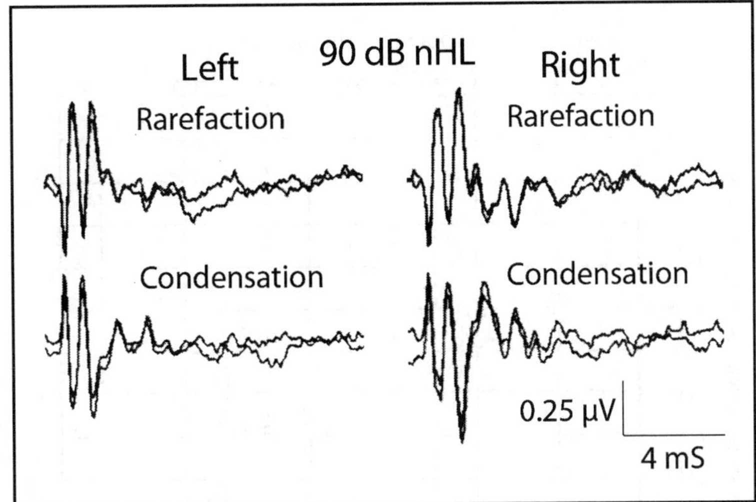

A

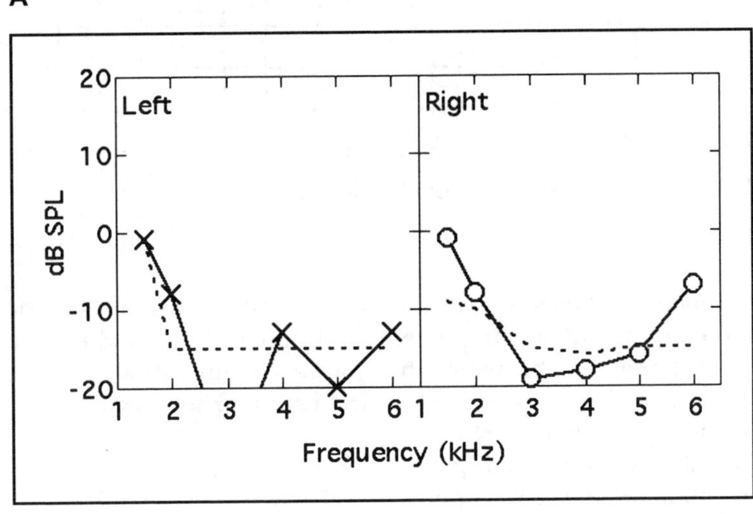

B

FIGURE 12–4. A. Auditory brainstem response for child in Case 1. Note large cochlear microphonic with reversal of waveform when stimulus polarity is inverted and lack of neural response. **B.** Otoacoustic emissions for Case 1.

present auditory nerves bilaterally. Subsequent behavioral audiometric testing at 10 months of age (7 months adjusted age) using VRA showed a moderate bilateral sensorineural hearing loss (Figure 12–5).

Once behavioral thresholds were obtained, the family decided to move forward with amplification, and the child was fitted with hearing aids appropriate for a moderate hearing loss. In addition to hearing aids, the family used a personal FM system at home once the child began to walk, and there was increasing distance between the child and the speaker. Aided speech perception measures showed aided benefit, and subsequent speech and language evaluations showed the child was making excellent progress in meeting communication milestones. At 3½ years of age, the child had recurrent middle ear problems and was scheduled for placement of tympanostomy tubes. ABR testing was repeated and again showed no neural responses to click stimuli at high intensity levels with only a CM present. The child is now 10 years old and has successfully completed fifth grade in a mainstream classroom. At the time of his most recent audiologic

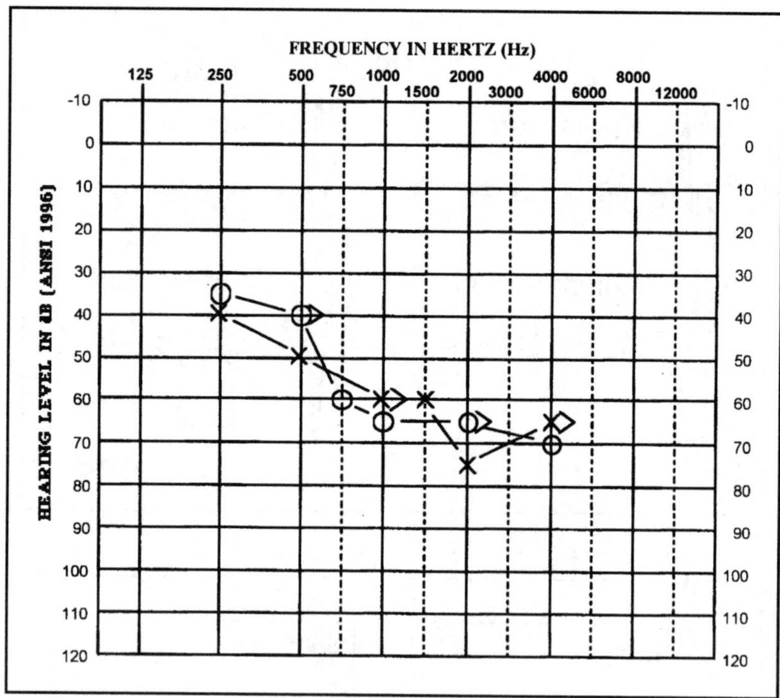

FIGURE 12–5. Audiogram for child in Case 1.

evaluation, his speech reception thresholds were 60 dB HL unaided and 30 dB HL aided, and his aided speech recognition score for recorded monosyllabic words in quiet was 86% for speech presented at 70 dB SPL. His most recent speech and language evaluation showed age-appropriate language skills with some mild speech production problems. He continues to receive support from a teacher of the deaf and a speech and language pathologist and uses FM in the classroom.

Key Points

In this case, the first ABR was done at a clinic that used alternating polarity rather than single polarity clicks. This resulted in an incorrect diagnosis of profound, bilateral sensory hearing loss. Fortunately, the family's move to another state resulted in the child having a repeat ABR study. The case illustrates the importance of asking the family about their observations of the child's auditory behaviors. Although the child was initially diagnosed with profound hearing loss, it was obvious to the family that their baby was responding to moderately loud sounds at home even without amplification—an unexpected finding with profound bilateral hearing loss. It also illustrates the importance of accurate initial diagnosis, as habilitative recommendations are often based on the initial diagnostic ABR evaluation. Finally, this is an example of a child who shows electrophysiologic findings that are characteristic of auditory neuropathy, yet receives significant benefit from acoustic amplification.

Case 2

The second case is a child who was born at full term in a hospital that used only otoacoustic emissions for their infant hearing screening program. The child passed his newborn OAE screen bilaterally. At age 3½ years, he subsequently developed recurrent middle ear problems and was scheduled for myringotomy and tube placement. His postoperative hearing evaluation showed normal hearing sensitivity for the right ear and a profound bilateral sensorineural hearing loss for the left ear (Figure 12–6A). Unexpectedly, with a profound hearing loss in one ear, OAEs were present bilaterally (Figure 12–6B).

The child was referred to our center for further evaluation. Diagnostic ABR testing showed, in the right ear, normal waveform morphology with responses consistent with normal hearing sensitivity. In the left ear, the ABR indicated absent neural responses with only a prolonged CM present at high intensity levels (Figure 12–7). MRI testing was completed and revealed

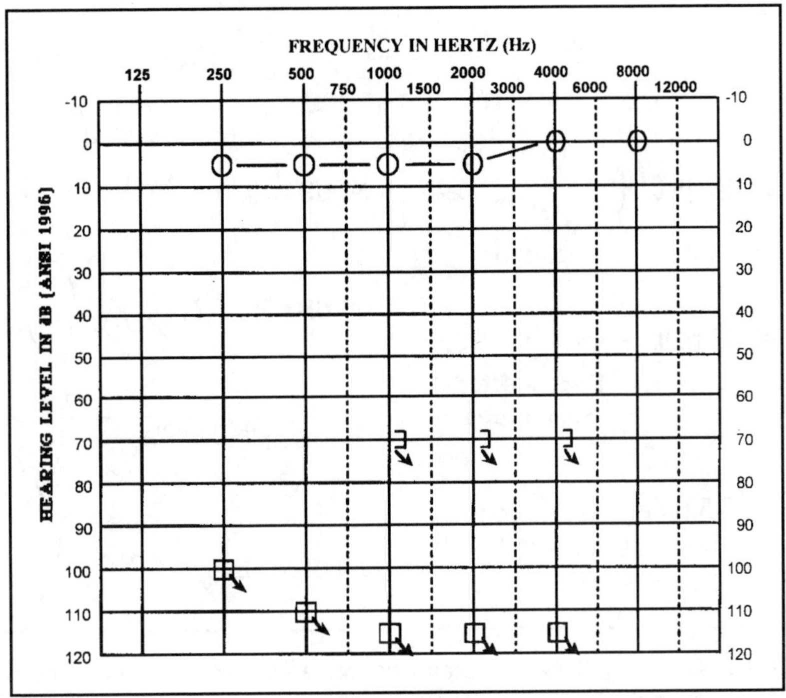

A

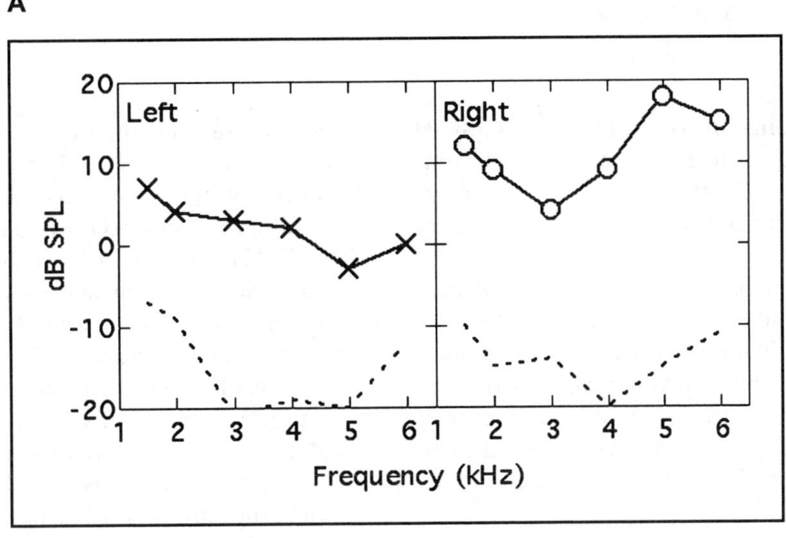

B

FIGURE 12–6. A. Audiogram for child in Case 2. **B.** Otoacoustic emissions for Case 2.

a normal study for the right ear and an absent auditory nerve for the left ear.

Key Points

As previously noted in this chapter, individuals who have cochlear nerve deficiency (small or absent VIII nerves) often present with the phenotype of ANSD (absent ABR, present CM, and present OAEs; Buchman et al., 2006). MRI is useful in identifying the site of lesion in these cases and will assist the audiologist and intervention specialist in making appropriate management recommendations. Use of radiologic imaging is particularly important when determining cochlear implant candidacy in cases of profound bilateral hearing loss when there is no evidence of residual hearing.

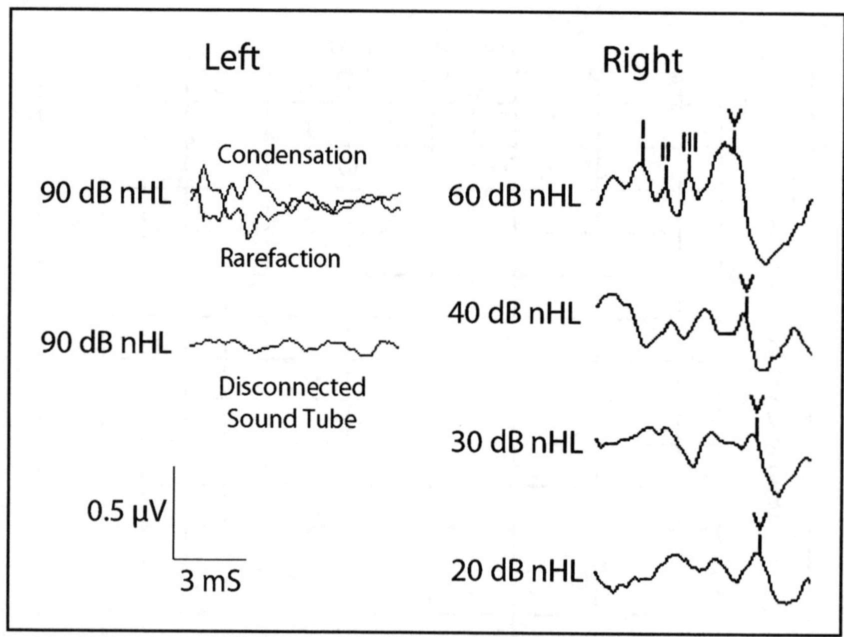

FIGURE 12–7. Auditory brainstem response for Case 2 showing normal response for right ear; left ear shows absent neural responses with only a cochlear microphonic present.

In this child's case, availability of MRI findings allowed the pediatric audiologist to make recommendations for management that were the same as those recommended for a child with profound, unilateral, sensory hearing loss.

Another key point is that it is possible to pass OAE-based newborn hearing screening and yet have a profound hearing loss in one or both ears. Professionals must be aware that passing newborn hearing screening does not ensure normal hearing, and further diagnostic study is warranted when there is concern about hearing status even when an individual has passed a newborn hearing screen.

Case 3

This is a child who was born prematurely at 24 weeks gestation. He was hospitalized in the newborn intensive care nursery (NICU) where he received ventilation. He did not pass his initial newborn hearing screen or a repeat screen using automated ABR. Subsequent diagnostic ABR testing at 4 months of age showed absent neural responses with only a CM present for single polarity clicks at a high intensity level (Figure 12–8A). OAEs were present bilaterally (Figure 12–8B).

Behavioral audiometry was attempted at regular intervals beginning at 7 months adjusted age. At 12 months of age (8 months adjusted age), a soundfield audiogram showed normal hearing sensitivity for 250 to 4000 Hz. At 13 months of age (9 months adjusted age), individual ear measures were completed with insert earphones and confirmed normal hearing sensitivity for each ear (Figure 12–9).

The results were discussed with the family, and the importance of monitoring the child's communication status in view of the abnormal ABR pattern was discussed. The child was enrolled in an early intervention program, and a teacher visited the home on a monthly basis. Because of reports of "recovery" in cases of ANSD, ABR testing was repeated at 17 months of age and test results again showed an abnormal ABR with no neural responses at maximum intensity levels for click stimuli with only a CM present.

It was recommended that the child return for audiologic evaluation every 6 months to monitor the stability of his thresholds and to obtain speech perception measures once he was developmentally able to perform this testing. At age 3 years, the child scored 100% on a closed-set monosyllabic word test (Early Speech Perception Test; ESP). The child developed spoken language, and at 3½ years of age he was able to

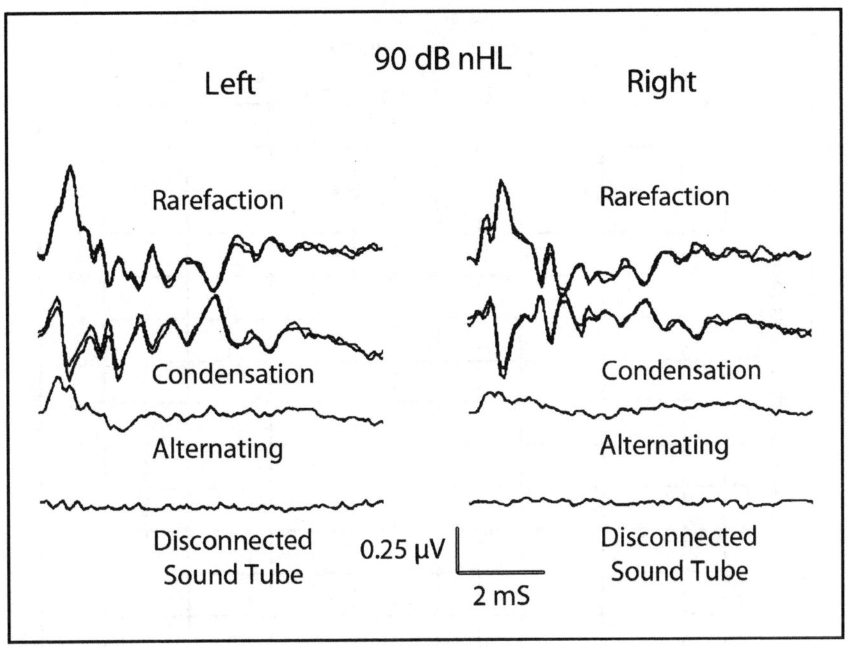

A

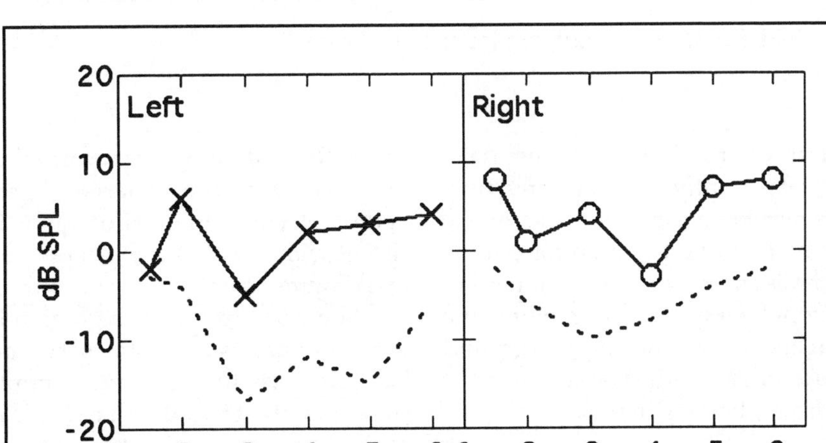

B

FIGURE 12–8. A. Auditory brainstem response showing no neural response with only a cochlear microphonic for child in Case 3. **B.** Otoacoustic emissions for child in Case 3.

comprehend speech and use multiple word sentences expressively. He was also able to repeat monosyllabic words in quiet without difficulty in an auditory-only condition.

Key Points

In this case, although the child's ABR was grossly abnormal showing absent neural responses, the child's

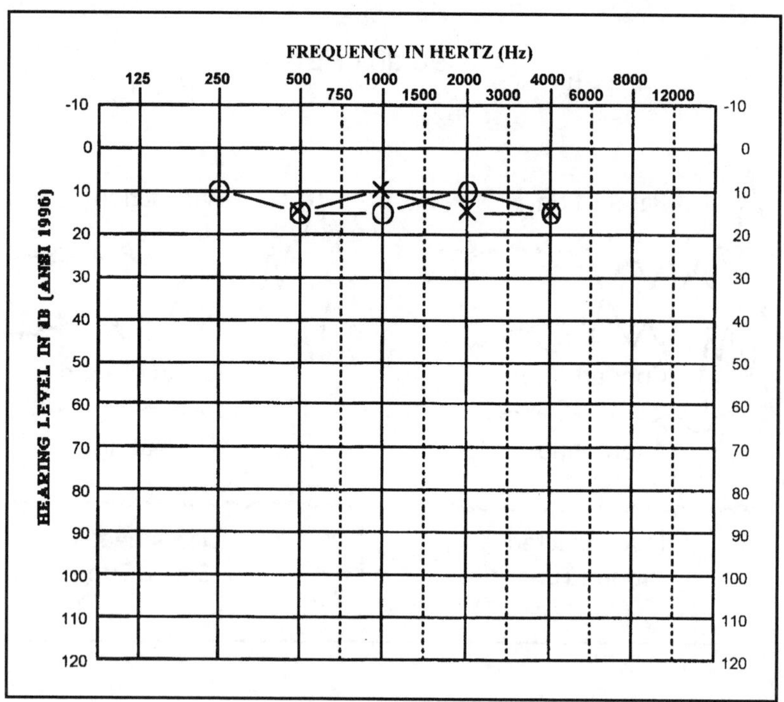

FIGURE 12–9. Audiogram for child in Case 3.

audiogram demonstrates normal hearing sensitivity. Although the child is not currently exhibiting any functional difficulty and is developing speech and language appropriately, it will be important to monitor performance at regular intervals and continue early intervention services. It also will be important to monitor the child's ability to hear in the presence of background noise and consider use of FM in the classroom if the child experiences difficulty hearing in noise.

Case 4

This child was born at full term without any significant complications. There was no family history of hearing loss. This child did not pass an automated ABR hearing screen at birth but passed a re-screen with otoacoustic emissions at an outside otolaryngologist office, and her parents were told she had normal hearing. At 8 months of age, her parents became suspicious that she was not hearing and brought her to our university hospital clinic for a diagnostic ABR. The results of the diagnostic ABR evaluation showed absent neural responses to clicks with only a CM present at high intensity levels (Figure 12–10A). OAEs were present bilaterally (Figure 12–10B).

MRI evaluation was normal and indicated the presence of auditory nerves bilaterally. Behavioral audiometry at 9 months of age using VRA was consistent with a profound bilateral sensorineural hearing loss (Figure 12–11).

She was fitted with high-gain hearing aids; however, her parents did not observe any improvement in her responses to sound with amplification. She was subsequently referred to the cochlear implant team for evaluation. She received a right cochlear implant at 21 months of age.

Key Points

In this case, the child's profound hearing loss would have been identified earlier if the outside clinic had recognized the importance of not rescreening with otoacoustic emissions when the child failed the ABR screen. Fortunately, the family obtained a second opinion in sufficient time for her to receive appropriate management. If a child does not pass a hearing screen with ABR, the child either should have a second level screen with ABR or a diagnostic ABR as a follow-up. In many clinics, ABR has replaced OAE screening in the intensive care nursery due to the high prevalence of ANSD in this population. However, screening with OAEs is still common

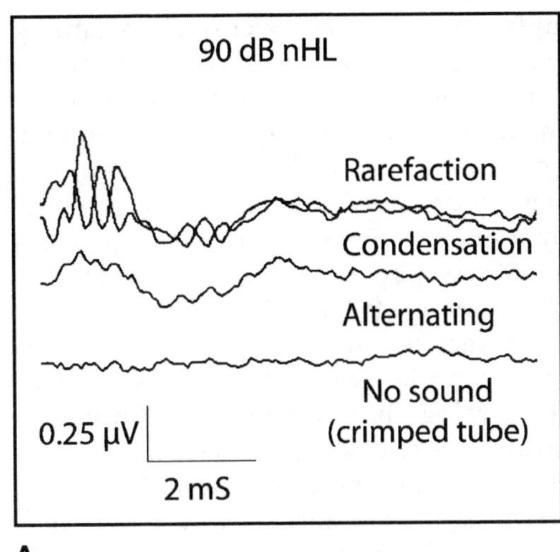

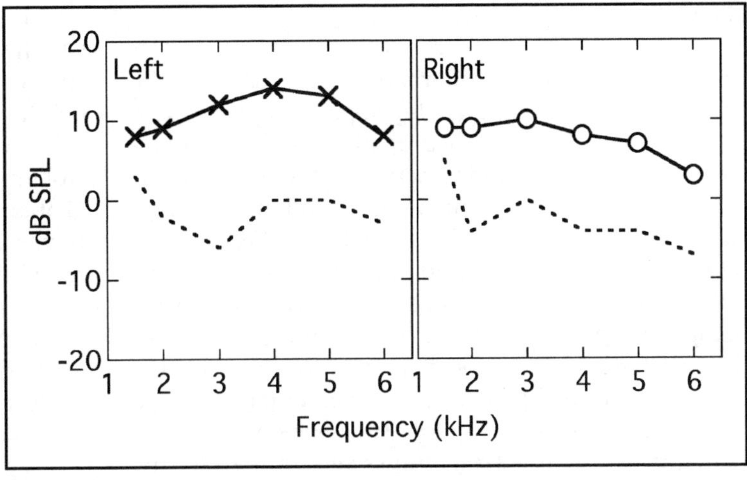

A B

FIGURE 12–10. A. Abnormal auditory brainstem response for Case 4 showing no neural response with only a cochlear microphonic. **B.** Present otoacoustic emissions for child in Case 4 with profound hearing loss.

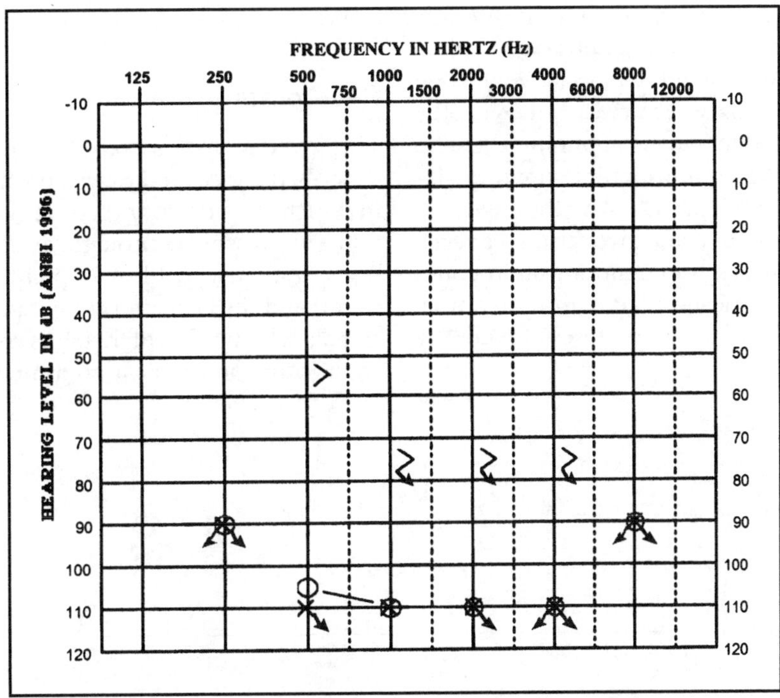

FIGURE 12–11. Audiogram for child in Case 4 showing profound hearing loss.

in many well-baby nurseries. Although the majority of cases of ANSD will be found in the NICU, it is possible to have a full-term birth without complications yet present with ANSD. Clinicians must be mindful of the possibility of ANSD when there is suspicion of hearing loss in a full-term infant who has passed a newborn hearing screen with OAEs. In some of these cases, a genetic basis for the ANSD might be the etiology of the disorder

Case 5

This is a child who had normal development for the first 2 years of life and then developed peripheral neuropathies including optic neuropathy. She was hospitalized at 3 years of age and underwent several diagnostic studies including electromyography and muscle biopsies. She has had numerous specialty medical consultations including otolaryngology, genetics, neurology, ophthalmology, and infectious disease. The etiology for her medical problems was never determined; Guillain-Barré, Charcot-Marie-Tooth, and mitochondrial disease were all ruled out. An audiogram obtained at age 6 years showed a bilateral low-frequency hearing loss with unaided speech recognition scores of 100% for the right ear and 84% for the left (Figure 12–12).

An audiogram at age 10 years showed a bilateral rising audiogram; mild on the right and moderate on the left with speech recognition scores using monosyllabic words of 40% for the right (presented at 65 dB HL) and 24% for the left (presented at 95 dB HL; Figure 12–13).

Subsequent hearing evaluations showed fluctuating speech recognition scores and a subsequent diagnostic ABR evaluation showed a pattern consistent with ANSD. Hearing aids were tried; however, the child and family reported they were of minimal benefit. By age 11 years, despite an audiogram showing significant residual hearing (Figure 12–14A), the child was unable to repeat any monosyllabic words on a speech recognition test and successful communication could only be accomplished at close range with lip reading. Robust otoacoustic emissions were present bilaterally (Figure 12–14B).

The family was counseled extensively regarding potential benefits and limitations of cochlear implantation, particularly in view of her history of multiple peripheral neuropathies. After careful consideration, the family decided to proceed with a left cochlear implant. After 1 year of device use, the child's monosyllabic word score with her cochlear implant was 32% on words and 66% on phonemes. Her parents reported that while she continued to have significant communication difficulty, they felt that the need for repetitions was reduced with the device on. After 4 years of device use, her speech recognition score while wearing her cochlear implant was only 20%, and she continued to have deterioration in her motor abilities. The parents reported that she had significant difficulty understanding anyone other than her family members with her implant. As the child still had significant residual hearing in her right ear, a decision was made to attempt hearing aid use again in the right ear. At the age of 17 years and after 6 years of implant use and with a hearing aid in the contralateral ear, this child only achieves a score of 20% for monosyllabic words.

Key Points

This child's case is complex and is similar to cases described by Arnold Starr and his colleagues in 1996 in which the auditory disorder occurs in combination with progressive neurologic disease. Despite the use of hearing aids, a cochlear implant, supplemental visual input, and the best effort of her parents and the professionals who work with her, this child continued to have significant communication difficulty.

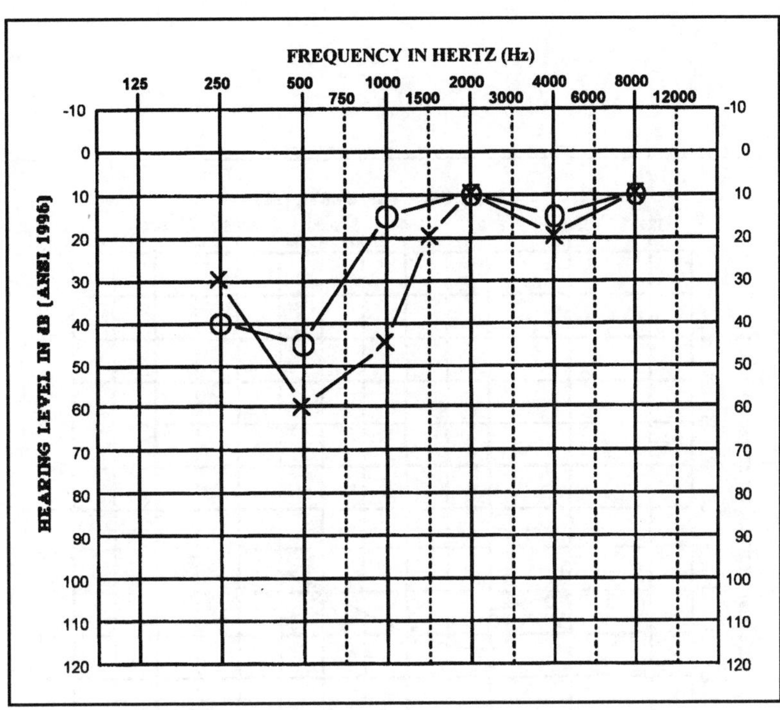

FIGURE 12–12. Audiogram showing rising low-frequency hearing loss for child in Case 5 (age 6 years).

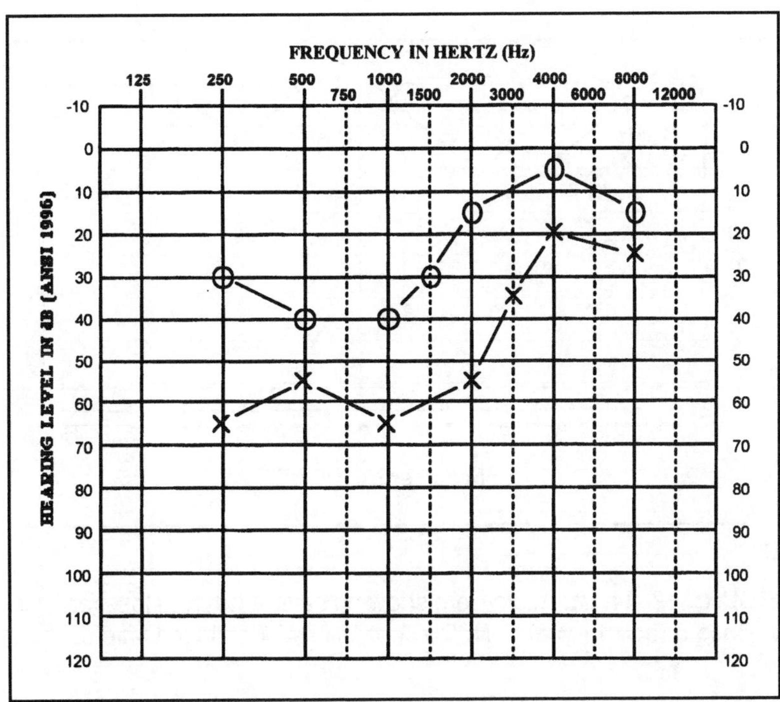

FIGURE 12–13. Audiogram showing left ear worse than right for child in Case 5 (age 10 years).

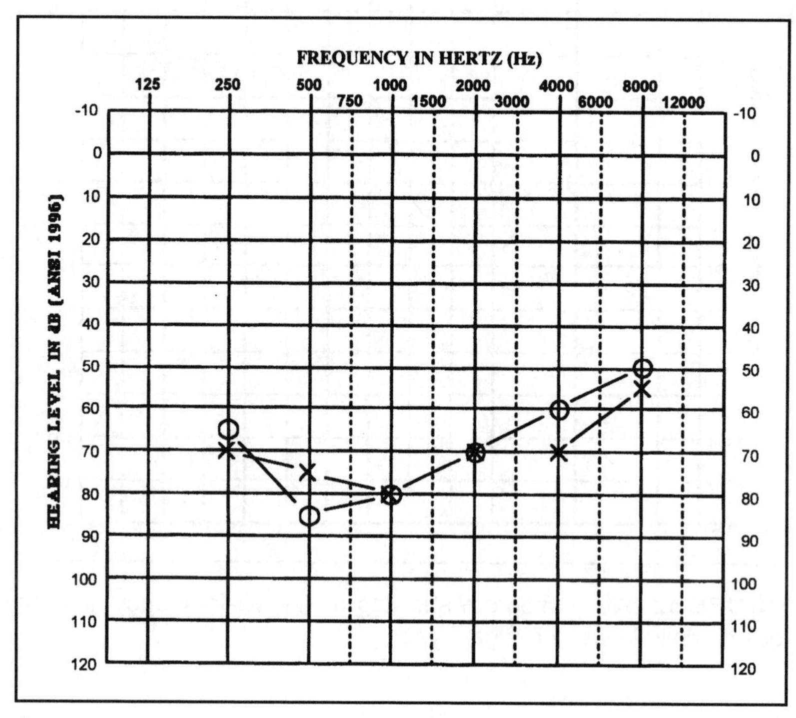

A

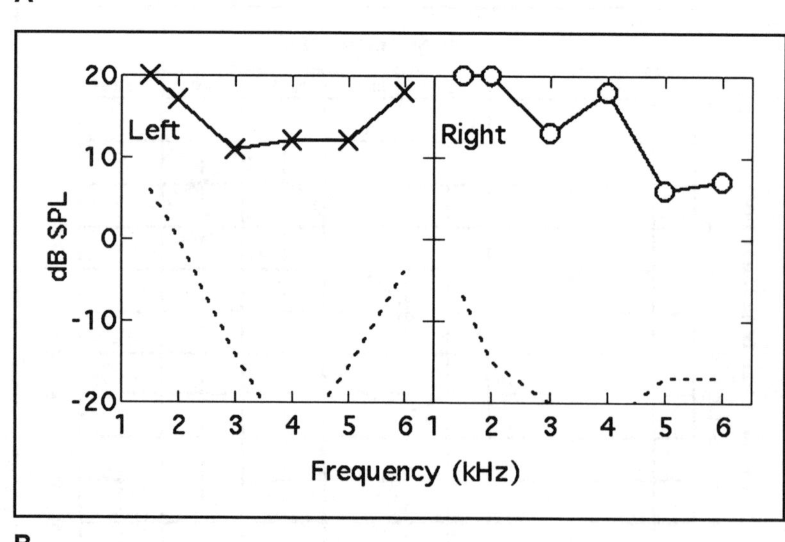

B

FIGURE 12–14. A. Audiogram showing severe hearing loss for child in Case 5 (age 11 years). **B.** Present OAEs for child in Case 5.

Conclusion

The disorder described as ANSD is more complicated than originally thought, and the patient population is more heterogeneous. Early recommendations were often based on findings in adults with other peripheral neuropathies. Hearing aids, cochlear implants, and other management strategies were both promoted and discouraged based on minimal evidence. There is now a considerable body of clinical evidence that indicates some children with ANSD are good candidates for amplification, but others obtain greater benefit from cochlear implantation. With either technology, a child's performance might differ from that expected in children with cochlear hearing loss, and in some cases neither strategy provides sufficient benefit. There is a growing body of literature, but the available evidence to guide clinical management of ANSD remains limited and more research is needed, especially with infants and young children. Considering the likelihood of varied etiologies, sites of lesion, age of identification, and risks of cognitive/developmental delays, it is unlikely that a single management strategy will apply to all infants and young children who present with this profile of audiologic findings. As with other types of sensorineural hearing loss, a continuum of multidisciplinary care is needed to provide optimal management of infants and children with ANSD.

References

American Academy of Audiology (AAA; 2013). *Clinical practice guidelines: Pediatric amplification.* Retrieved from http://galster.net/wp-content/uploads/2013/07/AAA-2013-Pediatric-Amp-Guidelines.pdf

American Academy of Pediatrics, Joint Committee on Infant Hearing (JCIH; 2007). Year 2007 position statement: Principles and guidelines for early hearing detection and intervention programs. *Pediatrics, 120*(4), 898–921. doi:10.1542/peds.2007-2333

Bagatto, M., & Scollie, S. D. (2014). *Ontario infant hearing program protocol for the provision of amplification.* Retrieved from http://www.mountsinai.on.ca/care/infant-hearing-program/documents/ihp_amplification-protocol_nov_2014_final-aoda.pdf

Berlin, C. I. (1996). Hearing aids: Only for hearing impaired patients with abnormal otoacoustic emissions. In C. I. Berlin (Ed.), *Hair cells and hearing aids.* San Diego, CA: Singular.

Berlin, C. I. (1999). Auditory neuropathy: Using OAEs and ABRs from screening to management. *Seminars in Hearing, 20,* 307–315.

Berlin, C. I., Hood, L. J., Morlet, T., Wilensky, D., St John, P., Montgomery, E., & Thibodaux, M. (2005). Absent or elevated middle ear muscle reflexes in the presence of normal otoacoustic emissions: A universal finding in 136 cases of auditory neuropathy/dys-synchrony. *Journal of the American Academy of Audiology, 16*(8), 546–553.

Berlin, C. I., Morlet, T., & Hood, L. J. (2003). Auditory neuropathy/dyssynchrony: Its diagnosis and management. *Pediatric Clinics of North America, 50*(2), 331–340, vii–viii.

Breneman, A. I., Gifford, R. H., & Dejong, M. D. (2012). Cochlear implantation in children with auditory neuropathy spectrum disorder: Long-term outcomes. *Journal of the American Academy of Audiology, 23*(1), 5–17. doi:10.3766/jaaa.23.1.2.

Buchman, C. A., Roush, P. A., Teagle, H. F., Brown, C. J., Zdanski, C. J., & Grose, J. H. (2006). Auditory neuropathy characteristics in children with cochlear nerve deficiency. *Ear and Hearing, 27*(4), 399–408. doi:10.1097/01.aud.0000224100.30525.ab

Buss, E., Labadie, R. F., Brown, C. J., Gross, A. J., Grose, J. H., & Pillsbury, H. C. (2002). Outcome of cochlear implantation in pediatric auditory neuropathy. *Otology and Neurotology, 23*(3), 328–332.

Ching, T. Y., Day, J., Dillon, H., Gardner-Berry, K., Hou, S., Seeto, M., . . . Zhang, V. (2013). Impact of the presence of auditory neuropathy spectrum disorder (ANSD) on outcomes of children. *International Journal of Audiology, 52*(S2), S55–S62. doi:10.3109/14992027.2013.796532

Cone-Wesson, B., Rance, G., & Sininger, Y. (2001). Amplification and rehabilitation strategies for patients with auditory neuropathy. In Y. Sininger & A. Starr (Eds.), *Auditory neuropathy: A new perspective on hearing disorders* (pp. 233–249). San Diego, CA: Singular Thomson Learning.

Deltenre, P., Mansbach, A. L., Bozet, C., Christiaens, F., Barthelemy, P., Paulissen, D., & Renglet, T. (1999). Auditory neuropathy with preserved cochlear microphonics and secondary loss of otoacoustic emissions. *Audiology, 38*(4), 187–195.

Dowley, A. C., Whitehouse, W. P., Mason, S. M., Cope, Y., Grant, J., & Gibbin, K. P. (2009). Auditory neuropathy: Unexpectedly common in a screened newborn population. *Developmental Medicine and Child Neurology, 51*(8), 642–646. doi:10.1111/j.1469-8749.2009.03298.x

Eisenberg, L. S., Johnson, K. C., & Martinez, A. S. (2005). Clinical assessment of speech perception for infants and toddlers. *Audiology Online,* 2005. Retrieved from http://www.audiologyonline.com/articles/pf_article_detail.asp?article_id=1443

Gravel, J. S., & Stapells, D. R. (1993). Behavioral, electrophysiologic, and otoacoustic measures from a child with auditory processing dysfunction: Case report. *Journal of the American Academy of Audiology, 4*(6), 412–419.

Guidelines Development Conference on the Identification and Management of Infants with Auditory Neuropathy. (2008, June). International Newborn Hearing Screening Conference, Como, Italy. Retrieved from http://www.childrenscolorado.org/health-professionals/clinical-resources/auditory-neuropathy-spectrum-disorder-guidelines

Haskins, H. (1949). *A phonetically balanced test of speech discrimination for children* (Unpublished master's thesis). Evanston, IL: Northwestern University.

He, S., Grose, J. H., Teagle, H. F., Woodard, J., Park, L. R., Hatch, D. R., . . . Buchman, C. A. (2015). Acoustically evoked auditory change complex in children with auditory neuropathy spectrum disorder: A potential objective tool for identifying cochlear implant candidates. *Ear and Hearing, 36*(3), 289–301.

He, S., Teagle, H. F. B., Roush, P., Grose, J. H., & Buchman, C. A. (2013). Objective hearing threshold estimation in children with auditory neuropathy spectrum disorder. *Laryngoscope, 123*(11), 2859–2861.

Humphriss, R., Hall, A., Maddocks, J., Macleod, J., Sawaya, K., & Midgley, E. (2013). Does cochlear implantation improve speech recognition in children with auditory neuropathy spectrum disorder? A systematic review. *International Journal of Audiology, 52*(7), 442–454. doi:10.3109/14992027.2013.786190

Kirk, K. I., Pisoni, D. B., & Osberger, M. J. (1995). Lexical effects on spoken word recognition by pediatric cochlear implant users. *Ear and Hearing, 16*(5), 470–481.

Kirk, K. I., Pisoni, D. B., Sommers, M. S., Young, M., & Evanson, C. (1995). New directions for assessing speech perception in persons with sensory aids. *Annals of Otology, Rhinology and Laryngology, 166*(Suppl.), 300–303.

Kovach, M. J., Lin, J. P., Boyadjiev, S., Campbell, K., Mazzeo, L., Herman, K., . . . Kimonis, V. E. (1999). A unique point mutation in the PMP22 gene is associated with Charcot-Marie-Tooth disease and deafness. *American Journal of Human Genetics, 64*(6), 1580–1593.

Kraus, N., Bradlow, A. R., Cheatham, M. A., Cunningham, J., King, C. D., Koch, D. B., . . . Wright, B. A. (2000). Consequences of neural asynchrony: A case of auditory neuropathy. *Journal of the Association for Research in Otolaryngology, 1*(1), 33–45.

Madden, C., Rutter, M., Hilbert, L., Greinwald, J. H., Jr., & Choo, D. I. (2002). Clinical and audiological features in auditory neuropathy. *Archives of Otolaryngology-Head and Neck Surgery, 128*(9), 1026–1030.

Mafong, D. D., Shin, E. J., & Lalwani, A. K. (2002). Use of laboratory evaluation and radiologic imaging in the diagnostic evaluation of children with sensorineural hearing loss. *Laryngoscope, 112*(1), 1–7. doi:10.1097/00005537200201000-00001

Margolis, R. H., Bass-Ringdahl, S., Hanks, W. D., Holte, L., & Zapala, D. A. (2003). Tympanometry in newborn infants —1 kHz norms. *Journal of the American Academy of Audiology, 14*(7), 383–392.

Mason, J. C., De Michele, A., Stevens, C., Ruth, R. A., & Hashisaki, G. T. (2003). Cochlear implantation in patients with auditory neuropathy of varied etiologies. *Laryngoscope, 113*(1), 45–49. doi:10.1097/00005537-200301000000009

Miyamoto, R. T., Kirk, K. I., Renshaw, J., & Hussain, D. (1999). Cochlear implantation in auditory neuropathy. *Laryngoscope, 109*(2 Pt. 1), 181–185.

Moog, J. S., & Geers, A. E. (2003). Epilogue: Major findings, conclusions and implications for deaf education. *Ear and Hearing, 24*(1 Suppl.) 121S–125S. doi:10.1097/01.AUD.0000052759.62354.9F

Narne, V. K., & Vanaja, C. S. (2008). Speech identification and cortical potentials in individuals with auditory neuropathy. *Behavioral and Brain Functions, 4*(15), 1–8.

Pearce, W., Golding, M., & Dillon, H. (2007). Cortical auditory evoked potentials in the assessment of auditory neuropathy: Two case studies. *Journal of the American Academy of Audiology, 18*(5), 380–390.

Psarommatis, I., Riga, M., Douros, K., Koltsidopoulos, P., Douniadakis, D., Kapetanakis, I., & Apostolopoulos, N. (2006). Transient infantile auditory neuropathy and its clinical implications. *International Journal of Pediatric Otorhinolaryngology, 70*(9), 1629–1637. doi:10.1016/j.ijporl.2006.05.005

Rance, G. (2005). Auditory neuropathy/dys-synchrony and its perceptual consequences. *Trends in Amplification, 9*(1), 1–43.

Rance, G., & Barker, E. J. (2008). Speech perception in children with auditory neuropathy/dyssynchrony managed with either hearing AIDS or cochlear implants. *Otology and Neurotology, 29*(2), 179–182. doi:10.1097/ mao.0b013e31815e92fd

Rance, G., Barker, E., Mok, M., Dowell, R., Rincon, A., & Garratt, R. (2007). Speech perception in noise for children with auditory neuropathy/dys-synchrony type hearing loss. *Ear and Hearing, 28*(3), 351–360. doi:10.1097/AUD.0b013e3180479404

Rance, G., Barker, E. J., Sarant, J. Z., & Ching, T. Y. (2007). Receptive language and speech production in children with auditory neuropathy/dyssynchrony type hearing loss. *Ear and Hearing, 28*(5), 694–702. doi:10.1097/AUD.0b013e31812f71de

Rance, G., Beer, D. E., Cone-Wesson, B., Shepherd, R. K., Dowell, R. C., King, A. M., . . . Clark, G. M. (1999). Clinical findings for a group of infants and young children with auditory neuropathy. *Ear and Hearing, 20*(3), 238–252.

Rance, G., Cone-Wesson, B., Wunderlich, J., & Dowell, R. (2002). Speech perception and cortical event related potentials in children with auditory neuropathy. *Ear and Hearing, 23*(3), 239–253.

Rance, G., McKay, C., & Grayden, D. (2004). Perceptual characterization of children with auditory neuropathy. *Ear and Hearing, 25*(1), 34–46. doi:10.1097/01.AUD.0000111259.59690.B8

Rance, G., Roper, R., Symons, L., Moody, L. J., Poulis, C., Dourlay, M., & Kelly, T. (2005). Hearing threshold estimation in infants using auditory steady-state responses. *Journal of the American Academy of Audiology, 16*(5), 291–300.

Rapin, I., & Gravel, J. (2003). "Auditory neuropathy": Physiologic and pathologic evidence calls for more diagnostic specificity. *International Journal of Pediatric Otorhinolaryngology, 67*(7), 707–728.

Rapin, I., & Gravel, J. S. (2006). Auditory neuropathy: A biologically inappropriate label unless acoustic nerve involvement is documented. *Journal of the American Academy of Audiology, 17*(2), 147–150.

Raveh, E., Buller, N., Badrana, O., & Attias, J. (2007). Auditory neuropathy: Clinical characteristics and therapeutic approach. *American Journal of Otolaryngology*, *28*(5), 302–308. doi:10.1016/j.amjoto.2006.09.006

Rea, P. A., & Gibson, W. P. (2003). Evidence for surviving outer hair cell function in congenitally deaf ears. *Laryngoscope*, *113*(11), 2030–2034.

Roche, J., Huang, B., Castillo, M., Bassim, M., Adunka, O., & Buchman, C. (2010). Imaging characteristics in children with auditory neuropathy spectrum disorder. *Otology and Neurotology*, *31*(5), 780–788.

Roush, P., Frymark, T., Venediktov, R., & Wang, B. (2011). Audiological management of children with auditory neuropathy spectrum disorder: A systematic review of the literature. *American Journal of Audiology*, *20*(2), 159–170.

Santarelli, R., Starr, A., Michalewski, H. J., & Arslan, E. (2008). Neural and receptor cochlear potentials obtained by transtympanic electrocochleography in auditory neuropathy. *Clinical Neurophysiology*, *119*(5), 1028–1041. doi:10.1016/j.clinph.2008.01.018

Simons, J. P., Mandell, D. L., & Arjmand, E. M. (2006). Computed tomography and magnetic resonance imaging in pediatric unilateral and asymmetric sensorineural hearing loss. *Archives of Otolaryngology-Head and Neck Surgery*, *132*(2), 186–192. doi:10.1001/archotol.132.2.186

Starr, A., McPherson, D., Patterson, J., Don, M., Luxford, W., Shannon, R., . . . Waring, M. (1991). Absence of both auditory evoked potentials and auditory percepts dependent on timing cues. *Brain*, *114*(Pt. 3), 1157–1180.

Starr, A., Michalewski, H. J., Zeng, F. G., Fujikawa-Brooks, S., Linthicum, F., Kim, C. S., . . . Keats, B. (2003). Pathology and physiology of auditory neuropathy with a novel mutation in the MPZ gene (Tyr145→Ser). *Brain*, *126*(Pt. 7), 1604–1619. doi:10.1093/brain/ awg156

Starr, A., Picton, T. W., Sininger, Y., Hood, L. J., & Berlin, C. I. (1996). Auditory neuropathy. *Brain*, *119*(Pt. 3), 741–753.

Starr, A., Sininger, Y., Nguyen, T., Michalewski, H. J., Oba, S., & Abdala, C. (2001). Cochlear receptor (microphonic and summating potentials, otoacoustic emissions) and auditory pathway (auditory brain stem potentials) activity in auditory neuropathy. *Ear and Hearing*, *22*(2), 91–99.

Starr, A., Sininger, Y. S., & Pratt, H. (2000). The varieties of auditory neuropathy. *Journal of Basic and Clinical Physiology and Pharmacology*, *11*(3), 215–230.

Teagle, H., Roush, P., Woodard, J., Hatch, D., Zdanski, C., Buss, E., & Buchman, C. (2010). Cochlear implantation in children with auditory neuropathy spectrum disorder. *Ear and Hearing*, *31*(3), 1–11.

Tsiakpini, L., Weichbold, V., Kuehn-Inacker, H., Coninx, F., D'Haese, P., & Almadin, S. (2004). *LittlEARS Auditory Questionnaire*. Innsbruck, Austria: MED-EL.

Varga, R., Avenarius, M. R., Kelley, P. M., Keats, B. J., Berlin, C. I., Hood, L. J., . . . Kimberling, W. J. (2006). OTOF mutations revealed by genetic analysis of hearing loss families including a potential temperature sensitive auditory neuropathy allele. *Journal of Medical Genetics*, *43*(7), 576–581. doi:10.1136/jmg.2005.038612

Walker, E. A., McCreery, R. W., Spratford, M., & Roush, P.A. (in press). Children with ANSD fitted with hearing aids using the AAA Pediatric Amplification Guideline: Current practice and outcomes. *Journal of the American Academy of Audiology*.

Widen, J. E. (1993). Adding objectivity to infant behavioral audiometry. *Ear and Hearing*, *14*(1), 49–57.

Widen, J. E., Folsom, R. C., Cone-Wesson, B., Carty, L., Dunnell, J. J., Koebsell, K., . . . Norton, S. J. (2000). Identification of neonatal hearing impairment: Hearing status at 8 to 12 months corrected age using a visual reinforcement audiometry protocol. *Ear and Hearing*, *21*(5), 471–487.

Wunderlich, J. L., & Cone-Wesson, B. K. (2006). Maturation of CAEP in infants and children: A review. *Hearing Research*, *212*(1–2), 212–223. doi:10.1016/j.heares.2005.11.008

Xoinis, K., Weirather, Y., Mavoori, H., Shaha, S. H., & Iwamoto, L. M. (2007). Extremely low birth weight infants are at high risk for auditory neuropathy. *Journal of Perinatology*, *27*(11), 718–723. doi:10.1038/sj.jp.7211803

Yasunaga, S., Grati, M., Cohen-Salmon, M., El-Amraoui, A., Mustapha, M., Salem, N., . . . Petit, C. (1999). A mutation in OTOF, encoding otoferlin, a FER-1-like protein, causes DFNB9, a nonsyndromic form of deafness. *Nature Genetics*, *21*(4), 363–369. doi:10.1038/7693

Zeng, F. G., & Liu, S. (2006). Speech perception in individuals with auditory neuropathy. *Journal of Speech, Language, and Hearing Research*, *49*(2), 367–380. doi:10.1044/10924388 (2006/029)

Zeng, F. G., Oba, S., Garde, S., Sininger, Y., & Starr, A. (1999). Temporal and speech processing deficits in auditory neuropathy. *NeuroReport*, *10*(16), 3429–3435.

Zimmerman-Phillips, S., Osberger, M. F., & Robbins, A. M. (1997). *Infant-Toddler: Meaningful Auditory Integration Scale (IT-MAIS)*. Sylmar, CA: Advanced Bionics.

(Central) Auditory Processing Disorders in Children

Prudence Allen

What Is Auditory Processing?

For many children, the understanding of complex sounds, particularly in difficult listening situations, is extremely difficult even though they have normal hearing sensitivity. They find it difficult to listen in noise, ignore competing signals, learn new sounds, or understand sounds that have been distorted in some way. This might lead to difficulty following orally presented directions, learning from what they hear, achieving well in school, and developing good communication skills. These children likely suffer from an auditory processing disorder.

The discussion of auditory processing disorders and the clinical evaluation and treatment of these disorders are probably some of the most controversial areas of contemporary audiology. In spite of over 50 years of research and discussion on the topic, there remains today no standard protocol for assessment or intervention. Our professional organizations have published recommendations (e.g., American Speech-Language, Hearing Association [ASHA], 1996, 2005a; British Society for Audiology [BSA], 2007; Jerger & Musiek, 2000), but the selection of clinical protocols remains under the discretion of individual clinicians. Test selection is difficult because there is no gold standard against which to evaluate the effectiveness of diagnostic tools. Most clinicians use a battery of tests for evaluation, but many of them report being unhappy with the contents of the battery (Chermak, Silva, Nye, Hasbrouck, & Musiek, 2007; Chermak, Traynham, Seikel, & Musiek, 1998; Emanuel, 2002; Noel, 2003). Rehabilitation protocols are not standardized, and a clear link between diagnostic outcomes and treatment recommendations does not exist. Yet there is nearly unanimous agreement on the existence of the problem and that the care of individuals suffering from an auditory processing disorder falls within the scope of practice of audiologists (e.g., ASHA, 2005b; BSA, 2007; Canadian Academy of Audiology [CAA], 2002).

Auditory processing is the hearing that takes place beyond the ability to sense or detect the presence of a sound. It includes the ability to perceive, interpret, and ultimately understand a sound, even when the sound is presented in less than optimal conditions. It allows a listener to recognize familiar sounds and learn new ones, to make meaningful associations between what is heard and what is known, to be selective and vigilant in listening, and to be able to monitor and understand multiple sounds at once. Familiarity and sound quality play important roles in the efficiency of auditory processing. Perceiving familiar sounds, especially in a quiet environment, is relatively effortless. Links to memory and language representations are made easily and rapidly even if signal clarity is reduced. When the signals are unfamiliar, substantially degraded, or presented in a background of noise or other competition, significantly greater processing resources and effort might be required for understanding. There is often a greater need for clear acoustic features under such conditions and as new sounds are learned. For a person with an auditory processing disorder, understanding unfamiliar sounds or those presented in noise can be very difficult, especially if his or her encoding skills are impaired. The consequences of difficulty understanding these sounds can be debilitating when the listener is a child trying to learn from what he or she hears and when much of what the child is learning includes new words that are presented in a noisy classroom.

Learning from our perceptions is a complex process. Early theories suggested that perception is constructive, that sensory experiences are impoverished, and that the mind is charged with the task of building mental representations from this impoverished information (see Gibson & Pick, 2003, for review). Children were thought to build their perceptions from their experiences, and the emphasis was not on the information from the sensory system but on that which the child brought to the experience—that is, their prior knowledge. Perception was thought to be very much a top-down, constructive process. Later theories argued that the sensory information and the environment in which it occurs are actually rich in detail and intimately linked (Gibson, 1991, 2000). During development, a child learns to perceive and appreciate a much finer level of that detail. Perception is achieved within the context of a vast array of multisensory information coming from the environment in which the perception is taking place. Therefore, to understand perceptual development and the learning that results from it, consideration must be made of the quality of the sensory encoding, of the ability to attend to and explore the information as it is encoded, of the prior experience and knowledge the individual brings to the experience, and of the environment in which the perception occurs. It is because of the intricate links between sensation, attention, and prior knowledge occurring within an environmental context that assessment of complex auditory processes is challenging.

What are the processes used by a child as perceptual ability is developed and as the (auditory) world is organized? There are several principles by which perceptual development unfolds (e.g., Goldstone, 1998). These principles are useful as we consider whether a child has the proper auditory skills to serve perceptual development. At the neural level, patterns of activation are developed and reinforced in response to frequently occurring stimuli. This allows the recognition of familiar stimuli to be rapid and resistant to degradation. It underlies auditory learning and the plasticity observed in response to auditory training and the introduction of assistive listening devices. With repeated exposure, the recognition of a stimulus is easier and quicker. The details become increasingly better perceived. As children mature, they become more adept at focusing attention on stimuli that are of interest to them and on the detail within a stimulus. Children are active and selective in their perception, and this skill improves with maturation. Because of the integration of information with that from the other senses and prior knowledge, the sensory experience strengthens such that when the stimulus occurs again, only some of the components might be necessary to bring about the perception of the entire event. This makes stimulus recognition and identification fast and efficient; thus, it is more reliable, even in the face of noise or stimulus degradation.

A stimulus will be most easily recognized or learned when it is clear. Signal clarity is governed by the quality with which it is produced, the media in which it is transmitted to the listener, and the integrity of the auditory system that receives it. A signal can lose clarity through interference from ambient noise or distortion as could occur from poor room acoustics or because the transmission medium has limited bandwidth, has reduced dynamic range, or produces harmonic distortion. The stimulus, when it is speech, can also appear to be distorted because the speaker has an unfamiliar accent, articulates poorly, or speaks at a very fast rate. Individuals with normal hearing are usually much less affected by reduced signal clarity than are individuals with auditory processing disorders. In fact, one way that audiologists traditionally test for the presence of an auditory processing disorder is to look for reduced recognition of noisy or distorted signals. Clinical tests have been developed that distort speech signals by adding noise, filtering, and time altering.

Signal clarity also will be affected by how well the auditory system of the listener receives and processes the stimulus. It is with this aspect of signal clarity that we are most concerned during clinical assessment. The processing of acoustic features generally occurs effortlessly through the responses and connections of brainstem nuclei (for a thorough review of the auditory system the reader is referred to the material available in the *Springer Handbook of Auditory Research*, e.g., Popper & Fay, 1992; Webster, Popper, & Fay, 1992). Ascending from the cochlea, which has already coded the complex spectral and temporal qualities of the stimulus, the tonotopic information is transmitted to multiple nuclei where it is further analyzed, and information about the frequency, phase, and level relations of the components is coded. For example, the cochlear nucleus codes fine structure and envelope cues, thus facilitating localization, aiding in signal-to-noise enhancement, and playing a role in pattern recognition, auditory attention, and learning. The superior olive, the first site of binaural convergence of information, codes interaural time, phase, and level differences essential for placing sounds in space. The inferior colliculus, as an obligatory relay, sees the convergence of auditory information from the lower brainstem nuclei. It also receives input from the visual, somatosensory, auditory, and motor areas of the cortex, making it a complex integrating center important for processing multisensory information, facilitating spectral coding, and sound localization. The medial geniculate body of the thalamus transmits information from the brainstem to the cortex. It is significant for its role in attention, behavioral readiness, gain control, and selective signal amplification or suppression. The medial geniculate body preserves tonotopic and binaural representation coded at lower nuclei and receives input from the superior colliculus enabling coordination of visual, motor, and acoustic representation of images in three-dimensional space. Furthermore, it aids in visual pursuit and plays a role in arousal through its links with the limbic system. At the level of the cortex, the integrated signal links to memory, and associations and meaning are determined. The auditory system is thus highly complex. As signals progress from the cochlea to the cortex, multiple aspects of their features are coded and integrated with information from other senses and from the cortex, as ecologic theories of perception suggest. What ultimately reaches the cortex is actively determined by attentive mechanisms working through the efferent system. The process of perceiving sound is rich and active. In the assessment of auditory processing disorders, we are interested in how the encoding of auditory signals takes place as a sound proceeds through the system and how encoding preserves the richness of information contained in those signals. Encoding can be evaluated through behavioral tests that measure discrimination and resolution abilities and through objective tests that measure the physiologic integrity of the neural pathways. A detailed review of auditory system anatomy and physiology as it relates to clinical pathology can be found in Musiek and Baran (2007). However, it is unlikely that with auditory processing disorders we will see a strong relationship between auditory skills and a specific locus within the central nervous system. Consideration of how the auditory system processes information should serve as a guide in how to think about auditory evaluation and what abilities are important, not as a way to determine a site of lesion. There is not a simple link between behavioral deficiencies and processing at specific levels of the auditory system.

Stimulus Encoding: Discrimination and Resolution of Acoustic Features

As with any audiologic assessment, one of the first areas to be examined is *detection*. It is critical to know what sounds are and are not audible. Assessment of detection typically includes the estimation of thresholds at octave intervals between 250 and 8000 Hz. Most children suspected of having disorders of auditory processing have normal pure-tone thresholds in this range. High-frequency thresholds (above 8000 Hz) can be used to evaluate the effects of ototoxic drugs, noise, and other conditions (e.g., Goldstein, Shulman, & Kisiel, 1987), but thresholds in this range have not been studied in children with auditory processing disorders (APDs), and the contribution of high-frequency hearing to auditory function is not well understood. It has been suggested that adults with poor high-frequency thresholds report more difficulty hearing in noise than do individuals with good high-frequency hearing (Liddell, Campbell, DePlacido, Owens, & Wolters, 2007), but whether the reduced high-frequency thresholds cause the difficulty hearing in noise or are comorbid is not clear. Although it is important that audibility be evaluated prior to any central auditory assessment, the presence of a peripheral hearing loss should not preclude an assessment of central auditory abilities if the child experiences difficulties that seem incommensurate with the degree of hearing loss.

Beyond the ability to detect signals, it is important to know how well stimulus features are discriminated or resolved. Discrimination of acoustic features can be measured by evaluating the smallest difference that can be perceived in an acoustic dimension. This is usually done by asking a listener to compare successively presented stimuli that vary in only one acoustic dimension. Resolution of features within a complex sound is slightly more complicated but also can be measured through discrimination tasks.

The minimum discriminable differences for frequency, level, and duration vary with the base value of the stimulus and with the age of the listener. In the region where the ear is most sensitive, the 1000 to 4000 Hz range, and at a comfortable listening level, adults generally are able to perceive frequency differences of about 1 to 2% (Sek & Moore, 1995), level differences of less than 1 dB for signals above 40 dB HL (Florentine, Buus, & Mason, 1987), and durational increments of 15 ms for a 100-ms signal (e.g., Abel, 1972). Young, normal-hearing children show improvements in basic discrimination abilities throughout the first few years of life, but large individual differences are seen (e.g., Jensen & Neff, 1993; Maxon & Hochberg, 1982). Improvements in the discrimination of intensity differences are fairly rapid with the discrimination of frequency and duration lagging behind and continuing to show variability into the school-aged years.

Poor *basic discrimination ability* has been observed in children with specific language impairment (Hill,

Hogben, & Bishop, 2005), auditory neuropathy (Zeng, Oba, Garde, Sininger, & Starr, 1999), and cortical damage (Thompson & Abel, 1992). Preliminary data from our laboratory with children suspected of having auditory processing disorders suggest they might require much larger differences for discrimination of simple features than normally developing children of the same age. Frequency and discrimination data from these individual children are shown by the filled diamonds in Figures 13–1 and 13–2, respectively. Open squares show data from normally developing children averaged within age groups (Jensen & Neff, 1993). Error bars show ±1 standard deviation. Note the large variability in the clinical group. Many children perform at age-expected levels, but many perform more like younger normally developing children or worse. Unfortunately, there are as yet no clinical procedures available for estimating frequency or intensity discrimination thresholds.

Most natural sounds are perceived as temporally changing spectral patterns. It is not the absolute energy at any one frequency that predicts a sound's identity, but the relative distribution of energy across frequencies, the spectral shape, and how it changes over the signal duration that is important. Green (1988) suggests that even simple tasks such as intensity increment detection are likely perceived by analysis of spectral content within, not between, sounds.

Spectral resolution can be investigated using a variety of psychometric procedures. Two common ways include evaluation of psychoacoustic tuning curves (Zwicker & Fastl, 1999) and estimates of detection thresholds in flat and notched-spectrum noises (Patterson, 1976). These measures tend to reflect the integrity of the auditory periphery, specifically the function of the basilar membrane mechanics and outer hair cells. Both give an estimate of auditory filter bandwidth and efficiency. Bandwidth reflects the sharpness of tuning

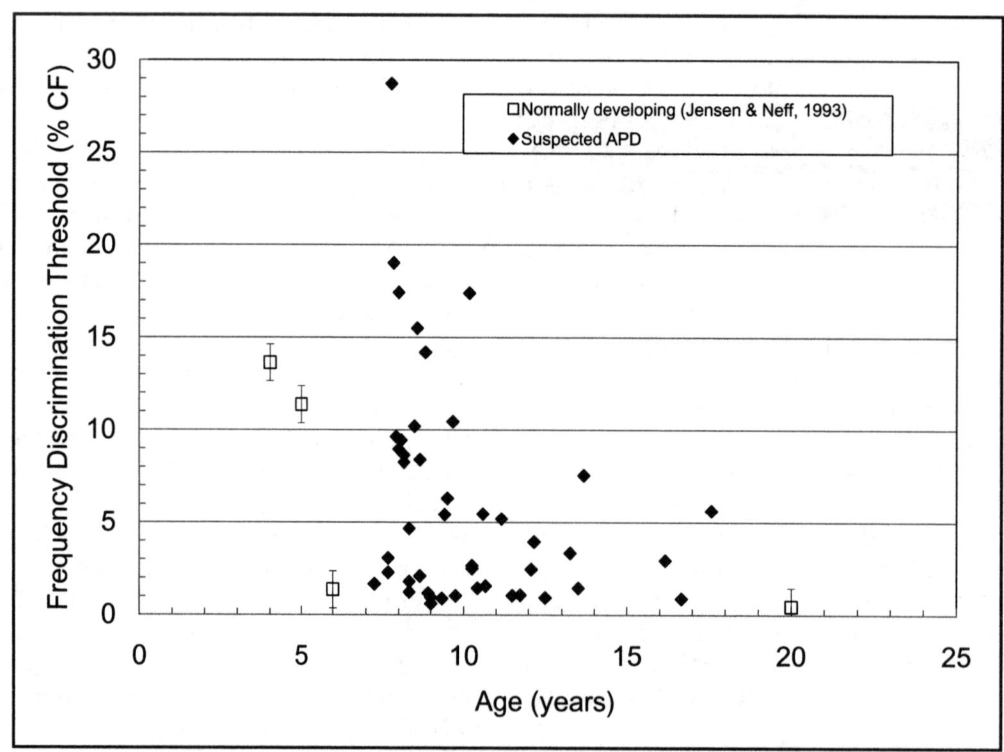

FIGURE 13–1. The frequency discrimination thresholds in normally developing children and in those suspected of having an auditory processing disorder. Open squares show averaged thresholds obtained from normal hearing preschool-aged children for a base frequency of 440 Hz (Jensen & Neff, 1993). Error bars show ±1 standard deviation. Filled diamonds show *individual* data obtained from children seen in our laboratory for auditory processing disorder (APD) assessment. Note the large variability in the performance of the children in the clinical sample. Many of the children performed at adultlike levels but many did not, performing consistent with younger children or much worse.

arising from basilar membrane mechanics and outer hair cell function, and efficiency reflects the signal-to-noise ratio at which detection occurs arising from a variety of likely more central factors. Psychoacoustic tuning curves are measured by presenting a tonal signal at near-threshold levels and measuring threshold shifts in the presence of narrowband noise maskers placed slightly above or below the signal. As the frequency of the masker moves away from the signal, more masker energy is required to eliminate signal audibility. The rate at which thresholds improve as the masker moves spectrally away from the signal can be used to estimate the tuning characteristics of the inner ear. Data from infants suggest that frequency resolution matures fairly rapidly, although efficiency remains immature for a prolonged period (Olsho, 1985). Data obtained from notched-noise masking procedures show a more protracted period of immaturity in frequency resolution extending through the preschool-aged years (Allen, Wightman, Kistler, & Dolan, 1989). With this procedure, the listener is asked to detect a signal in a broadband noise masker. A spectral notch is then placed in the masker around the signal frequency. The presence of the notch should improve audibility of the signal. The amount of improvement is thought to reflect the tuning characteristics of the periphery. Greater improvement reflects sharper tuning.

Figure 13–3, panel A, shows frequency resolution data obtained using the notched-noise masking procedure. Diamonds show data from the suspected APD population seen in our laboratory, and squares show data of normal-developing children from Allen et al. (1989). Filled symbols show threshold estimates in a flat spectrum masker, and open symbols show thresholds estimated in the presence of a notched spectrum masker. Panel B shows threshold differences (flat versus notched noise thresholds). Averaged data from normally developing preschool-aged children are shown by the open squares (Allen et al., 1989), and filled diamonds show individual data from the suspected APD population.

As Figure 13–3, panel A shows, with increasing age, thresholds for both conditions improve but the effect is more dramatic for the notched-noise masking

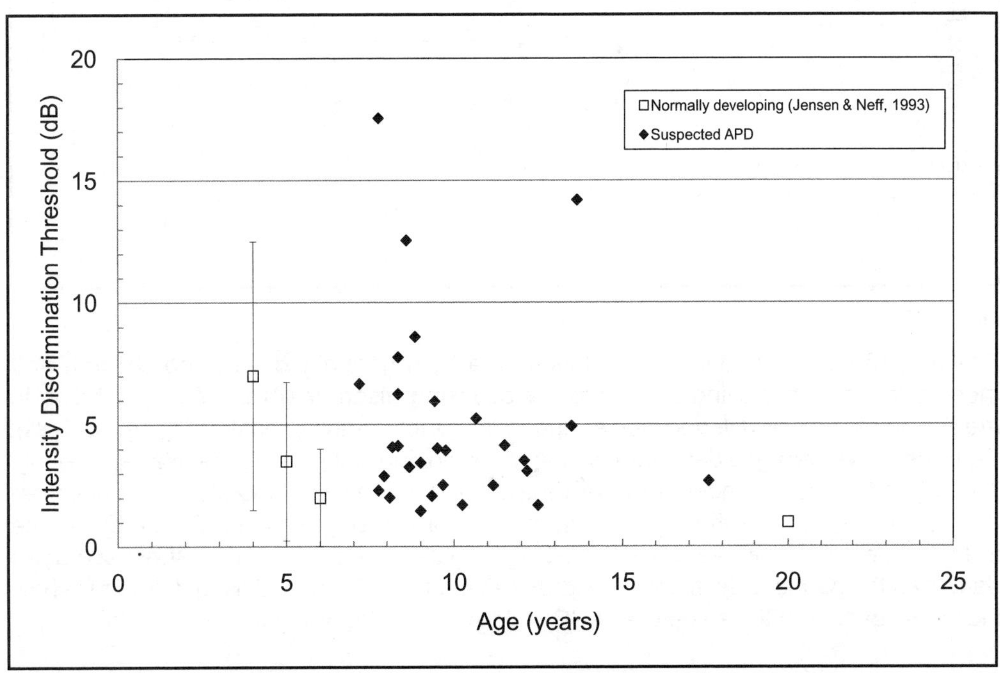

FIGURE 13–2. The intensity discrimination thresholds in normally developing children and in those suspected of having an auditory processing disorder (APD). Open squares show data from 4- to 6-year-old children, detecting an increment in a 440-Hz pure tone (Jensen & Neff, 1993). Error bars show one standard deviation. Filled diamonds show *individual* data from a group of children referred for testing for suspected APDs. Note the large variability in performance with some children performing at close to age-appropriate levels and some performing very poorly or consistent with the performance of younger children.

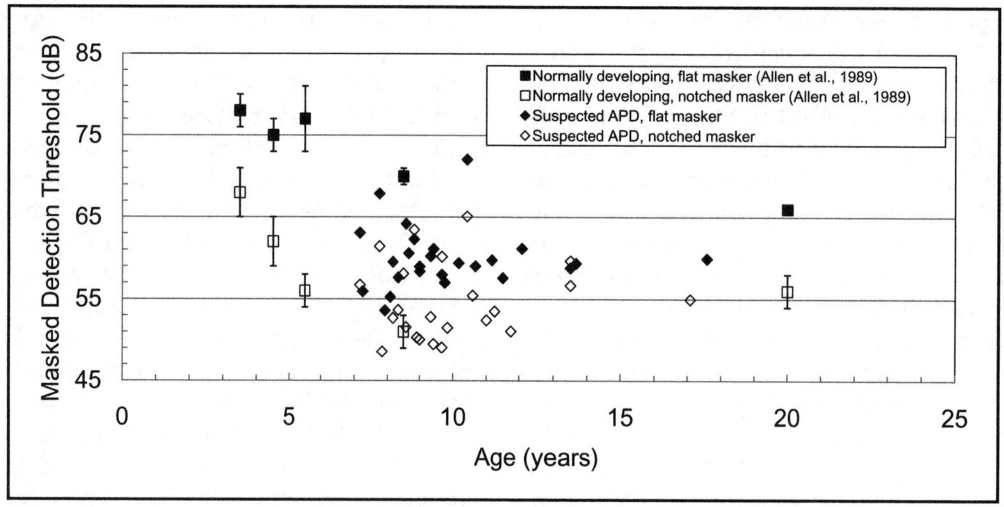

A

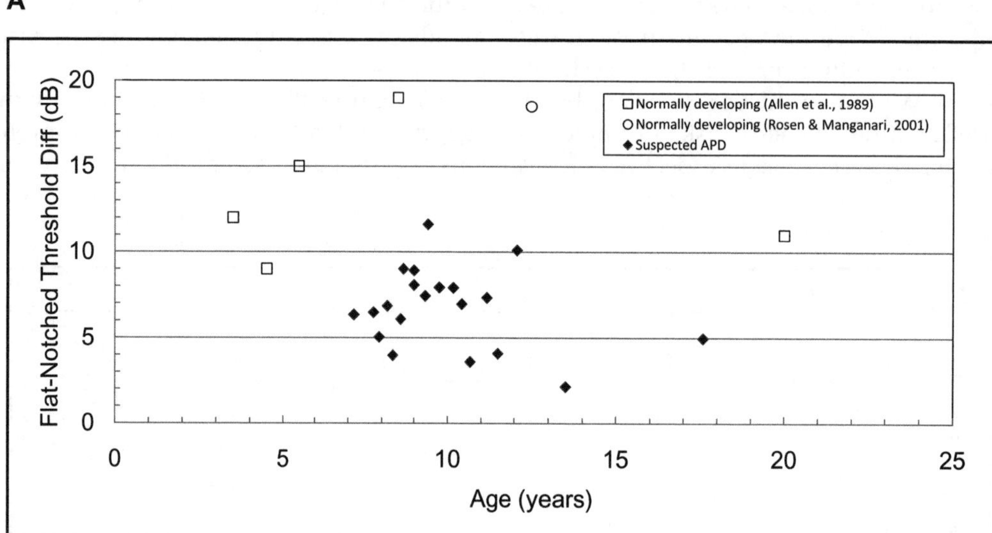

B

FIGURE 13–3. The frequency resolution data from normally developing children and those suspected of having an auditory processing disorder (APD). **A.** Thresholds in the flat noise masker (*filled symbols*) and in the notched-noise masker (*open symbols*). Squares show averaged data from normally developing children at 2000 Hz (Allen et al., 1989) Filled diamonds show *individual* data at 1000 Hz from our laboratory obtained from children suspected of suffering from an auditory processing disorder. **B.** The difference in thresholds in the flat versus notched noise masker. Open squares show averaged data from the normally developing children (Allen et al., 1989), and filled diamonds show individual data from the suspected APD children in our laboratory.

condition, suggesting a greater amount of frequency selective listening in the older subjects. For the children with suspected APD, there is a trend for better thresholds in the notched noise masker than in the flat noise. However, as can be seen in panel B, the difference in two thresholds is in many cases smaller than for younger children, possibly suggesting reduced frequency resolution. This procedure has not been used extensively with clinical populations. However, Rosen and Manganari (2001) reported adultlike frequency resolution data using the notched-noise procedure with a group of children with reading problems. Because thresholds in these masking conditions for younger children can be affected by attentional factors including the acoustic cues to which the child attends (Allen & Korpela, 1999), additional research using other procedures might be warranted before the APD data are interpreted. However, it remains that this clinical population, for whatever reason, does seem to do more poorly on this task than normally developing children. *Temporal resolution* has been studied extensively owing to the perceived importance to speech perception of the ability to perceive rapid changes in a stimulus. It is most frequently measured via gap detection thresholds. In this procedure, listeners are asked to discriminate between brief duration signals (usually noise samples) that are either continuous or that have a temporal gap in them. The ability to detect a gap of various durations is measured. A broadband background noise is usually presented to limit any cues provided by spectral splatter resulting from the sharp rise and fall times around the gap.

Normal hearing adults can, with practice, generally discriminate temporal gaps of less than 2 ms at higher frequencies. Children up to 6 years require much longer gaps for the same level of detection accuracy as adults (Irwin, Ball, Kay, Stillman, & Rosser, 1985; Wightman, Allen, Dolan, Kistler, & Jamieson, 1989). There is not only a change in gap detection threshold with age, but also a reduction in the variability between subjects.

Many individuals with auditory and learning disorders have been studied using gap detection tasks. Poor performance has been shown in children who have difficulties with reading or language (e.g., Wright et al., 1997), and in adults with auditory neuropathy spectrum disorders (ANSD; Zeng et al., 1999). Data from children with APDs seen in our laboratory also show larger gap detection thresholds as can be seen in the filled diamonds of Figure 13–4. Also shown are averaged data from groups of normally developing children from three different studies (Davis & McCroskey, 1980; Irwin et al., 1985; Wightman et al., 1989). Note the large developmental trend in performance and the large between-subject differences in the children with suspected APD. Many children perform at or

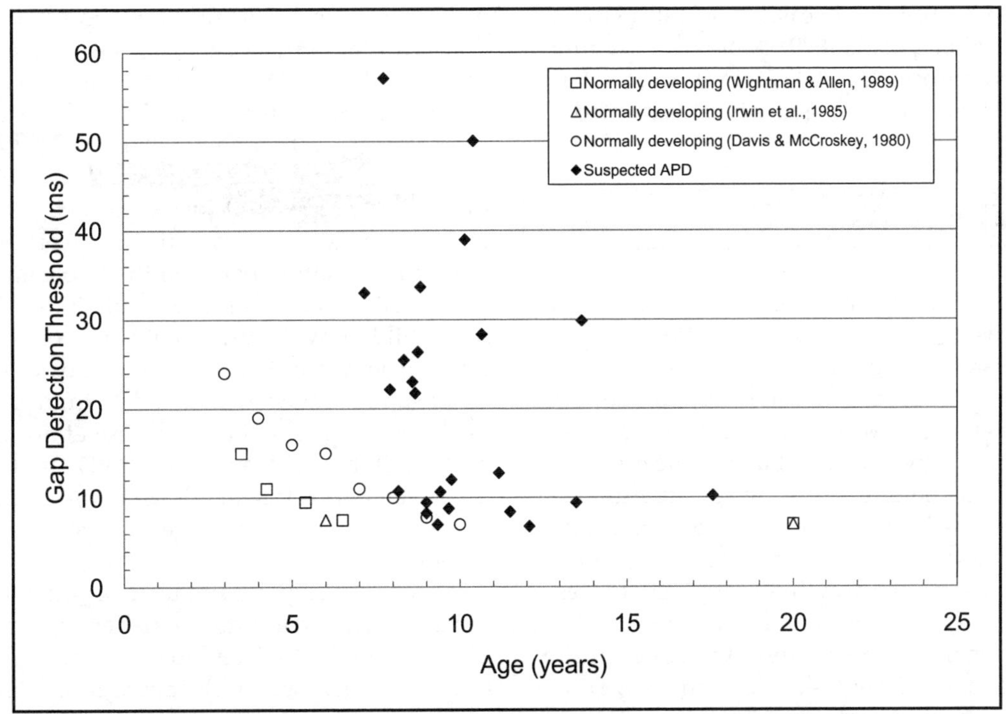

FIGURE 13–4. The gap detection thresholds in normally developing children and those who are suspected of having an auditory processing disorder (APD). Open symbols show averaged data from normally developing children. Open squares show data from Wightman et al. (1989) made using a 2000-Hz signal. Open triangles show data from Irwin et al. (1985). Open circles show data from Davis and McCroskey (1980). Filled diamonds show *individual* thresholds at 1000 Hz from children seen in our laboratory. Many of the children show thresholds falling with age-expected ranges, but many do not.

near age-appropriate levels, but many perform much more poorly, suggesting temporal processing deficits.

Because of the perceived importance of temporal resolution in speech processing, several tests of temporal resolution are available clinically, most assessing gap detection thresholds. These include, for example, the Auditory Fusion Test–Revised (McCroskey & Keith, 1996), the Random Gap Detection Test (Keith, 2000), the Gaps-in-Noise Test (Musiek et al., 2005), and the Adaptive Test of Temporal Resolution (Lister, Roberts, Shackelford, & Rogers, 2006).

Temporal resolution is likely a much more complex construct than is exemplified in a simple gap detection threshold estimate. Other measures that assess the ability of the auditory system to code sounds rapidly in time include nonsimultaneous masking (e.g., forward and backward masking) and estimation of the temporal modulation transfer function. Nonsimultaneous masking procedures have suggested abnormal temporal processing in children with language impairments (e.g., Marler, Champlin, & Gillam, 2002; Wright et al., 1997) and reading disorders (Rosen & Manganari, 2001). Abnormal temporal modulation transfer functions have been observed in cases of ANSD (Kumar & Jayaram 2005; Zeng et al., 1999). More data examining these temporal processing abilities in children referred for auditory processing assessment are warranted.

Binaural Processing

Once auditory features are encoded at each ear, the information is combined to form a single image. This allows the listener to place the sound in space creating a three-dimensional listening environment and facilitating the separation of real-world sound sources. There are many ways to study binaural hearing in the laboratory, and the effect of hearing impairment on performance has been of interest among researchers for some time (see Durlach, Thompson, & Colburn, 1981). Some assess the way interaural differences in time and level are perceived and how they affect perceived position or loudness. These studies can be done using headphones. Other tasks assess the way sounds are perceived in three-dimensional environments, asking listeners to discriminate between positions, detect perceived motion in a sound source, identify the sound source location, or perceive signals presented in noise that is spatially segregated from the signal. These free field studies take into account the frequency- and location-dependent spectral changes that occur as a result of the outer ear resonance. These cues can be modeled to create simulated three-dimensional sensations under headphones. The spectral transforms are the head-related transfer functions (HRTFs). Although a great deal is now known about how the adult auditory system functions in a binaural environment, somewhat less is known about children's capabilities (see Litovsky & Ashmead, 1997) and how children with auditory processing disorders perform.

Most of what is currently possible in clinic is done under headphones. One method through which we can gain clinical information on how the binaural system functions is through estimation of the masking level difference (MLD). In this procedure the threshold for the detection of a binaural signal is estimated in the presence of a binaural masker. The signal can be speech or low-frequency pure tones. The masker is noise. Threshold is measured when the signal and masker are presented in phase at the two ears (S_0N_0) and when either the signal ($S_\pi N0$), or the masker ($S_0N\pi$), is 180 degrees out of phase at the two ears. Thresholds can improve 10 to 15 dB with a shift in the binaural phase of the signal or the masker.

Developmentally, the MLD to speech stimuli has been shown to be adultlike in preschool-aged children (Nozza, 1987; Nozza, Wagener, & Crandell, 1988), whereas the MLD elicited to narrow-band stimuli showed a developmental trend until the age of 5 to 6 years (Grose, Hall, & Dev, 1997). The MLD in children with auditory processing disorders has been reported to be somewhat reduced (Sweetow & Reddell, 1978), possibly suggesting difficulties in the binaural integration of information between the two ears at the level of the brainstem (Olsen & Noffsinger, 1976). Data from children with suspected APD seen in our laboratory are shown in the filled diamonds of Figure 13–5. Open squares show averaged data from groups of normally developing children (Grose et al., 1997). Many of the children with suspected APD children show an improvement of thresholds when the signal is out of phase at the two ears suggesting good MLDs, others do not.

More recently, studies have begun to test children in simulated three-dimensional environments. In the Listening in Spatialized Noise-Sentence Test (LISN-S; Cameron & Dillon, 2008), speech reception thresholds are measured in the presence of competing noise that can be spatially separated from the signal allowing an estimate of the binaural advantage. The test creates a spatial perception through the use of head-related transfer functions and allows a perceived separation of speech and noise sources. Preliminary work with children having APDs suggests this procedure can be useful in measuring a child's ability to benefit from bin-

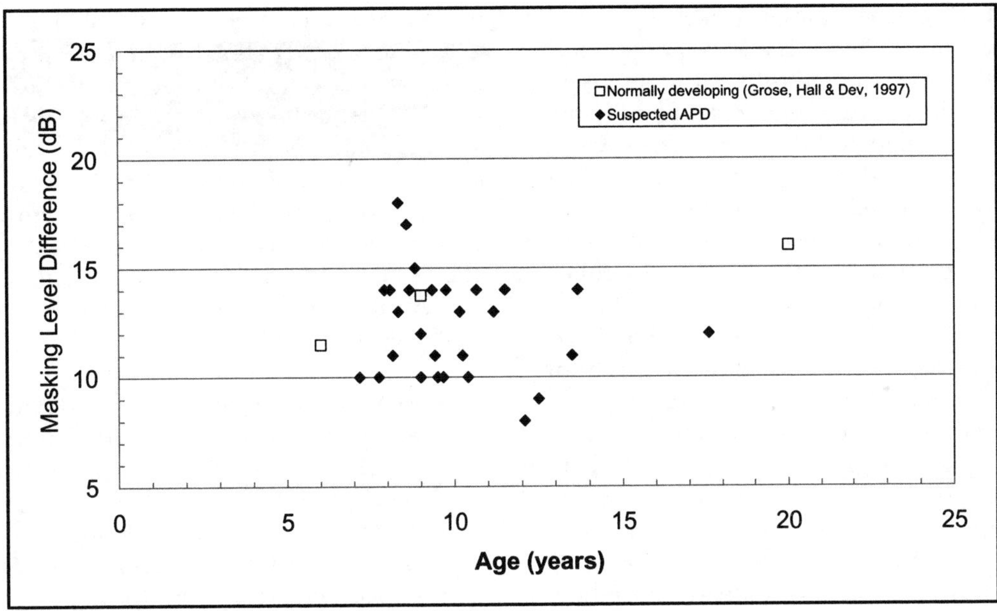

FIGURE 13–5. The average masking level differences for normally developing children in the open symbols (Grose, Hall, & Dev, 1997) and individual thresholds for children with suspected auditory processing disorders (APDs) in the filled diamonds.

aural cues in the perception of speech in noise and has shown that many children with APD fail to derive a binaural advantage.

Binaural integration has also been measured through the presentation of speech signals that are spectrally or temporally split between the two ears. In the test of binaural fusion (Matzker, 1959), a speech signal is filtered into two narrow frequency bands. A low-pass band, 500 to 800 Hz, is presented to one , and a high-pass band, 1815 to 2500 Hz, is presented to the other. Each band when presented alone does not permit good recognition of the signal. However, when both bands are presented, one to each ear, the signal is much more readily identified if the binaural system is intact. With central auditory processing disorders, specifically those originating in the brainstem, performance is reduced (Smith & Resnick, 1972). Recently, it has been shown that younger children require slightly wider frequency bands for the same level of speech recognition accuracy as adults, but that their ability to integrate the information from the two bands is similar to that of adults (Mlot, Buus, & Hall, 2010). Improvement in binaural fusion continues into the early school-aged years (Stollman, van Velzen, Simkens, Snik, & van den Broek, 2004). The speech stream can also be temporally split between the two ears using alternating segments (Bocca & Calearo, 1953). In the test of rapidly alternating speech perception (RASP; Willeford, 1976a), the speech signal is rapidly alternated between the two ears, often at a rate of 300 ms. The information arriving to one ear alone is unintelligible, but when both streams are presented to the intact system, the speech is easily understood. Adults with auditory processing deficits sometimes performed very poorly on these tests (e.g., Lynn & Gilroy, 1977; Musiek, 1983), and this is taken to suggest underlying difficulty at the level of the brainstem (Musiek & Geurking, 1982). Binaural fusion tests are available for clinical use through Auditec of St. Louis, although their use is falling out of favor as their sensitivity in detecting disorders is questionable.

Once signals reach the auditory cortex they can be recognized, and associations between what is heard and what is known can be made. Making these associations has a strong language and cognitive component. It is for this reason that central auditory evaluation should include a team of professionals and should include a pediatric speech-language specialist. There are numerous excellent tools available for assessing the phonologic and semantic aspects of hearing, the complete review of which is outside the scope of this chapter. Consultation with a qualified speech-language pathologist is an invaluable tool in APD assessments.

The discrimination and resolution skills discussed so far are meant to provide a representative, though not exhaustive, sample of encoding abilities that can be used to assess (central) auditory function. With recent advances in testing capabilities, it is likely that psychophysical procedures will become an important part of our diagnostic battery in the future. Interpreting the results will require a greater understanding of normal variability and developmental changes. The advantage of these procedures is that they use nonspeech signals that are easily calibrated and useful regardless of the child's first language. The procedures require relatively minimal language skills and therefore are useful even in cases of language problems. However, it should be noted that individual differences are common in complex listening tasks, and particularly so when children and clinical populations are tested. These differences most likely reflect characteristics of the listener, not error in the measurement. In some children, performance on a discrimination task, such as that described in these sections, can vary with their attention and motivation. In a study of masked detection thresholds, for example, Allen and Wightman (1994) showed individual differences in psychometric functions that persisted across conditions and over several months. Approximately one third of the preschool-aged children produced data with adultlike psychometric function slopes but elevated thresholds, one third showed poor thresholds and shallower slopes, and the final third showed variability between conditions and between repetitions (Allen & Wightman, 1994). Similar results were reported by Moore and colleagues in a study of discrimination learning. In the examination of performance changes over time they found that children were likely to fall into one of three general categories, those with consistently good performance, those with consistently poor performance, and those who showed more variability with a tendency to do well initially and more poorly thereafter, possibly because of lost motivation over time (Moore, Ferguson, Halliday, & Riley, 2007). It also has been suggested that a child with an untreated attention disorder might do poorly on an auditory discrimination task, suggesting, perhaps falsely, the existence of a hearing-related disorder (e.g., Sutcliffe, Bishop, Houghton, & Taylor, 2006). Because attention and motivation can affect performance, it is important that in any psychophysical measurement of performance, repeated measures be taken, especially when performance is not at age expectations.

Auditory Attention: Listening as an Active Process

Normal-hearing individuals generally are able to choose to what they will listen, at what level of detail, and for what duration. The ability to hear and understand signals in the presence of noise, the ability to concentrate on auditory information for extended periods, the ability to attend to multiple sources of information, and to switch attention quickly and efficiently between sources are important aspects of how individuals hear and listen. These abilities are frequently reported areas of difficulty for individuals suffering from auditory processing disorders. We cannot evaluate complex hearing abilities without consideration of auditory attention.

What is attention? According to William James (1890, reprinted in 1966),

> Everyone knows what attention is. It is the taking of possession by the mind, in clear and vivid form, of one out of what seem several simultaneously possible objects or trains of thought. Focalization and concentration of consciousness are of its essence. It implies withdrawal from some things in order to deal effectively with others. (p. 5)

What causes a stimulus to take our attention? Familiar signals often do so, such as when we hear someone call out our name. Very strong signals or components of signals will also capture our attention, as will unusual or unexpected signals. Once something has taken our attention, how well can we sustain it over time, and can we explore it with an increasing level of detail? Can we continue to focus on something of interest and with what ease and for how long? Can we focus on multiple items simultaneously? What causes us to lose our attention? How distractible are we and under what circumstances? Regardless of how well an auditory signal is encoded, the ability to listen to it can be greatly influenced by our auditory attention abilities. As such, auditory attention has occupied a major place in central auditory assessment. Auditory attention includes the ability to attend intentionally to a signal or portion of a signal in the presence of another stimulus (selective attention), the ability to monitor multiple messages and to switch between them at will (divided attention and executive control), and the ability to maintain focus on an auditory signal of interest (sustained attention).

Selective Attention

Signals of interest in everyday life are seldom presented in isolation. Instead, we are most often asked to attend to signals in the presence of irrelevant signals that are considered to be noise or competition, largely because we deem them to be of no or lesser importance than the signal of interest. Similarly, we sometimes wish to listen to more detail in a signal, an important aspect of perceptual learning. Our ability to attend to the signal of interest, or a portion of that signal, is termed *selective* or *focused attention*. When noise interferes with the perception of the signal of interest, it is deemed to be distracting, especially when there is unlikely to be peripheral masking from spectral or temporal overlap. Technologies that require a listener to repeat words as soon as they are heard (shadowing), retain the content of a message in the presence of competition, and avoid distraction (or intrusions) from a competing source suggest that auditory selective attention matures throughout the school-aged years (Davies, Jones, & Taylor, 1984).

One method used to study auditory selective auditory attention is the probe-tone method (Greenburg & Larkin, 1968). In this procedure, a listener is led to expect a signal of a given frequency. On a random, small portion of the trials, the signal frequency is different. Highly selective attention would allow a listener to detect the expected signal very well, but detection of the unexpected signal would be less reliable as attention is focused on the expected signal frequency. If the listener is not listening selectively but using a broader auditory filter, the expected and unexpected signals would be perceived with equal proficiency. Very young children appear to listen broadly and not in a frequency selective manner (Allen, Spencer, & Eskritt, 2001). It is not until school age that children listen with good frequency selectivity (Greenburg, Bray, & Beasley, 1970). Listening in a frequency selective manner can also be evaluated using a distraction paradigm. In this procedure, a signal at an off-frequency is presented simultaneously with a signal at an expected frequency. Frequency selective listening would eliminate any influence of the off-frequency distracter. As with attention band studies, distracter procedures also show that young children do not listen selectively. They are less able to "filter out" distraction, and detection accuracy for a signal that is otherwise readily detectable suffers in the presence of a distracter (Allen & Wightman, 1995; Bargones & Werner, 1994).

Direct measures of attention typically are not part of an audiologic battery, but some tests are included that indirectly assess selective attention. These include auditory figure ground tasks. In these tasks, recognition of a signal, usually speech, is measured in the presence of a masker, which might be broadband noise, multitalker babble, or continuous discourse. The disruption that occurs, which cannot be attributed to simple masking of the signal (limiting audibility of some or all of the components), is called *informational masking*. Tests of auditory figure ground for which the signal and masker are presented in the same ear include the Speech Perception in Noise (SPIN; Kalikow, Stevens, & Elliott, 1977), the Speech-in-Noise Test (Quick-SIN; Killion, Niquette, Gudmundsen, Revit, & Banerjee, 2004), the Hearing-in-Noise Test (HINT; Nilsson, Soli, & Sullivan, 1994), the Synthetic Sentence Identification with Ipsilaterally Competing Message (SSI-ICM; Speaks & Jerger, 1965), the Auditory Figure Ground subtest of the Screening Test for Auditory Processing Disorders for Children (SCAN-C; Keith, 2002), the Selective Attention Test of the Goldman-FristoeWookcock Auditory Skills Test Battery (GFW; Goldman, Fristoe, & Woodcock, 1970), an optional subtest on the Test of Auditory Processing Skills (TAPS-3; Martin & Brownell, 2005), the Words in Ipsilateral Competition test (WIC; Ivey, 1987), and the Selective Auditory Attention Test (SAAT; Cherry, 1980).

Selective attention also can be assessed with the noise masker presented to the opposite ear. For example, the Pediatric Speech Intelligibility test presents word and sentence length material to the listener with competition that can be presented in the contralateral as well as the ipsilateral ear (PSI; Jerger, 1987). Poor performance on these various tests of auditory figure-ground perception is frequently observed in children with auditory processing disorders.

Divided Attention

Hearing in the natural world is dichotic. That is, there are slight differences in the phase, level, time of arrival, and spectral shape of a signal arriving at the two ears. This is in contrast to diotic stimulation in which both ears receive identical stimuli. Dichotic listening has occupied a central position in central auditory assessments for over 50 years. Early dichotic listening work originated in the development of filter theories of attention (e.g., Broadbent, 1958; Cherry, 1958) that postulated that the system had a limited capacity for processing information requiring a filter that could switch between the various available stimulus inputs. In these studies, the stimuli in the two ears are very different (e.g., different consonant-vowel pairs, digits, words, or sentences). The application to auditory processing disorders began with the work of Kimura (1961) who used dichotic consonant–vowel stimuli to study processing in individuals with brain lesions. She noted that patients with cortical lesions had difficulty perceiving the syllable presented in the ear contralateral to the lesion but did well with that presented to the ipsilateral ear. Since then, many tests of dichotic listening have gained popularity in clinical use. These include, for example, the Staggered Spondaic Word Test (Katz, 1962), which uses dichotic spondees tested in both noncompeting and competing conditions, dichotic consonant vowel syllables (Berlin, Hughes, Lowe-Bell, & Berlin, 1973), and digits (Musiek, 1983). These tasks require stimuli in both ears to be reported. Children with APD show large reductions in dichotic listening tests.

Sustained Attention

Another important aspect of attention is the ability to attend consistently over time. This aspect is less frequently tested in the clinic but might be important in children with auditory processing disorders. The question is whether children have problems simply attending to auditory information or if they cease to attend to information that is hard to understand (as would be the case if auditory processing were reduced). Most tasks that assess sustained attention require the individual to detect or identify signals in a very boring task that lasts for an extended period of time. Identification accuracy over time in these vigilance tasks is taken as an estimate of sustained attention ability. Studies using vigilance procedures suggest that performance improves during the early school years (see Davies et al., 1984). Sustained attention can also be studied by measuring how long a listener or observer will focus on a stimulus at will. Studies with infants have shown that inspection of an unfamiliar visual stimulus is longer than for a familiar one (Richards, 2004). This suggests that the ability to sustain attention at will is an important element of perceptual processing.

Some common tests of auditory attention that assess sustained and selective listening include the Auditory Continuous Performance Test (ACPT; Keith, 1994), and the Test of Everyday Attention for Children (TEA-Ch; Manly, Robertson, Anderson, & Nimmo-Smith, 1998). The ACPT asks a child to listen to words over a 10-minute period and indicate when a target word occurs. The TEA-Ch has nine subtests that evaluate auditory and visual attention in simple and complex tasks, some of which are timed. It tests not only selective and sustained attention but also the extent to which a child can regulate his or her attention, switching between tasks and inhibiting responses. Performance across the subtests is different for individuals with a primary attention disorder (e.g., attention deficit disorder [ADD], attention deficit hyperactivity disorder [ADHD]) and those with traumatic brain injury (TBI). The TBI pattern shows general depression across all subtests examining selective and sustained attention as well as executive control. Interestingly, most children in our laboratory suspected to have an APD perform similarly to those with TBI, showing general depression across all subtests. Upper, middle, and lower panels of Figure 13–6 show individual composite scores on subtests examining sustained, selective attention, and executive control, respectively. Note that many children fall more than one standard deviation below expectations.

Note on Behavioral Indicators of Attention Disorders and Auditory Processing Deficits

Clinical identification of ADD is made by addressing behavioral manifestations as indicated by the *DSM-IV* (American Psychiatric Association, 2000). The indicators identify behavioral symptoms of inattention or hyperactivity-impulsivity. The presence of these symptoms is evaluated within the context of onset, severity, and persistence before a diagnosis is made. One tool that is often used to delineate problem behaviors consistent with an attentional disorder and the *DSM-IV* classification criteria is the Conners' Rating Scales–Revised (Conners, 2000). Interestingly, some of these behaviors are very like those used to describe children with auditory processing disorders (e.g., fails to give close attention to detail, difficulty sustaining attention, does not seem to listen to what is being said, and gets distracted when given instructions to do something). It also is interesting that when children meeting the diagnostic classification for inattention or impulsivity are evaluated on cognitive tests that assess these constructs, the correlations are not convincing, the performance is not predictable, and the performance deficits are not unique to children thought to suffer from attention disorders but are also seen in other clinical populations (see Swanson, Casey, Nigg, Castellanos, Volkow, & Taylor, 2004). This speaks to the importance of attention to most cognitive and learning abilities, including auditory processing.

Neural Integrity of the Auditory System Pathways

The ability of a listener to perceive subtle differences between sounds and hear the detail in complex sounds and attend to them will be a function of the underlying neurobiology of the auditory periphery and central mechanisms. Assessment of the neural integrity of the auditory pathways is therefore important in confirming the possible origins of the behavioral difficulties, in

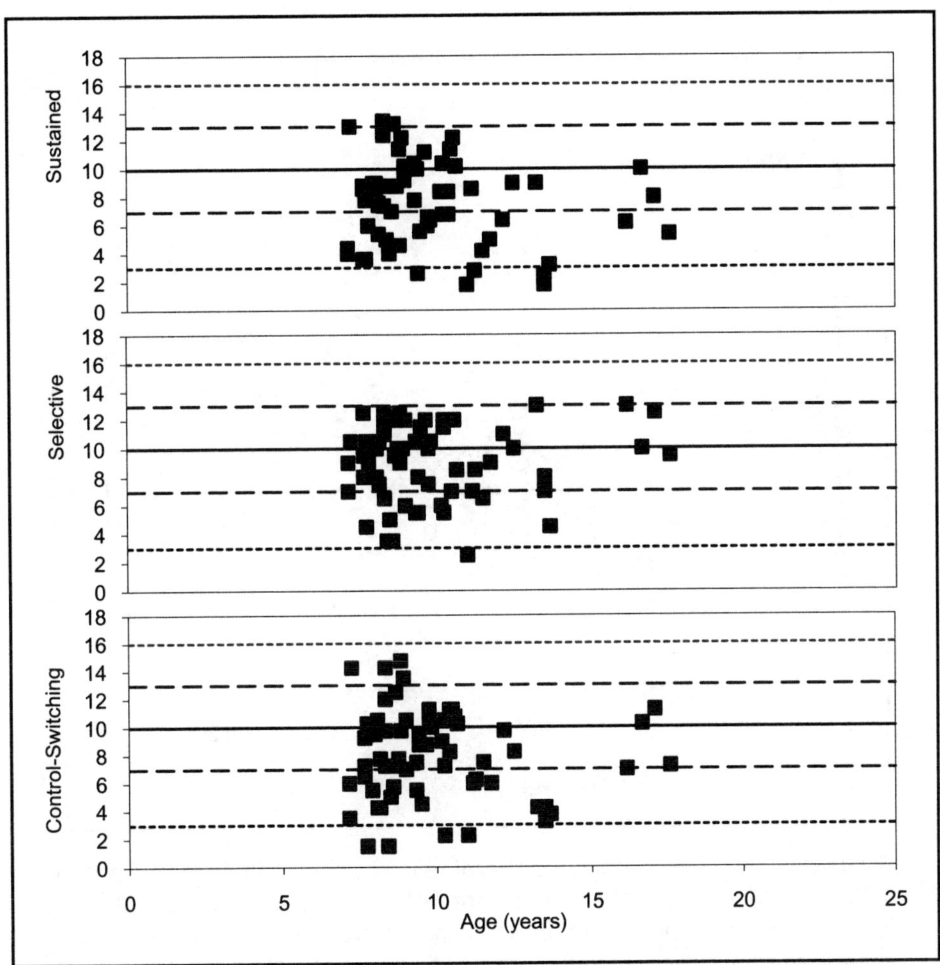

FIGURE 13–6. The composite scores on TEA-Ch (Manly et al., 1998) subtests measuring sustained (*top*), selective (*middle*), and execute control (*lower*) in our group of children with suspected auditory processing disorder (APD). Note that performance often falls one or more standard deviations below expectations on all types of attention.

predicting difficulties in young children or others who might not be able to perform behavioral tasks, and in advancing earlier diagnoses of potential problems. For a more thorough review of how objective techniques can be used to assess auditory system integrity, the reader is referred to Chapters 20 through 22 of this text. This section reviews only some areas of objective testing that can be particularly useful in assessing central auditory integrity.

Because of the significant encoding that takes place in the cochlea and brainstem pathways, it is important to conduct a thorough evaluation of the integrity of these structures. One useful measure is the acoustic reflex threshold, particularly when ipsilaterally and contralaterally stimulated and measured reflexes are compared. Elevated or absent reflexes can be seen in cases of disruption of low brainstem pathways. When ipsilateral reflexes are intact but contralateral reflexes are abnormal, it is an indication of pathology in the intra-axial brainstem, whereas a pattern of abnormalities both ipsilaterally and contralaterally more often are associated with extra-axial lesions (Jerger & Jerger, 1975, 1977). Although reflex abnormalities are common in cases of confirmed lesions, they have been reported to be less so in cases of suspected APD (Jerger, Johnson, & Loiselle, 1988). However, in our laboratory, we have observed a large proportion of the children showing abnormal crossed reflexes in the presence of normal ipsilateral responses. Figure 13–7 shows data from the children with suspected APD seen in our laboratory

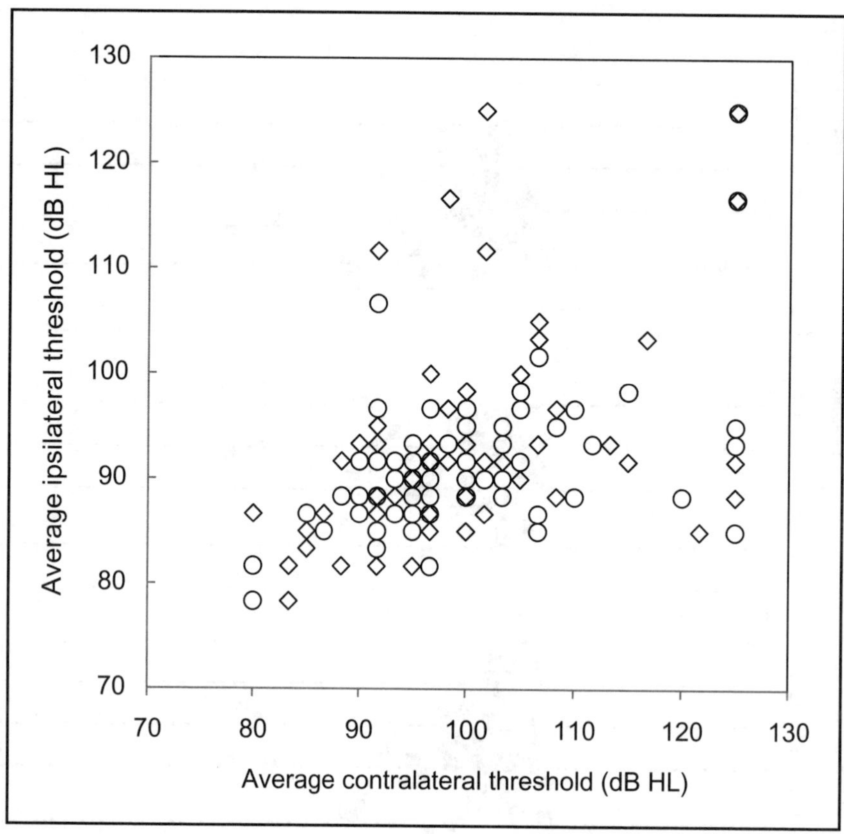

FIGURE 13–7. The average ipsilateral reflex threshold for 500, 1000, and 2000 Hz plotted against the same three frequency average for reflexes elicited with contralateral stimulation. Diamonds and circles represent data for left and right ear stimulation, respectively. Each data point represents data from one child. (Reprinted with permission from Allen and Allan, 2007, Figure 2. Copyright 2007 Phonak AG.)

(Allen & Allan, 2007). Average reflexes at 500, 1000, and 2000 Hz stimulated and recorded ipsilaterally are plotted against the average at those same frequencies stimulated in one ear and recorded in the contrateral ear. Individual data for right and left ears are shown by the circles and diamonds, respectively. Note the large numbers of children for whom ipsilateral thresholds are elicited at normal levels but contralateral responses are not. These children also tend to do quite poorly on clinical tests of central auditory processing disorders, suggesting a possible link between efferent system dysfunction and APD.

Another excellent measure of auditory brainstem integrity is the auditory brainstem response (ABR). Although auditory processing disorders are believed to be diffuse, in locus with peripheral function likely to be normal (e.g., Hood, 2007), we have observed a large number of abnormal ABRs in children referred for central auditory testing. This suggests poor neural integrity of the auditory nerve and brainstem in at least a portion of the children suffering from these disorders (Allen & Allan, 2007). Abnormalities include poor replicability, missing waves, low V/I amplitude ratios, and delayed latencies. Figure 13–8 shows ABR Wave V latencies in a group of children with suspected APD seen in our laboratory. Symbols show individual Wave V latencies from right and left ears plotted for both slow and fast repetition rates. Several of the children show latencies more than two standard deviations beyond expectations even at a slow repetition rate with rate dependent abnormalities common. Figure 13–9 shows sample waveforms from two of the children (Allen & Allan, 2007). The top panel shows responses with prolonged Wave V latencies and low V/I amplitude ratios.

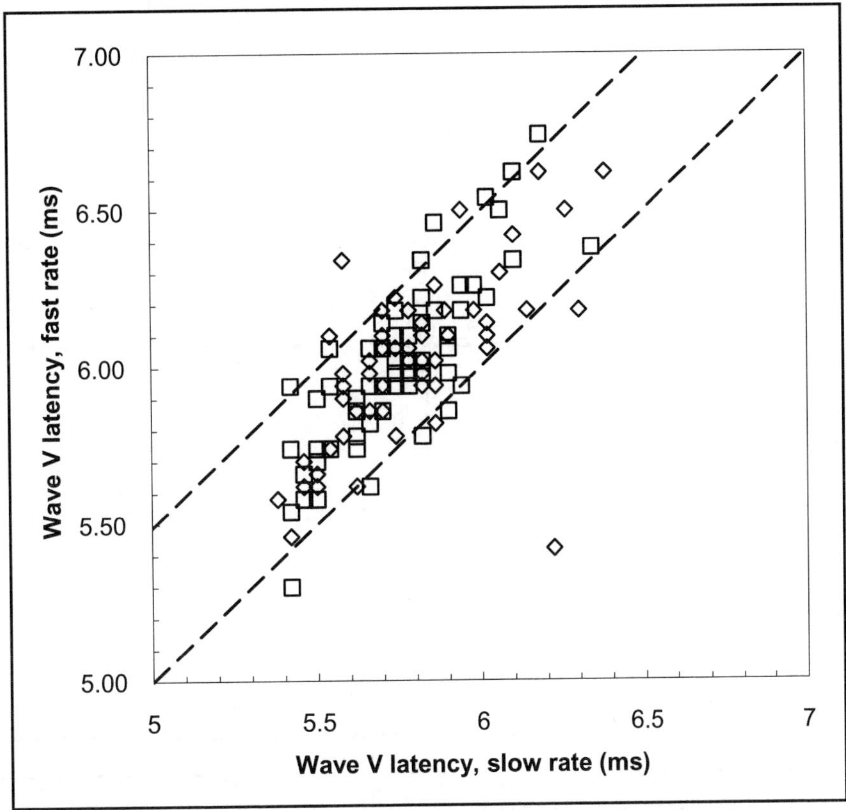

FIGURE 13–8. Wave V ABR latencies for individual children elicited to click stimuli at a faster repetition rate (57.7/s) plotted against Wave V latencies measured for a slower stimulation rate (11.1–31.1/s). Data for left and right ears are shown by diamonds and squares, respectively. (Reprinted with permission from Allen and Allan, 2007, Figure 4. Copyright 2007 Phonak AG.)

The bottom panel shows responses with only Wave V present and at a delayed latency. These results suggest that the neural integrity of the ABR can be reduced in children with APD. For a more detailed description of these two children and their other test results, see Allen and Allan (2007).

The auditory steady-state response (ASSR) can be one of the more useful potentials for evaluating neural correlates to suprathreshold hearing processes. The ASSR is an evoked response to stimuli that are frequency or amplitude modulated. The response is evaluated in the frequency domain rather than in the time domain. It has been used to estimate psychophysical tuning curves (Markessis et al., 2009), temporal acuity (Purcell et al., 2004), and complex stimuli such as speech (e.g., Aiken & Picton, 2006; Banai, Abrams, & Kraus, 2007; Dimitrijevic, John, van Roon, & Picton, 2001). It might prove to be a very useful tool for the clinical estimation of such processing skills in young children or those who cannot complete behavioral testing. To date, there is still only a small amount of data on children with suspected auditory problems and these potentials.

Integrity of the binaural pathways can also be measured using the ABR. The Binaural Interaction Component (Dobie & Berlin, 1979; Dobie & Norton, 1980) is obtained through a subtractive technique comparing the summed responses to monaural stimulation with the response elicited from binaural stimulation. A small negative going potential in the 7 to 9 ms range likely reflects the binaural activity in the brainstem (Polyakov & Pratt, 1994). A binaural response also occurs in the 20 to 40-ms range when evaluating middle latency responses (Berlin, Hood, & Allen, 1984). Neither procedure has enjoyed widespread clinical use,

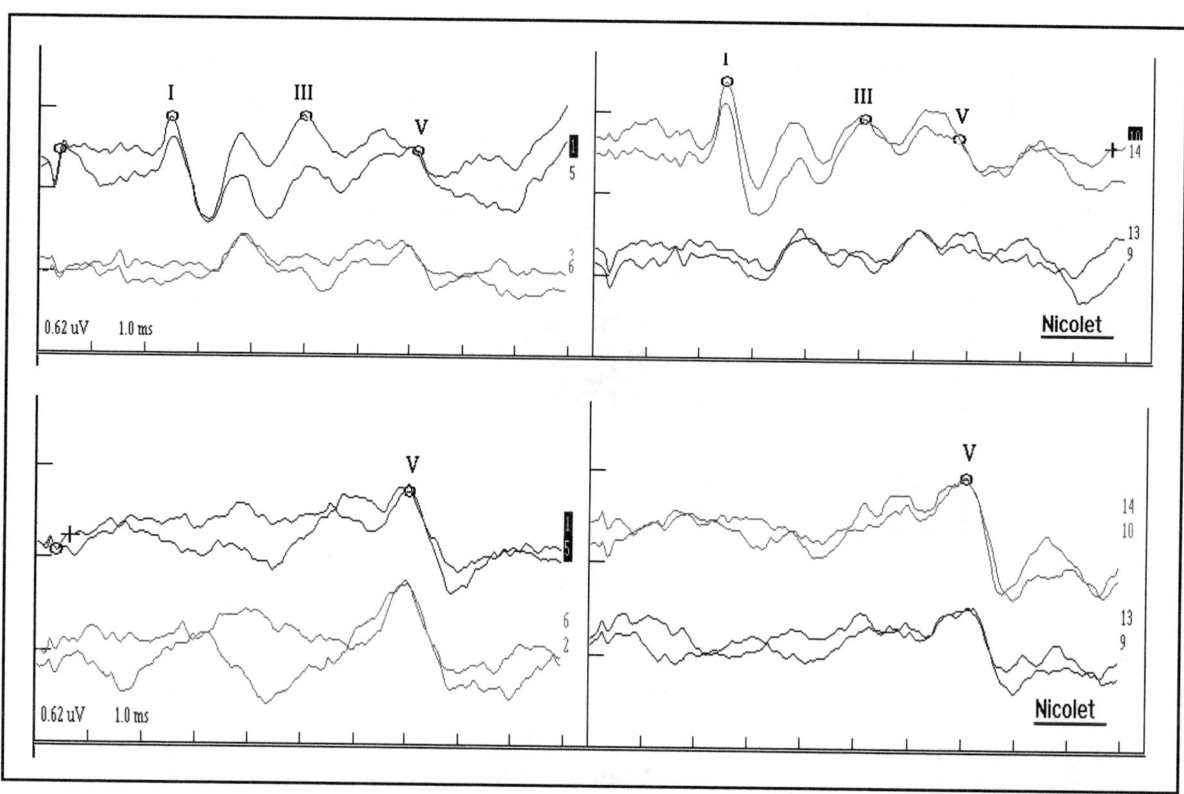

FIGURE 13–9. Auditory brainstem responses for two children with suspected auditory processing disorders seen at our laboratory. Left-most panels show left ear stimulation; right panels show right ear stimulation. Upper and lower traces show ipsilateral and contralateral recordings, respectively. *Top:* Auditory brainstem responses for subject CAFH show slightly delayed Wave III (4.18 ms and 4.10 ms for right and left ears, respectively) and V (5.94 ms and 6.27 ms for right and left ears, respectively) latencies producing a prolongated I–III and I–V interwave interval. The amplitude of Wave V relative to Wave I is also quite low. *Bottom:* Auditory brainstem testing with subject CACN using a slow rate of stimulation (27.7/s) shows significantly abnormal responses. Waves I–III are missing, and Wave V is significantly delayed in latency (6.18 ms bilaterally). (Reprinted with permission from Allen and Allan, 2007, Figures 12 and 13. Copyright 2007 Phonak AG.)

although there is a strong potential for yielding data on the integrity of the binaural auditory system. For example, reduced amplitudes of the binaural interaction component of the brainstem have been observed in children with suspected APD when compared to those of age-matched normal-hearing children (Delb, Strauss, Hohenberg, Plinkert, & Delb, 2003; Gopal & Pierel, 1999). The ASSR can also be useful in the evaluation of binaural processing (Schwarz & Taylor, 2005). Because we know that damage to higher auditory centers, such as the cortex, also has been known to produce abnormal discrimination abilities, it is important to examine auditory potentials evoked primarily from these regions. The middle and late evoked potentials are candidates for this analysis. Also, there have been several studies examining discrimination correlates in the cortex via event related potentials, most notably the P300 response, for which an infrequent stimulus is presented in a train of more frequent stimuli. The response to the different stimulus, when compared to the expected stimuli, can give an indication of discrimination for that change. Due to its variability between subjects, the P300 has not enjoyed a great deal of success in clinical application. The mismatch negativity response (Näätänen, Gaillard, & Mantysalo, 1978) is a cortical-evoked potential that might have some applicability to auditory attention as it appears to represent a preattentive response to discrimination. The potential is measured using an oddball paradigm in which an odd stimulus is interspersed in a train of expected stimuli. The response to this odd stimulus represents neural activity occurring prior to discrimination. It is measured using subtractive techniques, but like the P300, clinical use has been limited due to high between- and within-subject variability.

Professional Practice

ASHA, the American Academy of Audiology (AAA), and the BSA have published position papers on Auditory Processing Disorders (ASHA, 1996, 2005a; BSA, 2007; Jerger & Musiek, 2000). The Canadian professional associations are in the process of preparing a statement. It is clear from these initiatives that the associations are trying to meet the needs of their members in providing rigorous, evidenced-based solutions to the understanding, diagnosis, and treatment of hearing disorders that fall beyond sensitivity losses.

The documents from ASHA are noteworthy for their excellent review of scientific and professional issues surrounding auditory processing and its disorders as well as their treatment of clinical issues. ASHA suggests that central auditory processing refers to the "perceptual processing of auditory information in the CNS and the neurobiological activity that underlies that processing . . . " (ASHA, 1996, p. 145). It involves those mechanism that underlie "sound localization and lateralization, auditory discrimination, auditory pattern recognition, temporal aspects of audition including temporal integration, temporal discrimination, temporal ordering, and temporal masking; auditory performance in competing acoustic signals (including dichotic listening); and auditory performance decrements with degraded acoustic signals" (ASHA, 2005a, p. 2). A disorder is deemed to be present when there is an observed deficiency in any of these areas. Similarly, the BSA (2007) acknowledges the neural underpinnings of APD in their statement that an APD "results from impaired neural function and is characterized by poor recognition, discrimination, separation, grouping, localization, or ordering of nonspeech sounds" (p. 1). Their statement acknowledges that an APD might impact on speech sounds but that the label of APD should be applied only when nonspeech sound perception is impaired, in an attempt to avoid confusing language-based problems from those that arise from auditory processing deficits. The presenting problems of APD noted include "understanding when listening to speech, reading, remembering instructions or staying focussed while listening" (p. 3). The test battery approach is universally recommended for assessment although the specific tests are not named and the categories of tests are somewhat varied across recommendations. For some categories (e.g., localization and lateralization, basic discrimination), there are few tests commercially available. It generally is accepted that an evaluation begins with a thorough case history and information, and it is also important to obtain a description of the problem the child is experiencing. Issues such as understanding speech in difficult listening situations or noise, problems understanding and receiving auditory information, problems with auditory attention, and difficulties learning songs, reading, and spelling must be determined. A good way to get at these issues is through the use of behavioral checklists and questionnaires. These can help delineate the types of situations in which the child experiences difficulty and can guide the assessment protocol. Possible checklists include, for example, the Children's Auditory Performance Scale (CHAPS; Smoski, Brunt, & Tannahill, 1992), the Fisher Auditory Problems Checklist (Fisher, 1976), or the Screening Identification for Targeting Educational Risk (SIFTER; Anderson, 1989). These tools have normative data for children of various ages and grade levels. They also are useful for flagging the situations in which the child might have the most difficulty.

It also is clinical practice to begin an APD evaluation with a thorough evaluation of peripheral hearing status. This includes pure-tone thresholds, speech discrimination in quiet, otoacoustic emissions, and immittance testing. The goal primarily is to rule out a middle ear or cochlear problem, although comorbidity between peripheral and central auditory problems can exist. Acoustic reflex thresholds are also included in assessment recommendations, although interpretation of abnormal results is not addressed in the various task force or professional association reports other than in their use in evaluating peripheral system integrity and possibly ruling out ANSD. In the several surveys of professional practice in APD assessment mentioned earlier, acoustic reflex thresholds were used by the majority of clinicians in their assessment battery.

It is further recommended that evaluation include assessment of the reception of both speech and nonspeech signals. Many speech-type tests are available for APD evaluation. In one category, there are speech tests that attempt to degrade the signal in some way, such as by filtering, time altering, or presenting background noise or competition, either monaurally or dichotically. Also, it generally is agreed that tests of basic discrimination be included in any APD assessment. ASHA recommends tests that evaluate frequency and intensity discrimination, frequency resolution and temporal processes including gap detection, and forward and backward masking. Adaptive procedures embedded in a rigorous psychoacoustic paradigm generally are not available at this time, but given the improvements in signal processing capabilities, it is likely that such testing will be available in the future (e.g., Meng, 2009; Park, 2008).

Pattern recognition tests also figure quite prominently in test recommendations. Commercially available tests that are most popular include the Pitch Pattern Sequencing Test (Pinheiro & Musiek, 1985) and the Duration Pattern Sequencing Test (Musiek, Baran, & Pinheiro, 1990). In these tests, the listener is presented with a series of three tones and must report back the pattern they heard. In the Pitch and Duration Pattern test, the tones differ in frequency or duration, respectively. Children with APD tend to have a great deal of difficulty perceiving the patterns correctly. One of the interesting aspects of these patterning tests is their possible relationship to the processing of envelope information and the slower changing acoustic features of a signal so important to the perception of prosody, an area we have found difficult for many children with auditory processing disorders (McFaddden, 2006).

For the clinical interpretation of test results, it is recommended that performance be evaluated against age expectations to determine if a deficiency represents a clinical problem or a maturational delay and to examine performance within a child to determine areas of relative strength and weakness. This requires that a test have good normative data. It is recommended that for a diagnosis of APD, performance on at least two tests should be two standard deviations or more below expectations. Performance at least three standard deviations below age expectations on only one test also might be considered significant if there are significant behavioral indicators consistent with an APD (ASHA, 2005a). The specific tests to be used and the number of tests are not specified.

Objective measures are also strongly encouraged in APD assessment, although there is some controversy about how to interpret the results (Katz et al., 2002). Among the recommended procedures are OAEs and acoustic reflexes with decay, and evoked responses such as the ABR, middle and late responses, the 40-Hz response, ASSR, frequency-following responses, and event related potentials. Such tests are thought to prove most useful in the testing of young children for whom behavioral testing can be difficult, when a neurologic disorder is suspected, or to confirm behavioral findings that might be inconclusive. These tests likely are very important given the strong belief stated by our professional associations that the neurobiologic processes that underlie auditory processing are critical for proper functioning.

Because auditory processing difficulties most likely do not occur in isolation, and because success in academics and communication depends upon multiple skills, it is strongly encouraged that other areas of processing be evaluated when a child is referred for APD assessment. Specifically, the assessment of language, cognition, and memory are recommended.

Screening

The issue of screening is not addressed extensively in the documents by ASHA (1996, 2005a); however, it is addressed in some detail in the document from the AAA (Jerger & Musiek, 2000). This latter report suggests a screening tool is required and acknowledges that in seeking high sensitivity there will be a trade-off with specificity. However, the importance of a suitable screening tool is emphasized. The document suggests that screening can be done via a behavioral checklist and by testing. In agreement with ASHA, the suggestion is made that the behavioral checklists should tap the functions of interest in auditory processing—that is, perception of speech in noise or other difficult listening situations, the ability to follow oral instructions, discriminate between and identify speech sounds, and auditory inattention. A screening tool, they state, should include one measure of dichotic perception, specifically, the perception of dichotically presented digits, and a test of gap detection to assess temporal processing. In a more recent editorial, Jerger (2009) noted that the search for a "simple, quick, and easy to score screening test for APD . . . " (p. 160) might be inappropriate. He argued for a more thorough and systematic approach to assessment of this complex disorder, even though it can be more time consuming.

As a minimal test battery, the AAA recommends (Jerger & Musiek, 2000) evaluation of pure-tone thresholds, speech discrimination testing over a range of presentation levels, dichotic listening, duration pattern sequencing, and gap detection thresholds. Supporting this minimal battery is a recommendation for immittance including tympanometry, acoustic reflex thresholds, and otoacoustic emissions to rule out problems in the middle and inner ears. To evaluate the status of the brainstem and cortex, auditory brainstem and middle latency evoked responses are recommended.

Current Practice Patterns

What audiologists actually do in clinical assessment varies greatly between individuals and clinics and has changed over time. Chermak et al. (1998) reported the results of a survey taken in the United States just after the first ASHA task force report was published in 1998.

Responses were received from 183 audiologists. This same survey was also sent to audiologists in Canada to which 101 registered audiologists responded (Noel, 2003). Chermak's group reported that 48% of the audiologists responding conducted central auditory assessments, and most used a test battery approach but were unhappy with their choice of battery. The most common tests used included two objective procedures: acoustic reflexes and ABR. The behavioral test most frequently used varied by location of practice. Audiologists practicing in the school system used the SCAN (Keith, 2002), a screening tool that samples the perception of filtered speech, speech in noise, competing words, and competing sentences. Audiologists practicing in medical settings were most likely to use the Staggered Spondaic Word Test (SSW; Katz, 1962). Also used frequently were the Low-Pass Filtered Speech Test (FS; Willeford, 1976b) and the Synthetic Sentence Identification with Ipsilateral Competing Message (SSI-ICM; Speaks & Jerger, 1965). Binaural hearing was evaluated, although not frequently, using a test of binaural fusion (Calearo & Antonelli, 1973). Noel's results in Canada (2003) showed that the two most frequently used tests were acoustic reflexes and the SCAN. Infrequently, audiologists reported using frequency patterns, dichotic digits, and the SSW. As their American colleagues, most were dissatisfied with their protocols.

Emanuel (2002) reported the results of a survey a few years later suggesting that most clinicians continued to use the SCAN or the SSW as their primary behavioral assessment tool. Electrophysiologic measures remained in common use and included the ABR and acoustic reflexes. One change since 1998 was an increase in the use of systematic behavior questionnaires such as the Children's Auditory Performance Scale (CHAPS; Smoski et al., 1992), the Fisher Auditory Problems Checklist (Fisher, 1976), or the Screening Identification for Targeting Educational Risk (SIFTER; Anderson, 1989), a practice that had been suggested in the Task Force Report of 1996 (ASHA, 1996). An additional change in practice was the use of tests of auditory attention and memory, such as the Auditory Continuous Performance Test (Keith, 1994) or the Screening Auditory Abilities Test (SAAT; Cherry, 1980). In the category of monaural degraded speech tests, clinicians reported two subtests of the Test of Auditory Processing Disorders in Children–Revised (SCAN; Keith, 2000): Filtered Words and Auditory Figure Ground. Other low-redundancy speech tests used included filtered speech, time-compressed speech, and speech presented in the presence of ipsilateral noise or competing messages. Slightly less commonly used were tests of temporal processing in spite of their endorsement. The most commonly used test in that category was the Pitch Pattern Sequence Test (PPS; Pinheiro & Musiek, 1985). A few reported use of the duration pattern test and the Auditory Fusion Test (AFT-R; McCroskey & Keith, 1996), which tests gap detection. Few respondents reported using binaural tests, unlike the previous survey report. Of those that did, the Rapidly Alternating Speech Test (RASP; Willeford, 1976a) and the masking level difference (MLD) were the most common.

In a follow-up to their 1998 survey, Chermak and colleagues (Chermak et al., 2007) found that acoustic reflexes remained the most frequently used test but that the ABR had fallen in popularity. Some of the same procedures remained in use including dichotic tests (competing sentences, the SSW, dichotic digits) and filtered speech. However, pitch and duration pattern testing, speech in noise testing, and the Fisher's questionnaire emerged as more common procedures, and the use of reflex decay and middle latency responses became more popular.

Summary

It is unfortunate that in spite of so many years of interest and concern and volumes of research, we are still in a state of questioning over how to assess (and even what to call) auditory processing disorders. As the proceeding sections have attempted to show, the auditory system is extremely complex, and the unraveling of acoustic signals and the derivation of meaning from them that takes place holds many opportunities for disruption. Perhaps part of the problem in APD assessment lies in this complexity and in our inability to define patient populations easily that are similar enough to allow us to establish definitive tests that evaluate hearing and listening skills. Perhaps one of the most promising changes in audiologic assessment has come with the recognition of ANSD. In these individuals, we are able to see a wide range of hearing sensitivity levels with hearing problems that far exceed these thresholds. Through our study of these disorders, we are beginning to find new ways to assess hearing and new ways to understand auditory system pathology. Some of the behaviors seen in children with APD are not unlike those presented by individuals with ANSD. It is possible that some children with APD might be suffering from some form of neural disorder that is similar to ANSD, either in kind or in neural location. Still others might be suffering from similar neural disruptions that are occurring more central in the auditory nervous system, beyond the auditory nerve and lower brainstem.

It is clear from these reports that clinicians use a test battery approach and that they try to adhere to the recommendations of their professional associations. Limiting factors included the poor availability of materials for adaptive discrimination testing, lack of standardization in most available tests, limited access to electrophysiologic test equipment in some practices, lack of materials suitable for many different first languages, and poor availability of suitable procedures for very young children.

As is noted in our professional association reports (ASHA 1996, 2005a; Jerger & Musiek, 2000), much research is needed in the area of APD assessment. It is suggested that tests be developed that use rigorous psychophysical principles, validate these tests against individuals with known central nervous system problems, and make these tests commercially available. Techniques that use rigorous, adaptive psychophysical procedures to examine basic discrimination and resolution abilities in children with APD are much needed before they will be useful clinically. Laboratory psychometric measures have been used for a number of years with very young children (e.g., Allen & Wightman, 1992, 1994; Allen et al., 1989; Wightman et al., 1989), and coupled with new advancements in technology, these procedures might be adapted for clinical use in the very near future (Meng, 2009; Park, 2008). This will certainly enhance the ability of clinicians to evaluate the manner in which the child's auditory system preserves signal clarity.

Rehabilitation

Auditory processing disorders must not be thought of as a specific disease entity. The term more appropriately describes the types of problems an individual with a hearing loss might experience when there is difficulty hearing, but the cause cannot be attributed to a loss of audibility. Until such time as we have greater knowledge of the underlying causes of the problems, treatment will be limited to the amelioration of behavioral issues. This requires that we find ways to make listening easier, to help build the child's cognitive abilities so as to minimize the difficulties they experience, and to help them manage their hearing and learning more effectively through metacognitive strategies. The literature on aural rehabilitation for APD is vast, and there are many good texts giving strategies, treatment plans, and theories (Bellis, 1996; Chermak & Musiek, 2007; Katz, 2009; Masters, Stecker, & Katz, 1998; Sloan, 1991). Unfortunately, there is a relative paucity of efficacy research in most areas.

Categories of intervention strategies can be placed into a few broad areas. These include improving the quality of the signal, training the auditory system to recognize signals more effectively by taking advantage of neural plasticity, teaching the child to know when he or she will have difficulty and providing strategies to improve coping, and facilitating speech and language processing skills to enable better proficiency in general communication abilities. As with any treatment plan, the beginning is a comprehensive assessment protocol that will delineate the child's pattern of strengths and weaknesses. The treatment plan must be individualized, and the child's progress with any recommendations must be carefully monitored.

Improving Signal Quality

If the auditory system is compromised such that degraded signals or those presented in noise or competition are poorly perceived, one intervention is to improve the quality and clarity of the signal. This can be accomplished by improving the acoustics in the room such that signal transduction is better. Rooms in which there is significant noise and reverberation will degrade the quality of the signal. Allowing instruction to take place in rooms that are acoustically treated and quiet can help not only children with auditory processing disorders, but all children who are learning new or unfamiliar material. Recommendations for improving the acoustics of learning spaces have been published (ANSI, 2002). In many cases, it is difficult to achieve the recommended levels for noise, particularly since the children themselves will create a large amount of noise in any active learning environment. For children with APD, it can be useful to fit them with an FM device that will transmit to their ear a clear sound with a better signal-to-noise ratio (Rosenberg, 2002).

Auditory Training

Taking advantage of auditory plasticity and improving neural connections and efficiency is a key concept underlying another category of rehabilitative techniques. Generally, auditory training programs are intensive, requiring the child to work at them for extended periods of time several days each week. The difficulty of the tasks is generally presented in graded difficulty and most often target specific stimulus features or dimensions. Chermak and Musiek (2002) provide a fairly comprehensive review of remedial techniques in the area of auditory training for children based on their primary area of difficulty. For those whose primary problems are in basic discrimination, they recommend training in speech and nonspeech discrimination tasks in graded difficulty. For difficulties in temporal processing, they recommend sequencing tasks, prosody training, poetry reading, and following directions. For problems with the perception of speech in noise or degraded conditions, vocabulary building and practice listening in degraded or noisy conditions is recommended, and for those with binaural hearing deficits, a variety of dichotic listening tasks might be appropriate.

Speech and Language Training

Perhaps as much, or more, than any other area of pediatric audiology, the speech-language pathologist will be a valued asset in the intervention team for children with auditory processing disorders. A child will rely less on acoustic features when the sounds and words to which they listen are familiar and well learned. Exercises aimed at building a child's vocabulary, improving a child's knowledge of language structures, and predicting vocabulary content, will be key in minimizing the impact of an auditory processing disorder.

Metacognitive Strategies, Self-Advocacy, and Compensatory Strategies

It is important that we find ways to help children to cope with hearing difficulties. Tools to help them predict what situations will be most difficult and to aid them in minimizing the impact of being asked to work in difficult situations or tasks is very important. It is critical that intervention consider the child's self-esteem and minimize failures. To do so will require the involvement of parents, guardians, and teachers. Chermak (1998) outlines a management approach that is designed to allow children to help themselves. Key features include attribution training that motivates the child to continue to try to do well, cognitive behavior modification that is designed to promote active and self-regulatory listening behavior, reciprocal teaching that is aimed at promoting flexibility in the selection of appropriate strategies, and assertiveness training that is designed to build self-confidence and self-esteem.

Summary and Conclusions

Auditory assessment for auditory processing should consider the child's auditory skills within the context of adequacy for perceptual development and in support of learning and language development. The goal should be to assess the behavioral and neurologic integrity of the auditory system. What skills does the child have or not have? Can the child identify and discriminate between sounds and resolve features within sounds? Are acoustic components properly integrated into useful wholes that can be positioned in a three-dimensional space? Can the child selectively attend to sounds of interest and do so in a sustained manner even when the sounds are unfamiliar or presented in a difficult listening situation? Is the underlying neural integrity such that auditory skills are functional and mature according to age-matched peers, or is neural integrity showing reduced synchrony and transmission delays that could be expected to impair auditory processing? If we can answer these questions, then, as audiologists, we will have made a useful contribution to the team of professionals who are supporting the child's academic and social growth and development. We can then better prepare audiologic rehabilitation programs that are not general to all children with hearing difficulties, but that speak to the areas of strength and weakness in the individual child.

References

Abel, S. M. (1972). Duration discrimination of noise and tone bursts. *Journal of the Acoustical Society of America, 51,* 1219–1223.

Aiken, S., & Picton, T. W. (2006). Envelope following response to natural vowels. *Audiology and Neuro-Otology, 11,* 213–232.

Allen, P., & Allan, C. (2007). Putting the "neural" back into sensorineural hearing loss. In R. C. Seewald & J. M. Bamford (Eds.), *A sound foundation through early amplification 2007: Proceedings of the fourth international conference* (pp. 221–233). Stäfa, Switzerland: Phonak AG.

Allen, P., & Korpela, L. (1999). Notched-noise measures of frequency resolution in children revisited: What acoustic cues are available at children's threshold levels? Proceedings of the joint meeting of Acoustical Society of America and the European Acoustical Association, Berlin, Germany. *Journal of the Acoustical Society of America, 105,* 1152(A).

Allen, P., Spencer, D., & Eskritt, K. (2001). *Frequency selective listening in children as indicated by the measurement of auditory attention bands.* Association for Research in Otolaryngology MidWinter Meeting, St. Petersburg, Florida.

Allen, P., & Wightman, F. (1992). Spectral pattern discrimination by children. *Journal of Speech and Hearing Research, 35,* 222–233.

Allen, P., & Wightman, F. (1994). Psychometric functions for children's detection of tones in noise. *Journal of Speech and Hearing Research, 37,* 205–215.

Allen, P., & Wightman, F. (1995). Effects of signal and masker uncertainty on children's detection. *Journal of Speech and Hearing Research, 38,* 503–511.

Allen, P., Wightman, F., Kistler, D., & Dolan, T. (1989). Frequency resolution in children. *Journal of Speech and Hearing Research*, *32*, 317–324.

American National Standards Institute (ANSI; 2002). *Acoustical performance criteria, design requirements, and guidelines for schools*. New York, NY: Author.

American Psychiatric Association. (2000). *Diagnostic and statistical manual of mental disorders (DSM-IV-TR)* (4th ed., text revision). Washington, DC: Author.

American Speech-Language-Hearing Association. (ASHA; 1996). Central auditory processing: Current status of research and implications for clinical practice. *American Journal of Audiology*, *5*(2), 41–54.

American Speech-Language-Hearing Association (ASHA; 2005a). *(Central) Auditory processing disorders* [Technical report]. Retrieved from http://www.asha.org/policy

American Speech-Language-Hearing Association (ASHA; 2005b). *Scope of practice*. Retrieved from http://www.asha.org/policy

Anderson, K. L. (1989). *S.I.F.T.E.R: Screening Instrument for Targeting Educational Risk in children identified by hearing screening or who have known hearing loss*. Danvill, IL: Interstate.

Banai, K., Abrams, D., & Kraus, N. (2007). Sensory based learning disability: Insights from brainstem processing of speech sounds. *International Journal of Audiology*, *46*, 524–532.

Bargones, J. Y., & Werner, L. A. (1994). Adults listen selectively; infants do not. *Journal of the American Psychological Society*, *5*, 170–174.

Bellis, T. J. (1996). *Assessment and management of central auditory processing disorders in the educational setting: From science to practice*. San Diego, CA: Singular.

Berlin, C., Hood, L., & Allen, P. (1984). Asymmetries in evoked potentials. In C. I. Berlin (Ed.), *Hearing science*. San Diego, CA: College-Hill Press.

Berlin, C., Hughes, L. F., Lowe-Bell, S. S., & Berlin, H. L. (1973). Dichotic right ear advantage in children 5–13. *Cortex*, *9*, 394–403.

Bocca, E., & Calearo, C. (1953). Central hearing processes. In J. Jerger (Ed.), *Modern development in audiology* (pp. 337–370). New York, NY: Academic Press.

British Society for Audiology (BSA; 2007). *Position statement*. Retrieved June 24, 2010, from http://www.thebsa.org.uk/wp-content/uploads/2014/04/BSA_APD_PositionPaper_31March11_FINAL.pdf

Broadbent, D. E. (1958). *Perception and communication*. London, UK: Pergamon.

Calearo, M. D., & Antonelli, A. R. (1973). Disorders of the central auditory nervous system. In M. Paparella & D. Shumrick (Eds.), *Otolaryngology* (pp. 407–425). Philadelphia, PA: Saunders.

Cameron, S., & Dillon, H. (2008). The listening in spatialized noise-sentences test (LISN-S): Comparison to the prototype LISN and results from children with either a suspected (central) auditory processing disorder or a confirmed language disorder. *Journal of the American Academy of Audiology*, *19*, 377–391.

Canadian Academy of Audiology (CAA; (2002). *Position statement on audiology scope of practice*. Retrieved from https://canadianaudiology.ca/professional-resources/scope-of-practice/

Chermak, G. D. (1998). Metacogntive approaches to managing central auditory processing disorders. In M. G. Masters, N. A. Stecker, & J. Katz (Eds.), *Central auditory processing disorders: Mostly management*. Boston, MA: Allyn & Bacon.

Chermak, G. D., & Musiek, F. E. (2002). Auditory training: Principles and approaches for remediating and managing auditory processing disorders. *Seminars in Hearing*, *23*, 297–308.

Chermak, G. D., & Musiek, F. E. (Eds.). (2007). *Handbook of (central) auditory processing disorder: Comprehensive intervention, Vol II*. San Diego, CA: Plural.

Chermak, G. D., Silva, M. E., Nye, J., Hasbrouck, J., & Musiek, F. E. (2007). An update on professional education and clinical practices in central auditory processing. *Journal of the American Academy of Audiology*, *52*, 428–452.

Chermak, G. D., Traynham, W. A., Seikel, J. A., & Musiek, F. E. (1998). Professional education and assessment practices in central auditory processing. *Journal of the American Academy of Audiology*, *9*, 452–465.

Cherry, E. C. (1958). Some experiments on the recognition of speech with one and two ears. *Journal of the Acoustical Society of America*, *25*, 975–979.

Cherry, R. (1980). *Selective Auditory Attention Test (SAAT)*. St. Louis, MO: Auditec.

Conners, C. K. (2000). *Conners' Rating Scales-Revised*. North Tonawanda, NY: Multi-Health Systems.

Davies, D. R., Jones, D. M., & Taylor, A. (1984). Selectiveand sustained-attention tasks: Individual and group differences. In R. Parasuraman & D. R. Davies (Eds.), *Varieties of attention*. New York, NY: Academic Press.

Davis, S. M., & McCroskey, R. L. (1980). Auditory fusion in children. *Child Development*, *51*, 75–80.

Delb, W., Strauss, D., Hohenberg, G., Plinkert, P. K., & Delb, W. (2003). The binaural interaction component (BIC) in children with central auditory processing disorders (CAPD). *International Journal of Audiology*, *7*, 401–412.

Dimitrijevic, A., John, M. S., van Roon, P., & Picton, T. W. (2001). Human auditory steady-state responses to tones independently modulated in both frequency and amplitude. *Ear and Hearing*, *22*, 100–111.

Dobie, R., & Berlin, C. (1979). Binaural interaction in brainstem evoked responses. *Archives of Otolaryngology*, *105*, 391–398.

Dobie, R., & Norton, S. (1980). Binaural interaction in human auditory evoked potentials. *Electroencephalography and Clinical Neurophysiology*, *49*, 303–313.

Durlach, N. I., Thompson, C. L., & Colburn, H. S. (1981). Binaural interaction in impaired listeners: A review of past research. *Audiology*, *20*, 181–211.

Emanuel, D. C. (2002). The auditory processing battery: Survey of common practices. *Journal of the American Academy of Audiology*, *13*, 93–117.

Fisher, L. (1976). *Fisher's auditory problems checklist*. Bemidji, MN: Life Products.

Florentine, M., Buus, S., & Mason, C. R. (1987). Level discrimination as a function of level for tones from 0.25 to 16 kHz. *Journal of the Acoustical Society of America, 81,* 1528–1541.

Gibson, E. J. (1991). *An odyssey in learning and perception.* Cambridge, MA: MIT Press.

Gibson, E. J. (2000). Perceptual learning in development: Some basic concepts. *Ecological Psychology, 12,* 295–302.

Gibson, E. J., & Pick, A. D. (2003). *An ecological approach to perceptual learning and development.* New York, NY: Oxford University Press.

Goldman, R., Fristoe, M., & Woodcock, R. (1970). *Goldman Fristoe-Woodcock test of auditory discrimination.* San Antonio, TX: Pearson.

Goldstein, B., Shulman, A., & Kisiel, D. (1987). Electrical high frequency audiometry: Preliminary medical audiologic experience. *Audiology, 26,* 321–331.

Goldstone, R. (1998). Perceptual learning. *Annual Review Psychology, 49,* 585–612.

Gopal, K. V., & Pierel, K. (1999). Binaural interaction component in children at risk for central auditory processing disorders. *Scandanavian Audiology, 28,* 77–84.

Green, D. M. (1988). *Profile analysis: Auditory intensity discrimination.* New York, NY: Oxford University Press.

Greenberg, G. Z., Bray, N. W., & Beasley, D. S. (1970). Children's frequency selective detection of signals in noise. *Perception and Psychophysics, 8,* 173–175.

Greenberg, G. Z., & Larkin, W. D. (1968). Frequency-response characteristic of auditory observers detecting signals of a single frequency in noise: The probe-signal method. *Journal of the Acoustical Society of America, 44,* 1513–1523.

Grose, J. H., Hall, J. W., & Dev, M. B. (1997). MLD in children: Effects of signal and masker bandwidths. *Journal of Speech, Language, and Hearing Research, 40,* 955–959.

Hill, P. R., Hogben, J. H., & Bishop, D. M. (2005). Auditory frequency discrimination in children with specific language impairment: A longitudinal study. *Journal of Speech, Language, and Hearing Research, 48,* 1136–1146.

Hood, L. J. (2007). Auditory neuropathy and dys-synchrony. In R. F. Burkard, J. J. Eggermont, & M. Don (Eds.), *Auditory evoked potentials: Basic principles and clinical application.* Philadelphia, PA: Lippincott Williams and Wilkins.

Irwin, R. J., Ball, A. K. R., Kay, N., Stillman, J. A., & Rosser, J. (1985). The development of auditory temporal acuity in children. *Child Development, 56,* 614–620.

Ivey, R. G. (1987). *Words in ipsilateral competition (WIC)–Version 2.* Unpublished normative study.

James, W. (1966). Attention. In P. Bakan (Ed.), *Attention.* Princeton, NJ: Van Norstrand.

Jensen, J. K., & Neff, D. L. (1993). Development of basic auditory discrimination in preschool children. *Psychological Science, 4,* 104–107.

Jerger, J. (2009). Editorial: On the diagnosis of auditory processing disorder. *Journal of the American Academy of Audiology, 20,* 160.

Jerger, J., & Jerger, S. (1975). Extraand intra-axial brainstem auditory disorders. *Audiology, 14,* 93–117.

Jerger, J., & Jerger, S. (1977). Diagnostic value of cross vs. uncrossed acoustic reflexes: Eighth nerve and brainstem disorders. *Archives of Otolaryngology, 103,* 445–453.

Jerger, J., & Musiek, F. (2000). Report of the consensus conference on the diagnosis of auditory processing disorders in school-aged children. *Journal of the American Academy of Audiology, 11,* 467–474.

Jerger, S. (1987). Validation of the pediatric speech intelligibility test in children with central nervous system lesions. *Audiology, 26,* 298–311.

Jerger, S., Johnson, K., & Loiselle, L. (1988). Pediatric central auditory dysfunction: Comparison of children with confirmed lesions versus suspected processing disorders. *American Journal of Otology, 9,* 63–71.

Kalikow, D. N., Stevens, K. N., & Elliott, L. L. (1977). Development of a test of speech intelligibility in noise using sentence materials with controlled word predictability. *Journal of the Acoustical Society of America, 61,* 1337–1351.

Katz, J. (1962). The use of staggered spondaic words in assessing the integrity of the central auditory system. *Journal of Auditory Research, 2,* 327–337.

Katz, J. (2009). *Therapy for auditory processing disorders: Simple effective procedures.* Westminster, CO: Educational Audiology Association.

Katz, J., Johnson, C. D., Tillery, K. L., Brander, S., Delagrange, T. N., Ferre, J. M., . . . Stecker, N. A. (2002). *Clinical and research concerns—Regarding Jerger & Musiek (2000) APD recommendations.* Retrieved June 24, 2010, from http://www..audiologyonline.com/articles/pf_article_detail.asp?article_id=341

Keith, R. W. (1994). *The Auditory Continuous Performance Test.* San Antonio, TX: Psychological Corp.

Keith, R. W. (2000). *Random Gap Detection Test.* St. Louis, MO: Auditec.

Keith, R. W. (2002). *SCAN-C Revised. A Screening test for auditory processing disorders.* San Antonio, TX: Psychological Corp.

Killion, M. C., Niquette, P. A., Gudmundsen, G. I., Revit, L. J., & Banerjee, S. (2004). Development of a quick speech-in-noise test for measuring signal-to-noise ratio loss in normal-hearing and hearing-impaired listeners. *Journal of the Acoustical Society of America, 116,* 2395–2405.

Kimura, D. (1961). Cerebral dominance and the perception of verbal stimuli. *Canadian Journal of Psychology, 15,* 166–171.

Kumar, A. U., & Jayaram, M. (2005). Auditory processing in individuals with auditory neuropathy. *Behavioral and Brain Functions, 1,* 1–21.

Liddell, A., Campbell, P., DePlacido, C., Owens, D., & Wolters, M. (2007). *Can extended high frequency hearing thresholds be used to detect auditory processing difficulties in an ageing population?* Proceedings of the European Federation of Audiology, Heidelberg, Germany. Retrieved from http://www.cs.stir.ac.uk/~kjt/research/match/resources/documents/efas07-liddell.pdf

Lister, J. J., Roberts, R. A., Shackelford, J., & Rogers, C. L. (2006). An adaptive clinical test of temporal resolution. *American Journal of Audiology, 15,* 133–140.

Litovsky, R., & Ashmead, D. (1997). Development of binaural and spatial hearing in infants and children. In R. H. Gilkey & T. R. Anderson (Eds.), *Binaural and spatial hearing* (pp. 571–592). Hillsdale, NJ: Lawrence Erlbaum.

Lynn, G. E., & Gilroy, J. (1977). Evaluation of central auditory dysfunction in patients with neurological disorders. In R. W. Keith (Ed.), *Central auditory dysfunction*. New York, NY: Grune and Stratton.

Manly, T., Robertson, I. H., Anderson, V., & Nimmo-Smith, I. (1998). *Test of Everyday Attention for Children (TEA-Ch)*. Toronto, Cananda: Pearson Assessment, PsychCorp.

Markessis, E., Poncelet, L., Colin, C., Coppens, A., Hoonhorst, I., Kadhim, H., & Deltenre, P. (2009). Frequency tuning curves derived from auditory steady state evoked potentials: A proof-of-concept study. *Ear and Hearing, 30*, 43–53.

Marler, J. A., Champlin, C. A., & Gilliam, R. B. (2002). Auditory memory for backward masking signals in children with language impairment. *Psychophysiology, 39*, 767–780.

Martin, N., & Brownell, R. (2005). *Test of auditory processing skills* (3rd ed). Novato, CA: Academic Therapy.

Masters, M. G., Stecker, N. A., & Katz, J. (1998). *Central auditory processing disorders: Mostly management*. Boston, MA: Allyn & Bacon.

Matzker, J. (1959).Two methods for the assessment of central auditory functions in cases of brain disease. *Annals of Otolaryngology, Rhinology and Laryngology, 68*, 1155–1197.

Maxon, A. B., & Hochberg, I. (1982). Development of psychoacoustic behavior: Sensitivity and discrimination. *Ear and Hearing, 3*, 301–308.

McCroskey, R. L., & Keith, R. W. (1996). *Auditory Fusion Threshold Test-Revised*. St. Louis, MO: Auditec.

McFadden, M. (2006). *The receptive prosodic abilities of children with auditory processing disorders: A comparative study*. Unpublished master's thesis, University of Western Ontario.

Meng, Q. (2009). *Design and evaluation of portable psychoacoustic testing systems*. M.E.Sc. thesis. Department of Electrical and Computer Engineering, University of Western Ontario, London, ON, Canada.

Mlot, S., Buus, E., & Hall, J. W. (2010). Spectral integration and bandwidth effects on speech recognition in school-aged children and adults. *Ear and Hearing, 31*, 56–62.

Moore, D. R., Ferguson, M. A., Halliday, L. F., & Riley, A. (2007). Frequency discrimination in children: Perception, learning and attention. *Hearing Research, 238*, 147–154.

Musiek, F. E. (1983). Assessment of central auditory dysfunction: The dichotic digit test revisited. *Ear and Hearing, 4*, 79–83.

Musiek, F., & Baran, J. A. (2007). *The auditory system: Anatomy, physiology, and clinical correlates*. Boston, MA: Allyn & Bacon.

Musiek, F., Baran, J. A., & Piniheiro, M. (1990). Duration pattern recognition in normal subjects and in patients with cerebral and cochlear lesions. *Audiology, 29*, 304–313.

Musiek, F. E., & Geurking, N. A. (1982). Auditory brainstem response (ABR) and central auditory test (CAT) findings for patients with brainstem lesions: A preliminary report. *Laryngoscope, 92*, 891–900.

Musiek, F. E., Shinn, J. B., Jirsa, R., Bamiou, D. E., Baran, J. A., & Zaida, E. (2005). GIN (Gaps-In-Noise) test performance in subjects with confirmed central auditory nervous system involvement. *Ear and Hearing, 26*, 608–618.

Näätänen, R., Gaillard, A. W. K., & Montysalo, S. (1978). Early selective-attention effect on evoked potential reinterpreted. *Acta Psychologica, 42*, 313–329.

Nilsson, M., Soli, S. D., & Sullivan, J. A. (1994). Development of the Hearing in Noise Test for the measurement of speech reception thresholds in quiet and in noise. *Journal of the Acoustical Society of America, 95*, 1085–1099.

Noel, G. (2003). *Professional education and assessment practices in central auditory processing*. Canadian Academy of Audiology, Pre-conference workshop on Central Auditory Processing Disorders, Vancouver, CA.

Nozza, R. J. (1987). The binaural masking level difference in infants and adults: Developmental change in binaural hearing. *Infant Behavior and Development, 10*, 105–110.

Nozza, R., Wagener, E. F., & Crandell, M. A. (1988). Binaural release for masking for speech sounds in infants, preschoolers, and adults. *Journal of Speech and Hearing Research, 31*, 212–218.

Olsen, W. O., & Noffsinger, D. (1976). Masking level differences for cochlear and brainstem lesions. *Annals of Otology, Rhinology, and Laryngology, 85*, 820–825.

Olsho, L. W. (1985). Infant auditory perception: Tonal masking. *Infant Behavior and Development, 8*, 371–384.

Park, S. (2008). *The effectiveness of a handheld pocket PC in psychoacoustic measurements*. Seniors honors thesis. Department of Psychology, University of Western Ontario, London, ON, Canada.

Patterson, R. (1976). Auditory filter shapes derived with noise stimuli. *Journal of the Acoustical Society of America, 59*, 640–654.

Pinheiro, M. L., & Musiek, F. E. (1985). Sequencing and temporal ordering in the auditory system. In M. L. Pinheiro & F. E. Musiek (Eds.), *Assessment of central auditory dysfunction: Foundations and clinical correlates* (pp. 219–238). Baltimore, MD: Williams and Wilkins.

Polyakov, A., & Pratt, H. (1994). Three-channel Lissajous' Trajectory of the binaural interaction components in human auditory brainstem evoked potentials. *Electroencephalography and Clinical Neurology, 92*, 396–404.

Popper, A. N., & Fay, R. R. (Eds.). (1992). The mammalian auditory pathway: Neurophysiology. *Springer handbook of auditory research* (Vol. 2). Berlin, Germany: Springer.

Purcell, D. W., John, M. S., Schneider, B. A., & Picton, T. W. (2004). Human temporal auditory acuity as assessed by envelope following responses. *Journal of the Acoustical Society of America, 116*, 3581–3593.

Richards, J. E. (2004). The development of sustained attention in infants. In M. I. Posner (Ed.), *Cognitive neuroscience of attention*. New York, NY: Guilford Press.

Rosen, S., & Manganari, E. (2001). Is there a relationship between speech and nonspeech auditory processing in children with dyslexia? *Journal of Speech, Language, and Hearing Research, 44*, 720–736.

Rosenberg, G. G. (2002). Classroom acoustics and personal FM technology in the management of auditory processing disorder. *Seminars in Hearing, 23,* 309–317.

Schwarz, D. W. F., & Taylor, P. (2005). Human auditory steady-state responses to binaural and monaural beats. *Clinical Neurophysiology, 116,* 658–668.

Sek, A., & Moore, B. C. (1995). Frequency discrimination as a function of frequency, measured in several ways. *Journal of the Acoustical Society of America, 97,* 2479–2486.

Sloan, C. (1991). *Treating auditory processing difficulties in children.* San Diego, CA: Singular.

Smith, B. B., & Resnick, D. M. (1972). An auditory test for assessing brain stem integrity: Preliminary report. *Laryngoscope, 82,* 414–424.

Smoski, W. J., Brunt, M. A., & Tannahill, J. C. (1992). Listening characteristics of children with central auditory processing disorders. *Language, Speech, and Hearing Services in Schools, 23,* 145–152.

Speaks, C., & Jerger, J. (1965). Method for measurement of speech identification. *Journal of Speech and Hearing Research, 8,* 185–194.

Stollman, M. H. P., van Velzen, E. C. W., Simkens, H. M. F., Snik, A. F. M., & van den Broek, P. (2004). Development of auditory processing in 6–12-year-old children: A longitudinal study. *International Journal of Audiology, 43,* 34–44.

Sutcliffe, P. A., Bishop, D. V. M, Houghton, S., & Taylor, M. (2006). Effect of attentional state on frequency discrimination: A comparison of children with ADHD on and off medication. *Journal of Speech and Hearing Research, 49,* 1072–1084.

Swanson, J. M., Casey, B. J., Nigg, J., Castellanos, F. X., Volkow, N. D., & Taylor, E. (2004). Clinical and cognitive definitions of attention deficits in children with attention-deficit/hyperactivity disorder. In. M. I. Posner (Ed.), *Cognitive neuroscience of attention* (pp. 430–445). New York, NY: Guilford Press.

Sweetow, R., & Reddell, R. (1978). The use of masking level differences in the identification of children with perceptual problems. *Journal of the Acoustical Society of America, 4,* 52–56.

Thompson, M. E., & Abel, M. (1992). Indices of hearing in patients with central auditory pathology. *Scandanavian Audiology, 34*(Suppl.), 3–22.

Webster, D. B., Popper, A. N., & Fay, R. R. (Eds.). (1992). *The mammalian auditory pathway: Neuroanatomy. Springer handbook of auditory research* (Vol. 1). Berlin, Germany: Springer.

Wightman, F., Allen, P., Dolan, T., Kistler, D., & Jamieson, D. (1989). Temporal resolution in children. *Child Development, 60,* 611–624.

Willeford, J. (1976a). Differential diagnosis of central auditory dysfunction. In L. Bradford (Ed.), *Audiology: An audio journal for continuing education* (Vol. 2). New York, NY: Grune and Stratton.

Willeford, J. (1976b). Central auditory function in children with language disabilities. *Audiology and Hearing Education, 2,* 12–20.

Wright, B. A., Lombardino, L. D., King. W. M., Puranik, C. S., Leonard, C. M., & Merzenich, M. M. (1997). Deficits in auditory temporal and spectral resolution in language-impaired children. *Nature, 387,* 176–178.

Zeng, F-G., Oba, S., Garde, S., Sininger, Y., & Starr, A. (1999). Temporal and speech processing deficits in auditory neuropathy. *NeuroReport, 10,* 3429–3435.

Zwicker, E., & Fastl, E. (1999). *Psychoacoustics: Facts and models.* Berlin, Germany: Springer.

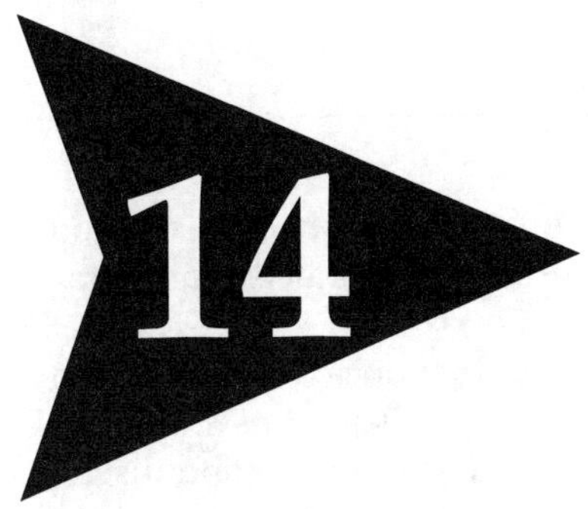

Pseudohypacusis: False and Exaggerated Hearing Loss

James E. Peck

Introduction

Although the incidence of childhood pseudohypacusis is low, it is not a rare condition to encounter in most audiological settings. Moreover, there is ample evidence that children who present a nonexistent or exaggerated hearing loss are at risk for having psychosocial problems. Beyond determining genuine hearing status, audiologists can play a key role in identifying the possibility of psychosocial problems and referring for evaluation of any underlying problems. This chapter deals with both the evaluation process and the psychological aspects.

The terms most used in regard to pseudohypacusis need scrutiny. *Nonorganic* and *functional* are synonymous and in medical usage mean apparent disorder in the absence of structural or anatomic explanation (*Mosby's Medical Dictionary*, 2009). Note they do not mean that the person really has no problem. Yet, when audiologists use these terms in regard to hearing, they mean just that, that there is no problem (or not as much as portrayed). "The loss either does not exist at all or does not exist to the degree that is indicated" (Roeser & Clark, 2007, p. 255). Contrast this to the condition of nonorganic failure to thrive, in which a baby is not gaining weight even with adequate nourishment, not from some organ failure but because of psychosocial disruptions within the family and extreme emotional neglect (Erikson & Egeland, 2011). Or, consider functional gastrointestinal disorders, such as irritable bowel syndrome, which are so common. To be sure, neither *nonorganic* nor *functional* in these examples means that there is no problem. Rather, they mean there is no problem in the organs, themselves, but in how the body is functioning. Hence, it is illogical to describe a hearing loss as nonorganic or functional when one means to say that there is actually no hearing loss to describe.

The other component included in *nonorganic* and *functional* is no known cause or medical explanation. In medicine, a disease or disorder, particularly one of rapid onset, with no detectable cause or explanation is labeled *idiopathic* (*Miller-Keane Encyclopedia and Dictionary of Medicine, Nursing and Allied Health*, 2003). An example familiar to audiologists is idiopathic sensory/neural hearing loss. In actuality, many a sensory/neural hearing loss has no demonstrable cause but is diagnosed on the basis of findings and history, such as age or noise exposure, which provide a reasonable explanation for the hearing loss. Surely, the implication in "idiopathic sensory/neural hearing loss" is not that the loss is not real.

Two other words are *malingering* and *psychogenic*. "Malingering is the intentional production of false or grossly exaggerated physical or psychological symptoms, motivated by external incentives" (e.g., money or avoiding undesired activity; American Psychiatric Association, 2013, p. 726). *Psychogenic* refers to producing or causing a symptom or illness by mental factors as opposed to organic ones (Shahrokh & Hales, 2003). Note that both *malingering* and *psychogenic* incorporate a state of mind, and because no audiologic test can determine what is in the patient's mind, they are not synonymous with pseudohypacusis and are not appropriate audiologically.

Pseudohypacusis means invalid hearing test results or untrue complaint of hearing loss in that a person responds "to stimuli only at levels well above their true organic thresholds" but without "implying an underlying causal factor" (Olsen, 1991, p. 40). Perhaps, equally logical—and more straightforward—would be the plain English *false hearing loss*. For situations with some degree of organic impairment, the more inclusive term is *false and exaggerated hearing loss* (FEHL).

Traditionally, false hearing loss has been considered to be either conscious or unconscious (or to lie along a continuum between the two poles). The classic examples of the two extremes are the aforementioned malingering and psychogenic, respectively. Many a psychogenic problem has been reclassified as a "conversion disorder," a sensory or motor symptom that causes significant impairment and is not compatible with or better explained by another condition. (The name came from the idea that psychological stresses were *converted* into symptoms, but a close temporal association between the onset of the symptom and some stress or trauma is no longer necessary for a diagnosis [American Psychiatric Association, 2013]).

In their landmark article, Austen and Lynch (2004) showed the conscious-unconscious dichotomy to be incomplete and simplistic. They asserted that not just the degree of consciousness but also the locus of the patient's need or goal must be taken into account. Thus, even though a malingerer consciously presents a symptom for an external goal, a person with a conversion disorder unconsciously exhibits a symptom for an internal need. Therefore, Austen and Lynch (2004) included "factitious disorder" in their model as something of an in-between in which a person intentionally produces a symptom but for an internal goal, such as making oneself sick to get medical attention. The Austen-Lynch model is as follows:

malingering	intentional and external need
factitious disorder	intentional and internal need
conversion disorder	unintentional and internal need

Audiologists cannot make these psychological judgments, but they can report relevant information about a patient's test behavior and background.

Here is this author's definition of his recommended designation, false or exaggerated hearing loss:

> A supposed hearing loss that does not exist or not to the degree presented regardless of psychological motivation, typified by inconsistencies and discrepancies but lacking medical explanation.

Characteristics

Demographics

The rate of FEHL among children and youth is unclear. Beagley and Knight (1968) estimated that it was substantially less than 1% in children seen for hearing evaluations. Leshin (1960) reported that 2.5% of 1,900 children who failed a state hearing screening later exhibited false hearing loss. Campanelli (1963) found 41 cases or 1.7% out of 2,300 screened in 1 year. Also in 1 year, Pracy, Walsh, Mepham, and Bowdler (1996) saw 10 children with FEHL out of approximately 1,000 for a rate of 1 per 100 children (1%). Saravanappa, Mepham, and Bowdler (2005) estimated that the incidence in their settings was about 220 per year or about 0.5%. In a German speech and hearing clinic over a 12-year period, 1.8% of child audiology patients had FEHL (Schmidt et al., (2013).

Reports on gender, age, degree of loss, type of loss, and ear(s) among FEHL children are remarkably similar across countries. Girls outnumber boys 2:1. The age span is 7 to 16 years with a consistent average around 11 years. The range of hearing loss presented is wide, typically 35 to 80 dB, with averages of 40 to 60 dB. For the most part the losses are sensory/neural in flat configurations and are bilateral 90% of the time.[1]

Causes and Maintaining Factors

The most frequently named causes of childhood FEHL are school difficulties, a history of ear disease, seeking attention, and psychosocial problems. Typically, school performance is low despite generally normal

[1]These data were gleaned from many reports. Because citing the articles for each characteristic would be repetitious and distracting, the sources are given here. Not every article had information on each aspect covered in this paragraph. The sources are Aplin & Rowson (1986, 1990); Bowdler & Rogers (1989); Campanelli (1963); Dixon & Newby (1959); Drouillard et al. (2014); Kothe, Fleischer, Breitfuss, & Hess (2003); McCanna & DeLapa (1981); Morita, Suzuki, & Iizuka (2010); Pracy et al. (1996); Psarommatis, Kontorinis, Kontrogiannis, Douniadakis, & Tsakanikos (2009); and Schmidt et al. (2013).

intelligence (Aplin & Rowson, 1990; Barr, 1960; Berger, 1965). The presumption is that the false hearing loss is adopted as an accepted excuse (Aplin & Rowson, 1990; Berger, 1965; McCanna & DeLapa, 1981), but inferring a causal relationship seems based more on supposition than on evidence. In this author's patients, there was often a point when grades declined, which coincided with a disturbing life event and sometimes with the onset of the supposed hearing loss. When one also considers reports that psychosocial problems are widespread among these children (discussed below), it seems equally or more likely that both the lowered school performance and the false hearing loss are cosymptoms of a third factor.

A history of middle ear problems is a frequent co-occurrence with FEHL (Aplin & Rowson, 1986; Barr, 1960; Lehrer, Hirschenfang, Miller, & Radpour, 1964). Many surmise that hearing loss is adopted as the symptom because that history affords first-hand experience with an ear problem, but this also lacks substantiation. As otitis media is so prevalent, it would not be unusual to find that numerous 11-year-old children had had otitis media. Furthermore, the great preponderance of children with a background of otitis media do not exhibit FEHL. Besides, ascribing the nonexistent loss to past ear trouble also sidesteps the question of why a child would feel a need to present a false disorder in the first place.

Displaying a hearing loss could be seen as a way to get attention and be attributed to a child being overly demanding or manipulative. It might well be true, but supporting empirical evidence is lacking. Children might be happy to miss school, but they might also have to miss after-school activities or risk being taken for medical care and getting a shot. Furthermore, seeking attention in this way, or learning to enjoy such attention, might well signal an underlying unmet need.

In stark contrast to the foregoing, there is considerable evidence that psychological difficulties are more common than not in childhood FEHL. Aplin and Rowson (1986) found introversion and neuroticism in most of their 30 subjects, especially in girls, whereas boys were more likely to be aggressive and antisocial. They also found that a greater degree of false impairment suggests greater psychological problems (Aplin & Rowson, 1990). Conflict is typical at home, school, or with friends (Barr, 1960; Berger, 1965). Lehrer et al. (1964) found several cases of insecurity, inadequacy, hostility, tension, and anxiety. In McCanna and DeLapa's (1981) study, 62% of the children with FEHL came from broken homes, and many were living with persons who were not their parents. In several instances, parental divorce occurred just prior to the appearance of the hearing concern. Eighty-six percent either were being seen by a psychologist or were described by their parents as being nervous, withdrawn, easily upset, or having peer problems or a disorganized personality. Similarly, 20 out of 26 Greek, pseudohypacusic children had positive histories for family or school problems (Psarommatis et al., 2009). In a clinical study (Peck, 2002), two thirds of children with FEHL had positive scores on the Pediatric Symptom Checklist, a screening test for psychosocial disorders. A group of German children with false hearing loss had a high prevalence of emotional and educational problems (Schmidt et al., 2013).

In short, the odds are that a child with FEHL has significant psychosocial burdens, and explaining away false test results could be misleading and hazardous.

Signs and Risk Factors

There are several signs and risk factors for invalid responding that can appear before and during testing.

Before Testing

Referral by Attorney

Almost always, this means a question of liability or compensation.

Reason for Visit

Litigation or eligibility determination, regardless of referral source, usually involves monetary benefit. This might not be evident at the outset, and the clinician might need to ask if eligibility determination is involved.

History

A report might lack credibility as to cause or onset or otherwise seem dubious. The history should cover a few important factors. A prime area is school problems, which are prevalent in children with FEHL. Changes in the child's behavior should be checked (e.g., gloomy, acting less mature, or spending more time alone). Abuse, neglect, and dysfunctional environment need to be considered. If the historian does not mention these, the clinician might need to inquire (techniques to do so are discussed later).

Observations and Behavior

The patient readily understands soft speech when the speaker's face is unseen. The person might exhibit behaviors that are out of the ordinary, such as having a flat affect, or being sullen, or argumentative.

During Testing

Behaviors

The patient understands speech that is softer than would be expected from the test results. Other suspicious behaviors are comments about being confused, looking uncertain, concentrating strenuously, radiating cooperation, acting bored, looking around the test room, and the like (McCanna & DeLapa, 1981).

Pure-Tone Audiometry

A hallmark of FEHL is inconsistent pure-tone thresholds. Test-retest reliability should be within 5 dB, and discrepancies should not exceed 10 dB at any frequency.

As compared to true responders, pseudohypacusics have more false-negative responses and especially fewer false-positive responses. The manner of responding can be significant, for example, slow, elaborate, or laborious. Such behavioral observations are not available from pressing a button for a response light, which might be a drawback for this sort of behavioral audiometry.

The audiometric configurations most common in entirely false hearing loss are flat and saucer shaped. However, if there is a coexisting organic loss with other than a flat pattern, that shape is added in to produce something other than the classic configuration. Furthermore, saucer and flat patterns are seen in purely organic hearing losses. Consequently, the audiogram configuration has no differential diagnostic significance whatsoever.

The absence of a shadow curve in severe unilateral losses, when the good ear is not masked, is highly indicative of invalid results. Usual interaural attention is on the order of 50 to 60 dB with typical supra-aural headsets (Snyder, 2001) but can be 70 dB. Accordingly, there should be responses due to crossover by about 75 dB HL. Insert-tube earphones in a foam plug tip generally add 15 dB of interaural attention; however, they might have a minimum interaural attention of 50 dB (Monro & Contractor, 2010). Thus, with insert earphones the lack of a crossover response above 60 dB HL is not a good indicator of invalid responding, and might only become so at about 85 dB HL.

Speech Audiometry

Perhaps, the most prominent of all signs of invalid performance is the speech recognition threshold (SRT) being significantly better than the pure-tone thresholds. The pure-tone average (PTA), whether the Carhart three frequency average of 500, 1000, and 2000 Hz or the Fletcher average of the two best thresholds of those frequencies, should agree with the SRT within about 6 dB, provided the audiogram is fairly flat. Differences beyond 10 dB are indicative of FEHL.

In addition to poor tone-speech threshold agreement, several telltale behaviors tend to mark FEHL and are much less often observed in true responders:

- Giving half-word responses during SRT (e.g., "ear" for "eardrum") (almost exclusively seen in false responders);
- Protesting, "You are too soft. I can't hear you," but otherwise responding to off-hand remarks at or below the SRT;
- Pressing the earphone to the ear;
- Claiming difficulty hearing the test signal;
- Giving a bizarre response or error of association: "boxcar" for "railroad," "dig" for "ditch";
- Making seemingly deliberate errors;
- Rising inflection, as if a question or uncertain: "sidewalk?," "pick?";
- Rhyming responses; and
- Displaying exaggerated straining to understand during the test.

Test Procedures

General Principles

With any patient, the clinician should be forming an idea during the interview of how much hearing loss a patient might have. In a real sense, the evaluation has begun before moving to the test area. Pure-tone and speech audiometry are different procedures, but several principles are applicable to both when it comes to FEHL testing as will be seen in a moment. If there is some reason to anticipate invalid responding, it is wise to begin with speech audiometry. Also, it can be worthwhile to make frequent changes in the test signal, such as type (speech/tone), frequency, intensity, interstimulus timing, and ear tested. The overarching principle is to disrupt a patient's loudness standard.

The literature routinely considers the subject's behavior, but that of the tester is also critical. It might call for some guile, certainly flexibility, and definitely agility in handling the controls. There is merit in some "acting," looking mystified or expectant, or telling the patient that the tester feels confused by the results. Many adjustments to normal procedures can be made on the spur of the moment. Creativity and ingenuity are invaluable. Paradoxically, FEHL testing calls for close adherence to sound audiologic principles, and not just "winging it" or going on "gut feelings." It might be helpful to think of FEHL testing as being unconventional with the conventional. Finally, to lend credibility to the clinician's impressions during the posttest counseling, it is valuable to have the parent observe the testing and witness the responses to very soft sounds.

Instructions

Instruct the patient face to face rather than through earphones to avoid providing a loudness standard for the patient. The person should be directed to respond to tones by a definite raising of an arm or finger, even to very faint sounds. In the case of speech, familiarize with the spondee test words prior to testing and urge the patient to repeat the word no matter how soft. During pure-tone audiometry, keep the patient's hands in sight to watch for the slightest finger or hand movements that are time-related to the stimulus. If discrepancies arise, offer a face-saving explanation, such as a misunderstanding, and reinstruct clearly and authoritatively but without putting the person on the defensive. Give the child an "out," a chance to "escape with honor." One could tell the person that inconsistencies might require much more time or necessitate a return session, and then invite the patient to continue. All the while, the clinician should give much encouragement and reinforce correct responses, especially those at or below the tentative threshold (Nilo & Saunders, 1976). At times, it might be appropriate to cajole and press the patient to respond, but tactfully.

Starting Levels

When there is a risk of FEHL, begin with low signal levels (0–20 dB) for both tones and speech, and proceed in ascending fashion to mitigate against the patient establishing a suprathreshold loudness reference. On the other hand, a good way to confirm preliminary results is to compare thresholds from ascending and descending intensity runs.

Ascending-Descending Threshold Comparisons

Comparing ascending thresholds with descending thresholds for tones or speech is a good screener. The reader should keep in mind that in this context of questionable validity, a *threshold* is necessarily tentative or preliminary. It might be the lowest level of response but not the lowest level that the subject can hear (i.e., a *pseudothreshold*). False responders yield substantially lower thresholds for stimuli starting from a low level and rising than for stimuli starting from a high level and decreasing, whereas true responders show no difference (Schlauch, Koerner, & Marshall, 2015). In pure-tone testing, a threshold difference greater than 5 dB is positive for FEHL (Harris, 1958). Testing at one frequency (1 kHz) takes about a minute and is a highly effective, simple screening tool (Woodford, Harris, Marquette, Perry, & Barnhart, 1997).

Another approach to rapid and accurate screening combines the ascending-descending threshold gap with the loudness effects of a pulsed tone (Martin, Martin, & Champlin, 2000). Because pulsed tones are off part of the time, they do not seem as loud as tones that are continuously on at the same decibel level. As a consequence, tones that are on for 500 ms and off for 500 ms tend to cause false responders to present poorer thresholds than continuous tones of 1- to 2-s duration (Rintelmann & Harford, 1967), and pulsed tones with a lengthened off-time of 700 ms are even more likely to yield a pulsed-continuous threshold difference (Hattler, 1970). Using a standard audiometer, one can obtain ascending and descending thresholds with a tone continuously on and with a pulsed tone having a lengthened off time of 700 ms to increase the chances of finding threshold gaps >10 dB (Martin et al., 2000).

Ascending SRTs obtained from normal-hearing subjects feigning a hearing loss have been found to be an average 9 dB lower than descending SRTs (Schlauch, Arnce, Olson, Sanchez, & Doyle, 1996). Similarly, the gap between SRT and PTA typically seen in false responders is magnified when the SRT is obtained in an ascending direction and the pure-tone thresholds are derived in a descending direction (the latter being higher). Schlauch et al. (2015) found that normal-hearing feigners produced an average difference of 31 dB between the ascending spondee threshold and the descending tone thresholds of 500 and 1000 Hz. Using combinations of a noise band and various frequencies produced significant ascending-descending differences, but they were smaller at 20 to 22 dB. When the spondee-two-frequency difference was used and compared to the initial audiogram, the result was 100% true positives and 0% false positives in identifying the false hearing loss. If there is a positive outcome, subsequent pure-tone threshold searches should be conducted with ascending approaches only (Schlauch et al., 1996).

Small Steps

Another variant of standard practice is to use 2- or 2.5-dB increments instead of the usual 5 dB, whether for tones or speech (Nilo & Saunders, 1976; Snyder, 2001). Indeed, a few presentations can be made at the same decibel interval (Nilo & Saunders, 1976). After some presentations of small or no increments, a patient apparently supposes that the signals are loud enough that it is time to respond. As a result, a much narrower intensity range is covered in an ascending series (Snyder, 2001). A good combination is a low starting point and small increment size (Nilo & Saunders, 1976).

Suggestibility

Clinicians can take advantage of their authority status and the element of suggestibility in various ways. Encourage the patient to be a bit bold. Give frequent prompts, "Go ahead. I think you got it," and similar ploys. Do not argue. If the child says he or she cannot hear it, either ignore it (i.e., do not reinforce the comment) and proceed, or deflect the comment saying something like, "sometimes they are soft, but that's OK, raise your hand/say the word anyway," or "the next ones are easier." For discrete-frequency testing, the next "easier" ones could be warble tones or narrow band noises. Employ much suggestibility and expectation. There is great value in the psychological tenet that people tend to behave in the direction in which they are expected to behave.

Pure-Tone Audiometry

Pure-tone audiometry can be modified in a few ways. For example, a simple way to check validity is to insert long silent intervals of 30 s between signals. Conscientious responders might make a few false-positive responses, but invalid responders are unlikely to make any (Chaiklin & Ventry, 1965).

A long-standing and remarkably successful approach is the "yes-no" test (Frank, 1976; Miller, Fox, & Chan, 1968). The child is instructed to say "yes" when he or she hears the tone and "no" when the child does not. Some children do not see the incongruity of acknowledging a supposedly inaudible signal by saying "no." The success of the test depends on responses coming within a normal time window after a signal, and also on "no response" when there is no signal or when the signal is below the child's true threshold. In this author's experience, some children spontaneously adopt a "no" response, which the clinician can exploit.

The variable intensity pulse count method (Ross, 1964) is presented to the child as a test of counting ability. In this test, the child is instructed to count how many times a tone was heard in a series of one to six pulses. Initially, a few series of tones are presented above admitted thresholds to be sure that the child can perform the task. Then, the intensity of one of the tones is given at 10 to 15 dB below the admitted threshold, and the succeeding tones are given above "threshold." A correct answer means the child most probably heard the lower tone. The intensity and number of tones are varied at random—that is, one or more tones below admitted threshold interspersed with one or more tones above admitted threshold. Intensity is varied until the lowest level of three consecutive correct responses is found. Even incorrect answers, intentional or not, can be informative when given just after the signal. If it happens that the signal is very near the true threshold, genuine errors might be expected. Also, an error could be intentional to mislead the tester. Hence, if a child does not answer during silent control periods but answers "on time," even if wrong, it is likely that the signal was heard.

Speech Audiometry

Familiarizing the patient with the spondee words prior to testing is always good practice. If a patient gives half-word responses during SRT testing, there are a few options. One is to accept the response and proceed; even a correct half-word means the spondee was heard. Or, the clinician can "remind" the patient that the words had been practiced beforehand; therefore, hearing "birth" could only be "birthday." Urge the patient to say what he or she *thinks* the word might be. Or, coax the patient to say the second syllable, "birth-what?" If the patient does not respond, sometimes waiting several seconds helps lend a sense of expectancy, which can elicit a response.

If a tentative SRT has been established, obtain a word recognition score at 10 to 15 dB SL. Alternatively, one could proceed directly to a soft conversational level (e.g., 35 dB HL). If hearing is actually quite good (i.e., 10 dB or better), recognizing the test words would be relatively easy. A countervailing caution is that a higher signal presentation level does help accustom the patient to greater loudness and goes against the notion of keeping signal levels low as much as possible. For normal hearers, word recognition scores reach 94% to 100% at about 27 dB SL re SRT (see Olsen & Matkin, 1991). In the case of FEHL, it is not unusual to obtain a high word recognition score at only 10 dB SL, which strongly suggests that the sensation level is actually greater than 10 dB. The SRT could be predicted to be at least 15 to 20 dB lower than the presentation level.

Additional Tests

Additional audiometric procedures beyond pure tone and speech audiometry can be very helpful in FEHL.

Stenger Test

The Stenger test is the most effective behavioral test for false, unilateral, or asymmetrical hearing losses. It is applicable when there is a difference in admitted thresholds between the two ears of at least 25 dB, but effectiveness increases sharply as the difference widens just another 10 dB. Not only does the Stenger test identify FEHL, but it can also help estimate true thresholds.

The test is based on the Stenger effect: when identical signals are introduced simultaneously to each ear, the signal is perceived on the side where it is louder. To reach the point that the perception of the two signals is in only one ear, the difference in sensation levels must be at least 10 dB (Hamill & Price, 2008). The test requires a single sound source to the two ears but with independent control of the intensities. A signal can be either a pure tone or speech.

To perform the Stenger test a signal is presented 10 dB above threshold to the "better" ear, and an identical signal is presented simultaneously 10 dB below supposed threshold to the "poorer" ear. If the threshold in the poorer ear is genuine, the patient will respond because of hearing the sound in the "better" ear (negative Stenger). In contrast, if there truly is no hearing loss in the "poorer" ear, the patient will hear the signal only in the "poorer" ear and not respond (positive Stenger). However, a patient becoming suspicious that a stimulus is going to both ears might do some clever guessing of when and when not to respond. Thus, now and then, one should withhold the signal to the "better" ear. If the patient responds, it must be because the person hears the signal in the "poorer" ear (also sometimes considered a positive Stenger). In addition, to check the validity of a negative Stenger, from time to time present the signal only to the "better" ear. Failure to respond shows that the patient is not responding validly.

This involved process highlights the need for the entire procedure to be performed seamlessly. During threshold testing, the audiologist can simply make a few control changes and apply the Stenger test. To the patient, it should seem that nothing has changed. Then, the Stenger can show almost instantaneously whether the "poorer" ear threshold is valid or not. The test can be employed in an ostensibly informal manner by making offhand remarks ("Tell me again how old you are.") or asking simple questions ("Do the earphones feel OK?").

A difference of 35 dB or more in admitted thresholds is advantageous because the test gives a 10-dB lower signal to the "poorer" ear and a 10-dB greater signal to the "better" ear. Consequently, any ear disparity in alleged thresholds is reduced by 20 dB. In other words, a large initial disparity helps absorb the reduction in the sensation level (SL) difference and still allows the Stenger effect to influence signal lateralization.

To estimate the true threshold of the "poorer" ear, find the lowest level to that ear at which the patient does respond. The interval just above that point where the patient does not respond is the lowest level in the "poorer" ear, which interferes with hearing the signal in the "better" ear, or the minimum contralateral interference level (MCIL). One can seek the MCIL either by lowering the signal to the "poorer" ear from a high starting point or raising the signal from 0 dB HL with the same result (Peck & Ross, 1970). The MCIL in the "poorer" ear roughly equals the SL in the "better" ear. For example, if the MCIL in the "poorer" ear is 40 dB HL and the signal in the "better" ear is 10 dB SL, one might infer that 40 dB HL is about 10 dB SL, and therefore, the threshold in the "poorer" ear is about 30 dB HL. This is merely an approximation because the range at which the MCIL occurs is somewhat broad. Tone MCILs have been found to be within 14 dB of the true thresholds, permitting some degree of threshold estimate of the "poorer" ear (Peck & Ross, 1970).

Evoked Otoacoustic Emissions

As a broad guideline, the presence of evoked otoacoustic emissions (EOAEs) argues against a hearing loss greater than 40 dB, whereas the absence of EOAEs denotes a hearing loss greater than 40 dB (provided a normal tympanogram). Screening for EOAEs can be done quickly and easily and is generally sufficient to corroborate or refute the audiometric results. However, EOAE testing provides little information about organic thresholds. Further details on EOAEs can be found in Chapter 20 of this volume.

Acoustic Reflex Threshold

In supposed hearing losses greater than 70 dB HL, absence of the acoustic reflex (presuming normal tympanograms) lends credence to the hearing test results. However, an acoustic reflex only 10 dB above a voluntary threshold makes that threshold highly suspicious, and an acoustic reflex lower than the voluntary threshold clearly indicates false test results (Rintelmann & Schwan, 1999). In the 1970s, attempts were made for sensitivity prediction from the acoustic reflex (SPAR test). For various reasons, it is rarely used, particularly to assess FEHL.

Auditory-Evoked Potentials

It is beyond the scope of this chapter to detail the various auditory-evoked potentials procedures; they are covered in Chapters 21 and 22. Suffice it to say that evoked potentials can confirm FEHL and quantify true sensitivity to a large degree.

Reporting

The report of any audiologic evaluation might well have legal ramifications, but especially reports regarding persons with FEHL. The language used in reports should be chosen with great care. It would be wise to avoid the word *diagnosis* and, instead, give descriptions, impressions, and recommendations. Audiologists should not use labels, such as *malingering*, *unconscious*, or similar words that refer to state of mind. Any label should be considered very carefully or avoided altogether (Martin & Clark, 2015; Rintelmann & Schwan, 1999; Snyder, 2001).

Protocol

Given the nature of FEHL and the need to be adaptable, it is difficult to lay out a routine test order. Flexibility is implicit in this outline. Here is a series of steps to consider as soon as there is a sign or risk of FEHL:

- Conduct OAE screening.
- Use visual indicators as deterrents, for example, picture of a tympanogram labeled "normal," or pointing out deflections on acoustic reflex meter or indication of "present;" similarly, showing display of normal OAEs or indication of "pass."
- Establish ascending SRT.
- Switch between speech and tones, and among frequencies and intensities from time to time.
- Find ascending-descending thresholds, preferably for ascending speech and descending tones.
- Employ Stenger test in unilateral loss or in bilateral loss with ≥35 dB ear difference.
- Obtain a low-level word recognition score.
- If necessary, perform diagnostic OAE or evoked potentials testing, particularly the auditory brainstem response.

Psychosocial Considerations

Nineteen percent of youth have a psychological or psychiatric problem at some time (Kashani et al., 1987). Major depressive disorder occurs in 4% to 8% of adolescents (see Birmaher & Brent, 2010), and lifetime prevalence by the end of adolescence is about 20% (see Brent & Weersing, 2007). Many of the precipitating factors and symptoms of depression are remarkably similar to characteristics of childhood FEHL—parental divorce, family discord, and lack of emotional availability of parents (Doebelling, 2000), along with a somatic complaint, decline in school performance, and behavioral problems (Sood & Sood, 2000; Waslick, Kandel, & Kakouros, 2002). Abuse and neglect are disturbingly common and contribute significantly to psychosocial problems, such as lowered academic achievement, poor social skills and relationships, low self-esteem, depression, and suicide risk (Devries et al., 2014; Hart et al., 2011). A number of instances of FEHL have been linked to abuse and neglect, either physical or psychological (Drake, Makielski, McDonald-Bell, & Atcheson, 1995; Lumio, Jauhiainen, & Gelhar, 1969; Riedner & Efros, 1995). Fortunately, rates of physical and sexual abuse have declined significantly since a peak in 1993, although the rates of neglect have not (Kaufman, 2007). In 2008, 3.3 million children in the United States were reported abused or neglected (Erikson & Egeland, 2011). At 2011 rates, one child in eight in the United States will have a verified event of maltreatment by age 18 years (Wildeman et al., 2014). Spurred by the prevalence and consequences of child maltreatment, the subspecialty of child abuse pediatrics was created in 2006 by the American Board of Pediatrics (Block & Palusci, 2006).

The 2:1 occurrence of FEHL in girls over boys has no clear explanation. Depression might play a role in the gender difference. The onset of puberty is accompanied by a disproportionate increased risk of depressive symptoms in girls, becoming twice as common in females as in males by the end of adolescence (Waslick et al., 2002). Also with puberty, sexual abuse rises sharply and occurs more often against females than males (Gordon & Schroeder, 1995). Approximately 20% to 25% of women have been victimized before adulthood (see Berliner, 2011; Gordon & Schroeder, 1995). Such treatment predisposes children to somatic complaints, depression, poor schoolwork, low self-esteem, and suicide.

Suicide deserves mention because it is often linked to depression and maltreatment (Waslick et al., 2002). Thoughts of suicide, suicidal gestures (Sood & Sood, 2000), and completions rise greatly during adolescence (U.S. Dept. of Commerce, 2004). At any moment in time, 15% to 25% of adolescents in the United States corroborate some degree of suicidal ideation, although ideation that is specific and active is far less common with estimates between 2% and 6% (see Goldstein & Brent, 2010). In 2007, the rate of suicide among 5- to 14-year-olds was 0.5 per 100,000, whereas among 15- to 24-year-olds, the rate was 9.7 per 100,000, a 19-fold increase (U.S. Dept. of Commerce, 2004). In 2010, suicide was the second leading cause of death among adolescents aged 12 to 17 years (Centers for Disease Control and Prevention, 2013).

Considering all the above, it seems most unlikely that by and large children with FEHL are emotionally well, clever swindlers out to cozen the system for some tangible benefit. Besides, the private nature of personal thoughts and motivations makes it difficult to be sure that a person is malingering (McCann, 1998). Even if a person is malingering, faking at any age is usually a poor way to handle adverse situations. What does seem likely is that children with FEHL are at much higher risk of having a psychosocial problem, indeed, one that could be painful and have serious consequences. Exhibiting a nonexistent disorder for whatever reason might be a symptom of something wrong and should not be dismissed out of hand (McCann, 1998).

Interviewing, Counseling, Referring

Should the false hearing loss resolve during the evaluation, still check for signs of psychosocial difficulty. The problem does not disappear just because the "hearing loss" disappears. Between extremes of referring no one or everyone for further evaluation, audiologists can reasonably expect to identify those most likely in need of referral by taking a few simple measures (Peck, 2011). Talk with the child and the parent separately. The clinician can begin by relating that every year one sees a few people who have trouble taking the test, and often they are preoccupied about something. If there is no reply after a moment, ask if that might apply to the patient. If not, ask a few, simple, open-ended questions tactfully. Is the person "bothered about something?" Follow up more specifically. Are there any problems with friends, school, or home? Ask the adult, does the child seem as well adjusted and as happy as other children? Has there been a change in behavior or mood?

An excellent aid in screening for psychosocial disorders is the Pediatric Symptom Checklist (PSC). The PSC is 35-item, pass-fail questionnaire completed by a caregiver and standardized for children 6 to 12 years of age (Jellinek et al., 1988). There is a briefer 17-item edition, as well as a pictorial and a youth self-report version, and translations into many languages (available from Massachusetts General Hospital Psychiatry, 2014).

If at some point one has sufficient information to warrant a referral, frame the overall situation, for example, "Based on the hearing testing, the reports of . . . [from history] . . . , and . . . [PSC score, other information,] . . . , I'm wondering if it would be worthwhile to talk to an expert about these things." Notice that the interviewing, counseling, and setting the stage for referral all blend together. For a more complete treatment of the entire process, see Peck (2011).

Before ending, explain to the parent that the child does not deserve punishment, and advise that there be little or no mention of hearing loss, so as not to reinforce the idea in the child. Leave the child with assurance that hearing is or will be getting better (taking advantage of suggestibility).

Sample Case

D.O., a 10-year-old female, was referred by pulmonology for concern about hearing loss. D.O. began to complain of and show signs of hearing loss 6 months previous, per mother and teacher. School grades dropped during the last school term. She was followed for a lung disorder. The mother and father divorced when she was 3 years old. Her father visited only occasionally, which caused the child to be resentful. By the mother's report, D.O. avoided peers, was withdrawn, was anxious about her overweight, and was "not happy." The mother, herself, was in counseling for "nerves." Initial pure-tone audiometry yielded inconsistent responses around 45 dB. Tympanograms were Type B, consistent with middle ear effusions. Nevertheless, when spondee words were presented to each ear separately at decreasing levels, D.O. repeated them at 15 dB. Similarly, she passed a pure-tone screening bilaterally at 15 dB for 500 to 4000 Hz. The Pediatric Symptom Checklist score was 46, far above the normal cutoff. Mental health evaluation was recommended and readily accepted.

Conclusion

Audiologists might be concerned that they will appear to be prying or inappropriate when screening for psychosocial disorders. Yet, almost invariably, patients and parents welcome the clinician's concern, empathy, insights, and suggestions. If an audiologist has reasonable suspicion of a psychosocial problem, refer to whoever can assure further evaluation and intervention. Follow-up is a matter of clinical judgment tailored to the individual case, depending on referral source, patient preference, distance, services available in the patient's locale, and so forth. Some audiologists might hesitate to refer, fearing the harmful stigma associated with mental health care. Yet, if there are already signs of a psychosocial difficulty, it is much more likely that greater harm will be done by *not* referring. By discounting the risk, an audiologist might delay badly needed help. By recognizing the risk, an audiologist can take the first step toward appropriate management.

References

American Psychiatric Association. (2013). *Diagnostic and statistical manual of mental disorders* (5th ed., p. 726). Washington, DC: Author.

Aplin, D. Y., & Rowson, V. J. (1986). Personality and functional hearing loss in children. *British Journal of Clinical Psychology, 25*, 313–314.

Aplin, D. Y., & Rowson, V. J. (1990). Psychological characteristics of children with functional hearing loss. *British Journal of Audiology, 24*, 77–87.

Austen, S., & Lynch, C. (2004). Non-organic hearing loss redefined: Understanding, categorizing and managing non-organic behavior. *International Journal of Audiology, 43*, 449–457.

Barr, B. (1960). Nonorganic hearing problems in school-children. Functional deafness. *Acta Oto-laryngologica, 52*, 337–346.

Beagley, H. A., & Knight, J. J. (1968). The evaluation of suspected non-organic hearing loss. *Journal of Laryngology and Otology, 82*, 693–705.

Berger, K. (1965). Pseudohypacusis in children. *Laryngoscope, 75*, 447–457.

Berliner, L. (2011). Child sexual abuse: Definitions, prevalence, and consequences. In J. E. B. Myers (Ed.), *The APSAC handbook on child maltreatment* (3rd ed., pp. 215–232). Thousand Oaks, CA: Sage.

Birmaher, B., & Brent, D. A. (2010). Depression and dysthymia. In M. K. Dulcan (Ed.), *Dulcan's textbook of child and adolescent psychiatry*. Arlington, VA: American Psychiatric Publishing. doi:10.1176/appi.books.9781585623921.md18

Block, R. W., & Palusci, V. J. (2006). Child abuse pediatrics: A new pediatric subspecialty. *Journal of Pediatrics, 148*, 711–712.

Bowdler, D. A., & Rogers, J. (1989). The management of pseudohypacusis in school-age children. *Clinical Otolaryngology, 14*, 211–215.

Brent, D. A., & Weersing, V. R. (2007). Depressive disorders. In A. Martin & F. R. Volkmar (Eds.), *Lewis's child and adolescent psychiatry. A comprehensive textbook* (4th ed., pp. 503–513). Philadelphia, PA: Lippincott Williams & Wilkins.

Campanelli, P. A. (1963). Simulated hearing losses in school children following identification audiometry. *Journal of Auditory Research, 3*, 91–108.

Centers for Disease Control and Prevention. (2013). Mental health surveillance among children—United States, 2005–2011. *MMWR, 62*(Suppl.), 1–35.

Chaiklin, J. B., & Ventry, I. M. (1965). Patient errors during spondee and pure-tone threshold measurement. *Journal of Auditory Research, 5*, 219–230.

Devries, K. M., Mak, J. Y. T., Child, J. C., Falder, G., Bacchus, L. J., Astbury, J., & Watts, C. H. (2014). Childhood sexual abuse and suicidal behavior: A meta-analysis. *Pediatrics, 133*, e1331–e1344. doi:10.1542/peds.2013-2166

Dixon, R. F., & Newby, H. A. (1959). Children with nonorganic hearing problems. *Archives of Otolaryngology, 70*, 619–623.

Doebelling, C. C. (2000). Epidemiology, risk factors, and prevention. In J. L. Levenson (Ed.), *Depression* (pp. 23–46). Philadelphia, PA: American College of Physicians.

Drake, A. F., Makielski, K., McDonald-Bell, C., & Atcheson, B. (1995). Two new otolaryngologic findings in child abuse. *Archives of Otolaryngology-Head and Neck Surgery, 121*, 1417–1420.

Drouillard, M., Petroff, N., Majer, J., Perrot, C., Quesnel, S., & François, M. (2014). Pseudohypacusis in children: Circumstances and diagnostic strategy. *International Journal of Pediatric Otorhinolaryngology, 78*, 1632–1636.

Erikson, M. F., & Egeland, B. (2011). Child neglect. In J. E. B. Myers (Ed.), *The APSAC handbook on child maltreatment* (3rd ed., pp. 103–124). Thousand Oaks, CA: Sage.

Frank, T. (1976). Yes-no test for nonorganic hearing loss. *Archives of Otolaryngology, 102*, 162–165.

Goldstein, T. R., & Brent, D. A. (2010). Youth suicide. In M. K. Dulcan (Ed.), *Dulcan's textbook of child and adolescent psychiatry*. Arlington, VA: American Psychiatric Publishing. doi:10.1176/appi.books.9781585623921.md35

Gordon, B. N., & Schroeder, C. S. (1995). *Sexuality: A developmental approach to problems*. New York, NY: Plenum Press.

Hamill, T., & Price, L. (2008). *The hearing sciences*. San Diego, CA: Singular.

Harris, D. A. (1958). A rapid and simple technique for the detection of nonorganic hearing loss. *Archives of Otolaryngology, 68*, 758–760.

Hart, S. N., Brassard, M. R., Davidson, H. A. Rivelis, E., Diaz, V., & Binggeli, N. J. (2011). Psychological maltreatment. In J. E. B. Myers (Ed.), *The APSAC handbook on child maltreatment* (3rd ed., pp. 125–144). Thousand Oaks, CA: Sage.

Hattler, K. W. (1970). Lengthened off-time: A self-recording screening device for nonorganicity. *Journal of Speech and Hearing Disorders, 35,* 113–122.

Jellinek, M. S., Murphy, J. M., Robinson, J., Feins, A., Lamb, S., & Fenton, T. (1988). Pediatric symptom checklist: Screening school-age children for psychosocial dysfunction. *Journal of Pediatrics, 112,* 201–209.

Kashani, J. H., Beck, N. C., Hoeper, E. W., Fallahi, C., Corcoran, C. M., McAllister, J. A., . . . Reid, J. C. (1987). Psychiatric disorders in a community sample of adolescents. *American Journal of Psychiatry, 144,* 584–589.

Kaufman, J. (2007). Child abuse and neglect. In A. Martin, & F. R. Volkmar (Eds.), *Lewis's child and adolescent psychiatry. A comprehensive textbook* (4th ed., pp. 692–701). Philadelphia, PA: Lippincott Williams & Wilkins.

Kothe, C., Fleischer, S., Breitfuss, A., & Hess, M. (2003). Diagnosis of psychogenic hearing disorders in childhood [in German] *HNO, 51,* 915–920. doi:10.1007/s00106-003-0892-0

Lehrer, N. D., Hirschenfang, S., Miller, M. H., & Radpour, S. (1964). Nonorganic hearing problems in adolescents. *Laryngoscope, 74,* 64–69.

Leshin, G. J. (1960). Childhood nonorganic hearing loss. *Journal of Speech and Hearing Disorders, 25,* 290–292.

Lumio, J. S., Jauhiainen, T., & Gelhar, K. (1969). Three cases of functional deafness in the same family. *Journal of Laryngology and Otology, 83,* 299–304.

Martin, F. N., & Clark, J. G. (2015). *Introduction to audiology* (12th ed.). Boston, MA: Pearson.

Martin, J. S., Martin, F. N., & Champlin, C. A. (2000). The CON-SOT-LOT Test for nonorganic hearing loss. *Journal of the American Academy of Audiology, 11,* 46–51.

Massachusetts General Hospital Psychiatry. (2014). *Pediatric Symptom Checklist.* Retrieved from http://www.massgeneral.org/psc

McCann, J. T. (1998). *Malingering and deception in adolescents: Assessing credibility in clinical and forensic settings.* Washington, DC: American Psychological Association.

McCanna, D. L., & DeLapa, G. (1981). A clinical study of twenty-seven children exhibiting functional hearing loss. *Language, Speech, and Hearing Services in Schools, 12,* 26–33.

Miller, A. L., Fox, M. S., & Chan, G. (1968). Pure tone assessments as an aid in detecting suspected non-organic hearing disorders in children. *Laryngoscope, 78,* 2170–2176.

Miller-Keane Encyclopedia and Dictionary of Medicine, Nursing and Allied Health (7th ed). (2003). Philadelphia, PA: Saunders.

Monro, K. J. & Contractor, A. (2010). Inter-aural attenuation with insert earphones. *International Journal of Audiology, 49,* 799–801.

Morita, S., Suzuki, M., & Iizuka, K. (2010). Non-organic hearing loss in childhood. *International Journal of Pediatric Otorhinolaryngology, 74,* 441–446.

Mosby's Medical Dictionary (8th ed.). (2009). St. Louis, MO: Mosby.

Nilo, E. R., & Saunders, W. H. (1976). Functional hearing loss. *Laryngoscope, 86,* 501–505.

Olsen, W. O. (1991). Special auditory tests: A historical perspective. In J. T. Jacobson, & J. L. Northern (Eds.), *Diagnostic audiology* (pp. 19–51). Austin, TX: Pro-Ed.

Olsen, W. O., & Matkin, N. D. (1991). Speech audiometry. In W. F. Rintelmann (Ed.), *Hearing assessment* (2nd ed., pp. 39–135). Boston, MA: Allyn & Bacon.

Peck, J. E. (2002). *Pseudohypacusis: Psychosocial issues and management.* Short course presented at the annual convention of the American Academy of Audiology, Philadelphia, PA.

Peck, J. E. (2011). *Pseudohypacusis: False and exaggerated hearing loss.* San Diego, CA: Plural.

Peck, J. E., & Ross, M. (1970). A comparison of the ascending and the descending modes for administration of the pure-tone Stenger test. *Journal of Auditory Research, 10,* 218–220.

Pracy, J. P., Walsh, R. M., Mepham, G. A., & Bowdler, D. A. (1996). Childhood pseudohypacusis. *International Journal of Pediatric Otorhinolaryngology, 37,* 143–149.

Psarommatis, I., Kontorinis, G., Kontrogiannis, A., Douniadakis, D., & Tsakanikos, M. (2009). Pseudohypacusis: The most frequent etiology of sudden hearing loss in children. *European Archives of Oto-Rhino-Laryngology, 266,* 1857–1861.

Riedner, E. D., & Efros, P. L. (1995). Nonorganic hearing loss and child abuse: Beyond the sound booth. *British Journal of Audiology, 29,* 195–197.

Rintelmann, W. F., & Harford, E. R. (1967). Type V Bekesy pattern: Interpretation and clinical utility. *Journal of Speech and Hearing Research, 10,* 733–746.

Rintelmann, W. F., & Schwan, S. A. (1999). Pseudohypacusis. In F. E. Musiek & W. F. Rintelmann (Eds.), *Contemporary perspectives in hearing assessment* (pp. 415–435). Boston, MA: Allyn & Bacon.

Roeser, R. J., & Clark, J. L. (2007). Pure-tone tests. In R. J. Roeser, M. Valente, & H. Hosford-Dunn (Eds.), *Audiology diagnosis* (2nd ed., pp. 238–260). New York, NY: Thieme.

Ross, M. (1964). The variable intensity pulse count method (VIPCM) for the detection and measurement of the pure-tone threshold of children with functional hearing losses. *Journal of Speech and Hearing Disorders, 29,* 477–482.

Saravanappa, N., Mepham, G. A., & Bowdler, D. A. (2005). Diagnostic tools in pseudohypacusis in children. *International Journal of Pediatric Otorhinolaryngology, 69,* 1235–1238.

Schlauch, R. S., Arnce, K. D., Olson, L. M., Sanchez, S., & Doyle, T. N. (1996). Identification of pseudohypacusis using speech recognition thresholds. *Ear and Hearing, 17,* 229–236.

Schlauch, R. S., Koerner, T. K., & Marshall, L. (2015). Effective identification of functional hearing loss using behavioral threshold measures. *Journal of Speech, Language, and Hearing Research, 58,* 453–465.

Schmidt, C. M., Am Zehnhoff-Dinnesen, A., Matulat, P., Knief, A., Rosslau, K., & Deuster, D. (2013). Nonorganic hearing loss in children: Audiometry, clinical characteristics, biographical history and recovery of hearing thresholds. *International Journal of Pediatric Otorhinolaryngology, 77,* 1190–1193.

Shahrokh, N. C., & Hales, R. E. (Eds.). (2003). *American psychiatric glossary* (8th ed.). Washington, DC: American Psychiatric Publishing.

Snyder, J. M. (2001). Audiological evaluation for exaggerated hearing loss. In R. A. Dobie (Ed.), *Medical-legal evaluation of hearing loss* (2nd ed., pp. 49–88). San Diego, CA: Singular Thomson Learning.

Sood, A. A., & Sood, R. K. (2000). Depression in children and adolescents. In J. L. Levenson, (Ed.), *Depression* (pp. 225–250). Philadelphia, PA: American College of Physicians.

U.S. Department of Commerce. (2004). Statistical abstract of the United States: 2004–2005. *The national data book* (124th ed.). Washington, DC: U.S. Department of Commerce.

Waslick, B. D., Kandel, R., & Kakouros, A. (2002). Depression in children and adolescents: An overview. In D. Shaffer & B. D. Waslick (Eds.), *The many faces of depression in children and adolescents* (pp. 1–36). Washington, DC: American Psychiatric Publishing.

Wildeman, C., Emanuel, N., Leventhal, J. M., Putnam-Hornstein, E., Waldfogel, J., & Lee, H. (2014). The prevalence of confirmed maltreatment among US children, 2004 to 2011. *JAMA Pediatrics, 168*, 706–713.

Woodford, C. M., Harris, G., Marquette, M. L., Perry, L., & Barnhart, M. (1997). A screening test for pseudohypacusis. *Hearing Review, 11*, 23–24, 26.

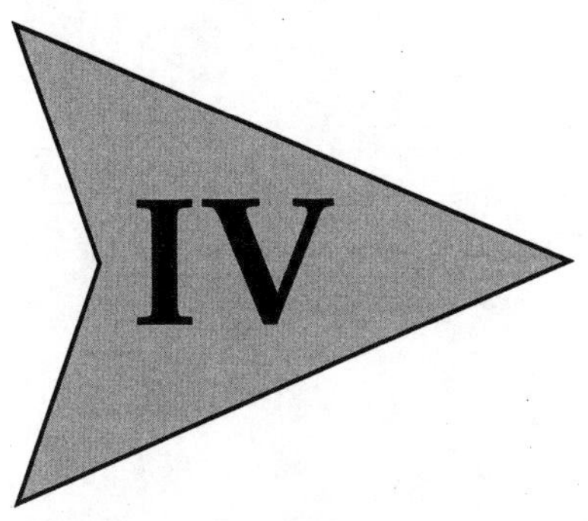

Early Identification of Hearing Loss

Principles and Methods of Newborn Hearing Screening

Martyn Hyde

Introduction

This chapter examines some issues that arise in population hearing screening. The main focus is on newborn hearing screening (NHS) within an early hearing detection and intervention (EHDI) program, but some of the principles and methods considered are common to almost any public health screening program. Many publications on EHDI and universal newborn hearing screening (UNHS) are available, so basic familiarity with the area is assumed. The intent here is to consider key aspects in some depth, to examine common assumptions critically, to identify challenges, and to consider alternative viewpoints and approaches.

The chapter is not a review of all possible NHS tests. It focuses exclusively on screening based on otoacoustic emissions (OAEs) and the auditory brainstem response (ABR), by far the most important techniques to date. The basic properties and applications of these phenomena have been described in numerous articles as well as in excellent review texts by Burkard and Don (2007) for the ABR and by Prieve and Fitzgerald (2009) for the OAE. Here, there is some further discussion of aspects of ABR and OAE that relate to their validity, effectiveness and efficiency as screening tools. Although references of special interest are cited throughout, many excellent articles are omitted, and there is no attempt at formal, systematic evidence review. Such reviews are essential, methodologically rigid, and typically tedious, if not indigestible. Rather, this chapter reflects the author's experience of screening and EHDI program design, development, evaluation, clinical support, critical appraisal of evidence, and clinical epidemiology over the last few decades. It is offered as food for thought.

A Conceptual Model of Early Hearing Detection and Intervention

Screening must be viewed in relation to its overall rationale and context. A conceptual model is a useful starting point. Readers will know that any EHDI program includes newborn screening, usually universal, followed by detailed (diagnostic) audiologic assessment of those who do not pass the screening and when permanent hearing loss (PHL) is identified, various types of communication with affected families, audiologic interventions, and other key components such as medical management. Rather than simply depict that procedural chain linearly, Figure 15–1 reflects some aspects of the *purpose or function* of various stages in the EHDI process.

Figure 15–1 looks like two filter funnels joined together. The lower, inverted funnel represents progressive filtering or selection of newborns. The starting baseline is some target population who are the defined candidates for screening; the proportion or percentage screened successfully and in a timely manner is referred to as *coverage*. The screening itself can have several stages, typically from one to three tests in series, in parallel, or a mixture. A small proportion of newborns screened successfully will fail the screening, and these are then input to more definitive diagnostic

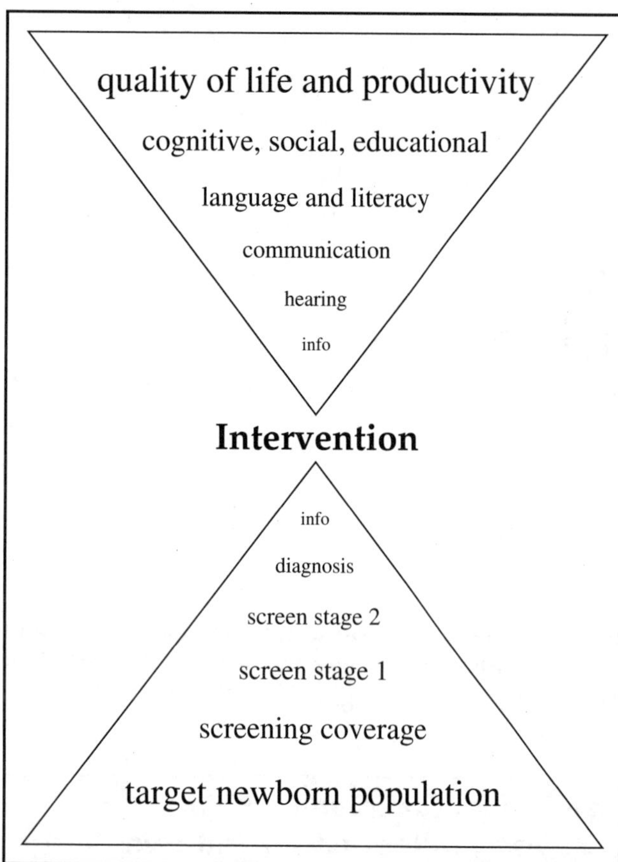

FIGURE 15–1. A conceptual model of EHDI. The bottom, inverted funnel represents a progressive filtering process that extracts babies with hearing loss from the newborn population and delivers them to interventions. The upper funnel represents an expanding array of personal, familial, and societal functioning that is facilitated by the interventions.

audiometry. In turn, some proportion of these will have confirmed hearing loss. The lower and upper funnels are linked by key procedures grouped under the term *intervention*, which receive input from below and deliver outputs above.

Although it has become common practice in the field to avoid using the term *fail*, the screening, substituting euphemisms such as *refer* or *no clear response*, it remains debatable whether such wordplay is appropriate, ill-conceived, or irrelevant. Babies do fail screens and despite screener actions that might reflect their own discomfort, an intention to reduce family anxiety, or to highlight follow-up testing, family members often use the word *fail* among themselves or with peers. A concern is that if screening personnel substitute less direct terms, family members might be confused or might not take the screening result as seriously as they might otherwise. Bear in mind that families often mistakenly believe that they can tell whether their baby's hearing is OK or not, or might view screening results with skepticism or denial for many other reasons.

The upper funnel represents not individuals but their levels of functioning. The processes of intervention are intended first to enhance hearing or other communication modes. These lead to an expanding array of functioning, including language, literacy, cognitive, social, and educational development, ultimately yielding a high quality of life and a full and productive participation in the family and in society at large. These are the ultimate endpoints that are the long-term purpose of the initial screening.

Consider this a little more quantitatively. Starting with the entire newborn population as a baseline, some proportion of that population will have the *target disorder*, which is the set of all hearing disorders that we wish to detect and then address by interventions. That proportion (p) is the population *prevalence* of the target disorder and is often quoted to be one to three per thousand (0.2%–0.3%) in developed countries, the true value depending on many variables, especially the breadth of target hearing loss criteria (see Chapter 5 in this volume for a detailed review). This is the *congenital* prevalence—that is, the prevalence of hearing loss at birth. Because we are primarily interested in *permanent* hearing disorders, prevalence increases with age. Note the distinction between prevalence and *incidence* of hearing loss, which is the number of new cases that arise in a given period of time, often expressed as a proportion of a given population subgroup size. Technically, the proportion of newborns that has congenital hearing loss is a prevalence, not an incidence, because it refers not to a time interval but to a population cross-sectional freeze-frame defined by the moment of birth. At first, we do not know who has the target disorder and who does not, so think of each newborn as having an invisible label stuck on the forehead. On each label is printed the same thing—the prevalence value 0.002, for example. That number can also be interpreted as the initial probability that any individual newborn selected at random will have the target disorder.

Newborns require levels of care ranging from routine or standard care in the well-baby nursery through to the highest levels of critical care in neonatal intensive care units (NICUs). Many babies in NICUs and some in well-baby nurseries have risk indicators for hearing loss. Each risk indicator increases the number on the baby's label to some level that is often not known exactly. For some groups, the probability might be quite large, and in some cases, such as babies with total ear canal atresia, the probability achieves certainty (1). Typically, most babies "at risk" based on the set of known indicators are considered as a group, in which the average level of hearing loss probability (high-risk prevalence) is about 1% to 2%, which is about 10 times that in the newborn population as a whole. Large variations of reported prevalence in entire populations or in high-risk groups are due to many factors, including sampling variation, epidemiologic, demographic, and socioeconomic features of the population, risk criteria, the effectiveness of risk determination, the quality of perinatal care, and the characteristics of special-care units.

The screening itself can be *selective* or *targeted,* which is usually directed at only the at-risk group or at some limited but convenient approximation to it, such as all graduates of an extended stay in a NICU. In developed countries, about 5% to 10% of the newborn population will be found to be at risk, given current methods of assessing hearing loss risk. Alternatively, the screening can be *universal,* directed at the entire population of newborns. Whichever is the case, it is not easy to access every newborn, and the coverage is always imperfect. In a good UNHS program, population coverage of at least 90% is usually achieved, and sometimes (generally in geographically smaller programs) it can be 99% or even higher.

When contemplating coverage reports, especially near-perfect values, the reader must understand precisely how the quoted value was calculated. For example, were families who were offered but declined the screen included as screened? What if the screen was attempted but not successful? What if the screen was not done until much later than the newborn period, and so on.

Those babies who are accessed successfully will receive screening and most, but not all, will have a successful screening test or tests. The imperfect coverage and success will lead to some babies with hearing loss being missed. In UNHS the proportion of babies with the disorder who will not be screened successfully typically is small. In a selective program, much larger losses will occur depending on the proportion of babies with hearing loss who are not identified as at risk. Many children with the disorder have no apparent, current risk indicator. Both the proportion of the newborn population found to be at risk and the proportion of all babies with the target disorder who are labeled as at risk are subject to many sources of variability. These include local population epidemiology and genetics, the quality of perinatal care, the risk indicator set used, the precise criteria for presence of individual indicators, the diligence with which the risk assessment is conducted, and the quality of the individual medical records. These many factors might explain why, for example, reported proportions of babies with hearing loss who are found to be at risk vary over a wide range, even though a value of about 50% is commonly quoted or assumed.

Although imperfect coverage and unsuccessful screening eliminate some small fraction of babies with hearing loss from consideration, the screening as a whole acts as a filter that increases the probability of the target disorder in those continue to the next step. Given screening with an appropriate protocol and good quality of testing, babies referred for diagnostic assessment will have a much higher number on their labels than the newborn population. Suppose the baseline prevalence were 0.002 and assume for simplicity that no baby with the target disorder was missed. If 5% to 10%, say, of newborns failed a Stage 1 screen (such as by OAE), then in the referred group the number on each baby's label increases by a factor of 10 to 20, to 0.02 to 0.04. A subsequent Stage 2 screen (such as an automated ABR; AABR) is likely to increase the label value further, typically to about 0.1 to 0.2 overall. This is a 50-fold to 100-fold overall enrichment of prevalence from that in the newborn population at large. The number of babies referred usually will be in the range 1% to 2% of the number of newborns screened.

Although the probability of disorder is greatly increased in babies who fail screening, a large majority of these babies *do not* have the target disorder. Therefore, it might be preferable to think of hearing screening tests not as tests that detect hearing loss, but as tests that classify babies into two groups: those with very low probability of loss and those with a much higher probability that demands follow-up action. This distinction is not as academic as it might seem. For example, screening personnel might fall into the trap of equating screening failure with hearing loss presence, which can result in misleading communications to families, needless levels of anxiety, and subsequent confusion when the diagnostic tests are within normal limits, which they will be in many cases.

Certain risk indicators, such as symptomatic congenital cytomegalovirus infection (CMV), can raise the prescreen probability of hearing loss to as high as 41% (NIDCD, 2002), well above the level generally associated with conventional hearing screening test failure. Should such babies be screened at all, or should they go directly to diagnostic hearing testing? Given that screening tests are far from perfect, as will be seen shortly, beyond a certain level of risk the direct route to diagnostics is more appropriate. In fact, the presence of specific risk indicators for hearing loss, such as congenital CMV, severe hypoxia, hyperbilirubinemia, and others, can be viewed as screening "tests" in their own right, because they serve to increase the probability of hearing loss, just as do conventional screening tests. Just to be crystal clear, a baby who has a risk indicator of congenital CMV infection already has a probability of hearing loss larger than that of a nil-risk baby who fails newborn screening that begins with automated OAE (AOAE) and proceeds to AABR if AOAE gives a fail result. If AOAE screening missed only 10% of babies with genuine PHL (which is realistic), then of those babies who had congenital CMV, about 4% (10% of about 40%) would be missed. The simple inference is—do not screen very high risk babies with AOAE. Whether you should screen them with AABR or send them straight to diagnostics is another story altogether.

The next step in Figure 15–1 is confirmatory and diagnostic audiometry. Although not the focus of this chapter, it should be noted that such testing is also imperfect in several respects, albeit less so than screening. In principle, high-quality diagnostic audiometry could be thought to yield post-test probabilities of either 0 (target disorder absent) or 1 (present). In practice, due to limitations of test access and delivery (diagnostic coverage), intrinsic accuracy, protocol appropriateness, and procedural quality, real diagnostic test performance will include errors of hearing loss confirmation and description. In principle, though, the bottom pyramid has filtered the newborn population down to only those babies who have the target disorder.

The entries in the upper part of Figure 15–1 are self-explanatory, and the details of their performance are beyond the scope of this chapter, except insofar as the relevant intervention services either are not delivered or have limited success. That aspect will be considered further in Chapter 16 on NHS program evaluation and quality. It is sufficient to say here that screening is not an end in itself. It is done to lay the groundwork to achieve the entire suite of functional outcomes outlined in Figure 15–1. Although this might seem obvious, it is worth noting that in the historical development of EHDI, attention and effort over many years were directed predominantly to screening itself, with rather less attention to the subsequent and much more complex procedures that translate screening failures into the desired short-term and long-term outcomes. The quality of diagnostic assessments and interventions has only emerged as a strong focus of attention in the decade or two, and a great deal of further effort will be required for many years to come.

Ground Rules for Population Screening

The starting point for most discussions of the principles of screening is the seminal text written many years ago by Wilson and Jungner for the World Health Organization (WHO; Wilson & Jungner, 1968). The report was commissioned because at that time, the WHO was facing a barrage of controversy and diverse efforts to implement early detection of many chronic diseases. The key propositions put forward in that text have become widely known as "the WHO principles of screening." They have been variously adopted or adapted by many authorities and agencies in the field of health services (see, for example, the 23 criteria of the United Kingdom National Screening Committee, 2009), as well as by many individuals manifesting variable levels of insight and interpretation. They are presented often enough that the reader might have met some version of them before and even be disappointed to see them again here. However, there is no better starting point, and it is hoped that the development here might include some features that are novel and informative, so the original wording is presented in Table 15–1, part A.

More recently, again under the auspices of the WHO, Andermann, Blancquaert, Beauchamp, and Dery (2008) reviewed the history and evolution of screening principles since the original publication. In an important update of the Wilson-Jungner criteria, they compiled a list of additional or modified criteria that reflect a modern approach to health programming in the age of evidence-based practice, genuinely client-centered or family-centered care, protection of privacy, and, above all, strong program accountability. These important additions are given in Table 15–1B. A reference of interest that addresses criteria for implementing population screening in this age of genomic medicine and of the potential to screen for not the actual presence of a disorder but the *susceptibility* to a disorder is Khoury, McCabe, and McCabe (2003). Genetic screening for hearing loss susceptibility as well as genetic testing for etiological purposes in young children with proven hearing loss are topics of great current interest that can radically affect the conduct of newborn hearing screening programs in the near future. See also Morton and Nance (2006) for a general review of newborn hearing screening with special reference to genetic causes of hearing loss.

The classical Wilson and Jungner criteria (Table 15–1A) have been criticized on several grounds. One issue is their susceptibility to variable interpretation

Table 15–1. Classical World Health Organization (WHO) Screening Criteria and Recent Enhancements

A. *Classical screening criteria* (Wilson & Jungner, 1968)	The condition sought should be an important health problem. There should be an accepted treatment for patients with recognized disease. Facilities for diagnosis and treatment should be available. There should be a recognizable latent or early symptomatic stage. There should be a suitable test or examination. The test should be acceptable to the population. The natural history of the condition, including development from latent to declared disease, should be adequately understood. There should be an agreed policy on whom to treat as patients. The cost of case-finding (including diagnosis and treatment of patients diagnosed) should be economically balanced in relation to possible expenditure on medical care as a whole. Case-finding should be a continuing process and not a "once and for all" project.
B. *Synthesis of emerging screening criteria proposed over the past 40 years* (Andermann et al., 2008)	The screening program should respond to a recognized need. The objectives of screening should be defined at the outset. There should be a defined target population. There should be scientific evidence of screening program effectiveness. The program should integrate education, testing, clinical services, and program management. There should be quality assurance, with mechanisms to minimize potential risks of screening. The program should ensure informed choice, confidentiality, and respect for autonomy. The program should promote equity and access to screening for the entire target population. Program evaluation should be planned from the outset. The overall benefits of screening should outweigh the harm.

Source: Reprinted with permission from Andermann, A., Blancquaert, I., Beauchamp, S., and Dery, V. (2008). *Revisiting Wilson and Jungner in the genomic age: A review of screening criteria over the past 40 years. WHO Bulletin, 86*(4), 241–320. Retrieved from http://www.who.int/bulletin/volumes/86/4/07-050112/en/index.html. Copyright 2010 World Health Organization.

and misinterpretation, using vague and subjective terms like "important," "accepted," and "suitable." Nevertheless, they have remained a cornerstone of the public health screening field. The propositions can be grouped and prioritized for the EHDI context specifically. First, there is the over-riding issue of identifying and quantifying the *important health problem* or *recognized need*. Why should newborns be screened for hearing loss? What problem or deficiency of previous approaches to early identification is being addressed by such screening? Why is early detection important? Is screening truly effective in the real world with all its messiness and complexity? Although the answers might seem apparent, important subtleties and complexities are often overlooked, such as the effects of hearing loss severity on the differential benefit from screening versus not screening, or the multiple sources of cumulative delay that can eat away at the time gained from newborn screening. There are also complications arising from the diversity, individuality, longitudinal trajectories, and interdependency of the cascade of benefits that can follow from early detection.

Second, the issues of latent period and natural history of hearing disorders are quite interesting, when considering congenital, permanent hearing disorders. At first sight, it seems obvious that congenital hearing loss clearly is *not* latent in the usual sense of "impending" or "waiting to happen." But, it will not be expressed symptomatically in a baby, and it is this lack of spontaneous and recognizable expression of an existing disorder that satisfies the key intent of the term *latency*. In fact, if we consider the accumulating and clinically silent, maladaptive neurodevelopmental effects of sensory deprivation, such as are revealed by dynamic imaging studies and the nondevelopment of cortical tonotopic mapping, it can be argued that there is, in fact, a latent period for the overall, negative effects of unidentified hearing impairment.

Delayed-onset hearing loss might well be truly latent in the affected infant at a molecular level, such as in a situation of cumulative, underlying cochleo-neural pathology that remains functionally subcritical, at least for a while. However, the intent of NHS is certainly not to detect hearing loss that is not yet present and failure to screen positive for a loss yet to be expressed is obviously not a false-negative screening error. Thus, the rationale for prompt detection of late-onset or progressive hearing loss is quite separate, qualitatively and quantitatively, from that for detection of congenital hearing loss.

Third, there must exist screening tests that are practicable, acceptable to its recipients, and reasonably accurate. Much of this volume addresses those issues, which have many facets, wrinkles, and challenges. Fourth, the question of an "accepted treatment" can be viewed through the stronger lens of evidence-based health care, which indicates that what should be required of an intervention is not its general acceptance but its proven effectiveness, given that what is historically generally accepted has often turned out not to be effective.

Last, there is the challenging question of cost justification, to be addressed later. Before delving into these specifics, some inherent attributes and peculiarities of screening are outlined, forming the basis for much of the ensuing discussion. These attributes of screening form the rationale underlying the WHO principles.

Population Screening Is Different From Ordinary Clinical Care

One reason why the WHO saw fit to commission the Wilson-Jungner (1968) report is that screening large numbers of people for some disorder of interest differs radically in many ways from the ordinary process of delivering health care to persons who seek it. People receiving public health screening usually are not actively seeking care because they perceive a specific sign or symptom of a disorder. Rather, screening is offered to them proactively, usually at some point when the disorder is unrecognized or occult. Although any medical or related intervention is guided by a basic principle of "first, do no harm," the proactive nature of screening leads to even stronger demands in terms of its justification and the balance of benefits and possible harms that might result. Although screening can become widely accepted and even sought out by the public as a perceived standard of care or as a right, the fact remains that the individuals being screened usually have no obvious expression of the disorder—if they did, then not screening but diagnostic investigation should be the usual action.

But what if the affected individual cannot be aware of a self-disorder and, therefore, cannot or will not seek care? Lack of care-seeking behavior has a different meaning when the behavior is impossible through no act of will of the affected individual. Although sudden hearing loss is perceptible by most adults, a newborn is unaware that such a sensory limitation is exceptional, and even if such awareness were possible, the newborn is incapable of directive complaint. Similarly, the elderly individual who has an insidious decline in auditory functioning might not recognize the extent of the disorder and impacts such as social withdrawal, dependency, isolation, or depression. It is this inability to recognize and act upon an impairment or an associated functional limitation that sets the stage for a "duty of care" viewpoint for population hearing screening. Whether such inability is intrinsic, such as for a baby, or is acquired, such as for many elderly persons, there is surely an increased onus on a productive and empathetic society to make detection and intervention services available proactively. Although such an onus does not negate the need for careful justification of real and the opportunity costs of screening (i.e., the cost of not being able to spend the money on something else), it can and should influence the search for a reasonable balance of benefits, harms, and resource expenditure.

A second facet of screening, related to the idea of a latent period noted earlier, is that it usually seeks to identify a disorder at an early stage, sometimes prior to its overt expression as a significant restriction in physical or psychological function. This usually has implications for the type of screening test that can be used and for the actions that typically follow when the test is positive for presence of the disorder. The screening test must be sensitive to the early or unrecognized stages of the disorder, and a screening failure must be followed by procedures that characterize the type, severity, impact, and probable time course of the disorder.

In the case of hearing disorders in newborns or infants, because the auditory periphery up to and including the cochlea is well developed at birth, many hearing disorders that do not immediately involve central auditory pathways are latent only in the sense that they are not accompanied by expressed symptoms, not in the sense that there is some occult precursor stage. In babies with severe or profound hearing losses, there might indeed already be signs of the disorder, such as lack of behavioral response to loud sounds. Remember that a *symptom* is typically something of which the subject complains, whereas a *sign* is some physical or behavioral manifestation of the disorder that might not necessarily precipitate any symptom.

A third aspect of population screening is that, by definition, it involves testing very large numbers of people, relatively few of whom might actually have the disorder of interest. This will involve major resource expenditure and organization to access the target population, explain the tests, perform the tests, document the findings, and ensure that appropriate follow-up services are delivered in a timely and effective manner. The resource expenditure itself implies that such programs should not be undertaken lightly and without a solid and well-documented expectation of sufficient benefit to the affected individuals and to society at large, especially given the major, economic constraints that exist for health care expenditures. Also, given the large numbers of individuals or families for whom the screening will prove negative, any harms or costs, even minor ones, are magnified by the large numbers involved. Typically, a large number of minor harms or inconveniences are balanced against a relatively small number of cases of major benefit from early detection.

The fourth key aspect is that no screening test is perfect at distinguishing those who do have the disorder from those who do not. Screening tests are typically cheap and relatively simple substitutes for more costly, more definitive tests that are often referred to as *gold standards*. Screening tests will make errors. They will miss (pass) some true cases of disorder (false-negative screens), and they will fail some persons who do not have the disorder (false-positive screens). For rare disorders, it is not unusual that the majority of screening failures are false positive. This raises important issues of credibility of screening results, labeling of persons who actually are free of disorder, as well as engagement of many persons in unnecessary diagnostic follow-up. Unnecessary interventions can also occur if the diagnostic tests are less than perfectly accurate.

Last, as already noted, preoccupation with screening appears to have been almost endemic over the last two decades, yet the real measures of success of screening relate to subsequent delivery of valued outcomes from diagnostic testing and from various types of intervention. A consequence is the frequently stated position that all the mechanisms needed to ensure adequate levels of follow-up care for babies who fail the screen should be in place before any screening program is implemented. This follows directly from the WHO principles. Basically, if you cannot deliver the benefits of screening, do not screen. Although such a view might be naïve in a political sense, it certainly expresses a necessity for overall success as well as reflects the ethical position that one should not impose on the public a health care process (screening) that cannot, for whatever reason, offer genuine benefit to its recipients. The naivety is that only the most far-sighted planners and sponsors would have the insight to invest in new services for individuals who are not yet detected by current systems, especially for an issue (hearing loss) that is not usually considered likely to win the hearts and minds of the average voter. In the developing world, especially, motivation to take advantage of the undeniable, global momentum for screening is understandable. By implementing universal or even targeted NHS, a growth in public demand for enhanced diagnostic and intervention services is created, and this might be seen in some contexts as the only viable way to generate the necessary pressure for professional and political action and funding.

A Viewpoint on the Real "Important Health Problem"

Over the last 30 years or so, many publications on newborn hearing screening (NHS) began with something like "Unrecognized hearing loss in young children compromises the development of speech and language . . . " usually leading to arguments in favor of screening. This focus on language development was understandable, but it is not the only viewpoint. One of its consequences was that the audiology community came to accept that the singular, important health problem to be addressed by screening was delay or limitation of language development. When the health services evaluation community subsequently set about seeking proof of screening effectiveness, it seemed natural to look for evidence of improved long-term language in screened versus unscreened groups. Such proof has been extremely hard to come by, as one might expect in view of the complex, multivariate, and longitudinal nature of language development trajectories.

To some, including the present author, the overwhelming focus on language development was always questionable. It treated hearing loss as a mere proxy for deficient language. An alternative viewpoint is that impaired hearing is a primary health condition. The cochlea is not an appendage (such as the appendix) but a primary sense organ, no less significant than the eyes or the organ systems of touch, smell, taste, or proprioception. Given that perspective, hearing loss is not a proxy for anything but a health condition that, if not acted upon, can have a wide range of potentially adverse effects on the affected child, family, and even society at large. It is also a causal or mediator variable that, along with other factors such as health care quality, concurrent sensory, motor, or cognitive conditions, parental educational level, home language environment, and socioeconomic and cultural factors, can have a strong influence on long-term language outcomes.

Using the language and conceptual framework of the WHO's International Classification of Functioning, Disability and Health (ICF, 2001) loss of hearing sensitivity in the young child is obviously an impairment and leads to activity limitation, unless it is detected promptly and managed effectively. It might or might not lead to significant restriction of participation in the usual range of human roles and choices, depending on the environmental demands, values, and preferences of the affected individual and family. On these issues, there is a myriad of viewpoints of varying rationality and depth, but persons who have experienced sudden, postlingual loss of hearing will tend to be uniquely informed about the vast functional diversity of hearing and the impact of hearing loss. The special role of hearing in facilitating oral language development cannot be disputed. More recent realizations include the crucial role of auditory input in early development of the central auditory nervous system (see, for example, the review by Kral, 2013), which might be crudely summarized as "use it or miss out on it" (dysgenesis or agenesis) and, at the other end of the experiential span, the crucial role of hearing in healthy aging, cognitive maintenance, and independent living (Institute of Medicine & National Research Council, 2014), which essentially is a matter of "use it or lose it"—atrophy. It will be a long time before the lifetime effects of auditory system adaptations to unaddressed hearing loss in early infancy are fully understood. Yes, of course hearing alone . . . is important.

As if direct effects of hearing loss on the infant were not enough, without screening, the family is likely to be unaware of hearing loss, use ineffective communication behaviors, experience frustration, and probably misinterpret the child's behaviors, and when the loss is finally recognized, might experience guilt and anxiety. Historically, the medical system would probably have dismissed any early parental concerns with the common "don't worry, she'll grow out of it" response. Believe it or not, even today (2015), in Western industrialized countries, there exist family physicians, even otolaryngologists, who still believe that hearing cannot be tested in a newborn (or, even worse, that it can be tested by whispering or clapping) and that hearing aids are unnecessary in the first year of life. Meanwhile, of course, the infant cannot hear, has no idea that the experience is not normal, adapts to anomalous communication patterns, and undergoes a period of explosive brain and behavior development without the proper range of sensory input.

Although analogies have limited validity, framing the infant hearing loss challenge and justification of hearing screening in terms of language measures is perhaps as curious as it would have been to frame an infant vision loss challenge and justification of vision screening in terms of reading measures at preschool. To some, the more rational course is to define the goal as one of detecting the primary impairment and fixing or ameliorating it. What this means is that the "important health problem" noted in the WHO principles is not language development but hearing loss itself. With this view, the crucial question in justification and evaluation of hearing screening would become the following: Does newborn hearing screening lead to improved hearing? This is a far more direct and answerable question than those involving language development causality. A possible, basic measure of effectiveness in addressing hearing loss would be loss-weighted hearing years gained, and any long-term advantage to language or literacy development would be viewed as icing on the cake or, in health services jargon, a collateral benefit. Of course, none of this makes any sense if you see nothing wrong with a question that the present author did in fact meet some years ago while defending universal newborn hearing screening. The question, seemingly posed quite seriously by a smart person, was, "What does it matter if a baby cannot hear for an extra year or two?" There is no end to the quirks of human opinion.

The Target Disorder and Population: What Do We Really Want to Detect, in Whom?

As noted earlier, the term *target disorder* refers to the set of all hearing disorders that the screening is intended to detect. Precise definition of this set is important but often lacking in published reports. Without such a definition it is difficult, if not impossible, to describe adequately the condition sought that is referred to in

Table 15–1A. The definition also is crucial for screening test and program design and evaluation, as well as for valid comparisons of program results. Would exactly the same screening test be appropriate for bilateral, moderate, average hearing loss and for unilateral, mild, frequency-specific hearing loss? *No, it would not.* How can you evaluate the success of a screening program if its targets have not been defined precisely? *You cannot.* How can you compare in a valid manner two or more screening programs that might not be seeking the same set of hearing disorders? *You cannot, except perhaps by sophisticated methods of meta-analysis.* How can you even develop a valid rationale for screening, without declaring exactly what is to be detected and why? *It is not possible.*

In the choice of the target disorder, three basic considerations arise directly from the WHO principles—all disorders in the target set must

- have a substantial negative impact on important hearing-related functioning;
- be detectable with reasonable accuracy by the screening tests; and
- be addressable by an effective intervention, with the cost of the endeavor being reasonable relative to health care costs more generally.

If detecting significant hearing loss is accepted as a rational objective of NHS and EHDI, the question becomes, what is meant by "significant"? With the traditional focus on long-term language as the metric of the health problem, significant hearing loss was actually a proxy target that might have been defined in terms of its quantitative relationship to long-term language itself, the real question being, what patterns of hearing loss in the newborn and young infant are sufficient to cause a meaningful decline in long-term language skills? But, the current state of knowledge was and still is unable to answer that question (if, indeed, there is any single, valid answer), so the various target levels of hearing loss adopted in various EHDI programs have emerged on some basis other than language-related evidence. Possibilities include a tendency to adopt choices advised or adopted by leaders in the field, a general sense of what is significant in relation to speech perception in adults, or a sense of the capabilities and limitations of current hearing screening methods.

If the alternative viewpoint that hearing disorders themselves are the primary issue is accepted, then "significant" must be defined in relation to hearing function directly, not to language development. Hearing sensitivity is an obvious starting point, so the target disorder could be defined in terms of the pure-tone audiogram. This generally is what has been done anyway, despite the emphasis on language and despite the additional irony that in adults, crucial, language-related functions such as speech perception have only a very limited correlation with simple audiometric thresholds. Notwithstanding these limitations, hearing loss itself has the advantage of relative simplicity and broad acceptance. The challenge of target disorder definition, then becomes to specify the least pure-tone hearing loss within the target disorder, plus other aspects such as frequency, type, and laterality. Clearly, all hearing losses above the least loss would also be targeted.

As for the target population, in the context of justifying or evaluating NHS, the target population includes neonates and young infants. It is desirable to be more precise with the definition of *young infant,* because the choice of appropriate screening techniques as well as their field performance might be different for older infants. Also, because the prevalence of hearing disorders increases with age (Fortnum, Summerfield, Marshall, Davis, & Bamford, 2001), difficulties will arise comparing programs with very different target population age limits. A reasonable definition might include neonates and infants under 3 months corrected age, but any upper age limit under about six months of age could be considered. At about six months of age, the possibility of behavioral screening emerges, and it becomes increasingly difficult to secure an adequate behavioral state (ideally, sleep) in which to conduct automated OAE or ABR screening quickly and accurately.

It makes no sense to include in the target set for NHS hearing losses that have later onset than the age limits just mentioned, and it is not reasonable to criticize NHS for not detecting hearing losses that are expressed later. These can only be detected by programmatic additions such as longitudinal surveillance of high-risk children, later population screening (prelingual or at school entry, for example), enhanced professional awareness and responsiveness to family concerns about hearing or language development, or by case-finding such as in medical visits unrelated to hearing. These represent an extension of the EHDI program target population to, for example, all children from birth to school entry, but they do not relate directly to NHS itself.

The reader will be aware that hearing loss categories relevant to screening targets include the following:

- bilateral hearing loss only or unilateral plus bilateral losses;

- the least severity (dB HL) or numerically lowest limit of the range of target losses;
- better ear or worse ear lowest limits of severity;
- average or worst-case lowest limits across frequencies;
- frequency range and the number of frequencies included;
- stability (transient, recurrent, permanent, acute, chronic, progressive, resolving);
- age at onset (congenital, early onset, late onset, acquired, pre- or postlingual, preschool, etc.);
- traditional audiometric type (conductive, sensory/neural, mixed);
- site of lesion (external ear, middle ear, OHC, OHC/IHC, IHC, cochleoneural, neural, ANSD, retrocochlear, mixed, etc.); and
- etiology (genetic, environmental, interactive, etc.).

There are many options to define the target disorder set. Should we include only bilateral losses or also unilateral losses? What is the minimum loss severity of interest? Should hearing losses of 40 dB HL or more, or down to 30 dB HL, or even less be included? Should the severity criterion chosen be applied to individual frequencies or to averages and over what range of frequencies? What types of hearing loss should be included? Should the focus be on "conventional" cochlear hearing loss that includes outer hair cell (OHC) pathology, or should the target include ANSD and other disorders of more central structures in the auditory system, even those that might not manifest a substantial pure-tone hearing loss component? Should conductive disorders be included, and if so, must they be permanent or chronic, or include transient or recurrent disorders?

For many of these questions, it is remarkable that there are not yet definitive or even compelling answers, and many different choices have been and continue to be made by program developers. In many current NHS programs, at least in developed countries, the target disorder is commonly assumed or stated to be permanent, unilateral, or bilateral and of 30 dB HL or more, either in terms of average hearing loss or worst-case loss at specific, key frequencies. ANSD is often but not always included in the target, even though it can occasionally present with normal pure-tone hearing sensitivity. *Permanent* is often defined to include sensory/neural loss or *structural* conductive loss, which is mostly conductive loss that is not attributable to transient middle-ear disorders. These decisions are not etched in stone, nor are they necessarily appropriate in situations of severely limited resources, such as in developing countries. In such situations, it might be reasonable to adopt more conservative target disorder definitions, such as bilateral loss only, moderate loss or worse, or losses not including ANSD. It is important to note that the program in England (NHSP), for many years arguably the world's model program, conservatively chose bilateral average hearing loss of at least moderate degree as the target disorder.

The choices made to date for the lower bounds of the target disorder have been made in the absence of a strong scientific evidence base about child impact and in many cases largely on the basis of clinical opinion, advocacy and some limited findings about long-term educational effects attributed to minimal, mild and unilateral hearing losses. A related factor is that there is little point in choosing lower bounds of target hearing loss that do not match appropriately with available stimulus and recording parameters of currently available screening devices. Common choices, therefore, have taken some account of what is readily accessible in terms of screening technology, as well as what seems reasonable on clinical grounds with respect to early intervention.

Unfortunately and quite understandably, there is limited information available on the short-term and longitudinal, functional impact of different degrees of hearing loss severity on the developing young child. The relationship between functional impact and pure-tone thresholds is multifaceted and likely to be highly nonlinear, with impact increasing rapidly at the low end of the moderate hearing loss range. If a reasonable, key element of the significance of the disorder is thought to be the effect of hearing loss on speech perception, then the Speech Intelligibility Index (SII; ANSI, 1997) could conceivably be a more useful impact quantifier than, say, an average pure-tone threshold.

Returning to the issue of the least hearing loss severity of interest, in general the lower the severity limit is set, the more cases will be defined as present in the population—that is, the prevalence of the target disorder will increase. This important effect is illustrated in Figure 15–2. Note that as the minimum target criterion hearing loss is lowered, the prevalence of the target disorder appears to increase ever more rapidly. If the limit of the standard definition of normal hearing were approached, it would increase exponentially because the number of individuals with slight hearing loss in the population will be large relative to the number with mild or moderate hearing losses. Bear in mind that the definition of normal hearing is essentially arbitrary, empirical, and based on a statistical distribution of hearing sensitivity in a select group.

When choosing lower limits of target hearing loss severity, several WHO criteria come into play forcefully—are those cases at or near the lower limit

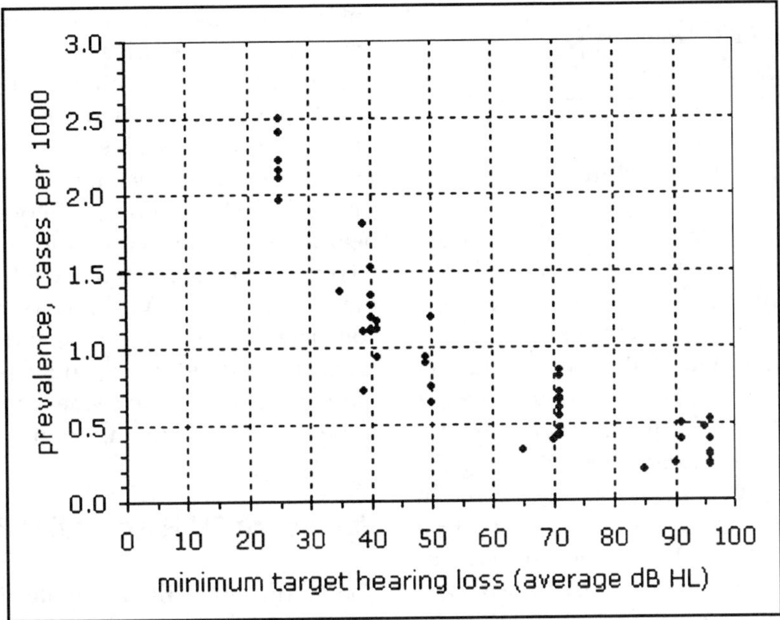

FIGURE 15–2. The prevalence of permanent hearing loss increases dramatically as the minimum (smallest) loss included in the target disorder is decreased. Note the accelerating rate of increase as the criterion is lowered. The data are extracted from studies reviewed by Fortnum (2003) and the Public Health Agency of Canada's Canadian Working Group on Childhood Hearing (CWGCH; 2005).

detectable reliably by current screening tests? That is very unlikely, at least with OAE screening, for targets lower than moderate severity. Even if they are detectable, given that program resources needed to deal with those who fail screening will increase rapidly as the lower limit decreases, are there sufficient resources available? Can the diagnostic tests accurately confirm and quantify the severity and type of hearing losses at, say, the low end of the mild category? Doubtful, for typical ABR-based assessment protocols, because click and tone-pip ABR threshold estimation becomes unreliable below about 30 dB nHL. Even if these concerns were addressed, what interventions are needed? Is there some evidence, or at least clinical consensus opinion, on what to do and whether it works? For example, should an infant with a 25-dB unilateral hearing loss at 4 kHz estimated by ABR receive amplification? Would such a child's family even believe such a loss existed or was important and, if they did not, would any such intervention be successful? Would such a child respond favorably to aiding, given the limited benefit that might ensue, or would the practical aspects of dealing with the device and its fitting cause the device to be abandoned? Would the medical community, including family physicians, pediatricians, and otolaryngologists, endorse and support such activities? What factors would modify or negate clinical candidacy for amplification? If these questions do not have clear, evidence-based answers, or if there is not at least some substantive clinical consensus opinion and practice, is it appropriate or even ethical to try and detect such hearing losses?

These concerns certainly do not mean that hearing losses that are, for example, slight and bilateral or at the low end of the mild range and unilateral are unimportant and do not have deleterious effects when undetected or unmanaged. What they do mean is that very careful consideration is required of whether such losses specifically can be addressed in a manner that satisfies the core WHO screening principles. The reader might find it interesting to search for evidence of such careful consideration, even in relation to the lower limits of hearing loss targeted by current EHDI programs. An interesting review of the question was presented by Gravel and her colleagues (2005). In that review, several concepts and issues covered in this chapter are addressed, mainly but not completely, with conclusions similar to those given here. See also Tharpe (2008) for a broad review of unilateral and mild bilateral hearing loss in children.

Do Acceptable and Suitable Screening Tests Exist?

What Do the Words Really Mean?

Wilson and Jungner's (1968) statement that there should be a screening test that is both acceptable and suitable is a deceptively terse summary of a large topic that is profoundly relevant to whether hearing screening should be undertaken and, if so, how it should be done. The word *acceptable* relates directly to the experience of the test by its recipients. This is a matter of whether the test is unduly onerous or carries significant risk of direct harm, either in fact or as perceived by the child's family. The commonly used screening tests such as automated OAE or ABR are not invasive by any sensible definition of the term, although reasonable care must be exercised in any skin preparation for ABR electrodes and whenever a transducer is inserted into an infant's ear canal. But these tests impose little, if any, discomfort so the acceptability requirement would seem to be easily satisfied. It is worth noting, however, that infection risk is a significant issue in some jurisdictions, but not in others, and there is much geographic variation in infection control practice and rigor. Debates still surround, for example, questions such as the following: Are mini-supra-aural or circumaural "disposable" earphones a justifiable cost relative to inserts with disposable eartips? Are acoustical or infection control factors more important? Does the external ear canal of a neonate constitute "intact skin"? How vigorous do probe and other equipment disinfection protocols have to be? And, how well are they followed in practice?

In contrast, suitability of the tests is a much more complex question. Although the word *suitable* seems vague, it covers many key aspects of any screening test, most importantly its validity and accuracy. In the original WHO document, validity was defined solely in terms of whether the test was accurate—that is, whether it made many errors. That definition of validity does not entirely match modern thinking. The position taken here is that validity is a deeper issue than accuracy and that the two are distinct but related—a valid test might or might not be accurate, because a valid measure could be subject to substantial random or systematic error. On the other hand, a highly accurate test is likely to be valid, because if it were not valid, the high accuracy would have to be serendipitous, which is inherently improbable. The reader might be wondering if the validity/accuracy distinction matters in our present context. Consider (a) AOAE screening in a crying baby, versus (b) AABR screening in a baby with severe hyperbilirubinemia. You cannot get an accurate screen in (a) consistently—there might be bias, imprecision, or both. In (b), because of the relatively high prevalence of ANSD in such babies, an AABR fail could be due to ANSD degrading or abolishing the ABR, even if hearing loss is not within the target severity range, or it could be due to moderate OHC sensory/neural hearing loss without any ANSD, or both could be present concurrently. The author would tend to say that case (a) is all about accuracy, and case (b) is more a matter of invalidity risk. The reader can think about whether these differences are important.

Validity of OAE and ABR Screening Tests

The OAE and ABR dominate the field of screening tests for newborns and infants under about six months developmental age. Evoked OAEs, whether of the transient (TEOAE) or distortion-product type (DPOAE), are generated by OHCs. Recording of a robust OAE by a miniature microphone in the ear canal generally is considered to reflect functioning OHCs. To evoke an OAE, there must be appropriate transmission of the stimulus through the middle ear to the cochlea and also back-transmission of the evoked emission through the middle ear. Thus, the OAE is an indicator of auditory functioning at the cochlear OHC level, but its recording is mediated by the external and middle ears, causing vulnerability to minor conductive disorders. In OAE screening devices, algorithmic decisions are made about the presence or absence of OAEs from several frequency regions of the cochlea. These are made directly, in the case of DPOAEs elicited by tone pairs at specific frequencies of interest, or indirectly, by decomposition of the complex TEOAE wave form elicited by a transient stimulus such as a click.

The relationship between OAE detectability and pure-tone audibility is not a simple one. OAE detection is inherently statistical and is a problem of recognizing a "signal" waveform that is reproducible, but not known exactly, within a background of acoustical "noise" that is largely random but with an energy density spectrum and autocorrelation structure that are also not known exactly. Physiologic variation is large, so in persons with classically "normal" hearing sensitivity or, more generally, in persons with thresholds outside the target disorder range, there is a wide distribution of OAE amplitudes elicited by standard, typical stimulus conditions that are chosen to yield on average the most detectable OAEs. Of course, groups of persons with a range of hearing losses that are within the target disorder set also show distributions of OAE amplitude. Substantial overlap between these target and nontarget distributions means that perfect discrimination of normal and impaired hearing is not possible, but separation of the distributions confers useful, binary discriminative ability. See, for example, the results reported by Gorga et al. (1997) for DPOAEs.

ABRs are electrical waveforms recordable with scalp electrodes after appropriate computer processing of minute responses to many transient acoustical stimuli presented rapidly. ABRs are usually complex waveforms that are the net result of superposition of thousands of synchronized action potentials and postsynaptic potentials elicited from the auditory nerve and brainstem pathways. The relationship between cochlear activity, bilateral brainstem pathway activity and the net ABR waveform recorded by a typical high-forehead-to-mastoid electrode derivation is extremely complex. However, there is a strong relationship between detectability of the ABR and the audibility of transient sounds such as clicks, tone pips, or chirps. Just as for the OAE in the acoustical domain, ABR detection is a statistical problem of signal recognition in noise, but in the electrical domain. Unlike the OAE, the ABR can be used to estimate directly the threshold of hearing, but this process is quite time-consuming. In the screening context, specific stimulus and recording parameters are applied in order to yield a binary (yes-no) decision about ABR presence or absence. See Sininger and Hyde (2009) as well as Sininger (2007) for detailed reviews and discussions. The ABR is not appreciably affected by minor middle ear disorders, but it *is* affected by disorders that reduce or abolish the volume or temporal synchrony of the action potential volley evoked by the stimulus. The most obvious such disorders include ANSD and space-occupying or demyelinating lesions affecting the auditory nerve.

Whatever the biophysical response to be used, population hearing screening demands that the process be objective and automated for speed, consistency and reliability of decision making. Although a highly skilled tester might be able to detect responses more reliably than a computer-based decision algorithm under some circumstances (such as in a diagnostic context), it is difficult if not impossible to maintain high subjective reliability over an enormous number of tests. Also, it is also virtually impossible to determine quickly who is highly skilled at ABR recognition and who is not, given that the only valid, evaluative method requires presenting or withholding stimuli with a wide range of parameters in a large population of subjects covering a wide range of severities and types of hearing disorders and under a wide range of measurement conditions and with repeated measures within subjects.

With respect to the intrinsic validity of OAE and ABR screening tests, the modern view of validity, originating in the field of psychometrics, is that it reflects the extent to which a test actually does measure what it is intended or purported to measure. The key questions are, does detection of an ABR or OAE obtained under some appropriate set of stimulus and recording conditions strongly imply absence of any target disorder? And, conversely, does failure to detect the ABR or OAE strongly imply presence of a target disorder? Neither the ABR nor the OAE are direct tests of hearing in the perceptual sense, because there are vast differences in the mechanisms underlying the three types of phenomena. Indeed, neither test possesses *intrinsic* validity. For example, in some subgroups of infants, a response (OAE or ABR) might be observed consistently in the absence of behavioral response to sound. Moreover, behavioral responses might be observed consistently in the absence of an ABR. The diversity and complexity of the auditory system are such that these situations are inevitable. The obvious example of physiologic response in the absence of auditory perception occurs in situations of pathologies that lie more centrally in the auditory pathway than the site of response generation. For example, a child with ANSD can have normal OAEs but severe loss of hearing sensitivity or highly disordered temporal processing, or both. It also is possible, although rarer, that a recordable ABR can occur in the presence of major central auditory disorder, as might occur due to pathologies at thalamic or cortical levels. Conversely, infants with hearing functions grossly within normal limits can have small or absent OAEs due to natural biologic variation or to minor middle-ear conditions. It is also possible to see absent or highly aberrant ABRs in the presence of normal hearing sensitivity and even normal open-set speech perception in quiet, in some cases of ANSD, for example.

For a slightly less obvious source of validity limitation, consider a screening test based on the click ABR. Is such an ABR a valid screening measure of the clinically important features of the pure tone audiogram that might be included in the target disorder definition? The answer is yes, but only as long as the pure-tone audiogram is flat. Even substantial hearing losses that are low-frequency, high-frequency, notched, or U-shaped can occur despite a detectable click ABR. Similar validity concerns arise with the OAE as implemented in current screening devices, especially in relation to low-frequency losses as well as losses restricted in frequency range. Note here the importance of the target disorder definition, when discussing this aspect of validity. For example, if average hearing loss at 1, 2, and 4 kHz was the chosen parameter of the target disorder, then the click-ABR would be more valid than it would be if hearing losses at individual frequencies were included in the target, one reason being that substantial losses at single frequencies would meet the target disorder criterion (with ABR present), whereas the averaged loss would be smaller and might not meet the criterion. Furthermore, the OAE becomes less valid if ANSD is included in the target, whereas the ABR is a valid screen for ANSD, even though it is not a valid measure of hearing thresholds when ANSD is present. These situations of invalidity are a significant concern. Although a screening test is not expected to equal the performance of any appropriate gold standard test of hearing, the existence of specific subgroups of infants for whom the target disorder will be systematically and consistently missed or for whom screening will consistently give false detection of disorder are challenging limitations of current hearing screening tests that are quite different from unpredictable instances of random error in screening outcomes.

Taking the screened population as a whole, lack of validity in specific subgroups will cause screening errors that will contribute to the overall frequency of errors. However, other types of error can arise from a variety of sources, such as the level of environmental acoustical noise, physiological noise, natural biological variations across infants in OAE or ABR amplitude, variations in efficiency of response detection methods, and so on, which will be explored in more detail shortly. These other types of error are considered to be sources of inaccuracy. Thus, the overall patterns of screening error are governed by sources of both invalidity and inaccuracy. Is the distinction between the two types of error important or useful? Most people would consider that the inability of OAE screening to detect ANSD is a far more fundamental limitation than the fact that OAE (or ABR) screening cannot be done in a baby who is agitated. Curiously, note that if the screening program did *not* have ANSD as a target disorder, then it would be the ABR that suffered the validity limitation, not the OAE.

The reader familiar with statistics might recall the difference between *bias* and *precision* when considering the overall quality of some estimator such as a sample mean or a sample proportion. The difference is that bias reflects a systematic, reproducible difference between the true value of some measure and the estimates of it from samples of observations, whereas precision reflects some amount of random error inherent in the estimates. The practical differences in the context of screening test evaluation lie in the interpretation of observed test performance and the steps that can be taken to improve performance. Suppose, for example, two studies of OAE screening came up with radically different rates of missed hearing loss. If it were found that the study with the higher rate was based on a sample with a much higher probability of ANSD, one source of bias is readily apparent. Improvements in the OAE detection method would have no effect whatsoever on the errors due to intrinsic invalidity, whereas they could improve the precision component substantially. This has clear implications for how screening should be done, how errors can be explained, and how test performance might be legitimately compared and improved.

It is worth noting that any limitations of screening test validity and accuracy that arise from the fact that OAE and ABR tests access different facets of auditory system activity are not in conflict with the increased ability for differential diagnosis of hearing disorders that arise from precisely those very differences. In the diagnostic context, as opposed to the screening context, the differences among the test measures are undoubtedly a source of increased insight into the location and nature of hearing disorders. An obvious example is the potential for disentanglement of a global term such as sensory/neural hearing loss into more precisely defined components relating to the outer hair cells, inner hair cells, synaptic junctions with primary auditory neurons, and the auditory brainstem pathways. However, those aspects are beyond the purview of this chapter on screening.

Classical Measures of Screening Test Efficacy

This section of the chapter addresses some standard measures and approaches to quantification of screening test efficacy (how well *can* it work?). The most important aspect of efficacy has to do with the accuracy of the test, because if a test is not acceptably accurate, it matters little how quick it is, how much it costs, how easy it is to do, how much expertise is required, and so on. This section has a didactic component, and some readers already might be less than delighted to embark on yet another explanation of sensitivity, specificity, and the like. But, no respectable chapter on the fundamentals of screening could omit such matters. Two arguments to stick with it here come to mind. First, there are many ways to explain the subject so there might be something new here or a light might go on where perhaps only darkness had been perceived. Second, in this chapter there are conceptual threads and terminology that are being developed. An effort has been made not to dwell on the simplest matters and to treat the subject somewhat critically.

Sensitivity and Specificity

The *efficacy* of a screening test reflects the extent to which the test is capable of discriminating cases from noncases. A *case* is a child with the target disorder and a *noncase* is a child without such a disorder. In the simplest version of this discrimination, the screening test yields a binary (pass-fail) result. Not all screening tests are binary, but those used in the EHDI context traditionally are used in a binary manner. For any given test on any given child, the disorder might be present or absent and the test might be positive (fail) or negative (pass) for the disorder, so four outcomes are possible:

- disorder present, test fail: a true positive (TP) event;
- disorder present, test pass: a false-negative (FN) event;
- disorder absent, test fail: a false-positive (FP) event; and
- disorder absent, test pass: a true negative (TN) event.

The performance of any binary screening test is commonly summarized by two numbers: the *sensitivity*, which is the probability of a positive test when the disorder is truly present, as well as the *specificity*, which is the probability of a negative test when the disorder is truly absent. When the disorder is truly present, the outcome of a successful screening test must be either a TP or FN event, so their combined probability is 1. Therefore, if we know the sensitivity, we can derive the false-negative probability, which is its complement (1 – sensitivity). Similarly, when the disorder is truly absent either a TN or FP outcome must occur, so their combined probability is also 1, and if we know the specificity we can derive the false-positive probability (1 – specificity). It follows that to quantify test performance in any given context of screening, *two and only two numbers are always needed*; knowing the sensitivity or the specificity alone is not enough. For example, we could adopt a ridiculous test strategy and simply call all screens positive, which would result in perfect sensitivity but useless (zero) specificity and no discrimination ability between cases and noncases. That is one of the reasons why the reader should regard skeptically any report that quotes only sensitivity or only specificity. A perfect test, which is virtually impossible except for a gold standard test itself, has unit (1) sensitivity and specificity. For a useless test, the sensitivity equals the false-positive rate, so the false-negative rate equals the specificity. In that case, the result gives no information about whether the disorder is present or not—that is, the test has zero discrimination ability. For a tabular illustration of test outcomes and related probabilities, test performance measures, and numerical examples, see Appendix 15–A

Screening Test Measures and Pass-Fail Criteria

The underlying measures for common screening tests are not naturally binary (yes-no) variables. Rather, the screening result arises by applying some numerical pass-fail criterion to a measure that is inherently continuous in nature. Consider Figure 15–3A.

In generic terms, the screening device takes a measurement of some kind of biophysical function. Such measures have inherent variability, both for repeated measures within any one subject and for measurements across subjects. For a large number of such measurements, there will be a statistical distribution of possible measured values, represented by the curves in Figure 15–3A. In such figures, the distributions are typically modeled as having a shape that is *normal* in the terminology of statistics and *Gaussian* in the terminology of engineering. Real measures, such as signal-to-noise ratios, can have other distributions but the normal distribution is typically used for illustration and approximation. Moreover, the distributions are standardized, meaning that the test measure is scaled (transformed) numerically such that mean value of the disorder-absent distribution is rescaled to zero and the standard deviation is set to unity (1). Conventionally, the left-hand distribution is that for disorder absence (D–) and the other distributions represent disorder presence (D+) for various different screening tests. The reader might imagine, for example, that the left-hand distribution represents possible blood pressure readings from a screening device in a normal population, whereas the other distributions represent such results in subjects with moderate hypertension, the tests differing in how sensitive they are to moderate hypertension. In general, for the screening measure to be useful, the distributions must be separated when the target disorder is present or absent. The more separated the distributions are, the better the test is likely to be at discriminating subjects with and without the target disorder.

The pass-fail criterion is some particular critical value of the screening measure, shown in Figure 15–3A with a numerical value of 1.64 standard deviations

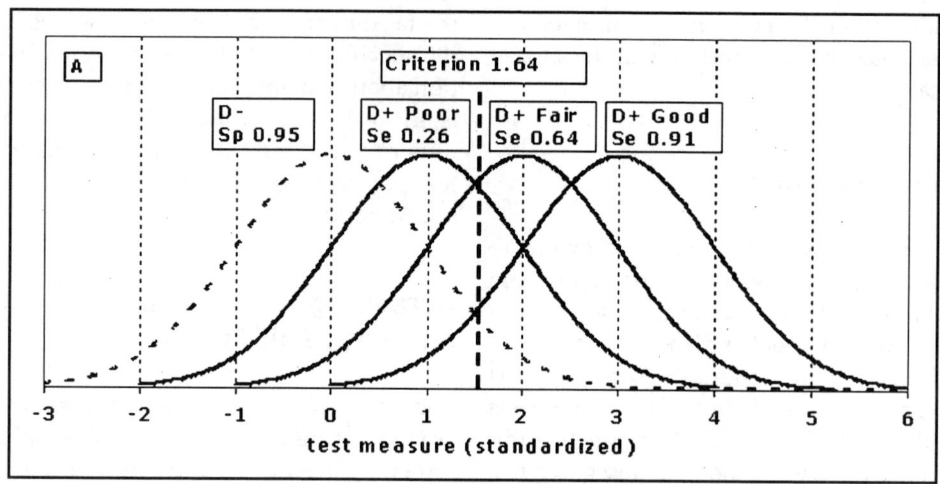

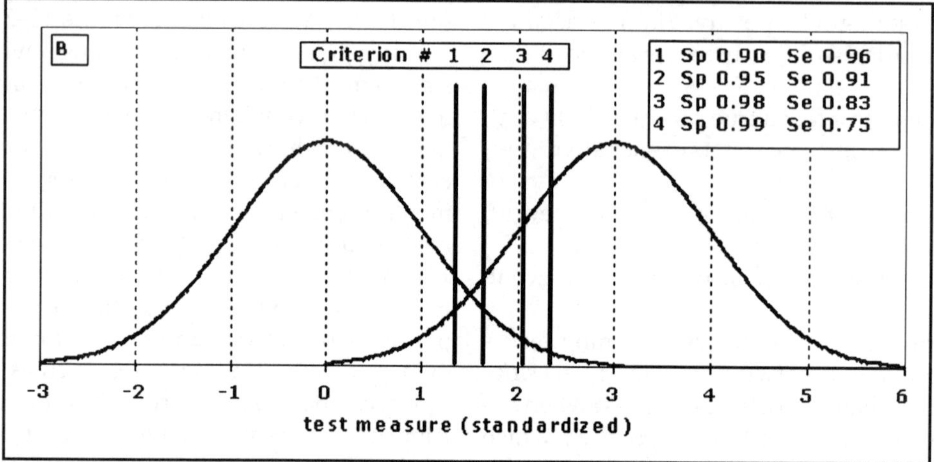

FIGURE 15–3. A. Statistical distributions of generic screening tests' underlying measures, for tests with different ability to discriminate presence or absence of the target disorder. The test measure has been "standardized" such that all distributions have unit standard deviation (SD) and the *x*-axis units are in standard deviations (SDs). The disorder absent (D−) distribution is always centered on zero but the disorder-present (D+) distributions can have any position. The greater the separation of the D− and D+ distributions, the better the test is. Three examples are shown for D+. Specificity is the area under D− left of the screening fail criterion, and sensitivity is the area under D+ to the right of the criterion. A criterion value is illustrated at 1.64 SDs above the D− mean, which would yield a specificity of 95% (0.95). The differing sensitivities of the various tests are shown. The distances in SD units between the D− and D+ distribution centers are the test performance parameter d′ (see text). **B.** For a given screening test and its associated, fixed pair of distributions, sensitivities, and specificities for various values of the failure criterion are shown and are seen to change inversely. Note that even with three SDs of distributional separation (d′ = 3), there is still substantial overlap. For a desired specificity of at least 0.98 (giving a screening fail rate of no more than about 2%), the sensitivity is barely acceptable.

above the mean of the D– distribution, as an example. Any measurement value arising from a single screening act will either be above or below the criterion and the task is to infer whether the observation came from the D– or D+ distribution. The usual approach is to decide that the measurement came from the D+ distribution if the observation equals or exceeds the criterion, otherwise it is deemed to have come from the D– distribution.

The reader might recall that probabilities can be represented as areas under statistical distributions. For any pair of distributions, one of which is the disorder-absent distribution, the test sensitivity equals the area under the D+ distribution for all values of the test measure that are to the right of the criterion, whereas the specificity is the area under the D– distribution for all values to the left of the criterion. In Figure 15–3A, the three different D+ distributions shown yield sensitivities of 0.26, 0.64, and 0.91, respectively, after applying the criterion that gives a specificity of 0.9 for the fixed D– distribution. The reader should note that only the rightmost D+ distribution could represent a screening test that would be acceptable or, in other words, that substantial separation of the D– and D+ distributions is required for a good screening test.

In Figure 15–3B, two distributions are shown, one is the D– distribution and the other is the D+ distribution for a good screening test. The two things that affect the values of sensitivity and specificity are the separation of the distributions and the chosen value of the criterion itself. For any given pair of distributions, if the criterion is changed, then the sensitivity and specificity will also change and *will do so inversely*—the higher the sensitivity, the lower the specificity, and vice versa. What this means is that an entire spectrum of values for sensitivity or specificity is obtainable, depending on where the criterion is set. What defines the quality of the screening test has far more to do with the distributional separation than with the criterion itself. The greater the separation, the better the test is intrinsically, regardless of which particular criterion is chosen. If two screening tests have the same distributional shape and separation on the standardized axis then they are essentially equivalent in terms of their intrinsic performance, even if they were based on different underlying measures or technologies.

In the specific case of automated OAE and ABR screening tests (AOAE and AABR), the measure underlying the tests is based either directly or indirectly on a signal-to-noise ratio (SNR), either acoustic (for the OAE) or electrical (for the ABR). The measure might be an actual SNR calculation, a variance ratio, a correlation coefficient, a probability estimate, or any of several other possible response detector functions. Although potentially confusing, it is important here to appreciate that response detection in typical screening devices is actually a variation on the illustrative schematics shown in Figure 15–3. In an automated ABR device, for example, the outcome or scoring algorithm decides that response is absent unless a specific numerical criterion is met or exceeded. The criterion is set such that the likelihood of it being exceeded by chance in the absence of response (due to noise fluctuations alone) is very small, typically less than 1% and sometimes much less, at least theoretically. Response absence equates to target disorder presence and vice versa, because hearing loss is assumed to abolish response. Thus, false-positive detection of a response leads to a false-negative screen, and conversely, false-negative response detection leads to a false-positive screen. Thus, by controlling the rate of false-positive response detection, the screening algorithm actually controls the false-negative screening error rate—that is, it effectively controls the (complementary) screening sensitivity and relates to the D+ distribution. Essentially, this amounts to a reversal of the conventional picture shown in Figure 15–3. In fact, proper performance analysis for OAE and ABR screening tests is somewhat complicated, and a full discussion is beyond the scope of this chapter. However, the principles discussed here and displayed in Figure 15–3 are entirely valid and useful as a basic conceptual model.

Returning to the general model of Figure 15–3, an obvious inference is that a given screening test might in effect become a different test (in terms of performance) if any change in its implementation or context of use were to alter the shape, spread, or location of the underlying distributions of the test measure. The crucial aspect is the extent of distributional overlap for D– and D+. There are many possible causes of such change, but two of them will be mentioned briefly, to illustrate how easy it is to alter such distributions. One example of a contextual change is a change in the target disorder definition, such as moving the lower limit of target hearing loss severity to a lower or higher value, which will be discussed further shortly. The other example is a procedural change in how the screening device works, such as a change in stimulus type or intensity, in the amount of averaging used in OAE or ABR measurement, or in the way in which the SNR is calculated. For instance, simply using more averaging sweeps or a more effective stimulus for the ABR can change the distributions and, therefore, could result in genuinely different test performance. This implies that there is not one but many substantively different versions of an ABR or an OAE screening test, even given a single, specific target disorder definition. This is important because there is a tendency to think that all OAE or all ABR screening tests have the same performance characteristics whereas, in fact, they do not.

Having clarified what is meant by two tests being equivalent or different in performance, there are three common, important questions:

1. Do the two sensitivity-specificity pairs being compared come from equivalent or genuinely different tests?
2. If they come from different tests, which test is better?
3. How should the optimal value for the criterion be chosen?

The Relative (Receiver) Operating Characteristic

A common method of evaluating and comparing tests makes use of the *relative operating characteristic* (also known as the receiver operating characteristic [ROC]). A definitive description of the application of ROCs to test evaluation was given by Swets (1988). An ROC is a plot of sensitivity on the *y*-axis or ordinate against the false-positive probability (1 – specificity) on the *x*-axis or abscissa, for various values of the test failure criterion. An example ROC plotted with linear probability axes is shown in Figure 15–4A. It can be seen that as the criterion is changed to make the test more liberal or lax (more likely to fail a child), both the sensitivity *and* the false-positive probability increase, which is reasonable intuitively. Figure 15–4A also shows a diagonal line, which represents the ROC for all useless tests that have no power to discriminate true positives from false positives, whatever their false-positive probability. Tossing a coin, for example, and calling the disorder present if a head came up, would give sensitivity and FP values of 0.5. Throwing a die and calling the disorder present if a six came up would make both the sensitivity and FP probability one in six (0.17). Both are tests with zero discriminant ability, and both yield a point on the diagonal ROC.

ROCs are often characterized by one of two common parameters, d′ and A. In graphical terms, d′ reflects how far the ROC is shifted from the diagonal line of the useless test (which has a d′ of zero), toward the upper left-hand corner (which has infinite d′). In terms of the underlying distributions of the test measure, d′ is the number of standard deviations by which the means of the D– and D+ distributions are separated. If those distributions are truly normal in shape, an entire ROC (known as a binormal ROC) is specified by a single value of d′. There is, of course, an infinite number of ROCs generated as d′ varies from zero to infinity. They all have the same general shape but with varying amounts of bulge toward the upper left corner of the ROC plane.

Note that an estimate of d′ can be calculated easily from any reported or observed sensitivity-specificity pair, simply by figuring out with statistical tables of the cumulative standard normal distribution (or using the Excel function [norminv(probability, 0, 1)]) what separation (number of standard deviations) of disorder-negative and disorder-positive distribution means would give the observed values (areas to the left and right of a criterion line). For example, a specificity of 95% (0.95), which equals an FP rate of 5% (0.05), would require the criterion to be at +1.64 above the (zero) mean of the D– distribution, and if the associated sensitivity were 90% (0.9) that criterion would have to be at −1.28 relative to the mean of the disorder-positive distribution, to give the correct area under the D+ curve to the right of the criterion. Thus, the value of d′ is 1.64 + 1.28 = 2.92, based on the binormal model. Remember, a completely useless test has a d′ of zero; that is, the two underlying distributions completely overlap, whereas good tests typically have d′ values of about 3 or higher, and excellent tests typically have d′ greater than 4.

The alternative measure A is the area under the ROC curve (AUC) when it is plotted with linear probability axes. Any useless test has an A of 0.5, whereas a (nonexistent) perfect test would have an A of 1. The measure A has some elegant and interesting properties. For example, if many pairs of babies were presented for testing, with one baby in each pair free from disorder and the other with the disorder, the quantity A actually equals the probability of correct detection of the baby with the disorder, which is approximated by the proportion correct over a large number of selections.

If the binormal model is actually correct in any given situation, d′ and A have a simple algebraic relationship. However, such a simple model is sometimes a poor approximation to the truth. But, perhaps the greatest limitation of the parameter A in the context of screening tests is that it reflects the area under the entire ROC. In screening for disorders with low prevalence, we are interested only in the test performance at very low values of the FP probability (high specificity); that is, toward the left-hand end of the ROC. An alternative measure of test quality is the "partial A," which can be denoted as A(max FP), for some particular acceptable maximum value of the false-positive probability. Because there is little interest in FP probabilities greater than, say, 10% or 0.1, the focus perhaps would be on A(0.1) and also on the values of the shift parameter d′.

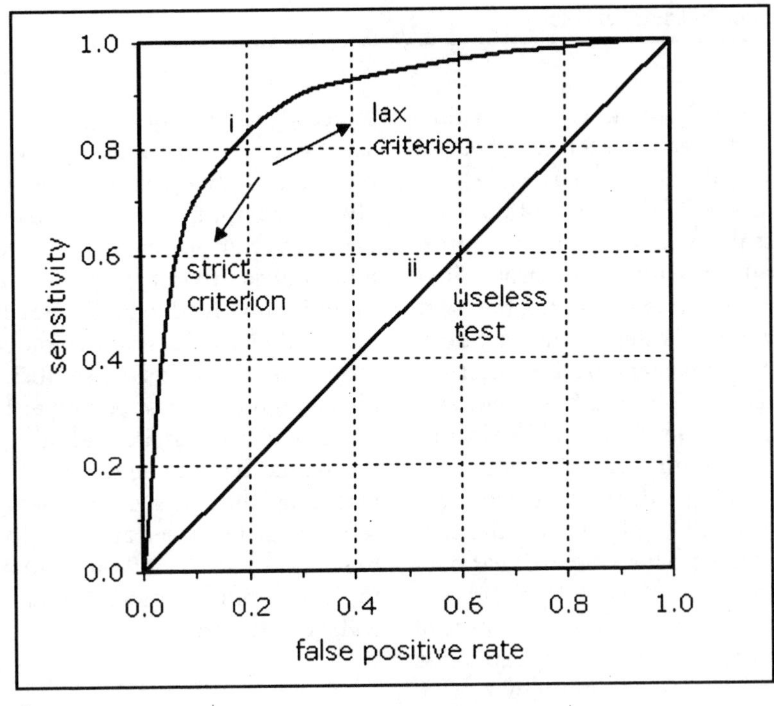

A

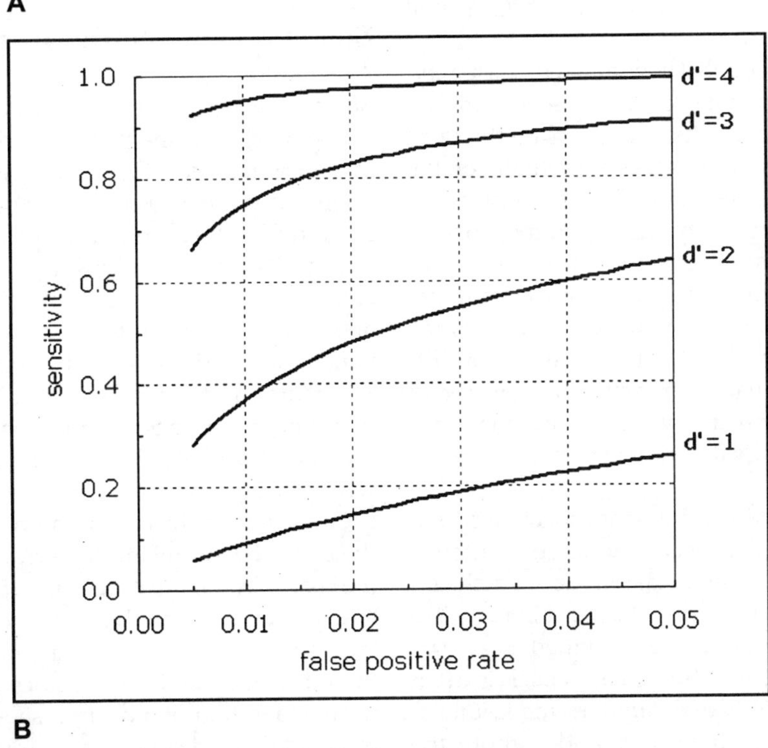

B

FIGURE 15–4. A. Relative (or receiver) operating characteristic (ROC) curves. The ordinate is the test sensitivity, and the abscissa is the false-positive probability (1 − specificity). As the screen failure criterion is changed, the sensitivity and specificity vary inversely, so the sensitivity and false-positive rate co-vary positively. The upper ROC curve (i) is typical for a "good" test. The diagonal (ii) is the ROC for a useless test with no ability to discriminate persons with and without the target disorder (such as tossing a coin or throwing a die), for which the sensitivity and false-positive rate are equal for any criterion. On this type of plot, d′ is the least distance from the ROC to the upper left corner. The measure A, the total area under the ROC, is 0.5 for the useless test and 1 for a perfect test. **B.** Segments of ROC curves for tests with different values of d′. Only the range of greatest interest for UNHS is shown, with false-positive rates less than 5% (0.05). The upper left box is the part of the ROC plane of interest for excellent test performance.

Figure 15–4B shows some ROCs with different values of d′. Only the FP range of greatest interest in hearing screening is shown, from 0.005 (0.5%) to 0.05 (5%).

It is worth noting that ROCs can be plotted using various different axis scales, including linear in probability (as shown here); logarithmic in probability, which is useful to zoom into interesting regions such as the region with very low FP rate; and normal deviate, which is basically linear in standard deviations of the standard normal distribution (and has mean zero and unit SD). Many real tests tend to yield ROCs that are straight lines when plotted on normal deviate axes. However, that property is less interesting if the focus is upon a small part of the ROC plane, as is the case here, because ROCs will tend to be close to linear over a small range of FP error, even when plotted with linear probability axes. There are many websites, some of them interactive, in which these matters are explained in more detail. They can be accessed simply by searching "receiver operating characteristic" or "ROC normal deviate" online.

Now consider two tests that have different sensitivity-specificity pairs such that neither test has both higher sensitivity *and* specificity. If the two points on the ROC plane corresponding to those values are actually on the same ROC, then neither test is intrinsically superior in terms of discrimination ability. The different sensitivity and specificity pairs reflect merely different values of the pass-fail criterion and, if the binormal model were operative, they would yield the same value of the underlying d′. In contrast, if the two tests fall on different ROCs they will have different values of d′ and if the differences are statistically significant, it is likely that the two tests are truly different in their discrimination ability.

A complication in this general approach occurs if the observed ROCs in the specificity range of interest do not follow the simple binormal model, which has equal SDs for the underlying distributions. In that situation, no single value of d′ can be assigned as a summary parameter for the test. If this happens, it is often the case that the variability of the underlying test measure differs in the populations with and without the target disorder, or because the shapes of the underlying distributions differ substantially from normal. In such a case, the decision between two tests is still straightforward if one of the ROCs always lies above (dominates) the other, but if the ROCs cross, then the decision about which test is better requires that a single, reference value or range of desired specificity (or sensitivity) be defined.

Unfortunately, there appears as yet to be no standard approach to the description and reporting of screening test performance. It is still not uncommon to see values of sensitivity or specificity calculated and reported singly (i.e., not in the required pairs) and not always computed in a valid manner. Evaluation or comparison of screening tests would be far easier and more informative if the clinical and technologic communities involved in NHS were to adopt a small range of specificity or a small number of key reference or index values such as the set [0.5, 1, 2, 5, and 10%]. The idea would be that screening test or screening protocol performance (estimates of both sensitivity *and* specificity) would have to be determined and reported for at least one value in such an index range or set, for any report to be taken seriously. Unfortunately, it is difficult to see how such a standardized approach would come to pass without impetus from a major funding agency collaborative group.

Selecting the Failure Criterion

Suppose a given test with a particular ROC is chosen; how should the pass-fail criterion be selected? In statistical decision theory, one way is to assign some quantitative cost to the test outcomes, usually to the FN and FP error events. The optimal criterion is the one that yields the least overall expected cost, which is the sum of error probabilities multiplied by their associated costs. However, it can be very difficult to assign valid, quantitative costs to FN and FP errors (especially FN errors), and the optimal criterion values so derived might be sensitive to changes in those numerical costs. A common viewpoint is that the cost of missing a child with hearing loss is much greater than that of a false-positive screen. In fact, it is only necessary to define the cost *ratio* for FN and FP errors in order to solve for the cost-minimizing criterion but, in fact, the ratio is no easier to define than the costs themselves.

If it is not possible to assign meaningful error costs, then the rationale for the choice of criterion is limited to consideration of a desired sensitivity or, more commonly, a desired specificity (or its complement, the FP probability). Typically, a very high specificity in the range 0.9 to 0.99 is desired, because of the preference to limit false-positive fails in order to control the refer rate to diagnostics, among other reasons. As already noted, there are no widely accepted standards for the choice of specificity. Moreover, screening devices usually offer limited or no flexibility in choice of the underlying pass-fail criterion. This renders optimization and valid comparisons of screening devices both limited and problematic.

Test Efficacy Depends on the Target Disorder Definition

The target disorder set for an NHS program clearly will include different severities and types of hearing loss, which complicates measurement of efficacy. There is no good reason to assume that the sensitivity and specificity of any given screening test will be the same for all degrees and types of hearing loss within the target disorder set. A simple example is offered by ANSD. If it were included in the target disorder, then the sensitivity of OAE screening, for example, would immediately decrease by 5% to 10%, that is, by the prevalence of ANSD in the screened population, because almost all such cases would be missed by OAE screening. As another example, small reductions (such as 10 dB or less) in the lower severity bounds of the target disorder range could have significant adverse effects on both sensitivity and specificity. It might be expected that close to the lower severity limit, the poorer the sensitivity will be, given that most tests are based on some kind of response SNR. A small hearing loss just within the target disorder range might not totally abolish the OAE or the ABR, which could in turn lead to reduced test sensitivity if the test criterion is such that small OAEs or ABRs will sometimes be detected and cause a screen pass. Conversely, the lower the hearing loss criterion, the higher is the likelihood of screen failure due to small hearing losses that might satisfy the numerical severity target but are due to transient (nontarget) conditions such as external ear debris or unresolved middle ear fluid. These will reduce the screen specificity. Although these potentially important effects are rarely described in published reports to date, they are especially relevant to the current, challenging issue of whether to screen for hearing losses at the lower end of the mild range. They also are relevant with regard to explaining some of the variability in reported accuracy of screening tests.

Sensitivity and Specificity Reporting

When a cohort of babies is studied in order to determine or verify sensitivity or specificity, it is common to have a few babies for whom a successful screen is not obtained. Sometimes, especially in studies of field performance of individual screeners, the proportion of unsuccessful screens might exceed 10%. How should these missing data be handled? The most common approach, and the least appropriate, is to count only the successful screens, as if there were no unsuccessful screens. This is misleading because the screened cohort is no longer a random sample or a sequential, complete sample. Rather, it is a subgroup that, for some reason, gave a successful screen. The minimum fix is to state the number or proportion of unsuccessful screens, describe any observable reasons for lack of success, and then analyze as if the sample with reduced number was complete. The first point is that the proportion of unsuccessful screens is potentially as important as the sensitivity/specificity estimates themselves. For example, if one device or protocol gave twice as many unsuccessful screens as another, the obvious question is whether this effect was random sampling variation or a consistent difference in testability with the two devices or protocols. The second point is that a device that essentially refines the test population, such as by having stricter ambient noise level criteria, might be expected to have different sensitivity or specificity than would a less picky but more practicable device.

A second point is reemphasis of the clear benefit to the audience of providing confidence limits on all proportions that are estimated, be they sensitivities, specificities, refer rates, case identification rates, and so on. A single point estimate of any such rate or proportion is not at all useful unless the sample size is stated. Better, though, is to report the point and interval estimates of the proportion, as would naturally be done when reporting noncount data such as sample means for continuous variables. Another benefit of calculating confidence limit on proportions is that it reminds the analyst about the remarkable variability of estimates of proportions. Perhaps that is one reason why such limits are still so often missing from reports. Bear in mind that Table 15–3 (ahead) can be used to inform this issue. At the risk of being repetitive, if you screened 20 babies and got two Refers, the Fail/Refer point estimate is about 10%, but the 90% confidence interval (CI) about the true value is 2.5% to 27%—almost no information. Even with 500 babies screened and a point estimate still of about 10%, the 90% CI is from 8% to 12.4%, useful now but still not impressive precision. A crude, general inference is that with binary proportions (percentages), at least 50 events of the less common type (Refers in this case) are required before the estimates begin to have sufficiently narrow confidence limits to be considered useful.

Impact of Fail and Pass Results: Positive and Negative Predictive Value

The sensitivity and specificity are *intrinsic* measures of the efficacy of the test itself; together, they tell us how good it is at separating cases from noncases. But, by themselves, sensitivity and specificity tell us little about the *meaning* or the *impact* of a given screening fail or pass result, such as how much confidence we can have that a baby who fails actually has hearing loss. The level of confidence is very important in relation to the amount of effort that is justifiable in pursuing high levels of follow-up, as well as in the proper explanation of the significance of screening outcomes to affected families. The actual pattern of fail and pass results expected when screening a large number of babies depends not only on the intrinsic performance of the screening test itself, but also on the context of test operation, most importantly, on the population prevalence of the disorder.

The probabilities of special interest that arise from the interaction of prevalence, sensitivity, and specificity are the *positive predictive value* (PPV) and *negative predictive value* (NPV). The PPV is the probability that any given baby who fails the screen (a positive screen) will turn out to have the disorder, whereas the NPV is the probability that any given baby who passes the screen (a negative screen) will turn out to be free of the disorder. The PPV is especially important because it governs the significance and the credibility of screening failure and these are the babies who require strong follow-up action. A test might have very good sensitivity but still result in a low PPV if the disorder is rare—that is, if the prevalence is small. If the general population prevalence of target hearing disorders in newborns is typically about two per thousand, the vast majority of any given sample of screened babies will not have the disorder. Consequently, the PPV is governed strongly not by *sensitivity* (which relates to the relatively few babies who do have the disorder) but by the *specificity* of the screen (which relates to the many who do not). It is essential that good screening tests for rare disorders have very high specificity. These effects are illustrated in Table 15–2. Given that the prevalence of hearing disorders is usually not controllable, the main strategy for enhancing PPV lies in increasing the specificity of screening, often by repeat testing or a serial protocol with different test technology. All serial screening reduces sensitivity to some degree, and the challenge is to minimize such sensitivity loss.

Table 15–2 shows PPV values for various combinations of disorder prevalence, test sensitivity, and specificity. Depending on the precise target disorder definition, a prevalence of about 0.001 (1/1,000) is typical in newborns who are not at traditional risk for hearing loss, and 0.01 (10/1,000 or 1%) is typical in high-risk newborns. Compare rows 1 and 2, 3 and 4, 5 and 6, and 7 and 8, to see the effect of specificity change from 0.9 to 0.99. In every case, the effect on PPV is very large. Now compare lines 1 and 3, 2 and 4, 5 and 7, and 6 and 8, to see the effect of sensitivity change by the same amount. In every case, the change in PPV is small. To see the effects of change in prevalence, compare lines 1 and 5, 2 and 6, 3 and 7, and 4 and 8. In each

Table 15–2. Examples of the Effect of Prevalence, Sensitivity, and Specificity of the Positive Predictive Value (PPV) of a Screening Test*

	Prevalence	*Sensitivity*	*Specificity*	*PPV%*
1	0.001	0.9	0.9	0.9
2	0.001	0.9	0.99	8.3
3	0.001	0.99	0.9	1.0
4	0.001	0.99	0.99	9.0
5	0.01	0.9	0.9	8.3
6	0.01	0.9	0.99	47.6
7	0.01	0.99	0.9	9.1
8	0.01	0.99	0.99	50.0

Note. *For large effects of prevalence, compare Rows 1 with 5, 2 with 6, 3 with 7, and 4 with 8. For small effects of sensitivity, compare Rows 1 with 3, 2 with 4, 5 with 7, and 6 with 8. For large effects of specificity, compare 1 with 2, 3 with 4, 5 with 6, and 7 with 8.

case, the effect on PPV is very large. Notice an important fact that is often not appreciated. Even when test sensitivity and specificity values are excellent (and better than those usually obtained with individual OAE or ABR screening tests), namely 0.99 in this example, the PPV for a relatively rare disorder like hearing loss in the nil-risk population does not exceed 9%, meaning that 91% of all nil-risk babies who fail the screen will *not* have the disorder, even with such excellent tests. What this suggests is that further efforts to bring the real-world false-positive rate down below 1% can be very worthwhile in terms of improving the credibility of screening failure and the efficiency of referral for diagnostic assessment. Given that missing babies with genuine PHL usually is assigned a high cost, reduction in false positives would only be acceptable if not accompanied by a substantial loss in sensitivity. That means that a screening method with truly better performance in the ROC false-positive probability region of 0.001 to 0.01 (0.1%–1%) would be a major advance. It also means that the benchmark value for the maximum acceptable false-positive probability for any screening protocol would be more reasonably set at 1%, not the much larger values commonly regarded as acceptable in the literature to date. With a 3% false-positive rate (specificity 0.97), for example, the PPV for prevalence 0.001 and excellent sensitivity of 0.99 is a mere 3.2%, which many might consider unacceptably low.

The NPV, in contrast, reflects the credibility that can be placed on a screening pass. If the target disorder has low prevalence, the NPV of any reasonable screening test inevitably is very high (close to 1.0) and so usually is of much less interest than the PPV. However, it is important to remember and to convey to families of screened newborns that a high NPV relates strictly to the absence of hearing loss at the time of the screen; it says nothing at all about the likelihood of subsequent hearing loss.

Likelihood Ratios Are Interesting and Useful

Although the PPV reveals the probability of target disorder presence given a screen failure, because its numerical value depends strongly on the prevalence (or, more generally, the pretest probability of the disorder) it must be recalculated for every possible pretest probability of interest. It is sometimes convenient to make use of test performance measures that are independent of pretest probability but that relate more directly and simply to the posttest probability of disorder than do sensitivity and specificity. The likelihood ratio (LR) is such a measure. It is a number associated with each screening outcome, so for a binary screen there are two LRs, one for a positive screen (fail) and one for a negative screen (pass). These are denoted as LR+ (LR positive) and LR− (LR negative), respectively. LR+ is simply the ratio of sensitivity to false-positive probability, whereas LR− is the ratio of false-negative probability to specificity. Referring back to Figure 15–4A, note that the LR+ is simply the ratio of areas to the right of the criterion, under the disorder-present and disorder-absent distributions of the test measure. The LR− is a similar ratio of areas but to the left of the criterion. These ratios are independent of the pretest probability.

If the LRs of a screening test pass and fail are known, then it is simple to calculate the postscreen probabilities of the target disorder (which is the PPV, given screening failure) for any specific value or range of prescreen probabilities. The latter can be either known or estimated values of the prescreen prevalence. Such estimates could be of baseline prevalence for the newborn population at large, or for any defined high-risk group, or even for individual babies with specific sets of risk indicators. The calculation involves not probabilities directly but odds for the disorder, which are easily converted to and from probabilities. The equation is

$$\text{Postscreen odds} = \text{prescreen odds} \times \text{likelihood ratio, where}$$

$$\text{Odds } (o) = p/(1-p) \text{ and, conversely, probability } (p) = o/(o+1).$$

For example, if the prevalence p is 0.002 or 2 per thousand, the sensitivity 0.9 and specificity 0.95, the LR+ is 0.9/0.05, which equals 18. The prescreen odds are 0.002/0.998, and it is easy to show that the postscreen probability is 0.035 or 3.5%. Referring back to the beginning of this chapter, this would mean that the number on the baby's forehead label changed from 0.2% to 3.5%. For a high-risk baby with a prescreen prevalence of 0.01, say, the result would be a probability change from 1% to 15%.

The postscreen probability can be calculated directly or by using tables that are easy to create using common spreadsheet software. There are also readily available graphical tools such as nomograms that are convenient for rough estimates. See the excellent website of the Centre for Evidence Based Medicine in Oxford, United Kingdom, for more details on this and many other aspects of test evaluation and critical appraisal of evidence, available at http://www.CEBM.net, or alternatively, Google "Likelihood Ratio Nomogram." Download the nomogram and play with it.

A pair of likelihood ratios is generated by each sensitivity-specificity pair. The advantages of LRs over sensitivity-specificity pairs are that LRs are easier to conceptualize in terms of the effect of the screening result on the pretest probability. In fact, for very small values of the pretest probability, a good approximation to the posttest probability is simply the product of the pretest probability and the LR. Thus, for the example prevalence above of 0.002 and typical LR+ of about 18, the posttest probability is crudely estimated at 0.002 × 18 = 0.036 (about 4%), whereas the exact value is 0.0348. Likelihood ratios are not commonly presented in the audiology literature but, after a little practice, they are simple and intuitively useful measures of screening test impact. They are more useful, in practical terms, than sensitivity and specificity, because when you are evaluating a screening test you are interested in sensitivity and specificity, but when you are considering individual babies or groups of babies, you are usually most interested in their current probability of having hearing loss.

Yield, Refer Rate (Fail Rate), Accuracy, and Number Needed to Screen (NNS)

The *yield* of a screening test reflects the number of true cases found, usually expressed as a proportion or percentage of the number of individuals screened. It is very important not to confuse screening yield with the prevalence of the target disorder. Screening program yields are (negatively) biased estimators of prevalence, because sensitivity is never perfect, and some babies will always be missed by real-world screening tests.

The refer rate reflects the number of screening tests that are positive, also usually expressed as a proportion or percentage of the number of individuals screened. It is made up of both true-positive and false-positive outcomes, usually with the latter dominating. It is of interest for two main reasons. First, if every screening failure must be followed up, the refer rate is related directly to the resources required to provide such follow-up, such as the number of initial diagnostic tests that will be needed. Second, the refer rate gives a sense of the number of families who will experience a screening failure, with its attendant stress and anxiety. Because for rare disorders the refer rate is usually dominated by false-positive outcomes, it also gives a sense of the number of families who experience a failure when in fact their child does not have the target hearing disorder.

Test *accuracy* is quite commonly listed in the literature on screening test measures, where the term is given a specific meaning—the estimated proportion of all screening tests that are correct, that is, are TP or TN. Not only is use of the term *accuracy* specific, but also the proportion so derived lumps all errors together and is uninformative when different importance is attached to FN and FP errors, which certainly is the case in NHS programs as well as in most screening programs more generally.

Finally, the reader might also meet the *number needed to screen* (NNS), which is simply the number of screens needed to yield one additional case. The lower the NNS, the more productive is the screening, in terms of new cases found per unit of screening resource expenditure.

Real-World Challenges of Screening Performance

The Elusive Gold Standard Hearing Test for Neonates and Young Infants

In the previous discussion of efficacy measures, reference was made to whether the screened persons did or did not have the target disorder, but nothing was said about how that truth can be determined. This is the issue of comparing a test under evaluation (called the "index test") to a gold standard test (or "reference test") of a baby's hearing. Comparing physiologic screening test outcomes in newborns with reliable, behavioral thresholds as soon as they can be obtained seems a plausible approach but the major threat to validity of the comparison is that the two tests are not concurrent—the interval between them might be at least 6 months, and there is no way of knowing whether the hearing has changed in the interim. For example, if the screen passes the baby but sensory/neural hearing loss is found at age 1 year, was the screen false negative? You can look for possible causes of progressive or late-onset loss, such as by doing a genetic mutation panel and molecular blood-spot analysis for asymptomatic cytomegalovirus infection, but not finding an obvious cause does not rule out late-onset loss, and finding a possible cause does not rule it in. So, the question of whether a screen was actually false negative is unanswerable in many situations.

It is possible to make a reasonable inference of false-negative screening if there is access to stored procedure and outcome records in a screening device or data upload repository. For example, well-designed screening protocols typically specify that an initial OAE screen should be repeated only once or twice if the first screen gives a fail result. Screeners who do not follow protocol might screen multiple times, apparently seeking a pass. Eventually, of course, they will succeed by chance alone even in the presence of significant hearing loss. This type of probable false-negative due to procedural error is often detectable by inspection and audit of the screening device. However, we have strayed a little from the question of screening efficacy (*can* it work under fairly ideal conditions) to screening effectiveness (*does* it work under real field conditions), which is addressed in more detail in Chapter 16.

The converse situation, in which the screen is positive but the reference audiometry is within normal limits, is so commonplace that the question really becomes a familiar one of how to reduce the usual mass of false positives. Conductive overlays can come and go, OAEs in particular are highly sensitive to them, and tympanometry has limited sensitivity and specificity as an adjunct test, even with high probe frequencies.

A second issue is error (bias or imprecision) or even invalidity of the reference test. VRA has natural face validity as a reference test because it is at least behavioral and it engages much more of the sensorimotor systems and pathways than does an OAE or an ABR. But, this very completeness exposes the technique to inaccuracy or invalidity. Behavioral response such as head-turning in a conditioned paradigm has several challenges. Visual reinforcement audiometry (VRA) minimum response levels (MRLs) are systematically higher than true, perceptual thresholds, by variable amounts across babies without nonauditory disorders, but what if there is a disorder of vision, sensory-motor integration, motor function, attention, and so forth? Moreover, these variables are graded in their effect on auditory response and, unless severe, might not be detected or even suspected. Clearly, therefore, VRA has substantial limitations as a reference test. High-quality VRA is more properly considered at best a "silver" standard, by virtue of its dependency on tester expertise and its limited applicability to a significant proportion of the target population, such as NICU graduates with multiple morbidities. Also, it can be speculated that the accuracy of VRA is more dependent on tester skill than is commonly realized, due to subjectivity of the task, a tendency to overrate one's own accuracy, the complexities of infant behaviors, and perhaps to a historically undemanding approach to behavioral test evaluation. More advanced, automated systems for VRA might address some of these problems of subjectivity and skill dependency, but automation alone cannot overcome neuromaturational, visual, or motor deficits, for example. What it might be able to do, though, is quantify more objectively and accurately the quality of test results in individual subjects.

An alternative to behavioral reference testing is to compare screening test results (OAE or ABR) to "manual" ABR. The reader might have read statements that high-quality, diagnostic ABR is a "gold standard hearing test" for infants under about six months of age. Manual ABR has the great advantage that it can be done in most newborns, almost concurrently with the screening, so change in hearing over time is much less of an issue. Detailed, manual ABR can estimate ear-specific, frequency-specific perceptual thresholds by air and bone conduction and does not require intact integrative, visual and motor systems, so many of the concerns that plague VRA as a reference test disappear. The problem is that although high-quality manual ABR testing has many useful attributes, it is questionable to equate the best available test (the test of choice) for some context with a genuine gold standard reference test for that context. The ABR is not a direct *measure* of hearing but a statistical *correlate* of it. Perhaps a better way to say it is that auditory perception and ABR detection are two possible outcomes of stimulus-related neural activity, mediated by completely different mechanisms. There is no particular reason why ABR detection thresholds should equal auditory perceptual thresholds, but they can be exploited as statistical *estimators* of them, within the limits of their mechanistic validity. A cause of large estimation error that could be seen as leading to invalidity is ANSD, in which pathologic changes in the volume and spatiotemporal distribution of afferent neural activity can lead to even completely absent ABRs at stimulus levels high above perceptual thresholds. There are also many variables of ABR measurement techniques that can affect the bias and precision of hearing threshold estimates based on the ABR.

When comparing screening ABR with manual ABR as the reference, the outcomes of both tests can be right or wrong with respect to actual hearing, but they will tend to be so in tandem; this is known as a problem of *correlated error*, and it causes the accuracy of the screen to be overestimated. Such comparisons do not assess screening test accuracy with respect to hearing per se, but they can be informative for other purposes, such as examining the relationship between click or chirp ABR screening and tone-pip ABR thresholds.

Frequency-specific, manual ABR testing with a well-designed, standardized test protocol remains the procedure of choice for prompt follow-up of newborns who fail screening but a distinction must be made from its use as a reference procedure to evaluate screening tests, which in a context of screening test evaluation is even more demanding in terms of accuracy and breadth of validity. Furthermore, the use of ABRs to estimate true, perceptual thresholds remains an immature field despite well over two decades of widespread clinical use follow-up from UNHS. If the optimal techniques for estimating the audiogram are not yet well-established, the potential for error or confusion in clinical management as well as in evaluation of screening tests using, for example, so-called frequency-specific ABR thresholds as a reference, is clear. An example is an apparent mismatch between the correction factors that convert observed ABR thresholds to pure-tone threshold estimates in decibel estimated hearing level (dB eHL) used in the Ontario Infant Hearing Program (IHP) and the British Columbia Early Hearing Program (BCEHP) and a recent report by McCreery et al. (2015). The primary caution is that audiologists must use only those correction factors that are normed with and specific to the stimulus and recording parameters they choose to use in the manual ABR. Using corrections derived for one type of stimulus when measuring ABRs with another is completely inappropriate. The second caution relates to taking the results of parametric statistical predictive techniques (such as regression analysis) at face value unless (a) they are clearly consistent with large-sample scatterplots of ABR and behavioral thresholds, (b) they are derived from precisely the clinically relevant range of predicted (dB eHL) and observed (dB nHL or dB ppeSPL) ABR thresholds, and (c) they are found to be clinically reasonable over a trial period of field use.

OAE and ABR Hearing Screening Sensitivity Are Not Well Understood

Values for automated OAE (AOAE) and automated ABR (AABR) screening test sensitivity are reported quite frequently, and there appears to be a tendency to believe that current screening tests detect all, or nearly all, hearing losses that are of moderate degree or greater. Unfortunately, less is known about the actual sensitivity of AOAE and AABR than the reader might imagine. There are several reasons for this. First, direct, prospective determination of sensitivity requires that *all* children screened be followed up by a definitive procedure to determine the true hearing status. It follows that sensitivity cannot be determined from a population screening program, because only screening failures are routinely followed up, usually by diagnostic ABR. To determine sensitivity, it is necessary to conduct a cohort study of the entire screened group, which means simply that all group members must have a described final outcome.

It might seem an obvious approach to compare screening program yield with independent estimates of prevalence, to estimate screening test sensitivity. Although valid in principle, the main problems are the availability and reliability of such prevalence estimates. Even if estimates were obtained for specific populations, for which there are many such examples, their generalizability across populations and over times is highly questionable. Prevalence is known to be subject to variation due to many facets of definition, measurement, and epidemiologic context.

Second, as noted earlier, there is no definitive hearing test that can be administered concurrently with the screen. When relying on later behavioral validation, late-onset or progressive loss in the intervening period can lead to underestimation of screening sensitivity, as can positive bias in VRA MRLs. Also, ear canal volume increase during early growth can reduce the effective SPL of a given stimulus dial level significantly, which might also cause sensitivity to be underestimated because the actual SPL at the screen is elevated relative to that for an equivalent nominal stimulus level at the subsequent behavioral audiometry. Fluctuating sensory/neural hearing loss and small levels of conductive overlay are also potential sources of bias or variability.

Third, there is a serious problem of insufficient sample size. Suppose that in any given study the screened group was a particular birth cohort, such as all children born in some date range at some screening location. The most common estimate of sensitivity obtained from follow-up of all screened babies is simply the proportion of all screened children found to have hearing loss at follow-up and who also failed the screen. There are readily available statistical tables or algorithms giving the variability of such proportions for various sample sizes (binomial confidence intervals). Examples of such confidence intervals are given in Table 15–3, derived using the *adjusted Wald* estimator calculator retrievable at http://www.measuringusability.com/wald.

The important issues are the maximum tolerable width of confidence interval for the estimate of sensitivity and the number of babies who need to be screened and followed up to achieve an interval of that width or less. For example, a sample that contained only 50 babies with genuine hearing loss and 45 of these failing the screen would yield a sensitivity estimate of approximately 0.9 and would have 90% confidence limits on that estimate from about 0.81 to 0.95. Remember that the true value of sensitivity can lie anywhere in that interval. Is such an estimate useful? Probably not, in that a value of 0.81 would be considered unacceptable, whereas a value of 0.95 would be considered excellent. It can be seen from Table 15–3 that perhaps 500 babies with hearing loss are needed

Table 15–3. Point Estimates and 90% Confidence Intervals (Adjusted Wald method) for True Sensitivity of About 0.9 (90%), for Different Numbers of True Cases*

Number of True Cases	20	50	100	200	500	1000
Number Failing Screen	18	45	90	180	450	900
Sensitivity Estimate (%)	86.4	88.5	89.2	89.6	89.8	89.9
Lower Confidence Limit	73.0	80.6	83.9	85.9	87.6	88.3
Upper Confidence Limit	97.5	95.3	94.0	93.0	92.0	91.5

Note. *The precision of the sensitivity estimate is not acceptable for samples containing fewer than at least 200 babies with hearing loss, and even then the range of plausible values is more than 7%. Higher, standard confidence levels such as 95% or 99% would require even larger numbers of true cases to achieve useful precision of sensitivity estimation. Note that the statistically preferred (point) estimator of sensitivity is not the simple proportion of true cases failing the screen but tends toward it as the sample size increases.

before the sensitivity estimate is sufficiently precise (0.88–0.92). In a natural, prospective screening sample with a prevalence of about 2 per 1,000, this would require follow-up of 250,000 babies, which is obviously prohibitive. One way around the difficulty would be to screen only NICU babies, for which the prevalence is much higher, perhaps as high as 2 per 100. This would lead to a natural sample requirement of 25,000 babies, which is still extremely demanding. Another problem with that approach is that the sensitivity in such a specialized sample might not be the same as it would be in the general population of all newborns. Despite the best effort to date (Norton et al., 2000), no prospective study has yielded the desirable precision on sensitivity estimates for OAE or ABR screening tests. It does not matter whether a single point estimate of sensitivity is derived or an ROC curve is used; the resulting confidence intervals for feasible, prospective studies are too wide to render typical estimates of much value in test development or evaluation. The more common 95% confidence interval, of course, would be wider still. Note also that these calculations take no account of any actual changes in true sensitivity for different degrees of hearing loss severity.

Fourth, there is the pervasive issue of differences between sensitivity estimates obtained from controlled trials and field sensitivity that occurs in actual practice. Laxity and diversity of screening practices in actual screening programs might have unpredictable effects on actual test performance, and there is very little published information available about such effects. It can be speculated that observed variations in specificity (see later) might also occur for sensitivity. The problem is that such effects are extremely difficult to demonstrate and quantify.

In practice, perhaps the only practicable approach to large-sample estimation of sensitivity is through so-called ascertainment studies. That is, for example, if all cases of hearing loss in a given geographical region are identifiable from a retrospective review of all audiologic records, then if all those cases had been screened, a reasonably valid and precise estimate of screening sensitivity might be derived. Such an estimate, however, will be affected by many challenges, including the completeness of the identification process, the quality of clinical records, the stability of the target population, the completeness of the screening, and, of course, the inherent problems of longitudinal validation just mentioned. Good ascertainment studies essentially demand regionally or nationally centralized, universal hearing health care programs based on consistent protocols, such as are implemented to some extent in, for example, England and Australia.

Given all of these concerns, the apparent ease and confidence with which sensitivities of NHS tests are reported and quoted is quite remarkable. In fact, there is very little hard data on sensitivity that is valid, precise, and generalizable across studies or program populations. We might believe that the sensitivity of a well-conducted AABR screen is "good," but we do not know, indeed we might never know, exactly what it is or how much it can vary across populations.

Intrinsic Sensitivity Limitations of OAE and ABR Screening

The complexity of hearing itself and of hearing screening tests raise many important issues that impinge directly on the ability to satisfy the Wilson-Jungner

(1968) criteria. Although there is no doubt that AABR screening as currently implemented is vastly superior to behavioral screening methods in newborns and young infants, what are the limits of this effectiveness, particularly with reference to its ability to detect all hearing disorders within the target disorder set? There are several substantial issues.

One reason for concern, or at least for curiosity, is that in the only multicenter, prospective, comparative study of OAE and ABR screening sensitivity to date by Susan Norton and her colleagues (2000), the ROCs for detection of average pure tone hearing loss showed that at a specificity of 0.95 the sensitivities of TEOAE, DPOAE, and ABR were in the range about 0.6 to 0.65. These are values that would be considered unacceptable for current screening programs. The main reason to doubt that such estimates apply to field performance of modern screening devices is that the yields of some screening programs (such as that in England) are broadly consistent with exceptionally well-characterized local prevalence data. However, one key to the difference might lie primarily in the fact that the hearing loss severity criterion used by Norton et al. was 30 dB HL by VRA, whereas the yield-prevalence match from the England data was based on an average loss criterion of at least 40 dB HL in the better ear. It was shown many years ago by Hyde, Riko, and Malizia (1990) that the predictive accuracy of the click ABR improves rapidly for hearing loss criteria in the 30 to 50 dB HL range, both by ROC and likelihood ratio measures.

Current AABR screening devices typically use wide-band stimuli, traditionally clicks but use of wide-band chirps is increasingly common. Chirps have been standard tools in dynamic analysis of physical structures in civil and aeronautical engineering for many decades, but their application to ABR is relatively recent and has unique relevance to cochlear mechanisms. Wide-band chirps are substantially more effective at ABR elicitation than are conventional click stimuli. They can be designed to have similar overall energy density spectra to clicks but a rapid sweep from low to high frequency (up-chirp) improves overall neuronal synchrony by at least partially compensating for predicted cochlear traveling wave delay (Cebulla, Stürzebecher, Elberling, & Müller, 2007). This tends to improve ABR detectability, especially at near-threshold stimulus levels, by essentially "stacking" the normally time-distributed and smeared ABRs from different parts of the cochlea on top of one another in time, increasing amplitude and sharpness of peaks. This is a significant technical advance.

Regardless of absolute ABR detectability, there are still concerns about screening test sensitivity, even validity. With any wide-band stimulus, a detectable ABR could be elicited from any cochlear region in the range from about 1 to 4 kHz, even from an isolated island of hearing around a specific frequency. Therefore, there is and there always has been a deep conceptual mismatch if a wide-band stimulus is used to detect a target disorder that is defined to include low-, mid-, or high-frequency hearing losses or notched losses. To the extent that such losses are present in the screened population, the sensitivity of AABR screening will be compromised and the false-negative rate increased. Essentially, ABR screening with clicks or wide-band chirps *de facto* targets flat, medium- to high-frequency hearing losses. Another way of expressing this problem is to say that wide-band stimuli "ask the wrong question" of the cochlea. They ask "is there any frequency region from about 1 to 4 kHz that has acceptable hearing sensitivity?" Perhaps a better question to ask is the following: "Is there any frequency in the target disorder range that does *NOT* have acceptable hearing sensitivity?" This question could only be answered by a more complex screening technique that measures response from several regions along the cochlear partition. The question would seem to be how many frequency regions, which ones and is there some way of measuring the ABRs from all the regions simultaneously or perhaps in some swept-frequency manner?

Any significant advance in ABR technique can have application both in screening and more detailed ABR-based assessments. It is reasonable to expect chirp-type stimuli to be explored in oto-neurologic ABR applications and also in frequency-specific threshold estimation. Are the improved responses and threshold clarity observed for wide-band chirps also seen when stimulus bandwidth is restricted? It might be expected that the chirp benefit would disappear if a stimulus such as a brief tone burst were used, but early indications are that the benefit might be sustained even for narrow-band chirps relative to tone pips (Ferm, Lightfoot & Stevens, 2013).

Another concern relates to screening stimulus levels. ABR thresholds in decibel normal hearing level do not necessarily equate directly to perceptual thresholds in decibel hearing level, so an adjustment must be made in order to relate screening stimulus levels correctly to the desired minimum hearing loss within the target disorder range. For a detailed explanation of relationships between ABR thresholds and perceptual thresholds, see Sininger and Hyde (2009). However, a deeper concern than simple correction for bias is the amount of variation among newborns in the actual sound pressure level (SPL) of the stimulus that results from use of a constant nominal stimulus level in decibel normal hearing level. The issue is not one of systematic average differences in stimulus levels across transducer types such as inserts versus supra-aurals, but of variation from baby to baby in the effective SPL at the tympanic membrane for a given nominal stimulus level and transducer type. The volume and geometry of the external ear canal affect the actual intensity of the stimulus at the tympanic membrane, and such effects differ over frequency (see, e.g., Bagatto, Scollie, Seewald, Moodie, & Hoover, 2002). It might be expected that SPL variations would be larger with inserts because of the smaller enclosed volume relative to that with "mini supra-aurals," but quantitative data on this issue are not available. At the very least, this means that with those AABR instruments that do not autocalibrate stimulus levels in individual ear canals, newborns are being screened at SPLs that might differ substantially from baby to baby. Such differences might in principle be as large as a range of 15 to 20 dB, with the highest SPLs generally occurring in those with the smallest canal volumes. Clearly, this might reduce the sensitivity of AABR screening in newborns with mild hearing losses who happen to have small canal volumes and, therefore, elevated effective stimulus SPLs. Conversely, it will increase sensitivity in newborns with unusually large volumes, because of lower effective SPLs. The size and scope of this effect on sensitivity are unknown, but it is a clear deficiency of measurement parameters that could be avoided by routine stimulus SPL autocalibration using a miniature microphone, as is commonly done for OAE stimuli. This is now becoming more widely available in the most recent generation of AABR screening devices.

Turning to response analysis, as noted earlier, AABR devices all implement some statistical test for response detection. Any such test will have an implicit or explicit significance level for response detection, usually expressed as the size of the probability of false-positive response detection. This equals the algorithmic screening false-negative probability, because false-positive response detection results in a screen pass in the absence of response, namely in the presence of hearing loss. The lower the false-positive response detection probability is set, the higher will be the (algorithmic) screen sensitivity and FP rate. Yet, again, there are no standards for setting such probabilities across screening devices, and the quantitative rationales that might guide choice of values do not seem to attract much attention. Where are the discussions, for example, of where an algorithmic false-positive response detection rate should be set and why; and, what are the consequences of different choices? Moreover, unless algorithmic false-positive response detection rates are known and controlled under standardized test time constraints, there can be no valid inferences made about how to optimize the statistical power and efficiency of response detection tests.

Notwithstanding the substantial recent advances in relation to stimulation techniques, including chirps, autocalibration, and steady-state methods, with very few exceptions current methods of ABR detection and analysis are actually not very sophisticated from a purely statistical perspective. There are several advanced statistical techniques that could improve SNR distributional characteristics for the ABR, but none of them is straightforward conceptually or technically and they tend to be published in rarefied engineering journals. Their implementation would require an extraordinary conjunction of statistical, clinical, and technological insight and cooperation, as well as strong commercial incentive and will. Given the apparently reasonable performance of existing devices, prospects for rapid development of much more efficient and powerful methods for ABR detection seem limited at present.

Taking a broader view, how might the sensitivity of AABR be significantly improved without concomitant increase in FP screens? The most obvious approach is to address the issue of false-negatives due to frequency-specific hearing losses. As just mentioned in the chirp discussion, this would require a frequency-specific, multiple-frequency method, and perhaps the most obvious approach is to use the multifrequency 80-Hz ASSR, which in essence is just a fast ABR with a simple, frequency-based response detection algorithm. The big question is the choice of the number and range of test frequencies. The time taken to screen with acceptable error rates will be governed by the lowest frequency chosen (e.g., 0.5 kHz or 1 kHz), because electroencephalogram (EEG) noise levels increase steadily at low frequencies. It remains to be seen whether such devices emerge in the near future. The pace of implementation might well be limited by problems of patent protection, a familiar issue in the history of newborn hearing screening.

Another approach would be to increase the separation between the case and noncase distributions, thereby increasing the value of d′. This boils down to reducing the distributional spread of the standardized SNR measure, by either increasing the signal or reducing the noise variability, under a constraint of constant average processing time across the target population. The constraint is necessary because it is easy to increase the separation if willing to take more time to do more averaging, but what we would prefer to do is somehow be more efficient rather than take longer to screen.

One of the challenges is the wide range of EEG noise levels in the target population. Averaging with a fixed number of stimuli would yield only a fixed reduction in noise level based roughly on the square root of the number of sweeps collected. Many screening units partially compensate for EEG noise levels by adjusting the number of sweeps in an attempt to stabilize the variance of the averaged noise, a strategy that makes total sense both for automated screening and for manual ABR. But, there are limits to the effectiveness of this technique because a fivefold range of EEG noise standard deviation (a conservative estimate of the true range) would require a 25-fold range of sweep counts, leading to impractically lengthy averaging times in some babies. So, for this reason among others, the higher the EEG noise level, the greater is the probability of both false-negative and false-positive response identification by the ABR detection algorithm, so the lower will be the sensitivity and specificity. The only obvious way to avoid this effect is for the device to declare the screen void beyond a given EEG noise level; some devices do versions of this, but the methods and criteria are not standardized. The practical challenge for manufacturers is that the tighter the control over required average noise levels is, the higher will be the incidence of voided screens and the longer will be the maximum screening times, both of which would not be welcomed by a user community acutely tuned to operational costs.

As is the case for the ABR, OAE screening currently only has empirical validity, based on observed correlations between OAE detectability and audibility. For the OAE, though, the correlations are smaller and have a more limited range of application than for the ABR. OAE measurements are more suited to binary categories of hearing loss than to estimation of hearing thresholds over the full range of possible values. Leaving aside the matter of ANSD, which AOAE screening intrinsically cannot detect, current test sensitivity is limited mainly by the wide natural distribution of AOAE amplitudes in subjects with hearing losses that are at or near the lower bound of a reasonable target disorder range. It is perfectly feasible to enhance AOAE specificity by improving the power of the emission detection algorithm, but improving sensitivity without concomitant increase in FP screens appears challenging. It seems clear that many children with hearing losses up to at least 30 dB HL can have detectable OAEs. Simply making the OAE detection criterion more conservative will increase sensitivity at the expense of already limited specificity. The prospects for accurate OAE screening for mild or minimal hearing losses seem constrained at best, because of underlying distributional overlap for the target and nontarget groups.

There are some indications that with more sophisticated OAE testing and analysis methods, OAEs might permit more accurate classification of individuals with and without hearing loss. For example, Kirby, Kopun, Tan, Neely, and Gorga (2011) confirmed previous reports that multivariate statistical methods applied to OAE signal and noise measurements at various frequencies improve discrimination between groups, which is the essence of screening test performance. Although conceptually quite straightforward and frequently superior in performance to the vastly more common univariate techniques, multivariate analysis has not yet achieved the widespread applications in audiology research and technical development that might have been anticipated. The sooner this occurs, the more rapidly will significant advances be realized in many areas related to early detection and intervention for hearing loss. The reader with even the slightest interest in data analysis is strongly urged to take a look at, for example, the book by Kachigan (1991). Note that in statistics, the word "multivariate" refers to joint or simultaneous consideration of multiple, measurable facets or components of a single variable, not to techniques that address a single (univariate) dependent variable affected by several independent variables, such as multiple linear regression.

Current AOAE devices, whether based on transient or distortion-product emissions, effectively test OAE SNR for several frequency regions. Frequencies below about 1 kHz are difficult to test accurately not because of absent OAEs but because of increasing environmental and body-generated acoustical noise levels at low frequencies. In principle, sensitivity could be increased by requiring response detection at *every one* of several test frequencies for an overall pass, somewhat analogous to the argument made earlier for multifrequency AABR. But, there is the ever-present issue of balance between sensitivity and FP rate. To the author's knowledge, there are limited efficacy and effectiveness data that adequately address the detailed effects of AOAE pass-fail criteria on actual test error rates in populations with diverse audiometric profiles and severities. Indeed, the scientific rationale underlying the nature and variety of current device pass-fail criteria is not readily apparent. Certainly, there is much room for evidence-driven, parametric improvement in OAE screening protocols.

OAE and ABR Screening Specificity Are Relatively Well Understood

The information available on specificity values for automated OAE and ABR screens is much greater than that for sensitivity. This is true simply because the population prevalence of hearing loss is low. Take a prevalence of, say, 2 per 1,000 live births. Because the vast majority of babies who fail the initial screening will *not* have hearing loss, the overall proportion of babies who fail (the refer rate) is actually quite an accurate estimate of the screen FP rate, given a substantial sample size that is relatively easy to obtain. No follow-up is required for this estimation. A modest screening program sample of 50,000 babies, for example, will yield a reasonably precise estimate of the refer rate and the specificity estimate is simply the complement of that rate. It is important to note that using the refer rate as an estimate of the true FP rate only works when prevalence is very low, which might not be a valid assumption when considering the performance of the later stages of a multistage screening process (see later).

Specificity Limitations of OAE and ABR Screening

In newborn hearing screening, the most common questions relate to which test(s) to use and should a one-, two-, or three-stage series of screens be used. The challenge is usually to increase specificity while suffering a minimal loss in sensitivity—that is, to reduce the net rate of screening failure without missing a significant additional number of babies with hearing loss. To understand how to do this, the various causes of false-positive and false-negative errors must be considered.

Some possible causes of false-positive screening failure, for automated OAE and ABR screens, are as follows:

AOAE	AABR
random algorithmic error	random algorithmic error
high environmental noise	high electromyogenic noise
minor middle ear conditions	substantial transient conductive loss
partially blocked probe	partially blocked insert phone
poor probe positioning	poor earphone positioning
naturally small OAEs	naturally small ABRs
suboptimal test methods	suboptimal test methods

These sources of false positives can be divided into categories that reflect different properties. First, there is algorithmic error. This is statistical error arising within the screening device response detection decision algorithm itself, because the pass-fail criteria are inherently statistical. Such errors are controlled in part by the choice of significance level of the response detection algorithm. The more conservative the test for response detection, the more reluctant the algorithm will be to conclude that response is present and, therefore, that the measurement comes from the disorder absent distribution; consequently, the higher the likelihood is of false-positive screens. Note also that the lower the statistical power of the detection algorithm, the less likely the algorithm will be to detect a genuinely present response, so the higher the FP rate will be. There are no standards yet in place for the statistical performance of screening devices and their associated response detection algorithms, and the algorithms themselves differ radically across devices and manufacturers. But, one important point about algorithmic error is that it is quite likely that such errors will be statistically random and independent of each other, so the probability that they will occur repeatedly declines dramatically with screen repetition.

The second group of errors that might be useful to identify could be called *transient*, for lack of a better term. These errors can arise from several sources, including temporary environmental, physiologic, or physical conditions that can readily change over a short time. For example, middle ear debris or fluid might resolve within a matter of hours. A blocked probe can be unblocked, or poor position avoided. Calming a baby can improve acoustic or electromyogenic noise levels, and so on. The key point about these error sources is that they can be changed readily. If, and only if, the source of potential error is recognized and addressed, then the errors will not persist across multiple screens and, therefore, they will become independent. If the sources persist, so will the errors. However, changing the test type might improve independence, because different tests tend to differ in their susceptibilities to various error sources.

The third error group might be called *sustained* errors. For these, little can be done and they will tend to persist across multiple tests of the same type, although they might not persist across different test types. For example, there is a natural distribution of OAE amplitude (and ABR amplitude) in babies who do not have significant hearing loss, so inevitably some babies will fail simply because they have small responses. Repeating an OAE screen would do nothing to reduce errors from that source, so the errors would persist, whereas changing to an ABR screen, for example, could avoid that error source completely (while introducing other possible sources, but possibly independent ones). Similar remarks could be applied to screening devices that have algorithms or stimulation/recording methods that are inherently inefficient at eliciting or detecting response.

The relative magnitudes of all the different possible sources of false-positive screening error are at present poorly understood and almost certainly are very different across locations, times, test populations, and test personnel. Some sources of error, such as poor probe positioning, can be addressed by better technique; the challenge there is how to detect the deficiency and remedy it. Probe blockage can sometimes be addressed by removal, cleaning, and immediate re-screening, but such rescreening will do nothing to abolish false positives due to middle-ear debris or infection; there is no choice but to wait or to rescreen on an outpatient or community basis. Debris or fluid issues can be addressed, if practicable, by delaying the test. For example, Figure 15–5 shows the effect of age in hours on the failure rate for DPOAE screening. Clearly, the more time that elapses from birth, the lower the OAE screening failure rate will be. However, the trend toward shorter perinatal hospital stays might limit options, if predischarge screening is the chosen mode. Movement noise, whether acoustical (AOAE) or electrophysiologic (AABR), is addressed by screening when the baby is in as quiet a state as possible but, again, this might or might not be achievable practically under the constraints of predischarge test scheduling. Moreover, high levels of such noise are not always readily apparent and accompanied by gross movement of the baby. In many ways, the predischarge hospital stay is not necessarily the most favorable situation with respect to false positives, but outpatient or community screening presents a common challenge of reduced access to the child, so the choice might be between high access and high FP rate versus poorer access and lower FP rate.

Refer Rate Variation: Is There a Unique Value for Screening Test Specificity?

Although test efficacy measures such as sensitivity and specificity reflect the extent to which the test *can* discriminate cases from noncases, *effectiveness* reflects the extent to which it *does* discriminate in actual field practice. Effectiveness is rarely, if ever, as good as efficacy studies lead us to expect. The reasons for this are many; some are obvious and some are more subtle. Test efficacy is typically established by controlled studies. Such

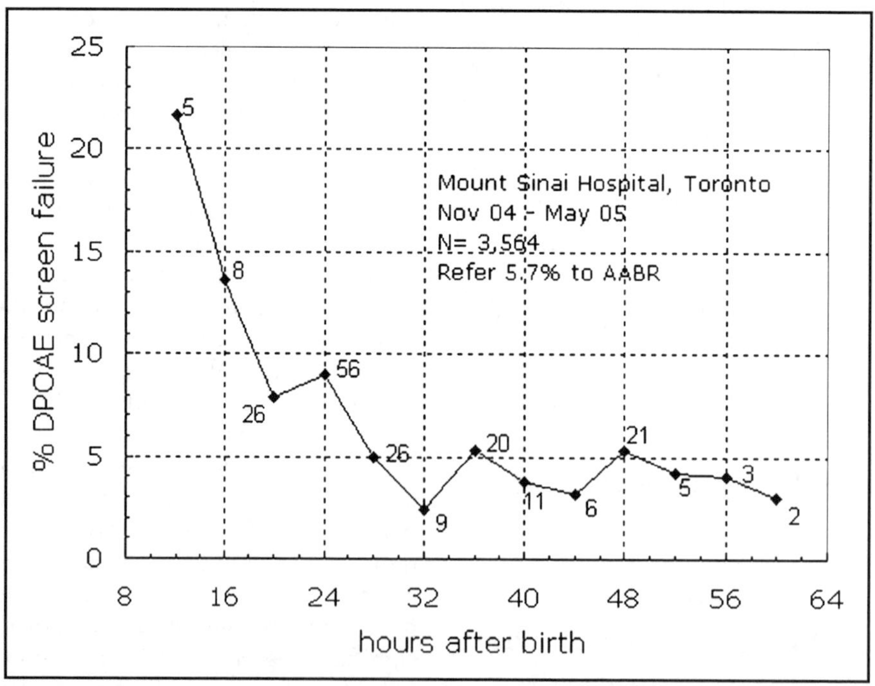

FIGURE 15–5. The fail (refer) rate from Stage 1 ADPOAE screening declines rapidly with age of vaginal-birth babies in hours, with an asymptotic value achieved at about 24 hours of age. The interval between birth and OAE screening is a strong source of variability in screening fail rates.

studies are usually undertaken with very careful optimization and standardization of procedures, instrumentation, and criteria. They are usually designed and implemented by experts in the specific area of interest, with training and oversight of practices. Moreover, studies almost always target specific populations of subjects that are filtered by clear inclusion and exclusion criteria.

In actual field practice, very few of these factors might operate. In contrast to the controlled study context, the populations are unfiltered and reflect the full range of natural variation in subject characteristics and behaviors. Instrumentation, protocols, and procedures can vary from place to place, tester to tester, subject to subject, and over time. The levels of understanding and expertise can vary substantially among testers and over time, perhaps improving with practice and perhaps deteriorating with carelessness or the development of idiosyncratic variations of practice. Every one of these factors will increase the variability of outcomes and will also tend to reduce test performance.

In the light of all of these concerns and sources of false-positive screens, it should be no surprise to the reader that reported screening refer rates for any given screening technology or specific device vary widely. What is remarkable is the large amount of variation in refer rates, not only across screening studies or service programs, but across regions, centers, and even screening personnel within centers. Figure 15–6 shows an example of such variation. Although there are few published reports of variation analysis, the author is aware of similar ranges of refer rate variation in several state and national programs.

What does screening refer rate variation, which is attributable primarily to variation in false-positive rates, really mean at a deeper level, with respect to program quality? First, it means that there is a loss of screening *equity*, in the sense that children can have radically different likelihoods of false-positive screening, depending on where they go for screening and who screens them. Second, there will be widely variable demand for follow-up services, such as diagnostic testing. These are important issues that have received little attention in published reports on EHDI programs.

Perhaps the most interesting implication of refer rate variation is that reports of screen test performance

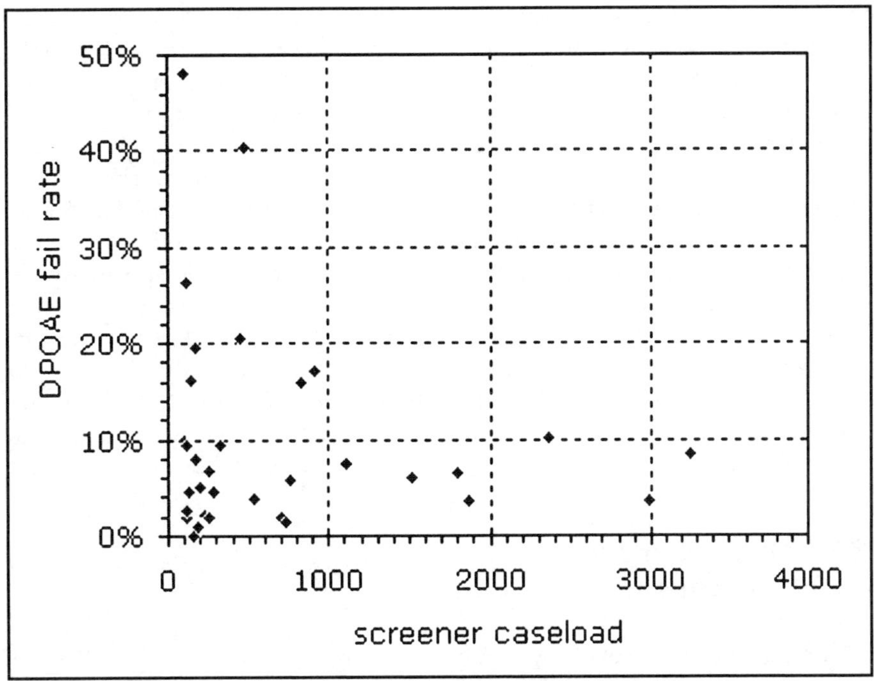

FIGURE 15–6. DPOAE Stage 1 screening fail (refer) rates for individual screening personnel can differ dramatically. Generally, the higher the caseload of any individual screener, the lower the fail (refer) rates tend to be, but it is also true that substantial differences that are massively significant statistically can occur even with very experienced, high-caseload screeners. These effects are dominated by false-positive screens.

must be viewed with great caution. Of course, there is the basic matter of sampling error, which is more important than commonly believed and are discussed shortly. But, more fundamentally, there is the question of whether it is actually meaningful to attribute a single, specific false-positive rate to a specific screening test technology or device. The reason is that FP rates are intimately dependent on a host of practical variables that have to do with technique, environment, and the precise characteristics of the screened population. For example, if two programs have different practices or constraints with respect to scheduling of initial screening tests, their FP rates will differ, perhaps substantially. Also, it is commonly reported that refer rates of screening programs decrease substantially over a period of years from program initiation. None of these reported rates is correct. In fact, it can be argued that there is no correct rate for any given screening test technology or device. There is a typical rate, a best rate, a median rate, and a range of rates, but it is the detailed procedures and factors that lead to the lowest rates that are of greatest interest in terms of screening program quality. They raise an important question of whether the common presumption that there exists a single fail (refer) rate for any given screening test has any real validity. The author's view is that the best performance by experienced, knowledgeable screeners under close to ideal conditions has meaning, but that most group data reports say more about uncontrolled sources of refer rate variation than they do about anything intrinsic to the screening test itself.

In summary, the challenge with specificity is not so much to obtain accurate estimates of it, but rather to make any valid use of those estimates, in light of the many sources of local variability in refer rates and, by implication, FP rates, which were discussed earlier. Note that it is the variation of observed FP rates across individual screeners, locations, and time, as well as the lowest observed rates that are of most interest in relation to screening program quality.

AOAE and AABR Combinations and Screening Protocol Performance

A *screening protocol* is defined here as a set of screening tests and decision rules that determine how the outcomes of individual screening tests are combined into an overall, pass-fail outcome for the whole protocol. Many screening programs make use of more than one screening test. The tests might be repetitions of a single test technology or mixtures of different test technologies, or both. Decision rules for combining test results into a pass or fail for the overall protocol can be *serial* or *parallel*. A common serial rule involves only those who fail a first (Stage 1) screen going on to another (Stage 2) screen, so an overall fail is a fail on both tests. An example of this is the use of AOAE as an initial screen, followed by AABR in AOAE failures. For a parallel rule, two (or more) tests are done on all subjects and an overall fail is a fail on any one of the tests. Such parallel protocols are less common, except for programs in which the nature of the screening follow-up differs depending on the pattern of failure. For example, newborns who fail an OAE and pass an AABR might be simply monitored by developmental questionnaire or interview, whereas those who fail AABR would go on to immediate diagnostic tests. Alternatively, those who pass OAE and fail AABR might be referred directly to a special follow-up for possible ANSD candidates. Finally, a *mixture* protocol can include different protocols for subgroups of the screening population. For example, babies who are not at risk might receive serial OAE/AABR, whereas babies at risk might receive only AABR. One rationale for that approach is that at-risk newborns will include the majority of ANSD cases, which is speculated but not yet proven and which might depend, as do so many aspects of screening, on local population epidemiology. A more traditional rationale is that the much higher prevalence of hearing loss in the at-risk group justifies the use of a more expensive test with higher intrinsic efficacy.

The purpose of using tests in combination is usually to control overall errors. Most commonly, it is to increase specificity—that is, to lower the net FP rate. What exactly is the effect of combining tests on the overall sensitivity and specificity? In the simplest case, the errors for each test are assumed to be statistically unrelated (independent), in which case probabilities can be calculated easily. For example, suppose we have two screens (S1 and S2) with sensitivities and specificities denoted as (se1, sp1) and (se2, sp2).

For S1 and S2 both with se and sp of 0.9 for simplicity, and with a serial decision rule:

$$\text{se (overall)} = \text{se1} \times \text{se2} = 0.9 \times 0.9 = 0.81\text{, and}$$

$$\text{sp (overall)} = 1 - [(1 - \text{sp1}) \times (1 - \text{sp2})]\ , = 1 - [0.1 \times 0.1] = 0.99,$$

so the sensitivity is reduced by 10% but the specificity increases dramatically, with a 90% reduction in false positives (from 0.1 to 0.01). This is a typical result—serial protocols usually improve specificity dramatically and reduce sensitivity slightly. In contrast, for S1 and S2 with a parallel decision rule:

$$se\ (overall) = 1 - [(1 - se1) \times (1 - se2)] = 0.99, \text{ and}$$
$$sp\ (overall) = sp1 \times sp2 = 0.81,$$

so the sensitivity increases to 0.99 and the specificity is reduced to 0.81. Parallel protocols usually increase sensitivity dramatically and reduce specificity slightly. One reason why they are less common is the high FP rates and the large workload involved if all protocol failures were to be followed up diagnostically. It is not possible to enhance sensitivity dramatically without FP cost.

In actual practice, the effects of multiple screens are not as dramatic as those just calculated, because the errors in the two screens are usually *not* completely independent. Suppose, for example, we took the extreme case of complete correspondence between the errors for S1 and S2. In the serial model, doing S2 will have no effect at all on the outcomes of S1, because all the FPs from S1 will also fail S2 and none of the FNs from S1 make it to S2. The overall performance equals that of S1 alone. In the parallel model, precisely the same subjects will be FP or FN so again the addition of S2 changes nothing. In the real world, neither the full independence or full dependence assumptions is true. There will be some degree of correlation between the errors for the two tests, and the amount of correlation will dictate the impact of adding the second screen.

Consider a situation in which about half of the false-positive screening errors arising in S1 were identical in S2. What that means is that the actual specificity of S2 in those subjects who fail S1 is very much poorer (sp2 = 0.5) than when S2 is used alone as a first screen (sp2 = 0.9) because half of all the false-positive errors from S1 were propagated by S2. Another way of putting this is that the *conditional specificity* of S2 given S1 failure is much lower than the unconditional (ordinary) specificity of S2. Redoing the above calculation example for the serial protocol now gives an overall specificity of 0.95, not 0.99. This is, however, still a 50% reduction in false positives, which is a big improvement.

AOAE and AABR Screening Device Parameter Options

Are Options Needed?

The effects of the intrinsic nature of the OAE and ABR on screening efficacy have been explored in some detail, but performance in the field is governed in part by the range of options for key test parameters made available by the manufacturers of screening devices, sometimes bundled into "protocols." Perhaps the first question is whether there is a real need for parameter options, or alternatively whether all screening devices using a specific bioacoustic phenomenon (AOAE or AABR) should do basically the same thing, albeit with different bells and whistles, ease of use, elegance of design, and perhaps with different underlying effectiveness and efficiency. If there are legitimate and substantial differences in screening objectives, parametric flexibility can be essential. Even if there are not such differences in objectives, do we yet know enough to achieve consensus on which are the crucial test parameters, what the most appropriate values for them are, and whether it is acceptable not to have some amount of control or choice? It seems reasonable to argue that whoever determines program funding has the right to decide, for example, whether the program will target only bilateral hearing loss or will include unilateral loss, as well as what frequency range and what minimum severity are of interest. These are big policy decisions that will affect screening yield, sensitivity, specificity, PPV, NPV, refer rates, practicability, efficiency, benefits, harms, and all manner of cost components.

Frequencies Targeted

Whether or not unilateral losses are to be included is not actually a question of technical device parameters but of overall screening protocol and decision rules. What frequency range of hearing losses is of interest is currently almost moot for AABR screening with a wide-band stimulus, because it is what it is as governed by the intrinsic properties of that stimulus paradigm, regardless of what you might want as a program designer. What you do know, though, is that if you say, as some programs do, that the target disorder includes hearing loss of a certain magnitude at "any frequency in the range 500 Hz through 4 kHz," you will immediately incur unknown loss of sensitivity with the AABR, because it cannot detect hearing loss below at least 1 kHz, and we do not have reliable data on the prevalence of such hearing losses.

For AOAE screening, in contrast, the range and specific frequencies of interest are directly controllable by the choice of technical parameters, most obviously and directly for distortion product paradigms. One could decide to push the envelope toward low frequencies, or toward high frequencies, or both, or neither. For example, for ADPOAE, should nominal F2 frequencies above 4 kHz be included in the pass/fail decision rule? Is there sufficient prevalence of isolated, high-frequency loss and an acceptable, effective intervention for such losses? Is it acceptable to have a decision rule that can pass a baby with no testing of any frequency below 2 kHz, or must lower frequencies be included? But are frequencies below 2 kHz even practicable given the low-frequency emphasis of OAE noise spectra and the implications for test duration or false-positive screens? Why should absence of an OAE at any single frequency be ignored, such as it is by the popular "2 of 3" or "3 of 4" frequency-pass decision rules? The reader might find it interesting to look for high-quality evidence that would answer any one of these questions. See, for example, the systematic review reported by Prieve, Sabo, Schooling, Culpepper, and Tharpe (2013). With the possible exception of Kirby et al. (2011), the author has not succeeded in finding such evidence from the last 15 years and is tempted to suggest that the current numbers of frequencies, range of frequencies, stopping rules, and pass criteria chosen by various manufacturers on some "best efforts" or opinion-driven basis with an extraordinary lack of solid rationale in either logic or experimental evidence. This is the kind of situation that can result in de facto "standards," things being done the way they are for no better reason than that is the way other people do them, or because some oracle plays the "this is how I do it" card. By the way, another example of that phenomenon is the popular but highly inefficient use of fixed 2,000-sweep averages in manual ABR. These are fertile areas for postgraduate studies. In the author's limited experience with various ADPOAE protocols, the results of parametric change can be unexpected and puzzling.

The choice of frequencies in AOAE screening is complicated further with certain multitest protocols. For example, if a series protocol for babies who are not at risk is ADPOAE followed by AABR when ADPOAE gives a fail/refer, the AABR with a click or wide-band chirp will probably pass any baby with a loss affecting a single OAE test frequency, whether it is low, medium, or high frequency. So, would there be any point in setting the OAE up to detect those frequency-specific losses in the first place? Why not just spend the test time getting more accurate AOAE at, say, 2 kHz, since only flattish losses will fail the AABR?

Severities Targeted

Turning to the question of the minimum target hearing loss severity, there is a totally different situation for AOAE and AABR. Here, for AOAE, there is reasonable consensus on a 65/55/1.22 parameter set for F1 SPL, F2 SPL, and the F2/F1 ratio, regardless of the minimum target disorder severity, so there is not much choice to be had, given the intrinsic properties of OAEs. In contrast, for AABR the stimulus level parameter is crucial, is strongly coupled to the target disorder limit, and has a powerful effect on all the key screening performance measures. If it is desired to detect 20 dB losses, the stimulus must be at about 25 to 30 dB nHL, whereas if losses of 30 dB or more are targeted, the level must be 35 to 40 dB nHL, and for losses that are moderate or more, an AABR at 45 to 50 dB nHL is appropriate. The sensitivity of a 40 dB AABR to 20 dB hearing loss will be very poor. Conversely, the specificity of a 35 dB AABR with respect to target losses of 40 dB or more is likely to be substantially lower than that of a 45 dB AABR. Parenthetically, this means that statements such as "OAEs are more sensitive than AABRs" have little meaning for at least two reasons, one of which is that the AABR stimulus level is not defined (the reader could look for another, if so inclined).

The grossly reasonable range of defensible options is not difficult to define, such as 20 to 50 dB in 5-dB steps. The program design issue is this: What are the desired target hearing losses, and what screening refer rates are considered acceptable and manageable within the available resource envelope? Suppose, for example, that screening AABR at 35 dB nHL was intended to detect hearing loss of 30 dB or greater and gave an overall 2% population refer rate to manual or "diagnostic" ABR assessment, for an expected case yield of 1 to 2/1,000. Is there an argument to change this to screen at 25 dB nHL in order to detect, say, a 3 to 4/1,000 case yield of losses of 20 dB or greater but with possible referral of 5% to diagnostic ABR? The change would identify 2/1,000 babies with slight or mild hearing loss that is likely to be transient and conductive in most cases but might possibly be sensory/neural. The downside is 150% increase in direct procedure costs for diagnostic ABR and there are the questions of management effectiveness for the incremental cases found. These are the kinds of basic issues that must be considered.

When discussing the stimulus level parameter, it is necessary to raise a question of credibility. Suppose a nominal 35 dB nHL is chosen. The word "nominal" is used because it is not clear that even a familiar stimulus such as a click at a specified dB nHL will actually be at that specified decibel normal hearing level, or will be acceptably similar across screening devices. The speculative hypothesis proposed here is that what is labeled by all as "35 dB nHL" could differ by a clinically significant amount such as 10 dB or more across manufacturers and screening devices, not because of differences in babies' ear canals, but because of deficiencies, errors, and procedural variability or even systematic bias in measuring dB nHL itself. It is not difficult to regret the existence of dB nHL in view of the overall confusion and error associated with it in audiology at large. In fact, the number and sizes of sources of variability in threshold measurement for small, so-called "normative" groups of subjects, together with some startling realities about the width of confidence intervals or tolerance intervals, render most statements involving dB nHL "local norms" at best unreliable and suspect.

False Positives and Test Time

Consider next the questions of false-positive rate and screening test time, which are major determinants of program cost, given that decisions about the desired target disorder set have been made (at least provisionally). Generally, the more inclusive the target disorder definition is, the higher the refer rate will be and it is to be anticipated that the PPV would decrease if the target were permanent hearing loss, because of the expected high prevalence of minor, transient conductive losses. Also generally, for any signal-in-noise problem involving time-domain averaging or some equivalent enhancement operation, the more averaging you do, the larger the SNR will be if there is genuine signal present, and the smaller the SNR will be (or the closer to unit value, depending on how it is formulated) if there is no signal present. So, other things being equal, the longer the averaging time, the lower the false-positive rate will be. This means that the maximum data collection time parameter can become highly relevant, yet we appear to know rather little about its effects in practice. The other side of this coin is that the time taken to do a screen depends on a host of variables, especially baby state and test environment, so it is not at all clear what the practical effect on screening test time of, say, doubling the maximum averaging time would be, or indeed, what is a reasonable maximum. Bear in mind that actual test run time is a rather minor part of the overall baby-contact-plus-administrative-overheads personnel time in screening.

Signal Detection Algorithms

The other obvious parameter that is often not made explicit is the algorithmic response detection criterion, is the prime determinant of false-positive rate. For ADPOAE, this is reflected in the SNR value required at any single F2 in order to consider the OAE present. Settings for this vary over a wide range, such as from about 5 to about 10 dB at individual frequencies. For AABR, this is an explicit statistical criterion value in some devices but in others is undisclosed and, therefore, unable to be evaluated. This is puzzling, because although proprietary details of an algorithm can justifiably be undisclosed, the algorithmic false-positive rate for signal identification is a basic performance parameter that any self-respecting program designer should require be known. Of course, such disclosure would render the statistic subject to experimental validation.

Device Evolution or Change Issues

There is one more practical reason to want some degree of technical, parametric control. A particular challenge for large, mature screening programs is the management of device changes over time, whether as a result of technical advances by the manufacturer, version changes in software, firmware, or hardware, or as a result of device obsolescence and new equipment procurement initiatives that might involve a complete change of device. Changing the device type is likely to change performance significantly even if protocols and parameters appear to be comparable. A major program cannot re-equip without careful consideration of continuity in refer rates, for example, largely because of the human resources chaos that would ensue from a significant increase in refer rates or major concerns about false negatives that would be prompted by major reduction in refer rates. Furthermore, large programs have, or ought to have, substantial quality control mechanisms in place and discrete changes in device performance wreak havoc with such activities, as screeners who are performing well suddenly appear falsely to perform poorly, or vice versa. Clearly, it is desirable for a program to conduct focused trials with new or modified devices, preferably with at least three screeners who have stable, exemplary refer rates, at sites with stable, large caseloads. One basic challenge with such trials is their size required to provide reasonable statistical power for testing the hypothesis of approximate refer rate equivalence. At least 25 refers would be required, typically, which implies trial screening of at least 500 babies at a nominal refer rate of about 5%. The immediate problem is a situation of substantial increase in refer rate, which might justify an immediate parametric change such as a modest increase in AABR click or chirp level, or a reduction in OAE SNR criteria followed by some kind of forensic investigation of the cause of the increase. This trial process is complicated by a frequent increase in refer rates when screeners use unfamiliar equipment for which there can be a learning effect that extends over at least 50 or more babies. Thus, longitudinal analysis of the trial cohort is desirable, to assess any trends of refer rate reduction over time.

A deeper question occurs if the new refer rates are much lower than expected, because two of the possible causes are that the new device is genuinely superior in an ROC sense and has not compromised sensitivity, or that the new device is not superior and has achieved a lower refer rate by effectively moving along an ROC to a point of lower sensitivity. These alternatives cannot be distinguished without careful verification of screening parameters and extensive data collection that includes re-screening of cases already identified.

Chaos or Opportunity?

What, then, are the downsides of having a number of options for technical parameters? The first objection stated is usually an appeal to chaos and ignorance. Will flexibility lead to chaos, defined as everyone using their own pet set of parameters, and will that situation make it impossible to compare data and derive generalizable inferences about how to do better? It is true that program leads might vary vastly in their understanding of the technologic, clinical, and epidemiologic consequences of their protocol selections. Some might have strong rationales and detailed, justifiable requirements for specific parameters, while others might have basically no idea what to choose other than to find some trustworthy advice and follow it. Guidelines issued by various individuals, groups, or agencies vary greatly in the extent to which their recommendations are evidence based and rational, but more importantly, they are rarely detailed enough technically and they usually lack any detailed justification and rationale. It is also true that manufacturers differ greatly in their insight, priorities, style, appreciation of, and responsiveness to the preferences, performance requirements, and contextual specifics of individual programs. As for choice leading to chaos, it is argued here that diversity, especially justifiable diversity, and chaos are two different things, and that known, parametrically controlled differences in practices are potentially a rich source of increased understanding of outcome determinants—quite the opposite effect from that of premature, inappropriate restriction of screening device operating characteristics, which as yet are necessarily based on insufficient evidence and which, conceivably, could be driven by marketing considerations.

Device Parameter and Protocol Options Are Necessary and Appropriate

The bottom lines for screening in practice are that (a) there are many good reasons for newborn hearing screening program leads to require an adequate range and selection of stimulation and response analysis operating parameters of screening devices; (b) screening program design can be and should be reflective of the operating context and the health care resource allocation priorities of the funding body, guided by the best available evidence and independent expert input; (c) the evidence necessary to fix on rigid parameter sets does not exist. Indeed, the lack of evidence on which to base rational parameter selection, especially for OAE screening, is both puzzling and disturbing; (d) quantitative stimulus and analysis parameters that are known to have a major effect on refer rates should be offered with reasonable options—limited default options with high fences for override are a reasonable approach; (e) absence of parametric flexibility and lack of explicit information about key operating parameters should be influential factors in device procurement; and (f) optimization of newborn hearing screening is in its infancy, and is fertile ground for high-quality research that has potential for profound impact.

References

American National Standards Institute (ANSI; 1997). *Methods for calculation of the Speech Intelligibility Index, ANSI S3.5-1997*. New York, NY: Acoustical Society of America.

Andermann, A., Blancquaert, I., Beauchamp, S., & Dery, V. (2008). Revisiting Wilson and Jungner in the genomic age: A review of screening criteria over the past 40 years. *WHO Bulletin, 86*(4), 241–320. Retrieved June 24, 2010, from http://www.scielosp.org/scielo.php?script=sci_arttext&pid=S0042-96862008000400018&lng=en&nrm=iso&tlng=en

Bagatto, M. P., Scollie, S. D., Seewald, R. C., Moodie, S., & Hoover, B. M. (2002). Real-ear-to-coupler difference predictions as a function of age for two coupling procedures. *Journal of the American Academy of Audiology, 13*(8), 407–415.

Burkard, R. F., & Don, M. (2007). The auditory brainstem response. In R. F. Burkard, M. Don, & J. Eggermont (Eds.), *Auditory evoked potentials—Basic principles and clinical application* (pp. 229–253). Baltimore, MD: Lippincott Williams & Wilkins.

Canadian Working Group on Childhood Hearing (CWGCH; 2005). *Resource document: Early hearing and communication development* (Chapter 3, Burden of the target disorder). Retrieved June 24, 2010, from http://citeseerx.ist.psu.edu/viewdoc/download;jsessionid=BE5867220F4917A95E7E991272B8FB92?doi=10.1.1.119.5306&rep=rep1&type=pdf

Cebulla, M., Stürzebecher, E., Elberling, C., & Müller, J. (2007). New clicklike stimuli for hearing testing. *Journal of the American Academy of Audiology, 18*(9), 725–738.

Ferm, I., Lightfoot, G., & Stevens, J. (2013). Comparison of ABR response amplitude, test time, and estimation of hearing threshold using frequency specific chirp and tone pip stimuli in newborns. *International Journal of Audiology, 52(6)*, 419–423.

Fortnum, H. M. (2003). Epidemiology of permanent childhood hearing impairment. *Journal of Audiological Medicine, 1*, 155–164.

Fortnum, H. M., Summerfield, A. Q., Marshall, D. H., Davis, A. C., & Bamford, J. M. (2001). Prevalence of permanent childhood hearing impairment in the United Kingdom and implications for Universal Neonatal Hearing Screening: Questionnaire based ascertainment study. *British Medical Journal, 323*, 536–539.

Gorga, M., Neely, S., Ohlrich, B., Hoover, B., Redner, J., & Peter, J. (1997). From laboratory to clinic: A large scale study of distortion product otoacoustic emissions in ears with normal hearing and ears with hearing loss. *Ear and Hearing, 18*(6), 440–455.

Gravel, J. S., White, K., Johnson, J., Widen, J., Vohr, A., James, M., . . . Meyer, S. (2005). A multisite study to examine the efficacy of the otoacoustic emission/automated auditory brainstem response newborn hearing screening protocol: Recommendations for policy, practice, and research. *American Journal of Audiology, 14*, S217–S228.

Hyde, M. L., Riko, K., & Malizia, K. (1990). Audiometric accuracy of the click ABR in infants at risk for hearing loss. *Journal of the American Academy of Audiology, 1*(2), 59–66.

Institute of Medicine (IOM) & National Research Council (NRC), (2014). *Hearing loss and healthy aging: Workshop summary.* Washington, DC: National Academies Press.

International Classification of Functioning, Disability and Health (ICF; 2001). Geneva, World Health Organization (WHO). Retrieved from the WHO Library Database June 24, 2010, from http://www.who.int/publications/en/

Kachigan, S. K. (1991). *Multivariate statistical analysis: A conceptual introduction*. New York, NY: Radius Press.

Khoury, M., McCabe, L., & McCabe, E. (2003). Population screening in the age of genomic medicine. *New England Journal of Medicine, 348*, 50–58.

Kirby, B., Kopun, J., Tan, H., Neely, S., & Gorga, M. (2011). Do "optimal" conditions improve distortion product otoacoustic emission test performance? *Ear and Hearing, 32(2)*, 230–237.

Kral, A. (2013) Auditory critical periods: A review from system's perspective. *Neuroscience, 247*, 117–133.

McCreery, R.W., Kaminski, J., Beauchaine, K., Lenzen, N., Simms, K., & Gorga, M. P. (2015). The impact of degree of hearing loss on auditory brainstem response predictions of behavioral thresholds. *Ear and Hearing, 36*(3), 309–319.

Morton, C., & Nance, W. (2006). Newborn hearing screening—A silent revolution. *New England Journal of Medicine, 354*, 2151–2164.

National Institute on Deafness and other Communication Disorders (NIDCD; 2002). *Report and recommendations: NIDCD workshop on congenital cytomegalovirus infection and hearing loss*. Retrieved June 24, 2010, from http://www.nidcd.nih.gov/funding/programs/hb/pages/cmvwrkshop.aspx

Norton, S. J., Gorga, M. P., Widen, J. E., Folsom, R. C., Sininger, Y., Cone-Wesson, B., . . . Fletcher, K. (2000). Identification of neonatal hearing impairment: Evaluation of transient evoked otoacoustic emission, distortion product otoacoustic emission, and auditory brain stem response test performance. *Ear and Hearing, 21*(5), 508–528.

Prieve, B., Beauchaine, K., Sabo, D., Schooling, T., Culpepper, B., & Tharpe A. M. (2013). *Evidence-based systematic review of newborn hearing screening using behavioral audiometric threshold as a gold standard.* Retrieved from http://www.asha.org/uploadedFiles/EBSR-Newborn-Hearing-Screening.pdf

Prieve, B., & Fitzgerald, T. (2009). Otoacoustic emissions. In J. Katz, L. Medwetsky, R. Burkard, & L. Hood (Eds.), *Handbook of clinical audiology* (6th ed., pp. 497–528). Baltimore, MD: Lippincott Williams & Wilkins.

Sininger, Y. S. (2007). The use of auditory brainstem response in screening for hearing loss and audiometric threshold prediction. In R. F. Burkard, M. Don, & J. Eggermont (Eds.), *Auditory evoked potentials—Basic principles and clinical application* (pp. 254–274). Baltimore, MD: Lippincott Williams & Wilkins.

Sininger, Y. S., & Hyde, M. L. (2009). Auditory brainstem response in audiometric threshold prediction. In J. Katz, L. Medwetsky, R. Burkard, & L. Hood (Eds.), *Handbook of clinical audiology* (6th ed., pp. 293–321). Baltimore, MD: Lippincott Williams & Wilkins.

Swets, J. (1988). Measuring the accuracy of diagnostic systems. *Science, 240*, 1285–1293.

Tharpe, A. (2008). Unilateral and mild bilateral hearing loss in children: Past and current perspectives. *Trends in Amplification, 12*, 7–15.

U.K. National Screening Committee. (2009). *Criteria for appraising the viability, effectiveness and appropriateness of a screening programme* (updated June 2009). Retrieved June 24, 2010, from http://www.screening.nhs.uk/criteria

Wilson, J. M. G., & Jungner, G. (1968). *Principles and practice of screening for disease.* Geneva: World Health Organization. Public Health Paper # 34. Retrieved June 24, 2010, from http://whqlibdoc.who.int/php/WHO_PHP_34.pdf

APPENDIX 15–A

Test Outcomes and Performance Measures

For any individual subject, the disorder must be either *present (D+)* or *absent (D–)* and any binary test for presence of the disorder will be either *positive (T+)* (i.e., Refer or Fail) or *negative (T–)* (i.e., Pass), on the basis of some underlying decision variable and a chosen criterion value. The four possible combinations of truth and test result are presented in a specific 2 × 2 table format that is shown below. The probability of each combination can be expressed in terms of the test sensitivity (se), test specificity (sp), and the prevalence (population probability) of the disorder (p). For each core cell, the probability of each cell event is the joint probability of its disease state and test result, which equals the probability of the disease state times the conditional probability of the test result given that disease state. This is usually expressed as *P(T & D) = P(D)*P(T | D)*. For example, for the cell (D+, T+), the P(D+) is the prevalence, p, and P(T+ | D+) is the test sensitivity, so the cell probability is p*se:

	D+	D–	sum
T+	p*se	(1–p)*(1–sp)	P(Refer)
T–	p*(1–se)	(1–p)*sp	P(Pass)
sum	p	1–p	1

Sensitivity se = P(T+ | D+)

Specificity sp = P(T– | D–)

Positive Predictive Value (PPV) =
P(D+ | T+) = p*se / [p*se + (1–p)*(1–sp)]

Negative Predictive Value (NPV) =
P(D– | T–) = (1–p)*sp / [(1–p)*sp + p*(1–se)]

Likelihood Ratio Positive (LR+) =
P(T+ | D+) / P(T+ | D–) = se / (1–sp)

Likehood Ratio Negative (LR–) =
P(T– | D+) / P(T– | D–) = (1–se) / sp

From a hypothetical study comparing the results of a screening protocol (AABR in at-risk babies and AOAE with Refers to AABR in nil-risk babies) with a (hypothetical) "gold standard" test in a sample of 10,000 babies, the expected cell counts for a prevalence of two per thousand, a presumed (protocol) sensitivity of 0.97 and a specificity of 0.99 (i.e., 1% net Refers to diagnostics), for example, are (rounded to the nearest integer):

	D+	D–	sum
T+	19	100	119
T–	1	9,880	9,881
sum	20	9,980	10,000

These values would yield the following estimates for key performance parameters:

Positive Predictive Value (PPV) = P(D+ | T+) = 19 / 119 = 0.16 or 16% (about one in six are D+).

Negative Predictive Value (NPV) = P(D– | T–) = 9880/9881 = 0.9999 or 99.99% (almost certainly D–).

Likelihood Ratio Positive (LR+) = P(T+ | D+) / P(T+ | D–) = se / (1–sp) = 0.97 / 0.01 = 97

Likehood Ratio Negative (LR–) = P(T– | D+) / P(T– | D–) = (1–se) / sp = 0.03 / 0.99 = 0.03

Although these parameters reflect very good screening test performance, the fact remains that we do not really know the sensitivity of our screening tests. To re-iterate, we ***do*** know that a broad-band transient stimulus for AABR will yield a detectable response if ***any*** frequency in the range from about 1 kHz to at least 4 kHz has normal or near-normal hearing sensitivity. So it is not just that ABR will miss frequency-specific hearing losses, *it will miss all hearing losses with frequency-specific near-normality*, which includes all frequency-specific hearing losses and many more possible configurations! This author, for one, would be a lot more comfortable with well-validated electrophysiologic screening devices that tested several frequencies, such as by ASSR or multifrequency AABR. Even AABR just with 1 kHz and 4 kHz chirps, for example, could be developed. It remains to be seen if this happens any time soon, the problem being that unless and until there is better evidence of the epidemiology of both frequency-specific hearing loss and frequency-specific hearing normality, there is limited commercial incentive for more sensitive screening technologies.

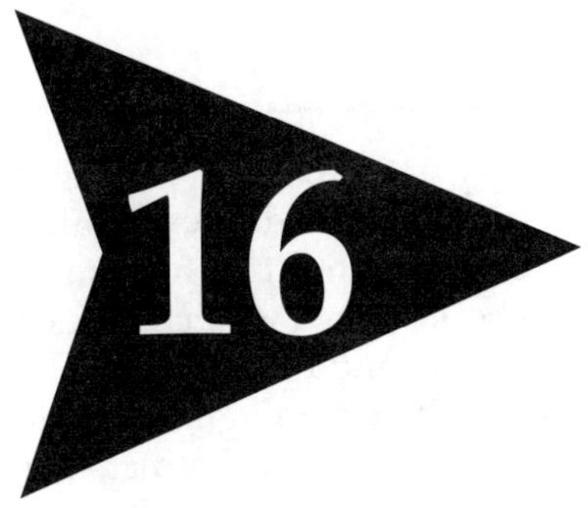

Newborn Hearing Screening Program Evaluation and Quality

Martyn Hyde

Introduction

This chapter follows on from the introductory overview of screening principles and methods in Chapter 15. Here, we look at concepts and techniques that are important in order to answer two fundamental questions: Is our screening program doing a good job? And, how do we make it even better? Here, when the term *newborn hearing screening* (NBHS) is used, it refers to universal newborn hearing screening (UNHS) within the context of an early hearing detection and intervention (EHDI) program.

Three Things Matter Most: Quality, Quality, and Quality

The Need for Excellence

It is an uncomfortable truth, perhaps verging on minor heresy, that if one is going to undertake universal NBHS, it had better be done very well or one should probably stick to targeted screening of newborns at risk, for all its limitations. There are particular pressures for excellence for NBHS. The first is that to justify its existence, systematic population screening for permanent hearing loss (PHL) must do substantially better than some alternative, baseline state. Several decades ago, the baseline state was no screening at all, but now there is no question that the only remotely acceptable alternative to NBHS is targeted screening of neonates and young infants at high risk of hearing loss, coupled with public education, and case-finding from well-informed primary care physicians. Although conventional wisdom is that only 50% of babies with congenital loss will be found by targeted screening, there is much variation in the quality of risk identification and the real figure may be substantially higher. The root objection, of course, is a perceived lack of fairness of such an approach.

The second pressure for excellence in UNBHS is that the point of screening is not just to screen but to enable hearing loss confirmation, diagnosis, and delivery of effective interventions for hearing and communication development. EHDI involves serial and parallel clinical procedures joined by linkages that promote effective movement of babies along the care pathway without dropout or other sources of loss. In any serial process, the overall performance of the pathway is no better than that of the worst-performing step and equals the product of the performance values (such as in percentage-success terms) of each serial step. Deficiencies cumulate rapidly; for example, think about a five-step process with 90% success at each step and what is 0.9 to the third, fourth, fifth power? In short, 90% success for a crucial procedural step such as screening is just not good enough for EHDI programs. Even 95% is really not that good when raised to the fifth power. And, how many steps are there in just the screening process? These include (a) become aware the baby was even born, (b) access the baby in a timely manner, (c) successfully screen the baby, (d) link the baby who fails to a second-stage screen, (e) do the second screen successfully, and (f) link the baby who fails again to a detailed audiologic assessment. There are more steps or opportunities for shortfall than maybe one first thought.

Given a congenital prevalence of hearing loss of about 2/1,000 live births in developed countries, one way to look at it is that if just one baby with PHL fails to receive the benefit of being identified early, then for starters, the screening effort for the 500 babies that on average it took to yield that one detected baby was largely wasted. The real cost to the child, family, and society is, of course, much greater.

The third pressure for excellence arises because EHDI is inherently about time and age; it is all about the differences in age at detection, confirmation, and intervention timelines with and without NBHS. For example, if it were to take 6 months to get a successful screening and 6 more months to confirm and diagnose a hearing loss, how much of the projected benefit of NBHS would actually be realized for that individual, relative to the age at diagnosis without screening of an identical individual? Thus, it is not enough simply to be screened, it must have been done in a timely manner.

The fourth pressure is that, as explained in Chapter 15 of this text, population screening causes costs, even minor harms, to all caregivers of newborns who are screened because they did not (even today) explicitly ask for the screening. It is something that society offers. There are several other pressures as well, but the idea is pretty clear by now.

What this all means is that, at least for the screening component of EHDI that is relevant here, we must quantify screening performance in a way that is valid, comprehensive, and incisive, and that such evaluation must lead to effective steps toward elimination or at least reduction of overall screening performance deficiencies. Not only that, but it is not good enough to initiate this endeavor once a year. There are so many challenges to achieving near-perfect performance that it has to be a continuous effort at improvement.

The importance of a subprogram for improvement of quality as a component of any EHDI program cannot be overstated. How well the program is working and whether it can be done more effectively and efficiently are *the* absolutely fundamental questions. They are certainly not new questions, but their current prominence has been driven by ballooning health care costs as well as the evidence-based, family-centered care revolutions. Over the years, it has also become painfully clear that many health care and social service initiatives were, and even might continue to be, poorly planned and operated as well as largely ineffective, nontransparent, and unaccountable. New programs will no longer get away with this—the microscope is ready and the light is on. Any self-respecting funding agency today would require some kind of evaluation and improvement plan. Few programs for which questions about quality cannot be answered will have much prospect of long-term survival, and opportunity cost (could we spend this money better doing something else?) is no longer an arcane economic construct. The overarching message here is that it is one thing to start an EHDI program and quite another for it to survive and flourish. Constant attention to evaluation and quality improvement is not only appropriate ethically, clinically, and socioeconomically, it is a program survival mechanism as well as *due diligence*.

What Is Quality, Exactly?

Quality is a construct that is used to express goodness, merit, worth, value (nonmonetary) or utility, value for money, "fitness for purpose," fulfilment of provider and consumer expectations, freedom from deficiencies, and so on. The obvious issues with quality are that it is subjective, fluid, and multifaceted. How it is defined can depend on whom you ask, what day it is, and what that person had for breakfast. To get anywhere, we need to do much better than that. Given that evaluating and improving quality are so important, we had better understand and agree on what we really mean by quality and choose a terminology with which to discuss it efficiently and without misunderstanding. This is the establishment of a "conceptual framework." Then, we can examine how best to measure and improve it. Here, this will be done from a standpoint of first principles of metrics as opposed to by reviewing available systems and software applications for NBHS program performance analysis. The main goals are to stimulate reflection and examine some challenges and possible advances. This chapter is not about what is done or available, so much as about what might make sense if you started from scratch with a blank slate.

Well, not really a blank slate—NBHS is a public health activity. Concepts, methodology, and the lexicon from the large field of health care quality management are appropriate here. Quality is a construct that has multiple facets (qualities). Generally, a thing might be said to be of high quality if it fulfils the needs and expectations of service recipients, but that is too simplistic. What if there are associated hazards or harms? What if perceived needs are ill-informed, irrational, or even merely different across recipients? What if the recipient is a family unit with internally conflicting needs, preferences, or values? What if the services are far more costly than they need be, and what if the access to service or the extent of need fulfilment differs substantially across recipient subgroups, geographically, culturally, ethnically, socioeconomically, and so on? These considerations help us to identify common components or dimensions of quality. But, this particular wheel has already been invented.

Avedis Donabedian was preeminent in the field of health care evaluation and quality measurement from the late 1960s through to the early 2000s. Of his many contributions, two will be outlined here: his analysis of care quality and his conceptual model of a health service program. His seminal work on defining and measuring quality is readily available and highly instructive (Donabedian, 1966). For those who prefer the abbreviated version, see Donabedian (1988). He defined seven "pillars of quality" that are shown in Table 16–1A, in his original wording. Each one of these "dimensions" of quality is itself a major area of inquiry, and some of these will be considered shortly. Much of Chapter 15 in this book has to do with measurement of the *efficacy* of NBHS, so it will not be considered further here.

As might be expected, over the years there have been many variations and much evolution of Donabedian's constructs and associated lists. For example, leading from a major publication by the U.S. Institute of Medicine (2001) on quality deficiencies in health care and recommendations to address this "quality chasm" in the United States, Berwick (2002) focused on six key dimensions of care quality that are listed in Table 16–1B. You can see that effectiveness, efficiency, and equity made it unchanged through the years, which is a testament to their underlying importance and relative purity as constructs.

Note that the Donabedian list is broad in scope, particularly in its inclusion of legitimacy, which engages the extremely challenging areas of cultural and social norms, mores, values, and behaviors. These areas are highly complex and diverse, intrinsically multivariate, even idiosyncratic and fractious in nature. Moreover, legitimacy is fickle, time-variant, and prone to sociopolitical manipulation. To some extent, the same might be

Table 16–1. Dimensions of Care Quality as Formulated by Donabedian (1988) and Berwick (2002)

A. According to Donabedian (1988)	
Efficacy	The ability of care, at its best, to improve health
Effectiveness	The degree to which attainable health improvements are realized
Efficiency	The ability to obtain the greatest health improvements at the lowest cost
Acceptability	Conformity to patient preferences regarding accessibility, the patient-practitioner relation, the amenities, the effects of care, and the cost of care
Optimality	The most advantageous balancing of costs and benefits
Legitimacy	Conformity to social preferences concerning all of the above
Equity	Fairness in the distribution of care and its effects on health

B. According to Berwick (2002)
Safety
Effectiveness
Patient-centeredness
Timeliness
Efficiency
Equity

said about acceptability, which has several highly subjective components mixed with some more quantifiable aspects such as effects and costs of care.

Donabedian took the interesting step of including both efficacy and effectiveness as key dimensions of quality. Effectiveness is derived from efficacy and upper-bounded by it. Basically, it is efficacy filtered through or degraded by the messy realities of human behavior and natural variation, both in service delivery and in recipient response to services. An advantage of including efficacy as a pillar is the explicitness and prominence it gives to what is possible and its relationship to what is actually achieved in field practice. For example, there is not much point in getting upset about limited effectiveness as reflected by an otoacoustic emission (OAE) screening refer rate of, say, 15%, if the babies are screened within 4 hours of birth, at which point two thirds of them could have substantial ear canal and middle ear fluid or debris. That issue is really best viewed as a problem of efficacy limitation, if you accept that the increase in OAE refer rates shortly after birth is a well-known and predictable phenomenon. Berwick, in contrast, focused exclusively on the performance actually achieved, namely, effectiveness, presumably incorporating knowledge of efficacy into evaluation of observed levels of effectiveness.

Overall, Berwick's list is more parsimonious and conceptually more straightforward than the Donabedian list, though its dimensions are far from simple in an absolute sense. Over the last decade, safety has come to the fore as a distinct, high-priority dimension of quality, whereas it was implicit in several other dimensions in the Donabedian list. Safety clearly reflects the longstanding principle of "first, do no harm." It also has the advantage of often being relatively easy to measure and improve. In the context of NBHS, which is an innocuous and noninvasive procedure, we do not dwell on safety. We have a choice to view family anxiety generated by false-positive screening failure as a safety issue, but that is a stretch and it makes more sense to consider false positives as a source of "harms" in the sense of negative benefit rather than a physical or mental hazard.

Patient-centeredness has also emerged as a distinct dimension that, like "evidence-based," has acquired the status of a totem, mantra, or *sine qua non*. What it often reflects is the rather obvious principle that if you are going to do things to people that depend for success on their understanding and cooperation, whether it is taking a pill or attending a follow-up appointment, it will work better if they or their peers are involved in determination of what you intend to do. It is often remarkable how the perceptions and priorities of the care recipient differ from those of even highly informed providers of care, let alone program administrators or sponsors. This is not rocket science, and the continued explicit emphasis on "family centeredness" is perhaps a lingering relic from overturning a longstanding, but hopefully near-extinct, medical tradition of authoritarianism.

Berwick has also broken out timeliness as a dimension of quality, which is understandable in the broad context of public access to care and concerns about waiting lists but is not really necessary in the specific context of NBHS and EHDI, for which timeliness is already an obvious and explicit part of the program purpose (e.g., *newborn* screening, *early* identification). From here on, we focus on what are often considered to be the deep dimensions of quality, namely, effectiveness, equity, and efficiency, with only passing comments on others in the Donabedian and Berwick lists.

Effectiveness

Effectiveness is unquestionably the most important single dimension of quality, in the sense that without some acceptable level of effectiveness (i.e., achievement of what was intended) everything else is moot. If the test or program of interest does not work well in real-world practice for most of its recipients, why do it? Especially in the context of screening programs that address disorders that are not commonplace, the balance of benefits and harms is likely to be unfavorable. From the *opportunity cost* perspective alone, resources expended on ineffective activity become obvious costs of not being available to employ them for better effect doing something else more useful. Activities with limited effectiveness are rarely justifiable unless benefit per affected individual is huge, which typically is considered plausible only if the target disorder for screening is perceived to be life-threatening or to confer massive morbidity and the resulting interventions are curative. Neither of these is true for NBHS. Opportunity cost discussions are sometimes unproductive because they have a tendency to awaken partisan opinion-venting, best quashed by appeals to focus on evidence-based process. The more productive path is usually on how to raise effectiveness to a defensible level.

Clearly, the effectiveness of a screening program must be quantified in terms such as the number and proportion of babies screened successfully. Also, because timeliness is crucial to early identification of hearing loss, not only the fact of being screened but the baby's age at successful screening is highly relevant. Furthermore, screening is ineffective, perhaps even pointless, unless it leads to prompt audiologic assessment of those babies who fail (refer), so it seems reasonable to include the linkage to diagnostics within the realm of screening effectiveness. One could include that linkage in the evaluation of effectiveness of diagnostic assessment, or perhaps treat the linkage as a separate, infrastructural tracking function that is separate from actual screening or diagnostics. But, stepping back from practices that are historical or specific to individual systems of care, the real job of a screening program is to deliver families to diagnostic audiologic assessment with screening test results in their hands and engagement in their heads. If any of these three pieces is missing, the value of the screening test is put in question. This viewpoint reflects the experience that the content and style of interactions between screening personnel and family members can affect whether and when families comply with follow-up recommendations, and even, to some extent, how they will respond to the results of diagnostic assessment. Another point is that separation of the establishment of need for detailed assessment and the actual delivery of that assessment makes no sense in terms of system integrity and transparency. To put it another way, the need for tight, longitudinal integration of critical EHDI phases is a "no-brainer" that really should be reflected in evaluations of program effectiveness. For further insight into this problem and some activities aimed at improving program quality in this regard, see the report by Russ, Hanna, DesGeorges, and Forsman (2010).

Equity

Equity belongs next to effectiveness in importance because it is so intimately connected to it. Equity relates to equality, uniformity, and homogeneity in the distribution of effectiveness over the entire target population. The original concept of equity was often described as having to do with *fairness* or *justice* in the distribution of the benefits of care. Are there identifiable groups for whom access to care or the improvement effected by the care is radically poorer than for others? Groups may be characterized in terms of care access barriers and facilitators, which may be factors intrinsic to the care recipient, or to the screening program, or to both.

Groups might be identified in many ways—by location, wealth, education, ethnicity, culture, behavior, attitude, and so on. Obvious groups that are frequently at risk of health care barriers are those who live in rural or remote communities, those with limited economic resources, those with little education, and those who otherwise tend to be socially disadvantaged or alienated. Of course, there are often interactions among these characteristics. Even apparently simple questions about equity can be challenging. For example, typically it will cost much more to provide accessible, expert services to persons in remote communities. Do you take the view that everyone is entitled to the service and the costs fall where they may? Or do you take the view that a given amount of resource is allocated in principle to each care recipient and whatever can be done within that limit is what is equitable? A related issue is the extent to which additional resources are expended in the interest of the child when the circumstances or behavior of the caregiver are not likely to lead to successful screening and follow-up linkage.

Efficiency

Efficiency seems simple conceptually but in practice can be more difficult than expected to quantify in a valid and accurate way. One approach is to monetarize all identifiable resources required to implement the screening program, decide on measures and units of effectiveness, and express the results as amount of effectiveness per unit cost (e.g., successful screens per $1,000) or, more commonly, dollar cost per successful screen. This is *cost-effectiveness analysis* (CEA). Some would argue that the measure should be chosen such that high efficiency is reflected in a bigger number, but lowering the production cost per unit of effectiveness seems to be entrenched as a measure of efficiency. Regardless of how the CE is expressed, the reader should view published cost and cost-effectiveness data and claims both skeptically and critically. Economic analyses published in clinical journals often do not achieve a high methodologic standard. It is not unusual for fixed costs to be underestimated or overlooked entirely, cross-program synergies to be discounted, infrastructural or other hidden costs to be ignored, and complex nonlinearities of input-output relationships overlooked (such as arise with remuneration schemes other than flat fee-for-service), quite apart from issues of capital equipment lifetime, depreciation, amortization, and changes in the value of money over time (discounting).

There are many ways to do screening program CEA other than simply counting screens per unit resource cost. For one thing, do all screens have the same value? Just counting screens makes no distinction between high-risk and low-risk screens, yet the former have on average about 10 times the expected yield of true PHL cases. It also makes no distinction between early and late screens, or between screens that have low or high probabilities of refers leading to timely follow-up. One might think intuitively that the higher the age at screening, the lower that screen should be valued; whereas the higher the risk and the higher the follow-up, the higher is the value. The underlying question here is what is legitimate to be incorporated as a component of effectiveness. For example, if Programs A and B both have the same overall screening costs and screen 90% of their target populations but A has a 90% refer follow-up rate and B has a 70% rate, do the two programs have different cost-effectiveness? Even more simply, if A and B have the same costs and numbers of babies screened, but A screens 95% of the target population and B screens only 85%, do they have the same CE?

If both costs and benefits are fully monetarized, this is cost-benefit analysis (CBA). Unfortunately, it is often extremely difficult to monetarize benefits in a valid and meaningful way, for many reasons. First, the benefit attributable directly to screening involves the advantages that accrue specifically from being screened versus other routes to hearing loss detection, such as case-finding through medical checks or parental concern. Counterintuitively, such benefits may be paradoxically smaller, the more severe the hearing loss, because infants with severe or profound losses are often more readily recognized without proactive measures such as screening, relative to those with lesser degrees of hearing loss. Second, there is enormous variation in cost-benefit across individuals because of the host of program and nonprogram variables that can affect resource expenditure (such as population density) and the overall benefit stream (such as the language environment at home). Third, some aspects of benefit are almost impossible to monetarize, such as socialization or the diversity and quality of employment opportunities. The cost-benefit relationship is especially complex if the trajectory of benefits of an early service program event flow imperfectly, longitudinally, and may or may not ramify over a lifetime depending on personal context and values, as is the case with childhood hearing loss.

For all these reasons and more, in the author's view CEA is by far the more useful tool for screening program design and evaluation directed at costs and efficiency. Although CBA can attempt to answer large questions such as, "under what conditions would universal NBHS within EHDI be likely to be a net cost saving to society?," it is less useful for decisions arising in the design, evaluation, or improvement of screening programs specifically . One reason is that the actual and expected flow of benefits accruing from screening are very difficult to observe or predict, being dependent on a whole host of performance variables and assumptions related to later steps in the EHDI care pathway. Even for the big questions, solutions to optimization problems can be unstable and strongly dependent on simplifying assumptions underlying monetarized benefits and true overall costs. However, in fairness, others might hold differing views about the utility of CBA; see, for example, Porter, Neely, and Gorga (2009).

What *Is* a Screening *Program*?

This question is not about the nuts and bolts of what make up an NBHS program. Most readers will already know that. What we are after here is another conceptual model, a generic paradigm of how to think about programs in the context of wishing to quantify, evaluate, and improve their quality. We can assume that a program is an organized matrix or network of activities that are integrated and that relate collectively to a defined goal and a set of explicit objectives. It is assumed that we are talking about population hearing screening programs on at least a moderate scale, though many of the concepts are widely applicable to almost any organized and goal-directed clinical or public health service activity or project.

We can infer some important generic attributes of screening programs from the World Health Organization's (WHO) two major sources on population screening program criteria (Andermann et al., 2008; Wilson & Jungner, 1968). But we need something more closely aligned to the measurement and improvement of quality.

The Structure-Process-Outcome (SPO) Model

We return to Donabedian, not surprising given that his analysis of healthcare quality was driven by the intent to measure and evaluate it. His Structure-Process-Outcome (SPO) model originated in the mid 1960s, and although it has been embellished, critiqued, and adapted over the years, it has endured as a leading paradigm underlying evaluation of care quality.

In the SPO model, a program is conceived as a system or entity that produces *outcomes*, which in essence are changes in the health state of care recipients. Outcomes are effects that are considered to be causally related, at least in part, to *processes*, which are actions or transactions that occur in encounters (direct or indirect) between the care recipient and program providers. In turn, these processes are enabled or actualized by contextual *structures*, which are physical or virtual objects necessary in order for the processes to occur. Structural elements include personnel, buildings, equipment, funding, supplies, and so on. So, for example, screening pass or refer results are outcomes delivered by the set of actions that comprise the process of screening, executed using a specific screening device and supplies in a specific facility. As a categorization scheme, the SPO model is helpful in thinking and talking about things such as the value of structure (such as number or locations of screening personnel) or process measures (such as number of screens performed per week) as proxies for real outcome measures (such as the proportion of all newborns who are screened). It is useful in clarifying exactly what structural elements are needed to enable the processes that are crucial to deliver the desired outcomes. It is also useful in examining, for example, whether a specific deficiency in outcome, such as missed screens before hospital discharge, is attributable to a structural element such as physical layout of a nursery or to process elements such as how each screen is carried out or how the screener is made aware of new births.

The SPO model can be applied at any level of program conceptualization. For example, an EHDI program as a whole can be thought of as a matrix of interlinked subprograms for screening, audiologic assessment, medical management, tracking, amplification, language development services, quality management, and so on. Each of these major activities can itself be viewed as a subprogram and analyzed in SPO terms. This can be taken down at least one more level, so for example, one might have a subprogram to optimize family adherence to recommendations for follow-up made by screening personnel.

Elaborations of this approach are many. For example, distinction is sometimes made among *outputs*, which are the items delivered by program processes (such as screened babies); *outcomes*, which are the effects of outputs upon recipients (such as better-informed families); and *impact*, which some define as outcomes that are directly and specifically attributable to the processes of the program. Others define impact in terms of ramifying, longer-term effects of immediate outcomes.

Program Logic Models

A related but different paradigm is called the *logic model*, a term that originated in the 1970s and has evolved into many alternative forms. At its core, logic modeling is a systematic approach, usually graphical or tabular, to identifying potential or actual causal relationships among the expenditure of resources or *inputs* to produce *activities* that in turn yield *outputs* that in turn might cause outcomes. Outcomes can be immediate, deferred, or even latent (expressed after a delay period); short-, medium-, or long-term; direct or indirect; intended or unintended; or desirable (benefits) or undesirable (harms). There might be unintended impacts that have little to do with the care recipients, such as changes in provider viewpoints and behaviors, changes in public perception and expectations, and so on. These side effects are sometimes called *collateral outcomes*. Logic models are, in essence, a way of thinking, organizing, and documenting systematically the input-output relationships of a set of defined operations or activities. They are useful in both planning and evaluation of new or modified programs. The obvious differences from the basic SPO model are the more explicit separation of structure and function in the latter and the more explicit elaboration of inputs and outputs in typical logic models.

One of the criticisms that might be made of the SPO model is that it is not explicit in its treatment of the care recipient as a transactional partner in the production of desired outcomes. It appears at first sight to treat the recipient as a passive object "operated upon" by the program of care. On reflection, that passive flavor is also apparent in the author's use of the term *care recipient* (so much for well-intended jargon, in an effort to avoid the overtones of *patient*, the commercialism of *client*, and the clumsiness of *affected family*). In fact, the characteristics of the recipient are woven into Donabedian's concept of the dimensions of care quality. The prevailing viewpoint is basically that the individual who is seeking or receiving health services ought to be an active, even dominant, partner in a transactional exchange of information that is geared specifically to their perceived needs, values, and preferences. This move away from authoritarian models of care inevitably raises the challenge of idiosyncratic and ill-informed recipient preferences and decisions, and hence, the prominence of "*informed* choice" in modern health services jargon.

One way in which care recipients can be given more obvious weight in conceptual models is to include recipient-centeredness (a.k.a. patient-, client-, family-, or child-centeredness) as an explicit dimension or facet of program quality, as did Berwick. Another way is to view the family, for example, as a program resource that has crucial characteristics that can affect outcomes. Family needs and capacities can be viewed as predisposing factors in response to program actions, as can features of the recipient or the context of care that are barriers or facilitators of the desired outcomes. These are often identified as components of program logic models.

Program Goals

Any program worthy of the name should have a clearly defined (documented) goal, and such goals are worth some careful crafting. Goal statements are usually large in scope and somewhat fuzzy, but they should not be transparently pie-in-the-sky. They are important in that usually they should reflect at least implicitly a compelling need for betterment of the *status quo*, offering the prospect of a major net benefit to a few individuals or at least a modest net benefit to many. A well-stated goal cannot only attract interest and sponsorship but also can help to bind program personnel who might come from various backgrounds and motivations together into a common overall rationale for their particular roles and activities. In large programs, it is not uncommon for those working on various parts of the program to lose sight of their overall purpose and as a result, to diverge into variable, idiosyncratic, and even misguided beliefs and practices. Goals should be uplifting, evocative, insightful, and frequently reinforced, in order to enhance and sustain commonality of understanding, motivation, and purpose among program personnel as well as the recipient community and program sponsors.

Core Values

The goal statement says in big picture terms what it is that the program is intended to achieve. Goal statements sometimes also reflect the "core values" of the program. For example, it might be stated that all components of a program will be designed and delivered in a manner that is evidence driven and family centered. Family-centered practice, for example, includes informed consent, informed choices, confidentiality of personal information, and respect for care recipient decision-making autonomy as key attributes. *Autonomy* basically is the right of a family to determine the services they wish to receive as well as the desired outcomes of those services, according to the dictates of their individual values and culture. What is critical is that the family be given full, timely, unbiased information about the implications of test results and the options available to them, in order to be in a position to exercise their autonomy in a meaningful way. Moreover, the information must be presented in a manner that is nondirective, comprehensible and acceptable, bearing in mind that overly compulsory, incomprehensible, or unacceptable information is actually no information at all. It is the service recipients' perception and understanding that matter, as distinct from those of service providers.

Appeal to an evidence-based approach can be a very useful tool. Not only is it appropriate that all pertinent evidence be brought to bear on program design, but the up-front explicitness can be helpful in cutting through the sea of personal opinion that can complicate and delay attempts to improve the current state of affairs in almost any field. Although the term *evidence-based* is vastly overused and abused, even the act of requiring a literature search with a declared search strategy, source materials, and selection strategy, followed by summarizing a few papers, can raise the level of discussion way beyond that of hurling mere opinions. On the other hand, family centeredness, while of great significance as a core value, is beyond the scope of this chapter. Suffice it to say that in the context of NBHS programs, contention between child-centered and family-centered approaches to service delivery is an area of challenge that seems resistant even to discussion, let alone to development of clear-sighted policy and procedure.

Objectives and Program Evaluability

Because program goals and core values are usually broad and thereby somewhat fuzzy, it is usually difficult or impossible to evaluate their achievement in quantitative terms. Therefore, the goals must be translated into a set of specific and measurable objectives. These objectives must be defined for the EHDI program as a whole as well as for every major subprogram. The importance of clear objectives is widely accepted and specifically stated in the expanded WHO guidelines.

The preferred objective is a concrete, explicit, and precise statement of a desired attribute of program structure, process, or outcome. A given objective can relate to an entire EHDI program, care pathway, subprogram, or individual S, P, or O element therein. *An objective is of little value if its achievement cannot be measured.* Collectively, the degree to which the set of objectives are measurable is what is meant by the term *evaluability*, which is the ability of a program to be evaluated in a valid, reliable, and useful manner.

Program Evaluation (PE)

The CDC Approach to Program Evaluation

In its self-study guide to program evaluation (available at http://www.CDC.gov/eval/guide), the Centers for Disease Control and Prevention (CDC, 2011) defines a program very broadly, as "any set of organized activities supported by a set of resources to achieve a specific and intended result." It defines PE as "the systematic collection of information about the activities, characteristics, and outcomes of programs to make judgments about the program, improve program effectiveness, and/or inform decisions about future program development." Although there are many alternative definitions of PE, commonalities among them reveal that it is *systematic* (as opposed to casual, haphazard, informal, or unstructured), that it involves measurement and data collection, that it relates to achievement of defined objectives and that it is oriented toward answering questions, assisting decisions, and improving program quality. Beyond that, it is neither necessary nor especially helpful to focus on coming up with an all-encompassing, one-size-fits-all definition. There is no such thing. The underlying purpose and operational context of any specific PE activity will govern its objectives, scope, methods, and impact. The most appropriate evaluation targets and approaches will differ in their context and purpose as a program evolves. What is most important is to define clearly and concisely what is being evaluated, why, how, and with what results and implications.

The CDC Framework for Program Evaluation (CDC, 1999) is influential and has been widely adopted. It is a cycle, the components of which can be summarized as (in this author's words) engage, describe, focus, collect, infer, justify, and use. In a nutshell, you engage collaboratively with all the program's major stakeholders, who may have different perceptions of what the program is for and what matters most. You describe, characterize, and document the program so that everyone agrees how it is supposed to work; you focus the evaluation activity on agreed targets, questions, or concerns, with a specific evaluative approach and method; you collect the required data; you make inferences and draw conclusions; you disseminate, explain, and justify your inferences to the key recipients; finally, you use the inferences to define further actions such as policy or procedure changes oriented toward quality improvement.

The evaluation should satisfy four key standards: utility (need, relevance, timeliness); feasibility (practicality, resources, expertise); propriety (provider and participant rights and welfare); and accuracy (validity, reliability). In essence, your evaluation must be useful, practicable, judicious, and accurate. Most good evaluations have a reflexive, self-evaluative component to assess the extent to which these standards of conduct have been met.

There are many other models of PE with associated terminology. For example, Kahan (2008) defined a process that could be summarized as clarify (the program), engage, resource, design, methods, plan (of the evaluation), collect, analyze. Darabi (2002) defined "Program Analysis and Evaluability Assessment" as the first steps in PE.

As the name suggests, evaluability assessment is a process that seeks to determine the extent to which a program is actually able to be evaluated, both in absolute terms and in relation to the feasible evaluation budget and available expertise. For example, are the program goals and objectives defined adequately? Are they agreed on and understood by all key stakeholders? If there are no well-defined, valid, quantitative, and measurable indicator variables for a specific program process, output, or outcome of interest, evaluation options are limited, perhaps severely. Even if the indicator exists and satisfies these desirable qualities in principle, has it been recorded with sufficient consistency (versus misunderstanding of the measure), completeness (versus missing data), and fidelity (versus data entry errors, carelessness, lack of timeliness, etc.). Is it necessary to enhance the measure itself or the related program processes in order to collect what is needed for the evaluation? To what extent can the available data be expected to be stable? Are the inferences to be drawn likely to be valid over time, space, structural changes, political variability, and so on? Are the current program processes sufficiently well defined and controlled that what it is that is causing the measured values to be what they are is likely to be identifiable? Are procedural protocols being followed, or are the processes actually occurring on the ground aberrant or idiosyncratic? Or is that issue itself a target of the evaluation? What, if any, partitions, subgroups, or heterogeneities of the dataset can be defined up front? Are there suspected sources of program performance limitation that could be defined in advance of data inspection? The reader will see that even just the evaluability assessment aspect of PE is far from trivial.

Implementation

One of the most important initial aspects of any program evaluation is to investigate the actual structure and process elements that are in place. Although a great deal of thought and planning might have gone into the design of a program, the details of how it is actually being executed on the ground are, in the author's experience, often surprising, sometimes ingenious, but more frequently alarming and clearly flawed. This has to be viewed as a deficiency of the initial implementation process control, but the point is that serving scrambled egg when an omelette was ordered is a fairly obvious candidate area for program improvement efforts.

One of the factors that can result in diverse implementation is the contention between central control and regional or local adaptation of structures and processes. On the one hand, in many jurisdictions there is a political *zeitgeist* that the local people on the ground know best how to do what needs to be done. Although this might be true in many endeavors, it is not the case for EHDI, for which centralized control is a profound force for quality. This is not to say that local adaptations are a bad idea—far from it. The challenge is to navigate the fine line between adaptation and transformation, or between order with flexibility on the one hand and something close to chaos on the other. Some of the possible results of idiosyncratic local adaptation are endless reinvention of the wheel, lack of program-wide sharing of solutions and lessons learned, as well as limited evaluability because of fragmentation of structures and processes.

Attribution

Suppose an evaluation has been conducted and certain deficiencies in program performance have been identified. After analysis of potential causes and possibly some quick trials of potential solutions, a program change is identified and implemented, perhaps in a local or exploratory manner, perhaps program-wide depending on the level of confidence about potential improvement. Now suppose that the postchange data indicate clear improvement that appears to be sustained. The big question is the following: What caused the improvement? There are several possibilities. First, the deficit in performance was actually caused by the identified S or P defect, and the change as implemented was genuinely remedial. Second, the deficit in performance was not caused by the identified S or P "defect" but by something else entirely, but there was a performance improvement that was actually a result merely of the fact that some process change (any process change could have worked) had been implemented and the simple fact of change-triggered attention or merely to being observed was what caused the performance improvement. The reader who is not aware of it might enjoy reading about the "Hawthorne" effect.

One aspect of attribution analysis, sometimes referred to as assessment of "change effect validity" or "causal analysis," is to watch carefully for reduction over time of the performance improvement, perhaps with return to the prechange levels. Another aspect is what might be called "360-degree effect review"—that is, collective brainstorming by all concerned of what actually happened during the change process, focusing specifically on possible alternative causes of the observed improvement. A side effect of such analysis can be generation of alternative strategies for beneficial change.

Continuous Quality Improvement

The reader has probably encountered several terms involving the word *quality* that relate to evaluation of program performance. These include quality assurance (QA), quality control (QC), quality management (QM), total quality management (TQM), quality improvement (QI), and continuous quality improvement (CQI). These terms will be briefly explained. A caveat is that there are differing views in the evaluation community on what some of these activities are and how they relate.

Quality assurance (QA) is a term that is less widely used in the health care field today than in the past. QA is inherently continuous, its goal being to assure recipients of program compliance with defined, usually static performance standards. It is retrospective and reactive. Its main orientation is toward avoiding, detecting, and fixing process or procedure deficiencies. It tends to use static standards for outcomes as a reference point against which to judge performance. Its investigative focus is usually the service provider As such, it is sometimes viewed as inherently negative, a sort of hunt for the responsible offender or even for "bad apples."

Quality control (QC) is a widely practiced procedure in the context of industrial production processes. Usually, it involves monitoring output, searching for deficiencies, and weeding out defective items. QC has a well-developed set of statistical and graphical tools that emphasize analysis of performance data as a time series, such as process control charts. The tools and concepts of QC, especially control charts and related statistical techniques, are relevant to screening program evaluation. For example, in the analysis of performance of hearing screening personnel, monthly refer rate data from a given screener can be viewed as a time-series process that can be examined for variation, discontinuity, and trend using control chart methods, among others.

Quality management (QM) is an umbrella term for a management process and style that may include planning for, assurance of, control of, or improvement of program quality. It is usually outcome oriented. QM encompasses all activities that have consistency and excellence of program performance as their focus, so it embraces not only measuring quality but structure and process design, planning, and implementation to deliver it as well as direct projects to improve it.

Total quality management (TQM), as its name suggests, is an all-encompassing, holistic approach to QM that views improvement in all aspects of an organization, program, or system as a continuous, transformative, core process. In principle, it engages everyone and includes everything (structures, processes, outcomes, contextual and infrastructural factors, attitudes, beliefs, behaviors, and so on) associated with the program.

Quality improvement (QI) is the term and activity that some believe should replace QA in the health care context. QI refers to any formal process that measures performance and systematically addresses its improvement. The approach is both retrospective and prospective. It specifically avoids assigning blame, and it usually involves system design or redesign that builds in proactive steps to prevent errors or omissions. It may make use of standards but treats them as a baseline for improvement, usually in a pre- to postmeasurement context of process change.

Continuous quality improvement (CQI) is a proactive, iterative, unending search for performance improvement. It is neither an action nor an event, nor is it simply a repetitive process or even a continuing series of QI projects. At its best, CQI is transformative. It is a participatory culture of engagement and empowerment. It involves all persons connected with a program, be they management, service providers, recipients of care, office workers, or janitors. *Everyone* is viewed as a potential source of insight and possible process improvement. It is positive in nature, with the implicit position that everyone is trying to do the best job they can, wants to do a better job, and if they look carefully at what they and others are doing, they will usually find a way. It is not naïve in that position, it is a deliberately constructive choice of viewpoint. It is a blend of "cup half full, not half empty," "treat others as you would wish to be treated," "carrots are more effective than sticks," "we're all in this boat together," "a journey of a thousand miles starts with a single step," "the Lorenz butterfly effect," and so on.

CQI had its origins in the work of Shewhart on statistical process control, at Bell Laboratories in the 1930s. As developed and applied by W.E. Deming, CQI philosophy and methods are considered by many to be highly instrumental in molding the highly successful postwar transformation of Japan's industrial processes.

A common paradigm for CQI is a four-step cycle (PDSA: plan-do-study-act or PDCA: plan-do-check-act) known as the "Deming (or Shewhart) wheel/cycle/circle" that is applied iteratively until the desired goal is achieved. In the author's experience, explanations of PDSA are variable and not always helpful, so Table 16–2A is the author's wording.

PDSA is only one of several popular paradigms applied to CQI, each with its own particular focus, style, procedures, and toolbox. But inevitably, there are common themes and components, and PDSA could be viewed as a basic CQI "macro" that, one way or another, is woven implicitly or explicitly into most CQI approaches. Some of the alternative paradigms are listed in Table 16–2B. The reader is urged to search on all of these terms, because each has a distinct flavor or might feel uniquely suitable for any specific quality improvement venture. Kaizen, for example, has "standardize" as an initial phase. This is very attractive because one of the truisms about program evaluation is that you cannot evaluate anything that you cannot describe, or anything that is basically a basket of different things.

One of the things that the reader might find on digging into CQI paradigms is that in service industries such as health care, the themes of human behavior and communication deficiency come up frequently as methodologic foci or as targets of CQI efforts. Individualism is deeply rooted in Western cultures, yet a key to success in the program context is consistency of processes, in order to operate continually in line with the best evidence, to guarantee minimum service standards and to promote equity of care. Left to themselves, humans will slowly but surely diverge in their beliefs and behaviors. We also forget things, we like to be respected, we have our idiosyncratic needs and fears, and almost everyone thinks his or her own opinion is "right." It is like the old saying, "90% of drivers think they are above average." Every one of these facets of human nature is a rich source of CQI projects in EHDI. Another truism in human service systems CQI is that if you want to improve process quality, look hard at what providers or recipients of care are actually believing and doing, not what you think they are thinking and doing. See, for example, Samson and Terziovski (1999), regarding the crucial role of people-oriented process facets in industrial TQM. For further insight into the nature and history of CQI, see, for example, Radawski (1999).

Basic Tools of PE/CQI: Measures, Indicators, Benchmarks, Targets, and Standards

As noted earlier, desired program processes, outputs, and outcomes are specified by documented program objectives. Every important facet of every objective requires one or more *indicator* variables or measures, if

Table 16–2. The Plan-Do-Study-Act (PDSA) Paradigm of Continuous Quality Improvement (CQI)

A. Part A: Steps in the PDSA Cycle for CQI	
Plan:	Identify an improvement need or opportunity, gather baseline data, analyze problem causes, select and define the change to be tried, performance targets, methods, and implementation plan. The identification of need for change may involve a program evaluation project or may arise from spontaneous emergence of challenges in structure, process, or outcome.
Do:	Execute the change plan, monitor the implementation, and collect new data on performance and on various aspects of response to change.
Study:	Analyze the postchange data to determine the effects and side effects of the change and extract lessons learned.
Act:	Decide whether to implement and standardize a successful change, to modify the change strategy and continue the cycle, or to turn to another area of need and restart.
B. Part B: Alternative Paradigms for CQI	
FADE	Focus, Analyze, Develop, Evaluate
Six Sigma: DMAIC	Define, Measure, Analyze, Improve, Control (existing programs/ processes)
Six Sigma: DMADV	Define, Measure, Analyze, Design, Verify (new programs/processes)
Kaizen:	Standardize, Measure, Innovate, Evaluate
Lean:	Purpose, Process, People; Value stream, Waste elimination

it is to be described and evaluated. When the focus is on processes or outcomes, the most core and influential of these indicators are sometimes called *key performance indicators* or KPIs. There is sometimes understandable confusion between an indicator and the underlying variable or *measure*, and there are various viewpoints. Sometimes the distinctions are more pedantic than substantive. In the author's view, all indicators are based, explicitly or implicitly, on one or more underlying measures. Any measure itself might be qualitative or quantitative in nature, but the measure is usually quantitative in our current context. Some indicators are the measures themselves, while other indicators are derived from their underlying measures by applying specific criteria to the values of the measure. Examples of measures that are also indicators include the proportion of families/caregivers who consent to NBHS, or the proportion of babies screened who yield a refer result. For an indicator such as the proportion of families who rate their overall satisfaction with the screening process as "satisfied" or "very satisfied," the measure is a family satisfaction rating, but the focus is on a specific value or values that in this example create a binary outcome indicator "acceptable or unacceptable" from the underlying level of satisfaction, so technically it would not be correct to refer to the original levels of satisfaction scale as the indicator.

Good KPIs are relevant, valid, specific, quantifiable, reliable, and referent to defined time periods. The best KPIs usually involve teamwork, not isolated individuals, and, furthermore, have a limited *dark side*. The dark side of a poor KPI is an unanticipated negative collateral effect of apparent improvement on the main thrust of the KPI. For example, suppose a high refer rate on initial screening was identified as a problem, and refer rate was identified as a KPI. Screeners can lower their refer rate by improving baby contact timing, calming techniques, probe insertion, electrode attachment, device operations, and retest tactics. They can also lower their refer rate by deciding more frequently that any given baby is not testable predischarge, which lowers their workload as well as running a risk of family nonattendance at a community screening visit. Furthermore, they might choose to immediately rescreen excessively, despite a protocol stipulation of a limited number of rescreens. This does not mean that lower refer rates cannot be sought or used as a KPI, but it does mean that steps must be taken to minimize obvious maladaptive behaviors.

Benchmarks are usually values of indicators that are derived from comparisons across programs that have comparable goals. They usually represent a level of performance that is indisputably high but that has been shown to be achievable in practice. Their derivation is not necessarily a formal, defined process and might not involve systematic evidence review. Benchmarks can even be opinion based or essentially pulled out of a face-valid hat. As such, it is not clear to the author how useful benchmarks really are except as a gross classifier of program performance. There is also the reservation that static benchmarks are conceptually at variance with a CQI viewpoint of the journey toward near-perfection.

Targets are values of indicators that are, or are anticipated to be, feasible to attain in the near future. Typically, and particularly for new screening programs, successive period targets can be set to improve serially and represent road marks on the way toward a standard. Insofar as targets should be set beyond current performance levels, they can be highly relevant to quality improvement, but they might also be set at or beyond benchmarks, if the latter are deemed insufficient. However, targets also can be exploited, in the obvious sense that if you want to look good you could set easily achievable targets. This is one defense of the need for valid benchmarks, because if the benchmark for something is, say, 95% achievement of a criterion on some indicator, it is difficult to argue that achieving an 85% target is a real success, except perhaps in the first year of a program.

Standards are variably defined. Some consider them interchangeable with benchmarks while others consider them to be essentially "best efforts" promises to the recipient that they will receive a certain level of service quality *now*, in quantitative or qualitative terms. For example, "Families of babies who refer on NBHS shall be offered an appointment for audiologic assessment that is within four weeks of the date of referral." Here, the outcome measure is the appointment interval, the indicator is the four week criterion, the performance benchmark might be 95% success in any one-month period, and the immediate target might be at least 90% success.

For basic information on performance indicators in NBHS, see the Joint Committee on Infant Hearing's 2007 Statement (JCIH, 2007), and for a good example of their application, see Uus and Bamford (2006). For a detailed explanation of program evaluation in public health programs, see the wealth of materials provided by the U.S. Centers for Disease Control and Prevention (CDC, 2012, available at http://www.CDC.gov/eval/framework.htm). See also the diverse materials on program evaluation and quality improvement available from the NCHAM (National Center for Hearing Assessment and Management at Utah State University), accessible at http://www.infanthearing.org/move-the-needle). For more in-depth reading, see the *Handbook of Practical Program Evaluation*, edited by Wholey, Hatry, and Newcomer (2004).

Reporting of Proportions

Before going any further, we must deal with an enduring, basic issue to do with reporting of any proportion, be it a coverage, a refer rate, a case yield, or anything else of interest. *Being told a proportion (or percentage) of anything is not useful without sample size information.* At least the numerator or the denominator of the observed proportion is required, and the latter gives the targeted caseload directly. So, for example, being told coverage was 90% is of little use, whereas being told it was 1,350 babies screened out of 1,500 consecutive live births is highly informative. Why? Mainly because knowing the denominator allows calculation of a confidence interval for the stated proportion; a small-sample *point estimate* of 90% with an *interval estimate* of, say, 80% to 99% is far less informative than, say, a large-sample interval of 88% to 92%. Of course, the best reports explicitly state both the point estimate *and* the interval estimate, but this should be a basic step that anyone would do without thinking about it. This is a rather obvious point, but the reader might be surprised at the number of reports even today that do not state confidence intervals on sample proportions, whatever the type of proportion reported and despite peer review. Yet, confidence intervals on proportions are at everyone's fingertips on the Web, such as at http://medepi.com/epitools/

Although giving at least the numerator and denominator of any proportion is always a good idea, caution might be required when actually deriving binomial CIs. For datasets that include small sample sizes (N) or values of the complementary sample proportions p or $(1 - p)$ such that $N \cdot p$ or $N \cdot (1 - p)$ is less than 30, the assumptions underlying approximations (such as the normal approximation) sometimes used to derive the confidence intervals might break down. This is not usually an issue when describing quantities such as screening coverage, for which N is usually very large (typically in the thousands) so only coverage values above about 0.95 (95%) could cause accuracy problems, but it might be an issue when analyzing screening refer rates, especially where the group size of interest can well be less than about 100 babies screened. For those interested in the challenging problem of accuracy of binomial confidence limits, the Wikipedia information on the matter is brief but quite solid and includes a discussion of various CI estimators. The author's favorite is known as the *continuity-corrected, modified Wilson score interval,* which looks complicated but is actually simple to calculate and has good statistical properties.

A related issue arises in the broader statistical analysis of multiple sample proportions, a common challenge in screening program evaluation, as later discussed. The issue arises because the error variance in an estimated proportion (such as a coverage, a refer rate, a follow-up rate, etc.) depends on the sample value of that proportion. This violates a common requirement of standard statistical analysis techniques based on normal distribution theory, such as analysis of variance (ANOVA), which is known as *homoscedasticity* or constancy of error variance. The interested reader should Google "variance stabilizing transformation binomial" for further information. Particular caution is needed when considering the commonly used *arcsine root* transformation.

Evaluation of Screening Program Effectiveness

The Real Goal of Screening

At first sight, it would appear that a screening program is intended to deliver screened babies as the primary outcome. This viewpoint is blinkered. The problem with it is that a screened baby is necessary but not sufficient to accrue any benefit from the screening. The real point of screening is not only to obtain a valid, accurate, and timely screening result but also to create an informed and engaged caregiver who will ensure at least that the baby with a refer result will move promptly to the next step in the screening or (diagnostic) audiologic assessment processes. The caregiver engagement is not icing on the screening cake or an ancillary issue—it is an integral part of the desired outcome, without which the act of screening is not only futile, but possibly even inappropriate when viewed from standpoint of the World Health Organization (WHO) screening criteria discussed in detail in Chapter 15 of this book.

The focus on the screening test itself is not surprising, just as the preeminence of the pure-tone audiogram in audiology at large is not surprising, because it is relatively easy to measure. But, it is easy to fall into the trap focusing exclusively on the doing of screening tests rather than the effects of doing them. This could provoke déjà vu in those readers who have worked within EHDI programs for a long time, in that for years the focus of meetings was at first all about screening technologies then all about diagnostic testing and technologies, rather than about the real business of EHDI, which is the delivery of timely, effective interventions to those who need them. As Richard Seewald remarked at the time, "the diagnostics were always in the Great Ballroom, whereas the intervention stuff was in a small room somewhere down a long, dark corridor." The parallel in screening is that it is all about performance of screening tests rather than about the impact that they might or might not have on what actually happens to the infant. Hopefully, our field has moved on from that phase. It clearly has evolved in the sense that the overall success of the EHDI care pathways is now a strong focus, but in the context of screening program per se, there remains an apparent preoccupation with coverage numbers in isolation.

At the risk of overdoing this point, insofar as the screening result determines the need for the caregiver engagement and follow-up, it is reasonable to be interested in counting screens, but it is only really useful if the delivery of the baby with a refer to the next program step is considered with at least equal weight and focus. A pass or refer screening result is not really an outcome in the sense of an impact on the baby—it can be viewed better as an *output* of a screening test or tests that is convertible to a real "child outcome" largely by the interaction and *messaging* between the screener and the caregiver.

What this means from an evaluation point of view is that there are at least two key processes going on, the screening itself and the caregiver engagement process. Of course, engagement does not guarantee that the baby with a refer will actually attend the next step promptly. All manner of events could interfere with that attendance, so what is relevant from the evaluation point of view is that the caregiver leave the screening refer appointment with a clear understanding of what the result means and a clear intention to attend the follow-up promptly. It is interesting that, at least to the author's knowledge, few programs actually attempt to measure those two variables—understanding and intent. In fact, it can be argued that actual attendance at a diagnostic assessment should be included as a component of real child outcome, a point that will be elaborated later.

To take this yet one step further, the hard-nosed view that is sometimes adopted in vertically integrated ("soup-to-nuts," screening-to-interventions) programs is that if a baby who refers from screening does not make it to timely diagnostics, then, excepting catastrophic causes, the overall screening process should not be counted as successful; it is as if it did not happen. This touches on a painful reality, in some but by no means all EHDI systems, of many babies who refer from screening being lost to follow-up (LTF) or lost to documentation (LTD). The argument for the distinction of these two "losses" is that in LTD the baby actually does receive the diagnostic assessment but the tracking system just does not know about it. The countervailing position is that if you do not even know that a baby has had a diagnostic assessment, in what sense can you be considered to be managing the baby's hearing and communication development effectively, and what, then, is the real merit of announcing, say, near-perfect delivery of screening tests to all live newborns? To some, LTD is essentially a speculative proxy for LTF, a viewpoint that others might vigorously contest.

The Measurement of Screening Coverage

NBHS programs within an EHDI context are usually intended to be universal, across all live births, but whether or not that is the case, there must be a clearly defined target population, together with a program goal of the type "To screen all babies who . . . " It seems natural to use the completeness with which screening is actually delivered across the target population as one measure of effectiveness. The simplest possible measure is whether or not screening was done, a binary outcome for each baby that can be counted over the target population. The obvious indicator is the sample proportion of targeted live births who are screened, usually called *coverage*.

Target Population Membership (Eligibility)

Consider the denominator of coverage, which is typically the number of live births that satisfy a set of screening eligibility criteria. In the event that the birth of every child in the program's area of operations is known in a timely manner, as is the case in many jurisdictions but certainly not in all, the ability to count births in any defined group offers enormous analytical flexibility. If that is not the case, the feasibility of calculating coverage accurately depends on the accuracy and the granularity over time and place of available birth statistics. It also depends on the timeliness with which such data become available. Jurisdictions with well-developed birth registration systems might have no issues here, but elsewhere, even in some "developed" countries or regions, it might be difficult to access reliable and timely birthrate data. In that situation, it is likely that estimated birthrate data will be used, with obvious vulnerability to error or bias. The bottom line is that coverage estimates are in many cases only as good as the more inaccurate of the numerator and denominator. Moreover, local birthrate data might be available at, say, a teaching hospital, but such data obviously do not address the issue of whether a given baby might have been screened elsewhere.

There might be systemic eligibility exclusions in some healthcare settings, such as on the basis of citizenship status, birthplace, ability to pay, alternative care pathways, and so on. These require adjustment of the denominator, so long as the position taken is that what really matters is the proportion of *eligible* live births screened. However, there is something fundamental about live births and something potentially messy about applying eligibility criteria that might be modified by simply a policy change.

Concerning consent, regardless of what is conventional, standard, or even regulated practice, the first-principles question here is whether babies for whom consent for screening is denied should be separated from the denominator of the birth cohort when reporting coverage. One view is that if consent is considered to be a standard process and the core program intent is screening of babies whose caregivers choose it to be done, then the proper denominator is based on the choice and not simply the live birth. Denial of consent to be screened is uncommon and could be treated as a valid cause of failure to screen. Furthermore, it might be deemed inappropriate even to attempt consent if the caregiver were highly anxious, distressed, or overwhelmed by events, though such events are not common and could be handled by deferral of the consenting. This gets more complicated because there is an array of consent options, ranging in strength from multipart, explicit, written consent through implied consent to standard-of-care screening and negative-option withdrawal. A different view is that babies denied consent should be left in the birth cohort denominator because they *were* live births and the consent process is a program action that is subject to scrutiny. It could and should be managed as a program deficiency if, for example, marked variation in the denial proportion across time or place is seen.

It becomes clear that what is important in coverage analysis and reporting is to make it crystal clear precisely who is and who is not included in the denominator and to list the numbers of babies who fall into distinct categories that caused them not to be screened.

Concerning medically eligibility, it is usually deemed inappropriate to screen if a baby were critically or seriously ill and this is not uncommon for babies in various types of special care units. It is not a coverage deficiency to not yet have screened such babies, so one option is to break out babies who are long-stay in special care from the coverage denominator and analyze them as a separate component of the birth cohort. Once again, who should be counted as a legitimate target is in question. Two things are clear: the longer you wait after the end of a birth cohort to report the coverage, the smaller the unscreened subgroup will be, for many reasons.

What Is Meant by "Screened," Exactly?

Turning to the numerator of the coverage ratio, perhaps the first questions are about what is meant by "screened." Exactness is crucial here, not a matter of nitpicking, because answers to evaluation questions can change dramatically depending on precisely how things are defined. If they are defined vaguely, then you do not know what the answer really means, and if they are defined differently for various programs or for different time periods, how can you compare? Explicitness, clarity, and exactness are essential for program performance evaluation of any kind to be much more than an empty exercise.

So, are we talking about a screen merely being *offered* to a caregiver but not necessarily done? Probably not, because the offer might be logged as a separate event, and similarly with consent being sought or presumed and, if sought, being given or withheld. Suppose consent were given; what if screening was attempted but without success? What qualifies as an attempt, and would an abort be counted? The number of attempts and the reasons for failure could be important information. Many evaluators might say that only successful screens should be counted in coverage estimates, but that attempts should also be counted because all substantial causes of nonsuccess should be examined forensically. What exactly qualifies as a successful screen? Does it matter if only one ear is successful if that ear gives a refer?

If there is a compound series or parallel screening protocol, does success mean completion of all tests in the protocol? If an OAE refer were the only successful test in an OAE-AABR series protocol, would that count as success? It is similar for only one test done in a parallel protocol. What happens in a protocol with repeat testing but the second test is missed?

A slightly deeper question relates to babies who are deliberately not screened. Some babies, such as those with congenital aural atresia, might be considered unscreenable and require bone-conduction ABR assessment. Some programs have protocols that require all babies at very high risk for permanent hearing loss to bypass screening and proceed directly to detailed ABR-based audiologic assessment. These can include babies with severe meningitis, branchiootorenal (BOR) syndrome, symptomatic cytomegalovirus (CMV) infection, or an affected sibling, for example. In the present author's view, any baby who has a known a priori probability of PHL exceeding about 10% or in whom there is a known a priori probability of frequency-specific PHL above about 1% should be routed directly to detailed audiologic assessment. Because of the potential for either false-negative screening or inappropriate caregiver overconfidence in a screening pass, it is probably better not to screen such babies. If this approach is followed, then clearly the bypassed babies should not be considered as missed by screening, and they should not be aggregated with screened babies except in regard to coverage, which is then reinterpreted to include "early hearing testing."

Binary Counts and Ratings

Typically, at least for programs based in hospitals, the majority of babies will be screened within a day or two of birth, but given the many causes of possible delay, there will be a distribution of babies' ages at screening. This distribution might extend for weeks, even months, given delay factors such as extreme prematurity, chronic illness, initial nonconsent, contact problems, caregiver challenges, and scheduling difficulties. It follows that coverage will increase over time, for a given birth cohort. The simplest approach to meaningful comparisons across programs, places, or times is to choose a criterion age for having been screened and define a binary cutoff. A common choice is 1 month of age, part of the 1–3–6 time course for screening, audiologic assessment, and starting intervention, recommended by the Joint Committee on Infant Hearing (JCIH, 2007). Why not 6 weeks or 2 months? There is no really good answer other than that a simple and reasonable choice that can be widely adopted as a standard measure is useful in itself. One month is somewhat arbitrary but is at least reasonable and simple.

With respect to popular coverage rating categories, there is usually clear satisfaction in having a point estimate of, say, 96% and being given a "very good" rating, though one could equally well call 93% "poor." The rating would have more meaning if it were based on a fairly current percentile ranking across comparable entities such as states or provinces, for example. Whatever the coverage value is that corresponds to the 90th percentile across the U.S. states, for example, is "very good" at least in a comparative sense.

The cynic might anticipate that favorable point estimates are more likely to be readily reported, whereas unfavorable estimates could be quietly buried in small-print tables, a selection bias that might be a motive for underreporting of confidence intervals. The fact is that if the confidence interval about a "very good" point estimate were wide enough to also embrace merely "good," or even to trespass into "fair," who knows what the category really is? The converse is also true, though. A point estimate that seems "fair" only could have an interval that extends well into the "good" or even the "very good" range, and you really do not know which to believe. The flaw in all this lies in trying to squeeze too much meaning out of the numbers given the artificiality and information loss inherent in imposing category labels upon essentially continuous numeric scales, combined with the variability that is inherent in sample measurement that are subject to error. The approach that cannot be criticized, if one must use a label, is to select the category that applies to the lower of the two confidence limits.

Cohort Definition

The definition of the baseline cohort to be analyzed is usually in terms of birth date, yielding a *birth cohort*. Although counting screened babies might be relatively straightforward, at least in principle, counting live births might not be, depending on the accuracy, granularity, and timeliness of birth data statistics reporting, as noted earlier. The period that defines the birth cohort for coverage calculation could be a week, month, quarter, or year, whatever is either mandated or best serves the purpose of the inquiry. Assuming adequate birthrate data, the choice of period involves a compromise between precision of the coverage estimate, which depends on the sample size, the temporal resolution, and the desired detail of any trend analysis over time. Quarterly data, if available, are usually appropriate for routine program-wide coverage reporting. Annual reports are typically obligatory for longer-term performance monitoring.

The basic questions that are asked about program-wide annual or quarterly coverage are typically, what is it, what rating (e.g., good, very good, excellent, etc.) has been achieved, how does it stack up in relation to comparable programs elsewhere, is it better or worse than the previous value, is there a long-term trend, and how can we do better? When comparing a single new estimate of coverage with a hypothesized value derived from theory, from historical data, or from any rationale whatsoever, the appropriate statistical test is just a one-sample binomial test. A simple comparison of two sample proportions usually requires the obvious binomial test for two independent samples. Multiple values over time should always be presented graphically as a time series with confidence interval and sample sizes either embedded or as an adjunct table. The first analysis act usually should be an *omnibus* test of the null hypothesis that all the proportions have an identical underlying true value. If that null hypothesis is accepted, then a valid, combined estimate can be derived. If it is rejected, then combination might be inappropriate and a deeper examination is needed, identifying oddball values, disjoint change over time, or some type of continuous underlying trend such as the asymptotic improvement often seen in the first few years of program implementation. For anything but the most basic analysis, well-validated statistical packages are needed. Ideally, the software should include apps specifically designed for proportions, which often include nonparametric exact tests (*permutation* tests) for small-sample data, such as the *Fisher exact test*. Large samples can usually be tested with an approach (called *asymptotic*) based on chi-square distributions.

Beyond Binary Cutoffs: Age Distributions

What do we *really* want to know about screening coverage? For most people, the first question that comes to mind is about *whether* a lot of babies were screened, but the immediate segue is about *when* were they screened, at what age, was it timely? In the context of an EHDI program, time is obviously of the essence, and the timeliness of the screening is part of its effectiveness.

In any given birth cohort, the actual ages of babies at screening typically will be statistically distributed over a period of weeks or months but with the vast majority screened in the first few days, for a program based mainly on predischarge hospital screening. A histogram of numbers screened by age in days allows easy visual appreciation of the distribution, but it is usually helpful to log-transform the ordinate because of the large range of daily counts. Although histograms technically are distribution functions and sometimes pretty, they are usually not as useful as empirical cumulative distribution functions (ecdfs), which are simply the sample proportion of all cases screened on or before age X days, as X goes from zero to the largest number of days of interest. The ecdf derived from a coverage sample is an estimate of the underlying true or *population* cdf. All ecdfs, being probability curves, are within the range from 0 to 1. For any value of age (X), running a vertical up to the ecdf allows you to read the proportion or percentage of babies screened by age X, so the ecdf includes the coverage estimate for the 1-month 1–3–6 cutoff as just one of many data points. Also, running a horizontal from any value on the Y-axis along to the ecdf and dropping a vertical allows you to read the age at which any desired percentile of the distribution is reached. The median age, interquartile range, and any other percentiles are immediately apparent, as is the probability of being screened between any two ages, by subtraction of the corresponding ordinates.

Even though binary cutoffs are much better than no standard criteria at all, they are best left for the most superficial, brief, and summary purposes of evaluation. In contrast, the ecdf requires very little more effort at data collection and analysis than does the binary value, yet it is vastly more informative and is the most elegant and powerful summarization of the entire picture of screening occurrence and timeliness. Screening age ecdfs should be the obligatory, primary tool for all coverage analysis. Moreover, ecdfs should be the main tool for any exploration of the temporal distribution of any key event, including ages at entry into audiologic assessment, completion of assessment, intervention events, intervals between key events, and the like, throughout the entire EHDI process. Examples of these analysis tools are shown in Figure 16–1.

Just to emphasize what is lost by binary cutoffs, note that no distinction is made between a baby who is screened at 1 month and 1 day versus 3 months, or between 1 month minus 1 day and at 1 day of age. Furthermore, a purpose of coverage analysis is to get a sense of the magnitude of any delays as well as how commonly they occur. Once that is done, the forensic audit for causes begins, and almost always this involves a prioritization of efforts toward addressing first those babies who have the largest delays. The ecdf is a simple and indispensable tool for the forensic audit process of target group identification.

If it is desired to place a confidence interval on any specific value of the ecdf at a given value of X, such as to answer properly a question such as "what is the coverage at one month of age," one way to do it is to take the Y value at 1 month and the number of babies in the overall cohort as the number of observations and simply look up the CI using any one of several Web apps (e.g., Google *binomial confidence interval calculator*). If you want to go deeper and place CI curves on an entire ecdf, you have to explore a commercial statistical package for the options or calculate the intervals using something like the Dvoretsky-Keifer-Wolfowitz (DKW) inequality, which is easier to do than it sounds, especially given access to a tame statistician.

Analysis Timing and Observation Period Censoring

Suppose the endpoints of a chosen birth cohort are dates A and B, and at a later date C it is desired to measure coverage using an extracted image of the required data at the time point C. Babies born at A will have the period A to C for database entry of their screened status, whereas those born at B will have the shorter period B to C. In fact, there is a continuum of data censoring, with the effect that *r* babies born earlier will tend to show larger coverage, simply because they had more opportunity to be screened and entered into the database. If a binary cutoff such as 1 month is used, then provided that C is at least 1 month later than B, the Yes or No status of every baby can be determined without censorship effects. If a cdf is to be used, then the maximum X-axis value for the cdf that is free from censorship bias is C-B because at the instant of C, all babies in the cohort have had an opportunity to be logged as screened. It follows, obviously, that if you are interested in large delays in screening, you cannot evaluate them in a stable and bias-free manner until after the last cohort birthdate plus the maximum delay of interest.

Whatever the maximum age limit of the age at screening distribution permitted by the coverage analysis, it is necessary to consider what is meant by "missed" or "not screened." It is one thing to have family lost without a trace after repeated contact attempts and with their baby not screened. But what about the baby whose family is initially not sure about screening but who turns up when the baby is 6 months old worried about hearing or speech delay and wanting a screen? What about the baby who is sick for 3 months but is screened on recovery? What this issue seems to require is a reasonable but essentially arbitrary cutoff that reflects an age limit for what can be called "newborn" hearing screening. One might choose 1 month, going with 1–3–6, but many would consider that too short and favor 3 months, say, or even 6 months. There is no obvious right or wrong age, but it is necessary to choose one because it determines when you stop counting for coverage.

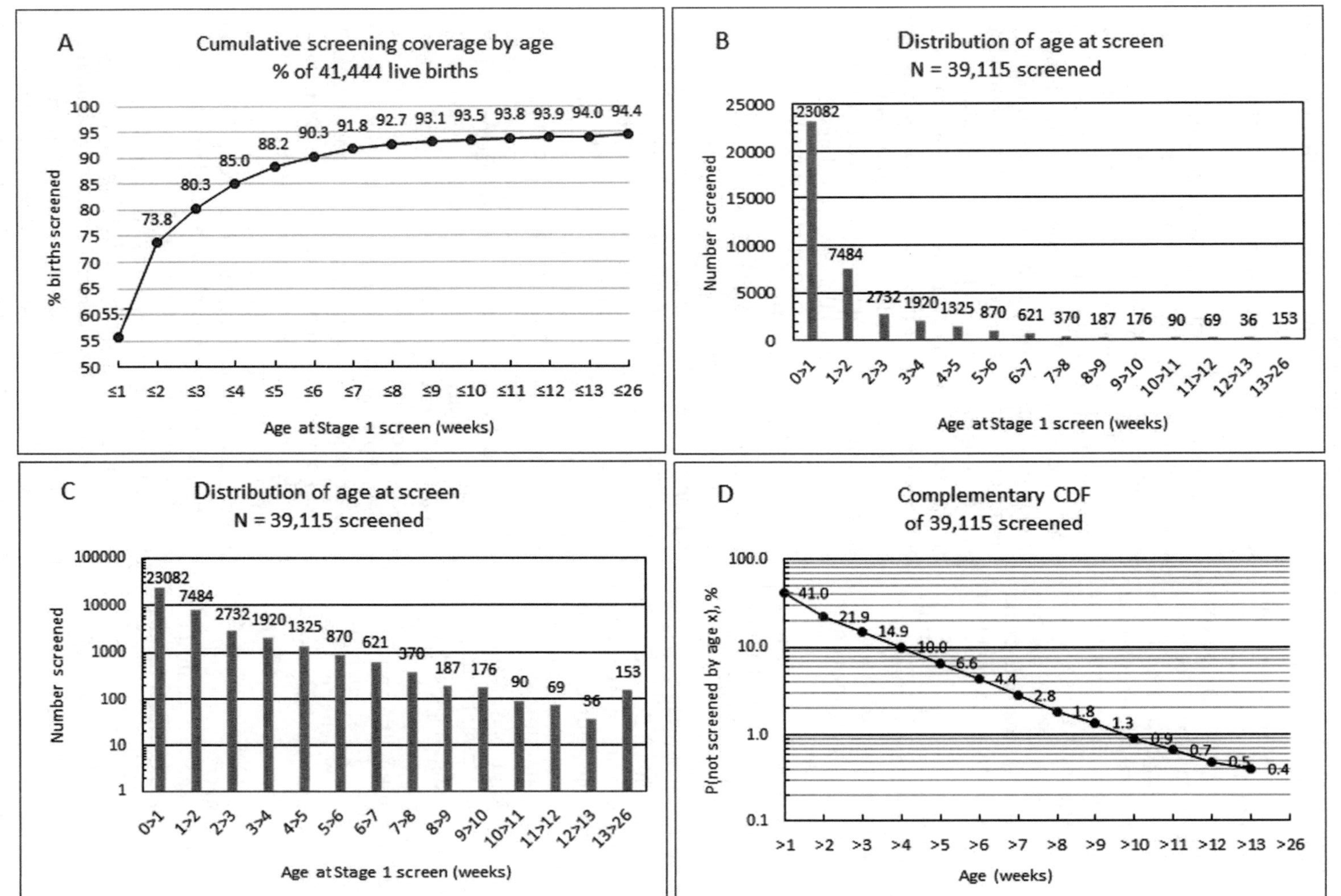

FIGURE 16–1. Real data examples. For simplicity, risk groups are not differentiated. **A.** Empirical cumulative distribution function (CDF) of live births screened by age at screen. The 1–3–6 one-month value is one point on the curve, at 4.3 weeks and 86%. The curve asymptote reveals 5.6% of births not screened even by 26 weeks. Causal audit of that subgroup is the logical continuous quality improvement project. **B.** Histogram of number of babies screened by age at screen in weeks. This shows, for example, that 1,325 babies were screened in the fifth week of age, as part of a smooth decline with no obvious discontinuity. This suggests multiple underlying contributors to delay. **C.** Conversion of B to a logarithmic *y*-axis clarifies the plot range and is roughly linear, suggesting an exponential decline up to about 13 weeks. **D.** Complementary CDF, showing the proportion of all babies screened who are *not* screened by age *x* weeks. This curve focuses strongly on the data aspect of greatest interest in continuous quality improvement, namely, the babies who are not yet screened. In this example, the curve is remarkably linear on a log *y*-axis.

Forensic Analysis

After the descriptive analysis of coverage, the next level of evaluation is to address the unscreened proportion and examine its component subgroups and individuals forensically, with a view to identifying distinct causes of nonscreening and practicable ways to increase coverage. In essence, the challenge is to take the selected birth cohort and pursue the screening-related outcome for every baby, particularly for those babies who are not screened. In this endeavor, it is important to be as careful as possible about assigning a cause; sometimes what appears to be the cause my not be the real cause, especially when exploring the reasoning and the behavior of families and of screening personnel for potential causal factors of delay.

As the most "delayed" members of the ecdf, truly lost babies are a natural priority for forensic analysis of cause, but such analyses can be very limited due to the noncontact, leaving only the issues of how the contact was lost and could anything have prevented it. One rather obvious step is routinely to seek two or more contact sources, at least the primary caregiver and at least one other person who is not a cohabitant and is likely to know where they are.

Great care is necessary in attributing cause to specific scenarios such as late screening. For example, a baby might be screened very late and miss predischarge because of logistical reasons, but the actual cause of delay might be lack of interest in screening on the part of the caregiver, a lengthy illness in early infancy, a family crisis of some kind, bad traffic and lack of parking at a community screening facility, and so on. In general, the deeper you dig, the greater the multiplicity of actual causes becomes and the more difficult it is to assign a specific cause with confidence. In fact, many situations in which causal analysis is attempted appear to be governed by what has been called the *critical incident* hypothesis, otherwise known as the *last straw* or *tipping point* hypothesis, wherein it is a cumulative body of factors that creates a context wherein a key behavior is triggered apparently by an event that is actually of little significance in itself. See Gremler (2004) for a review of the critical incident approach.

Equity of Coverage

Equity is all about fairness in the distribution of services across the population in need. A common metric of fairness is equality—equality of access to service and, arguably, equality of access to a given quality of services. If a baby is not screened, it is potentially an access issue. If a baby is screened late, then it can be viewed as a possible quality issue, in that the screening was accessed but not in a timely manner and early screening is associated with greater potential benefit than late screening.

Consider a baby who missed being screened, in the sense that screening had not been done by the criterion age defining screening as done acceptably early. If the cause was chronic illness and the baby was screened promptly upon recovery, there is no inequity. In contrast, consider a local population subset that is ethnically distinct and known to be largely unfamiliar with the majority language, say English, yet is not provided with appropriately compelling program information in a common language. If there were a high incidence of missed screening or ineffective contact in that subset, then there is a deficiency in program equity. The essence of inequity is that the individual did not receive a generally (on average) delivered level of service and that the program could and should have done better with reasonable effort.

Inequity can occur for individual care recipients or for groups that are discernably distinct. The larger and the more identifiable is the subgroup, the greater the sheer quantity of inequity. For example, if a constellation of individual and idiosyncratic factors caused a set of babies to be missed, there is no inequity unless some or all of those factors could and should have been addressed proactively by any reasonably competent administration. But if the subgroup has a readily identifiable and actionable common factor, then the potential inequity is increased. The usual suspects in evaluations of coverage equity are geographic, ethnic, and socioeconomic factors.

Some problems of inequity are relatively easy to solve or at least to ameliorate. Others are intractable, and still others are complex and difficult. Examples of relatively easy problems include ineffective communication or needless loss of contact. Intractable problems include missed screening due to severe socioeconomic of lifestyle challenge, such as a single mother with poor health and few resources. A complex problem, at least for program designers and managers, might be chronic shortage or unpredictability of resources; another might be the question of a trading relationship between resource expenditure for screening in remote communities or highly dispersed populations versus the quality of intervention services for many infants identified with hearing loss in urban concentrations.

At the end of the day, in the author's experience, so many challenges continually arise in the course of operating a large EHDI program that a great deal of time and effort is spent putting out obvious fires, solving urgent, local, off-the-wall problems, planning for looming major issues in communications, information technology, human resources, capital equipment, or operating supplies, all the while fighting pervasive forces of program fragmentation against a backdrop of stagnant budget, intensifying resource constraint, shifting political priorities, and not infrequently, a fairly constant groundswell of flavor-of-the-month thinking and ill-conceived revisionism in health systems organization. Although pursuit of improved gross effectiveness is frankly obligatory, serious pursuit of improved equity in key program areas is a more rarified activity, albeit important and rewarding.

Variations Analysis

Examination of equity addresses variation in an attribute of interest, in this case coverage, across groups or "areas" that are distinguishable by some measurable, common characteristic. This comparison of several proportions is a generic statistical problem that can be tackled using similar techniques to those mentioned earlier in the context of time-series analysis of coverage data, looking for trends. The areas that define the groups need not be physical or geographic, though they might be so. This type of activity is common in health services research, where it is often referred to as "small-area variations analysis" or "regional variations analysis." Although there are several sophisticated statistical methods that can be used, the basic idea is first to compare a set of coverage estimates to test the null hypothesis that they all come from an identical underlying binomial population with a constant true probability of having been screened. If this global or omnibus test rejects the null hypothesis, then any of several post hoc procedures can be used to locate the group or groups that differ and determine the size of the differences. The determination of whether statistically significant differences are of practical significance is a matter of clinical or operational judgment and is not a statistical matter. This analysis of variation clearly relates to questions of equity and inequity just mentioned. As noted earlier, for the specific case of coverage evaluation, the limitations of the analysis are likely to derive in part from what birth statistics and breakdowns are available from government agencies, institutions, or even from within programs.

Birthrate data are usually available from large birthing centers such as major teaching hospitals, so comparisons of at least predischarge screening coverage from at least some screening centers is often feasible. If there are many centers involved, it might be useful to present the data graphically ordered by increasing sample coverage and also by number of births. Ordering by coverage can reveal clusters of sites with similar coverage as well as possible outliers. Ordering by number of births looks at a common question, which is whether doing a lot of something tends to make you better at it.

Stratification in Coverage Analysis

Many audiologists will be familiar with what we might call the *fruit basket problem*, which is a name for the process of averaging or grouping dissimilar items together, treating them as homogeneous, and drawing inferences that might not be valid for any of the components individually or for any new basket of items. This is a common type of activity. Coverage is indeed a fruit basket, and there is risk in drawing overall conclusions without attention to the composition of the screened population, a sort of internal generalizability problem. Given institutional or program-wide birthrate data, one would expect, for example, that the coverage ecdf would be different for babies who did or did not attend a special care unit such as a neonatal intensive care unit (NICU), so it makes sense to view them separately for evaluation purposes, wherever feasible. Obviously, this requires that you know both the birth date and the stratification variable for every baby, as well as the age at screening. The general idea is that you should explore whether distinguishable groups are actually different on key measures or indicators before you lump them together.

If you do not stratify the analysis, you could derive an overall coverage by age ecdf, focus on a later-screened group, and analyze it forensically, only to discover that many members of that group were simply high-risk babies who were in intensive care for a long time. Or, up front you can divide the birth cohort into subgroups or strata, perhaps based on their highest level of care attended, derive the 1-month coverage or the ecdf for each group, and see if they are substantially different. The 1-month values can be compared statistically with a simple two-sample binomial test, as can the two coverage histograms or cumulative percentiles for any specific age at screening. A more global test of identity of ecdf shapes requires a test such as the Kolmogorov-Smirnov, also readily available. Although the stratification by actual PHL risk or by a risk proxy such as highest level of care attended (or a criterion such as NICU for 5 or more days) is an obvious one, there might be other variables that make sense in specific contexts, such as geographic birth location, ethnicity, and number of previous children.

Attendance in a special care unit is likely to yield a different pattern and a different overall proportion of coverage, but is this a matter of screening program inequity? It is not, because attendance in special care is medically indicated and beyond the purview of the NBHS program.

Screening Activity Analysis Versus Coverage Analysis

Consider any geographic "region" (country, state, county, district, set of screening sites, etc.) for which the total number of births in the defined birthdate cohort is known. Then for that region, coverage is simply the number of babies screened divided by the total number of live births, and this ratio constitutes a fixed scaling factor that applies only to the defined region. For that region, the ecdf of screening by age has exactly the same pattern as the ecdf of coverage by age, except that the former will range from 0 to 1, whereas the latter will range from 0 to the final proportion screened on or before the maximum permissible age criterion allowed for being counted as screening. None of the restrictions that apply due to birthrate data availability and granularity are relevant for screening activity analysis, but it is only for the region as a whole that the activity pattern can be scaled down to a coverage pattern using the region-cohort birth number. However, it is important not to lose sight of the question being asked; for the given region, the (screen by age) ecdf at 1 month, say, is the proportion of all babies screened by the maximum age criterion who are screened by age 1 month, whereas the (coverage × age) ecdf is the proportion of all live births in the region-cohort who are screened by age 1 month.

To emphasize further, suppose you were interested in statewide coverage by month in a 1-year birth cohort and you had 10 screening locations in the state. You can map the total number of screens at each location by month—an activity map. You can convert these numbers to actual coverages only if you know the number of births *at each location* by month. If you know only the total number of births by month, you can sum the screens across locations and get the coverage for each month; you can also compute the percentage contribution to the overall coverage per month from each location, but you cannot compute the location-specific coverage.

Evaluation of Screening Refer Rates

We have outlined basic approaches to evaluation of the yes-no occurrence of screening as well as its timeliness and group differences. The next step is evaluation of the *outputs* of screening. The usual ear-to-baby rule, at least for programs with unilateral loss included in the target disorder set for the program, is that a refer in either ear is a baby refer, while a baby pass requires a pass in each ear, and a "successful" screen is one that yield a baby pass or refer output. One passed ear does not equal success, on this definition, though it would if only bilateral loss were targeted. These rules must obviously be made clear when reporting or analyzing pass-refer data.

Unsuccessful Screens Matter

To put pass-refer analyses in proper context, we should not ignore the fact that some babies might not be screened successfully, even with multiple attempts. Quite often, published reports might not make clear the proportion of babies who are not successfully screened. For example, in evaluating a change in screening device design or operating protocol or firmware parameters, the proportion of screening attempts that were at the end of the day unsuccessful is every bit as important as the pass or refer rates, so actually there are three output values of interest from a screening test, not just two. Screening device immunity to acoustical or electrical noise is often an important issue in this regard. Notwithstanding these observations, the vast majority of screening output data are focused on refer rates, usually defined as the proportion of babies with successful screens who gave a refer.

Birth or Screening Date Cohorts

Suppose we wish to evaluate screening performance on a program-wide basis. The first question relates to the screened cohort definition; two distinct options are (a) all successful screens done in a particular range of dates, or (b) all successful screens done on a particular live birth cohort. The babies in the two cohorts are never all the same babies, though there might be some in common. For a given number of days in the observation epochs, the size of the two cohorts will not generally be the same, and Cohort (a) will usually be larger because even if there were entirely steady-state birth and screening activity, some babies in the birth cohort will not yield a successful screen. Cohort (a) addresses questions about what is happening over a completely specific screening epoch, such as a calendar month, quarter, or year. The results are smeared over a birth cohort date range governed, in a sense retrospectively, by the actual age distribution at successful screening.

Cohort (b) addresses questions about what happened to babies who were born in a completely specific birth epoch but whose screen dates were smeared in time, also by the age at screening distribution, but prospectively from the birth dates. Because most questions about refer rates are focused on looking for spontaneous time trends such as might arise due to learning effects or decay effects, or for effects of changes in screening structures or processes implemented at a specified date, Cohort (a) is the usual choice. Cohort (b) might be the better choice if the focus is on, for example, the overall EHDI program throughput characteristics experienced by a specific group of babies, especially if there is reason to suspect a change at a particular time in the population intake characteristics, perhaps within a specific region.

Overall and Risk-Stratified Refer Rates

Having chosen our cohort, we would start with the most basic descriptors, the overall point and interval estimates of the program-wide refer rate. What next? We might be concerned because we expect the percentage of refers to be higher in special care or at-risk babies, so again we might be confounding "apples and oranges" in the single, overall percent referred. We can stratify the refers by either level of care or risk status, and these two variables are not the same. At risk here means at risk for hearing loss; not all NICU attendees will be at such risk, and all babies who never attend a special care unit are not necessarily risk free. So now we might have two sets of summary statistics for overall percent refers, and it is easy to test for statistical significance of difference between them. If they are not different, then they can be aggregated, but if they are significantly different statistically, they can only be aggregated if there is an overriding judgment that the statistically genuine difference is of no material significance.

Area Variations and Subgroup Analyses

At this point, we might begin to think about regional or "small-area" variations analysis, especially for babies who are not at risk. Why? First because in UNBHS programs about 90% or more of babies will not be at risk on current risk registers, so samples will be large enough to support a substantial amount of subgrouping while retaining reasonable statistical power to detect subgroup differences in refer rates. That might not be the case for the much smaller refer groups at high risk, for which subgroup analysis capability will be much more limited. Second, almost certainly there will be area variations of some kind. The units of "area" between or among which refer rate variation may be found include individual screeners, categories of screening personnel (such as casual, part-time, full-time), screening devices, screening location types (birthing versus nonbirthing), individual hospitals or community clinics, population densities (urban versus rural versus remote), geoethnic regions, and so on. Most well-baby nursery or nil-risk refers are false positive. False positives waste program resources in unnecessary follow-up and cause both minor harms and direct costs to many families. The major underlying issue is that screening that is careless, unskilled, carried out in poor environments, at inappropriate times, or on babies in inappropriate behavioral states will tend to give refer rates that are unnecessarily high. They erode public and professional confidence when diagnostic assessments routinely find normal hearing in referred babies—a result of low positive predictive value (PPV, see Chapter 15 of this text). We might already be aware that individual screening personnel are a major source of variability in refer rates, even though they might have undergone standardized training. We might have a specific, a priori interest in examining refer rates for individual screening personnel, either as part of a general program of quality management or to evaluate specific individuals of interest, such as recently trained new screeners or screeners who have previously unusual refer rates or low caseloads.

One way to approach this for routine, as opposed to targeted, monitoring is to begin with a scatterplot or histogram of refer rates for all screeners. It is usually wise to inspect complex data visually prior to deriving summary statistics or plugging into statistical analysis packages. The *X*-axis might be screener ID in order of increasing refer rate, and CQI-oriented questions might include the following: who have the lowest and highest rates and why, is there clustering of rates with obvious outliers, are there clusters of similar rates, or is the distribution fairly uniform? They might also be ordered by increasing caseload (do screeners with the highest caseloads tend to do best?) or organized by site or site category (are some sites clearly better or worse than others? Do individual, peripatetic screeners do much better at some sites than at others?).

The Multiple-Comparisons Problem

One of the issues with nontargeted examination of refer rates, such as would be undertaken in routine continuous quality improvement programs, is multiplicity, sometimes known as the multiple comparisons problem. When looking at a lot of data points and asking the question, "Is any of these really different from the others?" the challenge is to distinguish genuinely different results from those that seem different but arise by chance just because there are multiple data points and sooner or later one or more are going to look different. One opinion is that you must preface any testing of seemingly unusual refer rates by an omnibus test as noted earlier. Thus, we are back to testing the identity of multiple proportions. If the answer is that the refer rates do not all come from the same, underlying binomial distribution, the we can proceed to use any of several common post hoc tests to identify differences for individuals or subgroups. If we do not use an omnibus test initially, we run a large risk of falsely identifying individuals or locations as poor performers, which might lead to auditing, retraining, or other quality improvement actions that are completely unjustified.

In-depth statistical analyses of screener performance in large screening program can become quite time consuming, yet to know whether individual screeners are performing well and consistently or not is very important to program management as well as in relation to both effectiveness and equity. Systematically high refer rates represent a deficiency in effectiveness, and large variability in refer rates is a clear deficiency in equity. For example, this means that whether or not you are likely to endure a false-positive screen is much higher if you get Screener A rather than Screener B.

Refer Rate Flag Levels and Screener CQI

One tool of practical value is a curve that is basically an upper confidence limit for a single sample refer rate taken from a population with a given "true" refer rate, computed as a function of number of babies screened in the sample, which can represent an individual screener or screening location. Because of the multiple comparisons issue, the chosen confidence probability must be adjusted to take approximate account of the number of individual screeners or "areas" being examined simultaneously. One can use a conservative adjustment procedure, such as the Bonferroni. What this means is that if you are routinely looking at, say, 50 individual screeners and you really intend to flag those who exceed a 95% confidence limit refer rate, you actually use a 0.001 level for the flag-level calculation. Because the Bonferroni adjustment of alpha is so conservative, you could also choose 0.005. An example of such flag curves is shown in Figure 16–2.

One purpose of flagging individual sites or individual screening personnel is to identify them as targets for performance monitoring. Because you are now watching a selected individual, the multiple comparisons problem goes away, and you can have much more confidence in statistical tests of whether the individual's observed refer rate is consistent with some assumed or measured "acceptable" refer rate. But, how do you choose this "target" or "true" refer rate? There are many options. The one that makes least sense to this author is to assume that the screening device manufacturers' published refer rates (if any) are applicable. Not much better is the use of published refer rates from research studies, because such studies frequently are not representative of performance under ordinary field conditions (remember—efficacy versus effectiveness?). One option that makes much more sense is to use the median refer rate obtained by a small group of skilled, knowledgeable, and experienced screeners who have high caseloads, over the course of several observation periods that yield no apparent trend over time and develop overall a substantial sample size, such as at least 50 refers. So, you answer the question, "What is a reasonable upper limit for the true refer rate?", then using that rate you compute the "upper flag curves" for the adjusted alpha and a range of caseloads such as 50 through 500. You then plug in your set of refer rates from an initial observation period and identify the target or targets for focused monitoring. When you have acquired a large enough sample, the period required for which you estimate beforehand, you test the new refer rate against the true rate. If it is significantly greater, you initiate a QI process, and when you believe the process is completed, you do another targeted observation to verify improvement.

Low Refer Rates

The other side of the coin is the challenge of individual screeners' refer rates that are too low. This is a less common problem than high refer rates, but it is more difficult to verify and fix. The concern is that whatever is causing the low refer rate might also be contributing to increased false-negative screens, for which the error cost is very high. A significant challenge is that reasonably low refer rates are desirable; screeners who are the most skilled and experienced, who follow well-designed protocols closely, tend to have the lowest rates. The issue becomes how low is too low? Another significant challenge is that the caseloads required to amass reliable estimates of low refer rates are very large, which means that the processes of initial monitoring, flagging, targeted monitoring, and verification of improvement can take too long to be practicable.

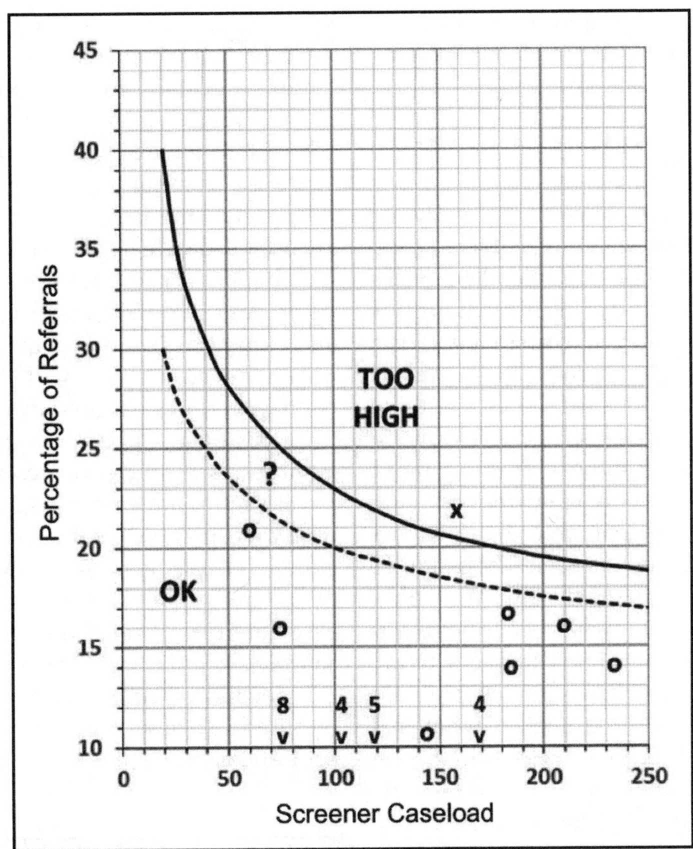

FIGURE 16–2. Examples of "flag curves" used in quality management to alert program managers to statistically extreme high refer rates in individual screeners. The challenges are to avoid chasing high rates that are illusory and due to either (a) natural, random refer rate variation over time, or (b) simultaneous inspection of multiple data points, such as from many screening personnel. The curves shown here are for introductory continuous quality improvement of automated distortion product otoacoustic emissions (ADPOAE) initial predischarge refer rates and are based on a nominal maximum acceptable true underlying binomial refer probability parameter of 0.12, which is liberal (high). The solid curve reflects a 0.1% upper limit and the dashed curve a 1% upper limit. Data points above the upper curve are high priority for prompt quality control intervention. Points below the lower curve are statistically acceptable. Points between the curves are questionable and are flagged for monitoring or for less urgent quality improvement initiatives. Illustrative 1-month data for 12 screeners from a Canadian program are shown. For ADPOAE screening in community centers postdischarge, the analogous curves have a lower binomial probability. The choices can be tailored to context and purpose and can be lowered as performance improves.

Multiple Rescreens

In the author's (and others') experience, the most common cause of very low refer rates is multiple, serial rescreening. For example, a screener might immediately rescreen a referred ear several times, seeking a pass. Eventually, a pass will occur by chance alone, although the exact probability of such events is difficult to determine because of the multiple, correlated potential causes. Nevertheless, *any* systematic departure from protocol that involves repeated testing of refers will at least change the basic performance characteristics of the screening test and increase the false-negative error rate. Good screening protocols, especially for OAE screening, allow or require a repeat screen after probe inspection for occlusion by debris or fluid following an initial refer, but set limits on the number of repeats permitted and the situations in which they can be done. One complicating factor is that protocol adherence in practice is imperfect, variable, and not always easy to detect. Another is that screening devices can provide ongoing visual information about signal and noise characteristics, which screeners might use to decide to terminate a data acquisition prematurely. This also can change device performance characteristics.

Screening Device Audits

Some OAE and ABR screening devices internally log useful data on the details of screening attempts and outputs for any given baby. For example, it might be possible to review an entire series of events that involve screen initiation, stimulus calibration, noise levels, run terminations, pass and refer outcomes, and the exact timing of these events. Such logs can be audited and are especially useful when a given screener is found to have a very low refer rate. One of the interesting things that can be revealed is that screening personnel can use a screen initiation attempt as a probe of baby behavioral conditions, sometimes repeating and aborting 10 times or more and thinking that this does not count as multiple rescreening. In fact, what is happening is that the range of noise conditions for which screens are run to completion is no longer the same as it would be without such practice, and it is unclear what that might do to overall screening error rates. This is yet another example of why it can actually have little or no meaning to claim that screening sensitivity, specificity, and refer rates have specific and generalizable values; screening performance is actually affected by a host of variables including all the minute details of exactly how the screen is conducted by the individual screener.

When auditing devices, it is regrettably necessary and appropriate that the device of interest be audited without prior notification, else one might encounter curiously absent or incomplete records, albeit rarely. Due diligence in performance management usually requires that interference with stored data be guarded against. Many readers might be aware of the exemplary New Zealand Ministry of Health (2012) report on quality management response to discovered anomalies in OAE screening data, including evidence of data falsification by self-screening. This spectrum of deficiency in practice must be assumed to be potentially present in any screening program. Worthy of note is that the events addressed by the New Zealand Quality Improvement Process initially came to light not through systematic QA or QI processes but by serendipitous observations of an unusually alert individual.

Monitoring Refers Over Time

Whatever is the source of a refer rate, a generic issue is to explore whether or not a set of values ordered in time is consistent and stable. This issue was touched on in the context of coverage analysis, but for refer rate evaluation it is even more relevant and diverse in application, especially to questions about the performance of individual screeners or screening sites. We might be interested, for example, in routine detection of aberration or of trend, or in targeted analysis of response to programmatic QI events or other interventions such as protocol or device changes, screener personnel changes, or indeed any other changes in structure or process. A detailed review of statistical method for such analyses is beyond the scope of this chapter, so only a few basic points will be mentioned. First, for the context of routine monitoring.

The most important first step is to inspect the data visually as a time-series control plot, easily done in Excel or in many custom applications. Both point and interval estimates should be shown, because the overriding concern is to guard against false identification of extreme values and trends. The amount of variation associated with refer rate values even for moderate sample sizes is routinely surprising to nonstatisticians. The second point is that special techniques are often required to draw valid inferences about binomial proportions data, which is what refer rates are.

Attendance for Audiologic Assessment

Increased understanding of hearing loss and engagement with program recommendations are positive outcomes of high-quality screener-caregiver interaction, but it is clear that the key valued outcome of screening is timely attendance at a diagnostic audiologic assessment. It could be argued further that the real point of screening is that babies thereby found to have hearing loss receive appropriate and successful interventions, but here we will draw a dividing line between screening and assessment for PE/CQI purposes. Obviously, attendance is essential, whereas successful assessment is not guaranteed and should be part of the evaluation of assessment itself, not of screening.

Basic Approach

In practice, the evaluation of "delivery" to diagnostics depends strongly on the health system context and EHDI program design; in "vertical" EHDI systems, logging diagnostic attendance is no more difficult than logging screening attendance, whereas for systems in which diagnostic services are not tightly linked into the EHDI program, which is a profound design flaw, tracking of diagnostics can be very challenging. At least in principle, however, it is not difficult to quantify diagnostic attendance. The indicators for linkage to assessment follow the same hierarchy as for screening itself: the proportion of refers that result in assessment attendance by a binary cut-point such as 2 months of age and the empirical cdf of ages at first assessment appointment attendance. If your purpose is to portray an overview of the birth cohort disposition, showing screening offers, declines, coverage, misses, bypasses, successes, and immediate outcomes, the count or cdf of age at assessment attendance are one endpoint of the birth cohort outcome tree. If, however, your intent is to answer the more specific question, "how are we doing with respect to linking refers to detailed assessment?" you might choose to increase the focus, sample size, and recency of the analysis by redefining the cohort of interest as the entire referred cohort in a given date range, as distinct from taking an earlier birth cohort for whom only perhaps 1% to 2% ended up being referred to assessment up to a month or more later.

Whether you take a birth cohort of referred cohort approach, for QI you will want to explore those who did not attend for assessment at an appropriate age, reflected either in a binary criterion age or as an upper percentile of an age at initial assessment ecdf. The first thing you are likely to find is that some of them were screened late and, consequently, referred late. If the high risk and no risk subpopulations have not been separated, these babies will include those with longer stays in special care units. In any such simple, age-based analysis, binary or cdf-based, age at the refer and the interval from refer to assessment attendance are confounded. A very informative way to display such data is a bivariate scatterplot with age at referral on the X-axis. The Y-axis can be age at first attendance for audiologic assessment, which yields an upper triangular display with the referral-attendance interval shown as a distance above the leading diagonal, with no points below the diagonal. This has the advantage that it shows directly the age at first assessment attendance.

An alternative is to plot the interval on the Y-axis, which yield a full-axis scatterplot and makes the delay explicit, with age at assessment implicit as $X + Y$. The preference depends on whether the primary focus is the sources of high age at assessment or the distribution of delay and its possible relationship to age at screening referral. It is, of course, a simple matter to convert the nondiagonal scatterplot to a two-way table with m rows and n columns, displayable as a bivariate histogram. One can also use a 2×2 table applying a dichotomous maximum acceptable age criterion to X and a dichotomous maximum acceptable interval criterion to Y, for summarization or tabulation purposes or to identify specific subgroups that might warrant further, forensic analysis. All these displays are easily done in Excel. If it is desired to focus on the postreferral events, then the ecdf of the delay from referral to attendance is the direct and complete tool, but what it does not explicitly reveal is any relationship between age at screening and delay to attendance, for which the bivariate scatterplot is uniquely informative.

Forensic Audit Group Selection

The purpose of displaying key indicators quantitatively is to understand their behavior and its causes, especially for indicator values considered as evidence of shortfall, deficiency, error, or quality improvement opportunity. The usual CQI action following an analysis such as an ecdf of age at screening or delay from referral to assessment attendance is to shine the audit microscope on the extremes of the cdf. Babies above the 90th or 95th percentile are potentially a rich source of structure or process shortcomings, which are revealed by a detailed case-by-case forensic audit of the events in the individual babies. Babies at the other end of the ecdf, such as below the 5th or 10th percentile, might be the poster children for program excellence and a rich source of lessons learned and deficiencies to avoid, but they might also arise for adverse reasons such as non-adherence to protocols and short-circuiting of desired process elements. Depending on the exact shape of the cdf, there might well be a group that is considered as typical, with large distributional concentration somewhere between the 25th and 75th percentiles. These are a good source for identifying the process performance "archetype" while encompassing a modest range of variability over cases that cannot be considered as extreme, exceptional, or oddball.

When examining the extremes of the ecdf, two patterns are interesting. One is that there is a frequent common element, be it a provider identity or location, or a recipient "barrier" characteristic such as a disadvantaged family. Another is that the cases in the distributional tail can show virtually unique, individual characteristics with almost nothing in common and a remarkable constellation of unanticipated causes for their tail membership.

Family Experience Surveys (FESs)

Exploration of the experiences of care recipients (families and other caregivers) is a standard methodologic element in the array of PE/CQI activities related to EHDI, and screening is no exception. Several examples of "parent surveys" are available from the NCHAM "move-the-needle" website.

Although adherence to screening program follow-up recommendations is a focused, quantitative indicator of effectiveness, there is much to be gained by asking families the much more general question: what was your experience of the screening process? One way to do this is to survey family experiences of the program routinely. Such surveys can be by snail mail, e-mail, Web-based, structured telephone interview, and so on. They can be brief and incorporated into the standard program process, or can be more detailed, sporadic, and theme focused. In a survey with which the author was involved as a program evaluator, over 500 families completed an FES through a telephone-structured interview and questionnaire with probability sampling stratified by risk (Y/N) and screening result (pass/refer). The questions included Likert scales (5-point), closed and open choice lists, contingent response elaboration, and free text comments. The domains of inquiry included

- understanding of UNBHS purpose, rationale, and what to expect (procedures);
- utility of program handouts and other information;
- convenience of screening process (pre- and postdischarge from hospital);
- screener knowledge, competence, empathy, respectfulness, patience, calmness, and baby handling;
- explanation and understanding of the meaning of the screening result (pass and refer);
- perceived hearing status of their baby;
- perceived credibility of the screening result;
- meaning of hearing loss risk;
- explanation and understanding of what to do next and why;
- intention with regard to attendance for detailed assessment (if indicated);
- overall satisfaction with the program;
- perceived importance and endorsement of NBHS;
- recommendations for program improvement (open ended); and
- needs for additional program information or contacts.

Results were analyzed quantitatively or qualitatively, as appropriate. A few results of note were as follows:

- Almost all families thought that NBHS was appropriate and worthwhile.
- Families did not find program brochures useful or did not remember receiving them; it was recommended that brochures be improved and that information be made more widely available, such as in prenatal classes. Materials provided shortly after delivery were mostly either not read or not recalled.
- Ratings of screener competence and conduct were generally favorable, with diverse, isolated concerns.
- Most families of babies who referred intended to attend promptly for audiologic assessment, even though they did not necessarily believe their baby had a hearing loss. Mostly, of course, they were actually correct as reflected in typically limited screening PPV grounds, but not for valid reasons.
- Many families believed that they could tell whether their child had a hearing loss. The reasons given were generally invalid.
- Most families were either moderately or very satisfied with their overall screening program experience.

As a result of these and other findings, screeners received enhanced training, including on key scripted messages to deliver and phrases to avoid. Families' limited ability to detect hearing loss observationally was explained much more fully in program information. Families' responses concerning needs, expectations, and concerns were fully explored. The next step in the CQI circle is to determine whether these program actions have had an impact on the pattern of attendance for assessment and the families' understanding of the meaning of a refer result.

One of the points of interest in this evaluation was that it was done in a context of a fairly high historical rate of prompt attendance for assessment (about 80%). Moreover, in the survey, several families commented that they intended to attend assessment even though they believed that they knew their baby's hearing was "OK." This suggests that while enhancing families' understanding of the challenges in detecting hearing loss reliably can be appropriate from a longer-term perspective, it might not be a key contributor to the limited shortfall in attendance. Of course, in a different context, the "credibility" of a screening refer can be a strong determinant. It is not yet established whether generalizable, useful predictors of attendance can be identified and explored at the point of first discussing the refer result, as part of a routine screening evaluation.

A related question is whether simple process elements such as "locking in" an assessment appointment date and time at the screening refer encounter, coupled with a bright yellow appointment card and a fridge magnet plus telephone and mailed reminders would be effective in a substantial number of cases who would not otherwise attend promptly. The author's speculation is that when major explanatory variables such as poor screener messaging, poor contact techniques, and inadequate tracking data systems (e.g., "lost to documentation") are dealt with effectively, what is left is likely to be an array of idiosyncratic, family-specific situation or events that have few, if any, common themes or factors.

Evaluation of Efficiency

What Is Efficiency?

There are many different facets of efficiency that might be the focus of program evaluation and CQI efforts. In general, efficiency has to do with some measure of achievement of a desired outcome for a given amount of resource utilization. The most obvious resource quantifier is money, though derivative structure or process measures such as number of screening personnel required for a given level of effectiveness, number of successful screens per screener per day, number of screening attempts needed for success, and so on, are alternatives. As is apparent in published literature, the distinction between effectiveness and efficiency is sometimes blurred, with effectiveness being referred to as efficiency. Insofar as people and time can be translated into numeric costs or *monetized*, by far the most relevant measure of efficiency is called, somewhat paradoxically, *cost-effectiveness*. One way or another, it is usually about *bang for the buck*, and the "bang" is some dyad of effectiveness and equity.

The importance of screening program cost is obvious, especially so in this era of accountability and economic concern. Cost can be viewed in several ways. In a *logic model* approach to program evaluation, cost is often treated as an input variable, expressed as required funding. In at least one classical approach to program evaluation, cost is treated as an element of program structure, just as are people, equipment, and buildings. In other models, cost might be treated as an outcome variable, so a program delivers both desired outcomes and costs. Whatever model is applied, cost basically is a negative attribute or parameter of any health services system and the associated health state of the population. Even to have no NHS program at all is one particular system choice, with an array of associated costs, such as the direct costs of the old medical referral system and the costs of special schooling to address compromised language development, for example.

Inevitably, the achievement of screening program objectives and desired clinical outcomes is constrained in the real world by consideration of the resources required. Program performance evaluation necessarily invokes the methods of *cost effectiveness* and *cost-benefit* analysis. In cost-effectiveness analysis (CEA), different programs or systems of care are compared in terms of the resources required to produce a given unit of desired outcome. For example, one might examine the communication skills of children at school entry in relation to three programs: a default program such as that historically based on medical referral for hearing services as and when suspicion of hearing loss arises, a system that includes targeted screening of newborns at high risk for hearing loss, and a system that includes universal screening of all newborns. Some of the outputs of each system might be desired, and these are positive benefits. Others might be undesirable, and these are negative benefits, more commonly referred to as *harms*. These benefits and harms might relate directly to the intended program goals, or they can be unanticipated side effects. The essence of CEA is computation of the costs of a given amount of net product or outcome of any given activity. Various methods are available for exploring quantitatively the values (positive or negative) that people assign to different outcomes or health states, broadly referred to as *health state utility analysis*, which leads naturally to cost-utility analysis.

Cost-benefit analysis (CBA) is a specific variant of CEA in which *all* of the inputs (resources) and outcomes (desired or not, targeted or side effects) are expressed in the same units, usually monetary and usually discounted for change in the value of money over time. The latter is especially important when calculating cost-benefit over periods of many years. A major challenge in applying CBA to NHS outcomes is to assign meaningful and valid monetary values to the variety of outcomes, be they benefits or harms. What is the monetary value, for example, of an earlier diagnosis or of an improved education readiness of a child? What is the cost of failure to achieve a valued societal goal for an individual child? Frequently, the cost values assigned are incomplete, approximate, or even speculative. This can render the conclusions of CBA very unstable, and at the very least, it is essential to explore how those conclusions might vary with changes in the monetary values assigned. This is known as *sensitivity analysis*, an unfortunate term that the reader should not confuse with the specific meaning of the word *sensitivity*, discussed earlier.

The reader interested in cost analysis of newborn hearing screening is encouraged to review carefully a landmark report by Keren, Helfand, Homer, McPhillips, and Lieu (2002), which included a substantial bibliography. This detailed and sophisticated study used well-founded estimates of program performance parameters, costs, and cost-savings to build a quantitative, comparative model of UNHS, selective screening and no screening. They included much sensitivity analysis, to test stability of the model's implications for ranges of assumed parameters. The bottom line was that UNHS is likely to result in long-term cost savings relative to selective screening or no screening, but that more evidence is required to substantiate the impact of EHDI on long-term language development, educational and occupational performance, and quality of life.

A significant, further limitation of many cost-oriented analyses of UNHS and EHDI to date has been a lack of separation of both absolute costs and changes in costs that can arise for different levels of hearing loss severity. Some cost analyses appeal to estimates of lifetime earnings with and without hearing loss, or special education costs with and without early interventions to improve hearing and language, but it cannot be valid to apply the same cost values to all children detected by screening and diagnosis. Different degrees of hearing loss cause different patterns not only of disadvantage and associated educational costs, but also of timing and delay in identification and intervention, both with and without screening programs. There might even be an unintended bias toward lines of argument that amplify the costs of undetected hearing loss as well as the cost saving attributable to UNHS programs. See, for example, an important report by Schroeder and her colleagues in 2006 and a commentary on it by Grosse and Ross (2006). Notwithstanding these benefit-inflationary concerns, it can also be said that most cost analyses to date have not taken into account the full array of potential benefits of EHDI to individuals, families, and society, both ethical and functional. It is hoped that higher standards of economic analysis such as those illustrated and recommended by Schroeder and colleagues will come to pass.

A Simple Example of Cost-Effectiveness Analysis

Here, we consider a rather basic issue in program design and evaluation: whether an additional screening test or stage should be interposed in the pathway from an initial screening test to the first detailed audiologic assessment. A specific example might be whether or not to use a serial second stage (re-)screening by AABR following an initial AABR refer in babies who are found to be at risk for PHL. The risk can be determined directly, such as by inspection of records for risk indicators such as those recommended by the US JCIH, for example, or the risk category could be based on an administrative process proxy of true risk, such as attendance in a Special Care Unit for a criterion number of days. The deficiency with the latter, of course, is that some babies in special care (such as those with feeding disorders) are not at genuine risk, and some not in special care are at risk (such as those with apparently nonsyndromic external ear anomalies).

Immediate repetition of a predischarge AABR that gives a refer result is often part of the standard AABR protocol and is aimed at reducing false positives due to short-term factors such as insert earphone occlusion, poor placement, or transient baby activity. In contrast, the use of a second AABR screening, typically on an outpatient basis after a few days, anticipates partial resolution of middle ear debris or fluid conditions as well as possible gains in baby state control in the outpatient, nonperinatal context. The intent, of course, is to reduce the demand for unnecessary, relatively expensive and burdensome diagnostic assessments.

The key question is whether this additional AABR leads to a substantive improvement in cost-effectiveness, relative to the single, predischarge AABR. The paths are shown in Figure 16–3, with plausible associated parameters. A small amount of simple algebra is required:

> Number of babies N, initial AABR cost C, expected refer rate $r1$, diagnostic cost D, PHL prevalence p, assumed AABR sensitivity approximately 1 (near-perfect sensitivity)
>
> Trial estimates: $C = \$25$, $r1 = 0.04$, $D = \$150$, $p = 0.01$ (overall for high-risk newborn). You can substitute any other cost values that seem reasonable, in your preferred currency units.
>
> Pathway A: Predischarge AABR only, refers directly to diagnostic audiologic assessment.
>
> Baseline operating cost: $N \cdot C + N \cdot r1 \cdot D$
> Yield: $N \cdot p$ true cases
>
> Pathway B: Outpatient repeat AABR for initial refers. Refer rate $r2$. Cost $C2$.
>
> Trial estimates: $C2 = 50$, $r2 = 0.5$.
>
> Operating cost: $N \cdot C + N \cdot r1 \cdot C2 + N \cdot r1 \cdot r2 \cdot D$
> Yield: $N \cdot p$ true cases.
>
> Cost difference $B - A$ per true case =
> $1/p \cdot [C + r1 \cdot C2 + r1 \cdot r2 \cdot D - C - r1 \cdot D] =$
> $r1/p \cdot [C2 - D(1 - r2)]$
>
> Difference is negative (saving) if: $C2 < D(1 - r2)$ or $C2/D < 1 - r2$
>
> For trial estimates, $C2/D = 50/150 = 0.33$ and $1 - r2 = 1 - 0.5 = 0.5$, so B costs less than A.
>
> Cost difference per true case identified =
> $4 \cdot (50 - 75) = -100$.

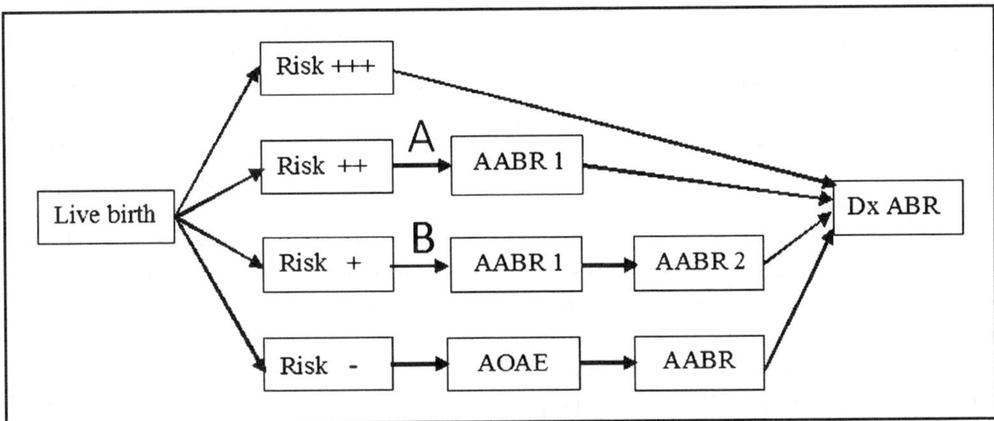

FIGURE 16–3. A risk-stratified screening protocol with four pretest risk categories. Risk+++ babies go directly to diagnostic audiologic assessment based primarily on ear-specific, frequency-specific auditory brainstem response (ABR) threshold estimation (diagnostic; Dx ABR). Risk ++ babies are screened once with automated ABR (AABR) predischarge (actually an immediate-repeated AABR), with refers going to Dx ABR. Risk+ babies have an additional AABR screen postdischarge, with refers in the second AABR going to Dx ABR. Babies with no identified risk indicator (R−) are typically screened predischarge with AOAE then AABR in the AOAE refers; this is usually followed by an outpatient AABR rescreen with overall refers going to Dx ABR. The simplified cost-efficiency analysis in the text addresses paths A and B as alternatives for a single risk group that is Risk+ and Risk++ combined. It illustrates an approach to the question of whether and under what conditions the repeated AABR is preferred.

With the parameters used, the baseline (Path A) operating cost per baby screened is $31. Because of the low refer rate (0.04 or 4%), only one in 25 babies refers to diagnostics and the average diagnostic cost per baby screened ($6) is less than 20% of this overall cost. If pathway cost reduction were part of a CQI focus on efficiency, the cost of the initial AABR seems a reasonable place to look. The simple analysis also shows that for every true case identified, the path with ABR rescreening saves on average $100 units of cost. To put this in perspective, to identify one case you must screen 100 high-risk babies (prevalence = 0.01) for an overall cost of $3,100. Saving $100 in $3,100 is about 3%, which seems to put the extra step into question. Note that we did not assume that the cost of an outpatient ABR equals that of a predischarge ABR; we assumed it cost more, because of contact and scheduling overheads. Another factor is cost to families, which were not included but arguably should be.

If direct costs to the family for test attendance were added into the equation, then because costs to families for the initial AABR are usually negligible but outpatient testing costs families in time off work, travel and other overheads, the effective, overall cost of second ABR and the diagnostic would go up, but the difference in those costs would probably increase because of the extra time needed for a diagnostic ABR. In effect, this means that the ratio $C2/D$ becomes smaller.

Typically, such calculations are followed by sensitivity analysis, which involves adjusting each parameter by some reasonable boundary of possible error, usually 10% to 20% in each direction. For example, obviously the saving would vanish if the second ABR cost 75 units or if two thirds or more of the babies referred on it. In contrast, if the initial AABR refer 10% ($r1 = 0.1$) and the second AABR passed four out of five of them ($r2 = 0.2$), then the saving is $600 on a base of $3,100, which is worth thinking about.

This simple example addressed at risk babies with a single AABR screening versus a series repeated AABR, but a more complex version would have to take into account the overall proportion of babies who bypassed screening per protocol. There might then be three paths of overall throughput to diagnostics for babies at risk: a direct path for those at highest risk (such as symptomatic CMV or an affected sibling) or for whom screening is unfeasible or inappropriate (such as bilateral atresia), a single, predischarge AABR for those at intermediate risk, and possibly a series repeated AABR for those at the lowest level of risk.

Babies at no known risk (the vast majority) might be subject to a different path entirely, typically one that involves initial OAE screening with AABR (single or repeated) in the OAE refers.

Whatever the efficiency question being addressed is, and regardless of whether it is being addressed in a program development phase or in a potential QI context of an established program, the analysis is going to be multiparametric, and it is crucial to take the most comprehensive possible view of costing and to employ stringent and careful sensitivity analysis and worst-case scenario development. In a fast PDSA CQI paradigm, a local trial of program pathways change would be absolutely obligatory and would probably be best done with at least two geographically distinct trial groups, given the strong dependence of program performance on context and behavior. One thing is certain: there is currently no single, optimal design that is applicable to all operational contexts. The other certainty is that the temptation to take published test efficacy data and assume that those data will apply in the real, field context must be resisted at all costs.

Program Oversight and Control

Adequate oversight and control are crucial to high, sustained program quality. Oversight refers to a mechanism by which overall program effectiveness, equity, and efficiency are monitored, with accompanying programmatic intervention if deficiencies in performance are detected. Thus, the oversight should embrace all aspects of quality as well as cost effectiveness and cost efficiency. Local or regional program management typically will not have the expertise or big-picture information necessary to detect or address quality shortfalls. Of course, oversight without teeth is somewhat pointless, and the most effective teeth are likely to be budgetary. Therefore, an effective oversight mechanism preferably should include some measure of budgetary and cost-control capability. The detailed mechanisms of oversight are beyond the scope of this chapter but can include statistical review of program inputs, activities, structures, processes, outputs, and real outcomes at the state, regional, or local level, even at the level of individual provider performance. Area variations analysis and cost-workload analysis are important tools. Some programs internationally also include adverse-event-driven or random performance audit of institutions', agencies', or individuals' performance. If done in a constructive manner, such audits can be accepted as beneficial, even necessary, for providers and recipients alike.

The word *control* applies not only to budget but to service practices. For the latter, control is not meant to be taken as meaning some kind of dictatorial restriction of freedom of professional practice. Rather, it refers to mechanisms that promote commonality of goals and practice styles, adoption of well-defined, evidence-driven procedural protocols and methods of ensuring and verifying achievement of desired clinical outcomes in an efficient and consistent manner. The best practice control mechanisms are those that are driven by professional integrity, consensus and drive for quality, putting quality of service above personal opinions and idiosyncrasy of viewpoints. The tendency toward adoption of evidence-based practices can be very helpful in this regard, provided that it is taken seriously and does not descend into a waving around of decision-makers' favorite, often discordant, pieces of published evidence.

In the author's experience, it is not unusual to encounter many kinds of passive or active resistance to detailed, mandatory practice protocols. Investment in one's own clinical opinion and perceived expertise is perfectly understandable. However, there is good reason why even expert clinical opinion is the lowest level of scientific evidence. In fact, rigorous, evidence-driven protocols are an important tool for enhancing program quality, provided it is realized that such protocols do not threaten freedom of practice. Rather, they can encourage easier achievement of minimum practice standards and focus professional skills on the unique characteristics and needs of individual patients or clients. Another objection often voiced is that protocols do not accommodate the diversity and individuality of children and families. Given a well-designed protocol, that is a misconception. People like their coffee in various ways, but boiling the water is a universally valid component, and attention can be directed at what blend, how strong, and how much sugar.

Finally, the author's quality-oriented lessons learned after decades of program design and evaluation are painfully simple despite the amount of time it took to really get it: (a) It is all about the people, not the devices. (b) It is not about what *you* think, but what *they* think. (c) Most people are trying their best, so do not pick holes in them, just help them. (d) Carrots or chocolate might work, sticks and stones never do. It all sounds a bit like a recipe for CQI, doesn't it?

Concluding Examples

Refer to Table 16–3.

Table 16–3. Screening Process Elements and Related Continuous Quality Improvement (CQI) Topic Examples

Preinformation	Public and professional information and engagement (websites, posters, handouts, articles, media events, physician office visits, prenatal classes, etc.). *CQI: Done? Family awareness, take-home messages received, perceived usefulness?*
Target identification	Program awareness of live birth, availability, currency, and accuracy of birth information *CQI: Were live births missed? Is birth-rate information adequate for coverage calculation? Are birth and screening data accurately matched for cohort dates?*
Candidature	Which, if any, babies are not screening candidates—demographically, administratively? *CQI: Are exclusion criteria justified, correctly implemented?*
Access	Logistical ability to access babies and families at the right time, especially predischarge. *CQI: Proportion of timely access? Barriers to access? Safety net for unaccessed babies?*
Explain need and process	Why should we screen your baby's hearing now? What does the screening involve? *CQI: Explained well? What did families understand? Scripts well-designed, followed?*
Consent and contact information	Obtain informed consent per protocol. Obtain primary and secondary contacts. *CQI: Was consent protocol followed? Was explicit or implied consent documented? What proportion did not consent? Was any nonconsent rescue procedure followed? Were two or more independent contacts obtained?*
Risk assessment	Determine defined permanent hearing loss risk indicators per protocol. *CQI: Were risk indicators missed or falsely identified? Can risk indicator wording, sources of risk information, or screener understanding be improved?*
Test pathway selection	If differential testing pathways (e.g., screening technology, direct to assessment, or test deferral) are specified, route baby to correct path. *CQI: Were path decisions correct?*
Explain testing	Tell the caregiver what is about to be done, what participation is desired, and why. *CQI: Did families feel that the testing was explained to their satisfaction?*
Conduct testing	Navigate through, and adhere to, single-stage or multistage screening protocol. *CQI: Multiple options related to test completion rate, success rate, refer rate magnitude and consistency, protocol adherence, test timing, number of screen attempts, aborts, repeats, technical skills (e.g., probe insertion, electrode attachment), baby handling skills (e.g., quieting), quality of interactions with family (e.g., calmness, respectfulness, empathy, knowledge, professionalism)*
Explain results	Explain what the results do and do not mean regarding presence of hearing loss now and in the future. If the baby has referred, manage and adapt to family's state of mind. The desired state is understanding, acceptance, constructive concern, and intent to follow through, not anxiety, denial, or dismissal. *CQI: Rate of assessment attendance, causes of nonattendance, timeliness of attendance, use of scripts at screening, avoidance of common explanatory errors, family perceptions of quality of explanation, and understanding of recommended actions and their rationale*
Documentation	Data entry and clinical report generation. *CQI: Timeliness, completeness, and correctness of entered data; match between entered data and clinical report; receipt of reports; tracking failures*

References

Andermann, A., Blancquaert, I., Beauchamp, S., & Dery, V. (2008). Revisiting Wilson and Jungner in the genomic age: A review of screening criteria over the past 40 years. *WHO Bulletin*, *86*(4), 241–320. Retrieved June 24, 2010, from http://www.ncbi.nlm.nih.gov/pmc/articles/PMC2647421/

Berwick, D. M. (2002). A user's manual for the IOM's "Quality Chasm" report. *Health Affairs*, *21*(3), 80–90. doi:10.1377/hlthaff.21.3.80

Centers for Disease Control and Prevention: U.S. Department of Health & Human Services. (1999). Framework for program evaluation in public health. *MMWR Recommendations and Reports*, *48*(RR11), 1–40.

Centers for Disease Control and Prevention: U.S. Department of Health & Human Services. (2012). *Introduction to program evaluation for public health programs: A self-study guide.* Retrieved May 2015, from http://http://www.cdc.gov/eval/guide/CDCEvalManual.pdf

Darabi, A. (2002). Teaching program evaluation: Using a systems approach. *American Journal of Evaluation*, *23*, 219–228.

Donabedian, A. (1966). Evaluating the quality of medical care. *Milbank Memorial Fund Quarterly*, *44*(2), 166–203.

Donabedian, A. (1988). The quality of care. How can it be assessed? *Journal of the American Medical Association*, *260*(12), 1743–1748.

Gremler, D. D. (2004). The Critical Incident Technique in service research. *Journal of Service Research*, *7*(1), 65–89.

Grosse, S. D., & Ross, D. S. (2006). Cost savings from universal newborn hearing screening. *Pediatrics*, *118*(2), 844a–845a.

Institute of Medicine (IOM; 2001). *Crossing the quality chasm: A new health system for the 21st century.* Washington, DC: National Academy Press.

Joint Committee on Infant Hearing (JCIH; 2007). Year 2007 position statement: Principles and guidelines for early hearing detection and intervention programs. *Pediatrics*, *120*, 898–921.

Kahan, B. (2008). *Review of evaluation frameworks.* Retrieved July 2015, from http://www.idmbestpractices.ca/pdf/evaluation-frameworks-review.pdf

Keren, R., Helfand, M., Homer, C., McPhillips, H., & Lieu, T. A. (2002). Projected cost-effectiveness of statewide universal newborn hearing screening. *Pediatrics*, *110*(5), 855–864.

Neumann, K., Nawka, T., Wiesner, T., Hess, M., Böttcher, P., & Gross, M. (2009). Quality Assurance of a universal newborn hearing screening. Recommendations of the German Society of Phoniatrics and Pediatric Audiology [Article in German]. *HNO*, *57*(1), 17–20. PMID:19145420

New Zealand Ministry of Health. (2012). *Quality improvement review of a screening event in the Universal Newborn Hearing Screening and Early Intervention Programme.* Wellington, New Zealand: Author. Published online January 31, 2013.

Porter, H. L., Neely, S. T., & Gorga, M. P. (2009). Using benefit-cost ratio to select Universal Newborn Hearing Screening test criteria. *Ear and Hearing*, *30*(4), 447–457.

Radawski, D. (1999). Continuous Quality Improvement: Origins, concepts, problems and applications. *Perspective on Physician Assistant Education*, *10*(1), 12–16.

Russ, S. A., Hanna, D., DesGeorges, J., & Forsman, I. (2010). Improving follow-up to newborn hearing screening: A learning-collaborative experience. *Pediatrics*, *126*(Suppl. 1), S59–S69.

Samson, D., & Terziovski, M. (1999). The relationship between total quality management practices and operational performance. *Journal of Operations Management*, 17(4), 393–409.

Schroeder, L., Petrou, S., Kennedy, C., McCann, D., Law, C., Watkin, P., . . . Ho, M. Y. (2006). The economic costs of congenital bilateral permanent childhood hearing impairment. *Pediatrics*, *117*(4), 1101–1112.

Uus, K., & Bamford, J. (2006). Effectiveness of population-based newborn hearing screening in England: Ages at identification and profile of cases. *Pediatrics*, *117*(5), e887–e893.

Wholey, J. S., Hatry, H. P., & Newcomer, K. S. (Eds.). (2004). *Handbook of practical program evaluation* (2nd ed., p. 720). San Francisco, CA: Jossey-Bass.

Wilson, J. M. G., & Jungner, G. (1968). *Principles and practice of screening for disease.* Geneva: World Health Organization. Public Health Paper # 34. Retrieved June 24, 2010, from http://whqlibdoc.who.int/php/WHO_PHP_34.pdf

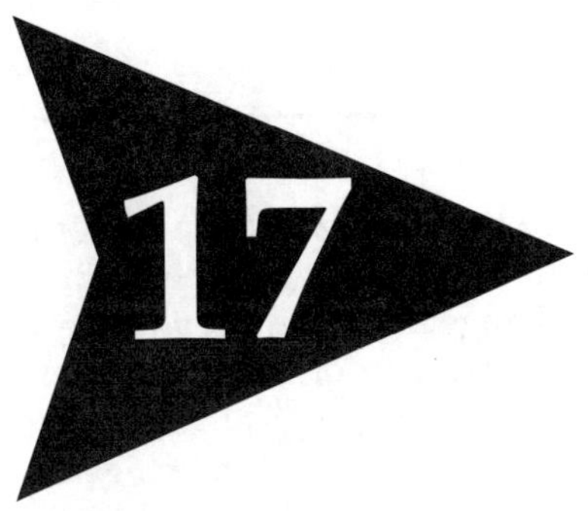

Screening for Hearing Loss and Middle Ear Disorders: Beyond the Newborn Period

Jackson Roush and Nicole E. Corbin

Introduction

Screening for hearing loss in children was among the first public health initiatives undertaken in the United States over 70 years ago. Schools, clinics, and health departments have employed a variety of hearing screening methods to identify children needing referral for comprehensive assessment. Methods have also been developed for detection of middle ear disorders. Considering the long history of screening for hearing loss and middle ear disorders, one would expect to find consistent and well-standardized protocols and procedures. Instead there remains considerable variability in screening procedures and, in many cases, limited evidence to support current practices. Some screening protocols appear to be guided more by history than by evidence. This chapter examines behavioral and physiologic screening for hearing loss and middle ear disorders in the months and years that follow the newborn period, with emphasis on older infants and children from preschool to school age. The chapter provides an evidence-based review of methodology and screening protocols as well as a review of instrumentation, personnel, follow-up, and other factors that must be considered in the design, implementation, and evaluation of a screening program. Where evidence is lacking, we highlight areas of need for future research.

Purpose of Screening

The purpose of screening is to identify children most likely to have a targeted disease or disorder in need of treatment. It is important to differentiate screening from diagnostic procedures. Screening is applied to populations with no apparent signs or symptoms of the target disorder. Diagnostic procedures, which are more time consuming and expensive, are applied only to a subset of individuals who are more likely to have the disorder. Thus, screening can be defined as an activity that separates individuals with high and low probability of a disease or disorder, from the general population. Decisions regarding whether to screen for a disease or disorder are guided by several considerations (Feightner, 1992; Hall, 2015; Roush, 2001):

- *Importance to society:* Each disease or disorder has a cost to society. The greater the societal cost, the greater is the justification for screening.
- *Diagnostic criteria:* There must be a clear and measurable definition of the disease or disorder and a gold standard diagnostic test.
- *Availability of treatment:* For those identified by screening, there must be treatment available that is known to be effective.
- *Access to those who will benefit:* The target population must be available and accessible.
- *Resources and compliance:* Resources needed for diagnosis and treatment must be available, and those referred must be willing to comply with recommendations for follow-up.
- *Feasibility of the screening test:* To be accepted by the public, by program administrators, and by those responsible for screening, the test must be rapid, inexpensive, easy to administer, and acceptable to the person screened.
- *Program evaluation:* The screening program must have a monitoring and evaluation process to determine

its efficacy and to allow for modifications based on experience and accumulated evidence.

- *Costs and benefits:* For each screening outcome, there are costs and benefits. Costs are determined by the number of individuals who actually have the condition in proportion to the total number screened and the expenses associated with the screening process; costs are also influenced by the number of incorrect screening outcomes. Benefits generally are associated with correct screening outcomes.

Screening Test Characteristics

A screening *test* result can be positive, suggesting increased risk for the target disorder and need for referral, or negative, suggesting no risk or reduced risk. However, a screening *outcome* can only be determined based on the results of a subsequent "gold-standard" diagnostic test. A positive screening test (fail) that subsequently results in a positive diagnostic test would be a *true positive*; that is, it occurs when the target condition is correctly identified. This outcome is likely to be beneficial because treatment that otherwise might have been denied or delayed can be provided. Screening can also result in a *true negative*—that is, a negative screening test (pass) confirmed by a negative diagnostic test in an individual who is truly free of the condition. A true negative is beneficial because the patient or the parents are reassured of the condition's absence at the time of the test. A *false positive* occurs when the screening results indicate the need for referral but a subsequent diagnostic test indicates absence of the condition. This outcome is costly from a financial standpoint because it entails unnecessary diagnostic procedures. It is also costly in human terms if patients or their families are needlessly concerned or inconvenienced. Finally, a *false negative* occurs when the screening procedure indicates a pass when the disorder is, in fact, present. This is considered the most serious error because the screening procedure fails to uncover an existing disorder. The costs associated with a false negative can include harm to the patient (exacerbation of the condition, delayed or inappropriate intervention or educational placement), increased cost to the health care system, and misinformation conveyed to the family.

To determine the performance of a screening protocol, it is necessary to calculate its *validity*. Several terms developed in the field of clinical epidemiology are useful in this regard. The first is *prevalence*, which is defined as the number of cases of a disease existing in a population during a specified time period. Prevalence rate is the proportion of the population that has the condition at a point in time. A related term sometimes mistakenly used interchangeably with prevalence is *incidence*. Incidence is the number of new cases identified over a given period of time, typically one year. Incidence rate is often reported as a fraction of the population at risk of developing the disease or condition of interest, for example, 1 per 1,000.

In addition to the incidence or prevalence of a disorder, determining the validity of a screening procedure requires calculation of *sensitivity* and *specificity*. Sensitivity refers to the percentage of people with a given disorder who screen positive—that is, the rate of correct classification for affected individuals. It is calculated by dividing the number of true positives by all those in the screened group with the disorder (the sum of the true positives and false negatives), or

$$Sensitivity = \frac{TruePositives}{TruePositives + FalseNegatives} \times 100$$

Thus, if 100 infants have a hearing loss and the screening is able to identify 90 of them as having the condition, the screening has a sensitivity of 90%.

In contrast, specificity refers to the test's accuracy in correctly identifying persons who *do not* have the condition—that is, the rate of correct classification for unaffected individuals. It is calculated by dividing the number of true negatives by all those in the screened group without the disorder (the sum of the true negatives and false positives), or

$$Specificity = \frac{TrueNegatives}{TrueNegatives + FalsePositives} \times 100$$

Thus, if 100 infants have normal hearing and the screening is able to classify 90 of them as normal, the test has a specificity of 90%.

The ideal screening test would have high sensitivity and high specificity, meaning that false negatives (misses) as well as false positives (unnecessary referrals) are few. However, there is an important trade-off between sensitivity and specificity, the extent of which is determined by the pass-fail criteria—that is, the rules that define a pass or a fail on a given screening test. The relationship between sensitivity and specificity is illustrated in Figure 17–1.

Figure 17–1 shows two hypothetical distributions, one representing individuals without the disorder of interest (nondisease curve) and the other representing those with the disorder (disease curve). In this example, the two groups have very different screening outcomes. As is typical of most screening scenarios, there

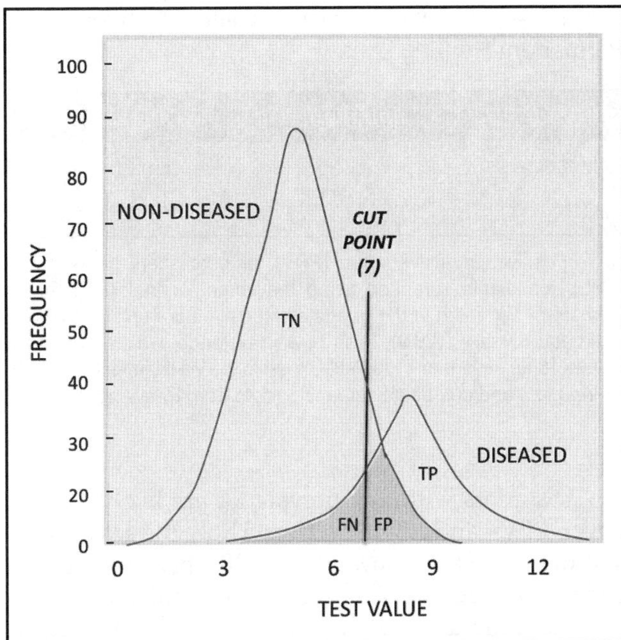

FIGURE 17–1. Hypothetical screening distributions showing the overlap of diseased and nondiseased populations. (TN, true negative; TP, true positive; FP, false positive; FN, false negative.)

are relatively fewer people with the disorder. Also, affected individuals show greater variability in their test results (i.e., wider range of results). For example, in Figure 17–1, the population without disease (nondisease curve) exhibits hypothetical screening results with test values ranging from approximately 0 to 9. In contrast, the population with disease (disease curve) exhibits hypothetical screening results with test values ranging from approximately 3 to 13. Note that the two distributions overlap from about 3 to 9, meaning that there are a few individuals without the disorder whose screening outcome measures were unusually high, and a few with the disorder whose measures were unusually low. This outcome, which is typical of most screening tests, shows overlapping distributions for those with and without the disease along the continuum of screening test outcomes. The outcome is illustrated by the shaded area where the false negatives (FN) and false positives (FP) overlap. If the two distributions were completely separated along that continuum, one could pick a test score that perfectly divides the two groups. But as illustrated in Figure 17–1, most screening procedures result in an area of overlap where the test cannot differentiate normal from abnormal. In this example, the clinician must choose a cut point (vertical black line) above which the screening is considered positive and below which the screening is said to be negative. The cut point will determine the number of true positives (TP; area under the disease curve, to the right of the cut point), false positives (FP; area under the nondisease curve to the right of the cut point), true negatives (TN; area under the nondisease curve to the left of the cut point), and false negatives (FN; area under the nondisease curve to the left of the cut point). Moving the cut point to the left would increase the sensitivity, but the trade-off would be lower specificity, as more nondisordered individuals would be referred. Conversely, moving the cut point to the right would increase the specificity at the expense of lower sensitivity. The cut point can be adjusted differently depending on the purpose of the screening and the implications of an incorrect outcome.

In assessing a screening procedure, it is also important to consider the *predictive value*. *Positive predictive value* (PPV) refers to the percentage of cases with positive screening outcomes that are found, by diagnostic evaluation, to actually have the disorder. Stated differently, PPV indicates the likelihood of the target condition being present when the screening test is positive. In contrast, *negative predictive value* (NPV) refers to the percentage of cases with negative screening outcomes that are found, by diagnostic evaluation, to be free of the disorder. A test's predictive value is especially important to clinicians because the goal of the practitioner is to apply a screening test to determine whether *an individual child* has the disorder (PPV) or does not have the disorder (NPV). The PPV is calculated by dividing the number of true positives by all positives, or

$$PPV = \frac{TruePositives}{TruePositives + FalsePositives} \times 100$$

The NPV is determined by dividing the number of true negatives by all negatives, or

$$NPV = \frac{TrueNegatives}{TrueNegatives + FalseNegatives} \times 100$$

Unlike sensitivity and specificity, which remain the same regardless of disease prevalence, predictive value is heavily influenced by the prevalence of the disorder being screened. This is illustrated in Figure 17–2, which includes calculation of sensitivity, specificity, and predictive value.

Note that prevalence has no effect on sensitivity or specificity, whereas predictive values are greatly affected by prevalence. This is because in the computing of predictive values the denominator represents the total number screened with a positive test (PPV) or

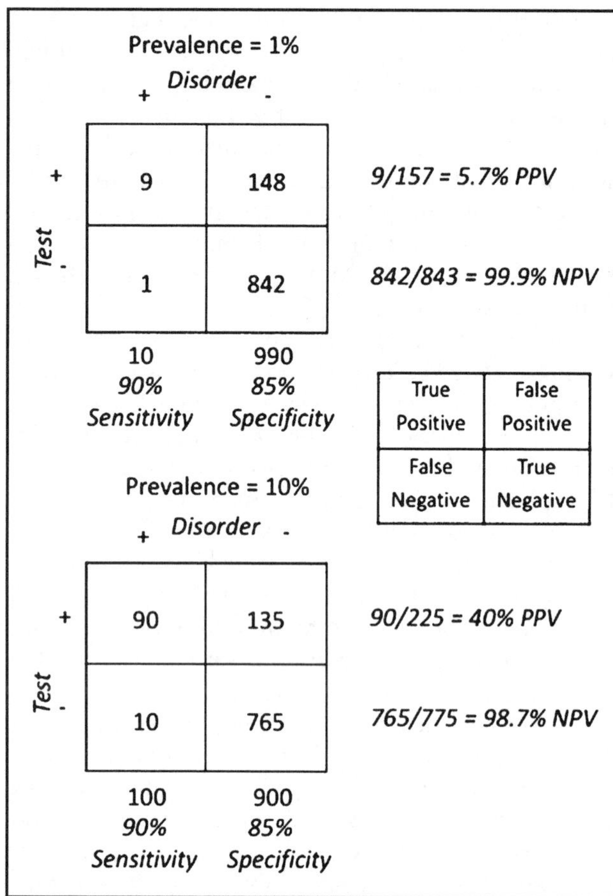

FIGURE 17–2. Two-by-two matrices of hypothetical data illustrating the effects of disease prevalence on test performance. In both cases, the test has sensitivity of 90% and specificity of 85%; however, positive predictive value (PPV) changes considerably with the increase in disease prevalence. NPV = negative predictive value; adapted from Nozza, 1996.

negative test (NPV), which will vary with prevalence even when sensitivity and specificity remain the same.

The effect of prevalence on PPV is illustrated in a study by Prieve et al. (2000) that compared hearing screening outcomes in the well-baby nursery (WBN) to those observed in the neonatal intensive care unit (NICU), where the prevalence of permanent hearing loss was approximately 10 times higher (Prieve & Stevens, 2000). Infants who did not pass an auditory brainstem response (ABR) screening were referred for diagnostic ABR assessment. As expected, the PPV for permanent hearing loss was significantly higher in the NICU than in the WBN for both inpatient and outpatient screening (Table 17–1).

Table 17–1. Positive Predictive Value (PPV) for Permanent Hearing Loss

PPV for PHL	*Inpatient Fail*	*Outpatient Fail*
NICU	12.5%	25.9%
WBN	2.2%	17.9%

Note. Positive predictive value (PPV) for permanent hearing loss (PHL), for infants screened using the same technology (auditory brainstem response) in the neonatal intensive care unit (NICU) and well-baby nursery (WBN). Note how prevalence, which is approximately 10 times higher in the NICU than in the WBN, affects the PPV for inpatient and outpatient screening (data from Prieve et al., 2000).

Disorders with low prevalence are likely to have lower PPVs and higher NPVs. Thus, the less prevalent the disease, the lower is the PPV because the proportion of true positives is smaller. Similarly, the less prevalent the disease, the higher is the NPV because of the larger proportion of true negatives. Because the status of each individual is unknown at the time of screening, knowledge of the predictive value for each screening procedure is vitally important. But despite their importance, predictive values are often among the least understood screening principles. Without them, however, a screening protocol cannot be properly evaluated. Moreover, consideration only of sensitivity and specificity without regard to predictive value can result in a distorted view of how well a screening protocol is performing. Measures of predictive value require an understanding of their relationship to sensitivity and specificity, and what can be done to improve them. In particular, it is important to remember that the vast majority of individuals screened in any program will *not* have the target condition. Hence, the false positives are derived from this relatively large pool of individuals. Consequently, low PPV is usually caused not only by the low prevalence of the disorder, but by low specificity as well. Even a small reduction in specificity can result in a large decline in PPV, because the proportion of individuals without the disorder is so great. Thus, the goal is to increase sensitivity with minimal effect on specificity. There are at least two ways this might be accomplished. One way is to limit screening to those individuals already known to be at increased risk. But the disadvantage of this approach in many screening contexts is that relatively few individuals have known risk factors. Thus, improving PPV might occur at the expense of lower sensitivity and delayed treatment. A more favorable approach might be to do repeated measures or a multiple-stage screening procedure. A rescreening or a two-stage approach might involve rescreening with the same technology or a different technology. In a two-stage protocol, the patient who fails the first screen is rescreened using the second technology and must also fail that test before being referred for diagnostic testing. If the number of referrals can be lowered by rescreening, the rate of false positives and the corresponding specificity and PPV will improve. It should be remembered, however, that multiple screening procedures increase the amount of clinical time and, in some cases, the instrumentation and space required, thus adding to the overall cost of the program. Multiple screening procedures also increase the burden on the child and family, at least for affected individuals who screen positive both times. Furthermore, multiple rescreenings can increase the possibility of a false-negative outcome. Each of these factors must be considered based on the goals of the screening program, the costs and benefits derived, and individual circumstances unique to each setting.

A key point here is that sensitivity and specificity must be known prior to implementing the screening program. This requires a comparison of screening test data with diagnostic test results in a controlled study representative of the population to be screened. Determination of disease prevalence requires diagnostic testing applied to a large number of cases in the target population. Even when accomplished, however, this only provides an *estimate* of the disorder's prevalence within a given population. Ideally, data on sensitivity and specificity will be monitored over time within the screening program, and adjustments will be made to pass-fail criteria as appropriate. Specificity is especially hard to monitor because those who pass the screening are typically not followed diagnostically. Furthermore, those who pass typically constitute a much larger group than those who fail. Following this large group to determine specificity is not practical within a screening program and, in fact, would defeat the purpose of screening. It is, however, possible to periodically check a small sample of those who pass to ensure that the false-negative rate is in line with the goals and objectives of the screening program.

Screening for Hearing Loss

Prevalence of Permanent Hearing Loss

Sensory/neural hearing loss is the most common abnormality affecting newborn infants in the United States and in most developed countries. Because of differences in data collection and reporting across the United States, prevalence estimates vary among studies and are often reported as a range. Population-based estimates of the prevalence for moderate-to-profound permanent hearing loss in one or both ears at infancy range from 1 to 3 per 1,000 (0.1 to 0.3%; CDC, 2013a; Finitzo, Albright, & O'Neal, 1998; Mauk & Behrens, 1993; Vohr, Carty, Moore, & Letourneau, 1998), whereas milder degrees of permanent hearing loss in infants account for a prevalence of approximately 0.55/1,000 (0.06%; Gravel et al., 2005). The prevalence of permanent hearing loss is at least 10 times higher for infants whose birth history required admission to the NICU, with a prevalence ranging from 8 to 20 per 1,000 or 0.8 to 2% (Gerber, 1990; Mauk, White, Mortensen, & Behrens, 1991; Prieve et al., 2000; Stein, 1999). Most permanent hearing losses detected in the NICU are cochlear in origin; however, NICU history is also an important risk factor for auditory neuropathy (Berg, Spitzer, Towers, Bartosiewicz, & Diamond, 2005), a condition characterized by absent or abnormal auditory brainstem response (ABR) in the presence of intact cochlear hair cell function (Starr, Sininger, & Pratt, 2000). The condition has also been called auditory neuropathy/dys-synchrony Joint Committee on Infant Hearing (JCIH, 2007) and more recently, auditory neuropathy spectrum disorder (ANSD) to account for its variable nature and etiology (Guidelines Development Conference on the Identification and Management of Infants with Auditory Neuropathy, 2008). ANSD is more prevalent than once thought and is now believed to affect 7% to 10% of all children with sensory/neural hearing loss (Madden, Rutter, Hilbert, Greinwald, & Choo, 2002; Rance, 2005).

Children with congenital *conductive* hearing loss comprise another special population of permanent hearing loss. Some of the congenital conditions associated with permanent conductive hearing loss, such as aural atresia, are apparent at birth. Others, due to ossicular fixation or other middle ear anomalies, can be more insidious and difficult to detect.

The overall prevalence of permanent hearing loss in children appears to increase during the preschool years. Bamford et al. (2007), in the United Kingdom, examined the prevalence of sensory/neural hearing loss at school entry, noting that among approximately 3.5 per 1,000 children known to have permanent hearing loss at school entry, nearly 1.9 in 1,000 required identification *after* the newborn screen. There is evidence of further increase in permanent hearing loss during the school years. Estimates vary based on methodological differences; however, two investigations published in

1998 (Bess, Dodd-Murphy, & Parker, 1998; Niskar et al., 1998) found a prevalence of sensory/neural loss ranging from 11% to 15% in school-age children when all types and degrees of hearing loss were included. Both studies reported a variety of audiometric configurations with more unilateral than bilateral hearing losses. For hearing losses greater than 20 dB HL in the "speech frequencies," Mehra, Eavey, and Keamy (2009) estimated a prevalence of 3.1% for all children and youth; the prevalence was relatively higher for Hispanic-American children and those from low-income households. Lack of standardized protocols for detecting, documenting, and reporting postnatal-onset hearing loss prior to school entry make it difficult to estimate the prevalence of delayed-onset hearing loss.

The reasons for the increasing occurrence of permanent hearing loss from birth to school age are not fully understood, but several contributing factors are evident. Some infants with congenital hearing loss are missed at newborn screening, possibly due to the degree, configuration, or nature of their hearing loss. Other contributing factors include illness during the neonatal period or birth at a facility that does not perform universal newborn hearing screenings (Bamford et al., 2007; Beswick, Driscoll, & Kei, 2012; Christensen, Thomson, & Letson, 2008). Others might be unreported, lost to follow-up, or lost to documentation (Mason, Gaffney, Green, & Grosse, 2008), and still others can have progressive or acquired sensory/neural hearing loss due to genetic disorders, infectious diseases, exposure to noise, ototoxic medications, or other environmental hazards. Additionally, errors by screening personnel can produce false negatives or lead to miscommunication of screening results (Thompson et al., 2001). A screening pass might also create a sense of false security among caregivers regarding later-onset hearing loss (Thompson et al., 2001). Of particular concern is the number of children with mild hearing loss who appear to be missed by newborn screening. In the study by Bess et al. (1998) cited earlier, the prevalence of mild permanent unilateral and bilateral hearing loss was estimated to be 54 per 1,000 (5.4%). These findings suggest that current screening outcomes do not account for the number of children who present with mild bilateral or unilateral hearing loss in later childhood (Gravel et al., 2005). Clearly, there is room for improvement in current surveillance protocols and a need to develop more uniform and reliable screening methods for early detection of postnatal-onset hearing loss in preschool-age children (Beswick, Driscoll, & Kei, 2012; Bhatia, Mintz, Hecht, Deavenport, & Kuo, 2013; Lü et al., 2014).

Justification for Hearing Screening Beyond the Newborn Period

The detrimental effects of hearing loss on speech, language, and educational development are well established (e.g., Moeller, Osberger, & Eccarius, 1986). Even minimal hearing loss, including mild or unilateral impairment, has been associated with psychosocial delays, poorer health-related quality of life, and compromised academic performance (Bess et al., 1998; Borton, Mauze, & Lieu, 2010; Porter, Sladen, Ampah, Rothpletz, & Bess, 2013). The estimated lifetime educational cost of moderate to profound permanent hearing loss was $115,600 in the year 2007 (Grosse, 2007), and the expected lifetime cost of prelingual deafness exceeds $1,000,000 (Mohr et al., 2000). Thus, it can be assumed that untreated or late-identified childhood hearing loss is costly not only to the affected individual, but also to society. As the prevalence of hearing loss in children increases over time, the societal and economic impacts of hearing loss after the newborn period are likely to increase as well (Vasconcellos, Colello, Kyle, & Shin, 2014). Moreover, there is the intrinsic right of children to hear and for families to be informed when their child's access to sound is compromised. Fortunately, there is growing evidence that early identification and intervention for young children with congenital hearing loss results in favorable developmental, societal, and economic outcomes (Moeller, 2000; Yoshinaga-Itano, Sedey, Coulter, & Mehl, 1998). Consequently, neonatal hearing screening is now considered a standard of care across the United States, and over 97% of newborns are screened for hearing loss prior to hospital discharge (Centers for Disease Control and Prevention [CDC], 2013a). It is important to emphasize, however, that even well-managed programs are unlikely to screen 100% of their newborns prior to hospital discharge. Furthermore, among those who are successfully screened but do not pass, an alarming number are lost to follow-up. In some states, the proportion of infants unreported or lost to follow-up is nearly 50% (CDC, 2013d). Also, as noted earlier, there is the potential for missed screenings, loss to follow-up, missing documentation, late-onset or progressive cochlear impairment, and undetected auditory neuropathy spectrum disorder. In addition, a substantial number of children experience chronic conductive hearing loss secondary to otitis media. For all of these reasons, ongoing surveillance of hearing status in children is essential.

Does this mean every child should undergo multiple hearing screenings after the newborn period, even if there are no hearing concerns or risk factors? This is an important question and one that has been answered differently by various professional organizations and public health agencies. Recommendations for hearing screening have been published by the American Speech-Language-Hearing Association (ASHA, 1997), the American Academy of Audiology (AAA, 2011), and the American Academy of Pediatrics (AAP; Harlor, Bower, & Committee on Practice and Ambulatory Medicine, and Section on Otolaryngology-Head and Neck Surgery, 2009). It is important to emphasize, however, that policies regarding implementation and management of hearing screening programs are determined at the state and local levels. All 50 states in the United States currently provide *newborn* hearing screening, but there is considerable variability in policies and procedures for screening that occurs after the newborn period. Some states have both legislative mandates and detailed protocols for hearing screening. Others have neither a legislative requirement nor statewide policies for screening beyond the newborn period, leaving decisions to individual health departments, school districts, and local educational agencies. Federal guidelines require that children in the United States receiving health care through the Medicaid program be monitored according to the guidelines established for Medicaid's Early and Periodic, Screening, Diagnosis and Treatment (EPSDT) well-child examination program. In 2004, the EPSDT screening guidelines committee recommended that hearing screenings be performed according to the methodology and periodicity guidelines established by the AAP. The most recent AAP guideline is titled, "Hearing Assessment in Infants and Children: Recommendations Beyond Neonatal Screening" (Harlor et al., 2009). Key points from this document call for periodic "objective screening" (e.g., otoacoustic emissions in the medical home of all children at 4 to 6 years, 8 years, and 10 years of age), and surveillance for children with one or more risk indicators. The document also calls for careful attention to parental concern regarding a child's hearing status; application of pneumatic otoscopy and tympanometry; referral to a pediatric audiologist for children who do not pass the screening; and comprehensive audiologic and otologic assessment for children with developmental abnormalities or behavioral conditions that preclude routine screening. The AAP recommendations emphasize the importance of interdisciplinary management and appropriate intervention for children with confirmed hearing loss. In summary, there is strong evidence to support screening after the newborn period whenever there are caregiver concerns or risk indicators for late-onset hearing loss. It is also recognized that hearing screening should be provided periodically for all children, even in the absence of concerns or risk indicators. States and municipalities vary substantially with regard to how and where screenings are performed and in the methodology employed. The recommendations of the AAP (Harlor et al., 2009) provide an important commitment from the medical community and a useful framework for physicians willing to conduct hearing screening in the medical home; however, implementation of these recommendations and evaluation of their efficacy will take time and additional research. In the meantime, programs for early hearing detection and intervention (EHDI), state health departments, and school-based hearing screening programs must work together to achieve functional, well-coordinated policies, procedures, and referral criteria. The process must consider the advantages and limitations of each screening method and the issues relevant to various special populations of infants and children.

Methods of Screening for Hearing Loss

Over the years, various institutions and professional organizations have published numerous guidelines and position statements related to high-risk and universal screening. Although the recommended protocols and procedures vary, there are certain characteristics required of any screening test. A good screening test is one that is simple and rapid to administer, safe, inexpensive, widely available, and acceptable for participants and their families (Association for Prevention, Teaching, & Research, 2015). Current methods of screening for hearing loss include behavioral procedures, physiologic procedures, and combined protocols that include both behavioral and physiologic methods. In the following sections we consider the advantages and disadvantages of each.

Behavioral Hearing Screening Procedures

It is well established that behavioral hearing screening cannot be reliably conducted in the newborn period (JCIH, 1971). Once infants reach a developmental age of 5 to 6 months, however, behavioral assessment is possible using visual reinforcement audiometry (VRA; Widen et al., 2000). For typically developing infants, VRA can be used for behavioral hearing screening or to estimate hearing threshold levels. Because the VRA technique requires specialized instrumentation and the expertise of a pediatric audiologist, however, it cannot be routinely applied as a tool for behavioral hearing screening outside the pediatric audiology clinic.

Screening children in the age range of 2 to 4 years can be challenging even for pediatric audiologists. The experienced clinician is often able to adapt behavioral methods to combine VRA with conditioned play procedures using a method known as *visual reinforced operant conditioning audiometry* (VROCA). As with VRA, however, the procedure cannot be used outside the pediatric audiology clinic because it requires specialized instrumentation and expertise. For these reasons, physiologic methods, described later in the chapter, are often preferred for routine screening of children in this age group.

Once a child reaches the chronological age of 3 to 4 years, pure-tone audiometry can be performed using developmentally appropriate assessment procedures. Behavioral pure-tone screening has been employed for decades by a variety of health care professionals. It is typically conducted at a fixed intensity of 20 dB HL at the frequencies 1000, 2000, and 4000 Hz (AAA, 2011; ASHA, 1997). Depending on the goals of the screening program and the target population, other frequencies can be included (AAA, 2011; Holmes, Niskar, Kieszak, Rubin, & Brody, 2004). However, when incorporating additional frequencies, it is important to establish the accuracy of instrument and environmental calibration and the sensitivity and specificity of test results obtained (Schlauch & Carney, 2011). A hearing screening pass requires repeatable responses in each ear to all stimuli (AAA, 2011; ASHA, 1997). It is recommended that children who do not respond at any frequency in either ear undergo an immediate rescreen by another tester with a different audiometer (AAA, 2011).

When accurate and reliable pure-tone screening is possible, there are several advantages. The portable audiometers typically employed are relatively inexpensive and uncomplicated, and because behavioral pure-tone screening involves the auditory system at all levels, it can be considered a true hearing test in the perceptual sense. There are, however, a number of limitations. First, behavioral screening requires an experienced examiner with the qualifications needed to select and apply developmentally appropriate methods and materials. It also requires a cooperative child capable of attending and responding appropriately to the test stimuli. Additionally, pure-tone screening necessitates an acoustic environment that is quiet enough to meet published standards for allowable levels of ambient noise (ANSI S3.1, 1999, 2008).

Considering the many prerequisites and potential pitfalls associated with behavioral pure-tone screening, it is not surprising that the procedure has resulted in mixed success. In a study of approximately 3,500 kindergarten and first-grade children using well-prepared examiners in a controlled acoustic environment, Fitz-Zaland and Zink (1984) reported sensitivity and specificity of 93% and 99%, respectively. A far less favorable outcome was reported by Halloran, Hardin, and Wall (2009) when pure-tone screening was conducted in a primary care medical setting. In the study by Halloran and colleagues, which involved approximately 1,000 preschool- and school-age children screened in eight pediatric medical offices using conventional pure-tone screening procedures, sensitivity and specificity was only 50% and 78%, respectively. Other investigators have encountered similar challenges including Sideris and Glattke (2006) who reported that nearly two thirds of the 2- to 5-year-old children referred from pure-tone screening could not be reliably conditioned to respond. Thus, pure-tone screening can be applied successfully for identification of hearing loss in preschool- and school-age children, but only under relatively ideal conditions. Because of the difficulties associated with behavioral pure-tone screening, there is growing interest in the use of physiologic measures, not only for newborns, but for screening older infants and preschool-age children.

Physiologic Screening Procedures

The physiologic procedures most commonly used to screen for sensory/neural hearing loss are based on the recording of ABR and otoacoustic emissions (OAE), including transient-evoked otoacoustic emissions (TEOAE) and distortion product otoacoustic emissions (DPOAE). Because these technologies are objective in nature, they can be applied to a variety of pediatric populations, including those too young for behavioral screening or those with developmental delays that preclude behavioral screening. There are important differences between the two technologies, and it is important to consider the advantages and limitations of each.

OAEs, recorded from a microphone placed in the external ear canal, are cochlear responses generated by the outer hair cells in response to acoustic stimuli. As such, they provide useful information regarding the *preneural* status of the auditory system. In contrast, ABRs, recorded from surface electrodes attached to the head, reflect neural activity in the auditory nerve and brainstem. Thus, OAEs provide an assessment of cochlear (outer hair cell) function, while ABRs provide a measure of neural integrity and synchrony beyond the level of the cochlea in the auditory nerve and brainstem. OAE screening with clicks or multiple frequencies provides a relatively broadband test of the cochlea, whereas click-evoked ABR screening is dominated by a more restricted range of frequencies in the region of 2000 to 4000 Hz. Although neither method is considered a true test of hearing in the perceptual sense, both ABRs and OAEs are sensitive to abnormalities at different levels of the auditory system making them useful for both screening and diagnostic assessment.

OAEs can be applied to awake children at any age using a variety of screening personnel. In contrast, ABR screening can be performed during natural sleep for the first few months of life. After 4 to 6 months of age, ABR often requires sedation or anesthesia, and thus is usually carried out in a clinical setting by an audiologist. The two technologies also differ with regard to the nature of the physiologic recording. Because OAEs require the conductive pathway for both delivery of the acoustic stimulus and for reverse transmission of the low amplitude cochlear emissions, middle ear status affects OAEs to a greater extent than ABR. Emissions are generally absent in the presence of middle ear effusion (Lonsbury-Martin, Martin, McCoy, & Whitehead, 1995; Margolis & Trine, 1997; Owens, McCoy, Lonsbury-Martin, & Martin, 1993) and even negative middle ear pressure can obscure their measurement (Marshall, Heller, & Westhusin, 1997; Prieve, Calandruccio, Fitzgerald, Mazevski, & Georgantas, 2008; Trine, Hirsch, & Margolis, 1993). Thus, a child with a normal cochlea can fail an OAE screening because of middle ear abnormalities.

Finally, the two technologies differ in their ability to detect disorders of the auditory pathway beyond the level of the cochlea. Because OAEs are generated by the outer hair cells in the cochlea, they are unaffected by disorders of the auditory nerve or brainstem pathway. Most permanent hearing loss in children is cochlear in origin with involvement of the outer hair cells. Hence, with appropriate test protocols and pass-fail criteria, OAEs provide a useful screening tool for even mild hearing losses. If the goals of the screening program include detection of ANSD, however, ABR is the screening procedure of choice (JCIH, 2007).

Although the focus of this chapter is on screening after the newborn period, a discussion of newborn hearing screening is relevant because the outcome at initial screening will impact the number of children requiring later identification and follow-up. In general, OAE screening in the newborn nursery has been considered faster than ABR and less costly with regard to consumable supplies needed for each screen (electrodes and ear couplers for ABR versus disposable probe tips for OAEs). In recent years, technologies using chirp stimuli have reduced ABR test time and eliminated the need for disposable supplies (van Dyk, Swanepoel, & Hall, 2015). Still, many newborn hearing screening programs employ both OAE and ABR using a two-step protocol that uses OAEs for the initial screen followed by automated ABR for infants who do not pass the OAE. The two-step protocol, whereby the child must fail both stages in order to be referred, is designed to improve specificity and reduce the number of infants requiring follow-up. Johnson et al. (2005) evaluated the sensitivity of a two-step protocol in a study that included VRA at 9 months as a gold standard for assessing the accuracy of OAE and ABR screening for infants who failed the initial screen. Their findings indicated that combining the two technologies resulted in a lower fail rate but at the expense of lower sensitivity. Specifically, nearly a quarter of the infants with confirmed hearing loss would have passed the ABR screening. Not surprisingly, most of those infants had mild cochlear hearing losses. Johnson and colleagues note that this finding is due, in part, to the fact that most ABR screening instruments are designed to identify infants with moderate or greater degrees of hearing loss. One of the fundamental principles of screening, that of defining the target disease or disorder, is relevant here. As typically applied in a screening environment, neither automated ABR or OAE screening is highly sensitive to mild cochlear hearing loss. As a result, audiologists responsible for infant screening programs must consider the feasibility of targeting mild hearing loss when relying on automated ABR or OAE screening (Gravel et al., 2005). There are trade-offs in screening that require balancing many factors including the nature of the disorder, the performance of the screening test, costs associated with screening/referral, and the implications of delayed identification and intervention. Most would agree, however, that missing over 20% of infants with congenital and early onset hearing loss in infancy (White et al., 2005) is an unacceptable scenario that places an even greater burden on screening after the newborn period (Gravel et al., 2005). Both ABR and OAE, as typically applied for infant hearing screening, are limited in their ability to detect mild degrees of hearing loss (e.g., 25 to 35 dB HL). A large multicenter study funded by the National Institutes of Health compared the relative sensitivity of TEOAEs with ABR (Gorga et al., 2000; Norton et al., 2000; Sininger et al., 2000). Each method performed well in the identification of moderate, severe, and profound hearing loss. The study also found similar pass rates for ABRs, TEOAEs, and DPOAEs but with mild hearing loss detected at a rate of only about 50% (Prieve, 2008). It is important to note, however, that there are important differences between OAE screening applied to the infant population compared to the same technology used with the preschoolers and school-age children. These differences are examined in the next section.

OAEs for Preschool- and School-Age Screening

Compared with the many studies of OAEs applied to newborn hearing screening, far fewer have investigated OAE screening in toddlers, preschoolers, and school-age children. The studies that have employed OAEs beyond the newborn period reveal generally good test characteristics, comparable to other methods. But the studies are difficult to compare because of differences in the degree of hearing loss targeted; the population of interest; stimulus and recording variables; pass-fail criteria; and test environment (Dille, Glattke, & Earl, 2007; Driscoll, Kei, & McPherson, 2001; Eiserman et al., 2008; Glattke, Pafitis, & Cummiskey, 1995; Lyons, Kei, & Driscoll, 2004; Nozza, Sabo, & Mandel, 1997; Shi et al., 2000; Sideris & Glattke, 2006). There is also evidence of differences in performance for TEOAEs and DPOAEs when applied to screening (Dille et al., 2007; Shi et al., 2000). Still, a growing body of evidence shows that OAEs can be applied successfully in primary care, preschool, and educational settings (Eiserman et al., 2008; Foust, Eiserman, Shisler, & Geroso, 2013; Sideris & Glattke, 2006; Taylor & Brooks, 2000). Foust et al. (2013) demonstrated that a multistep OAE hearing screening protocol with children 0 to 5 years of age in clinic settings was effective in identifying children with permanent hearing loss at a rate of 1.2 per 1,000, a rate similar to studies conducted with children 0 to 3 years of age in educational settings (Eiserman et al., 2008).

Those responsible for the screening of toddlers, preschool-, and school-age children are faced with an important decision regarding selection of physiologic versus behavioral screening methods. A recent evidence-based review of the literature is relevant here. In 2015, Prieve, Schooling, Venediktov, and Franceschini conducted a comprehensive review comparing the accuracy of pure-tone and OAE screening for identification of hearing loss in preschool- and school-age children. Eighteen studies published between 1975 and 2013 met the selection criteria which included measurement of behavioral hearing thresholds. Sensitivity and specificity, used to calculate positive and negative likelihood ratios for comparison of the two methods, revealed considerable variability among studies in reference to stimulus levels, response criteria, and definition of hearing loss. Acknowledging these limitations, the analysis revealed that both pure-tone and OAE screening were useful in identifying hearing loss in preschool- and school-age children; however, pure-tone screening was shown to have higher sensitivity. This is an important finding based on a rigorous and systematic review. But as stated by the authors, further research is needed to control for each of the variables noted above.

Considering the many challenges associated with behavioral pure-tone screening, improving the sensitivity of OAE as applied to preschool- and school-age children is an important priority. Dhar and Hall (2012) point out that the sensitivity of OAEs can be significantly increased by incorporating stimulus and recording parameters that are more rigorous than those typically applied in infant OAE screening. Citing the work of Gorga and colleagues at Boys Town National Research Hospital (Gorga, Neely, Dorn, & Hoover, 2003; Gorga et al., 2000), Dhar and Hall (2012) and Hall (2015) recommend a two-part criterion that includes a signal-to-noise ratio >6 dB *combined* with an absolute DP amplitude >0 dB SPL. Dhar and Hall (2012) and Hall (2015) note that this two-part criterion should result in detection of cochlear hearing loss at a level of sensitivity comparable to behavioral pure-tone screening at 20 dB HL, but with the advantages of reduced test time and greater overall efficiency. It should be noted that increasing the sensitivity of OAEs might occur at the expense of higher refer rates, but as Dhar and Hall (2012) point out, the consequences of a preschooler not passing an OAE screen are modest in comparison to those associated with a newborn screening failure. That is, *infants* who fail OAE screening generally require referral and follow-up with a pediatric audiologist, whereas preschoolers who do not pass OAE screening can simply be retested in the same session with behavioral pure-tone hearing screening.

The choice of behavioral pure-tone versus OAE screening requires careful consideration of many variables including the developmental age of the child and the skills of the screening personnel. Audiologists responsible for designing and implementing a screening program must be guided by the goals of the program, the target population, and available resources. If the program can ensure qualified and well-trained personnel combined with a suitable acoustic environment and children who are willing and able to respond appropriately, behavioral pure-tone screening might be the method of choice. But if one or more of these prerequisites is lacking, OAE might be preferable, although it must be kept in mind that successful OAE screening also requires qualified personnel, a suitable environment, and cooperation from the children. And as emphasized earlier, OAE sensitivity and specificity will be impacted by instrumentation variables and pass-fail criteria. Both pure-tone and OAE screening can be successfully employed for detection of hearing loss in preschool- and school-age children, but the advantages and limitations of the two methods, applied alone or in combination, must be well understood and fully appreciated.

Screening for Middle Ear Disorders

Prevalence of Middle Ear Disease

Otitis media is a highly prevalent disease that affects nearly all children at least once during early childhood. In fact, middle ear disease is cited as the most frequently diagnosed pediatric disease (Daly & Giebink, 2000). The incidence is affected by seasonal variation and other factors. However, it is estimated that over one third of preschool-age children experience recurrent otitis media and concomitant conductive hearing loss. Otitis media has its highest incidence before 2 years of age, although some pediatric populations are at risk throughout childhood (Daly et al., 2010). Those at highest risk include children in group daycare and those exposed to passive cigarette smoke. Others at risk include indigenous groups (e.g., American Indians) and children with predisposing conditions (e.g., Down syndrome, craniofacial anomalies).

Screening for Middle Ear Disorders: Is There Justification?

In contrast to hearing screening, which is widely accepted as necessary and appropriate, screening for middle ear disorders has been the subject of considerable discussion and debate for many years (Bluestone et al., 1986; Northern, 1992). From its inception as a clinical tool in the 1970s, tympanometric screening for asymptomatic otitis media with effusion (OME) has been questioned by the medical community and by some audiologists. Although single-frequency tympanometry using a single low-frequency probe tone has been shown to have good sensitivity for detection of middle ear effusion (MEE), the natural history of otitis media and lack of consensus regarding its sequelae have caused many to question its appropriateness for mass screening. Much of the controversy has been due to high false-positive rates when tympanometry is applied to large numbers of preschool- or school-age children. Early immittance screening protocols recommended medical referral based on abnormality of a single tympanometric screen (ASHA, 1979). This resulted in dissatisfaction from both pediatricians and parents when, by the time the child was seen for medical examination, many of the middle ear disorders had resolved (Bess, 1980; Bluestone et al., 1986; Roush & Tait, 1985).

It is now recognized that OME is usually a transient condition that resolves within a few weeks without treatment in over 50% of cases (Rosenfeld & Kay, 2003). It might or might not cause significant hearing loss, and its prevalence varies with age, time of year, and a variety of environmental factors (Bluestone & Klein, 2007; Daly & Giebink, 2000). If the decision is made to include screening for middle ear disorders, it must be applied judiciously as part of a comprehensive program designed to identify children with chronic or recurrent middle ear disorders, while minimizing false-positive medical referrals. The clinical practice guidelines for OME, revised by a subcommittee of the American Academy of Family Physicians, the American Academy of Otolaryngology-Head and Neck Surgery, and the American Academy of Pediatrics (2004), discourage mass tympanometric screening and recommend that population-based screening programs for OME not be performed in healthy, asymptomatic children. Screening for middle ear effusion is clearly justified, however, for children who are at high risk for otitis media. This would include children with predisposing conditions such as cleft palate or Down syndrome. Tympanometric screening also is justified for children likely to suffer adverse consequences from even a mild conductive hearing loss. Included in this group are children already experiencing developmental delays and those with concomitant sensory/neural hearing loss. Monitoring of middle ear status is especially important for children who use amplification because the benefits of hearing aid use can be seriously compromised by a transient conductive component.

Although population-based screening for OME is not recommended, tympanometric screening can be included in hearing screening programs as a second-stage screening method following the failure of a pure-tone hearing or otoacoustic emissions screening (AAA, 2011). When conducted in this manner, tympanometric screening can elucidate the nature of the failed hearing screen and inform the referral process (AAA, 2011). Decisions regarding inclusion of tympanometric screening in a preschool or school setting (i.e., as part of a hearing screening program) are often made by school administrators based on the advice of a consulting audiologist. It is incumbent upon audiologists responsible for these programs to consider the advantages and controversies associated with screening for middle ear disorders, as well as the epidemiological principles of screening in general. They should be familiar with local and state regulations pertinent to screening, and willing to consider the recommendations of the medical community as reflected in various practice guidelines and position statements. Where inconsistencies exist, it is important to communicate directly with health care providers in the community to achieve consensus on screening and referral criteria. Given their higher risk for hearing screening failure due to middle ear effusion, the AAA guidelines recommend consideration of tympanometric screening for children in preschool, kindergarten, and first grade (AAA, 2011).

Methods of Screening for Middle Ear Disorders

Tympanometry

If the decision is made to include tympanometric screening, it should be preceded by visual inspection of the external ear to detect observable signs of disease or malformation. The outer ear examination is followed by otoscopic inspection. Visual and otoscopic inspection are essential to identify conditions requiring immediate medical attention and to ensure that the ear canal is free of obstructions that might cause injury or affect screening results. Immittance screening criteria, protocols, and procedures have been outlined by several professional organizations. Although some of these recommendations were published over a decade ago, most are still applicable. AAA published a position statement in 1997 entitled *Identification and Diagnosis of Hearing Loss and Middle-Ear Dysfunction in Preschool and School-Age Children*; a similar document was issued by ASHA, *Guidelines for Audiologic Screening* (1997). The recent Childhood Hearing Screening Clinical Practice Guidelines published by AAA (2011) also address immittance screening. The recommendations contained in the AAA (1997, 2011) and ASHA (1997) screening documents are guided by two general tenets: (a) referral for medical examination should not be based on a single tympanometric screening; a follow-up test should occur at some later point in time, for example, in 4 to 6 weeks, to determine if there is evidence of persistent MEE, and (b) tympanometric data should be interpreted based on quantitative values rather than gross pattern detection. The latter recommendation is based on the fact that the A-B-C pattern-identification method of classification originated with tympanograms from impedance meters that used arbitrary units of measurement (Jerger, 1970; Liden, 1969). In 1987, standards for acoustic immittance instruments were developed (ANSI, 1987) that required direct measurement of acoustical admittance or impedance using absolute physical values to quantify, rather than qualify, the tympanogram. The resulting tympanometric patterns were not consistent with those from early impedance meters. Although many clinicians have developed their own criteria for classifying tympanograms according to A, B, and C patterns, there is no standard for such a classification and, therefore, is considerable variability among clinics and screening programs with regard to A-B-C classification. In addition, the pattern classification system gives weight to tympanometric peak pressure, a measure shown to be ineffective in the detection of MEE (Nozza, Bluestone, Kardatzke, & Bachman, 1994; Smith et al., 2006). Furthermore, the A-B-C classification system does not incorporate measures of tympanometric shape or gradient. In particular, tympanometric width (TW) has been shown to have good performance in identifying MEE. With current instruments, peak admittance and TW values are consistent across instruments, and there are data available relating these values to identification of MEE (Margolis & Heller, 1987; Nozza, 1998; Nozza et al., 1994; Roush, Drake, & Sexton, 1992; Smith et al., 2006). For these reasons, tympanometric screening should be interpreted quantitatively using evidence-based pass-fail criteria consistent with the goals of the middle ear screening program.

The tympanogram is quantified using four measures: equivalent volume (ml), tympanometric peak pressure (daPa), peak acoustic admittance (Peak Y in mmho), and TW (daPa). The pass-fail criteria recommended by AAA (1997, 2011) and ASHA (1997) are similar and are based on research designed to estimate sensitivity and specificity (Nozza, Bluestone, Kardatzke, & Bachman, 1992; Nozza et al., 1994; Roush, 1990; Roush & Tait, 1985; Silman, Silverman, & Arick, 1992). For example, the AAA (2011) Childhood Hearing Screening Clinical Practice Guidelines suggest that failure of a tympanometric screening for children ages 3 years and older be identified as TW > 250 daPa or Peak Y 0.2 < mmho. Tympanometric peak pressure greater than −200 daPa to −400 daPa might also result in a tympanometric screening failure; however, it does not warrant medical referral by itself. AAA (2011) states these criteria should not be applied to children who have abnormally large ear canal volumes with known pressure equalization tubes, or to children of Asian heritage who might have Peak Y < 0.2 mmho. ASHA Guidelines (1997) recommend a referral from an initial screening be made for children age 1 year through school age if Peak Y is less than 0.3 mmho or TW > 200 daPa. ASHA Guidelines (1997) recommend slightly different criteria for infants 6 to 12 months of age: Peak Y < 0.2 or TW

> 235 daPa (Roush, Bryant, Mundy, Zeisel, & Roberts, 1995). Chapter 19 in this volume provides a summary of several studies reporting normative data for various age groups.

The guidelines published by AAA (1997, 2011) and ASHA (1997) do not differentiate between the general population and high-risk groups in their recommended pass-fail criteria for MEE. For instance, the AAA (1997, 2011) and ASHA (1997) pass-fail criteria might not be appropriate for children who have a genetic disorder associated with smaller ear canal volumes such as Down syndrome. However, it is important to remember that the prevalence of the disorder in the population being tested will affect predictive values. Therefore, it is advisable to consider different criteria for different populations. Having good prevalence data for the target population is essential for estimating predictive values (Nozza et al., 1994). Current technology for tympanometric screening relies almost exclusively on measurement of acoustic admittance. A low-frequency (226 Hz) probe tone is commonly used for tympanometric screening in children over the age of 4 to 6 months. It should be noted that if tympanometry is used before 6 months of age, it is necessary to employ a high-frequency probe tone (e.g., 1000 Hz) and apply normative data for young infants (Kei, Mazlan, Hickson, Gavranich, & Linning, 2007; Margolis, Bass-Ringdahl, Hanks, Holte, & Zapala, 2003). See Chapter 19 of this volume for additional information regarding high-frequency and multifrequency tympanometry.

Clearly, there are many issues that need to be taken into account when tympanometry is used to screen for MEE. Decisions regarding pass-fail criteria must consider normative data and research findings on sensitivity and specificity, but they must also consider instrumentation variables, the population screened (especially age and prevalence of MEE), available resources for rescreening and follow-up, and most importantly, agreement between the screening fail criteria and the definition of the disorder according to the diagnostician. Referrals from a screening program that result in too many false positives according to the diagnostic practitioner will result in failure of the screening program.

When planning a program to screen for middle ear disorders, audiologists must determine if the goal is to detect *any* middle ear disorder or only MEE, and whether the program seeks to identify children with MEE at a single point in time or the subset of children with chronic conditions. Those responsible for the supervision of screening programs should monitor outcomes associated with screening, and communicate with local health care providers to determine if changes in referral criteria are needed. Achieving an acceptable balance between sensitivity and specificity requires thoughtful consideration of the issues noted above and careful evaluation of screening outcomes.

Is There a Dual Role for OAE in Screening for Middle Ear Disorders and Cochlear Hearing Loss?

In addition to their role in assessing cochlear function, OAEs provide a sensitive index of middle ear status that can provide useful clinical information in patients with a variety of middle ear abnormalities (Dhar & Hall, 2012; Koivunen, Uhari, Laitakari, Alho, & Luotonen, 2000; Lyons et al., 2004; Nozza et al., 1997). Because OAEs are typically abnormal in ears with hearing loss or middle ear disorders, a group of children screened with OAEs could produce referrals that include cochlear hearing loss, middle ear disorders with or without concomitant conductive hearing impairment, or a combination of these conditions. A few false positives would likely be included as well. Ears that pass the OAE screen would be assumed to have hearing threshold levels ≤25 to 35 dB HL and normal middle ear function. Those not passing the OAE screen would undergo tympanometry. This would be a small subset of the target population, making the number of children requiring both tests significantly reduced in comparison to a protocol requiring a hearing test (e.g., pure-tone screening or OAE) and tympanometry on all children. For example, even if 20% to 30% fail the initial OAE screening, 70% to 80% of the children would likely pass and not need a second screening test. Those who fail the initial OAE screening and demonstrate *abnormal* tympanometry would follow the protocol for immittance screening and return at a later date (e.g., 4 to 6 weeks) for tympanometric rescreening. If the child passes the tympanometric rescreening or is found by medical examination to be free of middle ear disease, a repeat OAE or behavioral hearing screening could be provided to rule out permanent hearing loss. A child referred from OAE screening who exhibits *normal* tympanometry would be considered at risk for cochlear hearing loss and referred to a pediatric audiologist for comprehensive assessment.

The suggestion that OAE might be useful for both hearing screening and detection of MEE was initially made in the context of school-age children (Nozza et al., 1997). Since then, the combined protocol has been explored with younger children (Hunter, Davey, Kohtz, & Daly, 2007). It is important to remember that this approach will be influenced by the age and demographics of the target population, the setting in which the screening is performed, and the skill of the examiners. Also, young children (4 years old) have a higher prevalence of MEE than school-age children, so a higher proportion will fail OAE screening. In nearly all cases, an OAE fail will be due to a middle ear disorder rather than cochlear hearing loss. This raises an important philosophical question regarding the use of OAE for detection of MEE. When normal cochlear function cannot be demonstrated, there is heightened concern regarding the possibility of permanent hearing loss even if the failed screen is likely due to a middle ear disorder. Thus, it is important to consider the potential for over-referring children for comprehensive audiologic assessment when the underlying cause is MEE. This issue comes down to the goals of the screening program as illustrated by Ho, Daly, Hunter, and Davey (2002). Ho and colleagues performed OAE and tympanometry in a group of children ranging in age from birth to 5 years, in a study designed to evaluate the concordance of tympanometry and TEOAE and how these measures compared to physician findings. Their results suggest that TEOAE screening is a useful complement to tympanometry screening and that the combination is more effective than either technique alone because both conductive and sensory/neural hearing loss, as well as middle ear effusion, can be detected with the combined measures. Ho and colleagues concluded that if the goal of a screening program is to detect sensory/neural and conductive hearing loss, then TEOAE screening alone would be effective in accomplishing that goal. However, if the goal is to detect OME, then both tympanometry and TEOAE screening are recommended.

It is important to emphasize that OAE screening is susceptible to environmental noise and noise generated by the child. When measuring OAEs in a clinical setting with a parent or caretaker present, movement and noise can often be controlled. In contrast, when OAEs are measured in a pediatrician's office or preschool setting, noise and other distractions can produce an excessive number of unsuccessful or false-positive results, thus diminishing the overall performance of the screening protocol (Nozza, 2001). This, in fact, was the outcome reported by Hunter et al. (2007) in a cohort of approximately 400 American Indian children followed prospectively from birth to 2 years of age. Hunter and colleagues found OAE screening to be challenging with these youngsters, even when employing well-trained examiners. A more favorable experience was reported by Eiserman et al. (2008) in a study that used "lay screeners" to assess 4,500 preschoolers in multiple child care settings and in the primary care setting.

Regardless of setting, the outcome of an OAE screening program will be influenced by several factors including the examiner's level of skill and experience with OAEs, the physical state of the child, noise levels, and the stimulus and recording parameters employed by the screening instrument.

Wideband Acoustic Immittance

Another method for assessing middle ear function that has undergone substantial refinement in recent years is based on analysis of acoustic reflectance. Sound introduced into the ear canal is reflected off the tympanic membrane in a manner that is influenced by the admittance characteristics of the middle ear. If the middle ear has normal admittance characteristics, sound will pass through easily and little will be reflected. Conversely, if the middle ear has low admittance, as with MEE, more sound will be reflected back into the ear canal. Different technologies use different means of quantifying reflectance; some measure the amplitude of the response, whereas others consider the broadband frequency response. A potential advantage of reflectance over traditional immittance testing is that it uses a wideband stimulus (e.g., a chirp) and therefore measures transfer of sound through the tympanic membrane across a range of frequencies, not just at a single probe frequency (e.g., 226 Hz).

There has been considerable research over the years on the potential role of acoustic reflectance for identification of MEE and other middle ear abnormalities (Babb, Hilsinger, Korol, & Wilcox, 2004; Hunter, Tubaugh, Jackson, & Propes, 2008; Lampe, Weir, Spier, & Rhodes, 1985; Teele & Teele, 1984; Vander Werff, Prieve, & Georgantas, 2007). An early device still commercially available, the *EarCheck Middle Ear Monitor*, is marketed to pediatricians and consumers for quick and easy screening for MEE; however, it has been met with mixed results. Data are limited on the sensitivity and specificity of the device, and it has reportedly lacked acceptance in the medical community because of difficulty setting standards and establishing pass-fail criteria (Waseem & Aslam, 2008). A study in Finland by Teppo and Revonta (2009) examined the diagnostic accuracy of the *EarCheck* monitor in a prospective study of preschool-age children that compared the results of acoustic reflectometry performed by parents, to otomicroscopic myringotomy conducted immediately following reflectometry. Their findings indicated good performance in identifying MEE. However, the authors emphasize, that parents performed the reflectance measures in the hospital shortly after being instructed in the use of the instrument and that all children in the study had chronic MEE or "glue ear." Thus, their findings might not easily be generalized to screening at home in the general population where various degrees of middle ear disease would be encountered. It should also be noted that the *EarCheck* instrument is not recommended for use with young infants or with children who have craniofacial abnormalities.

A more technically sophisticated and evidence-based approach to analyzing reflectance and absorbance of acoustic energy for middle ear assessment is known as *wideband acoustic immittance* (WAI). WAI has been studied in newborns (Abdala, Keefe, & Oba, 2007; Keefe et al., 2000; Hunter et al., 2010) and in typically developing infants and young children (Sanford & Feeney, 2008; Vander Werff et al., 2007). Although much of the research has been done in laboratory settings, two commercially available instruments designed for clinical use are now available. WAI has the potential to improve clinical diagnosis of auditory pathology in patients of all ages with various types of middle ear disease, and audiologists involved with screening for middle ear disorders should be familiar with this technology and aware of future developments. However, further research is needed before WAI is recommended for widespread implementation as a middle ear screening tool. See Chapter 19 in this volume for additional information on wideband acoustic immittance and related measures.

Special Populations and Settings

The issues outlined in the foregoing discussion apply to most settings where screening is conducted. There are additional considerations, however, that pertain to special populations of children based on age, risk factors, and setting. These include infants in the neonatal intensive care unit (NICU); older children with risk factors; and routine screening of preschool and school-age children.

Infants in the Special Care Nursery

The NICU provides specialized treatment in a hospital setting for infants with prematurity or serious illness. Special care facilities for infants are classified by the AAP as Level I Nurseries, which provide basic care to well infants; Level II Nurseries, which provide specialty care for infants at moderate risk of serious complications; and Level III Nurseries where infants receive specialty and subspecialty care including mechanical ventilation (Stark & American Academy of Pediatrics Committee on Fetus and Newborn, 2004). Infants requiring special care in the NICU represent approximately 10% of the newborn population or about 400,000 infants per year (JCIH, 2007).

Several reports have shown that infants whose birth histories include hospitalization in the NICU are at increased risk for both cochlear hearing loss and ANSD (Berg et al., 2005; D'Agostino & Austin, 2004). As noted earlier, the prevalence of sensory/neural hearing loss in the NICU population is at least 10 times higher than it is in the well-infant population, and studies have shown that NICU history is a significant risk factor for ANSD (Xoinis, Weirather, Mavoori, Shaha, & Iwamoto, 2007). Consequently, the JCIH recommends separate hearing screening protocols for the NICU and well-infant nurseries (JCIH, 2007). Specifically, for infants in the NICU who are at greatest risk for auditory impairment (defined as those admitted to the NICU for more than 5 days), ABR screening is recommended to avoid missing ANSD. JCIH further recommends that infants who do not pass an initial ABR screen in the NICU be referred directly to an audiologist for rescreening. The JCIH 2007 position statement also recommends that infants requiring readmission in the first month of life (NICU or well infant) for conditions associated with potential hearing loss (e.g., hyperbilirubinemia requiring exchange transfusion or culture-positive sepsis), undergo a repeat hearing screening with ABR prior to discharge.

Table 17–2 provides a summary of risk indicators for hearing loss in children including conditions that require surveillance for late-onset/progressive hearing loss.

Many of these conditions occur more frequently in infants with a NICU history. Of all the pediatric settings where screening is conducted, the prevalence of undetected sensory/neural hearing loss is likely to be the highest in the NICU. Thus, it is vitally important that hearing screening in the special care nursery be conducted with careful attention to optimal test protocols, and that infants who do not pass the ABR screening receive immediate referral to a pediatric audiologist.

Older Infants/Toddlers With Risk Factors

Although most permanent hearing loss in children can be detected at birth, some infants are at risk for later onset sensory/neural hearing impairment (e.g., Lü et al. 2011). Those infants pose a significant challenge for audiologists and EHDI personnel because once they are discharged from the hospital, access for rescreening becomes more difficult. In an earlier JCIH position statement (JCIH, 2000), it was recommended that infants at risk for postnatal hearing impairment be rescreened at intervals of approximately 6 months, until 3 years of age. This recommendation proved to be impractical because of the burden it placed on audiologists and

Table 17–2. Risk Indicators Associated With Permanent Congenital, Delayed-Onset, or Progressive Hearing Loss in Childhood

1. *Caregiver concern* regarding hearing, speech, language, or developmental delay
2. *Family history* of permanent childhood hearing loss
3. Neonatal intensive care of more than 5 days or any of the following regardless of length of stay: *ECMO*, assisted ventilation, exposure to ototoxic medications (gentamycin and tobramycin) or loop diuretics (furosemide/Lasix), and hyperbilirubinemia that requires exchange transfusion
4. In utero infections, such as *CMV*, herpes, rubella, syphilis, and toxoplasmosis
5. Craniofacial anomalies, including those that involve the pinna, ear canal, ear tags, ear pits, and temporal bone anomalies
6. Physical findings, such as white forelock, that are associated with a syndrome known to include a sensory/neural or permanent conductive hearing loss
7. *Syndromes associated with hearing loss or progressive or late-onset hearing loss*, such as neurofibromatosis, osteopetrosis, and Usher syndrome 131; other frequently identified syndromes include Waardenburg, Alport, Pendred, and Jervell and Lange-Nielson
8. *Neurodegenerative disorders*, such as Hunter syndrome, or sensory motor neuropathies, such as Friedreich ataxia and Charcot-Marie-Tooth syndrome
9. Culture-positive *postnatal infections associated with sensory/neural hearing loss*, including confirmed bacterial and viral (especially herpes viruses and varicella) meningitis
10. *Head trauma, especially basal skull/temporal bone fracture* that requires hospitalization
11. *Chemotherapy*

Note. *ECMO* = extracorporeal membrane oxygenation; *CMV* = cytomegalovirus. The risk indicators in *italics* are of greatest concern for delayed-onset hearing loss.

Source: Reproduced with permission from *American Academy of Pediatrics*, *120*(4), 898–921. Copyright © 2007.

referral sources, especially in regions where pediatric audiology services were limited. It was also recognized that there are infants with unknown risk factors who develop late-onset hearing loss. Thus, in the most recent position statement (JCIH, 2007), responsibility for surveillance is shifted to the pediatrician or family physician as part of the child's ongoing care within the medical home (AAP, 2002). According to this recommendation, surveillance does not occur through actual hearing screening but in conjunction with the use of a global developmental screening tool to be administered at 9, 18, 24, and 30 months to all infants or whenever there is parental concern. It is assumed that physicians will refer children with suspected hearing impairment to an audiologist. Unfortunately, there is evidence that some physicians do not encourage appropriate hearing screening and follow-up services, and might even undermine parental compliance with ongoing hearing surveillance (Serpanos & Jarmel, 2007). The JCIH (2007) position statement further advises that the timing and number of hearing reevaluations for children with risk factors be "customized and individualized" based on the likelihood of a subsequent, delayed-onset hearing loss. The JCIH (2007) position statement notes that early and more frequent assessment might be indicated for children with a history of cytomegalovirus infection, syndromes associated with progressive hearing loss, neurodegenerative disorders, trauma, or culture-positive postnatal infections associated with sensory/neural hearing loss. Closer surveillance is also justified for children who have received extracorporeal membrane oxygenation (ECMO) or chemotherapy, and whenever there are caregiver concerns or a family history of hearing loss (see Table 17–2). Finally, according to JCIH (2007), infants who pass the neonatal screening but have a risk factor should undergo at least one diagnostic audiology assessment by 24 to 30 months of age, even in the absence of hearing concerns. (This recommendation was also included in the AAP 2009 recommendations for screening after the newborn period.)

Most of the JCIH (2007) risk factors are not associated with postnatal hearing loss (Beswick, Driscoll, & Kei, 2012). Hence, ongoing hearing monitoring for children who have risk factors not linked to delayed-onset hearing loss is costly and unnecessary. A systematic review of the literature found that asymptomatic cytomegalovirus (CMV) infection, ECMO therapy, congenital diaphragmatic hernia, and persistent fetal circulation (PPHN) were strongly associated with postnatal onset hearing loss (Beswick, Driscoll, & Kei, 2012). There was insufficient evidence to suggest that neonatal toxoplasmosis, low birth weight (≤1,500 g), and preauricular skin tags and ear pits were strongly associated with delayed onset hearing loss (Beswick, Driscoll, & Kei, 2012). Combined with the finding that many children who develop hearing loss postnatally do not have risk factors, there is a need for systematic investigation into the extent to which risk factor registries are sensitive and specific to postnatal onset hearing loss (Beswick, Driscoll, & Kei, 2012; Wessex Universal Neonatal Hearing Screening Trial Group, 1998; Mehl & Thomson, 2002). Second-phase universal hearing screening programs, neonatal CMV screening, and neonatal genetic screening might improve surveillance and early detection of hearing loss in children who pass their newborn hearing screenings but develop hearing loss prior to school entry (Beswick, Driscoll, Kei, & Glennon, 2012). Further research is needed to establish the optimal method for genetic screening in newborns. However, many birthing facilities now perform neonatal CMV screenings, and at least one state, Utah, has passed legislation that directs medical practitioners to test infants who fail newborn hearing screening for congenital CMV and to inform the parents about the possible birth defects associated with CMV (Utah Department of Health, 2015).

The efficacy of a program that places responsibility for early detection of hearing loss in the medical home is yet to be determined. However, it has been shown that many primary care physicians, although concerned about hearing in children, have significant gaps in their knowledge (Moeller, White, & Shisler, 2006). Efforts to educate pediatricians and primary care physicians about risk factors and signs of hearing loss are ongoing, but few studies have prospectively investigated the efficacy of hearing screening in the primary care setting, especially for children under the age of 3 years. Now that most infants undergo hospital-based newborn hearing screening, detection of late-onset sensory/neural hearing loss in the medical home is an important priority for future investigation. Currently, there is no standard for physiologic hearing screening in the medical home, and it has been noted that surveillance through the sole use of questionnaires will only identify about half of children who have postnatal-onset hearing loss (Bhatia et al., 2013; Harlor et al., 2009). Permanent hearing loss in children is of primary concern, but it is also important to identify chronic or recurrent *conductive* hearing loss associated with otitis media. Otitis media remains the most common cause of hearing loss in this age group. In order for detection of hearing loss to occur in the medical home, primary care physicians must have the instrumentation and personnel needed for valid screening. They must also be willing to take the time needed to administer the global developmental screening tools mentioned earlier. These are not trivial expectations in a busy practice but when successful can lead to earlier identification and treatment.

Preschool Children and School-Age Children

Children over 3 years of age present a different set of challenges. Typically they are not seen as frequently in the primary care setting as younger children, but many are in daycare settings or preschools where hearing screening, and in some cases, screening for middle ear disorders, is provided. Many typically developing children 3 years of age and older can be screened using developmentally appropriate pure-tone procedures, but behavioral screening is susceptible to the challenges and limitations described earlier (Allen, Stuart, Everett, & Elangovan, 2004). If personnel from the daycare facility or preschool are involved in screenings, they should be thoroughly trained by an audiologist who also provides oversight and program evaluation. Children who are difficult to screen because of behavioral challenges or those already suspected of having a hearing impairment, developmental delays, or risk indicators for sensory/neural hearing loss, should be referred directly to a pediatric audiologist for comprehensive assessment.

Once children enter school, they are more accessible for screening purposes, but even then significant challenges remain. Hearing screening of school-age children has been conducted in the United States for decades, but despite the long history of school-based hearing screening programs, there is considerable variability in policies, procedures, and protocols. Some states have comprehensive and well-defined policies and procedures; some have even enacted legislation regarding school-age hearing screening. For example, one Midwestern state has a law that requires children to be screened for hearing loss before school entry, between 3 and 5 years. Although the cost-benefit of preschool hearing screening programs requires further evaluation, preschool hearing screening is likely to facilitate earlier diagnosis and intervention for delayed-onset permanent hearing loss in children 3 to 6 years of age (Lü et al., 2014). Upon reaching school age, children are screened in kindergarten and Grades 1, 2, 3, 5, 8, and 11. Annual hearing screening is also recommended for children with known hearing losses, those in special education classes, or those with one or more risk factors. In contrast to this state, which has both a legislative mandate and detailed protocols for implementation, many states have neither a legislative requirement nor statewide policies for screening beyond the newborn period, leaving decisions to individual health departments and local educational agencies. Furthermore, even among school districts that conduct hearing screening through adolescence, fewer than a quarter employ protocols that will detect noise-induced hearing loss (Meinke & Dice, 2007).

Regardless of whether preschool- and school-age screening are provided by legislative mandate or according to policies determined at the local or regional level, many programmatic elements must be considered in addition to the methodological issues reviewed earlier. These components, compiled from several sources (AAA, 2011; ASHA, 1997; Harlor & Bower, 2009; Roush, 1990, 2001) include screening personnel, when to screen, the screening environment, instrument calibration and maintenance, documentation, and follow-up.

Screening Personnel

In the United States and in many other nations, hearing screening must be conducted in accordance with licensing laws and regulations. In most states, a variety of health care providers, support personnel, and even volunteers are permitted to engage in hearing screening. However, it is essential that institutional screening programs be conducted under the general supervision of an audiologist. Although most instrumentation designed for screening is relatively uncomplicated, personnel must undergo comprehensive orientation and training. It is recommended that instruction be provided by an audiologist and that screening personnel be required to demonstrate proficiency in the administration of test procedures and the accurate recording of screening results. With appropriate training and supervision, hearing screening program protocols can provide consistent and accurate screening outcomes, referrals, and diagnoses (Richburg & Imhoff, 2008). Screening programs that involve teleclinical technology have additional requirements for audiological oversight (Lancaster, Krumm, Ribera, & Klich, 2008).

When to Screen

Recommendations vary with regard to age and screening intervals, but it is generally agreed that asymptomatic children without risk factors who passed newborn hearing screening should be screened for hearing loss at least once in the preschool years and at school entry. Most guidelines recommend screening at several different early elementary grade levels. For example, the AAP, in its Recommendations for Preventive Pediatric Health Care (Harlor & Bower, 2009), recommends that hearing screening be performed beyond the newborn period at the age of 4, 5, 6, 8, and 10 years, with yearly "risk assessment" for children who require screening on a more frequent basis. The AAA (2011) Childhood Hearing Screening Clinical Practice Guidelines recommend hearing screening be conducted in preschool, kindergarten, Grades 1, 3, 5, and either 7 or 9. AAA (2011) also recommends including Grade 2 in order to identify a greater proportion of children with new hearing loss rather than adding a higher grade level to the screening protocol. With regard to time of year, hearing screening can be conducted any time; however, for institutional programs, appropriate follow-up and intervention can be initiated early in the school year when screenings are conducted in the fall. Although prevalence rates vary, more children with transient hearing loss due to middle ear disorders are likely to be identified during the fall and winter months. The time of day is also important. Young children usually perform best from mid to late morning. Time of day is less critical for older children and likely will be dictated by instructional schedules.

The Screening Environment

Pure-tone screening requires a quiet environment, free of visual distractions and competing background noise. Table 17–3 provides a summary of permissible noise levels according to the American National Standards Institute (ANSI S3.1, 1999, 2008) for screening at 20 dB HL using supra-aural earphones and insert receivers.

The values shown are sound pressure levels for octave bands. Ambient noise levels must be at or below the levels indicated. It is important to note that ANSI S3.1 requires the measurement of octave or one-third octave bands within the inclusive range of 125 to 8000 Hz, regardless of the test condition or frequency range to be employed (Frank, 2000). It might be necessary for

Table 17–3. Maximum Permissible Ambient Noise Levels for Pure-Tone Screening at 20 dB HL, Using Supra-Aural and Insert Earphones, as Specified in ANSI S3.1-1999

	Supra-Aural Earphone			*Insert Earphone*		
Octave Band Intervals	***125–8000 Hz***	***Screening Level***	***Maximum Allowable Ambient Level***	***125–8000 Hz***	***Screening Level***	***Maximum Allowable Ambient Level***
125	35	20	55	59	20	55
250	25	20	45	53	20	45
500	21	20	41	50	20	41
1000	26	20	46	47	20	46
2000	34	20	54	49	20	54
4000	37	20	57	50	20	57
8000	37	20	57	56	20	57

Note. The ANSI standard requires measurement of octave (or one-third octave) bands within the inclusive range of 125 to 8000 Hz, regardless of the test condition or frequency range employed. If the test room is to be used for pure-tone screening at a fixed intensity, the screening level is added to the maximum permissible noise level at each octave band. Values are in decibel (dB), re: 20 μPa to the nearest 0.5 dB. Reprinted by permission of the Acoustical Society of America, New York, NY.

sound-level measures to be made by an audiologist or acoustic engineer. However, if screening personnel are properly trained and equipped, they can often perform these measures. It is essential that the screening environment meet ANSI specifications for acceptable noise levels. Unfortunately, two practical problems often arise. First, the equipment and personnel needed to accomplish sound-level measurements might be unavailable. Second, even if the measurements are made, ambient levels might vary over time. Screening personnel must exercise good judgment at all times in evaluating the adequacy of the acoustic environment. When sound-level measures are not available or if conditions vary, ANSI S3.1 includes a provision for applying a psychoacoustic check of ambient noise levels, using two listeners known to have normal hearing.

In any screening environment, the supervising audiologist must ensure that screening personnel are not tempted to increase the presentation level when screening is performed in a less than ideal environment. Attempts to compensate for a poor acoustic environment could result in failure to identify a child with a hearing loss whose thresholds are below the screening level. School administrators must understand the importance of an adequate acoustic environment and recognize that time and financial resources will be wasted if children are referred unnecessarily for diagnostic assessment. Research is ongoing to assess the efficacy of audiometric technology that would minimize the issues associated with conducting hearing screenings in nonacoustically treated environments such as school settings. For example, Swanepoel, Maclennan-Smith, and Hall (2013) determined that the use of real-time environmental noise monitoring and insert earphones enclosed by circumaural earcups during audiometric testing can improve reliability of air- and bone-conduction audiometry across acoustic environments. Further research is needed to investigate cost-effective methods to minimize environmental noise and increase the reliability of pure-tone hearing screenings.

Instrument Calibration and Maintenance

All instrumentation employed in the screening program requires calibration checks by a qualified technician at least once each year according to ANSI (1999, 2008) specifications. In addition to formal calibration measures, daily visual inspection and listening checks are essential. It is also important to ensure that equipment is carefully transported to and from screening sites and is well maintained when not in use. Time spent on proper maintenance and handling of equipment will be compensated by fewer repairs, less downtime, and perhaps most importantly, increased accuracy of hearing screening programs. Additionally, appropriate infection control protocols should be followed.

Documentation and Follow-Up

Screening itself does not improve the wellness of children; it is the action taken as a result of screening that leads to improved outcomes. A detailed examination of data management, reporting, and follow-up is beyond the scope of this chapter; however, it is essential that findings are accurately documented and promptly disclosed to parents and caretakers. It also is important to obtain parental consent, when required, and to inform the child's pediatrician or family practice physician of screening results. Communicating the hearing screening results to the child's physician can facilitate timely arrangement of follow-up testing and, potentially, intervention (Harlor & Bower 2009). For permanent conditions or those likely to be chronic or recurrent, it is important to notify school personnel and to make recommendations for environmental modifications when indicated. See DeConde Johnson and Seaton (2011) for additional information on screening and follow-up in the educational setting.

Adolescents and Teenagers: Prevention of Noise-Induced Hearing Loss

Several studies have suggested that adolescents and teenagers are at increased risk for noise-induced hearing loss (NIHL) and tinnitus from exposure to high-intensity sounds related to frequent and prolonged use of personal listening devices (Danhauer et al., 2012; Gilles & Paul Vde, 2014; Henderson, Testa, & Hartnick, 2011; Niskar et al., 1998, 2001; Schlauch & Carney, 2011; Shargorodsky, Curhan, Curhan, & Eavey, 2010; Vasconcellos, Kyle, Gilani, & Shin, 2014; Vogel, Brug, Hosli, Van der Ploeg, & Raat, 2008; Vogel, Brug, Van der Ploeg, & Raat, 2011). Methodological differences among studies make it difficult to determine the prevalence of NIHL in children and young adults, but some studies suggest estimates as high as 12.5% (CDC, 2013b; Niskar et al., 1998, 2001; Henderson et al., 2011). Further complicating an accurate estimate of prevalence is the insidious damage that noise exposure can have on hearing even before it is evident from routine audiometric assessment (Kujawa & Liberman, 2009; Liberman & Liberman, 2015; Schlauch & Carney, 2011). Other factors that confound the comparison and interpretation of studies include lack of case histories and baseline audiograms; inconsistent definitions of NIHL; calibration errors; and test-retest variability (Green, 2002; Schlauch & Carney, 2011). Also, current school hearing screening protocols rarely include additional high-frequency (above 4000 Hz) pure-tone screening to identify NIHL (Meinke & Dice, 2007; Schluach & Carney, 2011). Furthermore, calibration errors and poor test-retest reliability complicate the inclusion of additional high frequencies, such as 6000 Hz, that might be more sensitive to NIHL early in childhood than 1000, 2000, and 4000 Hz which are typically employed in school-based screening programs (Schlauch & Carney, 2011). There is clearly a need for additional research to examine the prevalence of NIHL among adolescents and young adults, and to determine how hearing screening can best identify NIHL in these populations. The CDC currently recommends that hearing screening be conducted at least once during middle school and at least once during high school (CDC, 2013c); however, specific guidelines are not included.

Prevention of NIHL through implementation of effective hearing conservation education constitutes an important and often overlooked component of hearing screening programs (Folmer, Griest, & Martin, 2002; Henderson et al., 2011; Lancaster et al., 2008). Education of students and staff about hearing health, hearing protection, and noise exposure as early as elementary school raises awareness about hearing loss and its prevention (CDC, 2013c; Henderson et al., 2011). Hearing loss prevention education has been shown to influence behavior positively, such that students will take precautions to preserve hearing when exposed to occupational and recreational noise (CDC, 2013c; Gilles & Paul, 2014; Henderson et al., 2011). Recreational noise sources to which children might be exposed include loud music, firearms, and fireworks, among others. The CDC recommends several topics for inclusion in a comprehensive hearing loss prevention program including normal hearing (auditory) function, types of hearing loss and their etiologies, noise sources that contribute to hearing loss, noise and its effects on hearing and quality of life, warning signs of NIHL, and recommendations for preventing hearing loss.

Tinnitus is a related topic that should be included in a comprehensive hearing loss prevention program. Teachers, health care professionals, and volunteers can be trained to provide this education to students and staff (CDC, 2013c). Hearing conservation programs can also include information about other risk factors for hearing loss that have been identified including passive exposure to tobacco smoke (Vasconcellos, Colello, Kyle, & Shin, 2014). By educating children and young adults about the dangers of noise at a young age, hearing screening and conservation programs can help prevent hearing loss and minimize the progression any preexisting impairment.

Screening Beyond the Newborn Period: Challenges, Emerging Technologies, and Future Needs

Hearing screening after the newborn period has existed in one form or another for decades, yet few large-scale prospective studies have addressed the efficacy of preschool- and school-based hearing screening programs. More research is needed to improve understanding of the validity of traditional screening practices as well as the advantages and disadvantages of replacing conventional methods, such as behavioral pure-tone hearing screening, with OAEs or other methods. Research is needed not only to validate hearing screening methods but also to better understand the causes of hearing loss in young children and the reasons for the increasing prevalence of permanent hearing loss after the newborn period. It is important to determine the proportion of children with hearing loss missed at the time of newborn hearing screening versus those added because of late-onset or progressive conditions. In addition to traditional analyses based on sensitivity and specificity, it is important to consider costs, benefits, and societal implications. Porter, Neely, and Gorga (2009) provide a useful framework for calculating benefit-cost ratios for evaluation of hearing screening protocols.

Improved detection of mild cochlear losses can be achieved by increasing the sensitivity of ABR or OAE screening protocols, but the implications of increasing the number of false-positive referrals need to be carefully considered (Gravel et al., 2005; White et al., 2005; Widen et al., 2005). Further research is needed to determine pass-fail rates associated with various OAE and ABR protocols alone and in combination, the impact of multilevel screens, the role of screening middle ear function, and the relative costs associated with each. ABR is not applicable for screening toddlers and preschoolers, but OAE remains a useful tool for detection of cochlear disorders when behavioral pure-tone screening is unfeasible or impractical, as long as stimulus and recording parameters are carefully selected to ensure adequate sensitivity (Dhar & Hall, 2012).

Broadly speaking, there remains a need for standards that pertain to the stimulus and recording parameters used in both OAE and ABR screening instruments as well as a need for more complete and uniform technical specifications (Durrant, Sabo, & Delgado, 2007; Burkard, 2010; 2011). As noted several years ago by Gravel and Kurman (2006) and still true today, the lack of ANSI standards for calibration of OAE and ABR devices has led to variability among commercially available screening instruments. Specifically, variation in acoustic stimuli and sound pressure levels at the tympanic membrane can result in different pass-fail criteria among devices. This is a particular issue with instruments designed for screening purposes, many of which are designed to restrict users from altering test parameters to meet recommended criteria. For example, among DPOAE screeners there are differences in the tonal pairs used, and among automated ABR screeners there are differences in stimulus levels (e.g., 35 dB nHL versus 40 dB nHL). These issues, according to Gravel and Kurman, not only affect calibration but create obstacles to the implementation of uniform pass-fail criteria. They also make it difficult to compare data across programs and settings, and they limit the ability to conduct prevalence estimates for various populations and geographic regions. This is a critical area of need, still unmet, with important implications for EHDI programs at the time of initial screening and for screening conducted after the newborn period.

There is also a need for continued efforts to decrease the number of infants unreported or lost to follow-up (Gaffney, Green, & Gaffney, 2010). This has been and remains a stubborn problem since the inception of newborn hearing screening. Data management systems that provide ongoing tracking and surveillance are vital components of EHDI programs. Unfortunately, they often are compromised by inaccurate recording or incomplete data entry (Allen et al., 2004; Gaffney et al., 2010). There is also a need for longitudinal prospective investigation of a large sample of infants who passed their newborn hearing screenings, with and without risk factors, to determine the relationship of various risk factors with delayed-onset hearing loss and to identify optimal screening intervals and test protocols.

In recent years there have been important strides in teleclinical technologies applied to hearing screening beyond the newborn period. Teleclinical methods can potentially provide considerable support to hearing screening programs especially in rural areas. For example, Lancaster et al. (2008) compared the results obtained from hearing screenings performed on-site and via telehealth technology for 32 children in a third-grade elementary school. Pure-tone screening outcomes differed between the audiologist on-site and from a distance via telehealth for 5 out of 32 children; this difference did not reach statistical significance (Lancaster et al.,

2008). Future research is needed to identify the need and define optimal protocols for audiologic screenings via teleclinical technology (Swanepoel et al., 2010).

Finally, and perhaps most pressing, there is a need for improved coordination of screening efforts and better communication among agencies and service providers. As new and updated guidelines and position statements emerge from various organizations, it is important to seek consensus at the state and local levels to achieve well-coordinated policies and procedures. Newborn hearing screening is mandated in most states, and the procedures employed are similar among hospitals. But screening *after* the newborn period involves a multitude of settings, service providers, public policies, and screening methods. Successful programs require evidence-based protocols and the concurrence of numerous stakeholders including those in health departments, hospitals, community clinics, and educational settings, working in partnership with clinicians and service providers in the public and private sectors. Without effective coordination and communication, screening can be insufficient or excessive. Responsibility will vary among states and municipalities based on legislative requirements, public policies, and local history, but the active engagement of pediatric and educational audiologists is needed at each level to achieve effective policies and procedures.

Summary and Conclusions

Hearing screening beyond the newborn period is supported by a substantial body of evidence that confirms the detrimental sequelae associated with undetected hearing loss. This includes speech, language, social development, and psychoeducational outcomes. Moreover, it is supported by the intrinsic right of all children to hear and for families to be informed if there is uncertainty regarding their child's access to sound. The role and efficacy of tympanometric screening is less clear, but it too remains vital for children at risk for middle ear disorders and those with concomitant sensory/neural hearing loss. The key points in this chapter are summarized as follows:

- Permanent hearing loss is the most common abnormality affecting newborn infants. Moreover, the prevalence appears to increase dramatically during the preschool and school years due to a variety of factors, including failure to detect mild hearing losses at the time of newborn screening, late-onset or progressive sensory/neural hearing loss, and an alarming number of young children lost to follow-up whose diagnosis inevitably will be delayed.
- The prevalence of permanent hearing loss is especially high among infants whose birth histories include special care in the NICU. In addition to higher prevalence of cochlear hearing loss, many infants with NICU histories are at increased risk for ANSD or delayed-onset/progressive cochlear hearing loss. ABR is currently the physiologic method appropriate for detection of sensory/neural hearing loss in the NICU because of its sensitivity to ANSD. Due to the relatively high incidence of sensory/neural hearing loss in this population, JCIH 2007 recommends that NICU infants who do not pass an initial ABR screening be referred to an audiologist for assessment and follow-up. Infants *readmitted* to the hospital after the newborn period for a condition that increases the risk of sensory/neural hearing loss should be rescreened with ABR prior to discharge.
- Screening ABR is an effective method for detection of hearing impairment, but as typically applied with newborns, can miss mild degrees of sensory/neural hearing loss. This inevitability increases the burden of accurate hearing screening after the newborn period.
- Routine behavioral hearing screening from birth to 3 years cannot be reliably conducted by nonaudiologists. Once a child reaches the age of 3 to 4 years, behavioral pure-tone screening might be feasible, but it requires capable and experienced examiners and cooperative children with the motivation and developmental maturity necessary to provide reliable responses. Behavioral pure-tone screening also requires a suitable acoustic environment, free of visual distractions and excessive noise. Challenges associated with these prerequisites have resulted in growing interest in the use of physiologic screening methods (e.g., OAE) as an adjunct or alternative to behavioral pure tone screening with preschool and school-age children.
- OAE screening can be applied to children at any age, and when used with preschool- and school-age children is generally easier to administer and more efficient than behavioral pure-tone screening. However, the stimulus and recording parameters typically employed in the newborn nursery might miss milder degrees of cochlear hearing losses. When used with preschool- and school-age children, the detection of mild cochlear hearing loss can be improved by applying a more sensitive OAE screening criteria (e.g., signal-to-noise-ratio >6 dB *combined* with an absolute distortion product amplitude >0 dB SPL) than is typically employed with newborns. Although

this can occur at the expense of lower specificity, preschool- and school-age children who do not pass OAE screening can be followed up immediately with behavioral pure-tone screening.

- OAEs are sensitive to otitis media *and* cochlear hearing loss. Applied judiciously in combination with tympanometry, they can be used to screen for both conditions. However, because OAE screening with not detect ANSD, it is best suited for screening asymptomatic children without risk factors for retrocochlear hearing loss.
- The use of tympanometry to screen for middle ear effusion in young children is widely practiced in the United States, although current recommendations from the medical community discourage mass tympanometric screening in healthy, asymptomatic children. Middle ear monitoring is justified, however, for children at increased risk for otitis media or for those with concomitant sensory/neural hearing loss.
- There is an urgent need for standards that define calibration of OAE and ABR screening devices and that set forth stimulus and recording parameters that make it possible to establish uniform pass-fail criteria among commercially available screening instruments.
- The AAP 2009 recommendations for screening after the newborn period represent an important commitment from the medical community and a useful conceptual framework. Effective screening in the medical home has the potential of facilitating earlier detection of hearing loss, especially among children who require surveillance because of a risk factor for late-onset or progressive hearing loss. However, the efficacy of hearing screening in the primary care setting has not been clearly established, and further research is needed.
- There is considerable variability among, and even within, states regarding screening policies and procedures employed with older infants, preschoolers, and school-age children. Inconsistencies exist in technology, personnel, pass-fail criteria, and surveillance of children with risk indicators for late onset-progressive hearing loss. Within most states and local communities, there is a need for better coordination of screening and follow-up, and improved communication with families and primary care providers. This requires the endorsement of many stakeholders, public and private, with the aim of achieving an effective continuum of screening, referral, and follow-up, balanced with a reasonable expenditure of public health resources.
- An important and often overlooked component of hearing screening programs is education regarding hearing protection and conservation. This component is especially important for adolescents and teens, many of who are at increased risk for noise-induced hearing loss.
- Because of limitations inherent in each of the screening methods currently available, children with known or suspected developmental delays, parental/caregiver concerns, educational concerns, risk indicators for sensory/neural hearing loss, or characteristics that make them "difficult to test" by conventional means, should be referred to a pediatric audiologist for comprehensive assessment.

The nationwide implementation of hospital-based, newborn hearing screening programs has been a remarkable achievement. But many challenges remain, among them the screening and follow-up needed in the months and years that follow the newborn period. The same level of commitment and advocacy that led to the successful implementation of neonatal hearing screening is needed on behalf of the infants and children who require screening and surveillance beyond the newborn period.

Acknowledgments. The authors acknowledge Dr. Robert Nozza, now retired, for his contributions as coauthor of this chapter in the first edition of this text.

References

Abdala, C., Keefe, D. H., & Oba, S. I. (2007). Distortion product otoacoustic emission suppression tuning and acoustic admittance in human infants: Birth through 6 months. *Journal of the Acoustical Society of America, 121*(6), 3617–3627. doi:10.1121/1.2734481

Allen, R. L., Stuart, A., Everett, D., & Elangovan, S. (2004). Preschool hearing screening: Pass/refer rates for children enrolled in a Head Start Program in eastern North Carolina. *American Journal of Audiology, 13*(1), 29–38.

American Academy of Audiology (AAA; 1997). *Identification of hearing loss and middle ear dysfunction in preschool and school-age children.* Reston, VA: Author.

American Academy of Audiology (AAA; 2011). *Childhood Hearing Screening.* Reston, VA: Author.

American Academy of Family Physicians (AAFP), American Academy of Otolaryngology-Head and Neck Surgery, & American Academy of Pediatrics (AAP) Subcommittee on Otitis Media With Effusion. (2004). Otitis media with effusion. *Pediatrics, 113*(5), 1412–1429.

American Academy of Pediatrics (AAP; 2002). Medical Home Initiatives for Children with Special Needs, Project Advisory Committee. The medical home. *Pediatrics, 110*, 184–186.

American National Standards Institute (ANSI; 1987). *Specifications for instruments to measure aural acoustic impedance and admittance (aural acoustic immittance).* ANSI S3.39-1987. New York, NY: Acoustical Society of America.

American National Standards Institute (ANSI; 1999, 2008). *American National Standard maximum permissible ambient noise levels for audiometric test rooms* (ANSI/ASA 3.1-1999, R 2008). Melville, NY: Acoustical Society of America.

American Speech-Language-Hearing Association (ASHA; 1979). *Guidelines for acoustic immittance screening of middle ear function.* Rockville, MD: Author.

American Speech-Language-Hearing Association (ASHA; 1997). Panel on audiologic assessment. *Guidelines for audiologic screening.* Rockville, MD: Author.

Association for Prevention, Teaching, and Research (APTR; n.d.). *Module 4: Screening.* Retrieved August 1, 2015, from http://www.aptrweb.org/?page=module4

Babb, M. J., Hilsinger, R. L. Jr., Korol, H. W., & Wilcox, R. D. (2004). Modern acoustic reflectometry: Accuracy in diagnosing otitis media with effusion. *Ear, Nose, and Throat Journal, 83*(9), 622–624.

Bamford, J., Fortnum, H., Bristow, K., Smith, J., Vamvakas, G., Davies, L., . . . Hind, S. (2007). Current practice, accuracy, effectiveness and cost-effectiveness of the school entry hearing screen. *Health Technology Assessment (Winchester, England), 11*(32), 1–168, iii–iv.

Berg, A. L., Spitzer, J. B., Towers, H. M., Bartosiewicz, C., & Diamond, B. E. (2005). Newborn hearing screening in the NICU: Profile of failed auditory brainstem response/ passed otoacoustic emission. *Pediatrics, 116*(4), 933–938.

Bess, F. H. (1980). Impedance screening for children. A need for more research. *Annals of Otology, Rhinology, and Laryngology Suppl., 89*(3 Pt. 2), 228–232.

Bess, F. H., Dodd-Murphy, J., & Parker, R. A. (1998). Children with minimal sensorineural hearing loss: Prevalence, educational performance, and functional status. *Ear and Hearing, 19*(5), 339–354.

Beswick, R., Driscoll, C., & Kei, J. (2012). Monitoring for postnatal hearing loss using risk factors: A systematic literature review. *Ear and Hearing, 33*(6), 745–756. doi:10.1097/AUD.0b013e31825b1cd9

Beswick, R., Driscoll, C., Kei, J., & Glennon, S. (2012). Targeted surveillance for postnatal hearing loss: A program evaluation. *International Journal of Pediatric Otorhinolaryngology, 76*(7), 1046–1056. doi:10.1016/j.ijporl.2012.04.004

Bhatia, P., Mintz, S., Hecht, B. F., Deavenport, A., & Kuo, A. A. (2013). Early identification of young children with hearing loss in federally qualified health centers. *Journal of Developmental and Behavioral Pediatrics, 34*(1), 15–21. doi:10.1097/DBP.0b013e318279899c

Bluestone, C. D., Fria, T. J., Arjona, S. K., Casselbrant, M. L., Schwartz, D. M., Ruben, R. J., . . . Rogers, K. D. (1986). Controversies in screening for middle ear disease and hearing loss in children. *Pediatrics, 77*(1), 57–70.

Bluestone, C. D., & Klein, J. O. (2007). *Otitis media in infants and children* (4th ed.). Philadelphia, PA: B.C. Decker.

Borton, S. A., Mauze, E., & Lieu, J. E. (2010). Quality of life in children with unilateral hearing loss: A pilot study. *American Journal of Audiology, 19*(1), 61–72. doi:10.1044/1059-0889(2010/07-0043)

Burkard, R. (2010). Update on a standard for the calibration of acoustic transients. *ASHA Audiology Connections*, p. 15.

Burkard, R. (2011). Update on several ANSI S3 standards. *ASHA Audiology Connections*, p. 24.

Centers for Disease Control and Prevention (CDC; 2007). *Annual EHDI Data, 2012.* Retrieved July 5, 2015, from http://www.cdc.gov/ncbddd/hearingloss/2012-data/2012_ehdi_hsfs_summary_b.pdf

Centers for Disease Control and Prevention (CDC; 2013a). *2013 Diagnosis and loss to follow-up/loss to documentation summary.* Retrieved September 14, 2015, from http://www.cdc.gov/ncbddd/hearingloss/2013-data/2013_lfu_summary_web.pdf

Centers for Disease Control and Prevention (CDC), Adolescent and School Health. (2013b). *Noise-induced hearing loss.* Retrieved from http://www.cdc.gov/healthyyouth/noise/

Centers for Disease Control and Prevention (CDC), Adolescent and School Health. (2013c). *Promoting hearing health in schools.* Retrieved from http://www.cdc.gov/healthyyouth/noise/promoting.htm

Centers for Disease Control and Prevention (CDC; 2013d). *Summary of 2013 National CDC Data.* Retrieved September 14, 2015, from http://www.cdc.gov/ncbddd/hearingloss/2013-data/2013_ehdi_hsfs_summary_a.pdf

Christensen, M., Thomson, V., & Letson, G. W. (2008). Evaluating the reach of universal newborn hearing screening in Colorado. *American Journal of Preventive Medicine, 35*(6), 594–597. doi:10.1016/j.amepre.2008.09.007

D'Agostino, J. A., & Austin, L. (2004). Auditory neuropathy: A potentially under-recognized neonatal intensive care unit sequela. *Advances in Neonatal Care, 4*(6), 344–353.

Daly, K. A., & Giebink, G. S. (2000). Clinical epidemiology of otitis media. *Pediatric Infectious Disease Journal, 19*(Suppl. 5), S31–S36.

Daly, K. A., Hoffman, H. J., Kvaerner, K. J., Kvestad, E., Casselbrant, M. L., Homoe, P., & Rovers, M. M. (2010). Epidemiology, natural history, and risk factors: Panel report from the Ninth International Research Conference on Otitis Media. *International Journal of Pediatric Otorhinolaryngology, 74*(3), 231–240.

Danhauer, J. L., Johnson, C. E., Dunne, A. F., Young, M. D., Rotan, S. N., Snelson, T. A., . . . McLain, M. J. (2012). Survey of high school students' perceptions about their iPod use, knowledge of hearing health, and need for education. *Language, Speech, and Hearing Services in Schools, 43*(1), 14–35. doi:10.1044/0161-1461(2011/10-0088)

Deconde Johnson, C., & Seaton, J. B. (2011). *Educational audiology handbook.* Independence, KY: Cengage Learning.

Dhar, S., & Hall, J. W. (2012). *Otoacoustic emissions: Principles, procedures, and protocols.* San Diego, CA: Plural.

Dille, M., Glattke, T. J., & Earl, B. R. (2007). Comparison of transient evoked otoacoustic emissions and distortion product otoacoustic emissions when screening hearing in preschool children in a community setting. *International Journal of Pediatric Otorhinolaryngology, 71*(11), 1789–1795.

Driscoll, C., Kei, J., & McPherson, B. (2001). Outcomes of transient evoked otoacoustic emission testing in 6-year-old school children: A comparison with pure-tone screening and tympanometry. *International Journal of Pediatric Otorhinolaryngology, 57*(1), 67–76.

Durrant, J. D., Sabo, D. L., & Delgado, R. E. (2007). Call for calibration standard for newborn screening using auditory brainstem responses. *International Journal of Audiology, 46*(11), 686–691.

Eiserman, W. D., Hartel, D. M., Shisler, L., Buhrmann, J., White, K. R., & Foust, T. (2008). Using otoacoustic emissions to screen for hearing loss in early childhood care settings. *International Journal of Pediatric Otorhinolaryngology, 72*(4), 475–482.

Feightner, J. W. (1992) Screening in the 1990s: Some principles and guidelines. In F. H. Bess & J. W. Hall (Eds.), *Screening children for auditory function* (pp. 1–16). Nashville, TN: Bill Wilkerson Center Press.

Finitzo, T., Albright, K., & O'Neal, J. (1998). The newborn with hearing loss: Detection in the nursery. *Pediatrics, 102*(6), 1452–1460.

FitzZaland, R. E., & Zink, G. D. (1984). A comparative study of hearing screening procedures. *Ear and Hearing, 5*(4), 205–210.

Folmer, R. L., Griest, S. E., & Martin, W. H. (2002). Hearing conservation education programs for children: A review. *Journal of School Health, 72*(2), 51–57.

Foust, T., Eiserman, W., Shisler, L., & Geroso, A. (2013). Using otoacoustic emissions to screen young children for hearing loss in primary care settings. *Pediatrics, 132*(1), 118–123.

Frank, T. (2000). ANSI update: Maximum permissible ambient noise levels for audiometric test rooms. *American Journal of Audiology, 9*(1), 3–8.

Gaffney, M., Green, D. R., & Gaffney, C. (2010). Newborn hearing screening and follow-up: Are children receiving recommended services? *Public Health Reports, 125*(2), 199–207.

Gerber, S. E. (1990). Review of a high risk register for congenital or early-onset deafness. *British Journal of Audiology, 24*(5), 347–356.

Gilles, A., & Paul Vde, H. (2014). Effectiveness of a preventive campaign for noise-induced hearing damage in adolescents. *International Journal of Pediatric Otorhinolaryngology, 78*(4), 604–609. doi:10.1016/j.ijporl.2014.01.009

Glattke, T., Pafitis, I. A., & Cummiskey, C. (1995). Identification of hearing loss in children and young adults using measures of transient evoked otoacoustic emission reproducibility. *American Journal of Audiology, 4*, 71–86.

Gorga, M. P., Neely, S. T., Dorn, P. A., & Hoover, B. M. (2003). Further efforts to predict pure-tone thresholds from distortion product otoacoustic emission input/output functions. *Journal of the Acoustical Society of America, 113*, 3275–3284.

Gorga, M. P., Norton, S. J., Sininger, Y. S., Cone-Wesson, B., Folsom, R.C., Vohr, B. R., Widen, J.E., & Neely, S. T. (2000). Identification of neonatal hearing impairment: Distortion product otoacoustic emissions during the perinatal period. *Ear and Hearing, 21*(5), 400–424.

Gravel, J., & Kurman, B. (2006, February). *Standards for newborn hearing screening equipment: What are we measuring in newborn hearing screening programs?* National Conference on Early Hearing Detection and Intervention, Washington, DC.

Gravel, J. S., White, K. R., Johnson, J. L., Widen, J. E., Vohr, B. R., James, M., . . . Meyer, S. (2005). A multisite study to examine the efficacy of the otoacoustic emission/automated auditory brainstem response newborn hearing screening protocol: Recommendations for policy, practice, and research. *American Journal of Audiology, 14*(2), S217–S228.

Green, J. (2002). Noise-induced hearing loss [Letter to the editor]. *Pediatrics, 109*, 987–988.

Grosse, S. D. (2007). Education cost savings from early detection of hearing loss: New findings. *Volta Voices, 14*(6), 38–40.

Guidelines Development Conference on the Identification and Management of Infants With Auditory Neuropathy. (2008). International Newborn Hearing Screening Conference, June 19–21, Como, Italy. Retrieved from http://www.childrenscolorado.org/health-professionals/clinical-resources/auditory-neuropathy-spectrum-disorder-guidelines

Hall, J. W. (2015, March). *Effective and efficient pre-school hearing loss identification and diagnosis: Essential for successful EHDI.* Presented at the Fourteenth Annual Early Hearing Detection and Intervention Meeting, Louisville, KY.

Halloran, D. R., Hardin, J. M., & Wall, T. C. (2009). Validity of pure-tone hearing screening at well-child visits. *Archives of Pediatrics and Adolescent Medicine, 163*(2), 158–163.

Harlor, A. D. Jr., Bower, C., Committee on Practice and Ambulatory Medicine, & Section on Otolaryngology-Head and Neck Surgery. (2009). Hearing assessment in infants and children: Recommendations beyond neonatal screening. *Pediatrics, 124*(4), 1252–1263.

Henderson, E., Testa, M. A., & Hartnick, C. (2011). Prevalence of noise-induced hearing-threshold shifts and hearing loss among US youths. *Pediatrics, 127*(1), e39–e46. doi:10.1542/peds.2010-0926

Ho, V., Daly, K. A., Hunter, L. L., & Davey, C. (2002). Otoacoustic emissions and tympanometry screening among 0–5 year olds. *Laryngoscope, 112*(3), 513–519.

Holmes, A. E., Niskar, A. S., Kieszak, S. M., Rubin, C., & Brody, D. J. (2004). Mean and median hearing thresholds among children 6 to 19 years of age: The third national health and nutrition examination survey, 1988 to 1994, United States. *Ear and Hearing, 25*(4), 397–402.

Hunter, L. L., Davey, C. S., Kohtz, A., & Daly, K. A. (2007). Hearing screening and middle ear measures in American Indian infants and toddlers. *International Journal of Pediatric Otorhinolaryngology, 71*(9), 1429–1438.

Hunter, L. L., Feeney, M. P., Lapsley Miller, J. A., Jeng, P. S., & Bohning, S. (2010). Wideband reflectance in newborns: Normative regions and relationship to hearing-screening results. *Ear and Hearing, 31*(5), 599–610. doi:10.1097/AUD.0b013e3181e40ca7

Hunter, L. L., Tubaugh, L., Jackson, A., & Propes, S. (2008). Wideband middle ear power measurement in infants and children. *Journal of the American Academy of Audiology, 19*(4), 309–324.

Jerger, J. (1970). Clinical experience with impedance audiometry. *Archives of Otolaryngology, 92*(4), 311–324.

Johnson, J. L., White, K. R., Widen, J. E., Gravel, J. S., James, M., Kennalley, T., . . . Holstrum, J. (2005). A multicenter evaluation of how many infants with permanent hearing loss pass a two-stage otoacoustic emissions/automated auditory brainstem response newborn hearing screening protocol. *Pediatrics, 116*(3), 663–672.

Joint Committee on Infant Hearing (JCIH; 1971). *Joint statement on neonatal screening for hearing impairment.* Retrieved January 23, 2010, from http://jcih.org/posstatemts.htm

Joint Committee on Infant Hearing (JCIH; 2000). Year 2000 position statement: Principles and guidelines for early hearing detection and intervention programs. *Pediatrics, 106*(4), 798–817.

Joint Committee on Infant Hearing (JCIH; 2007). Year 2007 position statement: Principles and guidelines for early hearing detection and intervention programs. *Pediatrics, 120*(4), 898–921.

Keefe, D. H., Folsom, R. C., Gorga, M. P., Vohr, B. R., Bulen, J. C., & Norton, S. J. (2000). Identification of neonatal hearing impairment: Ear-canal measurements of acoustic admittance and reflectance in neonates. *Ear and Hearing, 21*(5), 443–461.

Kei, J., Mazlan, R., Hickson, L., Gavranich, J., & Linning, R. (2007). Measuring middle ear admittance in newborns using 1000 Hz tympanometry: A comparison of methodologies. *Journal of the American Academy of Audiology, 18*(9), 739–748.

Koivunen, P., Uhari, M., Laitakari, K., Alho, O. P., & Luotonen, J. (2000). Otoacoustic emissions and tympanometry in children with otitis media. *Ear and Hearing, 21*(3), 212–217.

Kujawa, S. G., & Liberman, M. C. (2009). Adding insult to injury: Cochlear nerve degeneration after "temporary" noise-induced hearing loss. *The Journal of Neuroscience: The Official Journal of the Society for Neuroscience, 29*(45), 14077–14085. doi:10.1523/JNEUROSCI.2845-09.2009

Lampe, R. M., Weir, M. R., Spier, J., & Rhodes, M. F. (1985). Acoustic reflectometry in the detection of middle ear effusion. *Pediatrics, 76*(1), 75–78.

Lancaster, P., Krumm, M., Ribera, J., & Klich, R. (2008). Remote hearing screenings via telehealth in a rural elementary school. *American Journal of Audiology, 17*(2), 114–122. doi:10.1044/1059-0889(2008/07-0008)

Liberman, L. D., & Liberman, M. C. (2015). Dynamics of cochlear synaptopathy after acoustic overexposure. *Journal of the Association for Research in Otolaryngology, 16*(2), 205–219. doi:10.1007/s10162-015-0510-3

Liden, G. (1969). The scope and application of current audiometric tests. *Journal of Laryngology and Otology, 83*(6), 507–520.

Lonsbury-Martin, B. L., Martin, G. K., McCoy, M. J., & Whitehead, M. L. (1995). New approaches to the evaluation of the auditory system and a current analysis of otoacoustic emissions. *Otolaryngology-Head and Neck Surgery, 112*(1), 50–63.

Lü, J., Huang, Z., Ma, Y., Li, Y., Mei, L., Yao, G., . . . Wu, H. (2014). Comparison between hearing screening-detected cases and sporadic cases of delayed-onset hearing loss in preschool-age children. *International Journal of Audiology, 53*(4), 229–234. doi:10.3109/14992027.2013.858278

Lü, J., Huang, Z., Yang, T., Li, Y., Mei, L., Xiang, M., . . . Wu, H. (2011). Screening for delayed-onset hearing loss in preschool children who previously passed the newborn hearing screening. *International Journal of Pediatric Otorhinolaryngology, 75*(8), 1045–1049. doi:10.1016/j.ijporl.2011.05.022

Lyons, A., Kei, J., & Driscoll, C. (2004). Distortion product otoacoustic emissions in children at school entry: A comparison with pure-tone screening and tympanometry results. *Journal of the American Academy of Audiology, 15*(10), 702–715.

Madden, C., Rutter, M., Hilbert, L., Greinwald, J. H., Jr., & Choo, D. I. (2002). Clinical and audiological features in auditory neuropathy. *Archives of Otolaryngology-Head and Neck Surgery, 128*(9), 1026–1030.

Margolis, R. H., Bass-Ringdahl, S., Hanks, W. D., Holte, L., & Zapala, D. A. (2003). Tympanometry in newborn infants—1 kHz norms. *Journal of the American Academy of Audiology, 14*(7), 383–392.

Margolis, R. H., & Heller, J. W. (1987). Screening tympanometry: Criteria for medical referral. *Audiology, 26*(4), 197–208.

Margolis, R. H., & Trine, M. B. (1997). Effects of middle ear disease on otoacoustic emissions. In M. S. Robinette, & T. Glattke (Eds.), *Otoacoustic emissions: Clinical applications* (pp. 130–150). New York, NY: Thieme.

Marshall, L., Heller, L. M., & Westhusin, L. J. (1997). Effect of negative middle-ear pressure on transient-evoked otoacoustic emissions. *Ear and Hearing, 18*(3), 218–226.

Mason, C. A., Gaffney, M., Green, D. R., & Grosse, S. D. (2008). Measures of follow-up in early hearing detection and intervention programs: A need for standardization. *American Journal of Audiology, 17*(1), 60-67. doi:10.1044/1059-0889(2008/007)

Mauk, G. W., & Behrens, T. R. (1993). Historical, political, and technological context associated with early identification of hearing loss. *Seminars in Hearing, 14*(1), 1–17.

Mauk, G. W., White, K. R., Mortensen, L. B., & Behrens, T. R. (1991). The effectiveness of screening programs based on high-risk characteristics in early identification of hearing impairment. *Ear and Hearing, 12*(5), 312–319.

Mehl, A. L., & Thomson, V. (2002). The Colorado Newborn Hearing Screening Project, 1992–1999: On the threshold of effective population-based universal newborn hearing screening. *Pediatrics, 109*(1), E7.

Mehra, S., Eavey, R. D., & Keamy, D. G., Jr. (2009). The epidemiology of hearing impairment in the United States: Newborns, children, and adolescents. *Otolaryngology-Head and Neck Surgery, 140*(4), 461–472.

Meinke, D. K., & Dice, N. (2007). Comparison of audiometric screening criteria for the identification of noise-induced hearing loss in adolescents. *American Journal of Audiology, 16*(2), S190–S202.

Moeller, M. P. (2000). Early intervention and language development in children who are deaf and hard of hearing. *Pediatrics, 106*(3), E43.

Moeller, M. P., Osberger, M. J., & Eccarius, M. (1986). Language and learning skills of hearing-impaired students. receptive language skills. *ASHA Monographs, 23*, 41–53.

Moeller, M. P., White, K. R., & Shisler, L. (2006). Primary care physicians' knowledge, attitudes, and practices related to newborn hearing screening. *Pediatrics, 118*(4), 1357–1370.

Mohr, P. E., Feldman, J. J., Dunbar, J. L., McConkey-Robbins, A., Niparko, J. K., Rittenhouse, R. K., & Skinner, M. W. (2000). The societal costs of severe to profound hearing loss in the United States. *International Journal of Technology Assessment in Health Care, 16*(4), 1120–1135.

Niskar, A. S., Kieszak, S. M., Holmes, A., Esteban, E., Rubin, C., & Brody, D. J. (1998). Prevalence of hearing loss among children 6 to 19 years of age: The Third National Health and Nutrition Examination Survey. *Journal of the American Medical Association, 279*(14), 1071–1075.

Niskar, A. S., Kieszak, S. M., Holmes, A. E., Esteban, E., Rubin, C., & Brody, D. J. (2001). Estimated prevalence of noise-induced hearing threshold shifts among children 6 to 19 years of age: The Third National Health and Nutrition Examination Survey, 1988–1994, United States. *Pediatrics, 108*(1), 40–43.

Northern, J. L. (1992) Special issues concerned with screening for middle ear disease in children. In F. H. Bess & J. W. Hall (Eds.), *Screening children for auditory function*. Nashville, TN: Bill Wilkerson Center Press.

Norton, S. J., Gorga, M. P., Widen, J. E., Folsom, R. C., Sininger, Y., Cone-Wesson, B., . . . Fletcher, K. (2000). Identification of neonatal hearing impairment: Evaluation of transient evoked otoacoustic emission, distortion product otoacoustic emission, and auditory brain stem response test performance. *Ear and Hearing, 21*(5), 508–528.

Nozza, R. J. (1996). Pediatric hearing screening. In F. N. Martin & J. G. Clark (Eds.), *Hearing care in children* (pp. 95–114). Needham Heights, MA: Allyn & Bacon.

Nozza, R. J. (1998). Identification of otitis media. *Proceedings of the Fourth International Symposium on Childhood Deafness* (pp. 207–214). Kiawah Island, South Carolina, October, 1996. Nashville, TN: Wilkerson Center Press.

Nozza, R. J. (2001). Screening with otoacoustic emissions beyond the newborn period. In J. Durrant (Ed.), *Special topics in bases and applications of measurements of otoacoustic emissions. Seminars in Hearing, 22*(4), 415–425.

Nozza, R. J., Bluestone, C. D., Kardatzke, D., & Bachman, R. (1992). Towards the validation of aural acoustic immittance measures for diagnosis of middle ear effusion in children. *Ear and Hearing, 13*(6), 442–453.

Nozza, R. J., Bluestone, C. D., Kardatzke, D., & Bachman, R. (1994). Identification of middle ear effusion by aural acoustic admittance and otoscopy. *Ear and Hearing, 15*(4), 310–323.

Nozza, R. J., Sabo, D. L., & Mandel, E. M. (1997). A role for otoacoustic emissions in screening for hearing impairment and middle ear disorders in school-age children. *Ear and Hearing, 18*(3), 227–239.

Owens, J. J., McCoy, M. J., Lonsbury-Martin, B. L., & Martin, G. K. (1993). Otoacoustic emissions in children with normal ears, middle ear dysfunction, and ventilating tubes. *American Journal of Otology, 14*(1), 34–40.

Porter, H. L., Neely, S. T., & Gorga, G. (2009). Using benefit-cost ratio to select universal newborn hearing test criteria. *Ear and Hearing, 30*, 447–457.

Porter, H., Sladen, D. P., Ampah, S. B., Rothpletz, A., & Bess, F. H. (2013). Developmental outcomes in early school-age children with minimal hearing loss. *American Journal of Audiology, 22*(2), 263–270. doi:1059-0889_2013_13-0013 [pii]

Prieve, B. (2008). Otoacoustic emissions in infants and children. In J. Madell & C. Flexer (Eds.), *Pediatric audiology: Diagnosis, technology, and management*. New York, NY: Thieme Medical.

Prieve, B. A., Calandruccio, L., Fitzgerald, T., Mazevski, A., & Georgantas, L. M. (2008). Changes in transient-evoked otoacoustic emission levels with negative tympanometric peak pressure in infants and toddlers. *Ear and Hearing, 29*(4), 533–542.

Prieve, B., Dalzell, L., Berg, A., Bradley, M., Cacace, A., Campbell, D., . . . Stevens, F. (2000). The New York State universal newborn hearing screening demonstration project: Outpatient outcome measures. *Ear and Hearing, 21*(2), 104–117.

Prieve, B. A., Schooling, T., Venediktov, R., & Franceschini, N. (2015). An evidence-based systematic review on the diagnostic accuracy of hearing screening instruments for preschool and school-age children. *American Journal of Audiology*, doi:10.1044/2015_AJA-14-0065

Prieve, B. A., & Stevens, F. (2000). The New York State universal newborn hearing screening demonstration project: Introduction and overview. *Ear and Hearing, 21*(2), 85–91.

Rance, G. (2005). Auditory neuropathy/dys-synchrony and its perceptual consequences. *Trends in Amplification, 9*(1), 1–43.

Richburg, C. M., & Imhoff, L. (2008). Survey of hearing screeners: Training and protocols used in two distinct school systems. *Journal of Educational Audiology, 14*, 31–46.

Rosenfeld, R. M., & Kay, D. (2003). Natural history of untreated otitis media. *Laryngoscope, 113*(10), 1645–1657.

Roush, J. (1990). Identification of hearing loss and middle ear disease in preschool and school-age children. *Seminars in Hearing, 11*(4), 357–371.

Roush, J. (Ed.). (2001). *Screening for hearing loss and otitis media in children*. San Diego, CA: Singular/Thomson Learning.

Roush, J., Bryant, K., Mundy, M., Zeisel, S., & Roberts, J. (1995). Developmental changes in static admittance and tympanometric width in infants and toddlers. *Journal of the American Academy of Audiology, 6*(4), 334–338.

Roush, J., Drake, A., & Sexton, J. E. (1992). Identification of middle ear dysfunction in young children: A comparison of tympanometric screening procedures. *Ear and Hearing, 13*(2), 63–69.

Roush, J., & Tait, C. A. (1985). Pure-tone and acoustic immittance screening of preschool-aged children: An examination of referral criteria. *Ear and Hearing, 6*(5), 245–250.

Sanford, C. A., & Feeney, M. P. (2008). Effects of maturation on tympanometric wideband acoustic transfer functions in human infants. *Journal of the Acoustical Society of America, 124*(4), 2106–2122. doi:10.1121/1.2967864

Schlauch, R. S., & Carney, E. (2011). Are false-positive rates leading to an overestimation of noise-induced hearing loss? *Journal of Speech, Language, and Hearing Research, 54*(2), 679–692. doi:10.1044/1092-4388(2010/09-0132)

Serpanos, Y. C., & Jarmel, F. (2007). Quantitative and qualitative follow-up outcomes from a preschool audiologic screening program: Perspectives over a decade. *American Journal of Audiology, 16*(1), 4–12. doi:16/1/4 [pii]

Shargorodsky, J., Curhan, S. G., Curhan, G. C., & Eavey, R. (2010). Change in prevalence of hearing loss in US adolescents. *JAMA, 304*(7), 772–778. doi:10.1001/jama.2010.1124

Shi, S., Kei, J., Murdoch, B., McPherson, B., Smyth, V., Latham, S., & Loscher, J. (2000). Paediatric hearing screening in the community: A comparison of outcomes from transient evoked and distortion product otoacoustic emission measures. *Scandinavian Audiology, 29*(2), 83–92.

Sideris, I., & Glattke, T. J. (2006). A comparison of two methods of hearing screening in the preschool population. *Journal of Communication Disorders, 39*(6), 391–401.

Silman, S., Silverman, C. A., & Arick, D. S. (1992). Acoustic-immittance screening for detection of middle-ear effusion in children. *Journal of the American Academy of Audiology, 3*(4), 262–268.

Sininger, Y. S., Cone-Wesson, B., Folsom, R. C., Gorga, M. P., Vohr, B. R., Widen, J. E., . . . Norton, S. J. (2000). Identification of neonatal hearing impairment: Auditory brain stem responses in the perinatal period. *Ear and Hearing, 21*(5), 383–399.

Smith, C. G., Paradise, J. L., Sabo, D. L., Rockette, H. E., KursLasky, M., Bernard, B. S., . . . Colborn, D. K. (2006). Tympanometric findings and the probability of middle-ear effusion in 3686 infants and young children. *Pediatrics, 118*(1), 1–13.

Stark, A. R., & American Academy of Pediatrics Committee on Fetus and Newborn. (2004). Levels of neonatal care. *Pediatrics, 114*(5), 1341–1347. doi:10.1542/peds.2004-1697

Starr, A., Sininger, Y. S., & Pratt, H. (2000). The varieties of auditory neuropathy. *Journal of Basic and Clinical Physiology and Pharmacology, 11*(3), 215–230.

Stein, L. K. (1999). Factors influencing the efficacy of universal newborn hearing screening. *Pediatric Clinics of North America, 46*(1), 95–105.

Swanepoel de, W., Clark, J., Koekemoer, K., Hall, J. W., Krumm, M., Ferrari, D. V., . . . Barajas, J. (2010). Telehealth in audiology: The need and potential to reach underserved communities, *International Journal of Audiology, 49*(3), 195–202.

Swanepoel de, W., Maclennan-Smith, F., & Hall, J. W. (2013). Diagnostic pure-tone audiometry in schools: Mobile testing without a sound-treated environment. *Journal of the American Academy of Audiology, 24*(10), 992–1000. doi:10.3766/jaaa.24.10.10

Taylor, C. L., & Brooks, R. P. (2000). Screening for hearing loss and middle ear disorders in children using TEOAEs. *American Journal of Audiology, 9*, 1–6.

Teele, D. W., & Teele, J. (1984). Detection of middle ear effusion by acoustic reflectometry. *Journal of Pediatrics, 104*(6), 832–838.

Teppo, H., & Revonta, M. (2009). Consumer acoustic reflectometry by parents in detecting middle-ear fluid among children undergoing tympanostomy. *Scandinavian Journal of Primary Health Care, 27*(3), 167–171.

Thompson, D. C., McPhillips, H., Davis, R. L., Lieu, T. L., Homer, C. J., & Helfand, M. (2001). Universal newborn hearing screening: Summary of evidence. *JAMA, 286*(16), 2000–2010. doi:jrv10043 [pii]

Trine, M. B., Hirsch, J. E., & Margolis, R. H. (1993). The effect of middle ear pressure on transient evoked otoacoustic emissions. *Ear and Hearing, 14*(6), 401–407.

Utah Department of Health. (2015). *Children with special health care needs: Cytomegalovirus (CMV) Public Health Initiative.* Retrieved August 3, 2015, from http://www.health.utah.gov/cshcn/programs/cmv.html

Vander Werff, K. R., Prieve, B. A., & Georgantas, L. M. (2007). Test-retest reliability of wideband reflectance measures in infants under screening and diagnostic test conditions. *Ear and Hearing, 28*(5), 669–681.

Van Dyk, M., Swanepoel, D., & Hall, J. W. (2015). Outcomes with OAE and AABR screening in the first 48h—Implications for newborn hearing screening in developing countries. *International Journal of Pediatric Otorhinolaryngology, 79*(7), 1034–1040.

Vasconcellos, A. P., Colello, S., Kyle, M. E., & Shin, J. J. (2014). Societal-level risk factors associated with pediatric hearing loss: A systematic review. *Otolaryngology-Head and Neck Surgery, 151*(1), 29–41. doi:0194599814526561 [pii]

Vasconcellos, A. P., Kyle, M. E., Gilani, S., & Shin, J. J. (2014). Personally modifiable risk factors associated with pediatric hearing loss: A systematic review. *Otolaryngology-Head and Neck Surgery, 151*(1), 14–28. doi:0194599814526560 [pii]

Vogel, I., Brug, J., Hosli, E. J., Van der Ploeg, C. P., & Raat, H. (2008). MP3 players and hearing loss: Adolescents' perceptions of loud music and hearing conservation. *Journal of Pediatrics, 152*(3), 400–404. doi:10.1016/j.jpeds.2007.07.009

Vogel, I., Brug, J., Van der Ploeg, C. P., & Raat, H. (2011). Adolescents' risky MP3-player listening and its psychosocial correlates. *Health Education Research, 26*(2), 254–264.

Vohr, B. R., Carty, L. M., Moore, P. E., & Letourneau, K. (1998). The Rhode Island hearing assessment program: Experience with statewide hearing screening (1993–1996). *Journal of Pediatrics, 133*(3), 353–357.

Waseem, M., & Aslam, M., (2008). Otitis media: Differential diagnosis and work-up. *eMedicine, 2008.* Retrieved January 16, 2010, from http://emedicine.medscape.com/article/994656

Wessex Universal Neonatal Hearing Screening Trial Group. (1998). Controlled trial of universal neonatal screening for early identification of permanent childhood hearing impairment. Wessex Universal Neonatal Hearing Screening Trial Group. *Lancet, 352*(9145), 1957–1964. doi:S0140673698063594 [pii]

White, K. R., Vohr, B. R., Meyer, S., Widen, J. E., Johnson, J. L., Gravel, J. S., . . . Weirather, Y. (2005). A multisite study to examine the efficacy of the otoacoustic emission/automated auditory brainstem response newborn hearing screening protocol: Research design and results of the study. *American Journal of Audiology, 14*(2), S186–S199.

Widen, J. E., Folsom, R. C., Cone-Wesson, B., Carty, L., Dunnell, J. J., Koebsell, K., . . . Norton, S. J. (2000). Identification of neonatal hearing impairment: Hearing status at 8 to 12 months corrected age using a visual reinforcement audiometry protocol. *Ear and Hearing, 21*(5), 471–487.

Widen, J. E., Johnson, J. L., White, K. R., Gravel, J. S., Vohr, B. R., James, M., . . . Meyer, S. (2005). A multisite study to examine the efficacy of the otoacoustic emission/automated auditory brainstem response newborn hearing screening protocol: Results of visual reinforcement audiometry. *American Journal of Audiology, 14*(2), S200–S216.

Xoinis, K., Weirather, Y., Mavoori, H., Shaha, S. H., & Iwamoto, L. M. (2007). Extremely low birth weight infants are at high risk for auditory neuropathy. *Journal of Perinatology, 27*(11), 718–723.

Yoshinaga-Itano, C., Sedey, A. L., Coulter, D. K., & Mehl, A. L. (1998). Language of early- and later-identified children with hearing loss. *Pediatrics, 102*(5), 1161–1171.

Newborn Hearing Screening Program Implementation: Early Hearing Detection and Intervention

Kathryn L. Beauchaine, Jeffrey K. Hoffman, and Diane L. Sabo

Introduction

Early hearing detection and intervention (EHDI) is an approach to the newborn hearing screening process that goes beyond the initial screening and diagnosis to include the follow-up, management, and remediation of children found to have hearing loss, or who have risk factors for late-onset hearing loss. Contemporary benchmarks are include screening of hearing status prior to 1 month of age, confirmation of hearing status before 3 months of age, and the initiation of appropriate interventions by 6 months of age. Additionally, following diagnosis of hearing loss, amplification use should be initiated within 1 month. The 1-3-6 goals are the foundation for today's newborn hearing screening programs.

This chapter provides a practical discussion of the EHDI process. The roots and development of EHDI are reviewed, including the early, central role of pediatric audiologists. The interdisciplinary nature of EHDI and how pediatric audiologists play a pivotal role is discussed. The nuts and bolts of implementing and running a successful program are presented. Finally, future directions and challenges are addressed. At the outset, the reader is directed to Appendix 18–A for a list of acronyms used in this chapter. Appendix 18–B contains a brief list of EHDI-related documents and organizations.

EHDI Roots and Historical Perspective

It was not until technology developed to obtain objective measures of infant auditory status that there was impetus for widespread newborn hearing screening. However, attempts to identify hearing loss in children date back more than 200 years. Nisbet (1800) indicated that deafness was common in children and has three causes: "1. Cold. 2. induration of the secretion of the ear; or its deficiency; and, 3. diseased state of the auditory nerve" (p. 153). In early citations, health conditions known to be associated with hearing loss in children largely related to hearing loss caused by ear infections, syphilis, and meningitis. Thus, early efforts to identify hearing loss in young children focused on infants with specific diseases or disorders, and those in special care nurseries who were more likely to have significant hearing loss or deafness. Familial hearing loss was also recognized, though not fully understood. Recall that Mendel's work on the inheritance of traits was first presented in the 1860s, and published in 1865 (Mendel, 1865; Miko, 2008). Early diagnosis of permanent childhood hearing loss (PCHL) and its treatment seems rudimentary by today's standards, much in the way that today's technology someday will seem unrefined. Technology for screening, testing, and tracking, as well as the technology for remediation and (re)habilitation, continues to improve and change how we identify and treat PCHL.

As early as the 1940s, noisemakers were used to test hearing in infants and young children, based on the work of Ewing and Ewing (1944) and furthered by others (e.g., Richmond, Grossman, & Lustman, 1953). Although using uncalibrated noisemakers to screen hearing in infants seems crude by current standards, it was revolutionary and state-of-the-art at that time. This work provided the foundation of pediatric audiology.

In 1964, a group was appointed by the U.S. Secretary of Health, Education, and Welfare to study ways to improve the education of deaf students, and improve their educational opportunities and eventual employment options (Babbidge et al., 1965). Although education was the focus of the group's report, it is notable that they recognized the importance of early identification and intervention:

> The infant with a hearing deficit or a potential hearing deficit should have a better chance of being identified in the early months of life and put in touch with better and more generally available clinical facilities and multidisciplinary services for diagnosis and evaluation. Parents of deaf children need more readily available counsel, guidance, and instruction. (Babbidge, 1965, p. xvi)

In the United States, a group called the Joint Committee on Infant Hearing (JCIH) first organized in 1969. The member organizations included the American Speech and Hearing Association (ASHA), the American Academy of Ophthalmology and Otolaryngology, and the American Academy of Pediatrics (AAP). The beginning of JCIH was due largely to the efforts of Marion Downs, audiologist and advocate for children with hearing loss, who represented ASHA. The charge of the JCIH was to make recommendations about newborn hearing screening with the goal of identifying children at risk for hearing loss as early in life as possible. The first JCIH statement was published in 1971. It was one short page with four references, and it concluded that mass behavioral hearing screenings results were "inconsistent and misleading." Importantly, the recommendation was to increase research efforts in this area. The role of the audiologists as key professionals in newborn hearing screening was also established.

In the 1960s and early 1970s, hearing screening was done using behavioral observation of infants in response to noisemakers or using a handheld noise generator. One such handheld noise-generating device was called a Neometer. With this device, the screener presented a 90 dB SPL high-frequency (3000 Hz) signal approximately 6 to 12 inches from the infant's ear, and the infant's response was observed and noted. This subjective test was used in many hospitals, typically administered by trained volunteers. Due to the high level of the signal, only infants with severe or profound hearing loss would have been detected (Downs & Hemenway, 1969). Furthermore, the presence of a response was dependent on infant state/arousal, ambient stimuli (e.g., ambient noise, lights, vibrations), and the skill of the observers. As with all unconditioned behavioral responses, there are risks of high false-positive and false-negative results.

A newborn hearing screening method called the Crib-o-gram (Simmons & Russ, 1974) emerged in the early- to mid-1970s. For the Crib-o-gram, a motion-sensitive transducer was placed in the crib, typically under the mattress, to detect an infant's movement. A loudspeaker was placed in the crib that presented a 2500- to 4500-Hz noise with a center frequency of 3500 Hz at 92 dBA. The stimulus was presented more than 20 times during a 24-hour period, and the infant's motor activity was recorded on a strip chart before and after presentation of each stimulus. Recordings, at least in the early stages of device use, were scored by hand. Infants who did not pass the Crib-o-gram were seen for behavioral audiometry at 7 months of age. Like the Neometer, the Crib-o-gram was intended to identify only those infants with severe-to-profound hearing loss.

During this same period, the use of brainstem auditory-evoked potentials (AEPs) for the objective assessment of peripheral hearing sensitivity in humans was proposed and tested. Davis and Onishi (1969) did early work in human AEPs, and they voiced uncertainty as to whether brainstem AEPs would be feasible in infants, "This raises the practical question whether the V potentials can be observed in infants . . . " (p. 24). Their work on the clinical use of auditory brainstem response (ABR) paved the way to using ABR for infant hearing testing (e.g., Hecox & Galambos, 1974) and to the eventual development of automated ABR (Jacobson, Jacobson, & Spahr, 1990) to screen hearing in infants. Later in the 1970s, the development of clinical applications of otoacoustic emissions (OAEs) provided another objective test of hearing status. Early OAE work was done by David Kemp (1978), and this led to the application of OAEs as an approach to newborn hearing screening (e.g., Kemp, Ryan, & Bray, 1990).

By 1973, the JCIH had reconvened and recommended that a high-risk register be used to identify at-risk infants. It was recommended that at-risk infants be identified, tested, and followed. Five risk factors were recognized: a history of hearing loss that was known to be genetic; rubella or nonbacterial intrauterine infection; a defect of the ear, nose, or throat; a birth weight of less than 1,500 g; and a potentially toxic level of bilirubin. Importantly, the JCIH recommended that these children be followed even if hearing initially seemed to be normal, recognizing that some hearing loss has a delayed onset. In 1988, the then U.S. Surgeon General, C. Everett Koop, issued a challenge that by the year 2000 infants with permanent hearing loss would be identified prior to 12 months of age. This was part of the Healthy People 2000 initiative (Koop, 2010).

The National Institutes of Health (NIH) convened a task force in 1993 that endorsed universal newborn hearing screening in a consensus statement. The recommendation was to complete hearing screening by 3 months of age, and they recognized that the most effective way to achieve this goal was to test infants prior to hospital discharge. This groundbreaking document set the stage for contemporary screening programs (NIH, 1993). Additionally, the consensus statement emphasized the need for surveillance, recognizing the importance of identifying later-onset hearing loss. Bess and Paradise (1994) argued that more research was needed before proceeding with the recommendation for universal newborn hearing screening. They proposed that it would be more prudent and cost effective to continue with a high-risk register in combination with automated ABR rather than screening all infants. They were not alone in their concerns, but the wheels were in motion. Subsequently, evidence was presented suggesting that children whose hearing loss was identified early and who received early intervention before 6 months of age had better language outcomes than those identified after 6 months of age (Yoshinago-Itano, Sedley, Coulter, & Mehl, 1998).

The JCIH position statements continue to expand and be refined as new data become available. There were updates published in 1982, 1990, 1994, 2000, and 2007, and an update is currently underway. The JCIH has become increasingly interdisciplinary, with recommendations reflecting the growth of technology and knowledge about congenital and early-onset hearing loss and its effects on auditory and overall development. The current membership of the JCIH includes Alexander Graham Bell Association for the Deaf and Hard of Hearing, AAP, American Academy of Audiology, American Academy of Otolaryngology-Head and Neck Surgery, ASHA, Council of Education of the Deaf, and Directors of Speech and Hearing Programs in State Health and Welfare Agencies. Supporting organizations include Centers for Disease Control and Prevention (CDC), Maternal and Child Health Bureau, and National Institutes on Deafness and Other Communication Disorders (NIH-NIDCD). Thanks to New York Congressman James Walsh (NY-R), in 2000 there were federal monies allocated to Health Resources and Services Administration (HRSA), CDC, and NIDCD for development of newborn hearing screening programs, for development of data and tracking systems, and to support research in newborn hearing screening and intervention. Although these were not the first federal dollars supporting newborn hearing screening research and development, the "Walsh Act" provided the necessary backdrop for continued momentum.

Two U.S. Preventive Services Task Force (USPSTF) reports addressed the issue of universal newborn hearing screening. The conclusion from the 2001 USPSTF was that the evidence was not sufficient to recommend either for or against universal newborn hearing screening. The update in 2008 (Nelson, Bougatsos, & Nygren, 2008) concluded that children who had newborn hearing screening and were found to have hearing loss had better language outcomes at school age when compared to those not screened, and that these infants had significantly earlier identification, diagnosis, and intervention. The 2008 document is now inactive, and an update is not planned per the agency (USPTF, 2008). However, the Guide to Clinical Preventive Services (USPTF, 2014, see p. 72) endorses universal newborn hearing screening before 1 month of age, and for those not passing to have audiological and medical evaluations prior to 3 months of age.

International Momentum

Although much of the work described in this chapter originated in the United States, progress in universal newborn hearing screening programs has occurred in many developed and developing countries across the globe (Chen et al., 2012; Olusanya, 2012; Olusanya, Newmann, & Saunders, 2014; Sloot et al., 2015). The European Consensus Development Conference on Neonatal Hearing Screening convened in early 1998 and published their consensus statement endorsing neonatal hearing screening in 1999 (Grandori, 1998). Notably, the United Kingdom has had hearing screening programs for many years, with the policy recommendation for universal newborn hearing screening beginning in 2006 (Pimperton & Kennedy, 2012). Prior to 2006, hearing screening in the United Kingdom was done using the health visitor distraction test (HVDT). The HVDT is a behavioral hearing screening in which infants localize to sounds presented outside of their visual field, thus requiring the infants to be about 7 months old to participate reliably (Davis et al., 1997).

Although due for renewal and migrating to the http://www.gov.uk website as part of Public Health England, UK newborn hearing screening protocols and quality indicators are found currently at http://hearing.screening.nhs.uk/standardsandprotocols.

In Germany, the Institute for Quality and Efficiency in Health Care (IQWiG) produced the Neonatal Screening for Early Detection of Hearing Impairment: Final Report in 2007. The update of the IQWiG report was published by Wolff, Hommerich, Riemsma, Antes, Lange, and Kleijnen (2010) with the conclusion that high-quality evidence about all aspects of newborn hearing screening was lacking; however, they acknowledged that the early identification and intervention of children who were deaf or hard of hearing *may* be associated with improved language development.

The Universal Newborn Hearing Screening: Position Statement from the Canadian Paediatric Society was published in 2011(Patel & Feldman, 2011) and reaffirmed in 2014. The statement recommends universal newborn hearing screening using a comprehensive program of screening, diagnosis, and early intervention, encouraging all Canadian provinces to initiate comprehensive programs.

The World Health Organization (WHO) continues to address the issue of newborn and infant hearing screening. In Newborn and Infant Hearing Screening: Current Issues and Guiding Principles for Action (2009), the WHO recognized that each country and region has challenges implementing newborn hearing screening, with the largest challenges in remote and rural areas, especially in resource-poor countries. These same regions/countries are also those where most deliveries are at home rather than in a hospital or clinic. Although obstacles to universal newborn hearing screening are recognized, the WHO proposed six guiding principles for action to promote and support the development and implementation of universal hearing screening programs in a variety of settings with differing health care systems. These considerations and principles are summarized here:

1. Etiology of hearing loss in infants and children
   a. Etiology of hearing loss varies from country to country.
   b. About half of congenital and early-onset hearing loss is genetic.
   c. Hearing loss that is not identified (and treated) early adversely affects speech and language development.
   d. Without universal newborn hearing screening, children have later identification of hearing loss, with mild hearing loss and unilateral hearing loss not detected until children are 6 years of age or older.
   e. Identification of hearing loss and intervention in the first few months of life improves outcomes.
2. Use of "case definition" in newborn hearing and infant hearing screening
   a. Most current programs target permanent hearing loss of 30 to 40 dB or greater.
   b. There is increasing attention on identifying and treating milder degrees of hearing loss, as well as unilateral hearing loss.
   c. There is a need to use consistent definitions of the targeted population so that impact can be determined.
3. Approaches and methods used for screening
   a. The use of physiological screening tools, OAE or ABR, is well accepted; however, where not feasible, interim measures can be considered, such as family questionnaires or behavioral measures, to identify those in need of diagnostic audiological testing.
   b. Where universal newborn hearing screening is not feasible, a subset of infants may be the focus of the screening based on geography, those in intensive care units, or those with risk factors.
   c. The final goal, regardless of the interim approach, is universal physiological hearing screening of all neonates.
4. Program implementation components to foster success should
   a. clearly state program goals and the roles of those involved;
   b. specify a lead person who has oversight of the program;
   c. define the screening protocol;
   d. regularly monitor the program to insure correct implementation;
   e. specifically train the staff conducting the screenings;
   f. include training for informing parents of test findings, recording and reporting data, and related hospital/clinic procedures; and
   g. document quality indicators, including tracking infants who do not pass the screening and follow-up issues.
5. Cost-effectiveness
   a. approaches to determine cost and cost effectiveness vary from country to country; and
   b. each program needs to document its program adequately so that outcomes and costs can be correctly calculated.
6. Policy and legislation issues
   a. The primary goal is to provide the best possible timely care in a timely manner.

b. Each country has its own health care and screening policies.
c. Local and national professional associations set standards of care.
d. Local governments are responsible for the financing and quality monitoring of EHDI.
e. Public-private partnerships and nongovernmental organizations (NGO) should be explored to assist in the design and implementation of newborn hearing screening programs.

Details on other countries' development plans are in the WHO report (2013) entitled, Multi-Country Assessment of National Capacity to Provide Hearing Care. Although the focus of this report was on preventable or treatable hearing loss, identifying the main causes of hearing loss as chronic ear infections, meningitis, rubella, noise, and ototoxic drugs, the data provide insights into why some member states do not have national ear and hearing care programs; predictably, other health priorities and lack of financial resources were the most commonly cited reasons.

Contemporary Guidance for EHDI Programs

The overarching goal of successful EHDI programs is that *all* children who are deaf or hard of hearing (D/HH) have access to the resources that allow them to reach their full potential. In order to achieve this larger goal, there has to be a solid foundation, with specific steps in place that lead to fulfillment of that goal. The JCIH statement (AAP, 2007) provides guidance for EHDI programs with eight principles:

1. Every infant has access to a physiologic hearing screening by 1 month of age.
2. Infants who do not pass the first hearing screening or rescreening undergo audiological and medical testing to determine the presence of hearing loss by 3 months of age.
3. Those with confirmed permanent hearing loss are enrolled in early intervention (EI) by 6 months of age, or sooner, with a straightforward, single point of entry.
4. EHDI systems are family centered and abide by state and federal guidelines. All intervention and treatment options are provided to families.
5. There is immediate access to high-quality technology (hearing aids, cochlear implants, and assistive technology), if needed.
6. Communication development is monitored beginning at 2 months of age in the medical home regardless of risk factors for hearing loss.
7. Infants and their families receive interdisciplinary intervention from professionals with knowledge of hearing loss, and those interventions/programs reflect the family's strengths, choices, traditions, and cultural beliefs.
8. Information systems must interface with electronic health records, and data are used to assess outcomes, including reporting the effectiveness of services at all levels (individual, practice/clinic, community, state, and federal).

In addition to the eight principles, JCIH details the screening protocols for the well-infant nursery (WIN) and the neonatal intensive care unit (NICU) nurseries. Benchmarks and quality indicators are provided and are used to determine program effectiveness.

The success of newborn hearing screening programs has been measured largely by screening completion prior to 1 month of age, diagnosis prior to 3 months, and enrollment in early intervention by 6 months (Williams, Alam, & Gaffney, 2015). For those infants and children found to have hearing loss, meeting the 1-3-6 benchmarks is only the beginning of the journey for them and their families. To address the EI needs, a detailed supplement to the JCIH 2007 was published entitled, A Supplement to the JCIH 2007 Position Statement: Principles and Guidelines for Early Intervention After Confirmation That a Child Is Deaf or Hard of Hearing (JCIH, 2013). This comprehensive document provides an important level of detail about quality aspects of EI for infants and children who are deaf and hard of hearing (D/HH). Twelve goals are provided with rationales and recommendations for each:

1. There is access to EI programs, with a data management system that can track families and children from the identification of hearing loss to enrollment in services.
2. There is timely access to service coordinators with specialized knowledge and skills in serving individuals who are D/HH.
3. The EI providers have the professional qualifications, knowledge, and skills to optimize the child's development and the child/family's well-being.
4. For those children with additional disabilities, there are qualified specialists to optimize developmental outcomes.
5. Families from culturally diverse backgrounds and/or from non-English-speaking homes should have access to culturally competent care with the same

quality and quantity of information provided to families from the majority culture.

6. Children will have their progress monitored every 6 months from birth to 36 months of age, using a protocol with standardized, norm-referenced developmental evaluations, including language regardless of modality, social-emotional, cognitive, and fine and gross motor skills.
7. Those with hearing loss of any degree, including unilateral or *slight* hearing loss, with auditory neural hearing loss (auditory neuropathy, which is also called auditory neuropathy spectrum disorder or ANSD), and those with progressive or fluctuating hearing loss, receive monitoring and follow-up intervention services.
8. Families are active participants in the development and implementation of EHDI systems at all levels.
9. Families have access to other families who have children who are D/HH, and these families are trained to provide culturally and linguistically sensitive support, mentorship, and guidance.
10. People who are D/HH are active participants in the development and implementation of EHDI systems at all levels as integral members of the system.
11. Children and families have access to support, mentorship, and guidance from individuals who are D/HH.
12. There is fidelity in the services that they receive.

In this document, a benchmark of 90% was recommended to encourage each of the following:

1. A coordinated and timely system for access to EI services should be provided, with referral within 48 hours of confirmation of hearing loss, and an individual service plan (IFSP) completion within 45 days of the referral. (Note that the JCIH 2007 indicates that the U.S. federal guideline for referral to EI is within 2 days of the confirmation of hearing loss [CFR §303.21d]; however, the IDEA 2011 Part C regulations state that the child be referred as soon as possible, and not more than 7 days after identification [34 CFR §303.303- Referral Procedures]. Part C includes the U.S. federal regulations for serving 0- to 3-year-olds under the Individuals with Disabilities Act [IDEA].) The EI professionals should have the knowledge and skills to ensure positive outcomes for children who are D/HH, and there is a mechanism to track each child from confirmation to the end of EI services. A resource manual for families should be updated yearly.
2. Timely access to informed service coordination should exist with service coordinators specifically skilled in working with children who are D/HH 0 to 3 years of age and their families, and who are able to fulfill the Part C legal requirements.
3. EI service should be provided by providers who meet specific professional qualifications, with qualifications that are specified by each state/territory within 2 years of the document's publication. States/territories have a statement specifying professional development programs for EI providers within 5 years of the document's publication.
4. EI providers need specialized skills in listening and spoken language, sign language (American Sign Language, sign systems, or cued speech), and for integrated systems of visual communication and spoken language.
5. A system should be in place to ensure family involvement in EHDI programs at all levels, and families should have ongoing access to family-to-family supports.
6. Individuals who are D/HH participate in EHDI programs and families have access to these individuals.
7. A state/territory fidelity monitoring system for EI services is implemented within 5 years of the document's publication.
8. Each child's development is monitored annually.
9. A system should be in place to determine if EI providers have the skills and knowledge to provide intervention of children with additional disabilities (e.g., motor, vision, cognition).
10. A reporting mechanism exists to track the number and percentage of families who are served in nonnative English-speaking homes, specifying the home language(s).
11. Protocols should be in place for families who do not speak English or are culturally diverse, and there should be a system to monitor this aspect of care within 5 years of the document's publication.

On the international level, Moeller, Carr, Seaver, Stredler-Brown, and Holzinger (2013) delineated a best practices consensus statement that reflected input from 10 nations. The consensus panel included parents, researchers, deaf professionals, and EI program leaders and specialists. Ten best-practice principles were proposed, and within each of these, specific provider and program behaviors are specified. The best practice principles are summarized here:

1. There is immediate, timely, and equitable access to services and interventions.
2. There are balanced partnerships between families and professionals, and the partnerships should be

reciprocal, trusting, respectful and honest, with open communication.

3. Professionals support families to gain knowledge, information, and experiences so that they can make well-informed choices/decisions that are malleable.
4. Families have social and emotional supports, both formal and informal.
5. An optimal language-learning environment is created.
6. Providers are skilled to optimally support the child's language and communication development using assistive technologies and other tools.
7. Providers are qualified (with knowledge and competencies) to work with children who are D/HH and their families.
8. There is collaborative, interdisciplinary teamwork with team membership based on the needs of the family.
9. Child and family outcomes are routinely monitored.
10. Providers and programs are evaluated continuously.

Role of Audiologists in EHDI Programs

Audiologists should have a central role in newborn hearing screening and follow-up. Their skills, knowledge, and expertise and the best practice guidelines dictate that oversight of newborn hearing screening programs by audiologists is essential. Audiologists are the experts in hearing health care. The amount of involvement an audiologist has in newborn hearing screening and EHDI programs varies widely depending on program needs and regulations, as well as availability of audiologists. Audiologists' roles at the agency, hospital/clinic, state or federal level might include, but are not limited to, program manager, advisory board member, consultant, case reviewer, quality assurance manager, follow-up coordinator, and primary audiologist for children who are D/HH. For audiologists taking on the role of service coordination, their knowledge set extends well beyond the everyday program operations, and includes all other aspects of the EHDI process, including an in-depth working knowledge of all federal, state, and local rules and regulations that apply. In the upcoming section on Public Health, specifics of the various agencies and initiatives are detailed. For pediatric audiologists who are entering the EHDI world for the first time, there is much to learn because EHDI crosses many disciplines that require familiarization regardless of the audiologist's role.

In some states there are stipulations that screening programs *must* have oversight from an audiologist. Each state is unique, and the audiologist's role might or might not be specified. Thus, it is important to be well versed with the laws (statutes and regulations) where audiologists serve to ensure compliance. Some states require that audiologists serve on the state program's Newborn Hearing Screening Advisory Committee (e.g., Massachusetts, General Law, Section 67f). Kansas law specifies that "an audiologist on staff or a consulting audiologist to be responsible for overseeing the audiologic aspects of the facility's hearing screening program, including screening, tracking, referral for evaluation, and personnel training" (Kansas Administrative Regulations, p 163).

Oversight can be defined in different ways and encompass diverse responsibilities. It can be defined minimally as assisting to set up a screening program, having input into and/or choosing the equipment that is to be used and procedures to be followed. It can extend to training of personnel, but subsequently stepping back and becoming a resource for future issues and questions. A larger oversight role would be one wherein the audiologist helps to ensure sustainability of the program and assumes accountability for the program. The responsibilities can also extend into day-to-day oversight, and audiologists can assume the role of program manager.

Whether an audiologist or some other person is the screening program manager, that individual oversees the day-to-day activities related to screening. The daily activities include scheduling of the screeners or designating which nurses or key personnel will screen to cover births that occur throughout the day every day of the week. Other duties include monitoring hospital transfers, discharges, and ensuring that all births and admissions are screened prior to discharge. Supplies need to be monitored for consumption and ordered. The program manager needs to respond to equipment malfunctions and have policies and procedures for equipment down time or breakage. Equipment also needs to be scheduled for calibration, at minimal on a yearly basis.

Hospital policies and procedures vary and might specify screening location (e.g., nursery, mother's room, designated screening room), at what age to start screening, who talks to the families about the screening results, what specific information is shared, and how talk to the families. Guidelines for audiologists providing informational and adjustment counseling to families of infants and young children with hearing loss birth to 5 years of age can be found at http://www.ASHA.org (2008). In some hospitals, there might be a script for the screeners to use when talking with families. Additionally, procedures need to be in place to describe what is to be done when outer ear anomalies exist (e.g., when there is unilateral ear canal atresia, is the newborn screened or immediately referred to an audiologist for diagnostic testing?). Furthermore, are high-risk indicators collected and reported to the state, and who is responsible for follow-up of those children who have risk indicators? The proper documentation and dissemination of results are routinely required but can vary as to how the results are documented and where the results are sent. Other duties include monitoring quality indicators, generating and disseminating program reports, serving as a liaison between the hospital and state, and monitoring compliance with state guidelines. Besides the specific hospital policies and procedures for screening, knowledge of and adherence to confidentiality requirements, the patient Bill of Rights, nursery emergency procedures, universal/standard precautions, risk management and incident reporting, general safety issues, and effective communication to other hospital staff are essential.

The program manager needs to ensure that qualified individuals are hired to conduct the screenings. Some hospitals use nursing staff in this capacity as they are accessible to the babies during the infants' stay in the hospital. Some hospitals outsource the screening function. Regardless of who is screening, the program manager needs to ensure that the screening personnel are well trained, their competencies are assessed, and the staff have access to continuing education.

Screening Protocols and Equipment Acquisition

Decisions about equipment and the screening protocol are some of the largest decisions that need to be made by the audiologist. Factors to consider include who will be conducting the screening, the number of babies to be screened in the WIN and NICU, the availability of outpatient screening, and costs. In addition, it is necessary to define the targeted type and degree of hearing loss. Most manufacturers target identification of hearing losses of 40 dB and greater. However, there is equipment that allows adjustments to be made to the ABR screening level as well as parameters for OAE (see Chapter 20 of this volume) that can improve detection of milder degrees of loss. The ability to identify milder hearing losses is a worthwhile goal; however, there is a trade-off in increased failure rate. Community capacities to perform follow-up screenings, as well as resources to ensure follow-up of infants who do not pass, play a part in the decision of the screening level and other screening parameters.

Currently, automated ABR and OAEs are the primary test methods used in newborn hearing screening programs. There are five typical options: (a) ABR screening only for the NICU, (b) ABR screening only for the WIN, (c) OAE screening only, (d) OAE with ABR as the rescreen if OAE is failed, and (e) ABR and OAE. For the latter option, the infant must pass both tests. A flowchart for each option and the decision tree for each step are shown in Figures 18–1 through 18–5, and are found at http://www.ASHA.org in the Expert panel recommendations on newborn hearing screening section. ABR screening only can be used in the WIN (Figure 18–1) or NICU (Figure 18–2). OAE screening only is appropriate for the WIN (Figure 18–3). The OAE with ABR as the rescreen if OAE is failed can be used in the WIN (Figure 18–4), and the option for both ABR and OAE (Figure 18–5) can be applied in either nursery.

There are advantages and disadvantages to each method and test combination. Primary advantages of automated ABR include lower failure rates as compared to the OAE-only option and the potential to detect neural hearing loss. The primary advantages of OAE-only are the low cost, both initial equipment cost and ongoing supply cost as there are no electrode costs, test time is shorter with OAE, and OAEs are considered a reasonable screening tool in WINs (Berg, Prieve, Serpanos, & Wheaton, 2011). OAEs typically have a higher first-screen failure rate and overall higher failure rate compared to ABR because they are more sensitive to both middle ear problems and hearing loss. The easy availability of an outpatient rescreen is necessary if OAEs are the method of choice for the inpatient screen because more infants will require rescreening. OAEs have an additional disadvantage in that they do not detect neural hearing loss, if that is a goal of a screening program in the WIN. Identifying neural hearing losses is a must if the hospital has an NICU; therefore, the ABR is the method of choice for those infants.

If OAE testing is used, the decision has to be made as to which type of OAE to select—distortion product otoacoustic emissions (DPOAE) or transient-evoked otoacoustic emissions (TEOAE). Norton et al. (2000a), in a large-scale study, evaluated DPOAEs, TEOAEs, and ABR screening tests. Although some of the parameters used in that study were not the same as those some manufacturers employ, it is one of the few studies that evaluated performance across tests, and evaluated the hearing levels of the infants with behavioral test

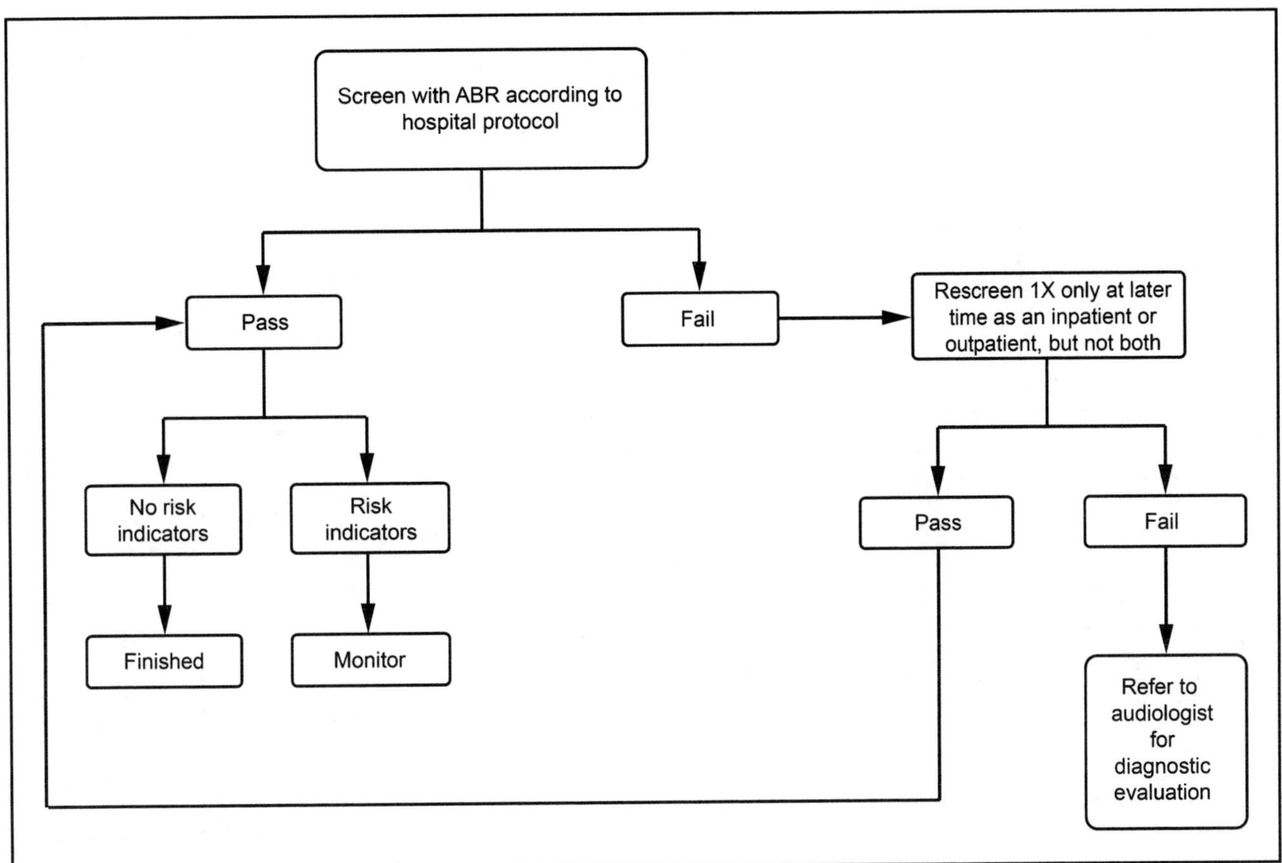

FIGURE 18–1. Auditory brainstem response (ABR) only protocol for well-infant nursery. (From American Speech-Language-Hearing Association. [n.d.]. *Professional Issues: Newborn Hearing Screening* [Practice Portal]. Retrieved June 2, 2015, from http://www.asha.org/PRPSpecificTopic.aspx?folderid=8589935234§ion=Key_Issues. Reprinted with permission.)

methods. The DPOAE stimuli levels were 65/50 (65/55 is more common in current clinical equipment), typical TEOAE click level was 80 dB pSPL, and a lower ABR click level of 30 dB nHL click ABR was used. The results showed a similar ability to identify hearing losses of 30 dB or greater as assessed by visual reinforcement audiometry (VRA) at 8 to 12 months corrected age (Norton et al., 2000b).

OAE technology might be a preferred option for those hospitals that have dedicated personnel who can become proficient at probe placement. Although probes can also be used for ABR testing, the necessary probe seal in the ear canal is different between ABR and OAE. The use of probes for ABR is not quite as problematic as it is for OAE because OAEs require a good acoustic seal and consistent signal in order to run properly, and that is not necessary for obtaining an ABR, which requires a consistent signal in the ear canal. Obtaining an adequate acoustic seal in a newborn's ear requires expertise, practice, and patience. For ABR, there is often the option to use disposable earphones/ear cups/muffs instead of probes.

Cost is also a factor in determining which equipment to use. Costs can make ABR prohibitive, especially for large birthing hospitals as there are costs associated with disposable electrodes and potentially disposable earphones (e.g., muffs, ear cup) if a probe is not used for the ABR screen. The costs of disposables vary among manufacturers.

Other equipment decisions that the audiologist needs to make has to do with how automated the equipment needs to be and the functionality of the equipment. Equipment needs to be automated when used by nonaudiology screeners. Equipment can include

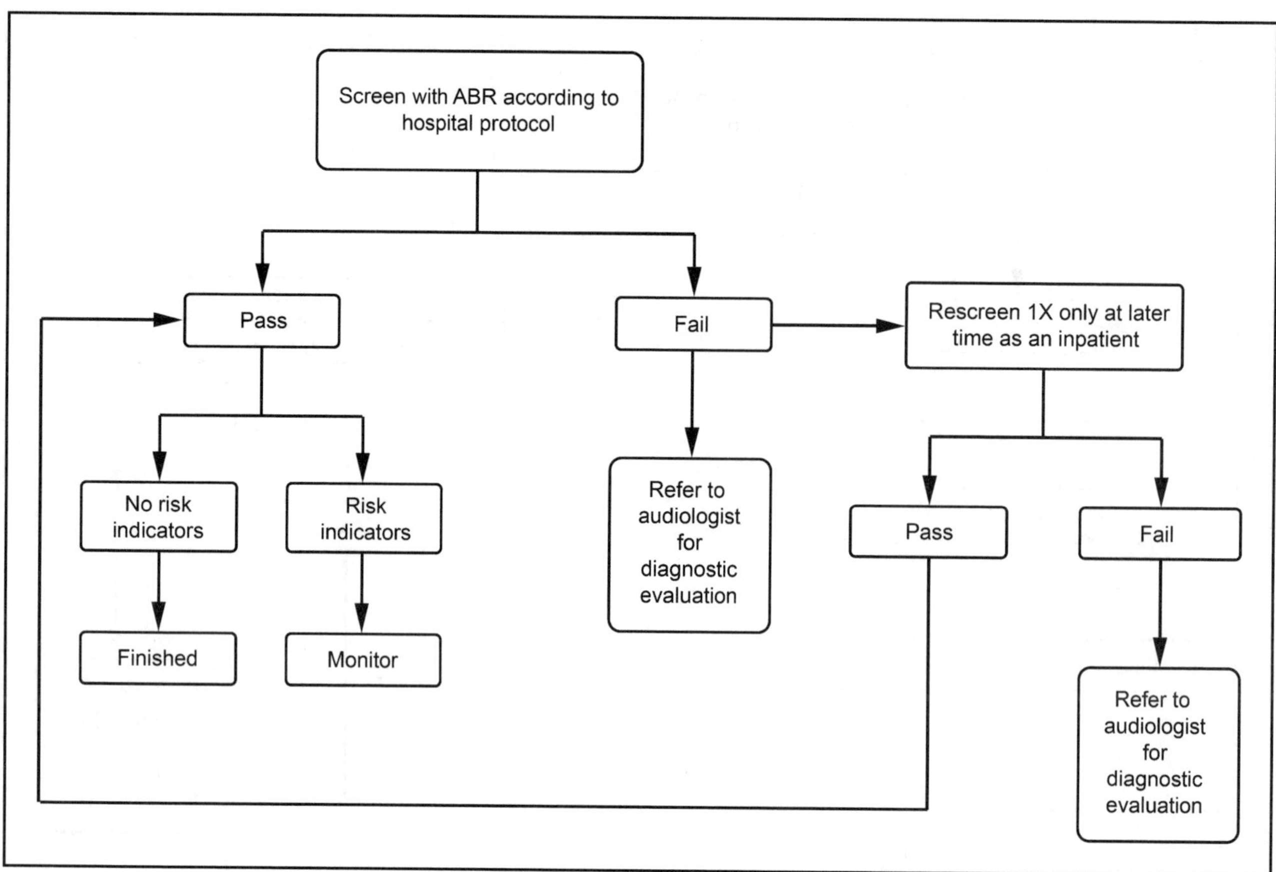

FIGURE 18–2. Auditory brainstem response (ABR) only protocol for neonatal intensive care nursery (NICU). (From American Speech-Language-Hearing Association. [n.d.]. *Professional issues: Newborn hearing screening* [Practice Portal]. Retrieved June 2, 2015, from http://www.asha.org/PRPSpecificTopic.aspx?folderid=8589935234§ion=Key_Issues. Reprinted with permission.)

a stand-alone OAE unit, a stand-alone ABR unit, or a combined OAE/ABR unit, all of which come in handheld as well as cart-based systems. Space and how the screenings are conducted can dictate which unit best fits the hospital space and practice (i.e., does the screener go room to room for screening, or are the infants transported to a designated screening room?). The current trend in the United States is for babies to be screened in the mother's room, necessitating taking the equipment from room to room. In addition to the type of equipment and test method chosen for the screening, another consideration is whether the state has a reporting system that allows for or requires that the screening results be downloaded at day's end. Some programs require that all data be reported, not just data for those who fail their newborn screen, and some programs want the raw data. The equipment and data fields need to be compatible with the state requirements. These factors influence which types of equipment need to be purchased.

All test equipment is not created equal even within a given test type. Knowledge of the test equipment will help determine which piece of equipment suits the environment. More specifically, it is important for audiologists to understand how the noise floors are calculated for OAEs, what determines response presence or absence, the algorithms that are used in the equipment, and which test parameters can be manipulated in the equipment. For example, to determine TEOAE response presence, several studies have shown that a signal-to-noise ratio (SNR) of at least 4 dB, with 6 dB preferred, is needed for response determination (Norton et al., 2000a; Wessex Universal Neonatal Hearing Screening Trial Group, 1998). An alternative method

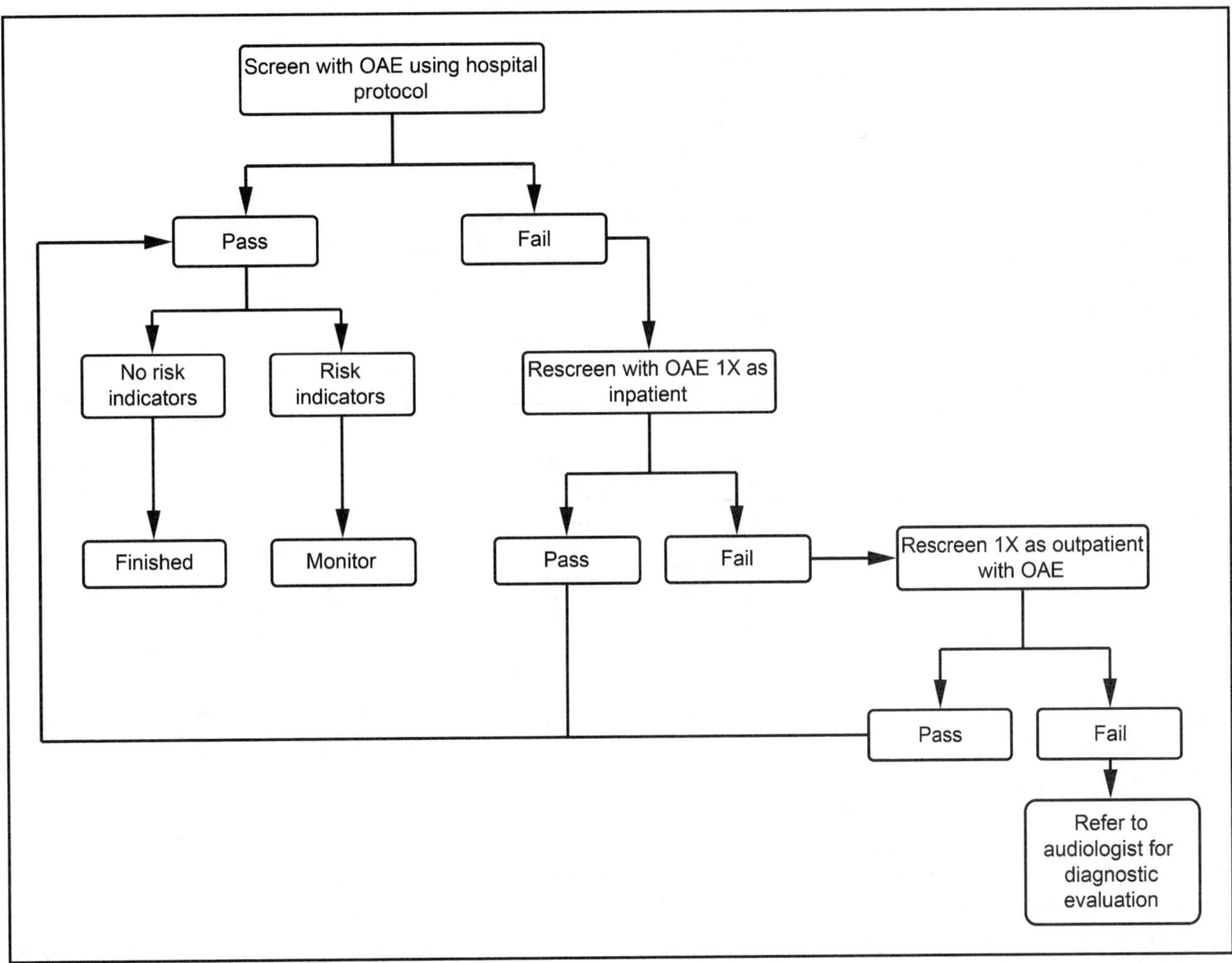

FIGURE 18–3. Otoacoustic emissions (OAEs) only protocol for well-infant nursery. (From American Speech-Language-Hearing Association. [n.d.]. *Professional issues: Newborn hearing screening* [Practice Portal]. Retrieved June 2, 2015, from http://www.asha.org/PRPSpecificTopic.aspx?folderid=8589935234§ion=Key_Issues. Reprinted with permission.)

for TEOAE response presence used by Vohr, Carty, Moore, and Letourneau (1998), was response reproducibility of 75% at 2000, 3000, and 4000 Hz. Equipment manufacturers might even use a combination of the two. More variability in response determination is seen with DPOAEs because of the differences in how the background noise is calculated. One method used is to measure the amount of noise in closely adjacent bins to where the DPOAE is being measured and determine the average or mean level. In this method, when compared to the mean, 6 dB is typically used, although it can be as high as 10 dB. Variations among manufacturers are found in the number of bins used to calculate the noise. Another common approach to calculating noise for DPOAEs is to use +2 SD above the mean noise floor (Whitehead, McCoy, Martin, & Lonsbury-Martin, 1993). For the mean plus 2 SDs method, 3 dB has been used (e.g., Norton et al., 2000a). Other approaches use the 90th percentile of the levels of the noise bins (Dorn, Piskorski, Gorga, Neely, & Keefe, 1999). Manufacturers will often have their own criteria programmed into the screening equipment and often also include an absolute minimum DP level. Thus, understanding the criteria used in the equipment is important for understanding differences seen in equipment and for changing parameters.

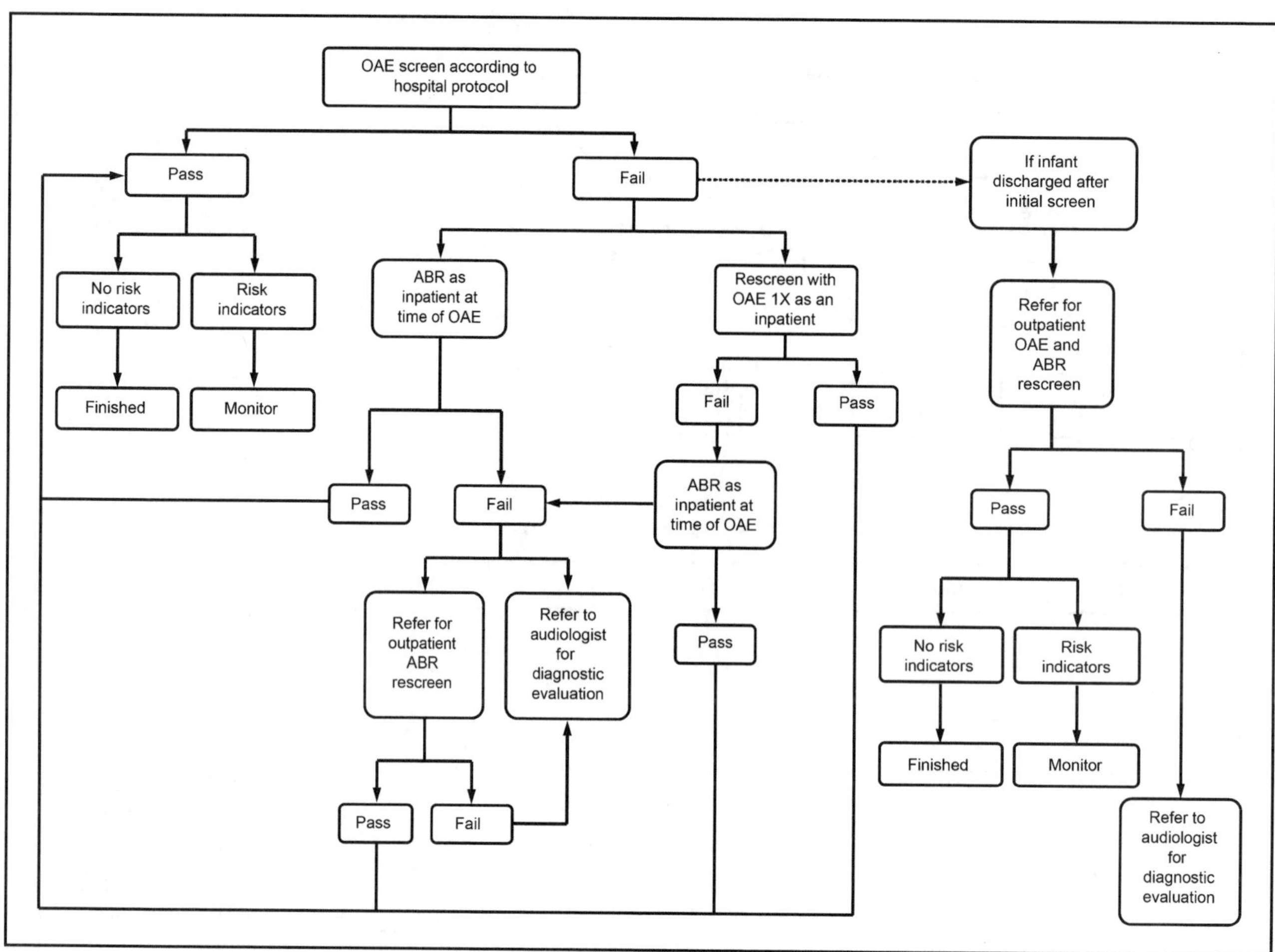

FIGURE 18–4. Two-tier protocol for well-infant nursery: otoacoustic emissions (OAE) followed by auditory brainstem response (ABR) when the OAE is not passed. (From American Speech-Language-Hearing Association. [n.d.]. *Professional issues: Newborn hearing screening* [Practice Portal]. Retrieved June 2, 2015, from http://www.asha.org/PRPSpecificTopic.aspx?folderid=8589935234§ion=Key_Issues. Reprinted with permission.)

Once technology is selected, the audiologist needs to determine the screening protocol. There are protocols that include a maximum of two inpatient screens and one outpatient screen prior to referral to audiology for a diagnostic evaluation. Regardless of screening method, repeated screenings are to be avoided with most recommended protocols calling for a maximum of three screens before a diagnostic evaluation is conducted. There are protocols that allow two inpatient screens with a referral straight to audiology for a diagnostic assessment when the inpatient screenings are not passed. Referral straight to an audiologist is more often recommended for infants in the NICU to avoid multiple follow-up appointments for infants who might still have some compromised health issues. Referral straight to an audiologist is also necessary when multiple screenings have already been conducted. The decisions with respect to setting the protocols also have to do, in part, with the resources available in the hospital or community. Are there audiology providers who can provide outpatient rescreens? Can the hospital provide outpatient rescreens? How far do the families have to travel for diagnostic audiology services, if not found locally? What is the wait time to get an appointment? These questions can help to formulate the best screening and follow-up protocol for a given program.

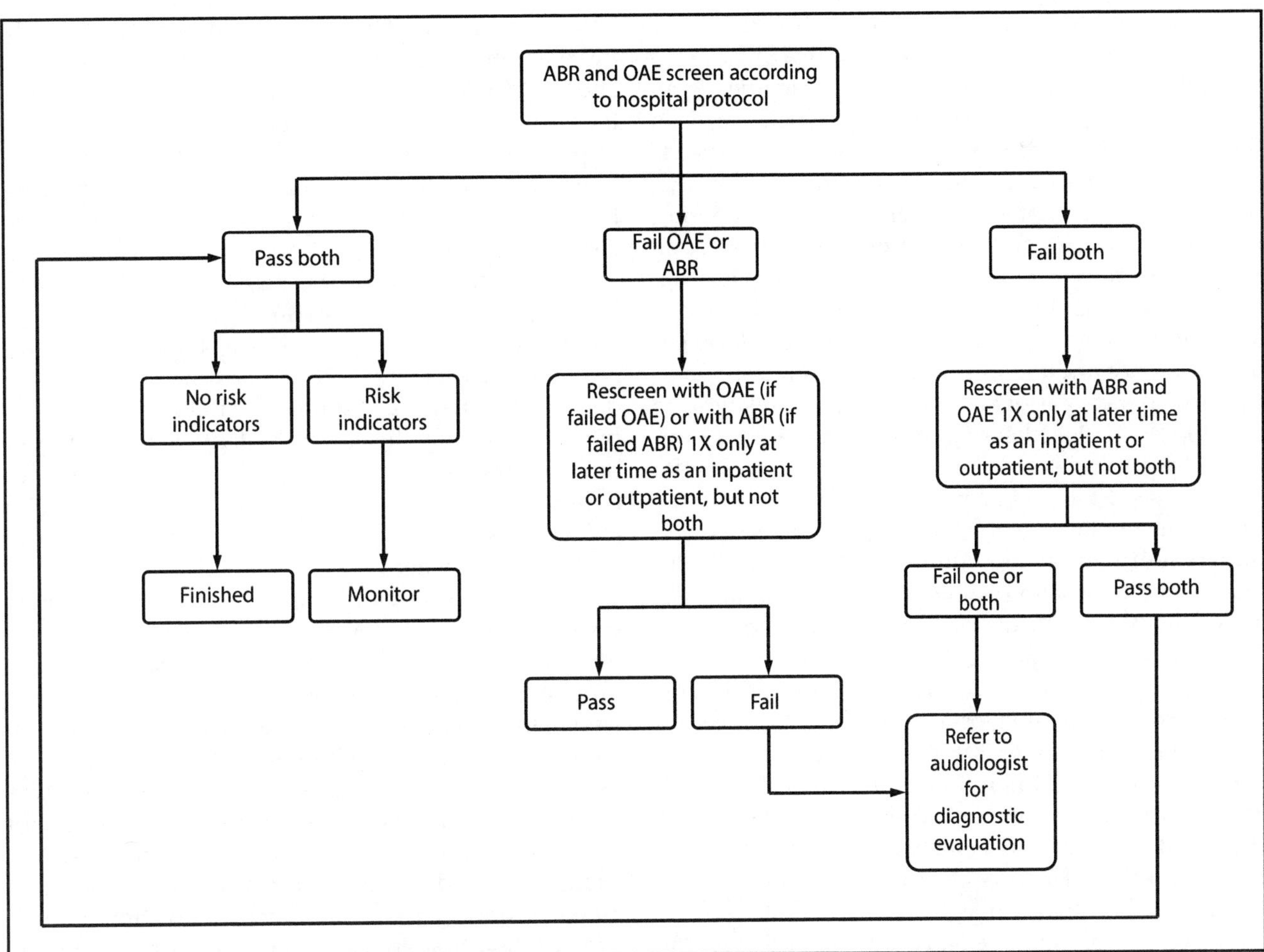

FIGURE 18–5. Two-technology protocol for well-baby and neonatal intensive care nurseries: auditory brainstem (ABR) and otoacoustic emissions (OAE). (From American Speech-Language-Hearing Association. [n.d.]. *Professional issues: Newborn hearing screening* [Practice Portal]. Retrieved June 2, 2015, from http://www.asha.org/PRPSpecificTopic.aspx?folderid=8589935234§ion=Key_Issues. Reprinted with permission.)

Follow-Up Procedures After Screening

Decisions about follow-up procedures are imperative in the screening process. Audiologists need to be knowledgeable about how to arrange follow-up appointment(s) and the timelines with which the follow-up must take place. To reiterate, the 1-3-6 benchmarks for timeliness are to screen (and rescreen, if indicated) by 1 month, diagnose by 3 months of age, with interventions in place by 6 months of age.

Knowledge of the method used to screen is important so that the outpatient rescreen method is the same. If an infant did not pass an ABR screening and passed a rescreen that was an OAE only, there is the possibility that neural hearing loss would be missed. The audiologist who is doing the follow-up testing needs to be skilled in evaluating infant hearing with physiologic methods to ensure timely diagnosis. If a hearing loss is found, the audiologist needs to understand and follow the next steps. Screening and diagnosis of hearing loss are useless if they occur in a vacuum. Test results must be communicated to the parents/caregivers and the primary care providers (PCPs), with a prompt referral to the EI program. The audiologist must be adept at management of infant hearing loss, as well as have familiarization of funding sources for amplification.

Building strong relationships with community PCPs (e.g., pediatricians or family practice physicians) as well as with clinics and audiology facilities is an important component of what the audiologist needs to do to ensure timely follow-up. In addition, there needs to be education of the stakeholders in the screening program. This is vital as there remain misconceptions, misunderstandings, and sometimes wrong information in the medical community regarding hearing, hearing loss diagnosis, and management. Education is needed to remind families and caregivers about developmental milestones and the importance of monitoring, particularly in the areas of auditory, speech, and language development. Once hearing loss is diagnosed, physician expertise becomes critical to the management process (see Chapters 7 and 8 of this volume). Their role in the etiologic evaluation, medical management, initiation of referrals for additional services or evaluations, and counseling is integral to guiding families smoothly through the maze of necessary appointments. The American College of Medical Genetics provides a guideline for the evaluation of newborns and infants with confirmed hearing loss (Professional Practice and Guideline Committee, 2014). Knowledge and good communication will help to ensure a team approach and, thus, potentially maximize favorable outcomes for the infant and family in a timely manner. In the United States, the Early Hearing Detection and Intervention-Pediatric Audiology Links to Services (EHDI-PALS) provides a database of pediatric audiologists who can provide timely follow-up (http://www.ehdi-pals.org).

In a 2012 survey, physicians' attitudes and knowledge of EHDI were explored (White, Behl, St. John, & Moeller, 2014). Approximately 54% of the respondents were pediatricians, and the remaining were family practice physicians, otolaryngologists, neonatologists, and a few obstetricians/gynecologists. The sample represented 26 states and mostly metropolitan areas (57%) but also small towns (26%) and rural areas (18%). Physicians were knowledgeable about the need for follow-up for infants who did not pass the newborn hearing screening, with over 93% specifying that the infant should be seen by or before 3 months of age. Most respondents knew that an infant can be diagnosed with hearing loss below 6 months of age (83%), but only 58% indicated that babies could be diagnosed below 3 months of age. These results suggest that there is still some misinformation about the age children can be diagnosed with hearing loss. Only about 12% of the responding physicians knew that infants can begin wearing hearing aids as early as 1 month of age or less, although 71% responded that infants can begin wearing hearing aids at less than 6 months of age. Only 12% of the respondents noted that referrals to early intervention should occur after 9 months of age, and about 62% responded such referrals could occur at less than 1 month of age. In an open-ended question, 73% of physician respondents noted that they would routinely refer a child with confirmed permanent hearing loss to otolaryngologists. In addition, there were misconceptions about what conditions put children at risk for permanent late onset hearing loss, with 26 % stating frequent colds, 30% stating hypotonia, and some reporting maternal age greater than 40 years (18%), and congenital heart disease (26%). Overall, 51% of respondents stated that their training did not adequately prepare them to meet the needs of infants with permanent hearing loss. These data suggest a continued need for audiologists to educate physicians and other health care professionals about hearing, hearing loss, diagnosis, and management.

Audiologists should employ evidence-based practices and follow national, state, and hospital guidelines for screening and follow-up. One document that helps programs to maintain consistency is the JCIH Position Statement (2007). Other documents that can inform consistent practice include regulatory guidelines, as well as hospital policies and procedures. Knowledge of the content of these documents is important to ensure accountability and quality of the program. Along with evidence-based practice, it is important to establish quality indicators for best practice. Knowledge of data that are collected by the state and CDC can guide which quality indicators should be gathered by programs. There are numerous quality indicators that can be used. Percent of babies screened is usually not an indicator that is of importance at this time as screening programs in the United States and Europe have reached high screening levels at this time (Sloot et al., 2015). However, indicators that describe quality of screening would be appropriate such as how many times infants are screened prior to discharge, failure rate, use of outpatient rescreens, and time required to complete outpatient rescreens. The ultimate measure of success are the positive outcomes from early identification and remediation of hearing loss in infants and young children.

Therefore, an important component of screening programs is reporting data to provide accurate tracking. Data reporting to the state is a key responsibility of those involved in the screening program. In addition to the screening results, ensuring that infants receive their diagnostic evaluations is part of the audiologist's responsibility, and reporting diagnostic results to the state is critical to state programs. Specifically, many states receive grant funding to operate their programs and must report accurate data to the granting agency. In addition, these data are reported to the CDC in the United States and territories, as CDC maintains national outcome data on state newborn hearing screening and follow-up programs. More details about tracking and reporting follow.

Stakeholders

Many states have established EHDI advisory committees (or boards) consistent with the CDC's recommended goals, objectives, and measures. Nearly half of the state EHDI programs are required by state statute to have an EHDI advisory committee (NCHAM, n.d.). Other state programs have established them on a voluntary basis. Of the 24 state EHDI programs with required EHDI advisory committees, only 10 specify the membership representation. Parents of children who are D/HH are the most common group representation specified in the state statutes consistent with the JCIH recommendations regarding advisory committee membership. Other commonly required advisory committee memberships include audiologists, physicians including pediatricians, otolaryngologists, and neonatologists, adults who are D/HH, hospital staff, and Part C/EI staff (JCIH, 2007).

The activities specified by state statutes for the EHDI advisory committees can include providing advice and recommendations for rules and regulations, implementation and oversight of the EHDI program, and reporting to the state legislature and governor. Typical areas of concentration include implementation and evaluation of the state EHDI program, collecting and reporting data, and developing screening and follow-up protocols. Some statutes specify the frequency of the advisory committee meetings, ranging from quarterly to annually.

The involvement of families of children who are D/HH in an EHDI program reaches far beyond membership on an advisory committee. The 2007 JCIH position statement suggests that parents can be instrumental in policy development and advocacy, resource development and dissemination, training of professionals, program assessment and quality improvement, and interaction with the Deaf community.

Henderson, Johnson, and Moodie (2014) conducted a scoping review of the literature focusing on parent-to-parent support for parents of children who are D/HH. Their goal was to identify the thematic concepts of key components of parent-to-parent support. Three themes were identified including well-being, knowledge, and empowerment. Key attributes of well-being included emotional, adaptational, and relational support for the family, and participation, autonomy, and goals for the child. The knowledge component included advocacy (legal rights, representation at many levels, and funding); system navigation of services, professionals, and transitions; and education regarding resources, skills, and unbiased information. The third component of the parent-to-parent conceptual framework was empowerment, which includes confidence and competence in parenting, decision making, self-awareness, problem solving, and parental engagement in the child's life. The results of this scoping review highlight the importance and relevance of parent engagement and parent-to-parent support.

Parent support groups have been created to provide education and emotional support to the parent(s) of a child who is D/HH. Some, such as the Alexander Graham Bell Association for the Deaf and Hard of Hearing and VOICE for Hearing Impaired Children, focus on a specific communication option, while Hands and Voices is inclusive of all communication options. Hands and Voices and VOICE for Hearing Impaired Children are both support groups that are parent driven. Hands and Voices has grown from a state parent-to-parent support organization in the 1990s to an international program with authorized or provisional chapters in the United States, Canada, Italy, and Kenya. Guide By Your Side, a licensed Hands and Voices program that employs parent guides who are trained to provide support to other parents, has been adopted by 23 Hands and Voices chapters.

Public Health and EHDI

Pediatric audiologists have an active role to play in EHDI programs and need to understand the intricate and larger world of EHDI and how it operates in their community. Even if an audiologist is acting solely in the role of providing diagnostic audiological services or amplification for infants and young children, understanding all aspects of EHDI is necessary to improve service delivery to an individual child and family, and to foster timely evaluations, interventions, and reporting.

EHDI is part of the public health system. Public health is defined by the WHO as "all organized measures (whether public or private) to prevent disease, promote health, and prolong life among the population as a whole. Its activities aim to provide conditions in which people can be healthy and focus on entire populations, not on individual patients or diseases. Thus, public health is concerned with the total system and not only the eradication of a particular disease"

(WHO, 2015). EHDI fulfills the three core public health functions of assessment, policy development, and assurance (CDC, 2014). Specifically, EHDI programs fulfill the core functions by assessing and monitoring community health problems and the effectiveness and quality of population-based health services; developing public policies to support community health efforts and priorities; and assuring that people are linked to appropriate care by ensuring the competency of both the public and private health care workforce, promoting health education, and forging collaborative efforts to solve health problems.

The disclosure of protected health information (PHI) to evaluate the effectiveness and quality of both personal and population-based health services is one example of how the core public health function of assessment is an integral component of the EHDI system. Privacy standards, developed in 2003 by the U.S. Department of Health and Human Services as required by the Health Insurance Portability and Accountability Act of 1996 (HIPAA), cover the use and disclosure of PHI by covered entities, such as health care plans, clearinghouses, providers, and business associates. Recognizing the need of public health programs, such as state EHDI programs, to collect individually identifiable PHI (screening and audiologic evaluation results) to conduct their activities, the privacy rule allows covered entities to disclose PHI to public health authorities without individual authorization when the public health authorities are legally permitted to collect the information (CDC, 2003b). Audiologists who are employed in medical settings are covered entities with regard to the privacy rule of HIPAA, and those who work in educational settings are covered under the Family Educational Rights and Privacy Act (FERPA), which has similar, though somewhat more stringent, safeguards for student information. As health records have steadily transitioned from paper records to electronic records, the issue of security has become increasingly critical and is also covered under HIPAA.

Two examples of the core function of EHDI policy development center on the provision of timely, affordable hearing aids for young children identified through newborn hearing screening programs to maximize their developmental outcomes. Following the lead of states with mandatory health insurance coverage for hearing aids, ASHA (2009) developed a model bill for insurance coverage for hearing aids for children, recommending a $2,000 hearing aid allowance per ear every 2 years. Another example of public health policy development occurs when bills are periodically introduced in the U.S. House of Representatives and Senate to provide a $500 tax credit per hearing aid once every 3 years for those purchasing a hearing aid (ASHA, 2015).

Because of audiologists' pivotal role in the EHDI system, the specification of audiologist qualifications and licensure are examples of the core public health function that assures a competent public health and personal health care workforce. Licensing is required in all states (Bureau of Labor Statistics, 2014) and the scope of practice for audiology might also be defined in statute. Medicaid, a U.S. public health insurance program for low-income individuals, is also an example of the assurance core function of public health. Medicaid regulations impact the audiology profession and EHDI programs by defining the qualifications necessary to receive reimbursement for services through Medicaid. A "qualified audiologist" is defined in the Centers for Medicare and Medicaid Services regulation 42 CFR 440.110(c; 3) as one who has a state license for audiology, if the license requirements meet or exceed ASHA's CCC-A requirements, or one who has a CCC-A in states with no licensure, lesser standards, or exemptions for practicing in certain settings (Office of the Federal Register, 2015).

In 2010, the WHO examined newborn hearing screening in the context of the accepted public health screening criteria that include

- an important health problem exists with an early symptomatic stage;
- a safe, suitable diagnostic test is available;
- acceptable and established intervention is available; and
- cost of diagnosis and treatment is balanced in relation to expenditure on medical care as a whole.

WHO recommended that universal newborn screening be adopted in all countries and communities if there were available rehabilitation services, and that the policy expand to additional countries and communities when rehabilitation services were available. This recommendation acknowledged that infrastructure development and capacity building of services and support are necessary to expand from newborn hearing screening to a comprehensive EHDI system that includes diagnostic, (re)habilitative, and other support services.

In the United States, the Healthy People initiative is the nation's health promotion and disease prevention agenda, and every 10 years objectives are set as part of the public health system. EHDI objectives were included for the first time in Healthy People 2000 (National Center for Health Statistics, 2001) and, therefore, required tracking and periodic reporting (White,

Forsman, Eichwald, & Munoz, 2010). In the current Healthy People 2020, Objective ENT-VSL-1 seeks to "increase the proportion of newborns who are screened for hearing loss by no later than age 1 month, have audiologic evaluation no later than age 3 months, and are enrolled in appropriate intervention services by no later than age 6 months" (U.S. Department of Health and Human Services, 2011).

The Government Performance and Results Act (GPRA) of 1993 (Public Law No. 103-62) specified that federal programs, including Maternal and Child Health Bureau (MCHB) and the CDC develop measureable goals to be reported annually. MCHB and CDC (DHHS, 2014) each award federal funding to state EHDI programs and have established measures to document the status of the EHDI system nationwide. These measures include efforts to increase the percentage of

- children with nonsyndromic hearing loss entering school with developmentally appropriate language skills;
- infants with hearing loss enrolled in early intervention before 6 months of age;
- infants suspected of having a hearing loss with a confirmed diagnosis by 3 months of age;
- infants screened for hearing loss prior to 1 month of age; and
- jurisdictions that collect, report, and use individually identifiable data in order to reduce the number of infants not passing hearing screening that are lost to follow-up.

The first state in the United States to pass newborn hearing screening legislation was Hawaii in 1990. Of the 43 states that have newborn hearing screening legislation, 34 were passed after 1998 (White et al., 2010). Examining the effect of legislation on newborn hearing screening rates, Green, Gaffney, Devine, and Grosse (2007) found that the average screening rate for states with legislation was 95% compared with 90% for those without legislation, and suggested that legislation was a causal difference in the screening rates. However, White (2015) indicated that legislation is not a necessary factor as some states without regulations have EHDI systems that are functioning well.

A recent analysis of legislation in 43 states (NCHAM, 2011) yielded the following findings:

- *Screening requirements*—All newborns are required to be screened in 28 states. Other states set the requirement as low as 85% and eight states provide exemptions for smaller birthing facilities.
- *Advisory committee established*—Of the 24 state EHDI programs with required EHDI advisory committees, only 10 specify membership representation.
- *Health insurance covered benefit*—Nineteen require health care providers to include newborn hearing screening as a covered benefit, but two require only that Medicaid includes coverage.
- *Reporting results to state health departments*—The reporting of newborn hearing screening results is required by 29 of the 43 states with legislation.
- *Educational materials for parents*—Twenty-three state statutes require parents of newborns to be educated about hearing screening, including two that specify educating parents who have out-of-hospital births. Five of those states require that members of the health care community receive education about newborn hearing screening.
- *Informed consent*—Statutes that require written parental informed consent for screening occur in only seven of the 43 states with legislation.
- *Liability immunity*—Nine states have statutes specifying that health professionals cannot be held criminally or civilly liable for reporting hearing screening results, and three states will not hold health care providers liable for not conducting a hearing screening.
- *Parental objection exclusion*—Parents can object to having a hearing screening conducted in 15 states for religious beliefs or tenets and five states permit parental objection without any reason specified.
- *Definition of hearing impairment*—The definition of hearing impairment in state statutes includes the degree of hearing loss for nine states (30 dB or greater in six states, 35 dB or greater in two states, and 40 dB or greater in one state), although four states include any hearing loss that is not sufficient to permit typical speech and language development. Five states define the frequency range of the hearing loss as 500 through 4000 Hz. Three states include both bilateral and unilateral hearing losses in the law.

U.S. Federal Legislation

The first U.S. federal legislation to support newborn hearing screening was written and sponsored by U.S. Representative James T. Walsh, and the Newborn and Infant Screening and Intervention Act, better known as the Walsh Act, was passed in 1999. The Walsh Act set up a system of discretionary grants to help states design and implement universal newborn hearing screening and statewide EHDI systems. Beginning in

2000, MCHB in the HRSA and the National Center for Birth Defects and Disabilities (NCBDD) at the CDC began awarding discretionary grants to states (Association of Maternal and Child Health Programs, 2005), which allowed states to screen newborns and track the results. Funding for projects was more narrowly focused with CDC cooperative agreements than with HRSA/MCHB grants that supported the development of statewide EHDI systems. The primary goals for CDC-funded projects were to develop comprehensive data reporting, tracking, and surveillance systems and to link or integrate those systems with other data systems. Funding was also provided to the NIH for research in the areas of screening and intervention. At the time of passage of the Walsh Act, only 34% of newborns had a hearing screening prior to discharge from birth admission. The act was later renamed the James T. Walsh Universal Newborn Hearing Screening Program.

The Early Hearing Detection and Intervention Act of 2010 expanded the scope of earlier federal legislation to include providing diagnostic services, recruiting and training personnel and providers, and fostering family-to-family support. A major emphasis of this legislation was to increase the rate of follow-up, in essence reducing the lost to follow-up (LTF) or lost to documentation (LTD; LTF/LTD) rate at each step in the EHDI protocol (42 USC § 280g-1). MCHB currently awards grants to EHDI programs in 58 states/jurisdictions (USDHHS, 2014), and CDC awards cooperative agreements to programs in 53 states/jurisdictions (DHHS, 2014). In 2015, new federal legislation was introduced to reauthorize the EHDI program.

Financial Resources: Funding and Budgets

An EHDI system consists of multiple components, each one contributing to the screening, medical, and audiological evaluations, early intervention, and family support services. As noted previously, federal funds have been available to each state EHDI program through grants from MCHB/HRSA and cooperative agreements with CDC. In a survey of state EHDI program coordinators in 2004, NCHAM found an average of 65% of EHDI program budgets were funded by federal sources through MCHB/HRSA and CDC. Other federal funding from MCHB Title V block grants, Medicaid, and Part C Early Intervention contributed an average of 16% of EHDI budgets. State funding through legislative appropriations was the source of an average of 14% of the reported budgets. The remaining 5% of the average state EHDI program budgets were from miscellaneous fees and state agencies (NCHAM, 2004).

Although no funding was reported from private foundations or donations for EHDI programs in the United States, Poland provides an example of an EHDI program that was initially totally funded through donations. Building on the success of an annual fundraiser to meet health care needs by collecting donations door-to-door, the Great Orchestra of Christmas Charity designated newborn hearing screening as the recipient of more than $6 million in 2001. With funding available, the lofty goal of setting up a universal newborn hearing screening in 440 hospitals in 30 days was achieved resulting in 99% of newborns receiving a hearing screening before leaving the birth hospital (Schillinger, n.d.). A variety of funding sources are reported for European Union countries, with primary funding from the government or health insurance (Sloot et al., 2015).

Developing a budget for the operations of an EHDI program is required for funders to know the projected use of the funds to be provided. Typical line items for an EHDI budget are as follows:

- *Personnel*—Often the largest expenditure for an EHDI program, personnel includes the wages and salaries of individuals employed by the EHDI program. For those funded by multiple sources, such as MCHB/HRSA and CDC for EHDI programs in the United States, each individual's time and salary or wages must be allocated to the funders' budgets in proportion to the planned amount of time to be obligated to the EHDI program.
- *Fringe benefits*—Fringe benefit costs include insurance, retirement, and all other employee benefits. Often the agency-wide cost of benefits is used to calculate a standard percentage that is applied to all personnel salaries.
- *Indirect costs*—Agency expenses that cannot be directly allocated to a particular program, such as space, utilities, and administrative costs, are considered to be indirect costs. The indirect cost percentage, which is calculated based on actual costs and approved by an outside entity, is applied to the salary or salary/fringe benefit totals.
- *Travel*—The costs of transportation and lodging for program staff and perhaps stakeholders to participate in meetings, attend conferences and seminars, and conduct on-site visits to hospitals and outpatient clinics is detailed in a budget.
- *Equipment*—Equipment costs could include computer equipment and hearing screening equipment that might be provided to screening sites, such as hospitals, audiology clinics, early care and educa-

tion programs, and health clinics. Some funders set a lower limit of equipment costs, with anything costing less than that amount being considered supplies.

- *Supplies*—Supplies are the smaller, miscellaneous items needed to run an EHDI program, such as paper and stamps. The cost of supplies might already be included in the indirect cost calculation if the program does not directly pay for these items.
- *Contractual*—Contracts for services are important mechanisms for EHDI programs, many of which are with state governments in the United States. By contracting with individuals for direct services within the EHDI program or for the development of products, such as software tracking systems, educational programs, and materials, the EHDI program can access expertise on an as-needed basis.
- *Interpreters*—The cost of providing interpreters to communicate with families and stakeholders who use a manual communication modality, or other language, might be a separate line item or can be included in the contractual line item.
- *Other*—Miscellaneous costs not specifically included in any of the other budget line items can be included here. Funders can request that certain types of costs be included in this category.
- *In-kind*—Some funders require a certain percentage of in-kind contribution by the provider of services, which is the value of goods, services, and donations that are given to the program. Determining the value of these contributions must be accurate because some funders disallow some in-kind, resulting in the program actually losing grant funds because the in-kind portion of the budget was not met.

A budget is an EHDI program's plan to use the funds provided by an outside funding entity. Actual expenditures will most likely differ from the budget as the program is implemented during the funding cycle. As costs are reallocated throughout a budget year, a request might need to be made to the funder for approval to move funds exceeding a predetermined amount from one line item to another.

Data Tracking and Reporting

As noted above, accurate tracking and reporting functions are essential to the success and improvement of any EHDI programs. In the United States, only 29 states have legislation that requires screening results be reported to the state EHDI program (NCHAM, 2011). Increasingly, states are developing systems that are either linked or integrated with public health data systems, such as metabolic/dried blood spot newborn screening, immunization, and vital records/birth records data systems. EHDI data systems that are integrated or linked with birth records can obtain identifying and demographic data for all births in the jurisdiction.

One of the national EHDI goals specifies that each state will have a comprehensive EHDI tracking and surveillance system for the purpose of minimizing loss to follow-up. The six tracking and surveillance system objectives (CDC, n.d.) include

- establishing a comprehensive data system with current hearing information on all infants birth to 3 years;
- developing written policies and procedures for the data system;
- developing data privacy and confidentiality policies, procedures, and informed consent requirements;
- ensuring that the system includes all live births;
- collecting hearing loss risk factors for all infants by linking with other state systems; and
- obtaining all hearing screening results within 1 week of discharge or transfer.

In 2009, 47 EHDI coordinators participated in a Strength-Weakness-Opportunity-Threat (SWOT) survey of their programs, identifying key factors in 12 program areas, including data management (Bradham, Hoffman, & Houston, 2011). The analysis of the coordinators' 242 responses in the data management area identified the following top themes:

- *strengths*: data collection practices, technology and Web-based systems, and resources;
- *weaknesses:* data collection practices, barriers with data management systems, and staffing concerns;
- *opportunities:* improving current data systems, data collection practices, and Web-based systems; and
- *threats:* funding, resources, and data collection practices.

A Threat-Opportunity-Weakness-Strength (TOWS) analysis of the SWOT data yielded three recommendations for EHDI programs:

1. address how to share data and/or link data systems;
2. maintain and/or upgrade existing systems so they are flexible and Web-based, streamline data entry, and make them accessible; and
3. implement a quality monitoring program from the data collected to improve systems.

A robust data tracking and surveillance system is a critical element of a quality EHDI system. A comprehensive data system supports the efforts of an EHDI program to document the hearing screening results of every child born in the state; the status of each child in the follow-up component of the program; details of audiologic evaluations, early intervention services, and specialty evaluations; and LTF/LTD status. These data support an EHDI program's in-depth analysis for quality improvement and reporting to stakeholders. CDC's funding for the development of data systems has been instrumental in the ability of state EHDI programs to develop systems that collect and process individually identifiable, rather than aggregate, data. As systems advance, data are transferred directly from screening equipment to the EHDI data system, reducing the need for paper results submission and/or data being input multiple times, which can result in errors (Hoff, Hoyt, Therrell, & Ayoob, 2006). Data that are Health Level Seven (HL7) compliant meet the standards for interoperability, permitting multiple health information systems to exchange data. Specific codes (using Logical Observational Identifiers, Names, Codes [LOINC] and Systematized Nomenclature of Medicine-Clinical Term [SNOMED-CT]) for newborn hearing screening, results, and risk factors have been developed (CDC, 2014).

EHDI programs fulfill part of public health's mission to prevent disability by maximizing language skills, communication competency, and literacy development for children who are D/HH. This requires EHDI programs to collect specific individually identifiable information in a timely manner and track the audiologic, medical, intervention, and support services for infants identified with PCHL. At a minimum, the screening provider should submit the following screening data:

- identifying information to include the infant's name, date of birth, place of birth, mother's name, address, phone numbers, and primary health care provider;
- date(s) of screening, type of screening, and ear-specific results; and
- recommendations, referrals, and follow-up plans.

An EHDI program might be tracking several hundred or thousand infants at any point in time, so it is important that sufficient identifying data be submitted with screening or evaluation results to accurately match the submitted report with the record in the EHDI data system. The EHDI data systems can be standalone; however, increasingly the systems are linked or integrated with other public health data systems, such as birth certificates, dried blood spot/metabolic, and immunization systems. By including a set of unvarying data elements (e.g., date of birth, place of birth, and mother's name) duplicate records can be merged even if infant names change. Basic information such as address, phone number, and primary health care provider's name assists the EHDI program to track all infants needing follow-up.

EHDI data systems in the United States continue to develop and expand the range of data being recorded and tracked, including the timeliness of provision of different services since EHDI 1-3-6 screening-evaluation-intervention goals are time-referenced. Information about risk factors or disabilities can provide information to the EHDI program about follow-up concerns. Data about the type, degree, and laterality of hearing loss, when combined with the child's age at diagnosis, provide the foundation for understanding factors that influence and contribute to longer-term linguistic, cognitive, and social-emotional developmental outcomes. Even submitting incomplete or inconclusive evaluation results allows an EHDI program to be aware of the current status and planned next steps. Identification of a transient conductive hearing loss due to middle ear dysfunction can necessitate the EHDI program prolonging follow-up activities until after medical management is completed. Similarly, reporting normal hearing evaluation results permits the EHDI program to record a definitive outcome and to cease follow-up efforts.

Nearly all of the state EHDI programs voluntarily complete CDC's Early Hearing Detection and Intervention Hearing Screening and Follow-up Survey (HSFS) each year. Aggregate numbers based on individually identifiable, unduplicated data about the screening, diagnostic, and early intervention components of the EHDI process are collected. HSFS is a snapshot of the birth cohort between 12 and 24 months of age. The survey, which began to collect information about screening, diagnostics, and early intervention outcomes in 2006, includes the following data:

- *screening data:* total screened and not screened, the reasons not screened, and the number and ages of screenings that were passed and not passed;
- *diagnostic data:* number with normal hearing and permanent hearing loss identified, ages at final evaluations, and the number with no diagnosis determined and the reasons;
- *intervention data:* number of referrals to Part C for EI services, numbers eligible and not eligible, age of enrollment in Part C or non-Part C services, and numbers with no services and reasons; and

- *type and severity of hearing loss:* numbers for each type, degree and laterality of PCHL.

The EHDI system in the United States continues to make improvements in all areas. In 7 years, the screened rate has increased by 2%, an increase of 664,539 infants screened as shown in Table 18–1. The overall failure rate has improved from 2.3% to 1.6%. The percentage of infants who completed an audiologic diagnostic evaluation after failing the final screening increased dramatically, from 34.1% to 58.7%, for a total of an additional 8,294 infants completing the diagnostic process. Improvements in the numbers and percentages of children receiving services at each step of the EHDI 1-3-6 protocol can be attributed to a major focus on reducing LTF/LTD. An emphasis on ensuring that transitions between and among service providers are effective, and, especially, better reporting at the diagnostic and early intervention levels have contributed to the improved outcomes. Additionally, the decrease in the screening failure rate suggests that screening has improved at the first step of the 1-3-6 protocol, thereby reducing the potential number of infants who do not complete the process. Improving the quality of services, tracking, and follow-up at any individual step of the EHDI process contributes to improved outcomes of the overall system.

The annual CDC survey requests that ear-specific evaluation results be reported for each child. As shown in Table 18–2, the percentage of bilateral and unilateral PCHL has remained relatively stable between 2006 and 2013. The reduction of numbers in the "unknown" category suggests that evaluations are more complete with better reporting to the EHDI programs.

The annual CDC survey also collects data about the type of PCHL (Table 18–3). The 2013 HSFS reports included an "unknown" category for type of hearing loss, accounting for 9% of those reported. This "unknown" category might account for the reduction of sensory/neural PCHL (72% and 66% in 2006 and 2013, respectively) and conductive PCHL (18% and 12% in 2006 and 2013 respectively). However, this would not account for the increase in neural hearing loss (auditory neuropathy spectrum disorder [ANSD]) that increased from 3% in 2006 to 5% in 2013. The increase in identification of ANSD could be attributed to several reasons. JCIH (2007) recommended the exclusive use of ABR for screening in the NICU because of the increased risk of neural hearing loss in this population (Norrix & Velenovsky, 2014). The higher rate of ANSD identification could result from more ABR screenings, especially

Table 18–1. Summary of National EHDI Data, 2006 and 2013

Description	2006	2013
Percent screened, including infant deaths and parental refusals	95.2%	97.2%
Percent not passing final/most recent screening	2.3%	1.6%
Percent diagnosed with hearing loss or normal hearing	34.1%	58.7%
Prevalence per 1,000 screened	1.1	1.5
Percent enrolled in early intervention (Part C and Non-Part C)	55.4%	62.1%

Note. Based on Annual Data Early Hearing Detection and Intervention (EHDI) Program (http://www.cdc.gov/ncbddd/hearingloss/ehdi-data.html).

Table 18–2. Laterality of Hearing Loss (by Ear)

Laterality of Hearing Loss	2006	2013
Unilateral	22.4%	21.4%
Bilateral	72.5%	78.0%
Unknown	4.5%	0.6%

Note. Based on CDC HSFS survey results. Based on Annual Data Early Hearing Detection and Intervention (EHDI) Program (http://www.cdc.gov/ncbddd/hearingloss/ehdi-data.html).

Table 18–3. Type of Hearing Loss (by Ear)

Type of Hearing Loss	2006	2013
Sensory/neural	72.3%	65.9%
Conductive	17.8%	11.5%
Mixed	7.1%	8.1%
Unknown	n/a	9.4%
Auditory neuropathy spectrum disorder	2.8%	5.1%

Note. n/a, not applicable. Based on Annual Data Early Hearing Detection and Intervention (EHDI) Program (http://www.cdc.gov/ncbddd/hearingloss/ehdi-data.html).

in the NICU. It could also be due to an increased incidence of ANSD or better identification of the condition. Rance (2005) suggested that approximately 7% of the PCHL in children could be attributable to ANSD, based on a review of the prevalence of ANSD in 10 studies. A more recent report suggests an incidence of 13% in children who have severe-to-profound hearing loss (Talaat, Kabel, Samy, & Elbadry, 2009). These data will become clearer as the EHDI system continues to evolve and as evaluation capabilities and reporting become more accurate and reliable.

Degree of hearing loss for each ear is also submitted by the state EHDI programs to the CDC (Table 18–4). Between 2006 and 2013, the classification system changed from one developed by the Directors of Speech and Hearing Programs in State Health and Welfare Agencies (DSHPSHWA) to the one developed by ASHA. The intensity range of the DSHPSHWA's moderate hearing loss (41–70 dB) is the same as ASHA's moderate (41–55 dB) and moderately severe (56–70 dB) hearing loss categories combined; therefore, the degree of hearing loss can be compared across the two surveys. The derived moderate degree of hearing loss for the 2013 HSFS would be 39% compared with 35% for the 2006 HSFS. The new slight degree of hearing loss (16–25 dB) for the 2013 HSFS is 2%, which minimally impacts the comparison between 2006 and 2013 (CDC, 2013). The increase in the unknown degree of hearing loss in 2013 might be the result of infants being identified with PCHL younger with reports being submitted to the EHDI program before degree is definitely determined. For example, "bone conduction testing was not reliable," or "neural hearing loss is suspected but unconfirmed." Reporting of subsequent audiologic evaluations likely would decrease the unknown percentage.

Lost to Follow-up/ Lost to Documentation

Although all U.S. states and jurisdictions have implemented newborn hearing screening programs, and there have been significant improvements in the outcomes from the screening, evaluation, and early intervention components, there are infants for whom follow-up results are unknown. Overall, there has been a steady reduction in the percentage of infants who are categorized as LTF or LTD. LTF occurs when an infant does not receive a recommended follow-up service after a failed newborn hearing screening and can occur at any point in the EHDI process. An infant who does not pass the birth admission screening might not receive the recommended outpatient rescreening or the recommended audiologic evaluations to determine if hearing is normal or a permanent hearing loss exists. Therefore, an infant who has been identified with a PCHL might not receive early intervention services.

Another group of infants with missing data is classified as LTD. Infants in this group are those who have received services but results have not been reported to the EHDI program and, therefore, cannot be documented. In a study of LTD in dried bloodspot screening programs Hoff, Hoyt, Therrell, and Ayoob (2006) found

Table 18–4. Degree of Hearing Loss (by Ear)

Degree of Hearing Loss, 2006 (DSHPSHWA)	*Percentage*	*Degree of Hearing Loss, 2013 (ASHA)*	*Percentage*
		Slight (16–25 dB)	1.7%
Mild (21–40 dB)	24.2%	Mild (26–40 dB)	19.5%
Moderate (41–70 dB)	34.8%	Moderate (41–55 dB)	27.7%
		Moderately severe (56–70 dB)	11.1%
Severe (71–90 dB)	16.3%	Severe (71–90 dB)	11.9%
Profound (91+ dB)	22.8%	Profound (91+ dB)	21.2%
Unknown	1.8%	Unknown	7.0%

Note. Directors of Speech and Hearing Programs in State Health and Welfare Agencies, DSHPSHWA; American Speech-Hearing-Language Association, ASHA. Based on Annual Data Early Hearing Detection and Intervention (EHDI) Program (http://www.cdc.gov/ncbddd/hearingloss/ehdi-data.html).

that name changes, data mismatches, incomplete or erroneous parent contact information, and unknown PCP contributed to loss to documentation. However, EHDI programs cannot identify which cases are LTF and which are LTD, as follow-up information is missing for both groups.

EHDI programs have different data requirements and reporting processes, based on the statutes, regulations, and protocols in each jurisdiction. Therefore, there have not been standard definitions of LTF/LTD across EHDI programs, although the CDC has standardized definitions for the annual HSFS survey. LTF/LTD includes infants who did not receive an audiologic evaluation because the parents or family were contacted but were unresponsive, parents or family could not be contacted, or other unknown reasons. Another definition, "no diagnosis," includes infants whose evaluations are ongoing at the time of the survey, are nonresidents or moved from the state of birth, cannot complete the evaluation for medical reasons, the PCP does not refer for evaluation because the baby has died, or the family refused services.

The results of the annual voluntary CDC HSFS have shown a steady decrease in the number and rate of both "no diagnosis" and LTF/LTD from newborn screening to audiologic evaluation between 2006 and 2013. The percentage of babies with no diagnosis after not passing the final hearing screening has decreased from 65.9% (44,466) to 41.3% (22,020). Similarly, the LTD/LTF rate has improved from 47.4% (32,189) to 32.2% (17,160; Table 18–5). However, the LTF/LTD rates vary considerably from state to state, ranging from 0% to 86.7% (CDC, 2015).

Determination of the percentage of infants who have not completed the EHDI 1-3-6 protocol is currently the major quality measure for EHDI programs and it is closely examined by stakeholders and funders. The current method to calculate LTF/LTD uses the total number of infants who did not pass the final hearing screening, regardless of whether it was a one-step screening during birth admission or a two-step method that includes an outpatient screening, as the denominator. There are alternative approaches to determining the percentage of infants who did not complete the protocol.

Three methods to determine the percentage of infants who have not completed the EHDI protocol from screening to diagnostic evaluation are shown in Table 18–6. In these examples, the number and percent of "incompletes" at two different times are calculated using the same total number of infants screened (10,000), number who failed the initial screening (1,000), and the number who failed on the final

Table 18–5. Lost to Follow-up/Lost to Documentation (LTF/LTD) of Infants Not Passing the Final Hearing Screening, 2006 and 2013

	2006	*2013*
Number LTF/LTD	32,189	17,160
Percentage LTF/LTD	47.7%	32.2%

Note. Based on Annual Data Early Hearing Detection and Intervention (EHDI) Program (http://www.cdc.gov/ncbddd/hearingloss/ehdi-data.html).

Table 18–6. Alternative Methods to Determine Incomplete (Lost to Follow-up/Lost to Documentation [LTF/LTD]) Rates

	Number Unresponsive, Unable to Contact, Unknown (Numerator)	*Total Screened (Denominator)*	*Refer on Initial Screening (Denominator)*	*Refer on Final Screening (Denominator) (Current Method to Determine LTF/LTD)*
Time 1: Number	40	10,000	1,000	100
Time 1: Percent incomplete		0.4%	4.0%	40%
Time 2: Number	25	10,000	1,000	100
Time 2: Percent incomplete		0.25%	2.5%	25%

screening (100). Reducing the number of infants with incomplete results typically is the result of a significant investment of resources to improve the follow-up, education, and outreach with families by health and audiology providers, and other collaborating stakeholders. However, the percentages that are calculated based on different denominators can present significantly different impressions of the overall level of effort and success of EHDI programs in the first two decades of universal newborn hearing screening.

Most EHDI programs have been able to develop and implement new data systems through funding of cooperative agreements with the CDC, moving toward systems that are linked or integrated with other public health databases, especially the birth registry, and that gather individually identifiable, rather than aggregate, data. Aggregate data often include duplicates, in which the same results are reported for the same child by different providers and are, therefore, counted twice. Conversely, aggregate numeric data can indicate a completion of services (one infant diagnosed with hearing loss and one enrolled in Part C early intervention) when, in reality, the numbers in an aggregate report might actually be two different infants, one of whom was diagnosed with a hearing loss and did not receive early intervention services (LTF) and the other might not have been reported as diagnosed with a hearing loss (LTD) but did receive early intervention services (Hoffman, Munoz, Bradham, & Nelson, 2011).

In 2008, ASHA published a technical report on LTF/LTD in the EHDI system, based on a systematic review of the evidence by the National Center for Evidence-Based Practice in Communication Disorders (N-CEP), consensus data, and policy statements (ASHA, 2008). Three types of issues were identified as contributing to LTF/LTD: systems issues, family issues, and quality assurance issues.

Systems issues contributing to improvement in LTF/LTD included accurate identification of the infant's PCP, communication of hearing screening results to the PCP, consistent and adequate timing of parent education about newborn hearing screening, and explanation of the results and recommended follow-up. Additional issues included the coordination of services (e.g., lack of integrated data systems) and potential communication barriers due to privacy laws and regulations. EHDI program funding and reimbursement rates for pediatric audiologic services were also identified as system issues contributing to LTF.

The second major category of concerns contributing to LTF involved family issues. These concerns included maternal demographics, such as educational and literacy levels, age, marital status, and substance abuse, as well as socioeconomic factors. The Massachusetts Department of Public Health studied maternal and child factors associated with an increased likelihood of LTF/LTD (Liu, Farrell, MacNeil, Stone, & Barfield, 2008). Factors that increased the risk of being LTF between newborn hearing screening and audiologic evaluation included maternal race/ethnicity, maternal smoking during pregnancy, public insurance coverage, and area of residence within the state. Factors associated with LTF between diagnosis and early intervention included degree of hearing loss (mild, moderate, and unilateral hearing loss), normal birth weight, and area of residence within the state.

The major quality assurance issue, to identify and minimize LTF/LTD at all stages of the EHDI process, can best be addressed with a comprehensive EHDI tracking and surveillance data system. Per the CDC Guidance Manual (2003), factors necessary to complete follow-up in an effort to reduce LTF/LTD include

- computerized systems that have information on all infants screened, diagnostic results on infants who failed the screening, and early intervention documentation;
- written policies and procedures for data tracking systems;
- policies and procedures to ensure privacy and the confidentiality of data, including informed consent requirements;
- inclusion of all births for the state matched with the birth certificate registry;
- identification of risk factors for progressive or later onset hearing loss by linking with other data systems;
- hearing screening results reported within 1 week of hospital discharge or transfer;
- mechanisms to report the results of any hearing testing and interventions available to all providers;
- programs that can identify all young children at each stage of the EHDI process on a weekly basis; and
- authorized case managers and health care providers with access to relevant information about an individual child's hearing status.

Beginning in 2006, HRSA/MCHB invited EHDI programs to participate in a learning collaborative to determine effective practices designed to reduce the LTF/LTD rate in the transition from newborn hearing screening to audiologic evaluation, and from diagnosis to early intervention (Russ, Hanna, DesGeorges,

& Forsman, 2010). The effective practices identified through a "small tests of change" improvement model for the National Initiative for Child Healthcare Quality (NICHQ) learning collaborative were to

- script the message given the parents when an infant does not pass the hearing screening;
- obtain a second point of contact for the family (e.g., a relative or friend);
- verify the identity of the infant's PCP before leaving the hospital;
- make the next appointment for the family before they leave the hospital and explain why it is important to keep the appointment;
- make reminder calls before appointments and again stress the importance of the appointment;
- make two consecutive audiology appointments so that the infant who cannot be completely tested at the first appointment is already scheduled to return in a reasonable time frame;
- "fax-back" to alert the PCP of screening results and the need for prompt follow-up;
- "fax back" between specialists, including the audiologist and PCP;
- obtain consent for release of information at first contact with early intervention so information can be entered in the state database; and
- provide clinically useful and timely early intervention reports to PCPs.

The SWOT survey in 2009 gathered 47 EHDI coordinators' perceptions of factors relating LTF (Hoffman et al., 2011). The analysis of the coordinators' 277 responses in the LTF area identified the following top themes:

- *strengths:* relationship building, coordinated tracking protocol, and program improvement;
- *weaknesses:* protocol, limited personnel, and access to care;
- *opportunities:* relationship building, data tracking systems, and access to state systems; and
- *threats:* funding, interagency cooperation, and family circumstances.

A TOWS analysis of the SWOT data yielded the following four recommendations:

1. Existing positive relationships with parents and professionals can be used to engage additional stakeholders in reaching out to other groups and individuals, adopting effective practices, linking families to the recommended services, and enlisting advocates.
2. Continual development of comprehensive data systems that are linked to other child data systems are easy to use and accessible by providers, efficiently support follow-up efforts, and provide for program and system evaluation.
3. Reporting, tracking, and follow-up protocols must be refined to incorporate effective practices, to focus on families most at risk of being categorized as LTF, and to maximize the efficiency of conducting follow-up to ensure that the recommended services are received and reported.
4. Health disparities must be reduced, especially for high-risk groups and those in unserved or underserved areas.

Surveillance for Later-Onset Hearing Loss

Morton and Nance (2006) reviewed the etiology of hearing loss in young children, estimating that 68% of PCHL at birth was caused by genetic factors, both syndromic, such as Pendred's syndrome, and nonsyndromic. Although many genes are implicated in genetic hearing loss, *GJB2*, which encodes connexin 26, is reportedly responsible for approximately 21% of all PCHL and 50% of nonsyndromic recessive hearing loss.

Environmental causes of PCHL differ by location. For example, congenital rubella infection in India is still a leading cause of PCHL, while in sub-Saharan Africa the indirect consequences of secondary infections resulting from HIV/AIDS can be the cause of congenital or acquired hearing loss (Swanepoel, 2010). Ototoxicity due to aminoglycoside sensitivity from a mitochondrial A1555G mutation causes up to 20% of familial nonsyndromic hearing loss in Spain, while only 10% of the people in the United States have hearing loss due to ototoxicity (Morton & Nance, 2006). In China, it is estimated that 21,600 infants annually are born with a A1555G mutation (Wang et al., 2011).

Congenital cytomegalovirus (CMV) is the most prevalent environmental cause of permanent childhood hearing loss in the United States, accounting for 10% of PCHL and 35% of moderate to severe late-onset hearing loss (Barbi et al., 2003). The incidence of congenital CMV ranges from 0.1% to 2% of newborns, depending on maternal demographic variables, and can be either symptomatic or asymptomatic (Morton & Nance, 2006). Morton and Nance (2006) reported that the presence of hearing loss with symptomatic CMV increases from 4% at birth to 36% by 6 years of age. PCHL is identified in 11% of children with asymptomatic congenital CMV by 6 years. PCHL caused by congenital CMV is variable and can be fluctuating, progressive, or both.

Screening newborns for congenital CMV is not yet routine in the United States, although the Canadian province of Quebec has been successful in the use of filter paper to collect urine samples for lab analysis during the first 3 weeks of life (Tvrdy, Johnson, Hoffman, Honaker, & Boney, 2011). As part of the public health system, EHDI programs have a role in the education of parents and professionals to reduce congenital CMV and possible PCHL. Vauloup-Fellous et al. (2009) reported that education focused on reducing transmission of CMV to women during pregnancy through hygiene counseling has reduced the seroconversion from 42% to 19%.

The JCIH 2007 position statement recommends surveillance of all young children, regardless of risk factors for PCHL, as not all risk factors for later onset hearing loss are known. Surveillance consists of monitoring for auditory skills, middle ear status, and developmental milestones during well-child visits consistent with the AAP periodicity schedule, with prompt referral for an audiologic evaluation for those who do not pass. For infants with any of the 11 risk factors associated with congenital, late-onset, or progressive hearing loss, at least one audiologic evaluation should be conducted by 24 to 30 months of age. The 11 risk factors (JCIH, 2007) are listed here; however, it is important to note that these risk factors continue to be updated:

- caregiver concern* regarding hearing, speech, language, or developmental delay;
- family history* of permanent childhood hearing loss;
- neonatal intensive care of more than 5 days or any of the following regardless of length of stay: extracorporeal membrane oxygenation (ECMO)*, assisted ventilation, exposure to ototoxic medications (gentamicin and tobramycin) or loop diuretics (furosemide/Lasix), and hyperbilirubinemia that requires exchange transfusion;
- in utero infections, such as CMV*, herpes, rubella, syphilis, and toxoplasmosis;
- craniofacial anomalies, including those that involve the pinna, ear canal, ear tags, ear pits, and temporal bone anomalies;
- physical findings that are associated with a syndrome known to have PCHL as part of the phenotype;
- syndromes associated with hearing loss or progressive or late-onset hearing loss*, such as neurofibromatosis, osteopetrosis, and Usher syndrome; other frequently identified syndromes include Waardenburg, Alport, Pendred, and Jervell and Lange-Nielson;
- neurodegenerative disorders*, such as Hunter syndrome, or sensory motor neuropathies, such as Friedreich's ataxia and Charcot-Marie-Tooth syndrome;
- culture-positive postnatal infections associated with sensory/neural hearing loss*, including confirmed bacterial and viral (especially herpes viruses and varicella) meningitis;
- head trauma, especially basal skull/temporal bone fractures that requires hospitalization; and
- chemotherapy.*

(Risk factors with an * carry a greater risk for hearing loss.)

For those with greater risk of late-onset or progressive hearing loss, early and frequent monitoring is recommended; however, the monitoring schedule is not specified (JCIH, 2007). For young children who have congenital CMV, Fowler (2013) recommended monitoring hearing every 6 months and more frequently before the child begins to talk or if hearing is changing. Chung et al. (2015) and Lanzieri et al. (2015) recommended ongoing audiologic monitoring based on their findings that sensory/neural hearing loss was identified as late as 10 years for children with symptomatic congenital CMV and 17 years for children with asymptomatic CMV.

Beswick, Driscoll, and Kei (2012) conducted a systematic literature review on the use of risk factors for postnatal hearing loss and reported that the most common risk factors were gestational age, low birth weight, TORCH (toxoplasmosis, other infections, rubella, cytomegalovirus, herpes simplex virus) infections, craniofacial anomalies, respirator support, and administration of aminoglycosides. Risk factors that were associated with late-onset hearing loss were CMV (symptomatic and asymptomatic), extracorporeal membrane oxygenation (ECMO), congenital diaphragmatic hernia, and persistent pulmonary hypertension of the newborn (PPHN). They suggested additional research to determine the relationship between late-onset hearing loss and three of the JCIH risk factors identified as having a greater risk of hearing loss: family history, syndromes associated with late onset hearing loss, and neurodegenerative disorders.

Hearing screening beyond the newborn period in the absence of risk factors for hearing loss is expanding the age range of interest for EHDI programs. Beswick, Driscoll, and Kei (2012) did not find any investigations that compared the use of risk factors with other approaches to monitor for late-onset hearing loss. However, several model protocols have been developed to conduct hearing screenings in health care settings and early care and education settings. Bhatia, Mintz, Hecht, Deavenport, and Kuo (2013) established an infant-toddler hearing screening program consisting of a risk factor questionnaire, OAE screening, and tympanometry in seven federally qualified health centers. They determined that screening in the primary care setting was effective and they identified five children with previously unidentified sensory/neural hearing loss ranging from mild to profound, yielding an identification rate of 3 per 1,000. Foust, Eiserman, Shisler, and Geroso (2013) also established a hearing screening program in three federally qualified health clinics consisting of a multiple step OAE screening for children birth to 5 years and older siblings upon request. The results showed that previously unidentified permanent hearing loss could be identified through screening in health care settings, yielding an identification rate of 1.2 per thousand for children less than 5 years old.

Hearing screening in early care and education settings is also a feasible approach to monitoring hearing of young children. Eiserman, Hartel, Shisler, Buhrmann, White, and Foust (2008) supported the creation of multiple step OAE screening and follow-up programs in Early Head Start programs by providing training and technical assistance. They reported that seven young children ages 0 to 3 years were identified with previously unidentified permanent hearing loss, yielding an identification rate of 1.5 per thousand. In addition, 2.2% of the children screened were identified with other hearing health concerns, primarily otitis media.

Screening for permanent hearing loss beyond the newborn period, regardless of whether it is targeted on specific risk factors or routinely conducted in health or early care and education settings, does identify late onset and progressive hearing losses. In addition, with timely reporting of the individually identifiable screening and evaluation results, whether normal or indicative of some type of hearing loss, to the state EHDI program, the potential exists to resolve the status of some of the children who have been categorized as LTF/LTD. See Chapter 17 for further discussion of screening beyond the newborn period.

Future Directions

The literature suggests several areas of need to continue improving EHDI programs. Prioritizing these needs is challenging. Although the overarching goal of EHDI programs is to minimize any negative consequences of PCHL, it could be argued that reducing preventable hearing loss could be considered a top priority. This is a particular area of need in under-resourced areas of the world where the main causes of hearing loss across the life span are chronic ear infections, meningitis, rubella, noise, and ototoxic medications (WHO, 2013). For neonates born in under-resourced areas, primary prevention is compromised by socioeconomic and health care limitations. Furthermore, genetic/hereditary issues are complicated by cultural and religious beliefs and by consanguinity in some cultures (Olusanya, 2012).

Other pressing areas of need include improving access to hearing screening and follow-up with high-quality diagnostic audiological services that are consistent across centers; reducing loss to follow-up and loss to documentation; improving access to hearing technology and early intervention services; enhancing communication between parents, between parents and professionals, and between professionals; and increasing the awareness of parents, family members, educators, and health care providers regarding the early diagnosis and treatment of hearing loss, and its link to communication development, social-emotional skills, academic achievement, and eventual gainful employment. The idea of a central repository for hearing health data and all related outcomes has been suggested and implemented in some states (NECAP, CDC, n.d.), and this would provide a valuable resource to better understand and highlight areas of progress and areas of need.

There are an increasing number of home births in the United States (CDC, 2009; Lewis, 2015) with a 29% increase in home births from 2004 to 2009. This speaks to a need for additional mechanisms to support hearing screening in the first month of life. Options that have been proposed include regional health clinics that provide hearing screening, hearing screening at the PCPs office, training midwives to perform hearing screening, and hearing screening by EI personnel.

There is a continued need for outcomes research; however, there are many roadblocks to acquiring meaningful data, in part due to the fact that infants who are D/HH are a highly heterogeneous group. Furthermore, there are differences in screening and follow-up protocols from program to program, target screening levels, and even how hearing loss is defined. There are inconsistencies in audiologic diagnostic testing and hearing loss management from clinic to clinic, discrepancies in when and how amplification is initiated, and differences in parent preferences for moving forward following the confirmation of hearing loss. Moreover, there are variations in the quality of EI services, and there are capacity issues at all levels. EHDI programs have come a long way, and there is a long way to go to improve programs and services.

References

American Academy of Pediatrics. (2007). Year 2007 position statement: Principles and guidelines for early hearing detection and intervention programs. *Pediatrics, 120*(4), 898.

American Speech-Language-Hearing Association (n.d.). *Expert panel recommendations on newborn hearing screening.* Retrieved May 25, 2015, from http://www.asha.org/Topics/Expert-Panel-Recommendations-on-Newborn-Hearing-Screening/#6

American Speech-Language-Hearing Association. (2008a). *Guidelines for audiologists providing informational and adjustment counseling to families of infants and young children with hearing loss birth to 5 years of age* [Guidelines]. Retrieved May 25, 2015, from http://www.asha.org/policy

American Speech-Language-Hearing Association. (2008b). *Loss to follow-up in early hearing detection and intervention.* Retrieved May 28, 2015, from http://www.asha.org/policy/tr2008-00302/

American Speech-Language-Hearing Association. (2009). *EHDI Phase II State Model Legislation.* Retrieved May 6, 2015, from http://www.asha.org/uploadedFiles/advocacy/federal/ehdi/EHDIStateModelBill.pdf#search=%22model%22

American Speech-Language-Hearing Association. (2015). *Hearing aid tax credit introduced in the House of Representatives, 2015.* Retrieved May 6, 2015, from http://www.asha.org/News/2015/Hearing-Aid-Tax-Credit-Introduced-in-the-House-of-Representatives/

Association of Maternal and Child Health Programs. (2005, March). Tune in to newborn hearing screening. *AMCHP Policy Brief.* Retrieved May 29, 2015, from http://www.amchp.org/programsandtopics/CHILD-HEALTH/projects/newborn-screening/Documents/Tune-In-to-NBS_Mar2005.pdf

Babbidge, H. (1965). *Education of the deaf in the United States. Report of the Advisory Committee on Education of the Deaf.* Washington, DC: Government Printing Office. Retrieved May 26, 2015, from http://files.eric.ed.gov/fulltext/ED014188.pdf

Babbidge, H. D., Dunning, L., Edwards, G., Godwin, W., Hardy, M., Hedgecock, L., . . . Rackley, J. (1965). Education of the deaf in the United States. The advisory committee's report. *Volta Review, 67*(5), 345–351.

Barbi, M., Binda, S., Caroppo, S., Ambrosetti, U., Corbetta, C., & Sergi, P. (2003). A wider role for congenital cytomegalovirus infection in sensorineural hearing loss. *Pediatric Infectious Disease Journal, 22*(1), 39–42.

Berg, A. L., Prieve, B. A., Serpanos, Y. C., & Wheaton, M. A. (2011). Hearing screening in a well-infant nursery: Profile of automated ABR-fail/OAE-pass. *Pediatrics, 27*(2), 269–275.

Bess, F. H., & Paradise, J. L. (1994). Universal screening for infant hearing impairment: Not simple, not risk-free, not necessarily beneficial, and not presently justified. *Pediatrics, 93*(2), 330–334.

Beswick, R., Driscoll, C., & Kei, J. (2012). Monitoring for postnatal hearing loss using risk factors: A systematic literature review. *Ear and Hearing, 33*(6), 745–756.

Bhatia, P., Mintz, S., Hecht, B. F., Deavenport, A., & Kuo, A. A. (2013). Early identification of young children with hearing loss in federally qualified health centers. *Journal of Developmental and Behavioral Pediatrics, 34*(1), 15–21.

Bradham, T., Hoffman, J., & Houston, K. T. (2011). Data management in the EHDI dystem. *Volta Review, 111*(2), 243–253.

Bureau of Labor Statistics. (2014). *Occupational outlook handbook, 2014–15 edition, audiologists.* Retrieved May 18, 2015, from http://www.bls.gov/ooh/healthcare/audiologists.htm

Centers for Disease Control and Prevention. (n.d.). *Annual data Early Hearing Detection and Intervention (EHDI) program.* Retrieved May 28, 2015, from http://www.cdc.gov/ncbddd/hearingloss/ehdi-data.html

Centers for Disease Control and Prevention. (n.d.). *National goals, program objectives, and performance measures for the Early Hearing Detection and Intervention (EHDI) tracking and surveillance system.* Retrieved May 28, 2015, from http://www.cdc.gov/ncbddd/hearingloss/documents/Goals.pdf

Centers for Disease Control and Prevention. (2003a). *Early hearing detection and intervention program guidance manual.* Atlanta, GA: Author.

Centers for Disease Control and Prevention. (2003b). HIPAA privacy rule and public health. *Morbidity and Mortality Weekly Report, 52,* 1–12. Retrieved May 6, 2015, from http://www.cdc.gov/mmwr/preview/mmwrhtml/m2e411a1.htm

Centers for Disease Control and Prevention. (2009). Home births in the United States, 1990–2009. Retrieved May 25, 2015, from http://www.cdc.gov/nchs/data/databriefs/db84.pdf

Centers for Disease Control and Prevention. (2011a). The public health system and the 10 essential public health services. Retrieved on May 6, 2015, from http://www.cdc.gov/nphpsp/essentialServices.html

Centers for Disease Control and Prevention. (2011b). *EHDI Hearing Screening and Follow-up Survey (HSFS): Explanations.* Retrieved May 28, 2015, from http://www.cdc.gov/ncbddd/hearingloss/2013-data/ehdi_hsfs_explanations_2013_verb.pdf

Centers for Disease Control and Prevention. (2014). *Early hearing detection and intervention and electronic health records technology.* Retrieved May 19, 2015, from http://www.cdc.gov/ncbddd/hearingloss/ehdi-hrt.html

Centers for Disease Control and Prevention. (2014). *The 10 essential public health services: An overview* [PDF document]. Retrieved May 28, 2015, from http://www.cdc.gov/nphpsp/documents/essential-phs.pdf

Chen, G., Yi, X., Chen, P., Dong, J., Yang, G., & Fu, S. (2012). A large-scale newborn hearing screening in rural areas in China. *International Journal of Pediatric Otorhinolaryngology, 76*(12), 1771–1774.

Chung, W., Lanzieri, T., Bialek, S, Flores, M., Caviness, C., Demmler-Harrison, G., . . . Miller, J. (2015, March). *18-Year audiologic follow-up of children with symptomatic congenital cytomegalovirus infection.* Podium paper presented at American Auditory Society Meeting, Scottsdale, AZ. Abstract retrieved May 28, 2015, from https://aas.memberclicks.net/assets/final_15_podium.pdf

Davis, A., Bamford, J., Wilson, I., Ramkalawan, T., Forshaw, M., & Wright, S. (1997). A critical review of the role of neonatal hearing screening in the detection of congenital hearing impairment. *Health Technology Assessment (Winchester, England), 1*(10), i–iv.

Davis, H., & Onishi, S. (1969). Maturation of auditory evoked potentials. *International Journal of Audiology, 8*(1), 24–33.

Department of Health and Human Services. (2014). *Justification of estimates for appropriations committees, the Centers for Disease Control and Prevention, fiscal year 2015.* 192. Retrieved May 22, 2015, from http://www.cdc.gov/fmo/topic/Budget%20Information/appropriations_budget_form_pdf/FY2015_CJ_CDC_FINAL.pdf

Dorn, P. A., Piskorski, P., Gorga, M. P., Neely, S. T., & Keefe, D. H. (1999). Predicting audiometric status from distortion product otoacoustic emissions using multivariate analyses. *Ear and Hearing, 20,* 149–163.

Downs, M. P., & Hemenway, W. G. (1969). Report on the hearing screening of 17.000 neonates. *International Journal of Audiology, 8*(1), 72–76.

Early detection, diagnosis, and treatment regarding hearing loss in newborns and infants. 42 USC § 280g-1. Retrieved May 28, 2015, from http://www.gpo.gov/fdsys/pkg/USCODE-2010-title42/pdf/USCODE-2010-title42-chap6A-subchapII-partP-sec280g-1.pdf

Eiserman, W. D., Hartel, D. M., Shisler, L., Buhrmann, J., White, K. R., & Foust, T. (2008). Using otoacoustic emissions to screen for hearing loss in early childhood care settings. *International Journal of Pediatric Otorhinolaryngology, 72*(4), 475–482.

Ewing, I. R., & Ewing, A. W. G. (1944). The ascertainment of deafness in infancy and early childhood. *Journal of Laryngology and Otology, 59*(9), 309–333.

Foust, T., Eiserman, W., Shisler, L., & Geroso, A. (2013). Using otoacoustic emissions to screen young children for hearing loss in primary care settings. *Pediatrics, 132*(1), 118–123.

Fowler, K. B. (2013). Congenital cytomegalovirus infection: Audiologic outcome. *Clinical Infectious Diseases, 57*(S4), S182–S184.

Grandori, F. (1998). European Consensus Statement on Neonatal Hearing Screening. Finalized at the European Consensus Development Conference on Neonatal Hearing Screening, May 15–16, Milan, Italy. *Scandinavian Audiology, 27*(4), 259–260. doi:10.1080/010503998420577

Green, D. R., Gaffney, M., Devine, O., & Grosse, S. D. (2007). Determining the effect of newborn hearing screening legislation: An analysis of state hearing screening rates. *Public Health Reports, 122*(2), 198. Retrieved May 28, 2015, from http://www.ncbi.nlm.nih.gov/pmc/articles/PMC1820423/

Hecox, K., & Galambos, R. (1974). Brain stem auditory evoked responses in human infants and adults. *Archives of Otolaryngology, 99*(1), 30–33.

Henderson, R. J., Johnson, A., & Moodie, S. (2014). Parent-to-parent support for parents with children who are deaf or hard of hearing: A conceptual framework. *American Journal of Audiology, 23*(4), 437–448.

Hoff, T., Hoyt, A., Therrell, B., & Ayoob, M. (2006). Exploring barriers to long-term follow-up in newborn screening programs. *Genetics in Medicine, 8*(9), 563–570. doi:10.1097/01.gim.0000237790.54074.3d

Hoffman, J., Munoz, K., Bradham, T., & Nelson, L. (2011). Lost to follow-up: Issues and recommendations. *Volta Review, 111*(2), 165–180.

Jacobson, J. T., Jacobson, C. A., & Spahr, R. C. (1990). Automated and conventional ABR screening techniques in high-risk infants. *Journal of the American Academy of Audiology, 1*(4), 187–195.

Joint Committee on Infant Hearing. (2007). Position statement: Principles and guidelines for early hearing detection and intervention programs. *Pediatrics, 120,* 898–921.

Joint Committee on Infant Hearing of the American Academy of Pediatrics. (2013). Supplement to the JCIH 2007 position statement: Principles and guidelines for early intervention after confirmation that a child is deaf or hard of hearing. *Pediatrics, 131*(4), e1324–e1349. doi:10.1542/peds.2013-0008

Joint Committee on Neonatal Screening for Hearing Impairment: Committee on Fetus and Newborn. (1971). *Pediatrics, 47,* 1085. Retrieved May 24, 2015, from http://pediatrics.aappublications.org/content/47/6/1085.full.pdf+html

Kansas Administrative Regulations 28-4-501. Retrieved May 25, 2015, from http://www.kssos.org/pubs/KAR/2009/2%20002_28-Department%20of%20Health%20and%20Environment%20Articles%201%20through%208,%202009%20KAR%20Vol%202.pdf

Kemp, D. T. (1978). Stimulated acoustic emissions from within the human auditory system. *Journal of the Acoustical Society of America, 64*(5), 1386–1391.

Kemp, D. T., Ryan, S., & Bray, P. (1990). A guide to the effective use of otoacoustic emissions. *Ear and Hearing, 11*(2), 93–105.

Koop, C. E. (2010). Foreword: Pursuing excellence in early hearing detection and intervention programs. *Pediatrics, 126,* S1–S2.

Lanzieri, T., Chung, W., Bialek, S., Grosse, S., Blum, P., Miller, J., . . . Demmler-Harrison, G. (2015, March). *18-Year audiologic follow-up of children with symptomatic congenital cytomegalovirus infection.* Podium paper presented at American Auditory Society Meeting, Scottsdale, AZ. Abstract retrieved May 28, 2015, from https://aas.memberclicks.net/assets/final_15_podium.pdf

Lewis, R. (2015). As home births increase, recent studies illuminate controversies and complexities. *Journal of the American Medical Association, 313*(6), 553–555.

Liu, C. L., Farrell, J., MacNeil, J. R., Stone, S., & Barfield, W. (2008). Evaluating loss to follow-up in newborn hearing screening in Massachusetts. *Pediatrics, 121*(2), e335–e343.

Massachusetts Newborn Hearing Screening Tests, Chapter 111, Sections 67F. Retrieved May 25, 2015, from https://malegislature.gov/Laws/GeneralLaws/PartI/TitleXVI/Chapter111/Section67F

Mendel, G. (1865). *Experiments in plant hybridisation. Mendel's Principles of Heredity* (W. Bateson, Trans.). Cambridge, UK: Cambridge University Press. (From German) Mendel Experiments in plant hybridization Mendel's Principles of Heredity 1909.

Miko, I. (2008). Gregor Mendel and the principles of inheritance. *Nature Education, 1*(1), 134.

Moeller, M. P., Carr, G., Seaver, L., Stredler-Brown, A., & Holzinger, D. (2013). Best practices in family-centered early intervention for children who are deaf or hard of hearing: An international consensus statement. *Journal of Deaf Studies and Deaf Education, 18*(4), 429–445.

Morton, C. C., & Nance, W. E. (2006). Newborn hearing screening—A silent revolution. *New England Journal of Medicine, 354*(20), 2151–2164.

National Center for Health Statistics. (2001). *Healthy people 2000 final review.* Hyattsville, MD: Public Health Service. Retrieved from http://www.cdc.gov/nchs/data/hp2000/hp2k01.pdf

National Center for Hearing Assessment and Management (NCHAM; n.d.). *Mandate provision: Advisory committee established.* [Date file]. Retrieved May 6, 2015, from http://infanthearing.org/legislative/provisions/committee.html

National Center for Hearing Assessment and Management. (2004). *State EHDI survey.* Retrieved from http://infanthearing.org/survey/2004statesurvey/index.html

National Center for Hearing Assessment and Management (NCHAM; 2011). *State EHDI/UNHS mandates: Summaries by provision.* Retrieved May 19, 2015, from http://infanthearing.org/legislative/provisions/index.html

National Early Childhood Assessment Project (NECAP). Retrieved May 24, 2015, from http://www.cdc.gov/ncbddd/hearingloss/transcripts/NECAP-Supplement.pdf

National Institutes of Health. (1993). *Early identification of hearing impairment in infants and young children.* NIH Consensus Statement Online 1993 Mar 1–3 [cited 2015 April 11], *11*(1), 1–24. Retrieved May 24, 2015, from http://consensus.nih.gov/1993/1993HearingInfantsChildren092html.htm

Nelson, H. D., Bougatsos, C., & Nygren, P. (2008). Universal newborn hearing screening: Systematic review to update the 2001 US Preventive Services Task Force Recommendation. *Pediatrics, 122*(1), e266–e276.

Nisbet, W. (1800). *The clinical guide; or, the concise view of the leading facts on the history, nature, and treatment of the state and diseases of infancy and childhood.* London, UK: J. Johnson, St. Paul's Church-Yard; and J. Watson, South-Bridge, Edinburgh.

Norrix, L. W., & Velenovsky, D. S. (2014). Auditory neuropathy spectrum disorder: A review. *Journal of Speech, Language, and Hearing Research, 57*(4), 1564–1576.

Norton, S. J., Gorga, M. P., Widen, J. E., Folsom, R. C., Sininger, Y., Cone-Wesson, B., . . . Fletcher, K. A. (2000a). Identification of neonatal hearing impairment: Evaluation of transient evoked otoacoustic emission, distortion product otoacoustic emission, and auditory brain stem response test performance. *Ear and Hearing, 21*(5), 508–528.

Norton, S. J., Gorga, M. P., Widen, J. E., Folsom, R. C., Sininger, Y., Cone-Wesson, B., . . . Fletcher, K. A. (2000b). Identification of neonatal hearing impairment: Summary and recommendations. *Ear and Hearing, 21*(5), 529–535.

Office of the Federal Register. (2015). Electronic Code of Federal Regulations §440.110 Physical therapy, occupational therapy, and services for individuals with speech, hearing, and language disorders. Retrieved May 17, 2015, from http://www.ecfr.gov/cgi-bin/text-idx?tpl=/ecfrbrowse/Title42/42cfr440_main_02.tpl

Olusanya, B. O. (2012). Neonatal hearing screening and intervention in resource-limited settings: An overview. *Archives of Disease in Childhood, 97*(7), 654–659.

Olusanya, B. O., Neumann, K. J., & Saunders, J. E. (2014). The global burden of disabling hearing impairment: A call to action. *Bulletin of the World Health Organization, 92*(5), 367–373.

Patel, H., & Feldman, M. (2011, and reaffirmed February 1, 2014). Universal newborn hearing screening. *Paediatrics & Child Health, 16*(5), 301. Retrieved May 24, 2105, http://www.cps.ca/documents/position/universal-hearing-screening-newborns

Pimperton, H., & Kennedy, C. R. (2012). The impact of early identification of permanent childhood hearing impairment on speech and language outcomes. *Archives of Disease in Childhood*, 97, 648–653.

Professional Practice and Guidelines Committee. (2014). American College of Medical Genetics and Genomics guideline for the clinical evaluation and etiologic diagnosis of hearing loss. *Genetics in Medicine, 16*(4), 347–355. doi:10.1038/gim.2014.2. Retrieved May 27, 2015, from https://www.acmg.net/docs/ACMG_Guideline_for_Clinical_Eval_and_Etiologic_Dx%20of_Hearing_Loss_GIM_Apr2014.pdf

Rance, G. (2005). Auditory neuropathy/dys-synchrony and its perceptual consequences. *Trends in Hearing, Winter, 9*(1), 10–11.

Richmond, J. B., Grossman, H. J., & Lustman, S. L. (1953). A hearing test for newborn infants. *Pediatrics, 11*(6), 634–638.

Russ, S. A., Hanna, D., DesGeorges, J., & Forsman, I. (2010). Improving follow-up to newborn hearing screening: A learning-collaborative experience. *Pediatrics, 126*(Suppl. 1), S59–S69. doi:10.1542/peds.2010-0354K

Schillinger, D. (n.d.). Newborn screening in Poland: A well-orchestrated success. *Hearing Health*, 22–24. Retrieved May 19, 2015, from http://www.infanthearing.org/ncham/publications/hearinghealth%28poland%29.pdf

Simmons, F. B., & Russ, F. N. (1974). Automated newborn hearing screening, the Crib-o-gram. *Archives of Otolaryngology, 100*(1), 1–7.

Sloot, F., Hoeve, H. L., de Kroon, M. L., Goedegebure, A., Carlton, J., Griffiths, H. J., . . . EUS€ REEN study group.

(2015). Inventory of current EU paediatric vision and hearing screening programmes. *Journal of Medical Screening, 22*(2), 55–64. doi:10.1177/0969141315572403

Swanepoel, D. W. (2010). The global epidemic of infant hearing loss—Priorities for prevention. *Proceedings from Sound Foundation Through Early Amplification Conference.* Retrieved May 29, 2015, from http://www.phonakpro.com/content/dam/phonak/gc_hq/b2b/en/events/2010/Proceedings/Pho_Chap_01_Swanepoel_final.pdf

Talaat, H. S., Kabel, A. H., Samy, H., & Elbadry, M. (2009). Prevalence of auditory neuropathy (AN) among infants and young children with severe to profound hearing loss. *International Journal of Pediatric Otorhinolaryngology, 73*(7), 937–939. doi:http://dx.doi.org/10.1016/j.ijporl.2009.03.009

Tvrdy, F., Johnson, T., Hoffman, J., Honaker, J., & Boney, S. (2011).Trends in congenital cytomegalovirus: A review of current screening methods and prevention strategies. *Seminars in Hearing, 32,* 321–331.

United Kingdom. (n.d.). *NHS newborn hearing screening programme quality standards.* Retrieved May 27, 2015, from http://hearing.screening.nhs.uk/standardsandprotocols

U.S. Department of Health and Human Services. (2011). *Hearing and other sensory or communication disorders.* Retrieved May 28, 2015, from http://www.healthypeople.gov/2020/topics-objectives/topic/hearing-and-other-sensory-or-communication-disorders/objectives

U.S. Department of Health and Human Services. (2014). *Justification of estimates for appropriations committees, health resources and services administration, fiscal year 2015* (pp. 237–240). Retrieved May 22, 2015, from http://www.hrsa.gov/about/budget/budgetjustification2015.pdf

U.S. Preventive Services Task Force. (2001). Newborn hearing screening: Recommendations and rationale. U.S. Preventive Services Task Force. *Internet Journal of Otorhinolaryngology, 1*(2). Retrieved May 23, 2015, from https://ispub.com/IJORL/1/2/8269

U.S. Preventive Services Task Force. (2008). *Hearing loss in newborns: Screening.* Retrieved May 27, 2015, from http://www.uspreventiveservicestaskforce.org/BrowseRec/InactiveTopic/218

U.S. Preventive Services Task Force. (2014). *The guide to clinical preventive services, 2014.* Recommendations of the U.S. Preventive Services Task Force, Agency for Healthcare Research and Quality, Rockville, MD. Retrieved May 27, 2015, from http://www.uspreventiveservicestaskforce.org/Home/GetFileByID/989

Vauloup-Fellous, C., Picone, O., Cordier, A. G., Parent-du-Châtelet, I., Senat, M. V., Frydman, R., & Grangeot-Keros, L. (2009). Does hygiene counseling have an impact on the rate of CMV primary infection during pregnancy?: Results of a 3-year prospective study in a French hospital. *Journal of Clinical Virology, 46,* S49–S53.

Vohr, B. R., Carty, L. M., Moore, P. E., & Letourneau, K. (1998). The Rhode Island Hearing Assessment Program: Experience with statewide hearing screening (1993–1996). *Journal of Pediatrics, 133*(3), 353–357.

Wang, Q. J., Zhao, Y. L., Rao, S. Q., Guo, Y. F., He, Y., Lan, L., . . . Shen, Y. (2011). Newborn hearing concurrent gene screening can improve care for hearing loss: A study on 14,913 Chinese newborns. *International Journal of Pediatric Otorhinolaryngology, 75*(4), 535–542.

Wessex Universal Neonatal Hearing Screening Trial Group. (1998). Controlled trial of universal neonatal screening for early identification of permanent childhood hearing impairment. *Lancet, 352,* 1957–1964.

White, K. (2015). *The evolution of EHDI: From concept to standard of care. The NCHAM eBook: A resource guide for early hearing detection and intervention,* 1–32. Retrieved May 19, 2015, from http://infanthearing.org/ehdi-ebook/2015_ebook/1b-Chapter1EvolutionEHDI2015.pdf

White, K., Behl, D., St. John, R., & Moeller, M. P. (2014). *Meeting the needs of physicains in support of EHDI.* Presented at 2014 EHDI conference. Retrieved May 3, 2015, from http://ehdimeeting.org/archive/2014/System/Uploads/pdfs/1314DianeBehl.pdf

White, K., Forsman, I., Eichwald, J., & Munoz, K. (2010). The evolution of early hearing detection and intervention programs in the United States. *Seminars in Perinatology, 34*(2), 171.

Whitehead, M. L., McCoy, M. J., Martin, G. K., & Lonsbury-Martin, B. L. (1993). Click-evoked and distortion-product otoacoustic emissions in adults: Detection of high-frequency sensorineural hearing loss. *Association of Research Otolaryngologists Abstracts, 16,* 100.

Williams, T. R., Alam, S., & Gaffney, M. (2015). Progress in identifying infants with hearing loss: United States, 2006–2012. *CDC: Morbidity and Mortality Weekly Report (MMWR).* Retrieved May 24, 2015, from http://www.cdc.gov/mmwr/preview/mmwrhtml/mm6413a4.htm

Wolff, R., Hommerich, J., Riemsma, R., Antes, G., Lange, S., & Kleijnen, J. (2010). Hearing screening in newborns: Systematic review of accuracy, effectiveness, and effects of interventions after screening. *Archives of Disease in Childhood, 95*(2), 130–135.

World Health Organization (WHO; 2010). *Newborn and infant hearing screening: Current issues and guiding principles for action.* Retrieved May 27, 2015, from http://www.who.int/blindness/publications/Newborn_and_Infant_Hearing_Screening_Report.pdf

World Health Organization (WHO; 2013). *Multi-country assessment of national capacity to provide hearing care.* Retrieved April 21, 2015, from http://www.who.int/pbd/publications/WHOReportHearingCare_Englishweb.pdf

World Health Organization (WHO; 2015). *Public health.* Retrieved May 27, 2015, from http://www.who.int/trade/glossary/story076/en/

Yoshinaga-Itano, C., Sedley, A. L., Coulter, D. K., & Mehl, A. L. (1998). Language of early- and later-identified children with hearing loss. *Pediatrics, 102*(5), 1161–1171.

APPENDIX 18–A

Acronyms List

American Academy of Audiology (AAA)

American Academy of Pediatrics (AAP)

American Speech and Hearing Association (ASHA)

Association of Maternal and Child Health Programs (AMCHP)

auditory brainstem response (ABR)

auditory-evoked potentials (AEPs)

auditory neuropathy spectrum disorder (ANSD)

Canadian Paediatric Society (CPS)

Centers for Disease Control and Prevention (CDC)

cytomegalovirus (CMV)

deaf or hard of hearing (D/HH)

Department of Health and Human Services (DHHS)

Directors of Speech and Hearing Programs in State Health and Welfare Agencies (DSHPSHWA)

distortion product otoacoustic emissions (DPOAE)

Early Childhood Technical Assistant Center (ECTA Center)

early hearing detection and identification (EHDI)

Early Hearing Detection and Intervention-Pediatric Audiology Links to Services (EHDI-PALS)

early intervention (EI)

Family Educational Rights and Privacy Act (FERPA)

Great Orchestra of Christmas Charity (GOCC)

Health Insurance Portability and Accountability Act (HIPAA)

Health Resources and Services Administration (HRSA)

Hearing Screening and Follow-up Survey (HSFS)

individual service plan (IFSP)

Individuals with Disabilities Act (IDEA)

Institute for Quality and Efficiency in Health Care (IQWiG)

Joint Committee on Infant Hearing (JCIH)

lost to follow-up (LTF)

lost to documentation (LTD)

Maternal and Child Health Bureau (MCHB)

National Center for Birth Defects and Disabilities (NCBDD)

National Center for Evidence-Based Practice in Communication Disorders (N-CEP)

National Center for Hearing Assessment and Management (NCHAM)

National Initiative for Child Healthcare Quality (NICHQ)

National Institute on Deafness and Other Communication Disorders (NIDCD)

National Institutes of Health (NIH)

neonatal intensive care unit (NICU)

nongovernmental organization (NGO)

otoacoustic emission (OAE)

permanent childhood hearing loss (PCHL)

primary care provider (PCP)

protected health information (PHI)

signal-to-noise ratio (SNR)

transient-evoked otoacoustic emission (TEOAE)

U.S. Preventative Services Task Force (USPSTF)

visual reinforcement audiometry (VRA)

well-infant nursery (WIN)

World Health Organization (WHO)

APPENDIX 18–B

Short List of Early Hearing Detection and Identification–Related Documents and Organizations

American Academy of Audiology (AAA)
- http://www.audiology.org/publications-resources/document-library/pediatric-diagnostics

American College of Medical Genetics and Genomics guideline for the clinical evaluation and etiologic diagnosis of hearing loss
- https://www.acmg.net/docs/ACMG_Guideline_for_Clinical_Eval_and_Etiologic_Dx%20of_Hearing_Loss_GIM_Apr2014.pdf

American Speech-Language-Hearing Association (ASHA)
- http://www.asha.org/public/hearing/Early-Intervention-for-Children-with-Hearing-Loss/

Association of Maternal and Child Health Programs (AMCHP)
- http://www.amchp.org/AboutAMCHP/Pages/default.aspx

Canadian Paediatric Society (CPA)
- http://www.cps.ca/documents/position/universal-hearing-screening-newborns

Centers for Disease Control and Prevention (CDC)
- http://www.cdc.gov/ncbddd/hearingloss/ehdi-programs.html

Directors of Speech and Hearing Programs in State Health and Welfare Agencies (DSHPSHWA)
- http://www.dshpshwa.org/

Early Childhood Technical Assistant Center (ECTA Center)
- http://ectacenter.org/

Early Hearing Detection and Intervention—Pediatric Audiology Links to Services (EHDI-PALS)
- http://ehdipals.org/

Health Resources and Services Administration (HRSA)
- http://www.hrsa.gov/

Joint Committee on Infant Hearing (JCIH)
- http://www.jcih.org/posstatemts.htm

National Center for Hearing Assessment and Management (NCHAM)
- http://www.infanthearing.org/

Neonatal Screening for Early Detection of Hearing Impairment: Final Report
- https://www.iqwig.de/download/S05-01_Final_report_Neonatal_screening_for_early_detection_of_hearing_impairment.pdf

Public Health England. Newborn Hearing Screening Programme
- http://hearing.screening.nhs.uk/standardsandprotocols

World Health Organization (WHO)
- http://www.who.int/pbd/deafness/WHO_GE_HL.pdf

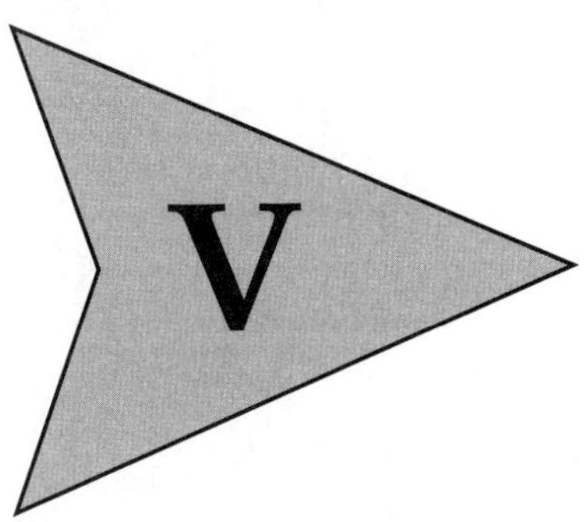

Audiologic Assessment of Children

Middle Ear Measurement

Lisa L. Hunter and Chelsea M. Blankenship

Overview

Middle ear measurement is a cornerstone of the basic audiologic test battery, and a physiologic measure that should be a part of all comprehensive audiologic assessments, particularly in infants and children. Middle ear measures provide a cross-check for other physiologic and behavioral measures, do not require behavioral response, are low cost, and require minimal time. Also known generically as acoustic immittance measures, these tests are simple to perform, yet complex to interpret in relation to the physical properties of the ear. The immittance battery contains three main components: single-frequency tympanometry, acoustic stapedial reflexes, and broadband or multifrequency immittance measures. The immittance battery is able to provide important diagnostic information about middle ear, cochlear, and neural functioning. Combined with other physiologic measures such as otoacoustic emissions and auditory brainstem response, useful diagnostic information can be gleaned even when behavioral tests are not possible.

Although single-frequency tympanometry and acoustic reflexes have comprised the standard immittance battery for the past 40 years, newer procedures using broadband stimuli have been developed recently, including broadband tympanometry and acoustic reflex measures, known collectively as wideband acoustic immittance (WAI; Feeney et al., 2013). To fully realize the diagnostic potential of these broadband measures, an understanding of the physical bases of aural acoustic immittance is useful. A brief overview is provided in this chapter, but for a more complete discussion, the reader is referred to Rosowski, Stenfelt, and Lilly (2013), Keefe and Feeney (2009), and Hunter and Shahnaz (2014).

Middle ear measurement is particularly important in infants and children, as the highest incidence of middle ear problems occurs in the first few years of life. In addition, as infants and young children are not able to provide their own perspectives about ear symptoms, and they are less able to provide us with behavioral test results, it is vitally important that sensitive and specific physiologic measures be available to provide information about functioning of the middle ear.

Middle Ear Characteristics and Postnatal Development

Although the cochlea is mature and adult in size at birth, the ear canal and middle ear are immature and undergo continued development, especially during the first 6 months after birth. Major changes that occur postnatally are depicted in Figure 19–1 and described here:

- There is an increase in diameter, length, and orientation of the ear canal, especially in the first 2 years of life.
- There is an increase in the rigidity of the ear canal. Initially, the neonate ear canal is relatively flaccid and collapsed, making visualization of the tympanic membrane difficult. The inner half of the infant ear canal begins ossifying prenatally and continues through the first year; thus, before this time, the ear canal is highly compliant (Holte, Margolis, &

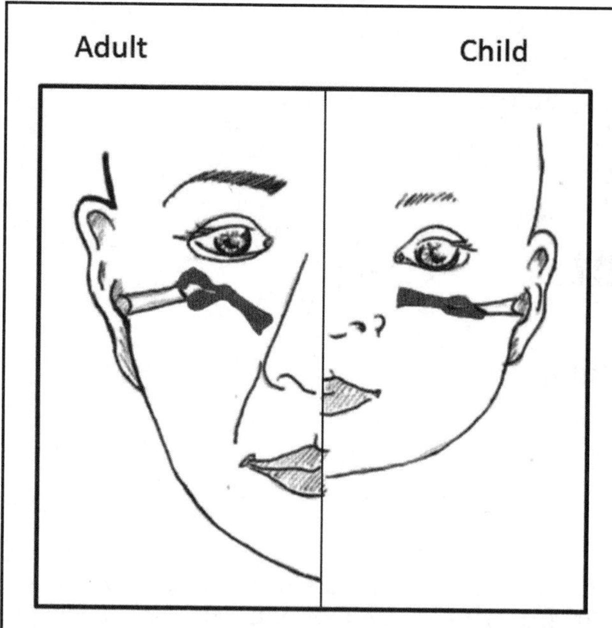

FIGURE 19–1. Adult (*left panel*) and child (*right panel*) ear canal, tympanic membrane, middle ear cavity, and eustachian tube showing changes in diameter, length, size, and orientation with development.

Cavanaugh, 1991). Stiffness of the ear canal increases as the medial bony portion ossifies and lengthens.

- As depicted in Figure 19–1, a change in orientation and thickness of the tympanic membrane (TM) occurs after birth. The TM is oriented horizontally with respect to the ear canal at birth and gradually becomes more perpendicular to the long axis of the ear canal, allowing better visualization. The appearance of the TM is normally dull, white, and thickened at birth. Over time, it thins due to loss of mesenchymal tissue (Ruah, Schachern, Zelterman, Paparella, & Yoon, 1991);
- There is an increase in aeration and size of the middle ear cavity, including pneumatization of the mastoid air cells; at birth, the middle ear may not be completely aerated. Based on temporal bone studies of deceased neonates, which likely are not reflective of normal newborns, contaminates in the middle ear space may be present including amniotic fluid, exudates, blood, desquamated epithelial cells and hair, keratinized cells, inflammatory cells, mucosal infiltrate, and reactive polyps (Palva, Northrup, & Ramsay, 1999). Estimates of the physical size of the middle ear and mastoid vary considerably among studies. A review of large consecutive planimetric studies by Cinamon (2009) revealed three distinct phases of mastoid pneumatization from birth to adult size. The mastoid bone and air cell compartments share a similar growth pattern, and bone expansion lags behind aeration. The mastoid antrum is well developed at birth with a volume of 1 to 1.5 cm^3. The mastoid cells are 3.5 to 4 cm^3 at age 1 year and grow linearly until the age of 6 years at a rate of 1 to 1.2 cm^3 per year. Thereafter, growth slowly continues, reaching adult size at puberty (approximately 12 cm^3). The mastoid bone expansion is about 0.6 to 0.9 cm per year in length and year, followed by half that rate until the age of 6 to 7 years. At puberty, there is a slower growth trajectory to adult size. Different ethnic groups share similar mastoid aeration and bone growth patterns. Interestingly, there were no differences between mastoid aeration measured in the preantibiotic era and after its widespread use (Cinamon, 2009).

  Physiologic studies of normal newborns using auditory brainstem response, otoacoustic emissions, video-recorded otoscopy, and multifrequency tympanometry are also consistent with the presence of fluid or other material in the middle ear space causing conductive hearing loss during the first few days after birth. Aeration normally occurs during the first 48 hr, but fluid and other materials may persist longer in some newborn ears. Infants born with meconium-stained amniotic fluid have a higher prevalence of material in the middle ear space (Piza, Gonzalez, Northrop, & Eavey, 1989). By the end of the first 24 hr after birth, approximately 50% of ears retain middle ear fluid, decreasing to 27% after 48 hr and 13% after 2 weeks (Roberts et al., 1995). In addition, the middle ear space is much smaller than that of an older child or adult. The length of the middle ear cavity increases in the first 6 months, from the tympanic membrane to the stapes footplate.
- Finally, the ossicles become less dense over the first 6 months as they resorb mesenchyme and ossify (Eby & Nadol, 1986), and the ossicular joints stiffen as well (Saunders, Kaltenbach, & Relkin, 1983).

Physiologically, these anatomic changes mean that at birth, the infant middle ear is more mass-loaded and less compliant than the adult ear. These developmental effects translate into lower static admittance, broader tympanometric width, appearance of notching at low frequencies (such as 0.226 kHz), transmission of low-frequency energy into the flaccid ear canal walls, and less energy transmission in middle to high frequencies into the middle ear due to the smaller and less aerated middle ear cavity and mastoid air cells. Thus, age-related normative values are important for middle ear measures.

Immittance Instrumentation

Most commercially available immittance instruments use a single probe tone frequency—usually 0.226 kHz, and measure the voltage delivered to the probe tone transducer that produces a constant sound pressure level in the sealed ear canal. As the ear canal is pressurized, it takes less voltage to produce the desired sound pressure level because some of the energy is reflected from the stiffened TM. Thus, when air pressure is high in the sealed ear canal, and the voltage to the probe tone transducer is low, the admittance is correspondingly low. This is indicated by the minimal admittance at the positive (A) and the negative (B) tails of the tympanogram (Figure 19–2). As air pressure in the sealed ear canal approaches ambient pressure (0 daPa), the admittance of the middle ear increases as the tympanic membrane assumes its normal flexibility and the voltage needed to maintain constant SPL in the ear canal increases. The peak of the tympanogram (TPP) corresponds to maximum admittance of the middle ear, which occurs at the ear canal air pressure that is approximate to the middle ear pressure (Figure 19–2C). This same principle holds for other probe tone frequencies, except that the physical volume relationship (in cm^3) to admittance (in mmho) is not 1:1 as it is at 0.226 kHz. For this reason, estimates of the volume of the tympanogram should be made when using a probe tone at 0.226 kHz.

The American National Standards Institute (ANSI) published the first standard for immittance instruments in 1987. Manufacturers generally adhere to this standard for design and calibration. The standard provides uniform terminology and plotting formats as well as calibration standards.

Single-Frequency (0.226 kHz) Tympanometry

Tympanometric Shapes

Two approaches have been used in the interpretation of 0.226-kHz tympanograms—qualitative and quantitative. Many of the early instruments that were used for tympanometry were uncalibrated and presented tympanometric results as "arbitrary compliance units." Because it was not appropriate to make quantitative measurements using uncalibrated instruments, qualitative measurements were based on the shapes of tympanograms. The most popular of these was the classification scheme originally described by Lidén (1969), Jerger (1970), and Lidén, Harford, and Hallen (1974). Tympanograms using the Lidén-Jerger classification scheme are qualitatively typed according to the height and location of the tympanogram peak. Type A tympanograms have normal peak height and location

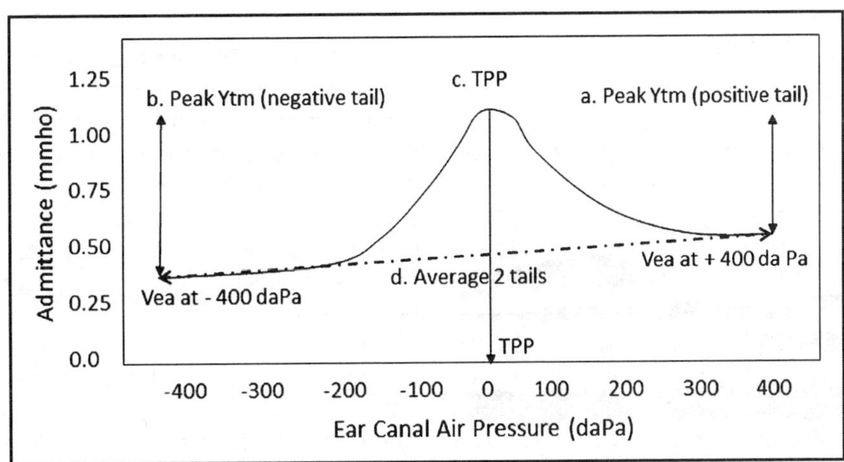

FIGURE 19–2. A single-frequency tympanogram (226 Hz), showing measurement of static compensated acoustic admittance (Y_{tm}). Compensated using positive (a), negative (b), and average (c), of two-tail compensation.

on the pressure axis. Type B tympanograms are flat with no discernable peak. A Type C tympanogram has a peak that occurs at negative middle ear pressure. Lidén also described a Type D tympanogram characterized by a double peak. Later, subtypes A_D and A_S were added (Feldman, 1976), indicating a high-peaked and shallow-peaked pattern, respectively. Although this qualitative approach was originally useful for identifying tympanometric shapes, and simplified interpretation, its lack of precision has led to clinical misinterpretations. For example, without quantitative criteria, no rule for distinguishing among Types A, A_D, and A_S exists. Even distinguishing between Types B and A is sometimes problematic when small or broad peaks occur, or shifts in the positive compared to the negative tails occur. Thus, it is recommended to use specific measurements that will be described in subsequent sections, rather than subjective typing.

After the publication of the ANSI (1987) standard, manufacturers began to conform to the requirement that immittance instruments provide calibrated physical units of measurement rather than arbitrary compliance units. Virtually all immittance instruments produced since then have been admittance meters. Quantitative analysis of tympanograms is preferable, especially when assessing infants and children, for which different normative values based on age are needed and the cut-points used for distinguishing normal and abnormal middle ear function require precise measurement of admittance and width. Four tympanometric features are used to quantify tympanograms. Table 19–1 provides age-related normative values for these measures.

Peak Compensated Static Admittance (Ytm)

The peak compensated static acoustic admittance, or Y_{tm}, is the most often used measurement of the 0.226-kHz tympanogram. The peak of the tympanogram includes the admittance due to the middle ear (Y_{tm}) and admittance of the ear canal. Compensation, or subtraction of the admittance of the ear canal, is necessary to determine Y_{tm}. There are three primary methods to compensate the tympanogram as shown in Figure 19–2: positive tail, negative tail, and the two-tails method. The positive tail method uses the value at +200 daPa to estimate the admittance of the ear canal, which is then subtracted from the peak admittance, as shown in Figure 19–2. The negative tail method uses the minimum tail value at −400 daPa, and the average two-tails method (d) uses the interpolated value of the positive and negative tail values, obtained by drawing a line between the two tails and measuring the value corresponding to the peak of the tympanogram (Baldwin, 2006). There are advantages and disadvantages for the three methods of compensation. The negative tail of the tympanogram presents some disadvantages for compensation. First, artifactual spikes are more common with extremes in negative pressure, which can affect measurements at the negative tail. Second, in newborns and infants, the ear canal may collapse with negative pressure, which complicates measurement of the minimum tail value. The positive tail overestimates ear canal volume and is less sensitive to the presence of middle ear effusion, and thus the average two-tails method has been recommended (Baldwin, 2006).

Static admittance is specific to many middle ear conditions, such as distinguishing otitis media with effusion (OME) and ossicular discontinuity from normal middle ear function. In a large study of children with OME, patients who had reduced static admittance on tympanometry had increased odds of bilateral hearing loss (Sidell, Hunter, Lin, & Arjmand, 2014). The mean preoperative tympanometric static admittance was 0.3 mmho. One unit less (0.2 mmho or less) in static admittance on tympanometry was associated with a 7.1 times increased odds of having bilateral hearing loss preoperatively. Sensitivity of Y_{tm} is poorer for conditions such as ossicular fixation or cholesteatoma that do not restrict mobility of the tympanic membrane because tympanometry is more affected by conditions that have close proximity to the measurement probe. Thus, other measurements have been suggested to complement Y_{tm}, specifically tympanometric width.

Tympanometric Width (TW)

A number of studies have demonstrated that the sharpness of the tympanometric peak is an indicator of middle ear pathology (Fiellau-Nikolajsen, 1983; Nozza, Bluestone, Kardatze, & Bachman, 1992, 1994). Brooks (1968) introduced the term *gradient* for this measurement. Methods for quantifying gradient were first proposed by Brooks (1968), Paradise, Smith, and Bluestone (1976), and Lidén (1969). Two studies have compared gradient measures obtained with the various techniques in normal children and adults (de Jonge, 1986; Koebsell & Margolis, 1986). These studies concluded that the preferred technique is the tympanometric width (TW). Figure 19–3 illustrates the measurement of TW based on the positive tail compensation method. Diagnostically, only broad TW is important in children for diagnosis of otitis media.

Table 19–1. Normative Data by Age for Single-Frequency Tympanometry

Study	Age Range	Probe Frequency (kHz)	Peak Compensated Static Admittance: Measurement Method	Peak Compensated Static Admittance: 5 to 95 Percentiles (mmho)	Tympanometric Width (daPa)	Pump Sweep: Direction	Pump Sweep: Speed (daPa/s)
Margolis et al., 2003	Birth to 4 weeks (CA)	1	−400 tail to peak	0.60 to 4.3	N/A	+200 to −400	At Tail: 600 At Peak: 200
Kei et al., 2003	1 to 6 days	1	+200 tail to peak	Right Ear 0.39 to 2.28 Left Ear 0.39 to 1.95	Right Ear 56.6 to 154 Left Ear 46.1 to 144.2	+200 to −200	50
Roush et al., 1992	6 to 12 months	0.226	+200 tail to peak	0.20 to 0.50	102 to 234 $Y_{tm} \geq 0.3$ mmho	+200 to −300	N/A
	12 to 18 months	0.226	+200 tail to peak	0.20 to 0.60	102 to 204 $Y_{tm} \geq 0.3$ mmho	+200 to −300	N/A
	18 to 24 months	0.226	+200 tail to peak	0.30 to 0.70	102 to 204 $Y_{tm} \geq 0.3$ mmho	+200 to −300	N/A
	24 to 30 months	0.226	+200 tail to peak	0.30 to 0.80	96 to 192 $Y_{tm} \geq 0.3$ mmho	+200 to −300	N/A
Sun et al., 2012	0 to 5 days	0.226 and 1 kHz	N/A	0.1 to 1.3	−56.5 to 136	+200 to −400	50 to 100
Mazlan et al., 2010	Birth (24–192 hr)	1 kHz	Baseline compensation at +200	0.65 ± 0.34*	N/A	+200 to −400	400
	6 weeks	1 kHz	Baseline compensation at +200	0.83 ± 0.49*	N/A	+200 to −400	400
Swanepoel et al., 2007	<1 weeks	1 kHz	N/A	1.2 to 3.4	N/A	+200 to −200	200
	1 to 4 weeks	1 kHz	N/A	1.5 to 3.8	N/A	+200 to −200	200
	0 to 4 weeks	1 kHz	N/A	1.4 to 3.7	N/A	+200 to −200	200

Note. *kHz* = kilohertz; *daPa* = decapascal; *mmho* = millimho; *CA* = chronological age; Y_{tm} = peak compensated static admittance; *Mean ± SD.

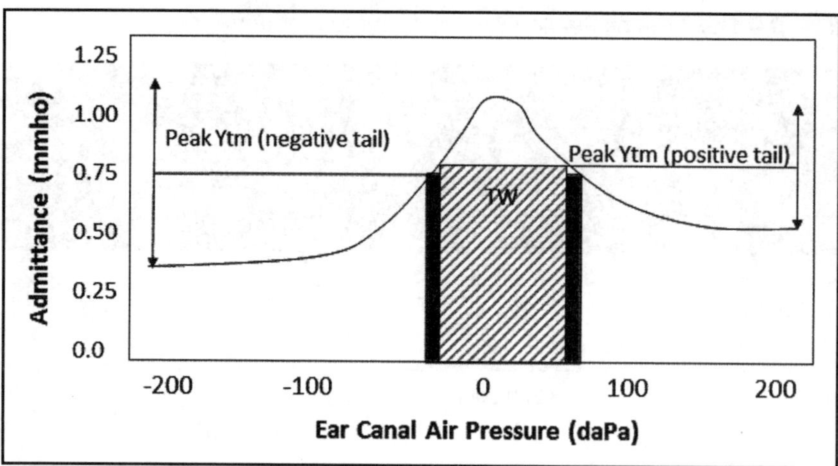

FIGURE 19–3. A single-frequency tympanogram (226 Hz), showing measurement of tympanometric width (TW), compensated using positive and negative tails.

Tympanometric Peak Pressure (TPP)

The ear canal air pressure at which the peak of the tympanogram occurs is the tympanometric peak pressure (TPP), as shown in Figure 19–2C. TPP is an indicator of the pressure in the middle ear space, although TPP overestimates the actual middle ear pressure, sometimes by as much as 100% (Elner, Ingelstedt, & Ivarsson, 1971; Renvall & Holmquist, 1976). A TPP of –300 daPa, for example, could occur with actual middle ear pressure of only –150 daPa. Negative TPP has not been shown to provide reliable diagnostic specificity or sensitivity to otitis media in children (Fiellau-Nikolajsen, 1983; Nozza et al., 1994; Paradise et al., 1976), and thus is not currently recommended as a reason to refer children for treatment (American Speech-Language-Hearing Association [ASHA], 2004).

Measurement of TPP can be useful for equilibrating ear canal air pressure to enhance acoustic-reflex and otoacoustic-emission responses (Trine, Hirsch, & Margolis, 1993). Hof, Anteunis, Chenault, and van Dijk (2005) compensated middle ear pressure while measuring transient-evoked otoacoustic emissions (TEOAEs) in 59 children and reported a mean amplitude increase of 1.9 dB between 1 and 2 kHz. Self-induced negative TPP has been shown to affect distortion product otoacoustic emission (DPOAE) responses below 1 kHz by about 4 to 6 dB (Sun & Shaver, 2009). However, Prieve, Calandruccio, Fitzgerald, Mazevski, and Georgantas (2008) measured TEOAE and noise levels in 18 children under two conditions: on a day when the tympanogram TPP was normal and on a day when the tympanogram TPP was negative. They reported that average TEOAE level was about 4 dB lower for all frequency bands from 1000 to 4000 when TPP was negative, but noise levels did not change between the two conditions. Importantly, the presence of negative TPP affected the pass rate in only 5% to 6% of cases.

Equivalent Ear Canal Volume (Veq)

Acoustic immittance measures using a 0.226-kHz probe tone are useful for estimating the volume of air in front of the probe (Lindeman & Holmquist, 1982; Shanks, Stelmachowicz, Beauchaine, & Schulte, 1992). In the presence of a flat tympanogram, an estimate of the volume of air in front of the probe can be useful for detecting eardrum perforations and evaluating the patency of tympanostomy tubes. Although a normal Veq does not rule out a perforation, a flat tympanogram with a large Veq is evidence of tympanic membrane perforation or a patent tympanostomy tube. In normal ears, the admittance at high positive or negative pressure is primarily determined by the ear canal volume. This measurement is the same as the tail value used to compensate the tympanogram, as shown in Figure 19–2. However, because the eardrum and ear canal walls are not perfectly rigid when the ear is pressurized, the admittance at 0.226 kHz, expressed as Veq, overestimates the actual ear canal volume by about 25% in adults, partly due to distension of the ear canal wall

(Shanks & Lilly, 1981). For this reason, the negative tail value is a more accurate estimate of Veq than the positive tail.

The average tympanometrically measured Veq is about 0.3 cm^3 in 4-month-old infants (Holte et al., 1991), 0.75 cm^3 in preschool children (Margolis & Heller, 1987), and 1.0 to 1.4 cm^3 in adults (Margolis & Heller, 1987; Wiley et al., 1996). An opening in the TM adds the volume of the middle ear space and contiguous mastoid air cells to the volume of the ear canal. On the basis of these tympanometric measurements, it should be possible to distinguish between ears with intact eardrums and those with perforations without difficulty. However, ears with perforations might have past or present middle ear disease that causes volumes to be decreased for several reasons. An ear with active middle ear disease may contain inflammation, fluid, granulation tissue, fibrosis, polyps, or cholesteatoma in the middle ear space. Mastoid air cells may be blocked by tissue or underdeveloped with poor pneumatization due to inflammation. Shanks et al. (1992) recommended an abnormal criterion of 1.0 cm^3 for children for equivalent volume. Another useful clinical application for equivalent volume is to monitor the course of middle ear disease after placement of tympanostomy tubes. It has been shown that equivalent volume correlates with disease severity (Hunter, Margolis, Daly, & Giebink, 1992) and with recurrence of otitis media (Takasaka et al., 1996). Progressively larger equivalent volume after tube insertion is an indication of recovery from otitis media. When equivalent volume remains small, it is an indicator of continued disease. In a prospective study of 157 children aged 6 months to 8 years, treated with tubes for OME, an equivalent volume of less than 1.5 cc was associated with greater OME recurrence (Hunter & Margolis, 1992). A large recent study by the MRC Multicentre Otitis Media Study Group (2003) provides equivalent volume measurements in 3- to 7-year-old children randomized to one of three interventions (tube insertion with or without adenoidectomy and nonsurgical observation). The study reported otoscopy for 336 ears with functioning tubes and 205 nonsurgery ears compared to equivalent ear canal volume (Veq) before and after tube insertion. Cutoff Veq was evaluated in terms of classification accuracy against otoscopy after intervention. Age range did not influence Veq, or the optimum Veq cutoff, but boys had significantly larger Veq (by 0.09 cm^3) than girls. The recommended mean cutoff for tube patency is greater than or equal to 1.13 cm^3, slightly higher than the 1.0 cm^3 recommended by Shanks et al. (1992). Another large recent study of children who had received PE tubes found that smaller equivalent volume obtained postoperatively had increased risk of hearing loss (Sidell et al., 2014).

Sensitivity and Specificity of Tympanometry

To gauge the clinical usefulness of any diagnostic test, a complete understanding must be developed of the test's performance in various populations at high and low risk for the disease of interest. Tympanometry is one of the most highly utilized diagnostic tests for diagnosing a specific condition in audiology. In most studies before 1990, tympanometry was measured with arbitrary units; therefore, qualitative types were compared with pneumatic otoscopy or with surgery. More recent studies have used quantitative analysis of tympanometry. Silman, Silverman, and Arick (1992) investigated several protocols for sensitivity and specificity of detection of OME in children. Children were identified with OME on the basis of pneumatic otoscopy. Combinations of static admittance, width, peak pressure, and ipsilateral acoustic reflex resulted in sensitivity varying from 76% to 95%.

Performance of two screening measures was also assessed by Roush, Drake, and Sexton (1992) in 374 ears of 3- to 4-year-old children in a preschool program. A "traditional" procedure, based on TPP less than −200 daPa or absent acoustic reflexes was compared with interim norms (ASHA, 1990) both against the gold standard of pneumatic otoscopy by an experienced, validated otoscopist. The traditional procedure had high sensitivity (95%) but low specificity (65%). The ASHA interim norms had high sensitivity (84%) and specificity (95%), with a positive predictive value of 69% and a negative predictive value of 98%. The interim 1990 ASHA screening guidelines have since been updated and are described in Chapter 17 by Roush and Corbin in this volume.

Nozza and colleagues (1992) studied two groups of children. One group (n = 61, aged 1 to 8 years) received tympanostomy tubes and thus was at high risk for OME. Tympanometry was performed no more than 30 minutes before surgery, and the surgeon was unaware of the results of tympanometry. Six different protocols were evaluated; three of these included ipsilateral acoustic reflex thresholds. Sensitivity (90%) and specificity (86%) were highest for gradient (width) combined with acoustic reflexes. Gradient combined with static admittance also produced relatively high sensitivity (83%) and specificity (87%). A second group of children who attended an allergy clinic (n = 77, aged 3 to 16 years) were unselected with regard to otitis media history and were reported in the same study with the same six protocols and gold standard. In that group, sensitivity was 78% for all protocols except ipsilateral acoustic reflex alone (sensitivity = 88%) and gradient or static admittance <0.1 mmho (sensitivity = 67%). Gradient + ipsilateral reflex and gradient + static admittance performed equally well for specificity (99%). Positive predictive value was higher for gradient + static admittance (88%) than it was for gradient + ipsilateral reflex (78%).

In a subsequent study (Nozza et al., 1994), a group of children (n = 171, aged 1 to 12 years) with recurrent or chronic OME, who were scheduled for myringotomy and tubes, received otoscopy by a validated otoscopist and tympanometry by a certified audiologist. The prevalence of OME in this group was 55%. Eleven criteria, with various cut-points for each criterion, were evaluated. As expected, there was a trade-off between sensitivity and specificity. Best overall performance was found for TW or Y_{tm} combined with pneumatic otoscopy (sensitivity and specificity = 80%), or for TW alone greater than 275 daPa (sensitivity = 78%, specificity = 82%). Interim norms (ASHA, 1990) showed high sensitivity (95%) but poor specificity (24%).

These studies demonstrate that the choice of cutoff criteria affects test performance greatly. It appears that combinations of criteria, such as otoscopy and TW, perform better than single criteria. Static admittance (Y) alone has poor sensitivity but good specificity, but this depends on the cutoff criteria selected. Use of either ipsilateral reflex or TW combined with Y provides good test performance, as does otoscopy combined with TW. If Y is used diagnostically, it should be combined with either pneumatic otoscopy, width, gradient, or ipsilateral acoustic reflexes.

It is important to note that all studies examining test performance of pneumatic otoscopy have used experienced otoscopists who have received specific training and have been validated, or compared to other expert otoscopists. Most OM is diagnosed by primary care physicians. In many cases, clinicians who use otoscopy to diagnose OME do not use pneumatic otoscopy and have not been validated against experienced otoscopists. In order for otoscopy to reach high levels of sensitivity and specificity, pneumatic otoscopy must be performed after ear canal cleaning by a highly experienced clinician. Due to these practical considerations, tympanometry is very useful as an alternative or a confirmatory test, especially when pneumatic otoscopy is unsuccessful or an experienced otoscopist is not available.

Screening Tympanometry

Tympanometry has been widely used in screening programs for identifying middle ear disease in pediatric populations. Principles underlying screening for hearing loss and middle ear disease in children after the neonatal period are described in Chapter 17 of this text. Mass screening programs for middle ear conditions such as OME in children have not been recommended (American Academy of Audiology [AAA], 1997, 2011; AAO-HNS OME Guidelines, 2004, Rosenfeld et al., currently in revision). Although various conferences, organizations, and agencies have been hesitant to recommend large-scale screening programs for OME, many programs for preschool- and school-age children have incorporated tympanometric screening into the protocol. Most programs combine audiometric screening with tympanometric screening to detect both hearing loss and middle ear disorders (AAA, 1997, 2011; ASHA, 1997).

Universal newborn hearing screening (UNHS) programs do not usually include middle-ear assessment in either well-baby nurseries (WBNs) or neonatal intensive care units (NICUs) for several reasons (Joint Committee on Infant Hearing [JCIH], 2007). Pneumatic otoscopy and bone-conducted ABR are impractical in UNHS due to the use of untrained personnel in many settings. Low-frequency tympanometry (e.g., 0.226 kHz) is insensitive to middle ear dysfunction in newborns (Hunter & Margolis, 1992; Paradise et al., 1976; Sprague, Wiley, & Goldstein, 1985), as described in more detail below.

Tympanometry in Newborns and Infants

0.226-kHz Tympanometry

Tympanograms recorded from normal ears of newborn infants are very different from those obtained from older infants, children, and adults. The earliest tympanometric recordings from neonate ears were made with single-component instruments that used a 0.22-kHz probe tone and expressed the results as "arbitrary compliance units" (Bennett, 1975; Keith, 1973, 1975; Poulsen & Tos, 1978). These studies reported a frequent occurrence of double-peaked tympanograms. Later studies recorded two-component tympanograms at two probe frequencies, 0.22 and 0.66 kHz (Himelfarb, Popelka, & Shanon, 1979; Sprague et al., 1985). These two-component recordings permit an analysis of the reactance and resistance of the infant ear. These studies indicated that at low frequencies, the newborn ear is highly resistive and has low negative reactance, suggesting a significant mass effect that offsets the stiffness of the middle ear system. These effects are probably related to developmental differences between infant middle ears and those of older children and adults. The reasons for differences in admittance characteristics between adults and newborns are not fully known. However, anatomical differences in the infant ear, such as a more compliant ear canal wall (Holte et al., 1991), smaller ear canal and middle ear space, tympanic-membrane thickening, middle-ear fluid and mesenchyme, and a more horizontal orientation of the tympanic membrane with respect to the axis of the ear canal, are the most likely contributors (Eavey, 1993; Ikui, Sando, Sudo, & Fujita, 1997; Ruah et al., 1991; Saunders et al., 1983).

In neonate ears with confirmed middle ear disease, 0.226-kHz tympanograms are not reliably different from those obtained from normal ears. In addition, the variability of 0.226-kHz probe-tone admittance tympanometry characteristics in young infants has led to conflicting interpretation of what tympanometric criteria define a normal infant middle ear, which casts doubt on the clinical utility of these measures for newborns (Keith, 1975; Paradise et al., 1976; Sprague et al., 1985). Infants with diagnosed middle ear fluid have been demonstrated to have normal 0.226-kHz tympanograms (Hunter & Margolis, 1992; Paradise et al., 1976; Zhiqi, Kun, & Zhiwu, 2010). For these reasons, 0.226-kHz tympanometry is not an effective test for middle ear measurement in newborns.

0.66- and 1-kHz Tympanometry

Evidence has accumulated that tympanometry using higher probe-tone frequencies (0.66 or 1 kHz) is more sensitive to changes in middle-ear status in infants less than 4 months old compared to 0.226-kHz tympanometry (Alaerts, Lutz, & Woulters, 2007; Baldwin, 2006; Calandruccio, Fitzgerald, & Prieve, 2006; Hoffmann et al., 2013; Marchant et al., 1986; Rhodes, Margolis, Hirsch, & Napp, 1999; Swanepoel et al., 2007). Some of these studies have reported normative data for a variety of ages, and some have investigated test performance of specific 1-kHz admittance criteria in predicting otoacoustic emission (OAE) screening results. A tympanogram measured at 1 kHz in a normal newborn is shown in Figure 19–4.

A normally shaped single or double peak is typical in newborns if the middle ear is aerated and the ear canal is not collapsed. An example of a tympanogram measured in a newborn with a collapsed ear canal is shown in Figure 19–5. To complicate matters, the tympanogram is also notched at the peak, which frequently occurs in newborns. Despite these considerations, Margolis, Bass-Ringdahl, Hanks, Holte, and Zapala (2003) recommend use of negative tail compensation because the tympanogram is often so asymmetric that the peak to positive tail difference is very small and therefore insensitive to fluid. The two-tail compensation method recommended by Baldwin (2006) averages or interpolates across the positive and negative tail, which offers a reasonable compromise over the use of one tail value alone.

Margolis et al. (2003) assessed 1-kHz tympanometric test performance in predicting whether a newborn infant passed or failed a DPOAE test. The 1-kHz tympanometry criterion had a specificity of 91% in predicting which ears passed the DPOAE test, but a sensitivity of only 50% in predicting which ears failed the DPOAE test. Kei et al. (2003) reported 1-kHz tympanometric data that were obtained from both ears of 106 infants (1 to 6 days old) who passed a click-evoked OAE hearing screening and presented with "single-peaked" tympanograms. Kei et al. (2003) suggested that a tympanogram representing normal middle-ear function should include a single peak (which was the case in 92.3% of their sample) and that its tympanometric variables (six were identified) should be within the 90% range of a population of normal-hearing infants (which would exclude at least 10% of their sample with single-peaked tympanograms). With their proposed six tympanometric variables, some normal-hearing infants would be within the 90% range on some variables and outside for others, but no procedure for choosing among these various criteria was described. Baldwin (2006) compared admittance tympanometry results at 0.226, 0.678, and 1 kHz between groups of infants (mean age of 10 weeks) classified as having either normal or disordered middle-ear function. Baldwin (2006) classified the infant tympanograms using a traditional visual classification scheme (Jerger, 1970; Liden, 1969), and a classification scheme proposed by Marchant et al. (1986). Comparisons of sensitivity and specificity values for the method after Marchant et al. (1986) revealed the best results for 1-kHz tympanometry (sensitivity of 0.99 and specificity of 0.89). Baldwin (2006) cautioned that these findings may not apply to neonates, as the youngest infant tested in her study was 2 weeks old. Swanepoel et al. (2007) reported sensitivity of 57% and specificity of 95% for 1-kHz tympanometry, 57% and 90% for acoustic reflex presence, and 58% and 87% for

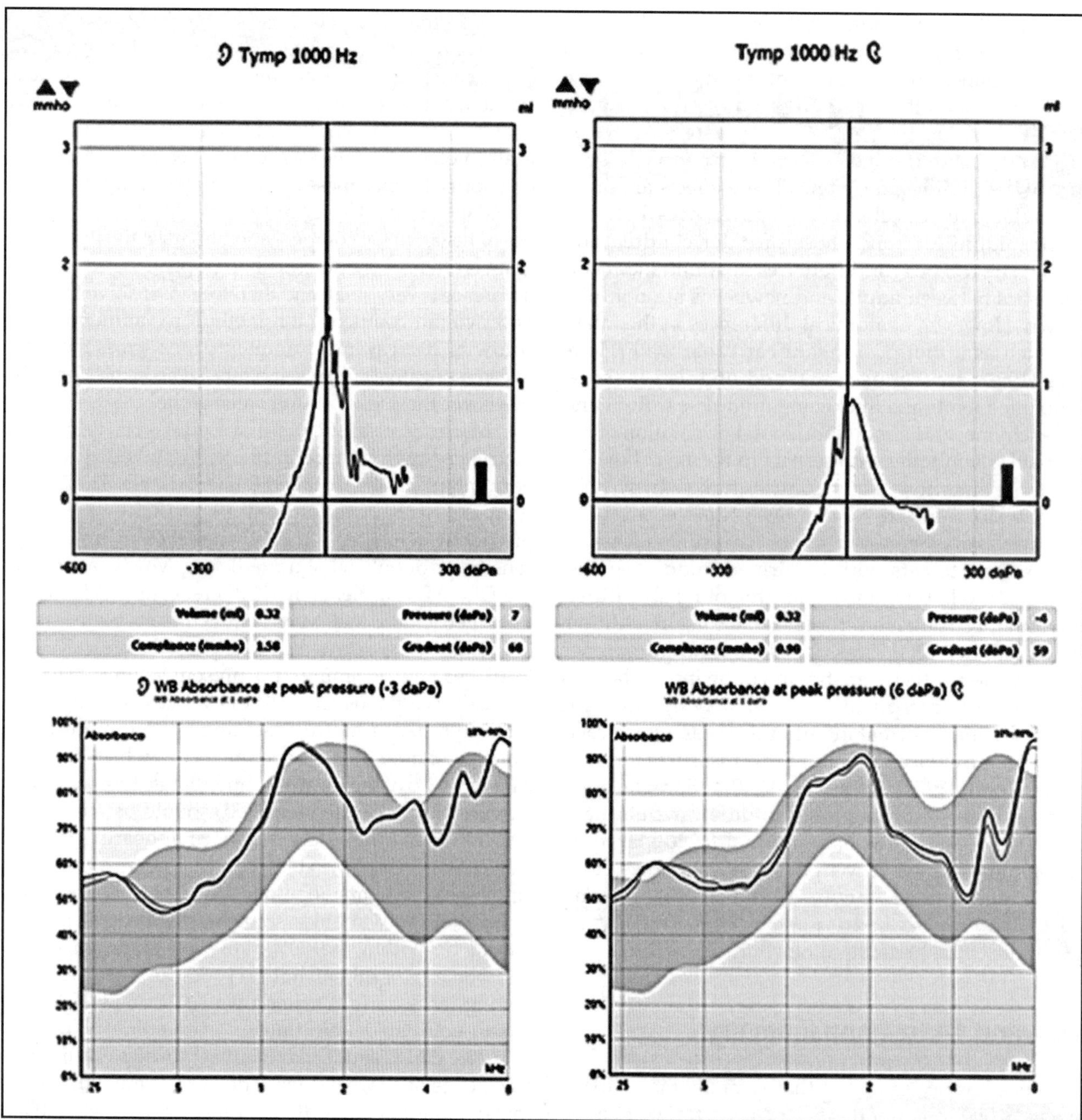

FIGURE 19–4. Single-frequency tympanometry at 1000 Hz for a 1-month-old infant with normal middle ear status (*top panels*), and corresponding wideband acoustic absorbance at TPP and ambient pressure in bottom panels, relative to normative ranges. Normal admittance magnitude, tympanometric width, and peak pressure are present. The tympanogram is asymmetric due to volume changes with positive versus negative pressure, characteristic of the newborn ear canal.

combined tympanometry and acoustic reflex results, respectively. Reliability of 1-kHz tympanometry has been studied by Mazlan, Kei, Hickson, Gavranich, and Linning (2010), showing high reproducibility for static admittance measures at birth and 6 weeks of age. The JCIH (2007) has recommended 1-kHz tympanometry for assessment of babies younger than 6 months on the basis of these studies.

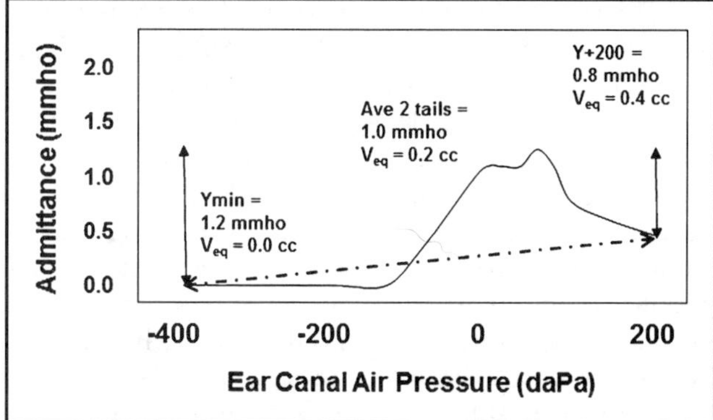

FIGURE 19–5. Example of a tympanogram measured in a newborn with collapsing ear canal, indicated by a sudden decrease to a volume of 0 cc with negative pressure. The collapsing volume measurement is reflected in the minimum tail value, and the notched peak of the tympanogram complicates measurement of peak admittance. The first peak was used to calculate static admittance. Note the differences in static admittance measured using the positive, minimum, and interpolated tail values, as well as the differences in equivalent ear canal volume.

Multifrequency Tympanometry

Earlier studies of multifrequency tympanometry give some clues as to why higher-frequency regions provide different results in neonates than in adults. For example, Holte et al. (1991) recorded multifrequency tympanometry (0.226 to 0.9 kHz) from newborns and followed them to 4 months of age. Tympanometric shapes were classified according to the model described by Vanhuyse and colleagues (Vanhuyse, Creten, & Van Camp, 1975). For newborns (1 to 7 days), at 0.226 kHz, all tympanograms conformed to the Vanhuyse model classifications. At higher frequencies, more tympanograms were classified as "other," meaning they did not adhere to the Vanhuyse classification model. At 0.9 kHz, none of the shapes conformed to the classification. With increasing age, more of the tympanograms became adult-like, following the Vanhuyse model. By 4 months of age, tympanometric patterns adhered to the Vanhuyse model, indicating that significant development had occurred. Reasons for the disorganized pattern of tympanograms in newborns are not entirely clear. Because the osseous portion of the ear canal of the newborn is not rigid, it has been suggested that ear canal wall motion influences the shape of the tympanogram (Paradise et al., 1976). There is evidence for and against this hypothesis. Holte, Cavanaugh, and Margolis (1990) found no relationship between canal wall movement of neonates measured with video otomicroscopy and their tympanometric patterns. Hsu, Margolis, and Schachern (2000) found similarly complex tympanometric patterns in newborn chinchillas despite the fact that their canal walls appeared to be fully ossified on histologic analysis. Keefe, Bulen, Arehart, and Burns (1993) measured complex impedance in infants at various ages and found a mass effect that was similar to the acoustic properties of soft tissue elsewhere in the body. Because this effect dominates at frequencies below 1 kHz, they argued that low frequencies are a poor choice for evaluating middle ear function in newborns. In addition to the flaccidity of the ear canal walls, the fluid and material found in newborn middle ears likely contributes to greater mass loading, which results in more complex, notched patterns at lower frequencies, consistent with the Vanhuyse model predictions. Thus, as a result of these studies, it has become apparent that higher-frequency probe tones are needed to adequately assess middle ear status in newborns, and that 0.226-kHz tympanometry becomes more adult-like by 4 months of age.

Wideband Acoustic Immittance (WAI)

Single-frequency admittance tympanometry contrasts with other tests of auditory function such as behavioral audiometry, OAE, and ABR tests. These tests all use stimuli over multiple octaves of the frequency range of human hearing. Techniques to classify such multifrequency admittance tympanometric patterns have been used to measure responses up to approximately 2 kHz (Colletti, 1977; Vanhuyse, Creten, & Van Camp, 1975; Wada, Koike, & Kobayashi, 1998) to measure the middle ear resonance frequency. Nevertheless, use of multifrequency tympanometry is not widely accepted in clinical settings, largely due to the complexity of the responses and uncertainty regarding interpretation. Thus, middle ear function is not currently adequately assessed at the higher frequencies important for audition. Single-frequency tympanometry and acoustic reflexes perform reasonably well for detection of middle ear effusion, but there are some ways these tests fall short:

- In babies under 6 months, 0.226-kHz tympanometry has very poor sensitivity to middle ear effusion.
- In infants less than 6 months, 1 kHz performs better, and other studies have shown it is less sensitive to middle ear problems with OAE screening failure.

- Single-frequency tympanometry does not accurately predict conductive hearing loss.
- Single-frequency tympanometry does not accurately detect otosclerosis.
- Single-frequency tympanometry cannot be realistically compared to broadband tests, such as otoacoustic emissions.

A relatively new immittance method known as wideband acoustic immittance (WAI), energy reflectance (WBA), or wideband absorbance (WBA; generically, wideband acoustic immittance or WAI) makes possible measurements at any frequency up to approximately 10 kHz through advances in calibration and measurement techniques that are relatively unaffected by standing waves in the ear canal. These newer WAI tests have the potential to improve clinical diagnosis of auditory pathology in infants, children, and adults with various types of middle ear disease. Two WAI instruments are commercially available: the Hear-ID ambient pressure system from Mimosa Acoustics, which is approved by the Food and Drug Administration (FDA) in the United States and can be combined with TEOAE and DPOAE in the same system, and the Titan (also FDA approved) system from Interacoustics, which includes wideband tympanometry, DPOAE, TEOAE, screening ABR, and acoustic reflexes. Figure 19–6 illustrates a normal ambient pressure and wideband tympanogram response.

The WAI technique was first developed to measure acoustic impedance in cats (Allen, 1986) and was later adapted for noninvasive clinical use in humans (Keefe, Ling, & Bulen, 1992). These wideband tests (ambient and pressurized reflectance and absorbance, admittance, impedance, and acoustic reflexes) have been shown to detect newborn hearing screening (NHS) failures associated with middle ear fluid in newborns (Hunter, Feeney, Lapsley Miller, Jeng, & Bohning, 2010; Keefe, Gorga, Neely, & Zhao, 2003; Keefe, Zhao, Neely, Gorga, & Vohr, 2003; Sanford et al., 2009) for early identification of infants with sensorineural hearing loss, and to detect middle ear dysfunction and conductive hearing loss in children and adults (Keefe & Simmons, 2003; Prieve, Vander Werff, Preston, & Georgantas, 2013). These tests use a wideband "chirp" stimulus that allows measurements over the range 0.200 to 10 kHz in a few seconds, are noninvasive, use a standard soft immittance probe tip, and provide a comprehensive set of measurements to assess the middle ear over the entire range of sound frequencies important to speech perception.

To perform the test, a calibrated click stimulus is presented to the ear canal from a speaker housed inside a probe, which is seated in the ear with a soft probe tip, just as in tympanometry or OAE tests. The test can be done with ambient ear canal air pressure or with varying pressure as in tympanometry. The SPL and phase of the sound in calibration cavities is compared to that of the sound recorded in the ear canal. The difference

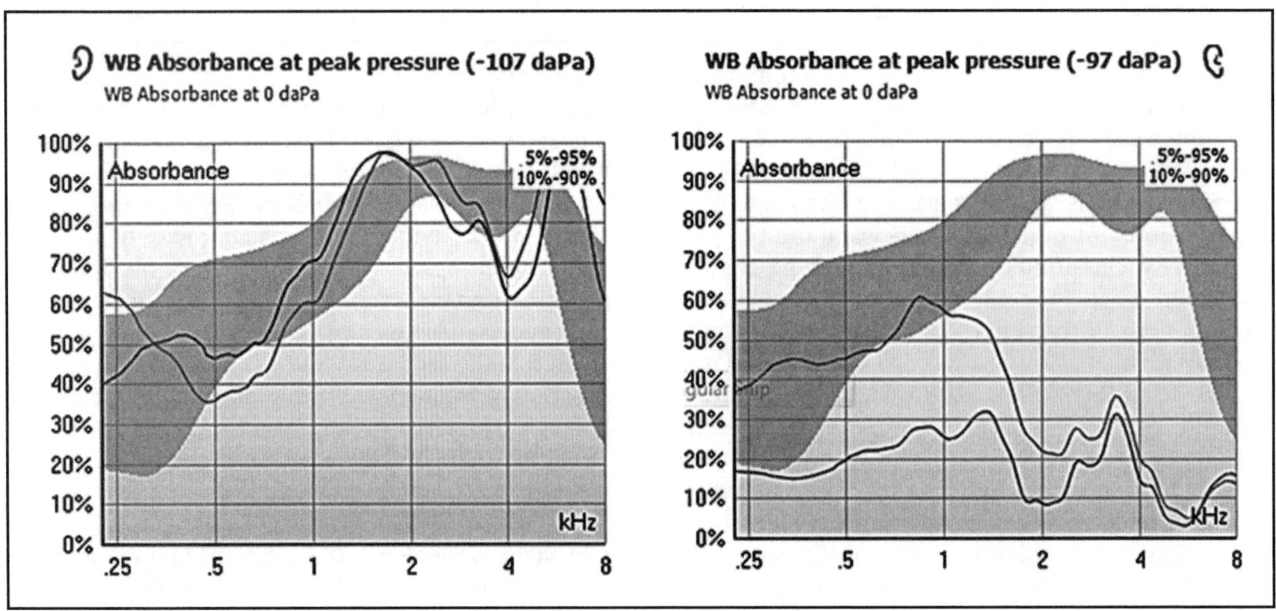

FIGURE 19–6. Wideband absorbance tympanogram and ambient pressure absorbance in a 1-month-old with normal hearing in the left ear and a conductive hearing loss in the right ear.

is energy that is absorbed by the middle ear structures. Energy reflectance (ER) is the ratio of the incident sound (input to the ear canal), and the reflected sound and varies between 0 and 1. Wideband immittance measurements can also be presented in terms of energy absorbance (EA), the inverse of ER. To the extent that the ear canal walls absorb no sound energy, EA is the fraction of incident energy absorbed by the middle ear (Keefe & Feeney, 2009); both EA and ER vary between 0 and 1 (assuming no OAE contribution). EA can also be converted into a decibel scale known as transmittance. Use of EA is more easily relatable to admittance, as measured in tympanometry. EA is largest at frequencies for which the middle ear is efficient in collecting sound energy (1 to 3 kHz). An EA tympanogram in a healthy adult middle ear, like a 0.226-kHz admittance magnitude tympanogram, has a single peak in its response across different air pressures.

The normal range for ambient pressure ER in infants and children reported by a number of studies in infants for several reference tests (DPOAE, TEOAE, AABR, 1-kHz tympanometry) was provided by Aithal, Kei, Driscoll, Khan, and Swanston (2015), and is shown in Figure 19–7. Computer algorithms for noise and artifact reduction, and calculation of impedance and admittance quantities such as admittance, impedance and their subcomponents, provide rapid, quantitative analyses of the acoustical response of the middle ear into the ear canal walls.

Wideband absorbance (WBA) and related measurements have been reported in normal children and infants (Keefe et al., 1993; Sanford & Feeney, 2008; Vander Werff, Prieve, & Georgantas, 2007), and newborns (Abdala, Keefe, & Oba, 2007; Aithal, Kei, & Driscoll, 2014; Aithal, Kei, Driscoll, & Khan, 2013; Aithal et al., 2015; Hunter et al., 2010; Keefe et al., 2000; Keefe & Abdala, 2007; Kei et al., 2003; Merchant, Horton, & Voss, 2010; Sanford et al., 2009; Shahnaz, Miranda, & Polka, 2008).

The first developmental study of WBA was reported by Keefe et al. (1993), who investigated middle ear maturation on wideband immittance measures in adults

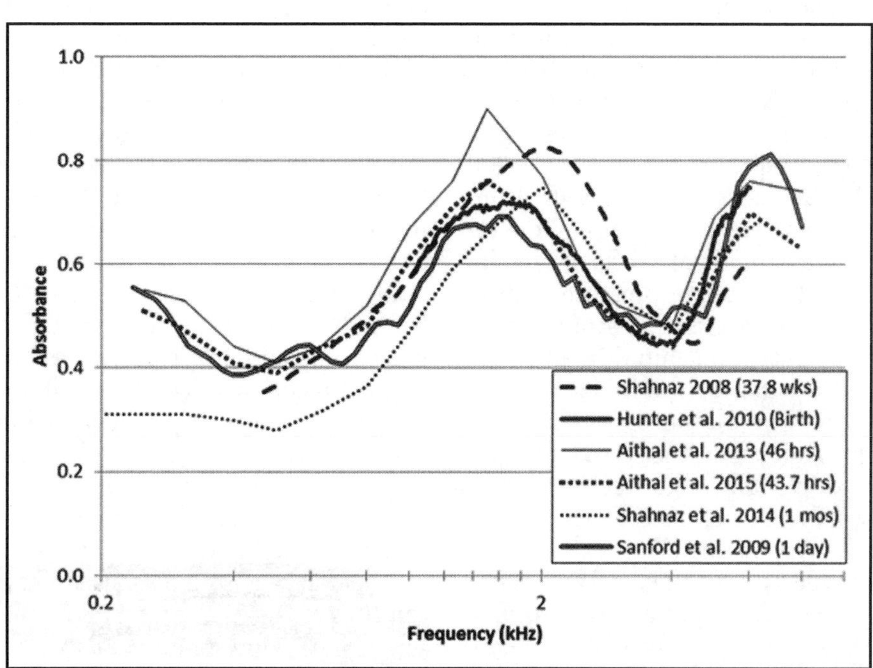

FIGURE 19–7. The normal range for ambient absorbance obtained from ears that passed various reference test standards plotted against frequency in comparison with published studies. From this comparison, there is agreement across studies for the normal absorbance shape, especially in the high frequencies. Two studies reported greater absorbance in the frequency region between 1.5 and 4 kHz. The comparison normal reference test standards had a minimal effect on the absorbance curve for ears that passed various reference standards.

and in five groups of infants and children (1, 3, 6, 12, and 24 months of age). This study reported that age-related variations in WBA over a frequency range of 0.125 to 10 kHz were most significant between 1 and 6 months of age. The greatest changes in WBA occurred at frequencies below 0.5 kHz, where WBA increased by up to 30% between 1 and 6 months of age. Keefe et al. (1993) concluded that greater energy transfer due to ear canal flaccidity was responsible for lower WBA in young infants and that these effects might account for the variability of 0.226-kHz admittance tympanograms and poor test sensitivity for detecting middle ear effusion in infants. Conversely, Hunter, Tubaugh, Jackson, and Propes (2008) did not find significant low-frequency effects from 1 month to 4 years of age using a different WBA measurement system and probe type but did find high-frequency development changes (specifically at 6 kHz), which may be due to mass effects at high frequencies. Another recent study (Sanford & Feeney, 2008) reported wideband tympanometry in infants, with 20 infants tested in each of three age groups (4, 12, and 24 weeks). Sanford and Feeney (2008) found developmental changes in WBA measurements varied as a function of frequency. For frequencies from 0.25 to 0.75 kHz there was as much as a 30% increase in mean WBA with changes in static ear canal pressure between 4 and 24 weeks of age. This change was hypothesized to be due to corresponding increases in stiffness of the external ear canal. The frequency region from 0.75 to 2 kHz was reported to be a developmentally stable frequency range with few age-related changes. Between 2 and 6 kHz, there were differential effects of pressure for the youngest infants, negative pressures caused increased WBA and Y, and positive pressures caused decreased WBA and Y, and the magnitude of this effect decreased with age. The authors hypothesized that the differential effects could be due to ossicular decoupling for negative pressure and increased coupling for positive pressure. Additionally, high-frequency WBA changes due to mass, possibly related to mesenchyme absorption, were also hypothesized.

Several recent studies of WBA normal and abnormal characteristics have been reported. Sanford et al. (2009) compared sensitivity and specificity of 1-kHz tympanometry to wideband absorbance tests using an experimental system combined with Interacoustics hardware, in 455 newborn ears (375 passed and 80 failed), and found excellent prediction of DPOAE screening results by WBA, while 1-kHz tympanometry was shown to produce poorer results. Of 80 infants who failed on Day 1, 67 infants were evaluated again after a second UNHS DPOAE test the next day (Day 2). Test performance was reported for wideband and 1-kHz tests in terms of their ability to classify ears that passed or failed, using DPOAE UNHS test outcomes as the "gold standard." This study found that the highest area under the ROC curve was 0.87 for an ambient WB test predictor, whereas the highest area under the ROC curve among several variables derived from 1-kHz tympanometry was 0.75. In general, ears that passed the DPOAE UNHS test had higher energy absorbance compared with those that failed, indicating that infants who passed DPOAE had a more acoustically efficient conductive pathway. The authors concluded that wideband immittance results in newborns ears that fail UNHS are related to transient conditions affecting the sound conduction pathway; that wideband data reveal changes in sound conduction during the first two days of life; and that wideband measurements are objective, quick, and feasible to consider implementing in conjunction with UNHS programs.

Hunter et al. (2010) reported normative data for wideband middle-ear power reflectance using the Mimosa Acoustics HEAR-ID system in a newborn hearing screening population in comparison to 1-kHz tympanometry for prediction of DPOAE-screening outcome in 324 infants. Normative frequency regions were reported, and receiver-operator characteristic (ROC) curve analyses showed that reflectance provides the best prediction of DPOAE status in the frequency ranges around 2 kHz. Power reflectance produced much better prediction of DPOAE status than 1-kHz tympanometry. Reflectance decreased with age over the first three days of age. Birth type and birth weight did not contribute to differences in reflectance. This study concluded that failures of OAE-based infant hearing screening can be evaluated by simultaneously measuring wideband power reflectance. The study authors recommended that newborns obtaining high reflectance scores be rescreened within a few hours to a few days, as most middle-ear problems are transient, whereas newborns with normal reflectance and who fail the OAE screen should be referred for immediate diagnostic testing with threshold ABR.

Because WBA provides reliable information of middle ear function in young infants, it could potentially be a useful tool in UNHS and EHDI programs. For example, Keefe et al. (Keefe, Gorga, et al., 2003; Keefe, Zhao et al., 2003) analyzed a subset of data obtained from two-stage hearing screening protocols (TEOAE/ABR and DPOAE/ABR) that had a 5% false-positive rate. They reported significant correlations between two ambient-pressure WBA variables and CEOAE responses, suggesting that WBA measures could be useful in interpreting TEOAE responses. Applying WBA factors identified in Keefe, Zhao, et al.

(2003) to a predictive test of middle ear dysfunction in infants, Keefe, Gorga, et al. (2003) showed that inclusion of the ambient-pressure WBA test decreased the false-positive rate from 5% to 1%. Thus, WBA is able to detect transient middle ear dysfunction in newborns. In a study of 192 neonates, Aithal et al. (2015) found that ears that passed a strong gold standard consisting of TEOAE, AABR, and 1-kHz tympanometry showed no significant differences in WBA among these test standards. However, for ears that failed each of the test standards, there were significant differences in WBA. The region between 1 and 4 kHz provided the best discriminability to evaluate the conductive status compared with other frequencies. Aithal et al. (2015) concluded that WBA is a desirable measure of conductive conditions in newborns due to its high performance in classifying ears with conductive loss as determined by the best performing surrogate gold standards.

Test-retest reliability has been reported in infants (Hunter, Tubaugh, et al., 2008; Vander Werff et al., 2007) and children (Hunter, Bagger-Sjoback, et al., 2008). In the study by Vander Werff et al. (2007), test-retest reliability and differences between WBA measures in an infant group receiving outpatient hearing screenings (mean age 7.6 weeks, SD = 5.3 weeks) was compared to an infant group receiving outpatient diagnostic hearing assessments (mean age 12.4 weeks, SD = 8.5 weeks). Lower (better) test-retest variability was reported for the diagnostic than the screening group, and the difference was attributed to decreased noise in the testing environment of the diagnostic group. Infants who failed the OAE screening had significantly higher WBA values (exceeding test-retest variability) for frequencies ranging from 0.63 to 2 kHz compared to infants who passed, suggesting the presence of a middle ear conductive component in infants who failed the OAE screening. In the Hunter, Tubaugh, et al. (2008) study, WBA showed high test-retest reliability in the same test session after removal and replacement of the probe tip. WBA was significantly higher in infants and children who failed a combination of otoscopy, OAE, and single-frequency tympanometry. A study of infants with unrepaired cleft lip and palate (Hunter, Bagger-Sjoback, et al., 2008) also demonstrated agreement between wideband reflectance and DPOAE that was higher than between otoscopy, 0.226 kHz, or 1-kHz tympanometry and DPOAE (Hunter, Bagger-Sjoback, et al., 2008). However, variability in WBA measurements can occur if the probe fit is loose. These studies overall show that infants and children with surgically confirmed otitis media with effusion have lower absorbance in the mid-frequency range (1 to 3 kHz) for the affected ear. Newborns who do not pass OAE screening at birth also have lower absorbance for frequencies from 1 to 3 kHz, suggesting that nonpass results are associated with middle ear issues at birth. Conclusions are limited by the fact that the true status of the middle ear and cochlea are not known for newborns and infants in studies that use OAE or tympanometry as the reference standard (Hunter, Prieve, Kei, & Sanford, 2013).

WB energy reflectance can be considered an alternative middle ear assessment technique to single-frequency admittance tympanometry (Sanford, Hunter, Feeney, & Nakajima, 2013). Wideband measurements of WBA tympanograms were first reported by Keefe and Levi (1996), and found in other studies to reveal more information than does a WBA test at ambient pressure (Margolis, Saly, & Keefe, 1999; Sanford & Feeney, 2008). Studies of tympanograms measured with a wideband stimulus predicted the presence of a wideband immittance measured at ambient pressure, indicating that pressurization may be important even if a wideband stimulus is employed (Keefe & Simmons, 2003). That study investigated the test performance of 0.226 kHz admittance tympanometry, ambient-pressure ER, and WB tympanometry as predictors of conductive hearing loss in children 10 years of age or older. Data were obtained from 42 normal-functioning ears and 18 ears with conductive hearing loss. The sensitivity of these measures to detect conductive hearing loss was only 28% for static acoustic admittance (0.226 kHz) but was higher (72%) for ambient-pressure WBA, and highest (94%) for WB tympanometry. In a study of specific middle ear conditions (Sanford & Brockett, 2014; Figure 19–8), average absorbance for ears in an OME group was reduced across the majority of frequencies; absorbance for ears with negative TPP was reduced in the 0.5 to 1.5 kHz, although to a lesser degree than in OME. Absorbance patterns for ears with PE tubes showed increases in absorbance below 1 kHz, with sharp peaks because of the effects of the tube and open middle ear cavity. WAI from ears with tympanoplasty and cerumen impaction was suggestive of middle ear dysfunction in the presence of normal single-frequency tympanometry. Thus, available research demonstrates that WB tympanometry is a useful diagnostic tool for detection of conductive hearing loss and is more sensitive than traditional tympanometry.

Middle Ear Muscle Reflexes (MEMRs)

Reflexive contraction of the stapedius muscle occurs in response to loud sounds and is mediated by the VII cranial nerve. The acoustically evoked stapedial reflex

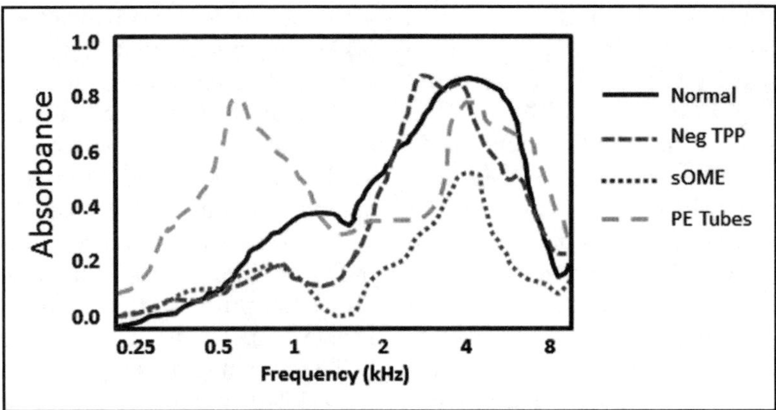

FIGURE 19–8. Average ambient absorbance obtained from ears with four conditions, modified from Sanford and Brockett (2014).

is a bilateral phenomenon, regardless of which ear is stimulated. An anatomical and functional review by Borg, Counter, and Rösler (1984) poses a protective role to attenuate sounds of high intensity, including one's own voice. These protective functions are also thought to assist in improving speech perception by attenuating low-frequency ambient noise. This theory was tested by Aiken, Andrus, Bance, and Phillips (2013) in patients with transected stapedial tendons by examining masking functions for speech intelligibility. These results demonstrated that indeed, the acoustic stapedial reflex offers a benefit by reducing upward spread of masking to improve speech intelligibility under adverse noise conditions. Historically, several methods have been used for measurement of the acoustic stapedial reflex (ASR), more accurately known as the middle ear muscle reflex (MEMR), but the method used in all commercially available instruments is monitoring of admittance changes evoked by a brief, loud pure-tone or broadband noise presented to the ear in which the admittance measurement is made (ipsilateral MEMR) or to the opposite ear (contralateral MEMR). The MEMR is present at birth, but because the impedance of the ear is very different in newborns as discussed earlier in this chapter, the MEMR is not reliably detected using low probe frequencies. Higher-frequency probe tones, at 0.66 kHz or higher, do evoke the MEMR reliably in newborns (McMillan, Bennett, Marchant, & Shurin, 1985; Weatherby & Bennett, 1980).

As in adults, the MEMR is useful in pediatric assessment to define middle ear problems, cochlear hearing loss, and problems beyond the outer hair cells, such as auditory neuropathy spectrum disorders (ANSDs), retrocochlear disorders, central auditory processing disorder, and facial nerve disorders. For a detailed review of MEMR measurement, and anatomy and physiology of the MEMR pathway, refer to Feeney and Schairer (2015). Studies of the acoustic reflex in the pediatric populations have focused on two fundamental issues: normative studies in various age groups and studies in middle ear disease. Studies of the MEMR in ANSD and auditory processing disorders consist primarily of cases or case series.

MEMR Normative Studies

A summary of normative studies of MEMR thresholds for infants and children for various probe and stimulus frequencies is shown in Table 19–2 for those that included probe tone frequency information. In newborns, three studies examined the effect of probe-tone frequency. Weatherby and Bennett (1980) studied broadband reflex thresholds with a series of probe-tone frequencies in 49 newborns from 10 to 169 hr old, and found that probe tones between 0.8 and 1.8 kHz provided the lowest MEMR thresholds. In a study of 95 well babies, McMillan and colleagues (McMillan, Bennett, et al., 1985; McMillan, Marchant, et al., 1985) found that ipsilateral and contralateral acoustic reflexes were detected three times more frequently with a 0.66-kHz probe tone than with a 0.22-kHz probe tone. Acoustic reflex thresholds were similar to adult values for activator stimuli at 0.5, 1, and 4 kHz and were 8 dB higher than adult values for a 2-kHz activator stimulus (0.66-kHz probe tone). Ipsilateral thresholds were lower than contralateral thresholds and were similar to adult thresholds for a 0.66-kHz probe tone.

Table 19–2. Summary of Acoustic Reflex Studies in Infants and Children

Study	*Age Range*	*Probe Frequency (kHz)*	*Test Stimuli*	*Presentation*		*Normative Values (dB HL)*
				Mode	*Intensity Level*	
Kankkunen & Lidén, 1984	N/A	0.66	0.5, 1, 2, 4 kHz and BBN	Ipsilateral	Up to limits of equipment: 0.5 kHz = 90 dB HL, 1 kHz = 110 dB HL, 2 kHz = 100 dB HL, and 4 kHz = 90 dB HL	Upper normal ART limits: 0.5 kHz = 95 1 kHz = 101 2 kHz = 102 4 kHz = 96
Gerber, Gong, & Mendel, 1984	12–36 weeks	N/A	0.5, 1, 2, 4 kHz and BBN	Contralateral	70 to 110 dB HL	12 weeks (μ ± SD) 0.5 kHz = 81 ± 7.8 1 kHz = 82 ± 9.3 2 kHz = 83 ± 8.5 4 kHz = 84 ± 8.8
Abahazi & Greenberg, 1977	1–12 months	N/A	0.5, 1, 2 kHz and low-pass, high-pass, and white noise	N/A	70 dB SPL ascending in 5-dB steps until AR elicited	Mean ART Values (dB SPL) 0.5 kHz = 105.3 1 kHz = 97.9 2 kHz = 98.9 low pass = 90.7 high pass = 88.3 white noise = 84.2
Attoni, Quintas, & Mota, 2010	5–7 years	0.22	0.5, 1, 2, 4 kHz	Ipsilateral and contralateral	N/A	ART Values (μ) Ipsilateral: R / L 0.5: 84.2 / 83.1 1: 82.8 / 82.2 2: 82.1 / 83.4 4: 84.2 / 82.6 Contralateral: R / L 0.5: 85.7 / 84.3 1: 83.2 / 82.4 2: 81.2 / 85.6 4: 82.3 / 81.4
Kei, 2012	1–16 days	1	0.5, 1, 4 kHz, BBN	Ipsilateral	70–100 dB HL in 5-dB steps	ART Values (μ) 500 = 81.4 2000 = 71.3 4000 = 65.3 BBN = 57.1

continues

Table 19–2. *continued*

Study	*Age Range*	*Probe Frequency (kHz)*	*Test Stimuli*	*Presentation* *Mode*	*Intensity Level*	*Normative Values (dB HL)*
Mazlan, et al., 2007	Birth	1	2 kHz, BBN	Ipsilateral	Starting from 60 dB SPL and ascending in 5-dB steps until AR response elicited with a maximum presentation at 90 dB SPL	ART Values (μ ± SD) Birth 2 kHz = 73.1 ± 10.3) BBN = 59.4 ± 10.3) 6–7 weeks 2 kHz = 79.6 ± 6.9) BBN = 65.8 ± 10.2)

Note. *AR* = acoustic reflex; *ART* = acoustic reflex threshold; *BBN* = broadband noise; *dB HL* = decibel hearing level; *dB SPL* = decibel sound pressure level; *kHz* = kilohertz; *SD* = standard deviation; μ = mean.

Sprague and colleagues (1985) studied 53 newborns who were 24 to 105 hr old, using probe tones of 0.22 and 0.66 kHz and evoked by 1-kHz pure tones and broadband noise presented both ipsilaterally and contralaterally. They reported that 80% of the newborns had observable MEMR for 0.66-kHz probe tones, whereas only 50% had observable MEMR with a 0.22-kHz probe tone. MEMR thresholds for broadband noise were significantly lower than for the 1-kHz pure tone. Ipsilateral presentation produced lower thresholds than contralateral presentation. They also reported that flat 0.66-kHz tympanograms were associated with absent MEMR. Thus, these studies taken together can be summarized as follows: The MEMR is measurable in a high proportion of newborns when a probe tone of 0.66-kHz or higher is used, the measured thresholds are similar to adults, and broadband stimuli provide lower MEMR thresholds than pure-tone stimuli. Limited information indicates a correlation between flat tympanometry at 1 kHz and absent MEMR at the same frequency.

Important data on test-retest reliability of the MEMR in neonates were reported by Mazlan, Kei, and Hickson (2009). In this study, 194 healthy neonates aged between 24 and 192 hours passed an automated ABR screening test and were assessed with TEOAE, 1-kHz tympanometry and MEMR using a 1-kHz probe tone with 2-kHz and broadband ipsilateral activators. The Madsen Otoflex diagnostic immittance system was used. Ipsilateral ASRs were present in 91% of neonates, whereas 9% showed flat tympanograms and absent MEMR as well as a failed result for the TEOAE test. The mean MEMR threshold was 76 dB HL for the 2-kHz activator and was 65 dB HL for the broadband noise (BBN) activator. MEMR thresholds did not differ significantly for the first test and second tests for either MEMR activator, and showed high intracorrelation coefficients (0.83). This study shows that 1-kHz probe tone ASRs are consistently elicited from healthy neonates who pass automated ABR and TEOAE screening and 1-kHz tympanometry, thus MEMR test holds promise as a useful diagnostic/screening instrument in ascertaining the hearing status in neonates.

Caution should be exercised when introducing high-level stimuli to the ear canal in infants and children for MEMR testing, due to the potential risk of permanent threshold shift and because SPL developed in a smaller ear canal can be at least 10 dB higher than in an adult ear (Hunter, Ries, Schlauch, Levine, & Ward, 1999). McMillan, Bennett, et al. (1985) measured ear canal SPL with a probe microphone compared to the level indicated on the immittance instrument. At maximum HL presentation permitted (generally 110 dB HL), the measured SPL in infant ears reached 126 dB and 130 dB SPL at 1 and 2 kHz, respectively. These levels are clearly a hazard, and despite this, levels on acoustic immittance instruments are not limited, so the audiologist must be aware of these potential hazards, especially when testing infants and children due to the smaller ear canal volumes and corresponding higher SPL. In general, acoustic reflex thresholds for infants and children are lower by 5 to 10 dB, and an upper limit of 90 dB HL is considered the normal range for pure-tone stimuli (Kankkunen & Lidén, 1984; McMillan, Marchant, et al., 1985). Gerber, Gong, and Mendel (1984) measured acoustic reflex thresholds for contralateral stimulation in 45 infants, ages 12 to 36 weeks, and found average thresholds between 81 and 84 dB HL for pure-tone stimuli at 0.5, 1, 2, and 4 kHz. Maximum presentation levels should be limited to no greater than 105 dB SPL (Hunter et al., 1999), but unfortunately this limits interpretation of the MEMR, as the upper limit of the MEMR in infants can exceed 105 dB SPL (see Table 19–2, note that many of these studies reported HL values). Broadband noise is recommended as an alternative stimulus to pure tones, as thresholds are lower, and the risk of iatrogenic hearing loss is lower since the energy is distributed across the basilar membrane, rather than concentrated as for pure tones.

MEMR in Otitis Media and Middle Ear Effusion

Other studies have examined the usefulness of the acoustic reflex test in children as an indicator of middle ear effusion. Studies suggest the presence of the acoustic reflex at normal levels can indicate an effusion-free middle ear. Freyss, Narcy, Manac'h, and Toupet (1980) used a 1-kHz stimulus to elicit the acoustic reflex in 99 ears for infants and children 6 months to 8 years of age immediately prior to myringotomy. They found that ears with an acoustic reflex threshold of 115 dB or lower were effusion free at the time of surgery. Conversely, those ears with an absent reflex above 115 dB were ears positive for MEE. This study did not specify if presentation levels were measured in decibels sound pressure level (dB SPL) or decibels hearing level (dB HL). Nozza and colleagues (1992) used myringotomy as a standard determination for middle ear effusion in a study of 264 ears for children 1 to 16 years of age. This study reported that up to 85% of ears without middle ear effusion had the acoustic reflex present at 1 kHz with a 100 dB HL presentation tone. Only 12% of ears with effusion had a measurable reflex. Marchant et al. (1986) found that an acoustic reflex at 100 dB HL or less for 1 kHz in infants was strongly associated with the absence of middle ear effusion and with a normal tympanometric peak.

The acoustic reflex is most reliable as a predictor of middle ear status when coupled with tympanometric measurements including static admittance (Casselbrant et al., 1985; Marchant et al., 1986) and gradient (Nozza et al., 1992). The acoustic reflex alone might not be the best predictor of middle ear effusion. Nozza et al. (1992) found 76% of ears without effusion had a measurable acoustic reflex. They concluded the absence of the acoustic reflex alone was not a sufficient predictor of middle ear effusion in children because 28% of ears had no reflex present and were also effusion free. However, coupled with tympanometric gradient of less than 0.1 mmhos, the absence of the acoustic reflex was a powerful indicator.

The suggested protocol for acoustic reflex measurement in infants less than 6 months of age includes ipsilateral presentation of a broadband noise or pure tones at 1 kHz and 2 kHz at levels that do not exceed 105 dB SPL and the use of a 0.66- or 1-kHz probe tone. At ages greater than 6 months, a standard 0.226-kHz probe tone is adequate for detection of the MEMR. These parameters should serve to elicit the acoustic reflex at the lowest possible sound pressure levels and provide reliable information regarding middle ear status complementary to tympanometric data for the detection of middle ear effusion.

MEMR in Auditory Neuropathy Spectrum Disorder (ANSD)

ANSD (previously known as auditory neuropathy/auditory dys-synchrony disorder or AN/AD) has been identified and described over the past 20 years but is still elusive in terms of etiology. It appears that multiple etiologies can be present, and there is a wide range of severity and clinical presentations; thus, a consensus conference at the International Newborn Hearing Screening Conference in 2008 recommended the addition of the qualifier "spectrum" to the disorder. Newborns can present with referral from ABR screening procedures, as ABR waveforms are markedly abnormal or absent by definition. Detailed descriptions of ANSD are beyond the scope of this chapter and are covered elsewhere in this text (see Chapters 11 and 12). However, it is important to recognize the value of MEMR measurements in infants and children suspected of having ANSD. MEMR is an effective, low-cost test that can be employed in the newborn nursery or the outpatient clinic to assess the possibility of ANSD, in combination with behavioral audiometry and otoacoustic emissions. Berlin et al. (2005) examined a subpopulation of 136 patients (from their database of 257 subjects with ANSD) in whom middle ear muscle reflexes had been measured. They found that none of the patients had normal acoustic reflexes for both 1 and 2 kHz, whether ipsilaterally or contralaterally elicited. Berlin and colleagues urged use of the ipsilateral MEMR at least at 1 and 2 kHz in any perinatal hearing screening that depends solely on otoacoustic emissions. If the emissions are present and the reflexes are absent or elevated, an ABR is recommended to determine whether ANSD is present.

Limitations of Pure-Tone Probe Acoustic Reflex Test

Although the acoustic reflex has been tested using the admittance method and a pure-tone probe of 0.226 kHz for many decades, there are some important limitations to consider. In addition to the limitations of low-frequency probe tones in young infants, current reflex tests employ subjective interpretation of the admittance change based on single responses to a pure-tone activator. This subjective methodology does not take advantage of modern methods of artifact rejection, signal averaging, and objective analysis of time-locked features that are part of other physiologic measures, such as OAE and ABR testing. Experienced audiologists can usually discern whether a legitimate reflex response has occurred, but accuracy of the test is improved with use of these techniques. Finally, as discussed previously, high-level reflex and decay test activators can result in temporary and permanent threshold shift, so a test that results in lower reflex thresholds is desirable. Fortunately, wideband acoustic reflex measures using absorbance methodology address all of these limitations (Feeney & Keefe, 1999; Feeney & Sanford, 2005; Schairer, Feeney, &Sanford, 2013).

Wideband Acoustic Reflex Measures

As in tympanometry, ASRs can be measured using wideband stimuli and reflectance measurements. This alternative method, known as wideband ASRT, uses shifts in absorbed or reflected power measured with broadband clicks rather than the standard 0.226-kHz pure tone (Feeney & Keefe, 1999, 2001). This procedure uses either broadband clicks (Feeney & Keefe, 2001) or pure-tone stimuli to evoke the MEMR (Feeney, Keefe, & Marryott, 2003), and threshold is about 12 dB lower in adults than the traditional 0.226-kHz probe-tone method (Schairer, Ellison, Fitzpatrick, & Keefe, 2007). Keefe, Fitzpatrick, Liu, Sanford, and Gorga (2010) studied a wideband aural acoustical test battery of middle ear status, including acoustic-reflex thresholds in comparison to newborn hearing screening results. Ipsilateral acoustic-reflex thresholds were assessed with a stimulus including four broadband-noise or tonal-activator pulses alternating with five clicks presented before, between, and after the pulses. This wideband absorbance method rejects transient high noise levels, averages the response across several clicks, examines the time-locked response, and measures correlation as well as increases in the reflex response with increases in stimulus intensity. Acoustic reflex thresholds were measured using maximum likelihood at both low frequencies (0.8 to 2.88 kHz) and high frequencies (2.8 to 8 kHz). The median low-frequency acoustic reflex threshold was elevated by 24 dB in NHS failures compared to passes. ATF and acoustic reflex threshold tests performed better than either test alone in predicting NHS outcomes, and WB tests performed better than 1-kHz tympanometry. Median ARTs reported by Keefe et al. (2010) in 1-day old infants who passed or failed the newborn screening are shown in Figure 19–9. At all frequencies, infants who failed had poorer (higher) thresholds, and the difference was greater for broadband compared to tonal activators. These wideband acoustic reflex tests are not yet commercially available but offer several advantages for clinical applications, so they will likely be on the horizon for clinical use.

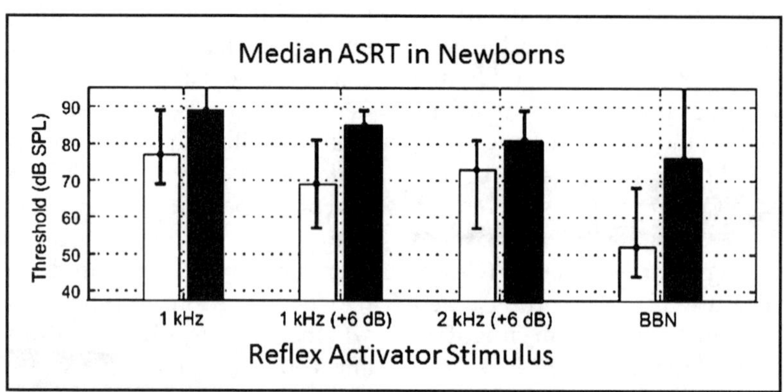

FIGURE 19–9. Median wideband ASRTs and interquartile ranges (in dB SPL) measured in newborns: pass (*white bars*) compared to failed ears (*black bars*) are plotted for low-frequency spectra. (Modified from Keefe et al., 2010.)

Summary

Acoustic immittance tests have long been a critical component of physiologic assessment for newborns, infants, and children. With significant advancements in the past few years that have brought multifrequency and now broadband measures into clinical and research use, it is now possible to diagnose newborns with middle ear problems more effectively, and to compare middle ear measures to cochlear measures in the same frequency range more directly.

Acknowledgments. Valued contributions of Robert Margolis to the first edition of this chapter are gratefully acknowledged.

References

Abahazi, D. A., & Greenberg, H. J. (1977). Clinical acoustic reflex threshold measurements in infants. *Journal of Speech and Hearing Disorders*, *42*(4), 514–519.

Abdala, C., Keefe, D. H., & Oba, S. I. (2007). Distortion product otoacoustic emission suppression tuning and acoustic admittance in human infants: Birth through 6 months. *Journal of the Acoustical Society of America, 121*(6), 3617–3627. doi:10.1121/1.2734481

Aiken, S. J., Andrus, J. N., Bance, M., & Phillips, D. P. (2013). Acoustic stapedius reflex function in man revisited. *Ear and Hearing, 34*(4), e38–51. doi:10.1097/AUD.0b013e31827ad9d3

Aithal, S., Kei, J., & Driscoll, C. (2014). Wideband absorbance in young infants (0–6 months): A cross-sectional study. *Journal of the American Academy of Audiology, 25*(5), 471–481. doi:10.3766/jaaa.25.5.6

Aithal, S., Kei, J., Driscoll, C., & Khan, A. (2013). Normative wideband reflectance measures in healthy neonates. *International Journal of Pediatric Otorhinolaryngology, 77*(1), 29–35. doi:10.1016/j.ijporl.2012.09.024

Aithal, S., Kei, J., Driscoll, C., Khan, A., & Swanston, A. (2015). Wideband absorbance outcomes in newborns: A comparison with high-frequency tympanometry, automated brainstem response, and transient evoked and distortion product otoacoustic emissions. *Ear and Hearing, 36*(5), e237–e250. doi:10.1097/aud.0000000000000175

Alaerts, J., Lutz, H., & Woulters, J. (2007). Evaluation of middle ear function in young children: Clinical guidelines for the use of 226- and 1,000-Hz tympanometry. *Otology and Neurotology, 28*(6), 727–732.

Allen, J. B. (1986). Measurement of eardrum acoustic impedance. In J. B. Allen, J. L. Hall, A. E. Hubbard, S. T. Neely, & A. Tubis (Eds.), *Peripheral auditory mechanisms* (pp. 44–51). New York, NY: Springer-Verlag.

American Academy of Audiology (AAA; 1997). Identification of hearing loss and middle-ear dysfunction in preschool and school-age children. *Audiology Today, 9*, 3.

American Academy of Audiology (AAA; 2011). *Childhood hearing screening.* Reston, VA: Author.

American Academy of Family Physicians (AAP), American Academy of Otolaryngology-Head and Neck Surgery (AAO-NHS), and American Academy of Pediatrics (AAP) Subcommittee on Otitis Media With Effusion. (2004). Otitis media with effusion. *Pediatrics, 113*(5), 1412–1429.

American National Standards Institute (ANSI; 1987). *American National Standard specifications for instruments to measure aural acoustic impedance and admittance (aural acoustic immittance).* ANSI S3.39-1987. New York, NY: Author.

American Speech-Language-Hearing Association (ASHA; 1990). Guidelines for screening for hearing impairment and middle-ear disorders. Working Group on Acoustic Immittance Measurements and the Committee on Audiologic Evaluation. American Speech-Language-Hearing Association. *ASHA Suppl.*(2), 17–24.

American Speech-Language-Hearing Association (ASHA; 1997). Panel on audiologic assessment. *Guidelines for audiologic screening*. Rockville, MD: Author.

American Speech-Language-Hearing Association (ASHA; 2004). *Guidelines for the audiologic assessment of children from birth to 5 years of age.* Retrieved from http://www.asha.org/policy

Attoni, T. M., Quintas, V. G., & Mota, H. B. (2010). Auditory processing, acoustic reflex and phonological expression. *Brazilian Journal of Otorhinolaryngology, 76*(6), 753–761.

Baldwin, M. (2006). Choice of probe tone and classification of trace patterns in tympanometry undertaken in early infancy. *International Journal of Audiology, 45*(7), 417–427. doi:N7780J87482990GN [pii] 10.1080/14992020600690951

Bennett, M. (1975). Acoustic impedance bridge measurements with the neonate. *Brazilian Journal of Audiology, 9*, 117–124.

Berlin, C. I., Hood, L. J., Morlet, T., Wilensky, D., St. John, P., Montgomery, E., & Thibodaux, M. (2005). Absent or elevated middle ear muscle reflexes in the presence of normal otoacoustic emissions: A universal finding in 136 cases of auditory neuropathy/dys-synchrony. *Journal of the American Academy of Audiology, 16*(8), 546–553.

Borg, E., Counter, S., & Rösler, G. (1984). Theories of middle-ear muscle function. In S. Silman (Ed.), *The acoustic reflex: Basic principles and clinical applications* (pp. 63–99). New York, NY: Academic Press.

Brooks, D. N. (1968). An objective method of determining fluid in the middle ear. *International Journal of Audiology, 7*, 280–286.

Calandruccio, L., Fitzgerald, T. S., & Prieve, B. A. (2006). Normative multifrequency tympanometry in infants and toddlers. *Journal of the American Academy of Audiology, 17*(7), 470–480.

Casselbrant, M. L., Brostoff, L. M., Cantekin, E. I., Flaherty, M. R., Doyle, W. J., & Bluestone C. D. (1985). Otitis media with effusion in preschool children. *Laryngoscope, 95*, 428–436.

Cinamon, U. (2009). The growth rate and size of the mastoid air cell system and mastoid bone: A review and reference.

European Archives of Otorhinolaryngology, 266(6), 781–786. doi:10.1007/s00405-009-0941-8

Colletti, V. (1977). Multifrequency tympanometry. *Audiology, 16*(4), 278–287.

de Jonge, R. (1986). Normal tympanometric gradient: A comparison of three methods. *Audiology, 25*(4–5), 299–308.

Eavey, R. D. (1993). Abnormalities of the neonatal ear: Otoscopic observations, histologic observations, and a model for contamination of the middle ear by cellular contents of amniotic fluid. *Laryngoscope, 103*(1 Pt. 2 Suppl. 58), 1–31.

Eby, T. L., & Nadol, J. B., Jr. (1986). Postnatal growth of the human temporal bone. Implications for cochlear implants in children. *Annals of Otology, Rhinology, and Laryngology, 95*(4 Pt. 1), 356–364.

Elner, A., Ingelstedt, S., & Ivarsson, A. (1971). The elastic properties of the tympanic membrane system. *Acta Otolaryngologica, 72*(6), 397–403.

Feeney, M. P., Hunter, L. L., Kei, J., Lilly, D. J., Margolis, R. H., Nakajima, H. H., . . . Voss, S. E. (2013). Consensus statement: Eriksholm workshop on wideband absorbance measures of the middle ear. *Ear and Hearing, 34*(Suppl. 1), 78S–79S. doi:10.1097/AUD.0b013e31829c726b

Feeney, M. P., & Keefe, D. H. (1999). Acoustic reflex detection using wideband acoustic reflectance, admittance, and power measurements. *Journal of Speech, Language, and Hearing Research, 42*, 1029–1041.

Feeney, M. P., & Keefe, D. H. (2001). Estimating the acoustic reflex threshold from wideband measures of reflectance, admittance, and power. *Ear and Hearing, 22*(4), 316–332.

Feeney, M. P., Keefe, D. H., & Marryott, L. P. (2003). Contralateral acoustic reflex thresholds for tonal activators using wideband energy reflectance and admittance. *Journal of Speech and Language Hearing Research, 46*(1), 128–136.

Feeney, M. P., & Sanford, C. A. (2005). Detection of the acoustic stapedius reflex in infants using wideband energy reflectance and admittance. *Journal of the American Academy of Audiology, 16*(5), 278–290.

Feeney, M. P., & Schairer, K. S. (2015). Acoustic stapedius reflex measurements. In J. Katz, M. Chasin, K. English, L. Hood, & K. Tillery (Eds.), *Handbook of clinical audiology* (pp. 165–186). Philadelphia, PA: Wolters Kluwer.

Feldman, A. S. (1976). Tympanometry—Procedures, interpretations and variables. In A. S. Feldman & L. A. Wilber (Eds.), *Acoustic impedance and admittance—The measurement of middle ear function* (pp. 103–155). Baltimore, MD: Williams and Wilkins.

Fiellau-Nikolajsen, M. (1983). Tympanometry and secretory otitis media. Observations on diagnosis, epidemiology, treatment, and prevention in prospective cohort studies of three-year-old children. *Acta Otolaryngologica Suppl., 394*, 1–73.

Freyss, G. E., Narcy, P. P., Manac'h, Y., & Toupet, M. G. (1980). Acoustic reflex as a predictor of middle ear effusion. *Annals of Otology, Rhinology, and Laryngology Suppl., 89*(3 Pt 2), 196–199.

Gerber, S. E., Gong, E. L., & Mendel, M. I. (1984). Developmental norms for the acoustic reflex. *Audiology, 23*(1), 1–8.

Himelfarb, M. Z., Popelka, G. R., & Shanon, E. (1979). Tympanometry in normal neonates. *Journal of Speech and Hearing Research, 22*(1), 179–191.

Hof, J. R., Anteunis, L. J., Chenault, M. N., & van Dijk, P. (2005). Otoacoustic emissions at compensated middle ear pressure in children. *International Journal of Audiology, 44*(6), 317–320.

Hoffmann, A., Deuster, D., Rosslau, K., Knief, A., Am Zehnhoff-Dinnesen, A., & Schmidt, C. M. (2013). Feasibility of 1000 Hz tympanometry in infants: Tympanometric trace classification and choice of probe tone in relation to age. *International Journal of Pediatric Otorhinolaryngology, 77*(7), 1198–1203. doi:10.1016/j.ijporl.2013.05.001

Holte, L., Cavanaugh, R. M., Jr., & Margolis, R. H. (1990). Ear canal wall mobility and tympanometric shape in young infants. *Journal of Pediatrics, 117*(1 Pt. 1), 77–80.

Holte, L., Margolis, R. H., & Cavanaugh, R. M., Jr. (1991). Developmental changes in multifrequency tympanograms. *Audiology, 30*(1), 1–24.

Hsu, G. S., Margolis, R. H., & Schachern, P. A. (2000). Development of the middle ear in neonatal chinchillas. I. Birth to 14 days. *Acta Otolaryngologica, 120*(8), 922–932.

Hunter, L. L., Bagger-Sjoback, D., & Lundberg, M. (2008). Wideband reflectance associated with otitis media in infants and children with cleft palate. *International Journal of Audiology, 47* (Suppl. 1), S57–S61. doi:902366002 [pii] 10.1080/14992020802294057

Hunter, L. L., Feeney, M. P., Lapsley Miller, J. A., Jeng, P. S., & Bohning, S. (2010). Wideband reflectance in newborns: Normative regions and relationship to hearing-screening results. *Ear and Hearing, 31*(5), 599–610. doi:10.1097/AUD.0b013e3181e40ca7

Hunter, L. L., & Margolis, R. H. (1992). Multifrequency tympanometry, current clinical application. *American Journal of Audiology, 1*, 33–43.

Hunter, L. L., Margolis, R. H., Daly, K. A., & Giebink, G. S. (1992). Relationship of tympanometric estimates of middle ear volume to middle ear status at surgery. In *Abstracts of the midwinter research meeting of the Association for Research in Otolaryngology*. St. Petersburg Beach, FL.

Hunter, L. L., Prieve, B. A., Kei, J., & Sanford, C. A. (2013). Pediatric applications of wideband acoustic immittance measures. *Ear and Hearing, 34*(Suppl. 1), 36S–42S. doi:10.1097/AUD.0b013e31829d5158

Hunter, L. L., Ries, D. T., Schlauch, R. S., Levine, S. C., & Ward, W. D. (1999). Safety and clinical performance of acoustic reflex tests. *Ear and Hearing, 20*(6), 506–514.

Hunter, L. L., & Shahnaz, N. (2014). *Handbook of acoustic immittance*. San Diego, CA: Plural.

Hunter, L. L., Tubaugh, L., Jackson, A., & Propes, S. (2008). Wideband middle ear power measurement in infants and children. *Journal of the American Academy of Audiology, 19*(4), 309–324.

Ikui, A., Sando, I., Sudo, M., & Fujita, S. (1997). Postnatal change in angle between the tympanic annulus and surrounding structures. Computer-aided three-dimensional reconstruction study. *Annals of Otology, Rhinology, and Laryngology, 106*(1), 33–36.

Jerger, J. (1970). Clinical experience with impedance audiometry. *Archives of Otolaryngology, 92*(4), 311–324.

Joint Committee on Infant Hearing (JCIH; 2007). Year 2007 position statement: Principles and guidelines for early hearing detection and intervention programs. *Pediatrics, 120*, 898–921.

Kankkunen, A., & Liden, G. (1984). Ipsilateral acoustic reflex thresholds in neonates and in normal-hearing and hearing-impaired pre-school children. *Scandanivian Audiology, 13*(2), 139–144.

Keefe, D. H., & Abdala, C. (2007). Theory of forward and reverse middle-ear transmission applied to otoacoustic emissions in infant and adult ears. *Journal of the Acoustical Society of America, 121*(2), 978–993.

Keefe, D. H., Bulen, J. C., Arehart, K. H., & Burns, E. M. (1993). Ear-canal impedance and reflection coefficient in human infants and adults. *Journal of the Acoustical Society of America, 94*(5), 2617–2638.

Keefe, D. H., & Feeney, M. P. (2009). Principles of acoustic immittance and acoustic transfer functions. In J. Katz, R. F. Burkhard, L. Medwetsky, & L. J. Hood (Eds.), *Handbook of clinical audiology* (pp. 125–156). New York, NY: Lippincott Williams & Wilkins.

Keefe, D. H., Fitzpatrick, D., Liu, Y. W., Sanford, C. A., & Gorga, M. P. (2010). Wideband acoustic-reflex test in a test battery to predict middle-ear dysfunction. *Hearing Research, 263*(1–2), 52–65. doi:10.1016/j.heares.2009.09.008

Keefe, D. H., Folsom, R. C., Gorga, M. P., Vohr, B. R., Bulen, J. C., & Norton, S. J. (2000). Identification of neonatal hearing impairment: Ear-canal measurements of acoustic admittance and reflectance in neonates. *Ear and Hearing, 21*(5), 443–461.

Keefe, D. H., Gorga, M. P., Neely, S. T., Zhao, F., & Vohr, B. R. (2003). Ear-canal acoustic admittance and reflectance measurements in human neonates. II. Predictions of middle-ear in dysfunction and sensorineural hearing loss. *Journal of the Acoustical Society of America, 113*(1), 407–422.

Keefe, D. H., & Levi, E. (1996). Maturation of the middle and external ears: Acoustic power-based responses and reflectance tympanometry. *Ear and Hearing, 17*(5), 361–373.

Keefe, D. H., Ling, R., & Bulen, J. C. (1992). Method to measure acoustic impedance and reflection coefficient. *Journal of the Acoustical Society of America, 91*(1), 470–485.

Keefe, D. H., & Simmons, J. L. (2003). Energy transmittance predicts conductive hearing loss in older children and adults. *Journal of the Acoustical Society of America, 114*(6 Pt. 1), 3217–3238.

Keefe, D. H., Zhao, F., Neely, S. T., Gorga, M. P., & Vohr, B. R. (2003). Ear-canal acoustic admittance and reflectance effects in human neonates. I. Predictions of otoacoustic emission and auditory brainstem responses. *Journal of the Acoustical Society of America, 113*(1), 389–406.

Kei, J. (2012). Acoustic stapedial reflexes in healthy neonates: Normative data and test-retest reliability. *Journal of the American Academy of Audiology, 23*(1), 46–56. doi:10.3766/jaaa.23.1.5

Kei, J., Allison-Levick, J., Dockray, J., Harrys, R., Kirkegard, C., Wong, J., . . . Tudehope, D. (2003). High-frequency (1000 Hz) tympanometry in normal neonates. *Journal of the American Academy of Audiology, 14*(1), 20–28.

Keith, R. W. (1973). Impedance audiometry with neonates. *Archives of Otolaryngology, 97*(6), 465–467.

Keith, R. W. (1975). Middle ear function in neonates. *Archives of Otolaryngology, 101*(6), 376–379.

Koebsell, K. A., & Margolis, R. H. (1986). Tympanometric gradient measured from normal preschool children. *Audiology, 25*(3), 149–157.

Liden, G. (1969). The scope and application of current audiometric tests. *Journal of Laryngology and Otology, 83*(6), 507–520.

Liden, G., Harford, E., & Hallen, O. (1974). Tympanometry for the diagnosis of ossicular disruption. *Archives of Otolaryngology, 99*(1), 23–29.

Lindeman, P., & Holmquist, J. (1982). Volume measurement of middle ear and mastoid air cell system with impedance audiometry on patients with eardrum perforations. *American Journal of Otology, 4*(1), 46–51.

Marchant, C. D., McMillan, P. M., Shurin, P. A., Johnson, C. E., Turczyk, V. A., Feinstein, J. C., & Panek, D. M. (1986). Objective diagnosis of otitis media in early infancy by tympanometry and ipsilateral acoustic reflex thresholds. *Journal of Pediatrics, 109*(4), 590–595.

Margolis, R. H., Bass-Ringdahl, S., Hanks, W. D., Holte, L., & Zapala, D. A. (2003). Tympanometry in newborn infants —1 kHz norms. *Journal of the American Academy of Audiology, 14*(7), 383–392.

Margolis, R. H., & Heller, J. W. (1987). Screening tympanometry: Criteria for medical referral. *Audiology, 26*(4), 197–208.

Margolis, R. H., Saly, G. L., & Keefe, D. H. (1999). Wideband reflectance tympanometry in normal adults. *Journal of the Acoustical Society of America, 106*(1), 265–280.

Mazlan, R., Kei, J., & Hickson, L. (2009). Test-retest reliability of the acoustic stapedial reflex test in healthy neonates. *Ear and Hearing, 30*(3), 295–301. doi:10.1097/AUD.0b013e31819c3ea0

Mazlan, R., Kei, J., Hickson, L., Gavranich, J., & Linning, R. (2010). Test-retest reproducibility of the 1000 Hz tympanometry test in newborn and six-week-old healthy infants. *International Journal of Audiology, 49*(11), 815–822. doi:10.3109/14992027.2010.493182

Mazlan, R., Kei, J., Hickson, L., Stapleton, C., Grant, S., Lim, S., . . . Gavranich, J. (2007). High frequency immittance findings: Newborn versus six-week-old infants. *International Journal of Audiology*, 46(11), 711–717. doi:10.1080/14992020701525858

McMillan, P. M., Bennett, M. J., Marchant, C. D., & Shurin, P. A. (1985). Ipsilateral and contralateral acoustic reflexes in neonates. *Ear and Hearing, 6*(6), 320–324.

McMillan, P. M., Marchant, C. D., & Shurin, P. A. (1985). Ipsilateral acoustic reflexes in infants. *Annals of Otology, Rhinology, and Laryngology, 94*(2 Pt 1), 145–148.

Merchant, G. R., Horton, N. J., & Voss, S. E. (2010). Normative reflectance and transmittance measurements on healthy newborn and 1-month-old infants. *Ear and Hearing, 31*, 746–754.

MRC Multicentre Otitis Media Study Group. (2003). The role of ventilation tube status in the hearing levels in children managed for bilateral persistent otitis media with effusion. *Clinical Otolaryngology and Allied Sciences, 28*(2), 146–153.

Nozza, R. J., Bluestone, C. D., Kardatzke, D., & Bachman, R. (1992). Towards the validation of aural acoustic immittance measures for diagnosis of middle ear effusion in children. *Ear and Hearing, 13*(6), 442–453.

Nozza, R. J., Bluestone, C. D., Kardatzke, D., & Bachman, R. (1994). Identification of middle ear effusion by aural acoustic admittance and otoscopy. *Ear and Hearing, 15*(4), 310–323.

Palva, T., Northrop, C., & Ramsay, H. (1999). Spread of amniotic fluid cellular content within the neonate middle ear. *International Journal of Pediatric Otorhinolaryngology, 48*(2), 143–153.

Paradise, J. L., Smith, C. G., & Bluestone, C. D. (1976). Tympanometric detection of middle ear effusion in infants and young children. *Pediatrics, 58*(2), 198–210.

Piza, J., Gonzalez, M., Northrop, C. C., & Eavey, R. D. (1989). Meconium contamination of the neonatal middle ear. *Journal of Pediatrics, 115*(6), 910–914.

Poulsen, G., & Tos, M. (1978). Screening tympanometry in newborn infants and during the first six months of life. *Scandinavian Audiology, 7*(3), 159–166.

Prieve, B. A., Calandruccio, L., Fitzgerald, T., Mazevski, A., & Georgantas, L. M. (2008). Changes in transient-evoked otoacoustic emission levels with negative tympanometric peak pressure in infants and toddlers. *Ear and Hearing, 29*(4), 533–542. doi:10.1097/AUD.0b013e3181731e3e

Prieve, B. A., Vander Werff, K. R., Preston, J. L., & Georgantas, L. (2013). Identification of conductive hearing loss in young infants using tympanometry and wideband reflectance. *Ear and Hearing, 34*(2), 168–178. doi:10.1097/AUD.0b013e31826fe611

Renvall, U., & Holmquist, J. (1976). Tympanometry revealing middle ear pathology. *Annals of Otology, Rhinology, and Laryngology, 85*(2 Suppl. 25 Pt. 2), 209–215.

Rhodes, M. C., Margolis, R. H., Hirsch, J. E., & Napp, A. P. (1999). Hearing screening in the newborn intensive care nursery: Comparison of methods. *Otolaryngology-Head and Neck Surgery, 120*(6), 799–808. doi:S019459989900234X [pii]

Roberts, D. G., Johnson, C. E., Carlin, S. A., Turczyk, V., Karnuta, M. A., & Yaffee, K. (1995). Resolution of middle ear effusion in newborns. *Archives of Pediatrics and Adolescent Medicine, 149*(8), 873–877.

Rosenfeld, R. M., Shin, J. J., Schwartz, S. R., Coggins, R., Gagnon, L., Hackell, J. M., . . . Corrigan, M. D. (in press). American Academy of Otolaryngology-Head and Neck Surgery. *Clinical Practice Guideline: Otitis media with effusion (Update).*

Rosowski, J. J., Stenfelt, S., & Lilly, D. (2013). An overview of wideband immittance measurements techniques and terminology: You say absorbance, I say reflectance. *Ear and Hearing, 34*(Suppl. 1), 9S–16S. doi:10.1097/AUD.0b013e31829d5a14

Roush, J., Drake, A., & Sexton, J. E. (1992). Identification of middle ear dysfunction in young children: A comparison of tympanometric screening procedures. *Ear and Hearing, 13*(2), 63–69.

Ruah, C. B., Schachern, P. A., Zelterman, D., Paparella, M. M., & Yoon, T. H. (1991). Age-related morphologic changes in the human tympanic membrane. A light and electron microscopic study. *Archives of Otolaryngology-Head and Neck Surgery, 117*(6), 627–634.

Sanford, C. A., & Brockett, J. E. (2014). Characteristics of wideband acoustic immittance in patients with middle-ear dysfunction. *Journal of the American Academy of Audiology, 25*(5), 425–440. doi:10.3766/jaaa.25.5.2

Sanford, C. A., & Feeney, M. P. (2008). Effects of maturation on tympanometric wideband acoustic transfer functions in human infants. *Journal of the Acoustical Society of America, 124*(4), 2106–2122. doi:10.1121/1.2967864

Sanford, C. A., Hunter, L. L., Feeney, M. P., & Nakajima, H. H. (2013). Wideband acoustic immittance: Tympanometric measures. *Ear and Hearing, 34*(Suppl. 1), 65S–71S. doi:10.1097/AUD.0b013e31829c7250

Sanford, C. A., Keefe, D. H., Liu, Y. W., Fitzpatrick, D., McCreery, R. W., Lewis, D. E., & Gorga, M. P. (2009). Sound-conduction effects on distortion-product otoacoustic emission screening outcomes in newborn infants: Test performance of wideband acoustic transfer functions and 1-kHz tympanometry. *Ear and Hearing, 30*(6), 635–652. doi:10.1097/AUD.0b013e3181b61cdc

Saunders, J. C., Kaltenback, J. A., & Relkin, E. M. (1983). The structural and functional development of the outer and middle ear. In R. Romand & M. R. Romand (Eds.), *Development of auditory and vestibular systems* (pp. 3–25). New York, NY: Academic Press.

Schairer, K. S., Ellison, J. C., Fitzpatrick, D., & Keefe, D. H. (2007). Wideband ipsilateral measurements of middle-ear muscle reflex thresholds in children and adults. *Journal of the Acoustical Society of America, 121*(6), 3607–3616. doi:10.1121/1.2722213

Schairer, K. S., Feeney, M. P., & Sanford, C. A. (2013). Acoustic reflex measurement. *Ear and Hearing, 34*(Suppl. 1), 43s–47s. doi:10.1097/AUD.0b013e31829c70d9

Shahnaz, N., Miranda, T., & Polka, L. (2008). Multifrequency tympanometry in neonatal intensive care unit and well babies. *Journal of the American Academy of Audiology, 19*, 392–418.

Shanks, J. E., & Lilly, D. J. (1981). An evaluation of tympanometric estimates of ear canal volume. *Journal of Speech and Hearing Research, 24*(4), 557–566.

Shanks, J. E., Stelmachowicz, P. G., Beauchaine, K. L., & Schulte, L. (1992). Equivalent ear canal volumes in children pre- and post-tympanostomy tube insertion. *Journal of Speech and Hearing Research, 35*(4), 936–941.

Sidell, D., Hunter, L. L., Lin, L., & Arjmand, E. (2014). Risk factors for preoperative and postoperative hearing loss in children undergoing pressure equalization tube placement. *Otolaryngology-Head and Neck Surgery, 150*(6), 1048–1055. doi:10.1177/0194599814529080

Silman, S., Silverman, C. A., & Arick, D. S. (1992). Acoustic-immittance screening for detection of middle-ear effusion in children. *Journal of the American Academy of Audiology, 3*(4), 262–268.

Son, E. J., Park, Y. A., Kim, J. H., Hong, S. A., Lim, H. Y., Choi, J. Y., & Lee, W. S. (2012). Classification of trace patterns of 226- and 1000-Hz tympanometry in healthy neonates. *Auris Nasus Larynx, 39*(5), 455–460. doi:10.1016/j.anl.2011.08.007

Sprague, B. H., Wiley, T. L., & Goldstein, R. (1985). Tympanometric and acoustic-reflex studies in neonates. *Journal of Speech and Hearing Research, 28*(2), 265–272.

Sun, X. M., & Shaver, M. D. (2009). Effects of negative middle ear pressure on distortion product otoacoustic emissions and application of a compensation procedure in humans. *Ear and Hearing, 30*(2), 191–202. doi:10.1097/AUD.0b013e31819769e1

Swanepoel de, W., Werner, S., Hugo, R., Louw, B., Owen, R., & Swanepoel, A. (2007). High frequency immittance for neonates: A normative study. *Acta Otolaryngologica, 127*(1), 49–56. doi:10.1080/00016480600740563

Takasaka, T., Hozawa, K., Shoji, F., Takahashi, Y., Jingu, K., Adachi, M., & Kobayashi, T. (1996). Tympanostomy tube treatment in recurrent otitis media with effusion. In D. J. Lim, C. D. Bluestone, M. Casselbrandt, J. O. Klein, & P. L. Ogra (Eds.), *Recent advances in otitis media* (pp. 197–199). Hamilton, Ontario, Canada: B. C. Decker.

Trine, M. B., Hirsch, J. E., & Margolis, R. H. (1993). The effect of middle ear pressure on transient evoked otoacoustic emissions. *Ear and Hearing, 14*(6), 401–407.

Vander Werff, K. R., Prieve, B. A., & Georgantas, L. M. (2007). Test-retest reliability of wideband reflectance measures in infants under screening and diagnostic test conditions. *Ear and Hearing, 28*(5), 669–681. doi:10.1097/AUD.0b013e31812f71b1

Vanhuyse, V. J., Creten, W. L., & Van Camp, K. J. (1975). On the W-notching of tympanograms. *Scandinavian Audiology, 4*, 45–50.

Wada, H., Koike, T., & Kobayashi, T. (1998). Clinical applicability of the sweep frequency measuring apparatus for diagnosis of middle ear diseases. *Ear and Hearing, 19*(3), 240–249.

Weatherby, L. A., & Bennett, M. J. (1980). The neonatal acoustic reflex. *Scandinavian Audiology, 9*(2), 103–110.

Wiley, T. L., Cruickshanks, K. J., Nondahl, D. M., Tweed, T. S., Klein, R., & Klein, B. E. (1996). Tympanometric measures in older adults. *Journal of the American Academy of Audiology, 7*(4), 260–268.

Zhiqi, L., Kun, Y., & Zhiwu, H. (2010). Tympanometry in infants with middle ear effusion having been identified using spiral computerized tomography. *American Journal of Otolaryngology, 31*, 96–103.

Otoacoustic Emissions in Infants and Children: An Updated Approach

Carolina Abdala, Margaret Winter, and Christopher A. Shera

Introduction

Otoacoustic emissions (OAEs), first reported by physicist David Kemp in the late 1970s (Kemp, 1978), are sounds created by the healthy cochlea, sometimes in response to external sounds and sometimes spontaneously. They offer a noninvasive window into cochlear function and associated hearing status without requiring any response from the patient. For these reasons and more, the field of audiology has been using OAEs in the assessment of hearing for the last 15 to 20 years. During this time, our understanding of how OAEs are generated has progressed, and these changes have implications for practice and diagnosis. For example, there are various types of OAEs, and although they all share a common dependence on outer hair cells (OHCs) and active cochlear processes, we now understand their generation mechanisms to differ in fundamental ways. These distinctions might render one OAE more (or less) sensitive to a given hearing loss or type of auditory deficit. Here, we present how OAEs fit into the subspecialty of pediatric audiology while considering an updated account of OAE generation and how this current knowledge might impact practice.

Although much of what we present is equally applicable to adults, we target pediatric factors and issues as much as possible. As with other objective tests of auditory function, OAEs are most useful and most commonly applied in pediatric patients where the behavioral response can be limited, unreliable, and embedded in an elevated noise floor.

In this chapter, we start with a brief background of OAE generation mechanisms, linking the current taxonomy to familiar types of OAEs. We summarize work defining the development of OAEs in human infants and describe how OAEs are applied and interpreted in a pediatric clinic. Much of this is based on literature but also on clinical experience at the Children's Auditory Research and Evaluation Center (of the House Ear Institute) and the Center for Childhood Communication at the University of Southern California. Our penultimate section considers clinical practice in light of an updated understanding of how OAEs arise and the properties they reflect. We present both human and mouse case studies to illustrate this approach and its potential benefits. Our final section considers advances on the horizon that will make their way into the audiology clinic sooner rather than later. Our goal is to provide the reader with background of how OAEs come about, an understanding of their basic features and distinctions, a description of how they are used in children, and ideas about how their effective application might be extended.

OAE Generation Mechanisms: Dual-Source Theory

Initially, all OAEs were thought to be generated by distortion related to OHC electromotility (Kemp, 1997). As a result, they were—and generally continue to be—used interchangeably for the assessment of hearing in clinics and laboratories. During the last decade, this unitary view of OAEs has been revised. Nonlinearity is only one of two basic mechanisms by which backward-traveling energy is initiated within the cochlea (Knight

& Kemp, 1999, 2000, 2001; Shera & Guinan, 1999; Shera & Zweig, 1993; Talmadge, Tubis, Long, & Piskorski, 1998). Research has revealed that OAEs arise via two principal mechanisms involving different cochlear processes (Shera & Guinan, 1999). Figure 20–1 provides a schematic illustration of this concept.

Reflection

The first of these mechanisms can be thought of as a kind of reflection. As traveling waves evoked by sound propagate down along the cochlear spiral, they encounter "irregularities" in the structure and mechanics of the organ of Corti (Figure 20–1A). These irregularities disturb the normal, forward flow of wave energy and produce reverse waves (reflections) that travel back along the spiral to the middle ear, and from there out into the ear canal, where they appear as OAEs.

Although the mechanical irregularities responsible for wave scattering and reflection can sometimes result from localized trauma (e.g., missing or damaged OHCs), irregularities are thought to arise predominantly from natural developmental variability (e.g., cell-to-cell variations in the orientation of OHC hair bundles or the security of their attachment to the overlying tectorial membrane). Although OAE models and measurements indicate that wave scattering occurs wherever irregularities are encountered, the strongest reflection occurs near the peak of the traveling wave. It is in this region at low sound levels that the OHCs contribute most to the cochlear response by boosting traveling wave amplitudes through mechanisms known collectively as the "cochlear amplifier."

Distortion

The second of the two principal mechanisms for creating OAEs is nonlinear distortion. Distortion of the traveling wave occurs at medium and high sound levels because the OHCs, like the amplifiers in a home stereo system, are limited in the amount of power they can provide. As a result, the gain of the cochlear amplifier depends on sound level, with smaller amounts of amplification and larger amounts of distortion generally occurring at higher levels. Distortion introduces components into the cochlear response that are not present in the original sound stimulus (e.g., components at combination-tone frequencies, such as $2f_1$-f_2, for stimuli consisting of tones at f_1 and f_2). These components propagate both forward and backward within

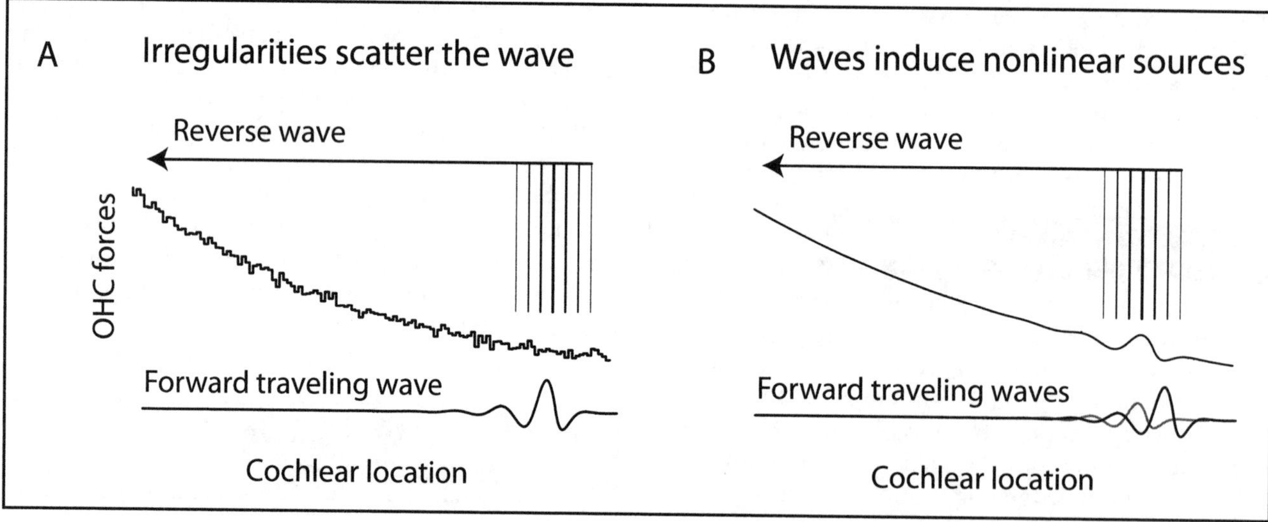

FIGURE 20–1. Mechanisms of intracochlear reflection and distortion. **A.** Intrinsic cell-to-cell irregularities in the strength of the forces produced by outer hair cells scatter the forward traveling wave, giving rise to multiple reflected wavelets. The wavelets combine to form a net reverse wave that propagates back out to the ear canal. The comb-like structure shows that scattering occurs over a broad region centered near the peak of the wave envelope. **B.** Nonlinearities in hair-cell transduction give rise to sources of wave energy that propagate away in both directions. In this case, nonlinearities driven by traveling waves at frequencies f_1 and f_2 induce sources at the combination-tone frequency $2f_1$–f_2. The sources are strongest in the region where the two waves overlap near their peaks.

the cochlea, some of it stimulating other hair cells and causing the sensation of sound, and some of it leaking out into the ear canal to be recorded as distortion product (DP) OAEs (see Figure 20–1B).

Although all physical materials behave nonlinearly when pushed to extremes, the most significant cochlear nonlinearities are thought to be those arising from the saturation of the current that flows through the transduction channels located near the tips of the OHC stereocilia. When the stereocilia are driven back and forth by sound-induced motions in the organ of Corti, the channels are alternately opened and closed via mechanical "gating springs." The alternating current that flows through the channels changes the voltage inside the OHC, causing the cell to move (i.e., electromotility), amplifying the motion of the whole structure. At low sound levels, the current increases in direct proportion to the stereocilia displacement, and so the amplified response grows linearly. However, at higher sound levels, the current begins to saturate once the hair bundle is bent far enough that most transduction channels are opened. Saturation both creates distortion and reduces the gain of the cochlear amplifier, causing the mechanical response of the cochlea to grow nonlinearly.

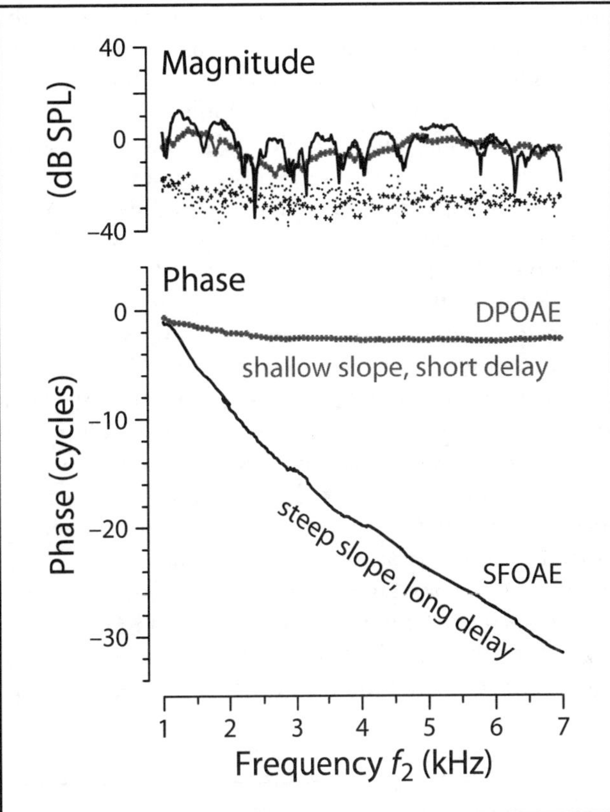

FIGURE 20–2. Measurements of human distortion product otoacoustic emissions (DPOAEs) and stimulus-frequency otoacoustic emissions (SFOAEs) under analogous stimulus conditions show that they have different phase slopes (delays), implying different mechanisms of generation. The black lines show SFOAE magnitude and phase versus frequency (probe level of 40 dB SPL). The gray lines show the $2f_1$-f_2 distortion product otoacoustic emission (DPOAE) measured in the same subject (f_2/f_1 = 1.2; L_1 ,L_2 = 50, 40 dB SPL). The dots in the upper panel show the approximate measurement noise floor (adapted from Shera & Guinan, 1999).

Different Signatures, Differential Sensitivities

OAEs generated by the two different mechanisms were first identified and defined theoretically but can be distinguished experimentally because they have different phase characteristics; their phases depend differently on emission frequency. What is OAE phase? Although accustomed to considering the magnitude or strength of a signal, some readers might be less comfortable with the phase or temporal elements of a signal. If we consider a sinusoidal waveform plotted as pressure versus time, the height of the peaks along the y-axis (pressure) provides a measure of magnitude. In an analogous fashion, the position of the peaks along the x-axis (time) defines the phase. The changes in OAE phase across frequency also provide a measure of the emission delay, which includes the time required for intracochlear generation of the OAE and round-trip propagation through the middle ear. Technically, the OAE delay is proportional to the slope of the phase-versus-frequency function, with a steep slope corresponding to a long measured delay. The lower panel of Figure 20–2 displays OAE phase versus frequency functions for both reflection and distortion emissions.

Based on their long delays or, what amounts to the same thing, the steep slope of their phase-versus-frequency function—click-evoked (CE) OAEs and stimulus-frequency (SF) OAEs are thought to arise predominantly via the reflection mechanism. By contrast, DPOAEs have shallow phase slopes and are thought to arise via the distortion mechanism. Figure 20–2 illustrates the striking differences between the phase slopes of human SFOAEs and DPOAEs; clearly, the mechanisms that give rise to these two emission types are very different. According to theory, the steep phase slope characteristic of reflection emissions (CEOAEs and SFOAEs) originates in the buildup time of the traveling wave as it reaches its peak, which in turn reflects the underlying sharpness of cochlear tuning with sharper tuning producing longer delays (Shera & Guinan, 2003; Shera, Guinan, & Oxenham, 2002, 2010). More details about the reflection and distortion mechanisms and how they give rise to different phase gradients can be found elsewhere (reviewed in Shera & Guinan, 2008).

Of course, the approximate correspondence between phase gradient and emission mechanism described above is only a rule of thumb deduced, for the most part, from OAEs in healthy ears. In practice, all emissions are thought to be mixtures of OAEs arising from both of these two basic mechanisms—and perhaps additional mechanisms awaiting discovery—with the relative magnitudes of the dual components depending both on stimulus parameters and on the particular ear being tested. For example, although DPOAEs are generally dominated by distortion generated in the region of overlap between the f_1 and f_2 waves (e.g., Kim, 1980), they often also include a significant "reflection component" arising from the DP place, which is near the peak of the wave at $2f_1$-f_2. The reflection component of DPOAEs arises because distortion at the overlap of the primary tones produces waves that travel in both directions along the cochlea (see Figure 20–1B); as they propagate apically, the forward waves emanating from the distortion overlap region encounter mechanical irregularities and are therefore partially reflected. As a result, the total DPOAE measured in the ear canal is made up of both distortion and reflection components (Kalluri & Shera, 2001; Knight & Kemp, 2000; Shera & Guinan, 1999; Talmadge, Long, Tubis, & Dhar, 1999). When DPOAEs are measured with adequate resolution across frequency, the resulting peaks and dips (termed *fine structure*) provide evidence of inference between the two components adding constructively and destructively in the ear canal. Figure 20–3 displays a high-resolution DPOAE recording (solid black line) to show this fine structure. The distortion and reflection components are also plotted.

Whereas the reflection mechanism for generating OAEs is a linear process, the distortion mechanism

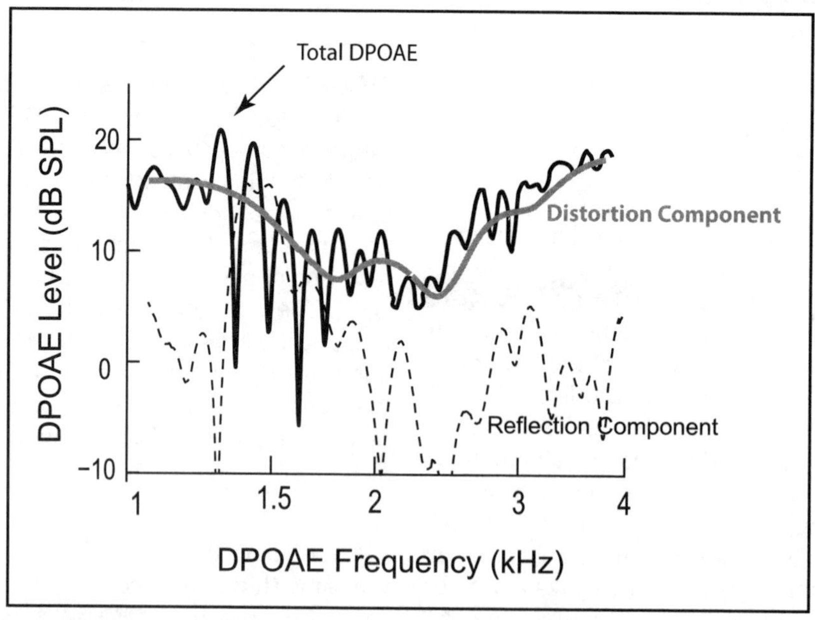

FIGURE 20–3. Distortion product otoacoustic emission (DPOAE) fine structure in a healthy ear (black line). DPOAE level (and phase though not shown here) shows quasi-periodic fluctuations across frequency due to constructive and destructive interference between distortion and reflection components, which make up the total DPOAE recorded at the microphone. The black line is the total DPOAE, and the gray and dashed lines are the individual distortion and reflection components that make up the total DPOAE. They have been separated using an inverse fast Fourier transform technique.

requires cochlear nonlinearity. Although the OAEs arising from both mechanisms require a healthy cochlear amplifier, distortion OAEs specifically depend on mechanisms that produce saturation of the cochlear responses observed at higher sound levels. Thus, the strongest distortion-type emissions tend to occur at moderate to high levels, where the amplifier gain is decreasing. By contrast, the strongest reflection-source emissions occur at lower levels, where the amplifier gain is maximal. For this reason, the two OAE types are thought to be especially sensitive to different aspects of cochlear function—reflection OAEs to the low-level gain of the cochlear amplifier and distortion OAEs to the form and strength of cochlear nonlinearities. Empirical support for these ideas exists in reports finding that DPOAE components mature and age independently and are differentially affected by various experimental variables such as aspirin and by medial efferent activation (Abdala & Dhar, 2010, 2012; Abdala, Mishra, & Williams, 2009; Deeter, Abel, Calandruccio, & Dhar, 2009; Rao & Long, 2011). In addition, large-scale studies have shown reflection emissions (CEOAEs) are sensitive to a more mild degree of hearing loss than distortion emissions (Gorga et al., 1993, 1997; Lapsley-Miller, Marshall, & Heller, 2004).

We do not yet know if the differences in the way reflection and distortion OAEs are generated make them uniquely sensitive or insensitive to specific sensory/neural hearing losses and deficits, but studies are currently underway to answer this important question (Abdala & Kalluri, 2015). At present, we do know that all OAEs require a relatively healthy cochlear amplifier, which imbues the cochlea with its hallmark sensitivity and sharp frequency tuning. When the amplifier is damaged, OAEs are diminished or eliminated altogether.

How Different OAEs Fit Into This Updated Taxonomy

To put this information in practical context, we can classify OAEs into predominantly distortion- or reflection-type emissions. The DPOAE is mostly a distortion OAE and provides evidence of cochlear nonlinearity (the aforementioned saturation of cochlear response growth). They are evoked when two primary tones, f_1 and f_2, are presented simultaneously. The most robust and reliably present DPOAE in mammals is the cubic distortion tone at $2f_1$-f_2, which is generated in both adults and infants at the overlap of traveling waves evoked by the primary tones (Abdala, 1996; Brown & Kemp, 1984; Kummer, Janssen, & Arnold, 1995; Martin, Lonsbury-Martin, Probst, Scheinin, & Coats, 1987). In the audiology clinic, DPOAEs are therefore used to assess the frequency region near the primary tones where they were generated (nearer f_2), not the frequency site of the DPOAE itself (i.e., $2f_1$-f_2). When the primary-tone region of the cochlea is damaged, DPOAEs are reduced or nonmeasureable (Konrad-Martin et al., 2002; Mauermann, Uppenkamp, van Hengel, & Kollmeier, 1999). Recall that DPOAEs are a mixture of distortion generated near the primary tones and reflection energy coming from the DP site. Although the DPOAE measured in clinic is the total DPOAE (including both components combined), there are signal-processing techniques that can separate the two and analyze their features independently as shown in Figure 20–3.

Click-evoked OAEs (CEOAE), sometimes referred to as transient OAEs or TEOAEs, are reflection-type emissions, and they were the first OAEs to make their way into the audiological repertoire. When a broadband click is presented to the ear, the healthy cochlea produces a slightly delayed response whose spectrum more or less resembles that of the click; hence, the term *cochlear echo*. The CEOAE is made up of many linear reflections produced by micromechanical irregularities along the cochlear spiral.

A less familiar reflection OAE is the SFOAE. SFOAEs, CEOAEs, and the reflection components of the DPOAE are generated in basically the same way within the cochlea (Kalluri & Shera, 2001, 2007). The SFOAE is perhaps the simplest reflection emission as it is evoked with a single low-level tone. The traveling wave produced by this tone backscatters off of micromechanical irregularities or "roughness" along the cochlea and reverse travels toward the base of the cochlea, through the middle ear, and into the ear canal. Because the cochlear irregularities are randomly distributed, the SFOAE has significant fine structure across frequency as shown by SFOAE magnitude displayed in the upper panel of Figure 20–2. Because the SFOAE occurs at the same frequency as the stimulus tone, it can be tricky to disentangle the two. One way involves a suppression paradigm. Briefly, two intervals are presented, one with the stimulus only and one with the stimulus plus a suppressor tone close to the stimulus frequency. Measurements from the first interval contain both stimulus and evoked SFOAE; ideally, measurements from the second interval contain only the stimulus because the SFOAE has been totally suppressed. By subtracting measurements from the two intervals, one is able to extract an SFOAE (Shera & Guinan, 1999). At present, no clinical instrumentation allows for measurement of the SFOAE though efforts in this direction are ongoing.

Both SFOAEs and CEOAEs are reduced as the degree of hearing loss increases and are no longer measurable when hearing loss exceeds 30 to 35 dB HL or so (Abdala & Kalluri, 2015; Collet, Levy, Veuillet, Truy, & Morgon, 1993; Ellison & Keefe, 2005; Harrison & Norton, 1999; Hussain, Gorga, Neely, Keefe, & Peters, 1998; Probst & Harris, 1993). Because they probe the lower-level, sensitive range of hearing, reflection OAEs appear to provide a better gauge of slight-to-mild hearing loss than DPOAEs (Gorga et al., 1993; Lapsley-Miller et al., 2004).

Finally, spontaneous OAEs or SOAEs are tones present in approximately 60% to 70% of normal-hearing adults and 70% to 90% of healthy newborns without any stimulating tone (Abdala, 1996). Many (although perhaps not all) SOAEs are initiated and perpetuated by a reflection mechanism (Shera, 2003). Because they are not present in all normal-hearing individuals, they are not especially helpful in the assessment of hearing though their presence is typically associated with cochlear health.

Development of Otoacoustic Emissions

Cochlear Morphology

OAEs require a functional cochlea. By term birth, the human cochlear anatomy is mostly adult-like though subtle immaturities seem to remain. The human otocyst is formed by the fifth embryological week (Sanchez-Fernandez, Rivera, & Macias, 1983). Approximately 3 to 4 weeks later, the otic capsule already includes three cochlear coils. Hair cells begin to differentiate around the ninth fetal week, and by Week 11, stereocilia form on the tops of both inner (IHCs) and outer hair cells (OHCs). The IHC acquires its flask-like shape quickly, whereas OHCs lag in attaining adult morphology, possibly until the onset of cochlear function (Pujol & Hilding, 1973). Lateral and tip links among stereocilia are apparent once bundle organization is established (Lavigne-Rebillard & Pujol, 1986; Lim & Rueda, 1992). By Weeks 20 to 22, adult-like stereocilia are observed on both types of hair cells, although the process begins earlier on IHCs. The apical regions of the cochlea are less regimented at this time and more irregular with fewer sensory cells and uneven development of ciliary bundles (Kaltenbach & Falzarano, 1994; Lavigne-Rebillard & Pujol, 1986; Tanaka, Sakai, & Terayama, 1979). The protracted course for OHC development in mammals is loosely correlated with the emergence of functional properties such as increased sensitivity, frequency tuning, and shifts in the tonotopic place code (Norton, Bargones, & Rubel, 1991; Pujol, Carlier, & Lenoir, 1980; Romand, 1987). The structural and physical features of the human organ of Corti have not been well characterized around the time of birth and during early postnatal life. Supernumerary hair cells have been identified (Bredberg, 1968; Igarishi, 1980; Lavigne-Rebillard & Pujol, 1986), but it is not clear how long they persist into the postnatal period. The physical properties and dimensions of the human basilar membrane and organ of Corti at birth are not known.

Overall, the anatomy of the cochlea appears mostly mature by term birth in humans. This is most evident in the midbasal and basal (mid- to high-frequency) regions, but the apical organization is less firm. Subtle immaturities in the innervation of OHCs by descending medial efferent fibers (Lavigne-Rebillard & Pujol, 1990), and in the mass/stiffness of the sensory epithelium, might persist. If any of these immaturities extend into the postnatal period, they could influence the generation of OAEs.

OAEs in Infants and Children

Both reflection- and distortion-type otoacoustic emissions are present and generally robust in newborns (Abdala, 1996, 1998, 2003; Abdala, Oba, & Ramanathan, 2008; Burns, Arehart, & Campbell, 1992; Kalluri & Abdala, 2015a; Lasky, Perlman, & Hecox, 1992; Smurzynski et al., 1993). Neonatal OAEs are higher in level than adult OAEs and show a broader, more ample spectral bandwidth. Spontaneous OAEs are often reported to be more prevalent in newborns, with estimates up to 90% (Abdala, 1996; Burns et al., 1992; Morlet et al., 1995). Newborns have higher-level SOAEs than adults (Qi, Cheng, En, Huang, & Zhang, 2014), and it is not uncommon to see spontaneous emissions as large as 20 to 30 dB SPL in a newborn ear. SOAEs are also more numerous per ear with reported averages as high as 6 to 7 per ear in premature newborns (Abdala, 1996). SOAEs tend to occur at higher frequencies in newborn ears. Figure 20–4 displays a rather typical SOAE spectrum from one prematurely born neonate with multiple high-level spontaneous emissions present.

Neonatal CEOAEs are also higher in level compared to adult OAEs (Bonfils, Uziel, & Narcy, 1989). Although amplitude decreases with increasing age, pediatric CEOAEs remain robust throughout childhood (Norton & Widen, 1990; Prieve, 1992; Prieve,

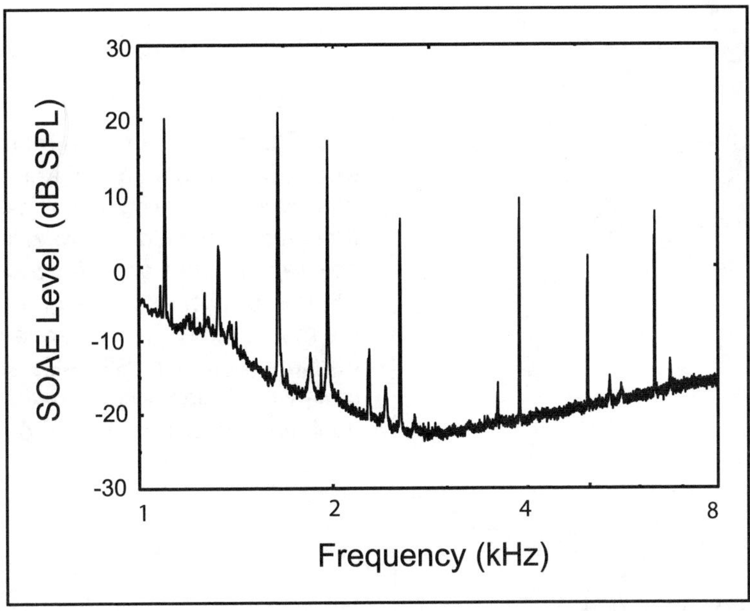

FIGURE 20–4. Spectrum showing numerous spontaneous otoacoustic emissions (SOAEs) recorded in the ear of a prematurely born neonate. These tones are present in this newborn's ear canal in the absence of any eliciting stimulus. SOAEs are thought to arise in the cochlea via a reflection-type mechanism.

Fitzgerald, & Schulte, 1997; Prieve, Fitzgerald, Schulte, & Kemp, 1997). CEOAEs, and reflection emissions in general, show greater adult-newborn level differences than DPOAEs. Both adult and pediatric ears show compressive growth of the CEOAE when recorded as a function of increasing stimulus level (Prieve, 1992; Prieve, Fitzgerald, Schulte, & Kemp, 1997); this reflects the nonlinear response of the cochlea. Developmental effects on the stimulus-frequency OAE (SFOAE), also a reflection-type emission, have not been widely studied. There is one published study indicating that the average newborn SFOAE is approximately 8 dB higher in level than adult SFOAE around the midfrequency region (Figure 20–5) and shows similarly compressive growth (Kalluri & Abdala, 2015a).

The reader will recall that DPOAEs, though generated at the region of wave overlap evoked by primary tones, also include a reflection component generated near the distortion frequency at $2f_1$-f_2. This reflection component has been studied in newborns and children (Abdala & Dhar, 2010, 2012). Like the CEOAE and SFOAE, the reflection component of the DPOAE is larger in newborns and older infants than adults by approximately 5 dB on average. Recall that reflection OAEs show rapid phase cycling across frequency and a steep phase slope (see lower panel of Figure 20–2). This is one of the signature features that allows us to classify OAEs as either reflection or distortion. In newborns, reflection-component delays derived from phase data are slightly longer than adult delays. Longer reflection emissions delays have been associated with sharper tuning (Oxenham & Shera, 2003). Therefore, large reflection OAEs and longer delays are consistent with a functional and robust cochlear amplifier in newborn ears, at least for mid-to-high frequencies where most of these measurements were taken.

DPOAEs are also present in nearly all normal-hearing newborns and children (Bonfils, Avan, Francois, Trotoux, Narcy, 1992; Lonsbury-Martin, Harris, Hawkings, Stagner, & Martin, 1990) and are slightly higher in level (~3–5 dB) compared to adults as shown by the mean age-group differences in Figure 20–6 (Abdala & Dhar, 2010, 2012; Lasky et al., 1992; Smurzynski et al., 1993). Prematurely born neonates appear to have temporarily reduced DPOAE levels compared to their term-born peers, but levels steadily increase until they reach the equivalence of term birth, around 40 postconceptional weeks (Abdala et al., 2008; Smurzynski, 1994). Halfway through the first year of life, DPOAE levels seem to peak, and they remain slightly higher than adult levels throughout childhood (Abdala & Dhar, 2012; Prieve et al., 1997).

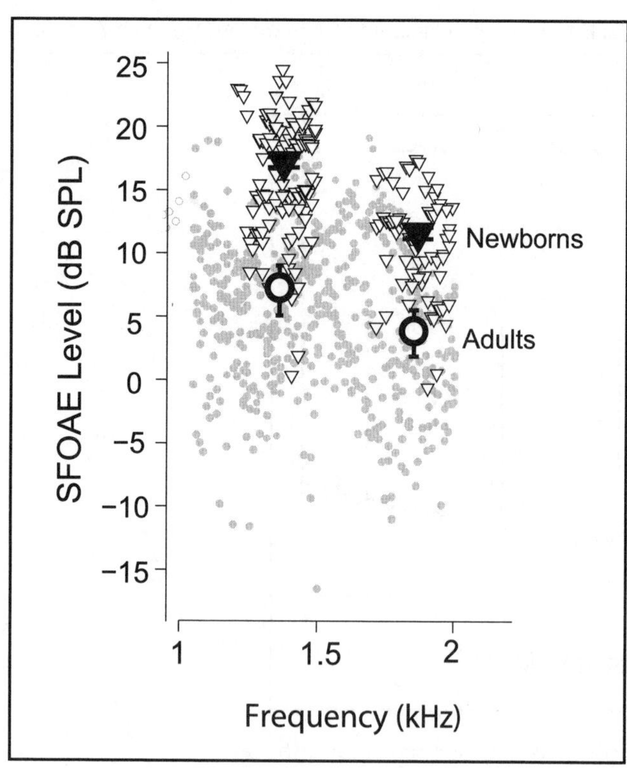

FIGURE 20–5. Stimulus-frequency otoacoustic emissions (SFOAEs) recorded from a group of adults (*small gray circles* = individual adult ears) and newborns (*open triangles* = individual newborn ears). The larger symbols (*open circles and filled triangles*) display the mean SFOAE level for each age group plus standard errors of the mean. Although data are available in only two mid-frequency regions, SFOAEs are on average approximately 8 dB higher in neonates than those recorded in adult ears (data from Kalluri & Abdala, 2015b).

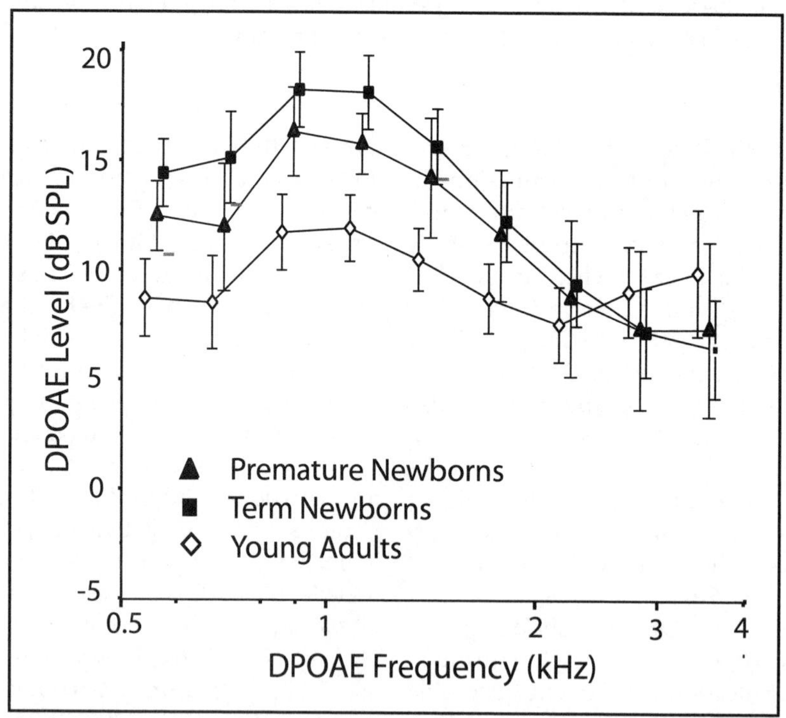

FIGURE 20–6. Average distortion product otoacoustic emission (DPOAE) level as a function of frequency in a group of premature and term-born neonates compared to a group of young adults. Primary tone levels were 65 (L_1), 55 (L_2) dB SPL and f_2/f_1 = 1.22. In general, newborns show an average of roughly 3 to 5 dB higher DPOAE levels than do adults. Error bars represent 95% confidence intervals (data from Abdala & Dhar, 2012).

When considering research on emission phase, DPOAE delays are not adult-like in newborns (Abdala, Dhar, & Mishra, 2011; Abdala & Dhar, 2010, 2012). All healthy adult or infant ears show a curious DPOAE phase pattern across frequency (when using a typical, fixed f_1/f_2 ratio around 1.2)—DPOAE phase is generally flat as shown in the lower panel of Figure 20–2 but shifts by a few cycles at lower frequencies (this shift is not apparent in Figure 20–2 because of the large scale). This phase shift suggests that cochlear motion is different in the apex compared to the base. Accumulating physiology and modeling research support the notion that unique, nonclassical patterns of vibration exist in the apical regions of the cochlea (Cooper & Rhode, 1995; Karavitaki & Mountain, 2007; Nowotny & Gummer, 2006). How does this aside on phase and the cochlear apex relate to auditory development and OAEs? In newborns, DPOAE delays in the apex (for frequencies below about 1.5 kHz) also shift as expected, but they are atypically long compared to adult delays, prolonged by nearly a full millisecond. Figure 20–7 shows mean DPOAE delays for newborn and adult age groups. This result cannot be easily explained by immaturities in the middle and outer ear because DPOAE phase is relatively insensitive to stimulus level. It is interesting to recall that the apex is the last region of the human cochlea to become anatomically mature. These results hint at the possibility of residual immaturities in the newborn cochlea.

Overall, OAE findings in newborns and children are generally consistent with a fully functional cochlea at birth across much of the human frequency range. In fact, one potential explanation for the higher OAE levels and longer delays is that the cochlear amplifier at birth is too strong for a brief developmental period, similar to what neonatal gerbils have shown (Mills & Rubel, 1996). Another possibility is that the adult cochlea undergoes subtle auditory "wear and tear" even in young adults, while the newborn cochlea is pristine and at its peak. Neither explanation can easily account for the persistent non-adult-like findings in the apical portions of the newborn cochlea. This could

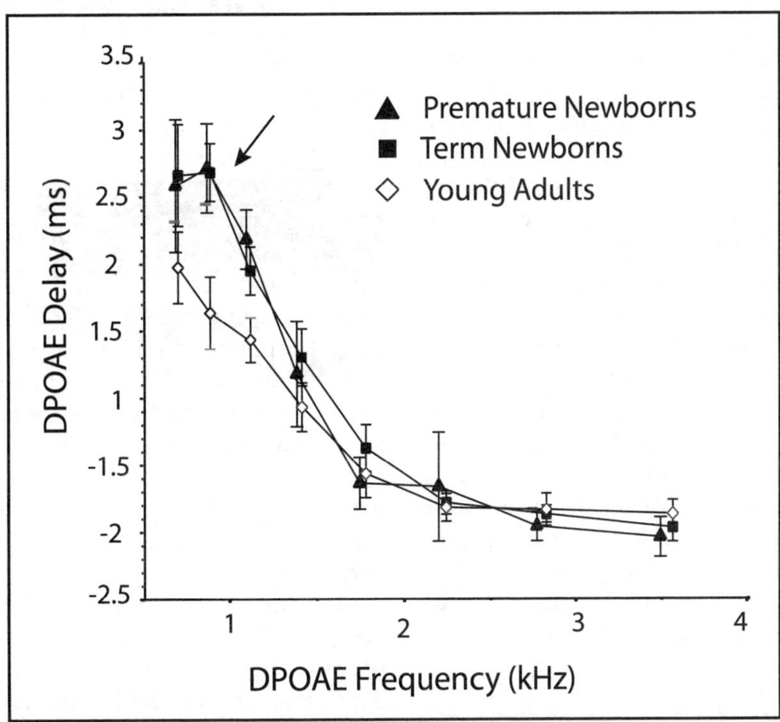

FIGURE 20–7. Distortion product otoacoustic emission (DPOAE) delay or latency (in milliseconds) as a function of frequency in the same group of newborns and adults shown in Figure 20–6. Below approximately 1500 Hz, newborn DPOAE delays are prolonged compared to adult delays. At the lowest frequencies, the average prolongation in newborns is approximately 1 ms (*see arrow*). Error bars represent 95% confidence intervals (data from Abdala & Dhar, 2012).

involve immaturity of the physical properties of the organ of Corti and basilar membrane, although this has not been systematically studied.

At this point in our developmental OAE journey, a strong caveat is in order. To generate evoked OAEs, the sound stimulus must travel through the ear canal and middle ear; to be recorded at the microphone, OAEs must travel in reverse from their point of generation through the middle ear and into ear canal. Any immaturities in the conductive pathway will impact this travel (see Abdala & Keefe, 2012, for a detailed review). In newborns, the ear canal is roughly two thirds of the adult length, it is softer, more cartilaginous, and has a reduced diameter (Keefe & Abdala, 2007). The tympanic membrane is thicker (Ruah, Schachern, Zelterman, Paparella, & Yoon, 1991), more horizontally oriented, and has an incomplete annular ligament (Saunders, Kaltenback, & Relkin, 1983). The middle ear cavity increases in size from birth through adolescence (Eby & Nadol, 1986). These changes impact the transmission of energy through the conductive system of infants and children.

As a result, even if equivalent sound pressure levels are presented to the adult and infant ear, the newborn cochlea receives an attenuated stimulus (compared to adults) because the middle ear is inefficient at transmitting the signal. This inefficiency affects the generation of OAEs, in particular reflection-type OAEs, which are sensitive to stimulus level and optimally generated at low levels. Also, the OAE coming from the cochlea and measured in the neonatal ear canal is effectively amplified by the smaller volume and reduced ear canal diameter. These factors can explain some of the non-adult-like pediatric OAE findings reported above. For example, the larger CEOAEs and SFOAEs, which are optimally evoked by lower stimulus levels, and even the longer reflection-OAE delays because cochlear delays are longest at low stimulus levels. However, DPOAE delays are not sensitive to stimulus level (Abdala, Dhar, & Kalluri, 2011; Mauermann & Kollmeier, 2004); therefore, the apical immaturities noted in newborns cannot be easily explained by simple attenuation from an immature middle ear.

OAEs and Otitis Media

In young children, a particular concern in the use and interpretation of OAEs is the high prevalence of negative middle ear pressure and otitis media. Otitis media is the second most common childhood illness after upper respiratory infection. By age 9 years, approximately 75% of children have experienced at least one episode of otitis media, with the prevalence being about 25% during the first five years of life (Stangerup & Tos, 1986). As noted in the previous section, alterations in either forward transmission of the stimulus toward the cochlea or backward transmission of the OAE to the ear canal can impact the resulting OAE measured at the microphone. Otitis media can produce such alterations in transmission.

Negative middle ear pressure typically reduces OAE levels but does not always eliminate them (Lonsbury-Martin, Martin, McCoy, & Whitehead, 1994; Owens, McCoy, Lonsbury-Martin, & Martin, 1993). Because normal OAEs in infants and young children are high in level, even with negative middle ear pressure, OAEs can be measurable though they might show lower levels. In children with already low-level OAEs due to slight or mild SNHL, negative pressure can push OAEs into the noise floor and make them undetectable. With otitis media of sufficient severity to affect mobility of the tympanic membrane and generate flat (no-peak) tympanograms, OAEs will likely be absent. In documented cases of otitis media, this outcome cannot provide any useful information about the health of the sensory organ because the result is the same with middle ear fluid or profound sensory/neural hearing loss: absent OAE.

In cases of recurrent or persistent otitis media, pressure-equalization (PE) tubes might be recommended in order to ventilate the middle ear and reduce the incidence of fluid accumulation behind the tympanic membrane. OAEs might still be present if the PE tubes are patent, although time after placement appears to be a factor. Although OAEs might be measureable in only half of patients immediately after tube placement (Cullington, Kumar, & Flood, 1998; Richardson, Elliott, & Hill, 1996), testing performed several weeks to months afterward can yield measurable emissions (Daya, Hinton, Radomskiej, & Huchzermeyer, 1996; Owens et al., 1993). Some work reports a higher noise floor in ears with patent PE tubes, although this has not been unequivocally observed (Owens et al., 1993). Because PE tubes can progress from patent to blocked or partially extruded over time, much of the variability in research and clinic reports is likely due to the shifting and uncertain status of the tubes during audiological assessment.

Here, we wish mostly to remind the reader that using OAEs to assess integrity of the cochlea requires a clear pathway in for the signal and a clear pathway out for the emission. Without this, an absent OAE cannot provide clear information about cochlear function.

Applying OAEs in a Pediatric Audiology Clinic

Typical Testing Parameters for Pediatric Audiology

Diagnostic protocols are conventionally implemented by measuring one (but not both) of the following OAEs as follows (with some wiggle room):

- CEOAEs are evoked with a broadband click presented between 80 and 84 dB pSPL, averaged using a nonlinear averaging technique (described in a later section) for approximately 20 ms after stimulus (corresponding to a frequency range roughly between 1000 and 4000 or 5000 Hz).
- The $2f_1$-f_2 DPOAE is recorded as a DP-gram (DPOAE level versus f_2 frequency) with primary tones presented at moderate levels (e.g., 60 or 65 dB SPL) and separated by perhaps 10 to 15 dB. The frequency ratio between primary tones is set to 1.22. Test frequencies might range from approximately 1500 to 6000 or 8000 Hz. If only one OAE is recorded, it is typically the DPOAE rather than CEOAE.

Why did these parameters come to define the typical OAE clinical protocol? An 80 to 84 dB pSPL click is roughly equivalent to a much lower-level pure tone, perhaps 40 or 45 dB SPL. (*Note*: Because of the transient and consequently broadband nature of the click stimulus and because it is measured at its instantaneous pressure peak, it is not comparable in effective level to an 84 dB SPL pure tone where pressure is averaged across time.) The CEOAE is recorded with these low stimulus levels because of how it is generated—reflection is strongest at low levels where the cochlear amplifier also functions optimally.

Overall, DPOAEs are largest in both adults and infants when the ratio of the two primary tone frequencies is around 1.22 (Abdala, 1996; Gaskill & Brown, 1990; Harris, Lonsbury-Martin, Stagner, Coats, & Martin, 1989). This ratio maximizes the nonlinear component of the DPOAE by optimizing the overlap between the primary traveling waves on the basilar membrane while maximizing the phase coherence of the distributed emission sources (Shera & Guinan 2008; Talmadge et al. 1988). Moderate to moderate-high primary tone levels are utilized because this is the level range where cochlear growth is compressive and nonlinearities become evident. Also, moderate levels are best at detecting hearing loss (Johnson et al., 2010; Stover, Gorga, Neely, & Montoya, 1996). The level separation between the tones is a little trickier and optimal separation differs across level, but strategies showing the most constant and strongest DPOAE typically include separations of 0 to 15 dB between the two primary tones (Boege & Janssen, 2002; Kummer, Janssen, & Arnold, 1998; Neely, Johnson, & Gorga, 2005).

This familiar set of OAE parameters has been used in audiology clinics rather universally for the last decade. In this format, the OAE test is essentially used as a screening tool. One brief test is conducted with fixed stimulus parameters, and the result is interpreted in a dichotomous manner—OAEs are either present or absent. In our Updated Approach section, we consider some modifications to this long-standing default protocol based on a current understanding of OAE mechanisms and a desire to move beyond this limited usage and maximize diagnostic information.

Indications for OAE Use in Pediatric Audiology

When might the measurement of OAEs be indicated in the clinical assessment of young infants and children who cannot participate reliably in behavioral audiometry? In addition to detecting hearing loss, OAEs are essential in formulating preliminary estimates of the degree, type, and configuration of hearing loss, which provides the foundation for the fitting of amplification. The auditory brainstem response (ABR) alone can, in many cases, be sufficient to formulate this estimate; however, OAEs serve to confirm ABR findings and in some cases contribute additional information. For example, a restless infant for whom only 500 and 2000 Hz tone-burst ABR thresholds could be measured might have absent OAEs for frequencies greater than 2000 Hz, providing information about high frequencies not otherwise obtainable that day. An infant with craniofacial anomalies might produce mildly elevated ABR thresholds but bone conduction ABR thresholds do not suggest a significant air-bone gap. He might be suspected of having a conductive component (undetectable by ABR) if DPOAEs are absent or reduced. A baby whose ABR shows poor morphology and questionable thresholds at 40 to 50 dB HL might have absent CEOAEs but present DPOAEs, suggesting a mild sensory/neural hearing loss (versus a severe loss). Auditory neuropathy spectrum disorder is indicated in a child with absent ABRs and present OAEs. Though only a handful of examples, in each case, OAEs were indicated and contributed to the overall diagnostic profile of the child's hearing and auditory health. They also contributed to decisions for further testing and directed initial steps toward appropriate intervention.

Although typically developing young children older than 6 months of age can be tested behaviorally through visual reinforcement audiometry (VRA) and conditioned play audiometry with excellent reliability, in some cases neither yields consistent responses. Children between ages 2 and 3 years of age, for example, are often bored by VRA but not yet developmentally ready to perform a conditioned play task to determine thresholds. A 2- or 3-year-old with speech and language delays should be assessed to rule out hearing loss as a contributing factor before he or she commences speech-language therapy. If this child is untestable in the test booth, OAEs can provide a rapid and clear indication of the urgency for intervention. If OAEs are present and robust, tympanograms are within normal limits, and acoustic reflexes are normal, it is highly unlikely that peripheral hearing loss accounts for the speech-language delay. If OAEs are absent or abnormal, immediate evaluation via ABR is indicated.

These real-life vignettes illustrate how and when OAEs might be effectively applied in the pediatric clinic and when they are indicated in infants and children. There are many more such examples, each unique and specific to a child's suspected auditory pathology, developmental ability to cooperate in testing, and the time available for such testing.

Applying OAEs to Assess Hearing

Click-Evoked OAEs

CEOAEs are measurable in 90% to 100% of normal-hearing individuals with healthy middle ear function (Bonfils, Uziel, & Pujol, 1988; Kemp, 1978; Kemp, Bray, Alexander, & Brown, 1986; Norton & Neely, 1987; Probst, Coats, Martin, & Lonsbury-Martin, 1986). Their incidence decreases with hearing loss; in general, the better the hearing threshold, the larger is the CEOAE (Bonfils et al., 1988; Collet et al., 1993; Kemp, 1978; Kemp et al, 1986; Probst & Harris, 1993). CEOAEs detect hearing loss well if the loss is greater than 30 dB HL (Harrison & Norton, 1999). Beyond this degree of hearing loss, they are likely to be absent. An ear with slight loss can still have measureable CEOAEs, but likely they will be reduced in level (Note that in children, slight loss is considered between 15 and 30 dB HL; Clark, 1981). CEOAEs are most reliable when measured in narrow frequency bands around the mid-frequency ranges, between approximately 1500 and 4000 Hz (Franklin, McCoy, Martin, & Lonsbury-Martin, 1992; Hussain et al., 1998). CEOAE tests at frequencies lower and higher than this optimal frequency range have reduced accuracy for the detection of hearing loss (Gorga et al., 1993). When multiple CEOAE outcome variables are considered in combination, test performance can be somewhat enhanced at the lower frequencies.

The clinical CEOAE can be analyzed in a number of ways. They are generally recorded using a "nonlinear averaging protocol" because they are susceptible to stimulus artifacts. Though the click begins as a brief electrical transient that should not interfere with the response, by the time it is transduced into an acoustical stimulus (at the earphone diaphragm) and further shaped by the outer and middle ear, it can overlap in time with the CEOAE and, in doing so, contaminate the recording. If the stimulus artifact gets into the averaged time waveform, there is danger of a false-negative result (i.e., a CEOAE is detected when there is none). The stimulus artifact can be a perilous confound. Figure 20–8 shows an example of a CEOAE waveform composed entirely of stimulus artifact. The child from whom it was measured is severely hearing impaired.

In the nonlinear protocol, the CEOAE is extracted by dividing the stimulus sequence into blocks, typically three plus one clicks—three identical clicks of one polarity followed by a single click with greater amplitude and opposite polarity (e.g., Kemp, Ryan, & Bray, 1990). When cochlear responses to the two blocks are summed, it theoretically eliminates linear elements thought to be stimulus, and retains nonlinear elements thought to be cochlear. This nonlinear technique produces CEOAEs that are less contaminated by stimulus artifact. However, we now understand the CEOAE to be generated by a linear reflection process. Consequently, the nonlinear protocol eliminates cochlear response as well as artifact, reducing CEOAE levels overall. In cases of slight or mild loss where the amplitude of the CEOAE is reduced already, nonlinear averaging might make it undetectable. If a linear CEOAE protocol is used, the OAE is obtained by averaging responses to identical clicks. This preserves linear elements of the cochlear response but is susceptible to stimulus artifact. At present, nonlinear averaging is the only technique available in most commercial instrumentation to avoid a stimulus-related artifact.

The time-averaged CEOAE waveform is sampled for approximately 20 ms after stimulus, which covers a frequency range from approximately 1000 to 4000 or 5000 Hz, and stored in two separate buffers, A and B.

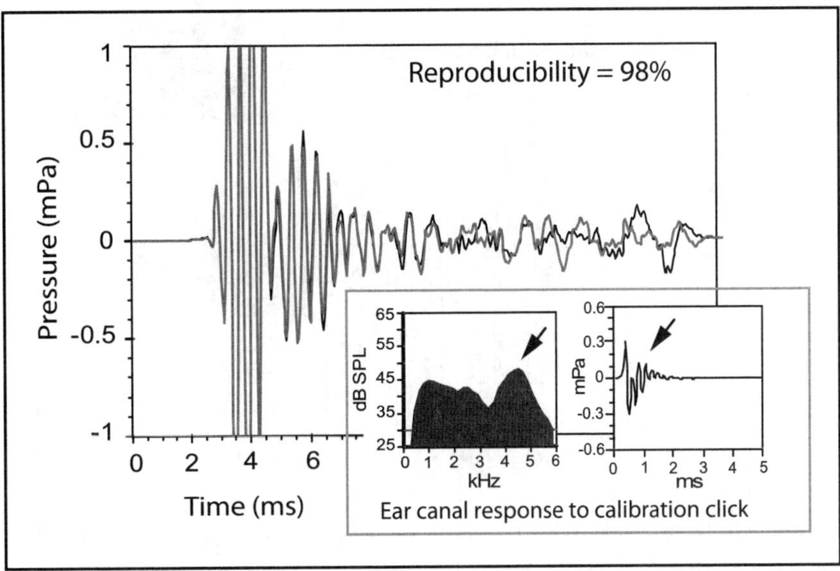

FIGURE 20–8. An apparent click-evoked otoacoustic emission (CEOAE) time waveform with excellent reproducibility recorded using linear averaging from the ear of a child with profound sensory/neural hearing loss. Note the inset calibration plots showing the ear canal response to a 82 dB pSPL click. The spectrum shows a prominent peak around 4500 Hz, and the time waveform shows persistent ringing (*see arrows*). The recorded waveform has been contaminated by a stimulus artifact and does not represent a true CEOAE.

The similarity of the two waveforms is assessed by a cross-correlation score, which determines whether the energy is random noise or repeatable and consistently present at given time intervals following the presentation of a stimulus. Figure 20–9 shows a normal CEOAE time waveform with strong reproducibility. Early studies of the CEOAE suggest that a reproducibility score equal to or greater than 50% indicates a present response (Kemp et al., 1986). A fast Fourier transform (FFT) is used to decompose the averaged time waveform into constituent frequency components and estimate overall CEOAE level. The noise floor is calculated using the difference between the two buffers. The CEOAE spectrum is also band-filtered, often in half-octave intervals, and amplitude and signal-to-noise ratio (SNR, defined as the difference between the OAE level and the noise floor) are calculated within these narrow bands as shown by the vertical black/gray bars across frequency shown in the Figure 20–9 inset. By combining observations of CEOAE reproducibility, overall level and narrow-band SNR values, the CEOAE is determined to be present or absent. Measures of SNR and waveform reproducibility are better diagnostic markers than overall amplitude (Gorga et al., 1993).

Distortion-Product OAEs

The *DP-gram*, as it is commonly called, plots DPOAE level as a function of f_2 frequency and includes a measure of the mean noise floor calculated at frequencies near the DPOAE (Lonsbury-Martin et al., 1990; Figure 20–10). The noise floor is often elevated in the low frequencies where biological and room noise are greatest as shown in Figure 20–10 by the gray shaded region that represents mean noise floor plus two standard deviations (s.d.). The overall level of the DPOAE (shown on the ordinate or *y*-axis) and the SNR are considered in establishing the response as present or absent. The clinical DP-gram is recorded by presenting six to eight pairs of moderate-level primary tones from ~1500 to 6000 or 8000 Hz. DPOAEs can be recorded at higher stimulus frequencies than CEOAEs because pure tones are not subject to the same stimulus artifacts as transients. The normal young-adult DP-gram generally peaks in the low-frequency range and shows a dip at

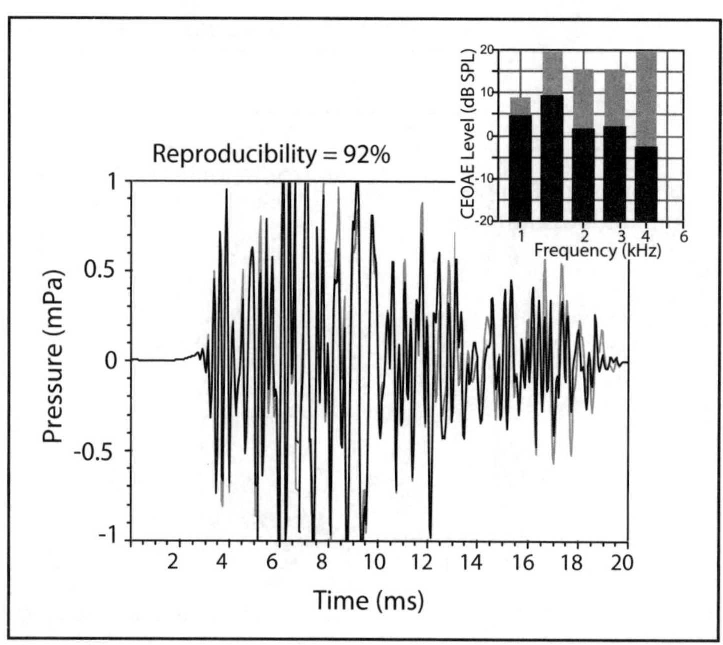

FIGURE 20–9. Click-evoked otoacoustic emissions (CEOAEs) recorded with 84 dB pSPL clicks and nonlinear averaging. The CEOAE time waveform shows the response from two buffers superimposed (*gray, black*). A cross-correlation analysis between buffers is conducted producing an excellent reproducibility score of 92%. (Note that it is difficult to distinguish between the two waveforms because they are so closely superimposed as reflected in the high reproducibility score.) The overall CEOAE level was 19 dB SPL. The response was further analyzed in half-octave bands as shown in the upper inset. The black portion of the bar represents noise, and the gray portions show CEOAE energy. As is evident, CEOAE levels and signal-to-noise ratios (SNR) were robust throughout the tested frequency range.

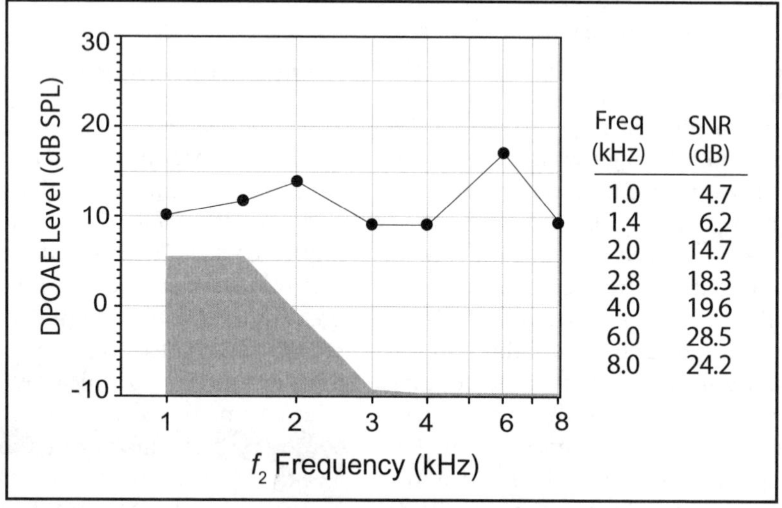

Freq (kHz)	SNR (dB)
1.0	4.7
1.4	6.2
2.0	14.7
2.8	18.3
4.0	19.6
6.0	28.5
8.0	24.2

FIGURE 20–10. A DP-gram recorded with default primary tone levels and frequency ratio (L_1, L_2 = 65, 55 dB SPL; f_2/f_1 = 1.22) in a normal-hearing ear. The gray area represents the noise floor. Distortion product otoacoustic emissions (DPOAEs) are present and robust across the tested frequency range despite higher noise at the lower frequencies. The signal-to-noise (SNR) for each test frequency is provided to the right of the DP-gram.

midfrequencies (Lonsbury-Martin et al., 1990; Lonsbury-Martin & Martin, 1990; Martin, Probst, Lonsbury-Martin, 1990). The infant DP-gram shows slightly higher DPOAE levels across frequency compared to adults, and a more flat configuration (Abdala et al., 2008; Lasky et al., 1992; Smurzynski et al., 1993).

In general, ears with hearing loss have lower-level DPOAEs than normal ears, although there is considerable overlap between groups, especially at low frequencies. DPOAEs are most accurate at detecting hearing loss between 1500 and 6000 Hz and show reduced detection accuracy for either lower or higher frequencies (Gorga et al., 1997). DPOAE level and SNR are good indicators of hearing loss and show "hit" rates (i.e., accuracy in detecting hearing loss) approximating 90% at mid-to-high frequencies, depending on how hearing loss is defined (Gorga et al., 1993). Measures of DPOAE SNR seem to perform better than absolute DPOAE level. Many audiology clinics apply a SNR criteria of at least 3 to 6 dB to consider DPOAEs present. The 3-dB criteria will likely result in some false-negative findings (no hearing loss identified when hearing loss is present), whereas higher SNRs can erroneously classify normal hearers as hearing impaired. A tester must decide which type of error he or she is willing to make. Test accuracy is slightly improved if multiple DPOAE outcome variables are considered (Dorn Piskorski, Keefe, Neely, & Gorga, 1998; Gorga et al., 2000, 2005).

A caveat must be included in any discussion characterizing the accuracy with which DPOAEs detect hearing loss. The DP-gram, as studied in previous research, recorded the total DPOAE at a fixed number of limited frequencies. The alternating pattern of DPOAE level known as fine structure, which comes from the interference between reflection and distortion components (see Figure 20–3) was not considered in the selection of test frequency. Therefore, whether the chosen test frequency fell at a peak or valley was not known. This uncertainty might have impacted much early research with DPOAEs, possibly affecting the conclusions. One relatively recent study showed that when DPOAE components are separated, no overall improvement is noted in accuracy of DPOAEs for detection of hearing loss; however, slight improvements were noted for ears with low-level DPOAEs or mild amounts of hearing loss (Johnson et al., 2007). For a normal-hearing or a profoundly hearing-impaired individual, the mixed nature of the DPOAE (and resulting fine structure) might not impact accuracy, but for those with mild-moderate degrees of hearing loss, it might. The possibility of using DPOAE component separation in the audiology clinic is further considered in Future Advances and Conclusions.

Interpretation of OAEs in Infants and Children

In general, if OAEs are not measurable in an ear (given very good test conditions), there is likely some degree of hearing loss present. Although the degree of loss cannot be precisely determined (i.e., an absent OAE can be consistent with both mild and profound hearing loss), preliminary clues about the degree and audiometric configuration can be gleaned from OAE tests if carefully examined. This idea is developed more fully under Updated Approaches. The interpretation of clinically recorded OAEs is most productive when the tester considers a combination of factors and extends his or her diagnostic conclusion beyond an absent or present determination. The following categories are often used to interpret OAE outcomes.

Absent OAE

The OAE is considered absent if it lacks adequate SNR across much of frequency range, and for CEOAEs, if whole-wave reproducibility is less than 50%. (*Note*: Because SNR can be improved with additional averaging, an absent OAE is only absent under the conditions of any particular test. That is, an "absent" OAE could become "present" if adequate SNR is achieved under alternative conditions (i.e., if more recording and averaging were conducted). As long as the test conditions were good and the middle ear healthy, an absent OAE can be associated with hearing loss of at least mild degree. Anecdotal comments from clinicians as well as a handful of research studies have shown that CEOAEs are more sensitive to slight and mild degrees of hearing loss than DPOAEs, which can be present even with mild-moderate sensory/neural hearing loss (Gorga et al., 1993; Lapsley-Miller et al., 2004). Combined with a good case history, clinicians can make some preliminary judgment about the severity of the hearing impairment. For example, an absent CEOAE combined with a present DPOAE might suggest mild (versus severe) sensory/neural hearing loss. An absent OAE result prompts additional testing to estimate hearing thresholds (e.g., ABR, conditioned play audiometry, etc.).

An OAE can be absent due to noncochlear factors such as a poor or unstable probe fit, which is common in restless infants and children, excessive room noise, or conductive problems. Therefore, this outcome cannot be reliably associated with hearing loss, and diagnostic follow-up should probably not be initiated based only on an unreliable OAE evaluation. If a clinician is lacking experience to judge the quality of an

OAE session adequately and distinguish between these two OAE "absent" outcomes, several indices can help such as the level of the noise floor (too high?), the number of rejected sweeps (too many?), the stability of the probe fit (changing throughout?), and the time elapsed during the test (too long?).

Normal OAE

An OAE is considered present if SNR is adequate; however, a present OAE should be further categorized as normal or abnormal. Normal indicates that SNR exceeded minimum criteria for most frequencies or frequency bands tested (an OAE is often not measurable at one frequency, especially in the low frequencies for children with elevated noise floors), and OAE levels were well within or at the high end of normative values for a pediatric population. Figures 20–9 and 20–10 illustrate normal CEOAE and DPOAE responses. The normal OAE is nonequivocal and can be associated with healthy cochlear function and good hearing except when an auditory-neural deficit is present.

Abnormal OAE

An OAE can be present because it meets SNR criteria, but its level does not conform to normative values. For example, a normal-hearing 6-month-old infant typically has robust DPOAE levels falling between 5 and 20 dB SPL; whereas a normal-hearing middle-aged adult can easily show OAE levels between −2 and 10 dB SPL and reduced (or absent) responses in the high-frequency range. Recognizing an abnormal-though-present OAE requires familiarity with normative ranges of OAE levels for different age groups (see Prieve, Fitzgerald, & Schulte, 1997; Prieve, Fitzgerald, Schulte, & Kemp, 1997 for children up to 17 years of age; and Abdala et al., 2008, Abdala & Dhar, 2012, for newborns). This familiarity will allow the tester to recognize that an infant or child (with healthy middle ear function) manifesting low-level OAEs is an abnormal outcome even if SNR is well within criteria. Figure 20–11 shows an abnormal DP-gram recorded from a school-aged child later confirmed to have mild-moderate sensory/neural hearing loss.

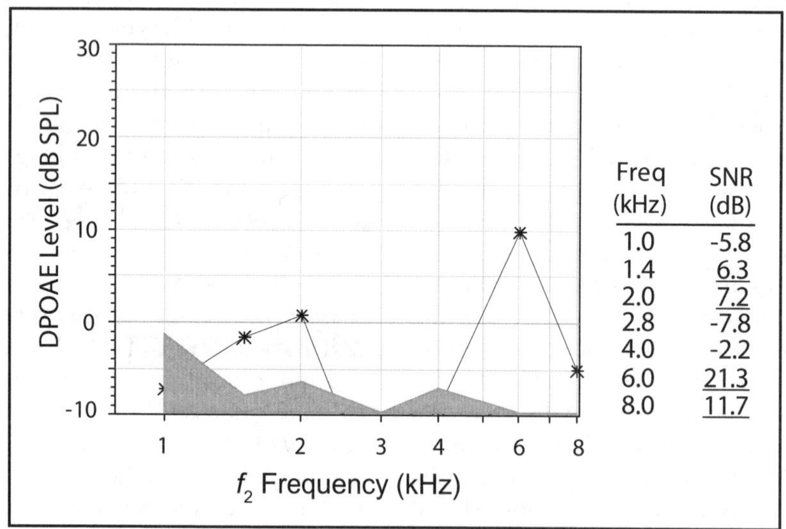

Freq (kHz)	SNR (dB)
1.0	-5.8
1.4	6.3
2.0	7.2
2.8	-7.8
4.0	-2.2
6.0	21.3
8.0	11.7

FIGURE 20–11. A DP-gram recorded with default stimulus parameters (L_1, L_2 = 65,55 dB SPL; f_2/f_1 = 1.22) in the left ear of a 9-year-old-boy. The gray area represents the noise floor. The right ear (not shown) has absent distortion product otoacoustic emissions (DPOAEs), but this ear shows low-level responses at four of seven test frequencies (see signal-to-noise-ratio [SNR] table to the right of the DP-gram; underlined numbers indicate a present DPOAE). The DPOAE is clearly present but is reduced in level and not measurable across the entire range of test frequencies. This young patient has a mild-moderate sensory/neural hearing loss in the left ear.

A second type of abnormal OAE outcome is a present response but only in a restricted frequency region. The OAE might be present from 2000 to 3000 Hz only, for example, indicating functional outer hair cells in the midfrequency region of the cochlea but perhaps not elsewhere. Although this result suggests a hearing loss with a trough-like audiometric configuration, the finding should prompt further testing. Familiarity with typical OAE levels and spectra from various age groups is helpful in recognizing when a present OAE is abnormal. A low-amplitude OAE might be the best indicator of mild hearing loss.

Other OAE Applications

OAEs and Newborn Hearing Screening

The objective of neonatal hearing screening differs from the objective of diagnosis and characterization of hearing loss. Screening is conducted to identify suspected hearing loss and not to confirm its presence or describe it. All 50 states mandate universal newborn hearing screening. The Joint Committee on Infant Hearing (JCIH) endorses goals that have become known as 1-3-6—screening by 1 month of age, appropriate audiologic and medical interventions before 3 months of age, and provision of appropriate interdisciplinary services by 6 months of age (JCIH, 2000). In the development of screening protocols, programs must be effective, affordable (considering equipment cost, personnel, administration, and pass-fail rates), implementable prior to hospital discharge and categorical, preferably using automated pass-refer criteria.

The typical OAE screening protocol is abbreviated and often automated to provide rapid testing and meet these mandates. Abbreviation is achieved in various ways. The OAE is recorded at only one stimulus level, or for CEOAEs, the time segment sampled poststimulus is shortened (to 12 ms, for example, from 20 ms), a fixed number of limited trials is recorded, and an automated pass-fail SNR criterion is applied. A DPOAE-based screening protocol might include testing at f_2 frequencies of 2000 and 4000 Hz only. The OAE screen is typically performed by a tester who is not a hearing specialist, thus necessitating an automated pass-refer outcome typically based on SNR values. By making the test short, simple, and rigid, testing time is minimized (but so are the potential benefits of tester expertise).

A large-scale, nationwide study involving seven research laboratories and data collection on nearly 5,000 newborns, the vast majority from neonatal intensive care units (NICU), compared the diagnostic performance of three tests for neonatal hearing screening: CEOAEs, DPOAEs, and ABR (Norton et al., 2000). DPOAEs were recorded at two levels: L_1, L_2 = 65, 55 dB SPL and 75, 75 dB SPL, while CEOAEs were recorded at 80 dB pSPL. Overall fail or "refer" rates were less than 4%, which is well within the stated goal of the JCIH (2000). All newborns screened with these three procedures were subsequently seen for behavioral audiological testing between the ages of 8 and 12 months. This follow-up provided the "gold standard" against which to assess the performance of each test.

Though performance was of course dependent on the specific testing parameters and criteria, overall the three screening procedures performed similarly as predictors of hearing at 2000 and 4000 Hz, with less accurate predictions by OAE tests at 1000 Hz. This was attributed to acoustic room noise. Overall, hit rates for all three tests were better than 80% when hearing loss was defined as audiometric thresholds greater than 30 dB HL. The DPOAEs recorded with 75 dB SPL provided slightly poorer detection of mild hearing loss compared to either moderate-level DPOAEs or CEOAEs. This finding is consistent with the notion that DPOAEs recorded at higher primary tone levels can be present with mild-moderate degrees of hearing loss (Whitehead, Stagner, McCoy, Lonsbury-Martin, & Martin, 1995). The sensitivity of OAEs was poorer for slight losses, but when the hearing impairment was severe, near 100% performance accuracy was achieved in detecting hearing loss.

One advantage of using an OAE procedure over ABR as a screening tool is that it is usually less expensive, does not require electrode application, is rapid to implement, and is generally effective in differentiating ears with normal hearing from those with hearing loss (Harrison & Norton, 1999; Lonsbury-Martin & Martin, 1990). However, there are some limitations. Babies screened via OAE in the first hours of life can have amniotic fluid or vernix in their ear canals that can impede the stimulus evoking the OAE and the measurement of the OAE at the ear canal microphone (Doyle et al., 1997). Most screening programs try to screen newborns as close to discharge as possible to allow this debris and fluid to resolve. Additionally, OAEs miss auditory-neural deficits because they are preneural indicators of cochlear health. The JCIH, therefore, mandates that high-risk newborns (i.e., those that have spent time in the NICU) must be screened with the ABR because they are at greater risk for neural dysfunction.

OAEs and Auditory Neuropathy

Individuals with auditory neuropathy show preserved cochlear receptor function combined with an impaired auditory nerve, IHC, or IHC-auditory nerve fiber synapse. The still poorly understood pathophysiology is thought to variously involve primary demyelization, postsynaptic axonal disease (Sininger & Starr, 2001; Starr et al., 2004), or gene mutations including the otoferlin gene (*OTOF, DFNB9*), which causes presynaptic dysfunction at the IHC synapse (Rodriguez-Ballesteros et al., 2003; Delmaghani et al., 2006). There are currently no clinical assessments that distinguish among the possible sites of lesion. Auditory neuropathy has more recently been termed *auditory neuropathy spectrum disorder* (ANSD) because of its multiple and mostly unknown etiologies.

In the pediatric population, significant risk factors for ANSD include low birth weight and prematurity, hyperbilirubinemia (especially when blood exchange transfusions are required), family history of ANSD or sensory motor neuropathies, and conditions such as Charcot-Marie-Tooth syndrome and Friedreich's ataxia (JCIH, 2007; Rance et al., 2008, 2012). Graduates of the NICU are particularly at risk for ANSD.

Clinically, a child with ANSD manifests with present OAEs (sometimes robust, sometimes reduced in level and spectral content), present cochlear microphonics, absent or grossly abnormal ABR, absent acoustic reflexes, and reduced medial olivocochlear reflexes, which traverse a descending brainstem pathway to the cochlea (Berlin, Morlet, & Hood, 2003; Starr et al., 1991; Starr, Picton, Sininger, Hood, & Berlin, 1996). Although the OAE might unaccountably disappear over time in patients with ANSD, the cochlear microphonic typically remains (Abdala, Sininger, & Starr, 2000; Deltenre et al., 1999; Starr et al., 2001; Starr et al., 1996). It is essential to recognize that the presence of OAEs upon early assessment and diagnosis of ANSD and their subsequent absence does not mean the pathology has resolved into a more conventional sensory/neural hearing loss. Combined with the ABR, OAEs form a critical component of the diagnostic battery by confirming a functional auditory periphery.

OAEs and Ototoxic Monitoring

Infants and young children might need to receive medical interventions that are toxic to the cochlea such as aminoglycoside antibiotics, platinum-based chemotherapeutic agents, and hemodialysis treatments. Hearing across the range of speech frequencies can be damaged by these ototoxins, though rarely after only one treatment (Bitner-Glindzicz & Rahman, 2007; Gooi, Hochman, Wellman, Blakley, & Blakley, 2008); the damage usually occurs over a period of time (Stavroulaki et al., 1999) and in some cases the onset of hearing loss is delayed for days or weeks after drug administration has begun (Beaubien et al., 1990). Monitoring the auditory status of children over the course of treatment can inform both choice of treatment and dosages, with the goal of preserving hearing in the speech frequencies and, where preservation is not possible, by facilitating early intervention through amplification and (re)habilitation.

Pediatric patients are more likely to develop hearing loss from some ototoxic agents than adults (Coradini, Cigana, Selistre, Rosito, & Brunetto, 2007; Li, Womer, & Silber, 2004). Detection of ototoxic hearing loss and early intervention are especially critical in the pediatric population because children are still developing speech and language skills. However, not all sick children can be tested behaviorally. Also, standard audiometry is not always sensitive to ototoxicity that affects cochlear function in the base first with initial signs appearing at frequencies above 8000 Hz (Blakley & Myers, 1993; Brock et al., 2012; Dreschler, Tange, & Urbanus, 1985; Fausti, Schechter, Rappaport, Frey, & Mass, 1984; Kopelman, Budnick, Sessions, Kramer, & Wong, 1988; Macdonald, Harrison, Wake, Bliss, & Macdonald, 1994). Much attention has been given to effective monitoring procedures that do not require a behavioral response. The ABR is one such procedure but might require the patient be sedated. OAE testing typically takes less time and can usually be performed even if the patient is awake as long as movement is minimized. Because natural test-retest reliability of OAE levels is generally good (Dreisbach, Long, & Lees, 2006; Franklin et al., 1992), changes due to otoxicity can often be differentiated from natural variations. Test-retest variations average ~3 dB for standard frequencies and ~5 dB for high frequencies above 8000 Hz (Dreisbach et al., 2006).

Both CEOAEs and DPOAEs are reduced in subjects receiving aminoglycoside antibiotics (Hotz, Harris, & Probst, 1994; Mulheran and Degg, 1997; Stavroulaki et al., 1999) and cisplatin for cancers (Lonsbury-Martin and Martin, 2001; Reavis et al., 2011; Ress et al., 1999). DPOAEs appear to show ototoxic effects earliest, possibly because they are more effectively measured at high frequencies than CEOAEs (Lonsbury-Martin & Martin, 2001). Also, in cases where mild sensory/neural loss preexists treatment, DPOAEs might be measureable at baseline, while CEOAEs might not (Norton, 1992;

Probst, Lonsbury-Martin, & Martin, 1991). Unfortunately, standard clinical instrumentation does not currently measure DPOAEs at ultrahigh frequencies.

Universal standards do not exist to determine significant OAE changes reflecting ototoxicity. As noted in Shera and Abdala (2012), conducting carefully controlled studies of the effectiveness of OAEs in monitoring ototoxicity, as well as determining criteria for significant change, can be problematic given that treatments and dosages are selected specifically for sick patients not for the purpose of a research protocol. Research (though most of it conducted in adults) as well as clinical practice suggest that DPOAEs in particular show promise as an effective monitoring tool for ototoxicity in children (Reavis et al., 2011). As is the case for diagnostic testing in general, OAEs are best used as one part of a more extensive battery of assessments whenever possible.

An Updated Approach

The conventional application of OAEs in the pediatric audiology clinic has been fruitful over the years as our above review of research and practice indicates. Here we offer some food for thought based on an updated understanding of the distinct and somewhat independent generation processes responsible for reflection and distortion emissions. Our objective is to consider how diagnostic information offered by OAEs might be exploited to the fullest extent in the pediatric audiology clinic.

Consider Recording Both CEOAEs and DPOAEs

We understand CEOAEs and DPOAEs to have independent mechanisms of generation. They are not identical markers of the same cochlear properties as initially thought. Recall that reflection emissions (e.g., CEOAEs and SFOAEs) are optimally generated by low-level sound and are produced by a reflection process occurring near the peak of traveling waves in the cochlea. This makes them sensitive to health of the cochlear amplifier, which is most active in this peak region, and consequently more sensitive to slight degrees of hearing loss. Distortion OAEs, such as the DPOAE, are best evoked by moderate-to-high-level sound and gauge cochlear nonlinearity. Some studies suggest that CEOAEs and DPOAEs have different sensitivities to hearing loss (Gorga et al., 1993; Lapsley-Miller et al., 2004), but this question requires more concentrated study.

We offer two good reasons to record both OAEs together when possible. First, consider our current ability to detect ANSD from a once paradoxical profile of results. Before OAEs were standard in the audiology clinic, it was perplexing to see absent ABRs coexisting with mild or only moderately elevated audiometric thresholds. By including an OAE, the enigma was resolved. Likewise, using a combination of CEOAEs and DPOAEs together could reveal other auditory pathologies with atypical profiles. In fact, deafness genes that present such atypical profiles and produce seemingly independent effects on reflection and distortion OAEs have been discovered (Cheatham et al., 2014; Goodyear & Richardson, 2002; Verpy et al., 2001). One such deafness gene is presented as a case study in a later section of this chapter.

Second (and perhaps the best reason for using both OAEs), CEOAEs disappear with slight-mild SNHL while DPOAEs can persist and are sometimes measured even with moderate amounts of sensory/neural hearing loss (especially if clinicians consider increasing primary tone levels for DPOAEs). By using both OAEs together, a clinician might get an outcome that helps differentiate between a mild sensory/neural hearing loss and a more severe one. With only an absent CEOAE, the audiologist knows there is some degree of hearing loss but cannot estimate the degree. However, if the ear has absent CEOAEs and present DPOAEs, it indicates that the cochlea is still able to generate nonlinearities even though the most sensitive part of the hearing range is lost. This outcome makes it more likely that the hearing loss is not severe.

Consider Using Higher Stimulus Levels for DPOAEs

If the DPOAE is not measurable at the standard moderate levels applied in clinic (50, 60, 65 dB SPL), the audiologist should consider presenting higher levels. Record the DPOAE with primary tone levels of 70 or 75 dB SPL. If time allows, the clinician might even record an abbreviated DPOAE input/output (I/O) function at one or more f_2 frequencies. To record an I/O function, the DPOAE is measured at one frequency for a series of stimulus levels. Figure 20–12 displays one such I/O function and shows that DPOAE response can continue to grow at primary tone levels beyond standard clinical levels (see asterisks). Therefore, increasing primary-tone levels will often increase the chance of measuring

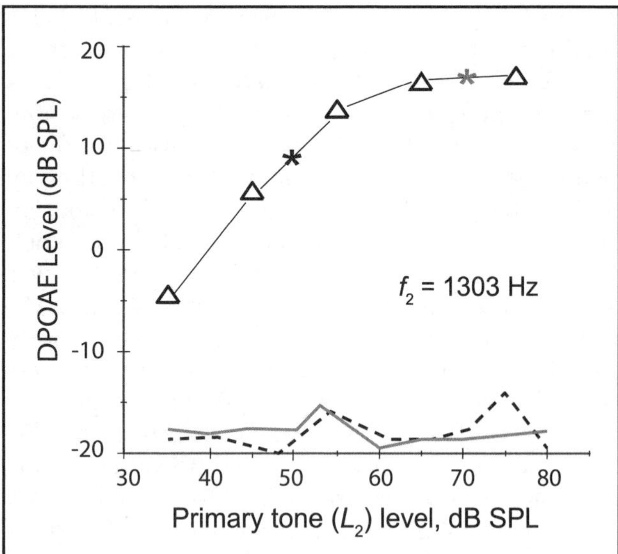

FIGURE 20–12. A distortion product otoacoustic emission (DPOAE) input/output (I/O) function in a normal-hearing ear. DPOAE amplitude is plotted as a function of primary tone level for one pair of stimulus frequencies (f_2 = 1303 Hz, f_1 = 1068 Hz). The solid and dashed lines represent the mean noise floor and system distortion. Note that for L_2 = 50 dB SPL (black asterisk re: *x*-axis), the DPOAE is approximately 10 dB SPL. When primary tone levels are presented 20 dB higher (gray asterisk re: *x*-axis), the DPOAE increases by about 7 dB, providing evidence of continued response growth beyond stimulus levels typically applied in the audiology clinic.

a DPOAE above the noise floor and a response that is well within the saturated portion of the dynamic range, which is where nonlinearities live. From the preceding paragraphs we understand that a measurable DPOAE, combined with a nonmeasurable CEOAE, might help us distinguish a mild from a more severe hearing loss.

Here we bring up an important concept. We wish to exploit the natural features and distinct diagnostic potential of each OAE. DPOAEs are best measured at higher levels where nonlinearity occurs, and where the distortion component of the DPOAE mixture dominates the recording. Recall that these two emission types do not come from a common generation process, and likely do not gauge the same underlying cochlear properties. Audiologists do not use the same stimulus to evoke both ABRs and behavioral audiograms, although both tests share the objective of determining auditory threshold. The stimulus used for each test is that which optimally evokes the target response and makes it most diagnostic. Why use low-to-moderate stimulus levels for both DPOAEs and CEOAEs when they each reflect different segments of our dynamic range of hearing?

A potential complication of using higher-level primary tones to elicit DPOAEs is that system-generated (versus ear-generated) distortion can become prominent. All OAE recording systems generate distortion at high enough levels. However, this type of equipment-related distortion can be measured by inserting the probe microphone in a coupler, which simulates the characteristics of the human ear canal, and running an OAE test. Because there is no biologically active component involved, the levels recorded at the microphone define distortion produced by instrumentation. Figure 20–12 displays a DPOAE I/O function and measured system distortion (gray line) as well as noise floor (dashed line). In this example, the system distortion is always at or below the noise floor.

Test Across a Broad Frequency Range

Diagnostic CEOAE tests sometimes restrict the time span of the recording epoch, and this accelerates testing. However, the range of frequencies tested is likewise restricted. Abbreviated DP-grams sometimes include only two f_1, f_2 frequency pairs (at 2000 and 4000 Hz, for example), again to save time. However, these abbreviated diagnostic protocols might not optimally inform (re)habilitation. Hints as to the configuration of the hearing loss, if present, will be derived from recording as broad a frequency range as possible.

Move Beyond Categorical "Absent" and "Present" Labels

If a patient shows a present OAE, as determined by reaching criterion SNR across a broad enough frequency spectrum, it provides important information; however, this is only a partial answer to the diagnostic question at hand. Presence or absence of the OAE can be determined by the separation between response and the noise floor (i.e., SNR) as described in the section on OAE interpretation. However, an OAE can be present and still abnormally low in level or restricted to an abbreviated frequency range. The low-level OAE can be signaling a mild hearing loss. Improving the detection of slight and mild hearing loss appears to be a realistic goal for OAEs. If one is satisfied with a simple categorical determination, there is a greater chance of missing mild hearing losses.

A Futuristic Goal: Consider Exploring OAE Phase as an Indicator of Cochlear Status

Emission abnormalities can occur in magnitude and phase, sometimes independently (Voss et al., 2010). They tell us different things about the emission. It is best to consider and measure both when designing and interpreting experiments and eventually, when conducting audiological evaluations. Analyzing possible changes along both magnitude and time coordinates can increase the sensitivity of the measurements. Also, SFOAE delays have been shown to be associated with cochlear frequency tuning, which might one day provide diagnostic clues to guide intervention. At present, the reality is that commercial systems do not allow for the accurate measurement of OAE phase or delay, and more studies are needed to link these measures to auditory health and pathology so as to confirm diagnostic value.

These five considerations have emerged from the OAE research and rely on important scientific concepts about how OAEs are generated in the cochlea. We recognize, of course, that implementing these guidelines can be impractical or unnecessary in many clinical situations. Test time with patients is limited and costly, and the implementation of these (or any other) protocols will vary from patient to patient at the discretion of the audiologist. However, when deciding whether the potential diagnostic gain might outweigh the time expenditure, an understanding of the concepts upon which these considerations are based is vitally important.

Case Studies

Here we present two case studies to illustrate application of an updated approach to OAE testing in the pediatric audiology clinic. One fictional case presents a rare form of deafness originally characterized in a genetically modified mouse but subsequently identified in humans. The second study describes an authentic clinical case involving hearing diagnosis with an infant.

A Mouse Case Study

The stereocilin protein is found almost exclusively in the hair bundle of cochlear sensory cells and specifically in the lateral links that join the stereocilia. These links allow the hair bundle to move in a coordinated fashion. When absent, the efficiency of the OHC as an agent of cochlear amplification and the effective coupling of OHC activity to IHCs, which are responsible for sending the auditory message upstream, are compromised. A genetic mutation resulting in the deletion of the stereocilin (STRC) protein produces nonsyndromic recessive sensory/neural hearing loss that has been traced to the human gene locus, *DFNB16* (Bitner-Glindzicz, 2002; Verpy et al., 2001, 2008).

The STRC mutation initially affects the nonlinearity of the cochlea then progresses to impact cochlear sensitivity and frequency tuning as well. Two-week-old mice have no DPOAEs or simultaneous masking, which is another hallmark of nonlinearity in the cochlea (i.e., if two sounds are presented simultaneously and are close enough in frequency, one can suppress the responsiveness of the cochlea to the other). Nevertheless, these mice show near normal compound action potential (CAP) thresholds and normal tuning. The effects of the mutation are progressive, and in the first two months of mouse life, thresholds are reduced by nearly 60 dB and cochlear frequency tuning becomes abnormally broadened.

Indulging in a thought experiment, what might we have seen if CEOAEs had been measured in these STRC mutant mice along with DPOAEs? Recall that CEOAEs do not necessarily require cochlear nonlinearity like DPOAEs do because they are generated by linear reflections and backscattering of wavelets. The normal tuning and sensitivity in the young STRC mouse suggest CEOAEs might have been present if measured in this mouse even though DPOAEs were absent. This cochlear deficit might be unlike any previously observed in the audiology clinic. Or is it? Given that a human analog of this genetic mutation exists, it is likely that audiologists have unwittingly encountered patients with this genetic complement (and odd OAE profile). Will clinicians be able to identify this deafness-related mutation using the current default OAE protocol? Perhaps we can answer this question by walking through a diagnosis for a fictional newborn with an STRC mutation.

Scenario 1

Baby boy Linkless is brought into the audiology clinic after failing a DPOAE hearing screening in the hospital. An ABR is conducted, and normal to near-normal thresholds are obtained. The diligent audiologist conducts a CEOAE test next, and they are present in both ears; therefore, she decides not to record DPOAEs. After all, the ABR is normal and CEOAEs are present, which suggests normal hearing. She believes the failed hearing screening in the hospital was a false positive and decides there is a high likelihood of normal hearing. She sends the family on their way.

One year later, Linkless develops normally in all other ways while the STRC deletion manifests its progressive effect on the cochlea. The parents bring him back to the audiology clinic just before his first birthday because he has stopped babbling and does not seem to startle anymore when pots crash to the floor at home. An audiological evaluation is scheduled. ABR thresholds are observed at 70 dB HL, and both CEOAEs and DPOAEs are absent. The child receives his initial (and unfortunately delayed) diagnosis of severe sensory/neural hearing loss at 1 year of age. There has been no preparation, no re(habilitation), and no warning to the family. At this point, the family is unaware of the gene mutation that produced the hearing loss, but a DNA test and genetic counseling will inform them shortly.

Scenario 2 (1 Year Earlier)

Here we invoke the services of a nearby wormhole and engage in a bit of time travel (because this is only a thought experiment, wormholes are conveniently located.) We regress to the initial diagnostic session during the newborn period. The audiologist, after recording a normal or near-normal ABR and present CEOAEs also records DPOAEs at various primary-tone levels. They are not present even at the highest levels. Clearly, something is wrong, and the results seem inconsistent—present CEOAE and absent DPOAE. A genetic test is conducted, and the STRC deletion is definitively identified. This leads to genetic counseling, very close monitoring of hearing status, family education, and appropriate habilitation, all initiated in the first months of his life.

Conclusion

The STRC deletion manifests an absence of cochlear nonlinearity but near-normal cochlear amplifier function (tuning and sensitivity) at birth. Soon after birth, sensitivity and tuning also become degraded. The hallmark signature for this form of deafness in its early stages would be normal ABR thresholds and present CEOAEs, with absent DPOAEs (the CEOAE part is conjecture, because they have not been measured in the STRC mouse). If the clinician records only CEOAEs or only ABRs, this hearing disorder will not be detected at birth. This delay could impact the child's success with auditory prostheses as well as educational, social, and linguistic advances (Yoshinaga-Itano, 2003).

A Human Case Study

Session 1

An 11-month-old infant fails his hearing screening in the hospital. A follow-up diagnostic audiology evaluation is conducted to confirm or rule out hearing loss. The infant presents normal tympanograms suggesting healthy middle ear function. CEOAEs measured with an 84 dB pSPL click and DPOAEs recorded with L_1,L_2 = 65,55 dB SPL were absent as shown in Figure 20–13A and Figure 20–13B. Click and tone-burst evoked ABR thresholds (not shown) in the left ear were 70 to 80 dB HL indicating a severe hearing loss. In the right ear, ABR thresholds were near normal at for low-frequency tone bursts, sloping to severe for high-frequency stimuli.

The astute audiologist, understanding that DPOAE level increases with increasing primary tone levels (and understanding why it might be important to detect a DPOAE with absent CEOAEs), decides to present one additional pair of primary tones at a higher level, 75,75 dB SPL. DPOAEs at these levels were present below 1400 Hz in the right ear, the same frequency region where ABR thresholds were also found to be near normal in the right ear (Figure 20–13C). Increasing primary-tone level provided additional information about this hearing loss: DPOAEs at low-mid frequencies are present, and CEOAEs are absent. Recording DPOAEs across a broad frequency range was also crucial in this case because an abbreviated DP-gram might have missed the functional regions of the cochlea below 1500 Hz.

Case Review

The right ear has a mild sloping to moderate severe loss. Let us consider the diagnosis in the absence of an ABR (perhaps the ABR schedule was full and the child had to wait 2 months for an appointment; or an ABR was attempted but sedation failed). What do we know from OAE results alone? The DPOAE (nonlinear distortion) is measurable at low frequencies, but the CEOAE is absent. This pairing should not come as a surprise given what we understand about the differences in CEOAEs and DPOAEs and their sensitivities. The DPOAE energy below 1400 Hz informs the audiologist that this child is not deaf in the right ear. The presence of a DPOAE suggests the ear is behaving nonlinearly, something an ear with profound sensory hearing loss is not expected to do. The measurable DPOAE in this case might guide the clinician's initial choice of an

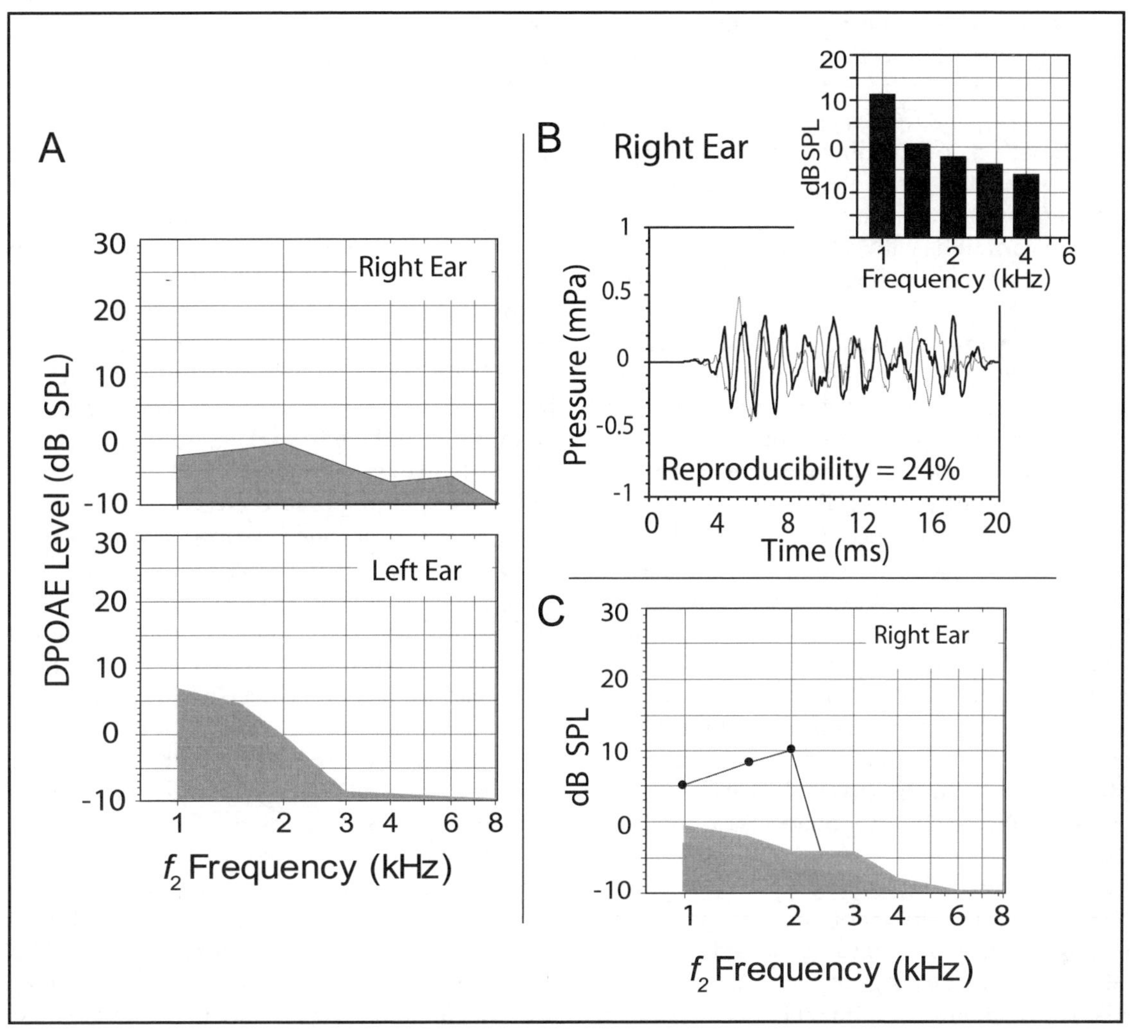

FIGURE 20–13. A. DP-grams recorded during an initial test session using default primary tone levels of L_1, L_2 = 65,55 dB SPL. The gray area represents the noise floor. The distortion product otoacoustic emission (DPOAE) is absent in both ears; **B.** Click-evoked otoacoustic emission (CEOAE) results recorded during the first test session (click = 84 dB pSPL). The CEOAE is absent in both ears although only one ear is shown. **C.** DP-gram recorded during the second test session in the right ear, applying higher than typical primary-tone levels (L_1, L_2 = 75, 75 dB SPL). Panel C shows measurable DPOAEs with normal response amplitude for frequencies below 2000 Hz. This DPOAE finding matches the normal auditory brainstem response (ABR) thresholds detected in the low-frequency range.

appropriately conservative hearing aid until the ABR is completed; it might also allow for some informative, though tempered counseling. Results suggest a sloping high-frequency loss with normal or near-normal hearing in the low frequencies. Had primary-tone levels not been increased while recording DPOAEs, this diagnosis would have remained murky for longer.

Future Advances and Conclusions

Although there has been much progress in OAE measurement over the years, many of the newest technical advances have yet to work their way into commercial instrumentation. For example, new calibration methods that allow much improved control over the stimulus levels presented to the ear at high frequencies are now available (for a recent summary see Souza, Dhar, Neely, & Siegel, 2014). These methods work by mitigating the effects of standing waves that form in the ear canal when the incident sound reflects off the tympanic membrane. Because standing waves create large pressure variations within the ear canal, they can seriously confound conventional, in-the-ear calibration procedures.

As another example, some of our laboratories no longer record DPOAEs using tones or pairs of tones presented at discrete frequencies. Rather, we present tones whose frequency varies continuously to cover the test frequency range rapidly allowing for more averaging and consequently better SNR as well as much improved frequency resolution (Abdala et al., 2009; Abdala & Dhar, 2010, 2012; Abdala et al., 2015; Kalluri & Shera, 2013; Long et al., 2008). These "swept-tone" protocols produce OAEs that are basically the same as conventional OAEs but their measurement is more efficient. Many of the parameters for swept-tone OAE recording have been defined in adults and infants but more research is needed to describe the most effective protocols and optimal analysis strategies (Abdala, Luo, & Shera, in press; Kalluri & Shera, 2013; Long, Talmadge, & Lee, 2008).

As a result of the added efficiency and speed provided by swept tones, OAEs not yet characterized for clinical application can now be studied and defined in normal-hearing and hearing-impaired subjects. The SFOAE is one such emission. It is the most direct and simple of the reflection-type OAEs because it is generated with one low-level pure tone. However, it is a low-level emission and has been difficult to measure using conventional techniques. Using a swept tone, we are able to average hundreds of individual observations rapidly to achieve excellent SNR (Abdala & Kalluri, 2015). SFOAEs are now being studied in newborns using swept-tone methods to determine their feasibility as a diagnostic tool. Integration of the SFOAE into the audiology clinic might improve the detection of slight and mild losses, which can impact academic success in school-aged children (Bess, Dodd-Murphy, & Parker, 1998).

Another clinical advance might be the separation of dual components of the DPOAE during an evaluation. The reader now understands the DPOAE to be a mixture of distortion energy generated around the overlap of the two primary tones and energy reflected from the $2f_1$–f_2 place. To record a metric of cochlear nonlinear distortion, contributions arising from reflection can be removed using signal-processing techniques. These "unmixing" techniques are routinely employed in many research laboratories (Abdala et al., 2009; Abdala & Dhar, 2010, 2012; Long et al., 2008; Poling, Siegel, Lee, Lee, Dhar, 2014) but are not yet available in the clinic. At present, it is not clear that separated components are any more diagnostic for hearing loss than the total DPOAE (Johnson et al., 2007), but this question warrants more study. It has been shown that separating DPOAE components reduces the variability of the OAE (Mauermann & Kollmeir, 2004; Moore, Hood, & Hornsby, 2014; Ortmann & Abdala, 2015).

Finally, most audiologists are comfortable thinking about response magnitude. Amplitude or level is an intuitive and well-taught concept in audiology programs. However, phase, which is measured along the time axis, is more obscure. Research has characterized OAE phase in normal-hearing newborns and adults (Abdala & Dhar, 2010, 2012; Abdala, Dhar, & Mishra, 2011; Dhar, Rogers, & Abdala, 2011; Shera, Talmadge, & Tubis, 2000) but its clinical utility remains mostly untested. Recent work suggests that DPOAE level and phase can show different sensitivities to certain pathologies, and phase might provide a noninvasive assay of changes in intracranial pressure (Voss et al., 2010). At present clinical OAE systems do not allow for measures of emission phase or delay.

The cochlea houses an exquisite yet inaccessible sensory organ encased in some of the hardest bone in the body. Otoacoustic emissions provide the only preneural gauge of its function, offering audiologists a critical diagnostic window. This objective probe of cochlear function is especially important in infants and children where the assessment of hearing by behavioral methods can be elusive, and the consequences of hearing loss great. Clearly, OAEs form an important part of the pediatric audiology assessment battery. They offer diagnostic information not provided by other audiological tests, detect hearing loss with high accuracy, and as part of a larger battery, can offer clues about degree of loss and configuration. By applying updated knowledge and understanding of OAEs and how they come about in the cochlea, it is likely that audiologists can optimize these diagnostic clues. Exciting advances are on the horizon, which will make OAE testing in a pediatric population more efficient and likely extend their clinical utility in detecting, describing, and understanding hearing loss.

Acknowledgments. The preparation of this chapter was supported by Grant Nos. R01 DC003552 (CA) and R01 DC003687 (CAS) from the NIDCD, National Institutes of Health, and by the University of Southern California.

References

Abdala, C. (1996). Distortion product otoacoustic emission (2 f1-f2) amplitude as a function of f2/f1 frequency ratio and primary tone level separation in human adults and neonates. *Journal of the Acoustical Society of America, 100*(6), 3726–3740.

Abdala, C. (1998). A developmental study of distortion product otoacoustic emission ($2f_1$-f_2) suppression in humans. *Hearing Research, 121*, 125–138.

Abdala, C. (2003). A longitudinal study of distortion product otoacoustic emission ipsilateral suppression and input/output characteristics in human neonates. *Journal of the Acoustical Society of America, 114*, 3239–3250.

Abdala, C., & Dhar, S. (2010). Distortion product otoacoustic emission phase and component analysis in human newborns. *Journal of the Acoustical Society of America, 127*(1), 316–325.

Abdala, C., & Dhar, S. (2012). Maturation and aging of the human cochlea: A view through the DPOAE looking glass. *Journal of the Association for Research in Otolaryngology, 13*(3), 403–421.

Abdala, C., Dhar, S., & Kalluri, R. (2011). Level dependence of distortion product otoacoustic emission phase is attributed to component mixing. *Journal of the Acoustical Society of America, 129*, 3123–3133.

Abdala, C., Dhar, S., & Mishra, S. (2011). The breaking of cochlear scaling symmetry in human newborns and adults. *Journal of the Acoustical Society of America, 129*, 3104–3114.

Abdala, C., & Kalluri, R. (2015). Exploiting dual otoacoustic emission sources. In D. P. Corey & K. D. Karavitaki (Eds.), *Mechanics of hearing*. Melville, NY: American Institute of Physics. Manuscript in preparation.

Abdala, C., & Keefe, D. H. (2012). Morphological and functional development of the ear. In L. Werner, A. Popper, & R. Fay (Eds.), *Springer handbook of auditory research: Human auditory development* (pp. 19–60). New York, NY: Springer.

Abdala, C., Luo, P., & Shera, C. A. (in press). Optimizing swept-tone protocols for recording distortion product otoacoustic emissions in adults and newborns. *Journal of the Acoustical Society of America*.

Abdala, C., Mishra, S., & Williams, T. (2009). Considering distortion product otoacoustic emission fine structure in measurements of the medial olivocochlear reflex. *Journal of the Acoustical Society of America, 125*(3), 1584–1594.

Abdala, C., Oba, S. I., & Ramanathan, R. (2008). Changes in the DP-gram during the preterm and early-postnatal period. *Ear and Hearing, 29*, 512–523.

Abdala, C., Sininger, Y., & Starr, A. (2000). DPOAE suppression tuning in subjects with auditory neuropathy. *Ear and Hearing, 21*, 542–553.

Beaubien, A. R., Dejardins, S., Ormsby, E., Bayne, A., Carrie, K., Cauchy, J., . . . St. Pierre, A. (1990). Delay in hearing loss following drug administration. A consistent feature of amikacin ototoxicity. *Acta Oto-Laryngologica, 109*(5–6), 345–352.

Berlin, C. I., Morlet, T., & Hood, L. J. (2003). Auditory neuropathy/dys-synchrony: Its diagnosis and management. *Pediatric Clinics of North America, 50*(2), 331–340.

Bess, F. H., Dodd-Murphy, J., & Parker, R. A. (1998). Children with minimal sensorineural hearing loss: Prevalence, performance, and status. *Ear and Hearing, 19*(5), 339–354.

Bitner-Glindzicz, M. (2002). Hereditary deafness and phenotyping in humans. *British Medical Bulletin, 63*, 73–94.

Bitner-Glindzicz, M., & Rahman, S. (2007). Ototoxicity caused by aminoglycosides. *British Medical Journal, 335*(7624), 784–785.

Blakley, B. W., & Myers, S. F. (1993). Patterns of hearing loss resulting from cisplatinum therapy. *Otolaryngology-Head and Neck Surgery, 109*(3 Pt. 1), 385–391.

Boege, P., & Janssen, T. (2002). Pure-tone threshold estimation from extrapolated distortion product otoacoustic emission I/O-functions in normal and cochlear hearing loss ears. *Journal of the Acoustical Society of America, 111*(4), 1810–1818.

Bonfils, P., Avan, P., Francois, M., Trotoux, J., & Narcy, P. (1992). Distortion-product otoacoustic emissions in neonates: Normative data. *Acta Oto-Laryngologica, 112*, 739–744.

Bonfils, P., Uziel, A., & Narcy, P. (1989). The properties of spontaneous and evoked acoustic emissions in neonates and children: A preliminary report. *Archives of Oto-Rhino Laryngology, 246*, 249–251.

Bonfils, P., Uziel, R., & Pujol, R. (1988). Evoked oto-acoustic emissions from adults and infants: Clinical applications. *Acta Oto-Laryngologica, 105*, 445–449.

Bredberg, G. (1968). Cellular pattern and nerve supply of the human organ of Corti. *Acta Oto-Laryngologica Supplementum*, 236, 1.

Brock, P. R., Knight, K. R., Freyer, D. R., Campbell, K. C., Steyger, P. S., Blakley, B. W., . . . Neuwelt, E. A. (2012). Platinum-induced ototoxicity in children: A consensus review on mechanisms, predisposition, and protection, including a new International Society of Pediatric Oncology Boston ototoxicity scale. *Journal of Clinical Oncology, 30*(19), 2408–2417.

Brown, A. M., & Kemp, D. T. (1984). Suppressibility of the 2f1 - f2 stimulated acoustic emissions in gerbil and man. *Hearing Research, 13*, 29–37.

Burns, E. M., Arehart, K. H., & Campbell, S. L. (1992). Prevalence of spontaneous otoacoustic emissions in neonates. *Journal of the Acoustical Society of America, 91*, 1571–1575.

Cheatham, M. A., Goodyear, R. J., Homma, K., Legan, P. K., Korchagina, J., Naskar, S., . . . Richardson, G. P. (2014). Loss of the tectorial membrane protein CEACAM16 enhances spontaneous, stimulus-frequency, and transiently evoked otoacoustic emissions. *Journal of Neuroscience, 34*, 10325–10338.

Clark, J. G. (1981). The uses and abuses of hearing loss classification. *ASHA, 23*, 493–500.

Collet, L., Levy, V., Veuillet, E., Truy, E., & Morgon, A. (1993). Click-evoked otoacoustic emissions and hearing threshold in sensorineural hearing loss. *Ear and Hearing, 14*, 141–143.

Cooper, N., & Rhode, W. (1995). Nonlinear mechanisms at the apex of the guinea pig cochlea. *Hearing Research, 82*, 225–243.

Coradini, P. P., Cigana, L., Selistre, S. G., Rosito, L. S., & Brunetto, A. L. (2007). Ototoxicity from cisplatin therapy in childhood cancer. *Journal of Pediatric Hematology/Oncology, 29*(6), 355–360.

Cullington, H. E., Kumar, B. U., & Flood, L. M. (1998). Feasibility of otoacoustic emissions as a hearing screen following grommet insertion. *British Journal of Audiology, 32*(1), 57–62.

Daya, H., Hinton, A. E., Radomskiej, P., & Huchzermeyer, P. (1996). Otoacoustic emissions: Assessment of hearing after tympanostomy tube insertion. *Clinical Otolaryngology Allied Science, 21*(6), 492–494.

Deeter, R., Abel, R., Calandruccio, L., & Dhar, S. (2009). Contralateral stimulation alters the magnitude and phase of distortion product otoacoustic emissions. *Journal of the Acoustical Society of America, 126*(5), 2413–2424.

Delmaghani, S., del Castillo, F. J., Michel, V., Leibovici, M., Aghaie, A., Ron, U., . . . Petit, C. (2006). Mutations in the gene encoding pejvakin, a newly identified protein of the afferent auditory pathway, cause DFNB59 auditory neuropathy. *Nature Genetics, 38*(7), 770–778.

Deltenre, P., Mansbach, A. L., Bozet, C., Christiaens. F., Barthelemy, P., Paulissen, D., & Renglet, T. (1999). Auditory neuropathy with preserved cochlear microphonics and secondary loss of otoacoustic emissions. *Audiology, 38*(4), 187–195.

Dhar, S., Rogers, A., & Abdala, C. (2011). Breaking away: Violation of distortion emission phase invariance at low-frequencies. *Journal of the Acoustical Society of America, 129*, 3115–3122.

Dorn, P. A., Piskorski, P., Keefe, D. H., Neely, S. T., & Gorga, M. P. (1998). On the existence of an age/threshold/frequency interaction in distortion product otoacoustic emissions. *Journal of the Acoustical Society of America, 104*, 964–971.

Doyle, K. J., Burggraaff, B., Fujikawa, S., Kim, J., & MacArthur, C. J. (1997). Neonatal hearing screening with otoscopy, auditory brain stem response, and otoacoustic emissions.00 *Otolaryngology-Head and Neck Surgery, 116*(6 Pt. 1), 597–603.

Dreisbach, L. E., Long, L. M., & Lees, S. E. (2006). Repeatability of high-frequency distortion-product otoacoustic emissions in normal-hearing adults. *Ear and Hearing, 27*, 466–479.

Dreschler, W. A., Tange, R. A., & Urbanus, N. A. (1985). The role of high frequency audiometry in early detection of ototoxicity. *Audiology, 24*(6), 387–395.

Eby, T. L., & Nadol, J. B. Jr. (1986). Postnatal growth of the human temporal bone: Implications for cochlear implants in children. *Annals of Otology, Rhinology, and Laryngology, 95*, 356–364.

Ellison, J. C., & Keefe, D. H. (2005). Audiometric predictions using stimulus-frequency otoacoustic emissions and middle ear measurements. *Ear and Hearing, 26*, 487–503.

Fausti, S. A., Schechter, M. A., Rappaport, B. Z., Frey, R. H., & Mass, R. E. (1984). Early detection of cisplatin ototoxicity. Selected case reports. *Cancer, 53*(2), 224–231.

Franklin, D. J., McCoy, M. J., Martin, G. K., & Lonsbury-Martin, B. L. (1992). Test/retest reliability of distortion-product and transiently evoked otoacoustic emissions. *Ear and Hearing, 13*(6), 417–429.

Gaskill, S. A., & Brown, A. M. (1990). The behavior of the acoustic distortion product, 2 f_1–f_2, from the human ear and its relation to auditory sensitivity. *Journal of the Acoustical Society of America, 88*, 821–839.

Goodyear, R. J., & Richardson, G. P. (2002). Extracellular matrices associated with the apical surfaces of sensory epithelia in the inner ear: Molecular and structural diversity. *Developmental Neurobiology, 53*(2), 212–227.

Gooi, A., Hochman, J., Wellman, M., Blakley, L., & Blakley, B. W. (2008). Ototoxic effects of single-dose versus 19-day daily-dose gentamicin. *Journal of Otolaryngology-Head and Neck Surgery, 37*(5), 664–667.

Gorga, M. P., Dierking, D. M., Johnson, T. A., Beauchaine, K. L., Garner, C. A., & Neely, S. T. (2005). A validation and potential clinical application of multivariate analyses of distortion-product otoacoustic emission data. *Ear and Hearing, 26*(6), 593–607.

Gorga, M. P., Neely, S. T., Bergman, B., Beauchaine, K. L., Kaminski, J. R., Peters, J., & Jesteadt, W. (1993). Otoacoustic emissions from normal-hearing and hearing-impaired subjects: Distortion product responses. *Journal of the Acoustical Society of America, 93*(4), 2050–2060.

Gorga, M. P., Neely, S. T., Ohlrich, B., Hoover, B., Redner, J., & Peters, J. (1997). From laboratory to clinic: A large scale study of distortion product otoacoustic emissions in ears with normal hearing and ears with hearing loss. *Ear and Hearing, 18*(6), 440–445.

Gorga, M. P., Nelson, K., Davis, T., Dorn, P. A., & Neely, S. T. (2000). Distortion product otoacoustic emission test performance when both $2f_1$-f_2 and $2f_2$-f_1 are used to predict auditory status. *Journal of the Acoustical Society of America, 107*, 2128–2135.

Harris, F. P., Lonsbury-Martin, B. L., Stagner, B. B., Coats, A. C., & Martin, G. K. (1989). Acoustic distortion products in humans: Systematic changes in amplitude as a function of f2/f1 ratio. *Journal of the Acoustical Society of America, 85*, 220–229.

Harrison, W. A., & Norton, S. J. (1999). Characteristics of transient evoked otoacoustic emissions in normal-hearing and hearing-impaired children. *Ear and Hearing, 20*(1), 75–86.

Hotz, M. A., Harris, F. P., & Probst, R. (1994). Otoacoustic emissions: An approach for monitoring aminoglycoside-induced ototoxicity. *Laryngoscope, 104*(9), 1130–1134.

Hussain, D. M., Gorga, M. P., Neely, S. T., Keefe, D. H., & Peters, J. (1998). Transient evoked otoacoustic emissions in patients with normal hearing and in patients with hearing loss. *Ear and Hearing, 19*, 434–449.

Igarishi, Y. (1980). Cochlea of the human fetus: A scanning electron microscope study. *Archivum Histologicum Japonicum, 43*, 195–209.

Johnson, T. A., Neely, S. T., Kopun, J. G., Dierking, D. M., Tan, H., Converse, C., Kennedy, E., & Gorga, M. P. (2007). Distortion product otoacoustic emission: Cochlear source contributions and clinical test performance. *Journal of the Acoustical Society of America*, *122*, 3538–3553.

Johnson, T. A., Neely, S. T., Kopun, J. G., Dierking, D. M., Tan, H., & Gorga, M. P. (2010). Clinical test performance of distortion product otoacoustic emissions using new stimulus conditions. *Ear and Hearing*, *31*, 74–83.

Joint Committee on Infant Hearing. (2000). Position statement: Principles and guidelines for early hearing detection and intervention programs. *Pediatrics*, *106*(4), 898–921.

Joint Committee on Infant Hearing. (2007). Position statement: Principles and guidelines for early hearing detection and intervention programs. *Pediatrics*, *120*, 898–921.

Kalluri, R., & Abdala, C. (2015a). Stimulus-frequency otoacoustic emissions in human newborns. *Journal of the Acoustical Society of America*, *137*(1), EL78.

Kalluri, R., & Abdala, C. (2015b). *Defining the combined reflection-distortion (SFOAE-DPOAE) distribution in normal ears.* Paper presented at the 36th Midwinter Meeting of the Association for Research in Otolaryngology, Baltimore, MD.

Kalluri, R., & Shera, C. A. (2001). Distortion-product source unmixing: A test of the two-mechanism model for DPOAE generation. *Journal of the Acoustical Society of America*, *109*(2), 622–637.

Kalluri, R., & Shera, C. A. (2007). Near equivalence of human click-evoked and stimulus-frequency otoacoustic emissions. *Journal of the Acoustical Society of America*, *121*(4), 2097–2110.

Kalluri, R., & Shera, C. A. (2013). Measuring stimulus-frequency otoacoustic emissions using swept tones. *Journal of the Acoustical Society of America*, *134*(1), 356–368.

Kaltenbach, J. A., & Falzarano, P. R. (1994). Postnatal development of the hamster cochlea: I. Growth of hair cells and the organ of Corti. *Journal of Comparative Neurology*, *340*, 87–97.

Karavitaki, K. D., & Mountain, D. C. (2007). Evidence for outer hair cell driven oscillatory fluid flow in the tunnel of Corti. *Biophysical Journal*, *92*, 3284–3293.

Keefe, E., & Abdala, C. (2007). Theory of forward and reverse middle-ear transmission applied to otoacoustic emissions in infant and adult ears. *Journal of the Acoustical Society of America*, *121*(2), 978–993.

Kemp, D. T. (1978). Stimulated acoustic emissions from within the human auditory system. *Journal of the Acoustical Society of America*, *64*(5), 1386–1391.

Kemp, D. T. (1997). Otoacoustic emissions in perspective. In M. S. Robinette & T. J. Glattke (Eds.), *Otoacoustic emissions: Clinical applications* (pp. 1–21). New York, NY: Thieme.

Kemp, D. T., Bray, P., Alexander, L., & Brown, A. M. (1986). Otoacoustic emission cochleography—Practical aspects. *Scandinavian Audiology Supplementum*, *25*, 71–95.

Kemp, D. T., Ryan, S., & Bray, P. (1990). A guide to the effective use of otoacoustic emissions. *Ear and Hearing*, *11*, 93–105.

Kim, D. O. (1980). Cochlear mechanics: Implications of electrophysiological and acoustical observations. *Hearing Research*, *3*, 297–317.

Knight, R. D., & Kemp, D. T. (1999). Relationships between DPOAE and TEOAE amplitude and phase characteristics. *Journal of the Acoustical Society of America*, *106*, 1420–1435.

Knight, R. D., & Kemp, D. T. (2000). Indications of different distortion product otoacoustic emission mechanisms from a detailed f1,f2 area study. *Journal of the Acoustical Society of America*, *107*, 457–473.

Knight, R. D., & Kemp, D. T. (2001). Wave and place fixed DPOAE maps of the human ear. *Journal of the Acoustical Society of America*, *109*, 1513–1525.

Konrad-Martin, D., Neely, S. T., Keefe, D. H., Dorn, P. A., Cyr, E., & Gorga, M. P. (2002). Sources of DPOAEs revealed by suppression experiments, inverse fast Fourier transforms, and SFOAEs in impaired ears. *Journal of the Acoustical Society of America*, *111*, 1800–1809.

Kopelman, J., Budnick, A. S., Sessions, R. B., Kramer, M. B., & Wong, G. Y. (1988). Ototoxicity of high-dose cisplatin by bolus administration in patients with advanced cancers and normal hearing. *Laryngoscope*, *98*(8 Pt. 1), 858–864.

Kummer, P., Janssen, T., & Arnold, W. (1995). Suppression tuning characteristics of the distortion-product otoacoustic emission in humans. *Journal of the Acoustical Society of America*, *98*, 197–210.

Kummer, P., Janssen, T., & Arnold, W. (1998). The level and growth behavior of the 2f1-f2 distortion product otoacoustic emission and its relationship to auditory sensitivity in normal hearing and cochlear hearing loss. *Journal of the Acoustical Society of America*, *103*, 3431–3444.

Lapsley-Miller, J. A., Marshall, L., & Heller, L. M. (2004). A longitudinal study of changes in evoked otoacoustic emissions and pure-tone thresholds as measured in a hearing conservation program. *International Journal of Audiology*, *43*(6), 307–322.

Lasky, R. E., Perlman, J., & Hecox, K. (1992). Distortion-product otoacoustic emissions in human newborns and adults. *Ear and Hearing*, *13*, 430–441.

Lavigne-Rebillard, M., & Pujol, R. (1986). Development of the auditory hair cell surface in human fetuses. A scanning electron microscopy study. *Anatomy and Embryology*, *174*, 369–377.

Lavigne-Rebillard, M., & Pujol, R. (1990). Auditory hair cells in human fetuses: Synaptogenesis and ciliogenesis. *Journal of Electron Microscopy Technique*, *15*, 115–122.

Li, Y., Womer, R. B., & Silber, J. H. (2004). Predicting cisplatin ototoxicity in children: The influence of age and the cumulative dose. *European Journal of Cancer*, *40*(16), 2445–2451.

Lim, D. J., & Rueda, J. (1992). Structural development of the cochlea. In Romand, R. (Ed.), *Development of the auditory and vestibular systems 2* (pp. 33–58). Amsterdam, the Netherlands: Elsevier.

Long, G. R., Talmadge, C. L., & Lee, J. (2008). Measuring distortion product otoacoustic emissions using continuously sweeping primaries. *Journal of the Acoustical Society of America*, *124*(3), 1613–1626.

Lonsbury-Martin, B., Harris, F., Hawkins, M., Stagner, B., & Martin, G. (1990). Distortion product otoacoustic emissions in humans: I. Basic properties in normal-hearing subjects. *Annals of Otology, Rhinology & Laryngology Supplementum, 147*, 3–14.

Lonsbury-Martin, B., & Martin, G. (1990). The clinical utility of distortion-product otoacoustic emissions. *Ear and Hearing, 11*(2),144–154.

Lonsbury-Martin, B. L., & Martin, G. K. (2001). Evoked otoacoustic emissions as objective screeners for oto-toxicity. *Seminars in Hearing, 22*(4), 377–391.

Lonsbury-Martin, B. L., Martin, G. K., McCoy, M. J., & Whitehead, M. S. (1994). Otoacoustic emissions testing in young children; Middle-ear influences. *American Journal of Otology, 15*(Suppl. 1), 13–20.

Macdonald, M. R., Harrison, R. V., Wake, M., Bliss, B., & Macdonald, R. E. (1994). Ototoxicity of carboplatin: Comparing animal and clinical models at the Hospital for Sick Children. *Journal of Otolaryngology, 23*(3), 151–159.

Martin, G. K., Lonsbury-Martin, B. L., Probst, R., Scheinin, S. A., & Coats, A. C. (1987). Acoustic distortion products in rabbit ear canal. II. Sites of origin revealed by suppression contours and pure tone exposures. *Hearing Research, 29*, 191–208.

Martin, G. K., Probst, R., & Lonsbury-Martin, B. L. (1990). Otoacoustic emissions in human ears: Normative findings. *Ear and Hearing, 11*, 121–127.

Mauermann, M., & Kollmeier, B. (2004). Distortion product otoacoustic emission (DPOAE) input/output functions and the influence of the second DPOAE source. *Journal of the Acoustical Society of America, 116*, 2199–2212.

Mauermann, M., Uppenkamp, S., van Hengel, P. W. J., & Kollmeier, B. (1999). Evidence for the distortion product frequency place as a source of distortion product otoacoustic emission (DPOAE) fine structure in humans. II. Fine structure for different shapes of cochlear hearing loss. *Journal of the Acoustical Society of America, 106*, 3484–3491.

Mills, D. M., & Rubel, E. W. (1996). Development of the cochlear amplifier. *Journal of the Acoustical Society of America, 100*, 428–441.

Moore, T. M., Hood, L. J. & Hornsby, B. W. (2014). Estimates of cochlear compression using distortion product otoacoustic emissions and growth of forward masking. *Ear and Hearing, 35*, 711–714.

Morlet, T., Lapillonne, A., Ferber, C., Duclaux, R., Sann, L., Putet, G., . . . Collet, L. (1995). Spontaneous otoacoustic emissions in preterm neonates: Prevalence and gender effects. *Hearing Research, 90*, 44–54.

Mulheran, M., & Degg, C. (1997). Comparison of distortion product OAE generation between a patient group requiring frequent gentamicin therapy and control subjects. *British Journal of Audiology, 31*(1), 5–9.

Neely, S. T., Johnson, T. A., & Gorga, M.P. (2005). Distortion-product otoacoustic emissions measured with continuously varying stimulus level. *Journal of the Acoustical Society of America, 117*(3), 1248–1259.

Norton, S. J. (1992). Cochlear function and otoacoustic emissions. *Seminars in Hearing, 13*, 1–14.

Norton, S. J., Bargones, J. Y., & Rubel, E. W. (1991). Development of otoacoustic emissions in gerbil: Evidence for micromechanical changes underlying development of the place code. *Hearing Research, 51*, 73–91.

Norton, S. J., Gorga, M. P., Widen, J. E., Folsom, R. C., Sininger, Y., Cone-Wesson, B., . . . Fletcher, K. (2000). Identification of neonatal hearing impairment: Evaluation of transient evoked otoacoustic emission, distortion product otoacoustic emission, and auditory brain stem response test performance. *Ear and Hearing, 21*(5), 508–528.

Norton, S. J., & Neely, S. T. (1987). Tone-burst evoked otoacoustic emissions from normal-hearing subjects. *Journal of the Acoustical Society of America, 81*, 1860–1872.

Norton, S. J., & Widen, J. (1990). Evoked otoacoustic emissions in normal-hearing infants and children: Emerging data and issues. *Ear and Hearing, 11*, 121–127.

Nowotny, M., & Gummer, A. W. (2006). Electromechanical transduction: Influence of the outer hair cells on the motion of the organ of Corti. *HNO, 54*, 536–543.

Ortmann, A., & Abdala, C. (2015). *Cochlear nonlinearity and aging: Preliminary results.* Paper presented at the 36th Midwinter Meeting of the Association for Research in Otolaryngology, Baltimore, MD.

Owens, J. J., McCoy, M. J, Lonsbury-Martin, B. L, & Martin, G. K. (1993). Otoacoustic emissions in children with normal ears, middle ear dysfunction, and ventilation tubes. *American Journal of Otology, 14*(1), 34–40.

Oxenham, A. J., & Shera, C. A. (2003). Estimates of human cochlear tuning at low levels using forward and simultaneous masking. *Journal of the Association for Research in Otolaryngology*, 4, 541–554.

Poling, G. L., Siegel, J. H., Lee, J., Lee, J., & Dhar, S. (2014). Characteristics of the 2f1-f2 distortion product otoacoustic emission in a normal hearing population. *Journal of the Acoustical Society of America, 135*(1), 287–299. doi:10.1121/1.4845415

Prieve, B. A. (1992). Otoacoustic emissions in infants and children: Basic characteristics and clinical application. *Seminars in Hearing, 13*, 37–52.

Prieve, B. A., Fitzgerald, T. S., & Schulte, L. E. (1997). Basic characteristics of click-evoked otoacoustic emissions in infants and children. *Journal of the Acoustical Society of America, 102*, 2860–2870.

Prieve, B. A., Fitzgerald, T. S., Schulte, L. E., & Kemp, D. T. (1997). Basic characteristics of distortion product otoacoustic emissions in infants and children. *Journal of the Acoustical Society of America, 102*, 2871–2879.

Probst, R., Coats, A. C., Martin, G. K., & Lonsbury-Martin, B. L. (1986). Spontaneous, click- and tone-burst evoked otoacoustic emissions in normal ears. *Hearing Research, 21*, 261–275.

Probst, R., & Harris, F. P. (1993). Transiently evoked and distortion-product otoacoustic emissions. Comparison of results from normally hearing and hearing-impaired human ears. *Archives of Otolaryngology-Head and Neck Surgery, 119*, 858–860.

Probst, R., Lonsbury-Martin, B. L., & .Martin, G. K. (1991). A review of otoacoustic emissions. *Journal of the Acoustical Society of America, 89*(5), 2027–2067.

Pujol, R., Carlier, E., & Lenoir, M. (1980). Ontogenetic approach to inner and outer hair cells functions. *Hearing Research, 2*, 423–430.

Pujol, R., & Hilding, D. (1973). Anatomy and physiology of the onset of auditory function. *Acta Oto-Laryngologica, 76*, 1–11.

Qi, B., Cheng, X., En, H., Huang, L., & Zhang, L. (2014). Characterization of spontaneous otoacoustic emissions in full-term newborns. *International Journal of Pediatric Otorhinolaryngology*, 78(12), 2286–2291.

Rance, G., Fava, R., Baldock, H., Chong, A., Barker, E., Corben, L., & Delatycki, M. B. (2008). Speech perception ability in individuals with Friedreich ataxia. *Brain, 131*(Pt 8), 2002–2012.

Rance, G., Ryan, M. M., Bayliss, K., Gill, K., O'Sullivan, C., & Whitechurch, M. (2012). Auditory function in children with Charcot-Marie-Tooth disease. *Brain, 135*(Pt. 5), 1412–1422.

Rao, A., & Long, G. R. (2011). Effects of aspirin on distortion product fine structure: Interpreted by the two-source model of distortion product otoacoustic emission generation. *Journal of the Acoustical Society of America, 129*(2), 792–800.

Reavis, K. M., McMillan, G., Austin, D., Gallun, F., Fausti, S. A., Gordon, J. S., . . . Konrad-Martin, D. (2011). Distortion-product otoacoustic emission test performance for ototoxicity monitoring. *Ear and Hearing, 32*, 61–74.

Ress, B. D., Sridhar, K. S., Balkany, T. J., Waxman, G. M., Stagner, B. B., & Lonsbury-Martin, B. L. (1999). Effects of cisplatinum chemotherapy on otoacoustic emissions: The development of an objective screening protocol. *Otolaryngology-Head and Neck Surgery, 121*(6), 693–701.

Richardson, H. C., Elliott, C., & Hill, J. (1996). The feasibility of recording transiently evoked otoacoustic emissions immediately following grommet insertion. *Journal of Clinical Otolaryngology Allied Sciences, 121*(5), 445–448.

Rodríguez-Ballesteros, M., del Castillo, F. J., Martín, Y., Moreno-Pelayo, M. A., Morera, C., Prieto, F., . . . del Castillo, I. (2003). Auditory neuropathy in patients carrying mutations in the otoferlin gene (OTOF). *Human Mutation, 22*(6), 451–456.

Romand, R. (1987). Tonotopic evolution during development. *Hearing Research, 28*, 117–123.

Ruah, C. B., Schachern, P. A., Zelterman, D., Paparella, M. M., & Yoon T. H. (1991). Age-related morphologic changes in the human tympanic membrane. A light and electron microscopic study. *Archives of Otolaryngology-Head and Neck Surgery, 117*, 627–634.

Sanchez-Fernandez, J. M., Rivera, J. M., & Macias, J. A. (1983). Early aspects of human cochlea development and tectorial membrane histogenesis. *Acta Oto-Laryngologica, 95*, 460–469.

Saunders, J. C., Kaltenbach, J. A., & Relkin, E. M. (1983). The structural and functional development of the outer and middle ear. In R. Romand & M. R. Romand (Eds.), *Development of auditory and vestibular systems* (pp. 3–25). New York, NY: Academic Press.

Shera, C. A. (2003). Mammalian spontaneous otoacoustic emissions are amplitude-stabilized cochlear standing waves, *Journal of the Acoustical Society of America, 114*, 244–262.

Shera, C. A., & Abdala, C. (2012). Otoacoustic emissions—Mechanisms and applications. In K. Tremblay & R. Burkard (Eds.), *Translational perspectives in auditory neuroscience: Hearing across the life span—Assessment and disorders* (pp. 123–159). San Diego, CA: Plural.

Shera, C. A., & Guinan, J. J., Jr. (1999). Evoked otoacoustic emissions arise by two fundamentally different mechanisms: A taxonomy for mammalian OAEs. *Journal of the Acoustical Society of America, 105*(2), 782–798.

Shera, C. A., & Guinan, J. J., Jr. (2003). Stimulus-frequency-emission group delay: A test of coherent reflection filtering and a window on cochlear tuning. *Journal of the Acoustical Society of America, 113*(5), 2762–7272.

Shera, C. A., & Guinan, J. J., Jr. (2008). Mechanisms of mammalian otoacoustic emission. In G. A. Manley, R. R. Fay, & A. N. Popper (Eds.), *Active processes and otoacoustic emissions* (pp. 305–342). New York, NY: Springer.

Shera, C. A., Guinan, J. J., Jr., Oxenham, A. J. (2002). Revised estimates of human cochlear tuning from otoacoustic and behavioral measurements. *Proceedings of the National Academy of Sciences USA, 99*, 3318–3328.

Shera, C. A., Guinan, J. J., Jr., & Oxenham, A. J. (2010). Otoacoustic estimation of cochlear tuning: Validation in the chinchilla. *Journal of the Association for Research in Otolaryngology, 11*, 343–365.

Shera, C. A., Talmadge, C. L., & Tubis, A. (2000). Interrelations among distortion-product phase-gradient delays: Their connection to scaling symmetry and its breaking. *Journal of the Acoustical Society of America, 108*, 2933–2948.

Shera, C. A., & Zweig, G. (1993). Noninvasive measurement of the cochlear traveling-wave ratio. *Journal of the Acoustical Society of America, 93*, 3333–3352.

Sininger, Y. S., & Starr, A. (2001). *Auditory neuropathy: A new perspective on hearing disorders*. San Diego CA: Singular/Thomson Learning.

Smurzynski, J. (1994). Longitudinal measurements of distortion-product and click-evoked otoacoustic emissions of preterm and full-term infants. *Ear and Hearing, 14*, 258–274.

Smurzynski, J., Jung, M. D., Lafreniere, D., Kim, D. O., Kamath, M. V., Rowe, J. C., . . . Leonard, G. (1993). Distortion-product and click-evoked otoacoustic emissions of preterm and full-term infants. *Ear and Hearing, 14*, 258–274.

Souza, N. N., Dhar, S., Neely, S. T., & Siegel, J. H. (2014). Comparison of nine methods to estimate ear-canal stimulus levels. *Journal of the Acoustical Society of America, 136*, 1768–1787.

Stangerup, S. E., & Tos, M. (1986). Epidemiology of acute suppurative otitis media. *American Journal of Otolaryngology, 7*(1), 47–54.

Starr, A., Isaacson, B., Michalewski, H. J., Zeng, F. G., Kong, Y. Y., Beale, P., . . . Lesperance, M. M. (2004). A dominantly inherited progressive deafness affecting distal auditory nerve and hair cells. *Journal of the Association for Research in Otolaryngology*, *5*, 411–426.

Starr, A., McPherson, D., Patterson, J., Don, M., Luxford, W., Shannon, R., . . . Waring, M. (1991). Absence of both auditory evoked potentials and auditory percepts dependent on timing cues. *Brain*, *114*, 1157–1180.

Starr, A., Picton, T. W., Sininger, Y., Hood, L. J., & Berlin, C. I. (1996). Auditory neuropathy. *Brain*, *119*(Pt. 3), 741–753.

Starr, A., Sininger, Y., Nguyen, T., Michalewski, H. J., Oba, S., & Abdala, C. (2001). Cochlear receptor (microphonic and summating potentials, otoacoustic emissions) and auditory pathway (auditory brain stem potentials) activity in auditory neuropathy. *Ear and Hearing*, *22*(2), 91–99.

Stavroulaki, P., Apostolopoulos, N., Dinopoulou, D., Vossinakis, I., Tsakanikos, M., & Douniadakis, D. (1999). Otoacoustic emissions—An approach for monitoring aminoglycoside induced ototoxicity in children. *International Journal of Pediatric Otorhinolaryngology*, *50*(3), 177–184.

Stover, L., Gorga, M. P., Neely, S. T., & Montoya, D. (1996). Toward optimizing the clinical utility of distortion product otoacoustic emission measurements. *Journal of the Acoustical Society of America*, *100*(2), 956–967.

Talmadge, C. L., Long, G. R., Tubis, A., & Dhar, S. (1999). Experimental confirmation of the two-source interference model for the fine structure of distortion product otoacoustic emissions. *Journal of the Acoustical Society of America*, *105*(1), 275–292.

Talmadge, C. L., Tubis, A., Long, G. R., & Piskorski, P. (1998). Modeling otoacoustic emission and hearing threshold fine structures. *Journal of the Acoustical Society of America*, *104*, 1517–1543.

Tanaka, K., Sakai, N., & Terayama, Y. (1979). Organ of Corti in the human fetus. Scanning and transmission electronmicroscope studies. *Annals of Otology*, *88*, 749–758.

Verpy, E., Masmoudi, S., Zwaenepoel, I., Leibovici, M., Hutchin, T. P., Del Castillo, I., . . . Petit, C. (2001). Mutations in a new gene encoding a protein of the hair bundle cause non-syndromic deafness at the DFNB16 locus. *Nature Genetics*, *29*, 345–349.

Verpy, E., Weil, D., Leibovici, M., Goodyear, R. J., Hamard, G., Houdon, C., ... Petit, C. (2008). Stereocilin-deficient mice reveal the origin of cochlear waveform distortions. *Nature*, *456*, 255–259.

Voss, S. E., Adegoke, M. F., Horton, N. J., Sheth, K. N., Rosand, J., & Shera, C.A. (2010). Posture systematically alters ear-canal reflectance and DPOAE properties. *Hearing Research*, *263*(1–2), 43–51.

Whitehead, M. L., Stagner, B. B., McCoy, M. J., Lonsbury-Martin, B. L., & Martin, G. K. (1995). Dependence of distortion-product otoacoustic emissions on primary levels in normal and impaired ears. II. Asymmetry in L1,L2 space. *Journal of the Acoustical Society of America*, *97*(4), 2359–2377.

Yoshinaga-Itano, C. (2003). From screening to early identification and intervention: Discovering predictors to successful outcomes for children with significant hearing loss. *Journal of Deaf Studies and Deaf Education*, *8*(1), 11–30.

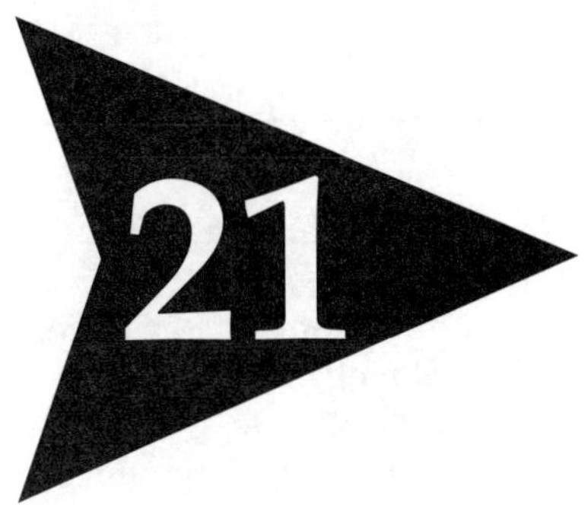

Threshold Assessment in Infants Using the Frequency-Specific Auditory Brainstem Response and Auditory Steady-State Response

Susan A. Small and David R. Stapells

Introduction

The importance of early identification and habilitation of hearing loss for improved access to auditory stimuli and for positive prognosis of speech, language, and psychosocial skills is well established in the literature (Hyde, 2005; Joint Committee on Infant Hearing [JCIH], 2007; Kennedy, McCann, Campbell, Kimm, & Thornton, 2005; Moeller, 2007; Yoshinaga-Itano & Gravel, 2001; Yoshinaga-Itano, Sedey, Coulter, & Mehl, 1998). As a result of the importance of early identification of hearing loss, many countries have established newborn hearing screening programs. Diagnostic audiologic assessment is required for follow-up of infants who do not pass newborn hearing screening, with the goal for most newborn hearing screening, follow-up and intervention programs, including the British Columbia Early Hearing Program (BCEHP), of confirmation and characterization of hearing loss (of a mild degree or worse) by age 3 months, and amplification by the age of 6 months (JCIH, 2007). An auditory-evoked potential (AEP) with high correlation to behavioral threshold is essential for the young infant population and for those older infants and children where accurate behavioral thresholds cannot be obtained. This chapter describes the two frequency-specific AEP methods currently considered appropriate for infant threshold measures: the tone-evoked auditory brainstem response (ABR), the current gold-standard measure, and the relatively new brainstem auditory steady-state response (ASSR).

Transient Versus Steady-State Responses

Auditory-evoked potentials such as Wave V of the ABR or N1 of the slow cortical potential are considered "transient" responses, where the response to one stimulus ends before the next stimulus occurs. An ASSR is a repetitive evoked potential, which is best considered in terms of its constituent frequency components rather than in terms of its waveform (Regan, 1989, p. 35). If stimulus rates are high enough, the resulting response often resembles a sinusoidal waveform whose fundamental frequency is the same as the stimulation rate, although it can be more complex (Regan, 1989, p. 35). In evoking an auditory steady-state response, stimulus rates are sufficiently rapid such that the transient response to one stimulus overlaps with responses to succeeding stimuli (Picton, John, Dimitrijevic, & Purcell, 2003).

With transient responses, longer latency responses tend to originate from sources higher in the auditory system; for example, Wave V, which occurs approximately 6 to 15 ms following a brief stimulus, originates in the brainstem, whereas N1 occurs 80 to 150 ms following a stimulus and has its main sources within the auditory cortex. It is relatively straightforward to relate stimulus timing with evoked potential measures for transient responses (i.e., amplitude and latency); however, the latencies and intracranial origins of ASSRs are more complicated because of the overlapped nature of ASSRs (Picton et al., 2003). Different stimulus rates result in ASSRs with different neural origins; ASSRs to faster rates tend to reflect earlier/lower processing. For example, the ASSR to a stimulus with an 80-Hz modulation rate has its main sources in the brainstem (and has thus been termed the *brainstem ASSR*), whereas the 40-Hz ASSR has its main source in the auditory cortex, but also has brainstem contributions (Herdman, Picton, & Stapells, 2002).

There also exist, in practice, differences between transient and steady-state responses in how they are detected (presence versus absence) and measured (timing and amplitude). As the ASSR typically resembles a sinusoidal waveform whose fundamental frequency is the same as the stimulation rate, it is best (and easily) measured using frequency-domain analyses, such as fast Fourier transform (FFT). Well-tested procedures exist to provide objective (computer-determined) measures of ASSR presence/absence as well as the amplitude and phase (timing) of the ASSR. In contrast, transient responses such as the ABR typically involve more subjective visual detection (e.g., is a peak replicable?) and measurement of peak latencies/amplitudes. The use of objective measures for the ASSR has been touted as an "advantage" of the ASSR over the transient ABR; however, this advantage might be less than commonly believed, as expert clinicians well trained in ABR measures can be accurate; also, objective statistical measures of the ABR are now available (see below).

What Information Is Required?

Many of the goals of AEP audiometry in infants are (or should be) the same as those of behavioral threshold estimation in older children and adults. Thus, as is routinely done in behavioral audiometry, AEP thresholds must be obtained for *frequency-specific* (i.e., tonal) stimuli, and to distinguish between sensory, conductive, and mixed hearing losses, AEP techniques must provide results for both air- and bone-conducted stimuli (Gravel, 2002; JCIH, 2007). Frequency-specific thresholds and identification of the type of hearing loss are necessary to make decisions regarding medical intervention and planning aural (re)habilitation. Uncertainty with regard to hearing loss type leads to large delays in medical treatment and audiological intervention (Gravel, 2002).

This chapter therefore assumes, as indicated by the 2007 JCIH Position Statement, that clinicians will use frequency-specific stimuli and, when thresholds are elevated, bone-conducted stimuli. Although frequency-specific (e.g., tone-evoked ABR) testing has been proven reliable for many years, surprisingly many clinicians today persist in using broadband click stimuli for ABR thresholds, even though the inadequacy of click-ABR threshold has been known and documented for several decades (e.g., Eggermont, 1982; Picton, 1978; Picton & Stapells, 1985; Stapells, 1989; Stapells & Oates, 1997). As a single "point" estimate, it is impossible for the click threshold to provide estimates for thresholds at each octave frequency of the audiogram. More importantly, as a broadband stimulus, the click stimulates most of the cochlea and one cannot say with certainty which frequency the click-ABR threshold represents—at best it represents the "best" hearing in the 500 to 8000 Hz range. Thus, the click-ABR should not be routinely used for threshold determinations. Interestingly, the use of broadband stimuli has never been an issue with the brainstem ASSR; ASSR threshold testing has always utilized frequency-specific stimuli. The ASSR and ABR share another problem in their use by many clinicians—although bone-conduction testing is known to be essential, many clinicians still continue to use only air-conducted stimuli when estimating thresholds in infants using the ABR (or ASSR).

A key difference between behavioral assessments in older children and adults and electrophysiological threshold assessments in infants concerns practical limits on the level of precision that is sought. In behavioral testing of adults, the threshold search is continued until actual threshold is obtained, even when well within normal limits (e.g., 0 or −10 dB HL). Furthermore, the search is typically ended using a 5-dB step size. Electrophysiological testing of infants does not have the luxury of time for such precision: Infants must be tested while sleeping and thus test time is limited. Modern, efficient protocols therefore limit the lowest level tested to those which will indicate the threshold is within normal limits. Most programs consider behavioral thresholds of 25 dB HL or better to be normal; thus, minimum ABR intensities are chosen to test no lower than required to indicate if thresholds are 25 dB HL or better. ABR minimum normal levels for air-conducted (AC) stimuli are currently 25 to 35 dB nHL (normal hearing level). Similarly, threshold searches normally end with a minimum stepsize of 10 dB, with the exception of hearing loss greater than 70 dB where 5 dB can be important given the much reduced dynamic range of hearing (BCEHP, 2012; Ontario Infant Hearing Program [OIHP], 2008).

"Response Present," "No Response," and "Could Not Assess"

As the above paragraph suggests, problems persist with the current practice of AEP audiometry. In addition to the above, misinterpretation of results, especially that of indicating a response is "present" or "absent" when the data are not of sufficient quality to make such a statement are not uncommon. In this case, an inaccurate threshold might result because an ABR Wave V was identified as "present" even though it was not significantly greater than the background noise (typically determined through replicability and/or flatness of tracings). As interpretation of the ABR usually relies on visual observation, ASSR thresholds based on statistical measures are thought by some to be more objective and thus better. However, even the ASSR is not immune to misinterpretation, as current clinical use of ASSR measures routinely violates statistical assumptions, and thus even "significant" ASSRs can sometimes be random noise (John & Purcell, 2008; Luts, Van Dun, Alaerts, & Wouters, 2008). Moreover, both ABR and ASSR current clinical practices are plagued by the common mistake of indicating a "no response" when the data are too noisy to say so (i.e., the amplitude of the residual EEG noise is larger than the amplitude of a typical threshold response, and thus a response might have been missed). Fortunately, for both ABR and ASSR testing, solutions to the above problems are relatively straightforward and are covered in the sections below.

Clinical Implementation of New Techniques

Wide-scale clinical implementation of a procedure requires evidence of reasonable quality in a sizable subject group that is similar to the population requiring the clinical testing. A history of successful clinical use over many patients and over a long enough time to indicate any problems also provides evidence of a procedure's usefulness. Preferably, these data have been published in peer-reviewed journals and by different research groups. In addition to numerous publications by many different investigators, the ABR to air- and bone-conducted brief tones has had a long history of successful clinical use (BCEHP, 2012; OIHP, 2008). In comparison, the brainstem ASSR has had a more limited history of clinical use. More importantly, ASSR stimulus and analysis procedures/parameters, published in the literature and used in the clinic have been much more diverse compared to the ABR, thus limiting the clinical history and amount of data for any one ASSR protocol. This lack of consistency in procedures/parameters is even greater since the first edition of this chapter.

The current considerable interest in the use of "chirps"—brief tonal stimuli rising in frequency—as stimuli to evoke ABRs and ASSRs presents a good example of the problems occurring with the implementation of new techniques. The rising-frequency chirp, with a timing of frequencies setup such that stimulation of each frequency place along the basilar membrane occurs simultaneously (theoretically, at least, for a normal adult cochlea), results in a Wave V with an amplitude some 50% to 100% larger than a standard click, at least for lower intensity levels (e.g., Cobb & Stuart, 2014; Dau, Wagner, Mellert, & Koomeier, 2000; Elberling & Don, 2008). The larger amplitudes in response to broadband chirps compared to clicks makes sense. However, as noted in the preceding section, thresholds for frequency-specific stimuli are required for evoked potential audiometry, not broadband click or chirp stimuli, although broadband chirps are likely useful for newborn screening purposes. Some researchers have been investigating use of narrowband (NB) chirps for ABR and ASSR threshold testing (e.g., Ferm, Lightfoot, & Stevens, 2013; Rodrigues & Lewis, 2014). Some research suggests that Wave V amplitudes are significantly larger than those in response to Blackman-windowed tone pips, in response to lower-intensity NB-chirps (e.g., Ferm et al., 2013). Unfortunately, there is very little research on NB-chirps in normal infants/children and almost none in children with hearing loss. Thus, many questions remain, including (a) what are the relative advantages/disadvantages of NB-chirps versus tone pips in infants with hearing loss, especially when testing at higher intensity levels (where amplitudes and frequency specificity of chirps can be significantly decreased); (b) what are the results for bone-conducted NB-chirps; (c) if they prove to be better than tone pips (e.g., faster due to larger amplitude), what are the normal infant ABR/ASSR thresholds for air- and bone-conducted NB-chirps, and what are the appropriate correction factors to estimate behavioral hearing threshold levels? Before clinical implementation of these new chirp (especially NB-chirp) stimuli, answers are necessary to these and other important questions, requiring considerable future research. Until then, clinicians must rely on the tone-pip ABR (and/or possibly the ASSR).

Estimating Behavioral Thresholds Using AEPs

The primary goal of frequency-specific ABR or ASSR audiometry is to estimate behavioral thresholds. Brief-tone ABR thresholds (typically in dB nHL) and ASSR thresholds (typically in dB HL) are not directly equivalent to perceptual thresholds in) decibels hearing level (dB HL), and there is no reason to expect them to be. Therefore, offset adjustments for bias of ABR or ASSR thresholds are required. There are several methods of obtaining this estimated behavioral hearing level (eHL; Bagatto, 2008; BCEHP, 2012; OIHP, 2008), with the most common methods being (a) application of a regression formula (e.g., McCreery et al., 2014; Rance et al., 2005; Stapells, Gravel, & Martin, 1995), or (b) subtraction of a correction factor (BCEHP, 2012; OIHP, 2008). Recording variables, such as averaging time and residual EEG noise (Picton et al., 2005), and subject factors, such as maturation, affect the accuracy of these methods. For example, because of the effects of ear-canal maturation, the observed relationships between ABR/ASSR and behavioral thresholds will incorporate the effects of maturational changes in sound pressure level (SPL) in the developing ear. Due to the effects of changing size/properties of the ear canal with age, less intensity is required to generate a given decibel sound pressure level (dB SPL) at the eardrum in a neonate as would be required in an older child. The actual SPLs in early infancy will be greater than those for the same stimulus at the time of later behavioral threshold measurement, especially at higher frequencies, so the results can give an impression of progressive impairment (Bagatto, 2008). Cognitive maturation also affects thresholds, such that behavioral visual reinforcement audiometry (VRA) thresholds in a 7-month-old are typically higher than a behavioral threshold obtained when the child is 3 years of age. ABR/ASSR threshold accuracy (and thus the estimated behavioral hearing level accuracy) is affected by procedural factors, including recording time (longer recording times per intensity typically equal less noisy recordings and thus more accurate thresholds) and final intensity stepsize (a 10-dB final stepsize could easily miss true threshold by 5 to 10 dB).[1] Finally, differences between AEP and behavioral thresholds typically show standard deviations of about 10 dB; thus, in about one in 20 subjects, behavioral thresholds are under- or overestimated by 20 dB (Picton et al., 2005). When using any thresholds obtained in infancy, and especially AEP thresholds, one must keep in mind that the estimated behavioral threshold is an estimate, and is often off by 10 dB and occasionally by 15 to 20 dB. Thus, eHL correction factors must take this possibility into account, as must any subsequent fitting of amplification.

Auditory neuropathy spectrum disorder (ANSD) or any significant neurologic dysfunction within the VIIIth nerve and/or brainstem will reduce or eliminate both the transient and steady-state brainstem responses. Thus, whenever no clear response is present at highest intensities (and for transient ABR, no *clear* Wave V), one must investigate the possibility that the elevated ASSR/ABR threshold is due to ANSD or a neurologic disorder. This is accomplished by recording the transient ABR to high-intensity monopolarity clicks as well as evoked otoacoustic emissions (EOAEs; see Chapter 11 in this volume on ANSD). When either ANSD or a neurologic disorder are present and Wave V is significantly degraded (or eliminated), or only earlier waves are present, neither the transient ABR nor the brainstem ASSR will provide accurate measures of hearing thresholds.

The Transient Tone-Evoked ABR

The first brief-tone ABR studies were published in the 1970s and have paved the way to successful threshold assessment for more than 30 years. Nevertheless, despite early and subsequent success, misinformation about the tone-evoked ABR has been published over the years. Many clinicians erroneously believed that tone-ABR thresholds lacked frequency specificity especially at low frequencies (i.e., they did not reflect the nominal frequency of the tone), that they did not provide accurate estimates of the behavioral audiogram, and finally, that they were too difficult and too time-consuming to obtain. In fact, there were relatively few research articles noting problems with tone-ABR, and most of these articles had significant technical problems or presented results from only a few cases. In contrast, our meta-analysis of the tone-ABR literature in 2000 (Stapells, 2000b) demonstrated that the great majority of research papers considering the tone-ABR for threshold estimation showed reasonably accurate results. As shown in Table 21–2, more recent studies have confirmed the utility and accuracy of the tone ABR and have expanded the results to even younger infants. Importantly, clinical programs have effectively used the ABR to air-conducted (and bone-conducted) tones for many years. Experience with province-wide universal early hearing programs in Ontario and British Columbia indicates that with appropriate training and use of efficient parameters and test sequences, a substantial amount of information is typically obtained within one test session, thus the tone-ABR is neither too difficult nor too time consuming (Janssen, Usher, & Stapells, 2010). Figure 21–1 shows typical tone-ABR recordings from a young infant in response to brief tones presented at "normal" levels (25–35 dB nHL, see below).

Tables 21–1 and 21–2 show how well the air-conduction tone-ABR threshold estimates threshold in

[1]However, due to test-time constraints imposed by the requirement that infants must sleep during ABR/ASSR testing, normally one uses a final stepsize of 10 dB for ABR/ASSR testing.

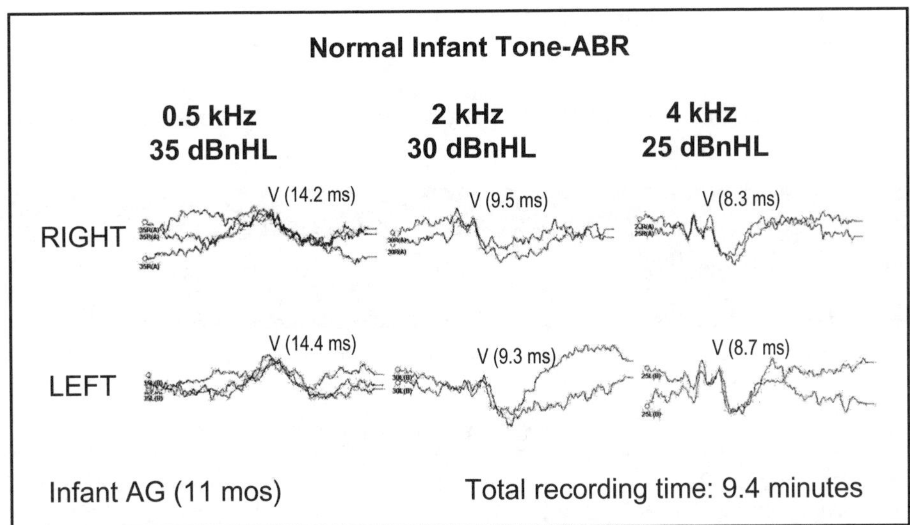

FIGURE 21–1. Tone-evoked ABR waveforms obtained from an infant (aged 11 months) with normal hearing. Brief-tone stimuli were presented at the "normal" intensity levels for each frequency. Replicable responses are clearly present for each waveform set, with Wave V location and latency indicated. Total time required to obtain these results was 9.4 minutes. The time base for waveforms is 25.6 ms. Results obtained in collaboration with Renée Janssen.

Table 21–1. Air-Conduction Tone-ABR Thresholds (in dB nHL) in Infants and Young Children With Normal Hearing

AC TONE-ABR STUDY	*500 Hz*	*1000 Hz*	*2000 Hz*	*4000 Hz*
*Weighted means of all **infant/child** data (1977–2014)*	*21 (571)*	*17 (167)*	*14 (211)*	*14 (327)*
*Meta-analysis of 1977–1999 **infant/child** data 9 studies (Stapells, 2000b)*	20 ± 9 (369)	17 ± 6 (78)	14 ± 7 (65)	15 ± 10 (209)
Infant/Child Research Since 1999				
Rance, Tomlin, & Rickards, 2006[a] (age 6 weeks data)	30 ± 7 (17)			15 ± 6 (17)
Lee, Hsieh, Pan, & Hus, 2007	18 ± 8 (88)	17 ± 7 (75)	13 ± 7 (69)	11 ± 6 (56)
Vander Werff, Prieve, & Georgantas, 2009	27 ± 8 (40)		14 ± 6 (40)	12 ± 6 (30)
Marcoux, 2011[a] (age 0–2 months data)	33 ± 6 (15)		9 ± 6 (15)	6 ± 6 (15)
Ferm, Lightfoot, & Stevens, 2014[a] (age <2 months)	27 ± 9 (19)	16 ± 8 (14)		
Valeriote & Small, 2015 (age 0–6 months)	25 ± 7 (23)		16 ± 9 (22)	
*Meta-analysis of 1977–1999 **adult** data 22 studies (Stapells, 2000b)*	*20 ± 13 (271)*	*16 ± 10 (271)*	*13 ± 8 (216)*	*12 ± 8 (258)*

Note. Adult results from Stapells (2000b) meta-analysis are shown for comparison. Mean (dB nHL) ± standard deviation; results rounded off to closest decibels; number of subjects in parentheses.

[a]Thresholds converted using nHL calibrations in Table 21–5.

Table 21–2. Air-Conduction Tone-ABR Minus Behavioral Threshold Difference Scores in Infants and Young Children With Hearing Loss

AC TONE-ABR STUDY	*HL Type*	*500*	*1000*	*2000*	*4000*
*Weighted means of all **infant/child** data (1977–2014)*	*SNHL*	*+6 (310)*	*+1 (510)*	*+2 (441)*	*−2 (368)*
Meta-analysis of 1977–1999 **infant/child** data six studies (Stapells, 2000b)	SNHL	+6 ± 14 (125)	+5 ± 14 (118)	+1 ± 11 (110)	−8 ± 12 (35)
Infant/Child Research Since 1999					
Lee, Jaw, Pan, Hsieh, & Hus, 2008[a] (Group with behavioral thresholds >40 dB HL)	SNHL	+5 ± 5 (135)	0 ± 5 (119)	−5 ± 8 (112)	−5 ± 8 (91)
Vander Werff et al., 2009	SNHL	+13 ± 12 (3)		0 ± 9 (7)	−3 ± 14 (6)
Rodrigues & Lewis, 2010[b]	SNHL	−2 ± 5 (17)	−13 ± 5 (13)	−8 ± 3 (13)	−11 ± 5 (13)
Stevens, Brennan, Gratton, & Campbell, 2013	SNHL or COND		2 ± 17 (32)		−9 ± 11 (49)
McCreery et al., 2015[b]	SNHL		−1 ± 11 (228)	7 ± 11 (173)	5 ± 10 (163)
Stapells & Gravel, unpublished (ABR and behavioral obtained on same day)	Otitis media	+10 ± 19 (30)		+1 ± 18 (26)	−11 ± 15 (11)
*Meta-analysis of 1977–1999 **adult** data eight studies (Stapells, 2000b)*	*ADULT SNHL*	*+13 ± 11 (85)*	*+10 ± 12 (167)*	*+8 ± 10 (100)*	*+5 ± 13 (84)*

Note. Adult results from Stapells (2000b) meta-analysis are shown for comparison. Difference score (dB) = tone ABR threshold (in dB nHL) minus pure-tone behavioral threshold (in dB HL). Mean (dB) ± standard deviation.

[a]Lee et al. results are median difference scores ±1 quartile.

[b]Results adjusted to stimulus calibrations shown in Table 21–4. Results rounded off to closest decibels. Number of subjects in parentheses.

infants with normal hearing or hearing loss. Results from the previous meta-analysis, as well as results from several more recent studies, and comparison to adults are included. As shown in Table 21–1, normal infants show mean thresholds of about 15 to 20 dB nHL for 500 through 4000 Hz, similar to adult thresholds. However, not all normal-hearing infants show responses at 20 dB nHL, and clinical programs are rarely interested in determining normal thresholds better than 25 to 30 dB eHL; thus, criteria for "normal" are higher than the mean thresholds. Typically, these normal levels are in the range of 30 to 40 dB nHL for 500 Hz, 25 to 35 dB nHL for 1000 Hz, 20 to 30 dB nHL for 2000 Hz, and 20 to 25 dB nHL for 4000 Hz. Currently, the BCEHP specifies normal levels of 35 dB nHL for 500 Hz, 30 to 35 dB nHL for 1000 and 2000 Hz, and 25 dB nHL for 4000 Hz (BCEHP, 2012). If a response is present at the normal level, the eHLs at that frequency are within the normal range.

The scatterplots presented in Figure 21–2 show tone-ABR (in dB nHL) and follow-up behavioral thresholds (in dB HL) for a relatively large group of infants with normal hearing and hearing loss (Stapells et al., 1995). Typical of the literature, correlations between infant tone-ABR and behavioral thresholds in this study were high: $r = .94$, $r = .95$, and $r = .97$ for 500, 2000, and 4000 Hz, respectively. Table 21–2 presents difference scores (i.e., tone-ABR threshold in dB nHL minus pure-tone behavioral threshold in dB HL) from many studies for infants and young children with hearing loss, and compares these to those from adults. Typically, tone-ABR thresholds are within 5 to 10 dB of the behavioral thresholds. Across most studies, standard deviations are typically on the order of 9 to 12 dB (see Table 21–2;

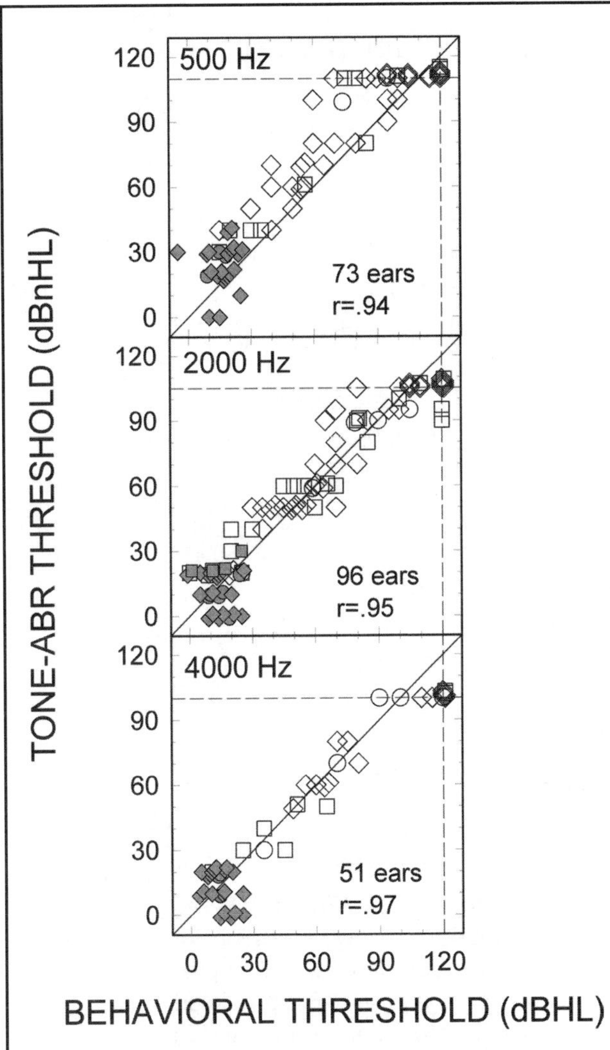

FIGURE 21–2. Threshold estimation using the ABR to 500 Hz (*top*), 2000 Hz (*middle*), and 4000 Hz (*bottom*) tones presented in notched noise. Results for normal-hearing (*gray symbols*) and sensory/neural-impaired (*open symbols*) ears are plotted with three age ranges (at time of ABR) identified: 0 to 6 months (*circles*); 7 to 48 months (*diamonds*); and 49 months or greater (*squares*). Shown also are the correlation coefficients for each frequency across all subjects and the number of ears involved. Dashed lines (- - - - -) indicate the no-response range for each frequency and test, equivalent to the equipment maximum output plus 10 dB. Points plotted at values greater than or equal to the dashed line indicate no-response for the measure. Points with multiple subjects have symbols offset (±1 dB per subject) to show clearly the overlapping data. Diagonals (*solid lines*) represent perfect ABR-behavioral threshold correspondence and are not regression lines. (Adapted from Stapells, Gravel, & Martin, 1995.)

Stapells, 2000b), and differences of 20 dB are occasionally found, although most (≥65%) thresholds are within 10 dB. Figure 21–3 shows ABR-predicted and behavioral audiograms for several infants. Table 21–2 also suggests there might be somewhat greater variability in tone-ABR minus behavioral threshold differences scores for infants with otitis media, highlighting the importance of obtaining bone-conduction results for these infants (Gravel, 2002; Stapells, 1989).

Although it is widely held that difference scores decrease (i.e., tone-ABR threshold is closer to behavioral threshold) as hearing loss increases (McCreery et al., 2014), many data do not support this (Sininger & Hyde, 2009). The slope of ABR versus behavioral threshold regression lines are typically close to unity, indicating thresholds are not closer with severe loss. For studies that suggest nonunity slopes, the issue is complicated by the fact that (a) most ABR measures in the normal range do not seek true thresholds; (b) accurate thresholds at lower intensities (e.g., mild loss) usually require longer averaging (more trials) due to the smaller size of the response—studies using an insufficient number of trials would show larger threshold differences for smaller hearing losses; and (c) for severe-profound hearing losses, the presence of no-response results for ABR occur at a lower intensity (in dB nHL) than for pure-tone behavioral (in dB HL), due in part to transducer limitations. It does appear that it is difficult to get close to true normal threshold (e.g., −5 to 10 dB nHL) in individuals with normal hearing, but this is complicated by acoustic noise (ambient noise in room) and electrical noise (room and subject) issues. Given near-unity slopes, estimation of behavioral thresholds (eHL) using either regression functions or correction factors should yield equivalent results. Importantly, as Table 21–2 shows, difference scores for infants and young children are clearly different from those of adults; it is therefore important that we use infant data to determine appropriate correction factors. The British Columbia Early Hearing Program currently uses conservative correction factors of −15, −10, −5, and 0 dB for estimating 500-, 1000-, 2000-, and 4000-Hz pure-tone behavioral thresholds (in dB HL) from air-conduction tone-ABR thresholds (in dB nHL; BCEHP, 2012, 2015).

ABR Assessment of Conductive Loss

The most common cause of elevated ABR (or ASSR) thresholds in young infants is conductive loss (Canadian Working Group on Childhood Hearing, 2005; Gravel, 2002). This is especially so for young infants referred for diagnostic ABR/ASSR testing after failing

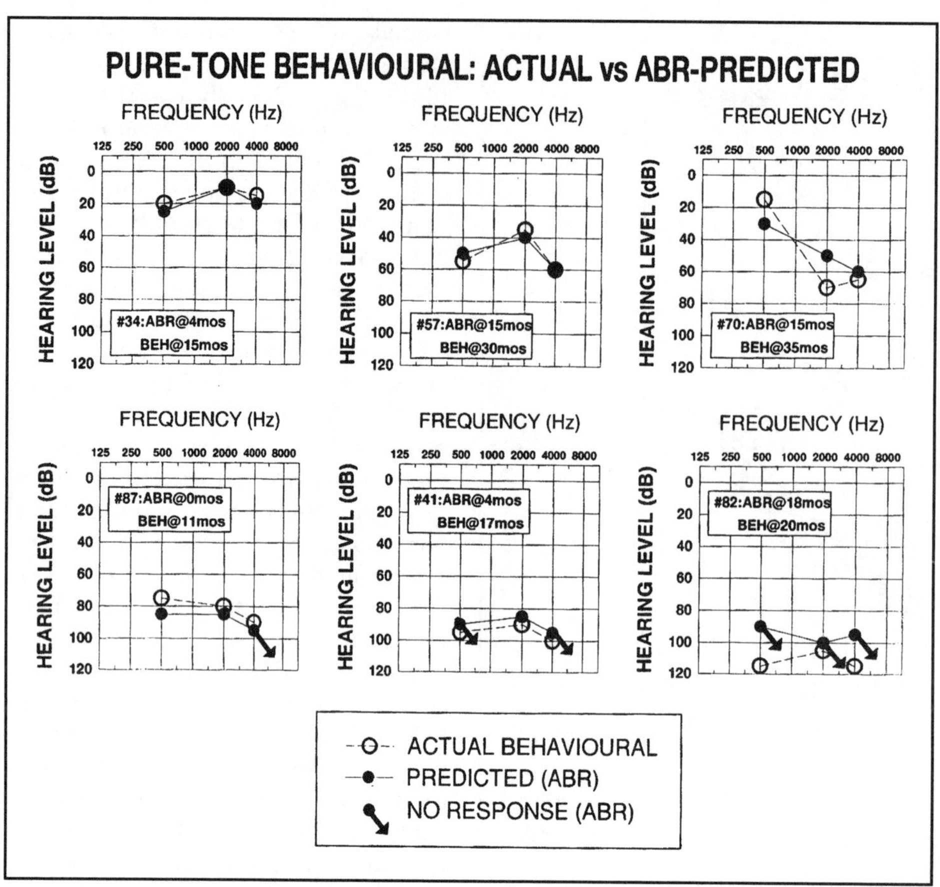

FIGURE 21–3. Comparison of auditory brainstem response (ABR)-predicted audiograms with actual behavioral audiograms obtained on follow-up testing for six infants. Results for individuals with normal hearing (*upper left corner*) to profound sensory/neural hearing loss (*lower right corner*) are shown. ABR-predicted thresholds were determined using the linear regression equations presented in Stapells, Gravel, and Martin (1995). Predicted thresholds with arrows were ABR "no response" results—note the ABR's inability to differentiate between 90 and 110 dB HL. Otherwise, most ABR-predicted thresholds are quite close to actual behavioral thresholds. BEH = behavioral. (Reprinted with permission from Phoank AG. Figure from Stapells, D. R. [2000a]. Frequency-specific evoked potential audiometry in infants. In R. C. Seewald [Ed.], *A sound foundation through early amplification: Proceedings of an international conference* [pp. 13–31]. Stäfa, Switzerland: Phonak AG.)

one or more newborn hearing screenings. Protocols, therefore, must be able to determine whether a significant conductive component is present. When testing older children and adults, this assessment is primarily achieved through comparison of air- versus bone-conduction thresholds to identify air-bone gaps of clinical significance (i.e., greater than 10 dB). This has not been the standard clinical practice when testing infants. Most of the infant ABR literature was obtained for either air- or bone-conducted stimuli but not both stimuli in the same infant, whether they had normal hearing or hearing loss. The typical practice, when air-conducted ABR thresholds are elevated, is to assess bone-conducted ABR thresholds at the normal level to distinguish between conductive and sensory losses. Two more recent infant ABR studies measured air- and bone-conducted thresholds in the same infants and reported that air-bone gaps in normal-hearing infants are often 15 to 20 dB compared to less than 10 dB in children and adults (Vander Werff et al., 2009; Valeriote & Small, 2015), similar to the "maturational" air-bone gap described for infant ASSRs (e.g., Casey & Small,

2014; Small & Stapells, 2008b), and predicted for infant behavioral testing (Hulecki & Small, 2011). These data suggest that conductive components could be overidentified using the criterion we use for older children and adults. Additional information about middle ear status can be gained from immittance and EOAE measures; however, these latter measures are unable to quantify the degree of conductive loss. In the presence of conductive pathology, they are typically abnormal whether the conductive component is relatively minor (e.g., only 5 dB) or substantial (e.g., 30 dB).

Others have suggested that analysis of ABR Wave V or Wave I latencies in response to air-conducted clicks can differentiate conductive from sensory losses, and perhaps can even quantify the conductive component (e.g., Fria & Sabo, 1979; McGee & Clemis, 1982; Yamada, Yagi, Yamane, & Suzuki, 1975). Our research, using click-ABR Wave I latencies, has indicated that although air-conduction latencies are indeed prolonged *on average* in infants with conductive hearing loss, latency-based measures of the conductive component are not reliable. Some infants with conductive loss showed normal latencies (Figure 21–4), whereas some infants with either sensory hearing loss or normal thresholds showed prolonged latencies (Mackersie & Stapells, 1994). The overlap between groups is even greater for Wave V latencies (Vander Werff et al., 2009). Given these overlaps, it should not be surprising that attempts to quantify the amount of conductive component using AC click-ABR Wave V or Wave I latency shifts have not proven reliable, with large errors in many infants (Eggermont, 1982; Mackersie & Stapells, 1994) and relatively low correlations between latency and the size of the air-bone gap (Vander Werff et al.,

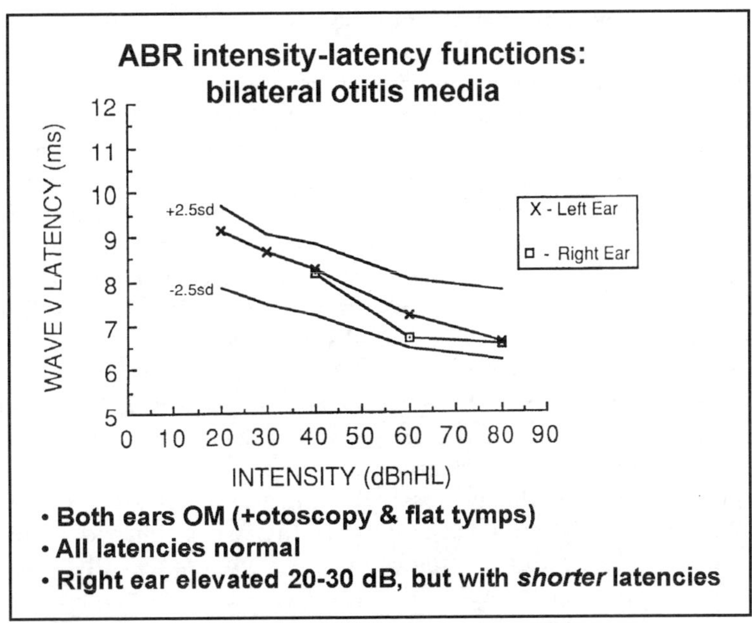

FIGURE 21–4. Click-evoked air-conduction auditory brainstem response (ABR) Wave V intensity-latency functions in an infant with bilateral otitis media (and normal bone-conduction hearing). Otitis media indicated by pneumatic otoscopy (i.e., presence of fluid) and flat tympanograms bilaterally. Despite bilateral otitis media and a 20 to 30 dB elevation for the right-ear ABR, all latencies are well within normal limits, with latencies for right-ear stimulation slightly shorter than for the left ear. Follow-up testing indicated normal ABR and behavioral thresholds, and normal middle ear function, indicating sensory/neural loss was not present and the elevation was conductive in nature. Thus, reliance on air-conduction ABR intensity-latency functions could have erroneously suggested no conductive loss, with the right-ear elevation being sensory/neural in nature. (Results obtained in collaboration with Judy Gravel.)

2009). Furthermore, latency-based measures typically require responses to air-conducted clicks (especially for Wave I measures). As discussed above, no frequency-specific information can be reliably obtained using clicks. Given the large amount of information required from sleeping infants, modern ABR protocols thus rarely use clicks, except when assessing infants suspected of ANSD or other neurologic problem that can disrupt the ABR.

The problems with latency-based measures are demonstrated in Figure 21–4, which presents results from an infant whose air-conducted click-ABR Wave V thresholds were normal (20 dB nHL or better) for the left ear but mildly elevated (40 dB nHL) for the right ear; Wave V latencies for both ears were well within normal limits. Latencies for the right ear with elevated thresholds were shorter in latency. Relying on latency shifts, one might interpret no conductive component was present in either ear, and the right-ear threshold elevation was a sensory loss. However, this infant had normal thresholds for bone-conducted stimuli, and otoscopic examination revealed bilateral otitis media; air-conduction thresholds returned to normal at a subsequent visit.

It is therefore not possible to reliably determine the presence or degree of a conductive component using air-conduction ABR latency information. With the exception of ABR assessment of ANSD and/or neurologic involvement, we do not use any ABR latency results when determining *threshold*.[2] Rather, we rely on the combination of air- and bone-conduction tone-ABR results. An elevated tone-ABR (or ASSR) threshold to air-conducted stimuli with tone-ABR responses to bone-conducted stimuli at normal levels clearly indicates the presence and degree of a conductive loss; if ABR thresholds to bone-conducted stimuli are elevated, a sensory component is present. Current comprehensive diagnostic protocols for infants emphasize the importance of obtaining bone-conduction information early in the process (i.e., as soon as an elevation in air-conduction thresholds is indicated)—this information is needed to determine the next test step and is important both for appropriate follow-up and for parent counseling. When bone-conduction thresholds turn out to be within normal limits, indicating a conductive loss, the thresholds for air-conducted stimuli in many cases are of less importance because, when resulting from fluctuating conditions such as otitis media, they can be quite different in the days following the assessment. Unfortunately, many clinicians still do not routinely obtain ABR results for bone-conducted stimuli after finding elevated air-conduction threshold(s), relying instead on immittance results. There is no need to omit this step for infant assessments as bone-conduction tone-ABR protocols, test parameters, and results are currently available for the assessment of conductive loss.

Bone-Conduction Tone-ABR

Bone-conduction tone-ABR has a history of over two decades of regular use in the clinic (Gravel, Kurtzberg, Stapells, Vaughan, & Wallace, 1989; Stapells, 1989; Stapells & Ruben, 1989), and protocols using bone-conducted tonal stimuli are currently routinely employed in large programs such as BCEHP (2012) and OIHP (2008).[3] Despite their history of clinical use and importance for clinical assessment, it is somewhat surprising that relatively few bone-conduction tone-ABR data in infants have been published in the peer-reviewed literature (Cone- Wesson, 1995; Cone-Wesson & Ramirez, 1997; Ferm et al., 2014; Foxe & Stapells, 1993; Hatton, Janssen, & Stapells, 2012; Nousak & Stapells, 1992; Stapells & Ruben, 1989; Vander Werff et al., 2009; Valeriote & Small, 2015), with most published for data in infants having normal hearing or conductive hearing loss. Recently, we published bone-conduction tone-ABR results from infants with sensory/neural hearing loss, as well as normal bone-conduction hearing (Hatton et al., 2012).

Infant thresholds for bone-conducted stimuli differ significantly from adults (Foxe & Stapells, 1993;

[2]We do not evaluate whether a tone-ABR Wave V latency is "normal" or "prolonged," as this typically provides no extra (or reliable) information over air- versus bone-conduction tone-ABR results. We do use latency differences when considering differences between Wave V recorded in ipsilateral and contralateral EEG channels (see below). Also, if a "Wave V" latency appears to be too early to be Wave V, we will be concerned the thresholds are unreliable (e.g., neurologic or ANSD concerns). Of course, for neurologic/ANSD assessment, we do consider normality of click-ABR latency measures.

[3]The ABR to bone-conduction clicks has also been used clinically, preceding the use of bone-conducted tones (e.g., Cone-Wesson, 1995; Cornacchia, Martini, & Morra, 1983; Hooks & Weber, 1984; Kavanagh & Beardsley, 1979; Mauldin & Jerger, 1979; Muchnik, Neeman, & Hildesheimer, 1995; Stuart, Yang, Stenstrom, & Reindorp, 1993; Yang, Rupert, & Moushegian,1987; Yang & Stuart, 1990). However, as with air-conducted clicks, bone-conducted clicks lack frequency specificity (Kramer, 1992); also, due to maturational issues, the "effective" spectra for air- and bone-conducted clicks differ (Small & Stapells, 2008b), making comparison between the two difficult in infants.

Small & Stapells, 2006, 2008b; Stapells & Ruben, 1989; Stuart, Yang, & Green, 1994; Stuart et al., 1993; Vander Werff et al., 2009; Yang et al., 1987), likely due primarily to the immaturity of the infant skull (Anson & Donaldson, 1981; Mackey, Hodgetts & Small, in press; Small & Stapells, 2008b; Yang et al., 1987). Table 21–3 shows normal infant bone-conduction tone-ABR thresholds obtained by several studies. There is some variability in the literature, but all show mean thresholds that are (a) better for low versus high frequencies, and (b) better than expected compared to those for adults. Thus, adult "normal" levels for bone-conducted stimuli do not apply to infants; criteria for infants must be determined directly from infant bone-conduction ABR results. We have found that to be considered "normal" (for bone-conduction hearing), infants should show ABRs to bone-conducted tones presented at 20 dB nHL for 500 Hz and at 30 dB nHL for 2000 Hz (Hatton et al., 2012; Stapells, 1989; Stapells & Ruben, 1989). Currently, there are too few infant ABR data for 1000- and 4000-Hz bone-conducted tones (see Table 21–3), so these frequencies are not routinely tested using bone-conducted stimuli. Because the upper limits (before distortion) of the most commonly used bone oscillator (B71) for brief tones is 51 dB nHL at 500 Hz and 63 dB nHL at 2000 Hz (Small & Stapells, 2003), a range of only 30 dB above these normal levels can be tested. Based on the results of our recent study of bone-conduction ABR in infants with sensory/neural (Hatton et al., 2012), the BCEHP recommends and uses the following correction factors for bone-conduction ABR nHL to dB eHL: 500 Hz: +5 dB (i.e., eHL threshold is 5 dB higher than threshold in dB nHL); 2000 Hz: −5 dB (i.e., eHL threshold is 5 dB better than threshold in dB nHL; BCEHP, 2012). Due to large differences in bone- versus air-conduction thresholds in young infants, calculation of the "air-bone gap" *must* be carried-out on eHL (i.e., corrected) values and not dB nHL values. It should be noted that even after eHL corrections have been applied, air-bone gaps as large as 10 dB (and occasionally 15 dB) might not be

Table 21–3. Bone-Conduction Tone-ABR Thresholds (in dB nHL) in Infants and Young Children With Normal Bone-Conduction Hearing

BC TONE-ABR STUDY	*500*	*1000*	*2000*	*4000*
Weighted means across all studies	*3 (140)*	*5 (14)*	*14 (94)*	*7 (20)*
Stapells & Ruben, 1989 (normal group)	2[a] (24)		6[a] (24)	
Stapells & Ruben, 1989 (all infants)	−2[a] (66)		4[a] (66)	
Foxe & Stapells, 1993	3 ± 10 (9)		14 ± 7 (8)	
Cone-Wesson & Ramirez, 1997 (age: 1–2 days) *Standard deviations estimated from graph in original study*	−15 ± 10[b] (24)			7 ± 7[b] (20)
Vander Werff et al., 2009	11 ± 8 (40)		17 ± 7 (40)	
Ferm et al., 2014 (age <2 months)[b]	3 ± 7 (19)	5 ± 8 (14)		
Valeriote & Small, 2015 (normal group, age 0–6 months)	10 ± 8 (24)		15 ± 10 (22)	

Note. Mean (dB nHL) ± standard deviation (where available). Results rounded off to closest decibels. Number of subjects in parentheses. Weighted means exclude Stapells and Ruben (1989) non-normal results (i.e., conductive loss).

[a]Threshold = 50% point on cumulative response-presence distribution for "normal" and "all" infants.

[b]Thresholds converted to decibels normal hearing level (dB nHL) using calibrations in Table 21–5.

clinically significant (Hulecki & Small, 2011; Valeriote & Small, 2015; Vander Werff et al., 2009). This deviation from the standard application of the air-bone gap used for adult audiometry stems from the following: (a) significant maturation differences in air- and bone-conduction thresholds, (b) use of a 10-dB stepsize for infants, (c) a limited bone-conduction dynamic range, (d) few published data for air-bone gaps in infants with hearing loss, and (e) the combined variability in normal infant air- and bone-conduction thresholds. Consequently, we do not routinely use the air-bone gap to indicate conductive loss versus sensory loss, unless it is >15 dB. Rather, the bone-conduction results are primarily used to indicate whether bone thresholds are "normal" or "elevated" and thus whether or not there is a sensory component (i.e., bone-conduction elevated) to an elevated air-conduction threshold. The approximately 30-dB dynamic range essentially only allows one to classify bone thresholds as "normal," "mild/moderate elevation," or "moderate or greater elevation" (Hatton et al., 2012). Figure 21–5 shows bone-conduction tone-ABR results from young children with conductive and sensory/neural hearing loss.

Bone-Conduction ABR: Isolating the Responding Cochlea

Masking of the contralateral ear, typically required with bone-conduction testing in adults, is somewhat difficult and often not necessary for ABR audiometry in young infants. Masking is difficult because only two studies have published infant effective masking levels for bone-conducted stimuli and only for ASSR stimuli (Hansen & Small, 2012; Small, Smyth, & Leon,

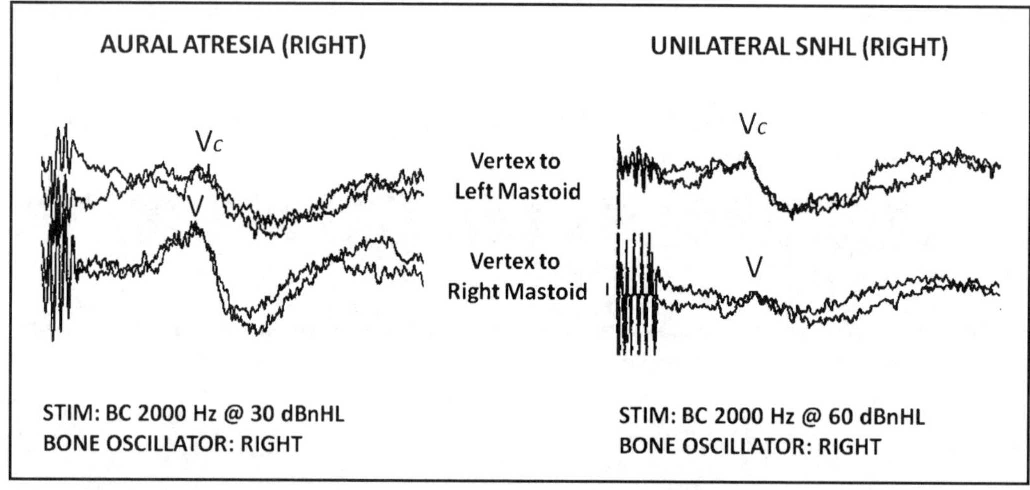

FIGURE 21–5. ABR to 2000-Hz bone-conducted tones in two children, one with conductive hearing loss (*left panel*) and one with unilateral sensory/neural hearing loss (*right panel*). Shown are the results for the left ("Vertex to Left Mastoid") and right ("Vertex to Right Mastoid") EEG channels, obtained simultaneously, with the bone oscillator placed on the right temporal bone. In the infant with conductive loss due to right-ear atresia, Wave V in the right EEG channel (i.e., ipsilateral to bone oscillator placement) is both earlier and larger than Wave V in the left (contralateral) EEG channel. This is a *normal asymmetry* and indicates the right cochlea is the primary contributor to the response to these bone-conduction tones at the normal (30 dB nHL) intensity. This indicates a normal 2000-Hz bone-conduction response for this ear. In the child with a unilateral (right-ear) sensory/neural loss, 60 dB nHL 2000-Hz bone-conduction tones presented to the right temporal bone resulted in a Wave V in the right EEG channel (i.e., ipsilateral to bone oscillator placement) that is much smaller and later than the Wave V seen in left (contralateral) EEG channel. This is an *abnormal asymmetry*, indicating the left ear is the primary contributor to the response, and thus indicating the presence of a sensory/neural hearing loss. Further ABR and behavioral testing indicated a severe unilateral sensory/neural hearing loss in the right ear. (Vc = wave V in contralateral EEG channel. Waveform timebase = 25 ms.)

2014). Also, time is too limited to record ABRs using several masking levels, when attempting plateau masking (Stapells, 2000a). However, because of their immature skulls, young infants show substantial interaural attenuation of bone-conducted stimuli, as much as 25 dB (Small & Stapells, 2008a; Yang et al., 1987). Thus, stimuli presented to the temporal bone at the low stimulus levels (20–30 dB nHL) required to demonstrate normal versus impaired cochlear function will stimulate primarily the cochlea ipsilateral to the oscillator placement, and masking might not be required. Furthermore, the laterality of ABR origin (i.e., which cochlea is resulting in the recorded ABR) can be reasonably inferred using two-channel EEG recordings, and observing the large ipsilateral/contralateral Wave V latency and amplitude asymmetries present in infants and young children (but not in older children or adults). As shown in Figure 21–5, in the infant with a normal ABR to bone-conducted tones, Wave V is larger and earlier in the EEG channel ipsilateral to the stimulated cochlea (Edwards, Durieux-Smith, & Picton, 1985; Foxe & Stapells, 1993; Stapells, 1989; Stapells & Mosseri, 1991); thus, if one sees this pattern in the channel on the same side as the bone oscillator, one can infer that stimulation of the cochlea on the same side has resulted in the ABR. However, if one sees the opposite pattern, as shown in the child with sensory hearing loss in Figure 21–5, then the opposite cochlea has produced the response, and a sensory impairment is present (Sininger & Hyde, 2009; Stapells, 1989). Although reasonably well-tested in infants with conductive loss (Stapells, 1989; Stapells & Ruben, 1989), the ipsi/contra technique requires further assessment in infants with sensory or mixed loss; the authors' clinical experience as well as that of larger programs (e.g., BCEHP, OIHP) indicates reasonable results in these latter groups (Hatton et al., 2012).[4] Nevertheless, when *significant* asymmetry in bone-conduction thresholds exists between ears, masking will be required to more accurately determine bone-conduction thresholds specific to each cochlea (BCEHP, 2012).

Tone-ABR Technical Details

Tables 21–4 and 21–5 present specific recording and stimulus parameters we recommend for tone-ABR, based on more than 30 years of research and 25 years of clinical application. The data supporting each choice are discussed in detail elsewhere (BCEHP, 2012; Stapells, 2000a; Stapells & Oates, 1997) and thus are not elaborated on here. Test sequences for tone-ABR are provided in a later section concerning clinical ABR/ASSR protocols.

Most clinical AEP equipment is reasonably capable of basic tone- and click-evoked ABR measures. However, not all systems are optimal, and some are not up to the task of brief-tone threshold estimation. Optimally, a wide *and flexible* range of stimulus and recording settings should be available. Currently, we consider that tone-ABR systems must be able to provide, as a minimum, the stimulus and recording setups outlined in Tables 21–4 and 21–5, *including* online calculation and presentation of the residual noise (RN) and signal-to-noise ratio (SNR) of a waveform (see below). An AEP system should provide additional features that allow for speedy changing of stimulus parameters, addition of waves, marking/measuring of waveforms, and subsequent printouts. We also strongly recommend that clinical AEP systems allow the recording of slow cortical potential to estimate hearing thresholds in infants with ANSD.

Interpretation of Tone-ABR Waveforms

Although the tone-ABR has the capability to provide reasonably accurate estimates of threshold, a continuing and substantial problem with the clinical use of the ABR today lies largely with the clinicians who carry out the testing and/or interpret the waveforms, rather than with the ABR itself. Currently, most clinicians determine response presence/absence and waveform noisiness "subjectively" by visually assessing the repeatability and noisiness of multiple "replicate" waveforms. Many clinicians become proficient at this and some become "experts"; however, there are some clinicians who do not acquire the skills necessary for accurate interpretation of the ABR. The differences are likely due to training, experience (e.g., number and diversity of cases), and inherent abilities. Fortunately, with modern systems, clinicians need not base their interpretation solely on their visualization of the responses (although for very experienced observers, this might currently be the best method). Objective measures of response replicability/signal-to-noise ratio and, importantly, response noisiness, are available and should be used.

[4]The normal infant ABR Wave V ipsi/contra asymmetries are also useful when recording responses to high-intensity air-conduction stimuli when one suspects a significant interaural difference in the degree of hearing loss.

Table 21–4. Recommended Recording Parameters for Tone-ABR

	Air Conduction	*Bone Conduction*
EEG channels	*Minimum:* One channel Cz- Mastoid-ipsi Preferred: Two channels[a] Cz- Mastoid-ipsi Cz- Mastoid-contra	*Minimum:* Two channels[a] Cz- Mastoid-ipsi Cz- Mastoid-contra
EEG filters (12 dB/oct slope)	30 Hz (high pass) to 1500–3000 Hz (low pass). (Note that the low-pass filter should be 3000 to 4000 Hz if assessing CM.)	
Gain	50,000 to 100,000	
Artifact rejection	Trials exceeding ±25 µV; ±10–15 µV acceptable if there are few rejections (<10%) Set artifact region to start *after* end of stimulus so that stimulus artifact does not trigger artifact rejection (if available)	
Number of accepted trials per replication	Typically 2,000 per replication; additional trials may be required to reduce noise (achieved either by increasing the number of trials per replication or by averaging together replications) • Minimum 1,000 per replication *After 1,000 trials, *if online residual noise measure available,* may stop when waveform noise reduced to < criterion (e.g., IHS RN <.05–.08 µV or Bio-Logic sp-variance <20–30 nV) *and* waveform appears flat	
Number of replications	At least two (very often three, sometimes four). *If* residual noise meets criterion and waveform is flat, one rep for "no response" is acceptable	
Recording (time) window and stimulus rate	Typically 24–25 ms which usually allows a rate up to about 39.1/s[b] *Some systems are slower, thus either a slightly shorter window (e.g., 23–24 ms) or a slightly slower rate (e.g., 37.1/s) must be used. Clinicians must check that their system averages at 39.1/s and does not skip stimuli. Then 2,000 trials should take about 51 seconds; if it requires much longer, it is skipping stimuli.*	
Visual display scale	Waveforms must be displayed with a sufficient display gain such that very small responses would not be missed. *A rule of thumb is to "blow-up" waves such that peak-to-peak height of largest wave is at least one quarter the length of the recording window (i.e., if ABR waveform displayed is 10 cm in length, then the display should be increased such that the peak-to-peak amplitude of Wave V-V′ is at least 2.5 cm in height; e.g., IHS Smart-EP amplitude scale of 0.5 µV and 20% plot size, split-page display)*	

[a]Laterality (cochlear origin) of BC-ABR determined from Wave V ipsi/contra asymmetries (infants/young children only). Consider this also for air conduction if a large difference in thresholds between ears exists.

[b]Although a 25-ms window works for all frequencies, infant responses to 2000- and 4000-Hz stimuli are shorter in latency; thus, a shorter time window (18–20 ms) *and a faster rate* (49.1/s) would be acceptable and faster.

Too often, clinicians indicate a response is "present" or "absent" when they do not have data of sufficient quality to make such a statement. As noted above, to conclude a response is present, the clinician must have evidence of a significant SNR. When assessed visually, a "present" response must contain a replicable waveform, one which is repeatable over its total duration, usually at least 3 to 4 ms for Wave V. To be sure it has a significant SNR, the waveform's peak-to-peak amplitude (from the average of all replications) must be at least three times the average difference between the replications (Don & Elberling, 1996; Picton, Linden, Hamel, & Maru, 1983; Picton & Maru, 1984). A decision that a wave is "absent" can only be made if replications are essentially flat and show little or no difference between them (i.e., repeatedly flat *for at least* a

Table 21–5. Stimuli for Tone-ABR Rise/Fall Times, Durations, Acoustic Calibrations for 0 dB nHL, and Signal-to-Noise (SNR) Regions

	Linear Window	Blackman Window	Acoustic Calibration for 0 dB nHL			SNR Region[a] (Begin to End, in ms)	
Frequency (Hz)	Rise/Fall (r/f) and Plateau (2-1-2 Cycles)	Total Duration (Five Cycles)	Insert (AC) ER-3A dB ppe SPL[b]	Supra (AC) TDH-49 dB ppe SPL	Bone (BC) B-71 dB ppe re: 1 µN RMS	Air (AC)	Bone (BC)
500	4-ms r/f 2-ms plateau	10 ms total	22	25	67	10.5–20.5	20 dB: 10.5–20.5 >30 dB: 14–24[c]
1000	2-ms r/f 1-ms plateau	5 ms total	25	23	54	7.5–17.5	7.5–17.5
2000	1-ms r/f 0.5-ms plateau	2.5 ms total	20	26	49	6.5–16.5	6.5–16.5
4000*	AC: 0.5-ms r/f [d] 0.25-ms plateau BC: 1-ms r/f 0.25-ms plateau	AC: 1.25 ms total BC: 2.25-ms total	26	29	46	5–15	5–15

Note. Rate = 37.1 to 39.1/s (assuming 23–25 ms averaging window); polarity = alternating; ppe = peak-to-peak equivalent dB ("peak" = ppe + 3 dB for brief tones).

[a]SNR region (for waveform noise and response presence measures) must not include stimulus artifact. May be a problem for high-intensity 500-Hz stimuli.

[b]Insert earphones calibrated using a DB0138 2-cc coupler (if using IEC 60711 occluded ear simulator, add 4.3, 5.8, 8.5, and 10.4 at 500, 1000, 2000, and 4000 Hz).

[c]Window later to exclude stimulus artifact but also excludes much of response. Valid for residual noise measures only (i.e., not CCR, SNR or Fsp).

[d]Bone conduction (BC) stimuli at 4000 Hz is slightly extended in total duration to reduce ringing by bone oscillator.

duration of 3 to 4 ms in the region of Wave V). If the waveform peak in question is not repeatable or if the replications are not flat (i.e., noisy), the clinician must obtain more replications. Otherwise, the result should be interpreted only as "could not evaluate" or "data incomplete" (BCEHP, 2012; Sininger & Hyde, 2009; Stapells, 2000a). Figure 21–6 shows examples of waveforms in each of these three categories. Much of the variability in ABR thresholds and the inconsistency with subsequent behavioral thresholds are the result of calling a response "present" when waveforms do not replicate sufficiently and calling a response "absent" when recordings are too noisy to make this judgement. Fortunately, the solutions to these problems are quite simple: obtain additional replications when needed (this assumes one has made every attempt to ensure the infant is quietly asleep), average together replications to increase the number of trials in an average and thus reduce residual noise in waveform, and do not interpret conditions with insufficient replications and/or noisy data.

As noted above, statistical measures of ABR SNR and waveform noisiness are currently available. Currently, of the two, an online measure of waveform noisiness is the most important and must be considered a requirement when considering any new clinical ABR system.[5] It is important that any system implementing these statistical measures must allow for flexibility in

[5]At the time of writing this chapter, appropriate statistical measures, especially waveform noise, were available on only a few clinical systems. However, several other manufacturers were in the process of implementing these measures.

their parameters, as they differ depending on stimulus and response characteristics (e.g., settings are different for 500 versus 2000 Hz tones; as well as Wave V versus later responses). Table 21–5 includes recommendations for latency windows ("SNR Regions," each 10 ms in duration) over which these measures are calculated. Exact parameters and especially criteria for statistical measures of waveform noisiness or response presence/absence (SNR) are not easily available; some information is provided below (further details are provided in BCEHP, 2012).

Waveform Noisiness (Residual Noise)

Single-point variance (sp variance; Don & Elberling, 1996; Don, Elberling, & Waring, 1984): This measure, available on only a couple of systems, estimates the trial (stimulus) by trial variance in amplitude of a single time point in the evoked potential waveform, usually in the region of the expected response and always beyond any stimulus artifact. As the number of trials averaged increases, the variance goes down. The location of the single point is typically placed in the middle of the SNR region. For threshold measures, in order to conclude "no response," the final sp variance must be down to 10 to 20 nV, a level smaller than a typical threshold Wave V response.[6]

Residual noise (Özdamar & Delgado, 1996; Picton et al., 1983): As with sp variance, residual noise is available on only one or two systems. The standard deviation of the plus-minus average is similar to that used on transient EOAE systems ("A-B" in dB). RN (from average of all replications) must be lower than a set value to conclude a "no response." Currently, BCEHP ABR protocols require the RN for the average waveform of all replications to be 0.08 μV *or less* before a "no response" is concluded (plus the waveforms must appear visually flat).[7] Details are available in the BCEHP protocols (BCEHP, 2012). Figure 21–6 shows RN values (calculated for the average of all replications) for results showing "response present," "no response," and "could not interpret" (i.e., too noisy to conclude no response).

Response Presence/Absence (Waveform Signal-to-Noise Ratio)

Correlation coefficient between replications (CCR; Hyde et al., 1998; Picton et al., 1983): Most current clinical ABR machines have the capability to calculate the correlation coefficient between two replications (Picton, Durieux-Smith, & Moran, 1994; Picton et al., 1983), a measure similar to the "reproducibility" measure used in transient EOAEs (Kemp, 1988; Picton et al., 1994). However, few systems calculate and update the correlation online as trials are averaged. Normally calculated using a 10-ms window centered on the typical response (see Table 21–5), a correlation of 0.5 and higher provides clinicians with an indication that a response is present—the higher the correlation, the more likely a response is present. Although it is not a perfect measure, individual clinicians can determine their own criterion correlation (over many sets of waves) and use this objective measure to aid in their response determination.

F-test using single-point variance (Fsp; Don et al., 1984; Elberling & Don, 1984; Hyde, Sininger, & Don, 1998): A somewhat better measure than correlation, the "Fsp," also provides an online/ongoing indication of response presence/absence. Unfortunately, Fsp (or the similar multipoint Fmp) is implemented on only a few clinical machines, and few published data are available. Also, typically calculated over a 10-ms window, "significant" Fsp values are typically in the range of 2.9 to 3.1 (Sininger & Hyde, 2009).

Signal-to-noise ratio or standard deviation ratio (SDR; Özdamar & Delgado, 1996; Picton et al., 1994; Picton et al., 1983)[8]: Also calculated over a 10-ms window (see Table 21–5), the SNR (or SDR) provides an online/ongoing calculation but is implemented on only a few clinical machines. SNR is nearly identical to the transient EOAE signal-to-noise measures. After a study of

[6]There is also a multipoint ("Fmp") version of this measure; it is not clear if it is superior to Fsp (Martin, Schwegler, Gleeson, & Shi, 1994).

[7]The Intelligent Hearing Systems (IHS) SmartEP calculation of "RN" does not divide the A-B difference wave by 2 (required to calculate the plus-minus average); thus, this measure overestimates the residual noise in the waveforms by a factor of 2. The BCEHP RN criterion of 0.08 μV is thus equivalent to 0.04 μV (i.e., 40 nanovolts). Other researchers (e.g., Don & Elberling, 1996), and our recent experience, indicate that a lower RN level of approximately 0.05 μV (equivalent to 25 nanovolts) is a more appropriate maximum noise level for no response.

[8]Due to overestimation of the residual noise by RN (see preceding footnote), the IHS SmartEP system's SNR measure is equivalent to SDR/2. Both SNR and SDR measures use a measure of the "signal" that contains both response and noise. One can estimate the true signal-to-noise ratio by $[(SNR * 2)^2 - 1]$ or $[SDR^2 - 1]$ (Picton et al., 1983).

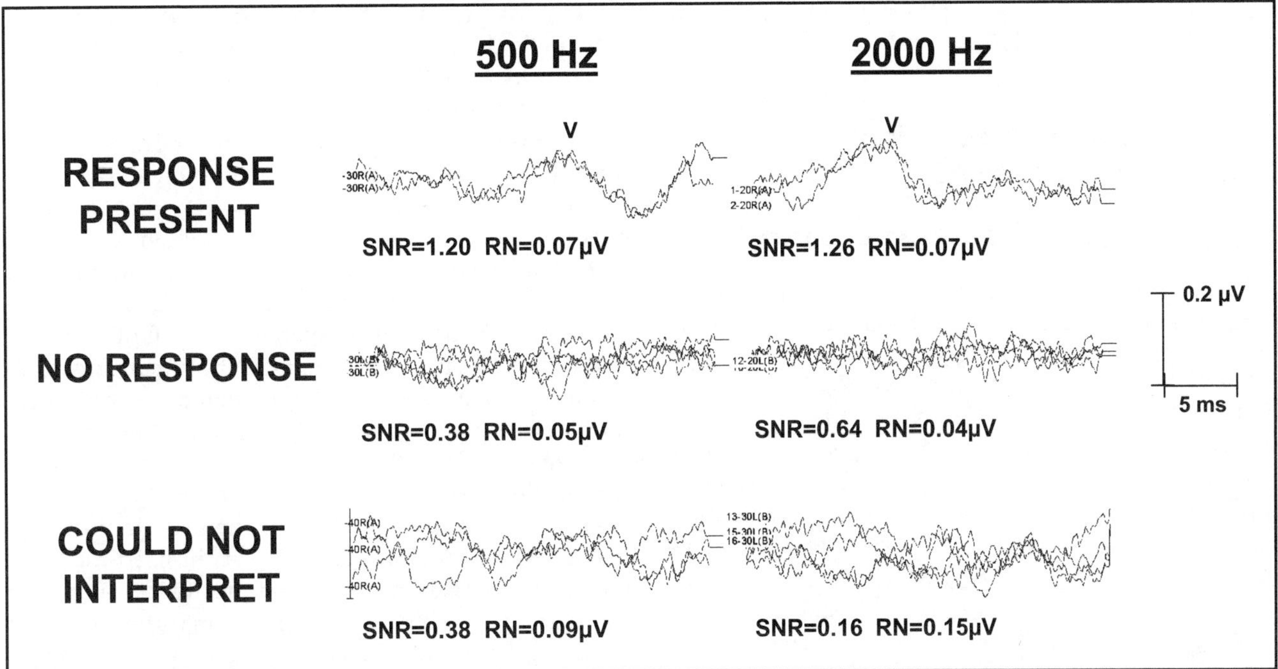

FIGURE 21–6. Interpretation of ABR waveforms. Infant ABR waveforms in response to 500- and 2000-Hz brief tones typical of "response present" (*top row*), "no response" (*middle row*), and "could not interpret" (*bottom row*) results. Shown also are the IHS Smart-EP "SNR" and "RN" measures calculated over a 10-ms window (see Table 21–5) on the average of all replications for a given set. The "response present" waveforms show a clear repeatable Wave V, the peak-to-peak amplitude of which is at least three times the average difference between the replications in the 3- to 4-ms region surrounding Wave V. The SNR measures are above 1, also consistent with response presence. Although not required for a present response, the RN values of 0.07 µV indicate reasonably quiet results. The "no response" waveforms do not show a repeatable waveform that is larger than the background noise (i.e., difference between replications is at least as large as any peak), and the waveforms are essentially flat. SNR values are well below 1 and thus consistent with no response. Most importantly, the waves are acceptably quiet (indicated both visually and by the low RN values which are less than the 0.08-µV criterion). The "could not interpret" waveforms do not show any repeatable peak and SNR values are well below 1; hence, they do not show any response. However, one cannot be sure a small, threshold-level response was not missed as these recordings are noisy. Thus, because the waves are too noisy (indicated by large differences between replications and nonflat waveforms and RN values that are above the 0.08-µV criterion) one must interpret these waves as "could not interpret." (SNR = IHS Smart-EP "signal-to-noise ratio"; RN = IHS Smart-EP "residual noise level"; waveform time base = 25.6 ms.)

SNRs of tone-ABRs in nearly 100 infants with normal or impaired hearing (Haboosheh, 2007), the BCEHP has recently implemented the use of SNR for determination of response presence in tone-ABR waves (BCEHP, 2012). Typically, SNR values of 1 or greater (or SDR ≥ 2) suggest a likely response (occasionally, "present" responses show SNR values <1). Figure 21–6 shows SNR values (calculated for the average of all replications) for results showing "response present," "no response," and "could not interpret" (i.e., too noisy to conclude no response).

None of the measures above are perfect and occasionally suggest "no response" when visual examination by experts conclude otherwise. Moreover, these measures are quite sensitive to the presence of stimulus artifact or 60-Hz (50-Hz in Europe) line noise; thus, care must be taken to ensure these are excluded from the SNR region. As noted above, measures of waveform noise (RN or sp-variance) are currently most important and essential. Statistical measures described above might be particularly helpful in training new clinicians and in ensuring consistency among clinicians within a facility or across multiple facilities within a larger program (such as the BCEHP).

Current Issues and Questions Concerning the Tone-ABR

Frequency Specificity of the Tone-ABR

To evoke ABRs of reasonable amplitude, brief tones with relatively short rise/fall times and durations must be used (Beattie & Torre, 1997; Brinkmann & Scherg, 1979; Kodera, Yamane, Yamada, & Suzuki, 1977; Stapells & Picton, 1981; Suzuki & Horiuchi, 1981). As shown in Table 21–5, we (as well as others) recommend brief tones with total durations of 5 cycles and rise/fall times of 2 to 2.5 cycles. Such brief tones demonstrate reasonable frequency specificity (Klein, 1983; Nousak & Stapells, 1992; Oates & Stapells, 1997a, 1997b; Purdy & Abbas, 2002; Stapells & Oates, 1997; Stapells, Picton, & Durieux-Smith, 1994), and many studies have shown these brief stimuli provide adequate estimates of the audiogram for all but very steep (≥50 dB/octave slope) hearing losses. When hearing losses are very steep, the tone-ABR threshold will indicate an elevated threshold but can underestimate the amount of hearing loss; this occurs as a result of the acoustic splatter to the better hearing at adjacent frequencies (Purdy & Abbas, 2002). Fortunately, hearing losses with such steep slopes (≥50 dB/octave) are relatively uncommon, especially in infants, thus the ABR threshold to brief (5-cycle) tones provides a good estimate of the audiogram for the large majority of infants.

It has been claimed that the frequency-specificity of the tone-ABR threshold estimate can be improved by using more complex nonlinear stimulus windowing functions, such as Blackman or exact-Blackman windows (Gorga, 2002; Gorga & Thornton, 1989). Although the acoustics based on the total duration of the stimuli might lead one to conclude these nonlinear windows would be better, such a claim assumes the ABR reflects the whole stimulus, whereas the "effective" portion of the stimulus is almost certainly less than the whole stimulus. The ABR appears not to be sensitive to the small differences in the temporal waveforms of the linear versus Blackman stimuli. Results published to date do not support the claim for superiority of these nonlinear windows, with at least five studies showing equivalent ABR results between linear and nonlinear (Blackman or exact-Blackman) windows (Beattie, Kenworthy, & Vanides, 2005; Johnson & Brown, 2005; Oates & Stapells, 1997a, 1997b; Purdy & Abbas, 2002). Thus, either linear- or Blackman-windowed stimuli can be used with equal accuracy.[9]

Another technique proposed to improve the frequency specificity of the ABR to brief tones, especially in the presence of very steep losses, is that of band-reject ("notched") noise masking (Picton, Ouellette, Hamel, & Smith, 1979; Stapells & Picton, 1981; Stapells et al., 1994). The notched noise restricts the region of the basilar membrane that is capable of contributing to the response to the frequencies within the notch. The noise has a one-octave-wide notch centered on the tone's nominal frequency; slopes of the noise filters must be quite steep (at least 48 dB/octave slope), and the intensity of the noise (before filtering) set 20 dB below the peak-to-peak equivalent SPL of the brief-tone stimulus. In recent years, we have de-emphasized the need for notched noise, as it adds complexity to equipment setup and test protocol, few clinical machines provide the capability for notched noise, and more importantly, results have shown the need for notched noise is limited to only very steep losses. Thus, ABR threshold results with and without notched noise masking are similar for more typical groups of individuals with hearing loss (Johnson & Brown, 2005; Stapells, 2000b).

It is important to remind readers that without special noise masking procedures, *no measure* is cochlear place specific when using moderate-to-high stimulus levels, not even a behavioral response to long-duration pure-tone stimuli. That is, when presented at 60 to 80 dB HL (and higher), even pure-tone stimuli result in fairly wide cochlear excitation (Moore, 2004). Thus, elevated thresholds obtained using behavioral pure-tone audiometry are affected by this broad cochlear excitation, and it is unreasonable to expect the ABR (or ASSR) at these intensities to exhibit any better frequency specificity (Picton et al., 2003).

Stimulus Onset Polarity: Alternating or Single Polarity?

Concern has often been expressed about the use of alternating onset polarity. Specifically, it has been suggested that response amplitudes with alternating polarity will be reduced due to phase cancellation, and thus thresholds are elevated (e.g., Gorga et al., 2006; Gorga, Kaminski, & Beauchaine, 1991). However, there is no evidence for this concern, especially

[9]There is little research on the frequency specificity of the ABR (or ASSR) to narrowband chirp stimuli.

concerning thresholds in infants. In an unpublished study in our lab, in nine normal hearing infants, we found no difference between single polarity (rarefaction or condensation onset polarity) and alternating polarity for Wave V amplitudes and thresholds for clicks, 500-Hz brief tones, or 2000-Hz brief tones (Wu & Stapells, unpublished). This is consistent with the fact that the majority of tone-ABR threshold studies have utilized alternating onset polarity, and, as noted above, threshold estimates have been quite accurate (see Tables 21–1 through 21–3). In fact, there are good reasons for employing alternating polarity tones: (a) at high intensities, electromagnetic stimulus artifact can significantly contaminate responses, especially at 500 and 1000 Hz. This artifact can make it difficult to recognize the physiologic response; if objective response detection measures are employed, the artifact can render these measures useless. Alternating polarity largely removes the artifact (though not completely at highest intensities); and (b) especially for moderate and higher stimulus intensities, there can be steady-state responses to each cycle of the tone's carrier frequency, such as the cochlear microphonic or the frequency following response, which often make it more difficult to recognize or measure the transient (e.g., Wave V-V′) response. Alternating the polarity, for the most part, removes these unwanted responses. Although we recommend routine use of alternating polarity for all brief-tone intensities, at lower stimulus intensities there is likely no difference and little concern about polarity, and either single polarity or alternating polarity are fine. It is important to note, however, that due to the very large electromagnetic stimulus artifact occurring with bone-conduction transducers, alternating polarity should always be used for bone-conducted stimuli.

Maximum Stimulus Intensities for ABR

For several reasons, there are limits to the maximum intensities of stimuli for the ABR. First, current transducers have limitations, beyond which significant distortion occurs. Insert earphones (ER-3A) typically are limited to a maximum of about 120 dB SPL. This limits 500- to 4000-Hz pure-tone stimuli to about 110 dB HL. Because behavioral and ABR thresholds for the brief stimuli used to elicit the ABR are in the 20 to 30 dB SPL range (see Table 21–5), maximum intensities are thus limited to about 90 to 100 dB nHL. This is not necessarily the maximum possible output for ABR stimuli, as other air-conduction transducers, including soundfield speakers, do have higher output. The maximum outputs (before distortion) are even more limited for the B-71 bone oscillator: about 70 dB HL for pure-tone stimuli, and 50 to 60 dB nHL for brief-tone stimuli (Small & Stapells, 2003).[10] A second reason there are maximum output limitations is the contamination of responses by large stimulus artifact at very high intensities. For the most part, the presence of stimulus artifact does not preclude interpretable recordings, as ABR Wave V-V′ usually occurs later than the artifact. Furthermore, stimulus polarity can be alternated to at least partially cancel stimulus artifact, and in extreme cases special shielding can reduce artifact. High-amplitude stimulus artifact has been shown to result in artifactual ASSRs (Gorga et al., 2004; Jeng, Brown, Johnson, & Vander Werff, 2004; Small & Stapells, 2004), although appropriate processing of the EEG largely removes these nonphysiologic spurious responses (Brooke, Brennan, & Stevens, 2009; Picton & John, 2004; Small & Stapells, 2004). A third cause of output limitation is the possibility of high stimulus levels producing nonauditory responses. Vibrotactile responses, especially to bone-conducted stimuli, place well-known limits for behavioral audiometry (Boothroyd & Cawkwell, 1970). Although vibrotactile responses are not likely to produce an ABR or brainstem ASSR, there is evidence that stimulation of the vestibular system can produce responses in the ABR and brainstem-ASSR time frame. Vestibular responses are especially problematic for interpretation of ASSRs to high-intensity stimuli in individuals with severe-to-profound hearing loss. This issue is discussed in the ASSR section below. Finally, a fourth cause of output limits is the real concern that maximum output stimuli might cause cochlear damage. This is of greatest concern for the ASSR where at least 10 minutes of averaging might be required to reduce the residual EEG noise to a level below that of the amplitude of a near-threshold response. As ASSR stimuli are continuous, stimulation at levels such as 90 to 110 dB HL must be regularly interrupted in order to rest the cochlea and protect it from damage. This is less of a concern for the transient ABR, as stimuli are already presented with a less than 50% duty cycle (a 500-Hz brief tone present using a 39 per second rate has at least a 15 ms quiet blank between each 10-ms stimulus). Similarly, damage from high-intensity stimuli is much less of a concern for behavioral testing, as stimuli are presented for only very brief durations.

[10] As with air conduction, there are other bone-conduction transducers with a higher maximum output (e.g., MAICO KLH96), but for which there are no published ABR (or ASSR) data.

How to Couple the Bone Oscillator to an Infant's Head

In our early research, we had an assistant hand-hold the bone oscillator to the infant's head during bone-conduction ABR testing, and found little difficulty with this procedure (Gravel et al., 1989; Stapells, 1989; Stapells & Ruben, 1989). However, other researchers expressed concern with this practice, so our subsequent bone-conduction research (Foxe & Stapells, 1993; Ishida, Cuthbert, & Stapells, 2011; Nousak & Stapells, 1992; Small & Stapells, 2003, 2004, 2005, 2006, 2008a, 2008b) utilized the technique described by Yang and colleagues (Yang, Stuart, Stenstrom, & Hollett, 1991; Yang, Stuart, Mencher, Mencher, & Vincer, 1993), which uses a wide elastic band with Velcro. However, we find this technique often awkward clinically, sometimes waking an infant and always requiring a longer time. Subsequently, we carried out research comparing the elastic-band and handheld procedures, and found the handheld procedure was at least as reliable (indeed, it was less variable) and accurate as the elastic band procedure, provided assistants were appropriately trained (Small, Hatton, & Stapells, 2007). For clinical use, we currently recommend (BCEHP, 2012) and use (Hatton et al., 2012) hand-holding the bone oscillator, given the relative ease and, importantly, speed and nonintrusiveness, of hand holding.[11]

Establishing Normative Data

Many popular textbooks instruct clinicians to obtain (a) normal hearing levels (nHL) for their ABR stimuli, and (b) their own normative latency data. Both of these practices have significant problems. Obtaining nHLs for click and brief-tone stimuli requires appropriate quiet sound booths, careful psychoacoustic procedures, and appropriate subjects (e.g., large number of normal young adults)—error in any of these can make a clinic's results uninterpretable, especially if no acoustic calibration of the obtained 0-dB nHL is made. Unless using a radically different stimulus for which little-or-no research exists, clinicians should use the acoustic calibrations of published research—in the same fashion as how they calibrate their equipment for behavioral audiometry but with different calibration values (see Table 21–5). The International Standards Organization (ISO) has proposed reference equivalent threshold sound pressure levels (RETSPLs) and reference equivalent threshold force levels (RETFLs) for AC and BC stimuli used for ABR testing (ISO 389-6:2007; Fedtke & Richter, 2007). However, the levels proposed (a) have not been universally accepted (e.g., they are not used in North America); (b) are not all based on actual measures on normal-hearing subjects (e.g., RETFLs for brief tones are derived from long-duration stimuli); and, importantly, (c) these "standards" fail to appropriately consider the many well-established large-group studies determining "nHL" for air- and bone-conducted brief tones. Even more important, as the bulk of the research on infant ABR thresholds has been based on these previously determined RETSPL/RETFL nHL values, and because several large discrepancies exist between these values and the ISO values, we continue to recommend our well-researched acoustic levels of normal thresholds for these stimuli. (Table 21–5 presents our recommended 0-dB nHL values for three transducers.[12])

Clinicians often ask for tone-ABR latency normative data. As noted above, we do not assess whether latencies are normal or prolonged when evaluating ABR thresholds. Thus, tone- ABR latency "norms" are not that helpful, other than to give an idea of where Wave V typically occurs. This information is available from the waveforms in Figures 21–1 and 21–5 (as well as other publications) and quickly comes after testing a few infants. On the more general question of clinicians obtaining their own latency norms (e.g., for click-ABRs), we strongly believe that the literature already contains excellent normative data, obtained for a greater number of subjects than is typically possible for most clinicians (good latency norms require large samples of subjects—sample sizes of 10–20 are too small). The most important click-ABR latency measures—the I–V interpeak interval and wave V interaural latency difference—are quite consistent across most studies and little affected by stimulus and recording factors (except for rates >20 per second), making it quite acceptable to use published norms. Thus, we do *not* recommend that clinicians determine their own norms; rather, we suggest they use published norms from a larger study

[11]The elastic-band technique is preferable when it is difficult to hand-hold the bone oscillator due to equipment setup or lack of a trained assistant.

[12]Differences between the ISO and Stapells (and other researchers) recommended AC RETSPLs, after corrections for type of ear occluder, are −2.7, **−9.5** (i.e., Stapells' reference is 9.5 dB SPL *higher*), 1.8, and −3.2 dB at 500, 1000, 2000, and 4000 Hz, respectively. Differences for BC RETFLs amount to 2.5, **4.5**, −1.5, and **7** dB (Stapells' reference is 7 dB SPL *lower*) at 500, 1000, 2000, and 4000 Hz, respectively. The large bolded differences (5–10 dB, after rounding) are problematic and likely clinically significant.

for reasonably similar parameters and subject population (for a listing of many normative samples, see textbook by Hall, 2007). To ensure their results are similar, clinicians can test a small group (e.g., test 10 subjects, after ensuring appropriate stimulus calibrations, test parameters, and procedures) and then make statistical comparisons between their results with the larger study. If no practically significant differences exist, clinicians can feel comfortable using the published norms for their clinical testing.

The Brainstem Auditory Steady-State Response

Auditory steady-state responses to stimuli presented using repetition, or modulation, rates in the 70- to 110-Hz range are referred to as the "80-Hz" or "brainstem" ASSR. These responses have attracted ongoing attention (and some excitement) by audiologists, especially by those involved in the assessment and subsequent hearing-aid fitting of very young infants identified with hearing loss. Equipment manufacturers have been marketing their ASSR systems for such testing. Readers will find comprehensive chapters about the brainstem ASSR in a text edited by Rance (2008a).

What Is the Auditory Steady-State Response?

First recorded in 1960 from the scalp of humans by Geisler (1960), ASSRs were subsequently recorded in response to clicks, to sinusoidally modulated tones, and to square-wave modulated tones by Campbell and colleagues (Campbell, Atkinson, Francis, & Green, 1977). Major audiologic interest in ASSRs came with the publication by Galambos, Makeig, and Talmachoff (1981) concerning the "40-Hz ASSR." Subsequent studies indicated frequency-based (Fourier) analyses could be used to accurately measure the ASSRs (e.g., Rickards & Clark, 1984; Stapells, Linden, Suffield, Hamel, & Picton, 1984). From 1981 through to the mid-1990s, the clinical audiology community went through its first phase of excitement concerning this new evoked potential threshold measure, with one manufacturer developing and marketing "the first objective infant audiometer" utilizing the ASSR to stimuli presented with a 40-Hz repetition rate. Unfortunately, subsequent research showed the 40-Hz ASSR was decreased in sleeping subjects (e.g., Cohen, Rickards, & Clark, 1991; Linden, Campbell, Hamel, & Picton, 1985), and, more importantly, it is very difficult to record in infants (e.g., Stapells, Galambos, Costello, & Makeig, 1988; Suzuki & Kobayashi, 1984). Interest and use of ASSRs by clinicians thus quickly disappeared. However, some researchers persevered and demonstrated that ASSRs to near-threshold stimuli presented with rates of 70 to 110 Hz—the brainstem ASSR—are easily recordable in sleeping infants (e.g., Lins & Picton, 1995; Lins, Picton, Picton, Champagne, & Durieux-Smith, 1995; Lins et al., 1996; Rance, Rickards, Cohen, De Vidi, & Clark, 1995), and today there is a growing body of data as well as availability of clinical systems that automatically stimulate and analyze these responses.

Discussion concerning the generators of the ASSR has thus far primarily focused on ASSRs evoked by stimulus rates in the 30- to 50-Hz range. Studies investigating the neural sources of the 40-Hz response have concluded the response has both brainstem and cortical generators (e.g., Herdman et al., 2002; Mauer & Döring, 1999). Studies investigating the neural sources of 80-Hz ASSRs in humans and animals indicate they originate primarily from brainstem structures (Herdman et al., 2002; Kuwada et al., 2002; Mauer & Döring, 1999). Although not yet confirmed, it is quite likely that 80-Hz ASSRs are actually ABR Waves V to rapidly presented stimuli. The ASSR stimulation and analysis techniques can differ, but the underlying physiology and interpretation of these brainstem ASSRs are likely similar to those for ABR Wave V.

ASSR Analysis Techniques

As noted above, an important feature of the ASSR is that frequency-domain analyses, such as the fast Fourier transform (FFT), provide excellent measures of the response, and there are clear procedures to determine response presence and absence. For example, similar to procedures for distortion-product otoacoustic emissions (DPOAEs), an FFT of the response provides the amplitude at exactly the stimulus modulation rate, which is compared to the amplitudes of "noise" frequencies immediately surrounding the modulation rate ("sidebins"; Figure 21–7). Thus, the amplitude and phase of the response at the rate of stimulation, as well as measures of response noise, are measured entirely objectively and automatically by a computer. However, in contrast to DPOAE measures, ASSR systems go a step further and determine the statistical probability of a response being present. A number of statistical tests have been employed, with most studies employing either a measure of phase variability ("phase coherence") or comparison of the amplitude at

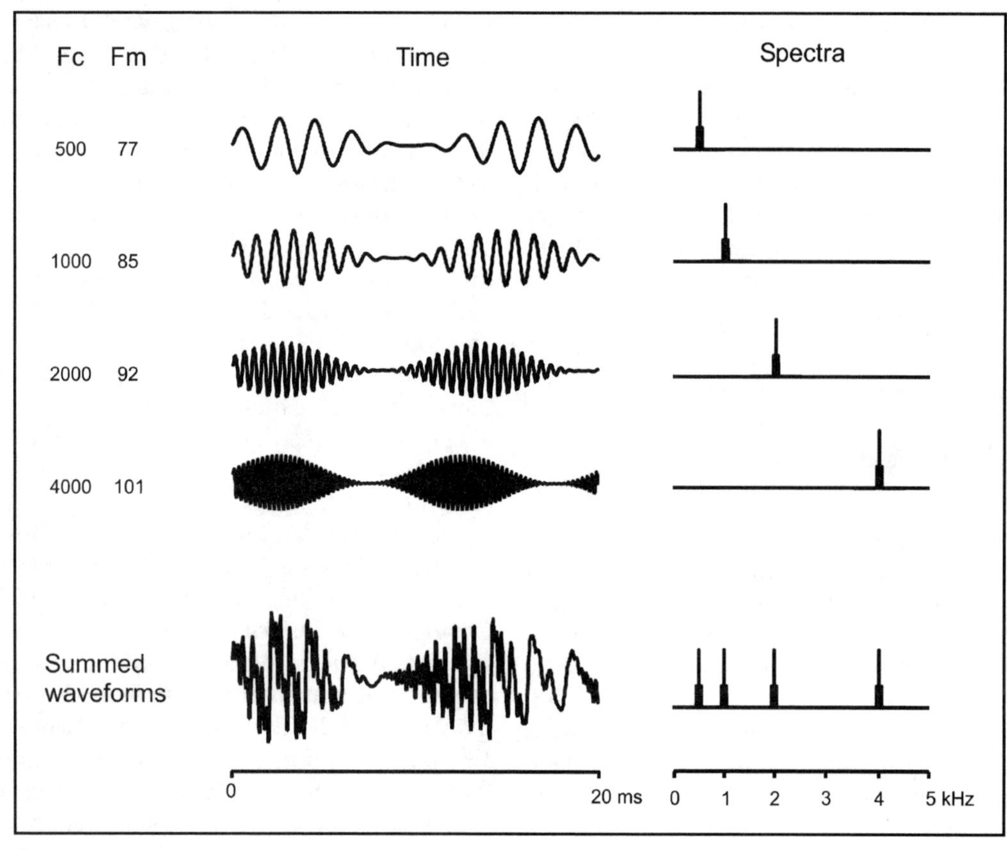

A

FIGURE 21–7. A. ASSR stimuli: Time and frequency spectra of multiple auditory steady-state stimuli. Four individual amplitude-modulated stimuli with carrier frequencies (Fc) ranging from 500 to 4000 Hz and modulation frequencies (Fm) ranging from 77 to 101 Hz are shown. Time waveforms spanning two cycles are shown (*left panel*). The corresponding spectra are shown in the right panel. The summed time and frequency spectra are shown at the bottom left and right panels, respectively. *continues*

the stimulus rate (or modulation frequency) to amplitudes of surrounding noise frequencies ("F-test"; for detailed reviews, see John & Purcell, 2008; Picton et al., 2003). Thus, with current ASSR systems, response determination is entirely objective; a human interpreter does not view waveforms or determine the replicability and location of peaks. This objectivity of response determination is a major advantage of the ASSR over the transient ABR, although as noted above, objective techniques are now available for the ABR.

As when interpreting the ABR, the "response noise" estimate is also an essential measure for ASSR interpretation. When concluding a "no-response" result, it is important that a clinician continues recording until the level of response noise is below the typical amplitude of a threshold-level response. That is, ensure that a small-amplitude response was not missed because of a noisy recording. Unfortunately, not all ASSR systems provide this noise measure and, importantly, not all research studies (or clinicians) have employed such noise measures. Furthermore, there remains some uncertainty concerning what is the appropriate noise criterion (e.g., what is an acceptably low level of noise?). Because near-threshold 80-Hz ASSRs have amplitudes of about 20 to 30 nV, mean noise levels (e.g., side-bin noise) of 10 nV or lower are typically required before one can conclude that no response is present, although this level appears to differ somewhat for different analysis methods (van Maanen & Stapells, 2009). The above notwithstanding, an appropriate noise criterion must be reached before concluding "no response."

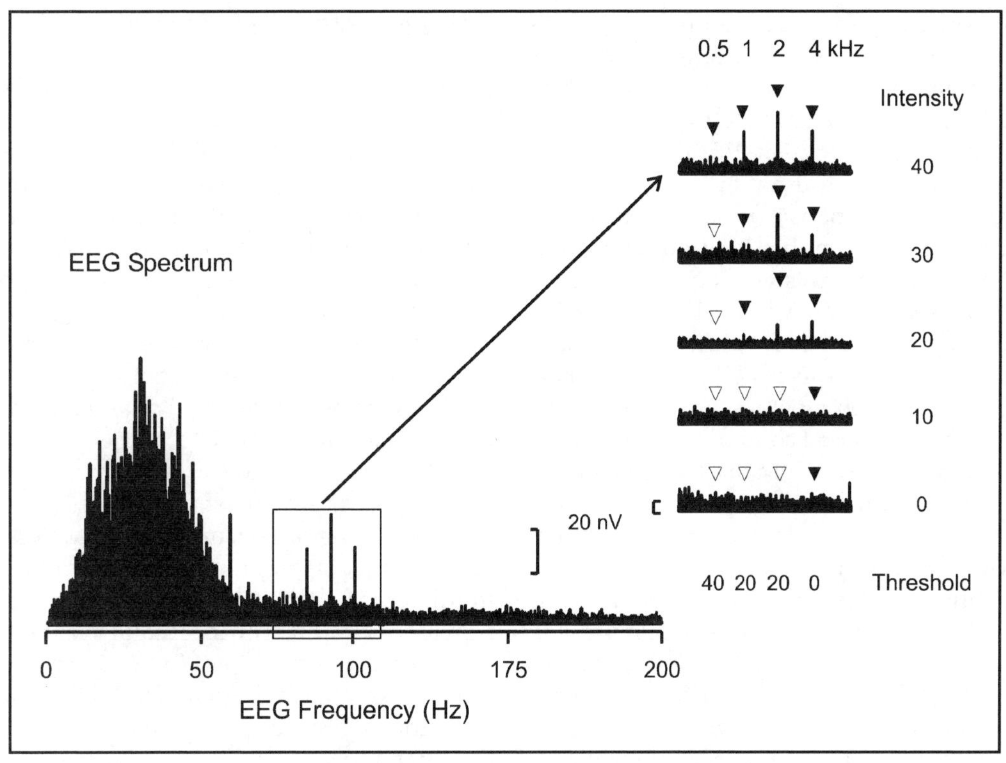

B

FIGURE 21–7. *continued* **B.** Response analyses: Threshold intensity series of multiple auditory steady-state responses recorded from an 11-week-old infant with normal hearing. Intensities are in dB nHL (Herdman & Stapells, 2001, 2003). Responses were elicited using the stimuli shown in Figure 21–7A. *Bottom right:* The entire EEG frequency spectra. *Right panel:* Spectra over the frequency range near the modulation frequency. Carrier frequencies corresponding to the four signals are shown on the top. Filled triangles indicate responses that reached significance ($p < .05$); open triangles indicate no-response ($p \geq .05$ *and* EEG noise < 11nV). Thresholds of 40, 20, 20, and 0 dB nHL at 500, 1000, 2000, and 4000 Hz are equivalent to 46, 29, 24, and 2 dB HL. (Reprinted with permission from Phonak AG. Figure from Stapells, D. R., Herdman, A., Small, S. A., Dimitrijevic, A., & Hatton, J. [2005]. Current status of the auditory steady-state responses for estimating an infant's audiogram. In R. Seewald and J. Bamford [Eds.], *A sound foundation through early amplification 2004: Proceedings of the Third International Conference* [pp. 43–59]. Stäfa, Switzerland: Phonak AG.)

As previously indicated, there is considerable research demonstrating the effectiveness of phase coherence and F-test response statistics, and some ASSR systems employ these well-tested measures (for review, see John & Purcell, 2008). Some recent ASSR systems, however, use modifications of these measures, or altogether entirely different algorithms. However, few studies have assessed these new or modified measures—it might be premature for individuals to consider purchase of these new and relatively untested systems.

ASSR Stimulus Paradigms

Although the earliest studies of ASSRs tended to use brief tonal stimuli, similar to those used to evoke the ABR, most recent research has focused on continuous sinusoidally amplitude-modulated (AM) tonal stimuli, sometimes with 10% to 25% frequency modulation (FM). Most current ASSR systems use such stimuli, as have most research studies. The acoustics of continuous sinusoidal AM stimuli are very frequency specific;

their spectra show energy at the carrier frequency plus two side lobes at frequencies equal to the carrier frequency plus-minus the modulation frequency. Thus, as shown in Figure 21–7, a 1000-Hz tone modulated at 85 Hz would contain energy at 915, 1000, and 1085 Hz. Because no energy is present at the modulation rate, interpretation of response presence-absence by the computer is less susceptible to stimulus artifact (assuming linear stimulus systems and appropriate EEG digitization; see below). Adding 10% to 25% FM results in somewhat larger ASSR amplitudes but also complicates the stimulus spectra (Purcell & Dajani, 2008). One possible reason most researchers studying the brainstem ASSR have used continuous stimuli (sine AM or AM/FM) might be because of a belief that these ASSRs are inherently different from the transient ABR. However, as discussed above, 80-Hz ASSRs are brainstem responses and thus can show similar stimulus-response limitations as ABR Wave V; for example, the transient ABR shows larger responses to stimuli with faster rise times (e.g., Stapells & Picton, 1981). Similarly, larger amplitude ASSRs are obtained using AM tones with more-rapid envelopes, such as brief-duration tones (Mo & Stapells, 2008) or exponential envelopes (John, Dimitrijevic, & Picton, 2002). One clinical ASSR system's default stimuli are Blackman-windowed brief tones (4–8 ms duration), which can result in larger-amplitude ASSRs. However, to obtain a significant improvement in ASSR amplitude (compared to longer stimuli), durations must be reduced to be quite brief (<4 cycles); such durations result in reduced frequency specificity as well as increased interactions (amplitude reductions) between responses to multiple simultaneous stimuli (Mo & Stapells, 2008).

As noted, stimuli with broader frequency spectra lead to larger-amplitude ASSRs. AM/FM stimuli show broader frequency spectra and result in larger amplitudes, and the small loss in frequency specificity has generally been considered acceptable. Some studies have investigated the use of stimuli with much broader frequency spectra (e.g., clicks or modulated noise; broadband chirps), specifically for the purpose of newborn hearing screening (Cebulla, Sturzebecher, Elberling, & Muller, 2007; John, Brown, Muir, & Picton, 2004). The broad frequency spectra result in large-amplitude ASSRs, making response detection (and thus screening) much faster. However, as with the click-ABR, there is no frequency specificity to this screening. Research into the use of more frequency-specific stimuli for newborn screening is also underway (Cone-Wesson, Parker, Swiderski, & Rickards, 2002; John et al., 2004; Savio, Perez-Abalo, Gaya, Hernandez, & Mijares, 2006; Sturzebecher, Cebulla, Elberling, & Berger, 2006).

The Multiple ASSR Technique

A unique feature of the ASSR is that responses to multiple stimuli can be separated and independently assessed, all simultaneously. Because the ASSR to a stimulus presented at a specific modulation rate has its major response energy at exactly the stimulus modulation rate, it is possible to present several stimuli each with different carrier frequencies and, importantly, different modulation rates (see Figure 21–7). Responses to each stimulus can then be evaluated by examining the response energy at each stimulus' exact modulation rate. First demonstrated by Lins and Picton in 1995, this multiple-stimulus ASSR technique has subsequently been developed to allow assessment of responses from both ears and four carrier frequencies (i.e., eight different modulation rates) simultaneously. Research to date suggests that (a) amplitudes are not reduced using the multiple-ASSR technique (compared to single stimuli) provided stimulus carrier frequencies (within an ear) are at least an octave apart in frequency and 60 dB SPL or less (Herdman & Stapells, 2001; John, Lins, Boucher, & Picton, 1998); (b) presenting multiple AM stimuli does not appear to reduce the frequency specificity of the stimulus-response pairing (Herdman et al., 2002; Herdman & Stapells, 2003); (c) at higher intensities (>60 dB SPL), amplitudes decrease due to interactions between responses to the multiple stimuli (John et al., 1998; Picton, van Roon, & John, 2009; Wood, 2009); and (d) the multiple-stimulus technique is more efficient (faster) than the single-stimulus technique, although not as much as initially expected. Issues such as sloping audiograms, smaller amplitudes at some frequencies compared to others, and amplitude reductions due to interactions at higher stimulus intensities (Ishida & Stapells, 2012; John et al., 1998; Mo & Stapells, 2008) all decrease the efficiency of the multiple stimulus technique such that it is, at best, only 1.5 to 3 times faster than the single-stimulus technique (Herdman & Stapells, 2001, 2003; John et al., 2002). Our recent research suggests that similar interactions are found in adults with sensory/neural loss as those with normal hearing (Ishida & Stapells, 2012).

Although many clinical systems employing the multiple ASSR are currently being marketed to clinicians, there are surprisingly few studies that have investigated the efficiency of the single versus multiple ASSR techniques. Our recent studies indicate that (a) normal infants show significant interactions with the multiple-ASSR, even at 60 dB SPL, but their thresholds are not affected and the multiple technique remains more efficient (Hatton & Stapells, 2011, 2013); (b) greater interactions are seen in response to higher-intensity stimuli (Ishida & Stapells, 2012; Mo & Stapells, 2008); and (c) stimuli with broader spectra, such as AM/FM, show significantly greater interactions, even at 60 dB SPL in adults, significantly reducing the efficiency of the multiple ASSR technique (Mo & Stapells, 2008; Wood, 2009).[13]

Frequency Specificity of the Brainstem ASSR

The *acoustic frequency specificity* of sinusoidally amplitude-modulated tones, even when combined with 10% to 25% frequency modulation (AM/FM), is reasonably narrow, a fact that is often touted as one advantage of the ASSR over the tone-evoked ABR. However, the *cochlear place specificity* and the *neuronal specificity* of the stimulus-response pairing must also be considered (Herdman et al., 2002; Picton, Dimitrijevic, & John, 2002). Use of acoustically specific stimuli does not always translate into responses that are more frequency specific, for example, as noted above, although Blackman-windowed tones show better acoustic specificity, the brainstem responses to these stimuli have the same frequency specificity as do those to brief tones shaped by linear windows (Oates & Stapells, 1997a, 1997b; Purdy & Abbas, 2002). Research into the frequency specificity of the brainstem ASSR is limited, especially for the ASSR to newer stimuli such as AM^2 stimuli or NB chirps. Nevertheless, using two distinct methods, (a) high-pass noise masking/derived response analyses in subjects with normal hearing (Herdman et al., 2002) and (b) assessment of thresholds in individuals with steeply sloping sensory/neural loss (Herdman & Stapells, 2003; Johnson & Brown, 2005), results indicate the ASSR to sine-AM tones has reasonably good frequency specificity. However, ASSR frequency specificity was not as good as would be expected from the acoustic specificity of the AM stimuli, with the ASSR frequency specificity being similar to that previously shown for the tone-evoked ABR (Herdman et al., 2002), a finding consistent with the view that ABR Wave V underlies the 80-Hz ASSR. Importantly, no difference in ASSR frequency specificity was seen for responses to multiple versus single stimuli (Herdman et al., 2002; Herdman & Stapells, 2003). It must be noted, however, that we currently know little of the frequency specificity of the brainstem ASSR to newer, more complex (compared to sinusoidal AM) stimuli, with no studies of the frequency specificity of brainstem ASSRs to exponential, NB-chirp or brief-tone stimuli, and only one such study for AM/FM stimuli (Johnson & Brown, 2005).

Calibration of Stimuli for the Brainstem ASSR

Similar to the long-duration pure-tone stimuli used for behavioral audiometry, the continuous nature of most ASSR stimuli makes them easy to measure using a sound-level meter set to "normal" (dB RMS) sound pressure level. Behavioral thresholds for continuous sinusoidal AM and AM/FM ASSR stimuli are close to those for long-duration pure tones; thus, most studies (and ASSR systems) have calibrated these stimuli in dB HL (ANSI, 1996). This is in contrast to the transient brief-tone stimuli used for the ABR, where calibrations are in dB "peak" or "peak-to-peak equivalent" SPL as well in "dB nHL." The nHL is employed because behavioral and ABR thresholds are elevated due to their brief duration (e.g., Stapells & Oates, 1997). However, as shown below, ASSR thresholds (in dB HL) are also significantly elevated compared to normal behavioral thresholds, especially in young infants. Interestingly, when expressed in decibel peak-to-peak equivalent SPL, air-conduction ASSR thresholds in normal infants are within about 5 dB of those for the tone-evoked ABR (e.g., Rance, Tomlin, & Rickards, 2006). Thus, similar to the situation for the ABR, brainstem ASSR thresholds likely reflect a brief portion of the stimulus rather than the long-term RMS SPL of the whole stimulus. Another problem for the use of dB HL is that there remain large gaps in our understanding of the relationship between ASSR thresholds (in dB HL) and pure-tone behavioral thresholds (in dB HL), especially in infants with hearing loss. Caution is thus required when interpreting infant ASSR thresholds in "dB HL."

The Problem of New ASSR Technology and Methodology

ASSR technology has evolved and expanded over the last 20 years. ASSR systems existed only in research labs until about 15 years ago when the first two clinical systems were developed: the single-stimulus Viasys/GSI "Audera" based on the Australian "ERA" system, and the multiple-stimulus Neuronic "Audix." Today,

[13]Spectra for 100% AM/25% FM tones are about three times wider (at −20 dB) than sine-AM and two times wider than AM^2 stimuli (Wood, 2009).

there are many commercial ASSR systems available,[14] yet the lack of standardization among the different systems is a concern. Some of these systems are closely based on the equipment and techniques used in much of the foundational ASSR research. However, many of the new systems employ new stimulation (e.g., AM^2 and NB-chirp stimuli) and analysis (e.g., Kalman filtering) techniques that are quite different from published research. There are few published studies to support these changes or, when available, the research has only been carried out in adults with normal hearing. With differing methodologies, new systems, and few published data (especially for infants with hearing loss), the current situation is one of "buyer beware," and caution must be advised. Individuals considering purchase of a particular ASSR system should ensure evidence (including clinical data) exists for that system's methodology. Preferably, such data would be available in the peer-reviewed scientific literature, be obtained in the target population (infants, especially hearing-impaired infants), and (at least some) be at arms-length from manufacturers and patent holders.

Artifactual ASSRs and Nonauditory Responses

One clear example of the pitfalls of using of a "new" response or technique (in this case, the 80-Hz ASSR), new system, or new technology, is demonstrated by the findings in our laboratory as well as others of spurious or artifactual ASSRs to high-intensity air- and bone-conducted stimuli (Gorga et al., 2004; Jeng et al., 2004; Nambi, & Vanaja, 2006; Picton & John, 2004; Small & Stapells, 2004).[15] In these studies, clear "responses" were shown to be present for individuals who were deaf and could not hear the stimuli. Some of these artifactual ASSRs are now known to be due to high-amplitude stimulus artifact contaminating the recorded EEG, and aliasing to mimic physiologic responses (Picton & John, 2004; Small & Stapells, 2004). By changing the analog-to-digital (AD) rate, filtering the EEG, and alternating the stimuli, thus removing any aliased energy, we showed that *most* of these artifactual ASSRs disappeared (Small & Stapells, 2004). This finding prompted an immediate change in at least one clinical ASSR system, but not until after many clinicians had reported ASSR responses to high-intensity stimuli for infants, some of which must have been due to technical error.

Although the artifactual ASSRs as a result of aliased stimulus artifact appear to have been solved through stimulus and analysis modifications—this has not been formally evaluated for many, if not most, clinical systems—there are, nevertheless, also physiologic but nonauditory ASSRs in individuals with severe or profound hearing loss (Nambi & Vanaja, 2006; Small & Stapells, 2004). In our 2004 study, we found that even when using an appropriate AD rate, anti-aliasing filter, and alternated-polarity stimuli, many of the deaf subjects still showed responses to 500- and 1000-Hz stimuli (no responses were seen at 2000 or 4000 Hz; Small & Stapells, 2004). We suggested these responses might be vestibular in origin, as suggested by other studies using transient-evoked potentials (e.g., Cheng, Huang, & Young, 2003; Kato et al., 1998; Murofushi, Iwasaki, Takai, & Takegoshi, 2005; Papathanasiou et al., 2004; Sheykholeslami, Kermany, & Kaga, 2000; Welgampola & Colebatch, 2001). At this time, we do not have a method to differentiate the auditory and nonauditory (vestibular) responses in an ASSR recording, and we do not know how this finding will impact audiologic decisions. The responses occur in response to high-intensity stimuli, usually low frequency, for air-conducted stimuli (at least 100 dB HL; Gorga et al., 2004; Nambi & Vanaja, 2006) and for bone-conducted stimuli (50 dB HL or higher; Nambi & Vanaja, 2006; Small & Stapells, 2004).

One drawback with ASSRs compared to transient-evoked ABRs is that ASSRs do not provide sensible time-domain waveforms to review when unexpected or questionable results are obtained. Sometimes, the time-domain waveforms can help differentiate auditory from nonauditory responses. Figure 21–8 shows ABR and ASSR results from an infant with profound hearing loss whose brainstem ASSR shows significant ($p < .05$) responses to 110 dB HL 500 to 4000 Hz air-conducted tones. However, his ABR waveforms to high-intensity air-conducted clicks and 2000-Hz brief tones are clearly abnormal, showing a clear early negative wave (3–4 ms poststimulus) with no Wave V following. Present even with alternating stimuli (i.e., not cochlear microphonic), this "N3" wave has been suggested to originate from stimulation of the vestibular system (Colebatch, 2001; Kato et al., 1998; Murofushi

[14]ASSR systems change and new systems appear regularly.

[15]Another clear example was the development and marketing of a 40-Hz ASSR "objective infant audiometer" in the 1980s before subsequent studies demonstrated the 40-Hz ASSR was not easily recorded in infants.

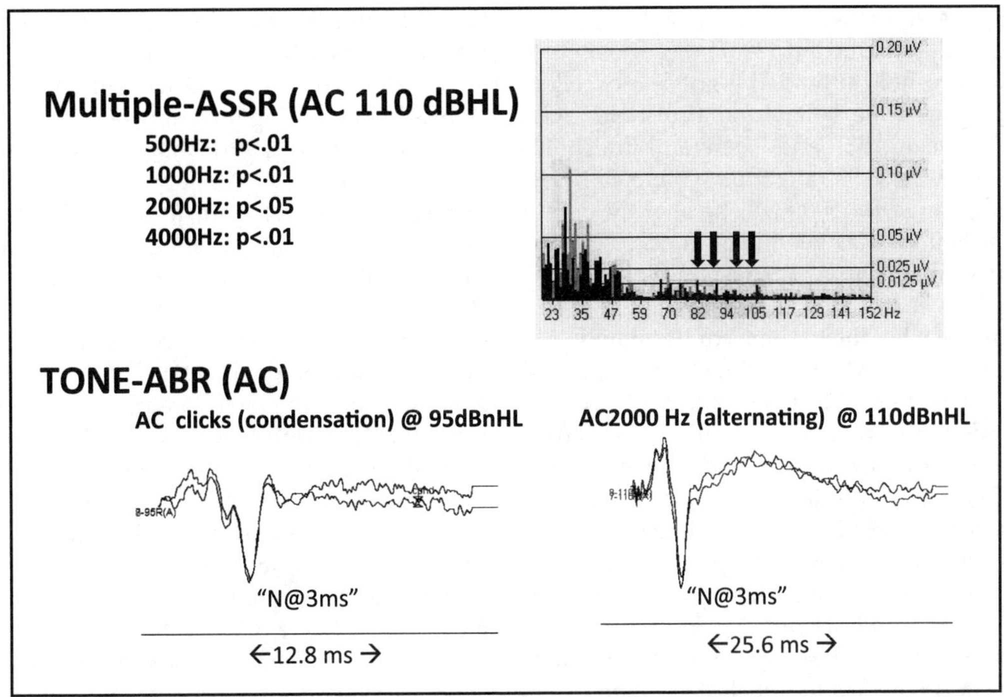

FIGURE 21–8. Air-conduction ASSR (*top panel*) and ABR (*bottom panel*) result in a 19-month-old infant with severe-to-profound bilateral sensory/neural hearing loss. The multiple-ASSR showed small-amplitude statistically significant responses (*arrows*) in response to all four frequencies presented at the system's maximum intensity. The click-evoked (*bottom left*) and tone-evoked (*bottom right*) ABR waveforms show a large negative wave at approximately 3 to 4 ms following stimulus onset, with no clear Wave V present. This "N3" wave is neural (i.e., not cochlear microphonic), as it remains present with the alternating-polarity tonal stimuli. N3 has been suggested to reflect a brainstem response originating from stimulation of the vestibular system. The presence of the significant ASSRs is likely due to repetition of the N3 to each stimulus modulation cycle—amplitudes are likely reduced due to a combination of (a) response refractoriness due to high modulation rates and multiple simultaneous stimuli, and (b) ASSR analysis focuses on energy at the modulation rate, which is lower than this short-latency response. These abnormal, vestibular, results are clearly evident in the time-domain waveforms of the ABR. It is much more difficult to differentiate vestibular from near-threshold auditory responses using current ASSR methodology (i.e., using frequency-domain analyses and/or multiple stimuli; Results obtained in collaboration with Renée Janssen.)

et al., 2005; Papathanasiou et al., 2004), and is likely the cause of the low-amplitude but significantly present ASSRs. Current ASSR methodologies typically do not provide the ability to view resulting waveforms in the time domain, and the use of rapid multiple stimuli (and thus overlapping responses) makes determination of response latency complicated. This highlights the importance of the transient ABR when thresholds are elevated.

Brainstem ASSR Thresholds to Air-Conduction Stimuli

Adults With Hearing Loss

There are now many studies of 80-Hz air-conduction ASSRs in adults and older children with sensory/neural hearing loss. Detailed review of these studies can be found in a chapter by Vander Werff, Johnson, and

Brown (2008) as well as the 2007 meta-analyses by Tlumak, Rubinstein, and Durrant (2007). For most studies, the ASSR threshold provided a good-to-excellent prediction of pure-tone behavioral threshold, with correlations between ASSR and behavioral thresholds typically in the 0.8 to 0.95 range for 1000 to 4000 Hz, and 0.7 to 0.85 range for 500 Hz. The slightly poorer correlation at 500 Hz has been suggested to be due to reduced neural synchrony for responses to 500-Hz stimuli (e.g., Lins et al., 1996), although the lower correlations could also be due to some studies having relatively few 500-Hz thresholds in the severe-profound range (i.e., a restriction of range problem). Nevertheless, 500-Hz ASSR thresholds do appear to be 5 to 10 dB worse than other frequencies, similar to those for the ABR (Stapells, 2000b; Vander Werff et al., 2008). As shown on the top of Table 21–6, Tlumak and colleagues' meta-analysis of nine studies showed mean difference scores (ASSR threshold minus behavioral threshold) for hearing-impaired adults ranging from 8 to14 dB, with individual studies showing standard deviations ranged from 7 to 18 dB (Tlumak et al., 2007). Some data suggest greater error (larger standard deviations) in estimating mild compared to more-significant hearing loss, especially at 500 Hz (D'Haenens et al., 2009; Rance et al., 2005). Studies using longer recording times (i.e., more averaging and thus lower residual EEG noise) tend to report better accuracy (Luts & Wouters, 2004; Picton et al., 2005; Vander Werff et al., 2008). In addition to estimating thresholds for individual frequencies reasonably accurately in adults, the brainstem ASSR appears to accurately estimate audiometric shape and configuration, as demonstrated by presentation of individual audiograms (e.g., Aoyagi et al., 1994; Herdman & Stapells, 2003) and through formal statistical analyses (Herdman & Stapells, 2003; Perez-Abalo et al., 2001). Thus, at least for adults with sensory and neural hearing loss, the 80-Hz ASSR provides a reasonably good estimate of behavioral threshold. Interestingly, these ASSR difference scores are similar to those shown in Table 21–2 for the tone-ABR (Stapells, 2000b).

Given that conductive loss is very common in young infants, the target population for the ASSR technique, very few published adult studies have investigated conductive loss (true or simulated), and none have estimated thresholds for mixed losses. The findings from the two studies that recorded ASSRs in adults with *simulated* conductive loss (produced by blocking the tubes of insert earphones) and the one study that assessed seven adults with true conductive loss (D'Haenens et al., 2009) suggest, overall, that difference scores (AC-ASSR minus behavioral thresholds) are somewhat larger in conductive loss than in SNHL (Dimitrijevic et al., 2002; Jeng et al., 2004). More research is clearly required to confirm these findings for conductive losses and to explore the accuracy of ASSRs in identifying mixed losses.

A number of studies have suggested that, compared to the ABR, the ASSR provides a better indication of residual sensitivity in individuals with profound hearing loss (Rance & Briggs, 2002; Rance, Dowell, Rickards, Beer, & Clark, 1998; Rance & Rickards, 2002; Rance, Rickards, Cohen, Burton, & Clark, 1993; Stueve & O'Rourke, 2003; Swanepoel & Hugo, 2004; Swanepoel, Hugo, & Roode, 2004). That is, ASSRs are present (especially for lower frequencies) when the ABR is absent. Although this can indeed be a real phenomenon, there are a number of issues with this suggestion. First, most studies used clicks to evoke the ABR. Clicks spread their energy over a wide frequency range (e.g., 100–8000 Hz), rather than concentrating their energy into a specific frequency region as do sinusoidal AM tones. The click-evoked ABR is well-known not to provide an accurate assessment for specific frequencies, especially for low frequencies. This is even worse when high-pass EEG filter settings of 100 Hz or higher are used (e.g., Stapells & Oates, 1997), which is the case of many of the above studies. Another problem is that the maximum click intensity of most studies was only about 90 dB nHL compared to 120 dB HL for the ASSR. Thus, for these two reasons (frequency spread and maximum intensity), the ASSR and ABR data have not been compared when the stimuli have equivalent energy at the frequency of interest. Second, the studies that compared 500-Hz tone-evoked ABR and the ASSR also had issues, such as lower maximum intensities for the ABR tones (in dB nHL) than the ASSR stimuli (in dB HL), incorrect (100 Hz) high-pass EEG filters, and waveform interpretation concerns (e.g., figures show clear ABR to 500 Hz but were indicated as "absent"). Third, and importantly, at least some of the ASSRs to high-intensity stimuli might have been artifactual, either due to stimulus artifact contamination or to a nonauditory physiologic response as previously discussed and shown in Figure 21–8 (Gorga et al., 2004; Jeng et al., 2004; Nambi & Vanaja, 2006; Picton & John, 2004; Small & Stapells, 2004).

In summary, although the ability to assess profound hearing losses is stated as a feature of the ASSR and an advantage over the ABR, there has yet to be an appropriate comparison that controls stimulus energy or artifactual (or nonauditory) responses. Further research and careful thought is required. Finally, it must be reiterated that presentation of high-intensity continuous tones for prolonged periods (at least 5 to 10 min might be required to reduce response noise below

TABLE 21–6. Air-Conduction Brainstem ASSR Thresholds and Maximum "Normal" Levels (in dB HL) in Infants and Young Children With Normal Hearing

AC ASSR Study	*STIM*	*Age*	*500*		*1000*		*2000*		*4000*	
			Mean ±SD	*Norm MAX*	*Mean ±SD*	*Norm MAX*	*Mean ±SD*	*Norm MAX*	*Mean ±SD*	*Norm MAX*
Weighted means across all studies (total number of subjects)			35 (297)		32 (239)		25 (272)		28 (258)	
Lins et al., 1996 (Ottawa data)	M:AM	1–10 months	40 ± 13	43	29 ± 10	43	23 ± 8	38	24 ± 10	35
Cone-Wesson, Parker, et al., 2002	S:AM/FM	<4 months		>71		>72		50		54
John, Brown, et al., 2004 (older group)	M:AM	3–15 weeks		>46		>50		>50		40
Rance et al., 2005[a]	S:AM/FM	1–3 months	32 ± 8	52	33 ± 7	47	24 ± 6	40	28 ± 8	43
Swanepoel & Steyn, 2005	M:AM/FM	3–8 weeks	37 ± 8	50	34 ± 10	>50	34 ± 11	>50	30 ± 11	40
Luts et al., 2006	M:AM/FM	<3 months	42 ± 10	>44	35 ± 10	>50	32 ± 10	42	36 ± 9	44
Rance & Tomlin, 2006	S:AM/FM	6 weeks	40 ± 7	50					33 ± 8	40
Van Maanen & Stapells, 2009	M:COS^3	≤6 months	39 ± 7	49	33 ± 5	45	29 ± 7	36	24 ± 10	32
Van Maanen & Stapells, 2009	M:COS^3	6.1–66 months	41 ± 7		37 ± 11		31 ± 8		22 ± 10	
Ribeiro et al., 2010 ("term" group; $p < .01$; 20 sweeps)	M:AM/FM	<2 weeks	39 ± 10	>40	28 ± 7	30	24 ± 6	30	27 ± 6	40
Casey & Small, 2014	M:AM^2	6.5–18 months	28 ± 8	40	22 ± 8	30	20 ± 8	30	22 ± 9	28
Valeriote & Small, 2015	M:AM^2	0–6 months	30 ± 9	40			20 ± 12	40		
*Meta-analysis of **adult** data 10 studies (Tlumak et al., 2007)*	*M*	*ADULT*	*17 ± 12*		*13 ± 12*		*11 ± 10*		*15 ± 10*	

Note. Adult results from Tlumak et al. (2007) meta-analysis are shown for comparison. STIM: S = single-stimulus ASSR; M = multiple-stimulus ASSR; AM = amplitude modulation (sinusoidal); FM = frequency modulation (sinusoidal); COS^3 = cosine^3-windowed tones 12-ms duration ; AM^2= exponential envelope modulation. Norm MAX: Maximum intensity (in dB HL) to be considered "normal" (i.e., level required for 90%–95% response presence); Individual studies: Mean ±SD: Mean threshold in dB HL and standard deviation; Results rounded off to closest decibels.

[a]Calculated from Figure 1 of Rance et al., 2005.

that required to state "no response") can result in noise-induced trauma to hair cells. Rest time for the cochlea must be provided by interrupting the stimuli.

Young Infants With Normal Hearing

As discussed above and shown in Table 21–1, there is a fairly reasonable database for the ABR to air-conducted brief tones thresholds in normal infants, as well as consensus as to what should be the criteria for "normal" in clinical testing (Stapells, 2000a, 2000b). The normative database for infant brainstem-ASSR thresholds is less well understood, and more recent. As noted above, this issue for the ASSR is complicated further because studies have used differing stimulus and analysis techniques. Nevertheless, there are now many studies providing normative thresholds for infants. Figure 21–7B presents air-conduction results for a normal 11-week-old infant, showing multiple ASSR thresholds of 46, 29, 24, and 2 dB HL at 500, 1000, 2000, and 4000 Hz, thresholds that are quite different from those of adults (see Table 21–6, bottom line). The detailed summary of normal infant thresholds from 11 studies shown in Table 21–6 indicates that mean infant thresholds range from 28 to 42, 22 to 37, 20 to 34, and 22 to 36 dB HL for 500, 1000, 2000, and 4000 Hz, respectively, with standard deviations less than or equal to 10 dB in most of the conditions tested. Importantly, infant air-conduction ASSR thresholds that are not corrected for ear-canal differences are elevated relative to those of adults by about 20 dB for 500 to 2000 Hz, and by 10 to 15 dB for 4000 Hz. Thresholds appear to be even more elevated in very young infants, especially those less than 3 to 6 weeks of age (John et al., 2004; Rance & Tomlin, 2006; Rance et al., 2006; Savio, Cardenas, Perez Abalo, Gonzales, & Valdes, 2001). However, results are variable; van Maanen and Stapells (2009)[16] reported no differences in thresholds between younger (≤6 months) and older (6.1–66 months) infants. Interestingly, the higher ASSR threshold in infants compared to adults contrasts with the similar tone-ABR thresholds (in dB nHL) for the two age groups (see Table 21–1). Rance and colleagues compared tone-ABR and ASSR thresholds in very young infants and showed elevated ASSR thresholds in 1-week-old infants that improved over at least 6 weeks; however, tone-ABR thresholds were better (lower) than the ASSR thresholds and did not change over the first six weeks of life (Rance et al., 2006). The reasons for these differences are not clear; one possible explanation is that very young auditory systems have reduced abilities to process the very rapid modulation rates (80–110 Hz) used for the brainstem ASSR, whereas the relatively slower rates (30–50/s) for the tone-ABR pose no problem (Burkard, Shi, & Hecox, 1990; Lasky, 1991; Rance, 2008a).

There has been some discussion, but no consensus, in the literature concerning what constitutes a "normal" versus an "elevated" ASSR threshold in infants. Given that mean air-conduction ASSR thresholds in normal infants are significantly elevated relative to adults (see Table 21–6), clearly "normal" levels typically used for adults (i.e., 20–25 dB HL) cannot be applied. To establish the criterion for "normal" for clinical testing, it is not advisable to use the mean or median thresholds because only ~50% of normal infants will demonstrate a response at these levels. Rather, the "normal" criterion must be a level where at least 90% to 95% of infants show a response. Table 21–6 presents "normal" levels using this definition for infant air-conduction ASSRs from 11 studies. It is evident that "normal" levels for air-conduction ASSRs range from 40 to 50 dB HL at 500 Hz, and 30 to 50 dB HL at 1000, 2000, and 4000 Hz, for the majority of these studies. Considering the results published up to 2010, van Maanen and Stapells (2010) recommended infant normal air-conduction ASSR levels of 50, 45, 40, and 40 dB HL for 500, 1000, 2000, and 4000 Hz, respectively, provided low-noise ASSR recordings are obtained in a quiet sound booth (see Table 21–6; van Maanen & Stapells, 2010).[17] More recently, Valeriote and Small (2015) investigated young infants with normal hearing (500 and 2000 Hz) and mild conductive loss (500 Hz) and found that a "normal" level of 40 dB HL more accurately identified normal hearing versus conductive loss than a level of 50 dB HL.

Young Infants With Hearing Loss

Perhaps the greatest concern for clinical implementation of ASSRs has been that there were few studies of ASSR thresholds in infants with hearing loss where ASSR thresholds have been compared with gold-standard frequency-specific measures of their actual thresholds (i.e., behavioral audiometry or tone-ABR). Although several studies of ASSR thresholds in children exist, the majority of these either compare ASSR

[16]The thresholds reported above are in decibels hearing level (dB HL; re: ANSI, 1996) and are not levels measured in the ear canal, which change due to maturation of the ear canal (Bagatto, Seewald, Scollie, & Tharpe, 2006; Rance & Tomlin, 2006; Seewald, Moodie, Scollie, & Bagatto, 2005; Sininger, Abdala, & Cone-Wesson, 1997).

[17]Interestingly, considered in ppe SPL, these normal ASSR levels are close, within 10dB, to those recommended for the tone ABR.

only to click-ABR thresholds; some study older children (e.g., 13 years old); and others have technical problems, especially with their tone-ABR methodology (for review see Stapells, Herdman, Small, Dimitrijevic, & Hatton, 2005). As shown in Table 21–7, there are now many studies that have published difference scores (AC-ASSR thresholds minus frequency-specific behavioral or tone-ABR thresholds) in infants and young children with hearing loss. The studies by Rance and colleagues, using the single-stimulus ASSR technique, have provided the largest sample size (285 with normal hearing and 271 with sensory/neural hearing loss; Rance et al., 2005). Five other studies used the multiple-ASSR technique and have a total sample size of approximately 350 ears (Chou et al., 2012; Han, Mo, Liu, Chen, & Huang, 2006; Luts, Desloovere, & Wouters, 2006; Rodrigues & Lewis, 2010; van Maanen & Stapells, 2010).[18] Unfortunately, as Table 21–7 also indicates, these studies employed a wide variety of stimulus and analysis paradigms (e.g., single versus multiple, or sine-AM versus brief tones), and there exists a large range in the resulting threshold difference scores.

As is the case with adult ASSR data, assessment of infants and children with conductive loss has received much less attention. There are only a few studies that

Table 21–7. Air-Conduction Brainstem ASSR Minus Behavioral Threshold Difference Scores (in dB) in Infants and Young Children (<7 Years) With Hearing Loss

AC ASSR STUDY	*STIM*	*Age*	*500*	*1000*	*2000*	*4000*
Weighted means across all studies (total number of subjects)		1–79 months	13 (508)	11 (594)	10 (481)	8 (466)
Rance & Briggs, 2002[a]	S:AM/FM	1–8 months	6 ± 9 (160)	6 ± 7 (232)	4 ± 8 (125)	3 ± 11 (131)
Han et al., 2006[b]	M:BLK	6–60 months	15 ± 9 (46)	9 ± 8 (45)	8 ± 8 (42)	11 ± 9 (27)
Luts et al., 2006	M:AM/FM	0–50 months	8 ± 13 (12)	6 ± 15 (25)	7 ± 13 (25)	9 ± 12 (20)
Van Maanen & Stapells, 2010[c]	M:COS³	1–79 months	14 ± 9 (50)	13 ± 9 (52)	9 ± 9 (54)	−3 ± 10 (56)
Rodrigues & Lewis, 2010[b]	M:BLK	1–36 months	−3 ± 6 (24)	0 ± 5 (24)	0 ± 6 (19)	−2 ± 4 (16)
Chou et al., 2012[b]	M:BLK	1–13 months	20 ± 14 (216)	17 ± 10 (216)	16 ± 11 (216)	14 ± 11 (216)
*Meta-analyses of **adult** data 9 studies (Tlumak et al., 2007)*	*M*	*Adults*	*14 ± 13 (327)*	*10 ± 13 (330)*	*9 ± 12 (328)*	*8 ± 13 (329)*

Note. Adult results from Tlumak et al. (2007) meta-analysis are shown for comparison. STIM: see Table 21–6; difference score (dB) = air-conduction ASSR threshold minus pure-tone behavioral threshold; mean (dB) ± standard deviation. Results rounded off to closest decibels; number of ears in parentheses.

[a]Rance and colleagues (2005) updated their 2002 results with additional infants; however, no difference scores were provided.

[b]Intelligent Hearing Systems' Smart-EP Blackman-windowed *brief-tone* stimuli, calibrated by manufacturer.

[c]Behavioral threshold (in dBHL) estimated from tone-ABR threshold using Stapells' (2000b) meta-analysis difference scores (Table 21–2).

[18] A study by Alaerts, Luts, Van Dun, Desloovere, and Wonters (2010) obtained both multiple-ASSR and follow-up behavioral thresholds in 50 young infants. However, details were not provided concerning (a) how many of these had hearing loss, (b) the type and range of hearing loss, or (c) the corresponding behavioral thresholds. It is also not clear if any of the infants (with normal or impaired hearing) were included in the earlier study (Luts et al., 2006) published by this research group.

have reported findings for either infants or children with conductive loss. Recently, we estimated air- and bone-conduction ASSR and ABR thresholds in infants with mild conductive loss at 500 Hz and found larger air-bone gaps for ASSR thresholds for confirmed conductive loss compared to normal-hearing infants; however, there was considerable overlap in air-conduction ASSR thresholds obtained at 500 Hz for these two groups (Valeriote & Small, 2015). This variability in 500 Hz ASSR thresholds was also found for adults with hearing loss, as mentioned earlier (D'Haenens et al., 2009; Rance et al., 2005). Nagishima et al. (2013) reported air- and bone-conduction multiple-ASSR and behavioral threshold data for nine infant/child cases with permanent and transient middle-ear involvement. They did not obtain complete sets of air- and bone-conduction data for each child; however, they provided some promising data. For one child, they showed similar air-bone gaps using each measure that supports that the ASSR has the potential to reflect similar diagnostic information to behavioral audiometry. For three children, they found an average bone-conduction ASSR minus behavioral difference of 11 to 16 dB, which is similar to data reported by Casey and Small (2014) that showed on average offset of 6 to 17 dB for a large group of infants with normal hearing. Nagishima and colleagues also assessed children before and after treatment for middle ear effusion (pretreatment bone-conduction ASSR thresholds only) and found that the air-bone-gap decreased by 10 to 25 dB after treatment. An earlier study estimated air-conduction ASSR thresholds in children with conductive loss (Swanepoel, Ebrahim, Friedland, Swanepoel, & Pottas, 2008) using single-stimulus ASSRs; however, the air-bone gap was not measured, and the conductive component was inferred from air-conduction click-ABR, EOAE, tympanograms, and otoscopy, none of which can provide an estimate of the amount of a conductive component.

Although the data to date are somewhat limited, the results in Table 21–7 could be used to provide preliminary difference scores (i.e., corrections) to convert air-conduction ASSR thresholds to eHL. Conservative air-conduction ASSR to eHL corrections (i.e., corrections less likely to overestimate the amount of hearing loss) appear to be about 10 to 15 dB (see Table 21–9 later in the chapter). These corrections apply to young children with sensory/neural hearing loss and will require elaboration and confirmation through further research.[19]

Brainstem ASSRs to Bone-Conduction Stimuli

Despite the need for bone-conduction ASSR threshold data for the full implementation of the brainstem ASSR as a clinical tool, this area of inquiry has not been studied as comprehensively as ASSRs elicited to air-conducted stimuli. Several studies have reported bone-conduction ASSR thresholds in adults with normal hearing (Dimitrijevic et al., 2002; Jeng et al., 2004; Lins et al., 1996; Small & Stapells, 2005, 2008a, 2008b). Table 21–8 also shows adult mean bone-conduction ASSR thresholds across four studies conducted by Small and colleagues using the same stimuli and response detection techniques (N = 58 adults). The pattern for bone-conduction ASSR thresholds in adults is similar across studies—poorer thresholds in the low frequencies compared to the high frequencies. As mentioned earlier, Jeng et al. (2004) assessed bone-conduction ASSRs in adults with simulated hearing loss. Ishida, Cuthbert, and Stapells (2011) simulated sensory hearing loss by presenting air-conducted masking noise and found reasonably high correlations (0.8–0.9) between bone-conduction ASSR and behavioral thresholds at 1000, 2000, and 4000 Hz, and somewhat poorer (0.7–0.8) correlations at 500 Hz. These findings support that, at least for 1000 to 4000 Hz, bone-conduction ASSRs should provide reasonable estimates of bone-conduction thresholds. Four additional studies have assessed the presence of spurious ASSRs in adults with severe-to-profound sensory/neural hearing loss (Gorga et al., 2004; Jeng et al., 2004; Nambi & Vanaja, 2006; Small & Stapells, 2004). Critically, however, results from infants with normal hearing and hearing loss are still required to confirm appropriate normal levels and determine corrections for ASSRs to bone-conducted stimuli.

To date, the majority of bone-conduction ASSR studies have investigated infants with normal hearing, as shown in Table 21–8. A major focus of these studies was to investigate the maturation of bone-conduction hearing sensitivity by estimating bone-conduction ASSR thresholds in groups of premature infants, young infants, older infants, and adults (Casey & Small, 2014; Small et al., 2007; Small & Hu, 2011; Small & Stapells, 2005, 2006, 2008a, 2008b; Valeriote & Small, 2015). Another aim has been to establish normal levels as a first step in evaluating bone-conduction ASSRs as a clinical measure to determine the nature of the hearing

[19]In reviewing the air-conduction ASSR normal levels (see Table 21–6) and the difference scores with hearing loss (see Table 21–7), it becomes clear that current information makes separation of normal hearing and mild hearing loss difficult, especially at 500 Hz. For example, even a 20-dB correction factor applied to the normal level of 50 dB HL at 500 Hz results in a predicted behavioral threshold of 30 dB HL, a result still in the elevated range.

Table 21–8. Bone-Conduction Brainstem Multiple ASSR Thresholds and Maximum "Normal" Levels (in dB HL) in Infants and Young Children With Normal Hearing

			500		*1000*		*2000*		*4000*	
BC ASSR Study	***STIM***	***Age***	***Mean ±SD***	***Norm MAX***	***Mean ±SD***	***Norm MAX***	***Mean ±SD***	***Norm MAX***	***Mean ±SD***	***Norm MAX***
Small & Stapells, 2006	M:AM/FM	32–43 weeks PCA[a]	16 ± 11 (29)	30	16 ± 10 (29)	30	37 ± 16 (26)	60	33 ± 13 (28)	50
Small, Hatton, & Stapells, 2007	M:AM/FM	32–43 weeks PCA[a]	16 ± 12 (15)	30	17 ± 9 (15)	30	35 ± 15 (13)	60	33 ± 15 (15)	50
Small & Stapells, 2008a	M:AM/FM	0–11 months	14 ± 13 (35)	30	5 ± 8 (35)	20	26 ± 10 (35)	40	14 ± 11 (35)	30
Small & Hu, 2011	M:AM/FM	0–7 months	18 ± 8 (9)	30	10 ± 7 (9)	20	26 ± 12 (9)	40	28 ± 10 (9)	40
Small, Hatton, & Stapells, 2007 (mastoid placement; ipsi EEG)	M:AM/FM	2–10 months	14 ± 14 (10)	40	6 ± 8 (10)	20	26 ± 10 (10)	40	13 ± 12 (10)	40
Small & Stapells, 2008b	M:AM/FM	2–11 months	13 ± 13 (11)	30	5 ± 5 (11)	10	20 ± 13 (11)	30	9 ± 8 (11)	10
Small & Hu, 2011	M:AM/FM	10–22 months	22 ± 10 (10)	30	17 ± 8 (10)	20	27 ± 13 (10)	40	19 ± 11 (10)	30
Small & Stapells, 2008a	M:AM/FM	12–24 months	22 ± 11 (13)	40	13 ± 6 (13)	20	26 ± 9 (13)	40	13 ± 9 (13)	20
Valeriote & Small, 2015	M:AM^2	0–6 months	17 ± 10 (33)	30			26 ± 14 (21)	40		
Casey & Small, 2014	M:AM^2	6.5–18 months	11 ± 11 (19)	30	9 ± 9 (20)	20	21 ± 11 (20)	40	15 ± 11 (20)	33
Adult data combined across four studies[b]	As above	*ADULT*	*26 ± 13 (58)*	40	*19 ± 13 (58)*	40	*18 ± 8 (58)*	30	*13 ± 10 (58)*	30

Note. Adult results combined across four studies are shown for comparison. STIM: see Table 21–6; norm MAX: Maximum intensity (in dB HL) to be considered "normal" (i.e., level required for 90%–95% response presence); individual studies: mean ±SD: mean threshold in dB HL and standard deviation; results rounded off to closest decibels.

[a]Postconceptional age.

[b]Adult results from Small and Stapells (2008a, 2008b); Hu and Small (2011); Casey and Small (2014).

loss when air-conduction ASSR thresholds are elevated (Casey & Small, 2014; Small & Stapells, 2005, 2006, 2008a, 2008b; Small et al., 2007; Small & Hu, 2011; Valeriote & Small, 2015). A detailed discussion of the time course of maturation of bone-conduction ASSR threshold and underlying mechanisms for infant-adult differences can be found in Small and Stapells (2008b). As shown earlier by ABR research (See Table 21–3), infant thresholds to bone-conducted stimuli are significantly different from those of adults, especially in the low frequencies. Bone-conduction ASSR research has significantly added to earlier ABR findings by providing a maturational trajectory across all four frequencies typically assessed clinically in young children. Our studies have shown that low-frequency bone-conduction ASSR thresholds are better (i.e., lower dB HL) in young infants than for older infants, and likewise, for older infants compared to adults. Thus, bone-conducted stimuli in infants are effectively more intense than the same stimuli in adults, likely due to infant skull maturation and other issues (reviewed in Foxe & Stapells, 1993; Mackey et al., in press; Small & Stapells, 2008b; Stuart, Yang, & Stenstrom, 1990). Overall, low-frequency bone-conduction ASSR thresholds increase (become worse) by about 15 to 20 dB from infancy to adulthood. ASSR thresholds to 2000- and 4000-Hz bone-conducted stimuli show little or no change (Small & Stapells, 2008b). Additionally, young infant ASSR thresholds to 500- and 1000-Hz bone-conducted stimuli are better than those to 2000- and 4000-Hz bone-conducted stimuli (Small & Stapells, 2008a, 2008b). These patterns are clearly different than those for air-conduction stimuli, and indicate that "normal levels" and bone-conduction ASSR-to-behavioral correction factors must be determined from infant data. The existing infant data are currently limited to research in our lab; based on this research, we have recommended normal bone-conduction ASSR levels of 30, 20, 40, and 30 dB HL for infants aged 0 to 11 months, and 40, 20, 40, and 30 dB HL for infants aged 12 to 24 months (see Table 21–8; Small & Stapells, 2008a; Valeriote & Small, 2015).[20]

We have also used ASSRs to investigate methodological issues, such as (a) bone oscillator placement (mastoid versus upper temporal bone versus forehead); (b) bone oscillator coupling technique (handheld versus elastic band); and (c) the occlusion effect (Small et al., 2007; Small & Hu, 2011). These infant studies indicate that a forehead placement should be avoided as thresholds are elevated and that upper temporal bone and mastoid results are similar although positioning on the upper temporal bone might be easier to accomplish. As noted in the ABR section, it was also demonstrated that either coupling by hand or an elastic band can be used, provided individuals are adequately trained (Small et al., 2007). These ASSR findings also indicate maturational changes in the occlusion effect which is routinely compensated for when estimating masked bone-conduction thresholds in adults. Our results support that the occlusion effect, on average, at 500 and 1000 Hz is negligible in young infants (0–7 months; 2–5 dB); however, the occlusion effect appears to be large enough to potentially affect the accuracy of bone-conduction threshold estimation in older infants (12–24 months; 8 dB). Consequently, insert earphones can be left in the ear canal when assessing young infants with no correction required at any frequency but should be removed for infants older than 1 year when estimating thresholds at 500 and 1000 Hz (Small & Hu, 2011). If bone-conduction thresholds are tested with occluded ears in older infants, we recommend that the bone-conduction threshold obtained be increased using a 10-dB correction factor.

Similar to the ABR two-channel EEG recordings of infant brainstem, ASSRs also show significant ipsilateral/contralateral asymmetries, with responses larger and earlier in latency in the EEG channel ipsilateral to the stimulated ear (Small & Stapells, 2008a; Small & Love, 2014). Our investigations indicated that asymmetries are most consistently present at 20 to 25 dB HL compared to higher intensities, similar to ABR findings (Stapells, 1989); however, we found that the asymmetries were consistently present only at 500 and 4000 Hz but not at 1000 and 2000 Hz (Small & Love, 2014). Published ABR findings show consistent asymmetries at 500 and 2000 Hz (Stapells, 1989). This ASSR phenomenon might be helpful clinically to determine the cochlea that is responding to the bone-conducted stimulus; however, further research is needed in infants with asymmetrical or unilateral hearing loss to test this theory. Clinical masking will be needed when the responses in the EEG channel ipsilateral and contralateral to the stimulated mastoid are not unequivocally asymmetric, as is also the case for the ABR. Effective masking levels (EMLs) appropriate for infants for the ABR and ASSR are needed to isolate the test ear in these cases. Our studies estimated EMLs for ASSRs elicited to bone-conducted stimuli at 500 to 4000 Hz in normal-hearing infants and adults and found maturational differences (Hansen & Small, 2012; Small, Smyth, & Leon, 2013). Based on these findings, we rec-

[20]We have also recommended normal levels of (a) 30, 30, 50+, and 50 dB HL for premature infants (Small & Stapells, 2006) and (b) 40, 30, 30, and 20 dB HL for adults (Ishida et al., 2011).

ommend the following EMLs in dB SPL for AM/FM ASSR stimuli presented at 35 dB HL for 500, 1000, 2000, and 4000, respectively; infant: 81, 68, 59, and 45 dB SPL; and adult: 66, 63, 59, and 55 dB SPL.[21] Further research is needed to confirm the accuracy of using these EMLs to isolate the test ear in infants with hearing loss before applying these methods clinically.

Currently, there are only three bone-conduction ASSR studies in infants with hearing loss, and only one study that confirmed hearing status using a standard measure, such as the tone ABR. As mentioned earlier, Valeriote and Small (2015) estimated 500-Hz thresholds in young infants with mild conductive loss using ASSR and ABR testing methods and found that mean bone-conduction ASSR thresholds were approximately 16 to 17 dB HL for infants with normal hearing and hearing loss (see Table 21–8). Swanepoel and colleagues (2008) found similar mean bone-conduction ASSRs thresholds in children ranging from 6 months of age to 11 years (mean age = 3.6 years) with elevated air-conduction click-ABR thresholds (Swanepoel et al., 2008). They also reported possible "spurious" responses using the single stimulus system, with results suggesting more spurious responses than studies using the multiple-ASSR technique (Jeng et al., 2004; Small & Stapells, 2004). Unfortunately, Swanepoel and colleagues did not confirm the hearing status or levels of their subjects. Nagashima et al. (2013) estimated air- and bone-conduction thresholds in a small sample of young children with middle ear effusion before and after surgery for the insertion of ventilation tubes and found that the air-bone gap in ASSR thresholds decreased by as much as 10 to 25 dB after tubes were inserted. Additional research comparing air- and bone-conduction ASSR thresholds in infants with greater degrees of hearing loss and different types of hearing loss confirmed by behavioral (or tone-ABR) thresholds to air- and bone-conduction stimuli is still required.

Current Status of the ABR and ASSR for Frequency-Specific Threshold Assessment in Infants and Young Children

The tone-evoked ABR is a long-standing and gold-standard clinical tool for the assessment of infants and young children that offers the possibility of obtaining ear- and frequency-specific (assuming brief-tone stimuli are used) air- and bone-conduction thresholds in one to two test sessions. There is ample evidence to support the use of this measure, but there remain a few gaps—limited published tone-ABR threshold data for both air- and bone-conducted stimuli collected in the same infant in order to allow accurate interpretation of air-bone gaps with different types and configurations of hearing losses, and no data regarding effective masking levels for bone-conduction testing when ipsilateral/contralateral asymmetries are equivocal about isolating the test ear. Since the first edition of this chapter was written, the ASSR has been investigated more extensively; however, some of the significant limitations previously identified remain: (a) new stimulus parameters, analysis methods, and clinical systems have received little assessment, with few peer-reviewed data supporting their use clinically, especially for infants with hearing loss; (b) data for ASSR estimation of threshold in infants with hearing loss are limited almost exclusively to air-conduction thresholds in infants with sensory/neural hearing loss and mild conductive loss; (c) the relationship of ASSR thresholds in individuals with profound hearing loss is not adequately studied; and (d) the impact of nonphysiologic (artifactual) or nonauditory physiologic (e.g., vestibular) "spurious" responses on results, especially in those with profound loss remains unclear.

Considering the current evidence, *the tone-evoked ABR remains the clinical tool of choice;* however, the motivation to utilize the ASSR remains strong due to somewhat easier training of clinicians on recording and interpretation of ASSRs, particularly in locations where infant ABR "experts" are not available (e.g., in areas where audiologist have low infant caseloads and find it difficult to maintain the high skill level to perform threshold ABRs, or in developing countries where there might be too few audiologists to provide ABR services). The much-needed ASSR evidence *might* be available within a few years—when considering the results of future ASSR studies, clinicians must critically appraise them to ensure they involve infants with hearing loss confirmed using frequency-specific gold-standard methods (i.e., behavioral or tone-ABR thresholds using air- and bone-conducted stimuli). Until then, only the tone-evoked ABR has the sufficient research, clinical database, and clinical history to recommend it as the *primary* technique for threshold estimation in young infants and children with conductive, mixed, and sensory hearing loss (i.e., accurate interpretation

[21]Effective masking levels for the BC ABR in infants have not yet been investigated.

of *both* air- and bone-conduction findings). However, there are sufficient data to support the use of the ASSR in conjunction with the ABR. The following sections will discuss recommended protocols for brainstem evoked potential assessment of hearing threshold in infants, whether the ABR or ASSR is used, and how the ABR and ASSR might be used in present-day clinical practice.

Protocols and the Sequence of Testing Using the ABR/ASSR

It is essential to use a test sequence that is fast and efficient, and provides the greatest increase in clinical information with each successive step.[22] Four principles guide the general strategy of stimulus conditions. The first is that test time is limited—the infant might wake up at any moment so the most important question must be assessed first. Second, the choice of stimulus condition should be based on what is the most probable outcome. For example, most infants coming to the diagnostic ABR stage after referral during the newborn period have normal hearing, most often due to a middle ear disorder that has resolved since the screening referral, although screening errors also occur. Thus, starting at a low intensity (i.e., at the "normal" levels discussed above) will quickly obtain the necessary results for most infants. Third, choice of stimulus condition should be based on provision of results that make a difference in management as well as information to the parents. For example, when no response is present at the air-conduction "normal" intensity, it is less useful to spend time collecting precise air-conduction threshold information than obtaining bone-conduction results because air-conduction thresholds in most infants with conductive hearing loss are "moving targets" (i.e., change over time). Having information about the type of impairment (i.e., air- and bone-conduction results) directs subsequent management, including medical management, and provides more certain information for the family. Four, efficient strategies require clinicians to frequently switch ears and mode (air versus bone) of stimulation—insert earphones should be placed in both ears at the beginning of testing, and the bone oscillator ready for application. For example, after obtaining a "no response" at the air-conduction screening intensity in the first ear, the clinician should switch to the other ear rather than seek threshold. Otherwise, too much time can be spent determining threshold for one ear, only to have the infant wake-up before determining that the other ear was normal (i.e., deferring diagnostic certainty to a subsequent ABR appointment). Obviously, it would have been better, both for management and for the family, to know that at least one ear was normal.

For most infants, therefore, the diagnostic ABR/ASSR assessment should aim to answer the following three questions, in order of priority: (1) Is an ear's air-conduction threshold normal or elevated? Is the other ear's air-conduction threshold normal or elevated? (2) If elevated, is the elevation conductive in nature or is there a sensory component? (3) If elevated, what are the specific thresholds (air- and/or bone conduction)? The first question is answered by testing *each ear* at the "normal" air-conduction level—that is, the minimum level required to conclude normal thresholds for that ear. Results for 2000 Hz are typically obtained first, and this step does not normally involve a threshold search. If the baby wakes up at the end of this, the clinician is still able to state whether one or both ears' thresholds are normal/elevated. If one has multiple-ASSR available, one can answer this question quite quickly by recording the ASSR to 500, 1000, 2000, and 4000 Hz air-conducted stimuli presented at the normal levels to both ears. Table 21–9 summarizes the normal levels currently recommended for air-conducted (and bone-conducted) stimuli for tone-ABR and ASSR.

The second question is answered by bone-conduction testing (at the minimum "normal" bone-conduction level) of the ear(s) with air-conduction elevation(s). Currently, this question can be answered accurately by the bone-conduction tone-ABR for 500 and 2000 Hz. Although normal levels have been proposed for bone-conduction ASSRs (Table 21–9), currently, bone-conduction ASSR data for only a small number of infants with hearing loss at 500 Hz are available, with none for 2000 Hz. Thus, the accuracy of the proposed normal bone-conduction ASSR levels requires verification for a larger group of infants with different degrees of hearing loss.

Bone-conduction testing should occur as soon as both ears have been tested in Step 1 at 2000 Hz and one or both ears show no-response to air-conducted stimuli (at the normal level). If the infant wakes up at the end of this bone-conduction stage, the clinician is able to state that the elevation in air-conduction thresh-

[22]Greater detail of our protocols and their rationale are provided in the BCEHP and OIHP protocol documents (BCEHP, 2012; OIHP, 2008), as well as in the chapter by Sininger and Hyde (2009).

Table 21–9. Normal Maximum Levels and Threshold Correction Factors for Infant Tone-ABR and ASSR

		500 Hz		*1000 Hz*		*2000 Hz*		*4000 Hz*	
		AC	*BC*	*AC*	*BC*	*AC*	*BC*	*AC*	*BC*
ABR	NORMAL MAX (dB nHL)	30–**35**	**20**	30–**35**	na	20–**30**	**30**	20–**25**	na
	eHL correction in dB	**10**[a]–15	**−5**	5–**10**	na	0–**5**	**5**	−5–**0**	na
ASSR	NORMAL MAX (dB HL)	40-50	30	40-45	20	40	40	40	30
	eHL correction in dB[b] *(preliminary, conservative)*	10–20	na	10–15	na	10–15	na	5–15	na

Note. NORMAL MAX = response must be present at this level to be considered "normal"; eHL = estimated behavioral hearing level (in dBHL); eHL correction: ABR (dB nHL) or ASSR threshold (dB HL) minus correction = estimated behavioral hearing threshold (in dB HL); "normal max" and "eHL corrections" used by BCEHP shown in **bold**. Na = not available or not applicable.

[a]In 2015, BCEHP adopted correction of 10 dB for AC ABR at 500 Hz.

[b]The eHL correction factors for AC-ASSR are preliminary. Further research is required. Corrections for BC-ASSR are not yet available.

old is either conductive in nature or has a sensory, and thus permanent, component. As the majority of infants referred from universal newborn hearing screening (UNHS) with elevated air-conduction thresholds will turn out to have conductive losses, this procedure will most often quickly identify an infant's elevation as conductive in nature, providing important information for subsequent management and for the parents.

The third question is answered by detailed determination of air-conduction (and bone-conduction) thresholds. Air-conduction thresholds for each required frequency are required for subsequent interventions, including amplification (when chosen by the family) when sensory hearing loss is present. Currently, this information must be provided by the tone-ABR. Given the relatively few bone-conduction ASSR data for infants with hearing loss, and uncertainties concerning appropriate ASSR-behavioral corrections, any threshold information obtained using the ASSR should come *after* completing the tone-ABR. The above does not clearly indicate the priority sequence of testing for stimulus frequencies. In general, greatest priority is given to 2000 Hz, and results for this frequency are normally obtained first. Next in priority is 500 Hz, then 4000 Hz following, and, if required, 1000 Hz following.[23] Prior information (excluding hearing screening results), history (e.g., ototoxic medications), and actual results obtained during the assessment might alter the relative priority of frequencies, but the above sequence should be appropriate for the majority infants requiring diagnostic ABR/ASSR assessment. Selecting the frequency test order is less of an issue for threshold searches carried out using the multiple-ASSR, as results are obtained for four frequencies simultaneously.

Generally, the regular use of intensity stepsizes smaller than 20 dB is inefficient; however, thresholds should be established using a *final* step-size of 10 dB (except, as noted above, when thresholds are greater than 70 dB nHL, where a 5-dB final stepsize might be helpful). It is inefficient to routinely use a 5-dB stepsize or to test at levels below the 25 to 35 dB nHL normal levels (with perhaps the exception of ototoxic monitoring) because the management of a "threshold" at the 25 to 35 dB nHL levels is unlikely to be different from a 10 to 20 dB nHL threshold (Sininger & Hyde, 2009). Intensities tested should bracket threshold; for example, if no response is seen at 30 dB nHL (2000 Hz), choosing the next level to be 40 dB nHL will give little information if there is no response at 40 dB nHL. A better compromise is 60 dB nHL. If both 30 and 60 dB nHL at 2000 Hz have been tested (as well as BC 2000 Hz at 30 dB) before the infant wakes up, then we know the following: (a) an impairment exists for one or both ears, (b) whether a sensory/neural component exists, and (c) whether the loss is mild or moderate (if 60 dB nHL response is present) or more severe (if 60 dB nHL

[23]Often, there is little gained in testing 1000 Hz if thresholds for 500 and 2000 Hz are within 20 dB of each other. Thus, testing at 1000 Hz should only be carried out (a) if 500 to 2000 Hz thresholds differ by more than 20 dB, or (b) all other required testing has been completed (BCEHP, 2012; OIHP, 2008).

is absent). Unfortunately, all too often, clinicians use smaller stepsizes, and follow a sequence that does not switch ears (and air/bone mode), with the end result that the infant wakes up before a clear picture of the status of *both* ears, as well as the type and severity of loss, has been obtained (BCEHP, 2012; OIHP, 2008).

ABR (and ASSR) assessment of young infants can be seriously compromised by ANSD and neurologic involvement (in such cases, especially in ANSD, ABR, and ASSR thresholds typically do not reflect cochlear or behavioral sensitivity; BCEHP, 2012; OIHP, 2008; Rance, 2005). As a rule, if a clinician sees a distinct wave that is *clearly* ABR Wave V (to a brief tone of any frequency, whether air or bone conduction), then they can be reasonably confident that an elevated ABR threshold is *not* due to ANSD or neurologic dysfunction. When Wave V is clear and the V/I amplitude ratio is normal, the finding of a prolonged Wave I-V interpeak latency should not be interpreted as suggesting any threshold elevation is due to neurologic dysfunction. The lack of a *clear* ABR Wave V in any waveform, even at the highest intensity, can be the result of profound peripheral (conductive and cochlear) impairment *or* ANSD/neurologic dysfunction. In such a situation (no tone-ABR response with a clear Wave V), the clinician must obtain recordings to high-intensity clicks (90–100 dB nHL, monopolarity, ~19 per second rate). Unfortunately, with ASSR one does not have interpretable time-domain waveforms; thus, for any elevated ASSR threshold, one requires confirmation by tone-ABR, and, if no clear Wave V is present to the brief tones, by click-ABR.[24]

The question is often asked, "How much time will this tone-ABR testing require?" It definitely takes longer than a simple air-conduction click-evoked ABR; after all, far more information is being sought. Because of this, clinicians must be skilled in carrying out and interpreting tone-ABR results, and they now must use appropriate and efficient test protocols. We recently reviewed 188 tone-ABR assessments (184 infants) carried out over a 20-month period in one of our clinical facilities utilizing tone-ABR protocols (BCEHP, 2012) similar to the sequence outlined above, and found that on average, we had 58 minutes of test time for sedated infants, during which we obtained about eight "measures" (e.g., four thresholds in each ear). Nonsedated infants, all aged under 6 months, had an average of 49 minutes of test time, with six "measures" obtained. Importantly, we obtained at least six measures (e.g., three frequencies per ear) for most infants (>80%), thus providing the required information in one session for most infants (Janssen et al., 2010). Nevertheless, even with efficient protocols, there will be infants for whom complete information is not obtained within one test session, and a second test session will be required. Although sedation provides, on average, about nine additional minutes of test time, our experience is that nonsedated appointments are much easier and flexible to schedule (no evaluation or monitoring by medical personnel need be arranged) and are typically more accepted by families. Importantly, with today's very early identification, many infants are now seen at a very young age when they sleep naturally, and sedation is rarely necessary or appropriate. There should be no hesitation in scheduling a second diagnostic ABR session.

What is the minimum information required from ABR/ASSR threshold assessment? Assuming results are deemed reliable and no neurologic/ANSD component to the threshold elevation is suspected (i.e., a clear Wave V is present), at a minimum, a "complete" tone-ABR evaluation should provide air-conduction thresholds for 500 and 2000 Hz (or, responses at the normal levels) and, if thresholds are elevated, bone-conduction tested at least for 2000 Hz and air-conduction thresholds for 4000 Hz (BCEHP, 2012; OIHP, 2008). Normally, additional information (EOAE, immittance) is also obtained (Janssen et al., 2010), but these additional measures are usually obtained *after* the tone-ABR testing is completed (i.e., they should not take up ABR test/sleep time; BCEHP, 2012). With this information, appropriate management can be initiated early, to be modified later as further information, especially behavioral thresholds, becomes available (Gravel, 2002; JCIH, 2007; Sininger, 2003).

Acknowledgments. This chapter is dedicated to the memory of our friend, colleague, and audiology mentor, Judith S. Gravel. We thank the many individuals with whom we have collaborated in this area, especially our colleagues at British Columbia's Children's Hospital Audiology Department/BCEHP: Jenny Hatton, Renée Janssen, Laurie Usher, and Anna Van Maanen. The research and preparation of this chapter were supported by funds from the Canadian Institutes of Health Research and the Natural Sciences and Engineering Research Council of Canada.

[24]It also is important to obtain other measures of auditory responsivity to cross-check the ABR/ASSR results, especially evoked otoacoustic emissions and behavioral responses.

References

Alaerts, J., Luts, H., Van Dun, B., Desloovere, C., & Wouters, J. (2010). Latencies of auditory steady-state responses recorded in early infancy. *Audiology & Neurootology, 15,* 116–127.

American National Standards Institute (ANSI; 1996). *American National Standard Specifications for Audiometers (ANSI S3.6-1996).* New York, NY: Author.

Anson, B. J., & Donaldson, J. A. (1981). The ear: Developmental anatomy. In B. J. Anson & J.A. Donaldson (Eds.), *Surgical anatomy of the temporal bone.* Philadelphia, PA: W.B. Saunders.

Aoyagi, M., Kiren, T., Furuse, H., Fuse, T., Suzuki, Y., Yokota, M., & Koike, Y. (1994). Pure-tone threshold prediction by 80-Hz amplitude-modulation following response. *Acta Otolaryngologica, Supplementum, 511,* 7–14.

Bagatto, M. (2008). Baby waves and hearing aids: Using ABR to fit hearing aids to infants. *Hearing Journal, 61*(2), 10–16.

Bagatto, M. P., Seewald, R. C., Scollie, S. D., & Tharpe, A. M. (2006). Evaluation of a probe tube insertion technique for measuring the real-ear-to-coupler difference (RECD) in young infants. *Journal of the American Academy of Audiology, 17*(8), 573–581.

Beattie, R. C., Kenworthy, O. T., & Vanides, E. L. (2005). Comparison of ABR thresholds using linear versus Blackman gating functions for predicting pure tone thresholds in hearing-impaired subjects. *Australian and New Zealand Journal of Audiology, 27*(1), 1–9.

Beattie, R. C., & Torre, P. (1997). Effects of rise-fall time and repetition rate on the auditory brainstem response to 0.5 and 1 kHz tone bursts using normal-hearing and hearing-impaired subjects. *Scandinavian Audiology, 26,* 23–32.

Boothroyd, A., & Cawkwell, S. (1970). Vibrotactile thresholds in pure tone audiometry. *Acta Otolaryngologica, 69*(6), 381–387.

Brinkmann, R. D., & Scherg, M. (1979). Human auditory on- and off-potentials of the brainstem. *Scandinavian Audiology, 8,* 27–32.

British Columbia Early Hearing Program (BCEHP; 2012). *Diagnostic audiology protocol* [pdf document]. Retrieved April 1, 2015, from http://www.phsa.ca/Documents/bcehpaudiologyassessmentprotocol.pdf

British Columbia Early Hearing Program (BCEHP; 2015). *ABR update October 31, 2015.* Retrieved from http://www.phsa.ca/Documents/bcehpaudiologyassessmentprotocol

Brooke, R. E., Brennan, S. K., & Stevens, J. C. (2009). Bone conduction auditory steady state response: Investigations into reducing artifact. *Ear and Hearing, 30*(1), 23–30.

Burkard, R., Shi, Y., & Hecox, K. E. (1990). A comparison of maximum length and Legendre sequences for the derivation of brain-stem auditory-evoked responses at rapid rates of stimulation. *Journal of the Acoustical Society of America, 87,* 1656–1664.

Campbell, F. W., Atkinson, J., Francis, M. R., & Green, D. M. (1977). Estimation of auditory thresholds using evoked potentials. A clinical screening test. *Progress in Clinical Neurophysiology, 2,* 68–78.

Canadian Working Group on Childhood Hearing. (2005). *Early hearing and communication development: Canadian Working Group on Childhood Hearing (CWGCH) resource document.* Ottawa, Ontario, Canada: Minister of Public Works and Government Services Canada. Retrieved September 20, 2009, from http://open.canada.ca/vl/en/doc/publications-270385

Casey, K.-A., & Small, S. A. (2014). Comparisons of auditory steady-state response and behavioural air-and bone-conduction thresholds for infants and adults with normal hearing. *Ear and Hearing, 35(4),* 423–439.

Cebulla, M., Sturzebecher, E., Elberling, C., & Muller, J. (2007). New clicklike stimuli for hearing testing. *Journal of American Academy of Audiology, 18*(9), 725–738.

Cheng, P.-W., Huang, T.-W., & Young, Y.-H. (2003). The influence of clicks versus short tone bursts on the vestibular evoked myogenic potential. *Ear and Hearing, 24,* 195–197.

Chou, Y. F., Chen, P. R., Yu, S. H., Wen, Y. H., & Wu, H. P. (2012). Using multi-stimulus auditory steady state response to predict hearing thresholds in high-risk infants. *European Archives of Oto-rhino-laryngology, 269*(1), 73–79.

Cobb, K. M., & Stuart, A. (2014). Test-retest reliability of auditory brainstem responses to chirp stimuli in newborns. *International Journal of Audiology, 53*(11), 829–835.

Cohen, L. T., Rickards, F. W., & Clark, G. M. (1991). A comparison of steady-state evoked potentials to modulated tones in awake and sleeping humans. *Journal of the Acoustical Society of America, 90,* 2467–2479.

Colebatch, J. G. (2001). Vestibular evoked potentials. *Current Opinion in Neurology, 14*(1), 21–26.

Cone-Wesson, B. (1995). Bone-conduction ABR tests. *American Journal of Audiology, 4,* 14–19.

Cone-Wesson, B., Parker, J., Swiderski, N., & Rickards, F. (2002). The auditory steady-state response: Full-term and premature neonates. *Journal of the American Academy of Audiology, 13*(5), 260–269.

Cone-Wesson, B., & Ramirez, G. M. (1997). Hearing sensitivity in newborns estimated from ABRs to bone-conducted sounds. *Journal of the American Academy of Audiology, 8,* 299–307.

Cornacchia, L., Martini, A., & Morra, B. (1983). Air and bone conduction brain stem responses in adults and infants. *Audiology, 22,* 430–437.

Dau, T., Wagner, O., Mellert, V., & Kollmeier, B. (2000). Auditory brainstem responses with optimized chirp signals compensating basilar membrane dispersion. *Journal of the Acoustical Society of America, 107,* 1530–1540.

D'Haenens, W., Dhooge, I., Maes, L., Bockstael, A., Keppler, H., Philips, B., & Vinck, B. M. (2009). The clinical value of the multiple-frequency 80-Hz auditory steady-state response in adults with normal hearing and hearing loss. *Archives in Otolaryngology-Head and Neck Surgery, 135*(5), 496–506.

Dimitrijevic, A., John, M. S., Van Roon, P., Purcell, D. W., Adamonis, J., Ostroff, J., . . . Picton, T. W. (2002). Estimating the audiogram using multiple auditory steady-state responses. *Journal of the American Academy of Audiology, 13*(4), 205–224.

Don, M., & Elberling, C. (1996). Use of quantitative measures of auditory brain-stem response peak amplitude and residual background noise in the decision to stop averaging. *Journal of Acoustical Society of America, 99*, 491–499.

Don, M., Elberling, C., & Waring, M. (1984). Objective detection of averaged auditory brainstem responses. *Scandinavian Audiology, 13*, 219–228.

Edwards, C. G., Durieux-Smith, A., & Picton, T. W. (1985). Neonatal auditory brainstem responses from ipsilateral and contralateral recording montages. *Ear and Hearing, 6*, 175–178.

Eggermont, J. J. (1982). The inadequacy of click-evoked auditory brainstem responses in audiological applications. *Annals of the New York Academy of Sciences, 388*, 707–709.

Elberling, C., & Don, M. (1984). Quality estimation of averaged auditory brainstem responses. *Scandinavian Audiology, 13*, 187–197.

Elberling, C., & Don, M. (2008). Auditory brainstem responses to a chirp stimulus designed from derived-band latencies in normal-hearing subjects. *Journal of the Acoustical Society of America, 124*(5), 3022–3037.

Fedtke, T., & Richter, U. (2007). Reference zero for the calibration of air-conduction audiometric equipment using "tone bursts" as test signals. *International Journal of Audiology, 46*, 1–10.

Ferm, I., Lightfoot, G., & Stevens, J. (2013). Comparison of ABR response amplitude, test time, and estimation of hearing threshold using frequency specific chirp and tone-pip stimuli in newborns. *International Journal of Audiology, 52*(6), 419–423.

Ferm, I., Lightfoot, G., & Stevens, J. (2014). Provisional stimulus level corrections for low frequency bone-conduction ABR in babies under three months corrected age. *International Journal of Audiology, 53*(2), 132–137.

Foxe, J. J., & Stapells, D. R. (1993). Normal infant and adult auditory brainstem responses to bone-conducted tones. *Audiology, 32*, 95–109.

Fria, T. J., & Sabo, D. L. (1979). Auditory brainstem responses in children with otitis media with effusion. *Annals of Otology, Rhinology, and Laryngology, 89*, 200–206.

Galambos, R., Makeig, S., & Talmachoff, P. (1981). A 40-Hz auditory potential recorded from the human scalp. *Proceedings of the National Academy of Sciences USA, 78*(4), 2643– 2647.

Geisler, C. D. (1960). Average response to clicks in man recorded by scalp electrodes. *M.I.T. Technical Report, 380*, 1–158.

Gorga, M. P. (2002). Some factors that may influence the accuracy of auditory brainstem response estimates of hearing loss. In R. C. Seewald & J. S. Gravel (Eds.), *A sound foundation through early amplification 2001. Proceedings of the second international conference* (pp. 49-61). Stäfa, Switzerland: Phonak AG.

Gorga, M. P., Johnson, T. A., Kaminski, J. R., Beauchaine, K. L., Garner, C. A., & Neely, S. T. (2006). Using a combination of click- and tone burst-evoked auditory brain stem response measurements to estimate pure-tone thresholds. *Ear and Hearing, 27*(1), 60–74.

Gorga, M. P., Kaminski, J. R., & Beauchaine, K. L. (1991). Effects of stimulus phase on the latency of the auditory brainstem response. *Journal of the American Academy of Audiology, 2*, 1–6.

Gorga, M. P., Neely, S. T., Hoover, B. M., Dierking, D. M., Beauchaine, K. L., & Manning, C. (2004). Determining the upper limits of stimulation for auditory steady-state response measurements. *Ear and Hearing, 25*(3), 302–307.

Gorga, M. P., & Thornton, A. R. (1989). The choice of stimuli for ABR measurement. *Ear and Hearing, 10*, 217–230.

Gravel, J. S. (2002). Potential pitfalls in the audiological assessment of infants and young children. In R. C. Seewald & J. S. Gravel (Eds.), *A sound foundation through early amplification 2001. Proceedings of the second international conference* (pp. 85–101). Stäfa, Switzerland: Phonak AG.

Gravel, J. S., Kurtzberg, D., Stapells, D. R., Vaughan, H. G. J., & Wallace, I. F. (1989). Case studies. *Seminars in Hearing, 10*, 272–287.

Haboosheh, R. (2007). *Diagnostic auditory brainstem response analysis: Evaluation of signal- to-noise ratio criteria using signal detection theory.* Unpublished M.Sc. thesis, The University of British Columbia, Vancouver, B.C.

Hall, J. W. (2007). *New handbook of auditory evoked responses.* Boston, MA: Pearson Allyn & Bacon.

Han, D., Mo, M., Liu, H., Chen, J., & Huang, L. (2006). Threshold estimation in children using auditory steady-state responses to multiple simultaneous stimuli. *O-R-L, 68*, 64–68.

Hansen, E., & Small, S. A. (2012). Effective masking levels for bone conduction auditory steady-state responses in infants and adults with normal hearing. *Ear and Hearing, 32*(2), 257–266.

Hatton, J. L., Janssen, R. M., & Stapells, D. R. (2012). Bone-conduction brief-tone ABR assessment of infants with conductive and sensorineural hearing loss. *International Journal of Otolaryngology, 2012*, 284864. doi:10.1155/2012/284864

Hatton, J. L., & Stapells, D. R. (2011). Efficiency of single- vs. multiple-stimulus auditory steady-state responses in infants. *Ear and Hearing, 32*(3), 349–357.

Hatton, J. L., & Stapells, D. R. (2013). Monotic versus dichotic multiple-stimulus auditory steady state responses in young children. *Ear and Hearing, 34*(5), 680–682.

Herdman, A., Lins, O., Van Roon, P., Stapells, D., Scherg, M., & Picton, T. (2002). Intracerebral sources of human auditory steady-state responses. *Brain Topography, 15*, 69–86.

Herdman, A. T., Picton, T. W., & Stapells, D. R. (2002). Place specificity of multiple auditory steady-state responses. *Journal of the Acoustical Society of America, 112*, 1569–1582.

Herdman, A. T., & Stapells, D. R. (2001). Thresholds determined using the monotic and dichotic multiple auditory steady-state response technique in normal-hearing subjects. *Scandinavian Audiology, 30*, 41–49.

Herdman, A. T., & Stapells, D. R. (2003). Auditory steady-state response thresholds of adults with sensorineural hearing impairments. *International Journal of Audiology, 42*(5), 237–248.

Hooks, R. G., & Weber, B. A. (1984). Auditory brain stem response of premature infants to bone-conducted stimuli: A feasibility study. *Ear and Hearing, 5*, 42–46.

Hulecki, L. R., & Small, S. A. (2011). Behavioral bone-conduction threshold for infants with normal hearing. *Journal of the American Academy of Audiology, 22*(2), 1–12.

Hyde, M. L. (2005). Newborn hearing screening programs: Overview. *Journal of Otolaryngology, 34*(Suppl. 2), S70–S78.

Hyde, M., Sininger, Y. S., & Don, M. (1998). Objective detection and analysis of auditory brainstem response: An historical perspective. *Seminars in Hearing, 19*(1), 97.

International Organization for Standardization (ISO; 2007). *Acoustics—Reference zero for the calibration of audiometric equipment. Part 6: Reference threshold of hearing for test signals of short duration* (ISO 389-6). Geneva, Switzerland: ISO.

Ishida, I. M., Cuthbert, B. P., & Stapells, D. R. (2011). Multiple-ASSR thresholds to bone conduction stimuli in adults with elevated thresholds. *Ear and Hearing, 32*(3), 373–381.

Ishida, I. M., & Stapells, D. R. (2012). Multiple-ASSR interactions in adults with sensorineural hearing loss. *International Journal of Otolaryngology*. Advance online publication. doi:10.1155/2012/802715

Janssen, R. M., Usher, L., & Stapells, D. R. (2010). The British Columbia's Children's Hospital tone-evoked ABR protocol: How long do infants sleep, and how much information can be obtained in one appointment? *Ear and Hearing, 31*, 722–724.

Jeng, F. C., Brown, C. J., Johnson, T. A., & Vander Werff, K. R. (2004). Estimating air-bone gaps using auditory steady-state responses. *Journal of the American Academy of Audiology, 15*(1), 67–78.

John, M. S., Brown, D. K., Muir, P. J., & Picton, T. W. (2004). Recording auditory steady-state responses in young infants. *Ear and Hearing, 25*(6), 539–553.

John, M. S., Dimitrijevic, A., & Picton, T. W. (2002). Auditory steady-state responses to exponential modulation envelopes. *Ear and Hearing, 23*(2), 106–117.

John, M. S., Lins, O. G., Boucher, B. L., & Picton, T. W. (1998). Multiple auditory steady-state responses (MASTER): Stimulus and recording parameters. *Audiology, 37*, 59–82.

John, M. S., & Purcell, D. W. (2008). Introduction to technical principles of auditory steady-state response testing. In G. Rance (Ed.), *The auditory steady-state response. Generation, recording, and clinical application* (pp. 11–53). San Diego, CA: Plural.

John, M. S., Purcell, D. W., Dimitrijevic, A., & Picton, T. W. (2002). Advantages and caveats when recording steady-state responses to multiple simultaneous stimuli. *Journal of the American Academy of Audiology, 13*, 246–259.

Johnson, T. A., & Brown, T. A. (2005). Threshold prediction using the auditory steady-state response and the tone burst auditory brain stem response: A within-subject comparison. *Ear and Hearing, 26*, 559–576.

Joint Committee on Infant Hearing (JCIH; 2007). Year 2007 position statement: Principles and guidelines for early hearing detection and intervention programs. *Pediatrics, 120*(4), 898–921.

Kato, T., Shiraishi, K., Eura, Y., Shibata, K., Sakata, T., Morizono, T., & Soda, T. (1998). A "neural" response with 3-ms latency evoked by loud sound in profoundly deaf patients. *Audiology and Neurotology, 3*(4), 253–264.

Kavanagh, K. T., & Beardsley, J. V. (1979). Brain stem auditory evoked response. Clinical uses of bone conduction in the evaluation of otologic disease. *Annals of Otology, Rhinology, and Laryngology, 88*, 22–28.

Kemp, D. T. (1988). Developments in cochlear mechanics and techniques for noninvasive evaluation. *Advances in Audiology, 5*, 27–45.

Kennedy, C., McCann, D., Campbell, M. J., Kimm, L., & Thornton, R. (2005). Universal newborn screening for permanent childhood hearing impairment: An 8-year follow-up of a controlled trial. *Lancet, 366*(9486), 660–662.

Klein, A. J. (1983). Properties of the brain-stem response slow-wave component. II. Frequency specificity. *Archives of Otolaryngology, 109*, 74–78.

Kodera, H., Yamane, H., Yamada, O., & Suzuki, J.-I. (1977). The effects of onset, offset and rise-decay times of tone bursts on brain stem responses. *Scandinavian Audiology, 6*, 205–210.

Kramer, S. J. (1992). Frequency specific auditory brainstem responses to bone-conducted stimuli. *Audiology, 31*, 61–71.

Kuwada, S., Anderson, J. S., Batra, R., Fitzpatrick, D. C., Teissier, N., & D'Angelo, W. R. (2002). Sources of the scalp-recorded amplitude-modulation following response. *Journal of the American Academy of Audiology, 13*, 188–204.

Lasky, R. E. (1991). The effects of rate and forward masking on human adult and newborn auditory evoked brain-stem response thresholds. *Developmental Psychobiology, 24*, 51–64.

Lee, C. Y., Hsieh, T. H., Pan, S. L., & Hsu, C. J. (2007). Thresholds of tone burst auditory brainstem responses for infants and young children with normal hearing in Taiwan. *Journal of the Formosan Medical Association, 106*(10), 847–853.

Lee, C. Y., Jaw, F. S., Pan, S. L., Hsieh, T. H., & Hsu, C. J. (2008). Effects of age and degree of hearing loss on the agreement and correlation between sound field audiometric thresholds and tone burst auditory brainstem response thresholds in infants and young children. *Journal of the Formosan Medical Association, 107*(11), 869–875.

Linden, R. D., Campbell, K. B., Hamel, G., & Picton, T. W. (1985). Human auditory steady-state evoked potentials during sleep. *Ear and Hearing, 6*(3), 167–174.

Lins, O. G., & Picton, T. W. (1995). Auditory steady-state responses to multiple simultaneous stimuli. *Electroencephalography and Clinical Neurophysiology, 96*, 420–432.

Lins, O. G., Picton, P. E., Picton, T. W., Champagne, S. C., & Durieux-Smith, A. (1995). Auditory steady-state responses to tones amplitude-modulated at 80–110 Hz. *Journal of the Acoustical Society of America, 97*, 3051–3063.

Lins, O. G., Picton, T. W., Boucher, B. L., Durieux-Smith, A., Champagne, S. C., Moran, L. M., . . . Savio, G. (1996). Frequency-specific audiometry using steady-state responses. *Ear and Hearing, 17*, 81–96.

Luts, H., Desloovere, C., & Wouters, J. (2006). Clinical application of dichotic multiple-stimulus auditory steady-state responses in high-risk newborns and children. *Audiology and Neurotology, 11*, 24–37.

Luts, H., Van Dun, B., Alaerts, J., & Wouters, J. (2008). The influence of the detection paradigm in recording auditory steady-state responses. *Ear and Hearing, 29*(4), 638–650.

Luts, H., & Wouters, J. (2004). Hearing assessment by recording multiple auditory steady-state responses: The influence of test duration. *International Journal of Audiology, 43*(8), 471–478.

Mackersie, C. L., & Stapells, D. R. (1994). Auditory brainstem response wave I prediction of conductive component in infants and young children. *American Journal of Audiology, 3*, 52–58.

Mackey, A., Hodgetts, W., & Small, S.A. (in press). Maturation of mechanical impedance of the skin-covered skull: Implications for soft band bone-anchored hearing systems fitted in infants and young children. *Ear and Hearing*.

Marcoux, A. M. (2011). Maturation of auditory function related to hearing threshold estimations using the auditory brainstem response during infancy. *International Journal of Pediatric Otorhinolaryngology, 75*(2), 163–70.

Martin, W. H., Schwegler, J. W., Gleeson, A. L., & Shi, Y. (1994). New techniques of hearing assessment. *Pediatric Otology, 27*, 487–510.

Mauer, G., & Döring, W. H. (1999). *Generators of amplitude modulation following response (AMFR).* Paper presented at the XVI Biennial Meeting of the International Evoked Response Audiometry Study Group. Tromso, Norway.

Mauldin, L., & Jerger, J. (1979). Auditory brainstem evoked responses to bone-conducted signals. *Archives of Otolaryngology, 105*, 656–661.

McCreery, R. W., Kaminski, J., Beauchaine, K., Lenzen, N., Simms. K., & Gorga, M. P. (2014). The impact of degree of hearing loss on auditory brainstem response predictions of behavioral thresholds. Advance online publication. *Ear and Hearing, 36*(3), 309–319. doi:10.1097/AUD.0000000000000120

McGee, T. J., & Clemis, J. D. (1982). Effects of conductive hearing loss on auditory brainstem response. *Annals of Otology, Rhinology, and Laryngology, 91*, 304–309.

Mo, L., & Stapells, D. R. (2008). The effect of brief-tone stimulus duration on the brain stem auditory steady-state response. *Ear and Hearing, 29*(1), 121–133.

Moeller, M. P. (2007). Current state of knowledge: Psychosocial development in children with hearing impairment. *Ear and Hearing, 28*(6), 729–739.

Moore, B. C. J. (2004). *An introduction to the psychology of hearing* (5th ed.). San Diego, CA: Elsevier Academic Press.

Muchnik, C., Neeman, R. K., & Hildesheimer, M. (1995). Auditory brainstem response to bone-conducted clicks in adults and infants with normal hearing and conductive hearing loss. *Scandinavian Audiology, 24*, 185–191.

Murofushi, T., Iwasaki, S., Takai, Y., & Takegoshi, H. (2005). Sound-evoked neurogenic responses with short latency of vestibular origin. *Clinical Neurophysiology, 116*(2), 401–405.

Nagashima, H., Udaka, J., Chida, I., Shimada, A., Kondo, E., & Takeda, N. (2013). Air-bone gap estimated with multiple auditory steady-state response in young children with otitis media with effusion. *Auris Nasus Larynx, 40*(6), 534–538.

Nambi, A., & Vanaja, C. S. (2006). *Reduction of stimulus artifacts in ASSR: An investigation of a stimulus approach.* Retrieved from http://www.aiish.ac.in/images/pdf/06-07aud.pdf

Nousak, J. K., & Stapells, D. R. (1992). Frequency specificity of the auditory brain stem response to bone-conducted tones in infants and adults. *Ear and Hearing, 13*, 87–95.

Oates, P., & Stapells, D. R. (1997a). Frequency specificity of the human auditory brainstem and middle latency responses to brief tones. I. High pass noise masking. *Journal of the Acoustical Society of America, 102*, 3597–3608.

Oates, P., & Stapells, D. R. (1997b). Frequency specificity of the human auditory brainstem and middle latency responses to brief tones. II. Derived response analyses. *Journal of the Acoustical Society of America, 102*, 3609–3619.

Ontario Infant Hearing Program (OIHP; 2008)., *Audiologic assessment protocol* [pdf document]. Retrieved December 26, 2010, from http://www.mountsinai.on.ca/care/infant-hearing-program/documents/IHPAudiologicAssessmentProtocol3.1FinalJan2008.pdf

Özdamar, Ö., & Delgado, R. E. (1996). Measurement of signal and noise characteristics in ongoing auditory brainstem response averaging. *Annals of Biomedical Engineering, 24*(6), 702–715.

Papathanasiou, E. S., Zamba-Papanicolaou, E., Pantziaris, M., Kleopas, K., Kyriakides, T., Papacostas, S., . . . Piperidou, C. (2004). Neurogenic vestibular evoked potentials using a tone pip auditory stimulus. *Electromyography and Clinical Neurophysiology, 44*(3), 167–173.

Perez-Abalo, M. C., Savio, G., Torres, A., Martin, V., Rodríguez, E., & Galán, L. (2001). Steady state responses to multiple amplitude-modulated tones: An optimized method to test frequency-specific thresholds in hearing-impaired children and normal-hearing subjects. *Ear and Hearing, 22*, 200–211.

Picton, T. W. (1978). The strategy of evoked potential audiometry. In S. E. Gerber & G. T. Mencher (Eds.), *Early diagnosis of hearing loss* (pp. 297–307). New York, NY: Grune & Stratton.

Picton, T. W., Dimitrijevic, A., & John, M. S. (2002). Multiple auditory steady-state responses. *Annals of Otology, Rhinology, and Laryngology Suppl., 189*, 16–21.

Picton, T. W., Dimitrijevic, A., Perez-Abalo, M. C., & Van Roon, P. (2005). Estimating audiometric thresholds using auditory steady-state responses. *Journal of the American Academy of Audiology, 16*(3), 140–156.

Picton, T. W., Durieux-Smith, A., & Moran, L. M. (1994). Recording auditory brainstem responses from infants. *International Journal of Pediatric Otorhinolaryngology, 28*, 93–110.

Picton, T. W., & John, M. S. (2004). Avoiding electromagnetic artifacts when recording auditory steady-state responses. *Journal of the American Academy of Audiology, 15*(8), 541–554.

Picton, T. W., John, M., Dimitrijevic, A., & Purcell, D. (2003). Human auditory steady-state responses. *International Journal of Audiology, 42*, 177–219.

Picton, T. W., Linden, R. D., Hamel, G., & Maru, J. T. (1983). Aspects of averaging. *Seminars in Hearing, 4*, 327–341.

Picton, T. W., & Maru, J. T. (1984). Comments on obtaining signals from noise. In A. Starr, C. Rosenberg, M. Don, & H. Davis (Eds.), *Sensory evoked potentials: An international conference on standards for auditory brainstem response (ABR)* (pp. 147–151). Milan, Italy: Amplifon.

Picton, T. W., Ouellette, J., Hamel, G., & Smith, A. D. (1979). Brainstem evoked potentials to tone pips in notched noise. *Journal of Otolaryngology, 8*, 289–314.

Picton, T. W., & Stapells, D. R. (1985). A "Frank's Run" latency-intensity function. In J. T. Jacobson (Ed.), *The auditory brainstem response* (pp. 410–413). San Diego, CA: College-Hill Press.

Picton, T. W., van Roon, P., & John, M. S. (2009). Multiple auditory steady-state responses (80–101 Hz): Effects of ear, gender, handedness, intensity and modulation rate. *Ear and Hearing, 30*(1), 100–109.

Purcell, D. W., & Dajani, H. R. (2008). The stimulus-response relationship in auditory steady-state response testing. In G. Rance (Ed.), *The auditory steady-state response. Generation, recording, and clinical application* (pp. 55–82). San Diego, CA: Plural.

Purdy, S. C., & Abbas, P. J. (2002). ABR thresholds to tonebursts gated with Blackman and linear windows in adults with high-frequency sensorineural hearing loss. *Ear and Hearing, 23*(4), 358–368.

Rance, G. (2005). Auditory neuropathy/dys-synchrony and its perceptual consequences. *Trends in Amplification, 9*(1), 1–43.

Rance, G. (2008a). Auditory steady-state responses in neonates and infants. In G. Rance (Ed.), *The auditory steady-state response. Generation, recording, and clinical application* (pp. 161–184). San Diego, CA: Plural.

Rance, G. (Ed.). (2008b). *The auditory steady-state response. Generation, recording, and clinical application*. San Diego, CA: Plural.

Rance, G., & Briggs, R. S. J. (2002). Assessment of hearing in infants with moderate to profound impairment: The Melbourne experience with auditory steady-state evoked potential testing. *Annals of Otology, Rhinology, and Laryngology, 111*(Suppl. 189), 22–28.

Rance, G., Dowell, R. C., Rickards, F. W., Beer, D. E., & Clark, G. M. (1998). Steady-state evoked potential and behavioral hearing thresholds in a group of children with absent click-evoked auditory brain stem response. *Ear and Hearing, 19*(1), 48–61.

Rance, G., & Rickards, F. (2002). Prediction of hearing threshold in infants using auditory steady-state evoked potentials. *Journal of the American Academy of Audiology, 13*(5), 236–245.

Rance, G., Rickards, F. W., Cohen, L. T., Burton, M. J., & Clark, G. M. (1993). Steady-state evoked potentials: A new tool for the accurate assessment of hearing in cochlear implant candidates. *Advances in Otorhinolaryngology, 48*, 44–48.

Rance, G., Rickards, F. W., Cohen, L. T., De Vidi, S., & Clark, G. M. (1995). The automated prediction of hearing thresholds in sleeping subjects using auditory steady-state evoked potentials. *Ear and Hearing, 16*(5), 499–507.

Rance, G., Roper, R., Symons, L., Moody, L.-J., Poulis, C., Dourlay, M., & Kelly, T. (2005). Hearing threshold estimation in infants using auditory steady-state responses. *Journal of the American Academy of Audiology, 16*, 291–300.

Rance, G., & Tomlin, D. (2006). Maturation of auditory steady-state responses in normal babies. *Ear and Hearing, 27*(1), 20–29.

Rance, G., Tomlin, D., & Rickards, F. (2006). Comparison of auditory steady-state responses and tone-burst auditory brainstem responses in normal babies. *Ear and Hearing, 27*, 751–762.

Regan, D. (1989). *Human brain electrophysiology: Evoked potentials and evoked magnetic fields in science and medicine*. New York, NY: Elsevier.

Ribeiro, F. M, Carvallo, R. M., & Marcoux, A. M. (2010). Auditory steady-state evoked responses for preterm and term neonates. *Audiology and Neurootology, 15(2)*, 97–110.

Rickards, F. W., & Clark, G. M. (1984). Steady-state evoked potentials to amplitude-modulated tones. In R. H. Nodar & C. Barber (Eds.), *Evoked potentials II* (pp. 163–168). Boston, MA: Butterworth.

Rodrigues, G. R., & Lewis, D. R. (2010). Auditory steady-state response in children with cochlear hearing loss. *Pró-Fono Revista de Atualização Científica, 22*(1), 37–42.

Rodrigues, G. R., & Lewis, D. R. (2014). Establishing auditory steady-state response thresholds to narrow band CE-chirps(®) in full-term neonates. *International Journal of Pediatric Otorhinolaryngology, 78*(2), 238–243.

Savio, G., Cardenas, J., Perez Abalo, M., Gonzales, A., & Valdes, J. (2001). The low and high frequency auditory steady-state responses mature at different rates. *Audiology and Neurotology, 6*, 279–287.

Savio, G., Perez-Abalo, M. C., Gaya, J., Hernandez, O., & Mijares, E. (2006). Test accuracy and prognostic validity of multiple auditory steady state responses for targeted hearing screening. *International Journal of Audiology, 45*(2), 109–120.

Seewald, R., Moodie, S., Scollie, S., & Bagatto, M. (2005). The DSL method for pediatric hearing instrument fitting: Historical perspective and current issues. *Trends in Amplification, 9*(4), 145–157.

Sheykholeslami, K., Kermany, M. H., & Kaga, K. (2000). Bone-conducted vestibular-evoked myogenic potentials in patients with congenital atresia of the external auditory canal. *International Journal of Pediatric Otorhinolaryngology, 57*, 25–29.

Sininger, Y. S. (2003). Audiologic assessment in infants. *Current Opinions in Otolaryngology-Head and Neck Surgery, 11*(5), 378–382.

Sininger, Y. S., Abdala, C., & Cone-Wesson, B. (1997). Auditory threshold sensitivity of the human neonate as measured by the auditory brainstem response. *Hearing Research, 104*, 27–38.

Sininger, Y. S., & Hyde, M. L. (2009). Auditory brainstem response in audiometric threshold prediction. In J. Katz,

L. Medwetsky, R. Burkard, & L. Hood (Eds.), *Handbook of clinical audiology* (6th ed., pp. 293–321). Baltimore, MD: Lippincott Williams & Wilkins.

Small, S. A., Hatton, J. L., & Stapells, D. R. (2007). Effects of bone oscillator coupling method, placement location, and occlusion on bone-conduction auditory steady-state responses in infants. *Ear and Hearing, 28*(1), 83–98.

Small, S. A., & Hu, N. (2011). Maturation of the occlusion effect: A bone-conduction auditory steady-state response study in infants and adults with normal hearing. *Ear and Hearing, 32*(6), 708–719.

Small, S. A., Smyth, A., & Leon, G. (2014). Effective masking levels for bone-conduction ASSRs to 500- and 2000-Hz stimuli in infants and adults with normal hearing. *Ear and Hearing, 35*(1), 63–71.

Small, S. A., & Stapells, D. R. (2003). Normal brief-tone bone-conduction behavioral thresholds using the B-71 transducer: Three occlusion conditions. *Journal of the American Academy of Audiology, 14*(10), 556–562.

Small, S. A., & Stapells, D. R. (2004). Artifactual responses when recording auditory steady-state responses. *Ear and Hearing, 25*(6), 611–623.

Small, S. A., & Stapells, D. R. (2005). Multiple auditory steady-state response thresholds to bone-conduction stimuli in adults with normal hearing. *Journal of the American Academy of Audiology, 16*, 172–183.

Small, S. A., & Stapells, D. R. (2006). Multiple auditory steady-state response thresholds to bone-conduction stimuli in young infants with normal hearing. *Ear and Hearing, 27*, 219–228.

Small, S. A., & Stapells, D. R. (2008a). Normal ipsilateral/contralateral asymmetries in infant multiple auditory steady-state responses to air- and bone-conduction stimuli. *Ear and Hearing, 29*(2), 185–198.

Small, S. A., & Stapells, D. R. (2008b). Maturation of bone conduction multiple auditory steady-state responses. *International Journal of Audiology, 47*(8), 476–488.

Stapells, D. R. (1989). Auditory brainstem response assessment of infants and children. *Seminars in Hearing, 10*, 229–251.

Stapells, D. R. (2000a). Frequency-specific evoked potential audiometry in infants. In R. C. Seewald (Ed.), *A sound foundation through early amplification: Proceedings of an international conference* (pp. 13–31). Stäfa, Switzerland: Phonak AG.

Stapells, D. R. (2000b). Threshold estimation by the tone-evoked auditory brainstem response: A literature meta-analysis. *Journal of Speech-Language Pathology and Audiology, 24*(2), 74–83.

Stapells, D. R., Galambos, R., Costello, J. A., & Makeig, S. (1988). Inconsistency of auditory middle latency and steady-state responses in infants. *Electroencephalography and Clinical Neurophysiology, 71*, 289–295.

Stapells, D. R., Gravel, J. A., & Martin, B. A. (1995). Thresholds for auditory brain stem responses to tones in notched noise from infants and young children with normal hearing or sensorineural hearing loss. *Ear and Hearing, 16*, 361–371.

Stapells, D. R., Herdman, A., Small, S. A., Dimitrijevic, A., & Hatton, J. (2005). Current status of the auditory steady-state responses for estimating an infant's audiogram. In R. Seewald & J. Bamford (Eds.), *A sound foundation through early amplification 2004: Proceedings of the third international conference* (pp. 43–59). Stäfa, Switzerland: Phonak AG.

Stapells, D. R., Linden, D., Suffield, J. B., Hamel, G., & Picton, T. W. (1984). Human auditory steady state potentials. *Ear and Hearing, 5*(2), 105–113.

Stapells, D. R., & Mosseri, M. (1991). Maturation of the contralaterally recorded auditory brainstem response. *Ear and Hearing, 12*, 167–173.

Stapells, D. R., & Oates, P. (1997). Estimation of the pure-tone audiogram by the auditory brainstem response: A review. *Audiology and Neurotology, 2*, 257–280.

Stapells, D. R., & Picton, T. W. (1981). Technical aspects of brainstem evoked potential audiometry using tones. *Ear and Hearing, 2*, 20–29.

Stapells, D. R., Picton, T. W., & Durieux-Smith, A. (1994). Electrophysiologic measures of frequency-specific auditory function. In J. T. Jacobson (Ed.), *Principles and applications in auditory evoked potentials* (pp. 251–283). Needham Hill, MA: Allyn & Bacon.

Stapells, D. R., & Ruben, R. J. (1989). Auditory brain stem responses to bone-conducted tones in infants. *Annals of Otology, Rhinology, and Laryngology, 98*, 941–949.

Stevens, J., Brennan, S., Gratton, D., & Campbell, M. (2013). ABR in newborns: Effects of electrode configuration, stimulus rate, and EEG rejection levels on test efficiency. *International Journal of Audiology, 52*, 706–712.

Stuart, A., Yang, E. Y., & Green, W. B. (1994). Neonatal auditory brainstem response thresholds to air- and bone-conducted clicks: 0 to 96 hours postpartum. *Journal of the American Academy of Audiology, 5*, 163–172.

Stuart, A., Yang, E. Y., & Stenstrom, R. (1990). Effect of temporal area bone vibrator placement on auditory brain stem response in newborn infants. *Ear and Hearing, 11*, 363–369.

Stuart, A., Yang, E. Y., Stenstrom, R., & Reindorp, A. G. (1993). Auditory brainstem response thresholds to air and bone-conducted clicks in neonates and adults. *American Journal of Otology, 14*, 176–182.

Stueve, M. P., & O'Rourke, C. (2003). Estimation of hearing loss in children: Comparison of auditory steady-state response, auditory brainstem response, and behavioral test methods. *American Journal of Audiology, 12*(2), 125–136.

Sturzebecher, E., Cebulla, M., Elberling, C., & Berger, T. (2006). New efficient stimuli for evoking frequency-specific auditory steady-state responses. *Journal of the American Academy of Audiology, 17*(6), 448–461.

Suzuki, T., & Horiuchi, K. (1981). Rise time pure tone stimuli in brain stem response audiometry. *Audiology, 20*, 101–112.

Suzuki, T., & Kobayashi, K. (1984). An evaluation of 40-Hz event-related potentials in young children. *Audiology, 23*, 599–604.

Swanepoel, D., & Hugo, R. (2004). Estimations of auditory sensitivity for young cochlear implant candidates using the ASSR: Preliminary results. *International Journal of Audiology, 43*(7), 377–382.

Swanepoel, D., Hugo, R., & Roode, R. (2004). Auditory steady-state responses for children with severe to profound hearing loss. *Archives of Otolaryngology-Head and Neck Surgery, 130*(5), 531–535.

Swanepoel, D. W., Ebrahim, S., Friedland, P., Swanepoel, A., & Pottas, L. (2008). Auditory steady-state responses to bone conduction stimuli in children with hearing loss. *International Journal of Pediatric Otorhinolaryngology, 72*(12), 1861–1871.

Swanepoel, D. W., & Steyn, K. (2005). Short report: Establishing normal hearing for infants with the auditory steady-state response. *South African Journal of Communication Disorders, 52*, 36–39.

Tlumak, A. I., Rubinstein, E., & Durrant, J. D. (2007). Meta-analysis of variables that affect accuracy of threshold estimation via measurement of the auditory steady-state response (ASSR). *International Journal of Audiology, 46*(11), 692–710.

Valeriote, H., & Small, S. A. (2015). Comparison of air- and bone-conduction auditory brainstem and multiple 80-Hz auditory steady-state responses in infants with normal hearing and conductive hearing loss. *Abstracts of the XXIV Biennial Symposium of the International Evoked Response Audiometry Study Group IERASG* (May 10–14; Busan, Korea). Retrieved April 4, 2015, from http://www.ierasg2015.org/

van Maanen, A., & Stapells, D. R. (2009). Normal multiple auditory steady-state response thresholds to air-conducted stimuli in infants. *Journal of the American Academy of Audiology, 20*, 196–207.

van Maanen, A., & Stapells, D. R. (2010). Multiple-ASSR thresholds in infants and young children with hearing loss. *Journal of the American Academy of Audiology, 21*, 535–545.

Vander Werff, K. R., Johnson, T. A., & Brown, C. J. (2008). Behavioral threshold estimation for auditory steady-state response. In G. Rance (Ed.), *The auditory steady-state response. Generation, recording, and clinical application* (pp. 125–147). San Diego, CA: Plural.

Vander Werff, K. R., Prieve, B. A., & Georgantas, L. M. (2009). Infant air and bone conduction tone burst auditory brain stem responses for classification of hearing loss and the relationship to behavioral thresholds. *Ear and Hearing, 30*(3), 350–368.

Welgampola, M. S., & Colebatch, J. G. (2001). Characteristics of tone burst-evoked myogenic potentials in the sternocleidomastoid muscles. *Otology and Neurotology, 22*, 796–802.

Wood, L. L. (2009). *Multiple brainstem auditory steady-state response interactions for different stimuli* (Unpublished M.Sc. thesis). The University of British Columbia, Vancouver, B.C.

Yamada, O., Yagi, T., Yamane, H., & Suzuki, J.-I. (1975). Clinical evaluation of the auditory evoked brain stem response. *Aurix-Nasus-Larynx, 2*, 97–105.

Yang, E. Y., Rupert, A. L., & Moushegian, G. (1987). A developmental study of bone conduction auditory brainstem responses in infants. *Ear and Hearing, 8*, 244–251.

Yang, E. Y., & Stuart, A. (1990). A method of auditory brainstem response testing of infants using bone-conducted clicks. *Journal of Speech Language Pathology and Audiology, 14*, 69–76.

Yang, E. Y., Stuart, A., Mencher, G. T., Mencher, L. S., & Vincer, M. J. (1993). Auditory brain stem responses to air- and bone-conducted clicks in the audiological assessment of at-risk infants. *Ear and Hearing, 14*, 175–182.

Yang, E. Y., & Stuart, A., Stenstrom, R., & Hollett, S. (1991). Effect of vibrator to head coupling force on the auditory brain stem response to bone conducted clicks in newborn infants. *Ear and Hearing, 12*(1), 55–60.

Yoshinaga-Itano, C., & Gravel, J. S. (2001). The evidence for universal newborn hearing screening. *American Journal of Audiology, 10*(2), 62–64.

Yoshinaga-Itano, C., Sedey, A. L., Coulter, D. K., & Mehl, A. L. (1998). Language of early- and later-identified children with hearing loss. *Pediatrics, 102*, 1161–1171.

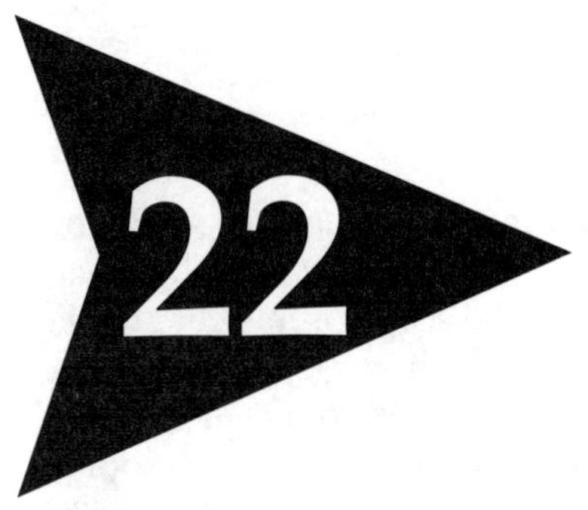

Electrophysiological Assessment of Hearing With Auditory Middle Latency and Auditory Late Responses

James W. Hall III and Anuradha R. Bantwal

Historical Perspective on Cortical Auditory-Evoked Responses

Cortical auditory-evoked responses were first reported nearly 80 years ago. The auditory late response (ALR) was described by Davis in 1939. Throughout the 1960s, the ALR was explored, and even relied on clinically, as an electrophysiologic index of auditory function, especially for objectively determining auditory thresholds in young children (Hall, 1992, 2007). About 20 years later, the auditory middle latency response (AMLR) was discovered by Geisler (Geisler, Frishkopf, & Rosenblith, 1958) and almost immediately applied by Robert Goldstein and colleagues at the University of Wisconsin (Goldstein & Rodman, 1967) in the assessment of auditory thresholds in young children, including newborn infants. With the emergence in the mid-1970s of the auditory brainstem response (ABR) as a clinical tool for pediatric auditory assessment, clinical use of the AMLR and ALR quickly diminished. However, within 10 years clinical audiologists and researchers (e.g., Hall, Huang-fu, & Gennarelli, 1982; Kraus, Özdamar, Hier, & Stein, 1982; Musiek, Geurkink, Weider, & Donnelly, 1984) began to recognize the need for an electrophysiological measure (or measures) of higher-level auditory function. Although the ABR clearly was valuable in the estimation of auditory threshold, and to document overt brainstem auditory dysfunction, it provided no information on suprabrainstem (e.g., thalamic and cortical) auditory dysfunction.

Within the past 25 years, reports of clinical application of cortical auditory-evoked responses, many of them case reports, periodically have appeared in the literature. However, neither the AMLR nor the ALR, or any other cortical auditory-evoked responses (e.g., the P300 response), are consistently included within the test battery for assessment of central auditory nervous system function. Until recently, cortical auditory-evoked responses were almost exclusively being employed by investigators in the laboratory setting for research rather than in the clinical setting by practicing audiologists. This trend is changing gradually with an increased awareness of the clinical applications of ALR, the most valuable being its demonstrated use as a biomarker of central auditory nervous system (CANS) maturation and as an objective index of intervention-related changes in the CANS. Dedicated instruments such as the HEARLab Cortical Auditory Evoked Potential Analyzer, which can be used for measuring ALR in children, are now available commercially. We predict that cortical auditory-evoked responses in the near future will play a more important, and regular, role in the assessment of central auditory function and processing.

Rationale for the Application of AMLR and ALR in Children

Several advantages of electrophysiological measures argue for inclusion of the AMLR and ALR in the diagnostic test battery for selected patient populations. Specific clinical advantages and limitations of the AMLR and ALR in the assessment of children are summarized in Table 22–1.

Electrophysiological measures are not influenced by the quality, validity, or feasibility of behavioral responses to sound. Valid and clinically useful AMLRs and ALRs can be recorded independent of listener (patient) variables that can confound traditional behavioral tests, such as motivation, fatigue, cognition, attention, motor function, and language. In addition, auditory-evoked responses offer a degree of site specificity not available from most behavioral auditory procedures. Some information on the site of dysfunction within the auditory system is gained from close analysis of auditory-evoked responses. Of course, some of these advantages apply also to electroacoustic auditory measures such as acoustic reflexes and otoacoustic emissions.

The following review focuses on clinical applications of the AMLR and the ALR in children. A complete review of the basic principles of the cortical auditory-evoked response, including anatomic and physiological underpinnings, and measurement techniques and procedures is far beyond the scope of this chapter. For more information and in-depth and current coverage of the topic, the reader is referred to recent textbooks devoted exclusively to auditory-evoked responses (e.g., Burkard, Don, & Eggermont, 2007; Hall, 2007, 2015; Picton, 2011).

Auditory Middle Latency Response (AMLR)

Measurement and Analysis

A protocol for clinical measurement of the AMLR, including major components Na, Pa, and Pb, is summarized in Table 22–2. For selected parameters in Table 22–2, changing the specific value does not affect

Table 22–1. Clinical Advantages and Disadvantages of Auditory Middle Latency (AMLR) and Auditory Late Response (ALR) in the Assessment of Children

Advantages	*Disadvantages*
AMLR	
• Accepted test protocols and procedures • Primary auditory cortex origins are known • Measurable in infants and young children • Analyses strategies are defined • Can be recorded with a clinical ABR system	• Influenced by sleep and sedatives • Requires hemispheric electrodes for neurodiagnostic information • Equipment must have three or more channels for simultaneous AMLR measurement with hemispheric and midline electrodes • Complex interaction among age, stimulus rate, and duration • Influenced by state of arousal and some medications • Few data available on relation between AMLR and behavioral findings (e.g., in APD)
ALR	
• Generally accepted test protocols and procedures • Can be recorded with a clinical ABR system • Measurable in infants and young children • Analysis strategies are defined • Can be elicited with speech stimuli • Provides information on integrity of secondary auditory cortical regions • Clinical findings for various clinical populations	• Influenced by sleep and sedatives • Influenced by state of arousal and some medications • Some confusion about appropriate test parameters

Note. Electrophysiologic assessment for auditory processing disorders (APDs) represents an example of a clinical application of these cortical auditory-evoked responses.

Table 22–2. Guidelines for Auditory Middle Latency Response (AMLR) Test Protocol

Parameter	Suggestion	Rationale/Comment
Stimulus Parameters		
Transducer	ER-3A	• Supra-aural earphones are acceptable for AMLR, but insert earphones are more comfortable and, because the insert cushions are disposable, contribute to infection control.
Type	Click	• For neurodiagnosis only. However, a more robust AMLR is usually recorded with longer-duration tone-burst signals.
	Tone burst	• For neurodiagnosis or frequency-specific estimation of auditory sensitivity • Detection of the Pb component of the AMLR is enhanced for lower-frequency tone-burst signals.
Duration		
Click signal	0.1 ms	• Click signals are less effective than tone bursts in evoking the AMLR.
Tone burst signal		
Rise/fall	Two cycles	• Rather abrupt tone-burst onset is important for AMLR as it is for the ABR.
Plateau	Multiple cycles	• Plateau durations of 10 ms or longer are appropriate for evoking the AMLR, and especially for detection of the Pb component.
Rate	≤7.1/s	• A slower rate of signal presentation is indicated for younger children, or for patients with cortical pathology. Signal presentation rates as low as 1/s, or 0.5/s (one signal every 2 s) are required to consistently record the Pb component.
Polarity	Rarefaction	• An AMLR can also be recorded for condensation or alternating polarity signals.
Intensity	≤70 dB HL	• For neurodiagnosis, a moderate signal intensity level is appropriate. Signal intensity is decreased, of course, for estimation of thresholds. High signal intensity levels should be avoided. Tone-burst signals should be biologically calibrated to dB nHL in the space where clinical AMLRs are recorded.
Number	≤1,000	• Signal repetitions vary depending on size of response and background electrical noise. Remember the signal-to-noise ratio is the key. Averaging may require as few as 50 to 100 signals at high-intensity levels for a very quiet and normal hearing patient.
Presentation ear	Monaural	• For estimation of auditory sensitivity and neurodiagnosis. There is no apparent clinical indication for binaural AMLR measurement.
Masking	50 dB	• Rarely required with insert earphones, and not needed for stimulus intensity levels of ≤70 dB HL.
Acquisition Parameters		
Amplification	75,000	• Less amplification is required for larger responses such as the AMLR.
Sensitivity	50 μvolts	• Lower sensitivity values are equivalent to higher amplification.
Analysis time	100 ms	• Long enough to encompass the Pa and Pb components
Prestimulus time	10 ms	• Provides a convenient estimate of background noise and a baseline for calculation of the amplitudes for waveform components (Na, Pa, Nb, and Pb)
Data points	512	
Sweeps	1,000	• See comments above for signal number.

continues

Table 22–2. *continued*

Parameter	*Suggestion*	*Rationale/Comment*
Filters		
Band-pass	10 to 1500 Hz	• For recording an ABR, and AMLR with an Na and Pa component.
	10 to 200 Hz	• For recording an AMLR with an Na and Pa component. Do not over-filter (e.g., high-pass setting of 30 Hz and low-pass setting of 100 Hz), as it may remove important spectral energy from the response, and it may produce a misleading filter artifact.
	0.1 to about 200 Hz	• Decrease high-pass filter to 1 Hz or less to detect the Pb (P50) component.
Notch	None	• A notch filter (removing spectral energy in the region of 60 Hz) is never indicated with AMLR measurement because important frequencies in the response (around 40 Hz or below for young children) may also be removed.
Electrodes		
Type	Disc	• Disc electrodes are applied with paste (versus gel) to secure the noninverting electrodes on the scalp. It is helpful to use red- and blue-colored electrode leads for the right and left hemisphere locations, respectively. Ear clip electrodes are recommended when an earlobe inverting electrode site is used.
Sites		
Channel 1	C3 to Ai/Ac or C3 to NC	• Hemisphere electrode locations are required for neurodiagnosis. A linked earlobe inverting electrode arrangement (Ai = ipsilateral ear; Ac = contralateral ear) or a noncephalic (NC) inverting electrode (on the nape of the neck) is appropriate, and reduces likelihood of PAM artifact.
Channel 2	C4 to Ai/Ac or NC	• C3 = left hemisphere site; C4 = right hemisphere site.
Channel 3	Fz to Ai/Ac or NC	• A third channel (3) is optional for neurodiagnosis. Only the midline noninverting electrode channel is needed for the estimation of hearing sensitivity.
Channel 4	Outer canthi of eye	• Optional for detection of eye blinks, and rejection of averages contaminated by eye blinks.
Ground	Fpz	

Note. The modifications in the test protocol are required for consistent detection of the Pb component. (Adapted from Hall, 2007.)

consistent detection of the AMLR. For example, altering the stimulus transducer from a supra-aural to an insert earphone or stimulus polarity from rarefaction to condensation has no impact on AMLR recordings. However, other measurement parameters are critical to ensure that an AMLR will be recorded or to minimize the likelihood of contamination of the waveform with artifact.

Although calculation of both latency and amplitude of wave components is routinely included in analysis of the AMLR, most clinical information is derived from amplitude values. Specifically, AMLR analysis relies on a comparison of the magnitude or amplitude of the three major wave components (Na, Pa, and Pb) among two or more channels of AMLR recordings. The most commonly reported and simplest analysis strategy calls for calculation of the amplitude of the Pa wave recorded simultaneously with a three-channel arrangement with noninverting electrodes located over the right hemisphere (C4 location), the left hemisphere (C3 location), and the midline (Fz location). The emphasis in AMLR analysis, therefore, is on the size of the response arising from auditory cortex in the left hemisphere versus the right hemisphere versus subcortical regions. A secondary concern is analysis of the amplitude of components of an AMLR elicited with right versus left ear stimulation, or with stimulation of the ear ipsilateral versus contralateral to the noninverting recording electrode.

Weihing, Schochat, and Musiek (2012) conducted a study with an aim to explore the clinical application of AMLR measures other than latency and amplitude. This study was prompted by the observation of high variability of traditional AMLR indices within normal individuals. Weihing and colleagues measured ear effects and electrode effects in normal adults and children. The pediatric sample consisted of 155 children ranging in age from 7 to 16 years, divided into five subgroups by age. The researchers found that electrode and ear effects did not change with age and that it was possible to have normative values for these relative difference measures. The mean ear effect was larger than the electrode effect. The within-group variability was significantly lower for these two relative difference measures compared to absolute measures. Ear and electrode differences were not significantly correlated, indicating that perhaps both measures could be incorporated in clinical settings as they did not appear to be overlapping. The authors concluded that acquiring relative differences in AMLR might be of clinical use in children suspected of CAPD, as abnormal inter-aural differences have been recorded by previous studies as well. This application of AMLR is discussed later in the chapter.

AMLR analysis in a hypothetical patient with dysfunction within the right primary auditory cortex is illustrated in Figure 22–1. The AMLR was recorded with a three-channel electrode array, as just described, with tone-burst stimuli presented separately to the right and then the left ears. Each replicated waveform was recorded or averaged minimally with 500 stimuli. Notice that for right and left ear stimulation, the amplitudes of the Pa and Pb components are normal (about 1 μvolt) when recorded with a noninverting electrode located over the left hemisphere and the midline site. Importantly, amplitude of these AMLR components is about two times the amplitude of the ABR Wave V under the same stimulus conditions. Whenever the AMLR is recorded with a noninverting electrode located over the right hemisphere, the site of dysfunction, amplitudes of the Pa and Pb components are markedly reduced in comparison to the AMLR detected over the opposite hemisphere and at midline. In fact, for the right hemisphere electrode condition, amplitude of the Pa and Pb components is smaller than even the amplitude for ABR Wave V (0.5 μvolt). For this case, localization of the AMLR amplitude abnormalities to the right hemisphere is compatible with auditory dysfunction within the thalamocortical pathways on the right side and, most likely, the right primary auditory cortex. This conclusion is unaffected by various patient characteristics that would interfere with analysis of behavioral measures of central auditory functioning including attention, motivation, cognitive variables, language level, or native language.

Nonpathologic Factors

Major nonpathologic factors influencing the AMLR, including measurement and subject variables, are summarized in Table 22–3. For children under 10 years, age must be considered in AMLR measurement and analysis. This is not to say that the AMLR cannot be recorded from young children but, rather, that adjustments must be made in the test protocol and expectations are altered for response parameters. In general, slower stimulus presentation rates are required for younger children. The use of relatively slow stimulus presentation rates of less than five stimuli per second is advised for children under the age of 10 years, and one or more per second for infants and very young children. Otherwise, AMLR measurement in children differs little from the approach taken with older children and adults. Given the well-documented influence of sleep on the AMLR, especially on amplitude, every attempt should be made to maintain a consistent state of arousal throughout the recording session. The challenge during pediatric AMLR recording is to prevent the child from falling asleep while keeping the child physically inactive. The most effective technique for accomplishing this goal is to encourage the child to view an engaging and age-appropriate DVD or videotape, preferably one chosen by the child or parents.

Auditory Middle Latency Response in Pediatric Populations

The term *middle latency response* (MLR) was coined following the discovery of ABR because the response follows the ABR in time and precedes the ALR. The term *auditory middle latency response* (abbreviated AMLR) is more accurate and preferred as it distinguishes the response from somatosensory-, visual-, and vestibular-evoked response components within the same time frame. AMLR components occur between approximately 10 ms and 50 ms after the presentation of a

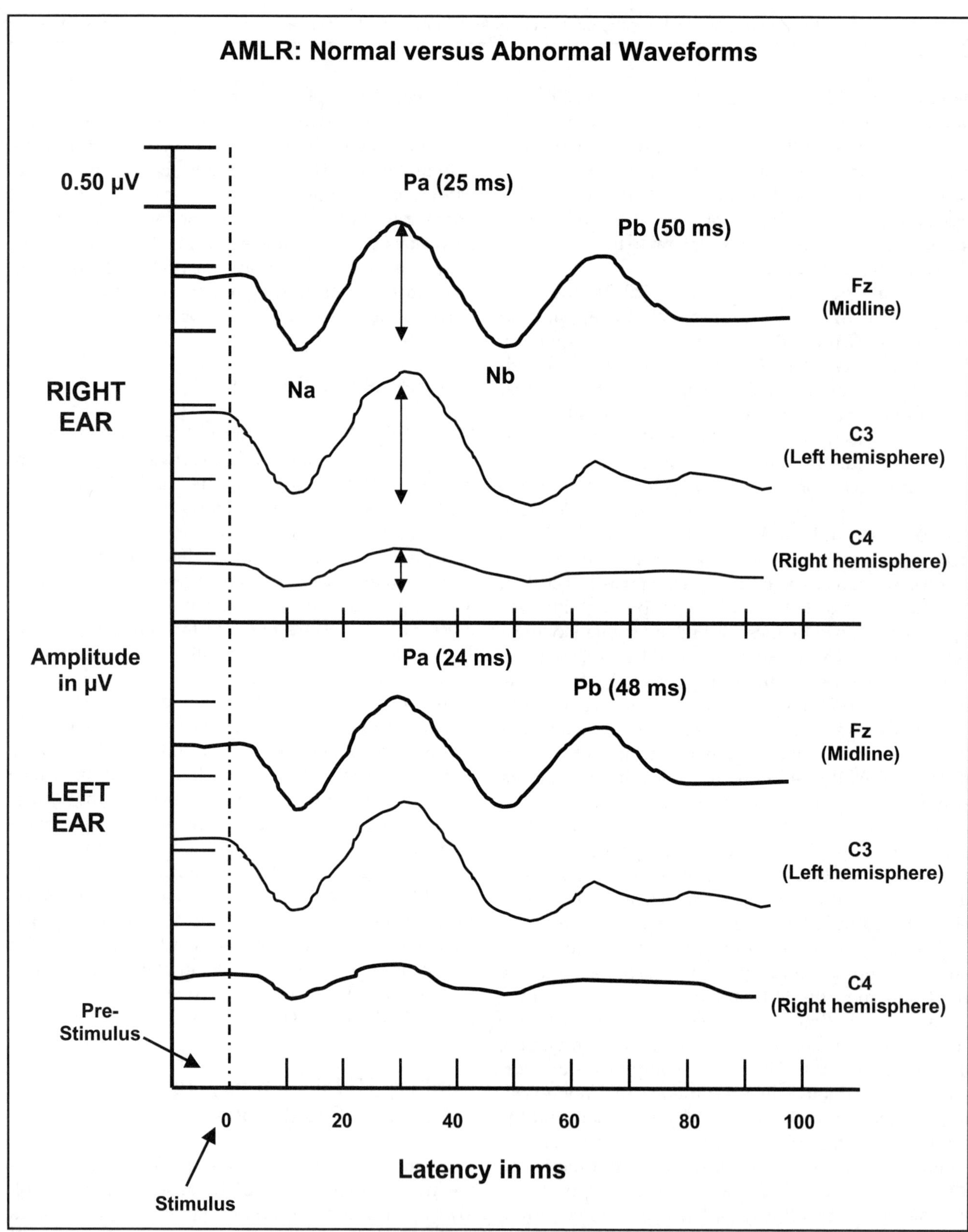

FIGURE 22–1. Auditory middle latency response (AMLR) waveforms elicited with tone-burst stimuli presented monaurally to the right and left ears and recorded with three noninverting electrode arrays from the left hemisphere (C3), right hemisphere (C4), and midline (Fz). The illustrative patient is a young adult with right-sided dysfunction within the primary auditory cortex. Note the abnormality of Pa and Pb amplitude as recorded with the C4 electrode, regardless of the side of stimulation.

Table 22–3. Major Nonpathologic Factors Influencing Measurement, Analysis, and Interpretation of the Auditory Middle Latency Response (AMLR)

Test Parameters
• Filtering: Avoid restricted high-pass filter setting (e.g., 30 Hz) and use HP setting of ≤1 Hz to detect the Pb component
• Stimulus intensity level: Avoid very high (>75 dB nHL) levels (PAM artifact)
• Stimulus duration: Longer (>10 ms) is better (avoid clicks)
• Stimulus rate: Slower rates for children and in pathology, with very slow rate (<1/s) to detect the Pb component
Subject Factors
• Age: Age is a factor for children under 10 years and interacts with stimulus rate
• Sleep: AMLR is more variable during sleep
• Postauricular muscle (PAM) artifact: Avoid if possible
• Sedation: Amplitude is reduced and variable
• Anesthesia: Typically suppresses AMLR activity (reticular formation generators)

stimulus (Cacace & McFarland, 2002; Hall, 1992; Kraus, Kileny, & McGee, 1994; Picton, Hillyard, Krausz, & Galambos, 1974).

AMLR in Children With Normal Hearing

Typical of other auditory-evoked responses, the human AMLR was first recorded in adults, and initial reported recording parameters and waveform descriptions were in the context of adult data. In the late 1970s, there were attempts to record AMLRs in infants and to apply them clinically as objective measures for threshold estimation. For example, Wolf and Goldstein (1978) described findings in five newborn infants in an attempt to validate the AMLR for threshold estimation. The authors did record responses and concluded that wave components were obtained at intensity levels "approaching voluntary adult behavioral thresholds" (Wolf & Goldstein, 1978, p. 513). Subsequent studies of AMLR in children were also conducted mostly to validate the response as a tool for threshold estimation. Although initial work on optimization of AMLR recording procedures and parameters was completed with healthy adults, the same parameters were then applied to pediatric auditory assessment. It is now known, however, that AMLR measurement in infants and children requires modification of stimulus and recording parameters from those used in adults (Hall, 1992, 2007). In order to optimize the test parameters for pediatric application of AMLR, one must understand the developmental changes in the response from infancy through adulthood. This, in turn, mandates knowledge of the anatomic generators of the AMLR because neurophysiologic development and neuromaturational status directly affect the morphology and characteristics of the response.

Developmental Changes in the AMLR and Anatomic Correlates

The AMLR in adult humans consists of scalp or vertex negative and positive peaks, including the Na, Pa, and Pb. The Pb wave is also sometimes referred to as the P50 because it occurs at approximately 50 ms. The Pb component of the AMLR is probably the same as the P1 of the ALR, but this point is debated in the literature. The AMLR components are widely distributed over the frontocentral scalp region and can be recorded using the same electrode array used for ABR (Kraus et al., 1994). The anatomic generators of the AMLR have been debated over the years, but it is now generally accepted that the Pa component is a reflection of activity in the central nervous system within pathways leading from, and including, the thalamus and the primary auditory cortex, specifically Heschl's gyrus. According to McGee and Kraus (1996), the AMLR seems to have a relatively long developmental time course and continues to develop through the first decade of life. AMLR components show developmental changes not only with respect to waveform morphology, but also with respect to response reliability. The likelihood of recording an AMLR consistently increases with age up to the age of 10 years (Hall, 2007).

In a review of literature on the development of the auditory system from the gestational period to adulthood, Moore and Linthicum (2007) report original findings and correlate various research findings on histologic examination with information on the development of AMLR components. These authors describe changes that take place during the prenatal, perinatal, and postnatal periods. During the perinatal period, myelination is observed in the axons that project through the brachium of the inferior colliculus to the medial geniculate body. These axons probably contribute to the AMLR component most easily detectible in infants, the Po-Na complex. This complex is barely detectible between the 25th and 27th fetal weeks but generally is present by the 33rd week and is even more pronounced in full-term neonates. The rate of detection of the Pa and Na components reaches 80% to 90% at about 30 weeks conceptional age (Rotteveel, Stegeman, de Graaf, Colon, & Visco, 1987). The latency of Na decreases from approximately 28 ms at the 30th fetal week to approximately 20 ms at term (Pasman, Rotteveel, de Graaf, Maassen, & Notermans, 1991; Rotteveel et al., 1987). Po and Na are the most consistent components in the AMLR wave sequence in 3-month-old babies (Rotteveel et al., 1986). The latency of Na decreases to 18 months by the age of 3 months and remains unchanged into adulthood (Kraus, Smith, Reed, Stein, & Cartee, 1985). According to Moore and Linthicum (2007), this early maturation follows that of the ABR closely; hence, it seems likely that the Po-Na components reflect transmission in the brachial pathway from the inferior colliculus to the thalamus.

There is an increasing prominence of the Na component of the AMLR across early childhood. This can be reflective of the newly maturing system of thalamocortical connections (Moore & Linthicum, 2007). The Pa component increases in detectability in early childhood with a latency of approximately 25 to 30 ms (Kraus et al., 1985). This increased likelihood of detecting Pa with age occurs regardless of whether the subject is a normally developing child or a child with any of a wide range of neurologic, cognitive, or speech and language disorders (Kraus et al., 1985).

According to McGee and Kraus (1996), the Pa component has a major dipole source in the temporal region. Moore and Linthicum (2007) speculate that as the Pa wave probably reflects activity in the pathway running from the medial geniculate body to the cortex because it matures in early childhood, and it closely follows the Na wave. The Pb component of the AMLR has a much longer course of development and reaches its adult value later than the Na component. The results of studies of AMLR maturation vary depending on whether the Pb component is considered part of the AMLR or it is the P1 wave in the ALR. Other major factors that seem to determine the age of maturation are the stimulus rate and state of consciousness. Detectability of wave Pa increases monotonically from 20% at birth to 90% at 12 years of age (Kraus et al., 1985), assuming the effect of sleep is ruled out. Other researchers also have reported that the variables of age, signal level, and site of recording significantly affect the peak amplitude and absolute latency of the Pa component (e.g., Tucker & Ruth, 1996).

Little information exists relating AMLR findings to those for behavioral measures of central auditory function. In a study conducted on 150 participants with normal hearing ranging from 7 to 16 years of age, Schochat and Musiek (2006) described relations between AMLR and data for the two behavioral tests of auditory processing—the duration pattern test and the pitch pattern test. There was improved performance with age on both the behavioral tests up to age 12 years. However, these authors did not find significant changes across this age range for either latency or amplitude measures on the AMLR. This finding seems to agree with the observation of Moore and Linthicum (2007) that the Pa component of the AMLR reflects activity in the pathways from the medial geniculate body to the cortex rather than solely in the cortical areas and, therefore, develops relatively early.

Frizzo, Funayama, Isaac, and Colafêmina (2007) studied AMLR components using tone-burst stimuli at 50, 60, and 70 dB HL in healthy children aged 10 to 13 years. These investigators found that the mean latencies of the Na, Pa, Nb, and Pb components at 70 dB HL were 20.8 ms, 35.3 ms, 43.3 ms, and 53.4 ms, respectively. The Na-Pa amplitude in their subjects ranged from 0.2 to 1.9 µV with a mean of 1.0 µV. Predictably, as the stimulus intensity increased, amplitude of the wave components increased and latency decreased. These findings indicate that within the age range of 10 to 13 years, AMLR patterns resemble those of adults.

Developmental Changes and Recording Parameters

Age and the Effect of Filter Settings. Although some early researchers did not observe the Pa component consistently in neonates and young children with normal hearing (Davis, 1976), other studies showed that the Pa could be recorded reliably in newborns and young children (e.g., McRandle, Smith, & Goldstein, 1974; Mendel, Adkinson, & Harker, 1977; Mendelson & Salamy, 1981; Wolf & Goldstein, 1980). Surprisingly, as noted by Hall (2007), the latency of Pa reported in the studies did not change as a function of age and, in some cases, was even shorter in infants than in adults. It is probable that the Pa reported by some of the studies was in fact an artifact caused by excessive bandpass filtering during the recording process. Removing the low frequencies with excessive high-pass filtering at 30 Hz versus a more appropriate setting of 10 or 15 Hz usually results in a loss of the actual Pa component and creates a positivity that mimics the Pa. Hence, an artifactual Pa can be recorded when there is no true response. Artifacts of this nature would obviously not show any change in latency across age groups.

Age and Stimulus Rate. Stimulus rate is another factor that probably contributed to differences in findings across developmental AMLR studies. Early studies on infants and children used stimulus rates of 10 per second or slightly faster rates in the interest of saving test time. This rate of stimulation is much too fast to elicit an AMLR from children (Fifer, 1985; Hall, 1992, 2007; Kraus, Reed, Smith, Stein, & Cartee, 1987). One principle of auditory-evoked response measurement bears repeating at this juncture. Slower stimulus rates are required for longer latency responses and for younger children. A stimulus rate as slow as one per second might be required to elicit the AMLR in infants and young children. When stimulus rates approach 11 stimuli per second, the proportion of children yielding a detectable AMLR reduces indirectly as age decreases (Hall, 2007).

Developmental Changes and State of Arousal

The AMLR can be recorded from adult subjects in sleep and even during sedation, but for infants and children, sleep, sedation, and attention are important variables that must be considered when interpreting the response (Hall, 2007). In general, there is an interaction between the AMLR response and all stages of sleep, but the response is more likely to be detected as stimulus rate is decreased (Hall, 2007). Kraus, McGee, and Comperatore (1989) recorded the AMLR in six normal-hearing children between the ages of 4 and 9 years in waking state and natural sleep. Sleep state was monitored during AMLR recordings that lasted for an average of about 2.1 hours per subject. The Pa component was consistently detected during wakefulness, alpha, Stage 1, and REM sleep. AMLR was inconsistently detected in sleep Stages 2 and 3, and rarely detected during Stage 4 sleep especially in younger children (within the tested age range). The probability of obtaining the Pa component during Stage 4 sleep increases steadily with age. The authors suggested that the differences in the effect of sleep on the adult versus child AMLR response could be arising from the difference in the neural generators at different developmental stages. The AMLR in children seems to be dominated by activity from the reticular formation and, thus, is more susceptible to sleep, whereas in adults, thalamocortical activity dominates the response, minimizing sleep effects.

Other studies reported similar findings. Collet, Duclaux, Challamel, and Revol (1988) recorded the AMLR, with two click-rates (1.3 stimuli/s and 8.9 stimuli/s) in 6- or 7-week-old infants in an attempt to define the effect of sleep on the amplitude of AMLR. The Na-Pa complex was always greater during waking states than sleep states regardless of stimulus rate. Okitsu (1984) reported the Na component was only 10% lower in sleep in young children, but the presence of Pa decreased considerably during sleep. Later waves such as Nb and Pb were rarely observed in both waking and sleep conditions. Contrary to these findings, Rogers, Edwards, Henderson-Smart, and Pettigrew (1989) found no change in wave latency or reproducibility of AMLRs recorded during different sleep states in infants between the ages of 3 to 5 days and 1 year. In summary, the majority of studies confirm an effect of the state of consciousness on the pediatric AMLR. There is a recent literature devoted to the application of the AMLR in documenting depth of anesthesia.

Clinical Applications of AMLR in Pediatric Populations

Threshold Estimation

The AMLR can be used to estimate hearing threshold objectively. AMLR offers several advantages for this clinical application. The amplitude of the major Pa component is about twice the size of the ABR Wave V. In theory then, the AMLR can be identified at lower signal levels and with less averaging. Another advantage is that the AMLR can easily be elicited using highly frequency-specific longer-duration tone bursts. In contrast, the ABR waves are not as robust when elicited with tone bursts, and stimulus duration must be shorter with a corresponding increase in spectral splatter. A third advantage is that AMLR measurement does not require specialized instrumentation and typically can be recorded with ABR instrumentation using a simple one-channel electrode montage for threshold estimation.

Despite these apparent advantages, there are compelling reasons why the AMLR is not as popular as the ABR for estimation of hearing threshold. AMLR is markedly affected by muscle and movement artifact, a major problem in pediatric populations. Sedation and anesthesia is the solution to the problem of movement interference for ABR measurement, but it greatly affects the AMLR. For this reason, AMLR has given way to ABR for electrophysiological auditory threshold estimation in children. ABR measurement with tone-burst stimulation and more recently the auditory steady-state response are the techniques of choice for frequency-specific estimation of auditory thresholds in infants and young children and are recommended for this purpose (Joint Committee on Infant Hearing [JCIH], 2007). For this reason, we do not review here the literature on this application of the AMLR.

AMLR as an Index of Depth of Anesthesia

The sensitivity of the AMLR to changes in sleep state has been exploited clinically to document and quantify level of consciousness (see Hall, 2007, for a detailed review). In an early study, Prosser and Arslan (1985) evaluated the AMLR and ABR in persons under general anesthesia. The authors found that ABR components remained normal under the effects of anesthesia, but AMLR was grossly abnormal as reflected by poor stability of the components and prolonged latencies of waves that were detectable. The study confirmed the role of the auditory cortex and perhaps the reticular formation in the generation of the AMLR response and the effect of drugs on these structures. Lamas et al. (2006) evaluated the utility of the AMLR in monitoring the level of sedation in six critically ill children. The level of sedation was measured using the COMFORT scale and the Bispectral Index (BIS). AMLR showed a correlation with the COMFORT scale and BIS in light and deep sedation and, in one patient, was effective in the early detection of brain death. In another patient who was chemically paralyzed, AMLR detected inadequate undersedation.

Documentation of Cochlear Implant and Hearing Aid Performance

The AMLR offers two distinct advantages for objective assessment of cochlear implant and hearing aid performance. AMLR provides information on higher regions of the auditory system, more closely related to "hearing," than the ABR because it is generated by suprabrainstem thalamocortical pathways. In addition, the AMLR with latency values far beyond the ABR is easy to record electrically without the problem of electrical or measurement artifacts. For these reasons, the AMLR has been applied clinically in the evaluation of cochlear implant users beginning with the investigation by Kileny, Kemink, and Miller (1989). Gordon, Papsin, and Harrison (2004, 2005) recorded electrically evoked AMLRs (EMLRs) in a series of 81 children with prelingual or perilingual deafness. Fifty of these children were studied longitudinally with repeated measures obtained first at the time of implantation, then at the initial device stimulation, and then again after 2, 6, and 12 months of implant use. EMLRs were measured only once in the remaining 31 children who had an average of 5.3 years (≥2.9 years) of experience with their implant. These investigators found that EMLRs were rarely detected at the time of implantation under anesthesia or sedation and were detected only in 35% of awake children on the day of device activation. The percentage of detection improved significantly with consistent implant use, reaching a detectability of 100% after at least 1 year after implantation. Older children had a greater likelihood of showing detectable EMLRs in the initial period of device use compared to younger children. However, with consistent use of the device, the younger children showed more rapid rates of increase in detectability of the evoked response compared to the older children. This observation might reflect the developmental plasticity of the thalamocortical pathways. Developmental plasticity and the deprivation effects of hearing loss on the central auditory system are discussed in detail in the following section on ALRs.

In a sample of 12 postlingually deaf and four prelingually deaf subjects, Groenen, Snik, and van den Broek (1997) found that the EAMLRs of both groups were remarkably similar though their speech perception skills were different. The researchers pointed out that the difference in speech perception ability between congenitally deaf and postlingually deaf cochlear implant users did not seem to be reflected in the EAMLR. Within the postlingually deaf subjects, there was more diversity in the amplitude of the EAMLR component peaks and a more diffuse EAMLR peak latency organization across the electrodes in individuals with poorer speech perception performance than those with better performance. Firszt, Chambers, and Kraus (2002) reported a link between EAMLR and speech perception in adults. Larger EAMLR amplitudes and lower thresholds for the Na-Pa complex were associated with higher speech perception scores. The authors proposed that this was as expected considering the role of the concerned neural generators (thalamus and primary auditory cortex) in speech perception.

Central Auditory Processing Disorder (CAPD) and Language/Learning Disabilities

In a review of AMLR research in children with CAPD, Hall (2007) noted that many of the early studies used recording parameters that have more recently proved to be inappropriate for children. A general finding across studies was latency prolongation and amplitude reduction for the Na and Pa components in children with CAPD. Purdy, Kelly, and Davies (2002) studied ABR, AMLR, and ALR in a small sample of 10 children in the age range of 7 to 11 years with "learning disability (LD)" and a control group of 10 age-matched children. They reported delayed Na latency and smaller amplitude of the Nb component in the LD group.

Based on close review of the behavioral findings for the LD group, it is difficult to verify whether the children would meet current diagnostic criteria for CAPD (American Academy of Audiology [AAA], 2010). Arehole, Augustine, and Simhadri (1995) reported that for certain recording conditions, latencies of AMLR for pediatric subjects with LD were significantly different from a group of normal hearing children. Again, criteria for definition of LD were neither well defined nor consistent with current criteria for CAPD.

AMLR was used by Cone-Wesson, Kurtzberg, and Vaughan (1987) as one of the tests to study auditory system integrity in a group of 59 infants at risk for subsequent hearing and language disorders due to low birth weight or perinatal asphyxia. In addition to the AMLR, these researchers recorded the ABR. They reported that 63% of their subjects had findings consistent with either normal peripheral hearing or slight unilateral impairment; 84% showed test findings reflecting normal auditory system functioning up to the level of the brainstem; 82% had normal AMLRs; and 81% showed normal ALRs. Some infants showed diverse patterns of peripheral, brainstem, and cortical abnormalities.

Topography of the ABR, AMLR, and "cortical-evoked responses (ACR)" was investigated by Mason and Mellor (1984) in children with normal speech and language development and those with either a language or motor speech disorder. They reported that AMLR amplitude in the group with motor speech disorders was significantly larger at the mastoid and temporal electrode sites than in either the control group or the group with language disorders. The authors interpreted that this pattern could be indicative of a larger myogenic response similar to brainstem reflexes that are known to be often more intense in individuals with congenital suprabulbar paresis. The cortical auditory-evoked responses showed significantly larger amplitudes in the motor speech group at the Cz site. This phenomenon was attributed to a possibility of less than normal levels of activity in the cortical inhibitory system. In the language-disordered children, cortical responses showed an abnormal hemispheric dominance in the left temporal region and a more inverted or "dissimilar" waveform at the site of the T3 electrode. The authors concluded that the AMLR findings suggested impaired functioning of the left temporal cortex in children who failed to develop language normally. Formal investigation of the AMLR in a series of children with CAPD as diagnosed with current criteria is certainly warranted. The findings would probably contribute to the inclusion of AMLR into the clinical CAPD test battery.

Recently, Schochat, Musiek, Alonso, and Ogata (2010) conducted a study in which pediatric subjects were tested using an accepted CAPD test battery in an investigation to explore pre- versus postauditory training effects on behavioral tests as well as on AMLR. The subjects were 30 children with CAPD and a control group of 22 children without CAPD ranging in age from 8 to 14 years. Each child underwent two dichotic and two monaural tests of CAPD before and after training to document auditory processing performance. The children with CAPD underwent an auditory training program that included frequency, intensity, and temporal training tasks and also dichotic interaural intensity difference training (Musiek, 2004). Post-training scores on the tests were improved, a finding supported with larger amplitude of AMLR components. The Na-Pa amplitude was significantly lower in the CAPD group and especially so over the left hemisphere (C3 electrode). The Na-Pa amplitude increased to the extent that there was no significant difference between the CAPD and control group after training. AMLR latency was not sensitive to CAPD as evidenced by no difference between the groups on this measure, even before training. The authors noted that the lack of significant test-retest difference in either latency or amplitude values for the control group confirm the stability of AMLR as a measure for evaluating change in auditory functioning. In a sample of 19 children aged 4 to 11 years with specific language impairment, Al-Saif, Abdeltawwab, and Khamis (2012) observed no difference in AMLR in comparison with a control group of 15 children with normal language development. The authors speculated that primary auditory cortex might not be the site of dysfunction in children with SLI.

Brain Injury

In contrast to the plentiful studies of AMLR in adults with brain injuries (e.g., Drake, Weate, & Newell, 1996; Gaetz & Weinberg, 2000; Hall, 1992), there are few studies in pediatric populations. A possible explanation for the limited neurodiagnostic application of AMLR in children is the concern that absence of an AMLR might not always be a manifestation of an auditory pathway dysfunction (Kraus et al., 1985).

Other Pediatric Populations

Kraus et al. (1985) investigated AMLRs as a function of age in 217 subjects aged 6 days to 20 years. All the subjects had normal auditory brainstem responses (ABRs). The researchers grouped the subjects into the following diagnostic categories: normal, communicative disorders (language delay, learning disability), mentally retarded, multiply handicapped, and postmeningitis. The authors examined age effects and effects of diagnostic category. They also compared AMLRs of males versus females and right versus left ears. Consistent with other studies, detectability of both Na and Pa components increased significantly as a function of age. There were no significant differences among diagnostic categories, and there were no gender and ear differences. Kraus et al. (1985) made an important point based on their findings—every clinician using the AMLR must keep in mind that "when responses are present, they might be useful indicators of hearing sensitivity, but the absence of [A] MLRs in children cannot be taken as an indication of hearing loss" (p. 343). Kraus and colleagues also concluded that if AMLRs are absent or abnormal, dysfunction of the auditory pathway cannot be conclusively inferred, as there was little difference between the AMLRs of normal subjects and those of patients with a "wide range of neurologic, cognitive, and speech and language disorders" (p. 343).

Children with autism spectrum disorders are selective to certain auditory stimuli while ignoring others who are not of interest. Kemner, Oranje, Verbaten, and van Engeland (2002) assessed sensory filtering in children with autism using the P50 (Pb) gating paradigm in 12 children with autism and 11 healthy controls. The authors found no differences in absolute P50 amplitude and P50 (Pb) suppression between the children with autism and the control children. Psillas and Daniilidis (2003) applied AMLR as an objective test to identify the presence of low-frequency hearing loss in 35 children with pervasive developmental disorder. Based on the observation that nine of the children had low-frequency hearing loss ranging from mild to severe, the authors strongly recommended the need for thorough audiological assessment in children with pervasive developmental disorder even in cases where caregivers did not suspect hearing loss.

A more recent study of children with autism spectrum disorder (Roberts et al., 2013) found delayed AMLR maturation in the clinical group compared with normal controls. Roberts and colleagues obtained AMLR data from 53 children with autism spectrum disorder and 39 typically developing children. In addition, they used diffusion tensor imaging to estimate white matter maturation through a method known as *fractional anisotropy*. The authors observed delayed M50 latency in the former group. In their control group, maturation of M50 latency was associated with age and maturation of white matter as estimated on fractional anisotropy. However, the same type of relation was not observed in children with autism. According to the authors, this was suggestive of uncoupling between the structure-function relationship of auditory cortex electrophysiology and thalamocortical white matter in autism spectrum disorder. Furthermore, they hypothesized that factors other than white matter conduction velocity might have a role in determining the time course of maturation of an auditory response.

Miliciç et al. (1998) recorded ABR and AMLR elicited with monoaural and binaural click stimulation in a group of 17 children with normal speech and 16 children with dyslalia. Eight of these children had systematic errors of speech, and eight had nonsystematic errors of speech. The authors hypothesized that auditory afferent control is an important feedback mechanism in speech generation and that a different organization of auditory afferent pathways in children with speech alterations exists. All subjects were approximately 7 years old. A latency prolongation of AMLR wave Na was recorded between the two groups. A difference between groups in the binaural interaction of the AMLR Na component was also reported, suggesting that children with dyslalia might have atypical organization in their auditory afferent pathway.

Auditory Late Responses (ALRs)

Introduction to the Family of Auditory Late Responses

More than a dozen specific components or responses can be recorded within the general latency region included within the rather vague term *auditory late responses*. Over the years, a variety of terms have been coined to refer to the responses in the ALR time frame. The general "late response" time frame extends approximately from 50 ms until 1000 ms after the presentation of the stimuli. Not surprisingly, a rather vast literature consisting of thousands of papers has accumulated since the discovery of the auditory late response in 1939. The focus of the following review is the ALR waveform consisting of an N1 and P2 component elicited with simple tonal or speech stimuli. The majority of the many publications on responses within the late latency region pertain to other components or responses, ranging from variations of the N1 component (e.g., N1a, N1b, N1c), the N150, N250, Nc, Nd,

N400, or positive peaks later than 200 ms and beyond the P2 component. Among the later components are the P3 and P3a waves as well as the mismatch negativity (MMN) response. For more detailed information on these many and varied responses, the reader is referred to textbooks (Hall, 2007, 2015; Picton, 2011) and also published review articles (search http://www.nlm.nih.gov).

Measurement and Analysis

A clinical protocol for recording N1 and P2 components of the ALR is summarized in Table 22–4. The literature contains many variations in the protocols for ALR measurement, in part due to development of more sophisticated instrumentation and evolution of measurement strategies over the past 70 years. Although as many as 20 or even 30 electrodes are often utilized in recordings conducted in laboratory experiments, ALR measurement is feasible with as few as two or three electrodes. A handful of clear differences between the protocols for measurement of AMLR versus ALR are readily apparent. Recorded with the protocols summarized here, both the AMLR and the ALR are generated by the onset of tonal or speech stimuli. Of course, analysis time is about five times longer for the ALR than the AMLR because latencies of the major ALR peaks are four or five times later than the Pb component of the AMLR. Stimulation differs considerably and in several ways for the ALR versus AMLR. Speech stimuli are now rather popular for elicitation of the ALR, whereas click or tone-burst stimuli are commonly used to elicit the AMLR. The rate of stimuli for the ALR is relatively slow at ≤1 stimulus per second, even when recording the response from older children and adults. The drastically different characteristics of subcortical responses such as the ABR versus cortical responses have traditionally meant the use of different recording parameters. Subcortical and cortical responses cannot be recorded with the same test protocol.

The frequency following response (FFR) component of the speech-evoked ABR has generated significant interest recently as a tool for evaluating speech processing in the brainstem (e.g., Banai & Kraus, 2008; Billiet & Bellis, 2011; Sinha & Basavaraj, 2010). A recent small sample study by Bidelman (2015) demonstrated a method to enable simultaneous measurement of the FFR as well as ALR using a single optimal recording paradigm. The stimulus was a synthetic /a/ presented in a "clustered stimulus presentation paradigm" in which 14 stimuli were presented at a rapid rate and then two stimuli at a slow rate to enable recording of the FFR and ALR, respectively. The responses were separately averaged for 3,500 sweeps to obtain the FFR and 500 sweeps to obtain the ALR. The possibility of collecting information about different portions of the central auditory nervous system within a single test is exciting from a perspective of clinical viability, especially in pediatric populations.

Table 22–4. Guidelines for an Auditory Late Response (ALR) Test Protocol

Parameter	*Suggestion*	*Rationale/Comment*
Stimulus Parameters		
Transducer	ER-3A	• Supra-aural earphones can be used for ALR measurement. Insert earphones are more comfortable for longer AER recording sessions, and they attenuate background sound.
Type	Tone-burst	• Longer-duration tonal signals are preferred for ALR elicitation.
	Speech	• The ALR can be effectively elicited with speech signals. Various features of speech signals (e.g., voice onset time) can be used in ALR stimulation.
Duration		
Rise/fall	~10 ms	• Longer-signal onset times are feasible and desirable to elicit the ALR.
Plateau	~50 ms	• Extended plateau durations are effective in eliciting the ALR.
Rate	≤1.1/s	• A slow rate of signal presentation is essential for the ALR, due to the long refractory time of cortical neurons.

continues

Table 22–4. *continued*

Parameter	*Suggestion*	*Rationale/Comment*
Polarity	Variable	• Signal polarity is not an important parameter for ALR measurement.
Intensity	≤70 dB HL	• Modest signal intensity levels are typical for ALR measurement.
Number	≤200	• Signal repetitions vary depending on size of response and background noise. Averaging may require as few as 20 to 50 signals at high-intensity levels for a very quiet and normal hearing patient.
Presentation ear	Variable	• Monaural or binaural signals are often used to elicit the ALR.
Masking	Variable	• Masking is rarely required with insert earphones, and not needed for stimulus intensity levels of ≤70 dB HL.
Acquisition Parameters		
Amplification	×50,000	• Less amplification is required for larger responses such as the ALR.
Sensitivity	25 or 50 μvolts	• Smaller sensitivity values are equivalent to higher amplification
Analysis time	500 to 600 ms	• An analysis epoch long enough to encompass the entire N1, P2, N2 sequence is required.
Prestimulus time	100 ms	• A prestimulus time provides a stable estimate of background noise and a baseline for calculation of the amplitudes for negative and positive waveform components (N1, P2, P3).
Data points	≤512	
Sweeps	1,000	• See comments above for signal number.
Filters		
Bandpass	0.1 to 100 Hz	• The ALR consists of low-frequency energy within the spectrum of the EEG.
Notch	None	• Notch filtering in the region of 60 Hz should be avoided with ALR measurement, because important frequencies in the response will be removed.
Electrodes		
Type	Disc or disposable	• Disc electrodes applied with paste (versus gel) are useful to secure the noninverting electrodes on the scalp. Red- and blue-colored electrode leads for the right and left hemisphere locations, respectively, are suggested. Disposable electrodes or a multiple-electrode cap are also appropriate with ALR measurement.
Electrode Sites		
	Noninverting	The Fz or Cz sites are appropriate for recording the ALR clinically. Many published studies include 20 or more electrode sites.
	Inverting	Linked earlobes are commonly used for inverting electrodes. A noncephalic electrode site (e.g., nape of the neck) is also appropriate.
	Other	Ocular electrodes (located above and below or to the side of an eye) are required for the detection of eye blinks, and rejection of averages contaminated by eye blinks.
	Ground (Fpz)	The common (ground) electrode can be located anywhere on the body. A low forehead (Fpz) or nasion (i.e., Nz—between the eyes) location is convenient and effective.

Note. Adapted from Hall (2007).

Nonpathologic Factors

Major nonpathologic or subject factors influencing the ALR that must be taken into account in the analysis, and interpretation of findings includes

- age and neurologic maturation,
- attention,
- sleep, and
- effects of intervention.

Given their importance in analysis of the ALR, these factors are reviewed in some detail in the following sections of this chapter. As with AMLR measurement, subject state of arousal is an important factor in ALR measurement. The strategy of encouraging the patient to view a video or DVD during recording noted in the AMLR section applies also when recording the ALR from young children. A typical ALR waveform with the P1, N1, and P2 components evoked with a tone-burst or speech signal and recorded with a single-channel electrode array is depicted in Figure 22–2.

ALR in Pediatric Populations

Morphology of the ALRs differs significantly for children versus adults. In addition, throughout childhood there are substantial maturational changes in ALR latency, amplitude, and morphology. The obligatory components within the ALRs, such as the P1, N1, and P2, are generated by portions of the auditory pathway beyond the medial geniculate body, more specifically, the thalamocortical and corticocortical pathways, primary auditory cortex, and different association cortices (e.g., Ceponienè, Cheour, & Näätänen, 1998; Eggermont & Ponton, 2003; Näätänen & Picton, 1987; Ponton, Eggermont, Khosla, Kwong, & Don, 2002; Ponton, Eggermont, Kwong, & Don, 2000; Sharma, Dorman, & Spahr, 2002a, 2002b). Axons of the geniculocortical system, an obligatory link in the ascending auditory pathway, mature between the ages of 6 months and 5 years. These centers are important for basic central auditory processing in childhood (Illing, 2004). The fibers of the corticocortical systems, which link the auditory cortex to other areas within the temporal, parietal, and prefrontal lobes, might not reach maturity until the age of 12 years or more (Illing, 2004). Besides the process of maturation of the axons themselves, synaptic maturation also plays a part in the scalp-recorded auditory responses from these generator sites. Hence, it is not surprising that the ALRs show significant changes with age and mature well into the teenage years. The differences between ALRs recorded at different stages of childhood and in adults are seen not simply in terms of the latency, amplitude, and relative amplitude of different components, but also in terms of refractoriness and the emergence of certain components only after a certain age (e.g., Gilley, Sharma, Dorman, & Martin, 2005; Moore, 2002) and complex changes in morphology and scalp distribution (e.g., Stapells, 2002). These morphologic differences are important to know as they guide the selection of test protocols, stimuli, acquisition parameters, and collection of normative data.

ALR in Children With Normal Hearing

The development of the obligatory subcomponents of the ALR has been the focus of a number of investigations. Results vary across studies due to methodological variables known to affect the waveform, such as the type of stimuli used, number of repetitions, rate and interstimulus interval, and acquisition parameters (Hall, 2007). The developmental course of the P1, N1, and P2 components of the ALR can be studied with respect to their latencies, absolute and relative amplitudes, and morphology. ALR components are easy to record even in young children who are not voluntarily responding to the stimulus. Because the P1, N1, and P2 components are objective measures of cortical auditory functioning, they are valuable in the audiologic test battery. ALR components have in recent years gained importance as markers of neuromaturation (e.g., Ceponienè et al., 1998; Sharma, Kraus, McGee, & Nicol, 1997; Sharma, Martin, et al., 2005) as well as their historical application as objective measures of hearing threshold (e.g., Barnet & Lodge, 1967; Rapin, Ruben, & Lyttle, 1970; Taguchi, Picton, Orpin, & Goodman, 1969).

General Developmental Changes in the ALR

In general, the P1 component of the ALR decreases in latency with increasing age. The latencies appear to decrease rapidly in the first decade of life, and then more gradually in the second decade of life (Cunningham, Nicol, Zecker, & Kraus, 2000; Ponton et al., 2000; Sharma et al., 2002b; Sharma et al., 1997). The ALR in children is characterized by prominent P1 and N2 waves. In adults, however, the N1-P2 complex is prominent (Gilley et al., 2005; Hall, 2007). The P1 component first appears developmentally, followed by an almost adultlike P2 and a clear and often robust N2 by the age of 3 to 6 years (Hall, 2007). In contrast, Ponton et al. (2000) suggests that the P2 does not emerge before

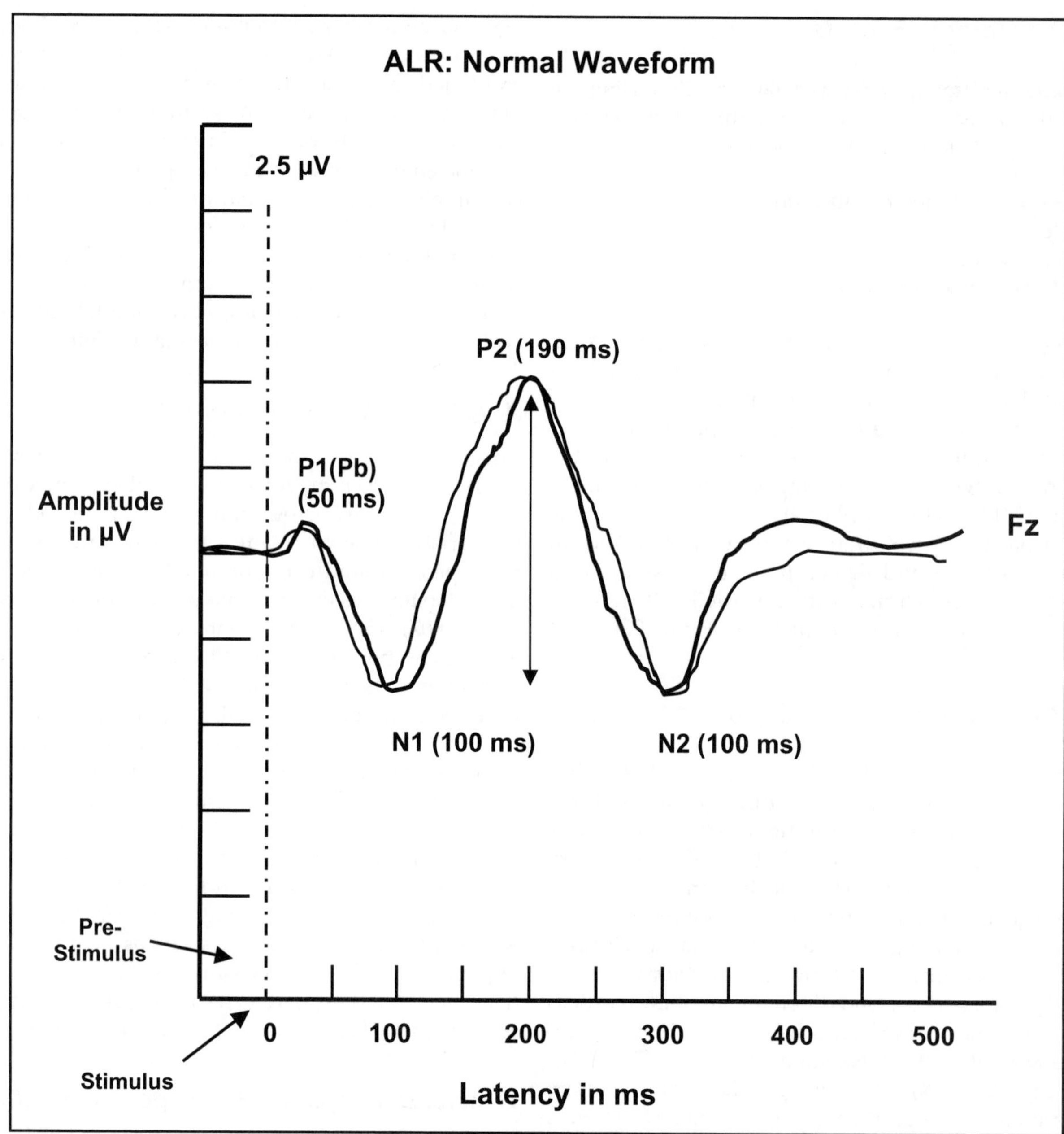

FIGURE 22–2. A typical auditory late response (ALR) waveform with the P1, N1, and P2 components evoked with a tone burst or speech signal and recorded with a single-channel electrode array with the noninverting electrode located at the Fz or Cz midline location, and the inverting electrode on the nape of the neck.

the age of 10 years. The N2 is often robustly present in the ALR of young normal hearing children even in the absence of a clear N1-P2 component (Almeqbel, 2013; Almeqbel & McMahon, 2015). The P1-N2 response appears to be responsive to changes in stimulus characteristics such as spectral content and voice onset time. Almeqbel (2013) observed latency and amplitude characteristics of P1 and N2 in normal children were different across three natural speech tokens (/g/, /m/, and /t/) indicating that the ALR could be an objective index of spectral processing at a cortical level.

Although the latency of all ALR components decreases and amplitude increases with age, age-related differences are not uniform across all the waves.

The P2 wave matures at a faster rate than the N1 wave. The latency of the P1 wave decreases from 96 ms at the age of 3 to 4 years to 76 ms at the age of 11 to 12 years for an interstimulus interval of 2000 ms (Gilley et al., 2005). Barnet, Ohlrich, Weiss, and Shanks (1975) and Ohlrich, Barnet, Weiss, and Shanks (1978) reported latency changes during the age range of 15 days to 3 years. Specifically, the latency of P2 shortens from 230 to 150 ms, N2 latency decreases from 535 to 320 ms, and P3 decreases from 785 to 635 ms. These latencies are highly prolonged compared to adult values for N1 (just under 100 ms), P2 (about 200 ms), and P3 (300 ms). Ponton et al. (2000) reported an increase in the latency of N2 with increasing age at some cephalic electrode locations. The N1/N2 amplitude ratio increases significantly with age (Ceponienѐ, Rinne, & Näätänen, 2002). The ALR N1 (N100) wave is actually a wave complex (Hall, 2007). Parameters of the N1 component, including its presence, latency, and amplitude, and the presence of subcomponents or other negative waves within the same time frame are determined by the physical properties of the stimulus and other factors such as alertness of the subject, attention, and memory (Alain, Woods, & Covarrubias, 1997; Picton, Woods, Baribeau-Braun, & Healy, 1977). Negativity of the N1 wave is enhanced when a subject attends to it or listens for a specific stimulus (Hall, 2007). Most studies report that the N1 is not apparent in very young children and in older children it is only observed at very slow stimulus rates (e.g., Ceponienѐ et al., 2002; Gilley et al., 2005; Ponton et al., 2000; Sussman, Steinschneider, Gumenyuk, Grushko, & Lawson, 2008). Eggermont and Ponton (2003) suggest that the emergence of the N1 component is reflective of the "maturation of the axons in layer II and upper layer III of the auditory cortex" (p. 249).

Cunningham et al. (2000) found that the N1 latency appeared adultlike by the age of 13 to 15 years with little additional age-related change. ALR N1 amplitude increased from age 5 years to well into the teenage years, and then was stable by adulthood. These researchers also found that N2 was measureable in 95% of children, 80% of young adults, and 20% of senior adults. Its latency decreased significantly between the ages of 5 and 10 years, was stable from 10 to 15 years, and decreased again in young adulthood. Data across studies can vary depending on the measurement conditions prevalent in a particular study as amplitude and latencies of the ALR components are additionally affected by state of arousal and sleep, stimuli used, and stimulus and recording parameters.

Purdy, Sharma, Munro, and Morgan (2013) recorded ALRs from normal-hearing infants aged 3 to 8 months using natural speech stimuli /m/ and /t/ at different stimulus intensity levels ranging from 30 to 80 dB SPL. The two speech sounds were chosen so as to represent low- and high-frequency acoustic information. Overall latencies of P1 were longer and amplitudes were smaller for /m/ compared to /t/. Amplitude growth functions were different for both stimuli. The latency of ALR components changed very little over the intensity range for /t/, but for /m/ the improvement in latency for low versus high stimulus levels was 50 to 60 ms. The authors noted that increasing stimulus levels above hearing threshold does result in shorter latency and higher amplitude of P1, but these improvements occur only over a small range of levels and appear to also be affected by the acoustic content of the stimulus. Comparing the findings of their study with other studies conducted on children after hearing aid fitting or cochlear implantation, Purdy et al. commented that the immediate improvement seen in P1 latency after device fitting appears to be reflective of "more than just improved audibility" (p. 479). Their reasoning was that latency changes in their study were small compared to large changes reported before versus after fitting of a device. Purdy and colleagues further suggested that the presence of ALR indicates stimulus audibility and adequate amplification. However, ALR is probably not useful in predicting where exactly the stimulus falls within the listener's dynamic range.

Developmental Changes in Scalp Distribution

Ponton et al. (2000) recorded ALR from 30 different scalp-electrode locations in 118 subjects between the ages of 5 and 20 years of age. For analysis, subjects were divided into groups so cross-sectional data for each year in between could be analyzed. Around the age of 10 years, the authors found sudden changes in P1, P1-N1b, and N2 peak amplitudes at the electrodes C3 and C4. No such changes were reported at the midline electrodes Cz and Fz. There were interhemispheric amplitude differences for the N1b peak. In all the age groups, except the 9- and 15-year-olds, the contralateral N1b measured at C4 was on average negative compared to the prestimulus baseline. The ipsilateral N1b amplitude did not become negative until the age of 16 years. The P2 also showed age-related difference in amplitude as a function of electrode location. Up to the age of 10 years, the P2 component was more clearly visible at electrode location Pz compared to more anterior locations such as Cz and Fz. For older children, the P2 became more prominent at anterior locations and less prominent at posterior locations. The N2 latency increased significantly as a function of age at electrodes

Cz, C3, and C4, but showed no changes with age at the frontal electrode Fz. Ponton et al. (2000) speculated that N2 might have several source components and "if the neural generators underlying N2 have different orientations toward the scalp, the distinct patterns of N2 maturation observed at central and frontal electrode locations might reflect the differential maturation of the generators contributing to this peak" (p. 232). These investigators also pointed out that differences in maturation observed for the components of ALR depended on recording electrode placement or the locations on the scalp. This is an important point to consider for the application of ALR in clinical populations such as children with hearing impairment, learning problems, or CAPD.

Gomes et al. (2001) investigated spatiotemporal maturation of N1 components recorded in central and lateral sites to tones in children ranging from 6 to 12 years of age and in adults. They found a developmental decrease in latency for the central N1 in children but no change in amplitude. The lateral N1 showed developmental changes in terms of both latency and amplitude. Gomes and colleagues speculated that the central component matures earlier because the generators of the response are closer in proximity to the primary auditory areas, and they mature before association areas.

According to Ceponienè et al. (2002), the N1 and N2 components of the ALR are generated by anatomically distinct generators in both adults as well as children. The scalp distributions of both N1 and N2 change with maturation. In adults and older children, the neural sources of the N1 and N2 appear to be the superior aspects of the temporal lobe. The sources for N1 are posterior to the sources for N2 (Ceponienè et al., 2002).

Developmental Changes in Morphology and Refractoriness

Every neuron has a refractory period—that is, the time required for the neuron to revert to its preconduction state. During this recovery period, the neuron's capacity to fire again is limited. The refractoriness of a neuron changes developmentally with factors such as myelination. The formation of myelin on the axon directly influences the speed of transmission or conduction velocity of a neuron and, thus, can affect the ability of the neuron to conduct successive stimuli at a high rate (e.g., Sabatini & Regehr, 1999). Neural refractory periods or recovery times for the ALR are relatively long. Hence, the interstimulus interval (ISI) rather than number of stimuli per second should be used to describe the rate factor for the ALR (Hall, 2007). Some of the early ALR studies confirmed that longer ISIs produced larger amplitudes of the N1 and P2 components but did not have a significant effect on the latencies (e.g., Davis, Mast, Yoshie, & Zerlin, 1966; Fruhstorfer, Soveri, & Järvilehto, 1970; Hari, Kaila, Katila, Tuomisto, & Varpula, 1982; Keidel & Spreng, 1965; Nelson & Lassman, 1968; Picton et al., 1977; Rothman, Davis, & Hay, 1970). This effect on the ALR was interpreted as a reflection of the time required by neurons to recover after being activated by a stimulus. However, refractory periods of individual neurons are significantly shorter than those for the N1 and P2 components of the ALR (Hall, 2007).

Gilley et al. (2005) studied developmental changes in refractoriness of responses within the ALR time frame. The ALR, or cortical auditory-evoked potentials (CAEPs), recorded with ISI conditions of 2000, 1000, 560, and 360 ms defined from offset to onset, were studied for 50 normal hearing children in the age range of 3 to 12 years and 10 adults ranging from 24 to 26 years of age. Results showed that P1 dominated the cortical response with a latency of about 100 ms for all the ISI conditions for ALRs recorded from children between the ages of 3 to 6 years. In the 7- to 8-year-old subjects, a "slight invagination" in the waveform began to emerge in the slowest ISI condition. This was labeled the N1. In the 11- to 12-year-old children, the N1-P2 complex was detected at all ISIs, although it was most robust in the slower ISI conditions. The N1-P2 complex was seen only in 20% of the 3- to 4-year-olds at the shortest ISI. In the adult group, Gilley et al. (2005) found the N1-P2 complex to be the most dominant regardless of the ISI condition. That study highlighted the importance of examining the interaction between stimulation rate and age-related development of the ALR. The finding that the N1 is only generated in children at ISIs of one second or longer has been observed in other studies, as well.

According to Sussman et al. (2008), slower stimulus rates can result in larger ALR amplitude, but they do not reflect the rates that occur in normal speech. Recording the ALR at higher rates might be more useful for understanding how the auditory system functions in a realistic auditory environment. These researchers studied the effect of ISI on the elicitation of the P1–N1–P2–N2 components to stimulus onset asynchrony of 200, 400, 600, and 800 ms calculated from onset to onset in children at ages 8, 9, 10, and 11 years, in adolescents at age 16 years, and in young adults at ages 22 to 40 years. Their findings showed that P1 and N2 components were the most robust of all components irrespective of stimulus rates in their youngest age group. N1, the dominant component in adults, emerged as a separate component only in adolescence. Although Sussman et al. (2008) described the P1–N1–P2 components as being more "adultlike" than "childlike" in the adolescent subjects, the N2 component typical of the child obligatory response was still present.

Ceponienè et al. (2002) attributed developmental change in N1 to its longer recovery cycle and its resulting overlap by the robust P1 and N2 peaks. The authors proceeded to record the ALR at different stimulus onset asynchrony times filtering out the slow N2 activity. Despite this maneuver, the N1 was only revealed at short stimulus onset asynchrony times in the 9-year-old children who were tested but not in the 4-year-olds. Sensitivity of the N1 wave to stimulation rates is reflected by the changes in amplitude of the components that occur with changes in stimulation rate (Näätänen & Picton, 1987). Components 2 and 3 of the N1 appear to be affected by attention and orienting responses, respectively. Unlike the N1, the N2 in children is largely unaffected by stimulus rate (Ceponienè et al., 1998).

With an aim to establish clinical protocols for ALRs in infants, Golding, Purdy, Sharma, and Dillon (2006) evaluated the effect of stimulus duration and ISI on the ALR of 3- to 7-month-old infants using natural speech stimuli (/m/ and /t/). They did not find a significant difference in either amplitude or latency across the limited range of stimulus durations used in the study. The authors offered an explanation for the difference between their study and previous reports, in particular that earlier studies were conducted with adults. Golding and colleagues suggested that the following might have contributed to the differences in findings: (a) methodological variables; (b) differences in auditory encoding in an adult auditory system versus that of an infant; and (c) responses to speech stimuli might be more complex compared to those for tonal stimuli.

Agung King et al. (2008) recorded ALRs elicited with speech stimuli of different voice onset times in 10 children between the ages of 4 and 8 years. They compared their results with those obtained on previous studies with adult subjects. The authors described a difference in findings for children and adults. Adult subjects, in previous studies, showed a "double on" pattern of the N1 response for longer voice onset times. Agung King and colleagues (2008) reported that their pediatric subjects only showed latency changes in the P1 and N2 components when stimulus voice onset times were changed. The authors concluded that changes in voice onset times in cortical responses of children in the age group of 2 to 8 years are represented by markers that are different from those in adults.

Anatomic and Physiologic Correlates of ALR Maturation

It would be plausible to assume that maturation of any neurologic component and the corresponding behavior should correlate with anatomic and physiologic changes that occur developmentally. Several researchers have described neuromaturation of the auditory cortex in normal hearing children and clinical populations using histologic evidence (Huttenlocher & Dabholkar, 1997; Kral, 2007; Moore, 2002; Moore & Guan, 2001; Moore & Linthicum, 2007; Shepherd & Hardie, 2001). In a rather innovative anatomical study, Moore and Guan (2001) examined the maturation of the auditory cortex posthumously from the second trimester of gestation to young adulthood using histologic and immunehistochemic data. They found a deep-to-surface sequence of maturation of the axons of the auditory cortex with deeper layers maturing first. Although axons are present in superficial layers of the cortex at a young age, their maturation as evidenced with the appearance of neurofilaments and development of a true axonal plexus actually begins as late as age 5 years and continues as late as age 11 to 12 years. Maturation of neurofilaments increases the conduction velocity of an axon. Moore and Guan (2001) suggested that late onset of neurofilament maturation and myelination in the superficial layers and the continued expansion of commissural and association pathways account for the changes in auditory processing abilities with age in children.

The ability to process speech in degraded acoustic environments is significantly enhanced in normal-hearing children beyond the age of 7 years. Eggermont and Ponton (2003) point out that it is not surprising for children under the age of 7 years to have no N1 component except at very slow stimulus rates of under one per second considering the timeline of development. Age-related alteration of the ALR and appearance of the N1 coincide with maturation of the upper cortical layers (Moore & Linthicum, 2007). The N1 component, as already mentioned, matures well into adolescence and seems to originate from the upper layer II of the cortex (Eggermont & Ponton, 2003). Huttenlocher and Dabholkar (1997) report synaptogenesis data suggesting that maturational differences persist for a shorter period in lower or deeper layers than in upper more superficial layers of the cortex. Also, cortical Layer IV that receives primary afferent input and contains the neurons giving rise to the efferent pathways in Layers V and VI develop faster than the areas responsible for information processing located in Layers II and III.

Eggermont and Ponton (2003) provided a detailed description of the structural, electrophysiological, and behavioral indexes of cortical maturation. Briefly, maturation of the neuronal structure continues nearly into the early teenage years. In infants below the age of 4.5 months, only axons of Layer I are mature. Neural activity at this stage is sufficient for generation of the ABR plus the P2 and N2 of the ALR. With behavioral measurement of auditory function, infants at this age are capable of responding differentially to changes in sounds. Between early infancy and 5 years of age, Eggermont and Ponton reported that axons in cortical Layers IV, V, and VI begin to mature. Electrophysiologically, this contributes to the generation of higher auditory responses such as the AMLR, mismatch negativity, and the T-complex. Behaviorally, auditory abilities resulting from this neuronal development enable the child to develop verbal language through the auditory mode. Cortical Layers II and III show maturation of axons with evidence of differentiation according to function between the ages of 5 and 12 years. This level of neural maturation enhances listening performance in increasingly challenging auditory environments. All cortical axons reach maturity above the age of 12 years. The rate of further change in behavioral and electrophysiological correlates slows and finally reaches a plateau.

Clinical Applications of ALR in Pediatric Populations

ALRs are effective noninvasive and objective tools for assessing central auditory nervous system maturation and processing (e.g., Arehole, 1995; Cunningham et al., 2000; Jerger, Martin, & McColl, 2004; Jerger et al., 2002; Ponton et al., 2000; Purdy, Kelly, & Thorne, 2001; Sharma et al., 2002b; Sharma et al., 1997; Sharma, Nash, & Dorman, 2009). Numerous studies have examined differences between ALRs in normal-hearing individuals and clinical populations using both life span longitudinal and cross-sectional experimental designs. Differences were described in latencies, presence versus absence of different components, and relative amplitude of different components. As with ABRs, aural immittance measures, and otoacoustic emissions, ALR is an attractive objective test for assessing the integrity of higher-order auditory processing, specifically at the level of the auditory cortex in pediatric populations. ALRs not only have proven diagnostic utility, but have also been effectively employed as objective outcome measures of successful hearing aid fitting or cochlear implantation (e.g., Bakhos et al., 2014; Ponton et al., 1996; Ponton, Don, Eggermont, Waring, & Masuda, 1996; Sharma, Dorman, & Kral, 2005; Sharma et al., 2002a; Sharma, Glick, Campbell, & Biever, 2013; Sharma, Martin, et al., 2005; Sharma et al., 2004; Silva et al., 2014), and auditory training in children with central auditory processing disorder (CAPD) and learning problems (e.g., Jirsa, 1992; Sharma, Purdy, & Kelly, 2014; Warrier, Johnson, Hayes, Nicol, & Kraus, 2004).

Central Auditory Processing Disorder

According to the 2010 AAA Clinical Practice Guidelines on (C)APD, "Auditory evoked responses (AER) from the auditory brainstem response (ABR) through higher level cortical auditory evoked responses have clinical value in the evaluation of (C)APD" (AAA, 2010, p. 19). Specifically referring to the ALR, the guidelines state:

> There is a growing literature describing many auditory evoked responses with latencies beyond 50 ms elicited with non-speech and speech signals. Those most relevant to clinical assessment of (C)APD include the auditory late response (ALR), which is comprised of the N1 and P2 evoked potentials and the P300 response. The cortical auditory evoked responses reflect the function of sites suspected of dysfunction in the majority of children with (C)APD. (AAA, 2010, p. 20)

This evidence-based and peer-reviewed document confirms the rationale for use of objective measures such as ALRs or event related potentials (ERPs) to diagnose CAPD. Every auditory behavior (or lack of it) should logically have a correlate in terms of presence (or absence) of a particular brain activity.

As noted earlier, obligatory components of the ALR arise from auditory thalamocortical and corticocortical pathways, primary auditory cortex, and different association cortices. These areas play an important role in central auditory processing. Measurement of the ALR P1, N1, and P2 components is recommended (AAA, 2010; American Speech-Language-Hearing Association, 2005) as part of the comprehensive test battery for diagnosing CAPD. This recommendation highlights the need for electrophysiological assessment of young children for whom behavioral measures of CAPD might not always yield reliable or valid findings. Another problem with behavioral auditory tests is the possibility of unpredictable learning effects among different patients that limit the usage of postdiagnosis follow-up tests necessary to track changes in auditory processing ability. Citing this disadvantage of behavioral speech-in-noise tests, Hassaan (2015) conducted a study to evaluate the viability of the P1-N1 complex as an objective index of the ability to listening in noise, a skill commonly affected in individuals with CAPD. Traditional behavioral tests for this auditory processing skill include presenting speech and competing signals together monaurally. The signal-to-noise ratio might be constant for calculation of a recognition score or it might be variable for calculation of a speech recognition threshold in noise. Individuals with CAPD do not necessarily have deficits in listening-in-noise. Other auditory processes can also be affected, such as temporal processing, binaural interaction, or dichotic listening.

Hassaan (2015) included two subgroups within the study sample of children with CAPD. There were 15 children with deficits on behavioral speech-in-noise tests and eight age-matched children with other auditory processing problems. A control group of 15 children without any auditory processing deficits was also included. Although all groups exhibited a suppression of P1-N1 complex in the presence of ipsilateral noise, the effects were greater for the group whose psychophysical measures indicated deficits listening in background noise. The author concluded that all measures of the ALR except threshold were sensitive to speech-in-noise deficits; therefore, cortical measurements could be considered objective equivalents of psychophysical speech-in-noise tests.

Correlations between auditory processing deficits and brain activity have been elegantly demonstrated through studies using topographic brain mapping. This strategy involves measurement of cortical responses from surface electrodes on multiple scalp locations to identify brain regions that are active while the subject performs certain tasks (Estes, Jerger, & Jacobson, 2002; Jerger, Moncrieff, Greenwald, Wambacq, & Seipel, 2000; Jerger et al., 2002). Jerger and colleagues (2000) reported their findings for a pair of fraternal twins. One child showed behaviors consistent with CAPD according to the Children's Auditory Performance Scale, or CHAPS, completed by the mother as well as schoolteacher (Smoski, Brunt, & Tannahill, 1998). The other child was essentially normal. Both twins were evaluated with the same audiological test battery. The findings were reported in two parts (Jerger et al., 2004; Jerger et al., 2002). The twin with symptoms of CAPD showed normal findings on traditional behavioral tests of CAPD. Event-related potential topographies for both girls were constructed from electrophysiological data obtained from 32 scalp locations during the performance of the tasks of visual gap detection, within-channel auditory gap detection, across channel auditory gap detection, dichotic listening for an acoustic target, and dichotic listening for a phonemic target.

Jerger et al. (2002) reported that the twins had comparable findings on the visual gap detection task, consistent with processing problems limited to the auditory system. For within-channel auditory gap detection, the nonaffected twin showed activation over both hemispheres, with greater activation on the left side. The affected twin showed only a limited activation pattern in the temporoparietal region on the left side. For across-channel gap detection, the nonaffected twin showed activation over both hemispheres with slightly greater activation over the right hemisphere, whereas the affected twin showed only a limited activation pattern in the C4 electrode (Jasper, 1958) region on the right side. For a dichotic listening task involving an acoustic target (sawtooth noise) with both right as well as left ear presentation, the nonaffected twin had an activation pattern that was asymmetric to the right of the midline—that is, greater activity on the right side. In contrast, the pattern was attenuated and asymmetric to the left of the midline for the affected twin. For a dichotic listening task involving a phonemic target, the nonaffected twin had an activation pattern that was asymmetric to the left of the midline with greater activity on the left side. In contrast, the pattern was asymmetric to the right of the midline for the affected twin. In other words, results for dichotic tasks suggested a reversal of hemispheric asymmetry and deficits in interhemispheric transfer of information via the corpus callosum. Interestingly, these researchers did not find any significant pattern of differences in the latencies of the corresponding ERPs between the twins. Hence, the brain activation patterns, rather than just latencies, brought out the differences between the twins. Jerger et al. (2002) concluded that activation patterns of ERPs for certain auditory tasks such as gap detection and dichotic listening might be especially effective in identifying CAPD. For the second study on the same set of twins, Jerger et al. (2004) analyzed their brain maps in response to presentation of dichotic stimuli. Three of the conditions involved the processing of real words for phonemic, semantic, or spectral targets, while one condition involved the processing of a nonword acoustic signal. The authors found marked differences in the cross-correlation functions between the twins. For the nonaffected twin, cross-correlation functions were uniformly normal across both hemispheres. For the affected twin, the findings suggested "poorly correlated neural activity over the left parietal region during the three word processing conditions and over the right parietal area in the nonword acoustic condition" (p. 79). Jerger and colleagues (2004) also analyzed the results on diffusion tensor magnetic resonance imaging (DTI). The affected twin (in comparison with the nonaffected twin) showed "reduced anisotropy over the length of the midline corpus callosum and adjacent lateral structures" (p. 79) and concluded that these findings indicated "reduced myelin integrity" (p. 84). They concluded that at least some children with CAPD might be unable to perform adequately on tasks involving activity in both hemispheres because ability to perform the task is dependent on interhemispheric transfer of information through the corpus callosum.

Changes in parameters of the ALR P1, N1, and P2 waves reflect neuromaturation (e.g., Gilley et al., 2005; Illing, 2004; Kraus & McGee, 1994; Sharma et al., 2002a). Jirsa and colleagues reported significant differences in the mean latencies of ALR N1 and P2 components and the P3 response in children with and without symptoms of auditory processing difficulties (Jirsa, 1992; Jirsa & Clontz, 1990). Jirsa (1992) found that the mean latencies of the components were significantly longer in children with behaviors consistent with processing problems. Jirsa and Clontz (1990) studied ALRs in children with auditory processing deficits and compared the findings with a control group of children with normal hearing, matched for age, intelligence, and gender. There was a significant latency increase for the ALR N1 and P2 waves, and the P3 response in the group with auditory processing disorder. In addition, the interpeak latency interval for P2-P3 was significantly longer in the CAPD group. Among the amplitude measures, only P3 amplitude differed significantly between the groups. It is possible, then, that children with CAPD might be reflecting the effect of an immature auditory nervous system. Findings of abnormalities in ALR were reported even in adults with auditory problems consistent with the presence of CAPD (Jutras, Lagacé, Lavigne, Boissonneault, & Lavoie, 2007). In contrast, however, other studies have found no relationship between the P1, N1, and P2 components of ALR and fine-grained speech sound perception (e.g., Cunningham et al., 2000).

Almeqbel and McMahon (2015) explored the possible clinical utility of the N2 component in identifying temporal processing problems in children. Their rationale was that the N1 component is an objective indicator of discrimination ability that is often not clearly present even in young children with normal hearing. The authors reported a significantly shorter N2 latency for the voiced consonant /d/ in comparison with its voiceless counterpart /t/. N2 latency also increased as signal to noise ratio became adverse. Further N2 latency did not show any consistent changes as a function of amplitude modulation depth. Overall, the authors concluded that the N2 had potential as an objective tool for identifying temporal processing problems in children, especially when behavioral test measures were not feasible.

ALR as an Index of Improvement in Central Auditory Processing

If ALR indices of amplitude, latency, and morphology can be used to assess auditory cortical functioning and developmental plasticity, then the ALR might also be an effective tool for objective assessment of change in cortical functioning as a result of either signal enhancement with, for example, FM technology or a training program targeted at improving auditory processing at the level of the cortex. Cunningham, Nicol, Zecker, Bradlow, and Kraus (2001) studied the effect of "cue enhancement" on behavioral auditory performance as well as electrophysiological measures in a sample of normal children and children with learning problems. They studied the effects of enhancing specific speech cues at the syllable level in order to examine which cues resulted in better auditory perception of the stop consonants /d/ and /g/ incorporated in the syllables /ada/ and /aga/. Cunningham and colleagues (2001) also examined corresponding differences in ABR, frequency following response [FFR], and ALRs. The authors reported that the differences between the normal control and the LP group on ALRs were eliminated by the use of cue-enhanced stimuli. This was an encouraging finding implying that ALRs might contribute to development of more effective therapy techniques and strategies.

Hayes, Warrier, Nicol, Zecker, and Kraus (2003) investigated changes in the central auditory pathways and cognitive skills of children with learning problems as a result of training. The subject sample consisted of children between the ages of 8 and 12 years. The group of 27 children with learning problems was subdivided into two groups. One group underwent the training program and one did not. Data from seven age-matched children without learning problems were collected for comparison to the control subjects with learning problems. Among the subjects, one of the subjects in the control group was on medication for ADHD and four in the trained group with learning problems were similarly medicated. The group that underwent training attended 35 to 40 one-hour training sessions over an 8-week period. The program consisted of the Steps I and II of the Earobics (http://www.cogcon.com)

computer-based program for development of auditory and prereading skills. The program uses interactive computer-based games to develop and improve skills such as phonological awareness and auditory language processing through interactive games. Behavioral measures for cognitive and perceptual performance were administered. ABR was recorded with click stimuli as well as the syllable /ga/. The ALR was elicited in quiet and in noise using the syllables /ga/ and /da/, respectively. Following intervention with the experimental group, all behavioral and electrophysiological measures were repeated.

Hayes and colleagues (2003) reported that the trained group showed significant improvements compared to the control group on the behavioral sound blending test. This improvement was independent of the subject's pretraining performance on the same test. The ABR showed no changes as a result of training. However, components of the ALR showed significant improvements in association with improvement on behavioral measures.

The large sample study by Warrier et al. (2004) is described in the following subsection on ALRs in children with learning difficulties. These investigators documented changes in the cortical auditory-evoked responses and corresponding improvements in speech perception in noise following training on the Earobics program.

Language and Learning Difficulties

Several studies have examined performance of children with language and learning disabilities on difficult auditory processing tasks and corresponding auditory-evoked responses (e.g., Arehole, 1995; Jerger, Martin, & Jerger, 1987; Kraus, 2001; Kraus et al., 1996; McArthur & Bishop, 2004; Moncrieff, Jerger, Wambacq, Greenwald, & Black, 2004; Warrier et al., 2004). Findings point to a possibility of altered auditory processing in at least some cases of learning disabilities (Wible, Nicol, & Kraus, 2002). Children with language-based learning problems show abnormalities in central auditory maturation (Gilley, Sharma, Dorman, & Martin, 2006).

Uhlén, Borg, Persson, and Spens (1996) recorded topographic maps from 20 children with learning impairment (LI) between the ages of 9 and 15 years and 20 normal age-matched children. The stimulus was a 500-Hz tone presented with an interstimulus interval (ISI) of 1 s. Focusing mainly on the ALR N1 response, these researchers found that the latencies of N1 were longer in the LI group, and there was no decrease in latency with increase in age. They speculated that the lack of improvement in latencies with age in the LI group might indicate the persistence of a processing disturbance, rather than just a delay in maturation. They further reported that the diagnostic sensitivity of N1 latency, amplitude, and topography in identifying LI subjects was 40% and the specificity was 90%.

Gilley et al. (2006) investigated ALRs recorded from 26 children with learning problems. The authors reported that a majority of the children had abnormal responses. They identified three atypical categories of responses in children with learning problems: Category 1 with delayed P1 latencies and absent N1/P2 components; Category 2 with a normal P1 component but delayed N1 and P2 responses; and Category 3 with overall low amplitude of all responses. A fourth subgroup had normal ALR responses. This research raises the possibility that differences in the obligatory ALRs between normal and learning-impaired children are evident only in difficult listening situations. A previous study by Cunningham et al. (2000) found no significant difference in the development of P1/N1 and N2 latency between normal children and children with learning problems. However, these authors did note that scores on auditory processing tests correlated better with latencies of the ALR N2 component indicating the possible value of the speech-evoked N2 response in identifying auditory processing deficits.

Listening in noise is a difficult auditory processing task. Comparison of a child's electrophysiological responses to auditory stimuli in quiet versus in noise might provide a direct estimate of the effects of noise on auditory processing. Cunningham et al. (2001) studied the ALRs in quiet and noise, for normal-hearing children and children described as learning impaired. The two groups had similar responses for the quiet situation, but in noise children with learning problems exhibited neurophysiologic abnormalities at both cortical and subcortical levels for auditory responses elicited by speech in noise. The authors also reported significantly lower amplitude of the ALR P1-N1 and P1′-N1′ components in children with learning problems for speech in background noise. This reduction in the presence of noise was larger for the P1′-N1′. The difference between the normal and learning impaired group was eliminated when the same stimulus /da/ was presented in quiet or with cue enhancement.

Large sample studies, though difficult to design and conduct, are a good experimental approach for establishing a link among auditory-evoked responses, behavioral auditory processing performance, and clinical entities involving the central nervous system. Warrier et al. (2004) conducted a relatively large sample study with children between the ages of 8 and 13 years. Eighty of the subjects had learning problems, and 32 were essentially normal (NL), as determined by standard tests. ALRs to the syllable /da/ were collected in quiet and noise conditions. The correlation of each subject's response in quiet versus that in noise was examined by shifting the waveforms for the latter with respect to time in order to achieve what the authors describe as a "best fit." The authors found some children in the learning-problem group whose correlation scores fell below the lowest NL score. Based on the cross-correlation of responses of the learning problem versus NL group, the learning problem group was further subdivided. The learning problem-out group consisted of those with poor correlation scores (below the mean −1 SD of the NL group's correlation scores) and the remaining were grouped under learning problem-in. In the quiet condition, the NL and learning problem groups were similar in terms of the morphology of the ALR P2-N2 complex, but in the noise condition the learning problem-out group had highly degraded morphology (compared to the NL and learning problem-in groups), particularly in the N2 region.

Warrier and colleagues (2004) postulated that the primary difference between the cortical responses of the NL and learning problem group was in terms of neural timing. Specifically, the difference between the groups was found for the ALR N2 component. In noise, the overall response activity in the learning problem group decreased to almost the same extent as the NL group, but in approximately one fourth of the learning problem group, the timing of the morphologic features of the waveform was altered due to noise. The latency of the N2 response in noise was earlier in the children with learning problems. As only a small later portion of the waveform conflicted morphologically with that obtained in a quiet condition, latency shift continued to produce a low quiet-to-noise correlation. In a second part of the experiment, some children from the learning problem group underwent intensive auditory training for 8 weeks on the Earobics program. Importantly, the ALRs showed postintervention improvement. The authors suggested that the subjects with learning problems and poor quiet-to-noise response correlations are especially able to benefit from auditory training and reported that the learning problem subjects, who previously demonstrated abnormal cortical responses in noise, showed improvement to the extent that their posttraining responses fell within the normal range. This improvement was reflected in improved speech perception scores.

More recent studies show that differences between normal and clinical populations, such as, for example, individuals with specific language impairment (SLI), might not be manifested in the typical measures of latency and amplitude. Examination of the hemispheric distribution using lexically meaningful and nonmeaningful speech tokens could add significant value (Helenius, Parviainen, Paetau, & Salmelin, 2009; Helenius et al., 2014). In a magnetoencephalography study, Helenius and colleagues (Helenius et al., 2014) found that children with SLI had abnormal hemispheric activation of the N400 component, although the latency and amplitude measures were no different from the normal control group. The typically developing children in their study displayed a reduction in amplitude of the response bilaterally over the temporal cortices when a word stimulus recurred during the test protocol. This suppression effect was not observed in children with SLI. Furthermore, meaningful words and pseudowords evoked equally strong activation in children with SLI, whereas in normal children, left hemisphere activation persisted for a longer time in case of pseudowords compared to meaningful words. The authors commented that the abnormally fast "decay of speech-evoked activation" and deviant N400 in the left hemisphere of children of SLI could contribute to difficulties in acquisition of language and vocabulary.

Vanvooren, Poelmans, Hofmann, Ghesquière, and Wouters (2014) studied the cortical responses to syllable and phoneme rate modulations in two groups of 5-year-old children. One group consisted of typically developing children and the other was at high hereditary risk for dyslexia having at least one family member with a confirmed diagnosis of dyslexia. There was no significant overall difference between the two groups with regard to hemispheric asymmetry of cortical responses. They concluded that for 5-year-old children who could be considered to be in a prereading stage, hemispheric specialization for syllable rate modulation is mature, whereas that for phoneme modulation rate is yet immature.

Davies, Chang, and Gavin (2010) recorded from normal adults and children the ALR in response to 1 and 3 KHz tones presented in blocks of tones. Additionally, they collected data from 5- to 12-year-old children with "sensory processing disorders." Within each block there were two tones of each frequency presented at one of two intensity levels. The purpose of the study was to establish whether the three groups could be differentiated based on their ALRs. The ALRs of adults displayed an organized pattern of responses to intensity and frequency changes compared to normal children. Children with sensory processing disorders showed the most disorganized ALR patterns. In response to stimulus frequency and amplitude changes, adults had greater peak-to-peak N1 and P2 amplitude compared to children, whereas the reverse was true for N2 and P3 components. Children with sensory processing disorders had large P3 amplitudes compared to their normal peers and to adult subjects. The authors speculated that children with sensory processing disorders actively processed each sensory event longer and more intensely than their peers. This finding could explain the sensory overload that such children face in day-to-day environments where there is a high demand for processing rapidly occurring sequential sensory information. Davies and colleagues (2010) proposed that sensory systems of children with sensory processing disorders might not be attuned to sensory experiences due to lack of maturation, even after they are repeatedly exposed to them. Therefore, the brain is unable to process a novel stimulus that requires intense processing even when the stimulus is repeated. The results further showed that children with sensory processing disorder could be identified with 97% accuracy based on the pattern of their ALR. The authors conclude with the statement that children with sensory processing disorders "exhibit less sensory detection of stimuli which is followed by more extended and intense processing than shown by their age-matched peers" (p. 8).

Brain Lesions and Injury

ALRs are a valuable approach for exploring the generators of different wave components in known cases of brain lesions. However, brain pathology can be diffuse and not localized to a small region, making it very difficult to attribute the presence, absence, or abnormality of the response to deficits in a particular cortical region. As Näätänen and Picton (1987) pointed out, a lesion in one location of the brain can result in loss or change of functions of other areas of the brain. Lesions can also alter the conductivity of the brain such that the electric fields produced by an active or unaffected neural generator are distorted. The effect of brain injury on the ALRs has been studied less for children than for adults. Also, components widely studied in adults, such as the N1 component, are difficult to study in children with brain lesions because the N1 component does not mature until late childhood and is often not recorded in younger children except at very slow stimulation rates.

One of the biggest problems in studying the immediate effects of brain injury is that the patient can be sedated or even in coma at the time of the initial electrophysiological measurement. The reduced state of arousal can seriously affect ALRs that are dependent on the state of consciousness. Young, Wang, and Connolly (2004) recommended the use of electrophysiological techniques such as the ABR and "cognitive" event–related potentials as prognostic indicators of recovery in patients who have been in coma. Liasis, Boyd, Rivera-Gaxiola, and Towell (2003) recorded auditory event-related potentials (ERPs) elicited by pure tones and syllables and detected with a 51-channel electrode array concentrated over the functional hemisphere. Subjects were 17 children (mean age 14.2 years) who had undergone hemispherectomy surgical procedures for intractable seizures of which eight had congenital brain damage and seven had acquired brain damage at or after the age of 1 year. The control group consisted of 10 children with a mean age of 13.5 years. These authors reported that topography of the ALRs in the children with hemispherectomy was localized to the centrotemporal regions of the functioning hemisphere as against the midline localization observed in the normal-hearing group. Regardless of the side of hemispherectomy, the clinical group showed longer latencies for cortical responses to syllables compared to tones. This finding was consistent with the pattern in the normal-hearing group. Furthermore, children with a left hemispherectomy showed delayed N1 and P2 responses to syllables, while those with right hemispherectomy did not. The authors suggested that the left hemisphere might be more efficient than the right hemisphere in processing tones as well as syllables. Furthermore, they surmised it might be more efficient than both hemispheres together when processing tones and syllables.

Klein et al. (1995) studied the ALR and the P3 response elicited with tones as well as consonant vowel stimuli using an oddball paradigm in six young adults who had verbal auditory agnosia since childhood. The ABRs and AMLRs for these subjects were normal. ALRs of the subjects with agnosia showed a delayed N1 component over the lateral temporal cortex. This was observed for both tones and speech sounds. The N1 component over the frontocentral region of the scalp was normal in latency. According to the authors, the findings indicate that processing of both speech as well as nonspeech stimuli was slower and that the abnormality is in the secondary auditory cortex.

Landau Kleffner syndrome (LKS) is a childhood-acquired epileptic aphasia. Most patients show complete recovery of epilepsy but persist in showing extinction of the ear contralateral to the affected hemisphere on dichotic tasks (Wioland, Rudolf, & Metz-Lutz, 2001). This syndrome and its associated auditory deficits have been documented in several studies (Baynes, Kegl, Brentari, Kussmaul, & Poizner, 1998; Metz-Lutz et al., 1997; Plaza, Rigoard, Chevrie-Muller, Cohen, & Picard, 2001; Seri, Cerquiglini, & Pisani, 1998; Wioland et al., 2001). Wioland et al. (2001) recorded ABRs, AMLRs, and ALRs from six children who had recovered from LKS. Recordings were compared with those of five normal children of the same ages. All five children with LKS had normal ABRs and AMLRs. However, there were abnormalities in the ALRs. Amplitude of N1c, reportedly arising from the association auditory areas, was significantly lower in amplitude in the temporal region on the side contralateral to the ear showing extinction. On the other hand, the N1b was within normal limits in terms of both latency and amplitude. The authors concluded that because these children had been medically declared "recovered" from the epilepsy, this persistence of an abnormal pattern of extinction in brain areas previously known to have been involved in the epileptic focus suggested that the damage to the association auditory cortex was permanent. The behavioral correlate of this dysfunction is unilateral dichotic extinction. In an earlier study, Metz-Lutz et al. (1997) also found that dichotic deficits and unilateral extinction in individuals with LKS persist several years after recovery from the epilepsy and normalization of the electroencephalogram (EEG).

Anatomical and Physiological Changes in Auditory Deprivation

Shepherd and Hardie (2001) reviewed several studies on the effects of auditory deprivation. Information on histological effects of hearing loss on the cochlea and nervous system are largely from animal studies. Most studies in humans focus on the effects of deprivation on behavioral and electrophysiological measures (Eggermont, Ponton, Don, Waring, & Kwong, 1997; Kral, Hartmann, Tillein, Heid, & Klinke, 2001; Ponton, Don, Eggermont, Waring, Kwong, et al., 1996; Sharma et al., 2002b; Sharma, Gilley, Dorman, & Baldwin, 2007). Postmortem studies are comparatively rare for obvious reasons (Huttenlocher & Dabholkar, 1997; Moore & Guan, 2001; Moore & Linthicum, 2007). Huttenlocher and Dabholkar (1997) suggested that early synaptogenesis is intrinsically controlled and, therefore, largely independent of a child's auditory experiences. However, they did point out that learning and memory affect the formation of synapses in later life and that onset of functions of the cerebral cortex seems to occur during the late phase of rapid synaptogenesis. Hence, cortical level auditory processing and ALRs should logically be dependent on auditory experience or lack of it due to hearing impairment.

Long periods of deafness can cause structural changes in the auditory system. Shepherd and Hardie (2001) in a review of studies on the subject highlighted some of these changes. Permanent sensorineural hearing loss causes "rapid and extensive loss of unmyelinated peripheral dendrites within the organ of Corti" (Terrayama et al., 1997 cited by Shepherd & Hardie, 2001, p. 305). Following these changes, there is a slow degeneration of myelinated dendrites in the osseous spiral lamina and cell bodies of the Type I spiral ganglion (Shepherd & Hardie, 2001, p. 305). Auditory nerve fiber responses to brief stimuli are affected. The nerve fibers exhibit bursting or chopping activity and periods of inactivity in response to a train of current pulses reflecting loss of temporal resolution (Shepherd & Javel, 1997, cited by Shepherd & Hardie, 2001). Furthermore, these authors based on their review of literature reported that neurons at the level of the brainstem and the cochlear nucleus are not susceptible to degeneration all throughout life, in contrast to the spiral ganglion cells. There is no loss of neurons in the brainstem with a period of stimulation before the onset of hearing loss. Cortical changes occurring as a result of deafness generally tend to affect secondary auditory areas rather than the primary auditory cortex (Giraud, Truy, & Frackowiak, 2001).

Cross-modal remapping at the level of the cortex can occur with reorganization leading to the takeover of one sensory area by another. Remapping after visual or auditory deprivation has been studied extensively in animal models. In humans, higher-order sensory areas are capable of cross-modality remapping (e.g., Giraud et al., 2001; Kral et al., 2001; Kral & Sharma, 2012). Inputs to one sensory area of the brain lost due to deprivation are replaced with inputs from other sensory systems (Kral et al., 2001). Kral and colleagues (2001) also suggested that continued deprivation due to congenital hearing loss results in the "unused or unstimulated" higher auditory areas in the cortex that are taken over by other sensory systems. "Congenitally deaf patients, implanted in adulthood show deficits in temporal auditory processing such as gap detection and auditory counting abilities" (Busby et al., 1992, 1993 cited in Kral et al., 2001, p. 348; Busby & Clark, 1999 cited in Kral et al., 2001, p. 348).

Literature reviews describe in detail the decoupling of neuronal connections between cortical areas as well as between cortical and subcortical areas resulting from untreated congenital deafness (e.g., Kral & Sharma, 2012; Sharma, Campbell, & Cardon, 2015). Synaptogenesis and synaptic specialization in the higher auditory system are vital for fine phonetic contrast perception in the brain. A "smeared central representation of auditory stimuli" due to poor development of synaptic connections in cases of long-term auditory deprivation, affects auditory discrimination of stimuli (Kral & Sharma, 2012, p. 117). The authors postulate that "partial decoupling of higher order areas from primary auditory cortex at the end of the sensitive period" is responsible for reduced top-down influences and also absence of the N1 components in affected individuals (Kral & Sharma, 2012, p. 119).

Effective amplification and cochlear implantation within a sensitive period can induce maturation of the auditory cortex (Kral et al., 2001; Ponton, Don, Eggermont, Waring, Kwong, et al., 1996; Ponton, Don, Eggermont, Waring, & Masuda, 1996; Sharma, Dorman, et al., 2005; Sharma et al., 2002a, 2002b; A. Sharma et al., 2007; Sharma, Martin, et al., 2005). The ALR has been used more than other responses to understand the effects of auditory deprivation in the auditory cortex and reorganization and plasticity of the cortex following reintroduction of sensory stimulation after a period of deprivation.

Effects of Audiologic Intervention on ALR in Children With Hearing Impairment

Sharma et al. (2002a) studied ALRs recorded from 22 prelingually deaf children managed with cochlear implants. The children who ranged in age from 1.25 to 5.65 years were divided into groups depending on the duration of stimulation with the implant. The authors found in congenitally deaf children who underwent implantation early that the cortical responses improved in the first 6 to 8 months postimplant and reached age-appropriate latencies within 8 months. The cortex can be adequately recruited for processing if adequate auditory experience is provided at an early age either through hearing aids or cochlear implants. Late intervention might result in irreversible effects on the ALRs and auditory behavioral correlates (Eggermont & Ponton, 2003; Ponton, Don, Eggermont, Waring, Kwong, et al., 1996; Ponton, Don, Eggermont, Waring, & Masuda, 1996; Ponton, Moore, & Eggermont, 1999; A. Sharma, Dorman, et al., 2005; Sharma et al., 2002b; Sharma et al., 2007).

Eggermont and Ponton (2003) noted that absence or immaturity of the ALR N1 indicates an "arrest or alteration in the maturation of the layer II axon neurofilaments" (p. 251). They further suggested that maturation of these layers coincides with improved processing of degraded and masked speech in normal children. Late-implanted children in their study reportedly had good to excellent open set word recognition in quiet, but they persisted in having difficulties in speech recognition in noise.

Gordon, Tanaka, Wong, and Papsin (2008) investigated in 16 children with cochlear implants the ALR using tone bursts of different frequencies. They found differences in the morphology of the P1-N1 response compared to children with normal hearing. The positive wave was dominant in all the participants of their study. Also, the N1 response in the participants who had fair speech perception skills did not show age-appropriate changes in amplitude with manipulation of stimulus frequency.

Dinces, Chobot-Rhodd, and Sussman (2009) studied event-related potentials in three late-implanted children and correlated the results with findings on behavioral tasks involving auditory discrimination of frequency, intensity, and duration. The child who was the highest performer with a cochlear implant showed better ability to discriminate contrasts behaviorally in comparison with another child who was a poor user. Similarly, there was faster improvement in the corresponding event-related potentials of this child compared to the poor user.

Based on research in children with hearing loss, Sharma and colleagues (Gilley, Sharma, & Dorman, 2008; Sharma et al., 2002b; Sharma et al., 2007; Sharma et al., 2009) suggested that the first 3.5 years of life are the most sensitive. During this time period, the human auditory cortex is maximally plastic. Between the ages of 3.5 and 7 years, the degree of plasticity is variable across children. Beyond 7 years plasticity is greatly reduced. Not only does the ALR P1 not reach normal latencies but the morphology of the waveform of the later developing ALR N1-P2 component is also affected in the long term. In young children with little or no prior auditory experience, the ALR waveform is often characterized by a deep negativity that Sharma and colleagues termed the "deprivation negativity." In the authors' words, the deprivation negativity is "the hallmark of an unstimulated or little-stimulated, yet plastic central auditory pathway" (Sharma et al., 2009, p. 276). An extreme situation could arise in which the auditory cortex has been left unstimulated well beyond the sensitive period resulting in its reorganization and re-recruitment for other sensory functions such as visual or somatosensory. This could be expected in cases of congenital deafness followed by late cochlear implantation and manifests as a "polyphasic waveform" (Sharma et al., 2009).

We must note that the clarity and/or quality of auditory signals, and specifically speech signals, as perceived through a cochlear implant is significantly dependent on factors that have no connection with central auditory processing. Some of these factors include the type of cochlear implant device, the number of functioning channels, the presence of cochlear deformities, the type of processing strategy used, the programming, and the reality that contemporary speech processing strategies do not necessarily provide 100% speech recognition in all including adverse listening situations. That later point is true even for postlingually deafened adults who have not had long periods of auditory deprivation. Friesen et al. (2009) observed a link between number of active channels in a cochlear implant and morphology of speech-evoked ALR in adult subjects. Amplitude of P1-N1-P2 increased and latency decreased as the number of channels increased. However, the growth functions of improved ALR morphology and behavioral speech recognition measures were not identical, leading the authors to theorize that factors other than acoustic transitions played a role in speech sound recognition.

Findings of studies such as those just reviewed are encouraging application of ALR in objective assessment of efficacy of hearing aid fittings. Dillon (2005) recommended speech stimuli for assessing the adequacy of amplification in different frequency regions. The phonemes /m/, /g/, and /t/ were chosen for their representation of the low-, mid-, and high-frequency regions in anticipation that the ALRs elicited for these sounds would reflect the child's perception of the sounds. Agung et al. (2004) investigated objective verification of speech perception using cortical auditory-evoked responses, including the ALR. These researchers found significant differences in the ALR (P1-N1-P2) for different speech stimuli, and concluded that cortical auditory-evoked responses can be used to objectively measure perception of different speech sounds. The reader is referred to reviews specifically on the applications of speech-evoked responses, including the ALR, in documenting performance with hearing aids and cochlear implants (Martin, Tremblay, & Korczak, 2008; Tremblay, Scollie, Abrams, Sullivan, & McMahon, 2014). A series of collaborative studies from Australia and New Zealand have also focused on ALR applications of various speech stimuli in infants and children (Golding et al., 2006; Purdy et al., 2013; Sharma, Johnson, Purdy, & Norman, 2013; Sharma et al., 2014).

Attention Deficit Hyperactivity Disorder (ADHD)

According to the Department of Health and Human Services, Centers for Disease Control and Prevention, ADHD is one of the most common neurobehavioral disorders of childhood, persisting through adolescence and into adulthood. The estimated prevalence of ADHD in the United States is 4% to 12% in school-aged children (Akinbami, Liu, Pastor, & Reuben, 2011; Brown, 2013). Inattention to sensory stimuli is a hallmark of ADHD. ADHD should be considered when diagnosing CAPD because children with both disorders can present with similar symptoms of poor attention to sound (Chermak & Bellis, 2013; Hamaguchi & Tazeau, 2007). However, children with ADHD can have inattention for more than the auditory sensory modality, whereas children with CAPD show deficits specifically for auditory tasks. Most research on cortical auditory-evoked responses in children with ADHD has focused on event-related responses such as the P300 and the mismatch negativity (MMN) response (e.g., Brown et al., 2005; Gumenyuk et al., 2005; Jonkman et al., 1997; Kemner et al., 2004; Oades, Dittman-Balcar, Schepker, Eggers, & Zerbin, 1996; Winsberg, Javitt, & Silipo, 1997). The reason for this wide interest in event-related responses rather than the obligatory components of ALR most likely is because event-related responses such as the P300 are highly dependent on attention.

Oades (1998) reported that one of the striking findings in cases with ADHD was a larger ALR P2 component. These authors also pointed out that previous studies actually reported a smaller P2 component that normalized after drug treatment. The discrepancy in outcomes among studies was attributed to the subgroups seen in children with ADHD. Children with ADHD are not a homogeneous group. Oades (1998) suggested that large P2 amplitudes were consistent with impulsivity. Hyperactivity is often treated medically. One of the drugs used in the therapy of ADHD is methylphenidate. Some researchers have measured ALRs and event-related responses before and after treatment with methylphenidate in an attempt to document objective evidence of neurophysiologic changes. Winsberg et al. (1997) investigated the P300 response and earlier occurring event related responses in children with ADHD treated with methylphenidate. These researchers did not find any changes in the traditional ALR components as a result of the treatment. They did report an increase in the amplitude of the P3 response suggesting that methylphenidate affects attention regulation.

Brown et al. (2005) studied auditory and visual event-related responses in the predominantly inattentive subtype of ADHD. They used an intermodal oddball task in which the target was a 2000-Hz tone and the nontarget stimulus was a counterphasing checkerboard. They considered two subgroups within the "predominantly inattentive type" of ADHD based on underlying EEG activity—cortically hypoaroused and maturationally lagged (with EEGs resembling those of younger children). Their sample consisted of 27 children identified as "cortically hypoaroused," 27 identified as "maturationally lagged," and 27 age-matched controls. They reported that the task successfully differentiated the children with ADHD from the age-matched controls with the former showing smaller amplitudes for ALR N1 and P2 components and for the P3 response elicited with the auditory targets. The only difference the authors found between the subtypes of ADHD was a relative increase in the left-frontal N1 amplitude in the cortically hypoaroused group. They concluded that in the group with maturational lag, the frontal lateralization of N1 was reduced. This supports the label for this group. These researchers also observed that the cortical hypoaroused group showed abnormal lateralization of the ALR. There is very little published research on the obligatory components of the ALR in children with ADHD in comparison to the numerous papers on event-related responses elicited by auditory and visual signals. Application of the ALR as an electrophysiologic index of auditory functioning in ADHD is a topic that warrants more research.

Autism Spectrum Disorder

Individuals with autism, more recently referred to by the term *autism spectrum disorder* (ASD) manifest behaviors that could range from mild to severe (American Psychiatric Association, 2013). ASD is often characterized by sensory inattention despite normal peripheral hearing abilities. One of the challenges encountered in conducting behavioral audiometry in populations with ASD is the tendency of these individuals to ignore auditory stimuli presented to them, and to demonstrate "selective attention" to sounds that they prefer. Faced with a child showing symptoms of autism spectrum disorder, an audiologist is well advised to ask the caregivers about the type of sounds the child usually ignores or consistently attends to. ASD is also characterized by communication problems and atypical language development (American Psychiatric Asso-ciation, 2013). Considering the type of auditory behaviors shown by these children, it would be logical to consider a neurobiological basis, and to explore this possible etiology through the measurement of electrophysiologic measures (e.g., cortical auditory evoked responses).

Echolalia is a common behavior seen in individuals with ASD. One of the goals in speech and language therapy is to reduce echolalia, a meaningless "echo" rather than communicative behavior. Wetherby, Koegel, and Mendel (1981) studied central auditory processing abilities through behavioral tests in six echolalic autistic individuals in the age range of 8 to 24 years. The subjects had a wide range of language abilities and different degrees of severity of echolalia. The researchers found in the subjects with echolalia, normal performance on monaural tests, but indications of central auditory dysfunction in the language dominant hemisphere on the dichotic tests (Staggered Spondaic Word Test and Competing Environmental Sound Test). Children who previously were diagnosed as autistic but no longer had echolalia yielded essentially normal findings.

Bruneau, Bonnet-Brilhault, Gomot, Adrien, and Barthélémy (2003) investigated the relation between ALRs recorded at temporal sites (the N1c wave or Tb) and verbal and nonverbal abilities in children with ASD. Subjects were 26 children with mental retardation and autism between the ages of 4 and 8 years. The researchers elicited ALRs with tone-burst stimuli presented at slow stimulation rates (interstimulus intervals of 3 to 5 seconds), and compared the findings for the autistic group with 16 normal-hearing children. ALRs recorded from both left and right temporal sites were smaller in amplitude for children with autism than for the normal subject group. Bruneau and colleagues reported a correlation between the amplitude of the right temporal N1c responses and the verbal and nonverbal communication abilities. The authors suggested that, in autism, there is an aberrant reorganization of the functions of the right and left hemispheres with activation of the right hemisphere for tasks in which the left hemisphere should be activated normally. This is especially so for tasks involving the secondary auditory areas, whose activation is reflected by the N1c and Tb wave components. One of the difficulties in such studies is the differential diagnosis of mental retardation versus autism spectrum disorders due to overlapping behavioral characteristics in both groups. Although mental retardation and autism spectrum disorders can coexist, it is often difficult to separate the effects of both when diagnosing a child with one or the other condition.

Orekhova et al. (2009) recorded event-related potentials to novel temporal gaps from 21 children with autism spectrum disorder and 21 typically developing children. They concluded that the cortical responses of children with autism indicated impairment in the right hemisphere tasks of processing temporally novel information. They also suggested that such findings are indicative of the neurobiological basis of autism. Orekhova et al. (2012) in a study of auditory magnetic fields in typical children and those with autism spectrum disorder reported differences in hemispheric distribution of P100m between groups for white noise click stimuli. In typically developing children, the P100m was lateralized over the right hemisphere, while left hemisphere dominance was recorded in children with ASD. The atypical findings were associated with severity of sensory abnormalities as evaluated on the Short Sensory Profile. Furthermore, these children had a history of hypersensitivity to sound in the first two years of life. The authors concluded that these aberrant dominance patterns of P100m indicate the possibility of a dysfunction in the ascending reticular brainstem pathways or thalamic and cortical projections in children with ASD. The authors also speculated that the left-sided dominance of the P100m component could reflect inadequate preattentive sensory processing in the right hemisphere, contributing to abnormal sensory perceptions in ASD.

Seri, Cerquiglini, Pisani, and Curatolo (1999) studied ALRs in 14 children with tuberous sclerosis complex, seven of whom fulfilled the *Diagnostic and Statistical Manual of Mental Disorders* (*DSM IV*) criteria for ASD.

As tuberous sclerosis complex is associated with autism and also with cortical and subcortical lesions of the temporal lobe, Seri and colleagues designed a study to explore the link between anatomic lesions of the tuberous sclerosis complex and functional mechanisms as exhibited by ALRs and event-related responses to auditory stimuli (Seri et al., 1999). All the subjects underwent high-resolution magnetic resonance imaging (MRI) and EEG. The cortical responses to different frequencies of sounds presented with different probabilities were recorded using 21 scalp electrodes. The same procedures were conducted on both groups of children with tuberous sclerosis complex (the group with and without autism spectrum disorder). Results indicated that the N1 component of the ALR had a significantly prolonged latency, and lower amplitude, in all the children with autism spectrum disorder. These children, as opposed to the children without autism, had MRI documentation of lesions on one or both temporal lobes. The MMN had a longer latency in the autistic subgroup.

Auditory Neuropathy Spectrum Disorder

Since the early 1990s when published reports first appeared in the literature, our understanding of the condition we now refer to as *auditory neuropathy spectrum disorder* (ANSD) has deepened considerably. The word *spectrum* in the term refers to the heterogeneity of clinical presentation although the hallmark absent ABR waves and present cochlear microphonics and otoacoustic emissions remain an unvarying feature of the condition. Multiple studies confirm that cortical auditory evoked potentials at conversational intensity levels are often recordable in infants, children, and adults with auditory neuropathy (e.g., Cone-Wesson & Wunderlich, 2003; Michalewski, Starr, Nguyen, Kong, & Zeng, 2005; Pearce, Golding, & Dillon, 2007; Rance, Cone-Wesson, Wunderlich, & Dowell, 2002).

Rance et al. (2002) conducted a study of 18 children with the diagnosis of auditory neuropathy. The purpose of the study was to investigate a relationship between the presence of ALRs and speech perception performance. They observed that seven of the children had no open-set speech perception ability, while the other eight exhibited performance levels comparable to children with a similar degree of sensorineural hearing loss. Approximately 50% of their subjects had cortical response morphology. A direct relation between presence versus absence of the ALR and speech perception abilities was evident. Poor speech perception was associated with absent ALR, whereas responses of children with better speech perception abilities were normal in latency. The authors suggested that obligatory cortical auditory evoked response test results "may offer a means of predicting perceptual skills" (p. 239) in young children diagnosed with auditory neuropathy. The presence of normal ALRs appeared to predict a possibility of some speech perception benefit with amplification. ALRs could be useful in deciding treatment options and hearing aid fitting strategies in infants with ANSD (Pearce et al., 2007)

Cochlear implants can be a viable treatment option for children with ANSD. However, speech perception outcomes can be variable. In recent years, studies have longitudinally tracked the progress of implanted children with ANSD using ALR as an outcome measure (Campbell, Cardon, & Sharma, 2011; Gardner-Berry, Purdy, Ching, & Dillon, 2015)

Miscellaneous Populations

There are a handful of studies on populations such as Down syndrome (e.g., Seidl et al., 1997) and Fragile X syndrome (Castrén, Pääkkönen, Tarkka, Ryynänen, & Partanen, 2003) that have found abnormalities in the latency and amplitude of the N1 component of the ALR. More systematic investigation of ALR in these populations is needed.

Acoustic Change Complex

Speech is a dynamic, ever-changing acoustic stimulus. Speech perception is dependent on the auditory system's ability to code and identify these constant changes in the stimulus. Evoked responses that can assess this ability of the auditory system objectively, especially in difficult-to-test populations, can add diagnostic value. One of the less discussed cortical responses that reflects this aspect of auditory functioning is the acoustic change complex (ACC). The ACC is a cortical auditory late response (P1-N1-P2) that occurs subsequent to a change in an ongoing stimulus. Studies describing the ACC date back to the late 1960s (Martin, Boothroyd, Ali, & Leach-Berth, 2010). Auditory-evoked responses such as the mismatch negativity and P300 have long been of research and clinical interest as objective measures of auditory discrimination. The ACC could therefore have potential applications in the assessment of infants and children with hearing loss, children with CAPD, or other clinical conditions in which the ability of the auditory areas to encode speech sounds is compromised in some way. Martin et al. (2010) have described in detail the advantages of the ACC over measures such as MMN. Martinez, Eisenberg, and Boothroyd (2013) recorded ACC recordings from a small sample of five children with normal hearing sensitivity and five with mild-to-moderate sensorineural hearing loss. They examined the response to vowel height (/u/–/a/) as well as vowel place (/u/–/i/) contrast. These authors concluded that the ACC could be recorded in children as young as 2 years and might have potential as an objective measure of "auditory resolution" in children. The authors added that further in-depth studies are warranted to understand all the factors that affect measurement and clinical interpretation of the ACC in the pediatric population.

Future Directions for Clinical Research

From the foregoing review, it is apparent that AMLR and ALR now have the potential to play an important role in the diagnosis of central auditory dysfunction in children, and in documenting the effectiveness of specific intervention strategies. More research is warranted, particularly in specific populations such as children with carefully defined and diagnosed patterns of CAPD. Nonetheless, there is ample research evidence to justify more widespread clinical applications of AMLR and ALR in the diagnosis and management of auditory dysfunction in children. Unfortunately, to date, most research findings have been generated in experimental investigations with sophisticated laboratory instrumentation, rather than clinical studies with commercially available equipment available to practicing audiologists. What is needed to facilitate the transition of cortical auditory-evoked response measurement from the laboratory to the clinical setting?

A handful of technologic advances and types of information would probably contribute to the inclusion of cortical auditory-evoked responses into the clinical test battery, at least for selected patient populations. First, consensus is needed on accepted test protocols for the measurement of cortical auditory-responses. Studies reported in the literature are characterized by diverse test protocols that consist of a wide range of stimulus and acquisition parameters. There is clear disagreement among authors on basic test parameters required for measurement of cortical auditory-evoked responses, such as the minimum number of electrodes required for valid detection of major components. Also, importantly, hearing scientists conducting research on cortical auditory-evoked responses invariably utilize complex and expensive instrumentation that is neither user friendly nor appropriate for clinical application. It would be very helpful to incorporate techniques, protocols, stimuli, and algorithms that have worked well in the laboratory into equipment that is accessible and clinically feasible for the clinical audiologist. Clinical instrumentation, for example, must include certain new features, such as software for producing an assortment of stimuli including speech signals and multiple channels (e.g., four to eight) for the minimum number of hemisphere electrodes, and the mandatory eye blink electrode(s). If recording methods, such as those described by Bidelman (2015) for simultaneous investigation of brainstem and cortical-level speech processing, could be incorporated into future clinical instruments, it would contribute toward more holistic objective audiological assessment. As mentioned in the AAA Clinical Practice Guidelines (AAA, 2010), there is no gold standard test for CAPD, but if such a test did become available, it would in all likelihood be an objective test based on evoked responses.

Protocols and algorithms are needed for measurement of the AMLR and ALR in children undergoing diagnostic assessment for CAPD, a major clinical application of auditory neurophysiology. Specifically, protocols are needed for cortical auditory-evoked responses elicited with a speech-in-noise stimulus paradigm, with dichotically presented stimuli, and with stimuli with modified temporal features (e.g., a gap detection paradigm) to assess temporal auditory processing. The option for rigorous, yet user-friendly statistical analysis of ALR findings would be very helpful and would contribute importantly to the acceptance by clinical audiologists of cortical auditory-evoked responses. Statistical calculation and confirmation of major response parameters such as latency, amplitude, and area under the curve should be available for the traditional components of the AMLR and ALR, with the possibility of statistically assessing differences in these parameters for cortical auditory-evoked responses recorded under various measurement conditions (e.g., left versus right hemispheres) have validated feasibility of inbuilt statistical algorithms for ALR. And, finally, regular and confident clinical application of cortical auditory-evoked responses is dependent on access to large sample and age-matched normative data collected with clinical instrumentation and various types of stimuli, and including maturational data on the AMLR and ALR from infancy to adulthood.

We confidently predict that research on clinical applications of cortical auditory-evoked responses will expand considerably before long and that technologic advances in clinical instrumentation will begin to catch up with the accelerating proliferation of research findings. The offspring of this marriage of laboratory and clinical technology and techniques might well be an internationally universal electrophysiological auditory test battery that can be employed in pediatric populations with unprecedented sensitivity and specificity for the identification, diagnosis, and treatment-related documentation of cortical auditory dysfunction and auditory processing. We are optimistic that an ever-increasing number of innovative researchers "thinking out of the box" as Jerger (2007) elegantly put it, will continue to develop novel audiological applications of the AMLR and ALR in infants and children.

References

Agung King, K., Campbell, J., Sharma, A., Martin, K., Dorman, M., & Langran, J. (2008). The representation of voice onset time in the cortical auditory evoked potentials of young children. *Clinical Neurophysiology, 119*(12), 2855–2861. doi:10.1016/j.clinph.2008.09.015

Agung King, K., Purdy, S., McMohan, C., Dillon, H., Katsch, R., & Newall, P. (2004). Objective verification of speech perception using cortical auditory evoked potentials (pp. 15–17). *National Acoustics Laboratories: Research and development annual report.* Chatswood, NSW Australia: Australian Hearing. Retrieved from http://www.nal.gov.au/pdf/Annual-Report-2003-04.pdf

Akinbami, L. J., Liu, X., Pastor, P. N., & Reuben, C. A. (2011). Attention deficit hyperactivity disorder among children aged 5–17 years in the United States, 1998–2009. *NCHS Data Brief, 70*, 1–8.

Al-Saif, S. S., Abdeltawwab, M. M., & Khamis, M. (2012). Auditory middle latency responses in children with specific language impairment. *European Archives of Oto-Rhino-Laryngology, 269*(6), 1697–1702. doi:10.1007/s00405-011-1901-7

Alain, C., Woods, D. L., & Covarrubias, D. (1997). Activation of duration-sensitive auditory cortical fields in humans. *Electroencephalography and Clinical Neurophysiology, 104*(6), 531–539. doi:10.1016/S0168-5597(97)00057-9

Almeqbel, A. (2013). Speech-evoked cortical auditory responses in children with normal hearing. *South African Journal of Communication Disorders, 60*, 38–43. doi:10.7196/sajcd.132

Almeqbel, A., & McMahon, C. M. (2015). Objective measurement of high-level auditory cortical function in children. *International Journal of Pediatric Otorhinolaryngology.* http://dx.doi.org/10.1016/j.ijporl.2015.04.026

American Academy of Audiology (AAA; 2010). *Clinical practice guidelines: Diagnosis, treatment and management of children and adults with central auditory processing disorder.* Retrieved from http://audiology-web.s3.amazonaws.com/migrated/CAPD%20Guidelines%208-2010.pdf_539952af956c79.73897613.pdf

American Psychiatric Association (APA; 2013). *Diagnostic and statistical manual of mental disorders* (5th ed.). Washington, DC: Author.

American Speech-Language-Hearing Association (ASHA; 2005). *(Central) auditory processing disorders* [Technical Report]. Retrieved from http://www.asha.org/policy

Arehole, S. (1995). A preliminary study of the relationship between long latency response and learning disorder. *British Journal of Audiology, 29*(6), 295–298. doi:10.3109/03005369509076747

Arehole, S., Augustine, L. E., & Simhadri, R. (1995). Middle latency response in children with learning disabilities: Preliminary findings. *Journal of Communication Disorders, 28*(1), 21–38. doi:10.1016/0021-9924(94)00004-J

Bakhos, D., Delage, H., Galvin, J., Lescanne, E., Roux, S., Bonnet-Brilhault, F., & Bruneau, N. (2014). Cortical electrophysiological markers of language abilities in children with hearing aids: A pilot study. *BioMed Research International.* http://dx.doi.org/10.1155/2014/198153

Banai, K., & Kraus, N. (2008). The dynamic brainstem: Implications for APD. In D. J. McFarland & A. T. Cacace (Eds.), *Current controversies in central auditory processing disorder* (pp. 269–289). San Diego, CA: Plural.

Barnet, A., & Lodge, A. (1967). Diagnosis of hearing loss in infancy by means of EEG audiometry. *Clinical Proceedings of Children's Hospital in Washington, DC, 23*, 1–18.

Barnet, A., Ohlrich, E. S., Weiss, I. P., & Shanks, B. (1975). Auditory evoked potentials during sleep in normal children from ten days to three years of age. *Electroencephalography and Clinical Neurophysiology, 39*, 29–41. doi:10.1016/0013-4694(75)90124-8

Baynes, K., Kegl, J. A., Brentari, D., Kussmaul, C., & Poizner, H. (1998). Chronic auditory agnosia following Landau Kleffner syndrome: A 23 year outcome study. *Brain and Language, 63*(3), 381–425. doi:10.1006/brln.1998.1955

Bidelman, G. M. (2015). Towards an optimal paradigm for simultaneously recording cortical and brainstem auditory evoked potentials. *Journal of Neuroscience Methods, 241*, 94–100. doi:10.1016/j.jneumeth.2014.12.019

Billiet, C. R., & Bellis, T. J. (2011). The relationship between brainstem temporal processing and performance on tests of central auditory function in children with reading disorders. *Journal of Speech, Language, and Hearing Research, 54*, 228–242. doi:210.1044/1092-4388(2010/1009-0239)

Brown, C. R., Clarke, A. R., Barry, R. J., McCarthy, R., Selikowitz, M., & Magee, C. (2005). Event-related potentials in attention-deficit/ hyperactivity disorder of the predominantly inattentive type: An investigation of EEG-defined subtypes. *International Journal of Psychophysiology, 58*(1), 94–107. doi:10.1016/j.ijpsycho.2005.03.012

Brown, P. (2013). ADHD and the DSM-5: Update on Revisions to Diagnostic Criteria. *Consultant for Pediatricians, 12*(10), 453–454.

Bruneau, N., Bonnet-Brilhault, F., Gomot, M., Adrien, J. L., & Barthélémy, C. (2003). Cortical auditory processing and communication in children with autism: Electrophysiological/behavioral relations. *International Journal of Psychophysiology, 51*(1), 17–25. doi:10.1016/S0167-8760(03)00149-1

Burkard, R. F., Don, M., & Eggermont, J. J. (2007). *Auditory evoked potentials: Basic principles and clinical applications*. Baltimore, MD: Lippincott Williams & Wilkins.

Cacace, A. T., & McFarland, D. J. (2002). Middle-latency auditory evoked potentials: Basic issues and potential applications. In J. Katz, R. F. Burkard, & L. Medwetseky (Eds.), *Handbook of clinical audiology* (5th ed., pp. 349–377). Baltimore, MD: Williams and Wilkins.

Campbell, J. D., Cardon, G., & Sharma, A. (2011). Clinical application of the P1 cortical auditory evoked potential biomarker in children with sensorineural hearing loss and auditory neuropathy spectrum disorder. *Seminars in Hearing, 32*(2), 147–155. doi:10.1055/s-0031-1277236

Castrén, M., Pääkkönen, A., Tarkka, I. M., Ryynänen, M., & Partanen, J. (2003). Augmentation of auditory N1 in children with Fragile-X syndrome. *Brain Topography, 15*(3), 165–171. doi:10.1023/A:1022606200636

Ceponienè, R., Cheour, M., & Näätänen, R. (1998). Interstimulus interval and auditory event-related potentials in children: Evidence of multiple generators. *Electroencephalography and Clinical Neurophysiology, 108*(4), 345–354. doi:10.1016/S0168-5597(97)00081-6

Ceponienè, R., Rinne, T., & Näätänen, R. (2002). Maturation of cortical sound processing as indexed by event-related potentials. *Clinical Neurophysiology, 113*(6), 870–882. doi:10.1016/S1388-2457(02)00078-0

Chermak, G. D., & Bellis, T. J. (2013). Differential diagnosis of central auditory processing disorder and attention deficit/hyperactivity disorder. In F. E. Musiek & G. D. Chermak (Eds.), *Handbook of central auditory processing disorder, Volume I: Auditory neuroscience and diagnosis* (pp. 557–590). San Diego, CA: Plural.

Collet, L., Duclaux, R., Challamel, M. J., & Revol, M. (1988). Effect of sleep on middle latency response (MLR) in infants. *Brain and Development, 10*(3), 169–173. doi:10.1016/S0387-7604(88)80022-6

Cone-Wesson, B., Kurtzberg, D., & Vaughan, H. G. J. (1987). Electrophysiologic assessment of auditory pathways in high risk infants. *International Journal of Pediatric Otorhinolaryngology, 14*(2–3), 203–214. doi:10.1016/0165-5876(87)90032-2

Cone-Wesson, B., & Wunderlich, J. (2003). Auditory evoked potentials from the cortex: Audiology applications. *Current Opinion in Otolaryngology and Head and Neck Surgery, 11*(5), 372–377. doi:10.1097/00020840-200310000-00011

Cunningham, J., Nicol, T., Zecker, S., Bradlow, A., & Kraus, N. (2001). Neurobiologic responses to speech in noise in children with learning problems: Deficits and strategies for improvement. *Clinical Neurophysiology, 112*(5), 758–767. http://dx.doi.org/10.1016/S1388-2457(01)00465-5

Cunningham, J., Nicol, T., Zecker, S., & Kraus, N. (2000). Speech-evoked neurophysiologic responses in children with learning problems: Development and behavioral correlates of perception. *Ear and Hearing, 21*(6), 554–568.

Davies, P. L., Chang, W. P., & Gavin, W. J. (2010). Middle and late latency ERP components discriminate between adults, typical children, and children with sensory processing disorders. *Frontiers in Integrative Neuroscience, 4*. doi:10.3389/fnint.2010.00016

Davis, H. (1976). Brainstem and other response audiometry. *Annals of Otology, Rhinology and Laryngology, 85*, 3–14. doi:10.3109/00016487709128823

Davis, H., Mast, T., Yoshie, N., & Zerlin, S. (1966). The slow response of the human cortex to auditory stimuli: Recovery process. *Electroencephalography and Clinical Neurophysiology, 21*(2), 105–113. doi:10.1016/0013-4694(66)90118-0

Dillon, H. (2005). So, baby, how does it sound? Cortical assessment of infants with hearing aids. *Hearing Journal, 58*(10), 10.

Dinces, E., Chobot-Rhodd, J., & Sussman, E. (2009). Behavioral and electrophysiological measures of auditory change detection in children following late cochlear implantation: A preliminary study. *International Journal of Pediatric Otorhinolaryngology, 73*(6), 843–851. doi:10.1016/j.ijporl.2009.03.002

Drake, M. E., Jr., Weate, S. J., & Newell, S. A. (1996). Auditory evoked potentials in postconcussive syndrome. *Electromyography and Clinical Neurophysiology, 36*(8), 457–462.

Eggermont, J. J., & Ponton, C. W. (2003). Auditory-evoked potential studies of cortical maturation in normal hearing and implanted children: Correlations with changes in structure and speech perception. *Acta Otolaryngolgica, 123*(2), 249–252. doi:10.1080/0036554021000028098

Eggermont, J. J., Ponton, C. W., Don, M., Waring, M. D., & Kwong, B. (1997). Maturational delays in cortical evoked potentials in cochlear implant users. *Acta Oto-Laryngologica, 117*(2), 161–163. doi:10.3109/00016489709117760

Estes, R. I., Jerger, J., & Jacobson, G. (2002). Reversal of hemispheric asymmetry on auditory tasks in children who are poor listeners. *Journal of the American Academy of Audiology, 13*(2), 59–71.

Fifer, R. C. (1985). *The MLR and SSEP in neonates*. Houston, TX: Baylor College of Medicine.

Firszt, J. B., Chambers, R. D., & Kraus, N. (2002). Neurophysiology of cochlear implant users II: Comparison among speech perception, dynamic range, and physiological measures. *Ear and Hearing, 23*(6), 516–531. doi:10.1097/01.AUD.0000042154.70495.DE

Friesen, L. M., Tremblay, K. L., Rohila, N., Wright, R. A., Shannon, R. V., Başkent, D., & Rubinstein, J. T. (2009). Evoked cortical activity and speech recognition as a function of the number of simulated cochlear implant channels. *Clinical Neurophysiology, 120*(4), 776–782.

Frizzo, A. C. F., Funayama, C. A. R., Isaac, M. L., & Colafêmina, J. F. (2007). Auditory middle latency responses: A study of healthy children. *Brazilian Journal of Otorhinolaryngology, 73*(3), 398–403. doi:http://dx.doi.org/10.1590/S0034-72992007000300016

Fruhstorfer, H., Soveri, P., & Järvilehto, T. (1970). Short-term habituation of the auditory evoked response in man. *Electroencephalography and Clinical Neurophysiology, 28*(2), 153–161. doi:10.1016/0013-4694(70)90183-5

Gaetz, M., & Weinberg, H. (2000). Electrophysiological indices of persistent post-concussion symptoms. *Brain Injury, 14*(9), 815–832.

Gardner-Berry, K., Purdy, S. C., Ching, T. Y., & Dillon, H. (2015). The audiological journey and early outcomes of twelve infants with auditory neuropathy spectrum disorder from birth to two years of age. *International Journal of Audiology, 27*, 1–12. doi:10.3109/14992027.2015.1007214

Geisler, C. D., Frishkopf, L. S., & Rosenblith, W. A. (1958). Extracranial responses to acoustic clicks in man. *Science, 128*(3333), 1210–1211. doi:10.1126/science.128.3333.1210

Gilley, P. M., Sharma, A., & Dorman, M. (2008). Cortical reorganization in children with cochlear implants. *Brain Research, 1239*, 56–65. doi:10.1016/j.brainres.2008.08.026

Gilley, P. M., Sharma, A., Dorman, M., & Martin, K. (2005). Developmental changes in refractoriness of the cortical auditory evoked potential. *Clinical Neurophysiology, 116*(3), 648–657. doi:10.1016/j.clinph.2004.09.009

Gilley, P. M., Sharma, A., Dorman, M., & Martin, K. (2006). Abnormalities in central auditory maturation in children with language-based learning problems. *Clinical Neurophysiology, 117*(9), 1949–1956. doi:10.1016/j.clinph.2006.05.015

Giraud, A. L., Truy, E., & Frackowiak, R. (2001). Imaging plasticity in cochlear implant patients. *Audiology and Neuro-Otology, 6*(6), 381–393. doi:10.1159/000046847

Golding, M., Purdy, S., Sharma, M., & Dillon, H. (2006). The effect of stimulus duration and inter-stimulus interval on cortical responses in infants. *Australian and New Zealand Journal of Audiology, 28*(2), 122–136. doi:10.1375/audi.28.2.122

Goldstein, R., & Rodman, L. B. (1967). Early components of averaged evoked responses to rapidly repeated auditory stimuli. *Journal of Speech and Hearing Research, 10*(4), 697–705. doi:10.1044/jshr.1004.697

Gomes, H., Dunn, M., Ritter, W., Kurtzberg, D., Brattson, A., Kreuzer, J., & Vaughan, H. G., Jr. (2001). Spatiotemporal maturation of the central and lateral N1 components to tones. *Developmental Brain Research, 129*(2), 147–155. doi:10.1016/S0165-3806(01)00196-1

Gordon, K. A., Papsin, B. C., & Harrison, R. V. (2004). Thalamocortical activity and plasticity in children using cochlear implants. *International Congress Series, 1273*, 76–79. doi:10.1016/j.ics.2004.08.026

Gordon, K. A., Papsin, B. C., & Harrison, R. V. (2005). Effects of cochlear implant use on the electrically evoked middle latency response in children. *Hearing Research, 204*(1–2), 78–89. doi:10.1016/j.heares.2005.01.003

Gordon, K. A., Tanaka, S., Wong, D. D. E., & Papsin, B. C. (2008). Characterizing responses from auditory cortex in young people with several years of cochlear implant experience. *Clinical Neurophysiology, 119*(10), 2347–2362. http://dx.doi.org/10.1016/j.clinph.2008.06.013

Groenen, P., Snik, A., & van den Broek, P. (1997). Electrically evoked auditory middle latency responses versus perception abilities in cochlear implant users. *Audiology, 36*(2), 83–97. doi:10.3109/00206099709071963

Gumenyuk, V., Korzyukov, O., Escera, C., Hämäläinen, M., Häyrinen, T., Oksanen, H., . . . Alho, K. (2005). Electrophysiological evidence of enhanced distractibility in ADHD children. *Neuroscience Letters, 374*(3), 212–217. doi:10.1016/j.neulet.2004.10.081

Hall, J. W., III. (1992). *Handbook of auditory evoked responses*. Needham Heights, MA: Allyn & Bacon.

Hall, J. W., III. (2007). *New handbook of auditory evoked responses*. Boston, MA: Allyn & Bacon.

Hall, J. W., III. (2015). *eHandbook of auditory evoked responses*. Kindle Direct Publishing. http://www.Amazon.com/dp/B0145G2FFM

Hall, J. W., III., Huang-fu, M., & Gennarelli, T. A. (1982). Auditory function in acute severe head injury. *Laryngoscope, 92*(8 Pt. 1), 883–890. doi:10.1288/00005537-198208000-00009

Hamaguchi, P. A., & Tazeau, Y. N. (2007). Comorbidity of APD with other "look-alikes." In D. Ross-Swain & D. Geffner (Eds.), *Auditory processing disorders: Assessment, management and treatment* (pp. 49–73). San Diego, CA: Plural.

Hari, R., Kaila, K., Katila, T., Tuomisto, T., & Varpula, T. (1982). Interstimulus interval dependence of the auditory vertex response and its magnetic counterpart: Implications for their neural generation. *Electroencephalography and Clinical Neurophysiology, 54*(5), 561–569. doi:10.1016/0013-4694(82)90041-4

Hassaan, M. R. (2015). Auditory evoked cortical potentials with competing noise in children with auditory figure ground deficit. *Hearing, Balance and Communication, 13*(1), 15–23. doi:10.3109/21695717.2014.998860

Hayes, E. A., Warrier, C. M., Nicol, T. G., Zecker, S. G., & Kraus, N. (2003). Neural plasticity following auditory training in children with learning problems. *Clinical Neurophysiology, 114*(4), 673–684. doi:http://dx.doi.org/10.1016/S1388-2457(02)00414-5

Helenius, P., Parviainen, T., Paetau, R., & Salmelin, R. (2009). Neural processing of spoken words in specific language impairment and dyslexia. *Brain, 132*, 1918–1927. http://dx.doi.org/10.1093/brain/awp134

Helenius, P., Sivonen, P., Parviainen, T., Isoaho, P., Hannus, S., Kauppila, T., . . . Isotalo, L. (2014). Abnormal functioning of the left temporal lobe in language-impaired children. *Brain and Language, 130*, 11–18. doi:10.1016/j.bandl.2014.01.005

Huttenlocher, P. R., & Dabholkar, A. S. (1997). Regional differences in synaptogenesis in human cerebral cortex. *Journal of Comparative Neurology, 387*(2), 167–178. doi:10.1002/(SICI)1096-9861(19971020)387:23.0.CO;2-Z

Illing, R. B. (2004). Maturation and plasticity of the central auditory system. *Acta Otolaryngologica Supplementum, 552*, 6–10. doi:10.1080/03655230410017157

Jasper, H. (1958). The 10–20 electrode system of the International Federation. *Electroencephalography and Clinical Neurophysiology, 10*, 371–375.

Jerger, J. (2007). Auditory evoked potentials in infants: Thinking out of the box. *Journal of the American Academy of Audiology, 18*(5), 356.

Jerger, J., Martin, J., & McColl, R. (2004). Interaural cross correlation of event-related potentials and diffusion tensor imaging in the evaluation of auditory processing disorder: A case study. *Journal of the American Academy of Audiology, 15*(1), 79–87. doi:10.3766/jaaa.15.1.8

Jerger, J., Moncrieff, D., Greenwald, R., Wambacq, I., & Seipel, A. (2000). Effect of age on interaural asymmetry of event-related potentials in a dichotic listening task. *Journal of the American Academy of Audiology, 11*(7), 383–389.

Jerger, J., Thibodeau, L., Martin, J., Mehta, J., Tilman, G., Greenwald, R., & Overson, G. (2002). Behavioral and electrophysiologic evidence of auditory processing disorder: A twin study. *Journal of the American Academy of Audiology, 13*(8), 438–460.

Jerger, S., Martin, R. C., & Jerger, J. (1987). Specific auditory perceptual dysfunction in a learning disabled child. *Ear and Hearing, 8*(2), 78–86. doi:10.1097/00003446-198704000-00004

Jirsa, R. E. (1992). The clinical utility of the P3 AERP in children with auditory processing disorders. *Journal of Speech and Hearing Research, 35*(4), 903–912.

Jirsa, R. E., & Clontz, K. B. (1990). Long latency auditory event-related potentials from children with auditory processing disorders. *Ear and Hearing, 11*(3), 222–232. doi:10.1097/00003446-199006000-00010

Joint Committee on Infant Hearing (JCIH; 2007). Year 2007 position statement: Principles and guidelines for early hearing detection and intervention programs. *Pediatrics, 120*, 898–921.

Jonkman, L. M., Kemner, C., Verbaten, M. N., Koelega, H. S., Camfferman, G., vd Gaag, R., . . . van Engeland, H. (1997). Event-related potentials and performance of attention-deficit hyperactivity disorder: Children and normal controls in auditory and visual selective attention tasks. *Biological Psychiatry, 41*(5), 595–611. doi:10.1016/S0006-3223(96)00073-X

Jutras, B., Lagacé, J., Lavigne, A., Boissonneault, A., & Lavoie, C. (2007). Auditory processing disorders, verbal disfluency and learning difficulties: A case study. *International Journal of Audiology, 46*(1), 31–38. doi:10.1080/14992020601083321

Keidel, W. D., & Spreng, M. (1965). Neurophysiological evidence for the Steven's power function in man. *Journal of the Acoustical Society of America, 38*, 191–195. http://dx.doi.org/10.1121/1.1909629

Kemner, C., Jonkman, L. M., Kenemans, J. L., Böcker, K. B. E., Verbaten, M. N., & van Engeland, H. (2004). Sources of auditory selective attention and the effects of methyl phenidate in children with attention-deficit/hyperactivity disorder. *Biological Psychiatry, 55*(7), 776–778.

Kemner, C., Oranje, B., Verbaten, M. N., & van Engeland, H. (2002). Normal P50 gating in children with autism. *Journal of Clinical Psychiatry, 63*(3), 214–217.

Kileny, P. R., Kemink, J. L., & Miller, J. M. (1989). An intrasubject comparison of electric and acoustic middle latency responses. *American Journal of Otology, 10*(1), 23–27.

Klein, S. K., Kurtzberg, D., Brattson, A., Kreuzer, J. A., Stapells, D. R., Dunn, M. A., . . . Vaughan, H. G., Jr. (1995). Electrophysiologic manifestations of impaired temporal lobe auditory processing in verbal auditory agnosia. *Brain and Language, 51*(3), 383–405.

Kral, A. (2007). Unimodal and cross-modal plasticity in the "deaf" auditory cortex. *International Journal of Audiology, 46*(9), 479–493. doi:10.1080/14992020701383027

Kral, A., Hartmann, R., Tillein, J., Heid, S., & Klinke, R. (2001). Delayed maturation and sensitive periods in the auditory cortex. *Audiology and Neuro-Otology, 6*(6), 346–362. doi:10.1159/000046845

Kral, A., & Sharma, A. (2012). Developmental neuroplasticity after cochlear implantation. *Trends in Neurosciences, 35*(2), 111–122. doi:10.1016/j.tins.2011.09.004

Kraus, N. (2001). Auditory pathway encoding and neural plasticity in children with learning problems. *Audiology and Neuro-Otology, 6*(4), 221–227. doi:10.1159/000046837

Kraus, N., Kileny, P., & McGee, T. (1994). Middle latency auditory evoked potentials. In J. Katz, W. L. Gabbay, S. Gold, L. Medwetsky & R. A. Ruth (Eds.), *Handbook of clinical audiology* (4th ed., pp. 387–405). Baltimore, MD: Williams and Wilkins.

Kraus, N., & McGee, T. J. (1994). Mismatch negativity in the assessment of central auditory function. *American Journal of Audiology, 3*, 39–51. doi:10.1044/1059-0889.0302.39

Kraus, N., McGee, T. J., Carrell, T. D., Zecker, S. G., Nicol, T. G., & Koch, D. B. (1996). Auditory neurophysiologic responses and discrimination deficits in children with learning problems. *Science, 273*(5277), 971–973. doi:10.1126/science.273.5277.971

Kraus, N., McGee, T. J., & Comperatore, C. (1989). MLRs in children are consistently present during wakefulness, stage 1, and REM sleep. *Ear and Hearing, 10*(6), 339–345. doi:10.1097/00003446-198912000-00004

Kraus, N., Özdamar, O., Hier, D., & Stein, L. (1982). Auditory middle latency responses (MLRs) in patients with cortical lesions. *Electroencephalography and Clinical Neurophysiology, 54*(3), 275–287. doi:10.1016/0013-4694(82)90177-8

Kraus, N., Reed, N., Smith, D. I., Stein, L., & Cartee, C. (1987). High-pass filter settings affect the detectability of MLRs in humans. *Electroencephalography and Clinical Neurophysiology, 68*(3), 234–236. doi:10.1016/0168-5597(87)90033-5

Kraus, N., Smith, D. I., Reed, N. L., Stein, L. K., & Cartee, C. (1985). Auditory middle latency responses in children: Effects of age and diagnostic category. *Electroencephalography and Clinical Neurophysiology, 62*(5), 343–351. doi:10.1016/0168-5597(85)90043-7

Lamas, F. A., López-Herce, J., Sánchez, P. L., Mencía, B. S., Borrego, D. R., & Carrillo, A. A. (2006). Middle latency auditory evoked potentials in critical care children: Preliminary study [Article in Spanish]. *Annals of Pediatrics (Barc). 64*(4), 354–359. Retrieved August 25, 2008, from http://www.ncbi.nlm.nih.gov/pubmed/16606573

Liasis, A., Boyd, S., Rivera-Gaxiola, M., & Towell, A. (2003). Speech and nonspeech processing in hemispherectomised children: An event-related potential study. *Cognitive Brain Research, 17*(3), 665–673. doi:10.1016/S0926-6410(03)00190-3

Martin, B. A., Boothroyd, A., Ali, D., & Leach-Berth, T. (2010). Stimulus presentation strategies for eliciting the acoustic change complex: Increasing efficiency. *Ear and Hearing, 31*(3), 356–366. doi:10.1097/AUD.0b013e3181ce6355

Martin, B. A., Tremblay, K. L., & Korczak, P. (2008). Speech evoked potentials: From the laboratory to the clinic. *Ear and Hearing, 29*(3), 285–313. doi:10.1097/AUD.0b013e3181662c0e

Martinez, A. S., Eisenberg, L. S., & Boothroyd, A. (2013). The acoustic change complex in young children with hearing loss: A preliminary study. *Seminars in Hearing, 34*(4), 278–287. doi:10.1055/s-0033-1356640

Mason, S. M., & Mellor, D. H. (1984). Brain-stem, middle latency and late cortical evoked potentials in children with speech and language disorders. *Electroencephalography and Clinical Neurophysiology, 59*(4), 297–309. doi:10.1016/0168-5597(84)90047-9

McArthur, G. M., & Bishop, D. V. M. (2004). Which people with specific language impairment have auditory processing deficits? *Cognitive Neuropsychology, 21*(1), 79–94. doi:10.1080/02643290342000087

McGee, T., & Kraus, N. (1996). Auditory development reflected by middle latency response. *Ear and Hearing, 17*(5), 419–429. doi:10.1097/00003446-199610000-00008

McRandle, C. C., Smith, M. A., & Goldstein, R. (1974). Early averaged electroencephalic responses to clicks in neonates. *Annals of Otology, Rhinology, and Laryngology, 83*(5), 695–702. doi:10.1177/000348947408300519

Mendel, M. I., Adkinson, C. D., & Harker, L. A. (1977). Middle components of the auditory evoked potentials in infants. *Annals of Otology, Rhinology, and Laryngology, 86*(3 Pt. 1), 293–299.

Mendelson, T., & Salamy, A. (1981). Maturational effects on the middle components of the averaged electroencephalic response. *Journal of Speech and Hearing Research, 24*(1), 140–144.

Metz-Lutz, M. N., Hirsch, E., Maquet, P., De Saint Martin, A., Rudolf, G., Wioland, N., & Marescaux, C. (1997). Dichotic listening performances in the follow-up of Landau and Kleffner syndrome. *Child Neuropsychology, 3*(1), 47–60. doi:10.1080/09297049708401367

Michalewski, H. J., Starr, A., Nguyen, T. T., Kong, Y. Y., & Zeng, F. G. (2005). Auditory temporal processes in normal-hearing individuals and in patients with auditory neuropathy. *Clinical Neurophysiology, 116*(3), 669–680. http://dx.doi.org/10.1016/j.clinph.2004.09.027

Miliciç, D., Alçada, M. N., Pais, C. L., Vecerina-Voliç, S., Jurkoviç, J., & Pais, C. M. (1998). A study of auditory afferent organization in children with dyslalia. *International Journal of Pediatric Otorhinolaryngology, 46*(1–2), 43–56. http://dx.doi.org/10.1016/S0165-5876(98)00135-9

Moncrieff, D., Jerger, J., Wambacq, I., Greenwald, R., & Black, J. (2004). ERP evidence of a dichotic left-ear deficit in some dyslexic children. *Journal of the American Academy of Audiology, 15*(7), 518–534. http://dx.doi.org/10.3766/jaaa.15.7.6

Moore, J. K. (2002). Maturation of human auditory cortex: Implications for speech perception. *Annals of Otology, Rhinology, and Laryngology Supplement, 189*, 7–10.

Moore, J. K., & Guan, Y. L. (2001). Cytoarchitectural and axonal maturation in human auditory cortex. *Journal of the Association for Research in Otolaryngology, 2*(4), 297–311. doi:10.1007/s101620010052

Moore, J. K., & Linthicum, F. H., Jr. (2007). The human auditory system: A timeline of development. *International Journal of Audiology, 46*(9), 460–478. doi:10.1080/14992020701383019

Musiek, F. E. (2004). The DIID: A new treatment for APD. *Hearing Journal, 57*(7), 50. doi:10.1097/01.HJ.0000293049.80297.cd

Musiek, F. E., Geurkink, N. A., Weider, D. J., & Donnelly, K. (1984). Past, present, and future applications of the auditory middle latency response. *Laryngoscope, 94*(12 Pt. 1), 1545–1553. doi:10.1288/00005537-198412000-00002

Näätänen, R., & Picton, T. (1987). The N1 wave of the human electric and magnetic response to sound: A review and an analysis of the component structure. *Psychophysiology, 24*(4), 375–425.

Nelson, D. A., & Lassman, F. M. (1968). Effects of intersignal interval on the human auditory evoked response. *Journal of the Acoustical Society of America, 44*(6), 1529–1532. doi:10.1121/1.1911292

Oades, R. D. (1998). Frontal, temporal and lateralized brain function in children with attention-deficit hyperactivity disorder: A psychophysiological and neuropsychological viewpoint on development. *Behavioural Brain Research, 94*(1), 83–95. doi:10.1016/S0166-4328(97)00172-1

Oades, R. D., Dittman-Balcar, A., Schepker, R., Eggers, C., & Zerbin, D. (1996). Auditory event-related potentials (ERPs) and mismatch negativity (MMN) in healthy children and those with attention-deficit or Tourette/tic symptoms. *Biological Psychology, 43*(2), 163–185. doi:10.1016/0301-0511(96)05189-7

Ohlrich, E. S., Barnet, A. B., Weiss, I. P., & Shanks, B. L. (1978). Auditory evoked potential development in early childhood: A longitudinal study. *Electroencephalography and Clinical Neurophysiology, 44*(4), 411–423. doi:10.1016/0013-4694(78)90026-3

Okitsu, T. (1984). Middle components of the auditory evoked response in young children. *Scandinavian Audiology, 13*(2), 83–86. doi:10.3109/14992028409043044

Orekhova, E. V., Stroganova, T. A., Prokofiev, A. O., Nygren, G., Gillberg, C., & Elam, M. (2009). The right hemisphere fails to respond to temporal novelty in autism: Evidence from an ERP study. *Clinical Neurophysiology, 120*(3), 520-529. doi:10.1016/j.clinph.2008.12.034

Orekhova, E. V., Tsetlin, M. M., Butorina, A. V., Novikova, S. I., Gratchev, V. V., Sokolov, P. A., . . . Stroganova, T. A. (2012). Auditory cortex responses to clicks and sensory modulation difficulties in children with autism spectrum disorders (ASD). *PLoS ONE, 7*(6), e39906. doi:10.1371/journal.pone.0039906

Pasman, J. W., Rotteveel, J. J., de Graaf, R., Maassen, B., & Notermans, S. L. (1991). Detectability of auditory evoked response components in preterm infants. *Early Human Development, 26*(2), 129–141. http://dx.doi.org/10.1016/0378-3782(91)90017-W

Pearce, W., Golding, M., & Dillon, H. (2007). Cortical auditory evoked potentials in the assessment of auditory neuropathy: Two case studies. *Journal of the American Academy of Audiology, 18*(5), 380–390. doi:10.3766/jaaa.18.5.3

Picton, T. W. (2011). *Human auditory evoked potentials*. San Diego, CA: Plural.

Picton, T. W., Hillyard, S. A., Krausz, H. I., & Galambos, I. (1974). Human auditory evoked potentials. I. Evaluation of components. *Electroencephalography and Clinical Neurophysiology, 36*(2), 179–190. doi:10.1016/0013-4694(74)90155-2

Picton, T. W., Woods, D. L., Baribeau-Braun, J., & Healy, T. M. G. (1977). Evoked potential audiometry. *Journal of Otolaryngology, 6*, 90–119.

Plaza, M., Rigoard, M. T., Chevrie-Muller, C., Cohen, H., & Picard, A. (2001). Short-term memory impairment and unilateral dichotic listening extinction in a child with Landau-Kleffner syndrome: Auditory or phonological disorder? *Brain and Cognition, 46*(1–2), 235–240. doi:10.1016/S0278-2626(01)80074-9

Ponton, C. W., Don, M., Eggermont, J. J., Waring, M. D., Kwong, B., & Masuda, A. (1996). Auditory system plasticity in children after long periods of complete deafness. *Neuroreport, 8*(1), 61–65. doi:10.1097/00001756-199612200-00013

Ponton, C. W., Don, M., Eggermont, J. J., Waring, M. D., & Masuda, A. (1996). Maturation of human cortical auditory function: Differences between normal-hearing children and children with cochlear implants. *Ear and Hearing, 17*(5), 430–437. doi:10.1097/00003446-199610000-00009

Ponton, C. W., Eggermont, J. J., Khosla, D., Kwong, B., & Don, M. (2002). Maturation of human central auditory system activity: Separating auditory evoked potentials by dipole source modeling. *Clinical Neurophysiology, 113*(3), 407–420. http://dx.doi.org/10.1016/S1388-2457(01)00733-7

Ponton, C. W., Eggermont, J. J., Kwong, B., & Don, M. (2000). Maturation of human central auditory system activity: Evidence from multi-channel evoked potentials. *Clinical Neurophysiology*. doi:10.1016/S1388–2457(99)00236-9

Ponton, C. W., Moore, J. K., & Eggermont, J. J. (1999). Prolonged deafness limits auditory system developmental plasticity: Evidence from an evoked potentials study in children with cochlear implants. *Scandinavian Audiology Supplement, 51*, 13–22.

Prosser, S., & Arslan, E. (1985). Does general anaesthesia affect the child's auditory middle latency response (MLR)? *Scandinavian Audiology, 14*(2), 105–107. doi:10.3109/01050398509045930

Psillas, G., & Daniilidis, J. (2003). Low-frequency hearing assessment by middle latency responses in children with pervasive developmental disorder. *International Journal of Pediatric Otorhinolaryngology, 67*(6), 613–619. doi:10.1016/S0165-5876(03)00071-5

Purdy, S. C., Kelly, A. S., & Davies, M. G. (2002). Auditory brainstem response, middle latency response, and late cortical evoked potentials in children with learning disabilities. *Journal of the American Academy of Audiology, 13*(7), 367–382.

Purdy, S. C., Kelly, A. S., & Thorne, P. R. (2001). Auditory evoked potentials as measures of plasticity in humans. *Audiology and Neuro-Otology, 6*(4), 211–215. doi:10.1159/000046835

Purdy, S. C., Sharma, M., Munro, K. J., & Morgan, C. L. (2013). Stimulus level effects on speech-evoked obligatory cortical auditory evoked potentials in infants with normal hearing. *Clinical Neurophysiology, 124*(3), 474–480. doi:10.1016/j.clinph.2012.09.011

Rance, G., Cone-Wesson, B., Wunderlich, J., & Dowell, R. (2002). Speech perception and cortical event-related potentials in children with auditory neuropathy. *Ear and Hearing, 23*(3), 239–253. doi:10.1097/00003446-200206000-00008

Rapin, I., Ruben, R. J., & Lyttle, M. (1970). Diagnosis of hearing loss in infants using auditory evoked responses. *Laryngoscope, 80*(5), 712–722. doi:10.1288/00005537-197005000-00003

Roberts, T. P., Lanza, M. R., Dell, J., Qasmieh, S., Hines, K., Blaskey, L., . . . Berman, J. I. (2013). Maturational differences in thalamocortical white matter microstructure and auditory evoked response latencies in autism spectrum disorders. *Brain Research, 6*(1537), 79–85. doi:10.1016/j.brainres.2013.09.011

Rogers, S. H., Edwards, D. A., Henderson-Smart, D. J., & Pettigrew, A. G. (1989). Middle latency auditory evoked responses in normal term infants: A longitudinal study. *Neuropediatrics, 20*(2), 59–63. doi:10.1055/s-2008-1071266

Rothman, H. H., Davis, H., & Hay, I. S. (1970). Slow evoked cortical potentials and temporal features of stimulation. *Electroencephalography and Clinical Neurophysiology, 29*(3), 225–232. http://dx.doi.org/10.1016/0013-4694(70)90135-5

Rotteveel, J. J., Colon, E. J., de Graaf, R., Notermans, S. L., Stoelinga, G. B., & Visco, Y. M. (1986). The central auditory conduction at term date and three months after birth III. Middle latency responses (MLRs). *Scandinavian Audiology, 15*(2), 75–84.

Rotteveel, J. J., Stegeman, D. F., de Graaf, R., Colon, E. J., & Visco, Y. M. (1987). The maturation of the central auditory conduction in preterm infants until three months post term. III. The middle latency auditory evoked response (MLR). *Hearing Research, 27*(3), 245–256. doi:10.1016/0378-5955(87)90006-2

Sabatini, B. L., & Regehr, W. G. (1999). Timing of synaptic transmission. *Annual Review of Physiology, 61*, 521–542.

Schochat, E., & Musiek, F. E. (2006). Maturation of outcomes of behavioral and electrophysiologic tests of central auditory function. *Journal of Communication Disorders, 39*(1), 78–92. doi:10.1016/j.jcomdis.2005.10.001

Schochat, E., Musiek, F. E., Alonso, R., & Ogata, J. (2010). Effect of auditory training on the middle latency response in children with (central) auditory processing disorder. *Brazilian Journal of Medical and Biological Research, 43*(8), 777–785. doi:10.1590/S0100-879X2010007500069

Seidl, R., Hauser, E., Bernert, G., Marx, M., Freilinger, M., & Lubec, G. (1997). Auditory evoked potentials in young patients with Down syndrome. Event-related potentials (P3) and histaminergic system. *Cognitive Brain Research, 5*(4), 301–309. doi:10.1016/S0926-6410(97)00008-6

Seri, S., Cerquiglini, A., & Pisani, F. (1998). Spike induced interference in auditory sensory processing in Landau-Kleffner syndrome. *Electroencephalography and Clinical Neurophysiology, 108*(5), 506–510.

Seri, S., Cerquiglini, A., Pisani, F., & Curatolo, P. (1999). Autism in tuberous sclerosis: Evoked potential evidence for a deficit in auditory sensory processing. *Clinical Neurophysiology, 110*(10), 1825–1830. doi:10.1016/S1388-2457(99)00137-6

Sharma, A., Campbell, J., & Cardon, G. (2015). Developmental and cross-modal plasticity in deafness: Evidence from the P1 and N1 event related potentials in cochlear implanted children. *International Journal of Psychophysiology, 95*(2), 135–144. doi:10.1016/j.ijpsycho.2014.04.007

Sharma, A., Dorman, M. F., & Kral, A. (2005). The influence of a sensitive period on central auditory development in children with unilateral and bilateral cochlear implants. *Hearing Research, 203*(1–2), 134–143.

Sharma, A., Dorman, M. F., & Spahr, A. J. (2002a). Rapid development of cortical auditory evoked potentials after early cochlear implantation. *Neuroreport, 13*(10), 1365–1368.

Sharma, A., Dorman, M. F., & Spahr, A. J. (2002b). A sensitive period for the development of the central auditory system in children with cochlear implants: Implications for age of implantation. *Ear and Hearing, 23*(6), 532–539. doi:10.1097/01.AUD.0000042223.62381.01

Sharma, A., Gilley, P. M., Dorman, M. F., & Baldwin, R. (2007). Deprivation-induced cortical reorganization in children with cochlear implants. *International Journal of Audiology, 46*(9), 494–499.

Sharma, A., Glick, H., Campbell, J., & Biever, A. (2013). Central auditory development in children with hearing impairment: Clinical relevance of the P1 CAEP biomarker in children with multiple disabilities. *Hearing, Balance and Communication, 11*(3). doi:10.3109/21695717.2013.812378

Sharma, A., Kraus, N., McGee, T. J., & Nicol, T. G. (1997). Developmental changes in P1 and N1 central auditory responses elicited by consonant-vowel syllables. *Electroencephalography and Clinical Neurophysiology, 104*(6), 540–545. doi:http://dx.doi.org/10.1016/S0168-5597(97)00050-6

Sharma, A., Martin, K., Roland, P., Bauer, P., Sweeney, M. H., Gilley, P. M., & Dorman, M. (2005). P1 latency as a biomarker for central auditory development in children with hearing impairment. *Journal of the American Academy of Audiology, 16*(8), 564–573. doi:10.3766/jaaa.16.8.5

Sharma, A., Nash, A., & Dorman, M. (2009). Cortical development, plasticity and re-organization in children with cochlear implants. *Journal of Communication Disorders, 42*, 272–279. doi:10.1016/j.jcomdis.2009.03.003

Sharma, A., Tobey, E., Dorman, M., Bharadwaj, S., Martin, K., Gilley, P. M., & Kunkel, F. (2004). Central auditory maturation and babbling development in infants with cochlear implants. *Archives of Otolaryngology-Head and Neck Surgery, 130*(5), 511–516. doi:10.1001/archotol.130.5.511

Sharma, M., Johnson, P. K., Purdy, S. C., & Norman, F. (2013). Effect of interstimulus interval and age on cortical auditory evoked potentials in 10–22-week-old infants. *Neuroreport, 25*(4), 248–254. doi:10.1097/WNR.0000000000000078

Sharma, M., Purdy, S., & Kelly, A. S. (2014). The contribution of speech-evoked cortical auditory evoked potentials to the diagnosis and measurement of intervention outcomes in children with auditory processing disorder. *Seminars in Hearing, 35*(1), 51–64. http://dx.doi.org/10.1055/s-0033-1363524

Shepherd, R. K., & Hardie, N. A. (2001). Deafness-induced changes in the auditory pathway: Implications for cochlear implants. *Audiology and Neuro-Otology, 6*(6), 305–318. doi:10.1159/000046843

Silva, L. A., Couto, M. I., Tsuji, R. K., Bento, R. F., Matas, C. G., & Carvalho, A. C. (2014). Auditory pathways' maturation after cochlear implant via cortical auditory evoked potentials. *Brazilian Journal of Otorhinolaryngology, 80*(2), 131–137. doi:10.5935/1808-8694.20140028

Sinha, S. K., & Basavaraj, V. (2010). Speech evoked auditory brainstem responses: A new tool to study brainstem encoding of speech sounds. *Indian Journal of Otorhinolaryngology and Head and Neck Surgery, 62*(4), 395–399. doi:10.1007/s12070-010-0100-y

Smoski, W., Brunt, M., & Tannahill, C. (1998). *C.H.A.P.S. Children's Auditory Performance Scale instruction manual.* Tampa, FL: Educational Audiology Association.

Stapells, D. R. (2002). Cortical event-related potentials to auditory stimuli. In J. Katz, R. F. Burkard & L. Medwetsky (Eds.), *Handbook of clinical audiology* (5th ed., pp. 378–406). Baltimore, MD: Lippincott Williams & Wilkins.

Sussman, E., Steinschneider, M., Gumenyuk, V., Grushko, J., & Lawson, K. (2008). The maturation of human evoked brain potentials to sounds presented at different stimulation rates. *Hearing Research, 236*(1–2), 61–79. doi:10.1016/j.heares.2007.12.001

Taguchi, K., Picton, T. W., Orpin, J. A., & Goodman, W. S. (1969). Evoked response audiometry in newborn infants. *Acta Otolaryngologica Supplementum, 252*(5–17).

Tremblay, K. L., Scollie, S., Abrams, H. B., Sullivan, J. R., & McMahon, C. M. (2014). Hearing aids and the brain. *International Journal of Otolaryngology, 2014*, 5. doi:http://dx.doi.org/10.1155/2014/518967

Tucker, D. A., & Ruth, R. A. (1996). Effects of age, signal level, and signal rate on the auditory middle latency response. *Journal of the American Academy of Audiology, 7*(2), 83–91.

Uhlén, I. T., Borg, E., Persson, H. E., & Spens, K. E. (1996). Topography of auditory evoked cortical potentials in children with severe language impairment: The N1 component. *Electroencephalography and Clinical Neurophysiology, 100*(3), 250–260. doi:10.1016/0168-5597(95)00256-1

Vanvooren, S., Poelmans, H., Hofmann, M., Ghesquière, P., & Wouters, J. (2014). Hemispheric asymmetry in auditory processing of speech envelope modulations in prereading children. *Journal of Neuroscience, 34*(4), 1523–1529. doi:10.1523/JNEUROSCI.3209-13.2014

Warrier, C. M., Johnson, K. L., Hayes, E. A., Nicol, T. G., & Kraus, N. (2004). Learning impaired children exhibit timing deficits and training-related improvements in auditory cortical responses to speech in noise. *Experimental Brain Research, 157*(4), 431–441. doi:10.1007/s00221-004-1857-6

Weihing, J., Schochat, E., & Musiek, F. (2012). Ear and electrode effects reduce within-group variability in middle latency response amplitude measures. *International Journal of Audiology, 51*(5), 405–412. doi:10.3109/14992027.2012.658970

Wetherby, A. M., Koegel, R. L., & Mendel, M. (1981). Central auditory nervous system dysfunction in echolalic autistic individuals. *Journal of Speech and Hearing Research, 24*(3), 420–429. doi:10.1044/jshr.2403.420

Wible, B., Nicol, T., & Kraus, N. (2002). Abnormal neural encoding of repeated speech stimuli in noise in children with learning problems. *Clinical Neurophysiology, 113*(4), 485–494. http://dx.doi.org/10.1016/S1388-2457(02)00017-2

Winsberg, B. G., Javitt, D. C., & Silipo, G. S. (1997). Electrophysiological indices of information processing in methylphenidate responders. *Biological Psychiatry, 42*(6), 434–445. doi:10.1016/S0006-3223(96)00429-5

Wioland, N., Rudolf, G., & Metz-Lutz, M. N. (2001). Electrophysiological evidence of persisting unilateral auditory cortex dysfunction in the late outcome of Landau and Kleffner syndrome. *Clinical Neurophysiology, 112*(2), 319–323. doi:10.1016/S1388-2457(00)00528-9

Wolf, K. E., & Goldstein, R. (1978). Middle component averaged electroencephalic responses to tonal stimuli from normal neonates. *Archives of Otolaryngology, 104*(9), 508–513. doi:10.1001/archotol.1978.00790090026006

Wolf, K. E., & Goldstein, R. (1980). Middle component AERs from neonates to low-level tonal stimuli. *Journal of Speech and Hearing Research, 23*(1), 185–201. doi:10.1044/jshr.2301.185

Young, G. B., Wang, J. T., & Connolly, J. F. (2004). Prognostic determination in anoxic-ischemic and traumatic encephalopathies. *Journal of Clinical Neurophysiology, 21*(5), 379–390.

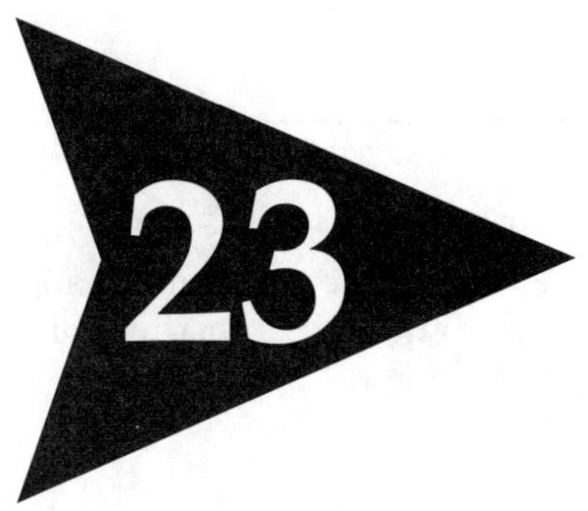

Behavioral Audiometry in Infants and Children

Allan O. Diefendorf and Anne Marie Tharpe

"Experience gained in the field of audiology for children during its rapid development in the past few decades has made it clearly evident that auditory disorders in children require more differential diagnosis than was formerly considered necessary and that the earlier this diagnosis is established the better. The pedagogic program that should be planned for the development of speech and put into effect from the first most formative years demands the detailed charting of the auditory range made possible by modern pure tone audiometry."

— Bengt Barr

Introduction

The importance of assessing hearing in children was recognized in 1928 when Alexander William Gordon (A.W.G.) Ewing advocated, "that the hearing of all children suspected of aphasia should be tested" (Ewing, 1930, p. 12). A.W.G. Ewing further recommended that reliable methods of testing young children's responses to sound are needed in the diagnosis of congenital aphasia and of other forms of defects that call for speech therapy (Ewing, 1930). This emphasis on threshold audiometry challenged clinicians to pursue the goal of developing valid and reliable techniques with young children. As such, the application of classical conditioning and instrumental conditioning facilitated the development of pediatric audiology as a subspecialty of audiology. Conditioned techniques would be pursued over the next 30 years with both physiologic (psychogalvanic skin response [PSR] audiometry) and behavioral (play audiometry) techniques evolving as approaches to hearing assessment in children.

When the authors were beginning their audiologic careers, current physiologic approaches (e.g., auditory evoked potentials, acoustic reflexes, evoked otoacoustic emissions) to infant and child hearing assessment were not available or just emerging. As such, audiologists were heavily reliant on careful and systematic behavioral observation for infant auditory assessment. There are limitations to relying exclusively on behavioral measures for accurate estimation of hearing thresholds in infants and young children (e.g., children with neurodevelopmental disabilities). However, although some might argue that physiologic approaches to hearing assessment have supplanted the need for behavioral audiometry with infants and young children, one must recognize that some of these approaches might not be effective in assessing hearing under certain clinical conditions (e.g., neural asynchrony, otitis media with effusion), and might not be possible without sedation in some cases (e.g., fragile medical conditions). Therefore, behavioral testing remains a crucial component of the audiologic test battery along with physiologic measures for the assessment of hearing in infants and children.

This chapter details the application and outcomes of behavioral audiometry with infants and children. To achieve this outcome, those issues that directly influence operant behavior (i.e., instrumental [operant] conditioning and reinforcement), and those that exert a secondary influence on behavioral audiologic outcomes (e.g., sensory and nonsensory factors, acoustic and other environmental factors, procedural adaptations, and resourcefulness of audiologists) are addressed.

Respondent Behavior

Behavior elicited by a stimulus is considered *respondent* behavior. Respondent behavior can be achieved through *classical* (or Pavlovian) *conditioning*, or through *instrumental* (or operant) *conditioning*.

Classical (Pavlovian) Conditioning

In the classical model, the response is *elicited* by the conditioned stimulus. The most familiar example of this paradigm is Pavlov's experiments in the 1880s in which he conditioned a dog to salivate at the sound of a bell. The bell initially is considered a neutral stimulus (NS), and food is considered the unconditioned stimulus (UCS). It is possible to transfer the power of an unconditioned stimulus to a neutral stimulus to elicit a conditioned response (salivation). That is, by pairing the sound of a bell with the presentation of food, Pavlov, after several trials, conditioned the dog to salivate in response to the bell. In classical conditioning, the neutral stimulus becomes the conditioned stimulus (NS→CS), and the unconditioned response becomes the conditioned response (UCR→CR). The power of the conditioned stimulus (the bell) to continue to elicit a conditioned response (salivation) diminishes over time through repeated trials unless the conditioned stimulus is restrengthened by occasional re-pairing with the unconditioned stimulus (food).

The application of the classical conditioning paradigm to the measurement of hearing in young children was achieved through the PSR technique (Bordley, Hardy, & Richter, 1948). In an attempt to measure hearing in young children, an auditory stimulus (neutral stimulus) and electric shock (unconditioned stimulus) are paired while measuring the amplitude and frequency of change in skin resistance (unconditioned response). In the initial trials of this procedure, the auditory stimulus is neutral and will not, of itself, elicit a response. However, after repeated trials, the response-eliciting power of the unconditioned stimulus (the electric shock) will be transferred to the neutral stimulus (the auditory stimulus). At this point, the neutral stimulus becomes the conditioned stimulus (NS→CS) and the resulting response (changes in skin resistance) becomes a conditioned response (UCR→CR). The PSR was used in the early evolution of pediatric audiology as an alternative to play audiometry for measuring hearing in children (Barr, 1955; O'Neill, Oyer, & Hillis, 1961; Statten & Wishart, 1956). However, the PSR was phased out of use when it was clearly demonstrated that the audiometric results and outcomes with children were less accurate, more time consuming, and traumatic when compared to the use of instrumental (operant) conditioning techniques.

Instrumental (Operant) Conditioning

Operant behavior is frequently spoken of as willful or purposeful behavior. In the instrumental model, a behavioral response elicited by a stimulus is *controlled* by the consequences of the behavior. Skinner (1953) stated, "the term 'operant' emphasizes the fact that the behavior *operates* upon the environment to generate consequences" (p. 65).

It is convenient to approach the behavioral assessment of hearing in infants and young children through an operant conditioning paradigm, specifically, through use of an operant discrimination procedure. In the operant conditioning paradigm, an auditory stimulus is introduced as a contingency to indicate the time interval during which an appropriate response will have a consequence. Thus, the auditory stimulus serves as a discriminative stimulus. In this paradigm, a response is defined as a single example of the appropriate behavior; an *operant* is defined as a range of responses that are controlled by their consequences. The consequence is an appropriately selected and appropriately applied reinforcement.

When a behavior generates a reinforcing consequence, there is an increased probability that similar behavior will reoccur. Operant behavior is increased or decreased in frequency by the changes it brings about in an organism's environment. The events in an environment can be classified as positive reinforcers, negative reinforcers, and neutral events. Neutral events have little or no specific effect on behavior. Depending on the application of negative or positive reinforcement, the response probability effect can be either increased or decreased (Table 23–1).

Additionally, response probability can be decreased by either of two punishment procedures: presenting an undesired consequence for completion of a required response, or removing a desired consequence for completion of a required response. It is important to understand the distinction between presenting and removing consequential stimuli on response behavior/probability. Decreasing unwanted behavior by removing the opportunity for receiving a desired stimulus is called time-out. Time-out is an effective punishment procedure for decreasing response probability. For example, if an unwanted behavior (false responding) from a child results in a delay (time-out) in the opportunity to receive positive reinforcement, the child will decrease the frequency of the unwanted behavior.

Because of a long-standing commitment to human/patient rights and to protecting patients through informed decision making, positive reinforcement procedures are preferred to increase response behavior, and the removal of a desired consequence (time-out) is the preferred punishment to decrease unwanted behaviors. In conventional, play, and visual reinforcement audiometry procedures, both positive reinforcement and time-out (punishment) are employed to shape and control response behavior (Figure 23–1).

In behavioral audiometry with children, behavioral responses (operants) are strengthened by positive reinforcement. This approach recognizes a view of infants and young children as active receptors of auditory stimuli who, when given the opportunity, will interact with their auditory environment to control subsequent consequences.

Table 23–1. Effects of Positive and Negative Reinforcement

	Present	*Remove*
Positive reinforcement	(Reinforcement) *Increases* response probability	(Punishment) *Decreases* response probability
Negative reinforcement	(Punishment) *Decreases* response probability	(Reinforcement) *Increases* response probability

Sequential Components in Operant Conditioning

Multiple stages make up the process of an operant discrimination procedure. It is important to note from Figure 23–1 that in addition to the identified components of the operant discrimination procedure, each component (interval) is defined by a temporal duration. Thus, examiners who employ the operant discrimination paradigm must be familiar with each component of the process, the examiner's role in each component, and the recommended time duration for each interval.

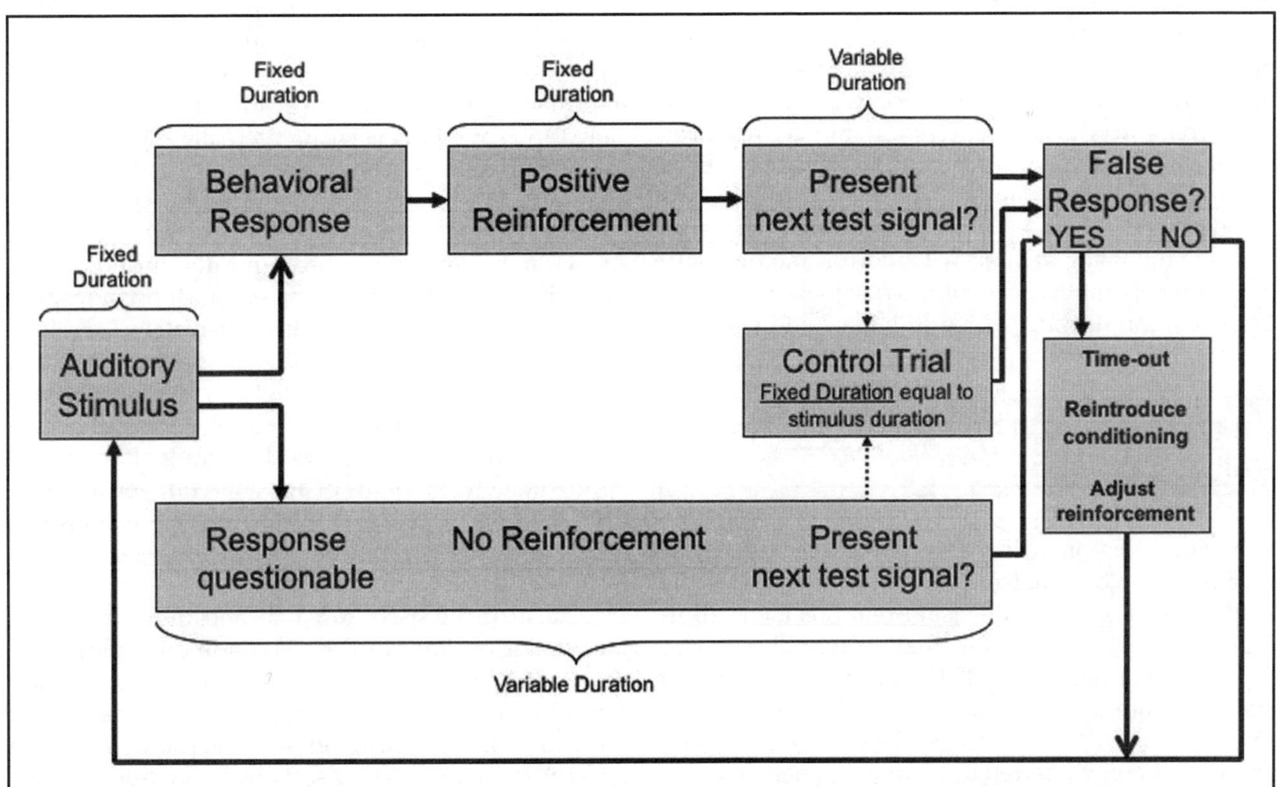

FIGURE 23–1. Test sequence in an operant discrimination procedure.

Interval Between Response and Reinforcement. Reinforcement in behavioral assessment with infants and young children is time related. That is, reinforcement should be presented immediately upon completion of the desired behavioral response (head-turn, play task, conventional hand-raising). Delays in reinforcement might suggest to the child that more than a single response is necessary to receive reinforcement. In turn, this behavior will increase false responding if the child receives reinforcement after an additional response has been initiated.

Sequencing the Time to Present the Next Test Signal. If a false response occurs during this interval, it might be necessary to implement time-out, reintroduce conditioning (depending on which phase of the operant procedure the examiner is engaged in), or adjust reinforcement. Responses during this interval (the nonauditory stimulus interval) should be followed by time-out (punishment by delaying opportunity for next auditory signal). This strategy provides differential consequential of the two intervals: auditory stimulus interval and deciding when to present the next test signal. When it is demonstrated that the desired response occurs during the presentation of the auditory stimulus and does not occur at other times, the child is considered to be under "stimulus control." At this time in the operant procedure, two levels of control have been demonstrated. The level of reinforcement control has been demonstrated (the response is under control of the reinforcer and an effective reinforcer has been established), and the level of stimulus control has been demonstrated (the stimulus controls discriminative responding).

The following sections will address, more specifically, how operant conditioning principles are applied to the clinical hearing testing of infants and children.

Behavioral Audiometric Measurements

Behavioral audiometric measurements include those that require volitional responses on the part of the listener (responder). For visual-reinforcement audiometry (VRA) with infants, the behavioral response (operant) is a head turn. The traditional response in standard pure-tone audiometry with children involves the raising of a finger or hand, or pressing a button and is commonly referred to as conventional pure tone audiometry. Modification of this procedure employs some form of "play" activity (pegs in a board, stacking blocks, placing blocks in a can) in establishing the conditioned response. This procedure is referred to as *play audiometry*.

Behavioral Observation

Behavioral observation procedures are not considered appropriate for the estimation of hearing in infants under the age of approximately 5 to 6 months because of the high inter- and intrasubject variability in responses (Hicks, Tharpe, & Ashmead, 2000; Moore & Wilson, 1987) and rapid response habituation (Diefendorf & Gravel, 1996; Widen, 1993). Habituation can be delayed if response reinforcement is used (e.g., VRA), as will be discussed in the following section. However, visual reinforcement has little effect on responsivity of infants under 5 months of age (Hicks, Tharpe, & Ashmead, 2000; Moore & Wilson, 1987). Therefore, the term *behavioral observation audiometry* is considered unsuitable because audiologists cannot use behavioral procedures in the absence of reinforcement to measure the range and sensitivity of a baby's hearing.

Nevertheless, in spite of these limitations, it is appropriate and useful to observe infant responses to sound to ensure general compatibility with other physiologic test results and confirm parent/caregiver observations, especially when physiologic testing is not informative or contributory because of middle ear effusion (OAE) or neural asynchrony (ABR). Because hearing or response thresholds are not being determined, a soundproof booth is not required for these observations. A quiet, nonreverberant room can be used. Awake and alert babies are typically curious about everything in a new environment and, thus, responsive to many different stimuli (visual, etc.). Therefore, it is often helpful to observe babies' responses to sound while they are in a drowsy or light state of sleep. Audiologists are then looking for gross behavioral responses to broadband noise or speech stimuli. For infants approximately 2 months of age and younger, audiologists should expect few, if any, behavioral responses to sound at intensity levels below those that elicit startle responses (Hicks et al., 2000).

Most of the early research and our subsequent knowledge of clinical VRA and conditioned play audiometry (CPA) procedures came from the dedicated and careful work of a team of developmental scientists at the University of Washington in Seattle in the 1970s and 1980s. The following sections will describe much of their work as well as other contemporary findings.

Visual Reinforcement Audiometry

A predecessor to VRA (conditioned orientation reflex) was first described by Suzuki and Ogiba in 1961. That procedure required an infant to orient (i.e., localize) to one of two sound sources (speakers) prior to being rewarded with a visual reinforcement. A short time later, Liden and Kankkunen (1969) coined the term *visual reinforcement audiometry* to describe a similar procedure but one that did not require a localization response for reward. Their procedure rewarded a change in behavior upon the presentation of an auditory stimulus. That is, VRA was designed as a detection, not a localization, task; for example, one could have a child look up at the ceiling for a reward whenever the auditory stimulus is perceived. However, as commonly practiced today, pediatric audiologists capitalize on a young child's ability and natural tendency to localize to the sound source as a way of clearly observing a child's response to sound (Figure 23–2).

Acceptable Behavioral Responses in VRA

About 20% of typically developing infants under 4 months of age are able to complete a VRA procedure successfully (Widen, 1993), but by approximately 4 to 5 months of age, reliable head-orienting responses to sound are observed in most infants (e.g., Muir, Clifton, & Clarkson, 1989). It is common to see audiology booths with speakers positioned at either 45° or 90°. There are at least two distinct advantages to having speakers placed at 90° versus 45°: (a) With speakers placed at ear level, a speaker at 45° will likely require that the reinforcer be placed on top of the speaker, making its position high relative to the infant's line of sight; when the speaker and reinforcer are positioned at 90°, they can be placed side by side at infant eye level. Also, (b) a robust head turn is required for an infant to look toward a speaker positioned at 90°; a 45° look can be obtained by a slight movement of the eyes without requiring a head turn at all. This can make it quite difficult for the examiner to determine whether or not a response occurred.

Another way to enhance an audiologist's ability to view a head turn is by having the child sit in a high chair where he or she is supported on three sides and is limited in ability to move around. By asking the parent or caregiver to place the child in the high chair after the child has had an opportunity to explore the room (e.g., during the taking of the history), the audiologist can avoid scaring the child. Furthermore, having a child in a high chair rather than a parent's or caregiver's lap, avoids the potential problem of the child being inadvertently cued by the adult to respond to the stimuli.

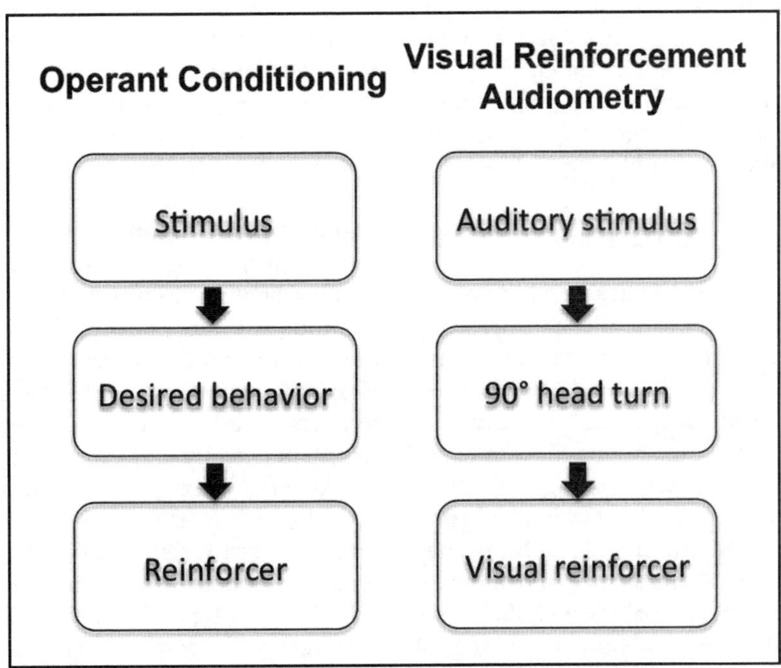

FIGURE 23–2. Test sequence in visual reinforcement audiometry.

Most audiologists prefer to initiate VRA in sound field to avoid frightening the child by placing earphones. However, ultimately, individual-ear information is required for both diagnostic purposes and, when indicated, hearing aid fitting. Children tend to tolerate insert earphones more readily than circumaural phones because they are lightweight and comfortable. Numerous audiologists have reported the successful use of insert phones for establishing ear-specific response thresholds with VRA (e.g., Widen et al., 2005). Furthermore, masking can be introduced to the nontest ear as needed. Infants initially turn to the onset of the masking noise but after a few seconds of not receiving reinforcement, they "ignore" the noise and return to conditioned responses to pure tones. For an excellent discussion of the impact of insert phones on sound pressure level in the infant ear canal and the use of a child's personal earmold for testing, see Chapter 25 of this volume.

Some pediatric audiologists prefer to test babies in a team with another audiologist present. However, several studies have confirmed that intra- and interjudge agreement of identifying a head-turn response is over 96%, respectively (Moore, Thompson, & Thompson, 1975; Moore, Wilson, & Thompson, 1977; Wilson, Moore, & Thompson, 1976); therefore, there seems to be no need to have two audiologists determine if a head turn has occurred. Moreover, in today's current health care climate with close attention to expenditures and a shortage of pediatric audiologists (Shaw, 2013), it appears that using two audiologists to test one baby might not be a good use of valuable resources. However, as will be discussed later in this chapter, having an assistant in the test booth to keep a child in the appropriate position and mood for testing, can be helpful if a parent or caregiver is not obliging.

Reinforcement Options for VRA

A challenge with VRA is that the head-turn response can extinguish or habituate before a full hearing assessment can be completed. Numerous investigators have used various strategies to prevent or delay response habituation, including examining a variety of reinforcement types. Moore et al. (1977) examined the number of head-turn responses of infants when using social reinforcement, simple reinforcement (light only), and complex reinforcement (lighted and animated toy). They found a positive effect (i.e., maintenance of responses) with all three reinforcement types; however, the use of complex reinforcement staved off habituation longest. Although it might seem obvious to practicing audiologists that complex reinforcement is the most effective, one should not overlook the power of social reinforcement. While using complex reinforcement, pediatric audiologists should consider witholding social reinforcement until such time that babies begin to habituate. Adding social reinforcement only when needed might extend the test session a bit longer.

More recently, another complex visual reinforcement has gained popularity, cartoons and pictures displayed on monitors from DVDs or online sources. Results have been mixed in terms of comparative strength of video and animated toy reinforcement (conventional), with some studies suggesting that video reinforcement is equal or superior to conventional reinforcement (Lowery, von Hapsburg, Plyler, & Johnstone, 2009; Schmida, Peterson, & Tharpe, 2003), and some suggesting the superiority of conventional reinforcement (Karzon & Banerjee, 2010). At this time, having both types of reinforcement available for VRA is advised, particularly when testing infants between the ages of 12 and 24 months of age.

Procedure

Unlike the widely accepted use of the modified Hughson-Westlake procedure to determine hearing thresholds in adults, there is no standard, accepted protocol for visual reinforcement audiometry. The three primary variants in protocols across clinics and laboratories are (a) the use of conditioning or training the baby's response at the start of the test session, (b) the starting level, and (c) the step size used in bracketing. Each of these factors can contribute to the overall efficiency of the behavioral test procedure. Given that behavioral test sessions are likely to last less than 30 min prior to a child's habituation (Primus, 1991), it is important to focus on test efficiency. Toward that end, these three factors will be discussed at some length below.

Training the Response for VRA. Clinicians differ in the use of training trials prior to initiating a VRA test session. That is, some audiologists present the auditory stimulus and the visual reinforcer *simultaneously* (pair the stimulus and reinforcer) to train the response (e.g., Gravel, 1989; Thompson & Folsom, 1984; note that the term *training* for purposes of this discussion of VRA, refers specifically to the act of pairing the stimulus and reinforcement for the purpose of showing the infant how the task works—this does not refer to the necessary and appropriate use of the operant process [stimulus → response → reinforcement]). Some examiners skip the training and visually reinforce the infant after a correct and spontaneous response (i.e., head turn; e.g., Eilers, Miskiel, Ozdama, Urbano, & Widen, 1991; Tharpe & Ashmead, 1993). There are abundant data to support the notion that it is not necessary to train typically developing infants the localization response as it is spontaneous by approximately 5 to 6 months of age (e.g., Hoversten & Moncur, 1969; Moore et al., 1975). However, exceptions might include those with unilateral hearing loss or neurodevelopmental disabilities, in which case training the appropriate response could be of value if no spontaneous head turn is observed. Or if a head turn occurs but localization is not accurate.

Another consideration with regard to training trials is that it is logical to assume that once a baby sees the visual reinforcer, false-positive responding will be initiated. That is, if an auditory stimulus is paired with a visual reinforcer, a baby is likely to start looking toward the reinforcer in search of the toy or video, whether or not the auditory stimulus is perceptible to the infant. If a baby has a significant hearing loss, it is feasible that the audiologist will waste a lot of time trying to sort out which are false positive responses and which are not when, otherwise, if a baby was not exposed to training trials at the beginning of the procedure, the baby would not be providing any responses until (or if) the auditory stimulus exceeded the baby's threshold.

Finally, some babies respond adversely (i.e., are scared) to the visual reinforcement, or they simply are fussy and will not provide more than a couple of responses before the test session is effectively over. In that scenario, the first responses are quite valuable in determining if a baby has any hearing. For example, imagine that the VRA session begins with a presentation of speech stimuli at 30 dB HL paired with the visual reinforcer. After a couple of head turns in response to the paired auditory stimulus and visual reinforcer, the baby starts crying and cannot be soothed to complete the test session. The audiologist in this situation cannot make any determination about the baby's hearing. However, if the audiologist had waited for a spontaneous head turn prior to reinforcing, there would be some general indication of hearing status for speech stimuli based on the child's initial response.

Starting Level. The starting level must also be determined prior to initiating a behavioral test procedure. There is ample evidence to suggest that the closer one starts to the subject's threshold before initiating the bracketing procedure, the more efficient and accurate the threshold estimation is (e.g., Eilers et al., 1991; Tharpe & Ashmead, 1993; Thompson & Folsom, 1984). This is logical when one considers that starting at too high or too low a level could result in wasting time and responses while trying to reach threshold. Of course, when an audiologist sees an infant for an initial evaluation, the baby's hearing status is unknown. However, given that most babies seen in general pediatric audiology practices are going to have normal to near-normal hearing (i.e., being seen because of otitis media with effusion or speech/language concerns), a start level of 30 dB improves the probability of starting close to threshold (as opposed to a start level of 50 dB or higher). Furthermore, if true threshold is in the moderate loss range or higher, and as long as one is looking for a spontaneous head turn (i.e., not training the response at the start of the session), it takes only a few seconds to increase the stimulus level by 20 dB steps until a head turn is noted, and the infant has wasted no responses in the meantime. Responses are wasted when starting at too high a level and then descending before an actual bracketing of threshold can begin.

Step Size and Trial Duration. The step size refers to the degree of intensity change in the stimulus level that is used throughout the behavioral test bracketing procedure. Again, although the step sizes associated with the Hughson-Westlake procedure are accepted by audiologists for use with adults, there is considerable variability in step sizes used for VRA (Gravel, 1989; Moore & Wilson, 1978; Nozza & Wilson, 1984; Primus, 1991). Step size is related to precision; that is, the larger the step size, the more imprecise the threshold estimation will be (Levitt, 1970, 1978). However, because of our need to be efficient when testing infants and estimate thresholds across the test frequency range for both ears, if possible, prior to infant habituation, most consider larger step sizes a compromise worth making.

Tharpe and Ashmead (1993) conducted computer simulations of VRA to examine these parameters (training versus no training, starting level, and step size) as well as false-positive (apparently responding when a sound was not really detected) and false-negative rates (failing to respond when a sound was presumably detectable), and the interaction of these factors with an extensive range of hearing capabilities of the "subjects." Numerous parameters were varied, resulting in 5,616 combinations, and for each combination 10,000 simulated subjects were tested at each of 13 hearing threshold levels, between 0 and 120 dB in 10-dB increments. The results suggested that the following parameters minimize the inherent test bias in this adaptive test procedure while maximizing efficiency:

- a start level of 30 dB, increasing in 20 dB steps, if no response occurs;
- after initial level is determined and replicated, a step size of 20 dB down, 10 dB up should be used on ascending and descending runs; and
- training (i.e., pairing stimulus and reinforcer) should not be utilized as a matter of routine but, rather, the examiner should begin testing without training.

Despite the need to maximize efficiency during VRA procedures, it is not appropriate to simply abandon the bracketing procedure and screen across test frequencies at, for example, 20 or 25 dB HL. An exception to this could be in situations where it is obvious that a child will not maintain attention long enough for the audiologist to establish response thresholds at each of the test frequencies. In that situation, one might choose to attempt obtaining two responses at a given screening level across each of the test frequencies. However, these results should be reported as *screening* results, not as response thresholds. And, it should be noted that such screenings can miss minimal hearing losses and can also miss the early stages of some progressive losses.

The recommended trial duration (incorporating the signal and response) in VRA is approximately 4 s (Primus, 1992). That is, although the signal duration is approximately 4 s, this 4-s duration also defines the interval of time during which a response should be judged to be present or not. Head-turn responses outside of the 4-s interval are typically not interpreted as valid responses, and therefore are not reinforced.

Recall that the term *threshold* refers to the level at which a listener detects a stimulus 50% of the time. However, it is common to refer to infant responses elicited via VRA as minimum response levels (MRLs), for reasons discussed thoroughly in Chapter 4 regarding infant auditory development and its impact on behavioral responsiveness in infants. This term is especially appropriate if the test procedure does not seek a threshold but, rather, has a specified stopping level within a normal hearing range. The term *response threshold* can be used when a 50% response level is used for behavioral assessment. For purpose of efficiency, it has been recommended that two responses at a given intensity level (whether while ascending or descending during bracketing) should constitute a stopping level (Tharpe & Ashmead, 1993).

Control Trials in VRA. After the first time a child sees the visual reinforcer, false-positive responses can begin. It is suggested that audiologists maintain a systematic method for inserting catch, or control, trials into the test procedure. Such trials are those in which conditions are acceptable for a stimulus to be presented (i.e., the infant is in a ready state), but instead of presenting a signal, an audiologist observes whether or not a false-positive response occurs. This process will assist audiologists in avoiding systematic or rhythmic presentations of stimuli. However, a false alarm rate estimate is not very accurate unless a considerable number of catch trials are obtained (i.e., 15 to 20), which is ambitious during the necessarily short time of a VRA session (Tharpe & Ashmead, 1993).

Although pediatric audiologists typically concentrate on ensuring that they recognize false-positive responses, there are times when an audiologist might not be sure if *lack* of an initial response is an indicator of hearing loss or an inability to condition the child to the VRA task (lack of initial head turn response). In that scenario, one might consider trying to condition the child to respond to a bone-conducted signal that produces a vibrotactile sensation (either with the bone vibrator on the child's head or held in his or her hand). If the child conditions to the vibrotactile stimulus, that would indicate the child is "conditionable" and suggest that the child cannot hear the auditory stimulus. If the child does not condition to the vibrotactile *or* auditory stimulus, it would suggest that the child is not conditionable to the VRA procedure, thus, indicating a need for a physiological procedure (e.g., ABR or ASSR) for threshold estimation.

Conventional and Conditioned Play Audiometry

Barr (1955) and Thompson and Weber (1974) tested children between the ages of 2 to 6 years and 2 to 5 years, respectively, by play audiometry and found that the percentage of successful completion of tests was directly related to age. When data between the two studies are compared based on similarities in subject demographics, conditioning procedures, and subject exclusion criteria, the outcomes are remarkably similar. In both studies, children age 3 years and older were successfully tested by play audiometry greater than 95% of the time. Thompson and Weber reported successful tests on 2.5- to 3-year-olds 90% of the time, whereas Barr reported success 61% of the time. For the 2- to 2.5-year-olds, Thompson and Weber reported success 70% of the time, whereas Barr reported success 20% of the time. Differences in the results from the two studies at the two age levels might be attributed to methodological differences studies relative to stimuli used, earphone (Barr) versus sound-field testing (Thompson and Weber), and the use of one examiner (Barr) versus the use of two examiners (Thompson and Weber) during conditioning and threshold measurements. Both studies support the use of play audiometry with children at developmental ages of 3 years, and carefully selected children beginning at age 2 years. When 2-year-olds are proficient with play audiometry, they are likely to provide more responses before habituation than they would if tested by visual reinforcement audiometry (Thompson et al., 1989). However, VRA has a greater likelihood of success as a test procedure in the sense that almost all typically developing 2-year-olds are certain to comply and learn the VRA procedure.

Eagles and Wishik (1961) demonstrated that in a sample public school system population, conventional pure-tone audiometry was successful down to at least 3 years of age. The total study sample consisted of 3,882 children ranging in age from 3 to 17 years. The significant points from this study included: (a) hearing sensitivity from 0 dB to 10 dB (corrected to current American National Standards Institute [ANSI], 2004, standards) for the frequencies 250 Hz through 8000 Hz, for the ages of children represented in the study; and (b) the auditory sensitivity in children below 6 years of age and as young as 2.5 to 3 years of age is not different from older, school-age children.

Experience with play audiometry indicates that reliable responses can be obtained when auditory stimulus → response control has been established and response criterion is maintained. Results from a clinical study (Diefendorf, 1981) of 40 preschool children, aged 30 to 48 months, revealed thresholds at an audiometric level of 10 dB HL or better. These findings were in close agreement with findings from other 4-year-old children (Gerwin & Glorig, 1974).

Acceptable Behavioral Responses With Conventional Audiometry or CPA

Selecting an appropriate response for children is critical to the success of conventional and play audiometry. A selected behavior must be clearly defined as the behavioral response, and the criteria limits of that behavior must be established. The response definition must explicitly differentiate the behavior from other random behavior. Additionally, the motor response must easily facilitate the procedure of operant conditioning and responding. If the physical demands are too great, the task will distract the child from maintaining a listening posture. If the task is too simple, the child will have less motivation to participate and will tire of the task.

Usually, a single task requiring a motor behavior to complete the response is sufficient to complete the acquisition of an audiogram. However, audiologists must be ready to switch to another play activity at the first sign of boredom. The learning of play-conditioning techniques starts at 2 years of age. Hodgson (1985) observed, however, "for successful play audiometry with a two-year-old, an exceptional child (and audiologist) is required." Northern and Downs (2002) commented, "one should not be deceived by the bright, talkative two-year-old who appears certain to be able to learn the procedure" (p. 183). That is, great care needs to be taken when differentiating "skill at completing the motor response" from "developmentally appropriate behavior and consistency within the operant conditioning paradigm."

With conventional and play audiometry, a response is defined as performance of the desired motor behavior within 3 s after stimulus onset of the auditory signal, and no later than 4 s. The rigorous definition of response latency (3–4 s after stimulus onset) is to minimize false-response behavior accepted as true-response behavior. By comparing the response behavior during the stimulus interval with response behavior during a control trial (see Figure 23–1), audiologists engage in a systematic protocol of comparing response behavior between the two intervals, leading to a quantification of false-response behavior.

Reinforcement When Using Conventional Audiometry or CPA

Many different types of reinforcement have been used with children during play audiometry. Dix and Hallpike (1947) introduced the "peep show" procedure where pictures were illuminated following a correct button-press response. Statten and Wishart (1956) adapted the peep-show idea of showing pictures by constructing a "movie screen" within an attractively colored doll's house. Rather than using single pictures, they used a color movie projector to show familiar animals and scenes from a farm. For young children who were frightened by the activity of a movie, Statten and Wishart also used a slide projector to show colored still pictures. Shimizu and Nakamura (1957) adapted their picture reinforcement from the peep-show idea. Their concern about the peep-show was that children must look at a picture in a box through a peephole; under Shimizu and Nakamura's technique, "no such complicated equipment is necessary and the children can enjoy the lantern slides in an easy and free posture" (p. 395). Miller (1963) also used slides as positive reinforcement. However, Miller recommended slide sets that tell a story as opposed to unrelated pictures. The Pediacoumeter is similar in principle to the peep-show. The basic difference is that instead of being rewarded for response to sound by a peep-show, the child might see any one of seven jack-in-the-box figures emerge from the testing apparatus (Guilford & Haug, 1952).

A common form of positive reinforcement used for young children during conventional audiometry or CPA is verbal praise ("that's good"; "good listening") or social reinforcement (pat-on-the-back; a smile and nod of the head; applause). Verbal praise and social reinforcement should be delivered naturally and meaningfully so that the child under test embraces this "consequential event" as positive reinforcement. If not viewed as positive reinforcement, the child eventually will become disinterested in the response behavior. In addition to verbal praise and social reinforcement, other forms of reinforcement have been suggested with children. Tokens that can be traded for small toys or stickers at the end of the test session, unsweetened cereal, or a changing computer display screen, all have been used successfully with play audiometry.

Importantly, play audiometry is not difficult to implement, but its successful application demands certain personal characteristics in the examiner. Examiners must be interested in children, comfortable with their actions and behavior, and able to relate to them well when delivering verbal praise and/or social reinforcement.

In general, a 100% reinforcement schedule (reinforcement for every correct response) results in more rapid conditioning, yet more rapid habituation. Conversely, an intermittent reinforcement schedule produces slower conditioning but also a slower rate of habituation. Consequently, most clinicians who conduct behavioral assessment of infants and young children recommend a protocol that begins with a 100% reinforcement schedule and then gradually shifts to an intermittent reinforcement schedule.

Intermittent reinforcement can be a fixed-ratio schedule, in which the child is required to complete a predetermined number of behavioral responses to receive reinforcement. Or reinforcement can be delivered on a variable-ratio schedule, in which the child receives reinforcement for a continuously varying number of responses. Certainly, the child's developmental level, motivation, enthusiasm, boredom, indifference, and shyness must be considered in presenting an appropriate schedule of reinforcement.

Reinforcement should be withheld when clinicians are uncertain about reinforcing delayed or ambiguous behavioral responses. The risk of reinforcing a false response is that it can lead to confusion for a child under stimulus control. However, failure to reinforce a correct response does not degrade performance. In this situation, withholding reinforcement is viewed as intermittent reinforcement, which will not interfere with subsequent behavioral responses. So, when in doubt, do not reinforce.

Conditioned Play Procedure

The audiologist is responsible for getting the child into a proper ready state (listening while holding a ring or peg next to the ear) and for teaching the child to respond (placing the ring on spindle or putting the peg in the board) at the onset of the auditory stimulus. Response shaping is critical to the success of the operant procedure for CPA. Moreover, this phase of testing is completely under the examiner's control. Thus, the examiner must be skilled in interacting with children, response training, delivering positive reinforcement, and be familiar with the process of response acquisition.

For some children, a period of pre-play is advisable to help comfort the child within a new environment, put the child at ease with unfamiliar faces, and to see to which toys the child might be naturally drawn. Once a toy is identified, it becomes the selected motor response for use in play audiometry.

Conditioning Process. As with VRA, the conditioning process for CPA consists of auditory stimulus → behavioral response → reinforcement. This description is accurate, but it minimizes the actual complexity of the process. The behavioral response requires the examiner to teach and engage the child to perform a motor task in response to the auditory signal. The examiner might use both verbal instruction ("put it on" or "drop the block") and physical assistance (taking the child's hand and helping the child perform the desired motor task) to guide the child. The response must be deliberate, consistent with the child's motor skill, and time efficient. As stated previously, a response is defined as performance of the desired motor behavior within 3 to 4 s after the onset of the auditory stimulus. Immediately following the required response, positive reinforcement is presented to strengthen subsequent responses. Once again, the duration of reinforcement should be short, but effective. When the listener cannot understand verbal (oral) instructions, some modification in the form of demonstration or training is employed.

Following several training (conditioning) trials, probe trials are used to determine if conditioning has been established. It is generally accepted that if the child responds appropriately during probe trials (e.g., two times out of three stimulus presentations), conditioning criteria have been met. If a child fails to meet the conditioning criteria, additional conditioning trials are employed until the conditioning criterion is met. It is recommended that when additional conditioning trials are required to teach the response, the stimulus intensity is raised to ensure that the child hears the stimulus. Failure to condition rapidly should alert the examiner to a potential calibration or auditory problem or other important factors (physical, cognitive, social) that might affect the child's behavior. After repeated unsuccessful attempts to condition a child to what is considered an age-appropriate behavioral technique (conventional or play audiometry), it might be necessary and prudent to drop back to a more developmentally appropriate behavioral technique (e.g., VRA).

Initial training can often be most easily accomplished with the audiologist seated directly beside the child. Importantly, the audiologist must be in close proximity to the child and maintain direct eye contact. Occasionally, instructions and demonstrations might be facilitated by the mother, a sibling, or a familiar caregiver. Use of pantomime, demonstration, and exaggerated gestures enhance teaching a child the desired task. For some children, having the parent play an active role in the play audiometry task is often very helpful in encouraging the child's behavior. The parent might need to play the game to encourage the child's participation and to model the correct response. Occasionally, some children prefer to use their parent's hand to play the game. Additionally, the parent might need to alternate taking turns with the child until the child is more comfortable in the test situation.

Threshold Exploration. For conventional testing or CPA with children, individual circumstances in hearing assessment will dictate the use of various starting intensities. Typically, the most efficient test is one that uses a low starting level (e.g., 30–40 dB HL) for reasons desribed earlier in the discussion of VRA.

Children who meet the conditioning criterion move to Phase 2 of the operant procedure, which is threshold exploration. Depending on response outcome during the test phase, signal intensity is either attenuated after every "yes" response or increased after every "no" response. An adaptive threshold search is initiated until a stopping criterion is met. For example, stimulus intensity is attenuated in 10-dB steps until the child makes the first "no" response to a signal trial. A "no" response is followed by an increase in signal (5 dB). A correct response is followed by a decrease in signal level. After a specific number of reversals, the threshold search has ended for that particular stimulus.

When two audiologists, or an audiologist and assistant, are used during testing (one with the child, one operating the equipment from the control room), the individual with the child must be able to hear all stimuli presented either by wearing an auxiliary intercom earphone or by wearing the bone oscillator with simultaneous presentation to the child (earphone) and audiologist (bone oscillator). In two-person play audiometry, precise timing of the stimulus presentation and resultant response is essential. Presenting reinforcement for correct responses is facilitated when the individual in the exam room is aware of signal trials versus control trials.

Play audiometry can be readily accomplished with only one examiner. The audiologist can position the child in a desk or chair next to the audiometer. All monitors and talkback microphones are turned off. The audiologist then manages the stimulus presentation, response, and social reinforcement independently and with total control. Having the child and the audiologist in the same room gives the audiologist an even better sense of when the child is truly in a listening posture, the time intervals for the stimulus presentation, the intensity level of the stimulus presentation, whether or not the response is reliable and consistent, and which responses should receive reinforcement.

Some children can certainly be categorized as "false responders." When confronted with false responders, the audiologist can place an open hand just in front of, or resting against the child's hand holding the response peg or block. The child then has to go around or through the audiologist's hand to complete the task once the sound is heard. This gentle visual and tactile reminder to wait is often sufficient to dramatically decrease a child's tendency to offer false positive responses.

Another difficulty encountered using play audiometry is the "reluctant responder." These children frequently wait until they are visually prompted to complete the task despite numerous training trials and reinforcement. In this event, the audiologist might want to identify if there is a definite facial response or reaction when the tone is presented. Some children look up at the audiologist for approval every time the tone is presented. The audiologist can then assist the child in completing the play task and watch for the child's reaction to the next stimulus.

For the child who is reluctant to respond, sometimes changing the game to something slightly more fun will be beneficial. If manual dexterity would suggest that placing a block in a large bucket might be the play activity of choice, then the play activity can be made more fun by moving the bucket away slightly and having the child "shoot a basket."

The major consideration for controlling the stimulus, regardless of mode, is the duration of the stimulus. The stimulus should be activated for at least 2 s and should remain on for no more than 4 s. Thompson, Thompson, and Vethivelu (1989) have demonstrated the effectiveness of a 2-s duration signal with young children engaged in play audiometry. In either presentation mode, latency factors help to validate a response; if the response occurs too early or too late, it is unacceptable.

There are two alternatives to stimulus presentation methods for acquiring response threshold in conventional and play audiometry—single-tone presentation (continuous mode) and pulsed-tone presentation (pulsed mode). Although little research data are available on differences in response behavior from children between these two modes, close observation on the part of the audiologist can facilitate which mode is most effective in maintaining stimulus-response control with children.

Some children can be categorized as "off responders." They prefer to wait until the stimulus has stopped prior to completing the task. For these children, utilizing a continuous tone can often assist them in feeling more confident in responding because there is a definite "off" to the signal.

Control Trials in Conventional and Conditioned Play Audiometry. The decision to "present the next test signal" (see Figure 23–1) is almost always longer in duration than the "auditory stimulus interval." Thus, a direct comparison between responses observed during these two periods is un-equated. Therefore, false-positive responses must be monitored by control trials when assessing children's hearing. Both signal trials (signal presented) and control trials (no signal presented) occur during threshold estimation. Either trial initiates an observation interval of approximately 4 s during which behavioral responses are judged. If the required behavioral response occurs during, or just after a signal trial, it is considered a correct detection, and reinforcement is presented. As noted previously in the section on VRA, a behavioral response occurring during a control trial is considered a false-positive response. Control trials are interspersed within the operant discrimination procedure to examine systematically the child's false-alarm rate. That is, the presence or absence of false-positive responses during control trials allows the audiologist to calculate the percentage of false-positive responses. The assumption is that children will produce a comparable number of incorrect behavioral responses during both signal and control trials. Therefore, it is possible to estimate chance responding (false responses during signal trials) during stimulus trials by monitoring false-response rate during control trials.

The purpose of the control trial is to assess the reliability of responses during behavioral audiometry. Test results on any child who reaches an unacceptable false-response rate (greater than 25 to 30% is suggested) should be excluded or interpreted with caution. If the criterion for false-response behavior is exceeded during conventional or play audiometry, audiologists should focus on four factors to rectify clinical outcomes: (a) reconditioning the desired behavioral response; (b) changing the desired behavioral response; (c) reconsidering the positive reinforcement utilized to maintain response behavior; and (d) increasing the duration of time-out as a form of punishment.

Acoustic and Other Environmental Factors

Audiometric testing as part of an audiologic assessment must be done in a room free of high levels of ambient noise or intermittent noises (cafeteria noise, noise from a hallway, telephone, pagers). Importantly, the environment in which the test is to be carried out must be evaluated. ANSI S3.1-1999 (ANSI, 1999) provides criteria for permissible ambient noise during audiometric testing. ANSI S3.1-1999 provides acceptable ambient noise values for threshold estimation at 0 dB HL, for one- and third-octave bandwidths, for use with supra-aural and insert earphones, and for sound-field and bone-conduction testing. In addition, it is imperative that the tester in the control room avoids using the loud speakers to talk with whoever is providing mid-line distraction for VRA in the test booth or serving as an assistant for CPA (e.g., student, parent). A system that allows the audiologist in the control room to speak with (instruct) the mid-line distractor or assistant via a personal headset or earphones is essential for ensuring that the test stimuli are the only auditory signals being introduced into the test booth. Otherwise, sounds coming through the speakers that are unrelated to the operant procedure will interrupt the conditioning paradigm and result in confusion for the child.

In addition to controlling the acoustic aspects, the test environment also should be free of distracting visual stimulation. Young children can be easily distracted by items such as pictures on the walls, games stored in the test area, and equipment stored in the room. Test rooms free of distraction help children focus on the conditioning task and subsequent response behavior. It is especially important to keep toys that will be used for mid-line distraction purposes (VRA) or play activities (CPA) out of sight until they are to be used to ensure that the child does not tire of them before the testing begins.

Prior to selecting the behavioral response activity and shaping stimulus-response behavior, it can be extremely helpful to position the child, if physically appropriate, in a student desk. The structure of the student desk assists the child in focusing on the task. If the child is enrolled in a school-based program, the desk might be a familiar reminder to pay attention and listen. Similarly, placement of a child in a high chair for

VRA is a gentle way of restraining the child and ensuring that he or she is facing forward and in line with the speakers and reinforcers.

Speech Perception

It is well known that infants begin life with a capacity to discriminate phonemes across all languages until about 6 months of age. Around that time, perceptual attunement to one's native language is exhibited by preferential attention to speech sounds in that language (Kuhl, 2004; Maurer & Werker, 2014). Furthermore, it is reasonably hypothesized that early infant phonetic perception plays a crucial role in language development. Specifically, some work has suggested that speech perception performance at 6 months of age can predict language at 2 years (Tsao, Liu, & Kuhl, 2004). Although infant phoneme perception research has utilized preferential looking and conditioned head turning tasks, such tests are not currently used clinically. See Chapter 3 in this volume by Houston for more information on infant speech perception.

As the range of sounds important for functional hearing is represented by phonemes, words, phrases, and sentences, tests that utilize speech stimuli are desirable for the evaluation of all children suspected of, and diagnosed with, hearing loss. Determination can be made of the extent to which hearing loss affects the ability to perceive, recognize, and discriminate speech stimuli. Such information is useful both in the diagnosis of the type and degree of hearing loss, and in the approach to assessing the development of auditory skills and subsequent functional listening behavior.

Audiologists concerned with assessing speech perception skills in children must consider several variables, both internal and external. Internal or subject factors include the child's developmental age, vocabulary, language competency, and cognitive abilities. External factors include the designation of an appropriate response task, the effective utilization of reinforcement, and controlling the memory load inherent in the task that can influence test performance.

Efforts to develop materials for testing speech perception in children date back to the late 1940s. Haskins (1949) developed *phonetically balanced* (PB) word lists based on the receptive vocabulary skills of children in kindergarten (PB-K). Clearly, test items must be in the vocabularies of the children tested. If not, the PB-K scores might be depressed reflecting vocabulary deficits, language deficits, or both, as well as deficits in speech perception. Sanderson-Leepa and Rintelmann (1976) indicated that normal-hearing preschoolers at 3.5 years of age yielded scores substantially lower on the PB-K words than did older children. Therefore, it is recommended that audiologists exercise caution in administering the PB-K test unless there is good assurance that the receptive vocabulary age of the child under test approaches at least that of a kindergarten-age child (Matkin, 1977). Verbal responses, as required by PB-K word presentation, can be limited not only by vocabulary deficits, but also by articulation deficits or lack of motivation. Yet, written responses on measures of speech perception are essentially out of the question for most young children. To bypass these problems and still test speech perception skills in children, picture discrimination tests can be used.

Ross and Lerman (1970) developed the Word Intelligibility by Picture Identification (WIPI) test that takes into consideration children who have restricted receptive vocabulary and cannot read. The WIPI test includes picture plates with six illustrations per plate. Four of the illustrations have words that rhyme, and the other two illustrations are presented as distractors to decrease the probability of a correct guess. The use of pictures rather than printed words adapts the test to those who cannot read.

Sanderson-Leepa and Rintelmann (1976) demonstrated that normal-hearing children at 3.5 years of age manifest a significant number of errors on the WIPI test due to words not being in their recognition vocabulary. Thus, the use of WIPI materials is appropriate for those children with receptive vocabulary ages of 4 years and greater. Moreover, Ross and Lerman concluded that the WIPI test is suitable for children with moderate hearing losses from ages 5 or 6 years and for children with severe hearing losses from ages 7 or 8 years.

Hodgson (1973) investigated the relationship between the WIPI words used as an open-set and as a closed-set test for normal-hearing children. Open-set tests are those in which the subject theoretically has an unlimited number of response possibilities. Upon hearing the test item, no response alternatives are given and, therefore, the listener is free to make any response. Closed-set tests restrict the subject to one of a fixed number of possible responses (e.g., as in a multiple choice test).

In the open-set version, children repeated the WIPI words. The closed-set version required the usual picture identification response task. Children also repeated the words of a PB-K list administered in the conventional open-set fashion. Although there was no reported difference between the intelligibility of the WIPI and PB-K words presented in the open-set format, use of the WIPI as a closed-set test improved the intelligibility scores by about 10%. Because the number of potential responses is limited, closed-set tests are easier and yield higher scores than open-set test procedures. Therefore, it is recommended that the audiologic record include intelligibility scores, the specific test materials used, and whether the test was presented in an open-set or closed-set format.

The Northwestern University Children's Perception of Speech (NU-CHIPS) test by Elliott and Katz (1980) was developed as a speech perception test appropriate for young children, and as a test designed to utilize a closed-set, picture-pointing response. The test items are representative of the most frequently occurring phonemes of English, with the exception of initial /r/. Additionally, test materials are limited to monosyllabic words that are documented to be in the recognition vocabulary of children with normal hearing as young as three years of age.

Children with hearing loss and a receptive language age of at least 2.5 years demonstrate familiarity with the words and pictures of NU-CHIPS. Children with language skills better than the target group for which NU-CHIPS was developed achieve higher scores on NU-CHIPS than on the WIPI test (Elliott & Katz, 1980). These findings are expected on the basis of the somewhat more difficult vocabulary on the WIPI test.

The development of the Pediatric Speech Intelligibility (PSI) monosyllabic word test by Jerger, Lewis, Hawkins, and Jerger (1980) was undertaken to create an instrument for use with children as young as 3 years of age. Initially, 30 monosyllabic words were chosen to represent an array of English phonemes in the initial and final positions. The responses to the 30 words by children sampled (normal hearing children ranging in ages from 3 to 7 years) did not differ as a function of chronologic age, vocabulary skill, or receptive language ability. However, for 20 words, a correct response was observed in more than 95% of the children. Thus, only those 20 words were selected for the PSI monosyllabic word test. The words are depicted on four response plates (five pictures per plate) in a closed-set format, and the child uses a picture-pointing response.

Finitzo-Hieber, Gerling, Matkin, and Cherow Skalka (1980) investigated the use of familiar environmental sounds as an alternative to speech stimuli for assessing auditory perception skills in children with very limited verbal abilities who are not capable of discriminating verbal stimuli. A measure of sound effects recognition is a unique approach to using environmental sounds to measure auditory recognition and perception. The Sound Effects Recognition Test (SERT) incorporates a closed-set format with a picture-pointing response. The SERT is composed of three equivalent sets, each containing 10 familiar environmental sounds (i.e., 30 different sounds, most of which are broadband in spectral content). The authors reported that by age 3 years, a child should be able to identify an average of 25 to 30 environmental test sounds. By the age of 5 years, a mean score of 29 of the 30 test sounds should be obtained.

The test contains four pictures on each of 10 response plates. Three of the pictures are foils, with one target item per page. The forms are equivalent in terms of item difficulty for children between the ages of 3 and 6.5 years. The SERT might be too easy for a large number of children with hearing losses who have measurable speech recognition. However, the SERT should be considered when other tests using verbal materials are inappropriate.

Conventional yet dated measures of word recognition in children provide descriptive information about word recognition performance, but yield limited information about the nature of underlying perceptual mechanisms contributing to word recognition. As traditional measures have considered receptive vocabulary and word similarity, a more systematic approach to speech perception can be achieved by identifying targets with similar acoustic-phonetic patterns, and selecting targets that occur with different word frequency.

Lexical characteristics, such as word frequency (i.e., the frequency of occurrence of words in the language) and lexical similarity (i.e., the number of phonetically similar items) have been shown to affect the accuracy of spoken word recognition in listeners with normal hearing. A measure of lexical similarity is the number of phonetically similar words or "lexical neighbors" that differ by one phoneme from the target word (Greenberg & Jenkins, 1964; Landauer & Streeter, 1973). For example, the following words are all lexical neighbors of the target word *cat*: bat, cap, cut, and scat. Words that occur frequently and have few lexical neighbors are considered "easy" words and are identified with greater accuracy than words that occur less frequently and have many lexical neighbors (i.e., "hard" words; Cluff & Luce, 1990; Elliot, Clifton, & Servi, 1983; Luce, Pisoni, & Goldinger, 1990).

The Lexical Neighborhood Test (LNT) and the Multisyllabic Lexical Neighborhood Test (MLNT) were developed by Kirk, Pisoni, and Osberger (1995) to assess word recognition and lexical discrimination in children with hearing loss. A primary goal in the development of the LNT and MLNT was to select words that were likely to be within the vocabulary of children with profound hearing losses. An initial pool of potential words was identified that are produced by children between the ages of 3 and 5 years of age with normal hearing. From the database, "easy" and "hard" word lists were developed for both the LNT and MLNT based on word occurrence and lexical density.

The LNT contains two lists of "easy" and two lists of "hard" monosyllabic words, and the MLNT contains one "easy" list and one "hard" list of two-to three-syllable words. The tests use an open-set response format, and are scored as the percentage of words and phonemes correctly identified as a function of lexical difficulty.

Kirk et al. (1995) assessed a group of pediatric cochlear implant users on the LNT and MLNT and compared their performance with individual scores from the PB-K word test. Results for both the LNT and MLNT demonstrated that word recognition was significantly better on the "easy" lists than on the "hard" lists, indicating that pediatric cochlear implant users are sensitive to acoustic-phonetic similarities among words. Moreover, these data suggest these children with cochlear implants organize words into similarity neighborhoods in long-term memory, consistent with children who have normal hearing. Additionally, word recognition was significantly higher on the lexically controlled lists than on the PB-K. Only 30% of the words on the PB-K are contained within the original database of words used for constructing the LNT and MLNT word lists. A reasonable explanation of these findings might be that restrictions imposed by creating phonetically balanced word lists such as the PB-K word lists result in the selection of test items that are unfamiliar to children with hearing loss.

Conclusion

The importance of assessing hearing in young children has been recognized for over 80 years. Adherence to two principles has been consistent during that period: balancing physiologic and behavioral approaches to hearing assessment results in the most optimal audiologic outcomes; and utilizing age-appropriate (based on developmental age) test techniques with children fosters efficiency and accuracy in audiologic measurement.

Consistent with these two principles is the recognition that behavioral test outcomes provide audiologists with data that reflect what children are actually "hearing." Therefore, the validity and reliability of behavioral test findings is of utmost importance. When principles of operant conditioning are maximized and when the operant discrimination protocol is applied to hearing assessment, audiometric data meet the high expectation of our patients, our health care colleagues, and our profession. Moreover, when operant principles are followed, the objectivity of our audiologic outcomes is quantified to the same level of precision achieved with our battery of physiologic measures.

References

American National Standards Institute. (1999). *Maximum permissible ambient noise for audiometric test rooms. ANSI S3.1-1999*. New York, NY: Author.

American National Standards Institute (ANSI; 2004). *About ANSI overview*. Retrieved from http://www.ansi.org/about_ansi/overview/overview.aspx?menuid=1

Barr, B. (1955). Pure tone audiometry for preschool children. *Acta Oto-Laryngologica Suppl., 121*, 5.

Bordley, J. E., Hardy, W. G., & Richter, C. P. (1948). Audiometry with use of galvanic skin-resistance response; preliminary report. *Bulletin of Johns Hopkins Hospital, 82*, 569.

Cluff, M. S., & Luce, P. A. (1990). Similarity neighborhoods of spoken two-syllable words: Retroactive effects on multiple activation. *Journal of Experimental Psychology: Human Perception and Performance, 16*, 551–563.

Diefendorf, A. O. (1981). *The effect of a pre-play period on play audiometry*. Paper presented at the annual convention of the Tennessee Speech-Language-Hearing Association, April. Memphis, TN.

Diefendorf, A. O., & Gravel, J. S. (1996). Behavioral observation and visual reinforcement audiometry. In S. E. Gerber (Ed.), *The handbook of pediatric audiology* (pp. 55–83). Washington, DC: Gallaudet Press.

Dix, M. R., & Hallpike, C. S. (1947). The peep show: A new technique for pure-tone audiometry in young children. *British Medical Journal, 2*, 719–723.

Eagles, E. L., & Wishik, S. M. (1961). A study of hearing in children. *Transactions of the American Academy of Ophthalmology and Otology, 65*, 261–282.

Eilers, R. E., Miskiel, E., Ozdamar, O., Urbano, R., & Widen, J. E. (1991). Optimization of automated hearing test algorithms: Simulation using an infant response model. *Ear and Hearing, 12*, 191–198.

Elliot, L. L., Clifton, L. B., & Servi, D. G. (1983). Word frequency effects for a closed-set word identification task. *Audiology, 22*, 229–240.

Elliott, L. L., & Katz, D. (1980). *Development of a new children's test of speech discrimination* [Technical manual]. St. Louis, MO: Auditec.

Ewing, A. W. G. (1930). *Aphasia in children*. Oxford, UK: Oxford Medical.

Finitzo-Hieber, T., Gerling, I. J., Matkin, N. D., & Cherow-Skalka, E. (1980). A sound effects recognition test for the pediatric audiological evaluation. *Ear and Hearing, 1*(5), 271–276.

Gerwin, K. S., & Glorig, A. (Eds.). (1974). *Detection of hearing loss and ear disease in children*. Springfield, IL: Charles C. Thomas.

Gravel, J.S. (1989). Behavioral assessment of auditory function. *Seminars in Hearing*, 10, 216–228.

Greenberg, J. H., & Jenkins, J. J. (1964). Studies in the psychological correlates of the sound system of American English. *Word, 20*, 157–177.

Guilford, R., & Haug, O. (1952). Diagnsosis of deafness in the very young child. *American Medical Association Archives of Otolaryngology, 55*, 101–106.

Haskins, H. (1949). *A phonetically balanced test of speech discrimination for children* (Unpublished Master's thesis). Northwestern University, Evanston, Illinois.

Hicks, C. B., Tharpe, A. M., & Ashmead, D. H. (2000). Behavioral auditory assessment of young infants: Methodological limitations or natural lack of auditory responsiveness? *American Journal of Audiology, 9*(2), 124–130.

Hodgson, W. R. (1973). *A comparison of WIPI and PB-K discrimination test scores*. Paper presented at the ASHA Convention, Detroit, MI.

Hodgson, W. R. (1985). Testing infants and young children. In J. Katz (Ed.), *Handbook of clinical audiology* (3rd ed., pp. 642–663). Baltimore, MD: Williams & Wilkins.

Hoversten, G. H., & Moncur, J. P. (1969). Stimuli and intensity factors in testing infants. *Journal of Speech and Hearing Research, 12*, 687–702.

Jerger, S., Lewis, S., Hawkins, J., & Jerger, J. (1980). Pediatric speech intelligibility test 1: Generation of test materials. *International Otorhinolaryngology, 2*, 217–230.

Karzon, R. K., & Banerjee, P. (2010). Animated toys versus video reinforcement in 16-24-month-old children in a clinical setting. *American Journal of Audiology, 19*, 91–99.

Kirk, K. I., Pisoni, D. B., & Osberger, M. J. (1995). Lexical effects on spoken word recognition by pediatric cochlear implant users. *Ear and Hearing, 16*, 470–481.

Kuhl, P. K. (2004). Early language acquisition: Cracking the speech code. *Nature Reviews Neuroscience, 5*(11), 831–843.

Landauer, T. K., & Streeter, L. A. (1973). Structural differences between common and rare words: Failure of equivalence assumptions for theories of word recognition. *Journal of Verbal Learning and Verbal Behavior, 12*, 119–131.

Levitt, H. (1970). Transformed up-down methods in psychoacoustics. *Journal of the Acoustical Society of America, 49*, 467–477.

Levitt, H. (1978). Adaptive testing in audiology. In C. Ludvigsen, & J. Barfod (Eds.). Sensorineural hearing impairment and hearing aids. *Scandinavian Audiology Supplement, 6*, 241–291.

Liden, G., & Kankkunen, A. (1969). Visual reinforcement audiometry. *Archives of Otolaryngology, 89*(6), 865–872.

Lowery, K. J., Von Hapsburg, D., Plyler, E. L., & Johnstone, P. (2009). A comparison of video versus conventional visual reinforcement in 7- to 16-month-old infants. *Journal of Speech and Hearing Research, 52*, 723–731.

Luce, P. A., Pisoni, D. B., & Goldinger, S. D. (1990). Similarity neighborhoods of spoken words. In G. M. Altman (Ed.), *Cognitive models of speech processing: Psycholinguistic and computational perspectives* (pp. 122–147). Cambridge, MA: MIT Press.

Matkin, N. D. (1977). Hearing aids for children. In W. Hodgson & P. Skinner (Eds.), *Hearing aid assessment and use in audiologic habilitation* (pp. 145–149). Baltimore, MD: Williams & Wilkins.

Maurer, D., & Werker, J. F. (2014). Perceptual narrowing during infancy: A comparison of language and faces. *Developmental Psychobiology*, 56(2), 154–178. http://doi.org/10.1002/dev.21177

Miller, A. L. (1963). The use of slide projectors in pure-tone audiometric testing. *Journal of Speech and Hearing Disorders, 28*, 94–96.

Moore, J. M., Thompson, G., & Thompson, M. (1975). Auditory localization of infants as a function of reinforcement conditions. *Journal of Speech and Hearing Disorders, 40*, 29–34.

Moore, J. M., & Wilson, W. R. (1978). Visual reinforcement audiometry (VRA) with infants. In S. E. Gerber, & G. T. Mencher (Eds.), *Early diagnosis of hearing loss* (pp. 177–213) New York, NY: Grune and Stratton.

Moore, J. M., & Wilson, W. R. (1987). Visual reinforcement audiometry (VRA) with infants. In S. E. Gerber & G. T. Mencher (Eds.), *Early diagnosis of hearing loss* (pp. 177–214). New York, NY: Grune and Stratton.

Moore, J. M., Wilson, W. R., & Thompson (1977). Visual reinforcement of head-turn responses in infants under 12 months of age. *Journal of Speech and Hearing Disorders, 42*, 328–334.

Muir, D. W., Clifton, R. K., & Clarkson, M. G. (1989). The development of a human auditory localization response: A U-shaped function. *Canadian Journal of Psychology, 43*(2), 199–216.

Northern, J. L., & Downs, M. P. (2002). *Hearing in children* (5th ed). Baltimore, MD: Lippincott Williams & Wilkins.

Nozza, R. J., & Wilson, W. R. (1984). Masked and unmasked pure-tone thresholds of infants and adults: Development of auditory frequency selectivity and sensitivity. *Journal of Speech and Hearing Research, 27*, 613–622.

O'Neill, J., Oyer, H. J., & Hillis, J. W. (1961). Audiometric procedures used with children. *Journal of Speech and Hearing Disorders, 26*, 61–66.

Primus, M. A. (1991). Repeated infant thresholds in operant and nonoperant audiometric procedures. *Ear and Hearing, 12*, 119–122.

Primus, M. (1992). Operant response in infants as a function of time interval following signal onset. *Journal of Speech and Hearing Research*, 35, 1422–1425.

Ross, M., & Lerman, J. (1970). Picture identification test for hearing-impaired children. *Journal of Speech and Hearing Research, 13*, 44–53.

Sanderson-Leepa, M. E., & Rintelmann, W. F. (1976). Articulation function and test-retest performance of normal-learning children on three speech discrimination tests: WIPI, PBK50, and NU auditory test No. 6. *Journal of Speech and Hearing Disorders, 41*, 503–519.

Schmida, M. J., Peterson, H. J., & Tharpe, A. M. (2003). Visual reinforcement audiometry using digital video disc and conventional reinforcers. *American Journal of Audiology, 12*, 35–40.

Shaw, G. (2013). Pediatric audiologist shortage leaves providers searching for a solution. *Hearing Journal, 66*(11), 18, 20, 22.

Shimizu, H., & Nakamura, F. (1957). Pure-tone audiometry in children: Lantern-slides test. *Annals of Otology, Rhinology, and Laryngology, 66*, 392–398.

Skinner, B. B. (1953). *Science and human behavior*. New York, NY: Macmillan.

Statten, P., & Wishart, D. E. S. (1956). Pure-tone audiometry in young children: Psychogalvanic-skin resistance and peep-show. *Annals of Otology, Rhinology, and Laryngology, 65*, 511–534.

Suzuki, T., & Ogiba, Y. (1961). Conditioned orientation reflex audiometry. *Archives of Otolaryngology, 74*, 192–198.

Tharpe, A. M., & Ashmead, D. A. (1993). A computer simulation technique for assessing pediatric auditory test protocols. *Journal of the American Academy of Audiology, 4*(2), 80–90.

Thompson, G., & Folsom, R. (1984). A comparison of two conditioning procedures in the use of visual reinforcement audiometry (VRA). *Journal of Speech and Hearing Disorders, 49*, 241–245.

Thompson, G., & Weber, B. A. (1974). Responses of infants and young children to behavioral observation audiometry (BOA). *Journal of Speech and Hearing Disorders, 39*, 140–147.

Thompson, M. D., Thompson, G., & Vethivelu, S. (1989). A comparison of audiometric test thresholds for 2-year-old children. *Journal of Speech and Hearing Disorders, 54*, 174–179.

Tsao, F.-M., Liu, H.-M., & Kuhl, P. K. (2004). Speech perception in infancy predicts language development in the second year of life: A longitudinal study. *Child Development, 75*(4), 1067–1084.

Widen, J. E. (1993). Adding objectivity to infant behavioral audiometry. *Ear and Hearing, 14*(1), 49–57.

Widen, J. E., Johnson, J. L., White, K. R., Gravel, J. S., Vohr, B., James, M., . . . Meyer, S. (2005). A multisite study to examine the efficacy of the otoacoustic emission/automated auditory brainstem response newborn hearing screening protocol: Results of visual reinforcement audiometry. *American Journal of Audiology, 14*(2), S200–S216.

Wilson, W. R., Moore, J. M., & Thompson, G. (1976). *Soundfield auditory thresholds of infants utilizing visual reinforcement audiometry (VRA).* Presented at the American Speech and Hearing Association Annual Convention, Houston, TX.

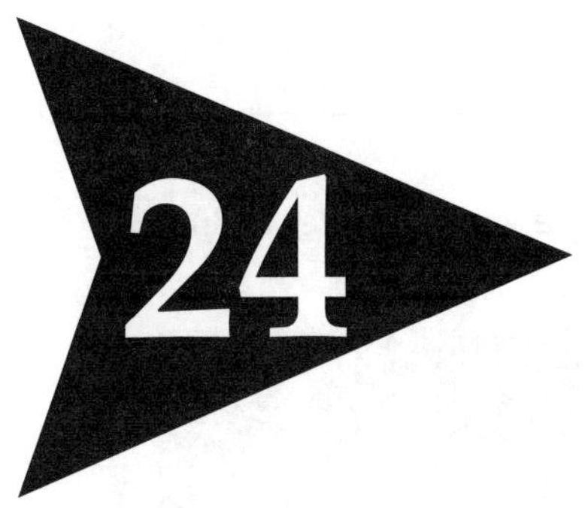

Audiologic Considerations for Children With Complex Developmental Conditions

Allan O. Diefendorf, Kathleen R. Corbin, Rebecca Trepcos-Klingler, and Amanda S. Weinzierl

Introduction

The etiology of congenital hearing loss can be derived from four major etiologic classifications including chromosomal origin, genetic origin, environmental teratogens, and low birth weight. Table 24–1 provides "frequent" selected examples within each classification. Usually, the most cited examples would be those that themselves are most frequently observed, with hearing loss being a variably occurring outcome of the etiology. However, for this table, the authors have chosen to define "frequent" as those patients seen at their home institution (James Whitcomb Riley Hospital for Children) having been diagnosed with hearing loss and also presenting with an additional chromosomal feature, genetic feature, or associated congenital clinical condition.

Historically, the past 25 years of demographic data (Fortnum & Davis, 1997; Gallaudet College Center for Assessment and Demographic Studies, 1983; Gallaudet Research Institute, 2005; Mace, Wallace, Whan, & Stelmachowicz, 1991) consistently have reported that 30% to 40% of children with hearing loss have one or more *additional* disabilities. Table 24–2 lists physical and cognitive/intellectual conditions that are most frequently reported to accompany hearing loss. Thus, Table 24–1 and Table 24–2 are complementary; that is, Table 24–1 identifies "etiology," and Table 24–2 identifies "outcomes" that can occur in a high percentage of children with congenital hearing loss. Additionally, the manner in which different etiologies *coexist* and the manner in which etiologic outcomes are *expressed* (by degree of involvement) contribute to each child's personal developmental outcome. Therefore, *every child* brings a unique combination of characteristics (hearing loss alone, hearing loss with diverse systemic involvement) to their individual developmental profile.

The fact that hearing impairment in children can be accompanied by additional challenging conditions emphasizes the importance of considering each child's developmental profile when implementing an audiologic assessment plan. Additionally, with the benchmark of audiologic diagnosis by 3 months of age (Joint Committee on Infant Hearing [JCIH], 2007), it is likely that many infants with hearing loss *and* multiple developmental conditions might not have had these conditions diagnosed at the time of the audiologic assessment. Therefore, audiologists face challenges when dealing with the diversity of individual characteristics that might be found among children suspected of hearing loss.

Clearly, the presence of physical and cognitive/intellectual conditions will add to the complexity of caring for children with multiple special needs. Furthermore, these conditions can influence audiologic test selection, audiologic outcomes, and subsequent recommendations which will undergird intervention planning. As such, audiologic test protocols must be, by necessity, flexible to accommodate individual child differences and preferences. As pointed out by Tharpe (2009), audiologists must be mindful of the possibility that unexpected or undiagnosed conditions might influence their testing and subsequent audiologic outcomes.

Table 24–1. Etiologic Classification of Congenital Hearing Loss and Selected Examples Within Each Classification

Etiologic Classification	*Selected Examples*	
Chromosomal origin	Trisomy 13 (Patua syndrome) Trisomy 18 (Edward syndrome) Trisomy 21 (Down syndrome) 5P (Cri-du-chat syndrome)	4P (deletion problem) Fragile X syndrome Turner syndrome
Genetic origin	Alport syndrome Branchiootorenal syndrome CHARGE association Chiari malformation Crouzon syndrome de Lange syndrome DiGeorge syndrome Hemifacial microsomia Jervell & Lange-Nielsen	Mitochondrial disorders Neurofibromatosis Type II Osteogenesis imperfecta spectrum Pendred syndrome Pierre Robin sequence Stickler syndrome Treacher Collins syndrome Usher syndrome Waardenburg syndrome
Teratogens[a]	Viral disease Bacterial disease Maternal smoking Thyroid disorders	Environmental toxins (lead, mercury) Fetal alcohol syndrome Drugs (substance abuse) Radiation
Low birth weight	Respiratory distress syndrome Bronchopulmonary dysplasia (BPD) Hyperbilirubinemia Neonatal sepsis	Patent ductus arteriosus Peri-/intraventricular hemorrhage Perinatal asphyxia

[a]Agents in the environment of the developing embryo and fetus that cause structural or functional abnormalities.

Thus, the purpose of this chapter is to focus on adaptations and enhancements in pediatric audiologic assessment when providing services to children with suspected or confirmed physical or developmental challenges.

Patient History

When assessing infants and young children with suspected or confirmed physical or developmental challenges, a thorough patient history is essential. Traditionally, acquiring patient history information has been completed by obtaining answers to a predetermined list of questions. However, this approach can limit audiologists to arbitrarily restricted personal information and prevent a more individualized patient-centered approach to acquiring relevant information. It is recommended that time for obtaining a patient history is viewed as a valuable opportunity to observe and interact with the child and family, build rapport, and instill confidence and comfort in the child and family, while acquiring specific personal history information. This is especially true when attempting to assess a child with special needs. Furthermore, these initial observations facilitate assessment planning and clinical strategies by determining how much independence, cooperation, communication, and physical ability can be expected.

Observation and Interaction

The patient history process begins as early as calling the child's name in the waiting room. Time spent observing

Table 24–2. Physical and Cognitive/Intellectual Conditions[a] Frequently Reported to Accompany Hearing Loss in Children

Physical Conditions
Asthma
Brain damage or injury
Cardiovascular defects
Cerebral palsy
Endocrine abnormalities (e.g., hypothyroidism, diabetes, kernicterus)
Epilepsy
Immunologic abnormalities
Kidney defects
Legal blindness
Neurologic abnormalities
Orthopedic abnormalities
Uncorrected or uncorrectable visual problem
Cognitive Intellectual Conditions
Intellectual disability
Specific learning disability that may include visual/auditory perceptual problems; fine motor coordination problems; attention deficit disorder; developmental delay
Emotional/behavioral problems that may include autism spectrum disorder; hyperactivity; passive/withdrawn behavior (social isolation); reduced self-esteem; aggressive/abusive behavior; unfounded physical complaints and symptoms

[a]There are 60% to 70% of children who present with no additional handicapping conditions, whereas 30% to 40% present with one (or more) additional handicapping conditions.

the child from the waiting room to the assessment area can provide cues about the child's physical and developmental status. Previous literature has stressed the importance of the "hallway conversation" or the history intake that is completed as the audiologist walks the family from the waiting room to the evaluation area (Renshaw & Diefendorf, 1998). However, in concert with increasingly stringent privacy laws (i.e., Health Insurance Portability and Accountability Act [HIPAA]), strict adherence to protecting confidential patient information in a public area is essential. A HIPAA compliant hallway conversation might be one where instead of asking personal questions regarding the child's medical history, the brief time is utilized for observation and for casual conversation intended to build rapport with the child and their family.

Observations can be made about behaviors such as, but not limited to

- temperament of the child;
- alertness of the child;
- clues about the developmental status of the child (e.g., walking, talking);
- clues about the interaction/communication between the child and their family;
- independence/shyness/fearfulness following introduction; and
- willingness of the child to engage/participate in conversation.

For example, a child older than 18 months of age who is not walking independently might signal delays in developmental status. If calling a child's name in the waiting room causes crying, this might suggest fearfulness, a low comfort level or a lack of willingness to engage.

Casual conversation allows the audiologist an initial opportunity to interact with the child for the purposes of building rapport with the child and family. The desired outcome is reducing their anxiety about a new environment, new adults, and entering a room with unfamiliar equipment. Some examples of rapport-building and anxiety-reducing strategies include

- introducing yourself to the child and family;
- complementing the child on attire or toys;
- asking about age or grade level;
- introducing positive reinforcements/rewards that might be used during or at completion of assessment (e.g., showing stickers/toys/high fives/blowing bubbles);
- informing the child and family about expectations of what is to come during the assessment in order to ease anxiety/fears (the benefit of this practice with the child should not be underestimated); and
- allowing the child to touch equipment (e.g., holding the otoscope, feeling the ear tips, touching the bone oscillator).

The most important factor that might determine the comfort level of the child is the communication between the family (caregiver) and the audiologist. Positive interactions are more likely to evoke positive feelings in the child about the assessment procedure (Northern & Downs, 2002). One preventable behavior that can lead to anxiety in the child is when the caregiver is negative about the examination prior to the start of the appointment. When caregivers report that their child does not like strangers and they do not believe their child will cooperate with your activities, this sends a negative signal to the child that might be irreversible. In turn, this negativity can cause lack of participation or reduced cooperation during the assessment. The audiologist's role is to ease parental and child anxiety and redirect negative comments in order to modify behavior that can influence assessment outcomes.

Interview

Audiologists need answers to some very direct and specific questions in order to accurately assess and diagnose hearing loss. One can find examples of various "case history questionnaires" published in audiology literature (ASHA, 2004; Beck, 2015). Even the most exhaustive of case history questionnaires essentially try to gather information regarding the same basic concepts including family history, birth history, developmental history (including hearing and speech/language development), and medical history. Each concept can be used to generate as many or as few questions as each child's situation might demand to create a meaningful history intake process. Each of these unique concepts should then be viewed collectively to integrate all the information obtained for the purpose of determining appropriate assessment and follow-up (Figure 24–1).

It is important to pose questions in a respectful and professional manner. It also is critical to rely on careful and active listening. Audiologists must be flexible enough to modify the order in which they

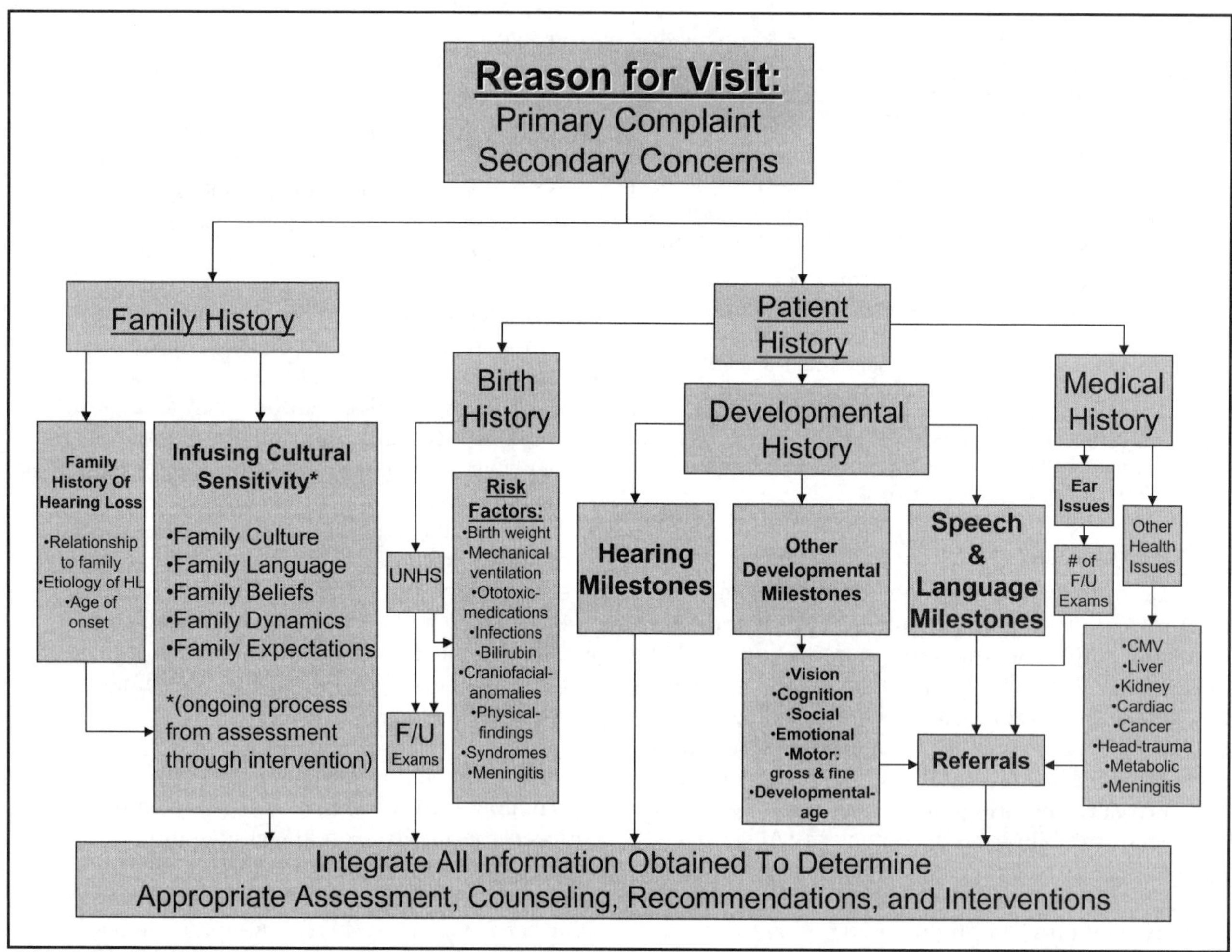

FIGURE 24–1. Flowchart demonstrating information management and integration from family and patient history for achieving optimal audiologic outcomes. (*F/U* = follow-up; *UNHS* = universal newborn hearing screening; *CMV* = cytomegalovirus.)

ask questions and be intuitive enough to ask appropriate follow-up questions (that might not be on the published questionnaire) based on initial observations and interactions. It also is important to clarify obtained information to ensure accuracy of reporting. Frequently, audiologists might need to ask sensitive questions about things such as visible physical characteristics, performance in school, achieving developmental milestones relative to other siblings, and ability of relatives, friends, and neighbors to understand their child's speech and language expression. Avoiding direct questions for fear of appearing insensitive can result in failure to learn relevant information about the child. Information that is acquired in a supportive, family-focused manner (ASHA, 2008) facilitates early diagnosis, early and appropriate referrals, and subsequent intervention plans.

The audiologist's challenge is to acquire sufficient information which, in turn, assists families in recognizing important information. When achieved, the interview process transforms parents and caregivers into informed consumers of complex diagnostic information.

All history intake questions that are asked should never lose track of the main goals of the interview process:

- child's individuality;
- family's culture and language;
- parent and caregiver concern;
- respect for family coping style;
- family's expectations from appointment; and
- support for the development of informed and empowered families.

Interview time also should be viewed as an opportunity to acknowledge the expertise of the caregiver or caregivers in their child's life. Caregivers should be viewed as experts about their child because they can provide unique insight about their child's personal preferences, personality, and other characteristics that constitute their individuality. "There are no magical instruments or questionnaires that can substitute for authentic understanding born of lengthy acquaintance, mutual trust, and rapport" (Turnbull, 1991, p. 39).

Multicultural Considerations

The U.S. population is becoming increasingly diverse as suggested by the U.S. Census data obtained over the last few years. According to data obtained in 2010, 36.3% of the U.S. population now belongs to racial and ethnic minority groups and approximately 20% of the population over age 5 years speaks a language other than English in the home. These population statistics are expected to increase over time.

The Institute of Medicine (IOM) published a report (2002) that reviewed over 100 studies that assessed the quality of health care for various ethnic and racial minority groups. The report highlighted existing disparities in quality of health care provided to minorities. The IOM committee concluded that very few of these differences in health care quality for minorities and nonminorities can be attributed to patient attitudes and preferences. More significant contributors to these disparities include

- ecology of health care systems and environmental factors. These include factors such as cultural or linguistic barriers (e.g., lack of interpretive services) and fragmentation of health care systems (e.g., minorities are less likely to access care at a private physician's office even when insured at the same level; IOM, 2002).
- discrimination: biases, stereotyping, and uncertainty. The report suggests that these disparities might originate from the provider—that is, prejudice against minorities, clinical uncertainty when interacting with minorities, and stereotypes held about minorities.

This increasing diversity poses unique challenges for health care professionals, including audiologists. Perceptions regarding hearing loss differ across cultures. Some cultures might not attribute much significance to hearing loss and, consequently, are less likely to seek hearing services. For example, individuals whose values and beliefs are representative of Deaf culture do not view hearing loss as a disability, but as a difference. As such, they might choose not to engage in "treatment and/or interventions" if recommendations are in conflict with personal or cultural views or their desired short- and long-term goals. People from other cultures might recognize hearing loss as a problem but choose to not follow recommended treatment or interventions due to religious or other societal beliefs.

Linguistic barriers and a lack of familiarity with accessing resources can prevent other minority groups from receiving quality care. In the case of a child who speaks any language other than English, testing materials in that language might not be readily available. This can compromise quality of service delivery, trust with the family, subsequent recommendations, and future appointments. Knowing a few key words or phrases in languages that are common in the community can help families feel comfortable, and often allows them to be more open about their concerns even in the presence of a language interpreter. Speaking to a child in the child's native language for phrases "how are you," "nothing hurts," "great job," "thank you," or having the child point to body parts in his or her native language during speech audiometry, demonstrates a level of compassion during the assessment that helps reduce the anxiety and stress of linguistic barriers.

Cultural Competence

As health care professionals, audiologists need to be respectful of and responsive to the needs of a diverse patient population by continually increasing their knowledge and skill in cultural competence. Being culturally competent is the ability to ensure that cultural disparities do not influence desired outcomes for patients. "Culturally competent professionals understand the power of culture in shaping family and professional beliefs, attitudes, and practices" (Kaufmann & McGonigel, 1991, p. 55). This skill is especially important during the history intake process. Audiologists should be proficient at the art of "ethnographic interviewing." Westby, Burda, and Mehta (2003) define ethnographic interviewing as the means for developing an appreciation of the "child and their family's perception of the communication disability and its effects." General principles for ethnographic interviewing as outlined by Westby et al. include

- ask for use instead of meaning;
- use open-ended questions rather than dichotomous questions;
- restate what the child or family says in exact words: do not paraphrase or interpret;
- summarize their statements and give them the opportunity to correct any misinterpretations;
- avoid multiple questions;
- avoid leading questions; and
- avoid using "why" questions because they tend to sound judgmental and assume that the person knows "why."

Interpreter Use

Another useful skill that audiologists must master is the effective use of interpreters when dealing with families that speak other languages. Some techniques to consider for ensuring successful exchange of information include using short concise sentences and pausing frequently between them to allow the interpreter to organize and effectively translate. It also is important to remember to speak directly to the child and family and avoid oversimplification of important explanations. It is necessary to be mindful of nonverbal gestures that can be interpreted differently by different cultures and certain words that might not have the same meaning when translated.

Revising our traditional views of the history intake procedures and implementing progressive strategies that are culturally sensitive and appropriate lays the foundation for providing high-quality health care to diverse patient populations. Additionally, these same principles should be applied throughout the EHDI process, and when children and families transition from EHDI programs to school-based services.

Visual Inspection of the Outer Ear and Otoscopy

Visual inspection of the outer ear, ear canal, and tympanic membrane is standard practice when evaluating hearing of infants and young children. Visual inspection of the outer ear does not usually require the use of magnification provided by an otoscope. Rather, visual inspection of the outer ear is typically performed by carefully looking at the outer ear and noting any abnormalities such as deformity of the pinna, unusual shape or position of the pinna, or preauricular skin tags or ear pits in front of the ear or upper neck area. In some cases, but certainly not all, these visual cues could be outer signs of other auditory system abnormalities and subsequent hearing loss, as well as concern for various genetic syndromes (e.g., Down syndrome, Treacher Collins syndrome, brachiootorenal syndrome). For example, Roth et al. (2008) studied the prevalence of hearing loss in a large cohort of infants with preauricular skin tags or ear pits in comparison to newborns without these outer ear abnormalities. Overall, they found a significantly higher prevalence of permanent hearing loss in the infants with preauricular skin tags or ear pits (8 per 1,000) when compared to infants without tags or pits (1.5 per 1,000).

Otoscopy is intended as a general inspection of the external ear canal for malformations, or blockage from atresia, stenosis, foreign bodies, cerumen, or other debris; and inspection of the tympanic membrane for obvious signs of disease including the presence of a perforation, pressure equalization tubes, or retraction of the eardrum. Moreover, because several audiologic assessment procedures require the insertion of a probe tip or insert earphone into the external auditory canal, the visual inspection serves to verify that there are no contraindications to placing a probe in the ear canal.

Children vary in their acceptance of an otoscopic exam. Some children will be resistant to the procedure and the audiologist will need to try to make the process as child friendly as possible. Suggestions for success include

- allowing the child to hold the otoscope;
- pointing the light in the child's hand;
- looking into the parent's or caregiver's ear to demonstrate the procedure; or
- gently touching the child's cheek with the head of the otoscope.

Optimizing Audiologic Assessment for Children With Complex Developmental Conditions: Physiologic Measures

Following observations, interactions, and a thorough patient history, an audiologist might decide that the child will not be able to participate in behavioral testing. Therefore, reliance on physiologic measures will be necessary.

Employing optimal test parameters with physiologic measures for children with complex developmental conditions should not be compromised, regardless of the child's disability. However, completing physiologic measures on children with additional disabilities can prove to be a challenge. As such, it is important to have a thorough familiarity with the child's medical history as it can offer insights into test selection, test order, test interpretation, and subsequent recommendations. Children who are behaviorally, developmentally, or cognitively challenged might be lethargic, hyperactive, combative, tactilely defensive, or unwilling to sit quietly. Additionally, they might be unwilling or unable to comply with instructions and unable to cooperate for a sufficient length of time for test completion. Although evidence-based protocols for administering physiologic measures remain the same with these children, there are several modified strategies that can easily be incorporated to maximize patient compliance.

Customizing your test battery and selection for the child is a skill that comes with experience. By paying careful attention to the subtle details of the child's behavior and demeanor, you might gain some insights regarding their capabilities and level of cooperation. This will save time in the limited window offered by the child. Choosing appropriate audiologic tests and deciding on the appropriate order of test presentation are essential to a successful outcome.

Acoustic Impedance Measures

Acoustic immittance measures are an integral part of the assessment battery when evaluating children with complex developmental conditions. Clinical decisions should be made on a quantitative assessment of the tympanogram, including consideration of equivalent ear canal volume, peak compensated static acoustic admittance, tympanometric width, and tympanometric peak pressure.

Frequently, a tympanogram is the first test attempted. However, there are times when tympanograms should be deferred until after behavioral testing. The rationale for deferring is that the positive interaction and overall compliance desired in behavioral testing might not be available if the child has found a tympanogram to be an unpleasant experience. Occasionally, children find the experience unpleasant due to the restraint that some parents initiate to hold their children, or due to the child's chronic ear pain where they fear anyone trying to touch their ears.

In addition to providing confirmation of middle ear status, acoustic reflex measurement is useful in the interpretation of other components in the audiologic test battery. That is, the acoustic reflex might provide supplemental information relevant to the functional status of the middle ear, cochlea, and brainstem pathway. The same distraction techniques used for obtaining tympanograms can be used while measuring acoustic reflexes.

Some suggestions for obtaining impedance measures include the following:

- Carefully observe the child.
  - Is there readiness to sit quietly or not at all?
  - Is the child calm or afraid?
  - Is the child crying?
- Tailor your approach accordingly.
- Enlist assistance from the parent. This could range from verbal reassurance to gentle restraint of the child. It is well established that involvement of families in the provision of clinical services is crucial for families' acceptance of hearing loss (Luterman, 1999). A family's presence and participation allow the audiologist to explain the purpose of each step of the assessment, which in turn improves the family's ability to understand the findings of an otherwise abstract and technical test process.

- Enlist your coworker as a participant (Table 24–3). A coworker can engage the child with positive comments or visual distractions such as bubbles.
- Use a bottle or a pacifier to comfort an infant who is crying.
- Select screening mode when possible rather than the diagnostic mode. This allows physical assistance by the audiologist in the maintenance of a proper seal and reduces the overall test time.

Otoacoustic Emissions

Otoacoustic emissions (OAEs) expand the pediatric audiology test battery by providing a physiologic means of assessing preneural auditory function. Knowledge of the physiology underlying the generation of OAEs makes them a powerful tool in the diagnostic test battery. Because they are indicative of mechanical, preneural activity of the outer hair cells, clinicians have an idea whether there is a "sensory" component to a more commonly described "sensory-neural" hearing loss (Lonsbury-Martin, McCoy, Whitehead, & Martin, 1993). Additionally, with the pediatric population, OAEs offer the clinician the opportunity to obtain ear specific data since behavioral audiometric measures obtained in sound field are not able to reveal individual ear information.

OAEs have the clinical capability to indicate normal cochlear function when it exists. As such, the presence of OAEs is consistent with normal or near-normal hearing thresholds in a given frequency region. For pediatric audiology this is particularly helpful when used in conjunction with other hearing assessment tools such as the ABR/ASSR and tests of middle ear function (tympanometry). For example, in children with neurologic involvement, an absent brainstem response can be the result of either severe cochlear involvement *or* lack of neural synchrony at the level of the brainstem. A finding of normal OAEs and normal middle ear function indicates normal peripheral (i.e., middle ear and cochlea) functioning, thus isolating the disorder to the brainstem auditory pathway. This finding illustrates an increasingly common audiologic challenge. Normal OAEs in combination with abnormal brainstem function represent the hallmark signs in infants and children of some form of auditory nerve pathology, brainstem neuropathy, or brainstem conduction defect.

Otoacoustic emissions also can provide an excellent tool for monitoring ototoxicity affects from aminoglycoside antibiotics such as tobramycin (Katbamma, Hommick, & Marks, 1999) or antitumor chemotherapy agents such as cisplatin (Ress et al., 1999). Stavroulaki et al. (2002) examined children receiving cisplatin. They concluded that OAEs (specifically distortion product OAEs) were sensitive indicators of cochlear damage and were superior to behavioral audiometry for identifying cochlear changes. When this audiological information is provided to the managing physician, it offers clinical evidence to the individual's susceptibility to potentially ototoxic agents and can result in an alternative plan of treatment or care. Additionally, because of their remarkable stability over time within the same ear, OAEs also are useful for monitoring the status of disease conditions that are progressive, including certain genetic disorders such as Usher syndrome (Meredith, Stephens, Sirimanna, Meyer-Bisch, & Reardon, 1992).

Schemes for trying to determine the degree of hearing loss and predicting thresholds using OAEs have been investigated (Boege & Janssen, 2002; Dorn et al., 2001; Gorga et al., 2003; Gorga, Neely, & Dorn, 2002; Gorga, Stover, & Neely, 1996). Although some strategies have met with success, variability is such that threshold predictions should be viewed cautiously. Although OAE testing should not be used to specify hearing thresholds, it can be used to establish an initial impression about hearing. These impressions determine if further assessments need to be completed (Evenhuis, 1996).

Table 24–3. Distraction Suggestions for Use During Acoustic Immittance Measurements

	Tactile	*Auditory*	*Visual*	*Visual*	*Visual*	*Visual*
Examining audiologist	Tickle the outer ear	Sing "one, two, three," as you "Take a picture"	"Watch the picture that your ear can draw"	—	—	—
Assisting coworker	—	—	—	Blow bubbles	Play "peek-a-boo"	Use puppets

Challenges in obtaining OAEs might arise if the child is unable to sit quietly or leave the probe tip in their ear for the duration of the test. Some considerations for obtaining OAE results include the following:

- Enlist parental support in holding the child on their lap and hold the child's hands as necessary.
- Place younger children in a high chair.
- Allow the child to quietly play with objects of distraction. Examples include Lego blocks, bubbles, Mr. Potato Head, pop beads, puzzles, and books.
- Sing children's songs to your patient. Children's favorites often include hand motions.
- Have a small DVD player available and allow the child to watch a cartoon or children's video without sound. This can help distract and quiet the child for an extended period of time.
- Consider your protocol selection. You might want to use a protocol that assesses a smaller range of frequencies, thus reducing overall test time.

Auditory Brainstem Response (ABR) and Auditory Steady-State Response (ASSR)

Achieving an audiologic diagnosis by 3 months of age (JCIH, 2007) necessitates detailed diagnostic assessment requiring frequency-specific thresholds *and* identification of the type of hearing loss including neural conduction deficits within weeks of referral. These outcomes are essential to inform decisions regarding medical follow-up, audiologic care planning, and early intervention services. Uncertainty with regard to hearing loss type leads to large delays in medical treatment and audiologic intervention (Gravel, 2002).

Therefore, auditory-evoked potentials (AEPs) with high correlation to frequency-specific behavioral thresholds are essential to facilitate confirmation and characterization of hearing loss (of a mild degree or worse). Moreover, measurements must include bone-conduction thresholds to frequency-specific stimuli to distinguish between sensory-neural, conductive, and mixed hearing losses, in turn facilitating early referral for medical or audiologic intervention.

The ABR to air- and bone-conducted (A/C and B/C, respectively) brief tones has a long history of successful clinical use. By comparison, the ASSR has a more recent history, but evidence continues to grow suggesting the ASSR has an emerging record of successful clinical use for infant threshold measurement by A/C, and as a cross-check with B/C ABR.

An important point to establish is that physiological thresholds rarely equal those measured behaviorally; after all, the procedures and measurements are fundamentally different. However, if a physiological method is to predict auditory status successfully across all age groups (with dynamic developmental considerations especially in infants), it is essential that a strong correlation exist between behavioral and physiological thresholds with appropriate supporting evidence. Comparisons between ABR- and ASSR A/C and B/C thresholds, as well as suggested corrections factors to estimate behavioral hearing thresholds in dB HL are presented in Chapter 21 of this volume.

Pediatric audiologic services rendered today should meet the patients' needs (and families' expectations), be based on the best scientific knowledge available, and be provided in an efficient manner that minimizes costs, resources, and time. Because test time might be limited, decisions about stimulus mode (A/C versus B/C), preferred frequencies and frequency order, and stimulus intensity levels must be made continuously in an assessment protocol. The reader is directed to Chapter 21 for a detailed analysis of best practice clinical decision making in frequency-specific threshold assessment with infants and young children referred for or suspected of congenital hearing loss.

Children presenting with complex developmental conditions often present challenges to the interpretation of AEP findings. For example, several studies have reported delayed conduction times in the ABR of children with autism (McCellend, Eyre, Watson, Calvert, & Sherrard, 1992; Rosenthall, Nordin, Brantberg, & Gillberg, 2003; Wong & Wong, 1991). Moreover, children with hydrocephalus can have elevated or absent ABR thresholds (Kraus, Ozdamar, Stein, & Reed, 1984). In children presenting with neurofibromatosis type I or II (NFI or NFII), involvement of the auditory system is indicated by abnormal middle ear muscle reflexes and abnormal ABRs (Pikus, 1995). Additionally, the ABR in children with Down syndrome reveals Wave V latency and amplitude differences at reduced intensity levels when compared to normal developing controls. However, at greater stimulus levels (e.g., 60 dB nHL) latency of the ABR is shorter than matched control subjects. Thus, the slope of the intensity-latency function is steeper for children with Down syndrome than for normally developing controls (Folsom, Widen, & Wilson, 1983). Dille (2003) concluded that ABR testing should be interpreted with caution, because it is likely that those with Down syndrome demonstrate a neural developmental time course that is uniquely different than the developmental time course of typically developing individuals. As such, it is important to note that AEP results should not be interpreted in isolation.

Additionally, children with auditory neuropathy/auditory dys-synchrony (AN/AD) present with absent and/or distorted AEPs, suggesting abnormal auditory pathway function beginning with the eighth nerve. The diagnosis of AN/AD requires an AEP test to assess the presence of a cochlear microphonic *and* tests of cochlear function, including otoacoustic emissions and acoustic stapedial reflexes. The JCIH (2007) has included neural hearing loss (e.g., AN/AD) in infants admitted to the neonatal intensive care unit (NICU) in their targeted definition of hearing loss. As such, the audiologic community must be vigilant concerning this disorder because intervention and management are different from those with sensory-neural hearing loss.

For children who are neurologically, cognitively, and/or behaviorally involved, interpretation of ABR waveform data must proceed with caution. Additionally, AEP findings should be considered as part of a test battery including behavioral audiometry, patient history, and other physiologic measures before developing a definitive diagnosis of the child's hearing status (Kaga, Ohuchi, Kaga, & Tanaka, 1984; Pijl, Stewart, & Laskowski, 1988; Siegenthaler, 1987).

To facilitate electrophysiologic recordings, a relaxed patient state is essential to improve response morphology and subsequent interpretation accuracy. In children with complex developmental conditions, this might be achieved during natural sleep or with the addition of sedation. Although the following suggestions work best for unsedated patients, they also might apply when sedation is administered:

- Request that the child arrive sleepy. This might require that parents awaken the child early. Prevent the child from taking a nap, and emphasize the importance of keeping the child awake while traveling to the appointment. Suggest bringing another caregiver, if possible, who can ride in the back with the infant/child in order to keep them awake if the distance to the appointment is far.
- Request that the bottle-fed or nursing child arrive hungry. Having the parent feed the child immediately prior to the test often facilitates sleep. If the infant/child is fed through alternative means, such as a G-tube, try to coordinate the appointment with feeding time, or have the parent arrive early to facilitate the increased time required for a feed.
- Reduce stimulation in the room. This might include dimming the lights or reducing the number of people present in the room. Request that parents and/or caregivers silence their cell phones or turn them off during testing.
- Make the setting more comfortable. Provide a recliner or rocking chair and allow the parent to hold the child during the test. Have a pillow or a blanket available and adjust the room temperature as needed.
- Allow the parent to bring any items that comfort the child. This could include a pacifier, bottle, blanket, stuffed animal, or special toy.

To gain the cooperation of some infants and young children during physiologic assessments of auditory function, sedation might be required. However, sedation of pediatric patients, with or without complex developmental conditions, might be contraindicated due to factors such as airway obstruction, apnea, cardiopulmonary impairment, and hypoventilation. As such, moderate sedation should only be administered by, or in the presence of, individuals skilled in airway management and cardiopulmonary resuscitation. Additionally, the oversight by a sedation team and the availability of age- and size-appropriate equipment, medications, and continuous monitoring are essential during procedures and for resuscitating the child should an adverse sedation event occur. When making a recommendation for a sedated AEP, audiologists can begin the process of determining eligibility by asking medical history questions related to sedation risks, such as the following: Does the child currently use oxygen? Does he or she have a history of sleep apnea? Has sedation ever been used in the past?

Optimizing Audiologic Assessment for Children With Complex Developmental Conditions: Behavioral Measures

The literature over the past 50 years has reinforced the widely held view that when children hear a sound, they will react in a deliberate manner that is consistent with their level of developmental/mental functioning (Barr, 1955; Eisenberg, 1969; Greenberg, Wilson, Moore, & Thompson, 1978; Hoversten & Moncur, 1969; Moore, 1995; Primus, 1992; Suzuki & Ogiba, 1960; Talbott, 1987; Thompson & Weber, 1974; Wilson, Moore, & Thompson, 1976). Scientific evidence coupled with clinical observations substantiate that predictable response behavior is characteristic of *typically developing children*. However, for children with complex developmental conditions (e.g., children with autism, Down syndrome, or other developmental conditions), auditory response behavior might not be as predictable, and it cannot be stereotyped (Tharpe et al., 2006). That is, children with complex developmental conditions might not orient to sound, might be hypersensitive to sound to the extent that they exhibit painful hearing, might have a preoccupation with or agitation to sound, cannot be conditioned to sound, or might demonstrate very poor test-retest reliability within a test session and between test sessions. Despite these challenges in behavioral assessment with children with complex developmental conditions, Tharpe (2009) advocates that, "we must bear in mind that behavioral tests provide an indication of how an individual uses his or her hearing, a very important factor when considering management needs."

Every effort must be made to ensure the comprehensiveness and accuracy of all audiologic results. For children with complex developmental conditions, audiologic results can be difficult to obtain, although no less important. With flexibility, patience, and determination, behavioral results can be obtained that provide valuable information regarding "hearing" in the child relative to their complex developmental profile.

Chapter 23 reviews behavioral assessment techniques for infants and children; however, physical conditions and cognitive/intellectual conditions (see Table 24–2) might have a significant influence on behavioral outcomes in audiologic assessment. That is, these conditions (e.g., cerebral palsy, neurologic abnormalities, blindness, and/or uncorrected visual problems) can influence reflexive and orienting responses, as well as "mask" conditioned responses. Additionally, cognitive/intellectual conditions can influence the child's operant conditioning, overall response behavior, response latency, dynamic range (threshold responses to loudness discomfort), and habituation to auditory stimuli. As such, the audiologic approach initiated (usually made on the basis of developmental age) must consider these variables on the specific protocol used (behavioral observation audiometry, visual reinforcement audiometry, and conditioned play audiometry).

When physical and cognitive/intellectual conditions are considered for each child's unique developmental profile, and appropriate modifications in behavioral protocols are implemented, confidence in behavioral results is improved. This confidence comes not only from experience, but also from the application of techniques and strategies that incorporate each child's abilities to the fullest potential in audiologic assessment.

Behavioral Observation Audiometry (BOA)

Although not a measure of auditory sensitivity, behavioral observation audiometry (BOA) is useful in conjunction with physiologic measures to provide additional insights into the response behavior of children with complex developmental conditions who might be unwilling or unable (cognitively and/or physically) to perform an audiologic procedure requiring a conditioned response. In fact, BOA is the only method of behavioral evaluation appropriate for individuals under approximately 6 months developmental age (a distinction between chronologic age and developmental age must be made, as chronologic age is often not an indicator of developmental age, especially in children with complex developmental conditions; additionally, subtraction of weeks of prematurity from chronologic age is necessary to compute an estimate of developmental age). Moreover, some children with complex developmental conditions are not good candidates for sedated procedures, and audiologists must rely on BOA as their only behavioral measure of a child's "hearing."

In BOA, a child's nonintentional responses to sound are observed by the audiologist. Diefendorf and Gravel (1996) placed these responses in two categories: (a) reflexive responses such as sucking, eye-blink, and startle; and (b) orienting responses such as eye widening, searching, a decrease in movement, and localization. Because of the nonintentional nature of these responses, and because they are often elicited by a suprathreshold level sound, Matkin (1977) suggested use of the term "minimum response level" to describe these responses rather than "auditory threshold." The difference in terminology implies that BOA responses simply provide information regarding suprathreshold auditory function, rather than auditory sensitivity.

Renshaw and Diefendorf (1998) listed three categories into which results of BOA testing might be placed: (a) no observable response to sound, (b) responses only to high-intensity stimuli (70–80 dB HL), and (c) responses to relatively soft and comfortable stimuli (30–50 dB HL). These categories provide some delineation about results obtained from BOA testing. In concert with BOA as a test of auditory responsivity (not sensitivity), the categories promote the use of BOA as a behavioral measure, useful to support physiologic findings and to verify the presence of a general level of functional hearing.

When attempting BOA with a child with complex developmental conditions, it is important to remain unbiased when judging the presence or absence of a response (Gans, 1987). Often, children with cerebral palsy or other neurologic conditions might elicit frequent involuntary movements or vocalizations, making it difficult to determine valid behavioral response patterns. As such, it often is beneficial to enlist the assistance of a second audiologist, who might be able to assess the child's responses from another perspective. Additionally, to reduce habituation, it also is recommended to alternate between several different types of stimuli, including narrowband noise, frequency-modulated tones, and speech. Using pulsed stimuli also seems to help reduce habituation. Enlisting the parent/caregiver's assistance in determining a response from children with complex developmental conditions also can be an invaluable strategy. Parents/caregivers typically know their child better than any other participant in the audiologic evaluation. Their input should be regarded as potentially very useful, although audiologists also must consider their input as potentially biased. Gravel (1992) suggests the parent/caregiver-participant wear earphones delivering a masking noise while involved in the test procedure to neutralize their potential bias. Conversely, Gravel also points out the benefit of allowing parents/caregivers to hear the intensity level at which the child responds to assist in counseling regarding any existing hearing loss. This also is beneficial for parents/caregivers who feel that their child's hearing is not the problem, and rationalize the developmental delay as the reason their child is not responding appropriately to sound and/or not vocalizing or talking.

Visual Reinforcement Audiometry (VRA)

As stated earlier, employing optimal test parameters with physiologic measures for children with complex developmental delay *should not be compromised* regardless of the child's disability. When employing behavioral measures for children with complex developmental delay, adapting test parameters might be necessary to match the physical and behavioral characteristics of the children under test. However, recognizing the impact that might result from these adaptations is essential.

Evidenced-based practice in pediatric audiology has a long history of defining clinical protocols in VRA. In most published studies, however, evidence-based protocols have been based on research data with typically developing infants. Examples include age appropriateness of VRA (Moore, Wilson, & Thompson, 1977), conditioning protocols (Primus & Thompson, 1985; Thompson & Folsom, 1984), use of reinforcement (Moore et al., 1977), types of reinforcement (Lowery, von Hapsburg, Plyler, & Johnstone, 2009; Moore, Thompson, & Thompson, 1975; Schmida, Peterson, & Tharpe, 2003), reinforcement novelty (Primus, 1987), reinforcement duration (Culpepper & Thompson, 1994), reinforcement schedules (Primus & Thompson, 1985), trial durations (Primus, 1992), use of control trials, and validity of findings from infants (Diefendorf, 1988; Nozza & Wilson, 1984; Primus, 1988). In fewer published studies, low-functioning children (Thompson, Wilson, & Moore, 1979), children with Down syndrome (Greenburg et al., 1978), children with autism spectrum disorders (Tharpe et al., 2006), and at-risk premature infants (Moore, 1995; Moore, Thompson, & Folsom, 1992; Widen, 1990) have been used as study subjects. For the most part, studies of children with hearing loss and complex developmental delay are missing in the literature. Yet, clinical experience suggests that VRA protocols *must be flexible and adapted* to accommodate children with complex developmental delay to establish behavioral audiologic profiles for these children. In doing so, the risks and benefits of modifying VRA protocols must be acknowledged.

The age at which VRA is optimally successful for the child with complex developmental delay must be considered. For example, Thompson, Wilson, and Moore (1979) found the VRA technique to be appropriate for children with Down syndrome beginning at a developmental age of approximately 10 to 12 months. Although these data serve as an excellent guideline, attempting behavioral audiologic evaluation on children presenting with any neurologic or developmental condition, including Down syndrome, under the age of 10 months is encouraged. In a clinical setting with a diverse and complex patient population, it is helpful to obtain any behavioral information that leads to more informed decision making and recommendations.

In a discussion that places its primary focus on assessments of typically developing children, Gravel (1992) lists additional factors necessary for optimization of the clinical VRA procedure: (a) judging true responses from false responses, (b) increasing attention and motivation, and (c) decreasing false alarm rate. These three factors also must be considered when utilizing VRA with children presenting with complex developmental conditions.

Judging Response Behavior

Judging the presence or absence of a head-turn response might be more difficult in children with complex developmental conditions (e.g., cerebral palsy, visual impairments, autism spectrum disorders, hyperactive behavior). These children might exhibit involuntary movements without purpose and/or random head turning that compromise the validity and reliability of the VRA procedure. Additionally, for children with hypotonia or problems with head or neck control, they might have increased difficulty turning their heads, in turn relying on eye shifts or movements as a response. For these behaviors, increasing the use of control trials (used to judge false-response behavior) must be considered. Additionally, the use of a second audiologist within the test room can be extremely helpful in determining the presence or absence of a response. The second audiologist also can assist in optimizing attention and motivation of the child under test.

It might be necessary to increase the trial duration (usually about 4 s) during which a true response is acceptable for children who have poor head control or are slow responders. However, by increasing trial duration, audiologists also risk an increase in judging false responses as true responses. When added control trials are necessary to verify valid response behavior, it is essential that the control trial duration is equal to the signal trial duration so that opportunities to judge false-response behavior are not biased.

Increasing Attention and Motivation

Initiating and maintaining the attention and motivation of children with complex developmental conditions is essential for establishing an accurate audiogram with VRA. For example, in the case of a child with autism, the presence of unusual sensory responses including preoccupation with or agitation to sound, abnormalities in auditory processing, and failure to condition are clinical features. These children might exhibit behaviors such as a disregard for speech stimuli, a fixation on one object, or an aversion for direct eye contact or physical contact. Additionally, children with attention deficits, cognitive delays, and vision impairment often need additional effort on the part of the examiner to ensure that they remain appropriately attentive and motivated throughout the evaluation that results obtained are representative of the child's hearing status.

Different strategies can be employed to increase a patient's attention during the VRA procedure. An obvious way to increase attention is to decrease distraction. When presenting stimuli for VRA, decreasing distraction might involve (a) darkening the control side of the booth, (b) keeping the child in an alert position (e.g., sitting up instead of leaning back on a parent's lap, sitting in a high chair, or sitting in a stroller), (c) keeping additional toys, picture boards, and other items that might cause distraction out of the child's line of sight, (d) allowing only one parent or caregiver to be in the booth with the child, and (e) involving a second examiner to serve not only as a second opinion regarding the presence/absence of a response, but also to provide centering distraction for the child, and to provide occasional social reinforcement to the child. In this role, the audiologist must stabilize behaviors that compromise true responses to the auditory stimulus. This can be achieved, although with some challenge, by maintaining the child's attention at midline and returning the child to this position once a response is made. The audiologist must be creative and proactive in keeping the child alert and in a listening posture without the child becoming too focused on the examiner or the activity. If the audiologist and distracting technique are not sufficiently interesting, the likelihood of random behavior will continue.

Audiologists also can influence attention and motivation by being flexible with the use of different auditory stimuli. Often, when a child becomes disinterested in a specific stimulus, response behavior can be increased by using a different (novel) stimulus. For example, head-turning to speech stimuli or narrowband noise after tiring to a pure-tone stimulus often results in the opportunity for further frequency-specific testing. The introduction of a novel stimulus, is a useful strategy to increase the child's attention to the VRA procedure. This strategy is especially useful when attempting to obtain ear-specific information.

For some children, a very brief presentation of the reinforcement toy/DVD video provides enough motivation to continue the evaluation until the audiologist has gathered all necessary information. Culpepper and Thompson (1994) studied the response behavior of 2-year-olds and found that habituation was delayed when subjects received very brief exposure to reinforcement (0.5 s) compared to those children who received longer exposure to reinforcement (4 s). For others, especially those with special needs, a longer presentation of the reinforcement might be necessary, possibly as a result of increased processing time, attention deficits, or visual deficits. Extending the reinforcement duration should only be considered when it is deemed necessary to allow the child with special needs longer access to the reinforcement. However, by increasing reinforcement duration, the audiologist also might observe more rapid onset of habituation.

One strategy to counteract the consequence of longer reinforcement durations is to employ the use of multiple reinforcers or DVD/video reinforcement. The use of conventional reinforcers permits the ability to only illuminate the colorful toys only, and select between animation/no animation for enhancing novelty and revitalizing motivation. This also might be necessary for children who are fearful of the animated conventional reinforcers.

Decreasing False Responses

Determining a true response from a false response is often one of the most challenging aspects of performing behavioral audiometry on a child with special needs. Decreasing the number of false responses is essential to have confidence in audiometric outcomes. Reliable audiologic data are achievable when attention is focused on response shaping, versatile midline distraction techniques, lengthening interstimulus intervals, and persistent monitoring of false-response behavior with control trials.

Response shaping is critical to the success of VRA. The examiner must be skilled in response training and sensitive to the various stages of response acquisition. Two different approaches that can be attempted in the conditioning phase are (a) pairing the stimulus with the reinforcer and (b) observing a spontaneous response from the infant followed by reinforcement. For the child with special needs, conditioning might take longer to establish the conditioned behavior. Successful completion of the conditioning stage occurs when the child is making contingent responses, and random head turning is at a minimum.

Excessive false responses suggest that the infant is not under stimulus control. As such, audiologists should focus on two factors to rectify clinical outcomes: (a) reinstitute response shaping or (b) increase the entertainment level of the midline distraction to engage the child's focus before presenting the auditory stimulus.

Northern and Downs (2002) suggest taking a "time-out" subsequent to false responses to permit the child time to relax and regain composure, as this can be a frustrating situation for many children with special needs. Taking "time-out" is essentially increasing the interstimulus interval (ISI). Increasing the ISI increases stimulus novelty, thereby increasing the likelihood of a correct response. Additionally, increasing ISI provides optimal time to bring the child to a midline gaze, thereby increasing the likelihood of obtaining stimulus-related head turn responses.

Tharpe et al. (2006) found that children with autism provided elevated and less reliable behavioral audiometric responses than their typically developing peers, with no significant difference in physiologic test results between the two groups. In this study, if the child became bored or distracted, the examiners would implement the following: (a) repeat the trial, (b) switch stimulus, or (c) switch transducer.

Although eliminating false responses altogether is not feasible or clinically desirable, these strategies serve to regain the child's focus when it might have lapsed. The desired outcome is achieved when the child's false-response rate during control trials is approximately 25% or less (Moore, 1995).

Conditioned Play Audiometry

Conditioned play audiometry (CPA) follows a model of auditory stimulus → response → reinforcement, in which a play activity (blocks in a bucket, pegs in a board) is the response and social praise is the reinforcement. Through conditioning, children learn to engage a response that is within their motor coordination ability and can be completed consistently.

Conditioned play audiometry is considered the most appropriate technique for obtaining ear- and frequency-specific information in children 3 years developmental age and above. Although this is an extremely useful guideline, the audiologist must always remain open to the behavioral test procedure that provides the most reliable responses coupled with facilitating the longest delay in habituation from the child. That is, a general knowledge of the child's developmental abilities will guide the audiologist to an *age-appropriate* test technique, whereas the child's physical abilities, developmental skills, and personal motivations will guide the audiologist to a *developmentally appropriate* test technique. For example, some 2-year-olds can be conditioned to play audiometry (Thompson, Thompson, & Vethivelus, 1989). Moreover, when 2-year-olds are conditioned for CPA, they are more likely to provide greater responses before habituation than they would if tested by VRA. For this reason, and for others discussed earlier in this chapter, the time the audiologist spends on history intake and building rapport with the child and the family is important in the determination of a test method with which to begin the evaluation.

When teaching children to perform CPA, it is usually not difficult to select a response behavior that children are capable of performing, as long as the audiologist is intuitive in matching the child's motor skill with an appropriate play activity. The challenge in CPA is teaching the child to wait, listen, and respond when the auditory signal is presented. In addition to teaching the child under test the conditioned response in the CPA task, the examiner also must be skilled in delivering social reinforcement at the appropriate time and interval.

Children with complex developmental conditions present unique challenges during audiometric evaluation using CPA. Response acquisition, identifying positive reinforcements, and response time are several challenges that must be carefully considered. Kile (1996) suggests that children with Down syndrome might require longer response intervals following the stimulus to ensure the child has adequate time to process and respond to the signal. The following suggestions will increase the likelihood of successful audiologic outcomes.

- Many factors should be considered prior to choosing an appropriate toy to be used during CPA. The audiologist must consider the child's gross/fine motor skills, vision, attention, developmental level, personal interests/motivators, and social interaction skills, to name several. If the physical demands of the game are too great, the child will give up prior to obtaining the necessary information. If the task is too simple, the child is less motivated and might fatigue earlier than the audiologist hopes (Diefendorf, 2003).
- Teaching the CPA task can be slightly more difficult in the child with complex developmental conditions. Holte et al. (2006) suggest using tactile cues (bone oscillator or simple touch), thereby physically training a child who is deaf-blind to perform the CPA task. The bone oscillator can be removed from the headband and held in the child's hand or rested against the child's arm. A 250-Hz signal is presented at the maximum output for the bone oscillator, and the vibratory stimulus is then paired with appropriate reinforcement following the desired response.
- Practicing the task together several times prior to beginning the formal evaluation is also extremely helpful. Northern and Downs (2002) suggest using animated facial cues and body language along with overtly demonstrating the task. Diefendorf (1981) demonstrated the positive effects of a "pre-play period" for facilitating response acquisition during conditioning. For example, the audiologist can place a block in the child's hand while also holding their hand, present the signal or imitate the signal such as repeating "beep-beep" and place the block in the bucket together. Practicing this procedure several times as part of a "pre-play period" allows the child to practice the task on his or her own. Not only does this help establish a reliable stimulus-response bond, it also builds conficence in the child when the child is able to successfully complete the task by himself or herself.
- Response patterns can differ greatly from child to child. Others might look to their parent or caregiver or the audiologist for confirmation they heard the stimulus at every presentation and wait for reinforcement prior to performing the play task (Renshaw & Diefendorf, 1998). Children with Down syndrome might elicit a sound mimicking the stimulus rather than perform the conventional CPA task. These behaviors (if consistent) should be considered valid and representative of reliable conditioned behavior.
- Often, in a busy clinic setting, using two audiologists to perform CPA (one in the test room playing with the child, one in the control room) is not always an option. Utilizing the parent as an assistant in this case often allows the evaluation to flow more quickly while also feeling more natural for the child.
- Even under headphones, pure tones might not be the stimulus that best holds the child's attention. Narrow-band noise or warbled tones might be found to be more interesting and novel by the child with special needs.

Conventional Audiometry

Once an audiologist has determined a child with special needs has developed the skills necessary to complete conventional audiometry (i.e., make a distinct and agreed-upon response to auditory stimuli), the audiologist must keep the evaluation upbeat, motivating to the child, and as comprehensive as time allows. Often, the window of opportunity to obtain this information is rather small when evaluating a child with special needs due to stress, tolerance, distractibility, habituation, or fatigue. Keeping the child motivated and attentive with intermittent social reinforcement, coupled with a response behavior that is physically easy for the child are key components for obtaining a valid and thorough audiogram. Air-conduction and bone-conduction data are desirable, and a trade-off between fewer air-conduction thresholds in favor of several bone-conduction thresholds can be important as the child begins to fatigue. For example, in the case of a suspected conductive hearing loss, it can be beneficial to complete speech testing under headphones first, utilizing techniques discussed later in this chapter and then attempting masked bone-conduction speech testing to establish the suspected conductive component. Discrete frequency information can then be attempted via air and bone conduction until the child fatigues.

The audiologist can introduce different options as fatigue sets in as an attempt to maintain or increase the child's motivation and continued response behavior. For example, the audiologist might need to become a more active participant in the evaluation. For a child with special needs, maintaining or increasing any of the conditioned responses for conventional audiometry can be made easier when the audiologist participates from the control side of the booth. That is, if the response option chosen is for the child to clap hands, the audiologist must be willing to clap hands *with* the child upon presentation of the stimulus. This not only aids in teaching the child the desired response, but also reinforces the child for the correct behavior.

Occasionally, the child with special needs might choose a unique response option as a modification of the task introduced by the audiologist. That is, a child might begin to smile and wave at the audiologist in response to auditory stimuli after being instructed to clap hands. As long as this alternate response is consistent and easily observable, the audiologist should be flexible and reinforce the behavioral response.

The following options have all been used successfully with children for whom conventional audiometry is physically or developmentally appropriate:

- raise hand,
- high-five to parent or caregiver,
- clap hands,
- nod head,
- push button,
- say "I hear it,"
- say "beep,"
- blink eyes, or
- give a thumbs up.

Social reinforcement such as nodding, smiling, and clapping on the part of the audiologist is often the only reinforcement necessary to obtain a standard audiogram for this age group. The audiologist evaluating a child with special needs must determine how much and how frequent social reinforcement needs to be provided to the child in order to motivate the child, without being overly praiseful (which might encourage false-positive responses from the child). Renshaw and Diefendorf (1998) also suggest using VRA toys as reinforcement in addition to social reinforcement for selected children who find this to be motivating.

Optimizing Audiologic Assessment for Children With Complex Developmental Conditions: Speech Audiometry

The inclusion of speech audiometry in the audiological evaluation of an individual with complex developmental conditions must be viewed as essential for developing a complete profile of auditory status and functional hearing ability. Because of the limitations of pure-tone or narrow-band noise thresholds in predicting functional efficiency for speech, additional clinical tests utilizing speech materials must be employed for a complete audiologic evaluation and follow-up description of auditory abilities. Additionally, although an individual's ability to understand speech is influenced by his audiometric threshold configuration, the former cannot always be predicted accurately from the latter, and it is this fact that makes speech audiometry an indispensable clinical tool.

Speech audiometry provides the audiologist with information that can only be obtained through the use of speech stimuli. Audiologists are acquiring information regarding the softest hearing level where speech can be detected, the hearing level at which speech can be recognized, or a percent score reflecting word, phrase, or sentence recognition when these materials are presented at a comfortable or optimal hearing level. All of these components help frame the diagnosis of an individual's hearing function or dysfunction.

Speech Detection/Awareness Thresholds (SDT/SAT)

The speech detection threshold (SDT) or speech awareness threshold (SAT) might be defined as the hearing level at which a listener might just detect the presence of an ongoing speech signal. A SDT/SAT can be obtained with a variety of stimulus words or phrases to gain the child's attention and cooperation. The audiologist often will call the child's name or "nickname," present words, present numbers, sing songs, or repeat syllables (bai-bai-bai; uh-oh) and look for a response from the patient. An acceptable response can be a preconditioned head nod, a hand raise, or a head turn toward the speaker when testing in sound field. Threshold is marked when a consistent response is given during approximately 50% of the test trials.

The signal selected is often delivered in repetition until a response is obtained. However, test trial duration should not exceed 5 s due to the risk of accepting a false response as a true response. The SDT/SAT often relates most closely to the best single pure-tone threshold within the frequency range of 250 to 4000 Hz. Considering this, the child will respond to the portion of this broad spectrum of frequencies at which hearing is most sensitive.

When obtaining SDT/SAT it is important to be versatile and flexible with the presented stimulus. The clinician will notice that some stimuli work better than others, reflecting the individual preferences of the child under test. Therefore, it might be helpful to consider using a familiar voice to present the stimulus.

Allowing a parent, sibling, or caregiver to speak into the microphone, while the audiologist is monitoring the VU meter, might facilitate the acquisition of speech awareness responses. It also might be necessary to enlist an interpreter or native language speaker to optimize speech awareness testing in the child's primary language. Regulating the VU meter and documenting strategies, as well as results, are essential.

Speech Reception Threshold (SRT)

Speech reception threshold, spondee recognition threshold, or speech recognition threshold are all appropriate terms referring to the lowest hearing level at which the patient can correctly identify spondaic words that are presented. The SRT is recognized as the intensity at which an individual is able to identify simple speech materials approximately 50% of the time.

The standard presentation involves the use of two-syllable words (spondees) where the child repeats back or points to the targeted word. However, the conventional protocol can be modified to meet the needs of any child, and particularly those with complex developmental conditions.

When developing a modified test protocol to use with a child with special needs, it is important to consider the familiarity of the words that are attempted. The child must have a familiarity with the words being considered, and eliminating those words that are not within the child's receptive vocabulary is crucial. The audiologist also must consider the child's ability to repeat the word. This includes accounting for possible speech or articulation disorders that can interfere with proper articulation and pronunciation.

The audiologist can use pointing tasks, game tasks, or classic repetition games. A picture board can be used for pointing tasks. Large, brightly colored, easily recognized images are recommended so there is no confusion with busy pictures. The use of either picture- or object-pointing rather than verbal response will require that the number of test items be limited to 12 or less (Olsen & Matkin, 1979). Otherwise, the visual scanning task, as well as the demands placed on memory and attention, become contaminating variables.

If a child is unable to view the picture board due to vision deficits, a "show me" game might be an effective alternative. The child might be able to point to body parts or a parent's body parts (e.g., "show me your nose," "eyes," "hair," "fingers," "toes," "shoes").

Some children might be more willing to play a game task. Their motor development must be considered to determine if they would be a successful candidate to participate in the game. A few options to choose between would include a familiar objects game or a "put it in" the bucket game. The familiar objects game would consist of placing known objects on the table and having the child point them out. Objects can be pulled from a parent's or child's belongings (e.g., toys, brush, phone, shoes, rings). When playing the bucket game, the child must have the dexterity and coordination to hold a ball, block, or peg and place it into a bucket during conditioning and testing.

The audiologist can play a simpler repetition game for children with compromised cognitive function. For example, the game might be enhanced by calling it "copycat," "mirror," "Simon says," or "being a parrot." The child mimics or copies the word that is being presented through the transducer.

Speech Perception

There are several challenges that must be considered when attempting to measure speech perception skills in children with complex developmental conditions. The selection of test materials within a child's receptive vocabulary competency, the designation of an appropriate response task, the utilization of reinforcement, and the reduction or alleviation of memory load are important factors that can affect the reliability and validity of speech perception measurement.

Clinicians must exercise caution in administering the phonetically balanced kindergarten (PB-K) word lists unless there is relatively good assurance that the receptive vocabulary age of the child approaches at least that of a normal-hearing kindergartner. Alternatively, the use of Word Intelligibility by Picture Identification (WIPI) test is appropriate for those children with receptive vocabulary ages of 4 years and older. The Northwestern University-Children's Perception of Speech (NU-CHIPS) test (Elliott & Katz, 1980) materials are documented to be in the recognition vocabulary of children with normal hearing as young as age 3 years. Kirk, Pisoni, and Osberger (1995) examined the effect of lexical characteristics on a group of pediatric cochlear implant users' spoken word recognition, and compared their performance on the Lexical Neighborhood Test (LNT) and Multisyllabic Lexical Neighborhood Test (MLNT) with their scores on the PB-K. Word recognition was significantly higher on the lexically controlled lists than on the PB-K.

When selecting appropriate speech perception measures for use with children (with or without complex developmental conditions), it is essential to match the developmental level of the child with a speech perception measure that reflects the vocabulary level of the child under test. Additionally, an appropriate response task that considers memory, attention, and physical capabilities also must be considered to ensure valid measures of speech perception that are not compromised by test protocols or vocabulary levels.

Conclusion

The standard of care in the United States for early hearing detection and intervention is articulated by the Year 2007 Joint Committee on Infant Hearing Position Statement. The 2007 statement advocates universal hearing screening by 1 month of age, audiologic diagnosis of hearing loss by 3 months of age, and intervention by 6 months of age. Compliance with this timeline is intended for *all* children with hearing loss.

For those children suspected of hearing loss who present with complex developmental conditions, meeting this timeline can be more challenging. Although there are evolving and ever-changing priorities for children with complex developmental conditions, optimal care coordination for these children is facilitated when an early and accurate diagnosis of hearing loss is established. Frequently, ruling out hearing loss is part of a global developmental evaluation of a child with complex developmental conditions. The definitive diagnosis of hearing loss is a crucial component of a child's coordinated, family-centered care plan, and the earlier hearing loss is established, the earlier a comprehensive intervention plan can be initiated. Therefore, an appropriate battery of audiologic tests coupled with appropriate protocols must be utilized to achieve a timely diagnosis of hearing loss in these children. When achieved, the goal of optimizing a child's communication development is positively influenced and significantly enhanced.

References

American Speech-Language-Hearing Association (ASHA; 2004). *Guidelines for the audiologic assessment of children from birth to 5 years of age* [Guidelines]. Retrieved from http://www.asha.org/policy

American Speech-Language-Hearing Association (ASHA; 2008). *Guidelines for audiologists providing informational and adjustment counseling to families of infants and young children with hearing loss birth to 5 years of age.* Retrieved from http://www.asha.org/policy

Barr, B. (1955). Pure tone audiometry for pre-school children [in Swedish]. *Nordisk Medicine, 51*(14), 464–468.

Beck, D. L. (2015). Case history. In J. Katz (Ed.), *Handbook of clinical audiology*. Philadelphia, PA: Wolters Kluwer.

Boege, P., & Janssen, T. (2002). Pure-tone threshold estimation from extrapolated distortion product otoacoustic emission I/O functions in normal and cochlear hearing loss ears. *Journal of the Acoustical Society of America, 111*, 1810–1818.

Culpepper, B., & Thompson, G. (1994). Effects of reinforcer duration on the response behavior of preterm 2-year-olds in visual reinforcement audiometry. *Ear and Hearing, 15*, 161–167.

Diefendorf, A. O. (1981). *The effect of a pre-play period on play audiometry*. Paper presented at the Tennessee Speech-Language-Hearing Association Annual Convention, Memphis, TN.

Diefendorf, A. O. (1988). Behavioral evaluation of hearing-impaired children. In F. H. Bess (Ed.), *Hearing impairment in children*. Parkton, MD: York Press.

Diefendorf, A. O. (2003). Behavioral hearing assessment: Considerations for the young child with developmental disabilities. *Seminars in Hearing, 24*, 189–200.

Diefendorf, A. O., & Gravel, J. S. (1996). Behavioral observation and visual reinforcement audiometry. In S. E. Gerber (Ed.), *The handbook of pediatric audiology*. Washington, DC: Gallaudet University Press.

Dille, M. F. (2003). Perspectives on the audiological evaluation of individuals with Down syndrome. *Seminars in Hearing, 24*, 201–210.

Dorn, P. A., Konrad-Martin, D., Neely, S. T., Keefe, D. H., Cry, E., & Gorga, M. P. (2001). Distortion product otoacoustic emission input/output functions in normal-hearing and hearing-impaired human ears. *Journal of the Acoustical Society of America, 110*, 3119–3131.

Eisenberg, R. B. (1969). Auditory behavior in the human neonate: Functional properties of sound and their ontogenetic implications. *International Journal of Audiology, 8*, 34–45.

Elliott, L. L., & Katz, D. (1980). *Development of a new children's test of speech discrimination* [Technical manual]. St. Louis, MO: Auditec.

Evenhuis, H. M. (1996). Dutch consensus on diagnosis and treatment of hearing impairment in children and adults with intellectual disability. *Journal of Intellectual Disability Research, 40*, 451–456.

Folsom, R. C., Widen, J. E., & Wilson, W. R. (1983). Auditory brainstem responses in Down syndrome infants. *Archives of Otolaryngology, 109*, 607–610.

Fortnum, H., & Davis, A. (1997). Epidemiology of permanent childhood hearing impairment in Trent Region, 1985–1993. *British Journal of Audiology, 31*, 409–466.

Gallaudet College Center for Assessment and Demographic Studies. (1983). *Annual survey of hearing-impaired children and youth, 1981–1982*. Washington, DC: Author.

Gallaudet Research Institute. (2005). *Regional and national summary report of data from the 2004–2005 annual survey of deaf and hard of hearing children and youth*. Washington, DC: Author.

Gans, D. P. (1987). Improving behavior observation audiometry testing and scoring procedures. *Ear and Hearing, 8*, 92–100.

Gorga, M. P., Neely, S. T., Dierking, D. M., Dorn, P. A., Hoover, B. M., & Fitzpatrick, D. (2003). Distortion product otoacoustic emission tuning curves in normal-hearing and hearing-impaired human ears. *Journal of the Acoustical Society of America, 114*, 262–278.

Gorga, M. P., Neely, S. T., & Dorn, P. A. (2002). Distortion product otoacoustic emissions in relation to hearing loss. In M. S. Robinette & T. J. Glattke (Eds.), *Otoacoustic emissions: Clinical applications* (2nd ed., pp. 243–272). New York, NY: Thieme Medical.

Gorga, M. P., Stover, L. T., & Neely, S. T. (1996). The use of cumulative distributions to determine critical values and levels of confidence for clinical distortion product otoacoustic emission measurements. *Journal of the Acoustical Society of America, 100*, 968–977.

Gravel, J. S. (1992). Audiologic assessment of infants and toddlers. In E. Cherow (Ed.), *Proceedings of the ASHA audiology superconference: ASHA Reports, 21*, 55–62.

Gravel, J. S. (2002). Potential pitfalls in the audiological assessment of infants and young children. In R. C. Seewald & J. S. Gravel (Eds.), *A sound foundation through early amplification (2001). Proceedings of the second international conference* (pp. 85–101). Stafa, Switzerland: Phonak AG.

Greenburg, D., Wilson, W. R., Moore, J., & Thompson, G. (1978). Visual reinforcement audiometry (VRA) with young Down syndrome children. *Journal of Speech and Hearing Disorders, 43*, 448–458.

Holte, L., Prickett, J. G., Van Dyke, D. C., Olson, R. J., Lubrica, P., Knutson, C. L., . . . Brenna, S. (2006). Issues in the evaluation of infants and young children who are suspected of or who are deaf-blind. *Infants and Young Children, 19*, 213–227.

Hoversten, G., & Moncur, J. (1969). Stimuli and intensity factors in testing infants. *Journal of Speech and Hearing Research, 12*, 687–702.

Institute of Medicine (IOM; 2002). *Unequal treatment: What health care providers need to know about racial and ethnic disparities in healthcare*. Retrieved December 14, 2009, from https://iom.nationalacademies.org/~/media/Files/Report%20Files/2003/Unequal-Treatment-Confronting-Racial-and-Ethnic-Disparities-in-Health-Care/Disparities hcproviders8pgFINAL.pdf

Joint Committee on Infant Hearing (JCIH; 2007) Year 2007 position statement: Principles and guidelines for early hearing detection and intervention programs. *Pediatrics, 120*, 898–921.

Kaga, M., Ohuchi, M., Kaga, K., & Tanaka, Y. (1984). Normalization of poor auditory brainstem response in infants and children. *Brain Development, 6*, 458–466.

Katbamma, B., Hommick, D. N., & Marks, J. H. (1999). Effects of chronic tobramycin treatment on distortion product otoacoustic emissions. *Ear and Hearing, 20*, 393–402.

Kaufmann, R. K., & McGonigel, M. J. (1991). Identifying family concerns, priorities, and resources. An overview. In M. J. McGonigel, R. K. Kaufmann, & B. H. Johnson (Eds.), *Guidelines and recommended practices for the individualized family service plan* (2nd ed., p. 55). Bethesda, MD: Association for the Care of Children's Health.

Kile, J. E. (1996) Audiologic assessment of children with Down syndrome. *American Journal of Audiology, 5*, 44–52.

Kirk, K. I., Pisoni, D. B., & Osberger, M. J. (1995). Lexical effects on spoken word recognition by pediatric cochlear implant users. *Ear and Hearing, 16*, 470–481.

Kraus, N., Ozdamar, O., Stein, L., & Reed, N. (1984). Absent auditory brain stem response: Peripheral hearing loss or brain stem dysfunction? *Laryngoscope, 94*, 400–406.

Lonsbury-Martin, B. L., McCoy, M. J., Whitehead, M. L., & Martin, G. K. (1993). Clinical testing of distortion-product otoacoustic emissions. *Ear and Hearing, 14*, 11–22.

Lowery, K. J., von Hapsburg, D., Plyler, E. L., & Johnstone, P. (2009). A comparison of video versus conventional visual reinforcement in 7- to 16-month-old infants. *Journal of Speech, Language and Hearing Research, 52*(3), 723–731.

Luterman, D. (1999). *The young deaf child*. Baltimore, MD: York Press.

Mace, A. L., Wallace, K. L., Whan, M. Q., & Stelmachowicz, P. G. (1991). Relevant factors in the identification of hearing loss. *Ear and Hearing, 12*(4), 287–293.

Matkin, N. D. (1977). Hearing sensitivity during preschool years. In F. H. Bess (Ed.), *Childhood deafness: Causation, assessment and management* (Chapter 10, pp. 127–133). New York, NY: Grune & Stratton.

McCellend, R. J., Eyre, D. G., Watson, D., Calvert, G. H., & Sherrard, E. (1992). Central conduction time in childhood autism. *British Journal of Psychiatry, 160*, 659–663.

Meredith, R., Stephens, D., Sirimanna, T., Meyer-Bisch, C., & Reardon, W. (1992). Audiometric detection of carrier of Usher's syndrome type II. *Journal of Audiological Medicine, 1*, 11–19.

Moore, J. (1995). Behavioral assessment procedures based on conditioned head-turn responses for auditory detection and discrimination with low-functioning children. *Scandinavian Audiology Supplement, 41*, 36–42.

Moore, J., Thompson, G., & Folsom, R. (1992). Auditory responsiveness of premature infants utilizing visual re-inforcement audiometry (VRA). *Ear and Hearing, 13*, 187–194.

Moore, J. M., Thompson, G., & Thompson, M. (1975). Auditory localization of infants as a function of reinforcement conditions. *Journal of Speech and Hearing Disorders, 40*, 29–34.

Moore, J. M., Wilson, W. R., & Thompson, G. (1977). Visual reinforcement of head-turn responses in infants under 12 months of age. *Journal of Speech and Hearing Disorders, 42*, 328–334.

Northern, J. L., & Downs, M. P. (2002). *Hearing in children* (5th ed.). Baltimore, MD: Lippincott Williams & Wilkins.

Nozza, R. J., & Wilson, W. R. (1984). Masked and unmasked pure-tone thresholds of infants and adults: Development of auditory frequency selectivity and sensitivity. *Journal of Speech and Hearing Research, 27*, 613–622.

Olsen, W. O., & Matkin, N. D. (1979). Speech audiometry. In W. F. Rintelmann (Ed.), *Hearing assessment* (pp. 133–206). Baltimore, MD: University Park Press.

Pijl, S., Stewart, I. F., & Laskowski, W. (1988). Limitations of ABR as a hearing test as exemplified in multiply handicapped adults. *Journal of Otolaryngology, 17*, 362–367.

Pikus, A. T. (1995). Pediatric audiologic profiles in type 1 and type 2 neurofibromatosis. *Journal of the American Academy of Audiology, 6,* 54–62.

Primus, M. A. (1987). Response and reinforcement in operant audiometry. *Journal of Speech and Hearing Disorders, 52,* 294–299.

Primus, M. A. (1988). Infant thresholds with enhanced attention to the signal in visual reinforcement audiometry. *Journal of Speech and Hearing Research, 31,* 480–484.

Primus, M. A. (1992). Operant response in infants as a function of time interval following signal onset. *Journal of Speech and Hearing Research, 35,* 1422–1425.

Primus, M. A., & Thompson, G. (1985). Response strength of young children in operant audiometry. *Journal of Speech and Hearing Research, 28,* 539–547.

Renshaw, J. J., & Diefendorf, A. O. (1998). Adapting the test battery for the child with special needs. In F. H. Bess (Ed.), *Children with hearing impairment: Contemporary trends* (Chapter 7, pp. 83–104). Nashville, TN: Vanderbilt Bill Wilkerson Center Press.

Ress, B. D., Sridhar, K. S., Balkany, T. I, Waxman, G. M. Stagner, B. B., & Lonsbury-Martin, B. I. (1999). Effects of cicplatinum chemotherapy on otoacoustic emissions. The development of an objective screening protocol. *Otolaryngology-Head and Neck Surgery, 121,* 693–701.

Rosenthall, U., Nordin, V., Brantberg, K., & Gillberg, C. (2003). Autism and auditory brainstem responses. *Ear and Hearing, 24,* 206–214.

Roth, D. A., Hildesheimer, M., Bardenstein, S., Goidel, D., Reichman, B., Maayan-Metzger, A., & Kuint, J. (2008). Preauricular skin tags and ear pits are associated with permanent hearing impairment in newborns. *Pediatrics, 122*(4), 884–890.

Schmida, M., Peterson, H., & Tharpe, A. M. (2003). Visual reinforcement audiometry using digital video disc and conventional reinforcers. *American Journal of Audiology, 12,* 35–40.

Siegenthaler, B. M. (1987). Auditory problems. In E. T. McDonald (Ed.), *Treating cerebral palsy: For clinicians by clinicians* (pp. 85–103). Austin, TX: Pro-Ed.

Stavroulaki, P., Vossinakis, I. D., Dinopoulou, D., Doudounakis, S., Adamopoulos, G., & Apostolopoulos, N. (2002). Otoacoustic emissions for monitoring aminoglycoside-induced ototoxicity in children with cystic fibrosis. *Archives of Otolaryngology-Head and Neck Surgery, 128*(2), 150–155.

Suzuki, T., & Ogiba, Y. (1960). A technique for pure-tone audiometry for children under three years of age: Conditioned orientation reflex (COR) audiometry. *Revue de laryngologie-otology-rhinologie (BORD), 81,* 33–45.

Talbott, C. B. (1987). A longitudinal study comparing responses of hearing-impaired infants to pure tones using visual reinforcement and play audiometry. *Ear and Hearing, 8,* 175–179.

Tharpe, A. M. (2009). Individuals with multiple disabilities. In J. Katz, L. Medwetsky, R. Burkard, & L. Hood (Eds.), *Handbook of clinical audiology* (6th ed., pp. 666–677). Philadelphia, PA: Lippincott Williams & Wilkins.

Tharpe, A. M., Bess, F. H., Sladen, D. P., Schissel, H., Couch, S., & Schery, T. (2006) Auditory characteristics of children with autism. *Ear and Hearing, 27*(4), 430–441.

Thompson, G., & Folsom, R. C. (1984). A comparison of two conditioning procedures in the use of visual reinforcement audiometry (VRA). *Journal of Speech and Hearing Disorders, 49,* 241–245.

Thompson, G., & Weber, B. (1974). Responses of infants and young children to behavioral observation audiometry (BOA). *Journal of Speech and Hearing Disorders, 39,* 140–147.

Thompson, G., Wilson, W. R., & Moore, J. M. (1979). Application of visual reinforcement audiometry (VRA) to low-functioning children. *Journal of Speech and Hearing Disorders, 44,* 80–90.

Thompson, M. D., Thompson, G., & Vethivelu, S. (1989). A comparison of audiometric test thresholds for 2-year-old children. *Journal of Speech and Hearing Disorders, 54,* 174–179.

Turnbull, A. (1991). Identifying children's strengths and needs. In M. J. McGonigel, R. K. Kaufmann, & B. H. Johnson (Eds.), *Guidelines and recommended practices for the individualized family service plan* (2nd ed., pp. 39–46). Bethesda, MD: Association for the Care of Children's Health.

Westby, C., Burda, A., & Mehta, Z. (2003, April 29). *Asking the right questions in the right ways: Strategies for ethnographic interviewing* [Online feature]. *ASHA Leader.* Retrieved from http://leader.pubs.asha.org/article.aspx?articleid=2292396

Widen, J. (1990). Behavioral screening of high-risk infants using visual reinforcement audiometry. *Seminars in Hearing, 11,* 342–356.

Wilson, W. R., Moore, J., & Thompson, G. (1976). *Sound-field audiometry thresholds of infants utilizing visual reinforcement audiometry (VRA).* Paper presented at the American Speech and Hearing Association Annual Convention, November 20–23, Houston, TX.

Wong, V., & Wong, S. N. (1991). Brainstem auditory evoked potential study in children with autistic disorder. *Journal of Autism and Developmental Disorders, 21,* 329–340.

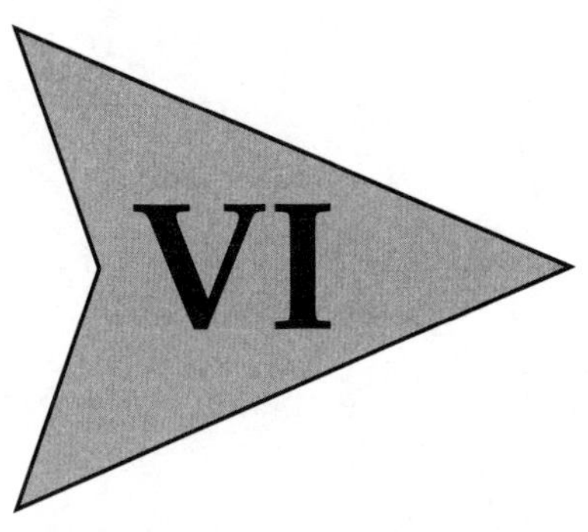

Hearing Technologies

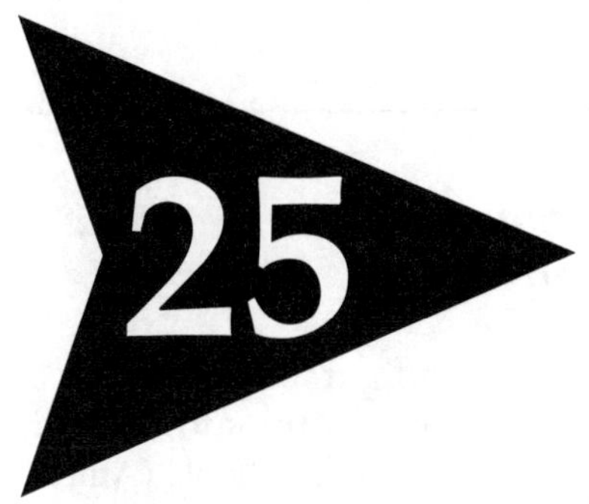

Current Approaches to the Fitting of Amplification to Infants and Young Children

Marlene P. Bagatto and Susan D. Scollie

Introduction

Many infants and children who have hearing loss use hearing aids to hear spoken language, and this is often their primary mode of communication. Early hearing detection and intervention programs allow us to assist families with hearing aid fitting even during infancy. In this chapter, we present current theories and practices that link hearing assessment to hearing aid fitting, with the goal of providing beneficial hearing aids to children of all ages.

Infants and young children bring unique qualities to hearing aid fitting, in at least three important ways. First, children who are born with hearing loss, or develop it early in life, have different listening needs from adults. In the context of universal hearing screening, a child's first hearing aid fittings can occur while in the process of learning speech and language during a critical period for the development of these skills (i.e., birth to 2 years of age). We therefore focus on providing full access to sound to support speech and language learning. Second, the ear canals of small children differ, acoustically, from those of the average adult and change as the child grows. We therefore focus on strategies to measure ear canal acoustics because they impact the level of sound delivered to the ear canal by the hearing aid. Finally, infants and young children are dependent upon a parent or other caregiver for their hearing aid use, monitoring, and maintenance. We therefore focus on child-friendly, family friendly, evidence-based techniques for pediatric hearing aid fitting, so that caregivers' efforts to mediate hearing aid use are supported by a beneficial and comfortable fitting.

This chapter is organized into sections that follow *the first three* of the five sequential stages that clinical audiologists follow when providing hearing aids to infants and children. The fourth and fifth sequential stages are covered in Chapters 26 and 28 of this volume. These sections follow the framework originally suggested by the Pediatric Working Group (PWG) in 1996:

1. The *assessment* provides information about the degree and configuration of the hearing loss in each ear from which candidacy for amplification is determined.
2. During *selection*, numerical values for the electroacoustic performance of the hearing aids are calculated, and the physical attributes of the hearing aid (size, shape, coupling to the ear) are chosen; a particular make and model of device (and typically, a custom earmold) is specified that meets both the electroacoustic and physical requirements.
3. *Verification* of the hearing aids is conducted to ensure that the desired electroacoustic performance is achieved.
4. In the *information and instruction* stage, hearing aid orientation is provided and hearing aid use is monitored.
5. *Outcome evaluation* occurs in the final stage where the child's aided auditory performance is assessed and compared with habilitative goals.

Each stage of this process provides feedback to previous and subsequent stages. This allows clinicians to monitor the patient in an ongoing and systematic way (Figure 25–1).

Assessment

Before we can determine whether a child is a candidate for hearing aids, we need a clear description of the child's hearing status in each ear. Therefore, audiological assessment precedes determination of hearing aid candidacy for patients of all ages. At the assessment stage, two variables affect directly the hearing aid prescription: (a) hearing thresholds and (b) ear canal acoustics. In the following sections, we review current knowledge of assessment considerations for infants or children who are possible hearing aid candidates. We also provide clinical strategies for ensuring that complete and valid assessment data are available for accurate pediatric hearing aid fittings.

Hearing Assessment in Infants and Young Children

A description of the degree, configuration, and type of hearing loss for each ear is necessary prior to proceeding with hearing aid fitting in young patients (American Academy of Audiology [AAA], 2013; American Speech Language Hearing Association [ASHA], 2004; Joint Committee on Infant Hearing [JCIH], 2007; Pediatric Working Group [PWG], 1996). Proceeding with amplification before these factors are known can result in improper assessment of candidacy or improper hearing aid recommendations, such as hearing aid provision rather than medical referral for medically treatable conductive hearing loss, or binaural amplification for monaural hearing loss (Gravel, 2002). Complete audiometric assessment is therefore an essential first step, including estimation of thresholds with air- and bone-conducted stimuli for *at least* two frequencies per ear, along with case history, otoscopic examination, immittance measures, and diagnostic otoacoustic emissions. When a clear audiologic picture is available,

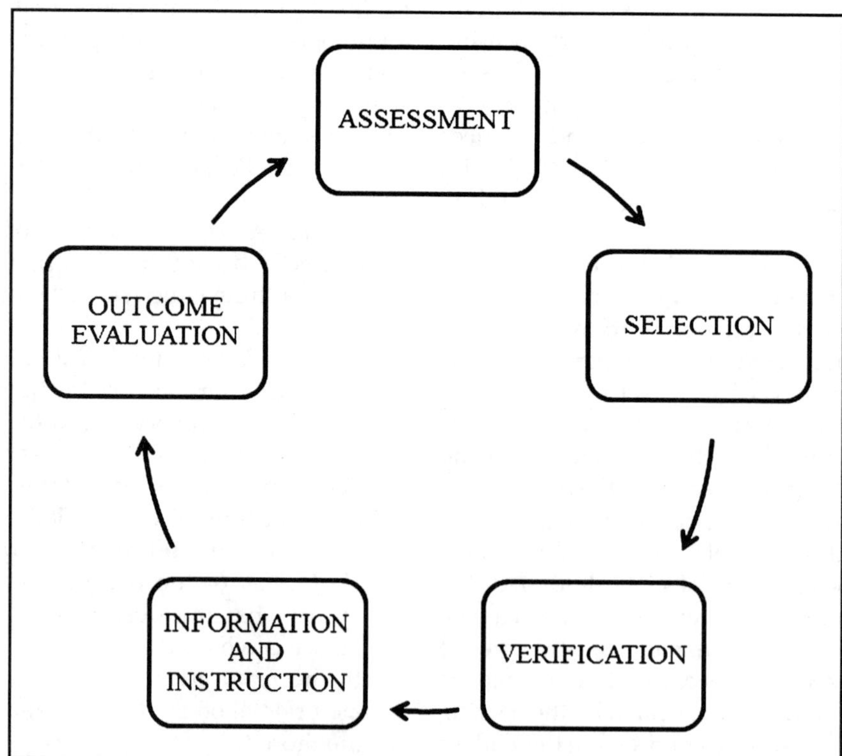

FIGURE 25–1. The five sequential stages involved in providing hearing aids to infants and children with hearing loss as suggested by the Pediatric Working Group (1996).

hearing aid candidacy evaluation and hearing aid prescription can begin. We refer the reader to Chapters 19 through 24 of this text for detailed information on hearing assessment in infants and children.

Clinical Application: Using Electrophysiologic Threshold Estimates for Hearing Aid Fitting in Early Infancy

To facilitate early assessment and intervention, electrophysiologic estimates of hearing sensitivity can be used as part of a complete audiologic test battery. These might be tests of the auditory brainstem response (ABR) or the auditory steady-state response (ASSR) in combination with ABR (see Chapter 21). Either approach can support the provision of hearing aids in early infancy.

The ABR can be measured using brief, yet frequency-specific stimuli, allowing the results from frequency-specific ABR (FS-ABR) to be used as the basis for infant hearing aid fitting. Threshold estimates from FS-ABR have been shown to be highly correlated with behavioral thresholds, for infants both with normal hearing and with hearing loss (Gorga, Kaminski, Beauchaine, & Bergman, 1993; Stapells, 2000a; Stapells, Gravel, & Martin, 1995). However, FS-ABR threshold estimates overestimate the behavioral audiogram by 5 to 30 dB across frequencies, depending on the patient's age and the calibration and stimulus parameters used. Some FS-ABR and ASSR procedures include this factor in their calibration (Gorga et al., 1993; Stapells, Herdman, Small, Dimitrijevic, & Hatton, 2004). Other FS-ABR procedures require correction of this overestimation prior to hearing aid prescription or fitting (Bagatto et al., 2005; Stapells, 2000b). As FS-ABR threshold estimates (normal hearing level [nHL]) are typically *higher* than behavioral thresholds (hearing level [HL]), the correction is *subtracted* from the nHL value to estimate behavioral thresholds (estimated hearing level [eHL]; Figure 25–2). This correction process is important for hearing aid prescription, because the prescribed targets will be too high (i.e., require too much gain in the hearing aid) if the corrections are inadvertently omitted. This could occur, for example, if one clinician conducts the FS-ABR evaluation and another prescribes the hearing aid, yet neither corrects the FS-ABR results to eHL. We recommend that correction protocols be in place to ensure that corrections are applied once, *and only once*. Otherwise, substantial over- or underamplification can occur.

The correction values are frequency specific and are generally larger in the low frequencies than in the high frequencies (Bagatto et al., 2005; Stapells, 2000a; Stapells et al., 1995). Clinics that follow Stapells' calibration and stimulus parameters (see http://www.courses.audiospeech.ubc.ca/haplab/HAPLAB_Download_Page.html) can use the following correction values: 20 dB at 500 Hz, 15 dB at 1000 Hz, 10 dB at 2000 Hz, and 5 dB at 4000 Hz. Figure 25–3 shows an example of applying these corrections to the results of an FS-ABR assessment. This FS-ABR correction approach is incorporated within the Desired Sensation Level (DSL) Method for hearing aid prescription and fitting (Bagatto et al., 2005; Scollie et al., 2005).

dB nHL – correction = dB eHL

FIGURE 25–2. A frequency-specific correction is subtracted from the threshold estimation, in dB nHL, obtained from the ABR system. The result is a dB eHL value that better predicts a behavioral threshold and denotes that the ABR (nHL) value has been corrected.

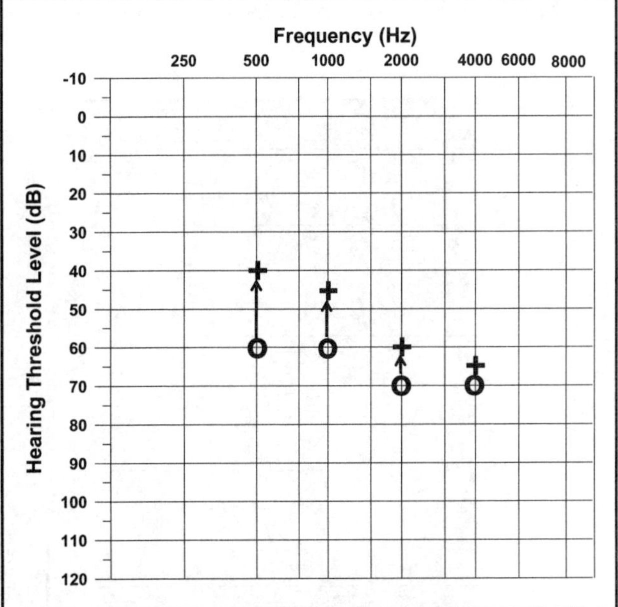

FIGURE 25–3. Correcting ABR threshold estimations in nHL to an estimated behavioral threshold in eHL. The circles (o) represent the nHL values obtained from the ABR system. The plus signs (+) represent the corrected ABR values that are now referenced in eHL.

Clinical Application: Obtaining Ear-Specific Thresholds in Behavioral Audiometry

In hearing assessments of infants and children, we place a high priority on obtaining ear-specific thresholds. For example, if using visual reinforcement audiometry (VRA) or conditioned play audiometry (CPA), we can obtain ear-specific thresholds under headphones or insert earphones. Insert earphones typically are preferred for their lighter weight and improved attenuation of sound from the room and between ears (ASHA, 2004). Some clinicians report difficulty in having young children accept insert earphones during hearing assessment, or that the insert earphones fall out of the child's ears during the VRA procedures. Erber (1973) suggested that a child's own button receiver earmold could be used during audiometry, within procedures for obtaining in situ estimates of thresholds in real-ear sound pressure level (SPL). Today, we maintain this general philosophy by coupling the child's behind-the-ear (BTE) earmold to insert earphones during VRA, CPA, or standard audiometry (Moodie & Moodie, 2004). In our experience, this unusual but helpful step permits better acceptance and retention of the insert earphones (Bagatto & Moodie, 2007). This approach can facilitate early assessment and intervention by supporting the measurement of ear-specific behavioral thresholds earlier and more consistently. A few clinical tips can help when using this strategy. First, clipping the insert earphones to the back of the child's shirt can help to keep the tubing and transducers out of view and reach. Second, if the BTE earhook has stretched the earmold tubing, the insert earphone might not couple well to the earmold. In these cases, a small amount of thin tubing from a standard insert earphone foam tip might be temporarily attached to the insert earphone, permitting a tight seal to the earmold. An example of this strategy is shown in Figure 25–4. Third, the use of a custom earmold is not the standard coupling type for insert earphone calibration. Therefore, the use of individualized HL to SPL transforms (discussed below) is of interest, to convert the resulting thresholds to either real-ear SPL or equivalent adult HL. Both scales have earmold acoustics removed in their calculations, allowing accurate comparisons to normative data over time.

Individual Ear Canal Acoustics

Accounting for the individual child's ear canal acoustics is the next step in improving the accuracy of pediatric hearing aid fitting. This affects both the assessment results and the hearing aid prescription and fitting. Individual ear canal acoustics vary by as much as 36 dB SPL, even in adults (Valente, Potts, Valente, Vass, & Goebel, 1994). Studies with children

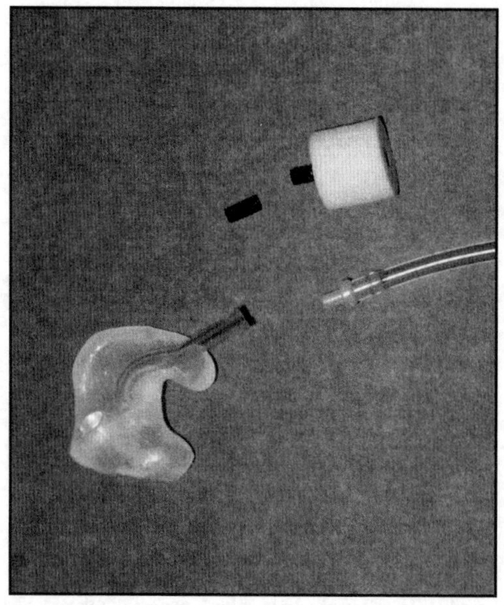
A

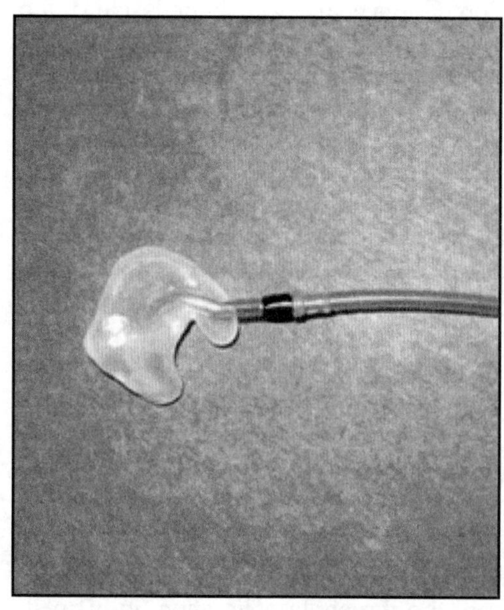
B

FIGURE 25–4. A technique for securely connecting an insert earphone to an earmold. **A.** A small portion is cut from the tubing of an insert earphone foam tip. **B.** The tubing is connected to the tip of the insert earphone and then inserted into the earmold tubing.

have shown a similarly large range of individual variability within and across age groups (Bagatto, Scollie, Seewald, Moodie, & Hoover, 2002; Feigin, Kopun, Stelmachowicz, & Gorga, 1989; Lewis & Stelmachowicz, 1993). To summarize, individual children of the same age vary substantially in their individual ear canal acoustics. Also, a given child's ear canal acoustics will change significantly over time as the ears grow and develop (Kruger, 1987). In general, smaller ear canal volumes are associated with larger resonant peaks in the ear canal's response, and these peaks likely occur at higher frequencies. Larger ear canal resonances associated with smaller volumes have been demonstrated in the literature for both infants and children, with values generally maturing when the pinna reaches adult size, at around age five or six years. The next section defines three clinical measurements of external ear canal acoustics, and reviews their normative properties in the pediatric population.

Clinical Measurements of External Ear Canal Acoustics

Three clinical measurements of external ear canal acoustics are available to capture the effects of individual ear canal acoustics in audiometry and hearing aid fitting. These are the real-ear unaided gain (REUG), the real-ear-to-coupler difference (RECD), and the real-ear-to-dial difference (REDD; ANSI S3.46, 1997; Mueller, 2001). The REUG is a derived measurement of the acoustic response of the *unoccluded ear canal*, with a characteristic 17-dB resonant peak that occurs just below 3000 Hz in the average adult (Shaw & Vaillancourt, 1985). Individual REUGs vary considerably from one another, particularly when the ear canal volume is small or the middle ear system is either stiff or flaccid. REUGs from young infants tend to peak at a higher frequency (up to 6000 Hz) and reach adult values by 2 years of age (Kruger, 1987; Figure 25–5A).

Finally, the REUG varies with signal azimuth; the average adult REUG peaks at a higher frequency when the source signal is to the side rather than to the front of the listener. In fact, this important variation provides one of the primary cues for localization of sound.

The RECD and REDD are measures of the acoustic response of the *occluded ear canal*. The RECD is measured with an insert earphone transducer, coupled either to a standard audiometric eartip or to the hearing aid wearer's earmold, and is referenced to the 2-cc coupler. The RECD is the *difference* between the real-ear SPL of a signal from the insert earphone transducer and the SPL of the same signal measured in a 2-cc coupler, across frequency. Typically, RECD values are positive and increase with increasing frequency (Figure 25–5B). Early investigations of age-related differences in the RECD demonstrated that pediatric RECDs were significantly higher than average adult RECDs, likely due to the smaller volume of the child's ear canal (Feigin et al., 1989). Test-retest reliability of the RECD is good, ranging from 0 to 2 dB in adults (Munro & Davis, 2003; Sinclair et al., 1996) to 1 to 4 dB in infants and children (Sinclair et al., 1996; Tharpe, Sladen, Huta, & Rothpletz, 2001).

In theory, the REDD could be measured as a comparison of the ear canal levels to those in a 6-cc coupler, rather than a 2-cc coupler. If this measurement was clinically feasible, it could serve a function as an audiometric transform for use with TDH headphones (discussed in detail in the next section). However, clinics do not typically have a 6-cc coupler. Therefore, the REDD was developed as an alternative measure of individual ear canal acoustics as they occur under TDH headphones. The REDD is the difference between the real-ear SPL produced by the audiometer and TDH phones and the dial level that produced it.

A key component of real-ear measurements is proper placement of the probe tube microphone in the child's ear canal. The goal is to place the probe tube far enough in the ear canal to represent the high frequencies accurately while avoiding standing waves. Placing the probe tube to within 5 mm of the eardrum is the typical clinical guideline (Dirks & Kincaid, 1987; Moodie, Seewald, & Sinclair, 1994). Although there are several methods for ensuring placement of the probe tube to the appropriate depth in the ear canal, a constant insertion depth strategy has been shown to be less time consuming and avoids contact with the tympanic membrane (Tharpe et al., 2001), which is preferred when working with the pediatric population. When measuring the RECD, different techniques can be used for young infants versus older infants and children.

For young infants, align the probe tube along the bottom of the earmold so the medial end of the tube extends 3 mm beyond the sound bore, and mark the tube on the portion of the earmold corresponding to the intertragal notch (Figure 25–6A). With young infants, it is often helpful to couple the probe tube to the foam eartip or earmold with plastic wrap or soft surgical tape (Figure 25–6B). This technique is helpful in coordinating insertion and ensuring a constant length of the probe tube remains at the tip edge, especially for active toddlers and very young infants with small ear canals (Bagatto, Seewald, Scollie, & Tharpe, 2006). The combined earmold/probe tube assembly is then inserted into the ear for the real-ear portion of the RECD measurement. Prior to the measurement, otoscopy is necessary to ensure that the ear canal is clear of

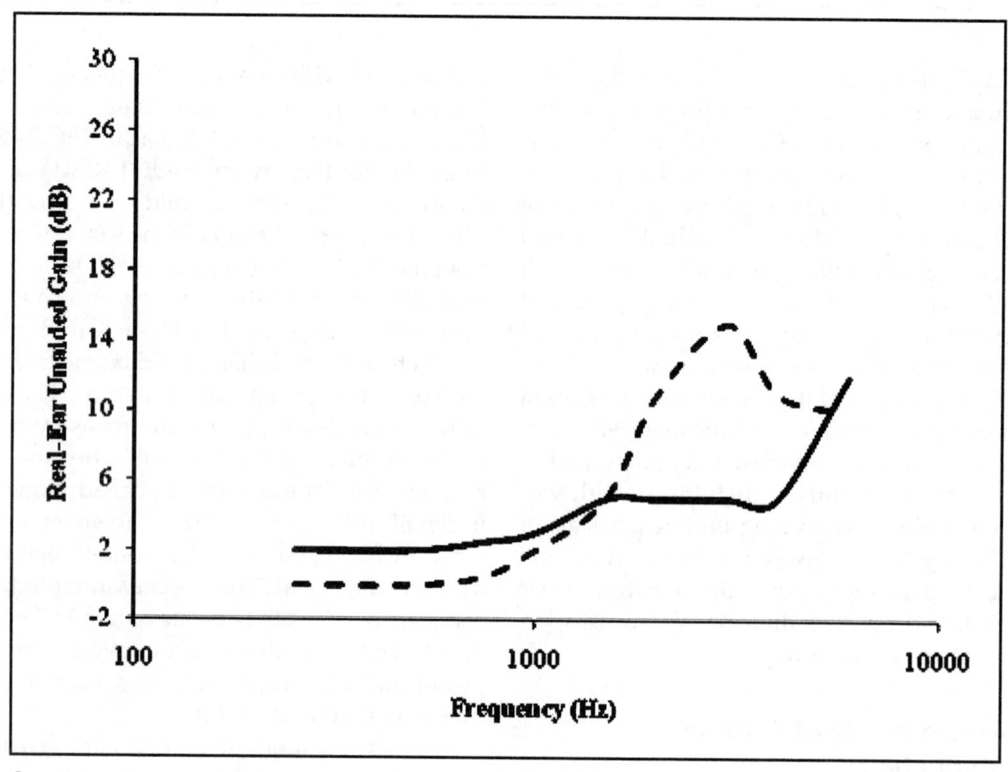

A

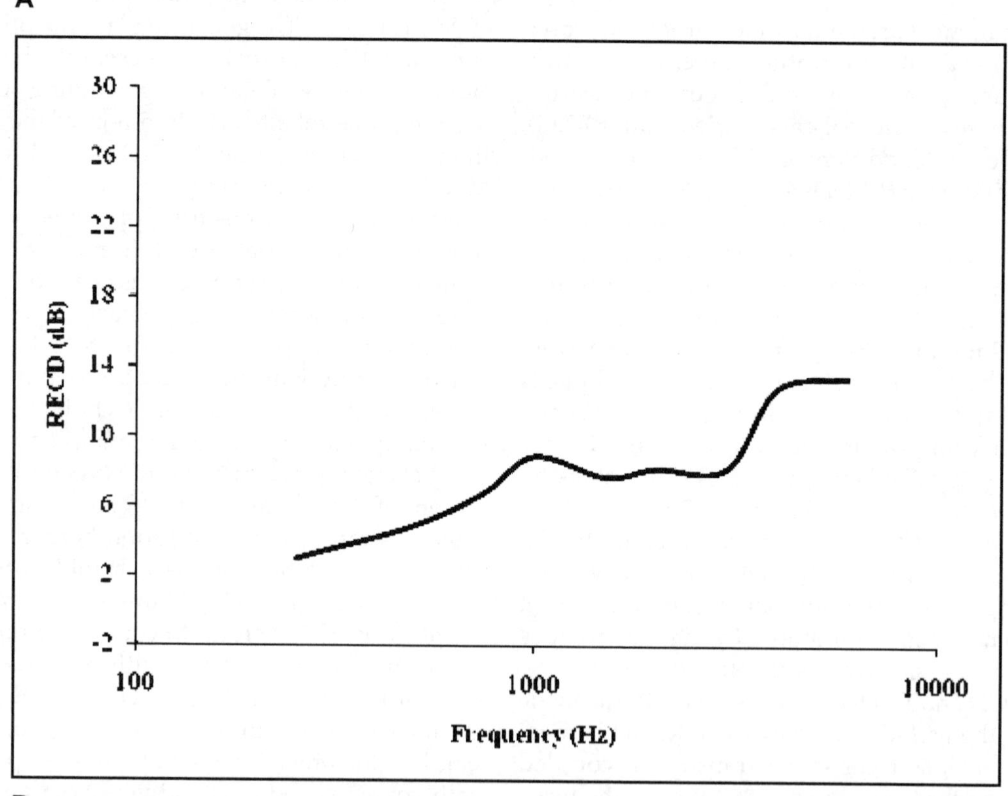

B

FIGURE 25–5. Examples of real-ear measurements. **A.** Real-ear unaided gain (REUG) across frequency for an infant (*solid line*) and an adult (*dashed line*). **B.** Real-ear-to-coupler difference (RECD) for an infant across frequency.

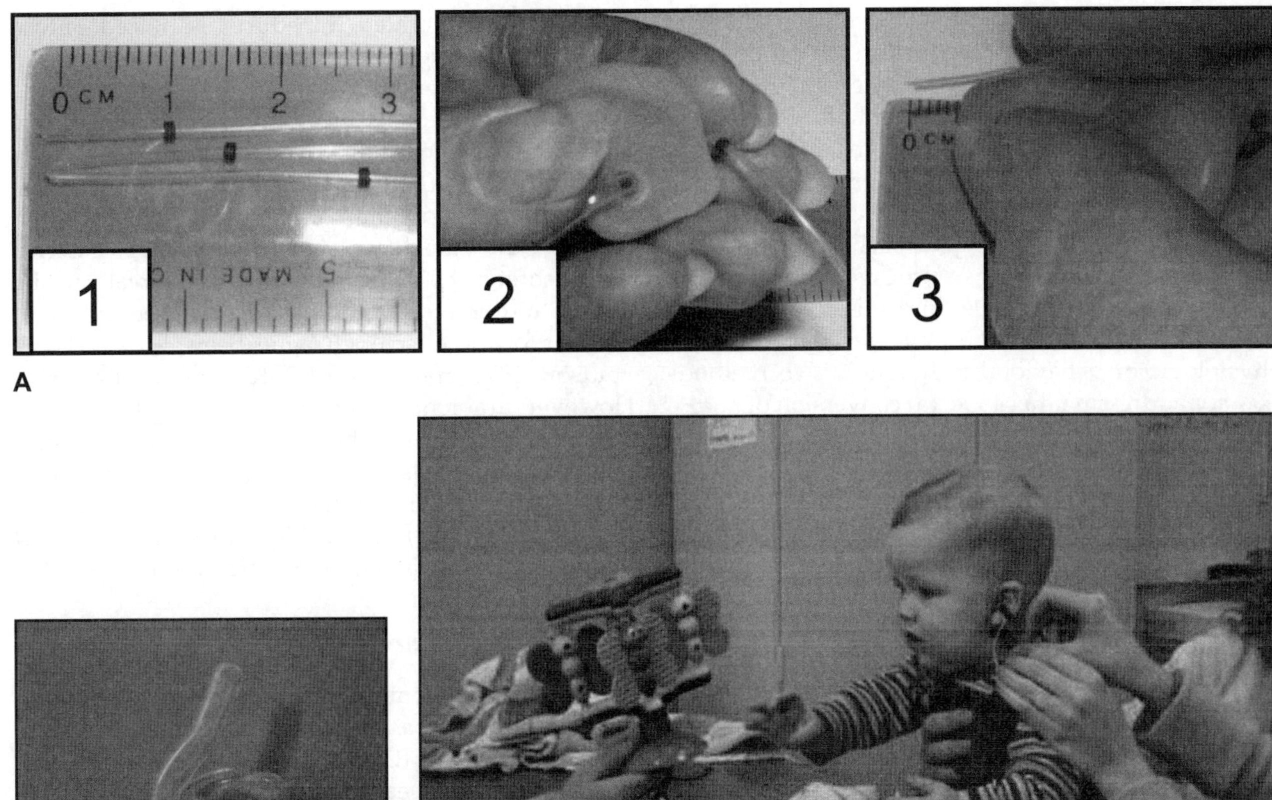

FIGURE 25–6. Customized probe tube insertion depth. **A.** (1) A constant insertion depth can be marked by using a ruler and following suggested insertion depth guidelines; (2) or, lay the probe tube microphone along the bottom of the earmold; (3) ensure the end of the tube extends a few millimeters beyond the sound bore, and mark the tube at the point corresponding to the intertragal notch. **B.** Attach the probe tube to the earmold with plastic wrap (*shown here*) or soft surgical tape for simultaneous insertion during RECD measures. **C.** Keep the child engaged during probe tube insertion.

debris. During the measurement, visual distraction of the infant (if awake) is often helpful.

For older infants and young children, the earmold can also be used as a guide. Align the probe tube along the bottom of the earmold so the medial end of the tube extends 5 mm beyond the sound bore and mark the tube on the portion corresponding to the intertragal notch (see Figure 25–6A). General insertion depth guidelines are 20 to 25 mm for children, with the mark meeting the intertragal notch (Moodie et al., 1994). The child's earmold is lubricated and inserted into the ear, taking care not to move the probe tube, and the real-ear portion of the RECD is measured. During probe insertion and measurement, the child is allowed to watch in a mirror or play with an engaging toy (Figure 25–6C).

Effects of the External Ear on Audiometry

The section above defined the REUG, RECD, and REDD as three different measures of individual ear canal resonance. All of these transforms vary across individuals, and some vary with development due to ear growth. This development has an impact on audiometry. Specifically, if the patient's hearing thresholds are stable, the real-ear SPL at threshold will remain the same across subsequent hearing tests. However, as the external ear grows, the HL required to generate a given real-ear SPL level will increase. Therefore, it is important to consider the impact of changing ear canal acoustics when comparing hearing assessment results at different ages for the same child; this occurs whether the assessment results were obtained using electrophysiologic or behavioral techniques. Two methods exist for addressing this issue: (a) conversion of audiometric data from HL to real-ear SPL; and (b) conversion of audiometric data from observed HL to equivalent adult HL.

Regardless of which method is used, understanding the corrections requires a review of how audiometric calibration relates to the HL values obtained during audiometry. Audiometric calibration sets the levels from each audiometric transducer so that a level of 0 dB HL approximates the normal threshold of hearing. These levels are the reference equivalent threshold sound pressure levels (RETSPLs) specified for each audiometric transducer (ANSI S3.6, 1997; R2010). The RETSPL values are defined by studies of the average normal hearing *adult* population and are often defined in a fixed test location (i.e., 6-cc coupler for TDH phones, 2-cc coupler for insert earphones and sound field for loudspeakers). Therefore, for any value of HL we can compute precisely the 6-cc, 2-cc, or sound-field SPL, but we cannot know the exact real-ear SPL unless further measures are made.

When a calibrated transducer is placed onto a human ear during audiometry, sound is delivered in different ways depending on the style of transducer. For instance, testing using sound-field loudspeakers leaves the ear unoccluded, whereas assessment using insert earphones occludes the ear. The resulting SPL at the eardrum will differ according to the specific combination of the transducer and the individual's external ear. Theoretically, a direct measure of the real-ear SPL during audiometry would be the preferred option to account for these factors (Gagné, Seewald, Zelisko, & Hudson, 1991; Hawkins, 1987; Kiessling, 1987, 1993). However, ambient or probe tube microphone noise floor, which can be higher than normal or near-normal threshold levels, and probe tube retention during audiometric assessment make this technique impractical. A more clinically feasible approach is to *predict* these values using an HL-to-SPL transform.

Clinical Application: HL-to-SPL Transforms

Because each audiometric transducer is calibrated differently, and uses a different set of RETSPL values, there is a different HL-to-SPL transform for each transducer. When insert earphones are used, the transform equals the 2-cc RECD plus the 2-cc RETSPLs for insert earphones (see Table 25–1 for case example calculations). When TDH headphones are used, the transform equals the 6-cc RECD plus the 6-cc RETSPL for TDH headphones. This is equivalent to the REDD. When loudspeakers are used, the transform equals the azimuth-dependent REUG plus the azimuth-dependent RETSPL for sound field. In summary, each HL-to-SPL

Table 25–1. HL-to-SPL Calculations for a 4-Month-Old Infant

	500 Hz	1000 Hz	2000 Hz	4000 Hz
dB eHL threshold	40	45	60	65
+	+	+	+	+
Insert earphone RETSPL	6	1	6	2
+	+	+	+	+
Measured RECD	8	13	15	23
=	=	=	=	=
dB SPL threshold	54	59	81	90

Note. dB = decibel; *HL* = hearing level; *eHL* = estimated hearing level; *RETSPL* = reference equivalent threshold sound pressure levels; *RECD* = real-ear-to-coupler-difference.

transform has a real-ear component and a calibration component. These are summed together with the audiogram to calculate the child's thresholds in predicted real-ear SPL. This HL-to-SPL approach is incorporated within the DSL Method for hearing aid prescription and fitting (Bagatto et al., 2005; Scollie et al., 2005). Several studies have found the HL-to-SPL transform approach, as implemented for insert earphones, to be valid for clinical use (Bentler & Pavlovic, 1989; Munro & Davis, 2003; Revit, 1997; Scollie, Seewald, Cornelisse, & Jenstad, 1998).

An alternative to the HL-to-SPL approach is the *equivalent adult HL* approach (Ching & Dillon, 2003; Marcoux & Hansen, 2003; Seewald, Ramji, Sinclair, Moodie, & Jamieson, 1993; Seewald et al., 1997). This approach corrects the audiogram for the difference between the child's ear canal and that of an average adult. It provides the HL audiogram that would have been measured on the ear of the average adult, assuming the same hearing sensitivity. The measured ear canal properties required for this correction are identical to the insert earphone, TDH, and sound-field requirements described for HL-to-SPL transforms. The main difference is that the equivalent adult HL approach does not convert the audiogram to real-ear SPL, and therefore does not make use of the calibration values, or RETSPLs. The equivalent adult HL approach is incorporated within the NAL-NL1 prescriptive software (Ching & Dillon, 2003), and the DSL Method (Scollie et al., 2005).

Regardless of the signal transducer used during audiometry, individual measurement of the real-ear component (e.g., RECD, REUG) is recommended to accurately define hearing thresholds for hearing aid fitting (Bagatto et al., 2002; Bentler, 1989). Sometimes, we cannot measure the real-ear component, such as when the child is too active or ear canal conditions prevent probe tube insertion (i.e., cerumen requiring management, discharge, objects requiring removal). In these cases, age-related normative values are available for both insert earphone and soundfield transforms (Bagatto et al., 2002, 2005; Kruger, 1987). Detailed information on normative data for the RECD is presented below. Transforms for TDH headphones exist on average, but evidence for age-related normative values do not exist (Lewis & Stelmachowicz, 1993).

Insert earphones are the only transducer that is calibrated in the 2-cc coupler. This allows a single real ear measurement, the RECD, to be used for the HL-to-SPL transform and also for hearing aid transforms (discussed separately below). This, combined with improved interaural attenuation, light weight, and ear-specificity, make insert earphones the preferred and recommended transducer type for use in assessments of children with hearing loss (ASHA, 2004). Therefore, the measurement of the RECD is more clinically relevant, in most cases, than measurement of the other real-ear transforms described above.

Clinical Application: Comparing Different Audiometric Test Sessions

The sections above have described two approaches that account for the effects of individual ear canal acoustics during audiometry. In pediatric audiology, it is common, and important, to see children for repeated assessments over time, and to compare results over time in order to evaluate stability of hearing thresholds. Sometimes, these results are compared across multiple assessment techniques and time points. For example, an infant whose hearing was assessed using FS-ABR techniques at the age of 4 months might have thresholds of 40, 45, 60, and 65 dB eHL at 500, 1000, 2000, and 4000 Hz, respectively. A behavioral hearing test session 5 months later, when the infant is 9 months of age, might yield thresholds of 45, 55, 70, and 80 dB HL at the same frequencies in the right ear (Figure 25–7A). A common misconception might be that the child's hearing loss has progressed. However, it is important to consider the change in ear canal acoustics from 4 to 9 months of age. This can be accomplished by measuring or predicting (using age-appropriate norms, as discussed in the following section) the RECD at the different audiometric test sessions. The thresholds from each session can be converted to real-ear SPL (or equivalent adult HL) for a more accurate comparison. This will account for the ear canal growth that occurred in the 5 months between test sessions (Figure 25–7B).

The example shown in Figure 25–7 reveals that a higher level of SPL was required to elicit a response in HL at age 9 months, compared to the assessment of eHL at 4 months of age. The likely cause of this change was ear canal growth, which was likely substantial between these two ages. Both sets of audiometric data were measured using insert earphones, so the relevant measure of ear canal acoustics for both is the RECD. By measuring or predicting the infant's RECDs at both points in time and applying them to each set of thresholds or threshold estimates, a more accurate comparison is available for interpretation. In this example, the real-ear SPL thresholds were 54, 59, 81, and 90 dB SPL at the test frequencies for the ABR assessment and 56, 62, 82, and 92 dB SPL for the behavioral assessment at the same frequencies. Therefore, the increase in HL level was not due to a progression in hearing but a change in individual ear canal acoustics over time.

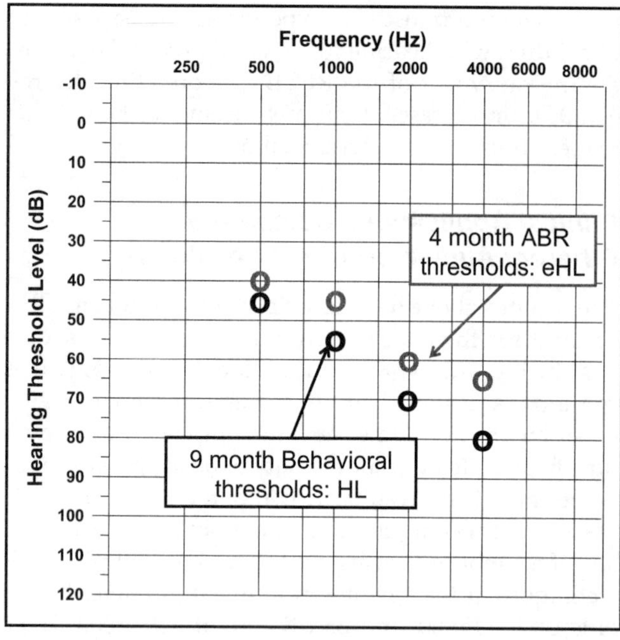

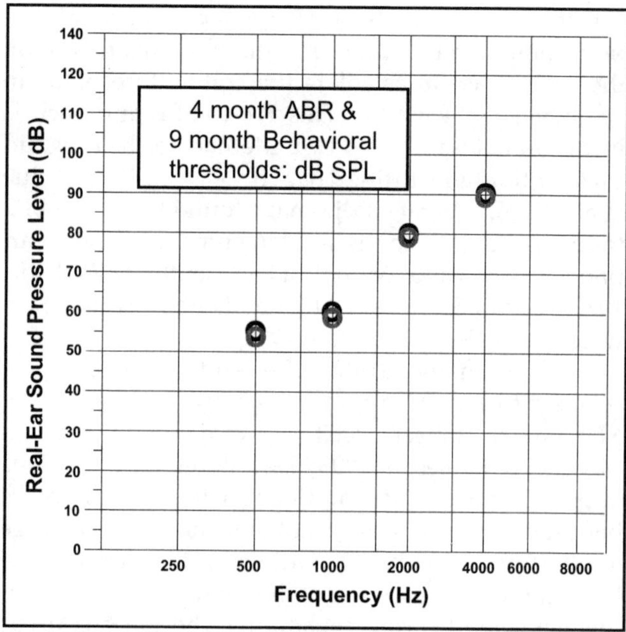

A B

FIGURE 25–7. When comparing HL thresholds for the two test sessions, an elevation in hearing levels from the auditory brainstem response (ABR) to behavioral assessments is noted (**A**). When the real-ear-to-couple-difference (RECD) is measured and used to convert the hearing level (HL) thresholds to real-ear SPL, thresholds are more similar because ear canal growth has been accounted for in the comparison (**B**; eHL = estimated hearing level.)

The absence of progression, in this case, is clarified by accounting directly for the acoustic effects of ear canal growth via the RECD.

For some clinicians, it might be preferable to account for ear canal acoustics in the dB HL scale when comparing audiometric test sessions in young children over time. This allows plotting of the test results over time on a standard audiogram and is easily accomplished by converting the infant's thresholds to equivalent adult HL. We have shown the required calculations for use with insert earphones in Table 25–2 for this case example. This calculation is implemented in some real-ear measurement systems by changing the scale from SPL to HL. This procedure might be helpful, in some cases, to account for the child's growing ear when comparing audiograms at different stages of the child's development to avoid inaccurate conclusions about the child's hearing sensitivity.

For these reasons, repeated measurements of a child's external ear canal acoustics over time are an important component of providing ongoing accurate care. In most cases, we can accomplish this by re-measuring the RECD using the child's own earmold, every time the earmold is re-made. This earmold RECD can be used as an HL-to-SPL transform as well as a 2 cc-to-real-ear transform (discussed further below), maximizing the customization of the prescription and fitting.

Normative RECD Values

There are times when individual measurement of the RECD is not possible on a young patient during a particular clinical appointment. An active toddler might not sit still for probe tube placement, or debris in the ear canal might prevent appropriate probe tube insertion. In these circumstances, age-appropriate normative values for the RECD are a reasonable alternative to individualized measures.

One current set of RECD normative data are available for infants through adulthood, and are implemented in the DSL Method, version 5.0 (Bagatto et al., 2002, 2005). These norms were derived from RECDs collected in the clinical environment, from infants and children of varying ages and are provided for both foam eartip and earmold coupling types. However, these values were derived from infants and children with normal middle ear status. Therefore, the predicted

Table 25–2. Equivalent Adult HL Audiogram Calculations for the Same Infant at 4 and 9 Months of Age

	500 Hz		*1000 Hz*		*2000 Hz*		*4000 Hz*	
	4 Months	*9 Months*	*4 Months*	*9 Months*	*4 Months*	*9 Months*	*4 Months*	*9 Months*
Measured RECD	8	5	13	7	15	9	23	12
−	−		−		−		−	
Average adult RECD	4		5		5		13	
+	+		+		+		+	
dB (e)HL threshold	40	45	45	55	60	70	65	80
=	=		=		=		=	
Equivalent adult HL threshold	44	46	53	57	70	74	75	79

Note. RECD = real-ear-to-coupler difference; *HL* = hearing level.

values might not reflect any acoustic changes that a fluid-filled middle ear or perforated eardrum will display, in the individual ear. For infants and children with normal middle ear status, tested with eartips, one can expect RECD prediction errors to fall within a range of ±5.6 dB (at 500 Hz) at best and ±10.9 dB (at 6000 Hz) at worst for children 24 months of age and younger. Predictions of earmold RECDs can span a range of accuracy from ±6.7 dB (at 2000 Hz) to ±12.4 dB (at 6000 Hz) for children 36 months of age and younger. Therefore, it is important to attempt an RECD measurement on an infant or child whenever possible.

Summary: Importance of Accurate Assessment Information

To this point, our chapter has described key factors to consider in the assessment stage of the hearing aid fitting process to infants and young children. The pediatric population differs from the adult population in several ways, and these differences warrant careful consideration. First, the hearing of infants is often assessed using electrophysiological techniques (i.e., ABR), which provides an estimate of behavioral thresholds if the appropriate correction is applied prior to the calculation of the hearing aid prescription. In addition, the ear canal acoustics of infants and young children are substantially different from the average adult and therefore will have an impact on the interpretation of HL thresholds if not accounted for. Finally, the acoustic characteristics of infant ear canals can be measured and applied regularly in the early stages of the hearing aid fitting process. Such dynamic and unique features are part of what makes fitting hearing aids to infants and young children a challenge. Individualizing the fitting for each child supports successful intervention with amplification. If key steps in the process are eliminated, error can be introduced into the fitting. Table 25–3 summarizes the procedures required for the assessment stage of the hearing aid fitting process, and the potential error introduced if each is eliminated.

Selecting Hearing Aids

Following the identification of a permanent hearing loss in an infant or child, hearing aids are a common device choice among families as part of a larger intervention program. The goal of amplification is to improve functional auditory capacity and participation in hearing- and communication-specific situations. Several published reports indicate that early improvement in hearing can facilitate the development of sensory and perceptual skills, receptive and expressive language, speech production and literacy, academic performance, and social-emotional growth (e.g., Carney & Moeller, 1998; Ching, Dillon, Day, & Crowe, 2007; Moeller, 2000; Vohr et al., 2008).

Table 25–3. Procedures Used for the Assessment Stage of the Hearing Aid Fitting Process and the Potential Error Introduced if Eliminated

Clinical Procedure	*Potential Error if Not Applied*
Audiometry with insert earphones	TDH uses 6-cc coupler for calibration; probe microphone systems do not allow for 6-cc coupler measures. Sound fields are not ear specific.
nHL to eHL correction	Threshold estimates will be 5 to 20 dB higher, depending on frequency
Measure the RECD	Up to 20 if average adult values are assumed.
Predict RECD using age-appropriate values	±15 dB

Note. RECD = real-ear-to-coupler difference.

The specific objectives of early amplification are to (a) provide an amplified speech signal that is consistently audible across varying input levels; (b) avoid distortion of varying inputs at prescribed settings; (c) ensure amplification of sounds in as broad a frequency range as possible; and (d) include sufficient electroacoustic flexibility to allow for changes in the required frequency/output characteristics related to ear growth or changes in the auditory characteristics of the infant (AAA, 2013; JCIH, 2007; PWG, 1996). Calculation of prescriptive targets based on accurate, ear-specific assessment information and the selection of the physical and electroacoustic elements of hearing aids are key aspects of the fitting process.

The prescription includes a specification of the type of hearing aid and earmold to be fitted, and appropriate settings and applications that will result in an amplification system that addresses the evolving needs of the individual infant and family. Prescription is followed by verification to ensure that the prescribed listening levels are produced by the hearing aids. This important step confirms that the real-ear performance of the selected hearing aid(s) provides output levels that are comfortable, safe, and without feedback. A scientifically based, generic fitting algorithm that takes into consideration the unique characteristics of infants and young children with hearing loss will provide fitting targets that, when matched appropriately, aim to meet these goals.

Prescriptive Algorithms

Prescriptive algorithms provide the foundation on which the hearing aid performance characteristics are selected for the infant to be fitted. Infants will wear their hearing aids at settings determined by their clinician for several months or years before being able to reliably express their preferences about the fitting (Scollie, 2004). It therefore is important to use a valid approach to selecting the hearing aid settings in order to facilitate speech and language development and maintain consistent treatment across children, clinicians, and clinics. The use of a systematic, objective prescriptive strategy has been recommended by several consensus statements (AAA, 2013; JCIH, 2007; PWG, 1996). Prescriptive algorithms provide objective and consistently derived targets for electroacoustic hearing aid performance that are acceptable and provide consistent benefit across patients. They are typically based on the hearing levels of the wearer to prescribe specific amplification characteristics. The resulting targets provide electroacoustic settings for the hearing aids that should result in appropriate detection, loudness, and intelligibility of amplified speech.

Generic Versus Proprietary Prescriptive Algorithms

Currently available prescriptive algorithms can be divided into two classifications: generic and proprietary. *Generic* prescriptive algorithms are based on published scientific evidence and are intended for use with any hearing aid. *Proprietary* prescriptive algorithms incorporate calculations developed by hearing aid manufacturers and are used with their specific brand of hearing aids. The lack of published information regarding the development of proprietary algorithms makes it difficult for clinicians to make an informed decision about which procedure will be best for their young patient.

Several investigators have compared different proprietary prescriptive algorithms to generic algorithms within manufacturer software. Differences in the amount of gain prescribed for adults were as much as 10 dB (Keidser, Brew, & Peck, 2003), and prescribed output ranged from 90 to 109 dB SPL (re: 2-cc coupler) for the same audiogram (Mueller, Bentler, & Wu, 2008). A study with pediatric algorithms from five different hearing aid manufacturers revealed differences of as much as 20 dB in the simulated real-ear aided response and 30 dB for the simulated real-ear saturation response (Seewald, Mills, Bagatto, Scollie, & Moodie, 2008). These large differences in prescriptions point to the importance of using an evidence-based prescriptive algorithm so that consistent amplification characteristics are applied across patients, regardless of the hearing aid being prescribed.

Current pediatric amplification guidelines recommend the use of a generic prescriptive algorithm that contains appropriate elements for use with infants and children (AAA, 2013; JCIH, 2007). Two prescriptive approaches have been suggested for use in deriving targets for pediatric hearing aid fittings: the DSL Method and the National Acoustics Laboratories' (NAL) prescription. Both formulae contain specific characteristics that are important for application with the pediatric population.

Characteristics of a Pediatric Prescriptive Method

There are several psychoacoustic and electroacoustic variables that impact the outcome of a hearing aid fitting for an infant or child with hearing loss. Relevant variables that should be included in a pediatric prescriptive algorithm include (a) implementation of auditory thresholds estimated from electrophysiological tests of hearing; (b) accounting for external ear canal acoustics in assessment data; (c) access to age-specific normative data for predicting ear canal acoustics; and (d) the methods to conduct coupler-assisted verification. Key functions of a prescriptive formula for pediatrics ensure that these variables are handled appropriately and are discussed in the following sections.

The prescriptive method should be able to compute targets based only on thresholds, and to handle partial audiometric data. Hearing thresholds, in dB HL, are the primary source used for computing gain and output targets. Although there can be large between-subject variability, loudness discomfort levels (LDLs) can be predicted from auditory thresholds (Bentler & Cooley, 2001; Dillon & Storey, 1998; Seewald, 1991) and used to define the auditory area for the listener. Predictions of LDL are computed conservatively when used with the pediatric population (Seewald, 1991) and typically are the only option when fitting hearing aids to an infant who cannot perform suprathreshold assessments. Therefore, a pediatric prescriptive formula should provide a prediction of the LDL for use in the common case that the LDL cannot be measured.

Hearing aid fitting should proceed based on electrophysiologic tests of hearing and not be postponed to obtain behavioral thresholds. For some electrophysiologic procedures, corrections are applied to facilitate an accurate estimation of behavioral thresholds (see Assessment section of this chapter). A prescriptive algorithm intended to be used with infants should have the capability to handle electrophysiologic assessment data appropriately and provide appropriate corrections, if necessary, prior to calculating targets.

The targets should account for the external ear canal acoustics. This is required in the assessment data, using HL-to-SPL transforms prior to calculating the prescription or by using the RECD to correct the assessment data to equivalent adult HL (see Assessment section). Additionally, the smaller size of the infant ear canal means that less coupler gain is required from the hearing aids, but also that the gain requirements must be revised as the ear grows. Therefore, target calculations should account for the child's RECD. Some clinical situations will prevent measurement of the RECD on a young patient, in which case the prescriptive formula should provide age-appropriate external ear normative data (Bagatto et al., 2002, 2005). Both the DSL and NAL prescriptive approaches integrate the child's RECD into target calculations, thereby updating the prescription as the child grows. Both accurately incorporate ear canal acoustics within prescription calculations, and make the prescribed targets available in 2-cc coupler format. This supports measurement and adjustment of the hearing aid response on the 2-cc coupler (see Verification section, below). Overall, these pediatric-friendly approaches to prescription ensure accuracy and consistency in the fitting for infants and young children.

Listening Needs of Infants and Children With Hearing Loss

In addition to accounting for the variables mentioned above, a pediatric prescriptive approach should take into consideration the specific listening needs of the population. Because children acquire hearing loss either before or during a period of speech and language learning, they must learn these skills through aided hearing rather than from prior experience with the language. This is different from adults who acquire hearing loss after many years of experience with language. Many investigators have demonstrated that children with hearing loss require more speech audibility than adults or children with normal hearing in order to perceive all speech sounds (Elliott, 1979; Elliott et al., 1979; Gravel, Fausel, Liskow, & Chobot, 1999; Hnath-Chisholm, Laipply, & Boothroyd, 1998; Kortekaas & Stelmachowicz, 2000; Nábělek & Robinson, 1982; Neuman & Hochberg, 1982). Age-related interactions with level, bandwidth, and sensation level in the perception of fricatives or the use of context for word recognition have been shown between children with normal and impaired hearing (Pittman, 2008; Pittman & Stelmachowicz, 2000; Pittman, Stelmachowicz, Lewis, & Hoover, 2003; Stelmachowicz, Hoover, Lewis, Kortekaas, & Pittman, 2000; Stelmachowicz, Pittman, Hoover, & Lewis, 2001, 2002). Therefore, children with hearing loss require more gain, a higher signal-to-noise ratio and a broader audible bandwidth of speech in order to have a better chance at acquiring speech and language. Currently, there are two prescriptive procedures that are widely recommended for use in pediatric fitting because they take into account these variables: the Desired Sensation Level Multistage Input/Output Method (DSL *m*[i/o]) v5.0a and the National Acoustics Laboratories Nonlinear Algorithm (NAL-NL2). The characteristics of each are described in the following sections.

The Desired Sensation Level Multistage Input/Output Algorithm (DSL m[i/o]) v5.0a

Richard Seewald and his colleagues developed the original DSL Method in 1985. Their review of research with adults and children with hearing loss indicated that speech must be amplified to a certain sensation level (SL) to maximize comfort and intelligibility (Erber & Witt, 1977; Kamm, Dirks, & Mickey, 1977; Macrae, 1986; Pascoe, 1978, 1988). The findings from these studies were used to define target SLs for amplified speech for children with hearing loss (Seewald, Ross, & Spiro, 1985) for various hearing levels. A long-standing goal of this prescriptive method is to amplify speech to these "desired sensation levels" across as broad a frequency range as possible to support auditory learning via audibility of speech cues. This has been described as an habilitative audibility approach (Scollie, 2004). Another goal of the DSL Method has been to provide targets that limit the maximum output, while still providing appropriate headroom and comfort for loud sounds. During this era, hearing aids with linear circuitry were available; therefore, the resulting DSL version 3.0 targets were developed for this type of processing.

With the advent of wide dynamic range compression (WDRC) circuitry in hearing aids, an updated version of the DSL Method was developed. In 1995, Leonard Cornelisse and his colleagues designed the "input/output formula" (DSL [i/o]) by using Steven's Power Law to map a wide range of input levels to target hearing aid output levels across various frequencies. The DSL [i/o] Method Version 4.1 prescribed targets for gain, output limiting, and compression ratios for use with both linear and WDRC hearing aids. The average speech SLs were equivalent to those recommended by earlier versions of the DSL Method (Cornelisse, Seewald, & Jamieson, 1995). A key feature of the DSL Method has been to display the characteristics of the hearing aid output together with the child's auditory characteristics in an "SPLogram" format. The SPLogram uses a real-ear SPL reference scale across frequencies to permit direct comparison of the performance of the hearing aid with the listener's thresholds and LDLs.

Several validation studies of the DSL [i/o] v4.1 algorithm were conducted in the late 1990s. The work showed that the preferred listening levels (PLLs) of children were 2 dB higher than the listening levels recommended by DSL, with about 70% of the PLLs falling within 5 dB of the DSL target (Scollie, Seewald, Moodie, & Dekok, 2000). In addition, WDRC hearing aids fitted to DSL [i/o] targets achieved comfort, intelligibility, and the perception of normal loudness of speech across a range of speech input levels (Jenstad, Pumford, Seewald, & Cornelisse, 2000; Jenstad, Seewald, Cornelisse, & Shantz, 1999). These studies indicate that the DSL algorithm (a) improves speech recognition scores in children over unaided performance; (b) improves low-level speech recognition and normalizes loudness when paired with WDRC; and (c) more closely approximates children's PLLs.

In 2005, the DSL Multistage Input/Output (DSL *m*[i/o]) v5.0a was released. Although the habilitative audibility goals are the same as previous versions of the DSL Method, DSL *m*[i/o] v5.0a provides compatibility with ABR data, updated RECD normative data for infants and children, infant-friendly RECD measurement techniques, targets for quiet and noisy environments, adjustments for conductive losses, and binaural fittings, and accounts for multichannel compression characteristics of modern hearing aids. Detailed descriptions of these modifications and additions can be found in Scollie et al. (2005) and Bagatto et al. (2005). This version of DSL is widely implemented in hearing aid fitting and verification systems.

The National Acoustics Laboratories Nonlinear Algorithm (NAL-NL2)

The National Acoustics Laboratories (NAL) originally developed a prescriptive formula for fitting hearing aids to adults by amplifying all bands of speech to the most comfortable level. Following a series of studies, it was noted that the NAL prescription did not achieve this goal and the algorithm was revised (Byrne, 1986a, 1986b). The revised formula, NAL-R, was evaluated and found to be superior to the original formula for measures of speech recognition and preference. However, the authors noted that the gain and frequency response might not be suitable for listeners with severe-to-profound hearing loss (Byrne & Dillon, 1986; Byrne & Murray, 1986). The PLLs of adults with severe-to-profound hearing loss wearing linear BTE hearing aids led to the release of NAL-RP (Byrne, Parkinson, & Newall, 1990). This formula was recommended for use with adult listeners wearing linear hearing aids whose thresholds exceed 95 dB HL at 2000 Hz.

More recent versions of the NAL formula advocate an effective audibility approach that attempts to limit the loudness of the fitting while optimizing speech recognition (Ching, Dillon, & Byrne, 1998). This approach assumes that additional high-frequency gain might not further improve word recognition performance in adults; therefore, provision of audibility across the full frequency range is not always a goal for this algorithm (Ching, Dillon, Katsch, & Byrne, 2001). In 2001, Byrne, Ching, Dillon, and colleagues released the NAL-NL1 prescriptive approach for fitting nonlinear amplification. This theoretically derived version of the formula prescribes targets for nonlinear hearing aids using an effective audibility approach. Empirical data were obtained to make adjustments to the theoretical predictions of NAL-NL1 in order to derive NAL-NL2 (Keidser, Dillon, Carter, & O'Brien, 2012). NAL-NL2 uses appropriate corrections for the acoustic properties of children's ear canals, including measured RECDs and age-appropriate averages. The formula prescribes more overall gain for children compared to adults and the limits to prescribed bandwidth derived from effective audibility predictions are applied for both adults and children, on the assumption that the limits of effectiveness in the adult population also apply to infants and children (Ching et al., 2001; Keidser et al., 2012).

Comparisons of NAL-NL1 and DSL Prescriptive Formulae

Because both NAL and DSL currently offer similar ranges of software support for pediatric hearing aid fitting, the clinician might debate over the choice between the two. In general, the choice of prescription for children might be informed by evidence, and by consideration of the theoretical principles of each prescription. The evidence for prescriptive difference might evolve as new information accrues. At the time of this writing, several sources of evidence exist. Older studies have compared children's listening preferences to prescribed listening response shapes or listening levels, but consistent findings have not been measured (Ching, Hill, Birtles, & Beacham, 1999; Ching, Newall, & Wigney, 1997; Ching et al., 2001; Scollie et al., 2000). In general, studies of children who were DSL users were more likely to prefer DSL, and studies of NAL users were more likely to prefer NAL, leading the authors to speculate that acclimatization might play a role in preferences. Older studies also compared the actual hearing aid frequency responses of successful pediatric hearing aid users to various targets. In general, these studies found that used gain was within ±5 dB of both the NAL and DSL prescriptions for speech-level inputs, and for the DSL targets for output limiting (Snik & Stollman, 1995; Snik, van den Borne, Brokx, & Hoekstra, 1995).

More recently, a collaborative study between the authors of the NAL and DSL prescriptions compared the performance of DSL[i/o] v4.1 and NAL-NL1 for a group of 48 school-aged children with up to moderately severe hearing losses. These children participated in a double-blind crossover study that evaluated both laboratory and real-world outcomes (Ching, Scollie, Dillon, & Seewald, 2010). The fittings in this study employed coupler-based verification and individualized measurement of RECDs, achieving a 7-dB difference in gain, overall, between the two prescriptions at an input level of 70 dB SPL (Ching, Scollie, Dillon, Seewald, Britton, & Steinberg, 2010). With these fittings, children carried out an 8-week trial with one prescription, then again with the other, and then completed another 8-week trial in which they wore both and compared the two. Loudness ratings for the two fittings changed significantly after the single-prescription trials, showing acclimatization-related changes that removed most of the baseline differences in loudness between prescriptions (Scollie et al., 2010a). Speech recognition measures in quiet indicated a high level of performance (average scores greater than 85% correct for nonsense syllables) across sites and prescriptions (Scollie et al., 2010a). Performance on this task varied with test level for the NAL prescription but not the DSL prescription. Real-world ratings from the single-prescription trials found that children have significantly more listening difficulty in noisy environments (Ching, Scollie, Dillon, Seewald, Britton, Steinberg, Gilliver, & King, 2010). These same performance ratings in noise were higher for the NAL fitting than for the DSL fitting. Australian children were more likely to prefer the NAL fitting overall in these trials. In the real-world trials comparing the two prescriptions, children at both sites rated the DSL fitting as preferable for speech in quiet or from behind (Scollie et al., 2010b). Children's preferences fell into two factors: quiet or low-level situations versus noisy or reverberant situations. Canadian children were more likely to prefer DSL overall in these trials. Many children expressed a preference for using both programs in a multimemory fitting, and described their strategic use of two memories in ways that were appropriate to each listening environment. The use of less gain to control excessive loudness or noisiness, and the use of more gain to enhance clarity of speech and perceived closeness of the talker were both important in many environments. Overall, of the objective and subjective measures in this study, individual children varied in whether they would perform best with or prefer the DSL or NAL prescription. Even when no difference existed on average, individual children demonstrated significant individual performance or preference advantages with one of the fittings.

Overall, this collaborative study provides strong evidence that hearing aid benefit is high when a systematic hearing aid prescription and fitting method is used with school-aged children. It also provides some insight into (a) the relative performance of DSL and NAL in different real-world environments; (b) the children's ability to use a multimemory strategy reliably and rationally; (c) the importance of evaluating outcome at the individual level; and (d) the importance of allowing a period of acclimatization prior to evaluation of outcome.

With some exceptions, the studies above have primarily evaluated children with up to moderately severe hearing losses: less information is available about children with severe to profound hearing losses. The studies mentioned above might also have been constrained, to some degree, by hearing aid flexibility in meeting precisely the prescriptive targets (Ching, Scollie, Dillon, Seewald, Britton, & Steinberg, 2010). Clinicians practicing hearing aid fitting today might frequently treat infants with severe to profound hearing loss, using instruments that are now capable of a more faithful representation of the prescriptions, and perhaps employing revised versions of these prescriptions. Therefore, current practice should consider the evidence for prescription choice, in addition to theoretical factors. First, if fitting an infant, is the prescription designed to compute targets based on electrophysiologic estimates of threshold? Second, if the fitting is steeply sloping and severe to profound, does the clinician wish to take a habilitative audibility approach or an effective audibility approach in fitting? Third, once fitted, does the infant's or child's behavior indicate an experience of sound awareness, comfortable loudness, and clear reception of speech cues? Although answers to this final question might take some time to obtain, we end this section by stressing the needs of the individual over the initial prescription. Fitting to a well-calculated target is an excellent beginning, but all prescriptive targets are best used within a larger program of care in which the child's responses and development are carefully considered.

Clinical Application: Deriving Prescriptive Targets

Prescriptive algorithms are available in real-ear measurement systems and hearing aid manufacturer's software so that clinicians can have easy access to the target calculations. This allows the clinician to determine the gain and output characteristics of the hearing aid based on the child's auditory thresholds and ear canal acoustics. Information to be entered into the applications typically consists of (a) hearing thresholds at each frequency for each ear, with an indication of the format (nHL, eHL, HL); (b) age of the child to be fitted; (c) type of transducer used during the assessment; (d) measured or predicted RECD values; and (e) style of the hearing aid to be fitted. Each piece of data is used in the calculation of targets for the individual.

Figure 25–8 shows the SPLogram for the case example shown in Figure 25–7. This includes targets for average conversational speech (large +) and maximum power output (small +) that were generated based on the hearing thresholds (o) and measured RECD from the child in this example. The graph also shows the patient's audiometric thresholds plotted against unaided average conversational speech (shaded region), all of which are referenced to real-ear SPL. In this case, when hearing aids are provided and adjusted to match the suggested targets, the child will have clear and safe access to speech at various levels. This explanation, in combination with the SPLogram display, becomes a useful counseling tool for parents to help them understand the goals of the hearing aid fitting.

Electroacoustic Characteristics

When choosing hearing aids for a young patient, consideration should be given to select devices that (a) avoid distortion; (b) allow frequency/output shaping and flexibility to provide audibility and prevent loudness discomfort; (c) apply wide dynamic range compression for most hearing losses (Jenstad et al., 1999, 2000); and (d) apply compression output limit-

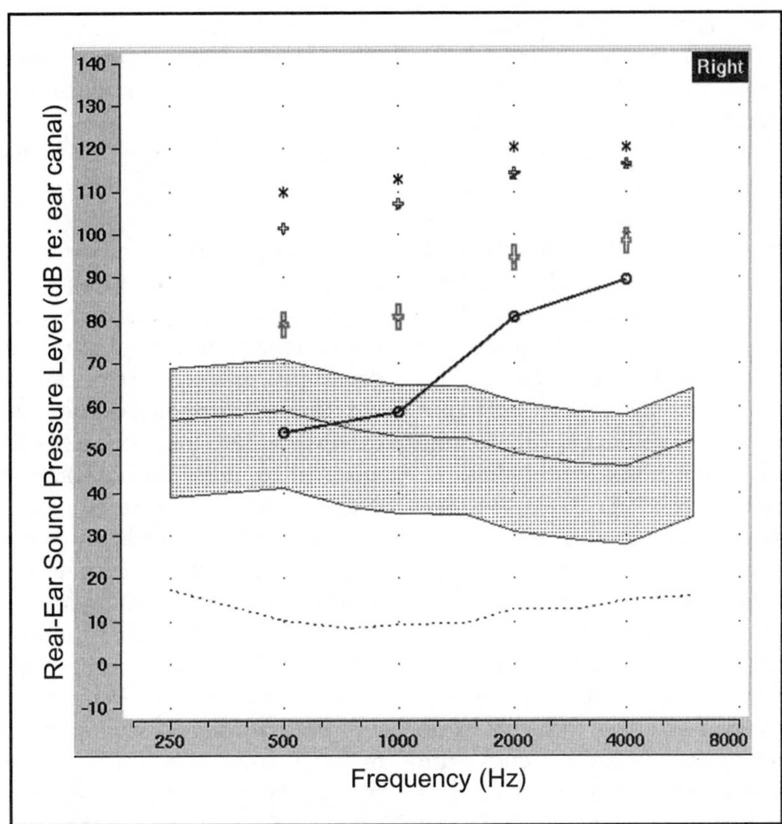

FIGURE 25–8. An SPLogram displaying the recommended targets for average speech (large +) and maximum power output (small +) for the infant in this case example. The circles (o) represent the child's hearing thresholds in real-ear SPL, and the shaded region represents unaided average conversational speech.

ing. Advanced signal processing schemes (e.g., expansion, multiple channels, frequency lowering, feedback cancellation/management, noise reduction, directional microphones and frequency lowering) are considered for each infant and child on an individual basis (AAA, 2013). For example, some feedback cancellation/management systems work effectively to control feedback without reducing high-frequency output. This might be a better option for controlling feedback while ensuring access to sound, compared to alternatives that reduce high-frequency output.

Audibility of high-frequency sounds can be limited by the bandwidth of conventional hearing aids, possibly impacting high-frequency speech sound recognition and production (see review in Stelmachowicz, Pittman, Hoover, Lewis, & Moeller, 2004). Possible solutions include the fitting of hearing aids with extended high-frequency bandwidths, or the use of frequency-lowering signal processing. Recent studies of certain forms of frequency lowering (e.g., frequency transposition; frequency compression) suggest that this technology can amplify high-frequency sounds (e.g., /s/, /ʃ/) for listeners who would otherwise have difficulty accessing such sounds (Auriemmo et al., 2009; Glista et al., 2009; Kuk, Keenan, Korhonen, & Lau, 2009; Miller-Hansen, Nelson, Widen, & Simon, 2003; Wolfe, Caraway, John, Schafer, & Nyffeler, 2009). Frequency transposition, frequency compression, and frequency translation provide different degrees and forms of frequency lowering. However, the specific audiometric range for frequency lowering, and for choosing among frequency lowering strategies is not yet entirely clear. Our knowledge in this area is rapidly evolving as new research emerges. Advantages of frequency lowering include improved detection and recognition of high-frequency speech sounds, and, in some cases, improved speech production. Some early evidence indicates that children and adults might respond differently to this type of signal processing, with children having stronger candidacy, at least for nonlinear frequency compression (Glista et al., 2009).

Adult-focused literature suggests that noise reduction algorithms can help to provide comfort and acceptance for listening in noisy environments (e.g., restaurant, vehicle) if the technology is activated and deactivated appropriately (see Bentler, 2005; Bentler, Yu-Hsiang, Kettel, & Hurtig, 2008; Mueller & Ricketts, 2005; and Palmer, 2006 for informative data and reviews). Noise reduction algorithms are beginning to be evaluated in the pediatric population. Recent work has demonstrated that the use of noise reduction in children's hearing aids does not affect speech recognition (Crukley & Scollie, 2014; McCreery et al., 2012; Pittman, 2011b; Stelmachowicz et al., 2010). Another recent study found increased rates of novel word learning with ANR in older children, but not with younger children (Pittman, 2011a). Pittman speculated that this was due to improved ease of listening, which is consistent with a recent study in adults (Sarampalis et al., 2009), and that older children were better able to take advantage of this versus younger children. More recently, children's performance and preference with directional-noise reduction systems was assessed, and in general children preferred systems that helped them perform well, including those with noise reduction activated (Pittman & Hiipakka, 2013). This emerging work demonstrates that the selection of a digital noise reduction (DNR) scheme that preserves audibility of speech and environmental sounds while reducing noisiness and loudness might help to provide comfort for children in a wider range of situations.

Directional microphones have been shown to provide benefit to older children and adults in noisy listening situations (Gravel et al., 1999; Ricketts & Tharpe, 2004). However, directional benefit is typically associated with communication situations in which the talker of interest is located in front of the listener. Infants and children do not always communicate in this situation, and might choose to manipulate their orientation to the talker or multiple talkers within a given situation. Some studies indicate that children can and do orient their heads at least some of the time to a talker of interest (Ching et al., 2009; Ricketts & Galster, 2008). Maintaining correct orientation in a classroom context might be challenging, particularly when taking notes while a teacher is speaking (Ricketts & Galster, 2008). Current research suggests that directional microphones provide a deficit for signals arising from the side or behind the child (Ching et al., 2009). This can cause a directional deficit in the frequent case where a child has not oriented toward the signal of interest (Ching et al., 2009). Importantly for the school environment, directional microphones provide less benefit than an FM system in simulated classroom environments (Ricketts, Galster, & Tharpe, 2007). Therefore, use of a directional microphone does not replace the FM system for management of room acoustics and classroom noise effects.

For infants or very young children, auditory access to the target talker and the potential contribution of overhearing on an infant's speech and language development should be considered along with the need for noise management. For many children, the most appropriate processing strategy can vary with the listening environment, just as it does for adults. An issue of controversy is how best to access this listening program, in order to avoid an inappropriate choice that could prevent the child from being aware of signals in the environment. Children who are about age 7 years and older might be able to take responsibility for the use of multiple hearing aid memories. In one study, children used two memories reliably and appropriately, indicating that children who can monitor their own listening performance can and do make technology choices that will benefit them in terms of communication performance (Scollie et al., 2010b). For younger children, a proxy strategy is required if noise management is to be utilized. Can we consider signal processing schemes that automatically enable directionality and noise reduction, and do they function appropriately? Can caregivers take responsibility for program manipulation? Strong evidence for either of these strategies is currently unavailable for the infant and toddler population. Clinicians are therefore advised to consider each child and each technology individually on respective needs and merits, applying solutions with caution, monitoring, and verifying of their effects electroacoustically (AAA, 2013). Empirical data regarding their effectiveness in the infant population are rare, and likely will continue to be rare, due to the challenges of evaluating such technologies in infants. Clinicians might choose to infer the possible needs, benefits, and limitations associated with these technologies from studies conducted on children in the absence of research on infants. In practice, consultation with the caregivers prior to introducing these technologies to the infant is critical to ensure accurate use and informed reporting of outcomes associated with the technology's use.

Physical Characteristics

The style of the hearing aid(s), monaural versus binaural fitting, deactivation of unnecessary signal processing, FM system compatibility, locking mechanism for the volume control, and tamper-resistant battery doors are important considerations when providing hearing aids to infants and young children (Table 25–4).

Behind-the-ear (BTE) hearing aids are the recommended style for infants and children for several reasons. Acoustic feedback is less of an issue, and greater electroacoustic flexibility is offered with this style of hearing aid. In addition, BTEs have direct audio input capabilities that are more compatible with the pediatric population. Finally, should the BTE aid require repairs from the manufacturer, a similar device from the loaner hearing aid stock can be coupled to the personal earmold so the infant is not without amplification while the device is being repaired.

A pediatric earhook is recommended to support secure retention on the ear. Unfiltered earhooks will add resonant peaks to the output response of the hearing aid, possibly causing feedback and making adjustment to maximum power output (MPO) targets difficult. A filtered earhook will smooth the response and allow for a better match to targets with less chance of feedback (Scollie & Seewald, 2002). Tamper-resistant battery doors should also be included on hearing aids for infants and children and a deactivation or locking system for the volume control and other automatic features should be available.

Direct audio input (DAI) should be included on the selected devices. This will enable coupling of assistive technology, such as FM systems, to the hearing aids. FM system use will enhance the benefits of hearing aids in infants and children and can be provided as an option to families for consideration. Other types of personal amplification such as implantable devices are considered on an individual basis. Further discussion regarding the use of other hearing technologies in the pediatric population can be found in Chapters 27, 29, 30, 31, and 32 of this volume.

Summary: Selecting Hearing Aids

Deriving electroacoustic targets, assessing the need for advanced signal processing schemes, and selecting the physical characteristics of hearing aid(s) is the second step in the hearing aid fitting process, following the collection of assessment information. When the hearing aid(s) have been received, confirmation that they are performing close to the prescriptive targets is the next essential step. The following sections describe the verification stage of the hearing aid fitting process for infants and children.

Table 25–4. Physical Characteristics of Hearing Aids Provided to Infants and Children

Characteristic	*Benefit*
Behind-the-ear (BTE) style	Reduces acoustic feedback Provides greater electroacoustic flexibility Provides direct audio input capabilities Allows loaner device to be easily used if needed Durable
Pediatric-sized filtered earhook	Supports secure retention on ear Reduces resonant peaks Allows for better match to targets
Tamper-resistant battery door	Prevents accidental ingestion of batteries
Deactivation or locking system for volume control	Prevents inadvertent increases or decreases to hearing aid output
Deactivation of advanced features	Allows for flexibility in the application of advanced technologies
Direct audio input (DAI)	Enables coupling of FM system
Choice of bright colors	For enjoyment

Verification of Electroacoustic Performance

Once we have defined the auditory thresholds, the acoustic characteristics of the ear canal, and the electroacoustic and nonelectroacoustic specifications of the hearing aid, we can proceed to verification of electroacoustic performance. In the verification stage, we adjust the hearing aids to match a set of targets for electroacoustic performance. This process provides a fitting that is expected to be comfortable, safe, and wearable without feedback. The following sections describe options and clinical procedures for the verification of hearing aids for infants and young children.

Real-Ear Measurements

Hearing aids can be measured in the context of the child's auditory area in order to evaluate the hearing aid fitting for audibility and comfort. This type of evaluation uses the SPLogram, on which we plot the thresholds and predicted LDLs, prescribed targets, and measured hearing aid responses in real-ear SPL as a function of frequency on the same graph (Figure 25–9). The advantage of using an SPLogram display for verification is that it allows electroacoustic evaluation of the hearing aid to serve as a proxy for the child's feedback regarding audibility and comfort of amplified sounds. This supports the fittings of hearing aids that provide a broad audible band of speech, yet avoids loudness discomfort. The primary verification format for an SPLogram is therefore the real-ear aided response (REAR). The REAR format is chosen over other real-ear measurement formats such as real-ear insertion gain (REIG). Most REIG insertion gain calculations assume average adult real-ear unaided responses (REURs), whereas measured insertion gain is calculated using the patient's measured REUR. Infants and young children are not likely to have average adult REURs; therefore, significant error is likely to be introduced into the hearing aid fitting if the insertion gain approach to verification is used. Even when these errors are removed by computing the REIG target using a child's own REUG, the measurement is made without any perceptual context: the REIG measurement cannot be directly compared to the patient's auditory thresholds or loudness discomfort levels.

There are two options for obtaining REAR measures using real-ear measurement equipment. One is to directly measure the output of the hearing aid while it is on the patient's ear. *Real-ear verification* protocols involve placement of a probe tube microphone in the ear canal prior to placing the hearing aid on the ear. While the patient faces a loudspeaker, stimuli of various input levels are delivered, and the output is measured directly in the ear canal. The hearing aid is adjusted using hearing aid fitting software in order to better approximate the prescriptive targets. Although this approach offers the advantage of directly measuring the output of the hearing aid in the ear canal and displays it within the context of the patient's auditory characteristics, there are some limitations of this approach for use with infants and children. First, care must be taken when selecting the levels of the test signals. Verification of the MPO of the hearing aid requires the use of a high-intensity (90–100 dB SPL) narrowband signal in order to saturate the hearing aid. This test level can be startling to the child and, depending on how the hearing aid was set prior to running the signal, might be uncomfortable for the listener. Second, passive cooperation is required during real-ear verification. The patient is required to sit still and quiet during the several minutes required to adequately adjust the hearing aid to meet targets. This typically is a challenge for children who are vocal and active. Young infants who do not have the head and neck control to face the loudspeaker without the assistance of a parent or caregiver will provide additional challenges for this approach. Their random head movements will introduce variability into the measurement.

For these reasons, an alternative strategy for measuring the real-ear performance of the hearing aid has been developed. This alternative approach requires measurements of coupler output, rather than the REAR. Then, the RECD is used, together with predictions of the acoustic effects of the hearing aid microphone's location (behind the ear or at various locations in the ear), to predict the REAR based on the coupler measures. This can be done using a measured or predicted age-appropriate set of RECD values. This *simulated or coupler* approach to real-ear verification generally is more compatible with the pediatric population, the details of which are described below.

Simulated Real-Ear Measurements

In the assessment stage, the RECD is used to convert HL thresholds to SPL. The same RECD values are used to convert real-ear gain and output requirements to 2-cc coupler targets for the purposes of selection. The

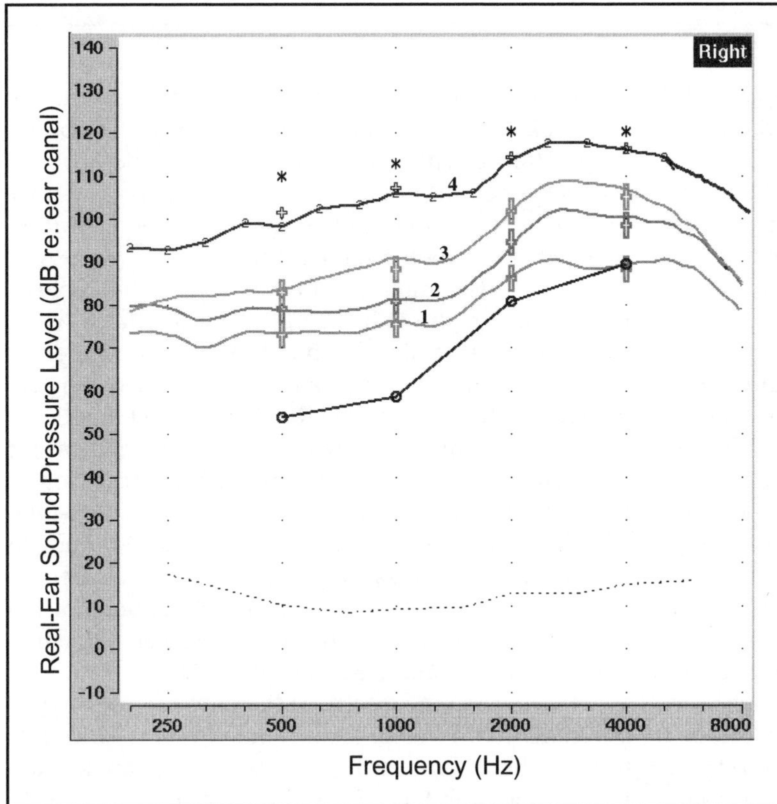

A

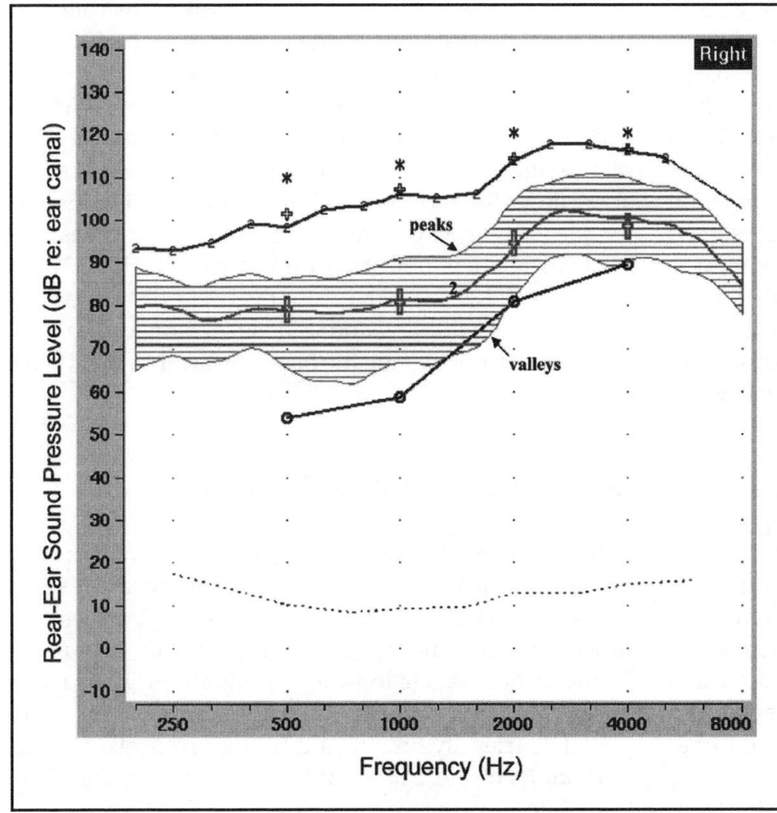

B

FIGURE 25–9. Verification of hearing aid performance displayed on an SPLogram. The solid lines represent the output of the hearing aid at soft (1), average (2), and loud (3) speech input levels as well as the maximum power output (MPO) (4). **A.** These are compared to the targets represented by the plus (+) signs or asterisks (*). **B.** Alternatively, the peaks and valleys of the output of average conversational speech can be viewed in this format.

third use of the RECD is to convert 2-cc coupler measurements of hearing aid output to predicted real-ear measurements. Simulated or coupler-based verification has the primary advantage of allowing clinicians to perform all electroacoustic response shaping of the hearing aid using an SPLogram format within the highly controlled acoustic conditions of a test box.

Simulating the REAR involves two main components: RECD values and coupler measures of hearing aid output. The RECD captures the child's individual ear canal acoustics across frequency and is applied to the coupler measures to *predict* the REAR, rather than measure it directly (Moodie et al., 1994; Seewald, 1991). Measuring the RECD takes little time and is unaffected by head movement, making it more accurate and reliable for the pediatric population than measuring the REAR (Seewald, Moodie, Sinclair, & Scollie, 1999; Sinclair et al., 1996).

In the coupler approach to real-ear verification, targets are generated for the 2-cc coupler. The hearing aid is attached to the 2-cc coupler and placed in a test box, and verification of hearing aid performance is conducted at various input levels representing soft, average, and loud speech (i.e., 55 to 70 dB SPL) in order to evaluate fit to targets and determine audibility of speech. The hearing aid's MPO is verified using high-level narrowband stimuli. In addition, a loud speech stimulus (75–80 dB SPL) can be measured to ensure that the peaks of speech fall at or below the upper limits of comfort (Scollie & Seewald, 2002). Figure 25–9A displays one example of this procedure. The solid lines represent the output of the hearing aid at various input levels. These are compared to the targets represented by the plus (+) signs or asterisks (*). Approximation of the output of the hearing aid to the calculated targets is important to ensure that speech is audible and loud sounds are not uncomfortable, across a broad frequency range. Figure 25–9B displays the same hearing aid fitting with the peaks and valleys for average conversational speech displayed.

The predicted REAR and RESR are plotted on an SPLogram so that performance of the hearing aid can be directly compared to thresholds, upper limits of comfort, and prescriptive targets. Using this display, the clinician can evaluate audibility, appropriate output limiting levels, and acoustic headroom across frequencies. If advanced signal processing was activated within the hearing aid(s), their electroacoustic characteristics as well as their impact on the audibility of speech should be verified (AAA, 2013).

Following simulated real-ear verification, the hearing aids are placed on the infant or child and the fit is checked for physical comfort and to ensure that they can be worn at the recommended settings without feedback. This is an essential step with coupler-based verification because the real-ear fit and the acoustic seal of the hearing aids are not assessed during coupler measures. It also does not assess any earmold venting that might be present in the fitting.

With these limitations in mind, simulated real-ear measurements are still the approach of choice when verifying hearing aids for infants and young children. Seewald and his colleagues (1999) examined the predictive validity of using the RECD to predict the REAG and real-ear saturation response (RESR) of hearing aids. They measured and predicted the REAG for 14 participants and results indicated that, on average, the REAG values were predicted using RECD values to within ±2.3 dB across frequency for 95% of cases. In addition, the average error for the predictions of the RESR was 4.4 dB. Similar findings were also noted in a study by Munro and Hatton (2000).

However, more recent studies have reported errors associated with this procedure due to impedance differences between hearing aids and some transducers used to measure the RECD (Munro & Salisbury, 2002; Munro & Toal, 2005). Resulting errors are exacerbated when the tubing in the custom earmold is longer, as it would be for adult earmolds, or when the earhook is unfiltered (Bagatto et al., 2005; Munro & Toal, 2005). In general, earmold tubing lengths typical of infants and young children, coupled with the use of filtered earhooks, result in accuracy of the RECD-based coupler verification procedure to within a clinically acceptable range (Bagatto et al., 2005). Recently, a protocol for measuring RECDs was included in the measurement of real-ear performance of hearing aids (ANSI S3.46, 1997; R2013) to address the potential impact of sound source coupling and its acoustic impedance. The update does not change the basic protocol of the RECD measurement.

Other Approaches to Verification

Behavioral evaluation (i.e., aided audiogram, functional gain measures) and insertion gain measures can be viewed as alternatives to the real-ear verification procedures for infants and young children discussed in the previous sections. With advances in hearing aid technology, real-ear measurement systems, and pediatric-friendly hearing aid fitting protocols, several limitations to these alternative approaches to verification have been noted.

Behavioral verification of the electroacoustic performance of the hearing aid is not compatible with young infants identified through early hearing and communication development (EHCD) programs. The first fitting of the hearing aid(s) is targeted to occur by 6 months of age, at which age many infants cannot perform conditioned tasks for behavioral tests of hearing. Therefore, relying on behavioral thresholds for hearing aid fitting is likely to delay the first fitting, thereby delaying intervention. In addition, aided sound-field measures require prolonged cooperation from the infant, provide information at only a few frequencies, and have poor test-retest reliability (Stuart, Durieux-Smith, & Stenstrom, 1990). Additionally, the narrowband stimuli used for aided sound-field measures are not representative of speech and they do not provide an estimate of the MPO of the hearing aid. Finally, the validity of aided sound-field thresholds is poor, especially with severe to profound hearing losses, or when nonlinear signal processing is used (Humes & Kirn, 1990; Macrae & Frazier, 1980; Seewald, Moodie, Sinclair, & Cornelisse, 1996; Stelmachowicz & Lewis, 1988). Aided sound-field threshold testing can be useful as an outcome measure and for counseling and educational purposes but is not the recommended procedure for use when verifying and fine tuning hearing aids for infants and children.

Summary

This chapter has described key considerations in the assessment, selection, and verification stages of providing hearing aids to infants and young children with hearing loss. Details regarding the use of ABR threshold estimates for hearing aid fitting, the importance of accounting for ear canal acoustics, the use of evidence-based generic prescriptive formulas, and pediatric-friendly electroacoustic verification procedures are just a few of the topics discussed. A systematic approach to the provision of amplification provides a framework with which clinicians can continuously monitor their young patients. This is especially important given the unique qualities that infants and young children bring to the hearing aid prescription process. Following the fitting of the devices to an infant or young child, it is important for the caregivers to be instructed on the care, use, and maintenance of the hearing aids. Furthermore, evaluating the impact of the hearing aids on the young child's auditory-related outcomes, especially in the early stages, is critical in order to provide a comprehensive management program. The University of Western Ontario Pediatric Audiological Monitoring Protocol (UWO PedAMP) is an example of a systematic, evidence-based approach for evaluating auditory-related outcomes in infants and young children who wear hearing aids (Bagatto et al., 2011). Further details about the information and instruction, and outcome evaluation stages of the hearing aid fitting process are addressed in subsequent chapters of this volume.

References

American Academy of Audiology. (2013). *Clinical practice guidelines on pediatric amplification.* Retrieved from https://audiology-web.s3.amazonaws.com/migrated/PediatricAmplificationGuidelines.pdf_539975b3e7e9f1.74471798.pdf

American National Standards Institute (ANSI; 1996). *Specification for audiometers.* ANSI S3.6–1996 (R 2010). New York, NY: Acoustical Society of America.

American National Standards Institute (ANSI; 1997). *Methods of measurement of real-ear performance characteristics of hearing aids.* ANSI S3.46-1997 (R 2013). New York, NY: Acoustical Society of America.

American Speech-Language-Hearing Association (ASHA; 2004). *Guidelines for the audiologic assessment of children from birth to 5 years of age.* Retrieved July 2, 2010, from http://www.infanthearing.org/coordinator_orientation/section2/10_asha_guidelines.pdf

Auriemmo, J., Kuk, F., Lau, C., Marshall, S., Thiele, N., Pikora, M., ... Stenger, P. (2009). Effect of linear frequency transposition on speech recognition and production of school-age children. *Journal of the American Academy of Audiology, 20*(5), 289–305.

Bagatto, M. P., & Moodie, S. T. (2007). Learning the art to apply the science: Common questions related to pediatric hearing instrument fitting. *Audiology Online.* Retrieved July 2, 2010, from http://www.audiologyonline.com/articles/learning-art-to-apply-science-933

Bagatto, M. P., Moodie, S. T., Malandrino, A. C., Richert, F. M., Clench, D. A., & Scollie, S. D. (2011). The University of Western Ontario Pediatric Audiological Monitoring Protocol (UWO PedAMP). *Trends in Amplification, 15*(1), 57–76.

Bagatto, M. P., Moodie, S. T., Scollie, S., Seewald, R. C., Moodie, S., Pumford, J., & Liu, K. P. R. (2005). Clinical protocols for hearing instrument fitting in the Desired Sensation Level Method. *Trends in Amplification, 9*(4), 199–226.

Bagatto, M. P., Scollie, S. D., Seewald, R. C., Moodie, K. S., & Hoover, B. M. (2002). Real-ear-to-coupler difference predictions as a function of age for two coupling procedures. *Journal of the American Academy of Audiology, 13*(8), 407–415.

Bagatto, M. P., Seewald, R. C., Scollie, S. D., & Tharpe, A. M. (2006). Evaluation of a probe-tube insertion technique for measuring the real-ear-to-coupler difference (RECD) in young infants. *Journal of the American Academy of Audiology, 17,* 573–581.

Bentler, R. A. (1989). External ear resonance characteristics in children. *Journal of Speech and Hearing Research, 54*(2), 265–268.

Bentler, R. A. (2005). Effectiveness of directional microphones and noise reduction schemes in hearing aids: A systematic review of the evidence. *Journal of the American Academy of Audiology, 16*, 473–484.

Bentler, R. A., & Cooley, L. J. (2001). An examination of several characteristics that affect the prediction of OSPL90 in hearing aids. *Ear and Hearing, 22*(1), 58–64.

Bentler, R. A., & Pavlovic, C. V. (1989). Transfer functions and correction factors used in hearing aid evaluation and research. *Ear and Hearing, 10*, 58–63.

Bentler, R., Yu-Hsiang, W., Kettel, J., & Hurtig, R. (2008). Digital noise reduction: Outcomes from laboratory and field studies. *International Journal of Audiology, 47*(8), 447–460.

Byrne, D. (1986a). Effects of bandwidth and stimulus type on most comfortable loudness levels of hearing-impaired listeners. *Journal of the Acoustical Society of America, 80*(2), 484–493.

Byrne, D. (1986b). Effects of frequency response characteristics on speech discrimination and perceived intelligibility and pleasantness of speech for hearing-impaired listeners. *Journal of the Acoustical Society of America, 80*(2), 494–504.

Byrne, D., & Dillon, H. (1986). The National Acoustic Laboratories' (NAL) new procedure for selecting the gain and frequency response of a hearing aid. *Ear and Hearing, 7*(4), 257–265.

Byrne, D., & Murray, N. (1986). Predictability of the required frequency response characteristic of a hearing aid from the pure-tone audiogram. *Ear and Hearing, 7*(2), 63–70.

Byrne, D., Parkinson, A., & Newall, P. (1990). Hearing aid gain and frequency response requirements for the severely/profoundly hearing impaired. *Ear and Hearing, 11*(1), 40–49.

Carney, A. E., & Moeller, M. P. (1998). Treatment efficacy hearing loss in children. *Journal of Speech, Language, and Hearing Research, 41*, S61–S84.

Ching, T. Y. C., & Dillon, H. (2003). Prescribing amplification for children: Adult-equivalent hearing loss, real-ear aided gain, and NAL-NL1. *Trends in Amplification, 7*(1), 1–9.

Ching, T. Y. C., Dillon, H., & Byrne, D. (1998). Speech recognition of hearing-impaired listeners: Predictions from audibility and the limited role of high-frequency amplification. *Journal of the Acoustical Society of America, 103*(2), 1128–1140.

Ching, T. Y. C., Dillon, H., Day, J., & Crowe, K. (2007). The NAL longitudinal study on outcomes of hearing-impaired children: Interim findings on language of early and later identified children at six months after hearing aid fitting. In R. C. Seewald, & J. M. Bamford (Eds.), *A sound foundation through early amplification: Proceedings of an international conference* (pp. 185–199). Stäfa, Switzerland: Phonak AG.

Ching, T. Y. C., Dillon, H., Katsch, R., & Byrne, D. (2001). Maximizing effective audibility in hearing aid fitting. *Ear and Hearing, 22*, 212–224.

Ching, T. Y. C., Hill, M., Birtles, G., & Beacham, L. (1999). Clinical use of paired comparisons to evaluate hearing aid fitting of severely/profoundly hearing impaired children. *Australian and New Zealand Journal of Audiology, 21*(2), 51–63.

Ching, T. Y. C., Newall, P., & Wigney, D. (1997). Comparison of severely and profoundly hearing-impaired children's amplification preferences with the NAL-RP and the DSL 3.0 prescriptions. *International Journal of Audiology, 26*(4), 219–222.

Ching, T. Y. C., O'Brien, A., Dillon, H., Chalupper, J., Hartley, L., Hartley, D., . . . Hain, J. (2009). Directional effects on infants and young children in real life: Implications for amplification. *Journal of Speech, Language, and Hearing Research, 52*(5), 1241–1254.

Ching, T. Y. C., Scollie, S. D., Dillon, H., & Seewald, R. C. (2010). A cross-over, double-blind comparison of the NAL-NL1 and the DSL v4. 1 prescriptions for children with mild to moderately severe hearing loss. *International Journal of Audiology, 49*(Suppl. 1), S4–S15.

Ching, T. Y. C., Scollie, S. D., Dillon, H., Seewald, R. C., Britton, L., & Steinberg, J. (2010). Prescribed real-ear and achieved real-life differences in children's hearing aids adjusted according to the NAL-NL1 and the DSL v. 4. 1 prescriptions. *International Journal of Audiology, 49*(Suppl. 1), S16–S25.

Ching, T. Y. C., Scollie, S. D., Dillon, H., Seewald, R. C., Britton, L., Steinberg, J., . . . & King, K. (2010). Evaluation of the NAL-NL1 and the DSL v. 4.1 prescriptions for children: Paired-comparison judgments and functional performance ratings. *International Journal of Audiology, 49*(Suppl. 1), S35–S48.

Cornelisse, L. E., Seewald, R. C., & Jamieson, D. G. (1995). The input/output formula: A theoretical approach to the fitting of personal amplification devices. *Journal of the Acoustical Society of America, 97*(3), 1854–1864.

Crukley, J., & Scollie, S. (2014). The effects of digital signal processing features on children's speech recognition and loudness perception. *American Journal of Audiology, 23*(1), 99–115.

Dillon, H., & Storey, L. (1998). The National Acoustic Laboratories' procedure for selecting the saturation sound pressure level of hearing aids: Theoretical derivation. *Ear and Hearing, 19*(4), 255–266.

Dirks, D., & Kincaid, G. (1987). Basic acoustic considerations of ear canal probe measurements. *Ear and Hearing, 8*(5), 60S–67S.

Elliott, L. L. (1979). Performance of children aged 9 to 17 years on a test of speech intelligibility in noise using sentence material with controlled word predictability. *Journal of the Acoustical Society of America, 66*(3), 651–653.

Elliott, L. L., Connors, S., Kille, E., Levin, S., Ball, K., & Katz, D. (1979). Children's understanding of monosyllabic nouns in quiet and in noise. *Journal of the Acoustical Society of America, 66*(1), 12–21.

Erber, N. P. (1973). Body-baffle and real-ear effects in the selection of hearing aids for deaf children. *Journal of Speech and Hearing Disorders, 38*, 224–231.

Erber, N. P., & Witt, L. H. (1977). Effects of stimulus intensity on speech perception by deaf children. *Journal of Speech and Hearing Disorders, 42*, 271–278.

Feigin, J. A., Kopun, J. G., Stelmachowicz, P. G., & Gorga, M. P. (1989). Probe-tube microphone measures of ear canal sound pressure levels in infants and children. *Ear and Hearing, 10*(4), 254–258.

Gagne, J. P., Seewald, R. C., Zelisko, D. L., & Hudson, S. P. (1991). Procedure for defining the auditory area of hearing-impaired adolescents with a severe/profound hearing loss. II: Loudness discomfort levels. *Journal of Speech-Language Pathology, 12*, 27–32.

Glista, D., Scollie, S., Bagatto, M., Seewald, R., Parsa, V., & Johnson, A. (2009). Evaluation of nonlinear frequency compression: Clinical outcomes. *International Journal of Audiology, 48*(9), 632–644.

Gorga, M. P., Kaminski, J. R., Beauchaine, K., L., & Bergman, B. M. (1993). A comparison of auditory brain stem response thresholds and latencies elicited by air- and bone-conducted stimuli. *Ear and Hearing, 14*, 85–94.

Gravel, J. (2002). Potential pitfalls in the audiological assessment of infants and young children. In R. C. Seewald, & J. S. Gravel (Eds.), *A sound foundation through early amplification 2001: Proceedings of the second international conference* (pp. 85–101). Stäfa, Switzerland: Phonak AG.

Gravel, J. S., Fausel, N., Liskow, C., & Chobot, J. (1999). Children's speech recognition in noise using omni-directional and dual-microphone hearing aid technology. *Ear and Hearing, 20*, 1–11.

Hawkins, D. B. (1987). Clinical ear canal probe tube measurements. *Journal of Speech and Hearing Research, 8*(Suppl.), 74–81.

Hnath-Chisolm, T. E., Laipply, E., & Boothroyd, A. (1998). Age-related changes on a children's test of sensory-level speech perception capacity. *Journal of Speech, Language, and Hearing Research, 41*, 94–106.

Humes, L. E., & Kirn, E. U. (1990). The reliability of functional gain. *Journal of Speech and Hearing Disorders, 55*, 193–197.

Jenstad, L. M., Pumford, J., Seewald, R. C., & Cornelisse, L. E. (2000). Comparison of linear gain and wide-dynamic range compression (WDRC) hearing aid circuits II: Aided loudness measures. *Ear and Hearing, 21*(2), 32–44.

Jenstad, L. M., Seewald, R. C., Cornelisse, L. E., & Shantz, J. (1999). Comparison of linear gain and wide-dynamic-range compression hearing aid circuits: Aided speech perception measures. *Ear and Hearing, 20*(2), 117–126.

Joint Committee on Infant Hearing (JCIH; 2007). Year 2007 position statement: Principles and guidelines for early hearing detection and intervention programs. *Pediatrics, 120*(4), 898–921.

Kamm, C., Dirks, D., & Mickey, M. R. (1977). Effect of sensorineural hearing loss on loudness discomfort level and most comfortable loudness judgements. *Journal of Speech and Hearing Research, 21*, 668–681.

Keidser, G., Brew, C., & Peck, A. (2003). How proprietary fitting algorithms compare to each other and to some generic algorithms. *Hearing Journal, 56*(3), 28–38.

Keidser, G., Dillon, H., Carter, L., & O'Brien, A. (2012). NAL-NL2 empirical adjustments. *Trends in Amplification, 4*, 211–223.

Kiessling, J. (1987). In situ audiometry (ISA): A new frontier in hearing aid selection. *Hearing Instruments, 38*, 28–29.

Kiessling, J. (1993). Current approaches to hearing aid evaluation. *Journal of Speech-Language Pathology, 16*(Suppl.), 39–49.

Kortekaas, R. W. L., & Stelmachowicz, P. G. (2000). Bandwidth effects on children's perception of the inflectional morpheme /s/. *Journal of Speech, Language, and Hearing Research, 43*, 645–660.

Kruger, B. (1987). An update on the external ear resonance in infants and young children. *Ear and Hearing, 8*(6), 333–336.

Kuk, F., Keenan, D., Korhonen, P., & Lau, C. (2009). Efficacy of linear frequency transposition on consonant identification in quiet and in noise. *Journal of the American Academy of Audiology, 20*(8), 465–479.

Lewis, D. E., & Stelmachowicz, P. G. (1993). Real-ear to 6-cm^3 coupler differences in young children. *Journal of Speech and Hearing Research, 36*(1), 204–209.

Macrae, J. (1986). *Relationships between the hearing threshold levels an aided speech discrimination of severely and profoundly deaf children.* NAL Report No. 107. Canberra: Australian Government Publishing Service.

Macrae, J., & Frazier, G. (1980). An investigation of variables affecting aided thresholds. *Australian Journal of Audiology, 2*, 56–62.

Marcoux, A., & Hansen, M. (2003). Ensuring accuracy of the pediatric hearing aid fitting. *Trends in Amplification, 7*(1), 11–27.

McCreery, R., Venediktov, R., Coleman, J., & Leech, H. (2012). An evidence-based systematic review of directional microphones and digital noise reduction hearing aids in school-age children with hearing loss. *American Journal of Audiology, 21*, 295–312.

Miller-Hansen, D. R., Nelson, P. G., Widen, J. E., & Simon, S. D. (2003). Evaluating the benefit of speech recoding hearing aids in children. *American Journal of Audiology, 12*, 106–113.

Moeller, M. P. (2000). Early intervention and language development in children who are deaf and hard of hearing. *Pediatrics, 106*, e43.

Moodie, K. S., Seewald, R. C., & Sinclair, S. T. (1994). Procedure for predicting real-ear hearing aid performance in young children. *American Journal of Audiology, 3*, 23–31.

Moodie, S., & Moodie, S. (2004). An approach to defining the fitting range of hearing instruments children with severe-to-profound hearing loss. In R. C. Seewald, & J. M. Bamford (Eds.), *A sound foundation through early amplification: Proceedings of the third international conference* (pp. 247–254). Stäfa, Switzerland: Phonak AG.

Mueller, H. G. (2001). Probe microphone measurements: 20 years of progress. *Trends in Amplification, 5*, 35–68.

Mueller, H. G., Bentler, R., & Wu, Y. (2008). Prescribing maximum hearing aid output: Differences among manufacturers found. *Hearing Journal, 61*(3), 30, 32, 34, 36.

Mueller, H. G., & Ricketts, T. A. (2005). Digital noise reduction: Much ado about something? *Hearing Journal, 58*(1), 10–18.

Munro, K. J., & Davis, J. (2003). Deriving the real-ear SPL of audiometric data using the "coupler to dial difference" and the "real ear to coupler difference." *Ear and Hearing, 24*, 100–110.

Munro, K. L., & Hatton, N. (2000). Customized acoustic transform functions and their accuracy at predicting real-ear hearing aid performance. *Ear and Hearing, 21*(1), 59–69.

Munro, K. J., & Salisbury, V. A. (2002). Is the real-ear-to-coupler difference independent of the measurement earphone? *International Journal of Audiology, 41*, 408–413.

Munro, K. J., & Toal, S. (2005). Measuring the RECD transfer function with an insert earphone and a hearing instrument: Are they the same? *Ear and Hearing, 26*, 27–34.

Nábělek, A. K., & Robinson, P. K. (1982). Monaural and binaural speech perception in reverberation for listeners of various ages. *Journal of the Acoustical Society of America, 71*(5), 1242–1248.

Neuman, A. C., & Hochberg, I. (1982). *The effect of reverberation on the phoneme discrimination of children*. Paper presented at the 1982 American Speech and Hearing Association convention, Toronto, Ontario, Canada.

Palmer, C. V. (2006). Amplification with digital noise reduction and the perception of annoying and aversive sounds. *Trends in Amplification, 10*(2), 95–104.

Pascoe, D. P. (1978). An approach to hearing aid selection. *Hearing Instruments, 29*, 12–16.

Pascoe, D. P. (1988). Clinical measurements of the auditory dynamic range and their relation to formulas for hearing aid gain. In J. H. Jensen (Ed.), *Hearing aid fitting: Theoretical and practical views* (pp. 129–151). Copenhagen, Amsterdam: Stougaard/Jensen.

Pediatric Working Group. (1996). Conference on Amplification for Children with Auditory Deficits. Amplification for infants and children with hearing loss. *American Journal of Audiology, 5*(1), 53–68.

Pittman, A. L. (2008). Short-term word-learning rate in children with normal hearing and children with hearing loss in limited and extended high-frequency bandwidths. *Journal of Speech, Language, and Hearing Research, 51*, 785–797.

Pittman, A. (2011a). Age-related benefits of digital noise reduction for short-term word learning in children with hearing loss. *Journal of Speech, Language, and Hearing Research. 54*, 1448–1463.

Pittman, A. (2011b). Children's performance in complex listening conditions: Effects of hearing loss and digital noise reduction. *Journal of Speech, Language, & Hearing Research, 54*(4), 1224–1239.

Pittman, A., & Hiipakka, M. (2013). Hearing impaired children's preference for, and performance with, four combinations of directional microphone and digital noise reduction technology. *Journal of the American Academy of Audiology, 24*(9), 832–844.

Pittman, A. L., & Stelmachowicz, P. G. (2000). Perception of voiceless fricatives by normal-hearing and hearing-impaired children and adults. *Journal of Speech, Language, and Hearing Research, 43*, 1389–1401.

Pittman, A. L., Stelmachowicz, P. G., Lewis, D. E. & Hoover, B. M. (2003). Spectral characteristics of speech at the ear: Implications for amplification in children. *Journal of Speech, Language, and Hearing Research, 46*, 649–657.

Revit, L. J. (1997). The circle of decibels: Relating the hearing test, to the hearing instrument, to the real-ear response. *Hearing Review, 4*, 35–38.

Ricketts, T. A., & Galster, J. (2008). Head angle and elevation in classroom environments: Implications for amplification. *Journal of Speech, Language, and Hearing Research, 51*(2), 516–525.

Ricketts, T., Galster, J., & Tharpe, A. M. (2007). Directional benefit in simulated classroom environments. *American Journal of Audiology, 16*(2), 130–144.

Ricketts, T., & Tharpe, A. M. (2004). Potential for directivity-based benefit in actual classroom environments. In R. C. Seewald & J. M. Bamford (Eds.), *A sound foundation through early amplification: Proceedings of the third international conference* (pp. 143–153). Stäfa, Switzerland: Phonak AG.

Sarampalis, A., Kalluri, S., Edwards, B., & Hafter, E. (2009). Objective measures of listening effort: Effects of background noise and noise reduction. *Journal of Speech, Language, and Hearing Research, 52*(5), 1230.

Scollie, S. D. (2004). Prescriptive procedures for infants and children. In R. C. Seewald, & J. M. Bamford (Eds.), *A sound foundation through early amplification: Proceedings of the third international conference* (pp. 91–104). Stäfa, Switzerland: Phonak AG.

Scollie, S. D., Ching, T. Y. C., Seewald, R. C., Dillon, H., Britton, L., Steinberg, J., & Corcoran, J. (2010b). Evaluation of the NAL-NL1 and DSL v4. 1 prescriptions for children: Preference in real world use. *International Journal of Audiology, 49*(Suppl. 1), S49–S63.

Scollie, S. D., Ching, T. Y. C., Seewald, R. C., Dillon, H., Britton, L., Steinberg, J., & King, K. (2010a). Children's speech perception and loudness ratings of children when fitted with hearing aids using the DSL v. 4.1 and the NAL-NL1 prescriptions. *International Journal of Audiology, 49*(Suppl. 1), S26–S34.

Scollie, S. D., & Seewald, R. C. (2002). Evaluation of electroacoustic test signals I: Comparison with amplified speech. *Ear and Hearing, 23*(5), 477–487.

Scollie, S. D., Seewald, R. C., Cornelisse, L. C., & Jenstad, L. M. (1998). Validity and repeatability of level-dependent HL to SPL transforms. *Ear and Hearing, 19*(5), 407–413.

Scollie, S. D., Seewald, R. C., Cornelisse, L. C., Moodie, S. T., Bagatto, M. P., Laurnagaray, D., . . . Pumford, J. M. (2005). The Desired Sensation Level Multistage Input/Output Algorithm. *Trends in Amplification, 9*(4), 159–197.

Scollie, S. D., Seewald, R. C., Moodie, K. S., & Dekok, K. (2000). Preferred listening levels of children who use hearing aids: Comparison to prescriptive targets. *Journal of the American Academy of Audiology, 11*(4), 230–238.

Seewald, R. C. (1991). Hearing aid output limiting considerations for children. In J. Feigin & P. Stelmachowicz (Eds.), *Pediatric amplification: Proceedings of the 1991 national conference* (pp. 19–35). Omaha, NE: Boys Town National Research Hospital Press.

Seewald, R. C., Cornelisse, L. E., Ramji, K. V., Sinclair, S. T., Moodie, K. S., & Jamieson, D. G. (1997). *A software implementation of the Desired Sensation Level (DSL[i/o]) Method for fitting linear gain and wide-dynamic-range compression hearing instruments, Version 4.1.* Hearing Health Care Research Unit, University of Western Ontario, London, Ontario, Canada.

Seewald, R., Mills, J., Bagatto, M., Scollie, S., & Moodie, S. (2008). A comparison of manufacturer-specific prescriptive procedures for infants. *Hearing Journal, 61*(11), 26–34.

Seewald, R. C., Moodie, K. S., Sinclair, S. T., & Cornelisse, L. E. (1996). Traditional and theoretical approaches to selecting amplification for infants and young children. In F. H. Bess, J. S. Gravel, & A. M. Tharpe, (Eds.), *Amplification for children with auditory deficits* (pp. 161–191). Nashville, TN: Bill Wilkerson Center Press.

Seewald, R. C., Moodie, K. S., Sinclair, S. T., & Scollie, S. D. (1999). Predictive validity of a procedure for pediatric hearing instrument fitting. *American Journal of Audiology, 8*(2), 143–152.

Seewald, R. C., Ramji, K. V., Sinclair, S. T., Moodie, K. S., & Jamieson, D. G. (1993). *A computer-assisted implementation of the Desired Sensation Level Method for electroacoustic selection and fitting in children: Version 3.1.* Hearing Health Care Research Unit Technical Report #02. London, Ontario, Canada: University of Western Ontario.

Seewald, R. C., Ross, M., & Spiro, M. K. (1985). Selecting amplification characteristics for young hearing-impaired children. *Ear and Hearing, 6*(1), 48–53.

Shaw, E. A. G., & Vaillancourt, M. M. (1985). Transformation of sound pressure level from the free field to the eardrum presented in numerical form. *Journal of the Acoustical Society of America, 78*(3), 1120–1123.

Sinclair, S. T., Beauchaine, K. L., Moodie, K. S., Feigin, J. A., Seewald, R. C., & Stelmachowicz, P. G. (1996). Repeatability of a real-ear-to-coupler-difference measurement as a function of age. *American Journal of Audiology, 5*, 52–56.

Snik, A. F., van den Borne, S., Brokx, J. P., & Hoekstra, C. (1995). Hearing-aid fitting in profoundly hearing-impaired children. *Scandinavian Audiology, 24*, 225–230.

Snik, A. F. M., & Stollman, M. H. P. (1995). Measured and calculated insertion gains in young children. *British Journal of Audiology, 29*, 7–11.

Stapells, D. R. (2000a). Threshold estimation by the tone-evoked auditory brainstem response: A literature meta-analysis. *Journal of Speech-Language Pathology and Audiology, 24*, 74–83.

Stapells, D. R. (2000b). Frequency-specific evoked potential audiometry in infants. In R. C. Seewald (Ed.), *A sound foundation through early amplification: Proceedings of an international conference* (pp. 13–32). Stäfa, Switzerland: Phonak AG.

Stapells, D. R., Gravel, J. S., & Martin, B. E. (1995). Thresholds for auditory brainstem responses to tones in notched noise from infants and young children with normal hearing or sensorineural hearing loss. *Ear and Hearing, 16*, 361–371.

Stapells, D. R., Herdman, A., Small, S. A., Dimitrijevic, A. & Hatton, J. (2004). Current status of the auditory steady-state responses for estimating an infant's audiogram. In R. C. Seewald & J. Bamford (Eds.), *A sound foundation through early amplification* (pp. 43–59). Staafa, SG: Phonak.

Stelmachowicz, P. G., Hoover, B. M., Lewis, D. E., Kortekaas, R. W. L., & Pittman, A. L. (2000). The relation between stimulus context, speech audibility, and perception for normal-hearing and hearing-impaired children. *Journal of Speech, Language, and Hearing Research, 43*, 902–914.

Stelmachowicz, P. G., & Lewis, D. E. (1988). Some theoretical considerations concerning the relation between functional gain and insertion gain. *Journal of Speech and Hearing Research, 31*, 491–496.

Stelmachowicz, P., Lewis, D., Hoover, B., Nishi, K., McCreery, R., & Woods, W. (2010). Effects of digital noise reduction on speech perception for children with hearing loss. *Ear and Hearing, 31*(3), 345–355.

Stelmachowicz, P. G., Pittman, A. L., Hoover, B. M., & Lewis, D. E. L. (2001). Effects of stimulus bandwidth on the perception of /s/ in normal- and hearing-impaired children and adults. *Journal of the Acoustical Society of America, 110*(4), 2183–2190.

Stelmachowicz, P. G., Pittman, A. L., Hoover, B. M., & Lewis, D. E. L. (2002). Aided perception of /s/ and /z/ by hearing-impaired children. *Ear and Hearing, 23*(4), 316–324.

Stelmachowicz, P. G., Pittman, A. L., Hoover, B. M., Lewis, D. E., & Moeller, M. P. (2004). The importance of high-frequency audibility in the speech and language development of children with hearing loss. *Archives of Otolarygology-Head and Neck Surgery, 130*, 556–562.

Stuart, A., Durieux-Smith, A., & Stenstrom, R. (1990). Critical differences in aided sound field thresholds in children. *Journal of Speech and Hearing Research, 33*(9), 612–615.

Tharpe, A. M., Sladen, D., Huta, H. M., & Rothpletz, A. M. (2001). Practical considerations of real-ear-to-coupler difference measures in infants. *American Journal of Audiology, 10*, 41–49.

Valente, M., Potts, L. G., Valente, M., Vass, W., & Goebel, J. (1994). Intersubject variability of real-ear sound pressure level: Conventional and insert earphones. *Journal of the American Academy of Audiology, 5*, 390–398.

Vohr, B., Jodoin-Krauzyk, J., Tucker, R., Johnson, M. J., Topol, D., & Ahlgren, M. (2008). Early language outcomes of early-identified infants with permanent hearing loss at 12 to 16 months of age. *Pediatrics, 122*(3), 535–544.

Wolfe, J., Caraway, T., John, A., Schafer, E. C. & Nyffeler, M. (2009). Study suggests that non-linear frequency compression helps children with moderate loss. *Hearing Journal, 62*, 32–37.

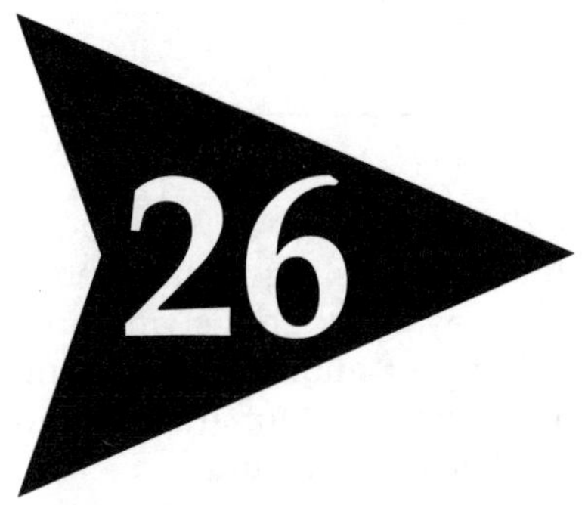

Hearing Instrument Orientation for Children and Their Families

Anne Marie Tharpe, Hollea A.M. Ryan, and Samantha J. Gustafson

Introduction

As established in previous chapters, the purpose of early identification of hearing loss in infants and children is the implementation of early intervention. And, the foundation of early intervention for children with hearing loss is the accurate and timely fitting of amplification. However, the fitting of amplification is only the first step. If families do not understand the importance of hearing aids or are not confident placing the devices on their children, our best efforts will be thwarted. Only when families are comfortable with and understand the importance of hearing aids will they be carefully cared for and worn consistently. Therefore, effective hearing aid orientation is fundamental to the long-term goals of consistent hearing aid use and care, and to the development of auditory and speech-language skills. This chapter describes the family support and education needed from audiologists throughout the hearing aid orientation process. Hearing aid orientation is referred to as a process because it does not occur only at the time when the child is fit with his or her first hearing aids. Rather, audiologists continue to educate families and children about hearing technology after the first fitting, as technology options change, and as the child's hearing needs change over time. This education extends to the child's other caregivers via interactions with daycare workers, teachers, and other qualified interventionists. Furthermore, although in many instances adults are the intended targets of the orientation information, as a child gets older and is able to participate in the care of and decisions about hearing technology, children also become direct recipients of this information.

Family Counseling and Education

A number of variables contribute to a family's ability to cope with the challenges of raising a child who has hearing loss. One of these variables is the level of support and education provided to the family by their audiologist throughout the various stages of intervention and management. The hearing aid orientation provides an opportunity for families to gain knowledge and, thus, confidence about the technology that can contribute to significant changes in their child's life. In other words, this knowledge can reinforce a family's confidence that they are making effective contributions toward their child's success.

Family Education

Following the initial diagnosis of hearing loss in children, it is typical for there to be a 2- to 3-week delay in the fitting of hearing aids after earmold impressions are made. This period of time can be an anxious one for families who want to start helping their newly diagnosed child. During this time, parents can either begin to grow in the knowledge that they are competent parents for their children or can begin to doubt themselves and their ability to parent their children effectively. This can be a key time for audiologists to contribute to parental confidence building. In 2002, Robbins published a list of things that parents can do in the weeks and months following the diagnosis of hearing loss in their child, including things that are likely to build confidence in parents by keeping them actively involved in their child's development. This information can be shared with parents at the time earmold impressions are made. Specifically, Robbins divided the time period after diagnosis into three phases with recommendations for actions parents can take in each phase. These phases and recommendations are outlined in Table 26–1.

Active participation in such activities prevents parents from spending time waiting for "professionals" to tell them what to do. Parents can proceed with the act of parenting, thus, gaining confidence in their own abilities and reducing family stress.

It is also during these early stages of hearing aid fitting that it is important to explain to family members how influential their attitudes are to their child's ultimate acceptance of hearing aids. If parents are obviously stressed during the process of making earmold impressions or during the hearing aid fitting, their child might interpret those signs as a reflection of their parents' attitudes about the hearing aids themselves. Recall that young children with hearing loss are likely to have language delays at the time of the hearing aid fitting and will be interpreting their parents' facial expressions as one way to judge the situation. Therefore, one responsibility of audiologists during this time is to maintain a calm, pleasant attitude and atmosphere—inform families beforehand that most children are reluctant to readily embrace wearing hearing aids for the first time, but assure them that they will be instructed on how to maximize their child's acceptance and hearing aid wearing time. Audiologists can remind parents to maintain pleasant facial expressions and demeanor while attempting to insert their child's earmolds and position the hearing aids.

Households today can be quite diverse with some consisting of a single parent and child, and others having multiple generations living under one roof. Audiologists can increase the likelihood that the information relayed during hearing aid orientation is heard and understood by inviting all of those directly involved in a child's care to participate—what one family member does not hear, another might. If additional family members or caregivers are not able to attend the hearing aid orientation appointment, audiologists can provide family members in attendance with the opportunity to demonstrate how they will teach those not present the required skills for daily care and maintenance. This is particularly important for children who

Table 26–1. Recommendations for Family Involvement Immediately Following Diagnosis

Phase I—From time of diagnosis to hearing aid fitting
• Continue to talk to your child—play gesture games, sing songs, be animated. • Begin a journal of your experiences. • Contact the John Tracy Clinic—they provide correspondence courses for families in more than 20 languages.
Phase II—Early weeks just following the hearing aid fitting
• Keep a weekly hearing aid calendar. • Refer to your child by name—always have a purpose for calling your child. • Use a hand-to-ear response when a sound is heard. • Tell your interventionists of changes in vocalizations as well as auditory responses.
Phase III—After the initial adjustment to hearing aids until formal intervention
• Imitate your child's vocalizations, using intonation, patterns, and sound. • Encourage an anticipatory response to sound—make clear to your child that you expect a response and wait for that response. • Select three common sounds in your home for your child to learn.

Source: Adapted from Robbins (2002).

spend the majority of their day at daycare or with a caregiver outside of the immediate family. The information conveyed can also be reinforced by the provision of written materials, including manufacturers' user guides. One must consider the clarity, complexity, organization, appearance, and cultural appropriateness of educational materials provided to families. Using tools such as the Flesch Reading Ease Formula (Kincaid, Fishburne, Rogers, & Chissom, 1975) can ensure that educational materials are written at a reading level appropriate for that of the average adult in the United States (eighth grade).

One of the first skills that parents must learn is the insertion and removal of the earmold and hearing aid from their child's ear. Parents should practice while with the audiologist and should demonstrate the ability to insert and remove the hearing aid and earmold for each ear before leaving the clinic with the hearing aids for the first time. Helpful insertion tips, such as using a thin layer of water-based lubricant on the canal portion of the earmold, can be useful for parents. Parents, and children if they are old enough, should be discouraged from removing the earmold by the tubing. Overtime, this practice can result in the tubing being torn or pulled loose from the mold. Either of these problems can result in acoustic feedback. Furthermore, if the earmold is not placed correctly, irritation and sores could develop in the child's ear. If possible, provide the parents with a photo, perhaps with the parent's camera phone, of how the earmold should look when properly inserted.

In addition to the expected benefits to a child upon receiving hearing aids, limitations of hearing aid use should be explained to families. Such discussions assist in setting appropriate and reasonable expectations, thus, reducing disappointment in families. Potential limitations, even temporary, that might warrant discussion include the following:

- Background noise—Although current hearing aids have circuits, microphones, and other features that can reduce the impact of background noise, background noise cannot be totally eliminated. The amount of difficulty one has listening in the presence of background noise is dependent on the degree and configuration of the loss as well as specific hearing aid features.
- Acoustic feedback—There are numerous reasons for feedback from hearing aids, especially in infants and young children whose pinnae and external auditory canals continue to grow until approximately 9 years of age. This problem can be addressed by feedback reduction technology, changes in hearing aid settings, new earmolds, or behavioral changes initiated by parents and children. However, at some point in time, parents should expect to experience the irritation of acoustic feedback on at least a temporary basis.

Despite the significant benefits that hearing aids can provide, additional communication strategies will likely be needed and should be discussed with the family. These include

- facing the child when speaking so he or she can see facial expressions and gestures for speech reading purposes;
- finding a quiet place to communicate whenever possible, away from background noise like televisions, and high-traffic areas in restaurants;
- considering alternative technologies like FM systems for use in classrooms or for recreational activities, when background noise is problematic; and
- considering assistive devices such as amplified or lighted alerting devices (e.g., doorbells, fire alarms, and alarm clocks), depending on the degree of hearing loss.

Child Education

As children get older, it becomes necessary and appropriate to include them in the hearing aid orientation process. This might start with something as simple as letting them put their hearing aids in a safe place for the night. Later, as children become more dependable, they can be taught skills and care tasks such as removing and inserting their own earmolds or hearing aids, changing hearing aid batteries, cleaning earmolds, and putting their hearing aids in drying kits.

A curriculum aimed at empowering school-age children by learning more about their hearing loss and hearing technology is the Knowledge is Power Curriculum (KIP; Mississippi Bend Area Educational Agency, 2009). KIP focuses on moving children along a continuum of knowledge from understanding the basics of anatomy and physiology of the ear to self-reliance and personal responsibility. Specifically, the following areas are reviewed in the KIP curriculum:

- anatomy and physiology of the ear,
- causes of hearing loss,
- hearing measurement,
- hearing technology,
- coping with hearing loss,
- rational emotive education,
- stories,

- legislation,
- transition, and
- resources.

KIP can be used with any school-age student with hearing loss if content and presentation adjustments are made to match the student's ability and language level. Worksheets and other handouts can be used to carry over information to parents and other family members.

The Physical Fit

Earmolds

As with adults, the earmold serves as a means to direct sound emitting from a hearing aid down the ear canal toward the tympanic membrane. A well-selected and well-fit earmold also accomplishes several other important objectives. First, a good earmold minimizes feedback by providing an acoustic seal. This seal primarily occurs at the first bend of the ear canal necessitating an earmold impression that extends beyond that point. Second, a good earmold helps to retain the hearing aid behind the ear. Third, a well-fit earmold should be worn comfortably by the child for the duration of the day. Finally, earmold filters can be used to alter the acoustics of the amplified signal. The effects of earmold features on the acoustics of the amplified signal are discussed in detail in other chapters of this book.

Earmold Material

Many considerations should be taken into account when selecting an earmold for infants or children. One of the first considerations is proper material for the earmold. Traditionally, a soft material is selected, both for a comfortable fit as well as for safety concerns. Soft materials, such as a poly-vinyl or silicone, typically provide a comfortable fit, a strong acoustic seal, are often hypoallergenic (if not colored), and are useful when fitting high-powered hearing aids as the material can help minimize feedback. For infants, a hypoallergenic material should be selected to minimize the risks of an allergic reaction, typically seen as redness in the concha or ear canal. Despite these positive reasons for using a soft material, there are also some negative considerations, including the following:

- Difficulty modifying—It can be difficult to buff down and smooth off areas of a soft earmold that are creating pressure points or a poor fit, thus, requiring the entire earmold to be remade.
- Difficulty getting cement to adhere—Cement used for adhering the tubing is traditionally not effective on soft material, resulting in the tubing being easily disconnected from the earmold. This is particularly relevant when children are becoming independent in their hearing aid care and maintenance, as they are likely to remove the hearing aids by pulling at the tubing. Retention rings, or tube locks, on the tubing can be used and help secure the tubing into the earmold. However, brass retention rings can reduce the high-frequency signals being emitted by the hearing aid. A compromise might be achieved by consulting the earmold laboratory and finding a balance between softness and ability to secure the tubing.
- Earmold color—Often, the type of material used will dictate what color options are available. Parents might initially select skin-colored or clear earmolds to minimize the appearance of the molds. However, children should be given the opportunity to select earmold colors once they are capable of making that decision. Allowing the child to select from colored, multicolored, swirled, or even glittered earmold options provides the child with ownership of the fitting process.

Earmold Tubing

The size and length of the tubing are important during the fitting of the hearing aid. In addition to acoustic effects, the length of tubing affects the placement of the hearing aids behind the ears. Proper placement ensures that the microphones are in the desired planes. In addition, the proper length of the tubing is essential to prevent sores or blisters resulting from too tight a fit of the hearing aid when the tubing is too short. Conversely, tubing cut too long will result in a loose fit and the hearing aid could dangle to the side of the ear rather than fitting snugly and comfortably behind the ear.

The tubing size is measured by the internal diameter of the tubing, with size #13 tubing being the most common. Smaller internal diameters have the potential to reduce the hearing aid response above 1000 Hz if not appropriately accounted for in the fitting process (Taylor & Teter, 2009). Older children often prefer more discrete, thin tubing. In this case, it is important for the audiologist to conduct proper verification procedures to take into account the reduced high-frequency response caused by the thinner tubing. Selecting a "thick" tubing size (e.g., #13 thick) will allow for additional attenuation of the amplified signal as it travels from the receiver of the hearing aid to the ear canal, and might reduce feedback for children requiring significant amounts of hearing aid gain.

Earmold Venting

A final consideration during the selection of the earmold is venting. Venting is provided to patients for pressure equalization between the ear canal and the environment and as a means of reducing low-frequency response. For infants, or children with very small ear canals, it might be impossible for any size vent to be added. When possible without introducing feedback, a small pressure vent can be appropriate even for severe losses. For those with milder losses, a medium or small vent can be appropriate but changes to the frequency response caused by the vent must be accounted for when verifying the hearing aid settings. For young children who cannot or will not sit for real-ear measures, this requires verification using simulated real ear measures obtained with the earmold coupled to an HA1 coupler.

Care and Maintenance

Care and maintenance of the hearing aid and earmold should be reviewed with parents at the time of dispensing, and as often as needed thereafter. As the child matures and is capable of keeping the hearing aid and earmold clean, the responsibility should be moved from the parent to the child, with parental supervision as needed. The primary components of the hearing aid should be noted and a demonstration provided on how to clean and protect those features. Caution should be advised when cleaning near the microphone and the receiver. A daily "wipe down" with a soft lint-free cloth should be recommended with periodic detailed cleaning as necessary. The difference between the vent and the sound bore of the earmold should be clearly defined in the event that the tubing disconnects from the earmold and requires reinsertion by the child's caregiver. Likewise, if the child's earmold has a "Y" vent, the parent should be instructed not to push the tubing all the way through to the end of the earmold so as to keep from occluding the vent opening. On a regular basis, the earmold should be cleaned in warm soap and water, never alcohol, as it can dry out some materials. Parents must be reminded that the earmold should be removed from the hearing aid prior to cleaning with water and allowed to dry thoroughly (usually overnight) prior to being reattached to the hearing aid. A live demonstration with opportunity to practice this process should be included in the first couple of hearing aid appointments following the fitting, as parents are likely to feel hesitant about taking apart this costly piece of medical equipment.

Often, when hearing aids are ordered for a child, the manufacturer also provides a care kit. Typically, this kit includes a listening stethoscope, battery tester, air blower, a cleaning tool, and some form of desiccant container. If a kit does not come from the hearing aid manufacturer, the dispensing audiologist should encourage the purchase of these items by the family. Effective use of each item in the kit should be reviewed with the parents and with the child when appropriate. When possible, an extra care kit can be provided to a school-age child's classroom teacher. Audiologists can help prepare parents to work with their child's teacher(s) to monitor hearing aid function in the classroom. The following points can be part of ongoing discussions about audiologic care for a school-age child with hearing loss:

- Introduce hearing aid technology and the accompanying care and maintenance to each of the child's teacher(s), including
  - hearing aid and additional technology, such as FM systems;
  - care kit;
  - general maintenance; and
  - troubleshooting.
- Discuss signs for parents and teachers that might indicate hearing aid malfunction or changes in hearing status, such as
  - child's attention or energy level has noticeably changed;
  - child does not respond to name;
  - child asks for things to be repeated;
  - child pulls at ear or takes hearing aid off; or
  - child's voice level changes.

A listening check via a stethoscope should be demonstrated at the initial orientation and reviewed at subsequent appointments as needed. Parents should be encouraged to listen to all programs (if applicable), and shown how to verify the t-coil function and any assistive listening devices. Parents should also be instructed on how and why to conduct the Ling-Six-Sound Test (Ling, 1976, 1989). The Ling-Six-Sound Test is a behavioral listening check to determine the effectiveness of amplification. The sounds /ah/, /ee/, /oo/, /sh/, /s/, and /mm/ are presented without visual cues, and the child indicates his or her ability to detect them. Obviously, this listening task cannot be completed with infants or very young children.

Hearing aids should be kept in their case or in a drying kit overnight with battery doors at least partially open. Storing hearing aids this way helps to prolong the life of both the battery and hearing aid. Furthermore, placing hearing aids in a case and out of reach of small children and pets, even when removed temporarily, helps to prevent accidental ingestion of the hearing aid or battery. The hearing aids should not be kept loose in the bottom of a diaper bag, backpack, purse, or pocket. A brief hearing aid orientation checklist is included in Appendix 26–A.

The importance of routine troubleshooting became apparent during the 1970s when several investigators examined the functionality of hearing aids in schools. Based on visual inspections and listening checks, a 20% to 60% range of inadequate hearing aid function was documented (Bess, 1977; Reidner, 1978; Ross, 1977; Zink, 1972). As a result of these studies, hearing aid monitoring programs in schools were implemented to address these problems. The documented number of hearing aids with problems in classroom settings appeared to decrease after initiation of monitoring programs (Kemker, McConnell, Logan, & Green, 1979). However, a more recent study showed that 17% of hearing aids (all behind-the-ear models) in a large metropolitan school system with a stringent monitoring program were defective, affecting roughly 27% of the hearing aid users (Smitherman, 2005). Improper earmold tubing (i.e., loose or torn tubing) and dead batteries accounted for the majority of the problems.

Another topic to review with parents during the initial fitting is extended hearing aid warranties. For the pediatric population, the chances are high that a hearing aid will be damaged or lost at some point. It is not unheard of for children's hearing aids to be thrown out car windows, flushed down toilets, dropped into cereal bowls, eaten by family pets, stepped on, and so on. Thus, the family might find it beneficial to purchase a warranty that covers both loss and damage.

Safety Features and Issues

Overamplification

Overamplification has been a long-standing concern among audiologists who work with young children (Berry, 1939; Humes & Bess, 1981; Jerger & Lewis, 1975; Kinney, 1961; Rintelman & Bess, 1988). Although the primary responsibility for avoiding overamplification will occur during the verification stage (see Chapter 25 by Bagatto and Scollie), there is an additional safety feature that can be implemented during hearing aid orientation. If the device has a volume control toggle or button, it can be deactivated or restricted to act within a limited range by the programming software of modern instruments. In some cases, one might want to order a remote control (available with certain brands) allowing for desired volume changes by parents or older children but with a reduced risk for accidental changes in volume level.

Battery Ingestion

In addition to overamplification, audiologists should demonstrate an appropriate level of concern about battery ingestion. Battery ingestion occurs at an estimated rate of 2,000 to 3,000 per year (Martin, 2009; National Capital Poison Center, 2006). Children under the age of 5 years, and particularly those between 1 and 2 years, are particularly prone to swallowing batteries, contributing to 62% of the reported battery ingestion cases per year in the United States (NCPC, 2006). Although "button batteries" are found in many items, such as toys and watches, 49% of ingested batteries are hearing aid batteries and of those swallowed by children, 33% come from their own hearing aids (Dire, 2013; NCPC, 2006).

At one time, hearing aid batteries were made out of mercury, but these types of batteries were banned in the United States in 1996 (H.R. 2024). Although most hearing aid batteries are currently made of alkaline or zinc—potentially less hazardous materials—they still can contain trace amounts of the heavy metal mercury that can be poisonous if ingested. Batteries can be dangerous even without leaking chemicals into the human system. Even more alarming is the fact that at least one infant death as a result of battery ingestion has been documented (Bronstein, Spyker, Cantilena, Green, Rumack, & Heard, 2007). Thus, for young children, it is important to consider ordering a locking mechanism on the battery door to reduce the likelihood of accidental battery ingestion. Different methods for locking the battery door are offered by different hearing aid manufacturers. It is important for audiologists to review with parents how to lock and unlock the tamper-proof battery door. The National Capital Poison Center in the United States or one's local poison control center should be contacted immediately if it is suspected that a child has swallowed a battery.

Proper Placement

Additional consideration needs to be given to ensure that each hearing aid is worn on the intended ear.

Although many children diagnosed with bilateral hearing loss will have symmetrical loss, this is not always the case. The first time a child is fit with a hearing aid, it is useful for the parents to have the right and left hearing aids differentiated, usually with stickers or tabs that are affixed to the hearing aids. Traditionally, a blue sticker is placed on the left hearing aid and a red to the right hearing aid. If a sticker or tab is not provided with the hearing aid from the manufacturer, a simple solution is to place a small red dot of fingernail polish, for the right hearing aid, on the side positioned against the head or on the bottom of the battery door. Likewise, it is important to remind parents that if they remove the earmold from the hearing aid for any reason, to do so one at a time until they are able to differentiate the left and right earmolds. This helps to ensure that the corresponding earmold and hearing aid are connected.

Retention and Use

Behavioral Retention

One of the most common exclamations by parents on the day that their child first receives a hearing aid is "How in the world am I going to keep that in!?!" This is when audiologists explain to parents that children are taught to wear hearing aids in much the same way as they learn to wear their shoes and their clothes. No new techniques are needed. Families have their own philosophies about following rules and their own forms of discipline. They should already have the skills and instincts to gain compliance from their children. If not, a discussion about behavioral modification techniques or even a referral to parenting classes might be appropriate. In any case, parents will need some assistance on determining wearing schedules.

When a child first receives a hearing aid, it is helpful if it is taken home at a day and time when the family can provide close supervision. In other words, one would not want to dispense a hearing aid to a child only to have the child dropped off at daycare for the rest of the day with those who have not been instructed in the care and retention of the device. The following guidelines might be useful to families receiving their child's first hearing aid:

- Insert and remove the hearing aid while the child is on a soft surface like a bed or carpeting. If the hearing aid should drop, it is not likely to be damaged.
- For infants and young children, adult caregivers should be the only ones who insert or remove the hearing aid. If the child purposefully or accidentally removes the hearing aid, the caregiver should immediately re-insert it, even if it is about time to remove the aid anyway. Like all other routines in a child's life, if an exception is made, the child is likely to remember it and might be encouraged to "challenge" the routine or caregiver. This re-insertion is likely to be required over and over again for the first few days after the initial fitting. However, with caregiver patience and consistency, most children will stop removing the hearing aid after 2 to 3 days.
- It is generally a good idea to insert the new hearing aids at a time when a child can be distracted and not as likely to investigate the aids. For example, a parent might insert the hearing aids right before sitting down to a meal, reading a book, or playing a game with the child.
- Unlike getting accustomed to wearing contact lenses, hearing aids do not require a graduated wearing time period. That is, if a child is willing to wear his or her hearing aids all day right after they are received, that is fine. However, more important than the length of time that a child initially wears the aids is that he or she learns to wear the hearing aids without trying to take them off. To accomplish that, for example, parents might determine that their child is willing to wear the aids for about an hour before getting fussy or restless. In that case, the parent might remove the hearing aids after an hour and then re-insert them after a short period of time, extending the wear-time period throughout the course of the first several days after receiving the aids. It should not be necessary to have a child adjust to wearing one hearing aid and then introduce the second hearing aid at a later time. We do not have children wear one shoe for a while and then introduce a second shoe. By the end of 1 to 2 weeks, a child should be wearing the hearing aids during all waking hours, removing them only rarely, if at all.

Physical Retention and Protection

Even when all behavioral techniques for retention have been implemented, sometimes the physical fit of the hearing aid is difficult to maintain, especially if the child is young and resistant to the aids or if the child is involved in activities that require considerable physical movement (e.g., sports activities). Devices have been created that help secure hearing aids in these conditions. For the smallest patients, sometimes the pinnae are not sturdy enough to support hearing aids.

A pediatric-sized earhook will help maintain the hearing aid behind the ear. Additionally, double-sided tape, such as wig or toupee tape, can be used to adhere the hearing aid to the head so that it will not fall off from behind the ear and dangle from the earmold.

Even if a hearing aid stays in place during most typical child activities, at some point parents might face a time when their child is purposely pulling the hearing aids out of their ears. To help prevent the loss of hearing aids, the use of a clip and cord (Figure 26–1A) will help. Essentially, the clip has a small plastic ring that slides onto the hearing aid. This ring is attached to a cord that is connected to a clip that is fastened to the upper back or shoulder area of the child's shirt, out of the child's reach. Thus, if a child pulls the hearing aids out of his or her ears, they are still attached to the child. A single clip can be used to secure one hearing aid, and a "Y" clip will secure two hearing aids.

When children are older, it might become necessary to secure the hearing aid when participating in physical activities. Specifically, children participating in sports like gymnastics need to have a means of keeping the hearing aid from falling off from behind the ear. They also need an effective way to minimize movement of the hearing aid during sporting events. One type of security device is a retention ring (Figure 26–1B). The retention ring consists of two small plastic rings that slide around the hearing aid. These thick, small rings are attached to a thinner, larger ring that is wrapped around the ear. The sizes of retention rings vary, accommodating infants to adults.

Another good alternative for active children or athletes is a specially designed headband. The headband has a pocket or a piece of elastic, depending on manufacturer, into which the hearing aid can slide and fit securely against the head. One headband can be used for one or two hearing aids.

Pilot caps or bonnets, hats that cover the entire head and tie under the chin, are also used for retention of hearing aids for infants and young children. The acoustically clear material allows sound to reach the microphone for proper amplification without feedback. The hat is a good way to keep young children from repeatedly pulling off their hearing aids.

An additional method to help reduce the likelihood of hearing aids being removed from the ear is to include a helix lock on the earmold. Although the addition of the helix lock makes the earmold slightly more difficult to properly insert, this modification provides a tighter, more secure fit that can make it just slightly more difficult for the infant or toddler to remove.

Finally, for children who need to protect their hearing aids from excessive moisture, such as perspiration generated during sports activities, there are options that completely cover the hearing aid, thus, preventing or minimizing the amount of moisture that can penetrate the hearing aid. These items, which function much like a slip cover for a hearing aid, are typically made of spandex or latex to reflect moisture or acoustically transparent fabric to absorb or repel moisture from the hearing aid (see Figures 26–2A and B for illustrative examples of such devices).

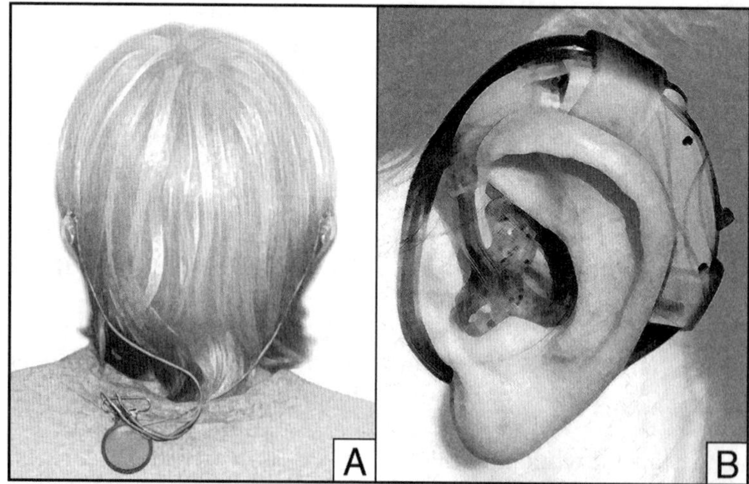

FIGURE 26–1. Hearing aid retention devices include a clip with a Y-cord (**A**), and a retention ring (**B**).

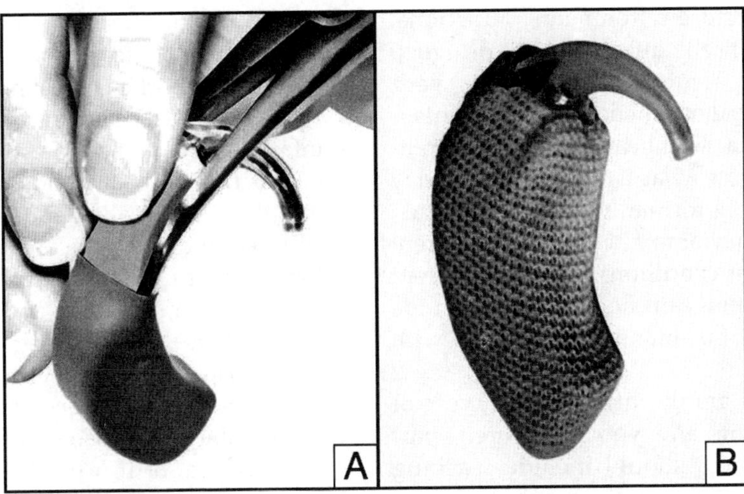

FIGURE 26–2. Protective covers for hearing aids that are designed to reflect moisture (**A**) or wick moisture (**B**).

Usage and Wear Time

A well-fit hearing aid does little to support the development of a child with hearing loss if it is not worn. There are a variety of factors that can potentially influence the consistency of hearing aid use for children with hearing loss. Daily hearing aid use time increases with age during the first seven years of life (Moeller, Hoover, Peterson, & Stelmachowicz, 2009; Walker et al., 2013). However, this use time is highly variable ranging from no use to 16 hours of use per day. Consistency of hearing aid use depends on a child's daily environments, with less supervised situations, such as riding in a car or playing outdoors, often resulting in reduced hearing aid use (Moeller et al., 2009). Audiologists can use these age- and situation-related changes in hearing aid use times to establish realistic expectations for hearing aid use with the family.

As might be expected, children with milder degrees of hearing loss are at higher risk of less hearing aid use compared to children with greater degrees of hearing loss (Munoz, Preston, & Hicken, 2014; Walker et al., 2013). Although parents might feel that their child with mild hearing loss has limited difficulty hearing without amplification, evidence suggests that the prolonged use of well-fit hearing aids provides children with mild hearing loss a better opportunity to achieve good speech and language outcomes when compared to children with similar hearing loss who have minimal use of a hearing aid (Tomblin, Oleson, Ambrose, Walker, & Moeller, 2014; Walker, Holte, McCreery, Spratford, Page, & Moeller, 2015). Moreover, children from families of lower socioeconomic status are also at risk for poorer hearing aid use than those of higher socialeconomic status (Walker et al., 2013).

As children enter adolescence, those with mild degrees of hearing loss appear to still be at increased risk for inconsistent or discontinued hearing aid use (Gustafson, Davis, Hornsby, & Bess, 2015). Furthermore, there are limited data to suggest that approximately 20% to 25% of adolescent and teenage children with hearing loss do not use their hearing aids routinely (Gustafson et al., in press; Jones & Feilner, 2014). As children age, audiologists can prepare families for potential changes in hearing aid use. One possible option for maintaining hearing aid use in adolescents includes transitioning children to smaller, more discrete hearing aids if appearance is of concern. Another alternative is allowing children to select the color of earmolds and hearing aids; decorating the casing with stickers, sequins, or glitter; or decorating the earmold tubing with tube twists or ear jewelry.

Validation

Validation of hearing aid performance involves a demonstration of the benefits and limitations of aided hearing abilities and can begin during orientation. As part of the follow-up and monitoring of hearing technologies, audiologists obtain measures of aided performance in clinical settings and functional auditory assessments in real-world environments. Functional assessment tools are typically questionnaires designed for administration to parents and other caregivers, such as teachers. The goal of functional assessments is to tell us not only *what* a child hears but, more importantly, how the child *uses* what is heard in everyday situations. In addition, information can be obtained about how listening behavior might change in different settings, under different conditions, or with different speakers. This information can then be used to guide our management plans for infants and children with hearing loss.

Insofar as families are the primary observers of behavior of their infants and young children, part of the orientation process should include teaching families how to observe their child's speech/language and auditory behavior with and without amplification. Such instruction needs to include warnings about potential visual cues that might be perceived by children that can result in a misinterpretation of what a child can actually hear, for example, the use of gestures during daily routine activities. Functional assessments are available for infants and children of all ages and with all degrees of hearing loss. See Appendix 26–B for a listing of commonly used functional assessment tools for children with varying degrees of hearing loss.

Follow-up and Monitoring

It is reasonable to expect that families will not remember all of the information provided to them on the day that hearing aids are dispensed. Furthermore, it is likely that an audiologist will not explain everything that families ultimately need to know about hearing aids at the first visit. Audiologists will provide the type and amount of information needed based on their interactions with the parents at the time. Therefore, it is important to review information already provided and add new information as needed on subsequent follow-up visits with families. Unless otherwise indicated, follow-up visits should occur at least quarterly (i.e., every 3 months) for the first two years of life. After 2 years of age, appointments can be scheduled every 4 to 6 months. Naturally, this schedule of appointments assumes that the parents, teachers, and child have not noticed a change in hearing ability, which would necessitate an immediate visit to the audiologist.

The allotted appointment times should allow for the following activities to be completed:

- Reevaluation of hearing function—This is especially important for infants and young children who are unable to report changes in their hearing.
- Remaking of earmold impressions—Especially for infants and young children, growth of the ear might necessitate new earmolds as often as every other month, but typically about every 4 to 6 months for children under the age of 5 years.
- Inspection of earmold and tubing—A brief visual inspection of earmolds and tubing helps to determine if there are any damage or tears present. Also, a visual inspection will determine if the vent or sound bore is blocked and needs to be cleaned. Inspection of the tubing will also determine if it fits tightly in the earmold, or if it has become loose or too stiff, affecting acoustics.
- Visual inspection of the ear—Audiologists can ensure at every follow-up visit that there are no sore spots in a child's concha, helix area, or ear canal resulting from earmold or hearing aid irritation. In addition, it is important to remember that properly cut tubing might become too short if the child experiences a growth spurt. Therefore, it is important to visually inspect the fit of the earmold and the hearing aid to ensure the best fit for the child.
- Electroacoustic analysis of the hearing aid(s)—Only through electroacoustic analysis can we verify appropriate hearing aid function. Electroacoustic analysis should be completed before the hearing aid is dispensed to ensure that it meets the specifications and desired settings. Electroacoustical analyses should also be completed at follow-up visits to verify hearing aid function and to confirm listening checks.
- Listening check of hearing aid(s)—Although audiologists will be conducting electroacoustic analyses of hearing aids, listening checks can reveal the presence of poor sound quality that might not be otherwise detected.
- Acquisition of real-ear-to-coupler differences (RECD) —Whenever a new earmold is received or when tubing is replaced with a longer or shorter length, it is necessary to remeasure the child's RECD. If a change is noted from the previous measurement, adjustments to hearing aid settings will need to be made.

During these follow-up visits, the audiologist will also focus on ensuring that the parents or caregivers have the necessary information and skills to care for the child's hearing needs. Table 26–2 provides information that can be shared with families about troubleshooting hearing aids when problems arise.

Table 26–2. Troubleshooting Common Hearing Aid Issues

Complaint	What to Do
"I don't hear any sound"	• Ensure that the device is turned on. • Ensure that the battery door is closed. • Ensure the volume control is set to the desired level. • Check battery function via a battery tester. • Check that battery contacts are clean. • Check that earmold bore is free of debris.
"Hearing aid has feedback"	• Ensure that the volume control is set to the desired level. • Check that the earmold bore is free of debris. • Determine if earmold or tubing is torn and needs to be replaced. • Verify that hearing aid casing does not have any damage. • Make sure microphone and receiver are free of debris.
"Hearing aid is weak or intermittent"	• Check battery function via battery tester. • Verify that hearing aid casing does not have any damage. • Check that earmold and tubing are free of moisture. • Recheck function of hearing aid after overnight use with desiccant container. • Check that earmold bore is free of debris. • Check that microphone and receiver are free of debris.

Conclusion

The day a child receives a first hearing aid can be one of the most memorable times in a family's experience. They come to this appointment with a myriad of emotions—anxiety, uncertainty, and in all likelihood, great hope and expectation. Audiologists can execute their finest work in this moment, families can find their greatest ally, and a new relationship can flourish.

Acknowledgment. The authors appreciate the graphic services of the Vanderbilt Kennedy Center for Research on Human Development, supported in part by NICHD Grant P30 HD15052.

References

Berry, G. (1939). The use and effectiveness of hearing aids. *Journal of Laryngology, 49*, 912–921.

Bess, F. H. (1977). *Condition of hearing aids worn by children in a public school setting* (Publication No. OE 77-05002). Washington, DC: DHEW.

Bronstein, A. C., Spyker, D. A., Cantilena, L. R., Green, J., Rumack, B. H., & Heard, S. E. (2007). 2006 Annual report of the American Association of Poison Control Centers' national poison data system. *Clinical Toxicology, 45*, 815–917.

Dire, D. J. (2013). *Disk battery ingestion: Treatment and management.* Retrieved from http://emedicine.medscape.com/article/774838-treatment

Gustafson, S., Davis, H., Hornsby, B. W. Y, & Bess, F. H. (2015). Factors influencing hearing aid use in the classroom. *American Journal of Audiology*, doi:10.1044/2015_AJA-15-0024

Humes, L., & Bess, F. H. (1981). Tutorial on the potential deterioration in hearing due to hearing aid usage. *Journal of Speech and Hearing Science, 46*, 3–15.

Jerger, J. F., & Lewis, N. (1975). Binaural hearing aids: Are they dangerous for children? *Archives of Otolaryngology, 101*, 480–483.

Jones, C., & Feilner, M. (2014). What do we know about the fitting and daily life usage of hearing instruments in pediatrics? In J. L. Northern (Ed.), *A sound foundation through early amplification 2013: Proceedings of the sixth international conference* (pp. 97–104). Stäfa, Switzerland: Phonak AG.

Kemker, F. J., McConnell, F., Logan, S. A., & Green, B.W. (1979). A field study of children's hearing aids in a school environment. *Language, Speech, and Hearing Services in Schools, 10*, 47–53.

Kincaid, J. P., Fishburne, R. P., Rogers, R. L., & Chissom, B. S. (1975). *Derivation of new readability formulas (automated readability index, fog count, and Flesch reading ease formula) for Navy enlisted personnel.* Research Branch Report 8–75. Chief of Naval Technical Training: Naval Air Station Memphis. Retrieved from http://www.readabilityformulas.com/flesch-reading-ease-readability-formula.php

Kinney, C. E. (1961). Further destruction of partially deafened children's hearing by use of powerful hearing aids. *Annals of Otology, Rhinology, and Laryngology, 70*, 828–835.

Ling, D. (1976). *Speech and the hearing-impaired child: Theory and practice.* Washington, DC: Alexander Graham Bell Association for the Deaf.

Ling, D. (1989). *Foundations of spoken language for the hearing-impaired child.* Washington, DC: Alexander Graham Bell Association for the Deaf.

Martin, R. L. (2009). In case of battery ingestion, act fast! *Hearing Journal, 62*(3), 64.

Mississippi Bend Area Educational Agency, Special Education Division. (2009). *Knowledge is power.* Retrieved from http://edaud.org/product/knowledge-is-power/

Moeller, M. P., Hoover, B., Peterson, B., & Stelmachowicz, P. (2009). Consistency of hearing aid use in infants with early-identified hearing loss. *American Journal of Audiology, 18*(1), 14.

Muñoz, K., Preston, E., & Hicken, S. (2014). Pediatric hearing aid use: How can audiologists support parents to increase consistency? *Journal of the American Academy of Audiology, 25*(4), 380–387.

National Capital Poison Center. (2006). *Swallowed a battery button? Battery button in the nose or ear?* Retrieved from http://www.hearingoffice.com/download/Swallowed_a_Button_Battery_Battery.pdf

Reidner, E. D. (1978). Monitoring of hearing aids and earmolds in an educational setting. *Journal of the American Auditory Society, 4*(1), 39–43.

Rintelman, W., & Bess, F. (1988). High level amplification and potential hearing loss in children. In F. Bess (Ed.), *Hearing impairment in children* (pp. 278–309). Timonium, MD: York Press.

Robbins, A. M. (2002, November). Empowering parents to help their newly diagnosed child gain communication skills. *Hearing Journal, 55*(11), 55–59.

Ross, M. (1977). *A review of studies on the incidence of hearing aid malfunctions* (Publication No. OE 77-05002). Washington, DC: DHEW.

Smitherman, S. (2005). *Evaluating amplification used by public school children: Hearing aids, FM systems, and cochlear implants* (Unpublished Au.D. capstone project). Vanderbilt University, Nashville, Tennessee.

Taylor, B., & Teter, D. (2009). Earmolds: Practical considerations to improve performance in hearing aids. *Hearing Review, 16*(10), 10–14.

Tomblin, J. B., Oleson, J. J., Ambrose, S. E., Walker, E., & Moeller, M. P. (2014). The influence of hearing aids on the speech and language development of children with hearing loss. *JAMA Otolaryngology-Head & Neck Surgery, 140*(5), 403–409.

U.S. Environmental Protection Agency. (1996). H.R. 2024. Mercury-Containing and Rechargeable Battery Management Act of 1996. Retrieved from http://www.epa.gov/mercury/regs.htm#act

Walker, E. A., Holte, L., McCreery, R. W., Spratford, M., Page, T., & Moeller, M. P. (2015). The influence of hearing aid use on outcomes of children with mild hearing loss. *Journal of Speech, Language, and Hearing Research, 58*(5), 1611–1625.

Walker, E. A., Spratford, M., Moeller, M. P., Oleson, J., Ou, H., Roush, P., & Jacobs, S. (2013). Predictors of hearing aid use time in children with mild-to-severe hearing loss. *Language, Speech, and Hearing Services in Schools, 44*(1), 73–88.

Zink, G. D. (1972). Hearing aids children wear: A longitudinal study of performance. *Volta Review, 74*(1), 41–51.

APPENDIX 26–A

Hearing Aid Orientation Checklist

1. Components of the hearing aid and earmold
   - ☐ Microphone, receiver, program switch, on/off control, volume control, battery door, earhook, tubing, soundbore, and venting
2. How to operate a hearing aid
   - ☐ Turn on/off, switch between programs, operate battery door, especially if tamper proof, and how to connect/disconnect earmold tubing from earhook
   - ☐ Insertion and removal of hearing aid and earmold
3. Retention of hearing aids
   - ☐ Use of retention devices
   - ☐ Behavioral retention strategies
4. How to differentiate the left from the right
   - ☐ Use of a sticker on one or both hearing aids
   - ☐ Use of red paint or permanent marker on only the right hearing aid
   - ☐ Orientation of earmold
5. Appropriate hearing aid settings
   - ☐ Volume control setting
   - ☐ How to switch between programs and how to confirm those settings
   - ☐ How to connect to assistive listening devices, when appropriate
6. How to care for hearing aid and earmold
   - ☐ Daily activities, including wiping hearing aids and earmolds off with soft cloth, opening battery door overnight, how to store hearing aids and earmolds especially overnight, use of desiccant container
   - ☐ Weekly cleaning of earmolds in soapy water
7. Troubleshooting guidelines
   - ☐ Troubleshooting kit for parents, and if possible, one for school use (by either teacher or child)
   - ☐ Demonstrate procedure, including how to do Ling-Six-Sound Test, to family
8. Battery information
   - ☐ Battery size
   - ☐ How to replace
   - ☐ Frequency of replacement
   - ☐ How to check battery function with and without a battery tester
   - ☐ Storage of batteries

- ☐ Dangers of battery ingestion
- ☐ Safe disposal of batteries

9. Warranty information
   - ☐ Earmolds
   - ☐ Hearing aids
     - ☐ Manufacturer
     - ☐ Extended warranty purchases

10. Clinical procedure for addressing hearing aid issues
    - ☐ Walk-in clinic schedule
    - ☐ Options offered by clinic if hearing aids need to be sent in for repair (e.g., loaner bank, etc.)

11. Additional information
    - ☐ Issuance of brochures from hearing aid and earmold manufacturer on care, maintenance, etc.
    - ☐ Troubleshooting tips for parents
    - ☐ Local, regional, and national organization and support group information
    - ☐ Websites pertaining to troubleshooting, pediatric hearing loss, and so on
    - ☐ Use and coupling of assistive listening devices

APPENDIX 26–B

Functional Auditory Assessment Tools

Test Name: ABEL: Auditory Behavior in Everyday Life

Age Range: 2 to 12 years

Purpose: Twenty-four item questionnaire with three subscales (Aural-Oral, Auditory Awareness, Social/Conversational skills) that evaluates auditory behavior in everyday life

Reference: Purdy, S., et al. 2002. ABEL: Auditory behaviour in everyday life, *American Journal of Audiology*, *11*, 72–82.

Test Name: CHILD: Children's Home Inventory for Listening Difficulties

Age Range: 3 to 12 years

Purpose: Questionnaire for the child and for the parent with 15 situations that rate how well the child understood speech

Reference: Anderson K. L., & Smaldino, J. J. (2000). *Children's Home Inventory for Listening Difficulties (CHILD).* Retrieved from http://home.earthlink.net/~karenlanderson/CHILD.pdf

---

Test Name: COW: Children's Outcome Worksheets

Age Range: 4 to 12 years

Purpose: Three worksheets (child, parent, and teacher) are requested to specify five situations where improved hearing is desired.

Reference: Williams, C. (2003), The Children's Outcome Worksheets—An outcome measure focusing on children's needs (Ages 4–12). *News from Oticon*, January 2005. Retrieved from http://www.oticon.com

---

Test Name: ELF: Early Listening Function

Age Range: 5 months to 3 years

Purpose: Twelve listening situations in which the parent and audiologist observe the child and record the distance the child responds to the auditory stimuli

Reference: Anderson, K. L. (2000). *Early Listening Function (ELF).* Retrieved from http://successforkidswithhearingloss.com/tests

---

Test Name: IT-MAIS: Infant Toddler Meaningful Auditory Integration Scale

Age Range: Birth to 3 years

Purpose: Parental interview with 10 questions that evaluate the meaningful use of sound in everyday situations (vocal behavior, attachment with hearing instrument, ability to alert to sound, ability to attach meaning to sound)

Reference: Zimmerman-Phillips, S., Osberger, M. F., & Robbins, A. M. (1997). *Infant-Toddler: Meaningful Auditory Integration Scale (IT-MAIS)*. Sylmar, CA: Advanced Bionics. Retrieved from http://www.amymcconkeyrobbins.com/PDF/it-mais_brochure.pdf

---

Test Name	LIFE: Listening Inventory for Education
Age Range:	6 years and up
Purpose:	Questionnaire that identifies classroom situations that are challenging for the child. There are two formats of the questionnaire: a teacher questionnaire with 16 items and a child questionnaire with 15 items.
Reference:	Anderson K. L., & Smaldino, J. J. (1996). *Listening Inventory for Education: An efficacy tool (LIFE).* Retrieved from http://successforkidswithhearingloss.com/tests

Test Name:	Little Ears
Age Range:	0 years and up
Purpose:	Questionnaire for the parent with 35 age-dependent questions that assess auditory development
Reference:	Kühn-Inacker, H., Weichbold, V., Tsiakpini, L., Coninx, S., & D'Haese, P. (2003). *Every step of the way: BRIDGE to better education.* Retrieved from http://www.medel.com/support-rehabilitation/

Test Name:	LSQ: Listening Situations Questionnaire
Age Range:	7 years and up
Purpose:	Questionnaire for the parent and child with eight situations. Responses focus on help of amplification, difficulty of understanding, and satisfaction of amplification.
Reference:	Grimshaw, S. (1996). *The extraction of listening situations which are relevant to young children, and the perception of normal-hearing subjects of the degree of difficulty experienced by the hearing impaired in different types of listening situations.* Nottingham: MRC Institute of Hearing Research. Retrieved from http://www.psych-sci.manchester.ac.uk/mchas/information/eval/quest/lsq.pdf

Test Name:	MAIS: Meaningful Auditory Integration Scale
Age Range:	3 to 4 years and up
Purpose:	Parental interview with 10 questions that evaluate meaningful use of sound in everyday situations (attachment with hearing instrument, ability to alert to sound, ability to attach meaning to sound)
References:	Robbins, A. M., Renshaw, J. J., & Berry, S. W. (1991). Evaluating meaningful integration in profoundly hearing-impaired children. *American Journal of Otolaryngology, 12*(Suppl.), 144–150. Robbins, A. M., Renshaw, J. J., & Berry, S. W. (1998). Meaningful auditory integration scale. In W. Estabrooks (Ed.), *Cochlear implants for kids* (pp. 373–386). Washington DC: AG Bell Association for the Deaf.

Test Name: PEACH: Parents' Evaluation of Aural/Oral Performance of Children

Age Range: Preschool to 7 years

Purpose: Interview with parent with 15 questions targeting the child's everyday environment. Includes scoring for five subscales (Use, Quiet, Noise, Telephone, Environment)

Reference: Ching, T. C., Hill, M., & Psarros, C. (2000). *Strategies for evaluation of hearing aid fitting for children.* Paper presented at the International Hearing Aid Research Conference, August 23, Lake Tahoe. Retrieved from http://outcomes.nal.gov.au/Assesments_Resources/PEACH%20ratings%20with%20coverpage%20260509.pdf

---

Test Name: P-APHAB: Pediatric Abbreviated Profile of Hearing Aid Benefit

Age Range: 10 to 15 years

Purpose: Questionnaire with 24 situations completed by the child in regard to use of a hearing aid and no use of a hearing aid. It includes scoring for four subscales (ease of communication, background noise, reverberation, and aversion)

Reference: Kopun, J., & Stelmachowicz, P. G. (1998). Perceived communication difficulties of children with hearing loss. *American Journal of Audiology, 7,* 30–38.

Test Name: Preschool SIFTER: Preschool Screening Instrument For Targeting Educational Risk

Age Range: 3 to 6 years

Purpose: Questionnaire with 15 items completed by the teacher which identifies children at risk for educational failure with five subscales (academics, attention, communication, participation, behavior)

Reference: Anderson, K. L., & Matkin, N. (1996). *Screening Instrument For Targeting Educational Risk in preschool children (age 3–kindergarten) (Preschool SIFTER).* Retrieved from http://successforkidswithhearingloss.com/catalog/sifters

---

Test Name: SIFTER: Screening Instrument For Targeting Educational Risk

Age Range: 6 years and above

Purpose: Questionnaire with 15 items completed by the teacher which identifies children at risk for educational failure with five subscales (academics, attention, communication, participation, behavior)

Reference: Anderson, K. L. (1989). *Screening Instrument For Targeting Educational Risk (SIFTER).* Retrieved from http://successforkidswithhearingloss.com/catalog/sifters

---

Test Name:	TEACH: Teachers' Evaluation of Aural/Oral Performance of Children
Age Range:	Preschool to 7 years
Purpose:	Interview with teacher with 13 questions targeting the child's everyday environment. Includes scoring for five subscales (Use, Quiet, Noise, Telephone, Environment)
Reference:	Ching, T. C., Hill, M., & Psarros, C. (2000). *Strategies for evaluation of hearing aid fitting for children.* Paper presented at the International Hearing Aid Research Conference, August 23, Lake Tahoe. Retrieved from http://www.nal.gov.au

Source: From Tharpe, A. M., & Flynn, T. S. (2005). *Incorporating functional auditory measures into pediatric practice: An introductory guide for pediatric hearing professionals.* Somerset, NJ: Oticon A/S.

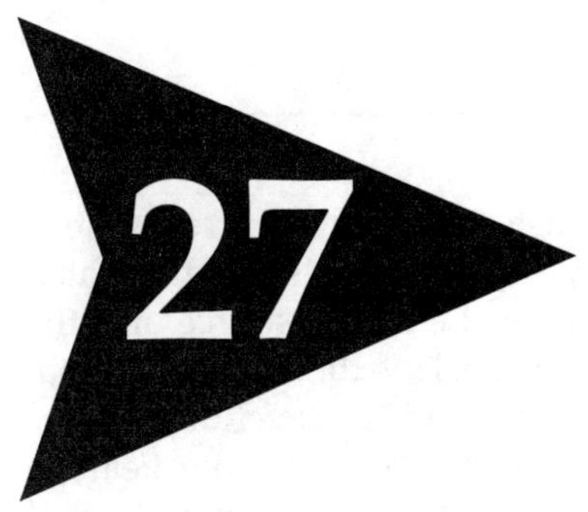

Remote Microphone Systems and Communication Access for Children

Jace Wolfe, Dawna Lewis, and Leisha R. Eiten

Introduction

Research has unequivocally indicated that children experience greater difficulty than adults in understanding speech in the presence of competing noise (Boothroyd, 1997; Wolfe, Morais, Neumann, et al., 2013). For more information on this topic, the interested reader is referred to Chapters 3 and 4 of this volume. Additionally, numerous studies have indicated that children with hearing loss are particularly likely to encounter difficulty with communication in noisy and reverberant situations and when the speech signal of interest originates from a distance (e.g., more than a meter) from the listener (Crandell, 1991, 1992, 1993; Crandell & Bess, 1986; Finitzo-Hieber & Tillman, 1978; Nabelek & Nabelek, 1985; Wolfe, Morais, Neumann, et al., 2013). The difficulties children with hearing loss experience with communication in challenging listening situations are discussed in Chapters 37, 38, and 39 of this book and will also be addressed briefly in this chapter. Pediatric audiologists are faced with the task of optimizing auditory performance across a wide range of acoustic settings in which the child must communicate. The objective of this chapter is to highlight the advantages and limitations of the use of remote microphone technology for improving hearing performance in challenging listening situations.

Communication Access

There is a paucity of published studies describing the typical acoustics of environments commonly encountered by infants and young children. Mulla (2011, 2013) measured the signal-to-noise ratio (SNR) across a variety of environments in which infants and young children commonly reside (e.g., rear-facing in car seat located in an automobile traveling 30 and 70 miles per hour, a city bus, a stroller, a shopping cart in a grocery store, a city park, etc.) and reported that it is common for the SNR to approach −5 to −10 dB. Crukley, Scollie, and Parsa (2011) measured noise and reverberation levels present in a preschool daycare where the age of children ranged from 3 months to 5 years. Median ambient noise levels exceeded 70 dBA, while classroom reverberation times (RT60) approached 0.7 s. The RT60 measured in the gymnasium setting was almost 1.5 s. Furthermore, Crukley et al. reported that competing noise was present throughout 80% of a child's day in the daycare setting. SNRs ranging from 0 to +5 dB SNR are typical for an environment possessing an ambient noise level exceeding 70 dBA (Pearsons, Bennett, & Fidell, 1977). Professional guidelines and research suggest that a SNR of at least +15 dB is imperative to allow for adequate communication for children with hearing loss (ANSI/ASA, 2010; ASHA, 2005).

Studies have demonstrated that unfavorable acoustics often exist in elementary, middle school, and high school classrooms. For example, Choi and McPherson (2005) reported that mean ambient noise levels in a group of typical occupied classrooms in Hong Kong were 61 dBA, and Massie and Dillon (2006) reported mean ambient noise levels in occupied classrooms in Australia ranging from 64 to 72 dBA. Sanders (1965) reported a mean SNR of −1 dB in 17 kindergarten classrooms and +5 dB in 24 elementary and high school classrooms. More recently, Crukley et al. (2011) reported median noise levels exceeding 60 dBA for elementary and high school classrooms with the SNR commonly approaching 5 dB. Again, Crukley and colleagues noted that elementary and high school students spend almost 75% of their day listening in noisy environments.

Reverberation times in typical classrooms range from 0.6 to 1.27 s (Knecht, Nelson, Whitelaw, & Feth, 2002). Furthermore, Knecht et al. found that 13 of 32 classrooms that were evaluated in their study possessed RT60s that exceeded the ANSI (2010) recommendation of 0.6 s. Of note, Crukley et al. (2011) reported that RT60 measured across a sampling of elementary and high school classrooms tended to fall below the recommended RT60 of 0.6 s. Many of the rooms in which these measurements were completed contained carpeted floors and curtains on the windows, both of which are examples of acoustic treatments that are certainly not found in all classroom environments. It should also be noted that the RT60 of the gymnasiums of the elementary and high schools were well in excess of 1 s.

The American National Standards Institute has published guidelines that indicate optimal acoustics for educational settings (ANSI, 2010). Specifically, maximum background noise levels should not exceed 35 dBA in unoccupied classrooms, and maximum reverberation times should be less than 0.6 s. A recently published study indicates that the ambient noise levels of many contemporary classrooms do not meet the ANSI recommendations. Ronsse and Wang (2013) measured background noise levels and reverberation times for 67 unoccupied elementary school classrooms in a Nebraska public school system. They found that only three of these classrooms contained unoccupied ambient noise levels below 35 dBA. In contrast, all of the classrooms possessed reverberation times below 0.6 s. Ronsse and Wang also found that student reading and language subject areas were adversely affected by higher ambient noise levels. Specifically, to meet the upper half of Nebraska state assessment targets, unoccupied ambient noise levels should not exceed 45 dBA. It should be noted that as the number of students in a classroom increases, one would expect the noise to most likely increase, while the reverberation time will decrease as the bodies partially absorb the sound. As a result, ambient noise levels of typical classrooms that are occupied by students are likely higher than what was measured in unoccupied classrooms in the Ronsse and Wang study.

Although it has not received as much attention in the peer-reviewed literature, the distance between a sound source and a listener can also have deleterious effects on hearing performance. It should be noted that the distance between the signal source and the listener affects both the level of the primary signal reaching the listener's ears and the level of that signal relative to background noise. For example, Pearson and colleagues (1977) reported that the overall level of a classroom teacher's voice 1 m from the listener is approximately 71 dB SPL, and at 4 m, it is approximately 61 dB SPL. Picard and Bradley (2001) summarized teacher voice levels across a number of studies and reported an average of 61 dBA at 2 m. Leavitt and Flexer (1991) used the Rapid Speech Transmission Index (RASTI) to examine the integrity of a speechlike signal at multiple seating positions in a classroom in relationship to a sound source at the front of the room. Perfect reproduction of the signal was only obtained 6 in (15.24 cm) from the sound source. The integrity of the signal reaching typical seating positions in the classroom was far from ideal. Although direct correlations between RASTI scores and speech perception were not examined, these results reveal that the signal reaching a hearing instrument or cochlear implant microphone will be significantly degraded at all but the closest listening distances.

When considering real-world speech understanding, the audibility of speech often is referenced to "conversational speech at 1 m," a reasonable conversational distance for adults. However, this reference point might not be as common for children as for adults. Any parent of a young child will be quick to report that the distance between a talker and a young listener can vary considerably in a very short period of time. In addition, there will be many times when the talker and listener will not be face-to-face. For infants and young children, there will be times when the level of speech reaching their ears will be higher than that of speech at 1 m. The level of speech at the near ear of an infant held in the cradle position is approximately 68 dB SPL and at the near ear of a young child held on the hip is approximately 76 dB SPL (Stelmachowicz, Mace, Kopun, & Carney, 1993). At other times, the level of speech reaching an infant or young child's ears can be lower, such as when the talker is farther away or the orientation of talkers is not face-to-face. For example, in the United States, infants up to 20 pounds or 1 year of age are placed in rear-facing infant seats in the back seat of cars. Even when they move to front-facing car seats, it is recommended that they remain in the back seat until they are 12 years of age (American Red Cross, 2007). In this environment, the combined effects of distance, orientation, and car noise may significantly impact the audibility of speech.

Communication Abilities and Related Difficulties Associated With Hearing Loss in Children

Children with hearing loss experience greater difficulty understanding speech in challenging listening environments when compared to children with normal auditory function (Finitzo-Heiber & Tillman, 1978; Nabelek & Nabelek, 1985; Neuman, Wroblewski, Hajicek & Rubenstein, 2010; Wolfe, Morais, Neumann, et al., 2013; Wroblewski, Lewis, Valente, & Stelmachowicz, 2012). For instance, Finitzo-Heiber and Tillman (1978) evaluated speech recognition of 12 children with normal hearing and 12 children with mild-to-moderate hearing loss at a variety of noise and reverberation levels and found that the children with hearing loss typically scored 20 to 30 percentage points poorer than their peers with normal hearing. Likewise, Wolfe, Morais, Neumann, and colleagues (2013) evaluated speech recognition of 10 adults with normal hearing, 15 school-age children with normal hearing, and 15 school-age children with hearing loss. At a 5 dB SNR, mean sentence recognition was 95% for the adults, 88% for the children with normal hearing, and 67% for the children with mild-to-moderate hearing loss. Deficits in hearing performance in noise are even observed for children with mild and unilateral hearing loss (Bess, Klee, & Culbertson, 1986; Crandell, 1993; Kenworthy, Klee, & Tharpe, 1990; Ruscetta, Arkmand, & Pratt, 2005; Wolfe, Morais, Neumann, et al., 2013). For example, Crandell (1993) reported that a group of children with minimal hearing loss scored 25 percentage points poorer than children with normal hearing when speech recognition was evaluated at a −6 dB SNR.

It is well known that childhood hearing loss can cause delays in speech, language/linguistic, and vocabulary development (Ching & Dillon, 2013; Geers, Strube, Tobey, & Moog, 2011; Tomblin, Oleson, Ambrose, Walker, & Moeller, 2014). Childhood hearing loss also has been associated with a higher incidence of academic failure (Bess, Dodd-Murphy, & Parker, 1998), literacy delays (Geers & Hayes, 2011), greater psychosocial and emotional problems (e.g., theory of mind, peer-to-peer relationships; Bess, Dodd-Murphy, & Parker, 1998; Cappelli, Daniels, Durieux-Smith, McGrath, & Neuss, 1995; Loeb & Sarigiani, 1986; Oyler, Oyler, & Matkin, 1988), higher levels of stress and fatigue (Bess, Gustafson, & Hornsby, 2014; Hornsby, Werfel, Camarata, & Bess, 2014), and greater cognitive load (Stiles, McGregor, & Bentler, 2012). Many of these nonaudiologic deficits accompanying childhood hearing impairment can be at least partially attributed to higher levels of fatigue present in children with reduced auditory function. Hornsby and colleagues (2014) reported on subjective fatigue in 10 children with normal hearing and 10 children with hearing loss (five who had mild-to-moderate hearing loss and used hearing aids, four who used cochlear implants, and one who had unilateral hearing loss). The children with hearing loss reported greater levels of general fatigue (e.g., "I feel tired"), sleep/rest fatigue (e.g., "I rest a lot"), cognitive fatigue (e.g., "It's hard for me to think quickly"), and total fatigue (composite score). Hornsby et al. noted that higher levels of fatigue are associated with poorer academic performance and a wide range of emotional and psychosocial deficits. The researchers also speculated that the increased fatigue observed in the children with hearing loss was likely due to the higher level of attention and cognitive load required to overcome hearing loss and to understand important audio information presented in the classroom.

Communication Difficulties of Children Who Have Normal Hearing Sensitivity

The negative effects of the poor acoustics present in many listening situations can also hinder communication for some children with normal hearing sensitivity (e.g., Bradley & Sato, 2004; Crandell & Smaldino, 1996; Jamieson, Kranjc, Yu, & Hodgetts, 2004; Nelson, Kohnert, Sabur, & Shaw, 2005). Boothroyd (1997) has shown that 5-year-old children with normal hearing require a SNR that is 5 dB more favorable than what is required for adult listeners for children to achieve performance that is similar to their adult counterparts. It is important to note that poor classroom acoustics can have an even greater effect on comprehension relative to the act of simple recognition of speech. Specifically, Valente, Plevinsky, Franco, Heinrichs-Graham, and Lewis (2012) measured speech recognition and discussion-based comprehension in a group of 8- and 11-year-old children who had normal hearing. Performance was assessed at a SNR of +7 dB and a reverberation time of 1.5 s. Although the mean speech recognition of the children was 95% correct, the mean discussion-based comprehension was only 15% correct. This finding exemplifies the deleterious impact poor acoustics can have on language and academic development of children with normal hearing and particularly for children with hearing loss.

Adverse room acoustics can be particularly detrimental for children who speak English as a second language or who have auditory processing disorders (APDs), learning disabilities, or other cognitive/neurological disorders, such as

- attention deficit disorders,
- auditory neuropathy spectrum disorder,
- autism spectrum disorders,
- developmental delays,
- dyslexia,
- recurrent middle ear dysfunction,
- speech and language disorders,
- history of conductive hearing loss, or
- hyperactivity.

For example, Schafer et al. (2013) evaluated speech recognition in noise for 11 children with attention deficit hyperactivity disorder (ADHD) and/or autism spectrum disorder (ASD) and 11 age- and gender-matched, typically functioning peers. The children with ADHD/ASD required a 5-dB improvement in the SNR to obtain similar levels of hearing performance in noise as their typically functioning peers. Furthermore, Bradlow, Kraus, and Hayes (2003) showed that children with normal hearing who have learning disabilities (LD) might also experience difficulties understanding speech in adverse environments. They compared sentence perception in noise (+4 and +8 dB signal-to-noise ratio) for children with and without LD. Children with LD performed more poorly than their peers and were more adversely affected by decreasing signal-to-noise ratio. Similarly, Johnston, John, Kreisman, Hall, & Crandell (2009) reported communication deficits in a group of 10 children with APD relative to a group of 13 children with normal auditory function. They reported that the children with APD reported significantly greater academic difficulty as indicated on responses for the Screening Instrument for Targeting Educational Risk (SIFTER; Anderson, 1989) and the Listening Inventory for Education (LIFE; Anderson, Smaldino, & Spangler, 2011) questionnaires. Also, the children with APD required a SNR that was 2 dB more favorable than their typically functioning counterparts in order to achieve similar levels of performance on the Hearing in Noise Test (HINT; Nilsson, Soli, & Sullivan, 1994).

Goals of Pediatric Amplification: Ensuring Consistent Communication Access

When attempting to alleviate the aforementioned difficulties and challenges related to childhood hearing loss, clinicians must promptly and aptly provide personal hearing technology that is individually optimized to meet the needs of each child. Children with mild-to-severe hearing loss typically receive substantial benefit from hearing aids that are properly selected and verified to meet the needs related to the child's hearing impairment (Ching & Dillon, 2013; Tomblin et al., 2014; Wolfe et al., 2010). Children with severe-to-profound hearing loss can achieve age-appropriate spoken language abilities with the use of cochlear implants (Geers et al., 2011).

In the American Academy of Audiology (AAA) Pediatric Amplification Clinical Practice Guideline (AAA, 2013), the goals of personal hearing technology fitted for a child with hearing loss are defined as follows:

> [T]o provide, to the degree possible given the hearing loss and limitations of hearing aid amplification, audibility across the long-term average speech spectrum (LTASS), without delivering any signal that is of an intensity that would be either uncomfortable or unsafe. Goals of amplification also include minimal distortion, appropriate signal-processing strategies for the listener, features that maximize audibility of the desired signal and, insofar as possible, reduction of undesired signals (noise), flexibility and ease of connection to external devices, and physical comfort such that consistent, daily use is possible. (AAA, 2013, p. 8)

Although the use of hearing aids and cochlear implants can support adequate hearing performance across many environments, communication access will continue to be negatively impacted in environments with competing noise, reverberation, and relatively greater distances between the sound source and the listener (Anderson & Goldstein, 2004; Anderson, Goldstein, Colodzin, & Iglehart, 2005; Schafer & Thibodeau, 2006; Schafer et al., 2013; Wolfe, Schafer, Heldner, Mulder, & Vincent, 2009; Wolfe, Morais, Neumann, et al., 2013; Wolfe, Morais, Schafer, Mills, & Mülder, 2013; Wolfe, Morais, Schafer, Mills, Peters, et al., 2013). As previously discussed, Leavitt and Flexer (1991) showed that ideal communication access required the listener to capture the audio signal 6 in (15.24 cm) from its source. Of course, it is impossible for a listener to consistently remain within 6 in (15.24 cm) of the signal source (e.g., 6 in [15.24 cm] from the mouth of the talker of interest). Without a doubt, use of remote microphone technology is the most effective solution for optimizing communication access in many challenging real-world listening situations. Remote microphone technologies can provide reproduction of close, undegraded input signals with minimal reverberation effects and reduced impact of noise.

Remote microphone technology has evolved substantially over the past several years, and as discussed in this chapter, there are many differences in the commercially available remote microphone systems currently offered by hearing technology manufacturers. In spite of these differences, contemporary remote microphone systems possess several common features. First, all remote microphone systems contain a microphone that is intended to be worn in close proximity (e.g., no more than 6 in [15.24 cm] to 8 in [20.32 cm]) to the primary talker's mouth. These microphones can be clipped to the talker's clothing or worn on the head (e.g., boom microphone). Remote microphones also can be handheld or placed on the table in front of the talker(s). The microphone is coupled to a transmitter that delivers the audio signal from the microphone to a receiver that is coupled to the listener's personal hearing technology or to a loudspeaker that is used to amplify the signal of interest. It is important to note that many transmitters also possess an audio input port that can receive audio input from consumer electronics (e.g., MP3 players, laptop computers, tablets, televisions, etc.) and allow for delivery of this signal from the transmitter to the receiver. For typical contemporary remote microphone systems, the signal of interest is wirelessly delivered to the listener's receiver. However, the mechanism of signal delivery differs across systems and can include electromagnetic induction, digital radio frequency transmission, frequency modulation radio transmission, and infrared transmission.

Methods for Signal Delivery in Remote Microphone Systems

Numerous modes of signal delivery are used for transmission of the audio signal conveyed in contemporary remote microphone systems. Figure 27–1 provides an illustration of the electromagnetic spectrum and an indication of the frequency range of transmission within that spectrum in which various modes of signal delivery reside. The following paragraphs provide a description of the various modes of signal delivery in remote microphone systems.

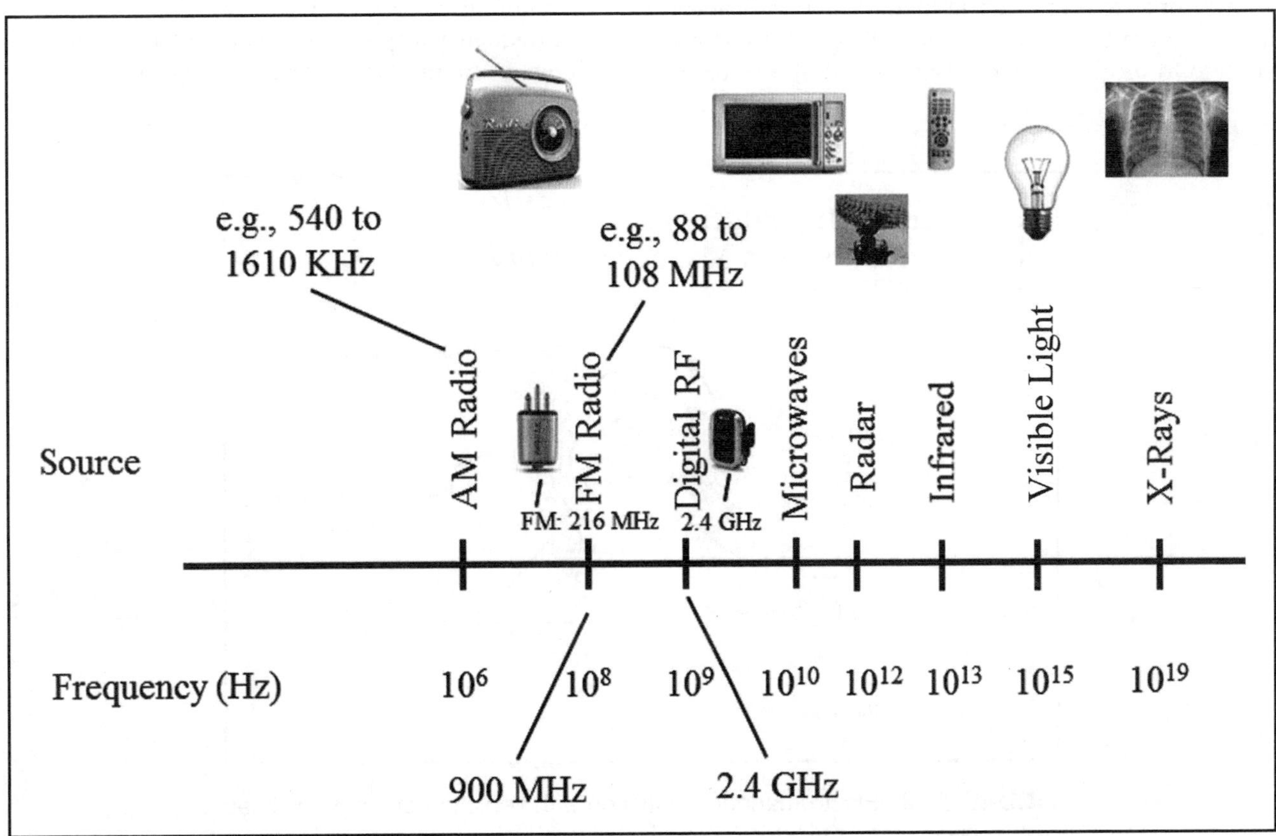

FIGURE 27–1. Electromagnetic spectrum as it relates to modern hearing technology.

Electromagnetic Induction

As the name implies, induction loop systems take advantage of the properties of electromagnetic induction to deliver an audio signal of interest to the telecoil of a user's hearing technology. Electromagnetic induction occurs in two basic forms. First, an electrical current is delivered through a conducting lead (e.g., copper or gold wire) generating magnetic lines of flux surrounding the lead (Figure 27–2). In practice, the conducting lead is typically arranged into the shape of a coil, which results in an enhancement of the strength of the magnetic lines of flux as current passes through the coil. Second, as magnetic lines of flux cross a conducting lead (e.g., copper wire or coil), an electrical current is induced through the conducting apparatus (Figure 27–3). With a conventional induction loop system, an audio signal is converted to an analogous electrical current, amplified, and delivered through a coiled, conducting wire (i.e., loop) that surrounds a room or a specific location within a room. Magnetic lines of flux are created as the electrical current travels through the loop, and these magnetic lines of flux emanate around the loop. Once again, these magnetic lines of flux are proportionally analogous (in frequency, intensity, temporal characteristics) to the original audio signal. If an appropriately selected induction loop is properly installed, these magnetic lines of flux will be strong enough to propagate across the telecoil of a listener's personal hearing technology. The magnetic line of flux will then induce an electrical current through the telecoil, and the current will be delivered to the analog-to-digital converter of the hearing instrument and processed according to the signal processing within the instrument and the individual programming completed by the user's clinician. It should be noted that electromagnetic induction can also be used with induction neckloop systems (described later in this chapter).

Advantages

- Equipment is relatively inexpensive in most cases (e.g., does not require the purchase of radio receivers for each hearing instrument), although additional expense can be incurred for installation.
- There is low power consumption.
- It is available to all users who have a telecoil in their personal hearing technology.

Disadvantages

- It requires a telecoil to be available in the user's hearing instrument.
- It can be susceptible to noise or interference from other electromagnetic sources (e.g., fluorescent lights, computer monitors, etc.).
- The frequency response of a hearing aid telecoil often differs from the standard frequency response of the

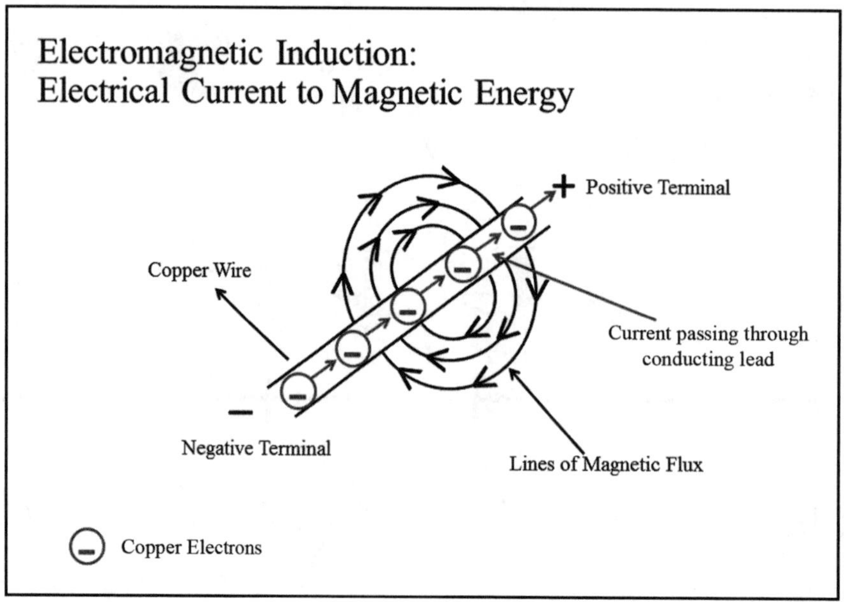

FIGURE 27–2. Electromagnetic induction with depiction of magnetic lines of flux developing as electric current is delivered through a conducting lead.

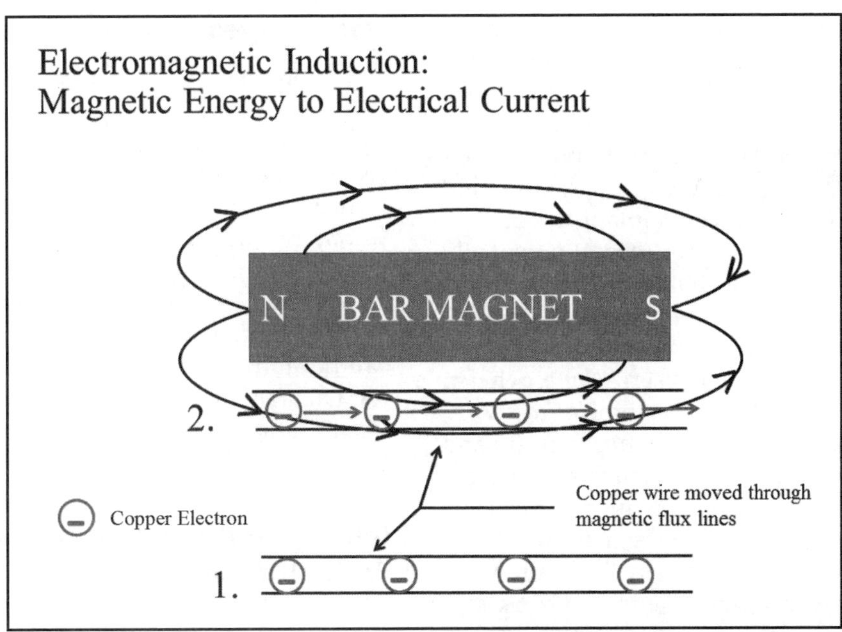

FIGURE 27–3. Electromagnetic induction with depiction of an electric current being induced within a conducting lead as the lead is passed through a magnetic field.

aid (e.g., less low- and high-frequency gain), which can negatively influence hearing performance.

- Signal strength might be insufficient depending on the strength of the installed loop system, the location of the listener relative to the loop, and the orientation of the telecoil in the user's hearing instrument. (This can adversely affect signal strength for room loops and also when a user moves his or her head while using a neckloop); many telecoils in modern hearing instruments are located in the horizontal plane in order to be maximally sensitive for telephone use. However, this orientation diminishes sensitivity to loop systems. Some hearing instruments allow the clinician to account for telecoil sensitivity via programming changes to suit the wearer's needs. Signal strength also can wax and wane depending on the distance between the loop and telecoil changes.

Near-Field Magnetic Induction

Several hearing instrument manufacturers have recently introduced near-field magnetic induction (NFMI) systems for wireless delivery of audio signals to a user's personal hearing technology. These systems have occasionally been referred to as audio streaming accessory devices and typically include a receiver that captures the audio signal of interest via Bluetooth digital radio frequency transmission and then delivers this signal to the user's hearing instrument via NFMI. Bluetooth digital radio transmission, which will be described later in this chapter, can be used to deliver an audio signal from a remote microphone or from Bluetooth-enabled personal consumer electronic devices (e.g., mobile telephone, tablet, computer) to the receiver that is coupled to an induction neckloop. The receiver processes the audio signal received via Bluetooth transmission and converts it to an electrical current that is delivered to the neck-worn loop. However, NFMI uses a more sophisticated process than conventional electromagnetic induction to deliver the signal of interest to the listener's personal hearing technology. The NFMI receiver converts the audio signal to a digital code that is delivered to the neck-worn loop via digital electromagnetic induction at a carrier frequency that varies by manufacturer and ranges from 4 to 14 MHz. Digitally modulated wireless transmission is described below. In short, the digitized signal is delivered in the form of electrical pulses to the loop creating magnetic lines of flux that emanate from the loop. These magnetic lines of flux elicit an electrical current in a NFMI receiver located within the hearing instrument, and this digitized electrical current is delivered to the hearing instrument for further processing. The NFMI receiver/

antenna is typically a small magnet that is surrounded by a copper coil. Figure 27–4 provides an illustration of a NFMI system. NFMI uses a lower carrier frequency than other wireless applications for a number of reasons. First, NFMI can also be used for interaural delivery of data and audio signals (e.g., from hearing aid to hearing aid or from cochlear implant to cochlear implant). This approach allows for several potentially beneficial applications such as binaural beamforming, binaural telephone reception, wind noise reduction, preservation of binaural cues, simultaneous bilateral control of volume, program, and so on (Wolfe, Schafer, Mills, John, & Hudson, 2015). At the time of this writing, it is not technically possible to stream audio and data interaurally using higher-frequency radio applications (2.45-GHz digital radio). Because of the short wavelength of these high-frequency signals, the signal is absorbed, reflected, and distorted by the head. Additionally, NFMI requires relatively low power consumption, and it is relatively immune to interference due to its short transmission range.

Advantages

- It allows for interaural exchange of data and audio signals between hearing instruments,
- It has relatively low power consumption.
- It is relatively immune to interference from other wireless devices.
- Its small antenna allows for inclusion into small hearing aids.

Disadvantages

- It requires a neck-worn or body-worn interface (i.e., does not allow for direct streaming from remote microphone to the receiver).
- NFMI does not allow for long-range transmission, which requires the interface device; as a result, Bluetooth transmission is often used to deliver the signal from external sources to the receiver in the body-worn interface. Transmission delays associated with Bluetooth can result in a dys-synchrony between audio and visual inputs or between the acoustic signal arriving directly from a talker and the Bluetooth signal.

Frequency-Modulated Radio Frequency Transmission

Frequency-modulated radio systems use an electromagnetic radio wave with a carrier frequency ranging from 30 to 230 MHz to deliver the signal of interest via radio frequency transmission. In the United States, FM radio stations broadcast on carrier frequencies ranging from 88 to 108 MHz. Also in the United States, personal FM radio technology for use with hearing instruments and cochlear implants broadcast at carrier frequencies that have been made available by the Federal Communications Commission for use with hearing instruments and range from 72 to 76 MHz and 216 to 218 MHz. It should be noted that the carrier frequencies

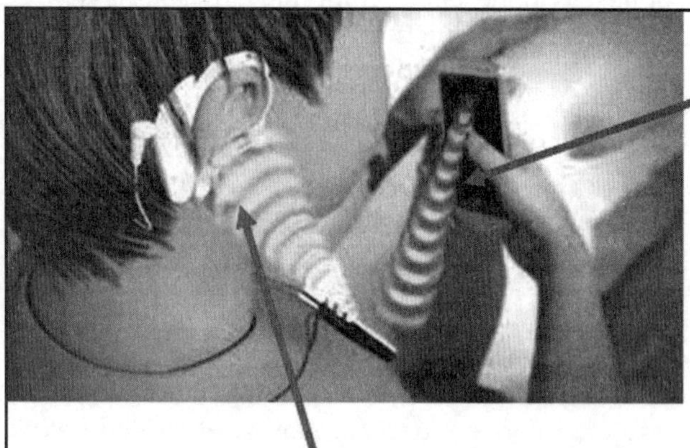

FIGURE 27–4. Hearing assistance technology that utilizes near-field magnetic induction (NFMI) to deliver a signal of interest to a cochlear implant sound processor. Image courtesy of Phonak.

allocated for use with systems designed for hearing aids and cochlear implants vary by country. In short, the audio signal captured by the remote microphone is used to modulate the carrier frequency in the frequency domain. The frequency of the audio signal is conveyed by the rate at which the signal modulates, and the intensity of the original audio signal is conveyed by the magnitude of the modulations. Figure 27–5 provides a visual representation of FM radio frequency transmission.

Advantages

- ➤ It has a long track record of proven benefit with personal hearing technology.
- ➤ It has relatively good transmission range.
- ➤ It is not susceptible to interference from light sources.
- ➤ It does not require direct line of sight between transmitter and receiver.

Disadvantages

- ➤ It is susceptible to interference and noise from other nearby radio signals.
- ➤ It has relatively high power consumption.
- ➤ Its antenna is larger than what is required for digital RF receivers.

Digital Radio Frequency Transmission

Digital radio frequency transmission utilizes ultra-high-frequency carrier waves to deliver digital information via radio frequency transmission. Digital radio frequency transmission is commonly broadcast at the 2.45-GHz band, but the 900-MHz band is also used for some applications. The 2.45-GHz band is particularly popular for commercial uses because the wide bandwidth coupled with frequency-/channel-hopping (explained below) reduces the chance for interference, and this band is globally licensed for use with industry, science, and medical (ISM) applications.

Digital radio frequency transmission can be accomplished via a range of different approaches, two of which are illustrated in Figures 27–6 and 27–7. Amplitude shift keying (ASK; see Figure 27–6) is one basic method of digital radio frequency transmission. Briefly, the audio signal captured at the remote microphone is converted to a digital code. Then, the digital code is used to modulate the absence or presence of the carrier frequency. In other words, a "0" is conveyed by the absence of the carrier frequency, and a "1" is conveyed by the presence of the carrier frequency (Grini, 2006).

Gaussian frequency shift keying (GFSK) is another method of digital radio frequency transmission. With GFSK, the cycles of the carrier frequency are shifted in order to convey the digital code (see Figure 27–7). Specifically, a cycle is "dropped" to convey a "0" and preserved to convey a "1." GFSK is the approach used with the most contemporary Bluetooth applications and also with many remote microphone audio streaming systems developed by manufacturers of hearing instruments. GFSK is more commonly used in contemporary systems, because it is less susceptible to noise. With both ASK and GFSK systems, the digital radio signal arriving at the radio receiver is converted to an electrical signal at the digital-to-analog converter and sent for processing by the hearing instrument (Grini, 2006).

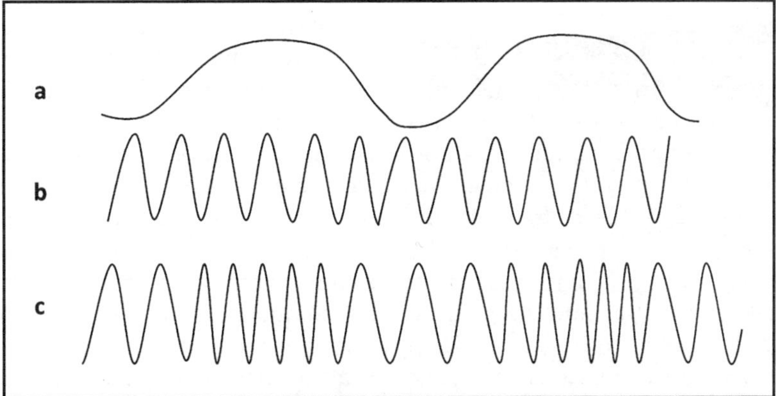

FIGURE 27–5. Frequency-modulated radio transmission. **A.** The original signal of interest. **B.** The radio carrier frequency. **C.** The carrier frequency as it is frequency modulated by the original signal of interest.

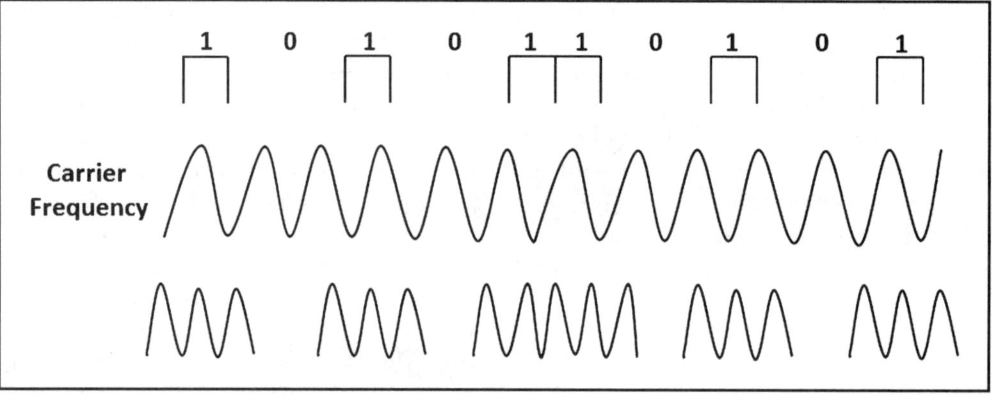

FIGURE 27–6. Digital radio frequency transmission using amplitude shift keying (ASK). **A.** The original digital code (e.g., the original speech signal after being digitized). **B.** The radio carrier frequency. **C.** The carrier frequency as its absence/presence is modulated by the digital code.

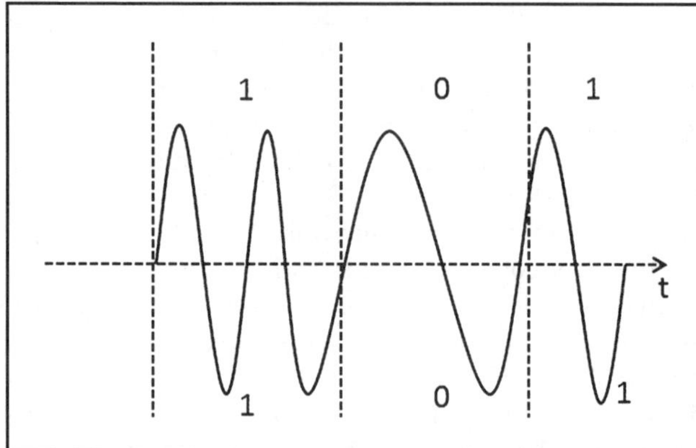

FIGURE 27–7. Digital radio frequency transmission using Gaussian frequency shift keying (GFSK).

Modern digital radio frequency systems deliver both data and audio information between the transmitter and receiver. It is important to note that this process is typically a bidirectional exchange (i.e., information is sent from the transmitter to the receiver and vice versa). The user must first "pair" together the transmitter and the receiver. This process essentially establishes a secure encrypted link (e.g., a security password) between the transmitter and receiver so that the receiver will only receive audio signals from the designated transmitter. This attribute is one of the primary advantages of modern digital radio frequency systems. In essence, once a transmitter and receiver are paired to one another, the system is immune from interference from other radio signals in the user's environment. Digital radio systems operate on a protocol, which is essentially a set of instructions that organizes and directs the exchange of information and audio signals between the transmitter and receiver. This protocol delineates the digital coding process that is utilized for data and audio signal delivery. During the transmission process, the first segment of the information that is transmitted is used to ensure that the receiver is communicating with the appropriate transmitter. Once the connection is confirmed, the digital protocol can be used to deliver audio information. Contemporary digital radio systems use a process known as frequency hopping spread spectrum, in which the exact carrier frequency of transmission within the 2.45-GHz band continuously and rapidly changes to prevent interference from other nearby radio devices. If conflicting information is simultaneously received from two different transmitters, then the receiver discards the signal to prevent the data. The rate of frequency hopping is so rapid, that momentary channel interference is typically imperceptible to the user. When conflicts exist, the receiver informs the transmitter, and that carrier frequency is avoided for future use. Some digital systems broadcast the same information simultaneously on multiple carrier frequencies in an effort to provide a redundant signal. As a result, if information on one carrier frequency is discarded, the user can still receive the information on another carrier frequency. Additionally, if all of the carrier frequencies used for transmission are occupied, then some of these systems utilize a technology referred to as package loss concealment (PLC) algorithm, which attempts to occupy the gap with the most likely fitting piece of audio.

It should be noted that variations exist among commercially available digital radio frequency systems. Bluetooth systems utilize digital radio frequency transmission on the 2.45-GHz band. The early versions of Bluetooth (versions 1.0–3.0) were plagued by high power consumption and long transmission delays, and as a result, they were unsuitable as a mode to directly transmit audio to a personal hearing instrument (Bluetooth, 2015). As a result, Bluetooth receivers were coupled with NFMI interfaces to allow for Bluetooth delivery of the signal from the transmitter to the interface and NFMI delivery from the interface to the hearing instrument.

Bluetooth 4.0 was recently introduced to allow for the wireless sharing of data with low power consumption. Bluetooth 4.0 was primarily developed to deliver data between personal electronic devices that operate on small, coin-size batteries (i.e., exchange of information from a wearable fitness armband to a mobile telephone). Bluetooth 4.0 cannot be used to stream audio signals (Bluetooth, 2015).

Hearing instrument manufacturers have recently introduced digital radio frequency systems that have overcome the problems typically associated with Bluetooth use with hearing aids. These systems use proprietary, closed platforms that exchange data and audio between transmitters and receivers that are designed to be coupled to the direct auditory input port of the hearing instrument or are integrated inside the hearing instruments (i.e., there is no need to couple an external radio receiver to the hearing instrument). Because these systems are not open platforms like Bluetooth, the power consumption and transmission delays are reduced. Most of these systems operate on the 2.45-GHz band, but one manufacturer also offers a proprietary system that operates on the 900-MHz band.

Finally, mobile telephone manufacturers have developed proprietary digital radio technology that can be used to transmit data and audio directly from a user's smart telephone to hearing instruments without the need for an external transmitter or interface device. These systems operate similar to low-power Bluetooth but also allow for the exchange of audio signals. Figure 27–8 provides an example of a "Made for iPhone hearing aid" (e.g., MFi) that utilizes this technology.

Advantages

- Modern systems are essentially immune to interference and noise from other systems.

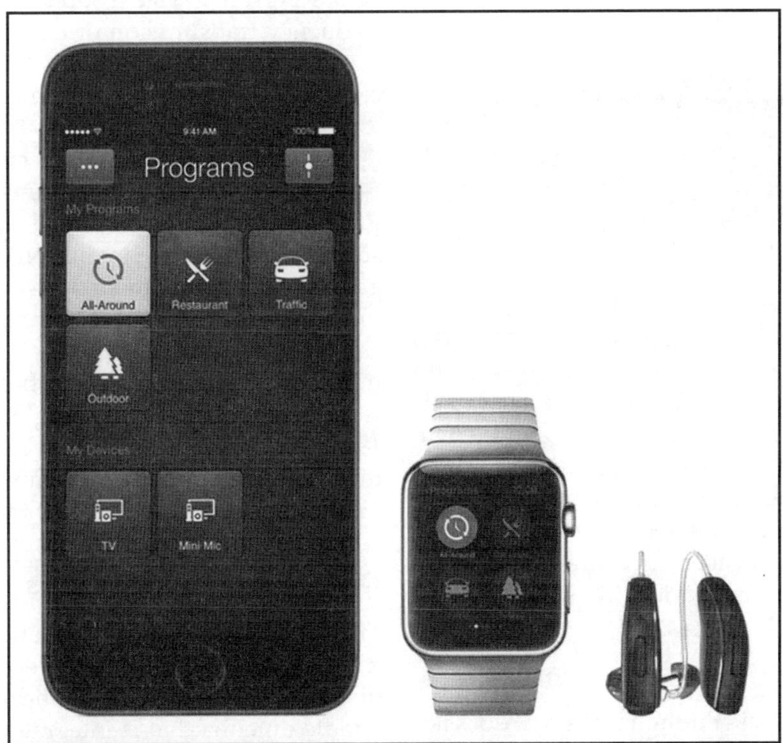

FIGURE 27–8. A Made for iPhone hearing aid and hearing assistance technology. Image courtesy of Resound.

- Digital control of the signal allows for an enhancement in the precision of the delivery of the audio signal of interest and also allows for refinement/manipulation of the signal; these characteristics allow for the potential to improve speech recognition and sound quality.
- These systems have wider bandwidth relative to analog FM systems.
- These systems enhance connectivity to personal consumer electronics such as mobile telephones, tablets, computers, and so on.

Disadvantages

- Digital RF systems are not universally available in public settings; in other words, induction neckloops are more likely to be found in public venues, because they are accessible to everyone who has a telecoil).
- The short wavelength of digital radio signals can cause signal dropouts when the system is used in areas without reflective surfaces (e.g., outside) and there is not a direct path between the transmitter and receiver.
- "Made for smartphone" technology is limited to certain models of mobile telephones.

Infrared Transmission

Infrared systems convert the audio signal captured at the remote microphone into an infrared light signal and transmit that signal to an infrared receiver where it is converted to an electrical signal suitable for processing by the hearing instrument or sound-field amplifier. Most infrared systems used with hearing technology operate on the 2.3- or 2.8-MHz carrier frequencies. Infrared technology is most commonly found in sound-field/classroom audio distribution systems. The audio signal captured at the remote microphone is delivered to a stationary infrared receiver that is strategically placed in the classroom (i.e., in a location where it can receive the infrared signal regardless of where the transmitter is located). Then, the signal is delivered from the infrared receiver to a receiver/amplifier that is hard-wired to loudspeakers that are strategically placed throughout the classroom.

Advantages

- The signal does not pass through walls so it does not produce interference across rooms; for this reason, infrared systems are often used in theaters and some classrooms.

Disadvantages

- Signal dropouts are possible in brightly lit environments.
- A direct line-of-sight is required between transmitter and receiver; for this reason, infrared systems are rarely used in contemporary personal remote microphone systems.

Types of Remote Microphone Systems

Remote microphone systems are available in several basic forms. There are two broad classes of remote microphone systems: personal remote microphone systems and sound-field remote microphone systems.

Personal Remote Microphone Systems

For personal remote microphone systems, the transmitted signal is delivered to a receiver that delivers the signal of interest directly to the user's personal hearing technology (e.g., hearing aid, cochlear implant, bone conduction device). The mode of delivery is variable across personal systems and typically includes radio frequency transmission or electromagnetic induction.

The primary objectives for use of a personal remote microphone system are to (a) improve the SNR, (b) reduce the deleterious effects of reverberation, and (c) compensate for the relatively long distance that often exists between the sound source and listener. Personal remote microphone systems provide substantial improvement in the SNR, ranging from as little as approximately 5 to 15 dB, when the remote microphones and hearing aid microphones are both active, to as great as approximately 15 to 25 dB when the remote microphone is active and the hearing aid microphone is disabled (Boothroyd & Iglehart, 1998; Hawkins, 1984). It should be noted that best practice for remote microphone use with children is to leave the hearing aid microphone active during remote microphone use.

Radio Frequency Systems

The signal of interest is delivered by radio frequency transmission to a radio receiver that is coupled to the direct auditory input of the hearing instrument or to a radio antenna that is integrated within the wearer's personal hearing technology. Figure 27–9 provides examples of personal remote microphone radio frequency systems.

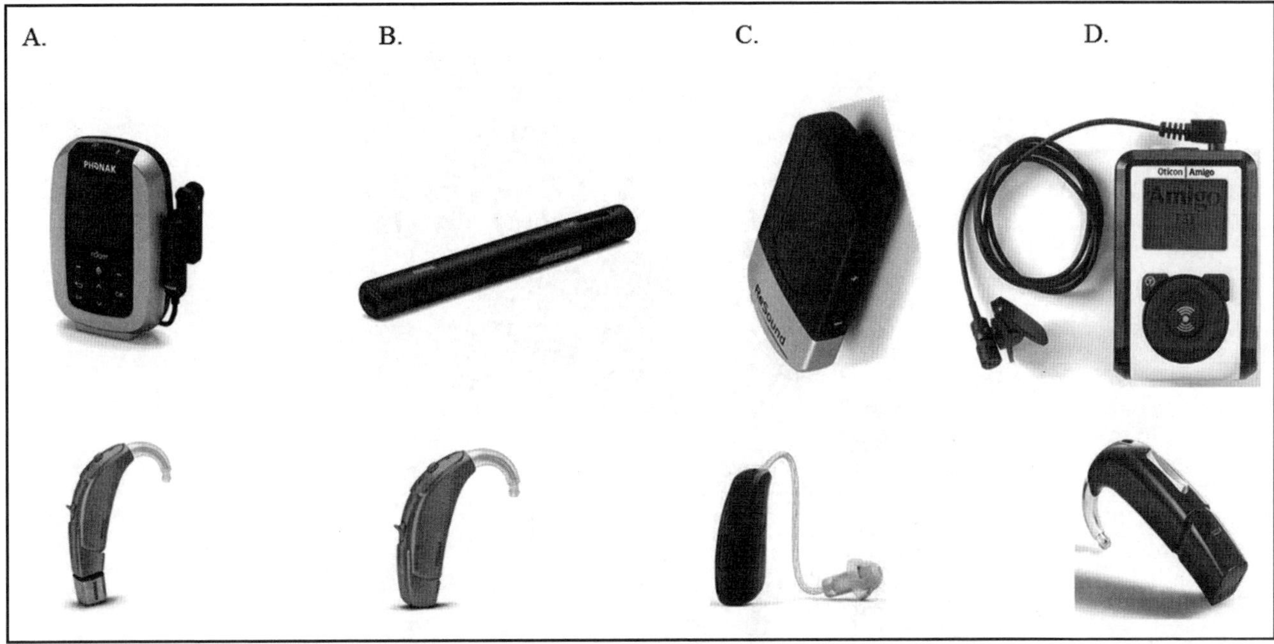

FIGURE 27–9. Personal remote microphone radio frequency systems. Image courtesy of Phonak and Oticon, Inc.

Electromagnetic Induction Systems

The audio signal of interest from the microphone or from another audio device (e.g., theatre sound system, television, computer, etc.) is delivered from a transmitter to a receiver via radio frequency or infrared transmission or by a hard-wired connection. The receiver amplifies the signal and delivers it in the form of an electrical current to a coiled loop that is installed around the periphery of the room. In some cases, the loop might only encompass a specific location within the room. As the electrical current, which is analogous to the audio signal, travels through the loop, electromagnetic lines of flux are emitted from the loop. These electromagnetic lines of flux propagate throughout the room and are captured by the telecoil of the user's personal hearing technology by way of electromagnetic induction. Figure 27–10 provides an example.

Personal Induction Neckloop Systems

The audio signal of interest is wirelessly delivered to a receiver (via radio frequency or infrared transmission) that is coupled to an induction loop that is worn around the neck. The personal receiver amplifies that transmitted signal of interest and delivers it to the neckloop where it is converted to electromagnetic lines of flux that are captured by the user's hearing instrument telecoil by way of electromagnetic induction. Figure 27–11 provides an example.

Sound-Field Remote Microphone Systems

Sound-field remote microphone systems/classroom audio distribution (CAD) systems deliver the audio signal from the remote microphone to a loudspeaker or loudspeakers that are strategically located throughout a room. The primary objective of a CAD system is to provide a uniform distribution of the audio signal of interest throughout the room. Achieving this objective can assist in overcoming the distance that might exist between the source of the signal of interest and the listener. Research has shown that CAD systems typically improve classroom SNR by 2 to 5 dB (Larsen & Blair, 2008; Massie & Dillon, 2006). Additionally, some studies have indicated that use of CAD systems can result in improvements in literacy development, standardized test scores, and classroom behavior, as well as a reduction in teacher absences (Chelius, 2004; Flexer & Long, 2003; Gertel, McCarty, & Schoff, 2004; Massie & Dillon, 2006; Massie, Theodoros, McPherson, & Smaldino, 2004). It should be noted that the audio signal delivered from a CAD system can originate from a remote microphone or from coupling to an audio output port of an electronic device in the room (e.g., classroom smart board, television, computer, etc.).

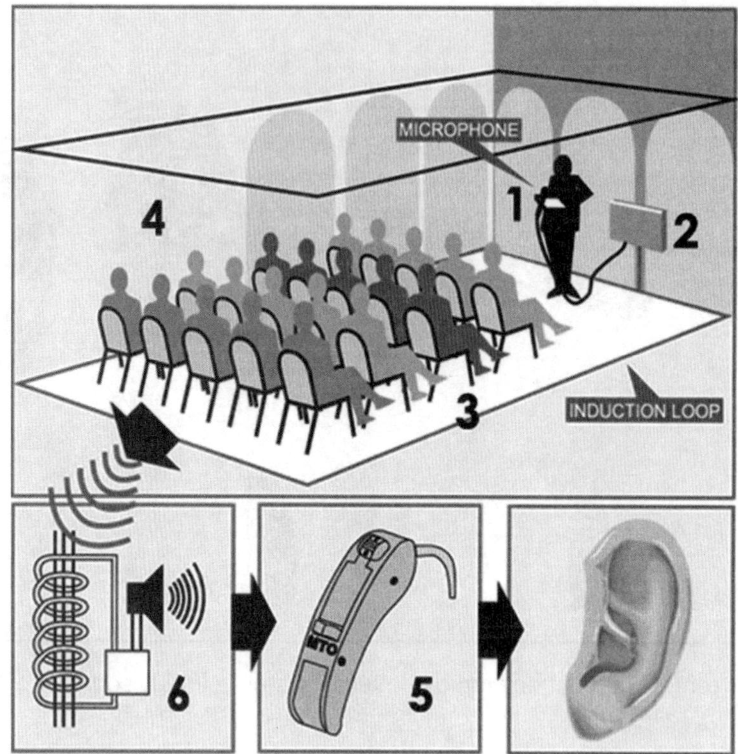

FIGURE 27–10. An induction room loop system. Image © copyright Ampetronic, Ltd. All rights reserved.

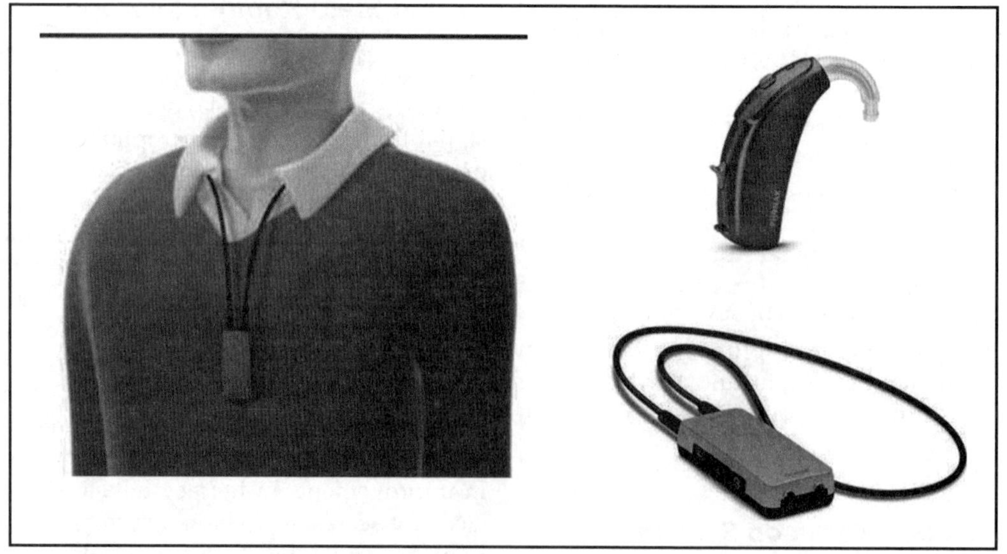

FIGURE 27–11. A personal induction neckloop system. Image courtesy of Lightspeed Technologies.

Examples of CAD systems are provided in Figure 27–12. As shown, CAD systems are available in several configurations. Some systems, like the examples shown in Figures 27–12A and 27–12B, contain a remote microphone, a receiver/amplifier, and several loudspeakers that can be strategically placed throughout

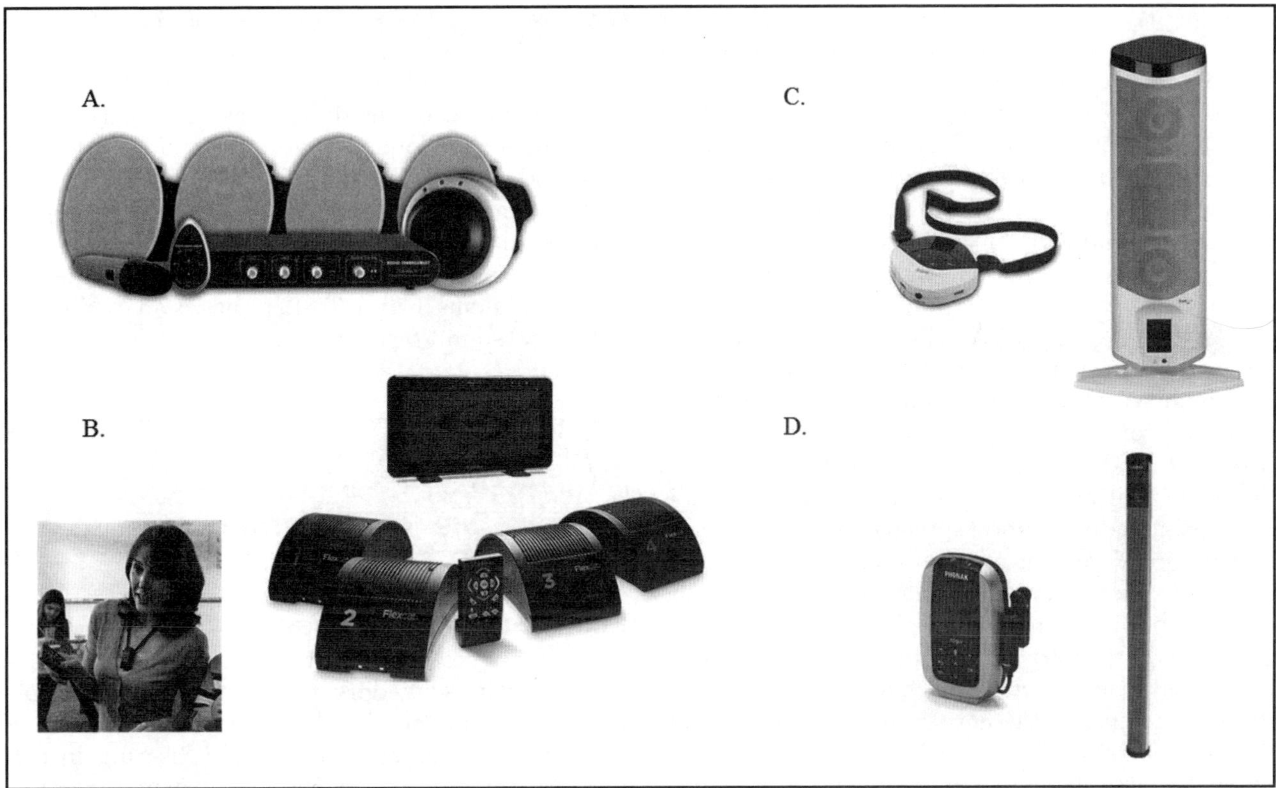

FIGURE 27–12. Commercially available classroom audio distribution systems. Image courtesy of Phonak and Audio Enhancement, Inc.

a classroom. Other CAD systems might contain only one or two loudspeakers (Figures 27–12C and 27–12D). It is important to clarify that some systems using one loudspeaker tower actually include an array of several loudspeakers within the tower. These loudspeakers are arranged in a manner designed to attempt to provide a uniform distribution of sound throughout a room with the use of the single tower. Single-tower CAD systems are intended to facilitate easier installation of the system in the typical classroom setting. Multiple loudspeaker systems require the loudspeakers to be anchored to the walls or ceiling, and cable must be run from the receiver/amplifier to the loudspeakers. This process is labor-intensive and requires technical expertise to yield an optimal outcome. CAD systems provide little to no improvement in speech recognition in classrooms with unfavorable acoustics (Wilson, Marinac, Pitty, & Burrows, 2011). The interested reader is referred to the American Academy of Audiology Clinical Practice Guideline for Remote Microphone Hearing Assistance Technologies for Children (Supplement B; AAA, 2011b) for more information on the proper selection, installation, and verification of CAD systems. The clinician should also refer to the CAD system manufacturer's installation instructions prior to installing a CAD system in a classroom.

It should be noted that a variety of different types of loudspeakers can be found in modern CAD systems including cone/piston-motion loudspeakers, flat panel/forced resonance loudspeakers, and line array loudspeakers. The interested reader is referred to an excellent article from Ostergren (2013) that nicely summarizes classroom acoustics and CAD systems. An example of a cone loudspeaker is shown in Figure 27–12A. A cone loudspeaker possesses a good dynamic range with a wide bandwidth, but it tends to be fairly directional in its projection of sound, particularly at higher frequencies. As a result, CAD systems using this type of loudspeaker typically include several cone loudspeakers positioned throughout the classroom in order to provide relatively uniform coverage of the speech frequency range throughout the classroom (Ostegren, 2013).

Flat panel/forced resonance transducers operate in a similar fashion to a tuning fork vibrating on the surface of a table. In other words, the entire surface oscillates across the speech frequency range. Flat panel/forced resonance transducers typically distribute the audio signal in a nondirectional manner. The latter property allows for a fairly uniform distribution of sound across the classroom, so multiple flat panel/forced resonance units are typically unnecessary. However, it should be noted that flat panel/forced resonance systems might not possess as wide a dynamic range as cone loudspeakers, and they might be limited in their delivery of audio signals in the very low-frequency and very high-frequency portions of the speech frequency range (Ostegren, 2013).

Line array systems actually possess several cone loudspeakers that are arranged in a straight line (typically in the vertical plane). Because they are composed of several cone loudspeakers, line array systems possess a wide dynamic range and wide bandwidth. The vertical arrangement of the cone loudspeakers is intended to reduce vertical spread of the audio signal, which should reduce reverberations introduced by the CAD system. At the same time, distribution of the audio signal in the horizontal plane should be sufficient. This property of a line array loudspeaker system is reported to allow for a long range of distribution of the audio signal in the horizontal plane throughout the classroom. Because vertical spread is limited, it is imperative that the height of the line array system be positioned near the head level of the students in the classroom (Ostegren, 2013).

Personal Sound-Field (Desktop) Systems

Personal sound-field systems (also referred to as desktop sound-field systems) are composed of a remote microphone that captures the audio signal of interest and delivers it (via radio frequency or infrared transmission) to a small loudspeaker that is positioned within a couple of feet from the listener. The loudspeaker of a desktop system, which is sometimes informally referred to as a "sound in a box" system, is typically placed on the desk of the listener. The close proximity of the loudspeaker to the child is intended to provide a more favorable SNR than a CAD system and to overcome the distance between the signal source and the child. There are no published studies that have formally examined the SNR improvement provided by desktop systems. Figure 27–13 provides an example of a personal sound-field system.

Remote Microphone Technology Characteristics That Influence Performance

Fixed-Gain Versus Adaptive Systems

Receiver gain is an adjustable parameter that controls the strength of the signal delivered from a remote microphone receiver to a listener's hearing instrument or from a CAD system loudspeaker. Generally, increases in receiver gain result in an increase in the output of the signal from the remote microphone system. Most remote microphone systems contain fixed-gain receivers meaning that the output of the remote microphone signal is static regardless of the ambient noise level. Typically, the gain of a fixed-gain remote microphone system is set so that the output of the signal captured at the remote microphone is higher than the output of the signal captured at the microphone of the hearing instrument. Prior to the advent of nonlinear (e.g., wide dynamic range compression) hearing aids,

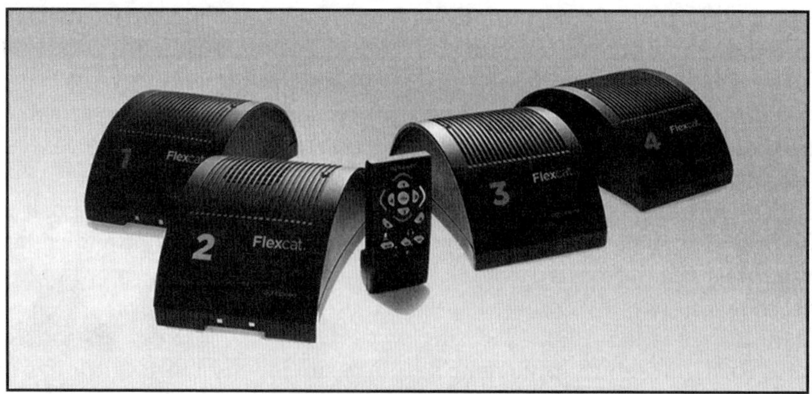

FIGURE 27–13. Example of a commercially available personal desktop loudspeaker system. Image courtesy of Lightspeed Technologies.

professional guidelines suggest that the output of a linear-gain hearing instrument should be 10 dB greater for an 85 dB SPL signal delivered to the remote microphone relative to the output measured for a 65 dB SPL signal delivered to the hearing instrument microphone (ASHA, 2002). This was often referred to as a +10 dB FM advantage. Because virtually every modern hearing instrument possesses nonlinear amplitude compression, the goal of obtaining a 10 dB FM advantage as measured with subsequent electroacoustic measurements is no longer appropriate. Electroacoustic verification of remote microphone systems will be discussed later in this chapter.

It should be noted that the 10 dB FM advantage is unlikely to be ideal for every situation a listener might encounter. Specifically, in a quiet environment, while listening to one's own voice or to speech that is not directed to the remote microphone, it is possible that the user might prefer less than a 10 dB FM advantage. In contrast, the listener might require an FM advantage that is much higher than +10 dB when listening to speech directed to the remote microphone in an environment with high-level noise (Lewis & Eiten, 2004). In other words, the desired FM receiver gain (or FM advantage) likely varies as a function of the competing noise level and the signal of interest.

In recognition of this dilemma, adaptive remote microphone systems were developed. Adaptive systems, which are also referred to as dynamic systems, automatically increase the receiver gain of the remote microphone system with increases in the ambient noise level. Figure 27–14 provides a visual representation of the function of an adaptive system. As shown, without a remote microphone system, the SNR systematically decreases with increases in the ambient noise level. The provision of a fixed-gain remote microphone system provides an improvement in the SNR, the magnitude of which is constant, regardless of the competing noise level. As can be seen in this example, when the ambient noise level approaches 65 dB SPL, the SNR reaches single-digit values. As previously mentioned, persons with hearing loss (especially children with hearing loss) require at least a 15 dB SNR for effective communication. As the ambient noise level exceeds 57 dB SPL, the adaptive system automatically increases receiver gain in an attempt to provide a robust SNR over a wide range of competing noise levels. Theoretically, the automatic increases in gain provided by adaptive

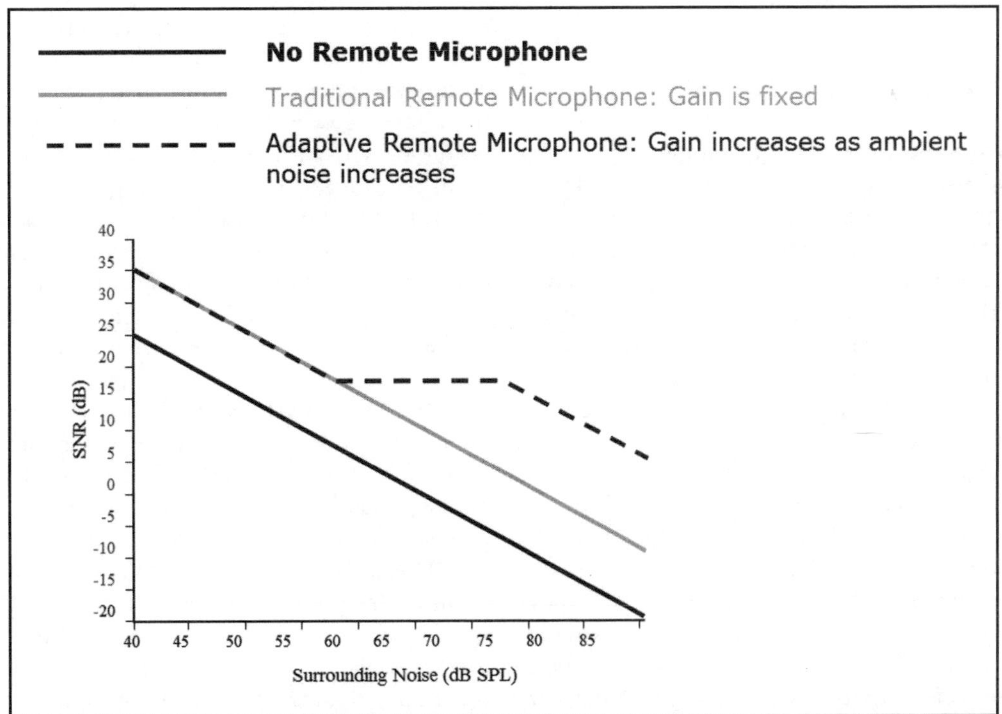

FIGURE 27–14. The SNR obtained without remote microphone use, with use of a fixed-gain personal remote microphone system, and the use of an adaptive personal remote microphone system. Image courtesy of Phonak.

systems should provide better speech recognition in moderate- to high-level noise when compared to performance obtained with fixed gain systems.

Adaptive remote microphone technology was first introduced in an analog FM system. Wolfe et al. (2009) evaluated sentence recognition in a group of 25 adult and pediatric cochlear implant recipients and reported mean improvements in sentence recognition of up to 50 percentage points at moderate-to-high noise levels with use of adaptive remote microphone systems relative to performance with fixed-gain systems. Likewise, Thibodeau (2010) compared sentence recognition in noise for fixed-gain and adaptive remote microphone systems used by five children and five adults who had moderate-to-severe hearing loss. She reported improvements in sentence recognition ranging from 20 to 40 percentage points when adaptive remote microphone technology was used rather than the fixed gain system. Furthermore, after a field trial in which subjects used the remote microphone during everyday activities (e.g., classroom, museum, etc.), eight of nine participants expressed a strong preference for using the adaptive system over the use of the fixed-gain personal system.

Take-home point: The use of adaptive remote microphone technology provides better speech recognition in moderate- to high-level noise when compared to performance with fixed-gain systems.

Digital Versus Analog Systems

The basic operation of digital and analog FM radio systems was discussed earlier in this chapter. There are only a handful of studies that have examined the potential performance differences obtained with digital versus analog FM personal remote microphone systems. Aslund, Olsson, Skagerstrand, and Dahlstrom (2011) evaluated 20 hearing aid wearers who were assessed with each of three personal remote microphone systems: (a) an adaptive, analog FM receiver that was directly coupled to the DAI of the hearing aid (i.e., Phonak ZoomLink+ transmitter with Phonak MLXi receiver); (b) an adaptive, analog FM receiver that was coupled to an electromagnetic induction neckloop that delivered the remote microphone signal to the telecoil of participants' hearing aids (Phonak ZoomLink+ transmitter with Phonak MyLink+ receiver/neckloop); and (c) a digital, fixed gain personal remote microphone receiver that was coupled to an electromagnetic induction neckloop that delivered the remote microphone signal to the telecoil of participants' hearing aids (Comfort Audio DC20 transmitter with DH10 receiver). Speech perception in quiet and in the presence of low-level noise was similar between the three systems. However, at higher competing noise levels (70 to 80 dBA), both of the adaptive, analog FM systems provided better performance than the fixed-gain, digital system. Additionally, the directly coupled adaptive system provided better performance than the adaptive, induction neckloop system at higher competing noise levels. The better performance observed with the adaptive systems is likely attributed to the automatic increases in receiver gain provided at higher competing noise levels. This finding indicates that digital radio systems do not necessarily provide better performance than analog FM radio systems.

Subsequent studies have evaluated speech recognition obtained with adaptive, analog FM systems versus adaptive digital systems. Wolfe et al. (Wolfe, Morais, Schafer, Mills, & Mülder, 2013; Wolfe, Morais, Schafer, Mills, Peters, et al., 2013) evaluated sentence recognition in quiet and in diffuse uncorrelated classroom noise with 44 cochlear implant recipients who were assessed in a classroom environment. Hearing performance was compared across four conditions: (a) cochlear implant alone (no remote microphone system); (b) a fixed-gain, analog FM personal system (Phonak MLxS); (c) an adaptive, analog FM personal system (Phonak MLxi); and (d) an adaptive, digital personal system (Phonak Roger). All three remote microphone systems provided better performance than what was obtained with the cochlear implant alone. At higher competing noise levels (70 to 80 dBA), the adaptive systems allowed for better performance than the fixed-gain remote microphone system. Finally, at moderate-to-high competing noise levels (65 to 80 dBA), the digital, adaptive system allowed for better speech recognition than what was obtained with the analog FM, adaptive system. For instance, at a competing noise level of 75 dBA, participants with Advanced Bionics cochlear implants obtained a mean improvement of 25 percentage points with use of the digital, adaptive system relative to their performance with the analog, FM system. The researchers attributed the better performance obtained with the digital system to the better precision of control over adaptive gain changes provided by digital signal processing.

Thibodeau (2014) also evaluated sentence recognition in quiet and in noise for a group of 11 adult hearing aid users with mild to severe hearing loss. Performance was evaluated across three conditions: (a) a fixed-gain, analog FM personal system (Phonak MLxS); (b) an adaptive, analog FM personal system (Phonak MLxi); and (c) an adaptive, digital personal system (Phonak Roger). Use of the adaptive systems provided significantly better speech recognition in high-level noise when compared to performance with the fixed-gain, analog FM system. Also, sentence recognition in noise was significantly better with use of the digital, adaptive system when compared to performance with the analog FM, adaptive system. At a competing noise level of 75 dBA, use of the digital system provided a mean improvement of 35 percentage points compared to performance with the analog FM, adaptive system.

Take-home Point: Research evaluating digital radio frequency remote microphone systems has shown the use of digital radio does not guarantee an improvement in speech recognition compared to performance obtained with analog FM systems. However, through the implementation of sophisticated signal processing, digital radio systems possess the potential to improve hearing performance beyond what is obtained with analog FM technology.

Advantages and Limitations of Personal, CAD Systems, and Personal Desktop Remote Microphone Systems

The relative merits of personal, CAD, and personal desktop remote microphone systems are as follows. Previous studies have suggested that personal remote microphone systems provide a greater improvement in the SNR relative to personal desktop and CAD systems (Anderson & Goldstein, 2004; Anderson et al., 2005; Schafer & Kleineck, 2009; Wolfe, Morais, Neumann, et al., 2013). However, personal remote microphone systems are often the most expensive option of the three, and they only are used by and provide benefit for the child with hearing loss. CAD systems most likely provide the poorest improvement in SNR of the three different types of systems, but one virtue of a CAD system is that it potentially provides better access to the primary audio signal of interest to every student in the classroom. Universal benefit associated with the use of CAD systems might reduce the negative stigma children with hearing loss might feel when a personal remote microphone system is only used to assist the child with hearing technology. Personal desktop systems are unlikely to provide an improvement in the SNR rivaling that provided by a personal system, but the improvement in SNR might be better that what is obtained with a CAD system. However, personal desktop systems do not benefit every child in the classroom, and the student might not have enough space in his or her work area (e.g., desk) to accommodate the small loudspeaker used in this system. Also, personal desktop systems might be awkward for the child to move from classroom to classroom, and CAD and personal desktop systems might not be as flexible for use across multiple activities (e.g., extracurricular activities at school or for home/outside-of-school use).

There are only a small number of peer-reviewed studies that have compared speech recognition obtained with CAD systems, personal desktop systems, and personal RF systems. Anderson and Goldstein (2004) evaluated speech recognition in noise for eight children (9–12 years old) who had mild-to-severe hearing loss and who used a personal FM system, a personal desktop system, and a CAD system. The researchers reported that the CAD system did not provide a significant improvement in speech recognition, but the personal desktop and personal FM systems each provided a statistically significant improvement in speech recognition in noise. Most subjects achieved ceiling-level performance with use of both the personal FM and personal desktop systems, and consequently, there were no differences in performance between the two.

Anderson et al. (2005) also compared speech recognition obtained with a personal FM, personal desktop, and CAD system for 28 children (8–14 years old) who used hearing aids or cochlear implants. Overall, the children performed better with the three different remote microphone systems than they did with their hearing aids or cochlear implant alone. However, subjects scored better with the personal FM and personal desktop systems than they did with the CAD system.

Schafer and Kleineck (2009) conducted a meta-analysis of studies that have examined speech recognition benefit obtained from personal systems, CAD systems, and personal desktop systems for cochlear implant recipients. They identified nine studies in which speech recognition of cochlear implant users was evaluated with and without the three different types of remote microphone technologies. They reported that use of CAD systems resulted in a nonsignificant 3.5 percentage point improvement in speech recognition when compared to performance with the cochlear implant alone. In contrast, speech recognition improved by a statistically significant 17 percentage points with use of personal desktop systems and by a mean of 38 percentage points with use of personal FM technology.

Wolfe, Morais, Neumann, and colleagues (2013) also evaluated speech recognition in 15 children with normal hearing, 15 children with mild-to-moderate hearing loss, and 10 adults using two different types of CADS, a fixed-gain infrared system with four loudspeakers located at the interquartile locations on the side walls of the examination room (Audio Enhancement

Elite II) and an adaptive (e.g., Dynamic), digital radio frequency, single-tower CAD system (Phonak Digimaster 5000 Dynamic Sound-Field System; Figure 27–15). The Phonak system contains a single tower array of 12 loudspeakers that are arranged along the vertical axis of the tower in an attempt to provide a uniform distribution of sound across the classroom and to reduce reverberation from the signal delivered by the CAD systems. The Audio Enhancement Elite II CAD system contains four wall-mounted double-cone loudspeakers that receive the signal of interest from an infrared sensor that is hard-wired to the loudspeakers. Sentence recognition in quiet and in noise was evaluated for all three groups of subjects with and without the use of the CAD systems. Additionally, the sentence recognition of the children with hearing loss was evaluated while they used a personal adaptive (e.g., Dynamic) FM system with Phonak MLxi FM receivers connected to the DAI of their hearing aids. Finally, hearing performance was also evaluated as these children simultaneously used the personal FM system along with each of the CAD systems. When the personal FM system was used with the Phonak CAD system, the Phonak inspiro transmitter was used to simultaneously deliver the audio signal from the transmitter to both the personal FM receiver and to the Phonak CAD system. When the personal FM system was simultaneously used with the Audio Enhancement CAD system, the test signals were delivered to the remote microphone of the Audio Enhancement CAD system and then presented through each of the four Audio Enhancement CAD system loudspeakers. Also, the Phonak inspiro transmitter was coupled to the audio output port of the Audio Enhancement receiver/amplifier, so that the test signals were also delivered to the personal FM receivers by way of the Phonak inspiro transmitter.

Several relevant findings were observed in the Wolfe, Morais, Neumann, et al. (2013) study. First, the adults with normal hearing performed better than both groups of children. In particular, at a +5 dB SNR, the adult group scored about eight percentage points better than children with normal hearing and almost 30 percentage points better than the children with hearing loss. Second, all three groups of participants obtained significant improvement in sentence recognition in noise with use of each of the CAD systems. Specifically, at a 0 dB SNR, sentence recognition was almost 30 percentage points better with use of the CAD system when compared to performance without remote microphone technology. Third, sentence recognition at moderate-to-high competing noise levels (65–75 dBA) was significantly better with the single-tower adaptive CAD system when compared to the multiple-loudspeaker, fixed-gain CAD system. The improvement in speech recognition obtained with the adaptive CAD system was primarily attributed to the increases in CAD system output level that automatically occur with increases in ambient noise level. Fourth, for the children with hear-

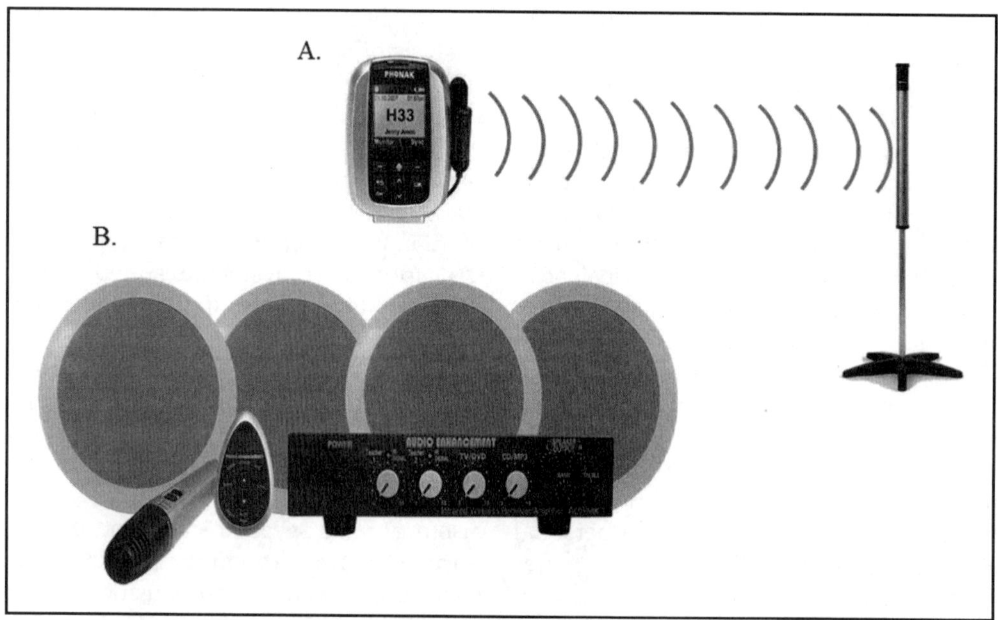

FIGURE 27–15. Classroom audio distribution systems evaluated in the Wolfe, Morais, Neumann, et al. (2013) study. Image courtesy of Phonak and Audio Enhancement, Inc.

ing loss, sentence recognition obtained with use of the personal adaptive FM system was significantly better than performance obtained with either of the CAD systems. For example, sentence recognition with the personal adaptive FM system exceeded performance with a CAD system by almost 20 and 50 percentage points at a 0 and −5 dB SNR, respectively. Fifth, no improvement in sentence recognition was obtained with simultaneous use of a CAD system and an adaptive personal FM system relative to performance with a personal FM system alone. Finally, performance with simultaneous use of the adaptive personal FM system and the Audio Enhancement CAD system was significantly poorer than performance with use of the personal FM alone. It was noted that the adaptive gain changes, and the directional properties of the microphone of the personal FM system were eliminated when the transmitter of the personal system was hard-wired to the receiver/amplifier of the multiple loudspeaker, fixed-gain CAD system.

The collective results of the aforementioned studies can be summarized as follows:

- CAD systems possess the potential to improve speech recognition.
- Adaptive CAD systems might provide better speech recognition in the presence of high-level noise than what can be obtained with fixed-gain CAD systems.
- Personal remote microphone systems provide better speech recognition than what might be obtained with use of a CAD system.
- The combined use of a personal remote microphone system and a CAD system provides very little improvement in speech recognition over the use of the personal system alone. However, simultaneous use of a CAD system and a personal system might be beneficial, because use of CAD systems has been associated with better classroom behavior and lower-levels of classroom ambient noise (Massie & Dillon, 2006; Rubin, Aquino-Rusell, & Flagg-Williams, 2007), factors that will likely improve the hearing performance of a child with hearing loss.
- Clinicians must exercise caution when endorsing the simultaneous use of a personal remote microphone system and a CAD system. Hard-wiring the transmitter of a personal remote microphone system to the audio output port of a CAD system might degrade the performance obtained with the personal system alone. When using a personal system and a CAD system that are designed by different manufacturers and specifically developed to interface with one another, the best solution might be for the teacher to use the microphone/transmitter of each system simultaneously (AAA, 2011). One manufacturer has created a system that allows for the output of an adaptive personal system to be simultaneously delivered to the personal receiver and to the audio input port of the CAD system of other manufacturers. This solution allows for the CAD system to function as an adaptive system.

Technology Present in the Transmitter of Modern Remote Microphone Systems

The technology present in the microphone and transmitter of modern remote microphone systems varies widely across manufacturers. The transmitters of most contemporary audio streaming accessories are coupled to an omnidirectional microphone (Figure 27–16). In contrast, many personal remote microphone systems available today possess directional microphones with the intent to focus on the speech signal from the primary talker and attenuate surrounding noise (Figure 27–17). Furthermore, some of the personal remote microphone systems allow for the user to switch between directional polar plot patterns to optimize performance for a variety of uses. For instance, an omnidirectional microphone response might be selected if the transmitter is going to be placed on a conference room table in an attempt to capture the speech of everyone in attendance around the table. In contrast, a highly directional response might be selected if the microphone is going to be pointed toward the mouth of a talker. Finally, remote microphone transmitters might also possess sensors that detect the transmitter's orientation in space (e.g., gyroscope, accelerometer) in order to select the microphone polar plot pattern that is most appropriate for a situation automatically. In other words, if the transmitter is laid flat on a table (i.e., "conference mode"), the omnidirectional response is selected. If the transmitter is positioned in the vertical plane (e.g., "lavalier mode"), the directional response is selected.

Numerous other signal processing differences exist in modern remote microphone transmitters. Some systems feature numerous signal processing options such as digital noise reduction, speech enhancement, and automatic voice activation, and others provide little to no processing to the input signal other than input compression limiting. Some transmitters contain manual volume/sensitivity controls that allow the user to adjust the emphasis that is placed on the signal captured at the microphone. Additionally, some transmitters allow the user to conduct diagnostic assessments

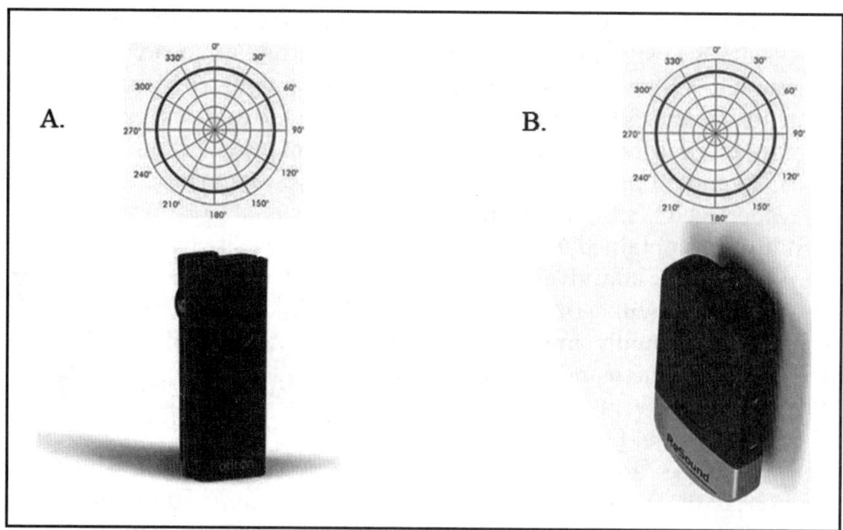

FIGURE 27–16. A remote microphone transmitter that possesses an omnidirectional response pattern. Image courtesy of Oticon, Inc. and Resound.

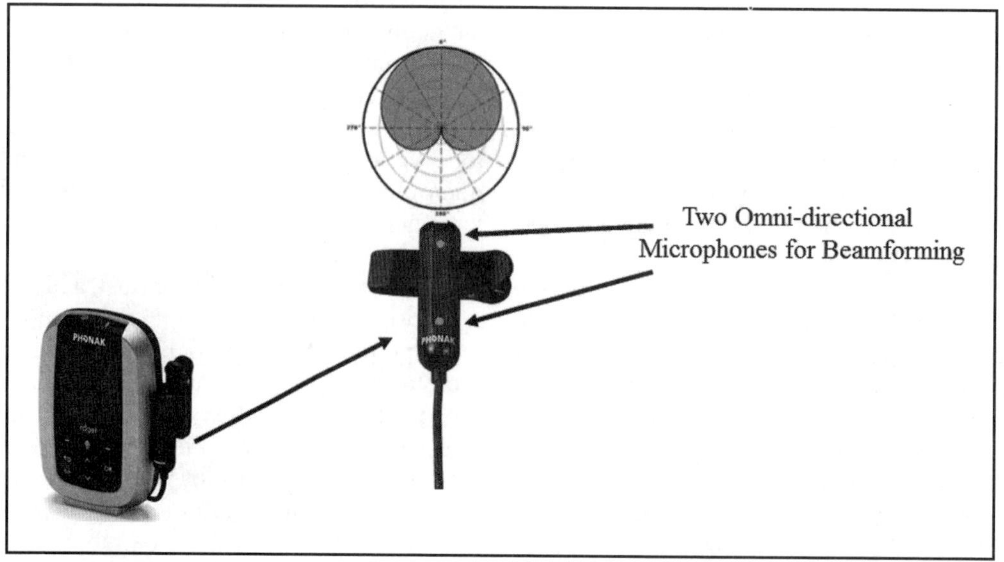

FIGURE 27–17. A remote microphone transmitter that possesses a directional response pattern. Image courtesy of Phonak.

in order to confirm that the signal is being delivered to and received from the remote microphone receiver. Furthermore, some transmitters operate on fixed, analog FM channels, and others allow the user to switch between a variety of analog FM channels. Many contemporary transmitters no longer use analog FM, but instead transmit only digital radio signals. In fact, there is at least one transmitter that allows for delivery of both digital and analog FM radio signals. Finally, some transmitters are programmable allowing the clinician to adjust settings to suit the unique needs of individual users, and other transmitters are not adjustable or can be adjusted through manual control of push buttons or screw-set potentiometers.

Remote microphone transmitters can also be configured with microphones designed to be worn in a variety of different positions. For many systems, the microphone is built into the body of the transmitter, and the entire unit is intended to be clipped on the talker's collar, lapel, or shirt pocket (e.g., lavalier style;

Figure 27–18A). It is important to remember that lavalier-worn microphones should be positioned no more than 6 to 8 in (15.24–20.32 cm) from the mouth. For directional microphones, care should be taken to orient the directional axis of the microphone toward the talker's mouth. Other systems contain a lavalier, clip-on microphone that is attached to the transmitter by a cable (Figure 27–18B). In many cases, this cable also serves as the antenna for the transmitter, which provides a longer transmission range. Finally, some transmitters are coupled by a cable to a "boom" microphone, which is positioned in close proximity to the mouth of the talker (Figure 27–18C). Boom microphones are advantageous because they capture the talker's voice near the source, preserving the integrity of the speech signal. They also reduce the likelihood that the microphone will be positioned too far away from the mouth. Furthermore, they are not susceptible to fluctuations in signal intensity as the talker's head moves, because the microphone moves with the head. Some talkers might be reluctant to use a boom mic, because they feel it is uncomfortable to wear on the head.

Many remote microphone systems feature access to multiple microphones to allow the listener to attend to multiple talkers. For instance, some systems include "pass-around microphones," that are typically hand-held microphones that accompany the primary microphone worn by the classroom teacher. Figure 27–19 provides examples of a "pass-around microphone." Pass-around microphones can be used in situations in

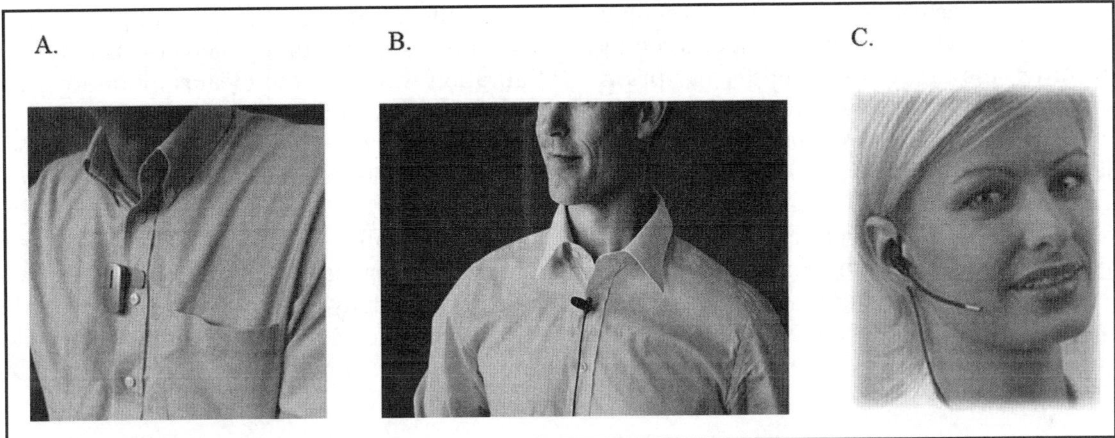

FIGURE 27–18. Examples of different wearing configurations for remote microphones. Image courtesy of Phonak.

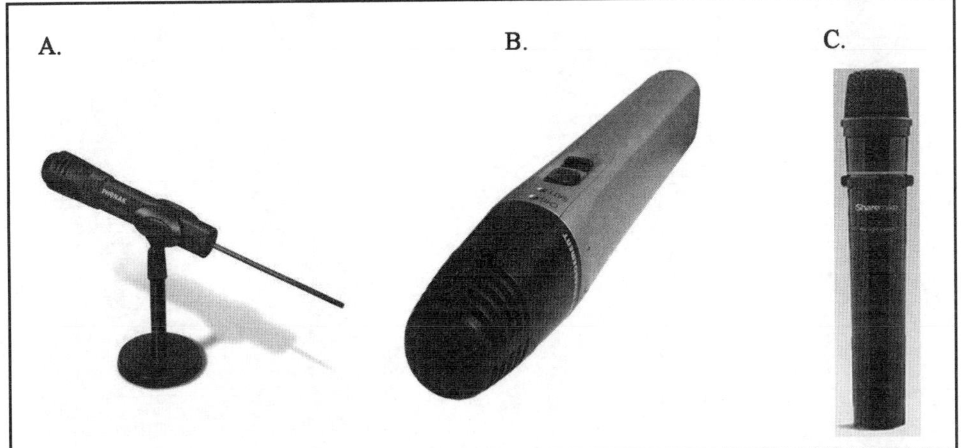

FIGURE 27–19. A "pass-around" microphone that may be used with remote microphone hearing assistance technology. Image courtesy of Phonak, Lightspeed Technologies, and Audio Enhancement, Inc.

which it is important to hear the speech of other students (e.g., group reading time). Pass-around microphones can also be used by a teacher's assistant or in situations in which classrooms have more than one teacher. Some manufacturers also have developed networks in which an array of transmitters can be used within one classroom or setting. Figure 27–20 provides an example of a "multi-talker network" that features several clip-on microphones that can be wirelessly grouped together to allow a listener to have access to multiple talkers in a room. Within a multitalker network, one transmitter is designated as the primary transmitter and is paired to the receiver of the listener's hearing technology. This primary transmitter is then paired to one or more secondary transmitters. Once pairing between the primary and secondary transmitters is complete, the signal captured at each transmitter can be delivered to the listener's receivers. When multiple signals are simultaneously present at more than one transmitter, the primary transmitter has priority in transmitting its signal. If multiple signals are simultaneously present across more than one secondary transmitter, then the transmitter that initially received a signal receives priority.

When discussing multitalker networks, it is important to mention that personal remote microphone systems can be configured in a number of ways. A "point-to-point" system is one that only allows for transmission of the audio signal from one transmitter to one receiver. A multipoint-to-point system allows for transmission of the audio signal from several transmitters/microphones to one receiver. This type of system might be advantageous in a classroom in which there is only one child with hearing loss who needs to hear multiple teachers or a teacher and multiple students/peers. As previously mentioned, this type of system has recently gained popularity in situations in which a child with hearing loss is included in a typical classroom setting with children with normal auditory function.

A point-to-multipoint system allows for transmission of the audio signal from one transmitter to multiple receivers. An example of this type of configuration would be found in a classroom where one teacher uses a microphone that transmits an audio signal to several children who are using personal receivers. Finally, a multipoint-to-multipoint system allows for transmission of the audio signal from multiple microphones/transmitters to multiple receivers. This type of configuration would be the ideal solution for classrooms with multiple children with hearing loss, as they could have access to the speech of multiple teachers as well as their peers who could also use remote microphones, as needed.

Additionally, some transmitters allow for access to signals other than what are captured at the remote microphone. Many transmitters possess an audio input port, which allows for the transmitter to receive audio signals from consumer electronics (e.g., computer, class-

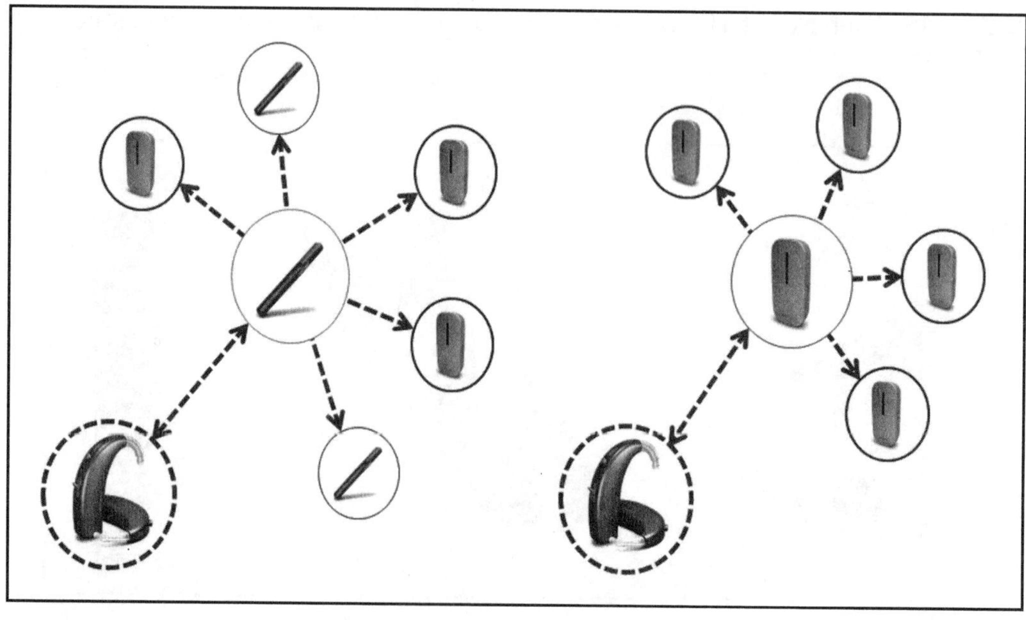

FIGURE 27–20. A remote microphone hearing technology multitalker network. Image courtesy of Phonak.

room smartboard, mobile telephone, etc.) by coupling to its audio output port via an auxiliary audio cable. Also, some transmitters are equipped with Bluetooth technology to allow for wireless coupling to Bluetooth-enabled consumer electronics. These systems allow the user to converse over smart mobile telephones through the remote microphone system or to wirelessly receive other audio signals from Bluetooth-enabled devices.

Technology Present in Receivers of Modern Remote Microphone Systems

There are also numerous differences in the technology present in modern remote microphone receivers available from different manufacturers. As previously mentioned, some receivers are fixed-gain systems, and others are adaptive. The gain of many contemporary fixed-gain receivers can be adjusted by the clinician via programmable software or adjustment of push buttons or screw-set potentiometers to meet a user's individual needs. Some transmitters possess fixed channels of transmission, and other receivers contain adjustable transmission frequencies. Additionally, some transmitters feature LED lights that alert caregivers to the function/status of the system. Receiver design can be universal—that is, intended to be coupled to the DAI of a hearing aid or cochlear implant sound processor by way of an interface known as a shoe or boot (Figure 27–21). In contrast, design-integrated receivers are developed for a particular make and model of hearing instrument in an attempt to enhance the aesthetics, size, and comfort of the receiver (Figure 27–22). Finally, some receivers are built completely into the body of the hearing aid or cochlear implant sound processor. These receivers typically operate at high carrier frequencies (e.g., 900 MHz, 2.45 GHz) and consist of a small strip of copper printed onto the casing of the processor/device.

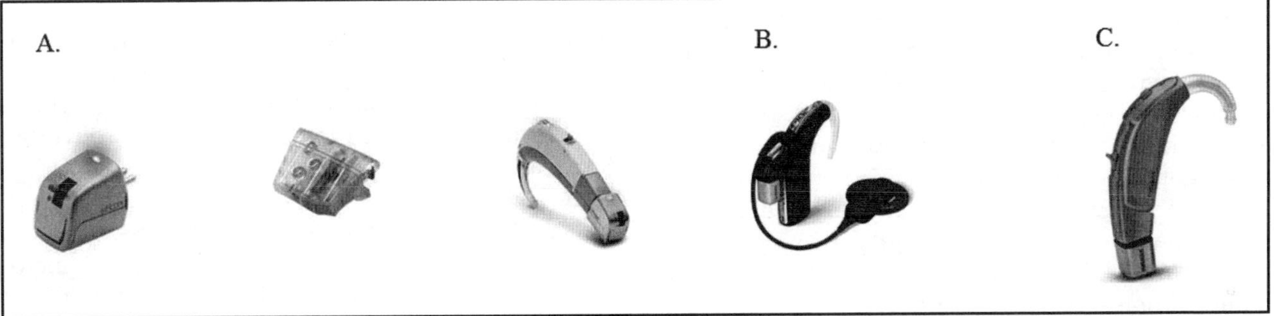

FIGURE 27–21. Universal radio frequency receivers coupled to personal hearing instruments by way of a boot/shoe. Image courtesy of Phonak and Oticon, Inc.

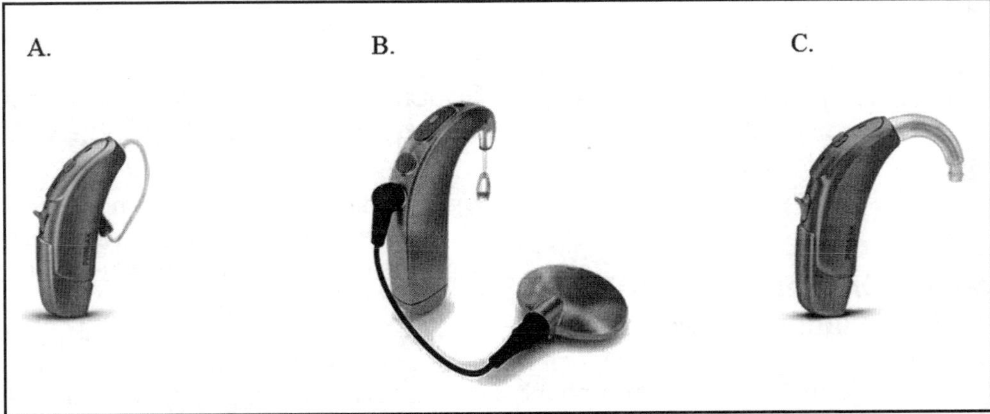

FIGURE 27–22. Design-integrated radio frequency receivers. Image courtesy of Phonak.

Additional Considerations Pertaining to the Design and Operation of Remote Microphone Technology

Advantages and Limitations of Personal Remote Microphone Systems and Audio Streaming Accessories

There are very few studies examining performance differences obtained between digital adaptive remote microphone systems, and digital remote microphone accessory devices. Wolfe, Duke, and Schafer (2015) evaluated speech recognition for a group of 18 adults with moderate sloping to severe to profound hearing loss with use of a digital adaptive personal remote microphone system and a digital audio streaming accessory remote microphone system. There were no differences in sentence recognition obtained with the two technologies in quiet or at low competing noise levels, but at competing noise levels of 65 and 75 dBA, use of the adaptive remote microphone system resulted in an average improvement in sentence recognition scores of 14 and 40 percentage points, respectively, relative to performance obtained with the digital accessory device. The better performance observed at higher competing noise levels was primarily attributed to the automatic increases in gain provided by the adaptive system but might also have been partially due to the directional microphone and digital noise reduction present in the adaptive system. Although performance at higher noise levels was better with use of the adaptive system, it is important to note that the digital audio streaming accessory system does possess its own relative advantages. The streaming accessory system is less expensive than most personal digital remote microphone systems, and the radio receiver is built into the hearing instrument and does not require a separate receiver to be coupled to the DAI. The proper choice of technology will depend on individual needs and a number of other personal factors, including difficulty with hearing performance in noise, frequency in which the user communicates in noisy situations, budget, ease of use, and acceptable cosmetics.

Directly Coupled DAI Receivers and Personal Neckloop Induction Systems

The use of directly coupled DAI remote microphone receivers allows for better hearing performance when compared to performance obtained with personal neckloop induction systems (Wolfe, Schafer, Parkinson, et al., 2013). These findings are most likely due to a loss in sensitivity of the signal when it is delivered from the induction neckloop to the telecoil of the hearing instrument. Many modern hearing aids are equipped with telecoils that are oriented to be most sensitive for telephone use, and as a result, they are less sensitive to loop systems. Also, use of telecoils and induction neckloop systems can increase the likelihood that the user encounters noise or interference from nearby electromagnetic sources (e.g., fluorescent lights, computer monitors, etc.). However, it should be noted that use of an induction neckloop requires the purchase of only one receiver (i.e., the receiver coupled to the neckloop) rather than two receivers that are typically coupled to the hearing instruments of binaurally aided users. This fact serves to make induction neckloop systems a financially attractive option.

Designated Programmable Audio Input

Most modern hearing instruments are equipped with two analog-to-digital (A/D) converters. In regular use, the output of each microphone of a dual-microphone hearing aid is delivered to a separate A/D converter. When an alternative input source is activated (e.g., telecoil, DAI, etc.), one of the microphones is disabled, so its A/D converter can be used to process the audio signal from the auxiliary source (e.g., remote microphone signal). As a result, most hearing aids revert to omnidirectional mode when remote microphone systems are enabled. In the future, manufacturers will likely designate a separate A/D converter for auxiliary inputs that will allow hearing aids to remain in adaptive directional modes during the use of remote microphone technology.

Special Considerations for Remote Microphone Use With Cochlear Implants

Research has unequivocally demonstrated the benefits of remote microphone technology for cochlear implant users (Schafer & Thibodeau, 2004; Wolfe et al., 2009; Wolfe, Morais, Schafer, Mills, & Mülder, 2013; Wolfe, Morais, Schafer, Mills, Peters, et al., 2013). However, there are several considerations clinicians must keep in mind while managing remote microphone use for cochlear implant recipients. First, cochlear implant sound processors typically have a higher input impedance at the direct auditory input relative to hearing aids. The default receiver gain of most remote microphone systems is set for hearing aid use. As a result, the receiver gain might be inappropriate for cochlear implant sound processors, and the clinician might need to select a setting that is optimized for cochlear implant use. Most manufacturers of remote microphone systems offer guidelines for determining receiver settings that are appropriate for a given cochlear implant sound processor. Clinicians should consult with manufacturers to determine what adjustments, if any, are necessary to optimize performance with use of a specific cochlear implant sound processor.

Second, many cochlear implant sound processors possess an adjustable parameter referred to as the mixing ratio, which controls the relative strength of the signals received from the remote microphone and sound processor microphone. The mixing ratio can be set so that equal emphasis is placed on signals from the remote microphone and sound processor microphone (e.g., 1:1 or 50/50), or the mixing ratio can be adjusted to attenuate the signal from the sound processor microphone in order to provide a greater emphasis on the signal from the remote microphone. Access to incidental sounds in the environment is critical for infants and children, so mixing ratios that do not result in significant attenuation of the sound processor microphone are most appropriate. In contrast, teenagers and adults can be equipped with multiple programs with different mixing ratios or given manual control of the mixing ratio so that the sound processor microphone can be more attenuated in noisy environments, relative to quiet environments, to allow for better access to the signal of interest arriving from the remote microphone.

Third, input signal processing within the cochlear implant sound processor can influence hearing performance obtained with a remote microphone system. For instance, Wolfe et al. (2009) showed that Nucleus cochlear implant recipients obtained poor speech recognition in noise with remote microphone use when autosensitivity control (ASC) preprocessing was disabled. However, activating ASC processing allowed for significant benefit from remote microphone use. Additionally, Wolfe, Morais, Schafer, Agrawal, and Koch (2015) evaluated the speech recognition in noise of Advanced Bionics Naida CI Q70 users who were equipped with the Phonak Roger digital adaptive remote microphone system. They found that the use of ClearVoice digital noise reduction processing resulted in better Roger hearing performance relative to speech recognition obtained with Roger and no preprocessing.

Remote Microphone System Verification

The development of ear-level remote microphone receivers has meant that the hearing instrument microphone acts as the local microphone of the remote microphone system. This allows the remote microphone system user to hear other talkers and sounds in the environment and monitor his or her own voice, while still receiving a consistent input from the main talker using the remote microphone/transmitter. With most current hearing instrument circuits incorporating some type of nonlinear compression processing, verification of remote microphone systems has been significantly impacted. Any verification of the function of the remote microphone system is dependent on accurate evaluation of the hearing instrument processing. Hearing instrument processing options include multiple channels, frequency compression/transposition, and active noise-reduction. Previous remote microphone system verification guidelines (ASHA, 1994, 2002) assumed local microphones functioned with single-channel linear circuitry. It has become clear in recent years that the rapid advances in hearing instrument and remote microphone technology require a reexamination of remote microphone system fitting and verification procedures.

Another technological advance that has impacted remote microphone system verification is the availability of hearing instrument test systems that offer speech-mapping using real speech inputs, rather than broadband noise or pure-tone inputs. As an input signal, real speech allows more accurate evaluation of how hearing instruments and remote microphone systems respond to typical inputs. Speech is one of the primary signals that both remote microphone systems and hearing instruments are designed to transmit and amplify. Advanced compression and noise reduction processing react differently to rapidly changing speech than they do to constant-level signals. Current guidelines recommend the use of calibrated real-speech inputs for the evaluation of hearing instrument and remote microphone responses.

Additionally, many modern remote microphone systems now use digital radio frequency technology rather than analog FM radio transmission. Speech-like signals should be used for verification measures conducted with digital remote microphone systems. In spite of the efforts to keep pace with the development of remote microphone technology, clinicians currently are not equipped with objective tests to evaluate many of the contemporary advanced features of remote microphone systems such as adaptive gain changes. The following section describes the current standard of care for verification of remote microphone systems.

Electroacoustic Remote Microphone System Verification

There are three assumptions that guide current verification processes and assist in prioritizing testing (AAA, 2011a).

1. Ear-level remote microphone systems use the microphone of the hearing instrument as the local microphone, and the input from the remote microphone is processed by the hearing instrument circuitry. All verification measures of the relationship between the remote microphone system and hearing instrument microphones are based on the assumption that the hearing instrument processing has been adjusted to provide appropriate audibility and output for the individual user (AAA, 2011a). Before verifying remote microphone system performance, audiologists must first verify that the hearing instrument is set appropriately and is meeting chosen prescriptive targets for a variety of speech input levels. True estimates of maximum output are obtained from input to the hearing instrument microphone, not the remote microphone. High compression ratios in the remote microphone/transmitter likely will prevent the hearing instrument from reaching its maximum output in response to remote microphone input. Audiologists must also confirm that the hearing instrument is able to accept a remote microphone input.
2. Most remote microphone systems are worn with both the remote microphone and hearing instrument microphone(s) active at the same time. Therefore, all verification should be completed with the remote microphone system and hearing instrument microphones active simultaneously. The remote microphone system output level can then be adjusted in relationship to the hearing instrument response so as to preserve as much of a speech-to-noise benefit as possible. Traditionally, it has been recommended that the signal from the remote microphone system maintain a 10-dB advantage over other signals coming to the local microphone. Although as stated previously, the preferred remote-microphone advantage of current systems can vary during use, this relationship is maintained for verification.
3. Because of the nonlinear characteristics of current hearing instrument and remote microphone system circuitry, different input levels to the two microphones will result in changing compression and gain results. This will create problems during electroacoustic verification measures as testing *only* can be completed sequentially, meaning that the hearing instrument microphone response is evaluated, followed by the remote microphone response. Current test systems do not allow for simultaneous inputs to both the microphone of the hearing instrument and the remote microphone system with separate outputs for the two inputs. Therefore, *if* the remote microphone response is evaluated using input levels that are typical for close microphone placements (80–95 dB SPL) and the hearing instrument microphone response is evaluated separately for conversational input levels (60–65 dB SPL), the compression parameters in response to these input signals will be significantly different than they will be when those signals reach both microphones simultaneously. Consequently, no valid comparisons could then be made between the remote microphone system and hearing instrument responses if different input levels were tested sequentially. A thorough discussion of the impact of nonlinear compression characteristics and the use of sequential versus simultaneous measurements can be found in Platz (2004, 2006).

Because current test systems do not allow simultaneous measures of the microphone of the hearing instrument and the remote microphone system, electroacoustic verification protocols require that input levels to the remote microphone be less than actual use inputs. This is required to ensure that the hearing instrument response to a remote microphone system input has the same compression characteristics as its response to input from the hearing instrument microphone. Verification of the relationship between remote microphone system and hearing instrument responses can be completed with equal inputs to the remote microphone system and hearing instrument microphones. The input level to both systems must be sufficiently low so that input compression in the remote microphone system's transmitter is not activated, and compression in the hearing instrument will act equally on both the remote microphone system and hearing instrument test signals. The goal is to achieve equal outputs for equal inputs to the two microphones. This new approach to FM system verification is defined as *transparency*.

With the remote microphone receiver set at its default remote microphone system gain position of +10 dB, the AAA Guidelines (AAA, 2011a) recommend a 65 dB SPL input to the hearing instrument microphone and a 65 dB SPL input to the microphone (in the HA+FM position) of the remote microphone system to evaluate for transparency (Figure 27–23).

If the remote microphone system output at this 10-dB setting is more than 2 dB different from the hearing instrument output, adjustments (offsets) are made to the remote microphone system level to achieve equal outputs, or transparency. When verified in this manner, the remote microphone system has been shown to maintain a 10 dB SNR advantage in relationship to the hearing instrument when typical use inputs are presented simultaneously to both microphones (Platz, 2006). This 10-dB recommendation is offered as a general starting point for selecting the remote microphone system level. It is based on the relationship between typical use inputs to the microphones of the remote microphone system and the hearing instrument and the kneepoint for compression in the remote microphone/transmitter. For step-by-step verification procedures, see AAA (2011a).

Because of the nonlinear nature of current hearing instrument and remote microphone system technology, functional gain or amplified sound-field threshold (ASFT) testing should never be used to verify remote microphone system function. With the changing compression characteristics of both remote microphone and hearing instrument microphones, no predictable relationship exists between amplified threshold information and remote microphone system performance at typical use input levels.

Real-Ear Remote Microphone System Verification

Real-ear verification of remote microphone systems can be completed for any hearing instrument plus remote microphone, or remote microphone-only combination.

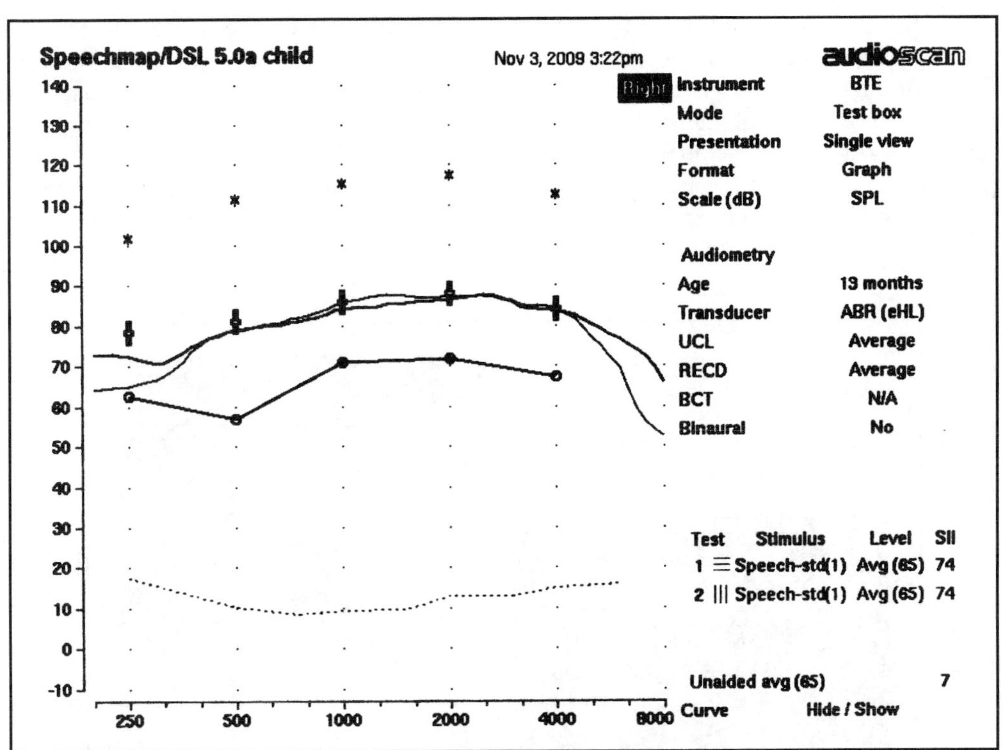

FIGURE 27–23. SPLogram graph illustrating transparency measures with 65 dB SPL input to the hearing instrument (Test 1) and 65 dB SPL input to the remote microphone (Test 2). Circles are hearing thresholds, crosses are long-term average speech spectrum targets, and asterisks are maximum output targets.

Due to the number of measures and possible adjustments needed when verifying remote microphone receivers coupled to hearing instruments, electroacoustic verification in a test box is typically the more efficient approach. However, verification of ear-level remote microphone-only systems requires special considerations. Ear-level remote microphone-only fittings are primarily used with children or students who have normal or near-normal hearing. The child's ability to hear himself or herself and others needs to be preserved; therefore, ear-level remote microphone-only fittings are designed to be nonoccluding. Electroacoustic verification in a test box with the remote microphone receiver coupled to a 2-cc coupler does not provide accurate information about how the system functions on the child's ear when open-ear acoustics are preserved. In addition to open-ear acoustic considerations, the remote microphone-only receiver is not coupled to personal hearing instruments and has no local microphone that amplifies other talkers. Using the same transparency approach previously described for remote microphone receivers coupled to hearing instruments is not appropriate when verifying ear-level remote microphone-only receivers.

When verifying any nonoccluding fitting, two sound pathways must be considered (Figure 27–24): (a) the amplified sound pathway, which is the transmitted signal from the remote microphone system, is the primary signal of interest for verification; and (b) the direct or unamplified sound pathway, which includes unamplified portions of the main talker's voice, other talkers, the remote microphone system user's own voice, and background noise. In a nonoccluding fitting, unamplified signals can move freely into and out of the ear canal. At the same time, much of the low-frequency regions of the amplified input signal leak out of the open ear canal (Hoover, Stelmachowicz, & Lewis, 2000). This will affect the expectations and targets for the remote microphone system response in the child's nonoccluded ear (Figure 27–25).

Verification priorities for ear-level remote microphone-only fittings are twofold. First, maximum output should be confirmed in the child's ear. Because most remote microphone-only devices are fitted on normal-hearing ears, it is critical to verify the maximum output of the system using a high-level pure-tone input. Output or volume control adjustments might be needed to prevent exposure to excessive sound pressure levels. Second, the remote microphone system should maintain consistent audibility and comfort for the main talker's voice. Recommended use settings are determined based on the response of the remote microphone-only system to close speech inputs (1–6 in [2.54–15.24 cm] from talker's mouth). Specific procedures for real-ear verification of remote microphone-only receivers will vary depending on the real-ear test system that is utilized. These procedures will be influenced by how the real-ear reference microphone is used during testing and whether remote microphone specific inputs and targets are available in the test system (AAA, 2011a; Eiten, 2008; Eiten & Lewis, 2008). For step-by-step real-ear verification procedures, see AAA (2011a).

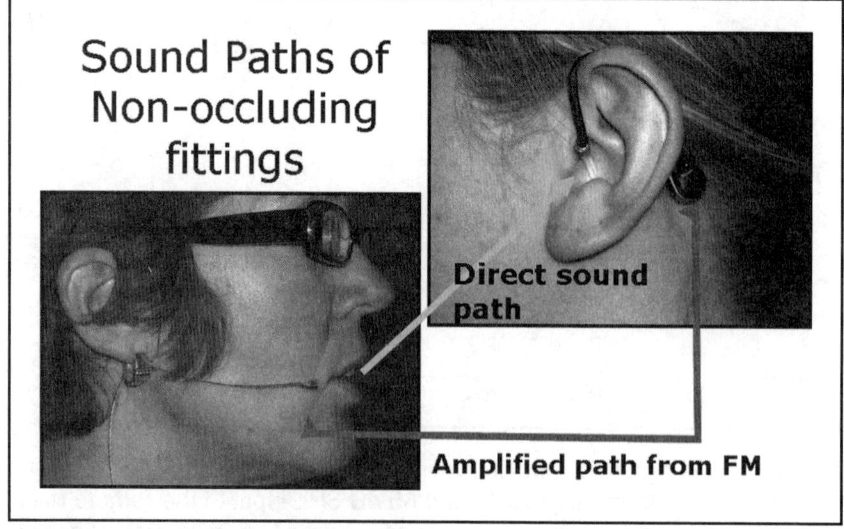

FIGURE 27–24. Two sound paths into the ear when wearing a nonoccluding remote microphone system.

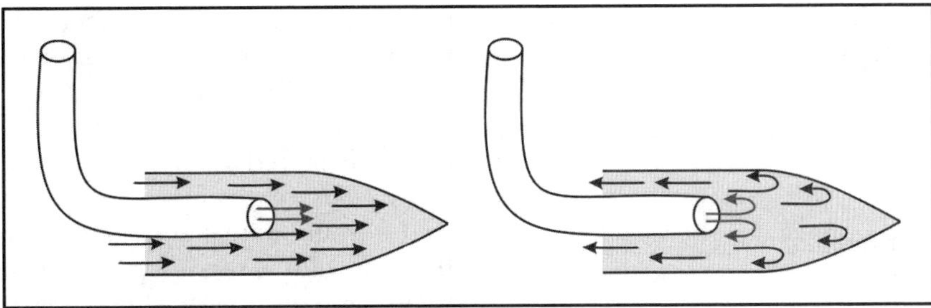

FIGURE 27–25. Amplified (*gray arrows*) and direct (*black arrows*) sound as it enters (*left*) and leaves (*right*) the nonoccluded ear canal.

Behavioral Remote Microphone System Verification

Behavioral verification of remote microphone systems using speech perception measures is a recommended option when an appropriate sound-field test environment is available (AAA, 2011a). Although behavioral verification is not a substitute for electroacoustic verification for HA, remote microphone, and ear-level remote microphone-only systems, it remains the primary method of verification for remote microphone systems coupled to cochlear implants. When using speech perception tasks to verify remote microphone system performance, testing should be completed under listening conditions that are representative of the child's typical listening environments. Priority is given to testing in noise. The child's performance when the remote microphone is not active (unaided, hearing instrument only, cochlear implant only) is compared to performance with the remote microphone active under the same noise conditions. The vocabulary and language level of the child must be considered when choosing this verification option.

Testing with adaptive or variable noise and speech levels is not recommended as part of the behavioral verification of remote microphone systems. When testing is conducted with varying speech levels and a fixed noise level, the input to the remote microphone will most likely be significantly lower than that found in normal use (Boothroyd & Iglehart, 1998). Similarly, when testing is conducted with varying noise levels and a fixed speech level at the remote microphone, the resulting noise levels might exceed typical classroom noise levels. For these reasons, the use of such testing to determine a threshold SNR is not recommended for behavioral remote microphone system verification. These types of procedures *are* appropriate when evaluating performance with personal hearing instruments or cochlear implants alone for determining hearing aid technology candidacy. Some currently available speech-in-noise tests that use adaptive or variable speech or noise levels include the BKB-SIN (Bamford-Kowal-Bench Speech-In-Noise Test; Etymotic Research, 2005) and HINT-C (Hearing-In-Noise Test-Child; Nilsson, Soli, & Gelnett, 1996). Finally, clinicians should always conduct a biologic listening check to evaluate the integrity and quality of the signal provided by the remote microphone system informally. These informal assessments can be completed with use of a listening stethoscope for hearing aids or with use of specialized monitoring earphones for cochlear implant sound processors. The caregivers of children (e.g., parents, daycare attendant, teachers, coaches, etc.) should also receive counsel on how to complete these informal listening checks. The interested reader is referred to the AAA Clinical Practice Guideline on Remote Microphone Technology for more detailed information pertaining to behavioral assessment and validation of remote microphone technology (AAA, 2011a).

Orientation and Outcome Measurement

Modern remote microphone technology systems are composed of sophisticated technology that can be quite intimidating to a new user, caregiver, or classroom teacher. As such, it is imperative that clinicians adequately orient the user and user's caregiver to the proper care, operation, use, function, and maintenance of remote microphone technology. The AAA Clinical Practice Guideline on Remote Microphone Technology explicitly lists several components that should be addressed during the orientation process:

Orientation and Training Topics for Children and Youth

Orientation and training topics for children and youth include the following:

- implications of hearing loss;
- basic function of device;
- appropriate use of device and features;
- expectations: benefits and limitations of the device including when to use and when not to use;
- care and maintenance;
- basic troubleshooting and reporting of a suspected malfunction;
- self-monitoring of function; and
- self-advocacy.

Training Topics for Parents/Caregivers/Teachers

Training topics for parents, caregivers, and teachers include the following:

- basic implications of hearing loss;
- basic function of device;
- appropriate use of device and features;
- when to use the device;
- expectations: benefits and limitations of the device including when to use and when not to use;
- listening check and basic troubleshooting (use of stethoscope, Ling-6-Sound Test, battery check, etc.);
- reporting of a suspected malfunction;
- advocacy; and
- classroom orientation to remote microphone technology.

Ideally, clinicians should discuss the aforementioned items, demonstrate appropriate use of the technology, provide the user or caregiver with the opportunity to operate the system with the clinician's support and assistance, and provide written, online, or video materials pertaining to the proper use of remote microphone technology and the specific features and functions of the technology provided to the user. Also, for educational or daycare settings, clinicians should assist the family in determining which personnel will support the child in day-to-day use of the remote microphone system. This support will include the facilitation of a daily listening check and inspection of basic function. Additionally, this person will assist the child in troubleshooting problems that might arise and will ensure that classroom teachers are comfortable with use of the system. This person will also assist the child in ensuring that the battery of the system is charged while not in use and that the components of the system are safely stored away while not in use.

Finally, clinicians should administer standardized questionnaires and conduct interviews to ensure that the child is receiving satisfactory benefit from the remote microphone system in real-world settings and that no detriment is associated with the use of the system. Again, the reader is referred to the AAA Clinical Practice Guideline on Remote Microphone Technology for more detailed information pertaining to questionnaires that are appropriate for the completion of outcome measurements with remote microphone technology in realistic situations (AAA, 2011a).

Conclusions

Research continues to support the need for hearing assistance technology in poor acoustic environments for children with hearing loss and for children with normal hearing who have special listening needs. Developments in remote microphone system technology have expanded their use and now provide audiologists with many options for addressing communication access needs. Miniature, ear-level remote microphone receivers are appropriate for children of all ages both in and out of school. Fitting and verification techniques have evolved to keep pace with technological developments in both hearing instruments and remote microphone systems, but additional advances are needed to allow for verification of modern features such as systems that adaptively change the gain of the remote microphone signal with increases in ambient noise level. It is important for audiologists who work with children to understand current methods for selecting and fitting remote microphone systems in order to address the specific communication needs of each child. Audiologists must also incorporate appropriate verification guidelines into their clinical practice and be aware of future advances as they become available.

References

American Academy of Audiology (AAA; 2011a). *AAA Clinical Practice Guidelines: Remote microphone hearing assistance technologies for children and youth birth–21 years (Includes Supplement A).* Retrieved June 9, 2015, from http://audi

ology-web.s3.amazonaws.com/migrated/HAT_Guidelines_Supplement_A.pdf_53996ef7758497.54419000.pdf

American Academy of Audiology (AAA; 2011b). *Supplement B. Classroom Audio Distribution Systems: Selection and verification.* Retrieved June 9, 2015, from http://audiology-web.s3.amazonaws.com/migrated/20110926_HAT_GuidelinesSupp_B.pdf_53996ef98259f2.45364934.pdf

American Academy of Audiology Task Force on Pediatric Amplification. (2013). Retrieved June 24, 2015, from http://audiology-web.s3.amazonaws.com/migrated/PediatricAmplificationGuidelines.pdf_539975b3e7e9f1.74471798.pdf

American National Standard Institute (ANSI)/Acoustical Society of America (ASA; 2010). *American National Standard acoustical performance criteria, design requirements, and guidelines for schools, Parts 1 and 2* (ANSI S12.60-2010). New York, NY: ASA.

American Speech-Language-Hearing Association (ASHA; 1994). Guidelines for fitting and monitoring FM systems. *ASHA, 36*(Suppl.), 1–9.

American Speech-Language-Hearing Association (ASHA; 2002). *Guidelines for fitting and monitoring FM systems* [Guidelines]. Retrieved September 28, 2015, from http://www.asha.org/policy/GL2002-00010/

American Speech-Language Hearing Association Working Group on Classroom Acoustics. (2005). *Acoustics in educational settings: Position statement.* Retrieved June 9, 2015, from http://www.asha.org/policy/PS2005-00028.htm

American Red Cross. (2007). *Health and safety tips: Car safety.* Retrieved December 21, 2007, from http://www.redcross.org/services/hss/tips/carsafety.html

Anderson, K. (1989). *Screening Instrument for Targeting Educational Risk (SIFTER).* Retrieved June 9, 2015, from https://successforkidswithhearingloss.com/uploads/SIFTER.pdf

Anderson, K., & Goldstein, G. (2004). Speech perception benefits of FM and infrared devices to children with hearing aids in a typical classroom. *Language, Speech, and Hearing Services in Schools, 35,* 169–184.

Anderson, K., Goldstein, H., Colodzin, L., & Iglehart, F. (2005). Benefit of S/N enhancing devices to speech perception of children listening in a typical classroom with hearing aids or a cochlear implant. *Journal of Educational Audiology, 12,* 14–28.

Anderson, K., Smaldino, J., & Spangler, C. (2011). *Listening Inventory for Education—Revised (L.I.F.E.-R). Teacher appraisal of listening difficulty.* Retrieved June 9, 2015, from http://successforkidswithhearingloss.com/wp-content/uploads/2011/09/LIFE-R-Instruction-Manual.pdf

Aslund, T., Olsson, J., Skagerstrand, A., & Dahlstrom, J. (2011). *Study report, assistive listening devices. Audiological Research Centre, Study Report.* Retrieved June 9, 2015, from https://www.phonakpro.com/content/dam/phonak/b2b/FM_eLibrary/Orebro_Study_Report_-_Assistive_Listening_Devices.pdf

Bess, F., Dodd-Murphy, J., & Parker, R. (1998). Children with minimal sensorineural hearing loss: Prevalence, educational performance, and functional status. *Ear and Hearing, 19,* 339–354.

Bess, F. H., Gustafson, S. J., & Hornsby, B. W. Y. (2014). How hard can it be to listen? Fatigue in school-age children with hearing loss. *Journal of Educational Audiology, 20,* 34–47.

Bess, F., Klee, T., & Culbertson, J. (1986). Identification, assessment, and management of children with unilateral sensorineural hearing loss. *Ear and Hearing, 7*(1), 43–51.

Bluetooth. (2015). *What is Bluetooth technology?* Retrieved June 9, 2015, from http://www.bluetooth.com/Pages/what-is-bluetooth-technology.aspx

Boothroyd, A. (1997). Auditory development of the hearing child. *Scandinavian Audiology Supplement, 46,* 9–16.

Boothroyd, A., & Iglehart, F. (1998). Experiments with classroom FM amplification. *Ear and Hearing, 19*(3), 202–217.

Bradley, J., & Sato, H. (2004). *Speech recognition by grades 1, 3 and 6 children in classrooms. Institute for Research in Construction.* Retrieved July 1, 2008, from http://irc.nrc-cnrc.gc.ca/pubs/fulltext/nrcc46871/nrcc46871.pdf

Bradlow, A., Kraus, N., & Hayes, E. (2003). Speaking clearly for children with learning disabilities. Sentence perception in noise. *Journal of Speech, Language, and Hearing Research, 46,* 80–97.

Cappelli, M., Daniels, T., Durieux-Smith, A., McGrath, P., & Neuss, D. (1995). Social development of children with hearing impairments who are integrated into general education classrooms. *Volta Review, 97,* 197–208.

Chelius, L. (2004). *Trost amplification study* (Unpublished report). Canby, OR, School District.

Ching, T. Y., & Dillon, H. (2013). Major findings of the LOCHI study on children at 3 years of age and implications for audiological management. *International Journal of Audiology, 52*(Suppl. 2), S65–S68.

Choi, Y. C., & McPherson, B. (2005). Noise levels in Hong Kong primary schools: Implications for classroom listening. *International Journal of Disability, Development, and Education, 52,* 345–360.

Crandell, C. (1991). Classroom acoustics for normal-hearing children: Implications for rehabilitation. *Educational Audiology Monograph, 2*(1), 18–38.

Crandell, C. (1992). Classroom acoustics for hearing-impaired children. *Journal of the Acoustical Society of America, 92,* 2470.

Crandell, C. (1993). Speech recognition in noise by children with minimal degrees of sensorineural hearing loss. *Ear and Hearing, 14*(3), 210–216.

Crandell, C., & Bess, F. (1986). Speech recognition of children in a "typical" classroom setting. *American Speech, Language, and Hearing Association, 29,* 87.

Crandell, C., & Smaldino, J. (1996). Speech perception in noise by children for whom English is a second language. *American Journal of Audiology, 5,* 47–51.

Crukley, J., Scollie, S., & Parsa, V. (2011). An exploration of nonquiet listening at school. *Journal of Educational Audiology, 17,* 23–35.

Eiten, L. (2008). *Assessing open-ear Edulink fittings.* Online presentation, First Phonak Virtual FM Conference: ACCESS 2, February.

Eiten, L., & Lewis, D. (2008). FM verification for the 21st century. *Perspectives on Hearing and Hearing Disorders in Childhood, 18*(1), 4–9.

Etymotic Research. (2005). *BKB-SIN Test, Version 1.03* [CD]. Elk Grove Village, IL: Author.

Finitzo-Hieber, T., & Tillman, T. (1978). Room acoustics effects on monosyllabic word discrimination ability for normal and hearing-impaired children. *Journal of Speech and Hearing Research, 21*, 440–458.

Flexer, C., & Long, S. (2003). Sound-field amplification: Preliminary information regarding special education referrals. *Communication Disorders Quarterly, 25*, 29–34.

Geers, A. E., & Hayes, H. (2011). Reading, writing, and phonological processing skills of adolescents with 10 or more years of cochlear implant experience. *Ear and Hearing, 32*(Suppl. 1), 49S–59S.

Geers, A. E., Strube, M. J., Tobey, E. A., & Moog, J. S. (2011). Epilogue: Factors contributing to long-term outcomes of cochlear implantation in early childhood. *Ear and Hearing, 32*(Suppl. 1), 84S–92S.

Gertel, S., McCarty, P., & Schoff, L. (2004). High performance schools equal high performance students. *Educational Facility Planner, 39*, 20–24.

Grini, D. (2006). *RF basics, RF for non-engineers.* Presented at MSP430 Advanced Technical Conference 2006, November 7, Dallas, TX.

Hawkins, D. B. (1984). Comparisons of speech recognition in noise by mildly-to-moderately hearing-impaired children using hearing aids and FM systems. *Journal of Speech and Hearing Disorders, 49*, 409–418.

Hoover, B., Stelmachowicz, P., & Lewis, D. (2000). Effect of earmold fit on predicted real ear SPL using a real ear to coupler difference procedure. *Ear and Hearing, 21*(4), 310–317.

Hornsby, B. W. Y., Werfel, K., Camarata, S., & Bess, F. (2014). Subjective fatigue in children with hearing loss: Some preliminary findings. *American Journal of Audiology, 23*(1), 129–134.

Jamieson, D., Kranjc, G., Yu, K., & Hodgetts, W. (2004). Speech intelligibility of young school-aged children in the presence of real-life classroom noise. *Journal of the American Academy of Audiology, 15*, 508–517.

Johnston, K. N., John, A. B., Kreisman, N. V., Hall III, J. W., & Crandell, C. (2009). Multiple benefits of personal FM system use by children with auditory processing disorder (APD). *International Journal of Audiology, 48*, 371–383.

Kenworthy, O., Klee, T., & Tharpe, A. (1990). Speech recognition ability of children with unilateral sensorineural hearing loss as a function of amplification, speech stimuli, and listening condition. *Ear and Hearing, 11*(4), 264–270.

Knecht, H., Nelson, P., Whitelaw, G., & Feth, L. (2002). Background noise levels and reverberation times in unoccupied classrooms: Predictions and measurements. *American Journal of Audiology, 11*, 65–71.

Larsen, J. B., & Blair, J. C. (2008). The effect of classroom amplification on the signal-to-noise ratio in classrooms while class is in session. *Language, Speech, and Hearing Services in the Schools, 39*, 451–460.

Leavitt, R., & Flexer, C. (1991). Speech degradation as measured by the Rapid Speech Transmission Index (RASTI). *Ear and Hearing, 12*, 115–118.

Lewis, D., & Eiten, L. (2004). Assessment of advanced hearing instrument and FM technology. In D. A. Fabry & C. DeConde Johnson (Eds.), *ACCESS: Achieving Clear Communication Employing Sound Solutions–2003. Proceedings of the First International FM Conference* (pp. 167–174). Stäfa, Switzerland: Phonak AG.

Loeb, R., & Sarigiani, P. (1986). The impact of hearing impairment on self-perceptions of children. *Volta Review, Feb/Mar, 88*(2), 89–100.

Massie, R., & Dillon, H. (2006). The impact of sound-field amplification in mainstream cross-cultural classrooms, Part 1: Educational outcomes. *Australian Journal of Education, 50*, 62–77.

Massie, R., Theodoros, D., McPherson, B., & Smaldino, J. J. (2004). Sound-field amplification: Enhancing the classroom listening environment for Aboriginal and Torres Strait Islander children. *Australian Journal of Indigenous Education, 33*, 47–53.

Mulla, I. (2011). *Pre-school use of FM technology* (Unpublished PhD thesis). School of Psychological Sciences, University of Manchester, UK.

Mulla, I. (2013, December). *FM technology: When to introduce to children.* Podium presentation at A Sound Foundation Through Early Amplification 2013, Chicago, IL.

Nabelek, A., & Nabalek, I. (1985). Room acoustics and speech perception. In J. Katz (Ed.), *Handbook of clinical audiology* (3rd ed.). Baltimore, MD: Williams and Wilkins.

Nelson, P., Kohnert, K., Sabur, S., & Shaw, D. (2005). Classroom noise and children learning through a second language: Double jeopardy? *Language, Speech, and Hearing Services in Schools, 36*, 219–229.

Neuman, A. C., Wroblewski, M., Hajicek, J., & Rubenstein, A. (2010). Combined effects of noise and reverberation on speech recognition performance of normal-hearing children and adults. *Ear and Hearing, 31*(3), 1–9.

Nilsson, M., Soli, S., & Gelnett, D. (1996). *Development and norming of a Hearing in Noise Test for children.* House Ear Institute Internal Report, Los Angeles, CA.

Nilsson, M., Soli, S. D., & Sullivan, J. A. (1994). Development of the Hearing in Noise Test for the measurement of speech reception thresholds in quiet and in noise. *Journal of the Acoustical Society of America, 95*(2), 1085–1099.

Ostegren, D. (2013). 20 questions: Improving speech understanding in the classroom—Today's solutions. *AudiologyOnline*, Retrieved July 1, 2015, from http://www.audiologyonline.com/articles/20q-classroom-acoustics-and-audio-12285

Oyler, R., Oyler, A., & Matkin, N. (1988). Unilateral hearing loss: Demographics and educational impact. *Language, Speech, and Hearing Services in Schools, 19*, 191–210.

Pearsons, K., Bennett, R., & Fidell, S. (1977). *Speech levels in various noise environments* (Report No. EPA-600/1-77-025). Washington, DC.

Picard, M., & Bradley, J. S. (2001). Revisiting speech interference in classrooms. *Audiology, 40*, 221–244.

Platz, R. (2004). SNR advantage, FM advantage and FM fitting. In D. Fabry & C. DeConde Johnson (Eds.), *ACCESS: Achieving Clear Communication Employing Sound Solutions,*

2003. Proceedings of the First International FM Conference (pp. 147–154). Stäfa, Switzerland: Phonak AG.

Platz, R. (2006). *New insights and developments in verification of FM systems.* Paper presented at the American Academy of Audiology Convention, Minneapolis, MN.

Ronsse, L. M., & Wang, L. M. (2013). Relationships between unoccupied classroom acoustical conditions and elementary student achievement measured in eastern Nebraska. *Journal of the Acoustical Society of America, 133*(3), 1480–1495.

Rubin, R. L., Aquino-Rusell, C. E., & Flagg-Williams, J. (2007). *Evaluating sound field amplification in New Brunswick Schools.* Podium presentation at the 2007 Conference of the Canadian Association of Speech-Language Pathologists and Audiologists, Moncton, New Brunswick, Canada.

Ruscetta, M., Arjmand, E., & Pratt, R., Sr. (2005). Speech recognition abilities in noise for children with severe-to-profound unilateral hearing impairment. *International Journal of Pediatric Otorhinolaryngology, 69*(6), 771–779.

Sanders, D. (1965). Noise conditions in normal school classrooms. *Exceptional Child, 31,* 344–353.

Schafer, E. C., & Kleineck, M. P. (2009). Improvements in speech-recognition performance using cochlear implants and three types of FM systems: A meta-analytic approach. *Journal of Educational Audiology, 15,* 4–14.

Schafer, E. C., Mathews, L., Mehta, S., Hill, M., Munoz, A., Bishop, R., & Moloney, M. (2013). Personal FM systems for children with autism spectrum disorders (ASD) and/or attention-deficit hyperactivity disorder (ADHD): An initial investigation. *Journal of Communication Disorders, 46*(1), 30–52.

Schafer, E. C., & Thibodeau, L. M. (2004) Speech recognition abilities of adults using cochlear implants with FM systems. *Journal of the American Academy of Audiology, 15,* 678–691.

Schafer, E. C., & Thibodeau, L. M. (2006). Speech recognition in noise in children with cochlear implants while listening in bilateral, bimodal, and FM system arrangements. *American Journal of Audiology, 15,* 114–126.

Stelmachowicz, P., Mace, A., Kopun, J., & Carney, E. (1993). Long-term and short-term characteristics of speech: Implications for hearing aid selection for young children. *Journal of Speech and Hearing Research, 36,* 609–620.

Stiles, D. J., McGregor, K. K., & Bentler, R. (2012). Vocabulary and working memory in children fit with hearing aids. *Journal Speech, Language, and Hearing Research, 55*(1), 154–167.

Thibodeau, L. (2010). Benefits of adaptive FM systems on speech recognition in noise for listeners who use hearing aids. *American Journal of Audiology, 19*(1), 36–45.

Thibodeau, L. (2014). Comparison of speech recognition with adaptive digital and FM remote microphone technology by listeners who use hearing aids. *American Journal of Audiology, 23,* 201–210.

Tomblin, J. B., Oleson, J. J., Ambrose, S. E., Walker, E., & Moeller, M. P. (2014). The influence of hearing aids on speech and language development of children with hearing loss. *JAMA Otolaryngology-Head and Neck Surgery, 140*(5), 403–409.

Valente, D. L., Plevinsky, H. M., Franco, J. M., Heinrichs-Graham, E. C., & Lewis, D. E. (2012). Experimental investigation of the effects of the acoustical conditions in a simulated classroom on speech recognition and learning in children. *Journal of the Acoustical Society of America, 131*(1), 232–246.

Wilson, W. J., Marinac, J., Pitty, K., & Burrows, C. (2011). The use of sound-field amplification devices in different types of classrooms. *Language, Speech, and Hearing Services in Schools, 42*(4), 395–407.

Wolfe, J., Duke, M. M., Schafer, E. C., Jones, C., Mülder, H. E., John, A., & Hudson, M. (2015). Evaluation of performance with an adaptive, digital remote microphone system and a digital remote microphone audio-streaming accessory system. *American Journal of Audiology, 24,* 440–450.

Wolfe, J., John, A., Schafer, E., Nyffeler, M., Boretzki, M., & Caraway, T. (2010). Evaluation of non-linear frequency compression for school-age children with moderate to moderately severe hearing loss. *Journal of the American Academy of Audiology, 21,* 618–628.

Wolfe, J., Morais, M., Neumann, S., Schafer E., Mülder, H. E., Wells, N., . . . Hudson, M. (2013). Evaluation of speech recognition with personal FM and classroom audio distribution systems. *Journal of Educational Audiology, 19,* 65–79.

Wolfe, J., Morais, M., Schafer, E. C., Agrawal, S., & Koch, D. (2015). Evaluation of speech recognition of cochlear implant recipients using adaptive, digital remote microphone technology and a speech enhancement sound processing algorithm. *Journal of the American Academy of Audiology, 26*(5), 502–508.

Wolfe, J., Morais, M., Schafer, E., Mills, E., & Mülder, H. (2013). Evaluation of speech recognition of cochlear implant recipients using a personal digital adaptive radio frequency system. *Journal of the American Academy Audiology, 24*(8), 714–724.

Wolfe, J., Morais, M., Schafer, E., Mills, E., Peters, R., Lianos, L., . . . Hudson, M. (2013). Better speech recognition with digital RF system in study of cochlear implants. *Hearing Journal, 66*(7), 24–26.

Wolfe, J., Schafer, E. C., Heldner, B., Mulder, H., & Vincent, B. (2009). Evaluation of speech recognition in noise with cochlear implants and dynamic FM. *Journal of the American Academy of Audiology, 20,* 409–421.

Wolfe, J., Schafer, E. C., Mills, E., John, A. B., & Hudson, M. (2015). Evaluation of the benefits of binaural hearing on the telephone for children with hearing loss. *Journal of the American Academy of Audiology, 26,* 93–100.

Wolfe, J., Schafer, E. C., Parkinson, A., John, A., Hudson, M., Wheeler, J., & Mucci, A. (2013). Effects of input processing and type of personal frequency modulation system on speech-recognition performance of adults with cochlear implants. *Ear and Hearing, 34*(1), 52–62.

Wroblewski, M., Lewis, D. E., Valente, D., & Stelmachowicz, P. G. (2012). Effects of reverberation on speech recognition in stationary and modulated noise by school-aged children and young adults. *Ear and Hearing, 33*(6), 731–744.

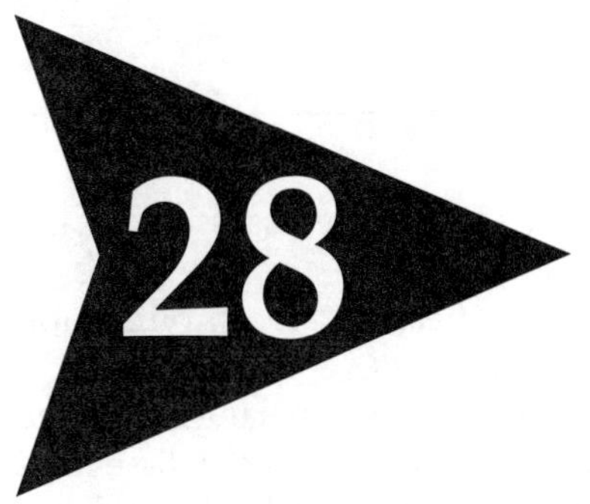

Measuring Outcomes of Infants and Children With Hearing Loss

Teresa Y.C. Ching, Sanna Y.L. Hou, and Vicky W. Zhang

Introduction

Many children with congenital permanent hearing loss experience outcomes that are often less than optimal, including poorer spoken language, reading, spelling, and math skills, and increased emotional and behavioral difficulties (Eisenberg, 2007; Moeller, 2007; Moeller, Tomblin, Yoshinaga-Itano, Connor, & Jerger, 2007; Petrou et al., 2007). Young people who are deaf or hard of hearing (DHH) are more likely than typically developing peers not to be in education or employment, and DHH adults report social isolation and anxiety (Kvam, Loeb, & Tambs, 2007). By implementing universal newborn hearing screening (UNHS) programs to detect deafness soon after birth, intervention can begin in infancy with the ultimate goal of improving long-term outcomes (i.e., minimizing the impact of hearing loss on limiting children's activities and full participation in real life [World Health Organization, 2007] so that they can fulfil their learning and development potentials).

A vital component of early intervention is the provision of effective amplification. To this end, procedures for selecting amplification and verifying that hearing devices match prescriptive targets have been established (see Bagatto and Scollie, Chapter 25). Despite this, evaluation of the effectiveness of amplification for infants and young children has received limited research. There are still many questions relating to how to determine whether the amplification provided is optimally effective, and how to judge what a child should be able to hear. Drawing on published literature and current research, this chapter addresses three key questions: (a) why evaluate? (b) what outcomes and how to evaluate? and (c) when to evaluate?

Why Evaluate?

After a clinician has verified that the prescribed response has been achieved in a hearing aid fitting, it is necessary to check, in each case, whether the hearing aids are effective in providing auditory information to a child. Ongoing monitoring of outcomes assists with fine-tuning the devices to meet the child's amplification requirements, and identifying children for whom hearing aids might not be the most appropriate treatment so that candidature for cochlear implantation might be considered in a timely manner.

Effectiveness for the Individual

Current hearing aid selection procedures widely used for children include the National Acoustic Laboratories (NAL) prescription (Byrne, Dillon, Ching, Katsch, & Keidser, 2001; Dillon, Keidser, Ching, Flax, & Brewer, 2011) and the Desired Sensation Level (DSL) procedure (Scollie et al., 2005; Seewald et al., 1997; Seewald, Moodie, & Scollie, 2005), both of which have been supported by research to prescribe amplification that on average, children prefer and with which they perform best (Ching, Scollie, Dillon, & Seewald, 2010). However, not all children are average, and some variation to the prescribed hearing aid characteristics could make it better for one child than for another (Ching, Newall, & Wigney, 1994; Ching, Scollie, Dillon, Seewald, et al., 2010; Eisenberg & Levitt, 1991), just as with adults. Whereas a verbal response from an adult to a question, "How does it sound?" can indicate whether fine-tuning is required and, if so, in which direction, the same cannot be applied for infants and young children. However, the need to evaluate is no less important because differences in gain and frequency response of hearing aids affect speech intelligibility and real-life functioning of children (Table 28–1).

Advances in digital signal processing in hearing aids have raised the clinical question of whether a child might benefit from technologies that are designed to adapt to the needs of the listener. In principle, the inability of young children to adjust hearing aid controls manually, the reduced speech reception at low levels, and the impracticability for a caregiver to monitor and adjust controls in the children's devices all support the use of automated controls in hearing devices for children. Nevertheless, decisions about whether to implement a certain processing scheme for children need to be guided by evidence of its efficacy (American Academy of Audiology [AAA], 2013; McCreery, 2014), and its effectiveness must be assessed for the individual child.

For some individuals, hearing aid amplification might not adequately support development of auditory skills and acquisition of spoken language. The earlier that this is revealed through systematic evaluation of the effectiveness of hearing aids, the earlier a child can be referred for alternative strategies, such as cochlear implantation, and the higher likelihood that maximal benefits can be obtained (Ching, Dillon, Marnane, et al., 2013).

Special Populations

Children with special needs, including those with auditory neuropathy spectrum disorder (ANSD) and those with additional disabilities, benefit from early fitting of amplification as do other DHH children (Ching, 2015; Ching, Day, Dillon, et al., 2013). In the general population of newborns identified with permanent childhood hearing loss, about 30% to 40% have additional disabilities and about 10% (some of whom also have additional disabilities) have ANSD. As ANSD is characterized by absent or abnormal auditory brainstem

Table 28–1. Evidence That Differences in Gain and Frequency Response in Hearing Aids Affect Outcomes

Evidence	*Number of Participants*	*Age (in Years)*	*Hearing Loss*	*Outcome*	*Citation*
Difference in hearing aid gain of more than 3 dB results in a difference in perceived loudness, preference for speech intelligibility, and real-life functioning	48	7 to 16 years	Mild to moderately severe	Loudness rating, Parent report (PEACH), self-report (SELF), paired-comparisons judgment	Ching et al., 2010; Scollie et al., 2010
Difference in hearing aid frequency response of >3 dB/octave results in a difference in real-life functioning	30	7 months to 5 years	Severe to profound hearing loss	Parent report (PEACH), teacher report (TEACH)	Ching, Hill, & Dillon, 2008
Difference in gain-frequency response led to a difference in sentence perception in quiet, but not in noise	7	7 to 17 years	Severe to profound	Sentence perception in quiet and in noise tests	Quar, Ching, Newall, & Sharma, 2013
Difference in gain-frequency response led to a difference in real-world functioning	16	7 to 17 years	Severe to profound	Parent report (PEACH), teacher report (TEACH), self-report (SELF)	Quar et al., 2013

Note. The subjective report measures include Parents' Evaluation of Aural/oral performance of Children (PEACH), Teachers' Evaluation of Aural/oral performance of Children (TEACH) ,and Self Evaluation of Listening Function (SELF).

response (ABR) with evidence of normal cochlear outer hair-cell function, the standard audiological procedure for estimating hearing sensitivity from ABR measures is not applicable (see Rance, Chapter 11). For this reason, clinical services in Australia (King, 2010) have based initial hearing aid fitting of infants with ANSD on a combination of behavioral observations and objective measurements of cortical auditory-evoked potentials (CAEPs) to speech stimuli, and outcomes evaluation by using a combination of aided CAEPs and parent reports (Parents' Evaluation of Aural/oral performance of Children or PEACH) to determine whether the amplification is optimal, and whether alternative strategies for rehabilitation are required for individual infants.

What Outcomes and How to Evaluate?

Hearing aid fitting delivered within the context of auditory rehabilitation for DHH children aims to provide an audible signal across as wide a frequency range as possible to maximize speech intelligibility, while keeping overall loudness within a comfortable loudness range. Determining whether this intervention makes a difference in terms of a child's auditory access to sounds to support language development, communicative function in real-world environments, and speech recognition is crucial to patient-level outcomes. It would be difficult to argue against this, in view of the dominant role of verbal communication in most human activities, and its importance for educational attainment and social adaptation. Related to these domains is the question of whether hearing aids are used, and whether the child experiences loudness discomfort when wearing the devices.

If the goal of evaluation is to assess whether hearing aids are effective for the child, and to indicate what changes to the settings might be required, it is appropriate to focus outcomes assessments on determining whether hearing aids are making speech and other sounds optimally audible for a child. The assessment can be based on speech recognition tests or on subjective reports.

Speech Recognition

Tests of detection and discrimination of speech sounds at suprathreshold levels provide information about a child's absolute performance with amplification that can be used to guide rehabilitation. One method to assess detection uses the Ling-6-Sounds as stimuli (Glista, Scollie, Moodie, Easwar, & Network of Pediatric Audiologists of Canada, 2014; Ling, 1989). Identifying the types of sounds that are not well perceived at a certain presentation level is useful for evaluating the benefit that hearing aids provide at the level tested. If two sounds are confusable due to audibility issues (e.g., /i/ and /u/ might sound similar to the impaired ear that does not perceive the higher formants of /i/), this might alert clinicians to consider adjusting the hearing aids to increase audibility of some frequencies. Once detection has been established, auditory discrimination can be assessed (Boothroyd, Eisenberg, & Martinez, 2010; Dawson, Nott, Clark, & Cowan, 1998; Eisenberg, Martinez, & Boothroyd, 2003).

The usual criterion for assessing whether amplification maximizes speech intelligibility is performance on a speech discrimination test. The problem arises as to deciding what kind of performance indicates that the individual is optimally fitted. The answers might then depend on which speech test is used as the criterion, and on particulars of the test condition such as choice of material, presentation level, signal-to-noise ratios, and location of a signal and noise source(s). Results based on special conditions chosen to demonstrate hearing aid "advantages" cannot be a general indicator of benefit. On the other hand, this approach might be logical if the benefit claim is specific because there is then no reason to expect the new device or algorithm to provide significantly better (or worse) speech discrimination or real-life performance. Table 28–2 summarizes findings from studies that examined the influence of variations in hearing aid characteristics on speech detection and discrimination. Even when conventional speech tests for evaluating variations in amplification characteristics do not reveal benefits for speech discrimination, there might be other potential benefits, such as increased perception of environmental sounds, enhanced self-monitoring of voice level and quality, or ease of listening. Furthermore, speech test results do not indicate how the hearing aid characteristics need to be changed to achieve better results. A low score can, for instance, reflect deficits with auditory processing or cognitive ability that are not directly related to the hearing aids (Tomlin, Dillon, Sharma, & Rance, 2015).

Speech tests can be used to help fine-tune hearing aids for a child if the tests help to identify the types of speech sounds that are not well perceived at a certain input level. As such, speech tests are useful for demonstrating aided benefits to parents. Speech tests can also be used within the context of an auditory rehabilitation program to determine the effectiveness of training, and to examine the difficulty that might be experienced by the child in different listening conditions.

Table 28–2. Evidence on the Use of Speech Tests for Hearing Aid Evaluation

Evidence	*Number of Participants*	*Age (in Years)*	*Hearing Loss*	*Outcome Measure*	*Citation*
Ling 6 (HL) thresholds can be reliably measured.	29	3 to 18	Mild to moderately severe	Ling 6(HL)	Glista et al., 2014
Speech tests are limited in sensitivity to differences in hearing aid gain-frequency responses.	48	6.6 to 19.8	Mild to moderately severe	Sentence perception in noise; vowel-consonant-vowel nonsense syllable test in quiet	Scollie et al., 2010
The consonant test did not distinguish between prescriptions.	15	7 to 17	Mild to severe	Consonant test	Quar et al., 2013
There was a significant difference in sentence perception in quiet between prescriptions.	7	7 to 17	Mild to severe	Sentences in quiet and in noise	Quar et al., 2013
Scores were significantly higher when nonlinear frequency compression (NLFC) was enabled in hearing aids than when it was disabled.	11	6 to 17 years	Mild to severe sloping loss	UWO Plurals test—detection of word final plural marker in English	Glista & Scollie, 2012
	11	6 to 13 years	Mild to moderate high-frequency hearing loss	UWO Plurals test	Wolfe, John, Schafer, et al., 2015
	15	5 to 13 years	Moderate high-frequency hearing loss	UWO Plurals test	Wolfe, John, Schafer, et al., 2010
No significant differences were found in speech perception scores between NLFC on and NLFC off conditions.	11	6 to 13 years	Mild to moderate high-frequency hearing loss	BKB test in noise	Wolfe, John, Schafer, et al., 2015
	15	5 to 13 years	Moderate high-frequency hearing loss	Identification of /s, sh, f, t, k, d/ in a vowel-consonant-vowel context, BKB sentence test in noise	Wolfe, John, Schafer, et al., 2010
	7	6 to 13 years	Cookie-bite audiograms	UWO Plurals test, distinctive feature test, nonsense syllable test; BKB sentence test in noise	John, Wolfe, Scollie, et al., 2014
	17	9 to 17 years	Mild to profound	12-alternative consonant-vowel identification test in quiet, 4-alternative spondee identification measure in noise	Hillock-Dunn, Buss, Duncan, et al., 2014

Preference: Paired-Comparison Tests

When the purpose of the evaluation is to determine whether an individual would do better with a frequency response that is different from the one prescribed, then comparisons of a prescribed frequency response with systematic variations (e.g., high-frequency emphasis) are warranted. Paired-comparison judgments of the intelligibility of speech in quiet and the pleasantness of speech in noise have been used in preference to word recognition testing because the former procedures were found to be more efficient for hearing aid evaluation (Byrne, 1986; Studebaker, 1991). A clinical procedure for adults has been published (Byrne & Cotton, 1988) and adapted for use with children (Ching, Hill, Birtles, & Beecham, 1999). When two alternatives are presented in quick succession, children older than about six years can reliably indicate which of the two hearing aid responses they prefer (Ching et al., 1994; Eisenberg & Dirks, 1995; Eisenberg & Levitt, 1991). The procedure has also been applied for comparing hearing aid prescriptions in school-aged children (Ching, Scollie, Dillon, Seewald, et al., 2010; Quar, Ching, Newall, & Sharma, 2013). Table 28–3 summarizes studies that have used paired comparison tests for hearing aid evaluation by children.

Effectiveness in Real Life: Subjective Report Measures

None of the available speech tests have been thoroughly validated by establishing how test performance relates to real-life functioning. Functioning across a range of everyday settings is not the same thing as a score on a speech discrimination test. If the aim of providing amplification is to improve functional auditory capacity and participation in real-world activities, then evaluation of device effectiveness in real life is essential. Subjective report tools have been designed for this purpose. Bagatto, Moodie, Seewald, Bartlett, and Scollie (2011) provided a critical review of the measures

Table 28–3. Use of Paired-Comparison Test for Hearing Aid Evaluation by Children

Evidence	*Number of Participants*	*Age (in Years)*	*Hearing Loss*	*Outcome Measure*	*Citation*
Paired-comparison judgments of clarity are used to evaluate variations in audible bandwidth.	16	8 to 16 years	Mild to severe	Compare three processing conditions for in terms of clarity	Brennan et al., 2014
Paired-comparison judgements can be used reliably with school-aged children to evaluate differences in gain-frequency response in hearing aids.	22	7 to 17 years	Severe to profound	Compare alternative gain-frequency responses in terms of speech intelligibility.	Ching et al., 1999
	15	6 to 16 years	Severe to profound	Compare alternative responses that varied by ±6 dB/octave in terms of speech intelligibility.	Ching et al., 2008
	48	School age	Mild to moderately severe	Compare the NAL with the DSL prescription in terms of speech intelligibility.	Ching et al., 2010
	16	7 to 17 years	Severe to profound	Compare the NAL with the DSL prescription in terms of speech intelligibility.	Quar et al., 2013

for assessing the performance of children from birth to 6 years of age who wear hearing aids.

Table 28–4 summarizes studies that have used subjective report measures for hearing aid evaluation. One of the parent report measures widely used in Australia is the Parents' Evaluation of Aural/oral Performance of Children or PEACH (Ching & Hill, 2007). The PEACH scale is a measure of functional communicative performance of children in everyday life as judged by parents or caregivers. The scale contains 13 questions, two of which address the child's use of sensory devices, and whether the devices cause loudness discomfort when worn. The remaining 11 questions solicit information about the child's ability to listen and communicate in quiet and in noisy situations, to use the telephone, and to respond to environmental sounds in everyday

Table 28–4. Use of Subjective Report Measures for Hearing Aid Evaluation in Children

Evidence	*Number of Participants*	*Age (in Years)*	*Hearing Loss*	*Outcome Measure*	*Citation*
Parent ratings agreed with children's preference on the best gain-frequency response.	15	6 to 17 years	Severe to profound	PEACH, paired-comparisons judgment of intelligibility	Ching et al., 2008
Parent and child ratings on functional performance in noisy situations were sensitive to difference in prescription.	48	School age	Mild to moderately severe hearing loss	PEACH, TEACH, SELF ratings, paired- comparisons	Ching, Scollie, Dillon, Seewald, Britton, Steinberg, et al., 2010
Ratings of parents, teachers, and children were sensitive to differences in hearing aid prescription.	16	7 to 17 years	Severe to profound	PEACH, TEACH, SELF	Quar et al., 2013
Parental ratings of children's real-world functional performance was significantly correlated with the children's language ability at 3 years of age.	133	3 years	Mild to profound	PEACH, PLS-4	Ching et al., 2010
Early functional performance was a significant predictor of language outcomes at 3 years.	102	3 years	Mild to profound	PEACH, PLS-4	Ching, Day, Seeto, et al., 2013
Early functional performance was a significant predictor of language outcomes at 5 years.	350	5 years	Mild to profound	PEACH, PLS-4	Ching, 2015
Parental report of children's functional performance in real-world situations was a significant predictor of psychosocial outcomes at 5 years.	356	5 years	Mild to profound	PEACH, CDI, SDQ	Wong et al., personal communication, June 24, 2015

Note. The measures include Parents Evaluation of Aural/oral Performance of Children (PEACH); Teachers' Evaluation of Aural/oral performance of Children (TEACH); Self- Evaluation of Listening Function (SELF); Pre-School Language Scale, version 4 (PLS-4); Child Development Inventory (CDI); and Strengths and Difficulties Questionnaire (SDQ).

situations. The scale gives an overall functional performance score based on ratings summed across 11 questions, a "Quiet" subscale score based on six items, and a "Noise" subscale score based on five items (http://outcomes.nal.gov.au/peach.html). Previous research has shown that overall PEACH scores were significantly related to measurements of cortical responses to speech stimuli in infants (Golding et al., 2007), and language development of children as measured by standardized language tests at 3 years of age (Ching, Day, Seeto, et al., 2013).

The PEACH tool has been adapted for self-report by older children—the Self Evaluation of Listening Function (SELF) scale (http://outcomes.nal.gov.au/self.html). In line with the PEACH scale, the SELF scale includes an item on usage of device and an item for rating loudness comfort, together with 10 items depicting different listening situations. Both scales have been used to evaluate alternative frequency responses for children with hearing loss (Ching, Hill, & Dillon, 2008; Ching, Scollie, Dillon, Seewald, et al., 2010). Normative data on the SELF scale have been collected from 48 typically developing children at 9 years of age in Australia. The mean overall score for the normative sample was 87.4% (SD = 10.5, Range = 81.25 to 95). The mean Quiet subscale score was 88.3% (SD = 10.6; Range = 85 to 95), and the mean Noise subscale score was 86.4 % (SD = 12.2; Range = 80 to 95). Figure 28–1A shows a template of norms suggested for evaluating overall and subscale scores, and Figure 28–1B shows a template for evaluating responses for individual item scores. The shaded areas depict the range of the middle 50% of the data for each score.

Audibility

Because signal audibility is a major goal of amplification, various approaches have been adopted in evaluation of audibility with hearing aids. A commonly used approach is to apply a predictive model for quantifying aided audibility. A second approach is to use objective measurement of evoked responses to speech sounds.

Speech Intelligibility Index

The Speech Intelligibility Index (SII) model, or its predecessor the Articulation Index theory, has been applied to determine the audibility of amplified speech, and for relating speech audibility to speech intelligibility (American National Standards Institute, 1969, 1997). This model quantifies how much signal will be audible under various acoustic conditions, and uses this information to predict understanding of speech. Signal audibility, in each frequency band, is determined by the extent to which the peak levels of speech exceed hearing thresholds or noise levels, whichever are greater. The SII is calculated by totaling the amounts of signal in each band. In principle, the SII considers the relative importance of different frequencies for understanding speech. However, when importance values are averaged over various types of speech, all octave bands from 0.5 to 4 kHz are about equally important (American National Standards Institute, 1969, 1997; Pavlovic, 1989).

The SII procedure assumes that a particular amount of signal makes a fixed contribution to SII (and hence speech intelligibility), regardless of hearing level. This assumption is erroneous when applied to moderate and more severe hearing loss. As hearing loss becomes greater at any frequency, a given amount of audibility contributes less to speech intelligibility (Dubno, Dirks, & Schaefer, 1989; Pavlovic, 1984). Therefore, SII calculations need to include a hearing loss desensitization (HLD) to take account of this (Ching, Dillon, Lockhart, Van Wanrooy, & Flax, 2012; Pavlovic, Studebaker, & Sherbecoe, 1986; Studebaker, Sherbecoe, McDaniel, & Gray, 1997). HLD is significant when considering what frequency response is best for severe hearing loss or sloping losses. Other things being equal, it will be better to provide more signal at the less impaired than at the more impaired frequencies. Calculations of SII for evaluation of hearing aids that do not take into account HLD will lead to wrong conclusions about the relative effectiveness of different frequency responses for audiograms with severe losses or sloping configurations (Byrne, 1992; Ching, Johnson, Hou, et al., 2013).

A higher SII can be achieved by simply increasing the gain in hearing aids. When hearing loss is severe, high audibility can contribute to loudness but very little to intelligibility (Ching, Dillon, Katsch, & Byrne, 2001; Ching, Johnson, Hou, et al., 2013). Previous research on examining how SII and subjective judgments of preference relate to each other have shown that SII predictions often disagreed with speech intelligibility ratings by adults. A frequency response that gave the higher SII because it provided more audibility at the higher frequencies was consistently judged to be the poorest out of a total of four frequency responses that were compared (Byrne, 1986, 1992). Rankovic (1991) found that subjects who had sloping high-frequency losses did not achieve the best speech recognition scores with a frequency response that maximized the SII.

Table 28–5 summarizes studies that have used the SII to quantify audibility with amplification for children. Comparisons of the NAL and the DSL prescription for children have revealed that on average, the DSL procedure provided higher overall gain than the NAL

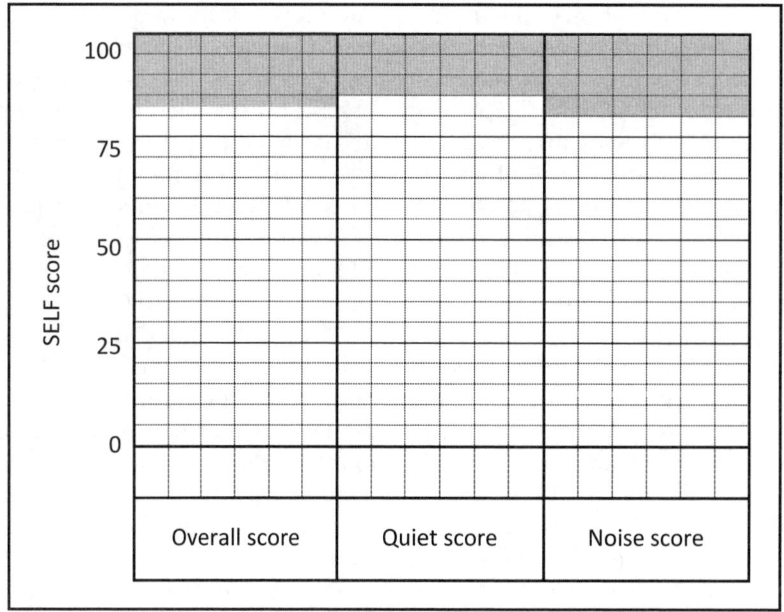

A

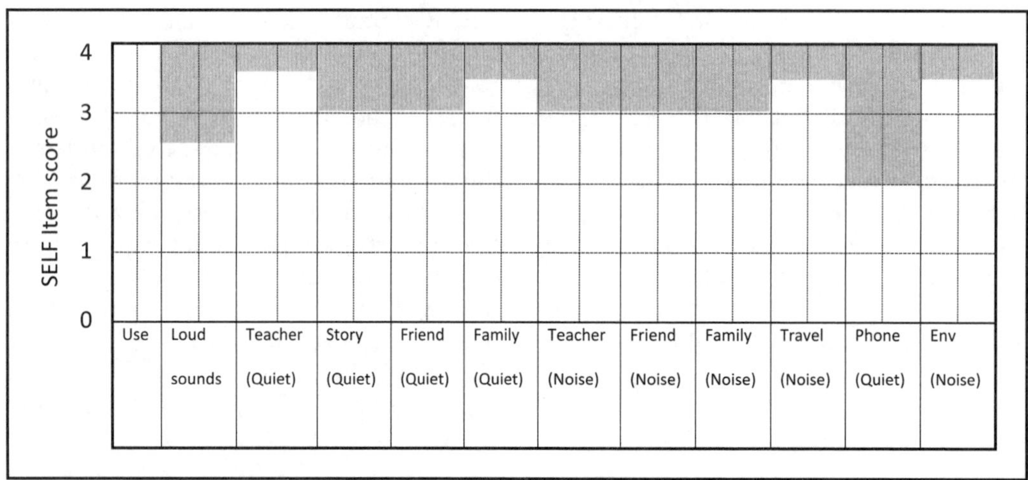

B

FIGURE 28–1. Template of norms to evaluate overall score and subscale scores (**A**), as well as template of norms to evaluate item scores (**B**) for the Self Evaluation of Listening Function (SELF) scale.

procedure, and hence higher SIIs and higher estimated loudness for the same audiograms. After incorporating HLD in SII calculations, the modified SIIs were similar between prescriptions despite differences in overall loudness (Ching, Johnson, Hou, et al., 2013; Ching, Quar, Johnson, Newall, & Sharma, 2015). Evaluations of school-aged children did not reveal differences in speech recognition scores between prescriptions, but there were differences in loudness ratings (Scollie et al., 2010). Also, a longitudinal study on infants and young children whose postdiagnostic fitting was randomly assigned to either the NAL or the DSL prescription has shown that the choice of prescription was not a significant factor influencing language development at 3 years of age, after allowing for the effects of communication mode, severity of hearing loss, and maternal education level (Ching, Dillon, Hou, et al., 2013).

The SII metric has also been used to reflect the goodness of fit to targets (McCreery, Bentler, & Roush, 2013), showing that the deviation of fit from prescribed targets was a significant predictor of aided audibility. Given that the calculated SII is related to hearing thresh-

Table 28–5. Studies on Aided Audibility for Children, Quantified Using the Speech Intelligibility Index (SII) Model With or Without Hearing Loss Desensitization (HLD)

Evidence	*Number of Participants*	*Age (in Years)*	*Hearing Loss*	*Outcome Measure*	*Citation*
Audibility of hearing aid prescriptions varied, depending on whether HLD was considered.	200	3 years	Mild to severe	SII, Modified SII that included HLD	Ching, Johnson, Hou, et al., 2013
	16	7 to 17 years	Severe to profound	SII, Modified SII that included HLD	Ching et al., 2015
SII overestimated speech recognition for children.	14	7.5 to 18 years	Mild to severe	SII, 21-consonant test in noise	Scollie, 2008
SII varied with goodness of fit and hearing loss.	195	5 to 85 months	Mild to severe	SII	McCreery, Bentler, & Roush, 2013

olds, hearing aid gains and the input speech spectrum or noise spectrum, a verification procedure that uses individual real-ear measurements would provide clinicians with a more direct assessment of whether the fitting matches prescriptive targets and how the hearing aid characteristics need to be adjusted to achieve an accurate fit (see Bagatto, Chapter 25).

Evoked Cortical Responses

A second approach to assessing how much speech is audible after fitting an infant is to use objective electrophysiological measurements. One technique that can provide information about the reception of sound is the measurement of CAEPs. The measurement does not require conscious attention of the child, although the child needs to be awake. Because CAEPs are generated at the auditory cortex, the detection of CAEPs to speech stimuli presented in the sound field indicates that neural signals initiated by the stimuli have traveled through the device (if a hearing device is worn) up the auditory pathway at least to the primary auditory cortex of the hearing aid wearer (Dillon, 2012). It might be expected that children with present cortical responses and normal latency when aided are more likely to derive benefit from hearing aids than those with absent or delayed responses. Previous research has indicated that the presence of CAEPs is significantly related to aided functional performance of infants with sensorineural hearing loss (Golding et al., 2007) and infants and children with ANSD (Cardon & Sharma, 2013; Gardner-Berry, Purdy, Ching, & Dillon, 2015; Sharma, Cardon, Henion, & Roland, 2011).

Table 28–6 gives a summary of studies that have measured evoked cortical responses for evaluation of hearing aids for children. In people with hearing loss, the amplitude of the cortical response increases with sensation level of the stimulus, which in turn, is determined by the level of the stimulus in the ear canal when aided. The relationship between sensation level and the detection rate of CAEPs in infants and young children with sensorineural hearing loss have been reported (Chang, Dillon, Carter, Van Dun, & Young, 2012; Van Dun, Carter, & Dillon, 2012). In children for whom hearing thresholds cannot be reliably estimated from ABR thresholds, as in the case of ANSD, measurement of evoked cortical responses has been used to assess detection of speech with and without amplification (Gardner-Berry, Purdy, et al., 2015). Extensive work on using the latency of CAEPs as a biomarker for auditory development in children who received cochlear implants has also been published (Sharma & Cardon, 2015; Sharma et al., 2005).

More recently, measurement of CAEPs has been used to evaluate signal processing in hearing aids. Glista et al. (2012) conducted a pilot study on measuring CAEPs evoked using tonal stimuli in five children when nonlinear frequency compression (NLFC) in hearing aids was enabled. Zhang et al. (2014) assessed the effect of NLFC by presenting /t/, /g/, and /s/ at 55 and 65 dB SPL in the sound field to young children using either hearing aids with NLFC or conventional amplification. The study found that /s/ presented at a low input level evoked a higher detection rate of CAEPs when NLFC was used. In a subsequent study that directly compared NLFC on and off conditions in the same hearing aids, Ching et al. (2015) found that the activation of NLFC increased the sensation level of /t/ and /s/ and the detection rate of CAEPs to these stimuli when they were presented at 55 dB SPL. These studies lend support to the technique of measuring CAEPs for assessing the detection of speech sounds with amplification.

Table 28–6. Studies That Used Measurements of Cortical Auditory-Evoked Potentials (CAEPs) for Hearing Aid Evaluation

Evidence	*Number of Participants*	*Age*	*Hearing Loss*	*Outcome Measure*	*Citation*
The detection rate of CAEP to speech stimuli increases with increase in sensation level.	25	8 to 30 months	Mild to severe	CAEPs to /m//g//t/	Van Dun et al., 2012
	18	2.7 to 10.5 months	Mild to moderate	CAEPs to /m//g//t/	Chang et al., 2012
	46	6 months to 2.5 years	29 SNHL, 17 ANSD	CAEPs to /m//g//t/	Gardner-Berry, Ching, Chang, & Hou, 2015
The presence of aided CAEP to speech stimuli is associated with better functional performance in real life in infants.	31	2 months to 3.5 years	Mild to severe; including 15 SNHL, 8 ANSD, and 8 MD	CAEPs to /m//g//t/; Parent report (PEACH)	Golding et al., 2007
The presence of CAEP to tonal stimuli is associated with receptive language and speech perception in children with ANSD.	18	6 to 92 months	ANSD	Oddball paradigm—400 Hz tone and synthetic /bæd/ and /dæd/ as stimuli; PBK Word test	Rance et al., 2002
CAEP latency is significantly correlated with functional ability of children with ANSD as observed by parents.	12	0 to 3 years	ANSD	CAEPs to /m//g//t/; parent report (PEACH)	Gardner-Berry et al., 2015
	21	9 months to 11 years	ANSD	IT-MAIS, CAEPs to synthetic /ba/	Sharma et al., 2011
Frequency lowering improved the audibility of specific frequencies for some listeners.	5	11, 14, and 18 years	High-frequency hearing loss	CAEPs to tone-bursts at 2 and 4 kHz	Glista et al., 2014
Frequency lowering improved the detection of /t/ and /s/ at low input levels.	27	6 to 16 years	Mild to severe hearing loss	CAEPs to /g//t//s/	Ching, Zhang, Van Buynder, Hou, & Burns, 2015
Frequency lowering improved the detection of /s/ at a low input level. A higher detection rate was associated with better speech intelligibility and functional performance in real life.	39	2.3 to 7.6 years	Mild to severe hearing loss	CAEPs to /g//t//s/; Speech Intelligibility rating, PEACH	Zhang et al., 2014

Note. Subjective report measures included the Parents Evaluation of Aural/oral performance of Children (PEACH), the Infant-Toddler Meaningful Auditory Integration Scale (IT-MAIS); and speech tests included the Phonetically Balanced Kindergarten (PBK) Words test and a Speech Intelligibility Rating scale.

Usage and Discomfort

No matter how accurately or optimally hearing aids have been fitted, they are not effective if they are not being used. Effective amplification for a DHH child requires the parents to ensure that the hearing aids are worn, and that the devices continue to function to provide maximal benefit to the child. Previous research has indicated that parents reported anxiety relating to maintaining consistent device usage in young children, and frustrations over not being able to tell if a device was working properly (Gilliver, Ching, & Sjahalam-King, 2013). Therefore, the correct operation of the devices also needs to be checked frequently until parents are confident with checking and troubleshooting the devices in the home environment. Challenging situations in which usage of device by young children might be compromised have also been identified (Moeller, Hoover, Peterson, & Stelmachowicz, 2009; Munoz, Preston, & Hicken, 2014; Walker et al., 2013).

Marnane and Ching (2015) have shown that higher device usage was positively associated with higher real-life functional performance in DHH children. In a longitudinal study of 413 children with hearing loss, usage of device from initial fitting to 3 years of age was examined. Based on parents' reports, full-time use of device was established for 75% of children by 3 years of age. The majority of children (87%) seldom or never experienced any loudness discomfort arising from the use of hearing devices. From 6 months after initial fitting to 3 years of age, 50% reported no change in device use, 36% reported a progressive increase in usage, and 14% reported a decline in usage. Decreased usage of device over time was reported more often for DHH children who have additional disabilities. Higher maternal education was associated with increase in usage over time for children with cochlear implants. In a similar vein, Walker et al. (2013) reported an increase of usage with older age, greater degree of hearing loss, and higher maternal education in children between 5 months and 7 years of age. Although data-logging capabilities in hearing devices might provide an accurate record of device activation (Walker et al., 2013), parent reports provide complementary information about the barriers to consistent hearing aid usage for their children in real life. Such information forms the basis for clinicians to support families to achieve consistent device usage.

Loudness comfort with amplification is an important factor that influences usage of hearing aids. The suitability of the prescribed maximum output for an individual child must be evaluated to ensure that the hearing aid does not cause loudness discomfort when worn. This is especially important for children as they are frequently exposed to intense noises in real-world environments (Crukley, Scollie, & Parsa, 2011); and especially more so for children with more than moderate degrees of hearing loss as the risk of temporary threshold shifts with hearing aid use increases with severity of hearing loss (Ching, Johnson, Seeto, & Macrae, 2013). To evaluate whether the maximum output prescribed in hearing aids is suitable for an individual, loudness ratings using face icons with simple descriptors can be used (Kawell, Kopun, & Stelmachowicz, 1988). For young children, parent observations can be solicited. In a previous study that compared hearing aid prescriptions, parents were asked to observe their children's auditory behavior in real-life situations when loud sounds occurred (Ching, Scollie, Dillon, Seewald, et al., 2010). The results revealed a higher incidence of loudness discomfort when the DSL prescription was used than when the NAL prescription was used for children who had previous experience with the NAL prescription, but the same was not found for children who had previous experience with the DSL prescription. An effect of acclimatization to a new prescription was revealed in loudness judgments over time (Scollie et al., 2010). Several children who were used to the NAL prescription declined using hearing aids matched to the DSL prescription due to loudness discomfort. The SELF questionnaire completed by the children further revealed a higher incidence of loudness discomfort compared to the PEACH ratings for the same hearing aid settings. Similar results were reported for children with severe-to-profound hearing loss (Quar et al., 2013). These findings support the need to evaluate loudness discomfort in infants and young children. In the clinic, intense noises should be made when the child is looking at the person making the noises, and the child's behavior should be observed for any visible signs of discomfort. This will ensure that the maximum output of the hearing aids is set appropriately to avoid loudness discomfort in real-world environments. Parents should also be advised to observe their child's auditory behavior in real life and communicate their observations in a systematic way to audiologists to guide audiological management of their child.

Summary of Measures to Assess Outcomes for Different Age Groups

A summary of measures applicable for different age groups is shown in Tables 28–7A and 28–7B, separately for behavioral tests and subjective report tools. As is apparent from the tables, methods for evaluating the effectiveness of hearing aids during the first year of

Table 28–7A. Measures for Assessing Outcomes of Children in Clinical or Laboratory Settings for Different Age Groups, Arranged by Minimum Applicable Age

			Age Group		
Type	**Measure**	**Citation**	**<3 Years**	**3–6 Years**	**>6 Years**
Detection	Aided audiogram[a]	Hawkins, 2004	✓	✓	✓
	Ling 6 (HL) test	Glista et al., 2014			✓
	UWO Plurals test	Glista & Scollie, 2012			✓
Discrimination	VRASPAC	Martinez, Eisenberg, Boothroyd, & Visserdumont, 2008	✓		
	PLAYSPAC, OLIMSPAC, VIDSPAC	Boothroyd, Eisenberg, & Martinez, 2010; Eisenberg, Martinez, & Boothroyd, 2007		✓	
	Early Speech Perception test (ESP) for profoundly hearing impaired children	Moog & Geers, 1990		✓	
	Phonetically Balanced Kindergarten Test (PBK)	Haskins, 1949		✓	
	The Lexical Neighborhood Test (LNT) and Multi-syllabic Lexical Neighborhood Test (MLNT)	Kirk, Eisenberg, Martinez, & McCutcheon, 1999		✓	✓
	Bamford-Kowal-Bench Sentences (BKB), BKB-SIN test	Bench, Kowal, & Bamford, 1979			✓
	CNC word list	Peterson & Lehiste, 1962			✓
	Hearing in Noise test–Children (HINT-C)	Nilsson, Soli, & Gelnett, 1996			✓
	Northwestern University Children's perception of speech (NU-CHIPS)	Elliott & Katz, 1980			✓
	PLOTT screening test and PLOTT sentence test	Plant & Moore, 1993			✓
	Word Identification by Picture Inventory (WIPI)	Ross & Lerman,1971			✓
Rating	Paired-comparisons judgement	Byrne & Cotton, 1988; Ching, Hill, Birtles, & Beecham, 1999			✓
	Loudness judgment	Kawell et al., 1988			✓

[a]Measurement of aided thresholds to tonal stimuli presented in the sound field is fraught with potential errors arising from the effects of room acoustics, hearing aid circuit noise, interaction between the hearing aid signal processing and the stimulus, and those relating to the ability of a child to respond reliably to sounds that are audible at low levels (Hawkins, 2004). Nevertheless, this method is applicable to verifying bone-conduction hearing aids for which real-ear measurements cannot be used.

Table 28–7B. Subjective Report Measures for Assessing Outcomes Suitable for Use With Children of Various Age Groups, Arranged by Minimum Applicable Age

			Age Group		
Respondent	***Measure***	***Citation***	***<3 Years***	***3–6 Years***	***>6 Years***
Parent	Functional Auditory Performance Indicator (FAPI)	Stredler-Brown & DeConde Johnson, 2001	✓		
	Infant-toddler Meaningful Integration Scale (IT-MAIS)	Zimmerman-Phillips et al., 1998	✓		
	LittlEARS	Kuehn-Inacker, Weichboldt, Tsiakpini, Conix, & D'Haese, 2003	✓		
	Family Expectations worksheet and Developmental Index of Auditory and Listening (DIAL)	Palmer & Mormer, 1999	✓	✓	✓
	Client Oriented Scale of Improvement for Children	National Acoustic Laboratories, 2011	✓	✓	✓
	Parents' Evaluation of Aural/oral performance of Children (PEACH)	Ching & Hill, 2007	✓	✓	✓
	Auditory Behaviour in Everyday Life (ABEL)	Purdy et al., 2002		✓	✓
	Children's Home Inventory of Listening Difficulties	Anderson & Smaldino, 2000		✓	✓
	Meaningful Auditory Integration Scale (MAIS)—for profound loss	Robbins, Renshaw, & Berry, 1991			✓
	Meaningful use of Speech Scale (MUSS)	Robbins & Osberger, 1990			✓
Teacher	Teachers' Evaluation of Aural/Oral performance of Children (TEACH)	Ching et al., 2008	✓	✓	✓
	Screening Instrument for Targeting Educational Risk (SIFTER)	Anderson & Matkin, 1996		✓	✓
	Teacher Opinion and Observation List	Smaldino & Anderson, 1997			✓
	Listening Inventory for Education	Smaldino & Anderson, 1997			✓
Child	Children's Abbreviated Profile of Hearing Aid Performance for Children (APHAP-C) – >10 years	Kopun & Stelmachowicz, 1998			✓
	Listening Inventory for Education	Smaldino & Anderson, 1997			✓
	Self-Evaluation of Listening Function (SELF)	Ching et al., 2008			✓

Note. These measures assess effectiveness of hearing aids in real-world environments.

life are scarce. Given that this is the time when there is greatest uncertainty about a child's hearing thresholds and how much signal is audible with amplification, the measurement of CAEPs to speech stimuli can provide valuable information to guide clinical management. As children grow, outcomes evaluation can be carried out using a wider range of behavioral tests and report tools.

When to Evaluate?

The effectiveness of hearing aids in providing auditory information to the child has to be established soon after the hearing aids have been verified to match prescriptive targets. Accordingly, the Australian Hearing (AH, the government-funded national hearing service provider in Australia) Protocol stipulates that measurement of CAEPs and PEACH assessments should be carried out around four to six weeks after the fitting appointment. Recent findings on the longitudinal outcomes of children with hearing loss have clearly indicated that children who receive cochlear implants have the best language outcomes at 5 years of age if they are implanted before 12 months of age (Ching, 2015; Ching et al., 2014). To streamline postdiagnostic hearing services and enable infants who need cochlear implants to get them early, evaluation of aided hearing during the first year of life by measuring CAEPs and conducting PEACH assessments is now routine in Australia (Punch, Van Dun, King, Carter, & Pearce, 2015). The following cases were drawn from a chart review to illustrate (a) management of ANSD in regard to decision for fitting [Case 1]; (b) validation of hearing aid fitting [Case 2]; and (c) management of ANSD for cochlear implant referral [Case 3].

Case Studies

To Fit or Not to Fit?

Case 1 was a full-term boy who was referred via the state UNHS program to AH for audiological management. There is no family history of hearing loss, and no complication at birth. As shown in Table 28–8, the diagnostic results are consistent with the presence of

Table 28–8. Case 1: Audiological Measurements

Age (Months)	*Assessment*	*Results*
1.5	Diagnostic ABR	No response at 0.5, 1, and 2 kHz; cochlear microphonics present bilaterally
	High-frequency tympanometry	Normal middle ear function bilaterally
	DPOAE	Present bilaterally
2.5	Diagnostic ABR (repeat)	No response at 1 kHz, cochlear microphonic present bilaterally
	High-frequency tympanometry	Normal middle ear function bilaterally
	DPOAE	Present bilaterally
2.5	BOA	Age-appropriate responses to noisemakers at moderate and high sound levels
3	Unaided CAEPs	CAEPs present for /m/, /g/, and /t/ at 65 dB SPL; CAEPs present for /g/ and /t/ at 55 dB SPL
4.5	PEACH	Within 1 SD of the normative mean for normal-hearing children at the same age
5	Unaided CAEPs to /m/	CAEPs present for /m/ at 55 dB SPL
22	VRA: sound field	Mild loss at high frequencies
34	VRA: ear specific	Mild loss at 4 kHz bilaterally

Note. Table includes auditory brainstem responses (ABRs), distortion product otoacoustic emissions (DPOAEs), behavioral observation audiometry (BOA), cortical auditory-evoked potentials (CAEPs), visual reinforcement audiometry (VRA), and Parents' Evaluation of Aural/oral performance of Children (PEACH).

ANSD. In accordance with AH clinical protocols, measurement of unaided CAEPs was carried out with /m/ /t/ /g/ presented at 65 and 55 dB SPL in the sound field. Between 3 and 5 months of age, the PEACH report and the cortical responses confirmed that the child was functioning within normal limits, and that speech sounds at conversational levels were audible to the child without amplification. Due to other non-hearing-related health issues, visual reinforcement audiometry (VRA) was not completed until 22 months of age, and ear-specific information was not available until 34 months of age. Figure 28–2 shows the audiogram of the child. The PEACH and CAEP results were useful for reaching the early decision of not proceeding with amplification. AH offered ongoing monitoring of hearing for the child, and the parents were advised that a wireless microphone system can be considered in the future.

Validation of Hearing Aid Fitting

Case 2 was born at 27 weeks gestation, weighing 1000 gm. He was admitted to a neonatal intensive care unit where he received antibiotic treatment (including gentamycin) for risk of infection. He had jaundice for 2 days, requiring phototherapy for 24 hr. There is no family history of hearing loss. He was referred to AH via UNHS, with diagnostic ABR results indicating severe hearing loss bilaterally (Table 28–9).

The child was first fitted with behind-the-ear hearing aids in both ears at 7 weeks (1.75 months) corrected age. The estimated behavioral audiogram based on diagnostic ABR results were used to derive prescriptive targets according to the NAL formula, and hearing aids were verified to match targets. The PEACH assessments were conducted at a postfitting appointment 2 weeks later, and again when the child was 3 months

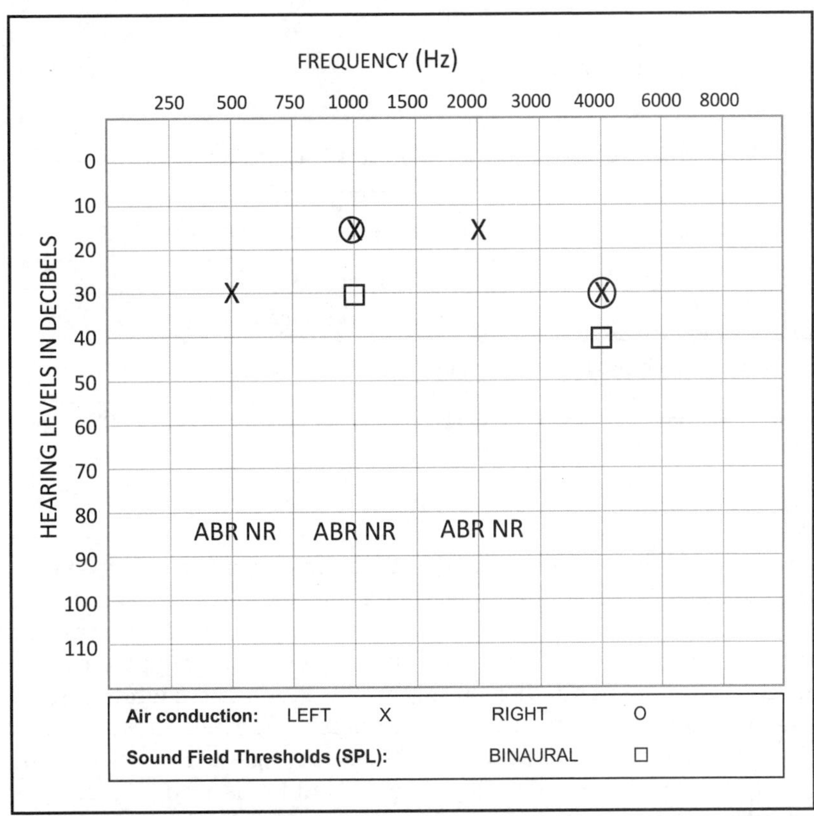

FIGURE 28–2. Audiogram of Case 1, showing no response (NR) at diagnostic auditory brainstem response (ABR) testing at 6 weeks, and behavioral hearing thresholds obtained using visual reinforcement audiometry (VRA) at 22 months (binaural) and 34 months (ear specific). Measurement of unaided cortical auditory-evoked potentials (CAEPs) at 3 months of age showed detection of responses to /m/ /g/ /t/ presented at 65 and 55 dB SPL in the sound field, before VRA testing could be attempted.

Table 28–9. Case 2: Audiological Measurements

Age (Months)	Assessment	Results
0.75	Diagnostic ABR	Left: 70 dBnHL at 0.5 kHz, 80 dBnHL at 2 kHz, 85 dBnHL at 4 kHz;
		Right: 60 dBnHL at 0.5 kHz, 80 dBnHL at 2 kHz, >90 dBnHL at 4 kHz;
		Cochlear microphonic present bilaterally
	High-frequency tympanometry	Normal middle ear function bilaterally
	DPOAE	Absent bilaterally
1.25	BOA	Responded at elevated levels to broadband and low-frequency noisemakers only
2	PEACH	Within normal range
3	PEACH	Within normal range
4.5	Diagnostic ABR	Left: 45 dBnHL at 2 kHz, 60 dBnHL at 4 kHz;
		Right: 55 dBnHL at 0.5 kHz, 60 dBnHL at 2 kHz; cochlear microphonics present bilaterally
	High-frequency tympanometry	Normal middle ear function bilaterally
	DPOAE	Absent bilaterally
6.5	Unaided CAEPs	Detected /m/, /g/, and /t/ at 65 dB SPL
		/m/ and /g/ at 55 dB SPL
	Aided CAEPs	Detected /m/ and /t/ at 55 dB SPL
11	VRA: ear specific	Left: mild to moderate loss
		Right: mild to moderately severe loss

Note. Table includes auditory brainstem responses (ABRs), distortion product otoacoustic emissions (DPOAEs), behavioral observation audiometry (BOA), cortical auditory-evoked potentials (CAEPs), visual reinforcement audiometry (VRA), and Parents' Evaluation of Aural/oral performance of Children (PEACH). "Age" depicts corrected age in months.

of age. The PEACH scores showed that the child's functional performance was progressing within the range of typically developing children of the same age. A subsequent ABR assessment conducted at the diagnostic hospital when the child was 4.5 months indicated a lesser degree of hearing loss than was indicated in the earlier test, attributable to neurological maturation. Subsequently, hearing aids were adjusted and verified to match new targets. However, the parents expressed uncertainties regarding whether the amplification was appropriate. Attempts to obtain behavioral responses using VRA testing at 6 months were not successful. Therefore, measurement of CAEPs was conducted in unaided and aided conditions at 6.5 months. It was found that /m/ /g/ /t/ presented at 65 dB SPL and /m/ /g/ presented at 55 dB SPL evoked CAEPs when the child was unaided. However, /t/ presented at 55 dB SPL evoked CAEPs only when the child was using hearing aids. At 11 months corrected age, reliable behavioral audiograms were obtained for each ear (Figure 28–3), consistent with the results on cortical-evoked responses. The measurements of PEACH and CAEPs at the earlier age were useful for fine-tuning the hearing aids, and for assuring the parents about the appropriateness of hearing aid settings for the child.

Referral for Cochlear Implant Candidacy Evaluation

Case 3 was born at 35 weeks gestation. She had jaundice and received phototherapy treatment. After bilateral referral from the UNHS program, diagnostic assess-

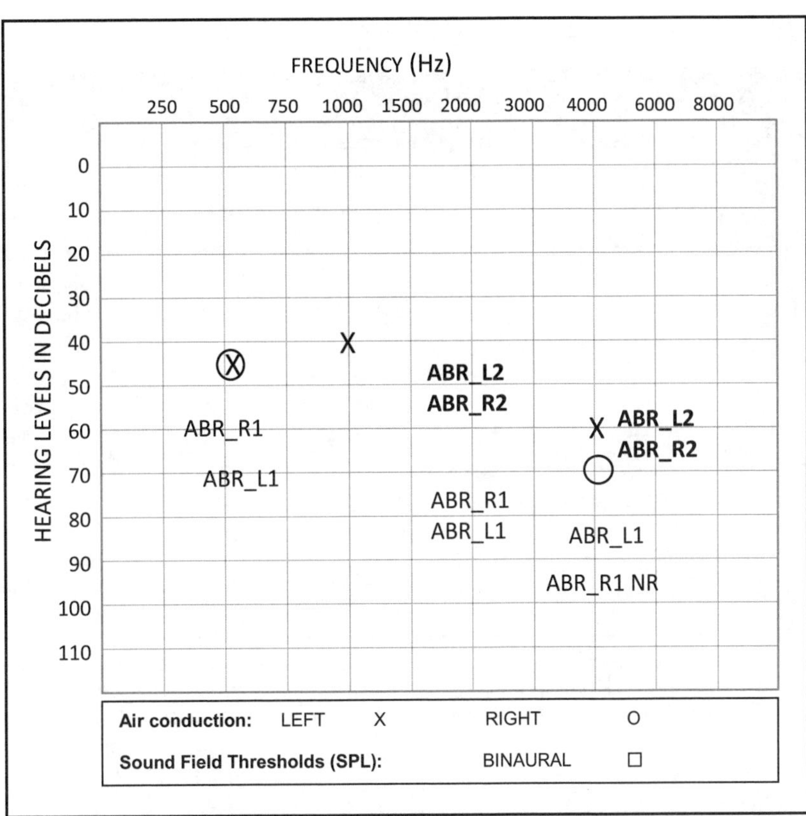

FIGURE 28–3. Audiogram of Case 2, showing results from the diagnostic auditory brainstem response (ABR) testing at 3 weeks corrected age that indicated severe-to-profound hearing loss (ABR_L1 and ABR_R1). A second set of ABR results conducted by the diagnostic hospital at 4.5 months corrected age indicated moderate hearing loss in the left and right ears (ABR_L2 and ABR_R2). Measurement of cortical auditory-evoked potentials (CAEPs) at 6.5 months corrected age indicated detection of /m/ /g/ /t/ presented at 65 dB SPL and /m/ /g/ at 55 dB SPL in the sound field when the child was unaided. CAEPs were detected for /t/ presented at 55 dB SPL only when the child was wearing hearing aids. Subsequent visual reinforcement audiometry (VRA) conducted at 11 months corrected age showed ear-specific hearing thresholds of mild to moderate degrees.

ment was completed at 1 week corrected age. As shown in Table 28–10, the diagnostic ABR assessments showed no measurable thresholds to a tone burst at 0.5 kHz and a click, but clear cochlear microphonics were indicated in both ears. Transient-evoked oto-acoustic emission testing (TEOAE) revealed that responses were present in both ears. These results were consistent with the presence of ANSD bilaterally. Once referred to AH, the child was assessed using behavioral observation audiometry (BOA) and measurement of unaided CAEPs, in accordance with the AH protocol.

The child was aided bilaterally at 5 weeks (1.25 months) corrected age. She was fitted to an estimated behavioral audiogram of 75 dB HL flat loss in both ears, based on the unaided testing of evoked potentials. The hearing aids were adjusted to match the NAL prescriptive targets. Four weeks later, aided measurement of CAEPs was carried out. As no responses were detected, the hearing aids were adjusted to meet targets for a flat loss of 85 dB HL. These results were explained to the parents. When the child was 6.5 months corrected age, VRA was carried out. The results indicated that the child

Table 28–10. Case 3: Audiological Measurements

Age (Months)	Assessment	Results
0.25	Diagnostic ABR	No response to click and tone-burst at 0.5 kHz Cochlear microphonics present bilaterally.
	ASSR	Left: 80 dB HL at 0.5 and 1 kHz, 60 dB HL at 2 and 4 kHz Right: no response between 0.5 and 4 kHz
	TEOAEs	Present bilaterally
0.25	BOA	No reaction to noisemakers at high level
0.5	Unaided CAEPs	No response to /m/, /g/, and /t/ at 65 dB SPL
2.25	Aided CAEPs for the right ear	No response to /m/, /g/, and /t/ at 65 dB SPL; no response to /g/ at 75 dB SPL
6.5	VRA: sound field	Severe to profound hearing loss in at least the better ear

Note. Table includes auditory brainstem responses (ABRs), auditory steady-state responses (ASSRs), transient-evoked otoacoustic emissions (TEOAEs), behavioral observation audiometry (BOA), cortical auditory-evoked potentials (CAEPs), and visual reinforcement audiometry (VRA). "Age" depicts corrected age in months.

has a severe-to-profound hearing loss in at least the better ear. The hearing aids were adjusted accordingly. At subsequent follow-up appointments, the parents reported that the child's reaction to sounds was inconsistent, and her speech and language development was delayed. In view of the aided CAEP results and parent reports, the family was advised to consider referral for cochlear implant candidacy evaluation. The family found the measurement of cortical responses to be useful in helping them to make a decision. At 14 months of age, the child received bilateral cochlear implants.

Developmental Outcomes

Hearing aid amplification is only a means to provide a DHH child with auditory access to sounds so that the child will not be handicapped by the hearing loss. The effectiveness of amplified hearing for development of spoken language is an important outcome for a DHH child.

There are many standardized measures for assessing receptive and expressive spoken language ability. However, an assessment of language outcomes does not indicate whether an optimal, or at least satisfactory, aid fitting has been achieved. Language ability is influenced by many factors including age at fitting, severity of hearing loss, nonverbal cognitive ability, and other environmental factors that are not related to hearing aid fitting (Ching, Dillon, Marnane, et al., 2013). Whereas an age-appropriate language outcome suggests that the hearing aid fitting and the educational intervention that a child receives provide adequate support for development, a below-average language outcome does not indicate what changes need to be made to hearing aid characteristics, whether other hearing devices (e.g., cochlear implantation) need to be considered, or whether alternative approaches to educational intervention need to be implemented. Table 28–11 gives a summary of studies that examined the relationship between language outcomes and hearing aid characteristics in children.

Nevertheless, the ultimate goal of early detection and early treatment is to improve long-term developmental outcomes of DHH children. Measurement of developmental outcomes has been considered as an integral part of the evaluation of the success of newborn hearing screening and early intervention programs (U.S. Centers for Disease Control and Prevention, Early Hearing Detection and Intervention Program Task Force). There is now concerted effort to collect and report developmental outcomes of infants and children identified through a hearing screening program in order to gain insight into the relationship

Table 28–11. Evidence on Relationship Between Language Outcomes and Hearing Aid–Related Factors

Evidence	Number of Participants	Age (in Years)	Hearing Loss	Outcome Measure	Citation
Choice of hearing aid prescription was not a significant predictor of language development.	218	3 years	Mild to moderately severe	Standardized language tests	Ching et al., 2013
Language outcomes were not affected by the use of nonlinear frequency compression in hearing aids.	66	3-, 4-, and 5-year-olds	Mild to severe	Standardized language tests	Bentler, Walker, McCreery, Arenas, & Roush, 2014
Higher hearing-aid gain was associated with better language and speech production.	180	3- and 5-year-olds	Mild and moderate-to-severe hearing loss	SII, standardized tests of language and articulation	Tomblin et al., 2014
Higher aided audibility was associated with better receptive vocabulary, but not with speech recognition.	18	6 to 9 years	Mild to moderately severe	SII, word recognition test, nonword repetition test, receptive vocabulary test	Stiles, Bentler, & McGregor, 2012

between developmental outcomes and the services provided at a population level. Standardized measures of developmental outcomes based on parent reports, including the Child Development Inventory and the McArthur Bates Communicative Development Inventory, have been proposed for assessing children up to 6 years of age (CDC and NCHAM Webinar: Collecting developmental outcome data on children who are deaf and hard-of-hearing, http://www.infanthearing.org/flashplayer/hd_videos.htm?file=http://www.infanthearing.org/flashvideos/webinars/cdc_ncham_webinar.mp4).

In Australia, a population-based study that examines the longitudinal outcomes of children with hearing impairment (LOCHI) found that at 5 years of age, children whose hearing loss was identified via UNHS and who received early intervention before 6 months of age had significantly better spoken language abilities than those whose hearing loss was discovered later than this. For children with severe or profound hearing loss, those who received a cochlear implant before 12 months of age had significantly better spoken language ability than those who received a cochlear implant at an older age. For children who do not have disabilities in addition to hearing loss, their receptive and expressive language scores, math reasoning skills, and real-world functional performance were within the normal range of their hearing peers. This evidence supports the efficacy of UNHS and early intervention for improving developmental outcomes of DHH children at a population level.

The LOCHI study has also found that PEACH scores obtained at 6 or 12 months after initial fitting uniquely accounted for 20% of total variance in language development at 5 years of age (Ching, 2015). Figure 28–4 shows the relationship between early PEACH scores and language scores of children at 5 years of age, separately for children using hearing aids and those using cochlear implants. This finding is consistent with the earlier results reported for children at 3 years of age (Ching, Day, Seeto, et al., 2013). The study also found that PEACH performance was a significant predictor of psychosocial outcomes of children measured using the Child Development Inventory and the Strengths and Difficulties Questionnaire at 5 years of age (Wong et al., personal communication, June 24, 2015). This finding supports the use of early functional performance evaluation based on parent reports (e.g., the PEACH scale) to assess outcomes of children during the first year of life as a monitoring tool to assist with identifying children who might be at-risk of language delays so that alternative strategies can be implemented early.

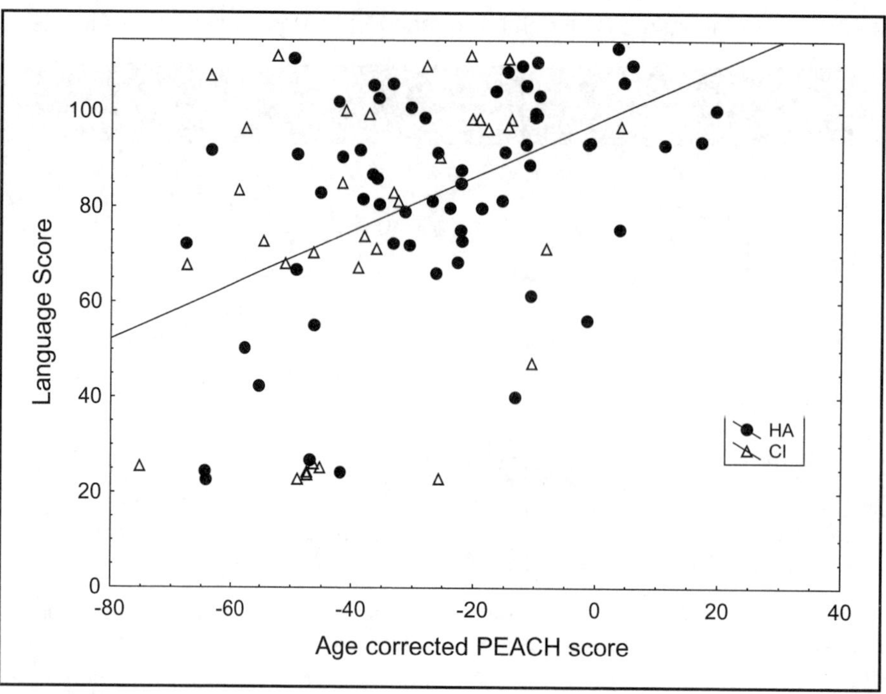

FIGURE 28–4. Standardized language scores at 5 years of age as a function of PEACH scores obtained at 6 or 12 months postfitting for children using hearing aids (*HA, filled symbol*) and children using cochlear implants (*CI, open symbol*). The solid line shows the regression function.

Conclusions

From early childhood into school age, the child outcomes of interest change over time. This chapter has focused on assessing outcomes that can be directly related to the provision of audiological intervention at a young age. After hearing aids have been verified to match prescriptive targets, outcome assessments should be performed to check that the amplification needs of individual children are met. Subjective reports by parents provide a reliable and sensitive method for evaluation of gain-frequency responses in hearing aids for young children. An infants' ability to detect speech sounds can be estimated by measuring the cortical potentials evoked by speech sounds when the child is wearing hearing aids or cochlear implants. This method is particularly useful for children who cannot provide reliable behavioral responses and children with ANSD. Ongoing monitoring of outcomes would assist with identifying children who might be at risk of language delay, and children who might require cochlear implantation as early as possible. As the child grows, so do listening needs and challenges, and different hearing technology will have to be solicited to meet the changing needs. Any use of new strategies or processing schemes for addressing specific needs of a child should be evaluated for its effectiveness in real life. For school-aged children, a range of measures including speech discrimination testing, paired-comparisons judgments, and self-reports can be used to evaluate outcomes. The routine collection of developmental outcomes data can also serve to evaluate the relative success of newborn hearing screening and early intervention services for children with hearing loss.

References

American Academy of Audiology (AAA; 2013). *American Academy of Audiology clinical guidelines: Paediatric amplification.* Retrieved from http://www.audiology.org

American National Standards Institute (ANSI; 1969). *Methods for the calculation of the Articulation Index* (ANSI S3.5-1969). New York, NY: Author.

American National Standards Institute (ANSI; 1997). *Methods for the calculation of the Speech Intelligibility Index* (ANSI S3.5-1997). New York, NY: Acoustical Society of America.

Anderson, K., & Matkin, N. (1996). *Screening instrument for targeting educational risk in preschool children (age 3–kindergarten; Preschool SIFTER)*. Tampa, FL: Educational Audiology Association.

Anderson, K. L., & Smaldino, J. J. (2000). *Children's home inventory of listening difficulties.* Retrieved from http://www.kandersonaudconsulting.com/uploads/child_questionnaire.pdf

Bagatto, M. P., Moodie, S. T., Seewald, R. C., Bartlett, D. J., & Scollie, S. D. (2011). A critical review of audiological outcome measures for infants and children. *Trends in Amplification, 15*(1), 23–33. doi:10.1177/1084713811412056

Bench, J., Kowal, A., & Bamford, J. (1979). The BKB (Bamford-Kowal-Bench) sentence lists for partially-hearing children. *British Journal of Audiology, 13*(3), 108–112.

Bentler, R., Walker, E., McCreery, R., Arenas, R. M., & Roush, P. (2014). Nonlinear frequency compression in hearing aids: Impact on speech and language development. *Ear and Hearing, 35*(4), 143–152.

Boothroyd, A., Eisenberg, L. S., & Martinez, A. S. (2010). An on-line imitative test of speech-pattern contrast perception (OlimSpac): Developmental effects in normally hearing children. *Journal of Speech Language and Hearing Research, 53*(3), 531–542. doi:10.1044/1092-4388(2009/08-0260)

Brennan, M. A., McCreery, R., Kopun, J., Hoover, B., Alexander, J., Lewis, D., & Stelmachowicz, P. G. (2014). Paired comparisons of nonlinear frequency compression, extended bandwidth, and restricted bandwidth hearing aid processing for children and adults with hearing loss. *Journal of the American Academy of Audiology, 25*(10), 993–998.

Byrne, D. (1986). Effects of frequency response characteristics on speech discrimination and perceived intelligibility and pleasantness of speech for hearing-impaired listeners. *Journal of the Acoustical Society of America, 80*(2), 494–504.

Byrne, D. (1992). Key issues in hearing aid selection and evaluation. *Journal of the American Academy of Audiology, 3*(2), 67–80.

Byrne, D., & Cotton, S. (1988). Evaluation of the National Acoustic Laboratories' new hearing aid selection procedure. *Journal of Speech Language and Hearing Research, 31*(2), 178–186.

Byrne, D., Dillon, H., Ching, T., Katsch, R., & Keidser, G. (2001). NAL-NL1 procedure for fitting nonlinear hearing aids: Characteristics and comparisons with other procedures. *Journal of the American Academy of Audiology, 12*(1), 37–51.

Cardon, G., & Sharma, A. (2013). Central auditory maturation and behavioral outcome in children with auditory neuropathy spectrum disorder who use cochlear implants. *International Journal of Audiology, 52*(9), 577–586. doi:10.3109/14992027.2013.799786

Chang, H. W., Dillon, H., Carter, L., Van Dun, B., & Young, S. T. (2012). The relationship between cortical auditory evoked potential (CAEP) detection and estimated audibility in infants with sensorineural hearing loss. *International Journal of Audiology, 51*(9), 663–670. doi:10.3109/14992027.2012.690076

Ching, T. Y. C. (2015). Is early intervention effective in improving spoken language outcomes of children with congenital hearing loss? *American Journal of Audiology, 24*, 345–348.

Ching, T. Y. C., Crowe, K., Martin, V., Day, J., Mahler, N., Youn, S., . . . Orsini, J. (2010). Language development and everyday functioning of children with hearing loss assessed at 3 years of age. *International Journal of Speech Language Pathology, 12*(2), 124–131.

Ching, T. Y. C., Day, J., Dillon, H., Gardner-Berry, K., Hou, S., Seeto, M., . . . Zhang, V. (2013). Impact of the presence of auditory neuropathy spectrum disorder (ANSD) on outcomes of children at three years of age. *International Journal of Audiology, 52*(Suppl. 2), S55–S64. doi:10.3109/14992027.2013.796532

Ching, T. Y. C., Day, J., Seeto, M., Dillon, H., Marnane, V., & Street, L. (2013). Predicting 3-year outcomes of early-identified children with hearing impairment. *B-ENT* (Suppl. 21), 99–106.

Ching, T. Y. C., Day, J., Van Buynder, P., Hou, S., Zhang, V., Seeto, M., . . . Flynn, C. (2014). Language and speech perception of young children with bimodal fitting or bilateral cochlear implants. *Cochlear Implants International, 15*(Suppl. 1), S43–S46. doi:10.1179/1467010014Z.000000000168

Ching, T. Y. C., Dillon, H., Hou, S., Zhang, V., Day, J., Crowe, K., . . . Thomson, J. (2013). A randomized controlled comparison of NAL and DSL prescriptions for young children: Hearing-aid characteristics and performance outcomes at three years of age. *International Journal of Audiology, 52*(Suppl. 2), S17–S28. doi:10.3109/14992027.2012.705903

Ching, T. Y. C., Dillon, H., Katsch, R., & Byrne, D. (2001). Maximizing effective audibility in hearing aid fitting. *Ear and Hearing, 22*(3), 212–224.

Ching, T. Y. C., Dillon, H., Lockhart, F., Van Wanrooy, E., & Flax, M. (2012). Audibility and speech intelligibility revisited: Implications for amplification. In T. Dau, J. C. Dalsgaard, M. L. Jepsen, & T. Poulsen (Eds.), *International Symposium on Auditory and Audiological Research* (pp. 11–19). Copenhagen, Denmark: Danavox Jubilee Foundation.

Ching, T. Y. C., Dillon, H., Marnane, V., Hou, S., Day, J., Seeto, M., . . . Yeh, A. (2013). Outcomes of early- and late-identified children at 3 years of age: Findings from a prospective population-based study. *Ear and Hearing, 34*(5), 535–552. doi:10.1097/AUD.0b013e3182857718

Ching, T. Y. C., & Hill, M. (2007). The parents' evaluation of aural/oral performance of children (PEACH) scale: Normative data. *Journal of the American Academy of Audiology, 18*(3), 220–235.

Ching, T. Y. C., Hill, M., Birtles, G., & Beecham, L. (1999). Clinical use of paired comparisons to evaluate hearing aid fitting of severely/profoundly hearing impaired children. *Australian and New Zealand Journal of Audiology, 21*(2), 51–64.

Ching, T. Y. C., Hill, M., & Dillon, H. (2008). Effect of variations in hearing-aid frequency response on real-life functional performance of children with severe or profound hearing loss. *International Journal of Audiology, 47*(8), 461–475. doi:10.1080/14992020802116128

Ching, T. Y. C., Johnson, E. E., Hou, S., Dillon, H., Zhang, V., Burns, L., . . . Flynn, C. (2013). A comparison of NAL and DSL prescriptive methods for paediatric hearing-aid fitting: predicted speech intelligibility and loudness. *International Journal of Audiology, 52*(Suppl. 2), S29–S38. doi:10.3109/14992027.2013.765041

Ching, T. Y. C., Johnson, E. E., Seeto, M., & Macrae, J. H. (2013). Hearing-aid safety: A comparison of estimated threshold shifts for gains recommended by NAL-NL2 and DSL m[i/o] prescriptions for children. *International Journal of Audiology, 52*(Suppl. 2), S39–S45. doi:10.3109/14992027.2013.847976

Ching, T. Y. C., Newall, P., & Wigney, D. (1994). Audio-visual and auditory paired comparison judgements by severely and profoundly hearing impaired children: Reliability and frequency response preferences. *Australian Journal of Audiology, 16*(2), 99–102.

Ching, T. Y. C., Quar, T. K., Johnson, E. E., Newall, P., & Sharma, M. (2015). Comparing NAL-NL1 and DSL v5 in hearing aids fit to children with severe or profound hearing loss: Goodness of fit-to-targets, impacts on predicted loudness and speech intelligibility. *Journal of the American Academy of Audiology, 26*(3), 260–274. doi:10.3766/jaaa.26.3.6

Ching, T. Y. C., Scollie, S. D., Dillon, H., & Seewald, R. (2010). A cross-over, double-blind comparison of the NAL-NL1 and the DSL v4.1 prescriptions for children with mild to moderately severe hearing loss. *International Journal of Audiology, 49*(Suppl. 1), S4–S15. doi:10.3109/14992020903148020

Ching, T. Y. C., Scollie, S. D., Dillon, H., Seewald, R., Britton, L., Steinberg, J., . . . King, K. A. (2010). Evaluation of the NAL-NL1 and the DSL v.4.1 prescriptions for children: Paired-comparison intelligibility judgments and functional performance ratings. *International Journal of Audiology, 49*(Suppl. 1), S35–S48. doi:10.3109/14992020903095791

Ching, T. Y. C., Zhang, W. V., Hou, S., & Van Buynder, P. (in press). Cortical auditory evoked potentials (CAEPs) reveal changes in aided audibility with nonlinear frequency compression in hearing aids for children: Clinical implications. *Seminars in Hearing*.

Crukley, J., Scollie, S., & Parsa, V. (2011). An exploration of non-quiet listening at school. *Journal of Educational Audiology, 17*, 21–35.

Dawson, P. W., Nott, P. E., Clark, G. M., & Cowan, R. S. (1998). A modification of play audiometry to assess speech discrimination ability in severe-profoundly deaf 2- to 4-year-old children. *Ear and Hearing, 19*(5), 371–384.

Dillon, H. (2012). Special hearing aid issues for children. In H. Dillon (Ed.), *Hearing aids* (2nd ed., pp. 502–504). Sydney, New South Wales, Australia: Boomerang Press.

Dillon, H., Keidser, G., Ching, T. Y. C., Flax, M., & Brewer, S. (2011). The NAL-NL2 prescription procedure. *Phonak Focus, 40*, 1–10.

Dubno, J. R., Dirks, D. D., & Schaefer, A. B. (1989). Stop-consonant recognition for normal-hearing listeners and listeners with high-frequency hearing loss. II: Articulation index predictions. *Journal of the Acoustical Society of America, 85*(1), 355–364.

Eisenberg, L. S. (2007). Current state of knowledge: Speech recognition and production in children with hearing impairment. *Ear and Hearing, 28*(6), 766–772. doi:10.1097/AUD.0b013e318157f01f

Eisenberg, L. S., & Dirks, D. D. (1995). Reliability and sensitivity of paired comparisons and category rating in children. *Journal of Speech and Hearing Research, 38*(5), 1157–1167.

Eisenberg, L. S., & Levitt, H. (1991). Paired comparison judgments for hearing aid selection in children. *Ear and Hearing, 12*(6), 417–430.

Eisenberg, L. S., Martinez, A. S., & Boothroyd, A. (2003). Auditory-visual and auditory-only perception of phonetic contrasts in children (Monograph). *Volta Review, 103*(4), 327–346.

Eisenberg, L.S., Martinez, A.S., & Boothroyd, A. (2007). Assessing auditory capabilities in young children. *International Journal of Pediatric Otorhinolaryngology, 71*(9), 1339–1350. doi: 10.1016/j.ijporl.2007.05.017.

Elliott, L., & Katz, J. (1980). *Northwestern University Children's Perception of Speech (NU-CHIPS)*. St Louis, MO: Auditec.

Gardner-Berry, K., Ching, T. Y. C., Chang, H. W., & Hou, S. (2015). Cortical auditory evoked potential detection rates at different sensation levels in infants with auditory neuropathy spectrum disorder and sensory/neural hearing loss. *Seminars in Hearing*. In press.

Gardner-Berry, K., Purdy, S. C., Ching, T. Y. C., & Dillon, H. (2015). The audiological journey and early outcomes of twelve infants with auditory neuropathy spectrum disorder from birth to two years of age. *International Journal of Audiology, 54*, 524–535. doi:10.3109/14992027.2015.1007214

Gilliver, M., Ching, T. Y. C., & Sjahalam-King, J. (2013). When expectation meets experience: Parents' recollections of and experiences with a child diagnosed with hearing loss soon after birth. *International Journal of Audiology, 52*(Suppl. 2), S10–S16. doi:10.3109/14992027.2013.825051

Glista, D., Easwar, V., Purcell, D., & Scollie, S. (2012). A pilot study on cortical auditory evoked potentials in children: Aided CAEPs reflect improved high-frequency audibility with frequency compression hearing aid technology. *International Journal of Otolaryngology, 2012*. doi:10.1155/2012/982894

Glista, D., & Scollie, S. (2012). Development and evaluation of an English language measure of detection of word-final plurality markers: The University of Western Ontario Plurals Test. *American Journal of Audiology, 21*(1), 76–81. doi:10.1044/1059-0889(2012/11-0036)

Glista, D., Scollie, S., Moodie, S., Easwar, V., & Network of Pediatric Audiologists of Canada. (2014). The Ling 6(HL) test: Typical pediatric performance data and clinical use evaluation. *Journal of the American Academy of Audiology, 25*(10), 1008–1021. doi:10.3766/jaaa.25.10.9

Golding, M., Pearce, W., Seymour, J., Cooper, A., Ching, T. Y. C., & Dillon, H. (2007). The relationship between obligatory cortical auditory evoked potentials (CAEPs) and functional measures in young infants. *Journal of the American Academy of Audiology, 18*(2), 117–125.

Haskins, J. (1949). *Kindergarten Phonetically Balanced Word List (PBK).* St. Louis, MO: Auditec.

Hawkins, D.B. (2004). Limitations and uses of the aided audiogram. *Seminars in Hearing, 25*(1), 51–62.

Hillock-Dunn, A., Buss, E., Duncan, N., Roush, P. A., & Leibold, L. J. (2014). Effects of nonlinear frequency compression on speech identification in children with hearing loss. *Ear and Hearing, 35*(3), 353–365.

John, A., Wolfe, J., Scollie, S., Schafer, E., Hudson, M., Woods, W., . . . Neumann, S. (2014). Evaluation of wideband frequency responses and nonlinear frequency compression for children with cookie-bite audiometric configurations. *Journal of the American Academy of Audiology, 25*(10), 1022–1033.

Kawell, M. E., Kopun, J. G., & Stelmachowicz, P. G. (1988). Loudness discomfort levels in children. *Ear and Hearing, 9*(3), 133–136.

King, A. M. (2010). The national protocol for paediatric amplification in Australia. *International Journal of Audiology, 49*(Suppl. 1), S64–S69. doi:10.3109/14992020903329422

Kirk, K. I., Eisenberg, L., Martinez, A., & McCutcheon, H. (1999). Lexical Neighborhood Test. Test-retest reliability and interlist equivalency. *Journal of the American Academy of Audiology, 10*, 113–123.

Kopun, J. G., & Stelmachowicz, P. G. (1998). Perceived communication difficulties of children with heairng loss. *American Journal of Audiology, 7*(1), 30–38.

Kuehn-Inacker, H., Weichbold, V., Tsiakpini, L., Coninx, F., & D'Haese, P. (2003). *LittlEARS auditory questionnaire manual—Parent questionnaire to assess auditory behaviour in young children.* Innsbruck, Austria: MED-EL.

Kvam, M. H., Loeb, M., & Tambs, K. (2007). Mental health in deaf adults: Symptoms of anxiety and depression among hearing and deaf individuals. *Journal of Deaf Studies and Deaf Education, 12*(1), 1–7. doi:10.1093/deafed/enl015

Ling, D. (1989). *Foundations of spoken language for hearing-impaired children.* Washington DC: Alexander Graham Bell Association for the Deaf.

Marnane, V., & Ching, T. Y. C. (2015). Hearing aid and cochlear implant use in children with hearing loss at three years of age: Predictors of use and predictors of changes in use. *International Journal of Audiology, 54*, 544–551. doi:10.3109/14992027.2015.1017660

Martinez, A., Eisenberg, L., Boothroyd, A., & Visser-Dumont, L. (2008). Assessing speech pattern contrast perception in infants: Early results on VRASPAC. *Otology and Neurotology, 29*(2), 183–188. doi:10.1097/MAO.0b013e3181625114

McCreery, R. W. (2014). Automatic hearing aid features and children: Stop and verify. *Hearing Journal, 67*(7), 22–23.

McCreery, R. W., Bentler, R. A., & Roush, P. A. (2013). Characteristics of hearing aid fittings in infants and young children. *Ear and Hearing, 34*(6), 701–710. doi:10.1097/AUD.0b013e31828f1033

Moeller, M. P. (2007). Current state of knowledge: Psychosocial development in children with hearing impairment. *Ear and Hearing, 28*(6), 729–739. doi:10.1097/AUD.0b013e318157f033

Moeller, M. P., Hoover, B., Peterson, B., & Stelmachowicz, P. (2009). Consistency of hearing aid use in infants with early-identified hearing loss. *American Journal of Audiology, 18*(1), 14–23. doi:10.1044/1059-0889(2008/08-0010)

Moeller, M. P., Tomblin, J. B., Yoshinaga-Itano, C., Connor, C. M., & Jerger, S. (2007). Current state of knowledge: Language and literacy of children with hearing impairment. *Ear and Hearing, 28*(6), 740–753. doi:10.1097/AUD.0b013e318157f07f

Moog, J. S., & Geers, A. (1990). *Early Speech Perception Test.* St. Louis, MO: Centeral Institute for the Deaf.

Munoz, K., Preston, E., & Hicken, S. (2014). Pediatric hearing aid use: How can audiologists support parents to increase consistency? *Journal of the American Academy of Audiology, 25*(4), 380–387. doi:10.3766/jaaa.25.4.9

National Acoustic Laboratories. (2011). *COSI-C: Client Oriented Scale of Improvement for Children.* Lovelock (unpublished). Retrieved from http://www.na.l.gov.au/outcome-measures_tab_cosi.shtml

Nilsson, M. J., Soli, S. D., & Gelnett, D. J. (1996). *Development of the Hearing in Noise Test for Chidlren (HINT-C).* Los Angeles, CA: House Ear Institute.

Palmer, C. V., & Mormer, E. (1999). Goals and expectations of the hearing aid fitting. *Trends in Amplification, 4*(2), 61–71.

Pavlovic, C. V. (1984). Use of the articulation index for assessing residual auditory function in listeners with sensorineural hearing impairment. *Journal of the Acoustical Society of America, 75*(4), 1253–1258.

Pavlovic, C. V. (1989). Speech spectrum considerations and speech intelligibility predictions in hearing aid evaluations. *Journal of Speech and Hear Disorders, 54*(1), 3–8.

Pavlovic, C. V., Studebaker, G. A., & Sherbecoe, R. L. (1986). An articulation index based procedure for predicting the speech recognition performance of hearing-impaired individuals. *Journal of the Acoustical Society of America, 80*(1), 50–57.

Peterson, G. E., & Lehiste, I. (1962). Revised CNC lists for auditory tests. *Journal of Speech and Hearing Disorders, 27*, 62–70.

Petrou, S., McCann, D., Law, C. M., Watkin, P. M., Worsfold, S., & Kennedy, C. R. (2007). Health status and health-related quality of life preference-based outcomes of children who are aged 7 to 9 years and have bilateral permanent childhood hearing impairment. *Pediatrics, 120*(5), 1044–1052. doi:10.1542/peds.2007-0159

Plant, G., & Moore, A. (1993). *The PLOTT screening test and PLOTT sentence test.* Sydney, New South Wales, Australia: National Acoustic Laboratories.

Punch, S., Van Dun, B., King, A., Carter, L., & Pearce, W. (2015). Clinical experience of using cortical auditory evoked potentials (CAEPs) in the treatment of infant hearing loss in Australia. *Seminars in Hearing.* In press.

Purdy, S. C., Farrington, D. R., Moran, C. A., Chard, L. L., & Hodgson, S. A. (2002). A parental questionnaire to evaluate children's Auditory Behavior in Everyday Life (ABEL). *American Journal of Audiology, 11*(2), 72–82.

Quar, T. K., Ching, T. Y. C., Newall, P., & Sharma, M. (2013). Evaluation of real-world preferences and performance of hearing aids fitted according to the NAL-NL1 and DSL v5 procedures in children with moderately severe to profound hearing loss. *International Journal of Audiology, 52*(5), 322–332. doi:10.3109/14992027.2012.755740

Rance, G., Cone-Wesson, B., Wunderlich, J., & Dowell, R. (2002). Speech perception and cortical event related potentials in children with auditory neuropathy. *Ear and Hearing, 23*(3), 239–253.

Rankovic, C. M. (1991). An application of the articulation index to hearing aid fitting. *Journal of Speech and Hearing Research, 34*(2), 391–402.

Robbins, A. M., & Osberger, M. J. (1990). *Meaningful use of speech scale (MUSS).* Indianapolis, IN: Indiana University School of Medicine.

Robbins, A. M., Renshaw, J. J., & Berry, S. W. (1991). Evaluating meaningful auditory integration in profoundly hearing-impaired children. *American Journal of Otology, 12* (Suppl.), 144–150.

Ross, M., & Lerman, P. (1971). *Word intelligibility by picture identification.* Pittsburgh, PA: Stanwix House.

Scollie, S. D. (2008). Children's speech recognition scores: The speech intelligibility index and proficiency factors for age and hearing level. *Ear and Hearing, 29*(4), 543–556. doi:10.1097/AUD.0b013e3181734a02

Scollie, S. D., Ching, T. Y. C., Seewald, R. C., Dillon, H., Britton, L., Steinberg, J., & King, K. (2010). Children's speech perception and loudness ratings when fitted with hearing aids using the DSL v.4.1 and the NAL-NL1 prescriptions. *International Journal of Audiology, 49*(Suppl. 1), S26–S34. doi:10.3109/14992020903121159

Scollie, S., Seewald, R., Cornelisse, L., Moodie, S., Bagatto, M., Laurnagaray, D., . . . Pumford, J. (2005). The Desired Sensation Level multistage input/output algorithm. *Trends in Amplification, 9*(4), 159–197.

Seewald, R., Cornelisse L. E., Ramji, K. V., Sinclair, S. T., Moodie, K. S., & Jamieson, D. G. (1997). *DSL v4.1 for Windows: A software implementation of the desired sensation level (DSL[i/o]) method for fitting linear gain and wide-dynamic-range compression hearing instruments. Users' manual.* London, Ontario, Canada: Hearing Health Care Research Unit.

Seewald, R., Moodie, S. T., & Scollie, S. D. (2005). The DSL method for pediatric hearing instrument fitting: Historical perspective and current issues. *Trends in Amplification, 9*(4), 145–157.

Sharma, A., & Cardon, G. (2015). Cortical development and neuroplasticity in auditory neuropathy spectrum disorder. *Hearing Research.* Advance online publication. doi:10.1016/j.heares.2015.06.001

Sharma, A., Cardon, G., Henion, K., & Roland, P. (2011). Cortical maturation and behavioral outcomes in children with auditory neuropathy spectrum disorder. *International Journal of Audiology, 50*(2), 98–106. doi:10.3109/14992027.2010.542492

Sharma, A., Martin, K., Roland, P., Bauer, P., Sweeney, M. H., Gilley, P., & Dorman, M. (2005). P1 latency as a biomarker for central auditory development in children with hearing impairment. *Journal of the American Academy of Audiology, 16*(8), 564–573.

Smaldino, J., & Anderson, K. (1997, September). *Development of the listening inventory for education.* Paper presented at the second Biennial Hearing Aid Research and Development Conference, Bethesda, MD.

Stiles, D. J., Bentler, R. A., & McGregor, K. K. (2012). The speech intelligibility index and the pure-tone average as predictors of lexical ability in children fit with hearing aids. *Journal of Speech Language Hearing Research, 55*(3), 764–778.

Stredler-Brown, A., & Johnson, C.D. (2001). *Functional auditory performance indicators: An integrated approach to auditory development.* Retrieved from http://www.tsbvi.edu/attachments/FunctionalAuditoryPerformanceIndicators.pdf

Studebaker, G. A. (1991). Measures of intelligibility and quality. In G. A. Studebaker, F. H. Bess, & L. B. Beck (Eds.), *The Vanderbilt Hearing Aid Report II* (pp. 185–194). Parkton, MD: York Press.

Studebaker, G. A., Sherbecoe, R. L., McDaniel, D. M., & Gray, G. A. (1997). Age-related changes in monosyllabic word recognition performance when audibility is held constant. *Journal of the American Academy of Audiology, 8*(3), 150–162.

Tomblin, J. B., Oleson, J. J., Ambrose, S. E., Walker, E., & Moeller, M. P. (2014). The influence of hearing aids on the speech and language development of children with hearing loss. *JAMA Otolarygology-Head and Neck Surgery, 140*(5), 403–409.

Tomlin, D., Dillon, H., Sharma, M., & Rance, G. (2015). The impact of auditory processing and cognitive abilities in children. *Ear and Hearing.* Advance online publication. doi:10.1097/AUD.0000000000000172

Van Dun, B., Carter, L., & Dillon, H. (2012). Sensitivity of cortical auditory evoked potential detection for hearing-impaired infants in response to short speech sounds. *Audiology Research, 2*(e13), 65–76.

Walker, E. A., Spratford, M., Moeller, M. P., Oleson, J., Ou, H., Roush, P., & Jacobs, S. (2013). Predictors of hearing aid use time in children with mild-to-severe hearing loss. *Language, Speech, and Hearing Services in Schools, 44*(1), 73–88. doi:10.1044/0161-1461(2012/12-0005)

Wolfe, J., John, A., Schafer, E., Hudson, M., Boretzki, M., Scollie, S., . . . Neumann, S. (2015). Evaluation of wideband frequency responses and non-linear frequency compression for children with mild to moderate high-frequency hearing loss. *International Journal of Audiology, 54*(3), 170–181.

Wolfe, J., John, A., Schafer, E., Nyffeler, M., Boretzki, M., & Caraway, T. (2010). Evaluation of nonlinear frequency compression for school-age children with moderate to moderately severe hearing loss. *Journal of the American Academy of Audiology, 21*(10), 618–628.

World Health Organization (WHO; 2007). *International Classification of Functioning, Disability and Health (ICF).* Geneva, Switzerland: Author.

Zhang, W. V., Ching, T. Y. C., Van Buynder, P., Hou, S., Flynn, C., Burns, L., . . . Wong, A. (2014). Aided cortical response, speech intelligibility, consonant perception and functional performance of young children using conventional amplification or nonlinear frequency compression. *International Journal of Pediatric Otorhinolaryngology, 78*(10), 1692–1700. doi: 10.1016/j.ijporl.2014.07.022

Zimmerman-Phillips, S., Osberger, M. J., & Robbins, A. M. (1998). Infant-Toddler: Meaningful Auditory Integration Scale (IT-MAIS). In W. Estabrooks (Ed.), *Cochlear implants for kids*. Washington, DC: AG Bell Association for the Deaf.

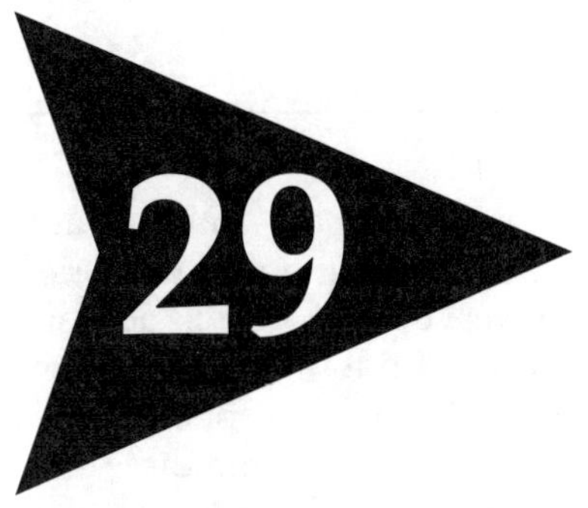

Cochlear Implants for Children: Promoting Auditory Development With Electrical Pulses

Karen A. Gordon

Introduction to Cochlear Implants

Cochlear implants allow individuals with severe-to-profound hearing loss to hear because they bypass any dysfunction in the inner ear (cochlea) and directly stimulate the auditory nerve with electrical pulses. Electrical stimulation of the auditory nerve was first attempted in an adult patient in the 1950s by surgeons Djourno and Eyries (1957; Djourno, Eyries, & Vallancien, 1957a, 1957b). Their work sparked scientific and clinical endeavors culminating in the development of commercial cochlear implants. The early recipients were almost entirely adults who had lost their hearing, and cochlear implants were first approved for adults in the United States in 1985.

Once the adult cochlear implant recipients began to show hearing benefits, children with acquired or even congenital deafness were considered for implantation. One hesitation in implanting children was the question of whether the completely abnormal auditory input from a cochlear implant would promote auditory development. There were some who felt that cochlear implants could never represent speech sounds clearly enough to allow children to develop oral speech and language. In 1990, cochlear implants were approved for children in the United States. Now, almost two decades later, it is clear that children with early onset deafness can learn to hear and understand speech with their cochlear implants and many have developed age-appropriate speech and language skills (e.g., Geers, 2006; Robinson, Davidson, Uchanski, Brenner, & Geers, 2012; Uziel et al., 2007). Not all children achieve the same outcomes of cochlear implantation, however, and most require considerable therapy and effort to learn to hear and speak. The child is part of a family and society, and with that in mind, it is not surprising that important factors contributing to outcomes of cochlear implantation involve the care and support of children as they grow and develop (Quittner et al., 2013). At the same time, it remains essential to understand how the mechanisms of hearing are established through cochlear implant use in children who are deaf. Continuing efforts of current research seek to enhance our understanding of how the many types of deafness that can occur in childhood affect the auditory system and how we might best promote auditory development in children with hearing loss. Auditory development can be measured in many ways, but in this chapter, we concentrate on the specific changes that occur along the auditory pathways with implant use measured using electrophysiological methods. By focusing on such objective measures of auditory activity, auditory function can be assessed in children of all ages even at early stages of device use. The value of this biological perspective of auditory development after cochlear implantation is multifold: (a) our understanding of the human auditory system can be compared to data in animal models; (b) the measures can be used to guide clinical decisions about fitting and managing auditory prostheses; (c) the data can help assess the variability in implant outcomes; and (d) there is potential to use these tools to monitor changes we make for implant users in areas such as education, therapy, and other sociological determinants of outcomes.

Basics of Cochlear Implant Structure and Function

Cochlear implants are designed to stimulate activity in the auditory nerve. This is done using electrical pulses delivered by electrodes that are typically placed in the cochlea close to the auditory neurons. Stimulation of the auditory nerve is normally accomplished by cochlear hair cells that send signals to auditory neurons regarding the frequency and the intensity of the incoming acoustic sound over time. Deafness is most commonly the result of dysfunction of the hair cells or the hair cell-neuron synapse and, consequently, the auditory nerve receives little or no information regarding the sounds passing through the ear. Current research has been focused on which types of dysfunction occur in the hair cells and hair cell-neuron synapses and why these abnormalities occur.

As discussed in Chapter 2, sound causes displacement of the tympanic membrane and middle ear ossicles. The last bone of the ossicular chain, the stapes, presses upon the round window causing fluid displacement in the cochlear, which, in turn, results in movement of the basilar membrane. The stiffness gradient of the basilar membrane sets up an organized arrangement of frequencies; high frequencies cause displacement at the base of the cochlea with progressively lower frequencies displacing the basilar membrane at more apical cochlear locations. The arrangement of frequencies by "place" provides an important basis for hearing pitch differences. Cochlear implants attempt to mimic this organization by sending electrical pulses from electrodes located in basal areas of the cochlea to represent high frequencies and from more apical electrodes for lower-frequency sounds. In a normal auditory system, the displacement of the basilar membrane activates a signaling pathway between hair cells and auditory neurons in the area of displacement. This signaling can occur in phase with the frequency of the incoming acoustic sound (when <4 kHz), allowing auditory neurons to fire at the same rate. The ability to hear frequency and pitch changes is based on these phase cues in addition to the place cues. Cochlear implants deliver electrical pulses at fixed rates from fixed electrode positions along the implanted array. Thus, cochlear implant users rely primarily on limited place cues to hear pitch differences. Acoustic amplitude cues, normally coded by the amplitude of basilar membrane movement, are converted to a range of current levels that represent very soft to loud sounds.

A typical cochlear implant, both internal and external components, is shown in Figure 29–1. In brief, the external components pick up and analyze acoustic sound and send this information to the internal components. Instructions are sent to an array of electrodes that are implanted in the scala tympani, and these electrodes deliver pulses of electricity. The internal component shown has no power source and cannot work without the external equipment.

A more detailed schematic of how cochlear implants function is shown in Figure 29–2 (Loizou, 1998). Sounds are picked up by the microphone and sent to the speech processor, as depicted in Figure 29–2A. At any one time, speech sounds are made up of a number of frequencies (pitches), each with its own intensity (amplitude). As shown in Figure 29–2B, the cochlear implant processor divides the sound into specific bands of frequencies and then analyzes the intensity within each band. Although four bands and four electrodes are shown in Figure 29–2, the number of bands and electrodes varies across different cochlear implant devices. Each frequency band typically is assigned to one implanted electrode. The intensity information for each frequency band is sent through FM wave transmission to the internal receiver-stimulator, which provides innstructions to the cochlear implant electrodes (depicted in Figure 29–2A). Each electrode is programmed to deliver pulses with a dynamic range of current intensity spanning from threshold of audibility to a percept of comfortably loud. The cochlear implant analyzes the quick changes in frequency and amplitude of running speech in real time. The plot in Figure 29–2C shows an example of how speech is converted into electrical pulses by the cochlear implant. Most implant users can track the rhythmic changes in amplitude of the incoming sound and learn to discriminate between different sound frequencies. With these cues, they can learn to understand speech sounds. For children with severe-to-profound bilateral hearing loss, this means that the cochlear implant provides access to sounds that they could not have received through conventional hearing aids and enables oral speech and language development.

Awakening the Deprived Auditory System

Electrical stimulation of the auditory nerve initiates a relay of activity along deprived auditory pathways. In children, these pathways might never have been stimulated before or might not have been active for a period of time. Cochlear implant stimulation therefore provides a unique

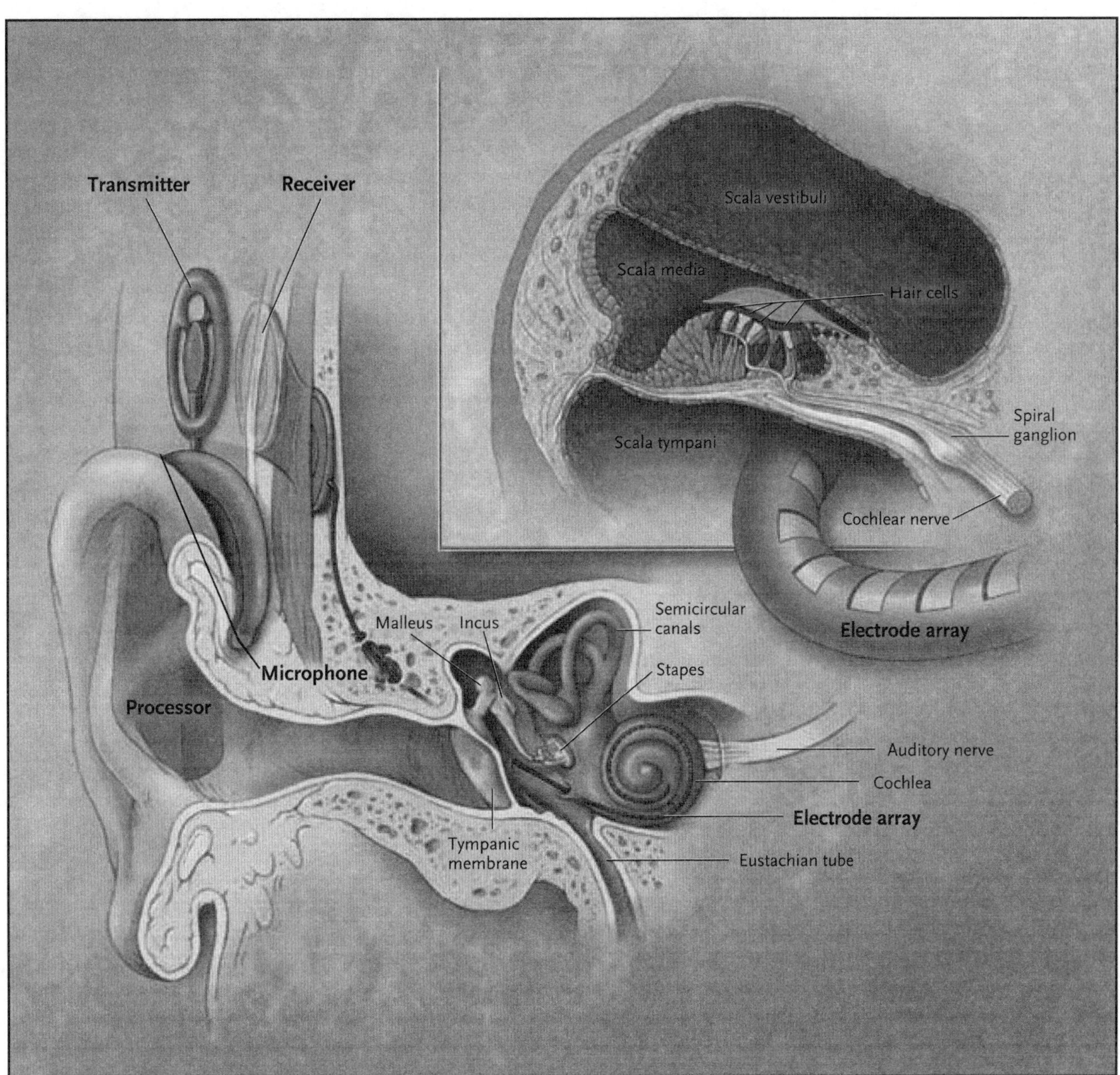

FIGURE 29–1. The cross section of the cochlea shows the electrode array surgically placed in the scala tympani. The implant converts acoustic sound to electrical pulses that stimulate the auditory nerve. Acoustic input enters the microphone, which is worn on the ear, and is sent to the speech processor for analysis of intensity in a number of set frequency bands. The resulting information is sent from the externally worn transmitting coil to the subcutaneous receiver-stimulator through FM waves. These components are held together by a pair of magnets so that they are separated only by the thickness of the skin flap. Each frequency band is assigned to a particular electrode along the implanted array (mimicking the normal basal-to-apical organization of high-to-low frequencies in the cochlea). If instructed, this array will provide a biphasic electrical pulse to stimulate the auditory nerve. The current level for the pulse provided by any one electrode will depend on the intensity of the frequency band and the dynamic range of the current level (minimum to maximum) programmed for that electrode. (Reprinted with permission from Papsin, B. C., and Gordon, K. A. [2007]. Cochlear implants for children with severe-to-profound hearing loss. *New England Journal of Medicine, 357*[23], 2380–2387. Copyright 2007 Massachusetts Medical Society.)

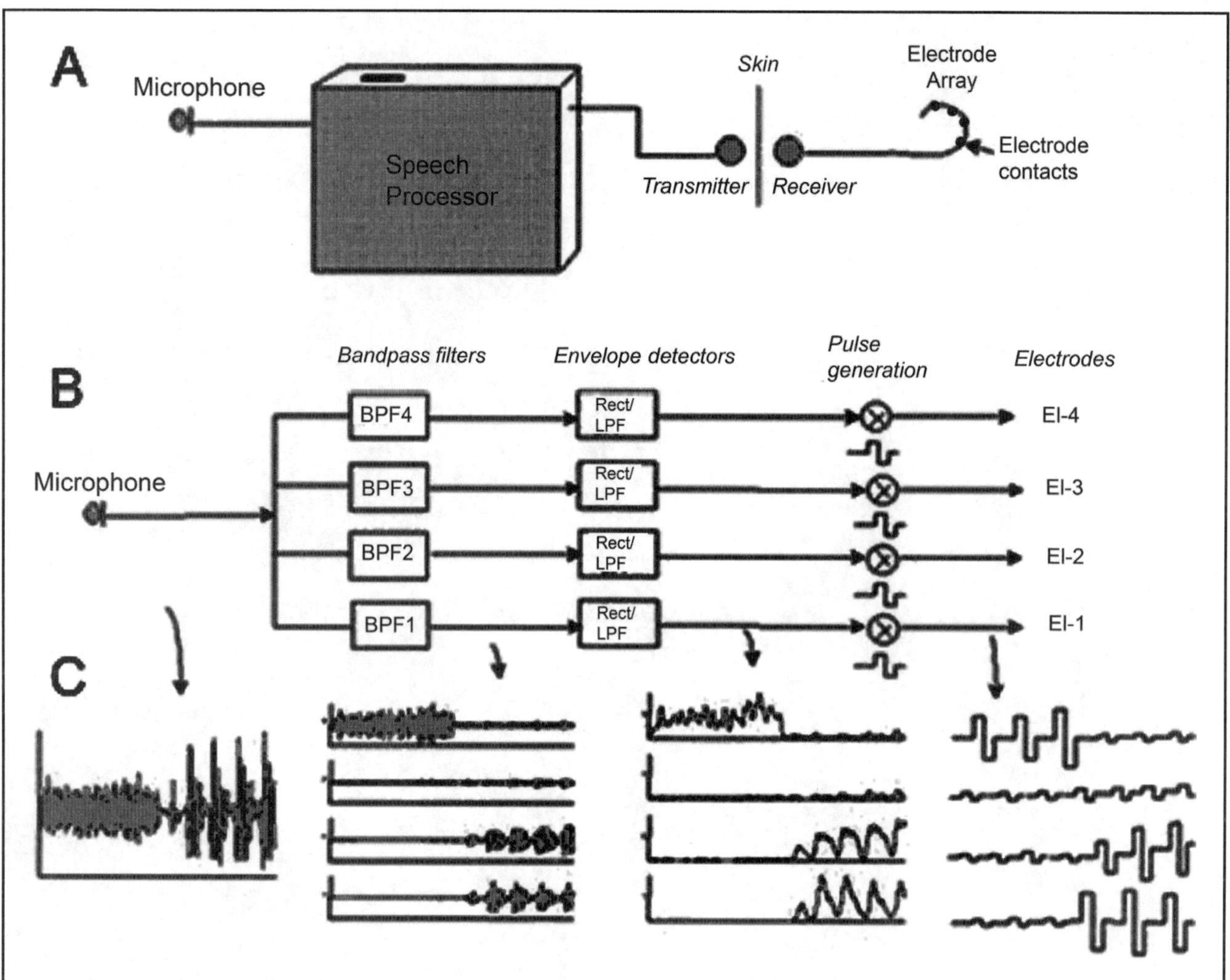

FIGURE 29–2. A. Sound is picked up by the microphone and sent to the speech processor for analysis. The transmitting coil (worn externally) sends this information to the receiver-stimulator (implanted under the skin) and provides instructions to the electrodes implanted in the cochlea. **B.** Further details of the speech processor analyses are shown. The frequency components of the sound are divided into a number of frequency ranges (bandwidths) using bandpass filters (BPFs). The intensity of each bandwidth over time (the envelope) is extracted by rectifying (Rect) and low-pass filtering (LPF) the signal. This information is then converted into electrical pulses delivered by one implant electrode (El). High-frequency bandwidths are assigned to electrodes at the basal end of the array and lower frequencies to more apical electrodes. The current level is customized for each implant user from very soft to comfortably loud. **C.** The process is shown for a particular sound. In this example, sound is divided into four bandwidths (BPFI, BPF2, BPF3, BPF4), and four electrodes (El-1, El-2, El-3, El-4) are available. There is little intensity in one of the four bandwidths, and thus the electrode assigned to this frequency range remains inactive while the others deliver biphasic electrical pulses. In current cochlear implants, electrical pulses are delivered by up to 22 electrodes. (Reprinted with permission from Loizou, P. [1998]. Mimicking the human ear. *IEEE Signal Processing Magazine, 15*(5), Figure 4. Copyright 1998.)

opportunity to study the functional consequences of deafness. The responses obtained in a naïve immature auditory system (one that has not been active before) are very important because they (a) confirm that neural pathways are present, can be stimulated electrically and are organized in an expected way; (b) provide a measure of the effects of deafness; and (c) are a baseline for any changes realized with ongoing cochlear implant use.

Electrophysiologic Responses Evoked by Initial Cochlear Implant Stimulation in Children

Even on the first day of cochlear implant activation in a child born with profound bilateral sensory/neural hearing loss, we can record electrophysiological responses from discrete areas of the auditory system. The cochlear implant is used to stimulate the auditory pathways; examples of responses are shown in Figure 29–3 with a rough approximation of where along the auditory pathways each is generated. The amplitude peaks of the responses evoked in children using cochlear implants are slightly different than those recorded from individuals with normal hearing. These differences can be explained to some extent by the direct stimulation of the auditory pathways with an electrical pulse. Cochlear implant stimulation results in shorter latencies of response peaks that are most evident in the early latency responses. Also, the rapid onset of the electrical pulse from the cochlear implant can result in an increase in the numbers of neurons that respond at the same time (neural synchrony; van den Honert & Stypulkowski, 1984) and are measured as larger and sharper response peaks than those generated by acoustic stimuli. The effects of deafness might also play a role in some of the differences between the cochlear implant and normal hearing responses.

Responses From the Auditory Nerve and Brainstem

The electrically evoked compound action potential (ECAP) of the auditory nerve can be recorded via the telemetry system of the cochlear implant, using a subtraction method to minimize stimulus artifact (Abbas et al., 1999). Electrodes along the cochlear implant array act to both stimulate and record, whereas responses occurring at longer latencies (as shown in Figure 29–3) are measured by recording electrodes placed on the head. The ECAP typically has a negative peak (eN1) at a very short latency (~0.30 ms) reflecting the direct stimulation of the auditory nerve. In a normal hearing individual, the auditory nerve is stimulated at ~1.5 ms, and the response can be recorded along with cochlear responses (see Figure 29–3) or as Waves I and II of the normal auditory brainstem response (ABR; Moller & Jannetta, 1982; Moller, Jannetta, Bennett, & Moller, 1981). As shown in Figure 29–3, the ABR is typically characterized by five positive amplitude peaks (I, II, III, IV, V). The electrically evoked brainstem response (EABR) usually occurs at latencies <5 ms and has three to four characteristic peaks (eII, eIII, eIV, eV) following the initial stimulus artifact. EABRs in our laboratory are often evoked using current levels at the upper part of the dynamic range in children. Waves eIII and eV are most commonly observed, and Wave eIV is rarely found. Comparisons between the ABR and EABR wave latencies and interwave latencies suggest that Wave eII comes from the auditory nerve (Gordon, Papsin, & Harrison, 2006). The EABR has shorter interwave latencies compared to the ABR. In particular, eII-eIII and eIII-eV are shorter than the ABR II-III and III-V, respectively. These measures indicate that neural activity is relayed more quickly through the electrically stimulated than the acoustically stimulated auditory brainstem. This likely reflects the high degree of neural synchrony evoked by the electrical pulse but could also mean that the EABR is generated by different populations of brainstem neurons than the ABR (Gordon, Papsin, & Harrison, 2006).

Responses From Auditory Thalamus and Cortex

The electrically evoked middle latency response (EMLR) ranges in latency from ~15 to 60 ms and is generated by thalamocortical pathways. The most commonly found peaks are eNa, ePa, and eNb. As shown in Figure 29–3, this response is similar to the middle latency response (MLR) recorded in a normally hearing adult. At this level of the auditory system, differences in peak latencies are no longer clear. The MLR in children below approximately nine years of age is known to be obscured in sleeping children (McGee & Kraus, 1996; McGee, Kraus, Killion, Rosenberg, & King, 1993) but is typically present when children are awake or in REM sleep (Rotteveel, Stegeman, de Graaf, Colon, & Visco, 1987). By contrast, we have found that detection of the EMLR at cochlear implant activation in children is variable even though all children were awake at the time of testing (Gordon, Tanaka, & Papsin, 2005). These differences suggest an immaturity of the thalamocortical pathways in children who are deaf. A normal late latency response is shown in the upper left of Figure 29–3 and reflects cortical activity. This response is characterized by three peaks (P1, N1, and P2) in normally hearing teenagers and adults, as well as in adults who received a cochlear implant after postlingual onset of deafness (Ponton & Eggermont, 2001). A typical cortical response in a child with early onset deafness is dominated by a large positive peak of variable latency (100–300 ms; Gordon, Papsin, & Harrison, 2005; Henkin et al., 2004; Ponton, 2006; Sharma, Dorman, & Kral, 2005). A similar response is found in children younger than about nine years of age (Pang & Taylor, 2000; Ponton,

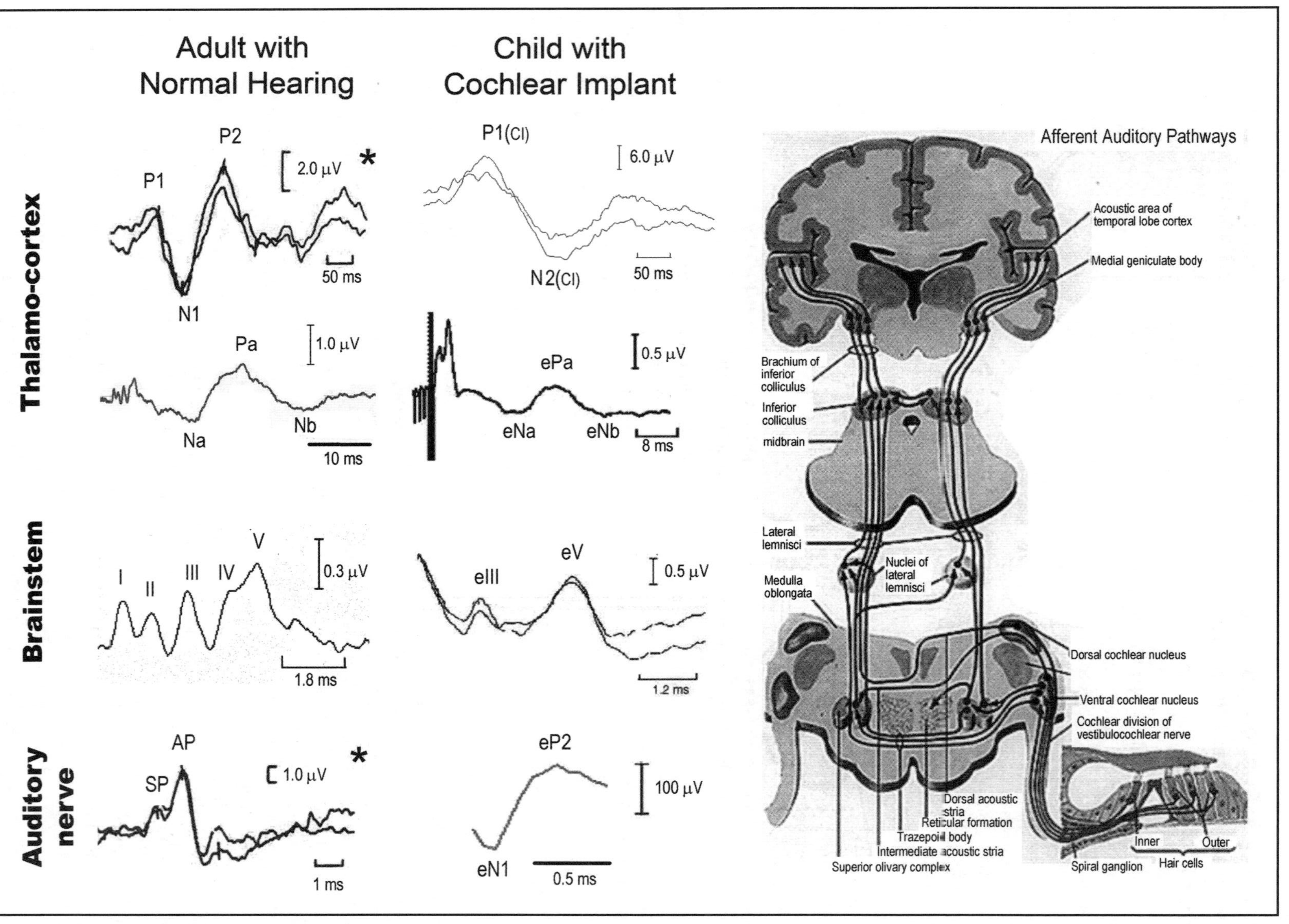

FIGURE 29–3. Electrophysiologic responses evoked by acoustic stimuli in a normal hearing adult and evoked by electrical pulses in a child using a cochlear implant. The responses are shown alongside the approximate areas at which they are generated in the central auditory system (as illustrated by Netter). The cortical response and auditory nerve response from the normal hearing adult (*) are from Hall (1992). (From Hall, J. W. [1992]. *Handbook of auditory evoked responses* (p. 4). Copyright 1992. Reprinted with permission by Pearson Education. AP = action potential; SM = summating potential.)

Eggermont, Khosla, Kwong, & Don, 2002; Sharma, Kraus, McGee, & Nicol, 1997). We have shown that the late latency response in children using cochlear implants can deviate substantially from the more typical waveform shown in Figure 29–3 (Gordon, Tanaka, Wong, & Papsin, 2008) and that this deviation might be particularly true at device activation. We recently showed that this response was strongly prevalent in the newly implanted ear of adolescents who recently received bilateral implants after using one cochlear implant for most of their lives with no stimulation in their opposite ear (Gordon, Jiwani, & Papsin, 2013; Jiwani et al., 2013; Jiwani, Papsin, & Gordon, 2015). Given the variability in cortical responses in children using cochlear implants, it has become essential to locate the neural generators underlying the peaks measured on the surface of the head. The effects of auditory deprivation on the auditory cortex are clearly linked to how the child will perform with his or her cochlear implant. Lee and colleagues (2001, 2007) show that speech perception scores decreased in those children with greater resting state activity in the right Heschl's gyrus and posterior superior temporal sulcus prior to implantation (measured by positron emission tomography). The increase in activity in these hearing areas of the brain in individuals who are congenitally deaf can be explained by the strengthening of other sensory inputs in these areas. The visual system plays a role in reorganization of the deprived and immature auditory cortex as evidenced by abnormally high activity in the auditory cortex when visual signals are shown to individuals who were deaf from an early age (Finney, Clementz, Hickok, & Dobkins, 2003; Finney, Fine, & Dobkins, 2001). This "cross-modal plasticity" likely supports a life with minimal access to sound but appears to be counterproductive to processing auditory input from a cochlear implant provided thereafter.

Bilateral Deafness in Childhood Changes the Auditory System Over Time

Electrophysiological measures recorded at initial cochlear implant activation provide a rare glimpse into the deaf auditory system and can be used to ask questions about the effects of deafness in childhood. We and several other investigators have shown that responses from the auditory nerve, brainstem, and cortex can be evoked in most children receiving cochlear implants at the first cochlear implant stimulation. This is true even for children who had severe-to-profound hearing loss from infancy or birth, which suggests that the central auditory pathways form despite the absence of normal auditory experience. These findings are consistent with recordings of electrically evoked auditory activity in the auditory nerve (Miller, Abbas, & Robinson, 1993; van den Honert & Stypulkowski, 1984), brainstem (Moore, Vollmer, Leake, Snyder, & Rebscher, 2002; Snyder, Rebscher, Leake, Kelly, & Cao, 1991; van den Honert & Stypulkowski, 1986; Vollmer et al., 1999), thalamus, and cortex (Hartmann, Shepherd, Heid, & Klinke, 1997; Klinke, Kral, Heid, Tillein, & Hartmann, 1999; Kral, Hartmann, Tillein, Heid, & Klinke, 2000) in deaf animals. The auditory nerve and brainstem respond in a very regular and predictable way, as shown by clear recording of ECAPs and EABRS at cochlear implant activation in most children who receive cochlear implants (Gordon, Papsin, & Harrison, 2004a, 2004b). Even children who have been bilaterally deaf from birth and implanted as teenagers can show clear ECAPs and EABRs at cochlear implant activation (Gordon, Papsin, & Harrison, 2003, 2007). Remarkably, ECAP and EABR amplitude and latency measures do not appear to be affected by the period of bilateral auditory deprivation (Gordon, Papsin, & Harrison, 2006, 2007). Yet, at the same time, the auditory nerve and brainstem pathways have not matured during the period of deafness, remaining at the same immature developmental stage in children who were deaf from infancy.

By contrast, thalamocortical responses are affected by an extended period of deafness in childhood. Although EMLRs were detected in the majority of older children with longer periods of early onset bilateral deafness, they were poorly detected in younger children (Gordon, Papsin, & Harrison, 2005). Work by Sharma and colleagues has shown some interesting parallels in late latency responses. Late-implanted children showed earlier latency cortical responses than early implanted children (Sharma et al., 2005). Shortened response latencies typically reflect a more mature system because latencies decrease as developing pathways become myelinated and as neural connections (synapses) become more efficient (Kral, 2013). Thus, both the EMLR and late latency responses suggest that the auditory thalamus and cortex undergo change during the period of bilateral deafness. One speculation is that this reflects the cross-modal changes occurring in deafness (discussed above). In support, cortical responses after long-term bilateral or unilateral deafness in childhood appear to be generated in nonauditory areas of the brain such as the parietal cortex (Gilley, Sharma, & Dorman, 2008; Gordon, Wong, & Papsin, 2010; Jiwani, Papsin, & Gordon, 2015).

Do Different Types of Childhood Deafness Affect the Auditory Pathways?

Responses from initial implant stimulation can be useful for studying effects of different types of deafness in children. The discoveries of multiple genetic mutations associated with hearing loss (see the Hereditary Hearing Loss Homepage at http://hereditaryhearingloss.org) have provided a major advance in our understanding of why some children are born without hearing and why others might develop hearing loss later in childhood. Genetic testing has become common in the clinical management of children with hearing loss. Each of these genetic changes might cause unique effects on the central auditory system. Whereas congenital deafness was once thought of as uniform, we now know that it is highly variable.

Cortical responses, shown in Figure 29–4 from 144 ears in 72 children with congenital deafness at initial cochlear implant use reveal impressive variability (Gordon, Tanaka, et al., 2011). It is possible that this variability in auditory activity is associated with differences in the onset and cause of deafness in the perinatal stage of auditory development. Might one etiology of deafness be more susceptible than another to brain changes (such as cross-modal reorganization) that are averse to cochlear implant hearing? Might one etiology be more likely to perform better with a cochlear implant than a hearing aid? These questions are becoming part of discussions in clinical assessments for cochlear implant candidacy as more is known about the etiology of deafness in individual children.

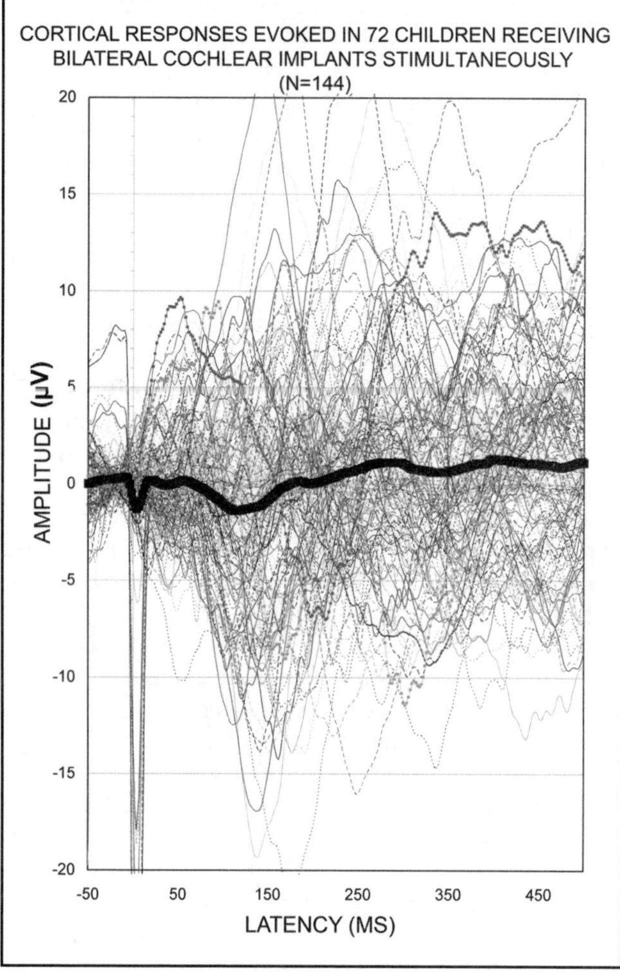

FIGURE 29–4. 144 cortical responses (*thin gray lines*) evoked by electrical pulses delivered by the left and right cochlear implants in 72 children with severe-to-profound deafness. There is a large degree of variability around the mean (*thick black line*). (Reprinted Figure 3 from Gordon et al., 2011b.)

Auditory neuropathy spectrum disorder (ANSD) provides an example of how we are beginning to take etiology of deafness into account when deciding whether to implant. Cochlear implantation in children with ANSD remains on a case-by-case basis as many, but not all, children with ANSD have been successful implant users (Humphriss et al., 2013). These types of hearing losses are characterized by an abnormal acoustically evoked auditory brainstem response and present otoacoustic emissions, indicating functioning outer hair cells but brainstem dys-synchrony. (See Chapters 11 and 12 of this volume for more information about ANSD.)

Etiologies of ANSD include neonatal risks such as hyperbilirubinemia, anoxia, and genetic mutations to *OTOF* and *DFNB59* genes or other hereditary conditions such as Friedreich's ataxia or Charcot-Marie-Tooth disease. Cochlear implantation is considered for these children because of functional hearing difficulties. However, candidacy can be complicated by pure-tone thresholds that can be better than traditional cochlear implant candidates, comorbidity with developmental delays, and questions of whether the site of lesion involves neuropathy of the auditory nerve or brainstem. The latter question is important because both behavioral and electrophysiological outcomes of cochlear implantation in children with hypoplasia of the auditory nerve are often poorer than their peers with normal radiological findings (Valero et al., 2012). Radiological assessments are thus essential to rule out structural deficits of the auditory nerve and brainstem in children with ANSD. Electrophysiological measures might also be helpful to indicate whether the lesion is pre- or postsynaptic and might predict poorer outcomes for the latter (McMahon et al., 2008). For children with ANSD who receive a cochlear implant, confirmation that synchronous activity of the auditory nerve and brainstem has been established can be determined by measurement of the ECAP and EABR. Further confirmation of cortical temporal processing after implantation has also been suggested (He et al., 2013).

Of the genetic determinants of hearing loss, mutations to the *GJB-2* gene that led to the disruption of the connexin 26 protein in the cochlea are most common. We have been interested in effects of homozygous *GJB-2* gene mutations. The auditory nerve (ECAP) response amplitudes recorded at initial device activation from an apical and basal electrode are shown in Figure 29–5A (top plot). The difference in response amplitudes evoked at the apical and basal ends of the array are shown in Figure 29–5A (middle plot). Minimal differences are found in children with homozygous *GJB-2* mutations compared with significantly larger differences in children with no such mutations (Propst, Papsin, Stockley, Harrison, & Gordon, 2006). We suggest that the disruption to cochlear gap junctions by a loss of connexin 26 is likely to occur randomly along the length of the basilar membrane. Any changes to the spiral ganglia as a result of connexin 26 depletion should then also be independent of cochlear location. In contrast, primary nerve responses in children without *GJB-2* mutations show more variable effects of deafness by place of electrical stimulation. Specifically, basal electrodes evoked lower amplitude responses with shallower amplitude growth than those evoked by apical electrodes. We have also found this response pattern in the auditory brainstem. As shown in Figure 29–5B, a large group of children with early onset deafness of primarily unknown etiology had reduced amplitudes and shallower amplitude growth of electrically evoked auditory brainstem responses (EABRs) when evoked by a basal implant electrode compared to responses evoked by an apical electrode (Gordon et al., 2007). These findings suggest that when the etiology of deafness is largely unknown, neural integrity is poorer in the basal than apical ends of the implanted array. This is consistent with evidence from temporal bone analyses that show lower spiral ganglion counts in the basal versus apical ends of the cochlea (Nadol, 1997) and perhaps with the tendency for poorer residual hearing in the high versus low frequencies. Thus, understanding subtle changes between different etiologies of childhood deafness is important as we strive to best promote auditory development in all children with hearing loss.

Clinical Use of Initial Electrophysiologic Responses

The responses shown in Figure 29–3 are objective measures that can be used both to evaluate the auditory system and to determine the current levels required to stimulate these pathways. Behavioral responses are not required for electrophysiological recording other than to monitor comfort. Thus, these objective measures might help to determine appropriate cochlear implant stimulation levels in children who provide limited reliable behavioral reactions to cochlear implant stimulation. Each child must be tested because the levels of current required for one implant user to hear can be quite different from another. In order to provide a dynamic range of intensities (loudness), current from the implant should range from the minimum level required to hear a very soft sound (threshold) to a maximum level that must be loud but comfortable for the user. Behavioral measures of thresholds remain the gold standard to determine these levels, but electrophysiological measures could help to predict these values (Kileny, 1991; Shallop, 1993). ECAP and EABR thresholds show significant correlations with behavioral measures of threshold, but these relationships are not exact (Gordon et al., 2004a, 2004b; Hughes, Brown, Abbas, Wolaver, & Gervais, 2000) and thus cannot be used to accurately predict optimal stimulus levels in all children (Brown, 2003). We have pointed out that maximum current levels are difficult to determine using behavioral responses in children with limited hearing prior to cochlear implantation (Gordon et al., 2004a, 2004b; Steel et al., 2014). The stapedius reflex provides a helpful alternative given that it is known to be elicited at loud levels in normal hearing individuals, that it can be evoked by electrical pulses in cochlear implant users (Almqvist, Harris, & Shallop, 2000; Shallop, 1993; Stephan, Welzl-Muller, & Stiglbrunner, 1990; van den Borne, Snik, Mens, Brokx, & van den Broek, 1996), and that the threshold of the reflex correlates with perceived loudness in adult cochlear implant users who acquired deafness after having normal hearing (Polak, Hodges, & Balkany, 2005; Shallop & Ash, 1995). In our clinic, we typically do not provide stimulation levels that exceed the stapedius reflex threshold so that the children do not experience these reflexes as part of their daily listening.

We have found that ECAP or EABR measures collected at the time of implantation in the operating room are very helpful for initial device activation. When clear responses are recorded, we can be confident that the device is working and that the auditory system is responsive. The stapedius reflex thresholds, measured

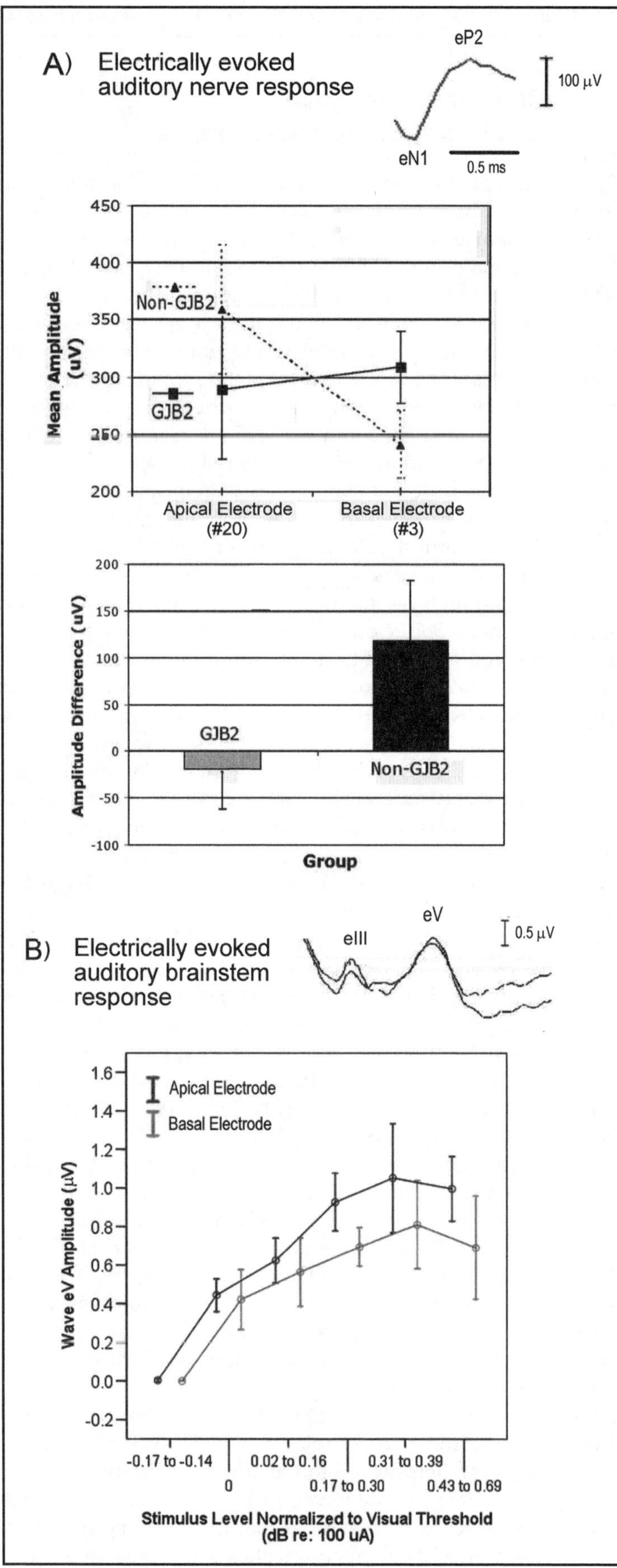

FIGURE 29–5. A. *Top plot:* An example of an auditory nerve response is shown. Auditory nerve responses were evoked by cochlear implant electrodes at the apical and basal ends of the array (#20 and #3, respectively). Estimated marginal mean amplitudes across electrodes are shown for groups with and without *GJB2* mutations. *Middle plot:* The difference in amplitude from apical to basal electrodes tended to be smaller in the *GJB2* group as compared with the non-*GJB2* group. (Reprinted with permission from Propst, E. J., Papsin, B. C., Stockley, T. L., Harrison, R. V., and Gordon, K. A. [2006]. Auditory responses in cochlear implant users with and without GJB2 deafness. *Laryngoscope*, 116[2], p. 323. Copyright 2006 John Wiley & Sons.) **B.** An example of a cochlear implant evoked auditory brainstem response is shown. Auditory brainstem responses were evoked by apical and basal cochlear implant electrodes (#20 and #3, respectively). Mean (1SE) wave eV amplitude obtained at initial stimulation in 50 children is plotted with respect to intensity (dB re:100 uV). Intensity is normalized to visual response thresholds; negative intensities are below visual threshold, 0 dB is equal to visual threshold, and positive values are suprathreshold measures. Amplitude growth appears slightly steeper when evoked by the apical versus basal electrode. (Reprinted with permission from Gordon, K. A., Papsin, B. C., & Harrison, R. V. [2007]. Auditory brainstem activity and development evoked by apical versus basal cochlear implant electrode stimulation in children. *Clinical Neurophysiology, 118*[8], p. 1676. Copyright 2007 Elsevier.)

by watching the stapedius muscle contract to electrical stimulation in the operating room, can be used to define the upper limits of this stimulation. Often children will only tolerate a limited dynamic range at initial stages of device use. As they become accustomed to the sound, however, we aim to increase the range of current intensities based on both objective and behavioral responses.

Objective measures might also be used to track changes in speech perception abilities over time. Cortical responses have been identified as the most likely candidates for this, and there has been some interest in measuring whether the auditory cortex can discriminate between two auditory inputs. Both the mismatched negativity (MMN) response (Groenen, Snik, & van den Broek, 1996; Kelly, Purdy, & Thorne, 2005; Kraus et al., 1993; Ponton & Don, 1995; Ponton et al., 2000; Roman, Canevet, Marquis, Triglia, & Liegeois-Chauvel, 2005) and the cortical "change" response (Brown et al., 2008; Friesen & Tremblay, 2006; Martin, 2007) have been recorded in individuals who use cochlear implants. These measures might help to monitor how the auditory cortex deals with changes in electrical input and to track improvements in hearing abilities (Cone-Wesson & Wunderlich, 2003; Singh, Liasis, Rajput, & Luxon, 2006; Wable, van den Abbeele, Gallego, & Frachet, 2000). Again, this is important for children who are not able to give reliable behavioral reactions to stimulation from their cochlear implant.

Summary of Findings at Initial Cochlear Implant Activation in Children

In general, the cochlear implant is very effective in stimulating the auditory nerve even immediately following implant surgery, although the responses might vary with different types of deafness. The activity evoked by cochlear implant stimulation in the primary auditory nerve is relayed through pathways that form in the absence of significant auditory experience but remain immature. Responses in children using implants can occur at shorter latencies than responses evoked by acoustic stimuli in normal hearing children and can have different amplitude peaks. These differences reflect the unique effects of electrical versus acoustical stimulation of the auditory pathways and also effects of deafness in the central auditory system. As the period of bilateral deafness lengthens, the thalamocortical areas of the pathways are vulnerable to competitive influences from nonauditory areas including the visual system. Responses from discrete areas of the auditory pathways, regardless of how they might differ from normal, indicate that the auditory system is responding to electrical pulses from the cochlear implant. They are thus useful for approximating the current levels required for an individual child to hear. When behavioral responses are not available, this information is particularly valuable.

Stimulating Auditory Development With a Cochlear Implant

The value of electrophysiological responses in children extends beyond the initial stimulation. As the child continues to wear and use the cochlear implant, responses can be monitored for change. The normal auditory system changes and develops throughout childhood (for review see Moore & Linthicum, 2007). Myelin forms around neural projections (axons); some of the connections (synapses) between neurons are strengthened (Ponton, Moore, & Eggermont, 1996), and others are pruned away (Huttenlocher & Dabholkar, 1997). The auditory nerve and brainstem are normally mature by 1 to 2 years of life, whereas the thalamocortical pathways take longer to develop. In the auditory cortex, axonal density increases over many years. As shown in Figure 29–6 from Moore and Guan (2001), deep cortical layers mature by ~6 years of age, while axons continue to form in superficial layers for another ~6 years. Children using cochlear implants allow us to explore whether this development requires activity or experience. The changes in auditory responses in children using cochlear implants reflect not only the ability of the auditory system to change in response to new input (auditory plasticity), but also the importance of activity in development. As discussed in the previous section, the auditory brainstem is formed but does not mature in children who are deaf. Moreover, cortical responses provide evidence of immaturity and even abnormal cortical organization after a period of bilateral deafness. This implies that auditory development does require stimulation, but a number of questions arise: (a) Can auditory development be promoted with cochlear implant stimulation? (b) Can the effects of deafness be overcome by cochlear implant use? And, (c) is electrically evoked auditory development different from normal?

Over time, children using cochlear implants learn to perceive speech with their cochlear implants (i.e., Geers, Brenner, & Davidson, 2003; Nikolopoulos, Archbold, & O'Donoghue, 1999; Papsin, Gysin, Picton, Nedzelski, & Harrison, 2000; Pulsifer, Salorio, & Niparko, 2003; Zeitler et al., 2008), although some children learn

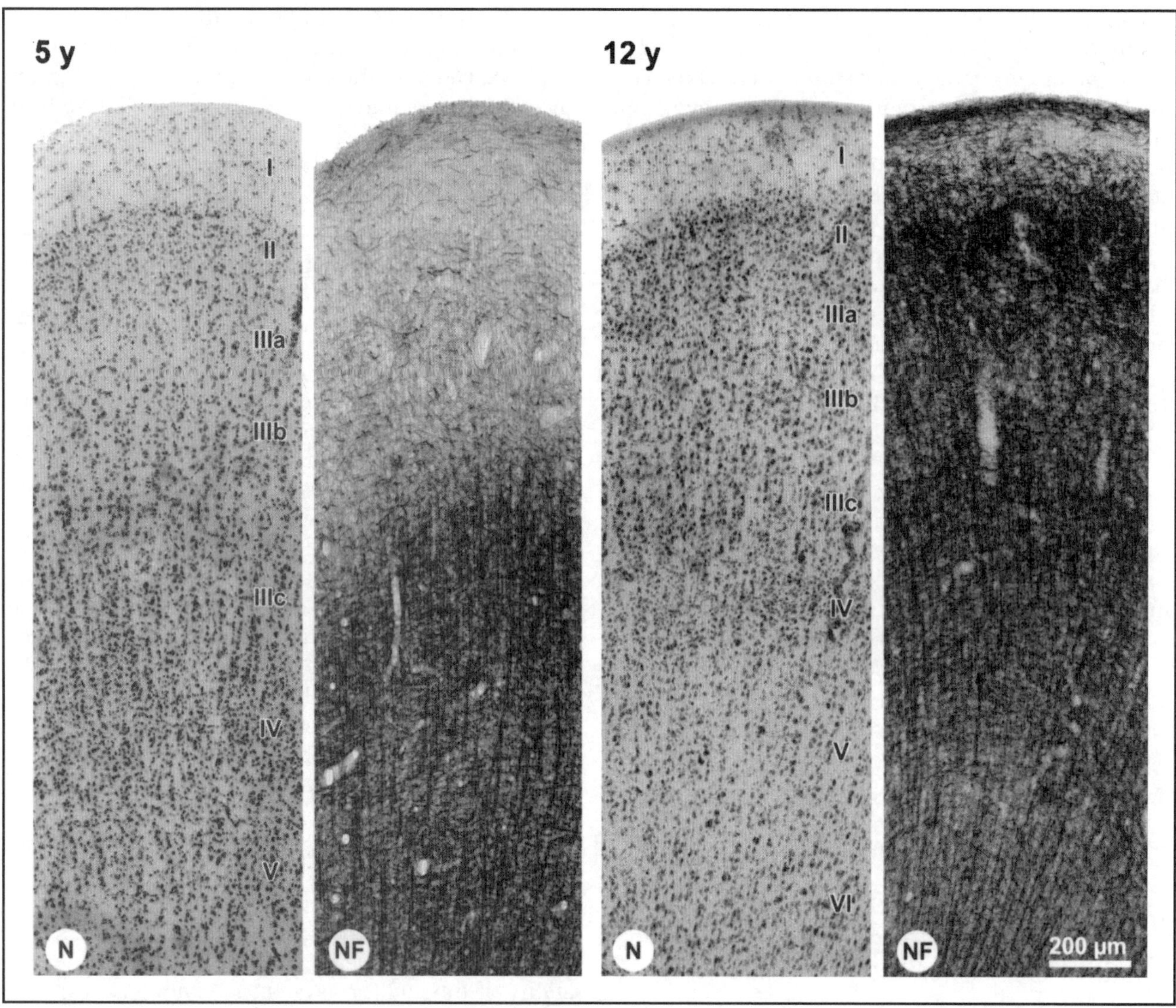

FIGURE 29–6. Cytoarchitecture and axonal maturation in later childhood: Roman numerals indicate cortical Layers I–VI. At ages 3 and 12 years (3 y, 12 y), the Nissl material (N) indicates that cortical depth and cytoarchitecture are similar to that seen at ages 1 to 3 years. Neurofilament (NF) immunostaining at 5 years (5 y, NF) showed that axonal density in Layers VI–IIIc is greater than at ages 1 to 3 years. By 12 years of age, Layers IIIb, IIIa, and II have become filled with a grid of horizontal and vertical immunostained axons (12 y, NF). At both 5 and 12 years, a limited number of NF-positive axons are present near the surface of the marginal layer. (Reproduced with permission from Moore, J. K., & Guan, Y. L. [2001]. Cytoarchitectural and axonal maturation in human auditory cortex. *Journal of the Association for Research in Otolaryngology, 2*[4], p. 306. Copyright 2001. Association for Research in Otolaryngology.)

to hear better and more quickly than others (e.g., Connor, Craig, Raudenbush, Heavner, & Zwolan, 2006; Geers, 2006; Harrison, Gordon, & Mount, 2005; Papsin, 2005). There can be many factors affecting how one child uses a cochlear implant compared with another, but the bases for any improvements in hearing are developmental changes that are promoted by the cochlear implant along the auditory pathways. We have used electrophysiological responses to detect small changes occurring at discrete areas of the auditory system in children using cochlear implants. These measures are also useful because they can be obtained in children of any age and done repeatedly without the use of sedation.

Figure 29–7 shows a typical example of ECAP and EABR recordings measured in one child over the first year of cochlear implant use. Responses are evoked by stimulation from an apical and a basal cochlear implant electrode. The auditory brainstem shows clear decreases in wave latencies over the first year of cochlear implant use. In a group of children, these changes are statistically significant and are not affected by the duration of bilateral deafness (Gordon et al., 2003, 2006, 2007). This has been confirmed by Thai-Van and colleagues (2007) who also showed that a period of normal hearing before the onset of deafness results in shorter EABR wave eV latency.

Decreasing EABR wave and interwave latencies reflect increasingly rapid neural conduction through the auditory brainstem with ongoing cochlear implant use. The ABR undergoes similar latency decreases over the first year of life in normal-hearing infants (Beiser, Himelfarb, Gold, & Shanon, 1985; Jiang, 1995; Ponton, Moore, & Eggermont, 1996; Ponton, Eggermont, Coupland, & Winkelaar, 1992). These changes have been explained by increased myelination and improved synaptic efficiency (Eggermont, 1985, 1988). The EABR changes suggest that once the auditory brainstem receives stimulation, similar processes can occur in children using cochlear implants. The developmental time course for decreasing EABR eIII-eV interwave latency in children with early onset deafness spans over the first year of implant use (Gordon et al., 2006). This means that the unilaterally electrically stimulated auditory brainstem should be approaching maturation at the first anniversary of implant activation. Thalamocortical responses in children also showed change with ongoing cochlear implant use; however, these changes were not consistent for all children (unlike the EABR latency decreases; Gordon, Papsin, & Harrison, 2005). Children implanted at older ages, who also had longer periods of bilateral deafness, showed slower and more subtle changes in both EMLRs (Gordon, Papsin, & Harrison, 2005) and late latency responses (Sharma et al., 2005) than their younger peers who demonstrated rapid changes in both responses during the first six months of implant use. Any limitations to change (or plasticity) of auditory responses in such children could be related to the changes found at initial stimulation. As discussed above, the EMLR was found to be better detected in late than early implanted children (Gordon, Papsin, & Harrison, 2005), late latency peaks were observed at shorter latencies (Sharma et al., 2005), and the auditory cortex was more active in children with longer periods of deafness likely due to cross-modal reorganization (Lee et al., 2001; Lee et al., 2007). It is possible that changes in thalamocortical

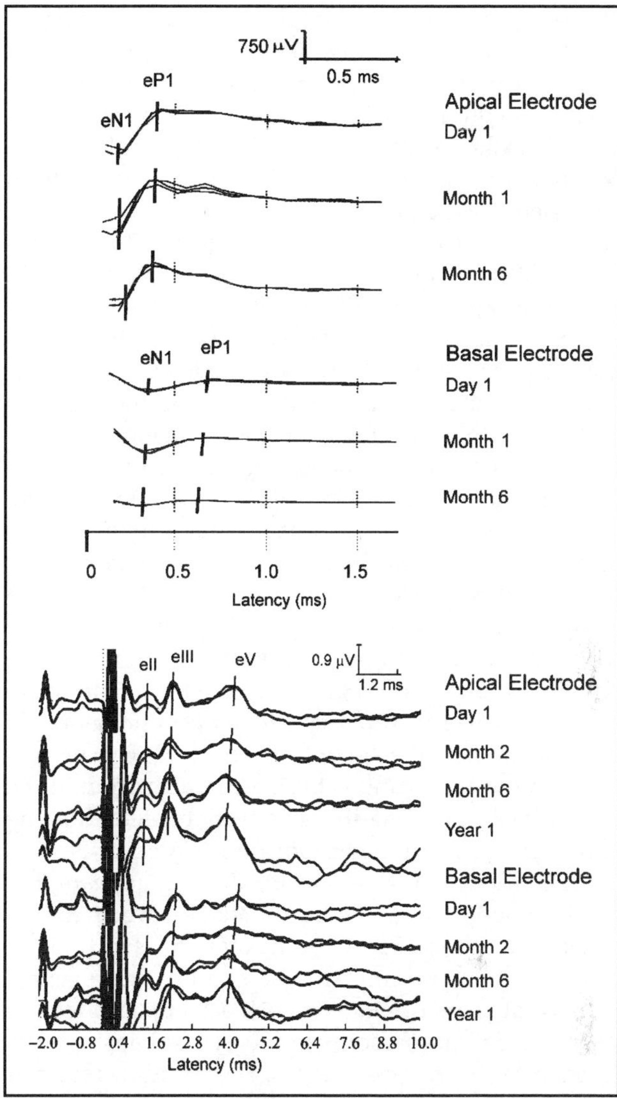

FIGURE 29–7. Measures completed over the first year of implant use in a child with prelingual deafness implanted at 3 years of age. The electrically evoked compound action potential is shown in the top panel and the electrically evoked auditory brainstem response in the panel below. Responses evoked by apical electrodes have noticeably shorter latencies than those evoked by basal electrodes. Decreasing latencies with implant use can also be seen. (Reprinted with permission from Gordon, K. A., Papsin, B. C., & Harrison, R. V. [2007]. Auditory brainstem activity and development evoked by apical versus basal cochlear implant electrode stimulation in children. *Clinical Neurophysiology, 118*(8), 1679. Copyright 2007 Elsevier.)

areas of the auditory pathways, occurring during the period of deafness, are not reversible or cannot be revised in a way that is meaningful for development of hearing. It has been suggested that this permanent effect of deafness is most likely to occur in children implanted after age 7 years and least likely to occur in children implanted before 3.5 years of age (Sharma, 2007; Sharma, Dorman, & Spahr, 2002). Based on these findings, the period of 0 to 3.5 years of age has been proposed to be a sensitive period in auditory development. What is not clear, however, is whether this age cutoff is related to the duration of bilateral deafness or the age of the child or both. Children born with bilateral deafness age at the same rate as their duration of deafness lengthens, which makes it difficult to separate these issues. Understanding the separate and interacting effects of increasing age and longer periods of deafness becomes important as we explore the optimal timing of bilateral cochlear implantation. Recent findings indicate that although long periods of unilateral cochlear implants promote mature looking cortical responses (Jiwani et al., 2013), both cortical hemispheres become abnormally preferential to stimulation from the stimulated ear (Gordon, Wong, & Papsin, 2013) and cortical regions involved in attention are abnormally recruited perhaps to support unilateral CI listening (Jiwani, Papsin, & Gordon, 2015). This reorganization has implications for later implantation of the opposite ear, reducing the benefits of bilateral hearing (Gordon & Papsin, 2009; Gordon, Jiwani, & Papsin, 2013; Gordon, Wong, & Papsin, 2013). It appears that some of these changes to the unilaterally driven immature auditory system occur quickly with as little as 1.5 years of unilateral implant use and are not reversed by several years of bilateral cochlear implant hearing (Gordon, Salloum, Toor, van Hoesel, & Papsin, 2012; Gordon, Wong, & Papsin, 2013). These findings suggest a sensitive period for bilateral input in development and also mean that asymmetric hearing loss in children should be treated as early as possible (Gordon, Henkin, & Kral, 2015). To this end, children with unilateral deafness are beginning to be provided with cochlear implants in an effort to stimulate bilateral hearing.

In sum, developmental change can be promoted with cochlear implant stimulation. Clear changes occur after very short periods of cochlear implant use (<12 months) in the auditory nerve, brainstem, and thalamocortical pathways as measured by electrophysiological responses. Thalamocortical responses showed more restricted degrees of change in children with early onset deafness and implanted at ages older than 7 years. This could be related to an inability to reverse the changes experienced by these areas of the pathway during the period of deafness. Cortical changes occur more quickly in children implanted at young ages, but an abnormal aural preference for the stimulated ear develops if the opposite ear is left deprived of hearing (Gordon, Jiwani, & Papsin, 2013; Gordon, Salloum, Toor, van Hoesel, & Papsin, 2012; Gordon, Wong, & Papsin, 2013; Kral et al., 2013; Kral, Heid, Hubka, & Tillein, 2013; Kral, Hubka, Heid, & Tillein, 2013).

Limitations to Auditory Development in Children Using Cochlear Implants

There are a number of reasons why children using cochlear implants might develop different listening skills than their hearing peers:

- Current cochlear implants do not replace normal hearing and do not perfectly represent acoustic sounds, leading to a loss of important cues.
- Effects of deafness in the auditory system might not be reversible.
- One cochlear implant provides unilateral stimulation only.

These issues are familiar to clinicians involved in cochlear implantation. In our program, parents and children receive counseling prior to implantation to expect that listening might challenging, and all children implanted in our program are required to enroll in auditory training therapy.

Limitations of Cochlear Implant Devices

Electrical pulses from a cochlear implant are highly effective in providing auditory percepts, but they cannot perfectly represent or code acoustic sound. For children, this means that although they are using the best signal currently available, they will not be able to hear as well as their normal-hearing peers. Because electrical pulses from a cochlear implant are presented at a fixed rate, the implant user has no access to the fine timing cues in speech. Efforts to increase the fine timing cues available have included the delivery of electrical pulses at rates of 4,000 pulses or greater. Unfortunately, higher rates of electrical stimulation do not appear to benefit speech perception (Verschuur, 2005) and cause degraded perception of auditory cues (Galvin & Fu, 2005; Pfingst, Xu, & Thompson, 2007). This might be related to neural adaptation that occurs in the auditory brainstem in response to high electrical pulse rates (Davids, Valero, Papsin, Harrison, & Gordon, 2008). In an attempt to mimic normal cochleotopic organization of place cues, cochlear implants assign low frequencies to apical electrodes and higher frequencies to progressively more basal electrodes. However, even the place cues are degraded relative to the normal cochlea because (a) there are a limited number of electrodes on each array; (b) most electrodes are located in the first basal turn of the cochlea; and (c) electrical current from one electrode can overlap with current from a neighboring electrode limiting the independence of each electrode (Bierer & Faulkner, 2010; Cohen, Richardson, Saunders, & Cowan, 2003; Hughes & Abbas, 2006).

Limitations Related to Deafness

As discussed above, the type and duration of deafness in childhood might promote changes in the auditory system that cannot be reversed by cochlear implant stimulation. Although the genetic origins of hearing loss in children are becoming clearer, there is still much to be learned about the mechanisms and effects of these abnormal changes. A better understanding of the effects of different types of deafness might help to improve the interface between the implant and the primary auditory nerve. Additionally, pharmaceutical approaches to reduce the inflammatory tissue response around the implant have been suggested (Lee et al., 2013) as have the use of growth factors to induce peripheral processes of auditory neurons to grow toward the implanted electrode array (Pettingill, Richardson, Wise, O'Leary, & Shepherd, 2007). Both lines of work show promise, but constant delivery of agents into the cochlea is required (King et al., 2013). This could be accomplished using the implant because it has the advantage of having close proximity to the auditory neurons (Pinyon et al., 2014). Remaining questions include whether growth factor–generated neural growth can provide sufficient place cues for better coding of pitch than possible with present cochlear implants.

Limitations Related to Unilateral Stimulation

Hearing with a cochlear implant is further compromised by the lack of binaural cues available when only one cochlear implant is provided. Asymmetric hearing, including hearing from one ear, can result in poorer than normal speech and language development and impaired educational outcomes (Bess, Tharpe, & Gibler, 1986; Klee & Davis-Dansky, 1986; Lieu, 2004; Lieu et al., 2010). Problems stem, in part, from the inability to localize sound and detect speech in noisy environments. Binaural integration, beginning at the level of the brainstem, mediates these functions by assessing interaural intensity cues (in the lateral superior olive) and interaural timing cues (in the medial superior olive). Children with bilateral severe-to-profound deafness can achieve very good speech and language perception in quiet situations using unilateral cochlear implants; however, they have difficulties hearing in noise (Battmer, Reid, & Lenarz, 1997; Luntz, Shpak, & Weiss, 2005), localizing sound (Ching et al., 2005; Figueiredo, Abel, & Papsin, 2001), and understanding emotion in speech (Hopyan-Misakyan, Gordon, Dennis, & Papsin, 2009).

Auditory Development in a Growing Child

Recently, there have been efforts to understand outcomes of cochlear implantation in context with the overall development of the child as a member of a family and society (Eisenberg et al., 2006; Fink et al., 2007; Quittner et al., 2013). The picture in Figure 29–8 is drawn by a child using bilateral cochlear implants who, when asked to draw a picture of himself, includes the color of his hair, the color of his eyes, his cochlear implants (also the correct color!), and other members of his family. He has also drawn his brother's bilateral cochlear implants. It is important to remember that although the primary goal of cochlear implantation in children is to promote auditory development so that speech and language skills can develop, these

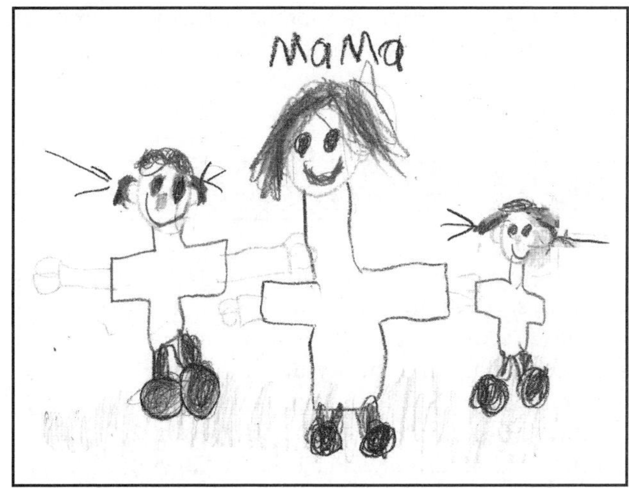

FIGURE 29–8. A portrait by a 7-year-old boy of himself, his mother, and his brother. All the main character traits are shown including the boys' bilateral cochlear implants (*arrows*).

changes will happen in a growing and changing child. The child's educational, emotional, and social development must press on with or without auditory input. Language development is closely intertwined in all of these areas; thus, the child could suffer delays in many areas if language is not attained.

Summary of Limitations to Auditory Plasticity in Children Using Implants

There are a number of factors that set up potential challenges to auditory development in children using unilateral cochlear implants. These include (a) limitations of the cochlear implant and of electrical stimulation; (b) effects of deafness on the auditory system; and (c) a lack of binaural cues. Children using cochlear implants are thus forced to expend greater than normal effort and attention to hear and understand speech in everyday listening environments including school. Our recent studies find that children with cochlear implants take longer than normal to respond in listening tasks (Hopyan et al., 2015) with increases in pupil dilation (Steel et al., 2015), which is thought to be a physiological marker of effort. Underlying changes are likely to involve brain areas including the prefrontal cortex (Lee et al., 2007). This additional effort is a reminder of the challenges that children with implants face. These challenges are important to keep in mind when assessing cochlear implant candidacy and counseling children and families regarding cochlear implant outcomes. Moreover, this means that the role of therapy, which emphasizes listening and speech-language skills and the use of supportive devices and personnel in school, continue to be vital for children using cochlear implants.

Bilateral Cochlear Implants

Of the issues raised in the previous section, the most viable to solve at present is the problem of single-sided listening. We are able to provide binaural cues and stimulate bilateral auditory development by implanting both ears (Gordon, Deighton, Abbasalipour, & Papsin, 2014; Gordon, Jiwani, & Papsin, 2011, 2013; Gordon, Salloum, Toor, van Hoesel, & Papsin, 2012; Gordon, Wong, & Papsin, 2013). Bilateral cochlear implantation is becoming more common in both adults and children. Data from adults who had normal bilateral hearing prior to becoming deaf and who received bilateral cochlear implants indicate that the use of the second device provides increased loudness of auditory input due to the summation of input between the ears (Litovsky, Parkinson, Arcaroli, & Sammeth, 2006). They also experience normal-like processing of level differences between the ears (Grantham, Ashmead, Ricketts, Haynes, & Labadie, 2008), which enables some improvements in sound localization (Litovsky et al., 2004) and speech perception in noise (Tyler, Dunn, Witt, & Noble, 2007). Unfortunately, these adults are not able to use interaural timing cues as effectively as normal-hearing adults (Grantham, Ashmead, Ricketts, Haynes, & Labadie, 2008; van Hoesel, 2007).

Bilateral cochlear implantation in children presents unique difficulties (Papsin & Gordon, 2008) because (a) processing of bilateral input might be complicated by the immaturity of the deprived central auditory system; (b) young children with limited auditory experience often cannot describe what they hear through the implant (Gordon et al., 2004a, 2004b); and (c) the two cochlear implants must be individually programmed and customized for each child, but as yet there are no standardized methods to "balance" or "calibrate" level, timing, and pitch information provided by the two devices (Gordon, Chaikof, Salloum, Goulding, & Papsin, 2012). Nonetheless, bilateral cochlear implantation is rapidly becoming the desired standard of care for bilateral deafness in both adults and children as indicated in position statements from American (Balkany et al., 2008), Canadian (Schramm, 2010), and European (Ramsden et al., 2012) groups. One of the strongest arguments for bilateral implantation in children is that there appears to be a sensitive period for bilateral auditory brainstem development that is missed if bilateral implants are not available for children with deafness in both ears (Gordon, Valero, van Hoesel, & Papsin, 2008; Gordon, Jiwani, & Papsin, 2013; Gordon, Wong, & Papsin, 2013). Cortical responses also suggest that older children with long periods of unilateral implant use prior to bilateral implantation can experience activation of nonauditory areas of the brain and limited auditory plasticity (Bauer, Sharma, Martin, & Dorman, 2006; Gordon et al., 2010; Wong, Papsin, & Gordon, 2010). Behavioral data indicate that children using two cochlear implants are better able to understand speech in quiet and in particular noise conditions (Galvin, Mok, & Dowell, 2007; Gordon & Papsin, 2009), and to discriminate between sound locations (Litovsky et al., 2006) than when using only one implant. Children receiving bilateral implants with limited implanted delays do not suffer from the aural preference that comes from listening from one side for long periods (Gordon,Wong, & Papsin, 2013). This allows for improved sound localization (Beijen, Snik, & Mylanus,

2007) and advantages for speech detection and perception in quiet and noise (Chadha et al., 2011; Gordon & Papsin, 2009; Illing et al., 2013; Mok, Galvin, Dowell, & McKay, 2007). Recent findings show that children with bilateral implants perceive interimplant level cues better than interimplant timing cues (Salloum, Valero, Papsin, van Hoesel, & Gordon, 2010), and long periods of bilateral implant use are required for children using bilateral implants to detect binaural timing cues (Gordon et al., 2014). They are thus more likely to use amplitude cues between the implants to achieve functional benefits. These benefits are achieved in unique ways as children using cochlear implants do not always fuse the input from the two devices into one common sound (Steel et al., 2015). The combined evidence thus far suggests that providing bilateral input to children during early development is essential for development of the auditory system from both ears but that further work is needed to ensure that the input each ear receives is better matched. Electrophysiological responses could be helpful to provide balanced levels (Gordon, Chaikof, Salloum, Goulding, & Papsin, 2012; Gordon Salloum, Toor, van Hoesel, & Papsin, 2012; Salloum et al., 2010) and matched places of stimulation (Gordon, Salloum, Toor, van Hoesel, & Papsin, 2012) between bilateral implants in children.

Conclusions

Cochlear implants allow children who otherwise would be almost completely isolated from sound to hear. Remarkably, cochlear implants have enabled such children to achieve excellent speech perception skills and to develop oral speech and language. We must realize, however, that these outcomes are variable and come with considerable effort on the part of child and family through therapy and educational support. There are multiple factors that contribute to successful cochlear implant use in children. Some issues relate specifically to the input provided by the implant and the auditory system as reviewed in this chapter.

The basic aim of cochlear implants is to stimulate the auditory nerve. However, electrical hearing through a cochlear implant cannot be equated to normal hearing because implants bypass normal processing by the external and middle ears and the cochlea; use fixed rate electrical pulses from limited cochlear locations, thus representing more limited acoustic cues than normal; stimulate auditory systems that might have been affected by deafness; and are often provided unilaterally. Bilateral cochlear implantation might ease listening for children and adults by addressing the latter point and making binaural cues available.

Going forward, cochlear implant research strives to provide the most effective input at optimal periods to promote auditory development that follows a normal auditory trajectory. Clearly, this is the first step for children who need this access to sound to acquire oral speech and language skills that they can use to pursue any educational, vocational, or other avenues of their choosing.

References

Abbas, P. J., Brown, C. J., Shallop, J. K., Firszt, J. B., Hughes, M. L., Hong, S. H., & Staller, S. J. (1999). Summary of results using the Nucleus CI24M implant to record the electrically evoked compound action potential. *Ear and Hearing, 20*(1), 45–59.

Almqvist, B., Harris, S., & Shallop, J. K. (2000). Objective intraoperative method to record averaged electromyographic stapedius muscle reflexes in cochlear implant patients. *Audiology, 39*(3), 146–152.

Balkany, T., Hodges, A., Telischi, F., Hoffman, R., Madell, J., Parisier, S., . . . Litovsky, R. (2008). William House Cochlear Implant Study Group: Position statement on bilateral cochlear implantation. *Otology and Neurotology, 29*, 107–108.

Battmer, R. D., Reid, J. M., & Lenarz, T. (1997). Performance in quiet and in noise with the Nucleus Spectra 22 and the Clarion CIS/CA cochlear implant devices. *Scandinavian Audiology, 26*(4), 240–246.

Bauer, P. W., Sharma, A., Martin, K., & Dorman, M. (2006). Central auditory development in children with bilateral cochlear implants. *Archives of Otolaryngology-Head and Neck Surgery, 132*(10), 1133–1136.

Beijen, J. W., Snik, A. F., & Mylanus, E. A. (2007). Sound localization ability of young children with bilateral cochlear implants. *Otology and Neurotology, 28*(4), 479–485.

Beiser, M., Himelfarb, M. Z., Gold, S., & Shanon, E. (1985). Maturation of auditory brainstem potentials in neonates and infants. *International Journal of Pediatric Otorhinolaryngology, 9*(1), 69–76.

Bess, F. H., Tharpe, A. M., & Gibler, A. M. (1986). Auditory performance of children with unilateral sensorineural hearing loss. *Ear and Hearing, 7*(1), 20–26.

Bierer, J. A., & Faulkner, K. F. (2010). Identifying cochlear implant channels with poor electrode-neuron interface: Partial tripolar, single-channel thresholds and psychophysical tuning curves. *Ear and Hearing, 31*(2), 247–258.

Brown, C. J. (2003). Clinical uses of electrically evoked auditory nerve and brainstem responses. *Current Opinions in Otolaryngology, Head and Neck Surgery, 11*(5), 383–387.

Brown, C. J., Etler, C., He, S., O'Brien, S., Erenberg, S., Kim, J. R., . . . Abbas, P. J. (2008). The electrically evoked auditory change complex: Preliminary results from nucleus cochlear implant users. *Ear and Hearing, 29*, 704–717.

Chadha, N. K., Papsin, B. C., Jiwani, S., & Gordon, K. A. (2011a). Speech detection in noise and spatial unmasking in children with simultaneous versus sequential bilateral cochlear implants. *Otology and Neurotology, 32*(7), 1057–1064.

Ching, T. Y., Hill, M., Brew, J., Incerti, P., Priolo, S., Rushbrook, E., & Forsythe, L. (2005). The effect of auditory experience on speech perception, localization, and functional performance of children who use a cochlear implant and a hearing aid in opposite ears. *International Journal of Audiology, 44*(12), 677–690.

Cohen, L. T., Richardson, L. M., Saunders, E., & Cowan, R. S. (2003). Spatial spread of neural excitation in cochlear implant recipients: Comparison of improved ECAP method and psychophysical forward masking. *Hearing Research, 179*(1–2), 72–87.

Cone-Wesson, B., & Wunderlich, J. (2003). Auditory evoked potentials from the cortex: Audiology applications. *Current Opinions in Otolaryngology, Head and Neck Surgery, 11*(5), 372–377.

Connor, C. M., Craig, H. K., Raudenbush, S. W., Heavner, K., & Zwolan, T. A. (2006). The age at which young deaf children receive cochlear implants and their vocabulary and speech-production growth: Is there an added value for early implantation? *Ear and Hearing, 27*(6), 628–644.

Davids, T., Valero, J., Papsin, B. C., Harrison, R. V., & Gordon, K. A. (2008). Effects of stimulus manipulation on electrophysiological responses of pediatric cochlear implant users. Part II: Rate effects. *Hearing Research, 244*, 15–24.

Djourno, A., & Eyries, C. (1957). Auditory prosthesis by means of a distant electrical stimulation of the sensory nerve with the use of an indwelt coiling. *La Presse Médicale, 65*(63), 1417.

Djourno, A., Eyries, C., & Vallancien, B. (1957a). Electric excitation of the cochlear nerve in man by induction at a distance with the aid of micro-coil included in the fixture [in French]. *Comptes Rendus des Seances de la Societe de Biologie et de Ses Filiales, 151*(3), 423–425.

Djourno, A., Eyries, C., & Vallancien, P. (1957b). Preliminary attempts of electrical excitation of the auditory nerve in man, by permanently inserted micro-apparatus [in French]. *Bulletin de Academie Nationale de Medecine, 141*(21–23), 481–483.

Eggermont, J. J. (1985). Evoked potentials as indicators of auditory maturation. *Acta Otolaryngologica Supplementum (Stockh), 421*, 41–47.

Eggermont, J. J. (1988). On the rate of maturation of sensory evoked potentials. *Electroencephalography and Clinical Neurophysiology, 70*(4), 293–305.

Eisenberg, L. S., Johnson, K. C., Martinez, A. S., Cokely, C. G., Tobey, E. A., Quittner, A. L., . . . Niparko, J. K.; CDaCI Investigative Team (2006). Speech recognition at 1-year follow-up in the childhood development after cochlear implantation study: Methods and preliminary findings. *Audiology and Neuro-Otology, 11*(4), 259–268.

Figueiredo, J. C., Abel, S. M., & Papsin, B. C. (2001). The effect of the audallion BEAM former noise reduction preprocessor on sound localization for cochlear implant users. *Ear and Hearing, 22*(6), 539–547.

Fink, N. E., Wang, N. Y., Visaya, J., Niparko, J. K., Quittner, A., Eisenberg, L. S., . . . Tobey, E. A.; CDaCI Investigative Team (2007). Childhood development after cochlear implantation (CDaCI) study: Design and baseline characteristics. *Cochlear Implants International, 8*(2), 92–116.

Finney, E. M., Clementz, B. A., Hickok, G., & Dobkins, K. R. (2003). Visual stimuli activate auditory cortex in deaf subjects: Evidence from MEG. *NeuroReport, 14*(11), 1425–1427.

Finney, E. M., Fine, I., & Dobkins, K. R. (2001). Visual stimuli activate auditory cortex in the deaf. *Natural Neuroscience, 4*(12), 1171–1173.

Friesen, L. M., & Tremblay, K. L. (2006). Acoustic change complexes recorded in adult cochlear implant listeners. *Ear and Hearing, 27*(6), 678–685.

Galvin, J. J., 3rd, & Fu, Q. J. (2005). Effects of stimulation rate, mode and level on modulation detection by cochlear implant users. *Journal of the Association for Research in Otolaryngology, 6*(3), 269–279.

Galvin, K. L., Mok, M., & Dowell, R. C. (2007). Perceptual benefit and functional outcomes for children using sequential bilateral cochlear implants. *Ear and Hearing, 28*(4), 470–482.

Geers, A. E. (2006). Factors influencing spoken language outcomes in children following early cochlear implantation. *Advances in Oto-Rhino-Laryngology, 64*, 50–65.

Geers, A., Brenner, C., & Davidson, L. (2003). Factors associated with development of speech perception skills in children implanted by age five. *Ear and Hearing, 24*(1 Suppl.), 24S–35S.

Gilley, P. M., Sharma, A., & Dorman, M. F. (2008). Cortical reorganization in children who are deaf. *Brain Research, 1239*, 56–65.

Gordon, K. A., Chaikof, M. H., Salloum, C., Goulding, G., & Papsin, B. (2012). Toward a method for programming balanced bilateral cochlear implant stimulation levels in children. *Cochlear Implants International, 13*(4), 220–227.

Gordon, K. A., Deighton, M. R., Abbasalipour, P., & Papsin, B. C. (2014). Perception of binaural cues develops in children who are deaf through bilateral cochlear implantation. *PLoS One, 9*(12), e114841.

Gordon, K. A., Henkin, Y., & Kral., A. (2015). Asymmetric hearing during development: The aural preference syndrome and treatment options. *Pediatrics, 136*(1), 141–153.

Gordon, K. A., Jiwani, S., & Papsin, B. C. (2011). What is the optimal timing for bilateral cochlear implantation in children? *Cochlear Implants International, 12*(Suppl. 2), S8–S14.

Gordon, K. A., Jiwani, S., & Papsin, B. C. (2013). Benefits and detriments of unilateral cochlear implant use on bilateral auditory development in children who are deaf. *Frontiers in Psychology, 4*, 719.

Gordon, K. A., & Papsin, B. C. (2009), Benefits of short interimplant delays in children receiving bilateral cochlear implants. *Otology and Neurotology, 30*(3), 319–331.

Gordon, K. A., Papsin, B. C., & Harrison, R. V. (2003). Activity-dependent developmental plasticity of the auditory brainstem in children who use cochlear implants. *Ear and Hearing, 24*(6), 485–500.

Gordon, K. A., Papsin, B. C., & Harrison, R. V. (2004a). Programming cochlear implant stimulation levels in infants and children with a combination of objective measures. *International Journal of Audiology, 43*(Suppl. 1), S28–S32.

Gordon, K. A., Papsin, B. C., & Harrison, R. V. (2004b). Toward a battery of behavioral and objective measures to achieve optimal cochlear implant stimulation levels in children. *Ear and Hearing, 25*, 447–463.

Gordon, K. A., Papsin, B. C., & Harrison, R. V. (2005). Effects of cochlear implant use on the electrically evoked middle latency response in children. *Hearing Research, 204*(1–2), 78–89.

Gordon, K. A., Papsin, B. C., & Harrison, R. V. (2006). An evoked potential study of the developmental time course of the auditory nerve and brainstem in children using cochlear implants. *Audiology and Neuro-Otology, 11*(1), 7–23.

Gordon, K. A., Papsin, B. C., & Harrison, R. V. (2007). Auditory brainstem activity and development evoked by apical versus basal cochlear implant electrode stimulation in children. *Clinical Neurophysiology, 118*(8), 1671–1684.

Gordon, K. A., Salloum, C.G., Toor, S., van Hoesel, R., & Papsin, B. C. (2012). Binaural interactions develop in the auditory brainstem of children who are deaf: Effects of place and level of bilateral electrical stimulation. *Journal of Neuroscience, 32*(12), 4212–4223.

Gordon, K. A., Tanaka, S., & Papsin, B. C. (2005). Atypical cortical responses underlie poor speech perception in children using cochlear implants. *NeuroReport, 16*(18), 2041–2045.

Gordon, K. A., Tanaka, S., Wong, D. D. E., & Papsin, B. C. (2008). Characterizing responses from auditory cortex in young people with several years of cochlear implant experience. *Clinical Neurophysiology, 119*, 2347–2362.

Gordon, K. A., Tanaka, S., Wong, D. D., Stockley, T. J., Ramsden, D., Brown, T., . . . Papsin, B. C. (2011). Multiple effects of childhood deafness on cortical activity in children receiving bilateral cochlear implants simultaneously. *Clinical Neurophysiology, 122*(4), 823–833.

Gordon, K. A., Valero, J., van Hoesel, R., & Papsin, B. C. (2008). Abnormal timing delays in auditory brainstem responses evoked by bilateral cochlear implant use in children. *Otology and Neurotology, 29*(2), 193–198.

Gordon, K. A., Wong, D. D. E., & Papsin, B. C. (2010). Cortical function in children receiving bilateral cochlear implants simultaneously or after a period of inter-implant delay. *Otology and Neurotology, 31*(8), 1293–1299.

Gordon, K. A., Wong, D. D., & Papsin, B. C. (2013). Bilateral input protects the cortex from unilaterally-driven reorganization in children who are deaf. *Brain, 136*(Pt. 5), 1609–1625.

Grantham, D. W., Ashmead, D. H., Ricketts, T. A., Haynes, D. S., & Labadie, R. F. (2008). Interaural time and level difference thresholds for acoustically presented signals in post-lingually deafened adults fitted with bilateral cochlear implants using CIS+ processing. *Ear and Hearing, 29*(1), 33–44.

Groenen, P., Snik, A., & van den Broek, P. (1996). On the clinical relevance of mismatch negativity: Results from subjects with normal hearing and cochlear implant users. *Audiology and Neurotology, 1*(2), 112–124.

Hall, J. W. (1992). *Handbook of auditory evoked responses*. Needham Heights, MA: Allyn & Bacon.

Harrison, R. V., Gordon, K. A., & Mount, R. J. (2005). Is there a critical period for cochlear implantation in congenitally deaf children? Analyses of hearing and speech perception performance after implantation. *Developmental Psychobiology, 46*(3), 252–261.

Hartmann, R., Shepherd, R. K., Heid, S., & Klinke, R. (1997). Response of the primary auditory cortex to electrical stimulation of the auditory nerve in the congenitally deaf white cat. *Hearing Research, 112*(1–2), 115–133.

He, S., Grose, J. H., Teagle, H. F., Woodard, J., Park, L. R., Hatch, D. R., & Buchman, C. A. (2013). Gap detection measured with electrically evoked auditory event-related potentials and speech-perception abilities in children with auditory neuropathy spectrum disorder. *Ear and Hearing, 34*(6), 733–744.

Henkin, Y., Kishon-Rabin, L., Tatin-Schneider, S., Urbach, D., Hildesheimer, M., & Kileny, P. R. (2004). Low-resolution electromagnetic tomography (LORETA) in children with cochlear implants: A preliminary report. *International Journal of Audiology, 43*(Suppl. 1), S48–S51.

Hopyan, T., Manno III, F.A.M., Papsin, B.C., & Gordon, K.A. (2015). Sad and happy emotion discrimination in music by children with cochlear implants. *Child Neuropsychology.* http://dx.doi.org/10.1080/09297049.2014.992400

Hopyan-Misakyan, T. M., Gordon, K. A., Dennis, M., & Papsin, B. C. (2009). Recognition of affective speech prosody and facial affect in deaf children with unilateral right cochlear implants. *Child Neuropsychology, 15*, 136–146.

Hughes, M. L., & Abbas, P. J. (2006). The relation between electrophysiologic channel interaction and electrode pitch ranking in cochlear implant recipients. *Journal of the Acoustical Society of America, 119*(3), 1527–1537.

Hughes, M. L., Brown, C. J., Abbas, P. J., Wolaver, A. A., & Gervais, J. P. (2000). Comparison of EAP thresholds with MAP levels in the Nucleus 24 cochlear implant: Data from children. *Ear and Hearing, 21*(2), 164–174.

Humphriss, R., Hall, A., Maddocks, J., Macleod, J., Sawaya, K., & Midgley, E. (2013). Does cochlear implantation improve speech recognition in children with auditory neuropathy spectrum disorder? A systematic review. *International Journal of Audiology, 52*(7), 442–454.

Huttenlocher, P. R., & Dabholkar, A. S. (1997). Regional differences in synaptogenesis in human cerebral cortex. *Journal of Comprehensive Neurology, 387*(2), 167–178.

Illg, A., Giourgas, A., Kral, A., Buchner, A., Lesinski-Schiedat, A., & Lenarz, T. (2013). Speech comprehension in children and adolescents after sequential bilateral cochlear implantation with long interimplant interval. *Otology and Neurotology, 34*(4), 682–689.

Jiang, Z. D. (1995). Maturation of the auditory brainstem in low risk-preterm infants: A comparison with age-matched full term infants up to 6 years. *Early Human Development, 42*(1), 49–65.

Jiwani, S., Papsin, B. C., & Gordon, K. A. (2013). Central auditory development after long-term cochlear implant use. *Clinical Neurophysiology, 124*(9), 1868–1880.

Jiwani, S., Papsin, B. C., & Gordon, K. A. (2015). Early unilateral cochlear implantation promotes mature cortical asymmetries in adolescents who are deaf. *Human Brain Mapping,* doi:10.1002/hbm.23019

Kelly, A. S., Purdy, S. C., & Thorne, P. R. (2005). Electrophysiological and speech perception measures of auditory processing in experienced adult cochlear implant users. *Clinical Neurophysiology, 116*(6), 1235–1246.

Kileny, P. R. (1991). Use of electrophysiologic measures in the management of children with cochlear implants: Brainstem, middle latency, and cognitive (P300) responses. *American Journal of Otology, 12*(Suppl.), 37–42; discussion, 43–47.

King, E. B., Hartsock, J. J., O'Leary, S. J., & Salt, A. N. (2013). Influence of cochleostomy and cochlear implant insertion on drug gradients following intratympanic application in Guinea pigs. *Audiology and Neurootology, 18*(5), 307–316.

Klee, T. M., & Davis-Dansky, E. (1986). A comparison of unilaterally hearing-impaired children and normal-hearing children on a battery of standardized language tests. *Ear and Hearing, 7*(1), 27–37.

Klinke, R., Kral, A., Heid, S., Tillein, J., & Hartmann, R. (1999). Recruitment of the auditory cortex in congenitally deaf cats by long-term cochlear electrostimulation. *Science, 285*(5434), 1729–1733.

Kral, A. (2013). Auditory critical periods: A review from system's perspective. *Neuroscience, 247*, 117–133.

Kral, A., Hartmann, R., Tillein, J., Heid, S., & Klinke, R. (2000). Congenital auditory deprivation reduces synaptic activity within the auditory cortex in a layer-specific manner. *Cerebral Cortex, 10*(7), 714–726.

Kral, A., Heid, S., Hubka, P., & Tillein, J. (2013). Unilateral hearing during development: hemispheric specificity in plastic reorganizations. *Frontiers in Systems Neuroscience, 7*, 93.

Kral, A., Hubka, P., Heid, S., & Tillein, J. (2013). Single-sided deafness leads to unilateral aural preference within an early sensitive period. *Brain, 136*(1), 180–193.

Kraus, N., Micco, A. G., Koch, D. B., McGee, T., Carrell, T., Sharma, A., . . . Weingarten, C. Z. (1993). The mismatch negativity cortical evoked potential elicited by speech in cochlear-implant users. *Hearing Research, 65*(1–2), 118–124.

Lee, D. S., Lee, J. S., Oh, S. H., Kim, S.-K., Kim, J.-W., Chung, J.-K., . . . Kim, C. S. (2001). Deafness: Cross-modal plasticity and cochlear implants. *Nature, 409*(6817), 149–150.

Lee, H. J., Giraud, A. L., Kang, E., Oh, S. H., Kang, H., Kim, C. S., & Lee, D. S. (2007). Cortical activity at rest predicts cochlear implantation outcome. *Cerebral Cortex, 17*(4), 909–917.

Lee, J., Ismail, H., Lee, J. H, , Kel, G., O'Leary, J., Hampson, A., Eastwood, H., & O'Leary, S. J. (2013). Effect of both local and. systemically administered dexamethasone on long-term hearing and tissue response in a Guinea pig model of cochlear implantation. *Audiology and Neurootology, 18*(6), 392–405.

Lieu, J. E. (2004). Speech-language and educational consequences of unilateral hearing loss in children. *Archives of Otolaryngology-Head and Neck Surgery, 130*(5), 524–530.

Lieu, J. E. C., Tye-Murray, N., Karzon, R. K., & Piccirillo, J. F. (2010). Unilateral hearing loss is associated with worse speech-language scores in children. *Pediatrics, 125*(6), e1348–e1355.

Litovsky, R., Parkinson, A., Arcaroli, J., & Sammeth, C. (2006). Simultaneous bilateral cochlear implantation in adults: A multicenter clinical study. *Ear and Hearing, 27*(6), 714–731.

Litovsky, R. Y., Johnstone, P. M., Godar, S., Agrawal, S., Parkinson, A., Peters, R., & Lake, J. (2006). Bilateral cochlear implants in children: Localization acuity measured with minimum audible angle. *Ear and Hearing, 27*(1), 43–59.

Litovsky, R. Y., Parkinson, A., Arcaroli, J., Peters, R., Lake, J., Johnstone, P., & Yu, G. (2004). Bilateral cochlear implants in adults and children. *Archives of Otolaryngology-Head and Neck Surgery, 130*(5), 648–655.

Loizou, P. (1998). Mimicking the human ear. *IEEE Signal Processing Magazine, 15*(5), 101–130.

Luntz, M., Shpak, T., & Weiss, H. (2005). Binaural-bimodal hearing: Concomitant use of a unilateral cochlear implant and a contralateral hearing aid. *Acta Otolaryngologica, 125*(8), 863–869.

Martin, B. A. (2007). Can the acoustic change complex be recorded in an individual with a cochlear implant? Separating neural responses from cochlear implant artifact. *Journal of the American Academy of Audiology, 18*(2), 126–140.

McGee, T., & Kraus, N. (1996). Auditory development reflected by middle latency response. *Ear and Hearing, 17*(5), 419–429.

McGee, T., Kraus, N., Killion, M., Rosenberg, R., & King, C. (1993). Improving the reliability of the auditory middle latency response by monitoring EEG delta activity. *Ear and Hearing, 14*(2), 76–84.

McMahon, C. M., Patuzzi, R. B., Gibson, W. P., & Sanli, H. (2008). Frequency-specific electrocochleography indicates that presynaptic and postsynaptic mechanisms of auditory neuropathy exist. *Ear and Hearing, 29*(3), 314–325.

Miller, C. A., Abbas, P. J., & Robinson, B. K. (1993). Characterization of wave I of the electrically evoked auditory brainstem response in the guinea pig. *Hearing Research, 69*(1–2), 35–44.

Mok, M., Galvin, K. L., Dowell, R. C., & McKay, C. M. (2007). Spatial unmasking and binaural advantage for children with normal hearing, a cochlear implant and a hearing aid, and bilateral implants. *Audiology and Neuro-Otology, 12*(5), 295–306.

Moller, A. R., & Jannetta, P. J. (1982). Auditory evoked potentials recorded intracranially from the brain stem in man. *Experimental Neurology, 78*(1), 144–157.

Moller, A. R., Jannetta, P., Bennett, M., & Moller, M. B. (1981). Intracranially recorded responses from the human auditory nerve: New insights into the origin of brain stem evoked potentials (BSEPs). *Electroencephalography and Clinical Neurophysiology, 52*(1), 18–27.

Moore, C. M., Vollmer, M., Leake, P. A., Snyder, R. L., & Rebscher, S. J. (2002). The effects of chronic intracochlear electrical stimulation on inferior colliculus spatial representation in adult deafened cats. *Hearing Research, 164*(1–2), 82–96.

Moore, J. K., & Guan, Y. L. (2001). Cytoarchitectural and axonal maturation in human auditory cortex. *Journal of the Association for Research in Otolaryngology, 2*(4), 297–311.

Moore, J. K., & Linthicum, F. H., Jr. (2007). The human auditory system: A timeline of development. *International Journal of Audiology, 46*(9), 460–478.

Nadol, J. B., Jr. (1997). Patterns of neural degeneration in the human cochlea and auditory nerve: Implications for cochlear implantation. *Otolaryngology-Head and Neck Surgery, 117*(3 Pt. 1), 220–228.

Nikolopoulos, T. P., Archbold, S. M., & O'Donoghue, G. M. (1999). The development of auditory perception in children following cochlear implantation. *International Journal of Pediatric Otorhinolaryngology, 49*(Suppl. 1), S189–S191.

Pang, E. W., & Taylor, M. J. (2000). Tracking the development of the N1 from age 3 to adulthood: An examination of speech and non-speech stimuli. *Clinical Neurophysiology, 111*(3), 388–397.

Papsin, B. C. (2005). Cochlear implantation in children with anomalous cochleovestibular anatomy. *Laryngoscope, 115* (1 Pt. 2 Suppl. 106), 1–26.

Papsin, B. C., & Gordon, K. A. (2007). Cochlear implants for children with severe-to-profound hearing loss. *New England Journal of Medicine, 357*(23), 2380–2387.

Papsin, B. C., & Gordon, K. A. (2008). Bilateral cochlear implants should be the standard for children with bilateral sensorineural deafness. *Current Opinions in Otolaryngology-Head and Neck Surgery, 16*(1), 69–74.

Papsin, B. C., Gysin, C., Picton, N., Nedzelski, J., & Harrison, R. V. (2000). Speech perception outcome measures in prelingually deaf children up to four years after cochlear implantation. *Annals of Otology, Rhinology, and Laryngology Supplement, 185*, 38–42.

Pettingill, L. N., Richardson, R. T., Wise, A. K., O'Leary, S. J., & Shepherd, R. K. (2007). Neurotrophic factors and neural prostheses: Potential clinical applications based upon findings in the auditory system. *IEEE Transactions on Biomedical Engineering, 54*(6 Pt. 1), 1138–1148.

Pfingst, B. E., Xu, L., & Thompson, C. S. (2007). Effects of carrier pulse rate and stimulation site on modulation detection by subjects with cochlear implants. *Journal of the Acoustical Society of America, 121*(4), 2236–2246.

Pinyon, J. L., Tadros, S. F., Froud, K. E., Wong, A. C. Y., Tompson, I. T., Crawford, E. N., . . . Housley, G. D. (2014). Close-field electroporation gene delivery using the cochlear implant electrode array enhances the bionic ear. *Science Translational Medicine, 6*(233), 233ra254.

Polak, M., Hodges, A., & Balkany, T. (2005). ECAP, ESR and subjective levels for two different nucleus 24 electrode arrays. *Otology and Neurotology, 26*(4), 639–645.

Ponton, C. W. (2006). Critical periods for human cortical development: An ERP study in children with cochlear implant. In S. G. Lomber & J. J. Eggermont (Eds.), *Reprogramming the cerebral cortex: Plasticity following central and peripheral lesions* (pp. 213–228). Oxford, UK: Oxford University Press.

Ponton, C. W., & Don, M. (1995). The mismatch negativity in cochlear implant users. *Ear and Hearing, 16*(1), 131–146.

Ponton, C. W., & Eggermont, J. J. (2001). Of kittens and kids: Altered cortical maturation following profound deafness and cochlear implant use. *Audiology and Neuro-Otology, 6*(6), 363–380.

Ponton, C. W., Eggermont, J. J., Coupland, S. G., & Winkelaar, R. (1992). Frequency-specific maturation of the eighth nerve and brain-stem auditory pathway: Evidence from derived auditory brain-stem responses (ABRs). *Journal of the Acoustical Society of America, 91*(3), 1576–1586.

Ponton, C. W., Eggermont, J. J., Don, M., Waring, M. D., Kwong, B., Cunningham, J., & Trautwein, P. (2000). Maturation of the mismatch negativity: Effects of profound deafness and cochlear implant use. *Audiology and Neurootology, 5*(3–4), 167–185.

Ponton, C., Eggermont, J. J., Khosla, D., Kwong, B., & Don, M. (2002). Maturation of human central auditory system activity: Separating auditory evoked potentials by dipole source modeling. *Clinical Neurophysiology, 113*(3), 407–420.

Ponton, C., Moore, J. K., & Eggermont, J. J. (1996). Auditory brain stem response generation by parallel pathways: Differential maturation of axonal conduction time and synaptic transmission. *Ear and Hearing, 17*(5), 402–410.

Propst, E. J., Papsin, B. C., Stockley, T. L., Harrison, R. V., & Gordon, K. A. (2006). Auditory responses in cochlear implant users with and without GJB2 deafness. *Laryngoscope, 116*(2), 317–327.

Pulsifer, M. B., Salorio, C. F., & Niparko, J. K. (2003). Developmental, audiological, and speech perception functioning in children after cochlear implant surgery. *Archives of Pediatric and Adolescent Medicine, 157*(6), 552–558.

Quittner, A. L., Cruz, I., Barker, D. H., Tobey, E., Eisenberg, L. S., & Niparko, J. K. (2013). Effects of maternal sensitivity and cognitive and linguistic stimulation on cochlear implant users' language development over four years. *Journal of Pediatrics, 162*(2), 343–348, e343.

Ramsden, J. D., Gordon, K., Aschendorff, A., Borucki, L., Bunne, M., Burdo, S., . . . Papsin, B. C. (2012). European Bilateral Pediatric Cochlear Implant Forum consensus statement. *Otology and Neurotology, 33*(4), 561–565.

Robinson, E. J., Davidson, L. S., Uchanski, R. M., Brenner, C. M., & Geers, A. E. (2012). A longitudinal study of speech perception skills and device characteristics of adolescent cochlear implant users. *Journal of the American Academy of Audiology, 23*(5), 341–349.

Roman, S., Canevet, G., Marquis, P., Triglia, J. M., & Liegeois Chauvel, C. (2005). Relationship between auditory perception skills and mismatch negativity recorded in free field in cochlear-implant users. *Hearing Research, 201*(1–2), 10–20.

Rotteveel, J. J., Stegeman, D. F., de Graaf, R., Colon, E. J., & Visco, Y. M. (1987). The maturation of the central auditory conduction in preterm infants until three months post term. III. The middle latency auditory evoked response (MLR). *Hearing Research, 27*(3), 245–256.

Salloum, C., Valero, J., Papsin, B. C., van Hoesel, R., & Gordon, K. A. (2010) Lateralization of inter-implant timing and level differences in children who use bilateral cochlear implants. *Ear and Hearing, 31*(4), 441–456.

Schramm, D. (2010). Canadian position statement on bilateral cochlear implantation. *Journal of Otolaryngology-Head and Neck Surgery, 39*(5), 479–485.

Shallop, J. K. (1993). Objective electrophysiological measures from cochlear implant patients. *Ear and Hearing, 14*(1), 58–63.

Shallop, J. K., & Ash, K. R. (1995). Relationships among comfort levels determined by cochlear implant patient's self-programming, audiologist's programming, and electrical stapedius reflex thresholds. *Annals of Otology, Rhinology, and Laryngology Supplement, 166*, 175–176.

Sharma, A. (2007). Special issue on central auditory system development and plasticity. *International Journal of Audiology, 46*(9), 459.

Sharma, A., Dorman, M. F., & Kral, A. (2005). The influence of a sensitive period on central auditory development in children with unilateral and bilateral cochlear implants. *Hearing Research, 203*(1–2), 134–143.

Sharma, A., Dorman, M. F., & Spahr, A. J. (2002). A sensitive period for the development of the central auditory system in children with cochlear implants: Implications for age of implantation. *Ear and Hearing, 23*(6), 532–539.

Sharma, A., Kraus, N., McGee, T. J., & Nicol, T. G. (1997). Developmental changes in P1 and N1 central auditory responses elicited by consonant-vowel syllables. *Electroencephalography and Clinical Neurophysiology, 104*(6), 540–545.

Singh, S., Liasis, A., Rajput, K., & Luxon, L. (2006). Event related potentials—Are they useful in pediatric cochlear implant patients? *Clinical Otolaryngology, 31*(3), 248–249.

Snyder, R. L., Rebscher, S. J., Leake, P. A., Kelly, K., & Cao, K. (1991). Chronic intracochlear electrical stimulation in the neonatally deafened cat. II. Temporal properties of neurons in the inferior colliculus. *Hearing Research, 56*(1–2), 246–264.

Steel, M. M., Abbasalipour, P., Salloum, C. A., Hasek, D., Papsin, B. C., & Gordon, K. A. (2014). Unilateral cochlear implant use promotes normal-like loudness perception in adolescents with childhood deafness. *Ear and Hearing, 35*(6), e291–e301.

Steel, M. M., Papsin, B. C., & Gordon, K. A. (2015). Binaural fusion and listening effort in children who use bilateral cochlear implants: A psychoacoustic and pupillometric study, *PLoS ONE, 10*(10), e0141945. doi: 10.1371/journal.pone.0141945.

Stephan, K., Welzl-Muller, K., & Stiglbrunner, H. (1990). Stapedius reflex growth function in cochlear implant patients. *Audiology, 29*(1), 46–54.

Thai-Van, H., Cozma, S., Boutitie, F., Disant, F., Truy, E., & Collet, L. (2007). The pattern of auditory brainstem response wave V maturation in cochlear-implanted children. *Clinical Neurophysiology, 118*(3), 676–689.

Tyler, R. S., Dunn, C. C., Witt, S. A., & Noble, W. G. (2007). Speech perception and localization with adults with bilateral sequential cochlear implants. *Ear and Hearing, 28*(2 Suppl.), 86S–90S.

Uziel, A. S., Sillon, M., Vieu, A., Artieres, F., Piron, J. P., Daures, J. P., & Mondain, M. (2007). Ten-year follow-up of a consecutive series of children with multichannel cochlear implants. *Otology and Neurotology, 28*(5), 615–628.

Valero, J., Blaser, S., Papsin, B. C., James, A. L., & Gordon, K. A. (2012). Electrophysiologic and behavioral outcomes of cochlear implantation in children with auditory nerve hypoplasia. *Ear and Hearing, 33*(1), 3–18.

van den Borne, B., Snik, A. F., Mens, L. H., Brokx, J. P., & van den Broek, P. (1996). Stapedius reflex measurements during surgery for cochlear implantation in children. *American Journal of Otology, 17*(4), 554–558.

van den Honert, C., & Stypulkowski, P. H. (1984). Physiological properties of the electrically stimulated auditory nerve. II. Single fiber recordings. *Hearing Research, 14*(3), 225–243.

van den Honert, C., & Stypulkowski, P. H. (1986). Characterization of the electrically evoked auditory brainstem response (ABR) in cats and humans. *Hearing Research, 21*(2), 109–126.

van Hoesel, R. J. (2007). Sensitivity to binaural timing in bilateral cochlear implant users. *Journal of the Acoustical Society of America, 121*(4), 2192–2206.

Verschuur, C. A. (2005). Effect of stimulation rate on speech perception in adult users of the Med-El CIS speech processing strategy. *International Journal of Audiology, 44*(1), 58–63.

Vollmer, M., Snyder, R. L., Leake, P. A., Beitel, R. E., Moore, C. M., & Rebscher, S. J. (1999). Temporal properties of chronic cochlear electrical stimulation determine temporal resolution of neurons in cat inferior colliculus. *Journal of Neurophysiology, 82*(6), 2883–2902.

Wable, J., van den Abbeele, T., Gallego, S., & Frachet, B. (2000). Mismatch negativity: A tool for the assessment of stimuli discrimination in cochlear implant subjects. *Clinical Neurophysiology, 111*(4), 743–751.

Wong, D. D. E., Papsin, B. D., & Gordon, K. A. (2010, February 5–10). *Hemispheric lateralization of cortical responses in children using bilateral cochlear implants*. Poster presentation at the Association for Research in Otolaryngology, Anaheim, CA.

Zeitler, D. M., Kessler, M. A., Terushkin, V., Roland, T. J., Jr., Svirsky, M. A., Lalwani, A. K., & Waltzman, S. B. (2008). Speech perception benefits of sequential bilateral cochlear implantation in children and adults: A retrospective analysis. *Otology and Neurotology, 29*(3), 314–325.

Care of Children Who Use Cochlear Implants

Marilyn Neault

Introduction

In the early 1990s, a child from halfway around the globe appeared in the otolaryngology clinic at Children's Hospital Boston, Massachusetts. "My son is deaf," said the father through an interpreter. "He had an operation last year in my country for his hearing, but he can't hear any better than before." Baffled, the resident sent the child to Audiology. The audiologist felt for a slightly raised area on one side of the child's head, behind his ear. "When he had the operation, were you given a box?" she asked. "Yes, it's in our hotel room," replied the father. "Nobody told us what to do with it, so we never opened it."

Absurd but true, this story is the antithesis of the preparation, teamwork, and follow-up steps that characterize most cochlear implant procedures at major pediatric implant centers today. A review of these steps, and the reasons for them, helps to clarify the factors that support a good outcome.

Overview of the Cochlear Implant

The cochlear implant is humankind's first artificial sense organ. It stimulates sensory neurons to fire in a pattern that mirrors aspects of the external environment. A thorough explanation of the function of a cochlear implant, both electrically and electrophysiologically, can be found in Chapter 29. An externally worn processor (Figure 30–1) transforms sounds picked up by a microphone into a complex series of pulses that are transmitted across the skin by radio waves to the implant (Figure 30–2). The processor's transmitting coil attaches to the receiver/stimulator portion of the implant by means of two magnets, one outside and one under the skin. If the child has been implanted with a magnetless internal device because of a projected need for future magnetic resonance imaging (MRI) tests, an adhesive retainer disk, changed weekly and containing a small magnet, can be worn on the scalp to hold the transmitting coil in place. The antenna of the receiver/stimulator under the scalp picks up the signal that has been sent across the skin and sends it to an array of electrodes in the cochlea.

Although the electrode arrays of current models can have 16 to 24 electrodes arranged into 12 to 22 channels, some electrodes might be deactivated in a particular user's program because they are not working (short circuit or open circuit), because they are not fully inserted in the cochlea, or because they elicit facial or vestibular stimulation. With present-day technology, the number of channels available for frequency encoding is limited by current spread and channel interactions. For some implants, additional virtual channels are made possible by current steering to achieve intermediate pitch percepts (Koch, Downing, Osberger, & Litvak, 2007), or by adding temporal encoding to the low frequency channels (Wilson et al., 2005). Although some users can identify more acoustically presented pitches than the number of channels of stimulation, other users might not be able to perceive pitch differences between all the channels employed, because of current spread, depleted neural survival, or learning effects.

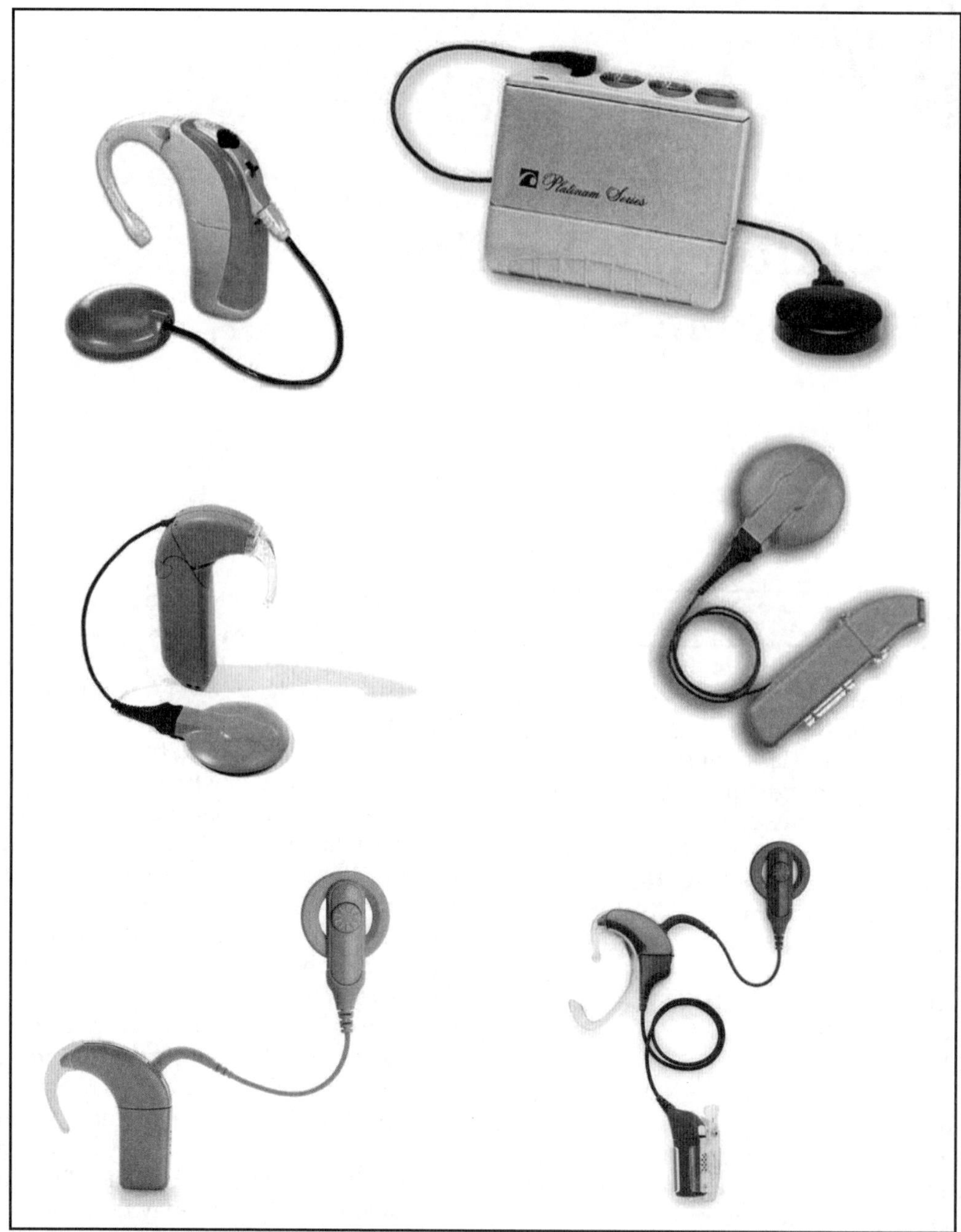

FIGURE 30–1. Examples of sound processors (photos are not depicted to scale). Configurations worn by older children are on the left, and configurations designed for toddlers are on the right. *Top row:* Advanced Bionics Harmony processor and Platinum Series Processor. *Middle row:* MED-EL OPUS 2 processor. *Bottom row:* Nucleus 5 (CP810) processor. (Photos provided courtesy of Cochlear Americas, © 2009 Cochlear Americas, MED-EL, and Advanced Bionics.)

The processor analyzes the incoming sound into the same number and boundaries of filtered frequency bands as there are channels included in the user's "map" or program.

Frequency bands are assigned to channels in tonotopic order from low frequency at the apical tip to high frequency at the basal end of the array. A cogent explanation of the differences in engineering among current

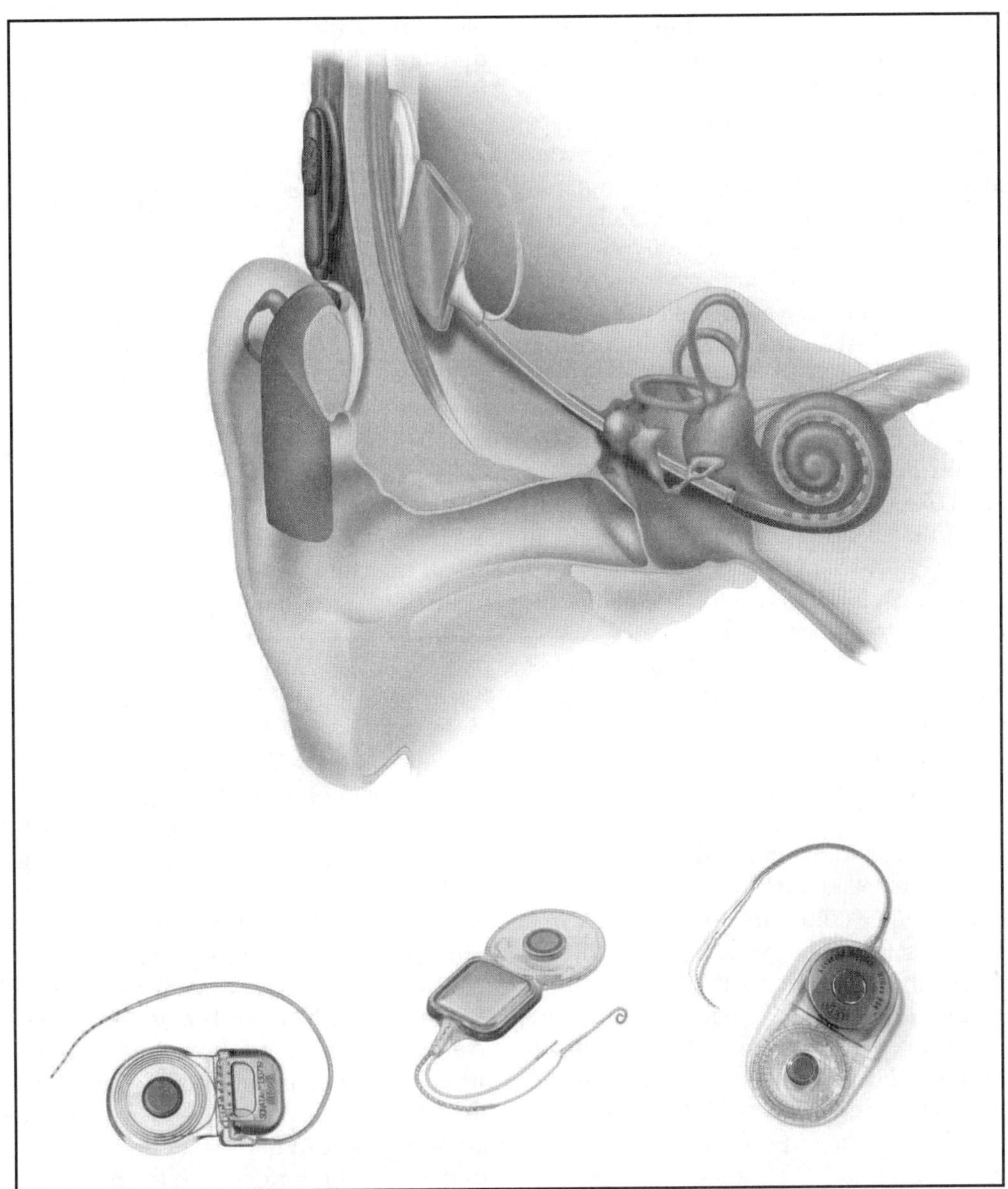

FIGURE 30–2. Examples of cochlear implants (photos are not depicted to scale). *Top:* Nucleus 5 implant and processor in. *Bottom left:* MED-EL SONATA 100 implant. *Bottom middle:* Nucleus 5 (CP512) implant. *Bottom right:* Advanced Bionics HiRes 90K® implant. (Photos provided courtesy of Cochlear Americas, © 2009 Cochlear Americas, MED-EL, and Advanced Bionics.)

implant models can be found in Zeng, Rebscher, Harrison, Sun, and Feng (2008). In the basic paradigm, biphasic pulses are delivered to the electrodes at an assigned stimulation rate. Depending on the implant's design and programmer's decisions, each electrode can function as an independent circuit, or might be grounded to another electrode inside the cochlea (bipolar mode) or outside the cochlea (monopolar mode). The pulses can be delivered to the channels simultaneously or sequentially, depending on the implant design and the coding strategy chosen by the programming audiologist. The pulses are amplitude-modulated according to the intensity of incoming sound in the assigned frequency band. These pulses replace the function of the inner hair cells and stimulate neural elements in the modiolus of the cochlea, causing the generation of compound action potentials in the auditory nerve. The input dynamic range, which used to be set to 30 dB in the 1980s and early 1990s to accommodate the 30-dB range from the weakest to the strongest phoneme, typically is now set to 40 to 60 dB or even larger to accommodate intensity variations in speech, environmental sounds, and music. In the amount of current delivered, the pulses are bound at the weaker limit by electrical threshold values (T levels) that are either measured behaviorally or determined by a formula used in the programming software. At the maximal limit, "comfort levels" (M or C levels) are determined based on psychophysical measures or estimated by measurement of the current required to elicit an electrically evoked compound action potential of the auditory nerve or an electrically evoked stapedial reflex. Although individuals with normal hearing experience changes in loudness over a 120-dB range, and the processor's input dynamic range typically is set to 40 to 60 dB, the dynamic range for nerve fiber discharge rates is only 4 dB (Kiang & Moxon, 1972). To code intensity changes adequately, therefore, very small increments in electrical current must be used to code greater changes in the intensity of the incoming sound. This amplitude compression is performed by the processor (Rubinstein & Miller, 1999).

Given the cochlear implant's limited number of channels for pitch percepts and its compressed dynamic range for intensity, one would think that its paltry display of auditory "pixels" would yield a grainy, incomplete picture of an incoming sound at best. Why, then, have cochlear implants become the standard of care for children with severe to profound bilateral sensorineural hearing loss whose parents have aspirations for them to speak? Why are legions of children who are congenitally deaf succeeding in transitioning to mainstream education using spoken language with the help of cochlear implants? The fact that cochlear implants work better than their electronics seemingly would allow is a testament to the power of neural plasticity in the young child's brain, with the support of the family and a team of professionals.

In the United States, the Food and Drug Administration (FDA) approved cochlear implantation starting at 24 months in 1990, at 18 months in 1998, and at 12 months for children with profound bilateral loss (24 months for severe loss) in 2002. Even younger infants are implanted when medically indicated. With each drop in age, cochlear implant clinicians strive to employ best practices based on available data. Until recently, however, studies of cochlear implant outcomes were limited to descriptions of small patient cohorts. Now that a substantial number of early implanted children are in high school and college, a body of literature is evolving that is helping to guide clinical decisions.

The Process of Getting an Implant

For the typical postlinguistically deaf adult, a cochlear implant team often consists only of the surgeon and audiologist, often with a single consultation with a social worker or mental health professional during the evaluation process. For a child, however, the team usually consists of the surgeon, audiologist, speech-language pathologist, psychologist, and deaf education specialist. All team members must be well-versed in working with children who are deaf and their families. If the child depends on sign language to communicate, then sign language should be accessible to the child during clinical encounters. The speech-language pathologist and psychologist in particular should be fluent to evaluate the child's language in sign. This same team, aided by an administrative coordinator, provides both evaluation and long-term care. A geneticist, ophthalmologist, radiologist, and neurologist also might see the child during evaluation of the potential benefit of an implant, because the implant evaluation might overlap with the etiologic workup for the hearing loss. For a child with motor disabilities, an occupational therapist can help optimize seating to participate in listening activities and headrest modifications so that the transmitting coil stays on the head. In addition to a sign language interpreter for a parent or child who primarily signs, an interpreter for a spoken language other than English must be provided when needed. A social worker can participate to assess family dynamics that might interfere with the outcome and to guide the family to resources that will help them to make appointments and support the child.

Although the order of events varies among teams, the evaluation begins with an intake questionnaire and a review of existing audiologic data to determine whether the hearing loss is severe enough for implant candidacy. The hearing aid fitting is optimized, and further audiologic evaluation is performed. If the child fits the general guidelines of the implant center for acceptance to the evaluation process, an informational consultation (audiologist with parents or guardians and with the child if older) is often the next step. At this session, parents relay what brings them to learn about the option of an implant, explain what they know about it thus far, share their aspirations for their child, and ask questions about the implant option. The audiologist in turn explains what an implant is and how it works, how the model is chosen, the process of evaluation and follow-up, the need for a concrete plan for expert auditory habilitation therapy postimplant, expectations for outcome in general and for their child. Internal device reliability and reimplantation likelihood are discussed. Printed and video materials are given to the family to keep. The parents' knowledge coming into the consultation varies from not knowing surgery is required to asking how different speech processing strategies are implemented. The audiologist's vocabulary level and rate of delivery during this important session should not exceed that of the parents, or the information will not be useful.

Most parents who seek consultation see the implant appropriately as an opportunity to open the auditory window for their child. Although hesitant parents never should be coerced into implants, those who wish to defer their decision should be familiarized with the better spoken language outcomes of children implanted at younger as compared to older ages. Common causes for parental hesitation to implant a good candidate are as follows: wishing to save the ears for future technology; misinformation from someone who opposes pediatric implantation for various reasons; guilt that implanting the child would mean not accepting the child as he or she is; viewing the implant as a failure of the hard-fought battle to make hearing aids work; reluctance to destroy residual hearing; lack of understanding how little the child hears now and how far behind his or her spoken language might become without auditory access; fear of the surgery; or a variety of cultural beliefs. It might be true that an ear with an implant will not benefit from some future technologies, but an ear with a long-unused auditory pathway also will not benefit. Accurate information must be presented about progress in spoken language development following implantation being supported by expert auditory habilitation, constant exposure to spoken language, and high auditory expectations. The audiologist should not decisively recommend implantation prior to team evaluation, as the other professionals on the team might discover reasons why an implant would not be a beneficial intervention. Particularly when the hearing loss is profound and computerized tomography (CT) scan and magnetic resonating image (MRI) have not yet been performed, one must keep in mind that the child might have no cochlea or no auditory nerve, rendering a cochlear implant useless. Parents often ask the audiologist questions best answered by the surgeon, such as how the risk of facial nerve damage is avoided and other details of the procedure. The audiologist can outline the topics that the surgeon will discuss, without giving details best left to the surgeon.

Candidacy for Benefit From Cochlear Implantation

Minimum Age for Surgery

The FDA (2010) issues approvals for cochlear implants that are device specific. The audiologic criteria and minimum age of implanation might be determined by the population of subjects and tests used in the clinical trial. Health insurance companies pay attention to these criteria and can question or deny authorization for surgery when the criteria are not met, unless medical necessity can be demonstrated. Current FDA criteria for minimum age are 12 months and up for bilateral profound sensorineural hearing loss and, for Nucleus devices, 24 months and up for severe (bilateral or better-ear) loss. Some surgeons implant infants well under 12 months, while others wait until 12 months, citing challenges including accuracy of audiologic diagnosis, increased anesthesia risks (lessened in the hands of a pediatric anesthesiologist), limited anatomical access during surgery, increased vulnerability of the facial nerve, blood loss, and temporal bone marrow development. However, when careful surgical techniques for infants are employed, risks are minimized (Birman, 2009; Vlastarakos, Candiloros, et al., 2010; Waltzman & Roland, 2005). Ossification following meningitis is one factor that many surgeons would agree constitutes medical necessity for implantation under 12 months, if the parents so desire. Although there is convincing evidence that implantation under age 18 months is associated with steeper learning curves for receptive and expressive spoken language than implantation at a later age (Niparko et al., 2010), there are not yet outcome data reported on enough infants to support a widespread policy change regarding implantation under age 12 months (Vlastarakos, Proikas, et al., 2010). Some parents might not be ready for their child to undergo surgery under 12 months. In no case should an implant team recommend that the surgery be scheduled to take place before the parents have an understanding of their child's hearing loss, habilitative therapy services are in place, and there is assurance that the implant offers the child an opportunity worthy of long-term commitment. The implant team should support the family in achieving readiness for surgery at an early age, if the family chooses implantation.

Candidacy and Preparation

Most children whose parents are inquiring about cochlear implants fall into certain categories that become familiar to the implant team. The most straightforward is the very young child with congenital severe-to-profound bilateral hearing loss and no other known developmental challenges. A second large category is that of older children who have acquired spoken language using hearing aids but have either experienced worsening of hearing in one or both ears, or have not found that hearing aids provide adequate access to speech at conversational intensity. A third category is that of children with auditory neuropathy spectrum disorder (ANSD), whose pure-tone audiogram might not be severe enough for typical guidelines but who would benefit from the increased synchrony of neuronal firing provided by the implant. A fourth category is the child with developmental disabilities for whom lack of hearing might not be the greatest challenge. A fifth group is that of older children who are deaf, do not use hearing aids, and use American Sign Language (ASL) to communicate.

The young child who presents under 4 years of age without significant medical or developmental issues other than hearing loss still poses major tasks for the implant team: determining whether the audiologic diagnosis is accurate; performing developmental and language assessments to foresee any previously unsuspected learning or behavioral concerns that should be addressed; and planning appropriate therapy services postactivation if the child is not already receiving expert auditory habilitation. The implant team typically performs auditory brainstem response (ABR) testing, otoacoustic emissions (OAEs) testing, and verification of the hearing aid fitting even if these have been performed elsewhere because of the diagnostic responsibility required for a surgical decision. It is helpful for the audiologist who is going to be activating and programming the implant to be the one who performs the last behavioral audiologic evaluation prior to surgery, so that the child's response style can be observed and familiarity and trust can be built.

By FDA guidelines, children who have not developed word recognition ability can meet audiologic criteria by showing lack of progress or developmental lag on a scale such as the Infant-Toddler Meaningful Auditory Integration Scale (IT-MAIS; Zimmerman-Phillips, Osberger, & Robbins, 2000) or Meaningful Auditory Integration Scale (MAIS; Robbins, Renshaw, & Berry, 1991). A 3- to 6-month period of hearing aid use and therapy is advised to determine adequacy of hearing aid use to support auditory development, but the waiting period is not advised in the case of profound hearing loss following meningitis because ossification can develop in the cochlea within weeks after the illness. With early diagnosis of hearing loss after newborn screening, most children have had a period of hearing aid use before the implant evaluation. Hearing aid use should not cause a delay in implantation if there is reason to believe that hearing aids will not provide benefit. The three models of implant most recently approved by the FDA (Cochlear Corporation's Nucleus System 5, Advanced Bionics Harmony HiResolution Bionic Ear System, and MED-EL Sonata TI100) have three different sets of approved indications, which are derived from the subjects and tests used in the clinical trials for each device. The FDA audiologic criteria for a young child include best-aided word recognition ability no greater than 20% for the Advanced Bionics and MED-EL devices and no greater than 30% for the Cochlear Corporation device using the Multisyllabic Lexical Neighborhood Test (MLNT) or Lexical Neighborhood Test (LNT; Kirk, Pisoni, Sommers, Young, & Evanson, 1995), whichever is developmentally appropriate. However, the implant team audiologist must judge whether the child is likely to receive more access to sound using an implant than a hearing aid in the ear being considered. Even if the child's word recognition skills are better than FDA guidelines for implantation, the audiologist should compare the child's performance with that of similar children from published data and consider the presentation level required to achieve best aided performance, when deciding whether to support implantation.

In addition to the speech-language evaluation and the developmental evaluation by a psychologist, the parents can meet with a psychologist or social worker to help prepare themselves for the surgery and follow-up, and learn how they can help prepare their child, as well. Even a toddler benefits from playing with surgical masks and stethoscopes, as it can be unnerving to see people with their mouths covered in the operating room area. Learning a few words or signs for the surgery (hospital, bandage, doctor, nurse, etc.) can help give the child confidence. Playing out the surgical experience with a doll or stuffed animal by placing a

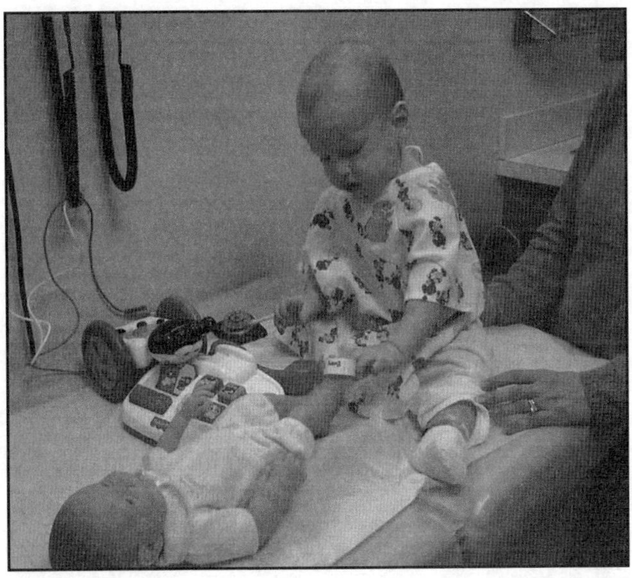

FIGURE 30–3. A 12-month-old boy, well prepared for cochlear implant surgery, places a hospital ID bracelet on his doll's ankle in the preop holding area. (Reprinted with permission by George Borhegyi.)

hospital identification bracelet, having it "breathe" in the anesthetic, go to sleep, and wake up with a head bandage can prepare the child for the experience (Figure 30–3). Parents (if there are two with whom the child feels equally comforted) can decide which parent goes into the operating room for a parent-present anesthesia induction based on which parent is less anxious, as the anxiety can be conveyed to the child.

A child over 4 years of age who has acquired spoken language using hearing aids, whether or not sign language also has been used, can receive great benefit from cochlear implantation to provide greater access to sound. Often these children present with an ear difference in hearing and the poorer ear is implanted first, because the better ear can continue to benefit from acoustic amplification. After the hearing aid fitting is optimized, aided word and sentence recognition tests should be given at 60 dB SPL and, if feasible, 50 dB SPL even if the aided performance would be better at a higher presentation level, because an implant affords perception of speech even at soft conversational intensities (Davidson, 2006). If a child does not have clear enough articulation to administer an open-set monosyllabic word test and does not yet write, closed-set word recognition tests can be given, with the caveat that closed-set tests are "easy" and the open-set test score on which candidacy is judged would be lower.

In the case of progressive hearing loss, the poorer ear often is implanted when the better ear does not yet meet candidacy criteria, rather than waiting until audition is a struggle for the child. Older children who can repeat sentences sometimes are judged by the implant audiologist using adult criteria—no more than 60% best-aided word score on a sentence recognition test such as the Hearing in Noise Test (HINT; Gelnett, Sumida, Nilsson, & Soli, 1995) given in quiet, or 50% in the ear to be implanted. Scores obtained with the test given at 60 dB SPL (average conversational level) or even 50 dB SPL (soft speech) with the hearing aids, rather than 70 dB SPL, often reflect the hearing aid user's struggles to hear speech at an average intensity, which could be improved with an implant. It is likely that the future holds increasing numbers of carefully considered implants for candidates with residual hearing, and eventually expanded FDA criteria for cochlear implantation, based on studies such as that by Dowell, Hollow, and Winton (2004) that showed that adults having up to 70% sentence recognition scores had greater than 75% chance of improvement with a cochlear implant.

Preparing a child over 4 years of age for surgery and activation includes the use of comic/coloring books about the implant, playing with a toy operating room set, and meeting other children who have implants and can explain their experience. The latter recommendation is particularly needed by adolescents, who might have helpful e-mail relationships with peers who use implants. The implant team must assist the parents in determining whether the child's school environment is conducive to learning to use the implant. If not, the team recommends changes in educational programming to foster the use of audition while nurturing language development. For most students, the appropriate environment uses spoken language as the mode of instruction, though some need sign support as well. Classroom acoustics should at least meet the background noise and reverberation requirements of ANSI/ASA S12.60-2002 (R2009), the American National Standard Acoustical Performance Criteria, Design Requirements, and Guidelines for Schools (Acoustical Society of America, 2009). There should be at least one member of the student's educational team, typically a speech-language pathologist or consulting teacher of the deaf, who is expert in language learning and classroom accommodations for children who use cochlear implants. The student should receive individual speech and language therapy specifically geared to auditory skill development. If the school speech and language clinician has little background in auditory development of children who use implants, mentoring by an experienced clinician is an option. Although in the United States the school is not obligated to pay for cochlear implant programming (mapping), the school is responsible for checking that the processor is functioning, providing assistive technology such as an educational amplification system, and providing needed support services (U.S. Department of Education, 2006).

Children with auditory neuropathy spectrum disorder (ANSD) might have pure-tone thresholds far better than typical implant candidacy requirements, yet could benefit from cochlear implantation (Roush, 2008). Children with ANSD undergoing cochlear implant candidacy evaluation should undergo MRI to determine the presence of normally sized cochlear nerves (Buchman et al., 2006). Accuracy of audiological diagnosis is critically important, as is determining whether hearing aids help and allowing an adequate time to determine whether neuronal synchrony and functional audition are developing. When the child's audition is holding back his or her communication development rather than helping it to move forward in a timely fashion, implantation should be considered. Filming a child's communication behavior in a spoken language interchange and watching it with the parents helps in making the implant decision. Functional auditory assessment scales are useful to catalog the child's everyday auditory skills (Can the child hear from front to back seat in the car? Understand words on the phone? Understand speech outdoors? etc.). Cortical-evoked potentials might prove to be useful as a correlate to functional speech perception ability (Rance, Cone-Wesson, Wunderlich, & Dowell, 2002). As yet there are inadequate data to know whether children with any particular genetic basis for ANSD, such as certain recessive mutations in the otoferlin (*OTOF*) gene, are immune from auditory recovery so that they can be implanted very young (Rodriguez-Ballesteros et al., 2003). Although Rance and Barker (2008) found that speech perception outcomes were lower in implanted children with ANSD than in implanted children with typical sensorineural hearing loss, Shallop (2008) reported no such difference between the two groups. However, because roughly half of children with ANSD have spent time in a neonatal intensive care unit (Bolajoko et al., 2008), many have medical and developmental problems apart from hearing loss that might slow their progress with an implant.

Ethical considerations become paramount when evaluating the child with developmental disabilities for cochlear implantation. Although the burning question of 1990 was, "How can you do this surgery *to* this child?" the question now is, "How can we *not* do this surgery *for* this child?" The child first must be healthy enough to undergo an elective surgery safely. The implant team must project what the child might do with some audition if he or she had access to it, and whether the child would be more participatory in family and peer interactions with access to sound. Children with physical but not cognitive disabilities make good progress in auditory skill development, whereas children with cognitive impairment make slower progress, might plateau in their spoken language development at the level of words and rote phrases without mastering grammar, and are more likely to use total communication (Edwards, Waltzman, & Scalchunes, 2007; Holt & Kirk, 2005; Waltzman, Scalchunes & Cohen, 2000; Wiley, Meinzen-Derr, & Choo, 2008). Children with autism spectrum disorder typically make only modest gains in communication function with the implant (Donaldson, Heavner, & Zwolan, 2004) and sometimes do not benefit from the implant, unless they already had spoken language development before becoming deaf.

Older children who use ASL to communicate, do not use hearing aids, interact primarily with signing Deaf peers and teachers, and have not developed awareness of the sounds of speech are at risk of becoming nonusers of their processors if they are implanted. Although the occasional older Deaf recipient enjoys having environmental sound awareness and basic speech pattern detection to support lipreading, most should be counseled that a cochlear implant will not change their communication modality or enable them to use a voice phone. If the older child who uses ASL to communicate has Usher syndrome or other risk for vision loss, cochlear implantation should be strongly considered, with careful counseling.

The use of a preimplant rating scale helps the implant team remember to weigh the input of all disciplines, to be objective in predicting benefit and to counsel the family regarding expectations. The original Children's Implant Profile (ChIP) developed by Hellman and colleagues (1991) has been adapted by different implant centers to suit their needs (e.g., Dava et al., 1999; Edwards, Thomas, & Raiput, 2009; Lazaridis, Therres, & Marsh, 2010). However, the sum of the ratings (no concern, some concern, great concern) for each category does not always predict the team's recommendation. For example, Lazaridis et al. (2010) found that the ratings predicted 75% of the team's recommendations to implant and 75% of their recommendations not to implant, in a group of 107 children for whom the ratings were completed. However, the rating scale does help to guide expectations and counseling. The rating scale currently in use at Children's Hospital Boston (O'Brien et al., 2007) is shown in Figure 30–4.

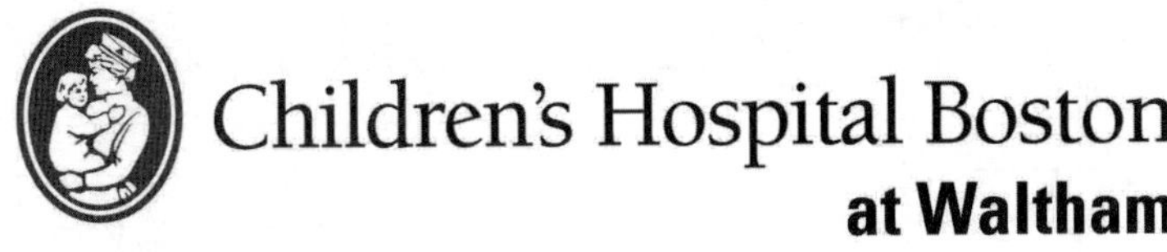

Cochlear Implant Program
9 Hope Avenue
Waltham, Massachusetts 02453
781-216-2250
www.childrenshospital.org

NAME:
CH#:
DOB:

I. Team Impressions of the Factors Important to Cochlear Implant Use and Success:					
	No Concern	Some Concern	Great Concern	Not Applicable	Comments
1. Chronological Age [Age:]					
2. Etiology [Cause:]					
3. Duration of Deafness [Age of onset:]					
4. Otolaryngology					
Medical					
Radiology					
5. Other Disabilities:					
6. Audiology					
Test Reliability					
Hearing Aid Use/Use of Residual Hearing (use of available auditory cues)					
Hearing Aid Fitting Optimized/Used					
7. Speech-Language Pathology					
Auditory Training—Past/Present					
Communication Ability—Parental Assessment					
Communication Ability—Clinician Assessment					
Formal Language Use/Comprehension					
Primary Language of the Family [Lang:]					
Primary Language of the Child [Lang:]					
Use of Voice to Communicate					
Speechreading (i.e. Lipreading) Skills					
Communicative Intent					
Parent-Child Language Interactions					
Vocabulary Measure [Score:]					
8. Psychology					
Cognitive Level [Score:]					
Developmental Level [Score:]					
Family Support					
Family System					
Behavioral Traits					
Behavioral Issues					
Behavioral Concerns—Parental					
Expectations (Parents)					
Expectations (Child)					
Adequate Information (Parents)					
Adequate Information (Child)					

FIGURE 30–4. Modification of the Children's Implant Profile used at Children's Hospital Boston to guide discussion, counseling, and expectations for the potential benefit of a cochlear implant (O'Brien et al., 2007; Reprinted with permission.) *continues*

9. Education					
Current Educational Placement					
Future Educational Placement (Transition)					
Access to Auditory-Oral Services					
Educational Staff CI Training					
Ability of Parent to Participate in Educational Process					
Overall impression of team					

II. **PREDICTORS OF HOW __________________ WILL BE COMMUNICATING IN THREE YEARS**
Based on communication continuum (Robbins, 2001; Circle one of each):

Expressive Communication Continuum

Fully Sign Communicator	Mostly Sign Communicator		Mostly Oral Communicator	Fully Oral Communicator
S	**S_O**	**SO**	**O_S**	**O**

Receptive Communication Continuum

Fully Visual Communicator	Mostly Visual Communicator		Mostly Auditory Communicator	Fully Auditory Communicator
V	**V_A**	**VA**	**A_V**	**A**

III. **EXPLANATORY NOTES:**

IV. **SIGNATURES:**

Team Members

____

____

____

____

Family Members

____

____

Date ____________________

Page 2

FIGURE 30–4. *continued*

Table 30–1. Definitions of No Concern, Some Concern, Great Concern, and Not Applicable for Audiologic Categories of the Form Depicted in Figure 30–4

Audiology	*No Concern*	*Some Concern*	*Great Concern*	*Not Applicable*
Test reliability	Good	Fair	Poor	No behavioral data
Hearing aid use/use of residual hearing	Developed some spoken language or detection/awareness of environmental sounds with limited auditory cues	Inconsistent responses, not clear; or may have too much useful hearing in other ear to appreciate sound of implant	Good amount of residual hearing with no auditory behaviors	Hearing loss too significant to derive any benefit
Hearing aid fitting optimized/used	Used consistently	Used inconsistently (e.g., couple of hours each day)	Never or infrequently used	

Table 30–1 shows the definitions of the categories that team audiologists need to determine in order to use the form consistently. For example, hearing status might be of concern because there is too much residual hearing or conversely, because there has been too little auditory experience for the candidate's age. A second rating scale, developed to guide expectations for outcome of sequential bilateral implantation (Neault et al., 2007) is shown in Figure 30–5. Such rating scales need periodic evidence-based revision as new data continue to emerge regarding factors that contribute to various outcomes.

Intraoperative Testing of the Cochlear Implant

Although some implant centers do not perform intraoperative tests of the function of the implant, many surgeons do elect for the audiologist to test the device following insertion while the surgical field remains sterile. A laptop computer loaded with the programming software, the patient interface box, programming cable, and sound processor are required. The processor and programming cable are inserted into a sterile plastic sleeve such as a camera drape. The surgeon places the transmitting coil over the receiver/stimulator. If the skin flap is not yet closed, either the unsutured flap, a spacer or gauze pads are required to simulate the thickness of the flap, rather than placing the coil directly on the exposed receiver/stimulator.

The audiologist typically performs two tests: impedance telemetry to check for short circuits or open circuits, and measurement of the action potential of the cochlear nerve upon stimulation of individual electrodes. High impedances on one or two electrodes sometimes improve postoperatively, whereas short circuits indicate electrodes that should not be included in the patient's map. The surgeon is advised of any malfunctioning electrodes so that a decision can be made about replacing the device. Following the impedance telemetry, the audiologist typically performs neural response measurements using the manufacturer's software. A good tutorial on neural response testing is found in Hughes (2006a, 2006b). If no interpretable response is seen in the automated version of the test, a more advanced version can be used with user-defined parameters and higher pulse widths available. The neural response should be measured on at least one apical, one medial, and one basal electrode. Lack of typical responses should be followed by an x-ray to check the placement of the electrode array. The impedance telemetry and neural response test can be accomplished while the surgeon is stitching the final layer of the flap, so that no time is added to the anesthesia. It is important for the surgeon to inform the audiologist whether the entire array was inserted into the cochlea, so that no extracochlear electrodes are activated postoperatively.

When a sufficient number of electrodes are tested for neural responses in the operating room, the results yield a contour that helps to predict the contour of the comfort levels of the map at activation of the device (Mason, Cope, Garnham, O'Donoghue, & Gibbin, 2001). Because the current levels required to measure the neural response are perceptually loud for a new user, these intraoperative measures are particularly valuable to have when activating a young child's implant.

Children's Hospital Boston

NAME:
CHB #
DOB:

BILATERAL CHILDREN'S HEARING IMPLANT PROFILE (BiCHIP)

Predictors for Use and Outcome of 2nd (Sequential Bilateral) Cochlear Implant

#	FACTOR	4	3	2	1	SCORE/DATE	SCORE/DATE
1	AGE AT 2ND CI	0-35 MONTHS	3-4 YEARS	5-8 YEARS	9+ YEARS		
2	GAP BETWEEN 1ST & 2ND CI	0-11 MONTHS	12-35 MONTHS	3-5 YEARS	6+ YEARS		
3	ANATOMY OF 2ND COCHLEA / AUDITORY NERVE	NO CONCERN	MILD CONCERN	MODERATE CONCERN	GREAT CONCERN		
4	COMMUNICATION MODE	AUDITORY/ORAL	AUD W/ VISUAL ASSIST	VISUAL W/ AUD ASSIST	VISUAL		
5	SPOKEN LANGUAGE DEVEL.	AGE APPROPRIATE	MILD DELAY/DISORDER	MODERATE DELAY/DISORDER	SEVERE DELAY/DISORDER		
6	WORD RECOGNITION AT 60 dBSPL WITH 1ST CI (PBK AT 5+ YEARS; NU-CHIPS <5 YEARS)	EXCELLENT 80-100%	GOOD 68-78%	FAIR 50-66%	LIMITED < 50%)		
7	SENTENCE RECOGNITION AT 60 dBSPL WITH 1ST CI (HINT-C IN QUIET AT 5+ YEARS; COMMON PHRASES TEST <5 YEARS)	EXCELLENT 91-100%	GOOD 80-90%	FAIR 50-78%	LIMITED <50%		
8	AUDIBILITY WITH HEARING AID IN 2ND EAR *	>30% OPEN-SET WORD RECOGNITION AT 60 dBSPL WITH HEARING AID	WORD RECOGNITION IN CLOSED SET OR AT HIGH INTENSITY WITH HEARING AID	ONLY SLIGHT BENEFIT FROM HEARING AID	HEARING AID GIVES NO USEFUL AUDIBILITY		
9	PREVIOUS AUDITORY EXPERIENCE OF 2ND EAR **	<100 dBHL WITH HX OF AIDED SPEECH RECOGNITION	<100 dBHL OR CONSISTENT HEARING AID USE	>105dBHL WITH SOME HEARING AID USE	NONE, OR >105 dBHL WITH LITTLE OR NO HEARING AID USE		
10	EQUIPMENT MANAGEMENT	NO CONCERN	MINIMAL CONCERN	MODERATE CONCERN	GREAT CONCERN		
11	EXPECTATIONS (PARENT)	NO CONCERN	MINIMAL CONCERN	MODERATE CONCERN	GREAT CONCERN		
12	READINESS (CHILD)	NO CONCERN	MINIMAL CONCERN	MODERATE CONCERN	GREAT CONCERN		
13	BEHAVIORAL TRAITS (CHILD)	NO CONCERN	MINIMAL CONCERN	MODERATE CONCERN	GREAT CONCERN		
14	COGNITIVE LEVEL	NO CONCERN	MINIMAL CONCERN	MODERATE CONCERN	GREAT CONCERN		
15	ACCESS TO EXPERT THERAPY	NO CONCERN	MINIMAL CONCERN	MODERATE CONCERN	GREAT CONCERN		
16	SUPPORTIVE EDUCATIONAL PROGRAM	NO CONCERN	MINIMAL CONCERN	MODERATE CONCERN	GREAT CONCERN		

* ALTHOUGH HEARING AID BENEFIT MAY PREDICT GOOD CI BENEFIT, CANDIDATES NEED GUIDANCE RE: CHOOSING TO LOSE RESIDUAL UNAIDED HEARING AND HEARING AID BENEFIT

** <100 dBHL MEANS 3-FREQ. PURE TONE AVERAGE BETTER THAN 100 dBHL IN 2ND EAR TO BE IMPLANTED

SCORES LOWER THAN 39 WITH CONCERN ON FACTORS 1, 2, 3, AND 9 WARRANT EXTRA CAUTION.

TOTAL SCORE

(HIGHER SCORE SUPPORTS BETTER CANDIDACY FOR INITIAL ADJUSTMENT, WEARING TIME, AND WORD RECOGNITION WITH 2ND CI)

COMMENTS:

DATE____________________ RATERS____

FIGURE 30–5. Bilateral Children's Hearing Implant Profile (BiChIP) used at Children's Hospital Boston to guide discussion, counseling, and expectations for sequential bilateral implant candidacy (Neault et al., 2007; Reprinted with permission.)

If a simultaneous bilateral implantation is performed, the audiologist might make two trips to the operating room, one to test each device before the patient is turned. When the audiology clinic is located far from the operating suite, remote testing is possible by means of a secure remote computer access program, provided that someone in the operating room can attach the processor to the laptop and place it over the implant.

Activation and Programming of the Cochlear Implant

One to 4 weeks after surgery, depending on the healing process and the philosophy and schedule of the implant team, the sound processor is programmed so that the child can begin to use it. Between surgery and activation, the child might play with a stuffed animal or doll with a toy processor, read a coloring book about implants, or get together with another child who has an implant. For a young child, the appointments should not be scheduled at naptime. Parents of a 1-year-old might wish to purchase a thin cotton "pilot cap" to bring to the activation, to help keep the processor on the ear and to keep little hands away from it while the child becomes accustomed to it. It is very helpful if the parents and older child have watched a video regarding how the processor works before the initial activation, even though the information will be reviewed in detail.

The initial activation and programming typically takes two visits, often scheduled in the same week. Simultaneous bilateral implants can be activated the same day or sequentially. The next visit is no more than a month later, with phone or e-mail contact in the interim, even if reliable measures are obtained in order to create a set of progressively louder maps (programs) to use as the child becomes accustomed to the new sound. Magnet strength should be adjusted and monitored carefully at each visit to avoid skin breakdown. The method used to determine the electrical threshold (T) levels and electrical comfort (C) levels varies with the characteristics of the device, as well as the child's ability to respond. It is in the activation and programming that it becomes clear once more, as it did in the preimplant counseling, that good pediatric audiology skills and a focus on the family spell success.

For a mapping strategy that does not require psychophysical thresholds on each channel, a default set of programming parameters sometimes is used and the processor, connected to the programming computer, is simply turned on at the minimum stimulation level and turned up very slowly while the child's behavior is observed. The contour of the comfort levels (the maximum levels set for each channel) can be determined by the contour of the neural response test results from the operating room, by behavioral observation, or by loudness scaling pictures (Figure 30–6) if the child is about 4 years or older. When the microphone of the processor is turned on, the room is kept quiet until the child begins to make sounds, whereupon a drum, little keyboard, and other musical toys are provided to explore (Figure 30–7). Parents are advised that the initial stage of learning to listen with an implant is to show awareness of sounds that the child is creating. In this phase, if the child is squeezing play-dough and the parent calls from behind, the child may think the sound has been created by the squeezing. When the parent does begin to speak during the session, it is wise to show the child the source of the sound.

For a map that will incorporate psychophysical thresholds on individual channels, the audiologist uses developmentally appropriate pediatric test measures.

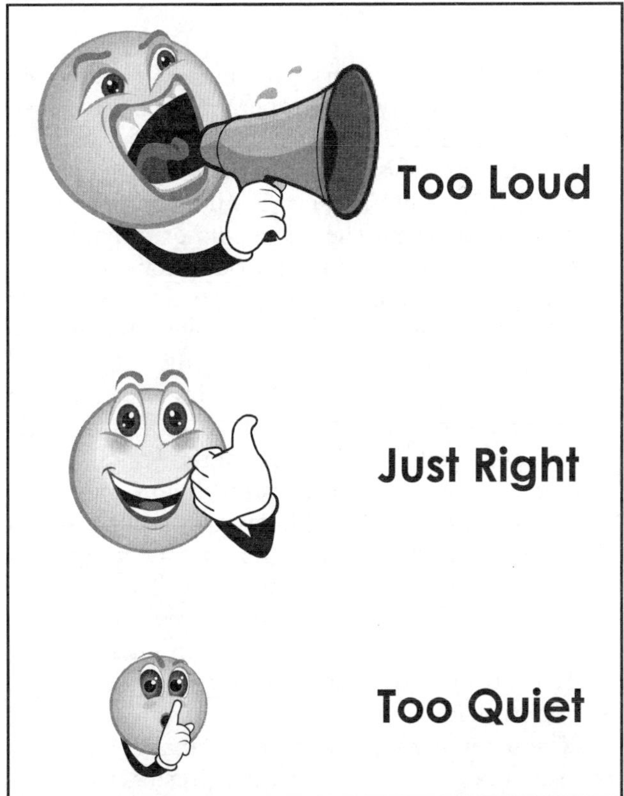

FIGURE 30–6. Example of loudness scaling pictures used by children to help in setting electrical comfort (C) levels when programming a cochlear implant processor.

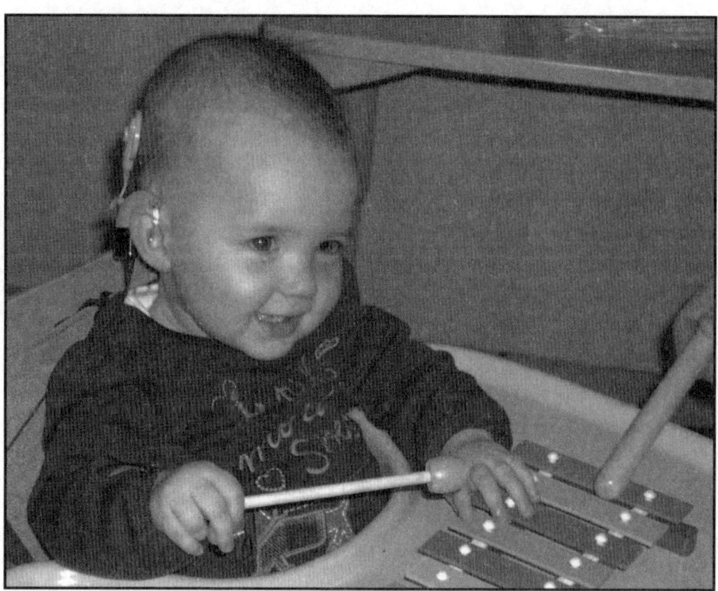

FIGURE 30–7. A 13-month-old girl whose implant was just activated at Children's Hospital Boston enjoys the sound of a xylophone. Her processor is attached to the mapping computer by a programming cable, and the processor microphone is activated following creation of the map. (Reprinted with permission.)

The young child can be on a parent's lap, or preferably in a chair with a tray and properly adjusted footrest. Electrical "beeps" are presented on individual channels to measure thresholds using visual reinforcement audiometry (VRA; Figure 30–8) or conditioned play audiometry (Figure 30–9). The older child or teenager can simply say "yes" or push a response button on hearing a beep. If VRA is used, initial responses might be closer to C levels than to T levels, so the overall levels are adjusted accordingly before activating the microphone. Interpolation of values on intervening electrodes is possible for some types of maps, if not all channels are measured individually. The overall levels should be reduced at least 30 current units below measured T levels, and a small range (no more than 20–30 units) set between T and C levels, before the microphone is activated to avoid an adverse response. Three or four progressively stronger maps are created and stored. The processor is detached from the computer, and the family is given instruction in the operation, care, and use of the device.

The parameters that constitute a map include the coding strategy, stimulation rate, pulse width, frequency allocation table, which electrodes are used, grounding (mode), and T and C levels. Preprocessing at the input stage, such as Adaptive Dynamic Range Optimization (ADRO), autosensitivity, and adjustments to the low end of the input dynamic range are part of the map. Output limits determined by voltage compliance may be displayed on the mapping screen. If the processor has an internal telecoil, the ratio of telecoil to microphone input is specified, as is the ratio of accessory input (FM receiver, audio cable, etc.) to microphone input.

It takes most cochlear implant users approximately 3 months to work up to the C levels they will use for the long term, with periodic fine tuning. It is a goal to achieve equal loudness across frequency bands. However, rate of loudness growth from T to C on the various channels might not be equally steep, so simply balancing the C levels for loudness might not always be enough. Occasionally there are channels with "T-tails" on which loudness begins to grow only partway up the range from T to C, in which case the T level should be reset to the level just below where loudness begins to grow. Likewise, if loudness stops growing below the C level, usually because of voltage compliance limitations, then the C level should be set where loudness stops growing as current units are increased. As speech sound perception develops, the map can be adjusted to optimize awareness and discrimination of individual phonemes. However, one must keep in mind that the child might not yet have developed the auditory skills necessary to recognize certain distinctions, even

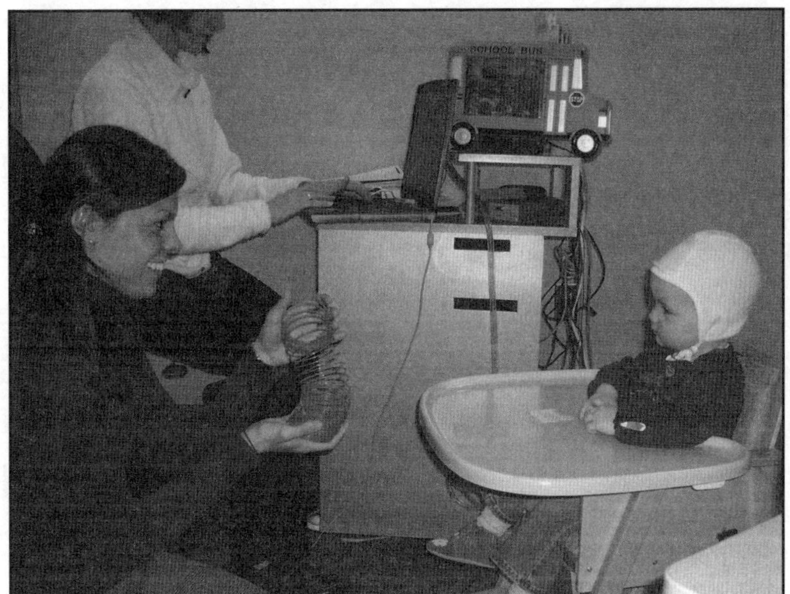

A

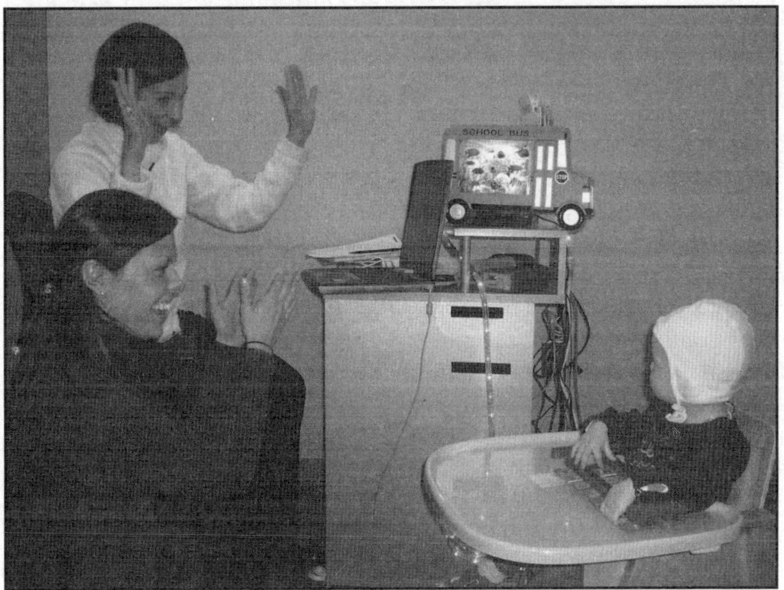

B

FIGURE 30–8. A. A graduate student enchants a 13-month-old girl, while the programming audiologist prepares to measure T levels using Visual Reinforcement Audiometry. The pilot cap worn by the child helps to keep the processor on her head. **B.** The child, whose implant is on the right ear, turns right toward the visual reinforcer in response to a sound. The programming audiologist operates the visual reinforcer with a foot switch. (Reprinted with permission.)

though the auditory information is accessible to him. Having achieved a phonemic distinction and then losing it might signal the need for a new map, if the processor microphone has not merely become muffled and distorted by moisture. Having mastered the production of a phoneme and then losing it also may signal

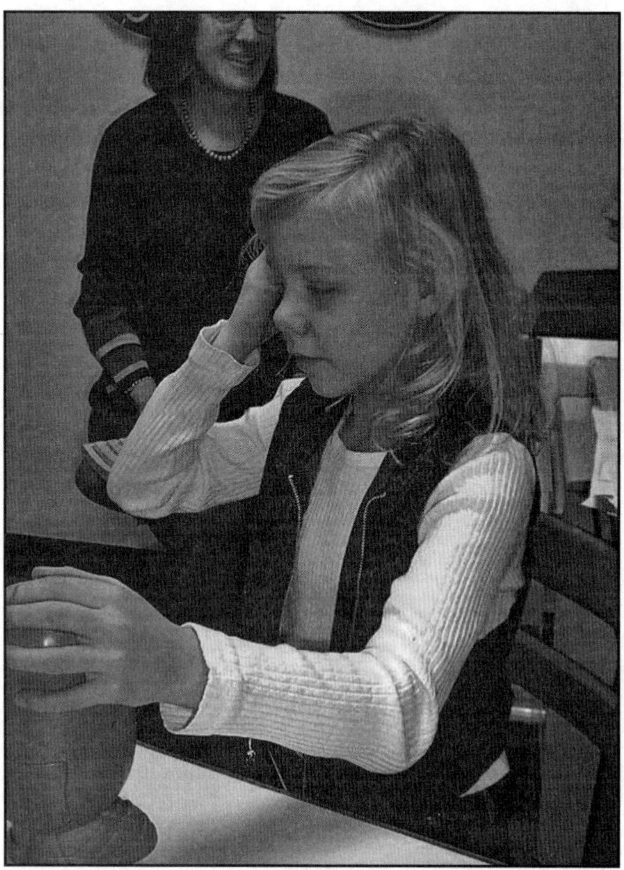

FIGURE 30–9. A child waits for a "beep" before she can place the toy piece, using conditioned play audiometry to measure T levels. Her cochlear implant processor is out of view on her right ear, attached to the computer by a programming cable and interface box. During this portion of the mapping, the processor microphone is not activated, and she cannot hear sounds in the room. (Reprinted with permission.)

the need for a new map, unless of course the phoneme is /s/ and the front teeth are missing in a 6-year-old.

Communication among the audiologist, speech-language pathologist, and parent (and the child if old enough) before and after a new map helps in determining needs and expectations. After the first 3 months, mapping typically takes place at 3-month intervals until the map seems fairly stable, then at 6-month intervals. After optimal loudness is achieved, maps are created and stored for different listening situations, such as quiet and noise environments, telephone, and music. Even for experienced users, regular visits are critical for monitoring progress, discussing educational, social, and therapeutic needs and informing the family about technology updates in processors or accessories. Children in an educational setting benefit from FM amplification when participating in group listening activities. Educational audiology support for the use of the processors and FM receivers is important for their benefit. Annual speech and language evaluation and psychological reevaluation at least every 3 years at the implant center maintains good monitoring of progress and adequacy of support services.

The Other Ear

For almost two decades of cochlear implantation, nearly all recipients used only one ear. They were, in fact, encouraged to remove the hearing aid from the other ear to promote adjustment to the implant. However, now the two ears are viewed as having both independent and interdependent needs. If the ear contralateral to the implant can benefit from traditional amplification without causing binaural interference, hearing aid use is encouraged. Ample evidence exists to support bimodal speech perception benefit for children who have residual hearing in the unimplanted ear (Ching et al., 2005; Holt, Kirk, Eisenberg, Martinez, & Campbell, 2005; Mok, Galvin, Dowell, & McKay, 2010). Particularly in the early stages of implant adjustment for a long-term hearing aid user, the child may rely on the hearing aid for intonational cues. In the words of a 10-year-old boy who received one implant at age 9 years, "With my cochlear implant, I hear the words; with my hearing aid, I hear the emotion." Unless the child can use the hearing aid independently to understand speech and use the aid on the phone, one might consider rolling off the high frequency gain of the hearing aid, as the implant will provide better access to high-frequency sounds. In this way a more comfortable earmold can be used, without feedback. A volume control is useful on the hearing aid in the initial stages of adjustment to bimodal input. When programming the hearing aid, the potential for FM system use should be considered, so that an FM plus environment setting can be accessed by the child. Although the child is more likely to use the cochlear implant than the hearing aid on the telephone, a telecoil setting should be included on the aid if the child might be using a neckloop FM receiver (needing an MT setting), or listening to music through inductive stereo earhooks.

If the contralateral ear does not have aided thresholds at a level that allows lateralization of sounds and does not have the potential for word recognition, a second implant should be considered to achieve bilateral implant use, which is discussed in depth in Chapter 29.

Bilateral cochlear implant use improves speech perception in noise, eliminates the head shadow experienced by unilateral implant users, improves perception of soft speech by binaural summation, and allows some localization ability to develop over time (Johnston et al., 2009). Although the processor on the originally implanted side is removed for some listening therapy sessions and for an hour or so per day at home so that the new ear can "practice," the ultimate goal is for the brain to integrate the input from the two sides. Using an FM receiver on the poorer performing side only, to "train" it, results in poorer hearing in background noise (Schafer & Thibodeau, 2006) and is not recommended.

Programming the two implants can be done at the same or separate visits. Even with slightly different insertion depths, having the frequency allocation tables start at the same frequency allows similar loudness of the user's own voice between the two sides. At the present time, there is no commercially available software that assists in programming the two sides to sound alike. It is hardly expected that they will sound identical and, in fact, the contribution of different bits of information from each side may add more "pixels" to improve the resolution of the grainy overall auditory picture. Each side is programmed as a separate entity, though both may be activated at once if two interface boxes and programming cables can be connected to the computer at the same time, so that adjustments can be made. If only one processor is connected to the programming computer at a time, then after the psychophysical measurements are completed, that processor's map can be adjusted "live," while the other processor is worn on its own battery power. The future might hold correlation of the two maps so as to allow the user to appreciate fine timing differences between sound arrivals at the two ears, which currently is a weakness of bilateral implant use, and to match pitch percepts on the two sides.

Monitoring Progress and Problems

Audiologic evaluation in the audiometric sound suite should occur at least at the 6-month interval and annually. For young children, these evaluations should take place at a separate appointment, not after a long bilateral mapping session. An unaided audiogram should be obtained annually for each ear, to assess any remaining residual hearing and to document the degree of loss in order to support the need for educational accommodations. Sound-field thresholds of detection for pulsed or pulsed warbled tones are measured at 250, 500, 1000, 2000, 4000, and 6000 Hz using each processor. Values poorer than 35 dB HL or uneven across the frequency range by more than 10 dB require an explanation. Thresholds typically average 20 to 30 dB HL (slightly better for narrowband noise stimuli than for pulsed tones) and are influenced by the sensitivity control setting, input processing, input dynamic range, and characteristics of the microphone. Unexplained poor thresholds warrant checking the processor function and reprogramming.

If a child is too young or not ready to point to pictures when they are named, early progress can be assessed using a scale such as the IT-MAIS (Zimmerman-Phillips, 2000), Auditory Skills Checklist (Meinzen-Derr, Wiley, Creighton, & Choo, 2007), MED-EL Corporation's LittlEars Auditory Questionnaire (Küehn-Inacker, Weichbold, Tsiakpini, Coninx, & D'Haese, 2003), or other functional auditory scales. Speech recognition testing is accomplished by developmentally appropriate measures, recorded rather than live voice when possible, starting with closed-set picture pointing tests graduating to open-set word recognition tests or another developmentally appropriate recorded sentence test in quiet and noise, given with optimized maps for each ear separately and together. If a hearing aid is used contralateral to the implant, the hearing aid should be checked and the fitting verified prior to speech recognition testing. A presentation level of 60 dB SPL is appropriate for speech recognition testing with a cochlear implant, with at least one test given at 50 dB SPL (soft speech level) if performance at 60 dB SPL is good, for comparison and counseling purposes. Careful sound-field calibration and placement of the head in the sound field are important. Decrements in performance should be taken seriously as they might signal a lapse in therapy or a device problem. Any suspicion of internal device malfunction triggers an alert to the surgeon and an integrity test, typically administered at the implant center by a manufacturer's clinical specialist.

Tympanometry should be performed at the first postoperative audiologic evaluation and then annually or as needed in otologic monitoring. The static admittance of the implanted ear typically is lower postoperatively than preoperatively and can remain lower than the unimplanted ear (Neault, O'Brien, Rimmer, Licameli, & Kenna, 2005), so a baseline measure with the implant in place when the ears are clear is helpful in the event of future need for the use of tympanometry to assess middle ear dysfunction. If vestibular-evoked myogenic potentials (VEMPs) were recorded and found to be present prior to surgery, the test can be repeated at the first postoperative audiologic evaluation. The VEMP threshold might be elevated and the amplitude reduced postoperatively (Licameli, Zhou, & Kenna, 2009). The use of cortical-evoked potentials to assess auditory response development is reviewed in Chapter 22.

Fostering Independence

Just as teenagers with hearing loss need to learn to wake themselves up in the morning with a vibrating or flashing alarm clock, they also need to begin to become independent users of their hearing technology. They might have been implanted when they were too young to understand the process or device and need progressive education about their hearing loss, how they access sound, and how their hearing differs from typical hearing. College preparation group meetings for students with hearing loss and other support groups, in person or online, foster independence. They can be independent in asking for captions to be turned on. They can begin to handle processor breakdowns independently before they graduate from high school. College preparation requires students with hearing loss to develop organizational skills and knowledge of accommodations including FM systems and real-time text support to access the curriculum at the same time as their classmates, not later by reading notes after class. Young adults who were implanted at age 2 years at the time of FDA approval of implantation for children are in college now, leading the way for a generation of children who have access to the world of sound using cochlear implants. Pediatric implant teams can anticipate the reward of watching them choose and become successful in their vocations.

References

Acoustical Society of America. (2009). ANSI/ASA S12.602002 (R2009). *American National Standard acoustical performance criteria, design requirements, and guidelines for schools* (reaffirmation of ANSI S12.60-2002). Retrieved from http://asastore.aip.org

Birman, C. (2009). Cochlear implant surgical issues in the very young child. *Cochlear Implants International, 10*(1), 19–22.

Bolajoko, O., Olusanya, A. B., Shiela, L., Wirz, C., Linda, M., & Luxon, A. (2008). Factors associated with auditory neuropathy/dys-synchrony in a developing country. *Audiological Medicine, 6*(2), 120–128.

Buchman, C. A., Roush, P. A., Teagle, H. F. B., Brown, C. J., Zdanski, C. J. & Grose, J. H. (2006). Auditory neuropathy characteristics in children with cochlear nerve deficiency. *Ear and Hearing, 27*(4), 399–408.

Ching, T. Y., Hill, M., Brew, J., Incerti, P., Priolo, S., Rushbrook, E., & Forsythe, L. (2005). The effect of auditory experience on speech perception, localization, and functional performance of children who use a cochlear implant and a hearing aid in opposite ears. *International Journal of Audiology, 44*(12), 677–690.

Dava, H., Figueirido, J. C., Gordon, K. A., Twitchell, K., Gysin, C., & Papsin, B. C. (1999). The role of a graded profile analysis in determining candidacy and outcome for cochlear implantation in children. *International Journal of Pediatric Otorhinolaryngology, 49*(2), 136–142.

Davidson, L. S. (2006). Effects of stimulus level on the speech perception abilities of children using cochlear implants or digital hearing aids. *Ear and Hearing, 27*(5), 493–507.

Donaldson, A. I., Heavner, K. S., & Zwolan, T. A. (2004). Measuring progress in children with autism spectrum disorder who have cochlear implants. *Archives of Otolaryngology-Head and Neck Surgery, 130*(5), 666–671.

Dowell, R., Hollow, R., & Winton, E. (2004). Outcomes for cochlear implant users with significant residual hearing. *Archives of Otolaryngology-Head and Neck Surgery, 130*, 575–581.

Edwards, L., Thomas, F., & Rajput, K. (2009). Use of a revised children's implant profile (GOSHChIP) in candidacy for paediatric cochlear implantation and in predicting outcome. *International Journal of Audiology, 48*(8), 554–560.

Edwards, L. C., Waltzman, S. B., & Scalchunes, V. (2007). Children with cochlear implants and complex needs: A review of outcome research and psychological practice. *Journal of Deaf Studies and Deaf Education, 12*(3), 258–268.

Gelnett, D., Sumida, A., Nilsson, M., & Soli, S. D. (1995). *Development of the Hearing in Noise Test for Children (HINT-C)*. Annual Meeting of American Academy of Audiology, Dallas, TX.

Hellman, S. A., Chute, P. M., Kretschmer, R. E., Nevins, M. E., Parisier, S. C., & Thurston, L. C. (1991). The development of a Children's Implant Profile. *American Annals of the Deaf, 136*, 77–81.

Holt, R. F., & Kirk, K. I. (2005). Speech and language development in cognitively delayed children with cochlear implants. *Ear and Hearing, 26*(2), 132–148.

Holt, R. F., Kirk K. I., Eisenberg, L. S., Martinez, A. S., & Campbell, W. (2005). Spoken word recognition development in children with residual hearing using cochlear implants and hearing aids in opposite ears. *Ear and Hearing, 26*(4 Suppl.), 82S–91S.

Hughes, M. L. (2006a). Fundamentals of clinical ECAP measures in cochlear implants. Part 1: Use of the ECAP in speech processor programming. *Audiology Online*, April 10, Article 1569. Retrieved April 10, 2006, from http://www.audiologyonline.com/articles/article_detail.asp?article_id=1569

Hughes, M. L. (2006b). Fundamentals of clinical ECAP measures in cochlear implants, Fundamentals of clinical ECAP measures in cochlear implants Part 2: Measurement techniques and tips. *Audiology Online*, November

6, Article 1717. Retrieved November 6, 2006, from http://www.audiologyonline.com/articles/pf_article_detail.asp?article_id=1717

Johnston, J. C., Durieux-Smith, A., Angus, D., O'Connor, A., & Fitzpatrick, E. (2009). Bilateral pediatric cochlear implants: A critical review. *International Journal of Audiology, 48*(9), 601–617.

Kiang, N. Y., & Moxon, E. C. (1972). Physiological considerations in artificial stimulation of the inner ear. *Annals of Otology, Rhinology, and Laryngology, 81*(5), 714–730.

Kirk, K. I., Pisoni, D. B., Sommers, M. S., Young, M., & Evanson, C. (1995). New directions for assessing speech perception in persons with sensory aids. *Annals of Otology, Rhinology, and Laryngology, 104*(Suppl. 106), 300–303.

Koch, D. B., Downing, M., Osberger, M. J., & Litvak, L. (2007). Using current steering to increase spectral resolution in CII and HiRes 90K users. *Ear and Hearing, 28*(2 Suppl.), 38S–41S.

Küehn-Inacker, H., Weichbold, V., Tsiakpini, L., Coninx, S., & D'Haese, P. (2003). *LittlEARS Auditory questionnaire: Parents questionnaire to assess auditory behavior*. Retrieved February 8, 2010, from http://www.medel.com/english/img/PDF/reha/MKT1070E_r20.pdf

Lazaridis, E., Therres, M., & Marsh, R. R. (2010). How is the children's implant profile used in the cochlear implant candidacy process? *International Journal of Pediatric Otorhinolaryngology, 74*(4), 412–415.

Licameli, G., Zhou, G., & Kenna, M. A. (2009). Disturbance of vestibular function attributable to cochlear implantation in children. *Laryngoscope, 119*(4), 740–745.

Mason, S. M., Cope, Y., Garnham, J., O'Donoghue, G. M., & Gibbin, K. P. (2001). Intra-operative recordings of electrically evoked auditory nerve action potentials in young children by use of neural response telemetry with the nucleus C124M cochlear implant. *British Journal of Audiology, 35*(4), 225–235.

Meinzen-Derr, J., Wiley, S., Creighton, J., & Choo, D. (2007). Auditory Skills Checklist: Clinical tool for monitoring functional auditory skill development in young children with cochlear implants. *Annals of Otology, Rhinology, and Laryngology, 116*(11), 812–818.

Mok, M., Galvin, K. L., Dowell, R. C., & McKay, C. M. (2010). Speech perception benefit for children with a cochlear implant and a hearing aid in opposite ears and children with bilateral cochlear implants. *Audiology and Neurotology, 15*(1), 44–56.

Neault, M., Kammerer, B., Clark, T., O'Brien, L., Kenna, M., & Licameli, G. (2007, April 12). *Pre-implant rating scale for prediction of outcome with sequential bilateral cochlear implantation in children*. Poster presentation at the 11th International Conference on Cochlear Implants in Children. Charlotte, NC.

Neault, M., O'Brien, L., Rimmer, D., Licameli, G., & Kenna, M. (2005, March 17). *Effect of cochlear implantation on static admittance of the middle ear*. Paper presented at the10th International Conference on Cochlear Implants in Children Dallas, TX.

Niparko, J. K., Tobey, E. A., Thal, D. J., Eisenberg, L. S., Wang, N.-Y, Quittner, A. L., & Fink, N. E. (2010). Spoken language development in children following cochlear implantation. *Journal of the American Medical Association, 303*(15), 1498–1506.

O'Brien, L., Kenna, M., Poe, D., Neault, M., Kammerer, B., Clark, T., . . . Licameli, G. (2007, April 12). *Validation of a modified cochlear implant profile (mChIP) tool for use in pediatric cochlear implant candidacy evaluation*. Poster presentation at the11th International Conference on Cochlear Implants in Children. Charlotte, NC.

Rance, G., & Barker, E. J. (2008). Speech perception in children with auditory neuropathy/dyssynchrony managed with either hearing aids or cochlear implants. *Otology and Neurotology, 29*(2), 179–182.

Rance, G., Cone-Wesson, B., Wunderlich, J., & Dowell, R. (2002). Speech perception and cortical event related potentials in children with auditory neuropathy. *Ear and Hearing, 23*(3), 239–253.

Robbins, A. M., Renshaw, J. J., & Berry, S. W. (1991). Evaluating meaningful integration in profoundly hearing-impaired children. *American Journal of Otolaryngology, 12*(Suppl.), 144–150.

Rodríguez-Ballesteros, M., del Castillo, F. J., Martín, Y., Moreno Pelayo, M. A., Morera, C., Prieto, F., . . . del Castillo, I. (2003). Auditory neuropathy in patients carrying mutations in the otoferlin gene (*OTOF*). *Human Mutation, 22*(6), 451–456.

Roush, P. (2008). Auditory neuropathy spectrum disorder: Evaluation and management. *Hearing Journal, 61*(11), 36, 38–41.

Rubinstein, J. T., & Miller, C. A. (1999). How do cochlear prostheses work? *Current Opinion in Neurobiology, 9*, 399–404.

Schafer, E. C., & Thibodeau, L. M. (2006). Speech recognition in noise in children with cochlear implants while listening in bilateral, bimodal, and FM-system arrangements. *American Journal of Audiology, 15*, 114–126.

Shallop, J. (2008). *Management of children with Auditory Neuropathy Spectrum Disorder: Cochlear implants. Guidelines for identification and management of infants and young children with auditory neuropathy spectrum disorder*. Guidelines Development Conference at NHS 2008, Como, Italy.

U.S. Department of Education. (2006). Final regulations to implement the Individuals with Disabilities Education Improvement Act of 2004 (IDEA). *Federal Register*, 71(56, August 14).

U.S. Food and Drug Administration (FDA; 2010). *Medical Device Premarket Approval (PMA) Database: Cochlear implants*. Rockville, MD: FDA. Retrieved April 30, 2010, from http://www.fda.gov/MedicalDevices/ProductsandMedicalProcedures/ImplantsandProsthetics/CochlearImplants/default.htm

Vlastarakos, P. V., Candiloros, D., Papacharalampous, G., Tavoulari, E., Kampessis, G., Mochloulis, G., & Nikolopoulos, T. P. (2010). Diagnostic challenges and safety considerations in cochlear implantation under the age of 12 months. *International Journal of Pediatric Otorhinolaryngology, 74*(2), 127–132.

Vlastarakos, P. V., Proikas, K., Papacharalampous, G., Exadaktylou, I., Mochloulis, G., & Nikolopoulos, T. P. (2010).

Cochlear implantation under the first year of age—The outcomes. A critical systematic review and meta-analysis. *International Journal of Pediatric Otorhinolaryngology, 74*(2), 119–126.

Waltzman S. B., & Roland, J. T., Jr. (2005). Cochlear implantation in children younger than 12 months. *Pediatrics, 116*(4), e487–e493. doi:10.1542/peds.2005-0282

Waltzman, S. B., Scalchunes, B., & Cohen, N. L. (2000). Performance of multiply handicapped children using cochlear implants. *American Journal of Otology, 21*(3), 329–335.

Wiley, S., Meinzen-Derr, J., & Choo, D. (2008). Auditory skills development among children with developmental delays and cochlear implants. *Annals of Otology, Rhinology, and Laryngology, 117*(10), 711–718.

Wilson, B. S., Schatzer, R., Lopez-Poveda, E. A., Sun, X., Lawson, D. T., & Wolford, R. D. (2005). Two new directions in speech processor design for cochlear implants. *Ear and Hearing, 26*(4 Suppl.), 73S–81S.

Zeng, F. G., Rebscher, S., Harrison, W., Sun, X., & Feng, H. (2008). Cochlear implants: System design, integration and evaluation. *IEEE Reviews in Biomedical Engineering, 1*, 115–142.

Zimmerman-Phillips, S., Osberger, M. F., & Robbins, A. M. (2000). *Infant-Toddler: Meaningful Auditory Integration Scale (IT-MAIS)*. Sylmar, CA: Advanced Bionics.

Other Hearing Devices: Bone Conduction

Bill Hodgetts

Overview

In the hearing sciences, two types of hearing are often described: air conduction (AC) and bone conduction (BC). Air-conduction hearing involves the entire auditory system. Tiny acoustic vibrations in the air molecules are funneled down the ear canal where they induce vibrations on the tympanic membrane. The tympanic membrane then vibrates the ossicular chain, which results in a traveling wave of fluid displacement in the cochlea. Sufficient displacement of the basilar membrane begins the electrochemical cascade from the inner hair cells through the auditory nerve, brainstem, and eventually the cortex where the sound is interpreted. Bone-conduction hearing largely bypasses the external and middle ear, delivering the mechanical vibrations directly to the cochlea. To hear by bone conduction, no matter how complex the actual physiology, vibrations from some location on the skull need to be sufficiently intense to generate a traveling wave in the cochlea. If that traveling wave is of sufficient magnitude, the cochlea-to-cortex pathway will be stimulated, and the perception of sound will occur. When we speak, we are actually hearing a blend of air-conducted and bone-conducted sounds. Some of our perception will come from the acoustic vibration of air molecules from our mouths that travel around our heads to the ear canals (air conduction). However, a portion of our speech will generate a mechanical vibration of the skull bones of sufficient magnitude to also contribute to our perception of our own voice (Reinfeldt, Ostli, Håkansson, & Stenfelt, 2010). This phenomenon is why we seldom recognize (and often dislike) our own voices on a recording such as voicemail—where only the air-conducted sound is available.

In the past few years, there has been a significant expansion in the clinical interest and acceptance of bone-conduction devices (BCDs) as successful treatment options for many individuals. Bone-conduction devices have transitioned from being considered a "last resort" with only one main option (direct bone conduction via a Bone Anchored Hearing Aid [BAHA]), to an almost confusing field with many new clinicians, researchers, companies, and technologies available. This expansion has made it difficult to even agree to a common terminology for all these devices. However, Reinfeldt, Håkansson, Taghavi, and Eeg-Olafsson (2015) provided a nice review of some of the current technologies, and they recommended a helpful method of categorizing these devices. A modified version of this categorization system can be seen in Figure 31–1. The aim of this chapter is to share what is known about the candidacy criteria and the audiological and surgical considerations of the bone-conduction systems available today. I will address some fundamental differences with the various options and, finally, will discuss some aspects of the fitting process.

Indications for Bone-Conduction Devices

BCDs were originally indicated for individuals with bilateral conductive hearing loss. These patients were often unable to wear a traditional air-conduction hearing aid due to chronic ear infections or malformed ear canals. In recent years, indications for BCD candidacy have expanded to include patients with unilateral conductive, mixed, and sensory/neural hearing loss.

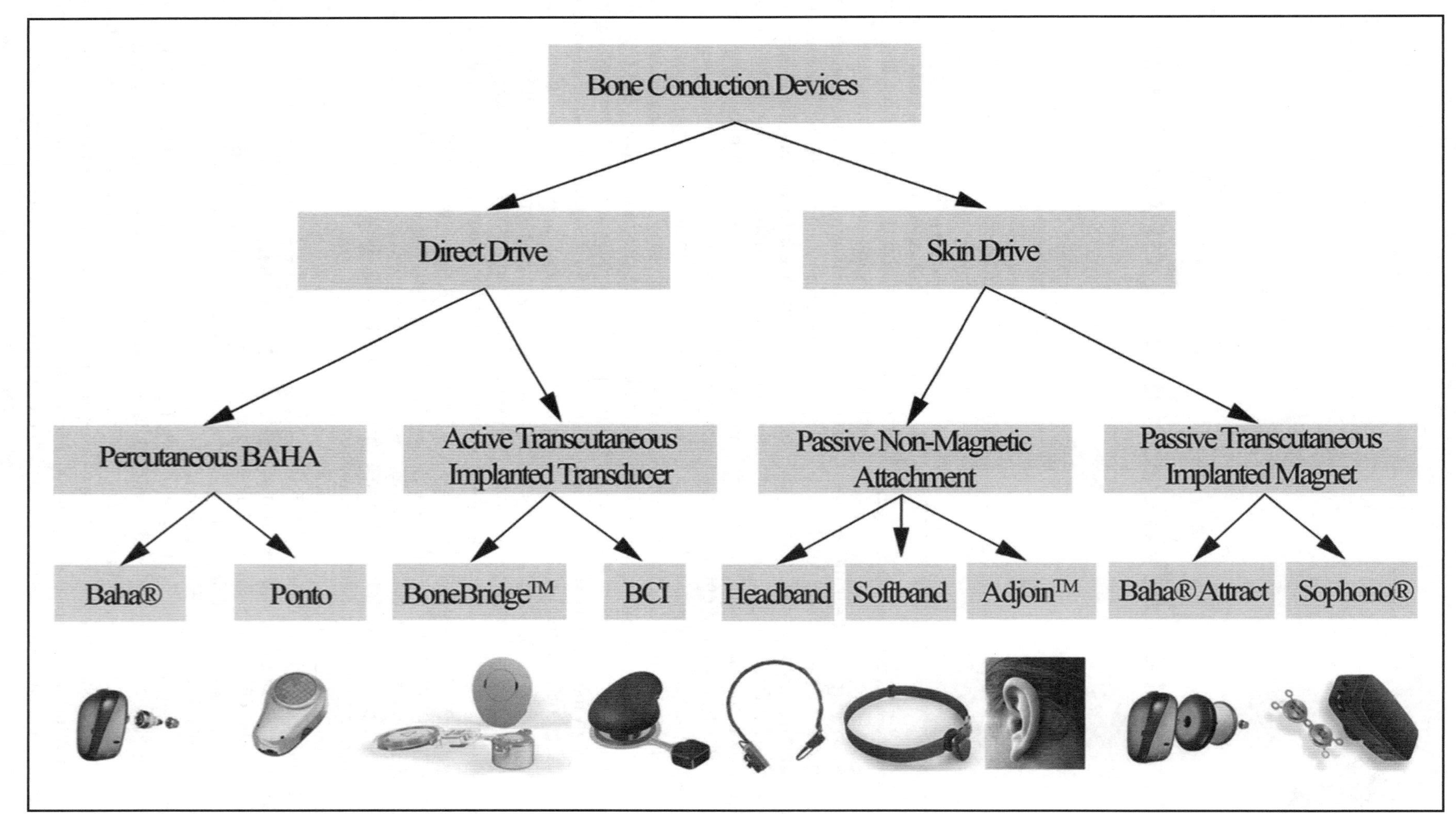

FIGURE 31–1. Categorization of current bone-conduction devices. (Modified from Reinfeldt, Håkansson, Taghavi, & Eeg-Olafsson, 2015; Images of BAHA, Headband, Softband, and BAHA Attract courtesy of Cochlear Ltd.; Ponto courtesy of Oticon Medical; Bonebridge courtesy of MED-EL; BCI courtesy of Håkansson; Adjoin courtesy of Otorix; and Sophono courtesy of Medtronic, Inc.)

BCD candidates can be broadly grouped into three categories:

1. those with conductive or mixed hearing loss who cannot wear an air-conduction hearing aid;
2. those with conductive or mixed hearing loss for whom surgery has been unsuccessful and/or future surgery is contraindicated; and
3. those with unilateral conductive, mixed, or sensory/neural hearing loss.

A summary of candidacy criteria and indications for BCD use related to these groups of patients is presented in Table 31–1.

Given the variety of etiologies and the associated difficulties with hearing in the unaided condition, not all BCD candidates can be expected to receive the same amount of benefit from the BCD (Dumper, Hodgetts, Liu, & Brandner, 2009). However, many BCDs are now a viable option for many individuals who would have otherwise gone untreated in the past.

Advantages of Direct-Drive Versus Skin-Drive Bone Conduction

In the 1960s, Per-Ingvar Brånemark discovered that living bone would connect to titanium through a process he coined "osseointegration" (Albrektsson & Wennerberg, 2005). Osseointegration was first applied to the field of dentistry. Titanium screws were implanted into the teeth of patients, and, after a period of healing, teeth could be connected to the implants. Researchers soon speculated that these same implants could possibly be used outside of the mouth to anchor facial prosthetics and BCDs. Broadly speaking, all BCD processors are similar to air-conduction hearing aids. They contain a microphone, battery, and internal digital signal processing (DSP) chips. The main difference between air-conduction hearing aids and all bone-conduction devices is the type of *output* delivered from each device. Air-conduction hearing aids deliver *acoustic vibrations*, and bone-conduction devices deliver *mechanical vibrations*. The main differences between the BCDs is the method by which the processor is connected to the patient and whether that connection allows for direct bone conduction (with no skin interference) or bone conduction with skin interference (Figure 31–2).

For many years the most available (and recommended) BCD was the BAHA. The principle behind the BAHA can be seen in Figure 31–2B. There are three components to the system, 1 = the processor, 2 = the abutment, and 3 = the implanted titanium screw. The system allows for the mechanical vibrations from the processor to be delivered to the skull bone without any skin interference. To date, it is estimated that more than 150,000 patients have been treated with this direct bone-conduction approach (Reinfeldt, Håkansson, Taghavi, & Eeg-Olafsson, 2015).

Table 31–1. Otologic and Audiologic Conditions That Might Have Indications for Bone-Conduction Device Use Divided Into Categories for Candidacy

Air-Conduction Hearing Aid Contraindicated	*Canal or Middle Ear Surgery Contraindicated*	*Unilateral Hearing Loss*
Congenital bilateral atresia	Repeated surgery fails to close air-bone gap; Baha reliably closes air-bone gap	Congenital unilateral atresia
Chronic draining ears that are unresponsive to treatment	Conductive or mixed hearing loss in only hearing ear; risk of damaging only remaining ear; Baha is a safe alternative	Acquired unilateral conductive or mixed hearing loss
External ear canal irritation	Total absence of ossicular chain and/or insufficient tissue to reconstruct ossicular chair	Congenital unilateral profound unilateral sensory/neural hearing loss (often called single-sided deafness in the Baha literature)
Large mastoid cavity resulting from mastoidectomy		Single-sided deafness resulting from VIIIth nerve tumor or tumor resection
Postoperative ear defects (absence of pinna, closure of ear canal) resulting from temporal bone resection		Sudden unilateral sensory/neural hearing loss
Excessive occlusion effect		

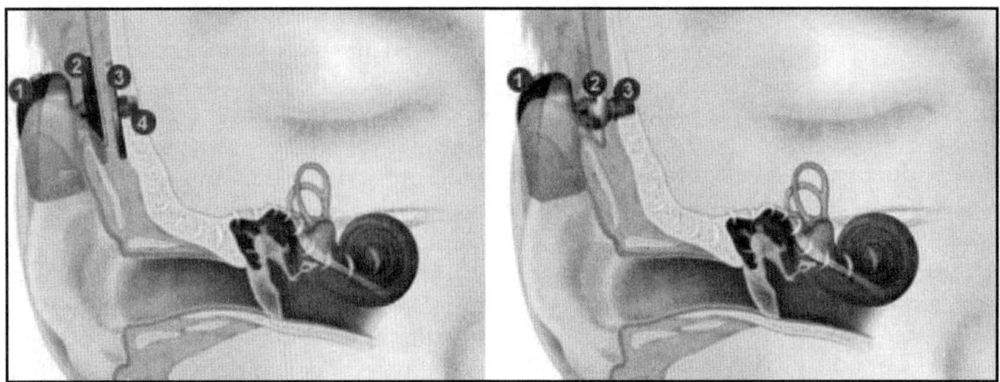

FIGURE 31–2. A. An example of passive magnetic skin-drive bone conduction (BAHA Attract; 1 = processor, 2 = external magnet, 3 = internal magnet, 4 = titanium screw.) **B.** A direct-drive bone-conduction solution (BAHA Connect; Image courtesy of Cochlear Corporation.)

There are several well-documented advantages to the direct bone-conduction systems. For example, there are differences in hearing sensitivity on the same patients when stimulated through the skin (transcutaneously) or directly to the bone (percutaneously; Håkansson, Tjellstrom, & Rosenhall, 1984, 1985; Mylanus, Snik, & Cremers, 1994; Stenfelt, & Håkansson, 1999). For example, Håkansson et al. (1984) used Bekesy audiometry to investigate the difference in voltage (dB) required to stimulate bone-conduction thresholds with a conventional Oticon bone-conduction transducer pressed against the skin or rigidly connected to an abutment. Of the 10 subjects tested, they found almost no difference in transcutaneous versus percutaneous bone-conduction thresholds in the low frequencies. However, they discovered a mean threshold improvement with the direct bone conduction of between 10 and 20 dB in the mid to high frequencies. Håkansson et al. (1985) found an even more dramatic improvement in thresholds by direct bone conduction when measuring the acceleration level at threshold. This time, the differences were large at all frequencies especially at 1000, 1500, and 2000 Hz, where the threshold improvements on the seven subjects averaged to 27, 25.5, and 27.5 dB, respectively. Stenfelt and Håkansson (1999) measured the voltage to the transducer for trans- and percutaneous thresholds and then converted these voltages to force as a reference quantity on nine subjects. They found that at 250, 500, and 1500 Hz, the force level required to generate a threshold was actually lower through the skin than when measured directly through the abutment (likely due to a skin resonance). At all other frequencies the direct bone-conduction thresholds required a lower force level. However, this time the average differences were only 7 dB or less. The threshold level shifts (±1 SD) for these three studies are graphed in Figure 31–3. Two things should be fairly obvious to the reader: (a) there are considerable differences in threshold shifts depending on the study and the method used to measure the threshold differences, and (b) the variability in responses at a given frequency appears to be fairly large. In fact, Håkansson et al. (1985) noted that: "The shapes and the absolute values of each threshold curve are highly individual and do not give any universally valid information" (p. 245).

In other words, we can be pretty sure that, on average, there is going to be an audiological advantage to direct-drive bone conduction, but the exact amounts for an individual patient are likely very difficult to determine or predict. To make matters worse, the differences in transcutaneous and percutaneous thresholds from subject to subject appear to be unrelated to what would seem to be an obvious variable. Mylanus et al. (1994) found no correlation between the thickness of the skin and subcutaneous tissue and the pure-tone average (PTA) threshold shift. An individual was just as likely to display a threshold shift of 10 dB with only 2 mm of skin and tissue as was an individual with 9 mm of skin and tissue. Conversely, they found an individual with only 2 mm of thickness had a PTA threshold shift of 16 dB, although someone else had 13 mm of thickness but a PTA threshold shift of only 3 dB (Figure 31–4).

Because direct bone conduction has superior high-frequency output capabilities and lower distortion (Cremers, Snik, & Beyon, 1992), it is no surprise that studies have revealed significant improvements in sound-field aided warble tone tests, speech-in-quiet, and speech-in-noise tests with the direct bone-conduction systems

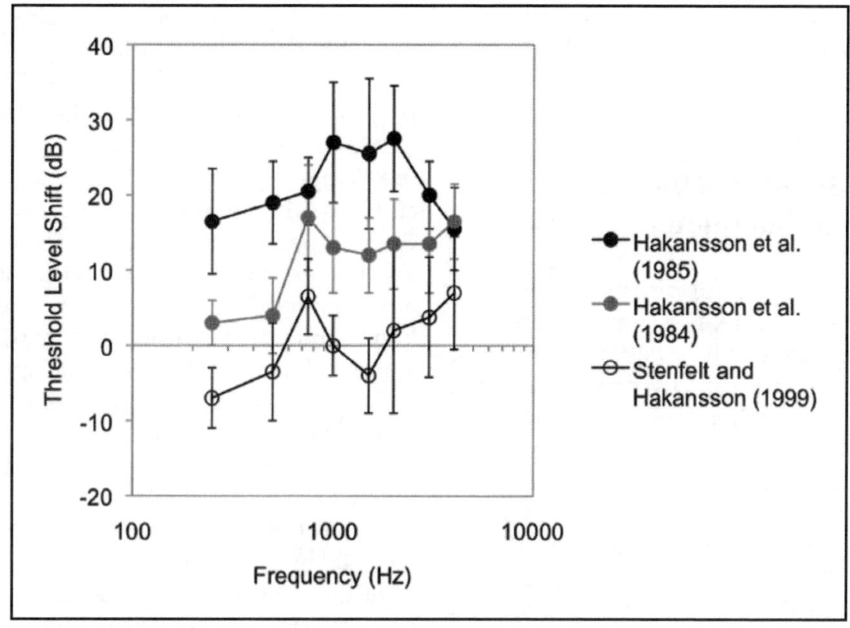

FIGURE 31–3. Difference in threshold level shifts measured three ways in three different studies (error bars = ±1 SD).

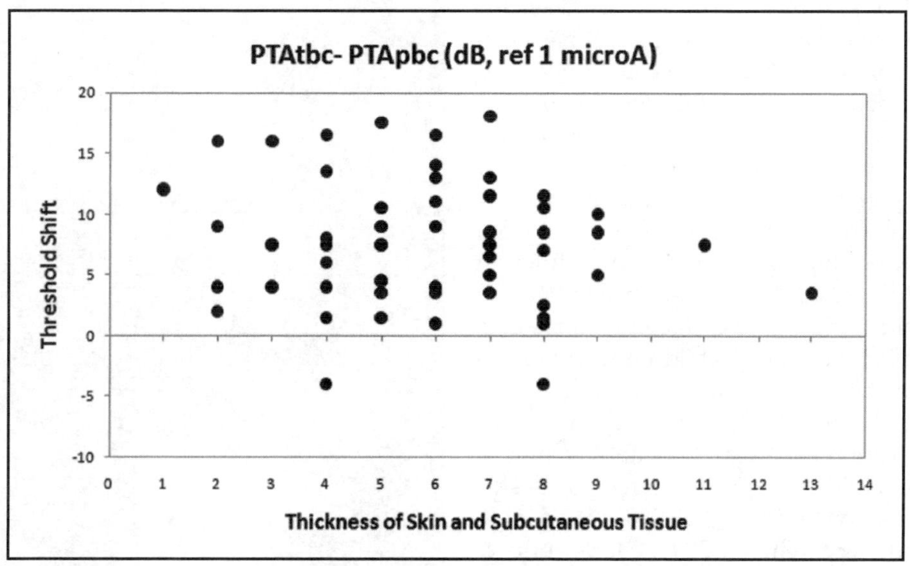

FIGURE 31–4. Pure-tone average threshold shift between skin-drive (PTAtbc) and direct-drive (PTApbc) thresholds as a function of skin thickness in millimeters.

over the skin-drive systems. These findings apply to both adults and children (Powell, Burrell, Cooper, & Proops, 1996; Tietze & Papsin, 2001; Tjellström & Håkansson, 1995). Long-term studies have also concluded that the majority of BAHA users were still using their systems daily and were quite satisfied with the device even 5 to 10 years after the BAHA fitting (van der Pouw, Snik, & Cremers, 1999). As with the pure-tone thresholds, the direct-drive hearing from a device like a BAHA (Ponto or BAHA) represents a superior audiological option compared to bone-conduction hearing aids that deliver the signal passively through the skin (Snik et al., 2005).

Advantages of Skin-Drive Versus Direct-Drive Bone Conduction

The audiological advantages for direct-drive hearing are quite clear in the literature. For a given individual with a given cochlea, there will be better sensitivity if the bone-conduction signal directly drives the skull. However, there are some primary challenges with the direct-drive approach. In the case of the BAHA (Ponto or BAHA), there is a surgery involved whereby a 3- to 4-mm screw is implanted in the head and a titanium abutment is installed onto which the audio processor can be connected. The titanium abutment protrudes through the skin essentially leaving an open wound that needs to be carefully maintained for the life of the abutment. Many children are not eligible for the surgery until they are around 4 or 5 years of age. (This varies slightly from country to country, but in the United States, the FDA requires the child to be 5 years old before the BAHA surgery.) The surgery itself for BAHA is less invasive than it used to be and has been simplified greatly in the past several years (Hultcranz, 2011). However, there are still well-known challenges with the surgery and aftercare. For example, a systematic review by Colquitt et al. (2011) revealed that implant losses range from 6.1% to 19.4%. In a review of pediatric studies only, implant losses ranged from 5.3% to 21.5% (McDermott & Sheehan, 2009). Although implant loss is significant, the day-to-day maintenance of the implant site can also be a challenge for some. This is especially true of young children who tend to have higher rates of infections around the implant site. McDermott and Sheehan (2009) reported on studies with skin complication as low as 2.4% and as high as 37%. The range of children requiring some type of surgical revision was from 7.7% to 25.9% (de Wolf, Hol, Huygen, Mylanus, & Cremers, 2008; McDermott & Sheehan, 2009).

Passive Nonmagnetic Skin-Drive Solutions

Clearly, some individuals do not wish to have an abutment sticking through their skin, and some clinicians are choosing technologies that carry fewer complications and risks of revisions/losses. A glance at Figure 31–1 shows that there are three options currently available or in clinical trials (e.g., Adjoin) for passive nonmagnetic skin-drive devices. For many years, the BAHA softband (an elastic headband that allows a BAHA device [Ponto or BAHA] to be attached; Figure 31–5) has been a highly effective solution for young children who are not yet eligible for surgery. In terms of aided hearing and language development, researchers have found that results with the BAHA Softband are comparable to the results obtained with traditional bone-conduction hearing aids connected to a steel tension headband (Hol, Cremers, Coppen-Schellekens, & Snik, 2005). The BAHA Softband is easier to wear and more comfortable than traditional bone-conduction hearing aids on a steel headband. Additionally, so long as the connection is not loose, the tension of the BAHA Softband is not a critical factor in the vibrations received by the child (Hodgetts, Scollie, & Swain, 2006). In fact, the newest (still under investigation at the time of writing) passive approach to skin-drive hearing, the Adjoin, takes advantage of this limited need for a high contact force. Essentially, the Adjoin is an adhesive-

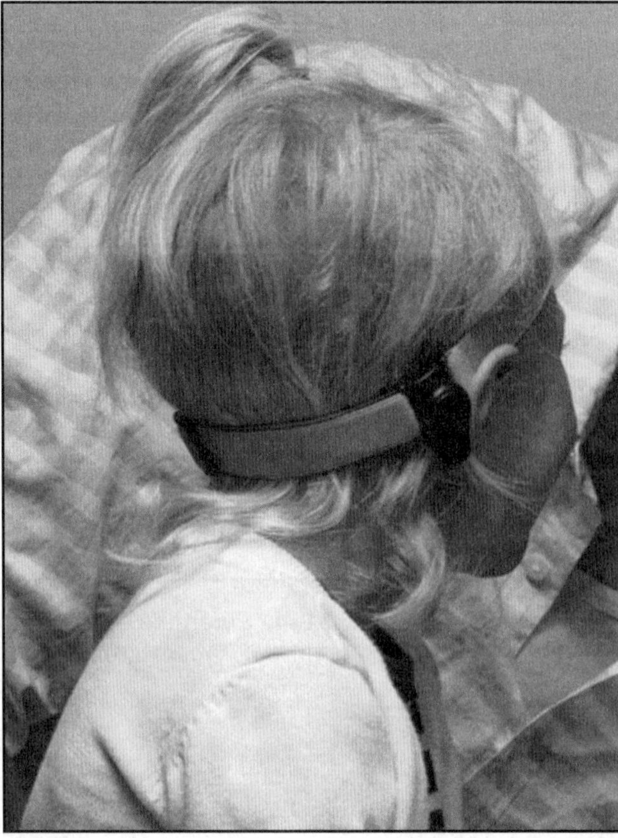

FIGURE 31–5. BAHA Softband connected to a young child.

based system that adheres to the skin for approximately 3 to 5 days behind the ear of a child (McDermott, Child, & Gill, 2015). A device can be connected and worn by a child without the need for surgery or any sort of headband. While still in the trial phases at the time of writing, this technology holds some distinct advantages over some of the other passive technologies from an aesthetic and practical perspective. However, there remain unanswered questions as to the long-term use of the adhesive as well as the ongoing maintenance costs and audiological outcomes (Figure 31–6).

Passive Skin-Drive Magnetic Solutions

Currently, there are two skin-drive magnetic solutions that are available on the market: The BAHA Attract and the Sophono (see Figure 31–1). Both of these technologies require a surgery for a magnet to be placed under the skin. Once healed, a second magnet is used on the outside of the skin to connect the processor to the patient. Because the vibrators (transducers) are inside the external processor that connects to the outside magnet, these devices function quite similarly to the skin-drive systems mentioned in the previous section. The vibrations need to travel through the skin and will therefore lose energy compared to the direct-drive systems like the BAHA (connect) and Ponto. To date, there have been some minor complications with the magnet systems related to skin pressure and magnet strength in the short term (O'Niel, Runge, Friedland, & Kerschner, 2014). There are not yet studies to show whether there are long-term negative consequences to the skin following extended use of these passive magnetic transcutaneous devices. One advantage of the BAHA Attact system over the Sophono is the ability to convert the magnet system to a direct-drive abutment if the patient does not tolerate the magnet well or their hearing thresholds worsen to a level where they require the greater sensitivity afforded by the direct-drive solution. The choice of which passive device might be best for a given child comes down to a lot of factors that will be dependent on what a particular clinic offers as well as a multitude of factors between the clinicians and the families considering these technologies.

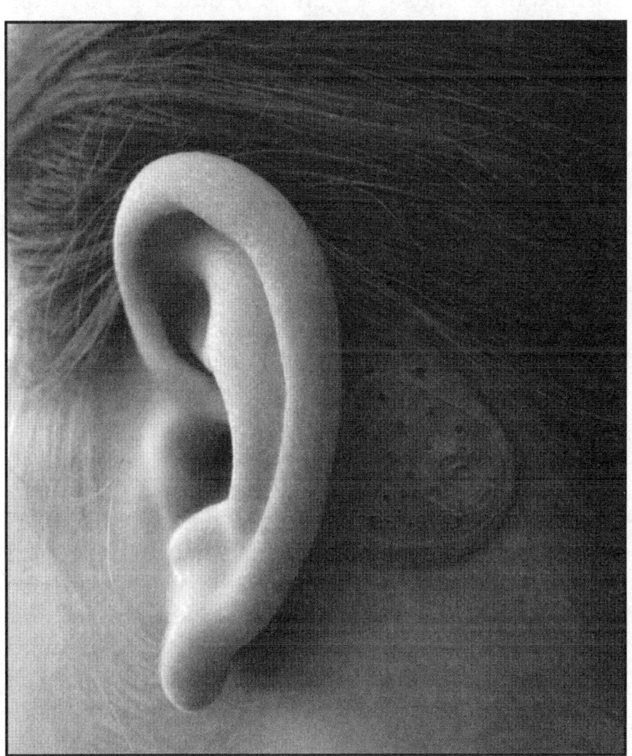

FIGURE 31–6. The Adjoin adhesive for connecting a bone-conduction device for skin-drive hearing. (Image courtesy of Otorix.)

The Best of Both Worlds?

Given the discussion to this point, it might be fairly clear to the reader that the best audibility or sensitivity for bone-conduction devices is available when the vibrator is directly coupled to the skull with no skin interference. However, there are definitely well-known challenges (especially in children) associated with having an implant protruding through the skin. For many years, there has been a push to develop bone-conduction technologies that have the benefits of direct drive on the skull, without skin penetration (Hakansson et al., 2010). At the time of writing there is currently one commercially available device (Bonebridge, MED-EL) and one device under clinical investigation (BCI; Reinfeldt, Håkansson, Taghavi, Jansson, & Eeg-Olafsson, 2015) that meets these criteria (see Figure 31–1). Both technologies have the active vibrator under the skin so they are direct- drive transducers. However, the signal from the processor is passed inductively across the skin to stimulate the vibrator so there is no skin penetration and, therefore, a *predicted* lower risk of skin complications. Recent trials are showing that audiological results obtained with these active transcutaneous devices are approximately on par with previous results from direct-drive BCDs (e.g., Reinfeldt, Håkansson, Taghavi, Jansson, & Eeg-Olafsson, 2015; Sprinzl et al., 2013).

The Bonebridge is approved at present for children over the age of 5 years. However, the transducer is quite large and the surgery is more complicated than traditional BAHA surgeries. In the case of a pediatric patient, there might be insufficient room to fit the vibrator as the skull thickness and mastoid space in children is smaller than in adults (Granstrom, Bergstrom, Odersjo, & Tjellstrom, 2001). Researchers recommend preoperative planning including computerized tomography (CT) scans to ensure that there is sufficient space to place the transducer (Manrique, Sanjhueza, Manrique, & de Abajo, 2014). The BCI has a smaller, thinner transducer than the Bonebridge and may prove to be easier to fit into pediatric mastoids. However, at present, the ongoing investigation of this device is on adults only (Reinfeldt, Håkansson, Taghavi, Jansson, & Eeg-Olafsson, 2015).

Device Considerations

It should be fairly clear that, at present, there are tradeoffs between all of these available BC devices audiologically and practically. For example, one device might be preferable from an audiology perspective (direct bone conduction), but the family might live a 10-hr drive from a clinic that might be able to look after any tissue problems that arise as a consequence of the abutment. In that case, it might make practical sense to consider a skin-drive system like a Sophono. However, what happens if the child's hearing worsens with time and there is insufficient output from the skin-drive magnet approach? Should the clinic have decided on the Bonebridge? Maybe, but what if there was not enough space in the mastoid cavity? Should they wait for the BCI? Which device is going to cost more? Who is paying? These hypothetical questions underscore how complicated and confusing the field has become.

Output Considerations

There are some things that can be addressed audiologically with respect to device differences. We already covered the differences in sensitivity between direct drive and skin drive. The differences are significant, but hard to predict on an individual basis. However, one method that can be used to provide some understanding of device output differences is to define their dynamic ranges in dB HL. Zwartenkot et al. (2014) and Reinfeldt, Håkansson, Taghavi, Jansson, and Eeg-Olafsson (2015) used the results of published studies to define the maximum dynamic range of output across a number of BCDs. They also argued that an aided pure-tone average threshold of 35 dB HL (500, 1000, 2000, and 4000 Hz) might be a reasonable target as that would likely result in word recognition of scores of approximately 75%, according to the articulation index (Mueller & Killion, 1990). Together, these values can be used to derive maximum inclusion criteria by device. Although these are somewhat limited assumptions, they at least provide a metric against which some comparisons can be made. (See Zwartenkot et al., 2014, and Reinfeldt, Håkansson, Taghavi, & Eeg-Olafsson, 2015, for a detailed explanation.)

Figure 31–7 shows the maximum dynamic range of hearing (in dB HL) and the maximum recommended pure-tone average unaided bone-conduction thresholds for a number of BCDs (Mertens et al., 2014; Reinfeldt, Håkansson, Taghavi, & Eeg-Olafsson, 2015; Zwartenkot, Snik, Mylanus, & Mulder, 2014). Of note, the BAHA Attract is likely to have similar values as the Sophono. Also, the maximum power output (MPO) of the Divino is similar to the MPO of the more recent devices (the Ponto Plus from Oticon Medical and the BAHA 4 from Cochlear Corporation). More powerful devices (e.g., Ponto Plus Power) are expected to have results in between the Divino and the Cordelle. Those familiar with this field might notice that the maximum unaided thresholds in Figure 31–7 differ slightly from many of the manufacturer's recommendations. These lower values are a conservative guide to ensure that sufficient output is available for a given user with a given BCD.

Device Fitting Considerations

One area that needs considerable attention in the field of BCDs is how to prescribe and verify the output of a given device on a given user's head. Broad considerations of candidacy like those presented in Figure 31–7 are a helpful guide; however, they do little to inform the clinician about the capabilities of a given device on a particular user in the clinic. Measures of aided soundfield thresholds, quite common in this field, do little to inform the clinician about the audibility of speech. (See Seewald, Moodie, Sinclair, & Cornelisse, 1996, and Hawkins, 2004, for reviews of these issues.) Hodgetts, Håkansson, Hagler, and Soli (2010) have argued that to properly fit and verify a given device on a given user, one needs to know the user's dynamic range of hearing and the output of the device with both measures being taken at a common reference point. The clinician can use these two pieces of information to assess the sensa-

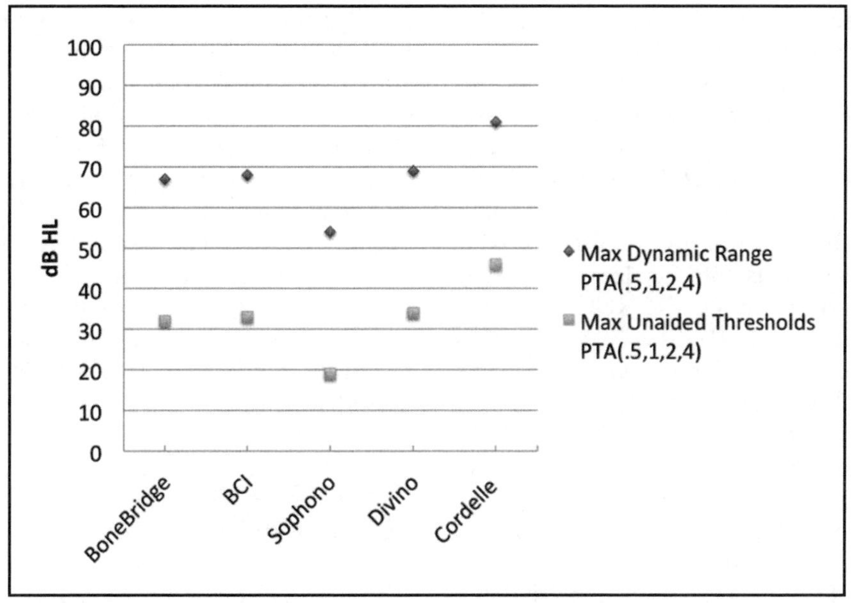

FIGURE 31–7. Maximum dynamic range of hearing and maximum recommended unaided bone-conduction thresholds for a variety of bone-conduction devices.

tion level or audibility of speech (Cornelisse, Seewald, & Jamieson, 1995). This is logically equivalent to the fitting of air-conduction devices. The dynamic range of hearing is defined in sound pressure level (SPL) at the eardrum and the device output (in response to real speech) is measured in SPL at the eardrum. Both measures share a common reference point (the eardrum SPL) and, therefore, sensation level of speech can be easily derived. In the following section, I discuss the fitting and verification considerations for direct-drive BCDs that have an abutment through the skin (e.g., BAHA and Ponto).

Fitting and Verification of Direct-Drive Percutaneous BCDs

As mentioned above, to make a comparison of aided speech output from a device, one needs to define the dynamic range of hearing and the output of the device in a common metric at a common reference point. In the case of percutaneous direct-drive BCDs (BAHA), the common reference is dB Force Level and the common measurement point is the abutment. Several important developments in recent years have made these measurements possible. First, modern BCDs have the capabilities of measuring thresholds, in situ, while connected to the patient. Second, in 2013, Interacoustics (Assens, Denmark) released a commercially available skull simulator (SKS10) that can be connected to a hearing aid test box to measure the force level of direct-drive BCDs. The skull simulator is a very close representation of the human head. Unlike a 2-cc coupler for air-conduction hearing aids, where the difference between the real ear and the coupler (RECD) can be quite large and variable, the differences between the patient's real head and the skull simulator (real-head-to-coupler differences; RHCDs) are quite small (Hakansson & Carlsson, 1989).

Illustrative Case

Imagine we have a patient who has already undergone surgery and has a BAHA abutment. We can use the device with the manufacturer's software to measure the patient's hearing through the abutment (unaided thresholds through the skin are no longer relevant). The manufacturer's software might display hearing levels (HL), but you can actually take the device off the patient and connect it to the Skull Simulator and measure the force level directly. For example, let us imagine that the in situ software threshold at 1000 Hz was 20 dB HL. If we placed that device on a skull simulator and presented the same tone, we might measure 50 dB Force Level. An alternative to measuring the force directly is to simply add the reference equivalent thresholds force levels for direct bone conduction (RETFLdbc; Carlsson & Hakansson, 1997) to the HL value from the software.

Table 31–2 shows the details of this approach. Row 1 displays the in situ HL values for our hypothetical patient. These are the values from the software when testing the user's thresholds with the device connected to the abutment. Row 2 shows the RETFLdbc from Carlsson and Hakansson (1997). Row 3 shows a measured RHCD for this particular patient (note the small difference between the real head and the skull simulator). Adding rows 1, 2, and 3 will provide us with this particular user's force level thresholds (row 4). Row 4 tells us directly, for this user, in order for any signal to be audible at each of these frequencies, the device will need to produce an output greater than the force listed in row 4. For example, at 4000 Hz, the direct-drive BCD will need to produce at least 69 dB in order for the signal to be audible. Row 5 of Table 31–2 shows the maximum power output (MPO) of the Ponto Pro Power (PPP). This was the device used in this case. Hodgetts (2008) showed that, in most cases, the MPO of the BCD are lower than the loudness discomfort level of the patient. Therefore, it was recommended that the device MPO be used to define the upper limit of the dynamic range. Whether the device MPO or the patient's measured loudness discomfort levels represent the most appropriate upper limit of the dynamic range of hearing is still an open question. However, for this case, the device MPO was used. Row 6 shows the dynamic range for this user into which the clinician might conceivably fit the aided speech output from a device. Finally, row 7 can be used by a clinician to "fit" speech into the dynamic range of hearing for this particular user. To do this, it is recommended that real calibrated speech (or equivalent) be delivered to the device on the skull simulator. Adjustments can be made to the output of the device in order to ensure that audibility of the speech is achieved. We are currently working on a new version of Desired Sensation Level Approach for Bone Conduction with plans for inclusion in both the manufacturers' software suites for BCDs as well as in hearing aid test box software to aid in both the prescription and verification of BCD output targets for clinics that own a skull simulator.

Prescription and Verification of Other BCDs

Although we have not solved all of the prescription and verification challenges for percutaneous direct-drive BCDs (e.g., fully validated prescription targets, skull simulators in all BCD clinics etc.), there are at least viable options to measure these devices. Unfortunately, with the new technologies, we will have to return to the development stages of verification. For example, the output of the Bonebridge and BCI can easily be measured using a skull simulator; however, once the implant is placed the output of the device can no longer be measured with this tool. Alternative verification approaches are needed that will still allow the clinician to define the dynamic range of hearing and measure the output of the device with a common metric at a common reference point. We are currently working on the development of new verification solutions that

Table 31–2. Hypothetical Case Showing How to Define Dynamic Range and Fitting in Decibel Force Level

	250	*500*	*750*	*1000*	*1500*	*2000*	*3000*	*4000*	*6000*	*8000*
In situ thresholds	20	20	25	25	30	30	35	40	45	45
RETFLdbc	64	53	52	47	37	29	31	29	28	27
RHCD	1	2	−3	−1	0	0	0	0	1	1
Force-level thresholds	85	75	74	71	67	59	66	69	74	73
MPO of PPP	100	114	121	118	107	100	101	99	98	97
Dynamic range	15	39	47	46	40	40	35	30	24	24
Fitting?										

Note. RETFLdbc = reference equivalent thresholds force levels for direct bone conduction; *RHCD* = real-head-to-coupler differences; *MPO* = maximum power output; *PPP* = Ponto Pro Power.

will hopefully allow for the measurement of all types of BCDs available today. The good news is that as long as the dynamic range is appropriately defined, the prescription of output targets will be possible regardless of how that dynamic range was measured. In other words, if we can develop a new way of verifying output for each of these new technologies, the prescription of aided output should be possible for all devices, not just percutaneous direct-drive BCDs (BAHA).

Conclusions

Over the past several years, the field of bone-conduction amplification has expanded tremendously. There are new technologies that connect to the patient in new ways. There are new clinics, researchers, and companies. There are magnetic skin-drive options that were once considered inadequate that have now returned and appear to be doing well. There are active vibrators that can provide the benefit of direct-drive stimulation without the complications of a skin-penetrating abutment. There is much to be learned about the short- and long-term benefits of these emerging technologies, including how to fit and verify them. Finally, there are constant improvements to the percutaneous direct-drive BCDs. For many years, these devices have been shown to be the best bone-conduction solutions from a hearing perspective. It is unlikely that they will be retired any time soon as they are a simple, effective solution for people who have conductive, mixed, and sensory/neural hearing loss.

References

Albrektsson, T., & Wennerberg, A. (2005). The impact of oral implants—Past and future, 1966-2042. *Journal of the Canadian Dental Association, 71*(5), 327.

Carlsson, P., & Håkansson, B. (1997). The bone-anchored hearing aid: Reference quantities and functional gain. *Ear and Hearing, 18*(1), 34–41.

Colquitt, J. L., Jones, J., Harris, P., Loveman, E., Bird, A., Clegg, A.j., . . . Welch, K. (2011). Bone-anchored hearing aids (BAHAs) for people who are bilaterally deaf: A systematic review and economic evaluation. *Health Technology Assessment, 15*(26), 1–200.

Cornelisse, L. E., Seewald, R. C., & Jamieson, D. G. (1995). The input/output formula: A theoretical approach to the fitting of personal amplification devices. *Journal of the Acoustical Society of America, 97*(3), 1854–1864.

Cremers, C. W. R. J., Snik, A. F. M., & Beyon, A. J. (1992). Hearing with the bone-anchored hearing aid compared to a conventional bone conduction hearing aid. *Clinical Otolaryngology, 17*, 275–279.

De Wolf, M. J. F., Hol, M. K. S., Huygen, P. L. M., Mylanus, E. A. M., & Cremers, C. W. R. J. (2008). Clinical outcome of the simplified surgical technique for BAHA implantation. *Otology and Neurotology, 29*(8), 1100–1108.

Dumper, J. D., Hodgetts, W. E., Liu, R., & Brandner, N. (2009). Indications for bone-anchored hearing AIDS: A functional outcomes study. *Journal of Otolaryngology-Head and Neck Surgery, 38*, 1, 96–105.

Granstrom, G., Bergstrom, K., Odersjo, M., & Tjellstrom, A. (2001). Osseointegrated implants in children: Experience from our first 100 patients. *Otolaryngology-Head and Neck Surgery, 125*, 85–92.

Håkansson, B., & Carlsson, P. (1989). Skull simulator for direct bone conduction hearing devices. *Scandinavian Audiology, 18*(2), 91.

Håkansson, B., Reinfeldt, S., Eeg-Olofsson, M., Ostli, P., Taghavi, H., Adler, J., . . . Granström, G. (2010). A novel bone conduction implant (BCI): Engineering aspects and pre-clinical studies. *International Journal of Audiolology, 49*, 3–215.

Håkansson, B., Tjellstrom, A., & Rosenhall, U. (1984). Hearing thresholds with direct bone conduction versus conventional bone conduction. *Scandinavian Audiology, 13*(1), 3.

Håkansson, B., Tjellstrom, A., & Rosenhall, U. (1985). Acceleration levels at hearing threshold with direct bone conduction versus conventional bone conduction. *Acta Oto-Laryngologica, 100*(3–4), 240.

Hawkins, D. B. (2004). Limitations and uses of the aided audiogram, *Seminars in Hearing, 25*, 51.

Hodgetts, W. E. (2008). *Contributions to a better understanding of fitting procedures for BAHA* (Doctoral thesis). Faculty of Rehabilitation Medicine, Edmonton, University of Alberta, Canada.

Hodgetts, W. E., Håkansson, B. E., Hagler, P., & Soli, S. (2010). A comparison of three approaches to verifying aided BAHA output. *International Journal of Audiology, 49*(4), 286–295.

Hodgetts, W. E., Scollie, S. D., & Swain, R. (2006). Effects of applied contact force and volume control setting on output force levels of the BAHA Softband. *International Journal of Audiology, 45*, 301–308.

Hol, M. K. S., Cremers, C. W. R. J., Coppen-Schellekens, W., & Snik, A. F. M. (2005). The BAHA Softband: A new treatment for young children with bilateral congenital aural atrisia. *International Journal of Pediatric Otolaryngology, 69*, 973–980.

Hultcranz, M. (2011). Outcome of the bone-anchored hearing aid procedure without skin thinning: A prospective clinical trial. *Otology and Neurotology, 32*, 1134–1139.

Manrique, M., Sanhueza, J., Manrique, R., & de Abajo, J. (2014). A new bone conduction implant: Surgical technique and results. *Otology and Neurotology, 35*(2), 216–220.

McDermott, A. L., Child, A., & Gill, J. (2015). *The Adjoin adhesive adaptor: New innovation in bone conduction hearing.* Presentation at the Fifth International Symposium on Bone

Conduction Hearing and Related Technologies, Lake Louise, Alberta, Canada.

McDermott, A. L., & Sheehan, P. (2009). Bone anchored hearing aids in children. *Current Opinions in Otolaryngology-Head and Neck Surgery*, *17*(6), 488–493.

Mertens, G., Desmet, J., Snik, A., & Heyning, P. (2014). An experimental objective method to determine maximum output and dynamic range of an active bone conduction implant: The Bonebridge. *Otology and Neurotology*, *35*, 1126–1130.

Mueller, H. G., & Killion, M. C. (1990). An easy method for calculating the articulation index. *Hearing Journal*, *43*(9), 1–4.

Mylanus, E. A., Snik, A. F., & Cremers, C. W. (1994). Influence of the thickness of the skin and subcutaneous tissue covering the mastoid on bone-conduction thresholds obtained transcutaneously versus percutaneously. *Scandinavian Audiology*, *23*(3), 201–203.

O'Niel, M. B., Runge, C. L., Friedland, D. R., & Kerschner, J. E. (2014). Patient outcomes in magnet-based implantable auditory assist devices. *Journal of the American Medical Association-Otolaryngology Head and Neck Surgery*, *140*(6), 513–520.

Powell, R. H., Burrell, S. P., Cooper, H. R., & Proops, D. W. (1996). The Birmingham bone anchored hearing program: Pediatric experience and results. *Journal of Laryngology and Otology*, *21*(Suppl.), 21–29.

Reinfeldt, S., Håkansson, B., Taghavi, H., & Eeg-Olafsson, M. (2015). New developments in bone-conduction hearing implants: A review. *Medical Devices* (Auckl), *8*, 79–93.

Reinfeldt, S., Håkansson, B., Taghavi, H., Jansson, K.-J., & Eeg-Olafsson, M. (2015). The bone conduction implant: Clinical results of the first six patients. *International Journal of Audiology*, *54*(6), 408–416.

Reinfeldt, S., Ostli, P., Håkansson, B., & Stenfelt, S. (2010). Hearing one's own voice during phoneme vocalization—Transmission by air and bone conduction. *Journal of the Acoustical Society of America*, *128*(2), 751–762.

Seewald, R. C., Moodie, K. S., Sinclair, S. T., & Cornelisse, L. E. (1996). Traditional and theoretical approaches to selecting amplification for infants and young children. In F. H. Bess, J. S. Gravel, & A. M. Tharpe (Eds.), *Amplification for children with auditory deficits* (pp. 161–191). Nashville, TN: Bill Wilkerson Press.

Snik, A. F. M., Mylanus, E. A. M., Proops, D. W., Wolfaardt, J. F., Hodgetts, W. E., Somers, T., . . . Tjellstrom, A. (2005). Consensus statements on the BAHA system: Where do we stand at present? *Annals of Otology, Rhinology, and Laryngology Supplement*, *195*, 2–12.

Sprinzl, G., Lenarz, T., Ernst, A., Hagen, R., Wolf-Magele, A., Mojallal, H., . . . Wolframm, M. D. (2013). First European multicenter results with a new transcutaneous bone conduction hearing implant system: Short-term safety and efficacy. *Otology and Neurotology*, *34*(6), 1076–1083.

Stenfelt, S. P., & Håkansson, B. E. (1999). Sensitivity to bone-conducted sound: Excitation of the mastoid vs the teeth. *Scandinavian Audiology*, *28*(3), 190.

Tietze, L., & Papsin, B. (2001). Utilization of bone-anchored hearing aids in children. *International Journal of Pediatric Otolaryngology*, *58*, 75–80.

Tjellström, A., & Håkansson, B. (1995). The bone-anchored hearing aid: Design principles, indications, and long-term clinical results. *Otolaryngologic Clinics of North America*, *28*(1), 53–72.

van der Pouw, C. T. M., Snik, A. F. M., & Cremers, C. W. R. J. (1999). The BAHA HC200/300 in comparison with conventional bone conduction hearing aids. *Clinical Otolaryngology in the Allied Sciences*, *24*, 171–176.

Zwartenkot, J. W., Snik, A. F. M., Mylanus, E. A. M., & Mulder, J. J. S. (2014). Amplification options for patients with mixed hearing loss. *Otology and Neurotology*, *35*, 221–226.

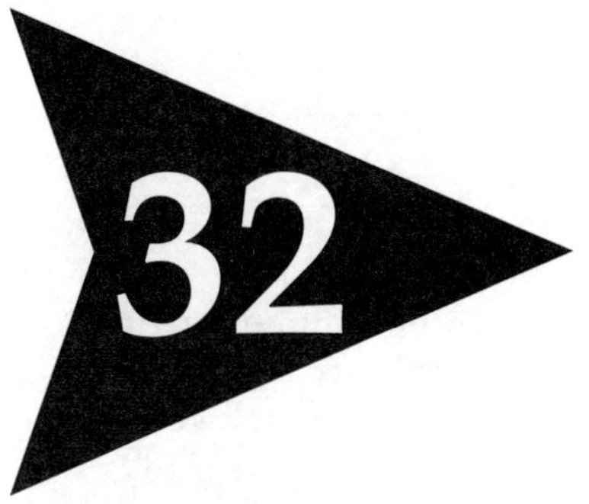

The Future of Auditory Implants

René H. Gifford

Introduction

Auditory implant technology has rapidly evolved in recent years such that there are a number of potential treatment options. Current options include middle ear implants, bone-anchored implants, cochlear implants, and auditory brainstem implants. Middle ear implants use mechanical energy to drive the inner ear with an implanted vibrational transducer attached to the ossicles, oval window, or round window membrane. For this reason, middle ear implants require a functional and intact middle ear system. Current labeled indications from the U.S. Food and Drug Administration (FDA) include individuals with sensory hearing losses ranging from a mild to severe-to-profound degree. Middle ear implants can be either semi-implantable (e.g., Ototronix Maxum, Houston, Texas; MED-EL Vibrant Soundbridge, Innsbruck, Austria) or fully implantable (e.g., Envoy Esteem, St. Paul, Minnesota). Middle ear implants are not currently indicated for use in the pediatric population and will thus not be covered further in this chapter.

Bone-anchored implants (BAIs) such as the Nucleus Baha hearing system and Oticon Medical bone-anchored hearing system have held long-standing application for individuals with conductive and mixed hearing losses. BAIs utilize direct bone conduction from the externally worn sound processor to the internal auditory system. The link between the external sound processor and the cochlea can be achieved via percutaneous coupling to an osseointegrated titanium implant/screw, transcutaneous magnetic coupling to an implanted titanium implant, or transcutaneous stimulus delivery via conventional oscillatory bone-conduction transduction with the sound processor placed on a soft band or hard band—similar to bone-conduction audiometry. The latter option is used for young children as osseointegrated BAIs are not approved for use in children under 5 years of age. As of 2002, bone-anchored hearing systems have been FDA approved for use in individuals with single-sided deafness (SSD), an indication that will be discussed in greater depth in this chapter.

Auditory brainstem implants (ABIs) are a class of implantable auditory prostheses that are designed to bypass the external, middle, and inner ear systems. An ABI is designed to directly stimulate the brainstem via an implanted electrode pad placed along the surface of the dorsal or ventral cochlear nucleus. ABIs are currently FDA approved for use in individuals 12 years of age or older with neurofibromatosis Type 2 (NF2). ABIs will be discussed throughout the chapter as expanded indications are currently being investigated in an FDA investigational device exemption (IDE) study for younger children with cochlear nerve deficiency (CND), a rare neural abnormality that is associated with an absent or hypoplastic auditory nerve.

To date, cochlear implants have been the most common of the implantable hearing systems used with both the adult and pediatric populations. Cochlear implants are designed to bypass the outer and middle ear directly stimulating the first order neurons located within the modiolus of the bony cochlea. Cochlear implant technology and patient management have both evolved rapidly since the FDA first approved multichannel cochlear implants for adults and children in 1985 and 1990, respectively. Despite this rapid evolution in technology, implant indications for adults, and audiologic practice, at the time of chapter preparation, FDA labeled indications for pediatric cochlear implant candidacy had remained unchanged since 2000. Given this evolution, it would follow that an expected element of our future is that clinical practices and patient management will most certainly change. It is also likely that we might be missing critical elements that are relevant to a patient's candidacy and postoperative assessment—even at present.

This chapter will discuss the components of auditory implant candidacy and postoperative assessment that we might be overlooking including cognitive status, listening effort, auditory related fatigue, and multisensory assessment. Just as with assessing initial candidacy for auditory implantation, these metrics can ultimately also prove useful for determining candidacy for a second implant or even perhaps for determining need for revision surgery—a decision that is not currently validated via clear-cut clinical or objective criteria. Given that pediatric indications for middle ear implants are not currently approved for use in children, and that cochlear implants are by far the most commonly utilized auditory implant in the pediatric population, the majority of the chapter will focus on cochlear implants; however, BAI, MEI, and ABI relevant information will be provided throughout.

Nontraditional Candidates for Auditory Implants

Cochlear Implants

There are a number of cochlear implant programs—typically housed within large academic medical centers—routinely implanting children with sensory hearing losses who might not meet the traditional candidacy profile. The reason this is generally considered common practice is that there is increasing evidence in support of expanding labeled indications for children with significant hearing loss who are not making expected progress for auditory, speech, and language skills with appropriately fitted hearing aids and recommended intervention. Historically speaking, there have been a number of reports advocating for the expansion of pediatric cochlear implant criteria (e.g., Cowan et al., 1997; Dettman et al., 2004; Gantz, Rubinstein, & Tyler, 2000; Mondaine et al., 2002; Tomblin, Spencer, Flock, Tyler, & Gantz, 1999). However, over the past decade, there have only been a handful of peer-reviewed articles dealing *specifically* with the issue of expanded criteria for pediatric cochlear implantation.

Yoshinaga-Itano, Baca, and Sedey (2010) studied repeated measures of auditory-oral language growth for 87 children with severe-to-profound hearing loss who had either been fitted with hearing aids (n = 38) or cochlear implants (n = 49). The children had been followed over time and the trajectory of language growth was tracked up to 7 years. Their findings demonstrated that cochlear implant recipients exhibited a steeper trajectory of receptive and expressive language than the children with hearing aids. Furthermore, they reported that children with cochlear implants closed the language gap relative to age-equivalent peers with normal hearing. Children with hearing aids, on the other hand, closed the gap at a much slower pace for receptive language and did not close the gap for expressive language. These data provided evidence for expanding implant criteria to include at least severe hearing losses for the youngest candidates.

In a comprehensive study examining expanded indications for pediatric cochlear implantation, Leigh, Dettman, Dowell, and Sarant (2011) evaluated speech recognition performance for 142 children with hearing loss who were fitted with either hearing aids (n = 62) or cochlear implants (n = 80). They demonstrated that for children with a pure-tone average (PTA) above 60 dB HL, there was a 75% chance of significant word recognition improvement with a cochlear implant. For sentence recognition performance, children with a PTA greater than 72 dB HL would have a 75% chance for significant improvement with an implant. Thus, they conservatively concluded that children with a PTA of 75 dB HL or greater should be recommended for cochlear implantation—at least unilaterally. Indeed one could interpret their findings to promote cochlear implantation for children with unaided PTA above 60 dB HL—provided that the child is not demonstrating *at least* year-for-year progress on speech, language, and auditory skills. It is also important to note that their recommendations were quite conservative as many children who might not have exhibited *significant improvement* still demonstrated improvement, and none exhibited a performance decrement following cochlear implantation. Thus, we could interpret these results as expanding pediatric implant criteria to at least the point of adult indications as the latter include moderate sloping to profound sensory hearing loss.

Carlson and colleagues (2015) described the results of a multicenter retrospective analysis of 51 children receiving the most recent generation implant system who did not meet labeled indications for implantation. Inclusion criteria required that a child have less severe hearing loss than specified in the current indications and open-set word or sentence recognition scores greater than 30%, excluding children with a diagnosis of auditory neuropathy. The children in this sample had, on average, moderate sloping to profound sensory hearing loss in the nonimplanted ear and a severe-to-profound sensory loss in the implanted ear. Carlson et al. (2015) reported a mean improvement in speech recognition of 63-percentage points in the implanted ear and 40-percentage points in the best-aided, bimodal condition—both of which were significant. Furthermore, there was a significant improvement in auditory and language development following implantation for this sample of nontraditional implant candidates. Perhaps the most powerful point in this paper was the fact that every one of the 51 children demonstrated improvement following implantation. That is, no one exhibited a decrement in performance for speech understanding, auditory skills development, and language development—consistent with Leigh and colleagues (2011). Thus, the point of diminishing returns—even for children with moderate sloping to profound sensory loss in the nonimplanted ear—has not been identified.

Auditory Brainstem Implants (ABIs)

FDA-labeled criteria for ABIs currently indicate use in individuals with neurofibromatosis Type 2 (NF2) for which it is anticipated that bilateral tumors will grow along cranial nerves VIII. Given that the cochleovestibular nerve is often, though not always, sacrificed during tumor removal, a CI would be contraindicated as a healthy functioning peripheral auditory system is required for use. Though ABIs are currently only approved for use in individuals with NF2, there is an FDA-approved investigational device exemption (IDE) clinical trial ongoing with children who have CND. For children with CND including an *absent* auditory nerve, cochlear implantation is contraindicated. The reason is that the primary auditory neurons (i.e., spiral ganglion cells located within the modiolus) are the neural stimulation targets for cochlear implant stimulation—and the cochleovestibular nerve is located distally to the stimulation targets. Given this, children with CND and auditory nerve hypoplasticity achieve poor postoperative outcomes, though there have been reports of cochlear implantation providing significant benefit (Breneman, Gifford, & Dejong, 2012; Buchman et al., 2011; Seymour et al., 2010; Teagle et al., 2010). For those children with CND who have not made any progress following cochlear implantation or for those with a confirmed absence of an auditory nerve—as documented via MRI and CT—ABI can be a viable treatment option. There are several peer-reviewed articles documenting the effectiveness of ABI for children with non-tumor-based hearing loss including severe cochlear ossification and various forms of 63-percentage points in the implanted ear and 40-percentage points including auditory nerve hypoplasticity, atretic internal auditory canal, and cochlear nerve aplasia. Children with non-tumor-based CND have been implanted with ABIs for over a decade across the globe (e.g., Bayazit et al., 2014; Choi, Song, Jeon, Lee, & Chang, 2011; Colletti, Colletti, Mandalà, Colletti, 2014; Colletti, Shannon, Carner, Veronese, & Colletti, 2010; Freeman et al., 2013; Kaplan et al., 2015). Thus, the ongoing multicenter IDE clinical trial in the United States is certainly timely as an alternative treatment option for children with non-tumor-based CND.

Despite the reports of success with ABI in children, there are certainly issues requiring careful consideration. First, there is always concern regarding nonauditory stimulation, particularly with respect to cranial nerve X. Cranial nerve X, or the vagus nerve, innervates a number of structures responsible for vital bodily functions including the pharynx, larynx, esophagus, heart, lungs, and intestinal tract. Given that the vagus nerve originates in the brainstem, the proximity of the ABI yields the possibility of vagal nerve stimulation. It is for this reason that ABIs are often initially stimulated in a conscious sedation center with pulse oximetry, heart rate, and blood pressure monitored throughout the activation session. Because this can be an involved process for young children, this has undoubtedly contributed to the conscientious ABI study design and rigorous study protocols well before the device protocol ever reached FDA submission for IDE.

Another issue for consideration is that children must be reliable reporters in order to manage electrodes and current levels eliciting noauditory stimulation. Experience with adult ABI recipients has shown that a particular electrode and current level can simultaneously provide auditory *and* nonauditory stimulation (e.g., Colletti et al., 2009, 2010). Given this, the use of electrical auditory brainstem response testing for identifying those electrodes eliciting auditory stimulation will not always be sensitive to those electrodes *also eliciting nonauditory stimulation*; however, the various clinical trials of pediatric ABIs in nontumor sensory hearing losses are being conducted at institutions of the highest surgical and audiological caliber. Thus, the teams of clinicians involved with this clinical trial will undoubtedly provide the field with valuable information regarding future applicability of pediatric ABI with nontumor deafness and optimized programming for managing nonauditory stimulation.

Hearing Preservation Cochlear Implantation

Considerable research and clinical attention has recently been placed on preservation of acoustic hearing with minimally traumatic cochlear implantation. Functional hearing preservation is possible both with short electrodes and associated shallow insertion depth (e.g., Büchner et al., 2009; Gantz, Turner, & Gfeller, 2006; Gantz et al., 2009; Gifford et al., 2013; Lenarz et al., 2013; Mowry, Woodson, & Gantz, 2012; Turner, Gantz, Karsten, Fowler, & Reiss, 2010) as well as for longer electrodes with deeper insertion (Arnolder et al., 2010; Gifford et al., 2013; Gstoettner et al., 2008; Helbig et al., 2011; Helbig et al., 2013; Kiefer et al., 2005; Obholzer & Gibson, 2011; Skarzynski, Lorens, Piotrowska, & Skarzynski, 2010; Skarzynski et al., 2012). By adding acoustic hearing to electrical stimulation, CI recipients can derive nonlinear, additive gains in speech understanding and basic auditory function (Ching, Incerti, & Hill, 2004; Dorman & Gifford, 2010; Dunn, Perreau, Gantz, & Tyler, 2010; Dunn, Tyler, & Witt, 2005; Gifford, Dorman, McKarns, & Spahr, 2007; Gifford et al., 2013; Gifford et al., 2014; Gifford et al., 2015; Morera et al., 2005; Morera et al., 2012; Schafer, Amlani, Seibold, & Shattuck, 2007; Sheffield & Zeng, 2012; Zhang, Spahr, Dorman, & Saoji, 2013). Furthermore, the benefit from acoustic stimulation can be added via the nonimplanted ear, the implanted ear in cases of hearing preservation, or both ears with binaural acoustic hearing. All three FDA-approved CI systems currently promote atraumatic electrodes for hearing and structural preservation. Further, all three manufacturers have hearing aid (HA) circuitry presently available within the implant sound processors. Current CI technology combined with HAs in the implanted and nonimplanted ear yields significant benefit for the vast majority of recipients. Mean benefit obtained via acoustic hearing in the implanted ear ranges from 10- to 15-percentage points or 2- to 3-dB improvement in the signal-to-noise ratio (SNR; Dorman & Gifford, 2010; Dorman et al., 2012; Dunn et al., 2010; Gifford, Dorman, & Brown, 2010; Gifford et al., 2013; Gifford et al., 2014; Gifford et al., 2015; Rader, Fastl, & Baumann, 2013; Turner et al., 2010). This benefit of 10- to 15-percentage points (or 2 to 3 dB) is beyond that obtained in the bimodal condition (CI + contralateral HA) for which the acoustic stimulation in the implanted ear is restricted.

The majority of the peer-reviewed literature focusing on hearing preservation and combined EAS has focused on adult CI recipients. However, there is a growing population of pediatric CI recipients with preserved acoustic hearing (e.g., Brown, Hullar, Cadieux, & Chole, 2010; Jayawardena, Kuthubutheen, & Rajan, 2012; Kuthubutheen, Hedne, Krishnaswamy, & Rajan, 2012; Skarzynski, Lorens, Piotrowska, & Anderson, 2007; Skarżyński, Matusiak, Furmanek, & Skarżyński, 2014) who have demonstrated similar significant electric-acoustic stimulation (EAS) benefits in speech understanding. Furthermore, a recent study of 153 ears has shown that younger age at implantation was a positive prognostic variable for acoustic hearing preservation with cochlear implantation (Anagiotos et al., 2015). Thus, we might expect to see an increase in children presenting for "hybrid/EAS" CI candidacy—particularly if high-frequency audibility is not attainable with conventional amplification or with frequency-lowering technology. It is important to note that FDA-approved indications for hybrid CI technology are currently limited to individuals aged 18 years and older. However, this is not to imply that atraumatic electrodes should not be used for children with low-frequency acoustic hearing that could be preserved and possibly aided for combined EAS. We can expect that future FDA-approved indications for hybrid/EAS hearing systems might include children younger than 18 years.

Infants Under 12 Months of Age

Current labeled indications for pediatric candidacy list children 12 months of age and older. However, this age restriction should not be interpreted as a lack of benefit for cochlear implantation in infants under 12 months. On the contrary, there is a growing body of literature demonstrating higher levels of word and language acquisition (Bergeson, Houston, & Miyamoto, 2010; Cuda, Murri, Guerzoni, Fabrizi, & Mariani, 2014; Houston & Miyamoto, 2010; Houston et al., 2012; Moog & Geers, 2010; Niparko et al., 2010), speech perception (Tajudeen, Waltzman, Jethanamest, & Svirsky, 2010), speech production intelligibility (Habib, Waltzman, Tajudeen, & Svirsky, 2010), gross motor development (De Kegel, Maes, Van Waelvelde, & Dhooge, 2015), and vocabulary development (Hayes, Geers, Treiman, & Moog, 2009; Houston & Miyamoto, 2010; Tomblin, Barker, Spencer, Zhang, & Gantz, 2005) for children implanted under 12 months of age—even when compared to children implanted in the second year of life.

One of the historical concerns regarding early implantation was related to specificity—or the risk of implanting a child *without* permanent sensory hearing loss. Given the audiologic tests at our disposal, including objective measures such as otoacoustic emissions and electrophysiology, as well as advanced behavioral audiometric techniques for use in children as young as 5 to 6 months, initial diagnostic and then confirmatory diagnostic testing can be easily accomplished by the seasoned pediatric audiologist for the infant without global developmental delay or other diagnoses that can impact motoric and cognitive development.

Cosetti and Roland (2010) provided a thorough review of the literature on the surgical and anesthetic-related risks associated with surgery in infants. Specifically, they reported that there is a higher incidence of morbidity, mortality, and life-threatening adverse surgical events for children undergoing surgery under 12 months. However, they also explained that the majority of concerns and complications reported in the literature have been confounded by emergency surgery for which there has been a lack of fasting and hence greater risk of aspiration as well as the risks of surgery in the very young and possibly medically fragile infant (under 1 month of age). Specifically related to cochlear implant surgery, there have been a number of studies demonstrating no greater anesthetic risk for infants under 12 months (Coletti et al., 2005; Dettman, Pinder, Briggs, Dowell, & Leigh, 2007; James & Papsin, 2004; Miyamoto, Houston, Bergeson, 2005; Miyamoto et al., 2008; Valencia, Rimell, Friedman, Oblander, & Helmbrecht, 2008; Waltzman & Roland, 2005). Cosetti and Roland (2010) outlined the pertinent surgical issues affecting this young population including intraoperative blood loss, facial nerve anatomy, skull thickness (<1 mm), fixation of the receiver/stimulator package, thin scalp flap, and device migration with skull growth. However, they reported that these are known variables and can be mitigated with a highly trained surgical team having extensive pediatric experience.

Given the favorable risk-benefit ratio for infants under 12 months, one might conclude that most children being identified at or near birth are routinely being implanted early. It is certainly the case that the request for insurance authorization is being submitted for infants as young as 6 months. The barrier to access for this population is that many insurance companies will at least initially deny coverage citing the FDA-labeled indications for children 12 months of age and older (Fitzpatrick, Ham, & Whittingham, 2015). Though it is *possible* to successfully appeal such denials—particularly in peer-to-peer review during which surgeons and audiologists advocate for their patients—most state Medicaid programs will generally deny authorization until the child reaches the 1-year mark based solely on the labeled indications that are not only over 15 years old, but are no longer in the best interest of the infant with bilateral severe-to-profound sensory hearing loss.

In addition to the growing number of peer-reviewed papers demonstrating significantly better outcomes for infants implanted under 12 months of age, another critical consideration is that infants with severe-to-profound sensory hearing losses are missing critical language learning opportunities occurring in the first year of life. This is true even for infants with appropriately fitted hearing aids given that audibility might not be sufficient to allow for consistent access to spoken language at average conversational levels. Developmental changes occurring rapidly in the first year of life include word segmentation, auditory memory, and phonological/lexical/semantic representation. Word segmentation is the process of dividing connected discourse into meaningful units, such as individual words. Research has shown that word segmentation develops rapidly between 7.5 and 10.5 months of age (e.g., Bortfeld, Morgan, Golinkoff, & Rathbun, 2005; Jusczyk, 2002). By 8 months of age, infants have the capacity for auditory memory and long-term storage of new words—both of which are important prerequisites for auditory-based language learning (Houston & Jusczyk, 2003; Jusczyk & Hohne, 1997). Development of phonological, lexical, and semantic representation also rapidly emerges during the first year of life (e.g., Gupta & MacWhinney, 1997; Hollich, Jusczyk, & Luce, 2002; Soja, Carey, & Spelke, 1991; Storkel, 2009). Given the remarkably rapid developmental changes occurring during the first year of life for the typically developing child, an infant with severe-to-profound sensory hearing loss and limited aided audibility is missing out on the development of critical auditory-based, language learning opportunities. It is actually possible that language-learning opportunities begin before birth, as research has shown that neural reorganization in response to speech is likely initiated in utero. Newborns have been shown to respond differentially to familiar sounds to which they were exposed as fetuses (e.g., DeCasper & Fifer, 1980; DeCasper & Prescott, 1984; Kisilevsky et al., 2003; Moon, Lagercrantz, & Kuhl, 2013) with greater brain activity observed in response to familiar sounds (e.g., Partanen et al., 2013). Thus, the future of cochlear implants for infants under 12 months of age is bright—provided that FDA-labeled indications are officially amended to include infants as young as 9 or perhaps even 6 months of age. It is likely that these changes to labeled criteria will occur in the very near future.

Unilateral and Asymmetric Sensory Hearing Losses

Implant candidacy has historically been based on bilateral sensory hearing loss as well as speech recognition in the bilateral, best-aided condition. To date, only one of the implant manufacturers makes reference to preoperative performance in the ear to be implanted in their labeled indications (Cochlear Americas physicians package insert for adult implant candidacy). The prevalence of unilateral sensory hearing loss in children is two to three times that of bilateral sensory hearing loss and has been estimated anywhere from 1 to > 3 per 1,000 births (Dalzell et al., 2000; Johnson et al., 2005; Watkin & Baldwin, 1999; White et al., 1994). For children with unilateral sensory hearing loss, it is reasonable to suppose that the best-aided condition might overestimate hearing and speech understanding abilities—particularly for typical listening environments including diffuse noise and reverberation in which the target stimulus might not always be directed toward the front of the listener or the better hearing ear. Furthermore, it has been known for decades that children with minimal hearing loss—including unilateral sensory loss—experience greater fatigue, stress, and increased academic risk as compared to their normal-hearing peers (e.g., Bess, Dodd-Murphy, & Parker, 1998; Lieu, Tye-Murray, & Fu, 2012; Lieu, Tye-Murray, Karzon, & Piccirillo, 2010; Tharpe, 2008).

Cochlear implantation in cases of SSD has been a hot topic for the past several years. There is a growing literature base including adults and children with highly asymmetric hearing losses as well as individuals with SSD receiving cochlear implants in the poorer ear. Firszt, Holden, Reeder, Cowdrey, and King (2012) described the outcomes for 10 adult recipients with asymmetric hearing loss for which implant candidacy was determined on the basis of the poorer hearing ear. In the nonimplanted ear, 4 of the 10 subjects had low-frequency audiometric thresholds in the normal to near-normal range. Even with the highly asymmetric nature of the hearing losses in their population, they showed significant improvement in speech recognition performance in quiet and noise as well as localization abilities. These findings suggest that we should consider implant candidacy on an individual ear basis even when the better hearing ear exceeds traditional candidacy criteria. However, they noted that adults with pre- or perilingual onset of deafness in the poorer hearing ear achieved modest benefit and thus might require more extensive counseling regarding realistic expectations.

Single-Sided Deafness (SSD)

A topic garnering increasing attention in the fields of otology, audiology, and hearing science is that of cochlear implantation in cases of true SSD. SSD is a special case of asymmetric hearing loss as one ear has *completely normal hearing*. Research has shown that a single hearing ear is sufficient for a child to develop speech and language within the age normative range; however, as documented previously herein, children with SSD have been shown to exhibit greater fatigue, stress, and increased academic risk as compared to their normal-hearing peers (e.g., Bess et al., 1998; Lieu, 2013; Lieu et al., 2012; Lieu et al., 2010; Tharpe, 2008).

In a study of 20 children with SSD who had received a CI, Arndt et al. (2015) assessed speech understanding in co-located and spatially separated noise conditions with and without the CI in place. They also obtained subjective reports of speech, spatial, and qualitative reports prior to and following CI surgery using the speech, spatial, and qualities (SSQ; Gatehouse & Noble, 2004) questionnaire administered to the parents. They documented significant improvements in speech understanding with the use of the CI for conditions in which the noise was presented to the normal-hearing ear. They further reported significantly improved qualitative reports on all subscales of the SSQ following cochlear implantation. Arndt and colleagues also mentioned that the speech and qualitative outcomes were better for children with postlingual onset of sensory hearing loss as well as an overall shorter duration of SSD as compared to the children with congenital sensory hearing loss and longer durations of SSD. Thus, it might ultimately be the case that cochlear implantation is recommended for cases of SSD with short durations of deafness or postlingual onset. However, what is unknown at this point in time, is whether or not the children with congenital sensory hearing loss would have fared better had they been implanted early in life minimizing the duration of unilateral auditory deprivation.

Tinnitus Suppression

Other cases of cochlear implantation with asymmetric hearing loss have been focused on tinnitus suppression rather than improving speech recognition. There are multiple published reports of the benefits of cochlear implantation for patients with unilateral hearing loss as a means for tinnitus suppression in CI recipients (Amoodi et al., 2011; Arndt et al., 2011; Arts, George, Stokroos, & Vermeire, 2012; Buechner et al., 2010; Gartrell et al., 2014; Kleinjung, Steffens, Strutz, & Langguth, 2009; Punte et al., 2011; Ramos et al., 2012; Ramos Macías, et al., 2015; van de Heyning et al., 2008; Vermeire & van de Heyning, 2009). Thus far, the majority of reports describing cochlear implantation for tinnitus relief in cases of SSD or asymmetric hearing loss have resulted in positive outcomes.

All reports of cochlear implants for tinnitus relief in cases of unilateral hearing loss, however, have investigated adult CI recipients. Despite the increased interest in this topic in recent years, it remains unclear whether cochlear implantation for tinnitus suppression in pediatric cases of asymmetric hearing loss or SSD is warranted. A primary issue is that the prevalence of tinnitus in children is not definitively known with reported estimates ranging from 3% to nearly 60% (Baguley et al., 2013; Nemholt, Schmidt, Wedderkopp, & Baguley, 2015).

Future Considerations Regarding Auditory Implants for SSD

Of great importance to note here is that at the time of chapter preparation, CIs were not FDA labeled as an approved treatment option for cases of SSD or as an intervention for a primary indication for tinnitus suppression in either adults or children. Before CIs are FDA approved for either indication, there are a number of issues that would need to be thoroughly investigated within the confines of an FDA-approved, multicenter IDE study. The most obvious issues demanding thorough investigation include efficacy, effectiveness, and safety. Furthermore, there are a number of factors that have yet to be rigorously investigated in this population—perhaps via randomized controlled trial (RCT)—including alternative treatment options such as CROS hearing aid systems, FM systems, and BAI. However, the issue with the use of CROS, FM, and BAI for SSD or asymmetric sensory hearing losses, is that none of these interventions will provide the individual with *binaural information*. The listener will be simply using assistive technology to deliver incoming sound stimulation to a single functioning cochlea. A CI would be the only of the mentioned intervention options that would provide the listener with bilateral auditory input with the *possibility* of binaural hearing restoration (e.g., Dorman et al., 2015). Thus, such interventions will leave an individual with asymmetric brainstem development that will result in abnormal and asymmetric reorganization of the central auditory system (e.g., Gordon, Wong, & Papsin, 2013; Polonenko, Papsin, & Gordon, 2015).

An industry-sponsored hearing symposium entitled "Asymmetric Hearing Loss" met in Toulouse, France, in November 2014 with the purpose of bringing together the world's leading experts on asymmetric hearing loss and implantable devices from otology, audiology, and hearing science. As a result of this symposium, a position statement was recently published that recommended that in cases of unilateral sensory hearing loss or SSD, an attempt should be made to provide the individual with access to alternative technology such as conventional air conduction CROS systems or BAI systems with or without osseointegration (Vincent et al., 2015). They also discussed the importance of assessing not only speech understanding abilities, but also localization and subjective reports of spatial hearing and disease-specific quality-of-life estimates such as that provided by the speech, spatial, and qualities (SSQ) questionnaire (Gatehouse & Noble, 2004) or generic health-related quality of life estimates. Clearly, there is much work to be done in this area prior to the determination of standard of care treatment strategy for individuals with asymmetric sensory hearing losses or SSD, though we can certainly expect this to remain an area of great interest and increased attention.

Cognitive Status

There are multiple reports of cognitive function—including general intelligence and working memory —influencing postoperative speech understanding, speech production, and language development for pediatric cochlear implant recipients (e.g., Geers, 2006; Geers, Brenner, & Davidson, 2003; Pisoni, 2000; Steven et al., 2011; Tobey, Geers, & Brenner, 2003). Most implant programs are not routinely assessing cognitive status of pediatric candidates with the exception of older children who might exhibit signs of global developmental delay. The primary reason is an increasing number of children with significant sensory hearing loss—in the absence of obvious comorbidities such as cerebral palsy and Down syndrome—are being implanted at such young ages that signs of impaired cognition might not yet be evident.

As compared to the growing literature base demonstrating the effects of cognition on postoperative speech understanding and production, there are some recent studies showing an inverse relationship between age at implantation and nonverbal intelligence (Colletti, Mandalà, Zoccante, Shannon, & Colletti, 2011; De Giacomo et al., 2013). Thus, it is possible that we might find that earlier auditory stimulation for children with severe-to-profound sensory hearing loss might benefit beyond auditory skills development and speech/language development. Kronenberger, Colson, Henning, and Pisoni (2014) theorized that expressive language development and earlier auditory exposure in children with severe-to-profound sensory hearing losses might strengthen the development of higher-order cognitive processes such as executive function; however, this is an area that will require further work before it is scientifically accepted and clinically recognized as motivation for earlier implantation.

Listening Effort and Fatigue

Hearing loss is known to increase the effort required for cognitive and linguistic processes (e.g., Hetu, Riverin, Lalande, Gety, & St-Cyr, 1988; Kramer, Zekveld, & Houtgast, 2009; Nachtegaal et al., 2009; Pichora-Fuller, 2007; Ronnberg, Rudner, Foo, & Lunner, 2008; Shinn-Cunningham & Best, 2008; Zekveld, George, Kramer, Goverts, & Houtgast, 2007). This has also been referred to as *listening effort,* which refers to the resources expended for attention and cognition that are required for speech understanding (e.g., Downs, 1982; Feuerstein, 1992; Fraser, Gagne, Alepins, & Dubois, 2010; Gosselin & Gagne, 2011; Hicks & Tharpe, 2002). Individuals with hearing loss commonly report that by the end of the day they experience significant fatigue. Thus, an obvious question is whether or not we should be including estimates of listening effort in our test battery for pediatric auditory implant candidacy? Although a child might be able to achieve above-criterion performance on a particular measure, this does not convey how much listening effort and attention was required to complete the task. Perhaps another way to phrase the question is, should children who happen to be better at top-down processing (i.e., filling in the gaps) be penalized by withholding auditory implant candidacy despite having significant communicative difficulty?

Children and Listening Effort

A child's academic performance is significantly influenced by degree of mental alertness. Sleep has historically been attributed as the primary underlying factor affecting a child's mental alertness in the classroom and has thus been the primary underlying mechanism driving research on mental alertness in school-aged children (e.g., Eliasson, Eliasson, King, Gould, & Eliasson, 2002; Gozal, 1998; Perez-Chada et al., 2007; Ravid, Afek, Suraiya, Shahar, & Pillar, 2009). However, for children with hearing loss, sleep is not the only factor, and it might not be the primary factor affecting academic performance. Evidence exists that children with hearing loss expend greater listening effort than their peers with normal hearing (e.g., Bess et al., 1998; Hicks & Tharpe, 2002; Stelmachowicz, Lewis, Choi, & Hoover, 2007). This translates to greater fatigue, stress, and increased academic risk for children with hearing loss—including children with milder degrees of hearing loss than those presenting for auditory implant candidacy (e.g., Bess et al., 1998; Tharpe, 2008). Furthermore, there are a growing number of reports documenting that children with sensory hearing losses experience significantly greater fatigue than their peers with normal hearing (e.g., Bess et al., 1998; Bess & Hornsby, 2014; Hornsby, Werfel, Camarata, & Bess, 2014). The deleterious effects of hearing loss on academic performance (Bess et al., 1998; Moeller, 2007; Most, 2004, 2006; Wake, Hughes, Hughes, Collins, & Rickards, 2004) coupled with the fact that fatigue—irrespective of hearing loss—further increases academic risk (e.g., Eliasson et al., 2002; Gozal, 1998; Perez-Chada et al., 2007; Ravid et al., 2009), then it would follow that an assessment of hearing-related listening effort and associated fatigue could provide a more comprehensive evaluation of a child's candidacy for implantable auditory prostheses. Thus, a clinical measure of listening effort and fatigue might ultimately become a part of the pediatric battery for implant candidate assessment. What will be needed in order for this to be adopted into clinical practice is a validated measure of listening effort for use in the pediatric population that is clinically feasible given the time and equipment constraints of the typical audiology clinic (Figure 32–1).

Physiologic Biomarkers of Stress and Listening Effort

There is currently no research available indicating how much auditory implants might be able to impact one's degree of listening effort—though the anecdotal reports from clinical patients are noteworthy. Studies using measures of listening effort such as pupillometry (e.g., Zekveld, Kramer, & Festen, 2010, 2011), heart rate variability (e.g., Dorman et al., 2012), or skin conductance (Mackersie & Cones, 2011) might provide assistance in determining the degree of benefit afforded by cochlear implantation for individuals with significant hearing loss. Furthermore, it is possible that measures of listening effort—objective or subjective—might also play a role in determining implant candidacy, particularly for patients who might be considered "borderline" candidates on the basis of audiometric testing.

Objective Estimates of Listening Effort

Pupillometry. There are a number of objective or physiologic correlates of listening effort. Pupils dilate in response to cognitive workload with peak dilation occurring approximately 1 to 2 s after demand onset.

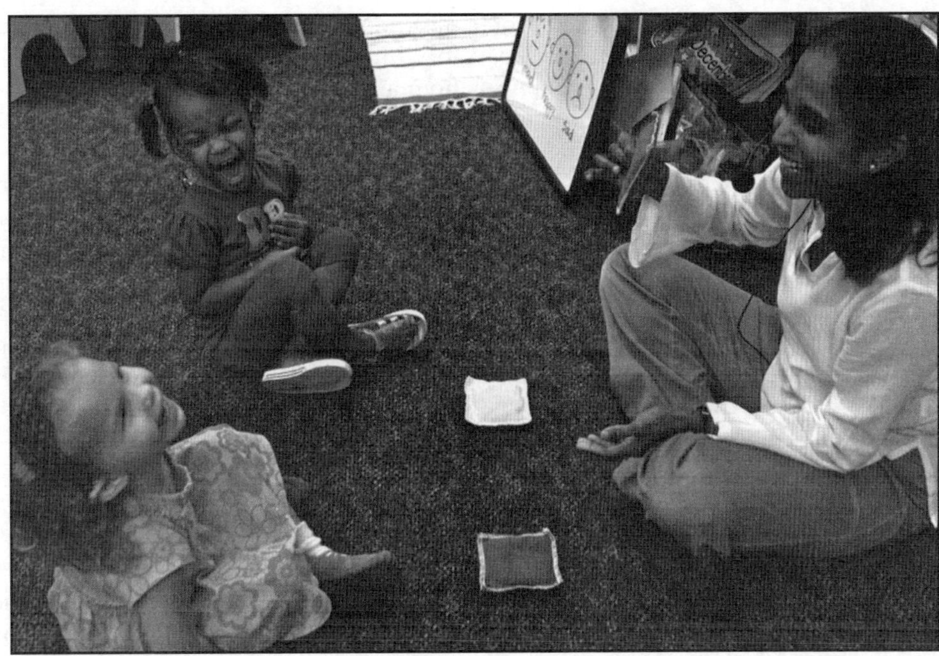

FIGURE 32–1. Auditory-based instruction is a vital part of a child's classroom experience. The effects of childhood hearing loss on listening effort and mental alertness can greatly impact learning and academic performance and might provide useful information in the assessment of candidacy for auditory implants.

Measuring degree and latency of pupil dilation has been used for a number of years to gauge cognitive processing load for tasks including mathematics and academic testing complexity (Ahern & Beatty, 1979; Klingner, Tversky, & Hanrahan, 2011) and memory recall (Granholm, Asarnow, Sarkin, & Dykes, 1996; Kahneman & Beatty, 1966; Klingner et al., 2011; Piquado, Isaacowitz, & Wingfield, 2010; Taylor, 1981). Pupil dilation has been used as a metric of listening effort for individuals with and without hearing loss (e.g., Koelewijn, Zekveld, Festen, & Kramer, 2012; Zekveld et al., 2010, 2011). Audiology clinics with integrated vestibular and balance programs will likely already have video eye-tracking systems that can calculate pupil position for assessing oculomotor function. However, pupillometry measures for gauging listening effort will likely not be included in the clinical software as the triggering programs for syncing speech stimuli and the measurement of onset and peak dilation latency include specialized coding that is currently customized by individual research labs. Moreover, it is questionable whether pupillometry would hold clinical applicability and efficacy for use in pediatric audiologic evaluation.

Heart Rate Variability. Heart rate variability (HRV) reflects beat-to-beat variation in the natural heart rate, created by the actions of the sympathetic and parasympathetic branches of the autonomic nervous system. When under stress, activity of the sympathetic nervous system activity is increased, thereby decreasing HRV. In less stressful conditions, there is greater activity of the parasympathetic nervous system, thereby increasing activity HRV.

Dorman and colleagues (2012) showed significant decreases in HRV with increases in background noise levels as related to speech understanding for normal-hearing listeners. Thus, it is possible that measures of HRV could be used to estimate the degree of auditory-related stress for individuals with hearing loss—and also potentially for supplementing the implant candidacy test battery. Though more research is clearly needed, the potential for clinical relevance is high. HRV measurement is rather simple and requires data from electrocardiogram (ECG) equipment already existing in most major medical centers—though its applicability and ease of use in the pediatric audiology clinic are questionable without the presence of medically trained staff.

Skin Conductance. Skin conductance—also referred to as galvanic skin response—is a measure reflecting the electrical conductance of the skin, and this varies with moisture level. Skin moisture is dependent upon activity of the sweat glands which are regulated by the sympathetic nervous system—primarily responsible for the body's fight-or-flight response. Thus, skin conductance provides an indirect estimate of physiologic stress.

Mackersie and Cones (2011) evaluated the sensitivity of a number of physiologic markers of stress for gauging listening effort and task demand for individuals with normal hearing. Though they incorporated four physiologic measures of stress including HRV, skin conductance, skin temperature, and electromyography, mean changes in skin conductance were found to be most sensitive to increasing task demand.

Skin conductance is currently measured best from the palm of the hand or the sole of the foot given that these areas have particularly dense populations of eccrine glands, which are involved in thermoregulation. Measurement of skin conductance is most generally achieved with electrodes placed on the palm of the hand such as that employed during polygraph, or lie detector testing. Thus, this is a noninvasive measurement and one that could be incorporated into a pediatric assessment. Unlike ECG and oculomotor equipment as discussed previously for the measurement of HRV and pupil dilation responses, skin conductance measurement and analysis equipment might not be widely available in a medical center environment. Furthermore, it is not fully understood how skin conductance might reflect physiologic stress related to listening effort for children with hearing loss. More research is necessary to address its clinical applicability and efficacy for use in pediatric audiologic evaluation.

Subjective Estimates of Listening Effort and Fatigue

As discussed, increased listening effort and auditory-related fatigue are known sequelae of hearing loss. Adults with severe-to-profound hearing loss frequently report increased anxiety, stress, and mental fatigue in response to the communication demands in both their professional and social lives. Additionally, children with sensory hearing loss have significantly greater fatigue than their peers with normal hearing (e.g., Bess et al., 1998; Bess & Hornsby, 2014; Hornsby et al., 2014). However, these reports are not considered in clinical audiology practice despite the large social, emotional, educational, and financial impact.

It would make sense to assess degree of auditory-related fatigue among individuals presenting for cochlear implant candidacy evaluation. It is possible that cochlear implantation might actually increase one's work productivity—though additional research is necessary. Thus, it would follow that attempts to gauge hearing-related fatigue would be a welcome addition to the pediatric assessment battery for determining auditory implant candidacy. There are a number of questionnaires that were designed specifically to address subjective fatigue. However, these questionnaires were not designed as disease-specific fatigue resulting from hearing loss. Rather, the majority of questionnaires have been designed to assess fatigue as related to chronic health conditions such as cancer, autoimmune disease, and sleep disorders. It is currently unclear what applicability such instruments would have for individuals with auditory-related fatigue—especially for children. There is one such instrument, the HEAR-QL (Umansky, Jeffe, & Lieu, 2011), which was designed as a disease-specific quality of life (QOL) questionnaire for children with hearing loss. The HEAR-QL is a validated instrument that has been shown to distinguish between children with hearing loss from their peers with normal hearing. However, this instrument seems to hold greatest appeal for evaluating the effectiveness of a particular intervention and thus might not hold diagnostic utility for assessing *hearing-related fatigue* or QOL as a criterion for auditory implant candidacy.

Multisensory Communication

Best practices for the assessment of speech understanding in the audiology clinic involve the use of recorded speech stimuli presented in the sound field via audition only. Though this currently represents the standard of care assessment for speech understanding in clinical audiology, it is not a realistic assessment of communication abilities, as we are rarely placed in situations during which all visual cues are absent. Audiovisual integration is a significant part of communication, as the majority of patients with whom we will work will have access to multiple sensory modalities for communication. For children with hearing loss, audiovisual integration is acquired via extensive early listening and communication experience.

Despite the audiovisual nature of speech communication, recent clinical practice has almost exclusively focused on speech testing in the auditory-only condition. The reason has primarily been to gauge listeners' abilities to understand speech in the most challenging condition. Clinical measures of audiovisual speech recognition already exist for both children and adults. For pediatric multimodal speech perception testing, there is the Children's Audio-Visual Enhancement Test (CAVET; Tye-Murray & Geers, 2001) and the Audiovisual Feature Test (Tyler, Fryauf-Bertschy, & Kelsay, 1991). Both tests allow for auditory alone, visual alone, and audiovisual administration of stimuli. The CAVET is an open-set test of word recognition and includes three lists of 20 words. The Audiovisual Feature Test is a closed-set test that assesses recognition of consonant features.

Holt, Kirk, and Hay-McCutcheon (2011) have proposed more widespread use of audiovisual speech recognition for children. They reported on the development and validation of the audiovisual version of the Lexical Neighborhood Sentence Test, which was adapted from the Lexical Sentence Test (Eisenberg, Martinez, Holowecky, & Pogorelsky, 2002). Holt and colleagues found that multimodal assessment of speech recognition was possible for children as young as 3 to 4 years for at least the auditory only and auditory + visual conditions. Holt and colleagues (2011) further reported that there are plans to ultimately adapt the audiovisual *Lexical Neighborhood Sentence Test* for use in clinical practice. We can be certain that as the field evolves, the assessment of the whole child—including multimodal speech perception abilities—will likely be integrated into the minimum pediatric speech recognition test battery.

Cross-Modal Reorganization: Helpful for Determining Implant Candidacy and Predicting Implant Outcomes?

In the presence of auditory deprivation, the auditory cortex can be recruited by other sensory modalities. This is commonly referred to as cross-modal reorganization or cross-modal plasticity. Cross-modal reorganization is not specific to auditory deprivation as it occurs in response to deprivation in any of the sensory modalities. Cross-modal reorganization of the auditory cortex has been well documented in individuals with severe-to-profound sensory hearing loss in response to visual stimuli (e.g., Buckley & Tobey, 2011; Fine, Finney, Boynton, & Dobkins, 2005; Finney, Clementz, Hickok, & Dobkins, 2003; Finney, Fine, & Dobkins, 2001), and somatosensory stimuli (e.g., Auer, Bernstein, Sungkarat, & Singh, 2007; Levanen, Jousmäki, & Hari, 1998; Sharma, Campbell, & Cardon, 2015).

A significant negative correlation has been demonstrated between degree of cross-modal plasticity of the auditory cortex and auditory-based outcomes with cochlear implants (e.g., Buckley & Tobey, 2011; Champoux, Lepore, Gagné, Théoret, 2009; Giraud & Lee, 2007; Lee et al., 2001; Lee, Truy, Mamou, Sappey-Marinier, & Giraud, 2007; Sandmann et al., 2012; Sharma et al., 2015; Strelnikov et al., 2013). The leading theory regarding the negative relationship between cross-modal reorganization and auditory CI outcomes is that these cross-modal changes either prohibit or hinder auditory cortical processing via the restored CI signal. That is, for deaf individuals with significant cross-modal reorganization, the auditory cortex continues to be recruited by other sensory modalities, and the presence of these shared resources leaves less processing capacity for auditory stimulation.

Given the relationship between cross-modal reorganization and auditory-based CI outcomes, preoperative assessment regarding the extent of cross-modal plasticity might hold significant clinical utility. To date, there is little preoperative information providing predictive value regarding auditory-only outcomes with the exception of age at implantation and an auditory-oral approach to communication. Thus, it is possible that preoperative neuroimaging might aid in the determination of CI candidacy for adults and children as well as in guiding expectations and recommendations for aural rehabilitation following implantation.

Bilateral Cochlear Implant Candidacy: When Is It Time to Consider a Second Implant?

One of the most frequently asked questions from both clinicians and families of implant recipients is focused on when they should consider a second implant for their child or patient. Despite the wealth of published research on both bimodal and bilateral function, there are currently no well-defined guidelines that can direct clinicians who are assisting with or recommending such decisions—especially for the youngest of implant recipients who have aidable hearing in the nonimplanted ear. More specifically, there are no definitive reports highlighting audiometric profiles, configuration of hearing loss, levels of speech perception performance, or levels of speech/language delay that can serve as preoperative indicators to determine whether an individual should pursue one or two implants.

Most children being considered for cochlear implantation will retain "bilateral" hearing in the sense that they will either hear bimodally with one cochlear implant and aided acoustic hearing in the nonimplanted ear or will receive two cochlear implants. At the time of chapter preparation, bilateral cochlear implantation was considered standard of care treatment for children with bilateral severe-to-profound sensorineural hearing loss for some of the largest of private health insurance companies in the United States including Aetna, Blue Cross Blue Shield, Cigna, Great West, Health Partners, Kaiser California, Medica, Priority Health, and TRICARE—though this list is in no way exhaustive. Furthermore, the William House Cochlear Implant Study Group (Balkany et al., 2008) and Papsin and Gordon (2008) have both recognized bilateral cochlear implantation as accepted medical practice and stated that it should be considered standard of care treatment for severe-to-profound sensorineural hearing loss.

To make data-driven recommendations for a second implant, one must recognize that the efficacy of a particular intervention—in this case, a second cochlear implant—depends heavily on the tests used for its measurement. Such tests must be sensitive enough to gauge the relevant speech information provided by acoustic hearing in the case of bimodal hearing as well as the information provided by a second cochlear implant for bilateral implant recipients. This is much easier said than done.

For children acquiring spoken language via implant technology, there are an increasing number of reports indicating that bilateral cochlear implantation—at a young age—yields higher levels of speech perception (Lovett, Kitterick, Hewitt, & Summerfield, 2010; Wolfe et al., 2007), rapid language acquisition achieving age-appropriate norms at younger ages (Wie, 2010), binaural summation (Buss et al., 2008; Dorman, Yost, Wilson, & Gifford, 2011; Koch, Soli, Downing, & Osberger, 2010; Litovsky, Parkinson, Arcaroli, & Sammeth, 2006), equivalent head shadow across ears (Buss et al., 2008; Litovsky et al., 2006), binaural squelch (Buss et al., 2008; Eapen, Buss, Adunka, Pillsbury, & Buchman, 2009), improved localization abilities (Beijin, Snik, & Mylanus, 2007; Godar & Litovsky, 2010; Grieco-Calub & Litovsky, 2010; Lovett et al., 2010; van Deun et al., 2010), and even significantly higher academic outcomes (Sarant, Harris, & Bennet, 2015).

For adults receiving a second cochlear implant, in addition to gains reported above for summation, squelch, and localization, there are large gains in health-related quality of life (QOL). On a dead/healthy scale of 0 to 1 —where 0 represents death and 1 represents perfect health—adult implant recipients report significant QOL improvement from 0.69 with one implant to 0.81 with a second implant (Bichey & Miyamoto, 2008). In fact, the improvement reported with the second implant was almost equivalent to the improvement seen with the first implant, a concept that can be difficult to understand given the much larger *relative* improvement in speech recognition observed with the first implant. Perhaps even more surprising is that the health-related QOL improvement observed with the second implant represents a favorable cost utility—much more favorable, and hence much less expensive at face value, than even estrogen replacement therapy and medical treatment for hypertension (Bichey & Miyamoto, 2008). Thus, one could conclude that recommending a second cochlear implant—when warranted—is truly a judicious use of health care funds. Despite these reports for adult bilateral users, we do not fully understand the value-added benefit of a second CI for pediatric recipients nor for their families as there have been few investigations (e.g., Sparreboom, Snik, & Mylanus, 2012).

Those assessments including the whole patient will be required in order to determine bilateral candidacy and to determine efficacy of bilateral cochlear implantation, as the current clinical measures of speech perception, as well as speech and language outcomes are not always sensitive to the effects of unilateral versus bilateral deafness. This is a fact that has been clearly outlined in the literature on minimal hearing loss (e.g., Bess & Tharpe, 1984, 1986; Klee & Davis-Dansky, 1986; Oyler, Oyler, & Matkin, 1988; Tharpe, 2008; Tharpe & Bess, 1991). In other words, as long as a single implant provides significant communicative improvement, standardized measures of speech perception and speech/language development will likely not provide the information needed to determine bilateral candidacy and to assess postoperative effectiveness of bilateral implantation.

Summary

Pediatric audiologists must strive constantly to challenge the status quo regarding standard of care assessment and question whether our current assessment battery is enough to identify patient and family concerns, to identify children who might continue to struggle with communication in typical everyday listening environments, and to identify the *global* effectiveness of a particular intervention. The latter concern, in particular, will certainly be considered by insurance and governmental agencies when proposing health care initiatives for cost containment. Though the field has made considerable strides in the management and assessment of children with sensory hearing loss, we still have much room for improvement. The future holds tremendous promise for children with various degrees and configurations of sensory hearing loss as we continue to see an increase in the selection of potential intervention options—particularly with respect to implantable auditory prostheses.

References

Ahern, S., & Beatty, J. (1979). Pupillary responses during information processing vary with Scholastic Aptitude Test scores. *Science, 205,* 1289–1292.

Amoodi, H. A., Mick, P. T., Shipp, D. B., Friesen, L. M., Nedzelski, J. M., Chen, J. M., & Lin, V. Y. (2011). The effects of unilateral cochlear implantation on the Tinnitus Handicap Inventory and the influence on quality of life. *Laryngoscope, 121,* 1536–1540.

Anagiotos, A., Hamdan, N., Lang-Roth, R., Gostian, A. O., Lüers, J. C., Hüttenbrink, K. B., & Beutner, D. (2015). Young age is a positive prognostic factor for residual hearing preservation in conventional cochlear implantation. *Otology and Neurotology, 36,* 28–33.

Arndt, S., Aschendorff, A., Laszig, R., Beck, R., Schild, C., Kroeger, S., . . . Wesarg, T. (2011). Comparison of pseudobinaural hearing to real binaural hearing rehabilitation after cochlear implantation in patients with unilateral deafness and tinnitus. *Otology and Neurotology, 32,* 39–47.

Arndt, S., Prosse, S., Laszig, R., Wesarg, T., Aschendorff, A., & Hassepass, F. (2015). Cochlear implantation in children with single-sided deafness: Does aetiology and duration of deafness matter? *Audiology and Neurotology, 20*(Suppl. 1), 21–30.

Arnolder, C., Helbig, S., Wagenblast, J., Baumgartner, Hamzavi, J. S., Riss, D., & Gstoettner, W. (2010). Electric acoustic stimulation in patients with postlingual severe high-frequency hearing loss: Clinical experience. *Advances in Otorhinolaryngology, 67,* 116–124.

Arts, R. A., George, E. L., Stokroos, R. J., & Vermeire, K. (2012). Review: Cochlear implants as a treatment of tinnitus in single-sided deafness. *Current Opinion in Otolaryngology-Head and Neck Surgery, 20,* 398–403.

Auer, E. T., Bernstein, L. E., Sungkarat, W., & Singh, M. (2007). Vibrotactile activation of the auditory cortices in deaf versus hearing adults. *Neuroreport,* 18, 645–648.

Baguley, D. M., Bartnik, G., Kleinjung, T., Savastano, M., & Hough, E. A. (2013). Troublesome tinnitus in childhood and adolescence: Data from expert centres. *International Journal of Pediatric Otorhinolaryngology, 77,* 248–251.

Balkany, T., Hodges, A., Telischi, F., Hoffman, R., Madell, J., Parisier, S., . . . Litvosky, R. William House Cochlear Implant Study Group: Position statement on bilateral cochlear implantation. *Otology and Neurotology, 29,*107–108.

Bayazit, Y. A., Kosaner, J., Cinar, B. C., Atac, A., Tutar, H., Gunduz, B., . . . Goksu, N. (2014). Methods and preliminary outcomes of pediatric auditory brainstem implantation. *Annals Otology Rhinology, and Laryngology, 123,* 529–536.

Beijin, J. W., Snik, A. F., & Mylanus, E. A. (2007). Sound localization ability of young children with bilateral cochlear implants. *Otology and Neurotology, 8,* 479–485.

Bergeson, T. R., Houston, D. M., & Miyamoto, R. T. (2010). Effects of congenital hearing loss and cochlear implantation on audiovisual speech perception in infants and children. *Restorative Neurology and Neuroscience, 28,* 157–165.

Bess, F. H., Dodd-Murphy, J., & Parker, R. A. (1998). Children with minimal sensorineural hearing loss: Prevalence, educational performance, and functional status. *Ear and Hearing, 19,* 339–354.

Bess, F. H., & Hornsby, B. W. (2014). Commentary: Listening can be exhausting—Fatigue in children and adults with hearing loss. *Ear and Hearing, 35,* 592–599.

Bess, F. H., & Tharpe, A. M. (1984). Unilateral hearing impairment in children. *Pediatrics, 74,* 206–216.

Bess, F. H., & Tharpe, A. M. (1986). Case history data on unilaterally hearing-impaired children. *Ear and Hearing, 7,* 14–19.

Bichey, B. G., & Miyamoto, R. T. (2008). Outcomes in bilateral cochlear implantation. *Otolaryngology-Head and Neck Surgery, 138,* 655–661.

Bortfeld, H., Morgan, J. L., Golinkoff, R. M., & Rathbun, K. (2005). Mommy and me: Familiar names help launch babies into speech-stream segmentation. *Psychological Science, 16,* 298–304.

Breneman, A., Gifford, R. H., & Dejong, M. D. (2012). Cochlear implantation in children with auditory neuropathy spectrum disorder: Long term outcomes. *Journal of the American Academy of Audiology, 23,* 5–17.

Brown, R. F., Hullar, T. E., Cadieux, J. H., & Chole, R. A. (2010). Residual hearing preservation after pediatric cochlear implantation. *Otology and Neurotology, 31,*1221–1226.

Buchman, C. A., Teagle, H. F., Roush, P. A., Park, L. R., Hatch, D., Woodard, J., . . . Adunka, O. F. (2011). Cochlear implantation in children with labyrinthine anomalies and cochlear nerve deficiency: Implications for auditory brainstem implantation. *Laryngoscope, 121,* 1979–1988.

Büchner, A., Schüssler, M., Battmer, R. D., Stöver, T., & Lesinski-Schiedat, A. T. L. (2009). Impact of low-frequency hearing. *Audiology and Neurotology, 14,* 8–13.

Buckley, K. A., & Tobey, E. A. (2011). Cross-modal plasticity and speech perception in pre- and postlingually deaf cochlear implant users. *Ear and Hearing, 32,* 2–15.

Buckner, R. L. (2004). Memory and executive function in aging and AD: Multiple factors that cause decline and reserve factors that compensate. *Neuron, 44,* 195–208.

Buechner, A., Brendel, M., Lesinski-Schiedat, A., Wenzel, G., Frohne-Buechner, C., Jaeger, B., & Lenarz, T. (2010). Cochlear implantation in unilateral deaf subjects associated with ipsilateral tinnitus. *Otology and Neurotology, 31,* 1381–1385.

Buss, E., Pillsbury, H. C., Buchman, C. A., Pillsbury, C. H., Clark, M. S., Haynes, D. S., . . . Barco, A. L. (2008). Multicenter U.S. bilateral MED-EL cochlear implantation study: Speech perception over the first year of use. *Ear and Hearing, 29,* 20–32.

Carlson, M. L., Sladen, D. P., Haynes, D. S., Driscoll, C. L., DeJong, M. D., Erickson, H. C., . . . Gifford, R. H. (2015). Evidence for the expansion of pediatric cochlear implant candidacy. *Otology and Neurotology, 36,* 43–50.

Champoux, F., Lepore, F., Gagné, J. P., & Théoret, H. (2009). Visual stimuli can impair auditory processing in cochlear implant users. *Neuropsychologia, 47,* 17–22.

Ching, T. Y., Incerti, P., & Hill, M. (2004). Binaural benefits for adults who use hearing aids and cochlear implants in opposite ears. *Ear and Hearing, 25*, 9–21.

Choi, J. Y., Song, M. H., Jeon, J. H., Lee, W. S., & Chang, J. W. (2011). Early surgical results of auditory brainstem implantation in nontumor patients. *Laryngoscope, 121*, 2610–2618.

Colletti, L., Colletti, G., Mandalà, M., & Colletti, V. (2014). The therapeutic dilemma of cochlear nerve deficiency: Cochlear or brainstem implantation? *Otolaryngology-Head and Neck Surgery, 151*, 308–314.

Colletti, L., Mandalà, M., Zoccante, L., Shannon, R. V., & Colletti, V. (2011). Infants versus older children fitted with cochlear implants: Performance over 10 years. *International Journal of Pediatric Otorhinolaryngology, 75*, 504–509.

Colletti, V., Carner, M., Miorelli, V., Guida, M., Colletti, L., & Fiorino, F. G. (2005). Cochlear implantation at under 12 months: Report on 10 patients. *Laryngoscope, 115*, 445–449.

Colletti, V., Shannon, R., Carner, M., Veronese, S., & Colletti, L. (2009). Outcomes in nontumor adults fitted with the auditory brainstem implant: 10 years' experience. *Otology and Neurotology, 30*, 614–618.

Colletti, V., Shannon, R. V., Carner, M., Veronese, S., & Colletti, L. (2010). Complications in auditory brainstem implant surgery in adults and children. *Otology and Neurotology, 31*, 558–564.

Cosetti, M., & Roland, J. T., Jr. (2010). Cochlear implantation in the very young child: Issues unique to the under-1 population. *Trends in Amplification, 14*, 46–57.

Cowan, R. S., DelDot, J., Barker, E. J., Sarant, J. Z., Pegg, P., Dettman, S., . . . Clark, G. M. (1997). Speech perception results for children with implants with different levels of preoperative residual hearing. *American Journal of Otology, 18*, S125–S126.

Cuda, D., Murri, A., Guerzoni, L., Fabrizi, E., & Mariani, V. (2014). Pre-school children have better spoken language when early implanted. *International Journal of Pediatric Otorhinolaryngology, 78*, 1327–1331.

Dalzell, L., Orlando, M., MacDonald, M., Berg, A., Bradley, M., Cacace, A., . . . Prieve, B. (2000). The New York State universal newborn hearing screening demonstration project: Ages of hearing loss identification, hearing aid fitting, and enrollment in early intervention. *Ear and Hearing, 21*, 118–130.

DeCasper, A. J., & Fifer, W. P. (1980). Of human bonding: Newborns prefer their mothers' voices. *Science, 208*, 1174–1176.

DeCasper, A. J., & Prescott, P. A. (1984). Human newborns' perception of male voices: Preference, discrimination, and reinforcing value. *Developmental Psychobiology, 17*, 481–491.

De Giacomo, A., Craig, F., D'Elia, A., Giagnotti, F., Matera, E., & Quaranta, N. (2013). Children with cochlear implants: Cognitive skills, adaptive behaviors, social and emotional skills. *International Journal of Pediatric Otorhinolaryngology, 77*, 1975–1979.

De Kegel, A., Maes, L., Van Waelvelde, H., & Dhooge, I. (2015). Examining the impact of cochlear implantation on the early gross motor development of children with a hearing loss. *Ear and Hearing, 36*, 113–121.

Dettman, S. J., D'Costa, W. A., Dowell, R. C., Winton, E. J., Hill, K. L., & Williams, S. S. (2004). Cochlear implants for children with significant residual hearing. *Archives of Otolaryngology-Head and Neck Surgery, 130*, 612–618.

Dettman, S. J., Pinder, D., Briggs, R. J., Dowell, R. C., & Leigh, J. R. (2007). Communication development in children who receive the cochlear implant younger than 12 months: Risks versus benefits. *Ear and Hearing, 28*, 11S–18S.

Dorman, M. F., & Gifford, R. H. (2010). Combining acoustic and electric stimulation in the service of speech recognition. *International Journal of Audiology, 49*, 912–919.

Dorman, M. F., Spahr, A. J., Gifford, R. H., Cook, S. J., Zhang, T., Loiselle, L., . . . Schramm, D. (2012). Current research with cochlear implants at Arizona State University. *Journal of the American Academy of Audiology, 23*, 385–395.

Dorman, M. F., Yost, W. A., Wilson, B. A., & Gifford, R. H. (2011). Speech perception and sound localization with bilateral cochlear implants. *Seminars in Hearing, 32*, 73–89.

Dorman, M. F., Zeitler, D., Cook, S. J., Loiselle, L., Yost, W. A., Wanna, G. B., & Gifford, R. H. (2015). Interaural level difference cues determine sound source localization by single-sided deaf patients fit with a cochlear implant. *Audiology and Neurotology, 20*, 183–188.

Downs, D. W. (1982). Effects of hearing aid use on speech discrimination and listening effort. *Journal of Speech and Hearing Disorders, 47*, 189–193.

Dunn, C. C., Perreau, A., Gantz, B. J., & Tyler, R. S. (2010). Benefits of localization and speech perception with multiple noise sources in listeners with a short-electrode cochlear implant. *Journal of the American Academy of Audiology, 21*, 44–51.

Dunn, C. C., Tyler, R. S., & Witt, S. A. (2005). Benefit of wearing a hearing aid on the unimplanted ear in adult users of a cochlear implant. *Journal of Speech Language and Hearing Research, 48*, 668–680.

Eapen, R. J., Buss, E., Adunka, M. C., Pillsbury, H. C., & Buchman, C. A. (2009). Hearing-in-noise benefits after bilateral simultaneous cochlear implantation continue to improve 4 years after implantation. *Otology and Neurotology, 30*, 153–159.

Eisenberg, L. S., Martinez, A. S., Holowecky, S. R., & Pogorelsky, S. (2002). Recognition of lexically controlled words and sentences by children with normal hearing and children with cochlear implants. *Ear and Hearing, 23*, 450–462.

Eliasson, A., Eliasson, A., King, J., Gould, B., & Eliasson, A. (2002). Association of sleep and academic performance. *Sleep and Breathing, 6*, 45–48.

Feuerstein, J. F. (1992). Monaural versus binaural hearing: Ease of listening, word recognition, and attentional effort. *Ear and Hearing, 13*, 80–86.

Fine, I., Finney, E. M., Boynton, G. M., & Dobkins, K. R. (2005). Comparing the effects of auditory deprivation and sign language within the auditory and visual cortex. *Journal of Cognitive Neuroscience, 17*, 1621–1637.

Finney, E. M., Clementz, B. A., Hickok, G., & Dobkins, K. R. (2003). Visual stimuli activate auditory cortex in deaf subjects: Evidence from MEG. *Neuroreport, 14*(11), 1425–1427.

Finney, E. M., Fine, I., & Dobkins, K. R. (2001). Visual stimuli activate auditory cortex in the deaf. *Nature Neuroscience, 4*, 1171–1173.

Firszt, J. B., Holden, L. K., Reeder, R. M., Cowdrey, L., & King, S. (2012). Cochlear implantation in adults with asymmetric hearing loss. *Ear and Hearing, 33*, 521–533.

Fitzpatrick, E. M., Ham, J., & Whittingham, J. (2015). Pediatric cochlear implantation: Why do children receive implants late? *Ear and Hearing, 36*(6), 688–694.

Fraser, S., Gagne, J. P., Alepins, M., & Dubois, P. (2010). Evaluating the effort expended to understand speech in noise using a dual-task paradigm: The effects of providing visual speech cues. *Journal of Speech, Language, and Hearing Research, 53*, 18–33.

Freeman, S. R., Stivaros, S. M., Ramsden, R. T., O'Driscoll, M. P., Nichani, J. R., Bruce, I. A., . . . Lloyd, S. K. (2013). The management of cochlear nerve deficiency. *Cochlear Implants International, 14*(Suppl. 4), S27–S31.

Gantz, B. J., Hansen, M. R., Turner, C. W., Oleson, J. J., Reiss, L. A., & Parkinson, A. J. (2009). Hybrid 10 clinical trial: Preliminary results. *Audiology and Neurotology, 14*(Suppl. 1), 32–38.

Gantz, B. J., Rubinstein, J. T., & Tyler, R. S. (2000). Long-term results of cochlear implants in children with residual hearing. *Annals of Otology, Rhinology, and Laryngology Supplement, 185*, 33–36.

Gantz, B. J., Turner, C. W., & Gfeller, K. E. (2006). Acoustic plus electric speech processing: Preliminary results of a multicenter clinical trial of the Iowa/Nucleus Hybrid implant. *Audiology and Neurotology. 11*(Suppl. 1), 63–68.

Gartrell, B. C., Jones, H. G., Kan, A., Buhl-Lawler, M., Gubbels, S. P., & Litovsky, R. Y. (2014). Investigating long-term effects of cochlear implantation in single-sided deafness: A best practice model for longitudinal assessment of spatial hearing. *Otology and Neurotology, 35*, 1525–1532.

Gatehouse, S., & Noble, W. (2004). The Speech, Spatial and Qualities of Hearing Scale (SSQ). *International Journal of Audiology, 43*, 85–99.

Geers, A. E. (2006). Factors influencing spoken language outcomes in children following early cochlear implantation. *Advances in Otorhinolaryngology, 64*, 50–65.

Geers, A. E., Brenner, C., & Davidson, L. (2003). Factors associated with the development of speech perception skills in children implanted by age five. *Ear and Hearing, 24*(1 Suppl.), 24S–36S.

Gifford, R. H., Dorman, M. F., & Brown, C. A. (2010). Psychophysical properties of low-frequency hearing: Implications for perceiving speech and music via electric and acoustic stimulation. *Advances in Otorhinolaryngology, 67*, 51–60.

Gifford, R. H., Dorman, M. F., McKarns, S. A., & Spahr, A. J. (2007). Combined electric and contralateral acoustic hearing: word and sentence recognition with bimodal hearing. *Journal of Speech Language and Hearing Research, 50*, 835–843.

Gifford, R. H., Dorman, M. F., Sheffield, S. W., Spahr, A. J., Teece, K., & Olund, A. P. (2014). Availability of binaural cues for bilateral cochlear implant recipients and bimodal listeners with and without hearing preservation. *Audiology and Neurotology, 19*, 57–71.

Gifford, R. H., Dorman, M. F., Skarzynski, H., Lorens, A., Polak, M., Driscoll, C. L., . . . Buchman, C. A. (2013). Cochlear implantation with hearing preservation yields significant benefit for speech recognition in complex listening environments. *Ear and Hearing, 34*, 413–425.

Gifford, R. H., Driscoll, C. L., Davis, T. J., Fiebig, P., Micco, A., & Dorman, M. F. (2015). A within-subject comparison of bimodal hearing, bilateral cochlear implantation, and bilateral cochlear implantation with bilateral hearing preservation: High-performing patients. *Otology and Neurotology, 36*, 1331–1337.

Giraud, A. L., & Lee, H. J. (2007). Predicting cochlear implant outcome from brain organisation in the deaf. *Restorative Neurology and Neuroscience, 25*, 381–390.

Godar, S. P., & Litovsky, R. Y. (2010). Experience with bilateral cochlear implants improves sound localization acuity in children. *Otology and Neurotology, 31*, 1287–1292.

Gordon, K. A., Wong, D. D. E., & Papsin, B. C. (2013). Bilateral input protects the brain from unilaterally driven reorganization in children who are deaf. *Brain, 136*, 1609–1655.

Gosselin, P. A., & Gagne, J. P. (2011). Older adults expend more listening effort than young adults recognizing audiovisual speech in noise. *International Journal of Audiology, 50*, 786–792.

Gozal, D. (1998). Sleep-disordered breathing and school performance in children. *Pediatrics, 102*(3 Pt 1), 606–620.

Granholm, E., Asarnow, R. F., Sarkin, A. J., & Dykes, K. L. (1996). Pupillary responses index cognitive resource limitations. *Psychophysiology, 33*, 457–461.

Grieco-Calub, T. M., & Litovsky, R. Y. (2010). Sound localization skills in children who use bilateral cochlear implants and in children with normal acoustic hearing. *Ear and Hearing, 31*, 645–656.

Gstoettner, W., Van de Heyning, P., O'Connor, A. F., Morera, C., Sainz, M., Vermeire, K., . . . Adunka, O. F. (2008). Electric acoustic stimulation of the auditory system: Results of a multi-centre investigation. *Acta Otolaryngologica, 128*, 968–975.

Gupta, P., & MacWhinney, B. (1997). Vocabulary acquisition and verbal short-term memory: Computational and neural bases. *Brain and Language, 59*, 267–333.

Habib, M. G., Waltzman, S. B., Tajudeen, B., & Svirsky, M. A. (2010). Speech production intelligibility of early implanted pediatric cochlear implant users. *International Journal of Pediatric Otorhinolaryngology, 74*, 855–859.

Hay-McCutcheon, M. J., Pisoni, D. B., & Kirk, K. I. (2005). Audiovisual speech perception in elderly cochlear implant recipients. *Laryngoscope, 115*, 1887–1894.

Hayes, H., Geers, A. E., Treiman, R., & Moog, J. S. (2009). Receptive vocabulary development in deaf children with cochlear implants: Achievement in an intensive auditory-oral educational setting. *Ear and Hearing, 30*, 128–135.

Helbig, S., Rajan, G. P., Stover, T., Lockley, M., Kuthubutheen, J., & Green, K. M. (2013). Hearing preservation after cochlear reimplantation. *Otology and Neurotology, 34*, 61–65.

Helbig, S., Van de Heyning, P., Kiefer, J., Baumann, U., Kleine-Punte, A., Brockmeier, H., . . . Gstoettner, W. (2011). Combined electric acoustic stimulation with the PULSARCI (100) implant system using the FLEX^{eas} electrode array. (2011). *Acta Otolaryngologica, 131*, 585–595.

Hetu, R., Riverin, L., Lalande, N., Getty, L., & St-Cyr, C. (1988). Qualitative analysis of the handicap associated with occupational hearing loss. *British Journal of Audiology, 22*, 251–264.

Hicks, C. B., & Tharpe, A. M. (2002). Listening effort and fatigue in school-age children with and without hearing loss. *Journal of Speech Language and Hearing Research, 45*, 573–584.

Hollich, G., Jusczyk, P. W., & Brent, M. R. (2001). How infants use the words they know to learn new words. In A. Do, L. Domínguez, & A. Johansen (Eds.), *Proceedings of the 25th Annual Boston University Conference on Language Development* (pp. 353–364). Somerville, MA: Cascadilla Press.

Hollich, G., Jusczyk, P., & Luce, P. (2002). *Lexical neighborhood effects in 17-month-old word learning.* Proceedings of the 26th Annual Boston University Conference on Language Development (pp. 314–323). Boston, MA: Cascadilla Press.

Holt, R. F., Kirk, K. I., & Hay-McCutcheon, M. (2011). Assessing multimodal spoken word-in-sentence recognition in children with normal hearing and children with cochlear implants. *Journal of Speech Language and Hearing Research, 54*, 632–657.

Hornsby, B. W., Werfel, K., Camarata, S., & Bess, F. H. (2014). Subjective fatigue in children with hearing loss: Some preliminary findings. *American Journal of Audiology, 23*, 129–134.

Houston, D. M., Beer, J., Bergeson, T. R., Chin, S. B., Pisoni, D. B., & Miyamoto, R. T. (2012). The ear is connected to the brain: Some new directions in the study of children with cochlear implants at Indiana University. *Journal of the American Academy of Audiology, 23*, 446–463.

Houston, D. M., & Jusczyk, P. W. (2003). Infants' long-term memory for the sound patterns of words and voices. *Journal of Experimental Psychology and Human Perceptual Performance, 29*, 1143–1154.

Houston, D. M., & Miyamoto, R. T. (2010). Effects of early auditory experience on word learning and speech perception in deaf children with cochlear implants: Implications for sensitive periods of language development. *Otology and Neurotology, 31*, 1248–1253.

James, A. L., & Papsin, B. C. (2004). Cochlear implant surgery at 12 months of age or younger. *Laryngoscope, 114*, 2191–2195.

Jayawardena, J., Kuthubutheen, J., & Rajan, G. (2012). Hearing preservation and hearing improvement after reimplantation of pediatric and adult patients with partial deafness: A retrospective case series review. *Otology and Neurotology, 33*, 740–744.

Johnson, J. L., White, K. R., Widen, J. E., Gravel, J. S., James, M., Kennalley, T., . . . Holstrum, J. (2005). A multicenter evaluation of how many infant with permanent hearing loss pass a two-stage otoacoustic emission/automated auditory brainstem response newborn hearing screening protocol. *Pediatrics, 116*, 663–672.

Jusczyk, P. W. (2002). Some critical developments in acquiring native language sound organization during the first year. *Annals of Otology, Rhinology, and Laryngology Supplement, 189*, 11–15.

Jusczyk, P. W., & Hohne, E. A. (1997). Infants' memory for spoken words. *Science, 277*, 1984–1986.

Kahneman, D., & Beatty, J. (1966). Pupil diameter and load on memory. *Science, 154*(3756), 1583–1585.

Kaplan, A. B., Kozin, E. D., Puram, S. V., Owoc, M. S., Shah, P. V., Hight, A. E., . . . Lee, D. J. (2015). Auditory brainstem implant candidacy in the United States in children 0–17 years old. *International Journal of Pediatric Otorhinolaryngology, 79*, 310–315.

Kiefer, J., Pok, M., Adunka, O. F., Stürzebecher, E., Baumgartner, W., Schmidt, M., . . . Gstoettner, W. (2005). Combined electric and acoustic stimulation of the auditory system: Results of a clinical study. *Audiology and Neurotology, 10*, 134–144.

Kisilevsky, B. S., Hains, S. M., Lee, K., Xie, X., Huang, H., Ye, H. H., . . . Wang, Z. (2003). Effects of experience on fetal voice recognition. *Psychological Science, 14*, 220–224.

Klee, T. M., & Davis-Dansky, E. (1986). A comparison of unilaterally hearing-impaired children and normal-hearing children on a battery of standardized language tests. *Ear and Hearing, 7*, 27–37.

Kleinjung, T., Steffens, T., Strutz, J., & Langguth, B. (2009). Curing tinnitus with a cochlear implant in a patient with unilateral sudden deafness: A case report. *Cases Journal, 18*, 7462.

Klingner, J., Tversky, B., & Hanrahan, P. (2011). Effects of visual and verbal presentation on cognitive load in vigilance, memory, and arithmetic tasks. *Psychophysiology, 48*, 323–332.

Koch, D. B., Soli, S. D., Downing, M., & Osberger, M. J. (2010). Simultaneous bilateral cochlear implantation: Prospective study in adults. *Cochlear Implants International, 11*, 84–99.

Koelewijn, T., Zekveld, A. A., Festen, J. M., & Kramer, S. E. (2012). Pupil dilation uncovers extra listening effort in the presence of a single-talker masker. *Ear and Hearing, 33*, 291–300.

Kramer, S. E., Zekveld, A. A., & Houtgast, T. (2009). Measuring cognitive factors in speech comprehension: The value of using the text reception threshold test as a visual equivalent of the SRT test. *Scandinavian Journal of Psychology, 50*, 507–515.

Kronenberger, W. G., Colson, B. G., Henning, S. C., & Pisoni, D. B. (2014). Executive functioning and speech-language skills following long-term use of cochlear implants. *Journal of Deaf Studies and Deaf Education, 19*, 456–470.

Kuthubutheen, J., Hedne, C. N., Krishnaswamy, J., & Rajan, G. P. (2012). A case series of paediatric hearing preservation cochlear implantation: A new treatment modality for children with drug-induced or congenital partial deafness. *Audiology and Neurotology, 17*, 321–330.

Lee, D. S., Lee, J. S., Oh, S. H., Kim, S. K., Kim, J. W., Chung, J. K., . . . Kim, C. S. (2001). Cross-modal plasticity and cochlear implants. *Nature, 409*, 149–150.

Lee, H. J., Truy, E., Mamou, G., Sappey-Marinier, D., & Giraud, A. L. (2007). Visual speech circuits in profound acquired deafness: A possible role for latent multimodal connectivity. *Brain, 130*, 2929–2941.

Leigh, J., Dettman, S., Dowell, R., & Sarant, J. (2011). Evidence-based approach for making cochlear implant recommendations for infants with residual hearing. *Ear and Hearing, 32*, 313–322.

Lenarz, T., Cuda, D., Fitzgerald, J., O'Connor, A., Frachet, B., Frijns, J. H., . . . Uziel, A. (2013). European multi-centre study of the Nucleus Hybrid L24 cochlear implant. *International Journal of Audiology, 52*, 838–848.

Levanen, S., Jousmäki, V., & Hari, R. (1998). Vibration-induced auditory-cortex activation in a congenitally deaf adult. *Current Biology, 8*(15), 869–872.

Lieu, J. E. (2013). Unilateral hearing loss in children: Speech-language and school performance. *B-ENT, Supplement, 21*, 107–115.

Lieu, J. E., Tye-Murray, N., & Fu, Q (2012). Longitudinal study of children with unilateral hearing loss. *Laryngoscope, 22*, 2088–2095.

Lieu, J. E., Tye-Murray, N., Karzon, R. K., & Piccirillo, J. F. (2010). Unilateral hearing loss is associated with worse speech-language scores in children. *Pediatrics, 125*, e1348–e1355.

Litovsky, R., Parkinson, A., Arcaroli, J., & Sammeth, C. (2006). Simultaneous bilateral cochlear implantation in adults: A multicenter clinical study. *Ear and Hearing, 27*, 714–731.

Lovett, R. E., Kitterick, P. T., Hewitt, C. E., & Summerfield, A. Q. (2010). Bilateral or unilateral cochlear implantation for deaf children: An observational study. *Archives of Disease in Childhood, 95*, 107–112.

Mackersie, C. L., & Cones, H. (2011). Subjective and psychophysiological indexes of listening effort in a competing-talker task. *Journal of the American Academy of Audiology, 22*, 113–122.

Miyamoto, R. T., Hay-McCutcheon, M. J., Kirk, K. I., Houston, D. M., & Bergeson-Dana, T. (2008). Language skills of profoundly deaf children who received cochlear implants under 12 months of age: A preliminary study. *Acta Oto-Laryngologica, 128*, 373–377.

Miyamoto, R. T., Houston, D. M., & Bergeson, T. (2005). Cochlear implantation in deaf infants. *Laryngoscope, 115*, 1376–1380.

Moeller, M. P. (2007). Current state of knowledge: Language and literacy of children with hearing impairment. *Ear and Hearing, 28*, 740–753.

Mondain, M., Sillon, M., Vieu, A., Levi, A., Reuillard-Artieres, F., Dequine, O., . . . Uziel, A. (2002). Cochlear implantation in prelingually deafened children with residual hearing. *International Journal of Pediatric Otorhinolaryngology, 63*, 91–97.

Moog, J. S., & Geers, A. E. (2010). Early educational placement and later language outcomes for children with cochlear implants. *Otology and Neurotology, 31*(8), 1315–1319.

Moon, C., Lagercrantz, H., & Kuhl, P. K. (2013). Language experienced in utero affects vowel perception after birth: A two-country study. *Acta Paediatrics, 102*, 156–160.

Morera, C., Cavalle, L., Manrique, M., Huarte, A., Angel, R., Osorio, A., . . . Morera-Ballester, C. (2012). Contralateral hearing aid use in cochlear implanted patients: Multi-center study of bimodal benefit. *Acta Otolaryngologica, 132*, 1084–1094.

Morera, C., Manrique, M., Ramos, A., Garcia-Ibanez, L., Cavalle, L., Huarte, A., . . . Estrada, E. (2005). Advantages of binaural hearing provided through bimodal stimulation via a cochlear implant and a conventional hearing aid: a 6-month comparative study. *Acta Otolaryngologica, 125*, 596–606.

Most, T. (2004). The effects of degree and type of hearing loss on children's performance in class. *Deafness and Education International, 6*, 154–166.

Most, T. (2006). Assessment of school functioning among Israeli Arab children with hearing loss in the primary grades. *American Annals of the Deaf, 151*, 327–335.

Mowry, S. E., Woodson, E., & Gantz, B. J. (2012). New frontiers in cochlear implantation: Acoustic plus electric hearing, hearing preservation, and more. *Otolaryngology Clinics of North America, 45*,187–203.

Nachtegaal, J., Kuik, D. J., Anema, J. R., Goverts, S. T., Festen, J. M., & Kramer, S. E. (2009). Hearing status, need for recovery after work, and psychosocial work characteristics: Results from an Internet-based national survey on hearing. *International Journal of Audiology, 48*, 684–691.

Nemholt, S. S., Schmidt, J. H., Wedderkopp, N., & Baguley, D. M. (2015). Prevalence of tinnitus and/or hyperacusis in children and adolescents: Study protocol for a systematic review. *BMJ Open, 5*, e006649.

Niparko, J. K., Tobey, E. A., Thal, D. J., Eisenberg, L. S., Wang, N. Y., Quittner, A. L., & Fink, N. E.; CDaCI Investigative Team. (2010). Spoken language development in children following cochlear implantation. *JAMA, 303*, 1498–1506.

Obholzer, R. J., & Gibson, W. P. (2011). Cochlear function following implantation with a full electrode array. *Cochlear Implants International, 12*, 44–47.

Oyler, R. F., Oyler, A. L., & Matkin, N. D. (1988). Unilateral hearing loss: Demographics and educational impact. *Language Speech and Hearing Services in Schools, 19*, 201–210.

Papsin, B. C., & Gordon, K. A. (2008). Bilateral cochlear implants should be the standard for children with bilateral sensorineural deafness. *Current Opinion in Otolaryngology-Head and Neck Surgery, 16*, 69–74.

Partanen, E., Kujala, T., Näätänen, R., Liitola, A., Sambeth, A., & Huotilainen, M. (2013). Learning-induced neural plasticity of speech processing before birth. *Proceedings of the National Academy of Sciences USA, 110*, 15145–15150.

Perez-Chada, D., Perez-Lloret, S., Videla, A. J., Cardinali, D., Bergna, M. A., Fernández-Acquier, M., . . . Drake, C. (2007). Sleep disordered breathing and daytime sleepiness are associated with poor academic performance in teenagers. A study using the Pediatric Daytime Sleepiness Scale (PDSS). *Sleep, 30*, 1698–1703.

Pichora-Fuller, M. K. (2007). Audition and cognition: What audiologists need to know about listening. In C. Palmer & R. Seewald (Eds.), *Hearing care for adults* (pp. 71–85). Stafa, Switzerland: Phonak.

Piquado, T., Isaacowitz, D., & Wingfield, A. (2010). Pupillometry as a measure of cognitive effort in younger and older adults. *Psychophysiology, 47*, 560–569.

Pisoni, D. B. (2000). Cognitive factors and cochlear implants: Some thoughts on perception, learning and memory in speech perception. *Ear and Hearing, 21*, 70–78.

Polonenko, M. J., Papsin, B. C., & Gordon, K. A. (2015). The effects of asymmetric hearing on bilateral brainstem function: Findings in children with bimodal (electric and acoustic) hearing. *Audiology and Neurotology, 20*(Suppl. 1), 13–20.

Punte, A. K., Vermeire, K., Hofkens, A., De Bodt, M., De Ridder, D., & Van de Heyning, P. (2011). Cochlear implantation as a durable tinnitus treatment in single-sided deafness. *Cochlear Implants International, 12*(Suppl. 1), S26–S29.

Rader, T., Fastl, H., & Baumann, U. (2013). Speech perception with combined electric-acoustic stimulation and bilateral cochlear implants in a multisource noise field. *Ear and Hearing, 34*, 324–332.

Ramos, Á., Polo, R., Masgoret, E., Artiles, O., Lisner, I., Zaballos, M. L., . . . Osorio, Á. (2012). Cochlear implant in patients with sudden unilateral sensorineural hearing loss and associated tinnitus. *Acta Otorrinolaringológica Española, 63*, 15–20.

Ramos Macías, A., Falcón González, J. C., Manrique, M., Morera, C., García-Ibáñez, L., Cenjor, C., . . . Killian, M. (2015). Cochlear implants as a treatment option for unilateral hearing loss, severe tinnitus and hyperacusis. *Audiology and Neurotology, 20*(Suppl. 1), 60–66.

Ravid, S., Afek, I., Suraiya, S., Shahar, E., & Pillar, G. (2009). Kindergarten children's failure to qualify for first grade could result from sleep disturbances. *Journal of Child Neurology, 24*, 816–822.

Ronnberg, J., Rudner, M., Foo, C., & Lunner, T. (2008). Cognition counts: A working memory system for ease of language understanding. *International Journal of Audiology, 47*, S99–S105.

Sandmann, P., Dillier, N., Eichele, T., Meyer, M., Kegel, A., Pascual-Marqui, R. D., . . . Debener, S. (2012). Visual activation of auditory cortex reflects maladaptive plasticity in cochlear implant users. *Brain, 135*, 555–568.

Sarant, J. Z., Harris, D. C., & Bennet, L. A. (2015). Academic outcomes for school-aged children with severe-profound hearing loss and early unilateral and bilateral cochlear implants. *Journal of Speech Language and Hearing Research, 58*, 1017–1032.

Schafer, E. C., Amlani, A. M., Seibold, A., & Shattuck, P. L. (2007). A meta-analytic comparison of binaural benefits between bilateral cochlear implants and bimodal stimulation. *Journal of the American Academy of Audiology, 18*, 760–776.

Seymour, F. K., Cruise, A., Lavy, J. A., Bradley, J., Beale, T., Graham, J. M., & Saeed, S. R. (2010). Congenital profound hearing loss: Management of hypoplastic and aplastic vestibulocochlear nerves. *Cochlear Implants International, 11*(Suppl. 1), 213–216.

Sharma, A., Campbell, J., & Cardon, G. (2015). Developmental and cross-modal plasticity in deafness: Evidence from the P1 and N1 event related potentials in cochlear implanted children. *International Journal of Psychophysiology, 95*, 135–144.

Sheffield, B. M., & Zeng, F. G. (2012). The relative phonetic contributions of a cochlear implant and residual acoustic hearing to bimodal speech perception. *Journal of the Acoustical Society of America, 131*, 518–530.

Shepherd, R. K., Shivdasani, M. N., Nayagam, D. A., Williams, C. E., & Blamey, P. J. (2013). Visual prostheses for the blind. *Trends in Biotechnology, 31*, 562–571.

Shinn-Cunningham, B. G., & Best, V. (2008). Selective attention in normal and impaired hearing. *Trends in Amplification, 12*, 283–299.

Skarzynski, H., Lorens, A., Matusiak, M., Porowski, M., Skarzynski, P. H., & James, C. J. (2012). Partial deafness treatment with the Nucleus Straight Research Array cochlear implant. *Audiology and Neurotology, 17*, 82–91.

Skarzynski, H., Lorens, A., Piotrowska, A., & Anderson, I. (2007). Partial deafness cochlear implantation in children. *International Journal of Pediatric Otorhinolaryngology, 71*, 1407–1413.

Skarzynski, H., Lorens, A., Piotrowska, A., & Skarzynski, P. H. (2010). Hearing preservation in partial deafness treatment. *Medical Science Monitor, 16*, CR555–CR562.

Skarżyński, H., Matusiak, M., Furmanek, M., & Skarżyński, P. H. (2014). Results of SRA Nucleus Freedom CI in population of children with functional residual hearing. *Cochlear Implants International, 15*(Suppl. 1), S24–S26.

Soja, N. N., Carey, S., & Spelke, E. S. (1991). Ontological categories guide young children's inductions of word meaning: Object terms and substance terms. *Cognition, 38*, 179–211.

Sparreboom, M., Snik, A. F., & Mylanus, E. A. (2012). Sequential bilateral cochlear implantation in children: Quality of life. *Archives of Otolaryngology-Head and Neck Surgery, 138*, 134–141.

Stelmachowicz, P. G., Lewis, D. E., Choi, S., & Hoover, B. (2007). The effect of stimulus bandwidth on auditory skills in normal-hearing and hearing-impaired children. *Ear and Hearing, 28*, 483–494.

Steven, R. A., Green, K. M., Broomfield, S. J., Henderson, L. A., Ramsden, R. T, & Bruce, I. A. (2011). Cochlear implantation in children with cerebral palsy. *International Journal of Pediatric Otorhinolaryngology, 75*, 1427–1430.

Storkel, H. L. (2009). Developmental differences in the effects of phonological, lexical and semantic variables on word learning by infants. *Journal of Childhood Language, 36*, 291–321.

Strelnikov, K., Rouger, J., Demonet, J. F., Lagleyre, S., Fraysse, B., Deguine, O., & Barone, P. (2013). Visual activity predicts auditory recovery from deafness after adult cochlear implantation. *Brain, 136*, 3682–3695.

Tajudeen, B. A., Waltzman, S. B., Jethanamest, D., & Svirsky, M. A. (2010). Speech perception in congenitally deaf children receiving cochlear implants in the first year of life. *Otology and Neurotology, 31*, 1254–1260.

Taylor, J. S. (1981). Pupillary response to auditory versus visual mental loading: A pilot study using super 8-mm photography. *Perceptual and Motor Skills, 52*(2), 425–426.

Teagle, H. F., Roush, P. A., Woodard, J. S., Hatch, D. R., Zdanski, C. J., Buss, E., & Buchman, C. A. (2010). Cochlear implantation in children with auditory neuropathy spectrum disorder. *Ear and Hearing, 31*, 325–335.

Tharpe, A. M. (2008). Unilateral and mild bilateral hearing loss in children: Past and current perspectives. *Trends in Amplification, 12*, 7–15.

Tharpe, A. M., & Bess, F. H. (1991). Identification and management of children with minimal hearing loss. *International Journal of Pediatric Otorhinolaryngology, 21*, 41–50.

Tobey, E. A., Geers, A. E., & Brenner, C. (2003). Factors associated with development of speech production skills in children implanted by age five. *Ear and Hearing, 24*(1 Suppl.), 36S–45S.

Tomblin, J. B., Barker, B. A., Spencer, L. J., Zhang, X., & Gantz, B. J. (2005). The effect of age at cochlear implant initial stimulation on expressive language growth in infants and toddlers. *Journal of Speech Language and Hearing Research, 48*, 853–867.

Tomblin, J. B., Spencer, L., Flock, S., Tyler, R., & Gantz, B. (1999). A comparison of language achievement in children with cochlear implants and children using hearing aids. *Journal of Speech, Language, and Hearing Research, 42*, 497–509.

Turner, C. W., Gantz, B. J., Karsten, S., Fowler, J., & Reiss, L. A. (2010). Impact of hair cell preservation in cochlear implantation: combined electric and acoustic hearing. *Otology and Neurotology, 31*, 1227–1232.

Tye-Murray, N., & Geers, A. (2001). *Children's Audio-Visual Enhancement Test*. St. Louis, MO: Central Institute for the Deaf.

Tyler, R. S., Fryauf-Bertschy, H., & Kelsay, D. (1991). *Audiovisual Feature Test for Young Children*. Iowa City: University of Iowa.

Umansky, A. M., Jeffe, D. B., & Lieu, J. E. (2011). The HEAR-QL: Quality of life questionnaire for children with hearing loss. *Journal of the American Academy of Audiology, 22*, 644–653.

Valencia, D. M., Rimell, F. L., Friedman, B. J., Oblander, M. R., & Helmbrecht, J. (2008). Cochlear implantation in infants less than 12 months of age. *International Journal of Pediatric Otorhinolaryngology, 72*, 767–773.

van de Heyning, P., Vermeire, K., Diebl, M., Nopp, P., Anderson, I., & De Ridder, D. (2008). Incapacitating unilateral tinnitus in single-sided deafness treated by cochlear implantation. *Annals of Otology, Rhinology, and Laryngology, 117*, 645–652.

Van Deun, L., van Wieringer, A., Scherf, F., Doggouj, N., Desloovere, C., Offeciers, F. E., . . . Wouters, J. (2010). Earlier intervention leads to better sound localization in children with bilateral cochlear implants. *Audiology and Neurotology, 15*, 7–17.

Vermeire, K., & Van de Heyning, P. (2009). Binaural hearing after cochlear implantation in subjects with unilateral sensorineural deafness and tinnitus. *Audiology and Neurotology, 14*, 163–171.

Vincent, C., Arndt, S., Firszt, J. B., Fraysse, B., Kitterick, P. T., Papsin, B. C., . . . Marx, M. (2015). Identification and evaluation of cochlear implant candidates with asymmetrical hearing loss. *Audiology Neurotology, 20*(Suppl. 1), 187–189.

Wake, M., Hughes, E. K., Hughes, Z. P., Collins, C., & Rickards, F. W. (2004). Outcomes of children with mild-profound congenital hearing loss at 7 to 8 years: A population study. *Ear and Hearing, 25*, 1–8.

Waltzman, S. B., & Roland, J. T., Jr. (2005). Cochlear implantation in children younger than 12 months. *Pediatrics, 116*, 487–493.

Watkin, P. M., & Baldwin, M. (1999). Confirmation of deafness in infancy. *Archives of Disease in Childhood, 81*, 380–389.

White, K. R., Vohr, B. R., Maxon, A. B., Behreus, T. R., McPherson, M. G., & Mauk, G. W. (1994). Screening all newborns for hearing loss using transient evoked otoacoustic emissions. *International Journal of Pediatric Otorhinolaryngology, 29*(3), 203–217.

Wie, O. B. (2010). Language development in children after receiving bilateral cochlear implants between 5 and 18 months. *International Journal of Pediatric Otorhinolaryngology, 74*, 1258–1266.

Wolfe, J., Baker, S., Caraway, T., Kasulis, H., Mears, A., Smith, J., . . . Wood, M. (2007). 1-year postactivation results for sequentially implanted bilateral cochlear implant users. *Otology and Neurotology, 28*, 589–596.

Yoshinaga-Itano, C., Baca, R. L., & Sedey, A. L. (2010). Describing the trajectory of language development in the presence of severe-to-profound hearing loss: A closer look at children with cochlear implants versus hearing aids. *Otology and Neurotology, 31*, 1268–1274.

Zekveld, A. A., George, E. L. J., Kramer, S. E., Goverts, S. T., & Houtgast, T. (2007). The development of the text reception threshold test: A visual analogue of the speech reception threshold test. *Journal of Speech Language and Hearing Research, 50*, 576–584.

Zekveld, A. A., Kramer, S. E., & Festen, J. M. (2010). Pupil response as an indication of effortful listening: The influence of sentence intelligibility. *Ear and Hearing, 31*, 480–490.

Zekveld, A. A., Kramer, S. E., & Festen, J. M. (2011). Cognitive load during speech perception in noise: The influence of age, hearing loss, and cognition on the pupil response. *Ear and Hearing, 32*, 498–510.

Zhang, T., Spahr, A. J., Dorman, M. F., & Saoji, A. (2013). Relationship between auditory function of nonimplanted ears and bimodal benefit. *Ear and Hearing, 34*, 133–141.

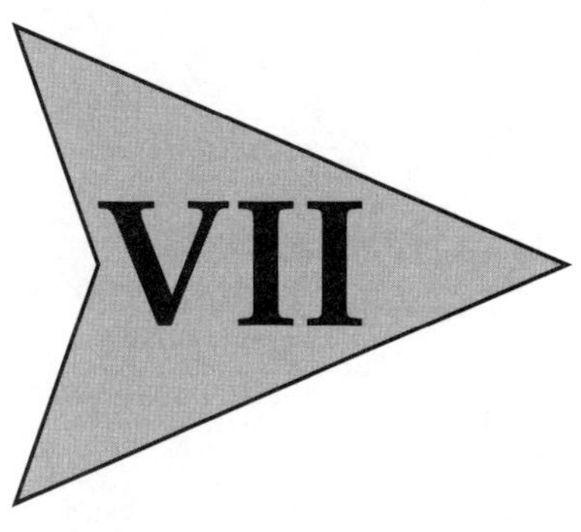

Management of Childhood Hearing Loss

History of the Management of Hearing Loss in Children

Andrée Durieux-Smith and Elizabeth M. Fitzpatrick

Deaf Children: Historical Perspective

Permanent bilateral hearing loss, if undetected, can lead to significant delays in the development of speech, language, and literacy, which in turn can limit educational and occupational options. The consequences of hearing loss have been known for centuries although not clearly understood. Misconceptions abounded particularly in relation to individuals with severe-to-profound hearing loss. One such misconception concerning "the deaf" was that these individuals could not speak because they had no vocal folds (Davis & Silverman, 1970). This inaccurate information led to the unfortunate term of *deaf mute* suggesting that deafness and muteness depended on some common organic abnormality. In addition, it was acknowledged even at that time that speech was the vehicle to transmit thought and was essential for education. The term *deaf and dumb* reflected the belief that the deaf could not be educated because they could not hear or speak. This implied that the deaf had limited mental capacity that in turn influenced their legal and civil status. Roman law (Silverman, 1970) classified individuals who were deaf with those who were considered mentally incompetent.

Deafness was clearly seen as an educational barrier because hearing was the normal channel through which speech is perceived and was considered essential for learning. Although information on the education of the deaf is relatively sparse prior to the 15th century, it is clear that during this period some thought was given to providing the deaf with other means so that they could express their thoughts. Agricola wrote a book that was not published until the 16th century in which he proposed that the deaf could express themselves by putting their thoughts down in writing (Silverman, 1970). Little information is available on the method that was used to achieve this goal. In the 16th century as well, Cardano, an Italian physician and father of a deaf child became interested in Agricola's work and promoted the notion that the deaf could be taught to comprehend written symbols by using pictures (Silverman, 1970). At that time, the belief that the deaf could learn to express themselves using words or gestures was introduced. This was a turning point as it was realized that deafness was a barrier to communication and not an intellectual deficit. The key, therefore, was to find ways to help the deaf communicate and learn.

In 1555, the first school for the deaf was established in Spain by Pedro Ponce de Leon, a Catholic monk. The goal of this school was to teach "deaf mutes" to speak. The first book exclusively on the deaf was produced by Juan Pablo Bonet in 1620 (Silverman, 1970) and promoted the teaching of language and articulation supplemented by sign language and a manual alphabet. Several other books followed, and it is clear that, in this period, there was recognition that the deaf could be educated and that they were equal to normal-hearing individuals. In the latter part of the 17th century, two individuals in particular developed different methods to educate deaf children and both made significant contributions to this field. In France, the Abbe de l'Epee founded the first public school for the deaf in Paris, and students were educated using sign language. In Germany, Heinicke founded a public school for the deaf and advocated for the use of speech and speech reading. De l'Epee and Heinicke disagreed about the merits of sign language and oralism as methods of instruction, a controversy that was repeated in many countries and still persists today. Regardless of the methods used, by the end of the 17th century, it was clear that the deaf were capable of instruction, and it was also recognized that this was a legal and moral obligation. In the United States, the first permanent school for the deaf was founded in 1817 in Hartford, Connecticut, by Thomas Hopkins Gallaudet who had traveled to France and learned the methods of de l'Epee. The school at Hartford was known as the American Asylum for the Education and Instruction of the Deaf and Dumb, which later became the American School for the Deaf. In 1872, a Canadian educator of the deaf and inventor, Alexander Graham Bell, whose wife was deaf, opened a training school for teachers of the deaf in Boston. Bell was a strong believer of lipreading and speech in the education of deaf children.

Technologic developments were taking place at this time that eventually had a great impact on the management of hearing loss in children. This was also the era of the advent of electricity, and Bell started experimenting with ways to make speech visible and audible to the deaf. This led to the invention of the telephone that laid the firm foundation for the electrical transmission of sound. The development of devices that had the potential to increase the audibility of sound for the deaf was a critical milestone in the management of deaf children. Bell founded the Volta Bureau in 1887 to disseminate information about deafness. In 1897, Max Goldstein, an otologist who was also a strong advocate for the importance of residual hearing, founded the St. Joseph's School for the Deaf in St. Louis, Missouri. Instruction included a series of exercises to give children practice with sound stimulation. In 1924, Goldstein established the Central Institute for the Deaf in St. Louis. In the late 19th century and at the beginning of the 20th century, deafness was viewed as a problem that belonged to the field of education. Many schools for the deaf developed programs predominantly for school-age children. Over the years, with the advent of electricity and the development of technology, a better understanding of deafness took place.

Technologic Developments That Have Influenced the Management of Hearing Loss in Children

The Profession of Audiology

Prior to the advent of electricity and the development of the audiometer, it was very difficult to obtain precise information on the degree, configuration, and nature of hearing loss. The importance of obtaining information about a child's hearing loss was recognized, and methods using various environmental sounds and speech were used. Itard in the 19th century (Silverman & Lane, 1970) developed a classification based on children's responses to bells, drums, and flutes. Urbantschitsch (Silverman & Lane, 1970) used a harmonica with specific frequency ranges and known intensities for the same purpose. These efforts led to classifications of types of hearing loss based on children's responses that were not unlike those used a half century later.

In 1929, the National Research Council in the United States sponsored a conference to address the problems of the deaf and hard of hearing (Hirsh, 1952). The need to accurately measure the degree and type of hearing loss was identified as an important priority together with the standardization of methods.

During World War II, audiology became the recognized discipline with expertise in the science of hearing. Audiology was best defined by its multidisciplinary origins as it included knowledge from physics, psychology, education, and otolaryngology. This new specialty was created because of the numerous war casualties who suffered from hearing loss and deafness. Audiology provided a much needed professional service that had not been available. Since the work of Hirsh (1952), considerable information has been collected about sound and hearing measurement. The developments of the electric audiometer and audiometric standards have made it possible to measure auditory thresholds at frequencies important for speech perception. In addition, the medical field of otology contributed to the identification of the site of lesion and to the medical management of hearing loss in children. Hearing aids were developed and could provide some deaf children with access to sound. In these early days of technologic developments, the professions of audiology, otology, and education worked together to develop the most appropriate rehabilitation and educational programs for children with hearing loss.

The ability to measure hearing led to some interesting classifications of hearing loss in children. The terms *deaf* and *hard-of-hearing* were based predominantly on the degree of hearing loss and age of onset, and were used to guide the educational process and also, indirectly, to set expectations. It also was recognized that some children who had developed speech and language prior to the onset of severe to profound deafness had very different needs and therefore were considered to fall into the hard-of-hearing category. The deaf child was defined as one who did not have sufficient residual hearing to understand and develop speech even with a hearing aid, without special instruction. The sense of hearing for the deaf child was thought to be nonfunctional for everyday functioning. Systematic and laborious procedures were necessary in order for the deaf child to learn to communicate (Silverman & Lane, 1970). As in North America, a similar trend took place in England under the School Health Regulations, whereby children were described as deaf and partially deaf (Ewing & Ewing, 1954). The deaf had no "naturally" acquired speech when they were admitted to school, whereas the hard-of-hearing had begun to talk naturally although with some imperfections. The hard-of-hearing child was thought to have a sense of hearing, which although defective, was somewhat functional with or without a hearing aid. Deaf children were described as having pure-tone average hearing losses of 91 dB or greater, and as not being able to rely on the auditory channel as a primary avenue of communication. It was believed that hearing losses of such severity could not be overcome. Although the terms *deaf* and *hard of hearing* were used extensively at that time, the need to define children with hearing loss in terms of their educational and psychological potential was also identified. In fact, it came to be recognized that some "totally deaf" individuals could benefit from the use of appropriate amplification (Silverman & Lane, 1970).

Early Identification

Although the technologic developments of the 1940s to the 1960s clearly contributed to enhancing the management of children with hearing loss, many challenges still needed to be addressed. One such challenge was the late identification of hearing loss in children. The importance of early education of children with hearing loss had been identified, and it was recognized that infants needed to be exposed to sound. The period from birth to age 5 years was identified as being particularly critical to learning. At the same time, however, it was acknowledged that it was difficult to evaluate a young child's hearing reliably, and there was a lack of awareness by physicians of hearing loss in children. The average age of identification for hearing impairment in children was reported as 3 to 4 years (Bess, 2000; Wong & Shah, 1979), and there were significant delays between identification of hearing loss and hearing aid fitting. In addition, there was *no consensus* on when a child was ready to wear a hearing aid and whether hearing aids could damage hearing.

Several individuals and events influenced the development of early identification initiatives. In the United Kingdom, the Ewings (Ewing, 1957), who stressed the importance of early identification, parental involvement, and early amplification, had an enormous impact on the management of hearing loss in children. In 1964, an international conference, "The Deaf Child" took place in Toronto, Canada, bringing together more than 30 experts from North America, Great Britain, Scandinavia, and the Netherlands (Davis, 1965). Participants were already sensitized to the importance of the early identification and early management of hearing loss in children. The purpose of the meeting was to find ways to alleviate the handicap to auditory communication imposed by early hearing loss. Considerable discussion took place on definitive tests of hearing for very young children, which were not available at that time. Systematic reviews of available tests were presented at the meeting, and these included new electrical techniques that detected cortical-evoked responses to sound in young children. This was seen as a breakthrough that might make it possible to eventually identify hearing loss in newborns and infants. Neonatal tests of hearing and the age at which reliable, reasonably valid, and definite tests of hearing could be performed were seen as crucial, but the technology was not yet available. For this reason, the screening of high-risk groups of infants was recommended, although the concept of universal neonatal screening, in fact, was also discussed. Participants felt that it was too early to form an opinion about auditory-evoked cortical responses as a test, and some were skeptical that an inexpensive, uncomplicated instrument could be developed to satisfy the requirements for clinical applications. All felt that more research was needed to determine the validity and reliability of tests to identify hearing loss early. Interestingly, at this conference, consensus was not reached on the age at which the use of amplified sound should be initiated, and opinions ranged from 2 weeks to 2 months. The majority agreed, however, that 2 years was the maximum acceptable delay. Generally, participants felt that it would be ideal if hearing impairment was detected and confirmed by 6 months of age.

In 1969, in the United States, because of a concern with the current procedures available for newborn hearing screening, a National Joint Committee on Newborn Screening (JCNS) was established. This committee at that time included representatives of the American Academy of Ophthalmology and Otolaryngology, the American Academy of Pediatrics, and the American Speech and Hearing Association. The committee was mandated to make recommendations with regard to the early identification of hearing loss. Over the years, the Joint Committee on Newborn Screening became the Joint Committee on Infant Hearing, and several position statements were published (JCNS, 1970; JCIH [supplementary statement], 1976, 1982, 1990, 1994, 2000, 2007; Statement of Endorsement, 2013) and addressed the populations to be screened, the methods and protocols to be used for screening, and more recently, guidelines for early hearing detection and intervention (EHDI).

In the first statement (JCNS, 1970), after reviewing the data from a small number of controlled studies on the screening of infants for hearing loss, the committee did not recommend the routine screening of newborns because of a lack of accurate screening methods. At that time, screening methods were limited to behavioral responses to the presentation of relatively loud broadband stimuli (Mencher, 1976). These techniques had evolved from the behavioral responses obtained to auditory stimuli by Ewing and Ewing (1944) and Wedenberg (1956) to name a few. At the same time, and similar to the recommendations made by the 1964 Conference on the Deaf Child, the JCIH started to identify certain children who were at significant risk of developing hearing loss. This gave rise to the use of the high-risk register, which was introduced as a supplement to the 1970 JCNS statement (Joint Committee on Infant Screening, 1976). Between 1982 and 1994, the high-risk register was further refined to include additional factors (JCIH, 1982, 1990, 1994). The approach was therefore to screen children on the high-risk register because it was felt this would lead to the identification of the majority of children with permanent hearing loss. At the same time, it became more evident that behavioral screening, even in its most sophisticated and automated form such as the Crib-O-Gram (Simmons & Russ, 1974), was neither reliable nor valid (Durieux-Smith, Picton, MacMurray, & Goodman, 1987; Wright & Rybak, 1983).

In the last 35 years, considerable technologic developments have taken place, making it possible to identify abnormal auditory function accurately in newborns and infants. Two physiological measures, the auditory brainstem response (ABR) and otoacoustic emissions (OAEs), have clearly revolutionized early hearing detection and have led to the early identification and intervention of children with permanent hearing loss. In the late 1970s, Schulman-Galambos and Galambos (1979) recommended the ABR for newborn hearing assessment. Subsequently, several studies continued to investigate the usefulness of the ABR, particularly with high-risk infants (Durieux-Smith, Picton, Edwards, Goodman, & MacMurray, 1985; Galambos, Hicks, & Wilson, 1982, 1984; Hyde, Riko, & Malizia, 1990; Kileny, 1987). Follow-up studies of infants screened by this technique also showed good validity (Durieux-Smith et al., 1987; Hyde et al., 1990). The 1982 JCIH Position Statement recommended that the initial screening include the observation of behavioral or electrophysiological responses to sound, although the committee did not recommend any specific testing method. In the 1990 Position Statement, the JCIH recommended the use of ABR using clicks as the screening method for high-risk neonates. One of the problems at the time was that the equipment used to assess the ABR was costly, required considerable expertise to operate, and was not readily portable and therefore not really appropriate for screening. In the late 1980s and early 1990s, another technique, OAEs, was introduced as a promising method to assess cochlear function in newborns and infants. In 1978 in England, Kemp was the first to show that OAEs could be detected in the human external ear in response to stimulation with clicks. The recording of these OAEs was viewed as evidence of normal cochlear function and more specifically of outer hair cell integrity (Kemp, 1980). Kemp's discovery and the development of equipment to record OAEs gave rise to an entirely new approach to newborn and infant screening (Bonfils, Uziel, & Pujol, 1988; Kennedy et al., 1991; Stevens et al., 1989; Stevens et al., 1990; White & Behrens, 1993). Studies that followed infants screened with this technique reported that OAEs could identify infants with hearing loss of approximately 30 dB HL and greater (Kennedy et al., 1991).

In 1993, the National Institute of Deafness and other Communication Disorders (one of the National Institutes of Health [NIH]) held a consensus development conference, "Early Identification of Hearing Impairment in Infants and Young Children," in the United States (NIH, 1993). The objective of this conference was to develop an improved approach to identifying hearing loss in infants. The 1993 Consensus Statement recommended that all infants be screened for hearing loss by 3 months of age. This recommendation was made after reviewing compelling evidence that clearly demonstrated that screening infants on a high-risk register missed 50% of children with a permanent hearing loss (Jacobson & Jacobson, 1990; Mauk, White, Mortensen, & Behrens, 1991; Watkin, Baldwin, & McEnery, 1991); this was subsequently confirmed by other studies (Durieux-Smith & Whittingham, 2000; Korres et al., 2005; Uus & Bamford, 2006). This was the first recommendation for universal newborn hearing screening. In addition, a screening protocol was proposed that included a two-stage screening process, namely, OAEs followed by ABRs for children who were referred by the OAE screen. In 1994, the JCIH gave careful consideration to the recommendations of the NIH conference and endorsed universal hearing screening while recommending additional research on the evaluation of the electrophysiological techniques that were now established to assess auditory function in newborns and infants. Since 1994, several investigators (Finitzo, Albright, & O'Neal, 1998; Mason & Hermann, 1998; Prieve & Stevens, 2000; Vohr, Carty, Moore, & Letourneau, 1998) have documented the validity, reliability, and effectiveness of both electrophysiological measures for universal newborn hearing screening. In 2000, the JCIH issued a new position statement describing the principles underlying effective EHDI programs and providing guidelines for their successful implementation. In 2007, the JCIH reiterated its support for universal hearing screening, recommending that all infants be screened by 1 month of age, have a complete audiological evaluation by 3 months of age, and receive appropriate intervention no later than 6 months of age. The definition of the target disorder was refined together with protocols for screening, diagnostic audiologic evaluation, and medical evaluation.

New developments in newborn screening such as auditory steady-state responses (ASSRs) are being investigated and might become helpful in screening for hearing impairment in infancy (Savio, Perez Abalo, Gaya, Hernandez, & Mijares. 2008). In addition, considerable progress has taken place in methods for audiologic diagnosis (Ackley & Decker, 2006; Picton, 2011). Tonepip ABRs have supplemented click ABR and can now yield clinically acceptable estimates of pure-tone thresholds by air conduction (Stapells, 2000). Recent studies have investigated the use of different stimuli such as CE-chirps to further improve the recording of ABRs (Rodrigues, Ramos, & Lewis, 2013).

Bone-conduction (BC) frequency-specific ABR threshold estimates can be obtained, although the dynamic range of BC stimulation is limited, and the possibility of error still exists (Campbell, Harris, Hendricks, & Sirimanna, 2004; Stapells & Oates, 1997). An assessment of infant middle ear systems using high-frequency probe tones can also contribute to differential diagnosis (Alaerts, Lutz, & Woulters, 2007; Meyer, Jardine, & Deverson, 1997). Technologic developments in the last 30 to 40 years now make it possible to accurately identify hearing loss in infants and proceed with management for those with a permanent hearing loss.

Amplification

One of the preoccupations in the management of permanent hearing loss in children has been to expose the deaf child to sound stimulation through the use of amplification. Before the advent of electricity, mechanical hearing devices were developed. The ear trumpet dating from the 17th century was initially used by sailors to communicate with each other over long distances. Only in the 19th century did this device become an option for the deaf together with smaller versions known as cornets and auricles (Niemoller, Silverman, & Davis, 1970). The first electric hearing aid was designed in the late 1800s, and it is thought that this invention was related to Alexander Graham Bell's work on the development of the telephone. This first prototype amplified sounds by mechanically funneling sound to the ear by electronic magnification. The first amplification device contained a battery-operated carbon transmitter and earphones, and subsequently a carbon transmitter model hearing aid became commercially available. In the 1920s, the carbon transmitter was replaced by the vacuum tube. The device now consisted of a microphone, an ear receiver, amplifier, and two batteries. Batteries only lasted for 1 day. One of the main challenges of the early hearing aids was to deliver sufficient energy. Over the next several decades, improvements were made with batteries becoming smaller, and in 1947 a major breakthrough came with the development of the transistor (Northern & Downs, 1974). Silicon transistors allowed hearing aids to shrink in size so that they could become "body aids." Even with these developments, early hearing aids were still very large, unattractive, provided limited bandwidth, and produced high levels of harmonic distortion (Killion, 1997). During that time, hearing aids primarily were designed for adults and not children. Binaural fittings were impossible with these cumbersome instruments, and monaural fittings became an established practice. Because hearing aids were so large, a single Y-cord was often used to provide "binaural" amplification.

The main difficulty with these early electrical instruments continued to be the high power requirements and the size. Nevertheless, these early electronic aids revolutionized opportunities for deaf children, as they provided sound stimulation. Due to their large size, the earliest electric models were not portable and were used exclusively in classrooms. The portable or desk-type hearing aid was used as it had more power and provided a better-quality signal (Niemoller et al., 1970). The teacher spoke into a free-standing microphone and the listener with hearing loss received the amplified sound through headphones. This type of system therefore required that the child remain in one place. The microphone and headphones were connected to an amplifier by means of cables, and the child's movements were restricted by the radius of the cord connecting the amplifier and the headphones. This system was used for individual speech training. Systems were capable of reproducing a wider range of frequencies than individual hearing aids, few of which could provide significant amplification beyond 3500 Hz (Ling & Ling, 1978). For some children, hard-wired systems helped to provide acoustic cues not available through personal hearing aids.

Another type of system was the group hearing aid with one or more microphones, an amplifier and as many as 10 pairs of over-the-ear or insert receivers. The use of electromagnetic transmission eliminated the need for connecting wires from amplifier to the listeners. Because the speaker wore the microphone, a better signal-to-noise ratio was achieved. Another method used an induction loop around the classroom that received electric energy from the amplifier of the group hearing aid. The magnetic field created by the loop current was sensed by a telephone pickup. This allowed the child to receive speech at the same level anywhere within the loop. In addition, the movements of the child were not restricted, and loops could be used in settings outside of the classroom such as the child's home. One of the disadvantages was that loops could not be used in adjacent classrooms because of overspill, whereby the electromagnetic field would extend outside the loop area. Group hearing aids were used in schools for the deaf and the technology at that time required that the management of children with permanent hearing loss take place predominantly in an educational setting. Today, special amplification systems such as radio frequency–modulated systems (FM) make it possible for children to wear their personal hearing aids with an FM system. This ensures teacher and child mobility and consistent favorable signal levels and has facilitated the inclusion of children with a permanent hearing loss in the regular school system (Sanders, 1993). Furthermore, the use of such systems is not restricted to the classroom setting.

With the advent of transistor circuitry and resulting miniaturization of hearing aids, it became recognized that the greatest advantage of personal hearing aids was that the child could have access to amplification at all times. It was acknowledged that the management of hearing loss should not only take place in the classroom setting, but that children should benefit from auditory experience in everyday life. In the early 1950s, it became possible to wear two body aids, and by 1955 hearing aids were worn in a harness around the body worn over clothing. The superiority of true binaural fittings was recognized as providing an increased directional sense and better perception of speech in noise (Carhart, 1958; Harris, 1965; Jordan, Greisen, & Bentzen, 1967; Ross, 1969). Furthermore, it became recognized that in most instances binaural hearing aids should be the standard treatment in every case of bilateral hearing loss. It also was acknowledged that it was more natural to receive sound at ear level, and since the early 1960s, ear-level hearing aids have become more widely used (Northern & Downs, 1974). Because behind-the-ear aids were not as powerful as body hearing aids, it was recommended that behind-the-ear aids be fitted on all hearing losses below 80 dB HL and that two body aids be used for children with hearing losses greater than 80 dB HL (Jordan et al., 1967). The other advantage of body hearing aids was the separation of microphone and receiver that diminished the probability of acoustic feedback.

Tremendous technologic advances have been made with regard to hearing instruments in the past five decades. Digital technology developments have led to signal processing that allows the provision of a uniform and high-quality signal, but it is beyond the scope of this chapter to review these in detail. Furthermore, there have been advances in hearing aid selection and verification methods. Much research and discussion have taken place addressing the appropriate selection of frequency responses, gain, and output characteristics of hearing aids for children (Stelmachowicz, 2005). In the 1970s and early 1980s, systematic hearing aid fitting algorithms began to emerge, although these were based solely on average adult data. One major development has been the use of clinical probe-microphone systems in the 1980s, which facilitated the fitting of hearing aids to children. Through the use of these systems, Seewald and colleagues (Moodie, Seewald, & Sinclair, 1994) developed the innovative real-ear-to-coupler difference (RECD) procedure that facilitates real-ear measures in infants as young as a few weeks of age. (See Chapter 25 of this volume.)

Despite these developments with hearing aids, there remained a population of profoundly deaf children who received very limited auditory information with conventional amplification. Cochlear implants were developed on the premise that in sensory deafness, although hair cells are damaged or depleted, some cochlear neurons could be stimulated directly by the application of an externally produced electric current. Cochlear implants were developed from a single-channel analog device in the 1960s, and in the 1980s multichannel implants were introduced (Owens & Kessler, 1989). Initially, the use of cochlear implants was restricted to adults who were postlingually deafened. In 1990, cochlear implants were approved by the U.S. Food and Drug Administration (FDA) for use with children. The single analog channel cochlear implant such as the 3M/House single-channel implant provided little more than sound awareness, prosody, or rhythm of speech. Improvements also were observed in speech recognition as determined on closed-set auditory only tests. Multichannel cochlear implants, with each channel uniquely programmable, provide sufficient frequency discrimination capability to facilitate speech perception and understanding (Thoutenhoofd et al., 2005). Language and literacy improvements in children with cochlear implants have been reported as being comparable to the results obtained with children who use hearing aids and who have less severe hearing loss (Fitzpatrick et al., 2012; Moog & Geers, 2003). In fact, language scores of some children with implants have been documented as being within the range of children with normal hearing (Fitzpatrick, Crawford, Ni, & Durieux-Smith, 2011; Geers, Moog, Biedenstein, Brenner, & Hayes, 2009; Geers & Nicholas, 2013; Geers, Nicholas, & Sedley, 2003). Consequently, cochlear implants have become standard practice for children with bilateral severe to profound hearing loss (Berg, Ip, Hurst, & Herb, 2007). In fact, bilateral cochlear implantation has become the desirable standard of care for children (Balkany et al., 2008)

Advances in technology have fundamentally altered the way we think of the development of communication skills in deaf children. The early, appropriate fitting of hearing aids was probably the most important tool in the management of the child with permanent hearing loss (Ross, 1977). Technologies for early identification and audiologic diagnosis of permanent hearing loss have made it possible to fit amplification to babies. Technologies for digital and programmable hearing aids have substantially improved sound quality for children. Cochlear implants have made it possible for children with profound hearing losses to have access to sound and to spoken language. These advances have significantly altered our expectations of spoken language development for deaf children. However, these technologies, on their own, are of little use if not followed by "individualized, targeted and high quality intervention programs" (JCIH, 2013, p. e1324).

Intervention for Children With Hearing Loss

Educational Options

Historically, there has been considerable difference of opinion about the most effective methods for developing communication. However, there is a consensus that the overall goal of (re)habilitative and educational management for children with hearing loss is to overcome or minimize the barriers to communication imposed by hearing loss in order to enable learning and participation in society. The extent to which permanent hearing loss affects typical spoken communication development and the need for specialized management will depend on characteristics of the hearing loss, such as time of onset and severity, as well as characteristics specific to the child, family, and learning environment. These factors undoubtedly influence decisions related to language learning and educational approaches for facilitating communication development. However, it is clear that management approaches have also been extensively influenced by technologic limitations, practitioners' experiences, and philosophical views of what constitutes appropriate communication for a child with hearing loss (Beattie, 2006; Marschark & Spencer, 2006; Spencer & Marschark, 2010). It is perhaps these views, more than empirical data, that have contributed to the rich history of the (re)habilitation and education of children with hearing loss, one characterized by a mosaic of intervention methods.

As outlined in the previous sections of this chapter, prior to the availability of modern-day hearing aids and particularly cochlear implant technology, children with hearing loss fell essentially into two broad categories based on hearing potential: those who had considerable access to acoustic speech signals, and those who had limited or no access to speech despite the best available hearing technology at that time. Two parallel (re)habilitation and educational management philosophies evolved, both with a focus on equipping the child with communication skills. One philosophy described as a manual approach supported the development of communication through a visual-based sign language system as the natural language of individuals who were deaf. In contrast, the oral philosophy adopted spoken communication and participation in the hearing community as a primary goal of intervention. Numerous variants of these two primary philosophies were developed throughout the world. A detailed review of the many approaches is beyond the scope of this chapter, but a brief description of some of the most common intervention methods that fall under the manual and oral philosophies will be described briefly in the following sections. The interested reader is referred to more comprehensive historical perspectives and critical reviews in such writings as by Spencer and Marschark (2006), Schick, Marschark, and Spencer (2005), and Lynas, Huntington, and Tucker (1989).

Although hearing loss begins as a health issue, the management of children with hearing loss has its roots in education and, historically, service provision was viewed as the "field of education of the hearing-impaired," with teachers of the deaf responsible for educating children (Clark, 1997). This was likely because most children were not identified with hearing loss until late, and there were no or limited intervention programs in the preschool years. As audiologic services and better technology became available, earlier identification and early intervention services provided the foundations for changes in practice. Accordingly, responsibilities for the management of children expanded to include not only educators, but also speech-language pathologists, audiologists, and other specialists in the management of children with hearing loss.

Traditionally, the educational systems for children with hearing loss consisted primarily of special schools for the deaf that provided services in either sign language or oral communication methods. Two important notions underlie the support for manual communication. One fundamental concept is that sign language systems such as American Sign Language (ASL) or its international counterparts constitute the natural language of individuals who are deaf. Accordingly, ASL is a visual language composed of signs with its own grammatical structure that is distinctly different from that of spoken English grammar. Visual-manual systems such as ASL are consistent with a cultural view of deafness in which the Deaf individual is viewed as belonging to a linguistic minority with a distinct language and culture (Lynas, 2005). Essentially, ASL and other manual languages are structured for visual rather than auditory learning. The second important concept that led to support for sign language, particularly for children with profound deafness (prior to cochlear implantation), is that strong visual input is a requirement to overcome the barriers to communication imposed by reduced access to the acoustic patterns of speech.

More recently, programs referred to as bilingual-bicultural or sign-bilingualism (Lynas, 2005) have also emerged. The premise of these educational methods is that from the time of diagnosis of hearing loss, children should be exposed to a language such as ASL as their first language in an educational model that meets not only their linguistic but also their cultural needs as a participant in the Deaf community. Subsequently, written English is taught as a second language. These programs may also teach spoken English as a second language to enable the child to participate in everyday situations as a bilingual child (Lynas, 2005).

In contrast to visual-based approaches, the oral communication philosophy has been supported on the basis that more than 90% (Marschark, Lang, & Albertini, 2002) of children with permanent hearing loss have normal-hearing parents who participate in a hearing society where spoken communication is central to the child's development, education, and employment opportunities. Central to this philosophy is the notion that despite reduced auditory access to the natural acquisition of spoken language, children can learn oral communication through systematic teaching methods. As noted, prior to the widespread availability of hearing instruments, access to hearing through vacuum tube hearing aids and group amplification systems was necessarily limited to classroom settings. Oral educational options, therefore, consisted primarily of special schools with special classroom programs for children with hearing loss. Unquestionably, a major breakthrough occurred with the availability of wearable transistorized hearing aids in the 1950s to 1960s. These hearing instruments dramatically affected the variety of educational environments that became available for children with hearing loss (Clark, 1997), ranging from special schools to special classrooms in schools for normal-hearing children and eventually to integration into typical classrooms with normal hearing peers (Clark, 1997; Northcott, 1990).

The limited, part-time access to speech sounds dictated the methods that evolved for teaching children spoken communication. Until the 1960s, oral communication methods consisted primarily of oral-visual methods with a strong focus on speech-reading and a related spoken language curriculum that concentrated on didactic methods of teaching through the teaching of words and sentence patterns (Clark, 1997). Speech skill teaching developed as a separate activity aimed at improving the quality of the child's articulation. Certain practitioners also believed that the written text was an effective method for teaching children spoken language, and thus, structured writing approaches as a visual means to teaching spoken communication supplemented traditional oral methods to provide the learner with increased access to communication (Clark, 1997; Marschark & Spencer, 2006).

As hearing technology and early identification services progressed and as new knowledge was acquired about speech and language development, traditional oral communication methods were modified. Several variants of the oral communication philosophy were developed to capitalize on these new opportunities. Overall, the ultimate goal of oral education of children with hearing loss remained the development of speech and language as similar to hearing models as possible. The oral approaches are based on the premise that despite reduced input, the overwhelming majority of children have residual hearing and essentially acquire language along the same developmental trajectory as children with normal hearing, although they may reach milestones at a slower pace. Improved access to hearing led to the development of models of rehabilitation that differed in their focus on audition, and natural language acquisition, inclusion with hearing peers, and parental involvement. Known under terms such as auditory-oral, aural-oral, and auditory-verbal therapy, the defining difference between these variants of the oral philosophy to rehabilitation appears to relate primarily to the emphasis on the use of residual hearing. As noted above, traditional oral methods involved significant emphasis on speech-reading. At the other end of the spectrum lies auditory-verbal therapy, an approach that gained momentum in the 1980s and continued to grow as hearing technologies improved. The approach, which is fundamentally based on the premise that even small amounts of hearing can be tuned to acquire spoken language, has grown in popularity with the increased access to hearing provided by cochlear implants for children with severe to profound hearing loss. This approach relies heavily on language learning through the development of residual hearing. Characteristics of auditory-verbal practice include individual teaching of language via a primary caregiver and the early inclusion of children with hearing loss with their normal hearing peers. However, until the advent of cochlear implants, a significant proportion of children with profound hearing loss who required specialized care had minimal access to acoustic speech signals (Boothroyd, 2008). Therefore, support continued for auditory-oral methods that also use speech-reading in teaching spoken language. The primary differences between auditory-verbal and other oral-based approaches are related to the emphasis placed on audition as the primary learning channel for speech reception and on the view that optimal development of communication and social functioning requires that children with hearing loss interact in learning environments with children with normal hearing.

The general assumption of oral language approaches is that exposure of the child to visual-based systems will delay or prevent the acquisition of spoken communication skills. In addition to auditory-based learning methods, other teaching approaches have evolved that can be viewed as aligned with manual or oral communication methods depending on the ultimate communication development goals of the rehabilitation program. Cued speech is one method that is consistent with the oral philosophy but involves the addition of a systematic system of hand signals or cues to facilitate speech-reading and therefore speech reception. Cued speech involves the use of hand cues to code the phonemes of speech (Cornett, 1967).

Total communication is another teaching method that gained widespread recognition, particularly in the United States in the 1970s and 1980s. The method promotes the use of all input modalities including audition, speech-reading, and signs in order to enhance comprehension of speech. The approach essentially involves manually coded speech with visual symbols intended to compensate for reduced access to speech sounds through hearing. Other terms such as *simultaneous communication* and the *combined approach* have been used to describe manually coded speech systems. These multimodal communication approaches were promoted by some experts as a response to improve the low language and academic outcomes documented for children with hearing loss educated through oral communication approaches (Babbidge, 1965; Geers & Moog, 1989; Schildroth & Karchmer, 1986).

Despite much expert opinion and considerable research on communication development outcomes for children with hearing loss, there is no good-quality evidence to support specific intervention methods (Brennan-Jones et al., 2014; Fitzpatrick et al., 2015; Schachter et al., 2002). This appears to be due to the inherent difficulty in conducting controlled studies in view of the many child, family, and environmental factors that affect the development of children with hearing loss (Fitzpatrick et al., 2015; Schachter et al., 2002) Nevertheless, it is clear that there is a great need to strengthen the evidence base supporting specific early intervention approaches (JCIH, 2013).

New Influences on (Re)habilitation

As described above, developments in newborn hearing screening, hearing aid, and cochlear implant technology have had a significant impact on current thinking and management approaches. Cochlear implantation has had a significant impact on the quantity and quality of auditory information available to children with profound hearing loss and represents the most important development in auditory (re)habilitation for these children in recent years. Early and appropriate hearing aid fitting or cochlear implants coupled with early identification of hearing loss resulting from universal newborn hearing screening initiatives have created a dramatic shift in the approaches and expectations for all children with hearing loss. Early identification through newborn hearing screening combined with advanced hearing technology has shifted rehabilitation from a remedial to a developmental model whether the choice of rehabilitation is sign language or oral language. Early access to spoken language patterns has created opportunities for children to acquire language in more naturalistic contexts and to participate in the educational system with hearing peers. Previous rehabilitation models such as auditory-verbal therapy emphasized spoken language acquisition following typical language developmental models, and efforts were made to develop spoken language in natural home and learning environments (Simser, 1993). However, due to late identification and limited access to auditory information, particularly for children with severe-to-profound hearing loss, many approaches included structured speech and language teaching that included remedial components, particularly as children grew older (Ling, 2002).

The possibilities afforded by early identification, management through hearing technology, and the developmental model are aligned with a model of family-centered care. The notion of family-centered care has dominated the management of children with hearing loss for many years but is now growing due to the need to manage hearing loss in infancy and the new opportunities for enhancing language development in more natural and everyday contexts (Tattersall & Young, 2006; Young & Tattersall, 2007). Studies indicate that families want to be involved as partners in the process of language development and to make informed choices (Eriks-Brophy et al., 2006; Fitzpatrick, Angus, Durieux-Smith, Graham, & Coyle, 2008; Robinshaw & Evans, 2003).

There is a body of research documenting that some children with various degrees of hearing loss who receive early intervention have the potential to develop age-appropriate spoken communication skills (Ching et al., 2013; Fitzpatrick, Durieux-Smith, Eriks-Brophy, Olds, & Gaines, 2007; Geers et al., 2009; Nicholas & Geers, 2008; Yoshinaga-Itano, Sedley, Coulter, & Mehl, 1998). Nevertheless, despite the many technologic advances and improvement in communication outcomes, studies continue to show that children with hearing loss, as a group, have spoken language abilities below their hearing peers (Ching et al., 2013; Kennedy et al., 2006; Niparko et al., 2010; Wake, Poulakis, Hughes, Carey-Sargeant, & Rickards, 2005).

These findings suggest that management through hearing technology alone is insufficient to attain age-appropriate skills. Accordingly, children with hearing loss continue to require professional management in developing communication and parents are required to make decisions about which intervention approach is best suited to their needs and desired outcomes.

In its recent statement of endorsement (2013), the JCIH stressed that all deaf and hard-of-hearing children and their families should have access to timely and coordinated entry into early intervention programs. These programs should be part of comprehensive systems including data management and tracking so that families are not lost to follow-up. Equally important is the need to assess progress on a regular (annual) basis. The JCIH also emphasized that early intervention providers need to have professional qualifications and core knowledge and skills regardless of the route chosen by parents to facilitate their children's development and language skills.

In summary, there is a wide range of management approaches for children with hearing loss. Many of these constitute different routes to a common objective, that of developing competent spoken communication. Other approaches focus on the development of a strong communication system through sign language, which is viewed by supporters as the natural language of children who are deaf. The intervention approach and type of amplification selected depend partly on the severity of the hearing impairment and on the characteristics of the child and family but also largely on the families' choice of communication mode for the child. Advances in hearing technology and newborn hearing screening, combined with research documenting the benefits of these interventions, have increased the demand for spoken communication approaches for children with hearing loss. However, there is an understanding that families should have the right to make a fully informed decision based on the best available evidence and their long-term objectives and values for their child and family (Jerger, Roeser, & Tobey, 2001; Joint Committee on Infant Hearing, 2007).

Much progress has been made in hearing loss identification and intervention in the last decades; however, there are still many remaining questions. We need more research on the best way to assess hearing impairment, which in turn will facilitate decisions on what therapies are most appropriate for children and their families. We need the evidence base to support specific early intervention approaches.

References

Ackley, R. S., & Decker, N. T. (2006). Audiological management and the acquisition of spoken language in deaf children. In P. E. Spencer & M. Marschark (Eds.), *Advances in the spoken language development of deaf and hard of hearing children* (pp. 64–84). New York, NY: Oxford University Press.

Alaerts, J., Lutz, H., & Woulters, J. (2007). Evaluation of middle ear function in young children: Clinical guidelines for the use of 226- and 1000-Hz tympanometry. *Otology and Neurotology, 28*(6), 727–732.

Babbidge, H. (1965). *Education of the deaf. A report to the Secretary of Health, Education, and Welfare by his Advisory Committee on the Education of the Deaf.* Ref. No. 0-765-119. Washington, DC: Government Printing Office.

Balkany, T., Hodges, A., Telischi, F., Hoffman, R., Madell, J., Parisier, S., . . . Litovsky, R. (2008). William House Cochlear Implant Study Group. *Otology and Neurotology, 29*(2), 107–108. doi:10.1097/mao.0b013e318163d2ea

Beattie, R. G. (2006). The oral methods and spoken language acquisition. In P. E. Spencer & M. Marschark (Eds.), *Advances in the spoken language development of deaf and hard-of-hearing children* (pp. 103–135). New York, NY: Oxford University Press.

Berg, A. L., Ip, S. C., Hurst, M., & Herb, A. (2007). Cochlear implants in young children: Informed consent as a process and current practices. *American Journal of Audiology, 16*, 13–28.

Bess, F. (2000). Early amplification for children: Implementing change. In R. C. Seewald (Ed.), *A Sound Foundation Through Early Amplification: Proceedings of an international conference* (pp. 247–251). Stäfa, Switzerland: Phonak AG.

Bonfils, P., Uziel, A., & Pujol, R. (1988). Screening for auditory dysfunction in infants by evoked otoacoustic emissions. In K. Gerkin & A. Amochaev (Eds.), Hearing in infants: Proceedings of the national symposium. *Seminars in Hearing, 8*, 165–168.

Boothroyd, A. (2008). The acoustic speech signal. In J. R. Madell & C. Flexer (Eds.), *Pediatric audiology: Diagnosis, technology, and management* (pp. 159–167). New York, NY: Thieme Medical.

Brennan-Jones, C. G., White, J., Rush, R. W., & Law, J. (2014). Auditory-verbal therapy for promoting spoken language development in children with permanent hearing impairments. *Cochrane Database System Review, 3*, Cd010100.

Campbell, P. E., Harris C. M., Hendricks S., & Sirimanna T. (2004). Bone conduction auditory brainstem responses in infants. *Journal of Laryngology and Otology, 118*(2), 117–122.

Carhart, R. (1958). The usefulness of the binaural hearing aid. *Journal of Speech and Hearing Disorders, 23*, 41–51.

Ching, T. Y., Dillon, H., Marnane, V., Hou, S., Day, J., Seeto, M., . . . Yeh, A. (2013). Outcomes of early- and late-identified children at 3 years of age: Findings from a prospective population-based study. *Ear and Hearing, 34*(5), 535–552.

Clark, M. (1997). An overview of educational provision for hearing-impaired children from 1950 to present day. *Seminars in Hearing, 18*(3), 229–239.

Cornett, R. O. (1967). Cued speech. *American Annals of the Deaf, 112*, 3–13.

Davis, H. (Ed.). (1965). The young deaf child: Identification and management. *Acta Oto-Laryngologica Suppl., 206*(5), 1–258.

Davis, H., & Silverman, S. R. (1970). Forward to the first edition (1947). In H. Davis & S. R. Silverman (Eds.), *Hearing and deafness* (3rd ed., pp. XV–XV1). New York, NY: Holt, Rinehart and Winston.

Durieux-Smith, A., Picton, T. W., Edwards, C. G., Goodman, J. T., & MacMurray, B. (1985). Brainstem electric-response audiometry in infants of neonatal intensive care unit. *International Journal of Audiology, 26*, 284–297.

Durieux-Smith, A., Picton, T., MacMurray, B., & Goodman, J. (1987). The Crib-o-gram in the NICU and evaluation based on brainstem electric response audiometry. *Ear and Hearing, 6*, 20–24.

Durieux-Smith, A., & Whittingham, J. (2000). The rationale for neonatal hearing screening. *Journal of Speech-Language Pathology and Audiology, 24*, 59–67.

Eriks-Brophy, A., Durieux-Smith, A., Olds, J., Fitzpatrick, E., Duquette, C., & Whittingham, J. (2006). Facilitators and barriers to the inclusion of orally educated children and youth with hearing loss in schools: Promoting partnerships to support inclusion. *Volta Review, 106*(1), 53–88.

Ewing, A. W. G. (Ed.). (1957). *Educational guidance and the deaf child.* Washington, DC: Volta Bureau.

Ewing, J. R., & Ewing, A. W. G. (1944). The ascertainment of deafness in infancy and early childhood. *Journal of Laryngology and Otology, 59*, 309–333.

Ewing, J. R., & Ewing, A. W. G. (1954). *Speech and the deaf child.* Washington, DC: Volta Bureau.

Finitzo, T., Albright, K., & O'Neal, J. (1998). The newborn with hearing loss: Detection in the nursery. *Pediatrics, 102*(6), 1452–1460.

Fitzpatrick, E., Angus, D., Durieux-Smith, A., Graham, I., & Coyle, D. (2008). Parents needs following identification of childhood hearing loss. *American Journal of Audiology, 17*, 1–12.

Fitzpatrick, E., Crawford, L., Ni, A., & Durieux-Smith, A. (2011). A descriptive analysis of language and speech skills in 4- to 5-yr-old children with hearing loss. *Ear and Hearing, 32*(5), 605–616.

Fitzpatrick, E., Durieux-Smith, A., Eriks-Brophy, A., Olds, J., & Gaines, R. (2007). The impact of newborn hearing screening on communication development. *Journal of Medical Screening, 14*, 123–131.

Fitzpatrick, E. M., Hamel, C., Stevens, A., Pratt, M., Moher, D., Doucet, S. P., . . . Na, E. (2015). Sign language and spoken language for children with hearing loss: A systematic review. *Pediatrics*, 137(1), e20151974.

Fitzpatrick, E. M., Olds, J., Gaboury, I., McCrae, R., Schramm, D., & Durieux-Smith, A. (2012). Comparison of outcomes in children with hearing aids and cochlear implants. *Cochlear Implants International, 13*(1), 5–15.

Galambos, R., Hicks, G. E., & Wilson, M. J. (1982). Hearing loss in graduates of a tertiary intensive care nursery. *Ear and Hearing, 3*, 87–90.

Galambos, R., Hicks, G. E., & Wilson, M. J. (1984). The auditory brain stem response reliably predicts hearing loss in graduates of a tertiary intensive care nursery. *Ear and Hearing, 5*, 254–260.

Geers, A. E., & Moog, J. (1989). Factors predicting the development of literacy in profoundly hearing-impaired adolescents. *Volta Review, 91*(2), 69–86.

Geers, A. E., Moog, J. S., Biedenstein, J., Brenner, C., & Hayes, H. (2009). Spoken language scores of children using cochlear implants compared to hearing age-mates at school entry. *Journal of Deaf Studies and Deaf Education, 14*, 371–385.

Geers, A. E., & Nicholas, J. G. (2013). Enduring advantages of early cochlear implantation for spoken language development. *Journal of Speech, Language, and Hearing Research, 56*, 643–653.

Geers, A. E., Nicholas, J. G., & Sedley, A. L. (2003). Language skills of children with early cochlear implantation. *Ear and Hearing, 24*, 46S–58S.

Harris, J. D. (1965). Monaural and binaural speech intelligibility and the stereophonic effect based on temporal cues. *Laryngoscope, 75*, 428–446.

Hirsh, I. J. (1952). *The measurement of hearing*. New York, NY: McGraw-Hill.

Hyde, M. L., Riko, K., & Malizia, K. (1990). Audiometric accuracy of the click ABR in infants at risk for hearing loss. *Journal of the American Academy of Audiology, 1*, 59–66.

Jacobson, C. A., & Jacobson, J. T. (1990). Follow-up services in newborn hearing screening programs. *Journal of the American Academy of Audiology, 4*, 181–186.

Jerger, S., Roeser, R. J., & Tobey, E. A. (2001). Management of hearing loss in infants: The UTD/Callier Center position statement. *Journal of the American Academy of Audiology, 12*, 329–336.

Joint Committee on Infant Hearing (JCIH; 1982). Position statement 1982. *Pediatrics, 70*(3), 496–497.

Joint Committee on Infant Hearing (JCIH; 1990). 1990 Position statements. *ASHA, 33*(Suppl. 5), 3–6.

Joint Committee on Infant Hearing (JCIH; 1994). 1994 Position statement. *Pediatrics, 95*(1), 152–156.

Joint Committee on Infant Hearing (JCIH; 2000). Year 2000 Position statement: Principles and guidelines for early hearing and intervention programs. *Pediatrics, 106*(4), 798–817.

Joint Committee on Infant Hearing (JCIH; 2007). Year 2007 Position statement: Principles and guidelines for early hearing detection and intervention programs. *Pediatrics, 120*(4), 898– 921.

Joint Committee on Infant Hearing (JCIH; 2013). Supplement to the JCIH 2007 position statement: Principles and guidelines for early intervention after confirmation that a child is deaf or hard of hearing. *Pediatrics, 131*(4), e1324–e1349. doi:10.1542/peds.2013-0008

Joint Committee on Infant Screening (JCIS; 1976). The supplementary statement of the Joint Committee on Infant Screening. In S. E. Gerber & G. T. Mencher (Eds.), *Early diagnosis of hearing loss* (Appendix 1, pp. 12–13). New York, NY: Grune and Stratton.

Joint Committee on Newborn Screening (JCNS; 1970). Statement on neonatal screening for hearing impairment. In J. Northern, & M. P. Downs (Eds.), *Hearing in children* (1974, pp. 108–109). Baltimore, MD: Williams and Wilkins.

Jordan, O., Griesen, O., & Bentzen, O. (1967). Treatment with binaural hearing aids. *Archives of Otolaryngology, 85*, 319–326.

Kemp, D. T. (1980). Toward a model for the origin of cochlear echos. *Hearing Research, 2*, 533–548.

Kennedy, C. R., Kimm, L., Dees, D. C., Evans, P. I., Hunter, M., Lenton, S., & Thorton, R. D. (1991). Otoacoustic emissions and auditory brainstem responses in the newborn. *Archives of Diseases in Childhood, 66*, 1124–1129.

Kennedy, C. R., McCann, D. C., Campbell, M. J., Law, C. M., Mullee, M., Petrou, S., & Stevenson, J. (2006). Language ability after early detection of permanent childhood hearing impairment. *New England Journal of Medicine, 354*, 2131–2141.

Kileny, P. R. (1987). ALGO-1 automated infant hearing screener: Preliminary results. In K. P. Gerkin & A. Amochaev (Eds.), Hearing in infants: Proceedings from the National Symposium. *Seminars in Hearing, 8*, 125–131.

Killion, M. C. (1997). Hearing aids: Past, present and future: Moving toward normal conversations in noise. *British Journal of Audiology, 31*, 141–148.

Korres, S., Nikolopoulos, T. P., Komkotou, V., Balatsouras, D., Kandiloros, D., Constantinou, D., & Ferekidis, E. (2005). Newborn hearing screening: Effectiveness, importance of high-risk factors, and characteristics of infants in the neonatal intensive care unit and well-baby nursery. *Otology and Neurotology, 26*(6), 1186–1190.

Ling, D. (2002). *Speech and the hearing-impaired child: Theory and practice* (2nd ed.). Washington, DC: Alexander Graham Bell Association for the Deaf.

Ling, D., & Ling, A. H. (1978). *Aural habilitation: The verbal foundations of learning in hearing-impaired children*. Washington, DC: A. G. Bell.

Lynas, W. (2005). Controversies in the education of deaf children. *Current Paediatrics, 15*, 200–206.

Lynas, W., Huntington, A., & Tucker, B. (1989). *A critical examination of different approaches to communication in the education of deaf children*. Manchester, UK: Department of Audiology, University of Manchester.

Marschark, M., Lang, H. G., & Albertini, J. A. (2002). *Educating deaf students: From research to practice*. New York, NY: Oxford University Press.

Marschark, M., & Spencer, P. E. (2006). Spoken language development of deaf and hard-of-hearing children: Historical and theoretical perspectives. In P. E. Spencer & M. Marschark (Eds.), *Advances in the spoken language development of deaf and hard-of-hearing children* (pp. 3–21). New York, NY: Oxford University Press.

Mason, J. A., & Herrmann, K. R. (1998). Universal infant hearing screening by automated auditory brainstem response measurement. *Pediatrics, 103*(3), 670–672.

Mauk, G. W., White, K. R., Mortensen, L. B., & Behrens, T. R. (1991). The effectiveness of screening programs based on high-risk characteristics in early identification of hearing impairment. *Ear and Hearing, 2*, 312–319.

Mencher, G. (Ed.). (1976). *Early identification of hearing loss*. New York, NY: Basel, Karger.

Meyer, S. E., Jardine, C. A., & Deverson, W. (1997). Developmental changes in tympanometry: A case study. *British Journal of Audiology, 31*, 189–195.

Moodie, S., Seewald, R. C., & Sinclair, S. T. (1994). Procedure for predicting real-ear hearing aid performance in young children. *American Journal of Audiology, 3*, 23–31.

Moog, J. S., & Geers, A. E. (2003). Epilogue: Major findings, conclusions and implications for deaf education. *Ear and Hearing, 24*, 1215–1255.

National Institutes of Health (NIH; 1993). Early identification of hearing impairment in infants and young children. *NIH Consensus Statement, 11*, 1–24.

Nicholas, J. G., & Geers, A. E. (2008). Expected test scores for preschoolers with a cochlear implant who use spoken language. *American Journal of Speech-Language Pathology, 17*, 121–138.

Niemoeller, A. F., Silverman, S. R., & Davis, H. (1970). Hearing aids. In H. S. Davis (Ed.), *Hearing and deafness* (3rd ed., pp. 280–317). New York, NY: Holt, Rinehart and Winston.

Niparko, J. K., Tobey, E. A., Thal, D. J., Eisenberg, L. S., Wang, N. Y., Quittner, A. L., & Fink, N. E. (2010). CDaCI Investigative Team. Spoken language development in children following cochlear implantation. *JAMA, 303*(15), 1498–1506.

Northcott, W. H. (1990). Mainstreaming: Roots and wings. In M. Ross (Ed.), *Hearing-impaired children in the mainstream* (pp. 1–25). Parkton, MD: York Press.

Northern, J. L., & Downs, M. P. (1974). *Hearing in children*. Baltimore, MD: Williams and Wilkins.

Owens, E., & Kessler, D. K. (Eds.). (1989). *Cochlear implants in young deaf children*. Boston, MA: College-Hill Press.

Picton, T. (2011). Infant hearing assessment: Opening ears. In T. Picton (Ed.), *Human auditory evoked potentials* (pp. 449–492). San Diego, CA: Plural.

Prieve, B., & Stevens, F. (2000). The New York State universal newborn hearing screening demonstration project: Introduction and overview. *Ear and Hearing, 21*, 85–91.

Robinshaw, H., & Evans, R. (2003). Service provision for preschool children who are deaf: Parents' perspectives. *Journal of Social Work in Disability and Rehabilitation, 2*, 3–39.

Rodrigues, G., Ramos, N., & Lewis, D. (2013). Comparing auditory brainstem responses (ABRs) to toneburst and narrow band CE-chirp® in young infants. *International Journal of Pediatric Otorhinolaryngology, 77*(9), 1555–1560. doi:10.1016/j.ijporl.2013.07.003

Ross, M. (1969). Changing concepts in hearing aid candidacy. *Eye, Ear, Nose and Throat Monographs, 48*, 27–34.

Ross, M. (1977). Hearing aids. In B. Jaffe (Ed.), *Hearing loss in children—A comprehensive text* (pp. 676–698). Baltimore, MD: University Park Press.

Sanders, D. A. (1993). *Management of hearing handicaps* (3rd ed.). Englewood Cliffs, NJ: Prentice-Hall.

Savio, G., Perez Abalo, M., Gaya, J., Hernandez, O., & Mijares, E. (2008). Auditory steady state responses in screening. *Clinical Neurophysiology, 119*(9), e109. doi:10.1016/j.clinph.2008.04.055

Schachter, H. M., Clifford, T. J., Fitzpatrick, E., Eatmon, S., MacKay, M., Johnston, C. J., & Moher, D. (2002). Systematic review of interventions for hearing loss in children. Submitted to Health Canada; Contract #03055–HT091-010001.

Schick, B., Marschark, M., & Spencer, P. E. (Eds.). (2005). *Advances in the sign language development of deaf children*. New York, NY: Oxford University Press.

Schildroth, A. N., & Karchmer, M. A. (Eds.). (1986). *Deaf children in America*. San Diego, CA: College-Hill Press.

Schulman-Galambos, C., & Galambos, R. (1979). Brain stem evoked response audiometry in newborn hearing screening. *Archives of Otolaryngology, Head and Neck Surgery, 105*, 86–90.

Silverman, S. R. (1970). From Aristotle to Bell. In H. Davis & S. R. Silverman (Eds.), *Hearing and deafness* (3rd ed., pp. 375–383). New York, NY: Holt, Rinehart and Winston.

Silverman, S. R., & Lane, H. S. (1970). Deaf children. In H. Davis & S. R. Silverman (Eds.), *Hearing and deafness* (3rd ed., pp. 384–425). New York, NY: Holt, Rinehart and Winston.

Simmons, B., & Russ, F. N. (1974). Automated newborn hearing screening, the crib-o-gram. *Archives of Otolaryngology, 100*, 1–7.

Simser, J. (1993). Auditory-verbal intervention: Infants and toddlers. *Volta Review, 95*(3), 217–229.

Spencer, P. E., & Marschark, M. (Eds.). (2006). *Advances in spoken language development of deaf and hard-of-hearing children*. New York, NY: Oxford University Press.

Spencer, P. E., & Marschark, M. (2010). *Evidence-based practice in educating deaf and hard-of-hearing students*. New York, NY: Oxford University Press.

Stapells, D. R. (2000). Threshold estimation by tone-evoked auditory brainstem response: A literature meta-analyses. *Journal of Speech Language Pathology and Audiology, 24*, 74–83.

Stapells, D. R., & Oates, P. (1997). Estimation of the pure-tone audiogram by the auditory brainstem response: A review. *Audiology and Neuro-Otology, 2*, 257–280.

Stelmachowicz, P. G. (2005). Pediatric amplification: Past, present, and future. In R. C. Seewald & J. M. Bamford (Eds.), *A Sound Foundation Through Early Amplification: Proceedings of the third international conference* (pp. 27–40). Stäfa, Switzerland: Phonak AG.

Stevens, J. C., Webb, H. D., Hutchinson, J., Connell, J., Smith, M. F., & Buffin, J. T. (1989). Click evoked otoacoustic emissions compared with brain stem electric response. *Archives of Diseases in Childhood, 64*(8), 1105–1111.

Stevens, J., Webb, H., Hutchinson, J., Connell, J., Smith, M., & Buffin, J. (1990). Click evoked otoacoustic emissions in neonatal screening. *Ear and Hearing, 11,* 128–133.

Tattersall, H., & Young, A. (2006). Deaf children identified through newborn hearing: Parents' experiences of the diagnostic process. *Child: Care Health and Development, 32,* 33–45.

Thoutenhoofd, E., Arhbold, A., Gregory, S., Lutman, M., Nikilopoulos, T., & Sach, T. (2005). *Pediatrics cochlear implantation: Evaluating outcomes.* London, UK: Whurr.

Uus, K., & Bamford, J. (2006). Effectiveness of population-based newborn hearing screening in England: Ages of interventions and profile of cases. *Pediatrics, 117*(5), e887–e893.

Vohr, B. R., Carty, L. M., Moore, P. E., & Letourneau, K. (1998). The Rhode Island Hearing Assessment Program: Experience with statewide hearing screening (1993–1996). *Journal of Pediatrics, 133*(3), 353–357.

Wake, M., Poulakis, Z., Hughes, E. K., Carey-Sargeant, C., & Rickards, F. W. (2005). Hearing impairment: A population study of age at diagnosis, severity, and language outcomes at 7–8 years. *Archives of Disease in Childhood, 90,* 238–244.

Watkin, P. M., Baldwin, M., & McEnery, G. (1991). Neonatal at risk screenings and the identification of deafness. *Archives of Disease in Childhood, 66*(10 Spec. No.), 1130–1135.

Wedenberg, E. (1956). Auditory tests on newborn infants. *Acta Otolaryngologica, 45,* 446–461.

White, K. R., & Behrens, T. R. (Eds). (1993). The Rhode Island Hearing Assessment Project: Implications for universal newborns hearing screening. *Seminars in Hearing, 14,* 1–119.

Wong, D., & Shah, C. D. (1979). Identification of impaired hearing in early childhood. *Canadian Medical Association Journal, 121*(5), 529–546.

Wright, L. B., & Rybak, L. P. (1983). Crib-o-gram (COG) and ABR effect of variables on test results. *Journal of the Acoustical Society of America, 74,* 540–544.

Yoshinaga-Itano, C., Sedley, A. L., Coulter, D. K., & Mehl, A. L. (1998). Language of early- and later-identified children with hearing loss. *Pediatrics, 102,* 1161–1171.

Young, A., & Tattersall, H. (2007). Universal newborn hearing screening and early identification of deafness: Parents' responses to knowing early and their expectations of child communication development. *Journal of Deaf Studies and Deaf Education, 12,* 209–220.

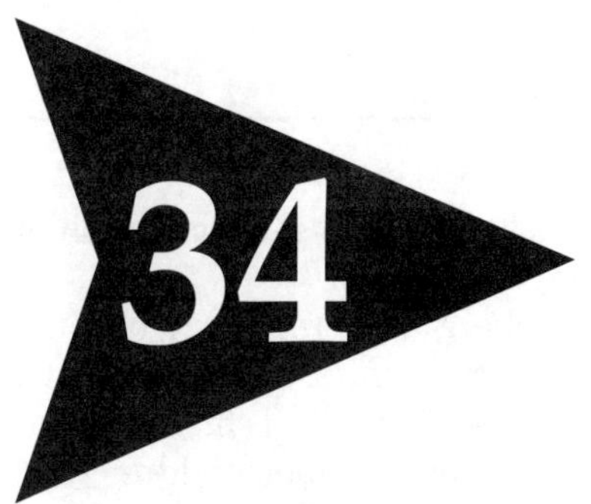

Facilitating Communication in Infants and Toddlers With Hearing Loss

Melody Harrison

Introduction

Early identification of hearing loss was motivated by the goal to prevent, or at least ameliorate, the effects of hearing loss on auditory development and subsequent language learning. Early identification programs have been successfully established in many developed countries, implementation has begun in some developing countries, and attention to follow-up after screening is steadily improving (Bamford, Uus, & Davis, 2005; Kennedy, McCann, Campbell, Kimm, & Thornton, 2005; Morton & Nance, 2006; Shulman et al., 2010; Swanepoel, Störbeck, & Friedland, 2009). The success of these programs and ongoing advances in hearing technologies has facilitated the development of audition, speech, and language among children with a wide range of hearing levels. However, even with the availability of early screening and sophisticated technologies, many children are unable to attain the goal underlying newborn hearing screening (NHS). Coexisting anatomical, sensory, medical, or developmental conditions present barriers to listening and spoken language development that are difficult, and in some cases, impossible to overcome. Some families will choose not to pursue spoken language for their child, and others will be impeded by an inadequate level of professional support for families to establish the practices that have been shown to produce the best child language outcomes.

As efforts to identify hearing loss in infants have become more successful, stresses on early intervention (EI) programs in the United States have both increased and changed. The demographic shift that occurred in an EI program in Kansas between 2002 and 2006 is representative of changes occurring across the United States. Following implementation of NHS, the number of children who were deaf or hard of hearing (DHH) enrolled in the program doubled, the average age at enrollment decreased from 12 to 3.7 months, and children with mild-to-moderate hearing levels were enrolled in equal numbers to those with severe and profound hearing levels. Prior to NHS, the majority of the children had hearing in the severe-to-profound range (Halpin, Smith, Widen, & Chertoff, 2010). Clearly, the early age of identification has altered the skills required of professionals who must now be knowledgeable about multiple aspects of development from the earliest months of infancy to adolescence or later. Additionally, they must be able to mentor and coach families in learning skills they never expected or wanted to acquire.

As clinical experience has indicated and research has demonstrated, children with the best language outcomes by school age are those whose parents have been involved in their EI (Moeller, 2000). Calderon and her colleagues have reported that early parental involvement resulted in improved reading skills (Calderon & Naidu, 2000) and better communication between parent and child (Calderon, Bargones, & Sidmans, 1998). Spencer (2004) investigated language performance in a group of children who received cochlear implants before their third birthday. Age of implantation and family involvement were the two variables associated with differences in language outcomes. Watkin et al. (2007) investigated outcomes of two groups of children who were DHH, one was identified before 9 months and the other was identified after. The authors reported that teacher ratings of parents' level of involvement and the language outcomes of their children who were DHH were strongly correlated. When two groups of children with later-confirmed hearing losses were compared, those with highly involved families had higher speech and language scores than those with families who were less involved. The investigators concluded that a high level of family involvement can serve to mitigate the consequences of later identification.

A related factor contributing to child outcomes appears to be parental self-efficacy. Jean Desjardin and her colleagues have studied the concept of maternal self-efficacy and its effect on child outcomes among children with hearing loss for more than a decade. They have repeatedly shown that higher levels of maternal self-efficacy result in better child outcomes. The concept of self-efficacy was originally described by Bandura (1986) as the beliefs people have about their ability to organize and perform a course of action needed to successfully manage a task. Bandura demonstrated that individuals' beliefs about their abilities powerfully affect they ways in which they behave. Knowledge, skill, and prior accomplishments alone are often poor predictors of the ability to affect outcomes. A self-efficacious person has not only the knowledge and skills, but also the confidence to persist in a behavior or set of behaviors until a goal is attained. Another individual might have access to the same knowledge but be unable to implement or persist to attain a goal. Judgments about self-efficacy are task and domain specific, and thus an individual might be highly competent and self-efficacious in one area but not in another, even when the two seem to be related.

In 2005, Desjardin investigated the effects of maternal self-efficacy on child language outcomes between two groups of preschool children who were DHH. One was composed of children with cochlear implants (CIs) and the other of children who had hearing aids (HAs). The mothers of children with CIs reported feeling more involved in their child's intervention programs and more competent adjusting the CI, conducting daily checks of their child's listening skills, and making a difference in their child's learning new sounds and words. Conversely, mothers of children with HAs rated themselves as less involved in their child's EI program, and they had lower ratings of self-efficacy related to care and maintenance of the HAs. One possible explanation for these differences was that the mothers of children with CIs reported the EI professional routinely invited them to participate in the sessions. This finding supports research by Woods, Kashinath, and Goldstein (2004), who found that a mentorship model emphasizing hands-on training and practice with constructive and encouraging feedback enhanced generalization of newly learned knowledge and skills.

DesJardin and Eisenberg (2007) investigated the relationships between maternal contributions (linguistic input, involvement, and self-efficacy) and children's language skills. Thirty-two mothers and their children with CIs participated. Level of maternal involvement and their self-efficacy scores regarding their ability to affect speech-language development were positively related to both the quantity and quality of the mothers' linguistic input. The authors suggested that incorporating goals promoting involvement in EI and mothers' self-efficacy could enhance child outcomes. In 2015, Stika et al. studied the developmental outcomes of early identified children with mild-to-severe hearing levels between 12 and 18 months of age. One of the measures used was the Scale of Parental Involvement and Self-Efficacy (SPISE) developed by Desjardin (2003). The results indicated that greater maternal self-efficacy was associated with better language skills, social-emotional competence, adaptive behaviors, and fewer problem behaviors.

The notion of self-efficacy is crucial in understanding how we can best support parents achieve goals for their child. As professionals, we often believe we have completed the counseling aspect of our job when we have provided parents with the information we believe they need. Yet, for most parents, information is only one step. For families to be able to implement agreed-upon goals fully, they must have opportunities to practice the techniques and skills with hands-on mentorship from knowledgeable professionals. When access to EI professionals who are prepared to guide families in developing spoken language is unavailable, they are likely to turn to the audiologist as the expert regarding all things related to their child's hearing, including oral language development. This chapter has been designed primarily to be a resource for audiologists who find themselves in this unexpected role. It is not a step-by-step guide to auditory, speech, and language development, but aims to provide a framework the practicing audiologist can use to support families and to collaborate with other professionals in the child's sphere to create an accessible and responsive communication environment that will maximize the hearing technology that has been fitted.

A growing body of research indicates that early and well-fitted hearing aids that are worn consistently to provide access to audition and exposure to a rich linguistic environment are necessary to achieve optimal language. Although a growing number of EI professionals, especially teachers of the deaf and hard of hearing and speech-language pathologists, receive specialized preparation to work with children who are DHH, some EI providers have little or no preparation in this area. In a study of factors affecting EI services, one area in which many EI professionals expressed the least amount of comfort was related to HA use and management (Harrison et al., 2015). Regardless of their level of preparation to work with young children who are DHH, forming a collegial working relationship with EI professional(s) is an essential step in ensuring the goal of consistent auditory access is achieved as soon as possible after HA fitting and CI mapping is completed. Reaching out to the family's EI professional to introduce yourself and suggest working together to help the family achieve the best outcomes for their child will almost always be welcomed.

In those cases when working collaboratively with the EI provider is not possible, creating a collaborative relationship with the family becomes even more important. As parents learn about their child's hearing loss, they not only gain knowledge, but they also acquire a sense of mastery over a body of information that initially seemed alien and overwhelming. Most parents want to be actively involved in providing solutions to the challenges and limitations created by their child's hearing loss. Engaging the family in the process of habilitation, including consistent device use and maintenance, management of the child's listening environment, and promotion of early communication and auditory development provides excellent opportunities for parents to understand the hearing loss and to accept and even promote device use.

This chapter is divided into two primary sections. The first covers topics related to helping families learn to manage their child's hearing instruments to develop consistent auditory access for their child. The second section is devoted to the fundamentals of facilitating early language development.

Developing Consistent Access to Audition

Hearing aids and cochlear implants are interventions that have the potential to mitigate the effects of hearing loss on speech and language development. However, to achieve their potential, two critical conditions must be met. First, the devices must be worn consistently; second, they must be in good working condition. These might seem to be too obvious to address, and as a result receive only cursory attention in the form of a brief demonstration and printed information. Because consistent auditory access is necessary for a child to optimally benefit from a device, one of the key roles that audiologists and EI professionals can play is to help families achieve that goal. The research described in this section focuses primarily on HA use; however, the clinical suggestions are applicable to CIs as well.

Establishing Hearing Aid Use

Understanding the factors that influence HA use is essential to providing the information, problem-solving support, and coaching that a family might require in the months following HA fitting or CI activation. When a child is fitted as an infant and the HAs are worn consistently, challenges to use might be minimized. Unfortunately, although some babies easily accept HAs, others might be initially accepting but begin to remove them as they become more coordinated, and some will resist them from the beginning. Parents and audiologists frequently report that HA use by infants and toddlers is a challenge, and so it is important to be proactive about potential problems rather than assuming all will go well. Acknowledging that it can be a challenge and strategizing with parents about consistent use creates a team approach to the problem and can help to reduce the sense of failure experienced by some families.

In recent years, several investigators have studied HA use among children. Moeller, Hoover, Peterson, and Stelmachowicz (2009) followed seven families longitudinally to learn about the challenges they faced in establishing consistent HA use among their early identified infants with mild to moderate hearing loss. The parents reported that factors such as the child's state (ill, hungry, fussy) and the context (book sharing, outside playing, in a car seat, etc.) influenced HA use. Unhappy babies or babies who were isolated in a car seat or who were unable to interact with others were much more likely to resist or remove their HAs. The investigators also found that as the infants aged into toddlerhood, HA use increased and became much more consistent. Jones and Feilner (2013) used data logging information from clinics serving approximately 5,000 children, ages birth to 19 years, to assess the amount of time HAs were worn. These investigators defined full-time use as 12 or more hours per day. Similar to the finding of Moeller et al. (2009), data logging information indicated HA use increased with age. However, only 10% of all of the children in this large sample were full-time users, and 40% used their HAs 4 hours per day or less. These results indicate a wide range of hearing aid use among children.

Walker and her colleagues (2013) investigated the factors that predict HA use among children enrolled in a longitudinal study, Outcomes of Children with Mild to Severe Hearing Loss (OCHL). Parents of 272 children responded annually to a HA use questionnaire, adapted from the one developed by Moeller et al. (2009). The investigators compared data logging to the parents' responses. Three factors influenced the amount of time that children wore their HAs during the week and on the weekends; these were the child's age, better-ear pure tone average, and mother's level of education. There was almost a 2-hr daily difference in the amount of HA use time reported by mothers with a college education as compared to the amount reported by mothers with a high school education. This difference was supported by data logging information. Holte et al. (2012) reported that among these same mothers, maternal education was the only factor that predicted the age of the first diagnostic audiology evaluation. These two factors together, later confirmation of hearing loss and less HA use time, illuminate the need for families within this demographic to receive a higher level of counseling and hands-on demonstration and coaching. Another important finding was that older children wear their HAs more than younger children even in challenging situations. For example, when children 12 months to 24 months old were in less immediately supervised situations such as the car, parents reported they almost never had HAs on. Yet by the time the children were preschoolers (3 to 4 years old), parents reported they almost always wore their HAs in the car. Thus, age and situation both contributed to HA use.

Understanding the potential effects of these factors on device use can be very useful in working with a family to achieve consistent auditory access. When families struggle with HA use, striking a balance between letting them know that it is likely to become easier following infancy, and simultaneously working to help them establish consistent use during their baby's infancy can be a challenging balancing act. A concern is that they will simply give up and wait until the child is older. Working with families to identify times when they are most likely to be successful is important. It can be helpful to reassure parents that a consistently constructive response to their baby's negative behaviors will eventually extinguish their attempts to remove the hearing devices. In part, this is because the devices and the auditory signal they provide will no longer be novel. Conversely, the less consistently the instruments are worn, the more likely the child will be to remove them. Some of the barriers to device use in infancy, such as feedback because of head positioning in infant seats and car seats, decreases as head control and mobility develop. Persistence will pay off over time. It can be just as important to help parents explore when it would *not* be a good time to attempt repositioning the hearing instruments, such as the baby's fussy times or in the car when feedback is likely to occur and the child is unable to engage with the adult. Try to include the child's speech-language pathologist, teacher of the deaf and hard of hearing, or other EI specialist in planning how to achieve the goal of consistent device use at the time of confirmation of hearing loss, or as soon after as feasible.

Talking with a family about their daily schedules and identifying situations that can develop into predictable routines can provide initial successes upon which they can build. For example, suggest having the HAs in close proximity to the baby's clothing so that the HAs can be put on *before* beginning to dress the baby each morning. Once the HAs are on, the parent or caregiver can talk about what the child will wear. Although some parents are very skilled at talking with their infants, others will need to be coached to identify the article of clothing, describe the textures and colors of the items, and talk about the process of putting the article on the baby. *"Let's wear your yellow shirt today. It is so soft. Here it goes over your head ... there you are! Now, one arm in a sleeve, where's your other arm? Here it is. Where are your warm blue pants? Here they are."* Mealtimes also provide rich opportunities several times each day for monitored HA use. The colors, tastes, temperatures, and names of the foods are all topics for conversation. Virtually all babies prefer interacting with an attentive adult to any other activity. Remind parents to speak at a normal conversational level and to minimize background noise created by television or radio so that the child is not overly stimulated. If the child is still an infant, help the family learn how to position the infant during monitored HA use so that the baby can easily see and interact with the adult, and the instruments are comfortable in the child's ear and not creating feedback. Families engage in multiple activities with their children every day. Helping them identify those times as opportunities for HA use and engaging in rich linguistic interactions with their child can support families in developing the perception that they can manage their child's HAs and they are helping develop their child's speech and language. As DesJardin (2005) noted, parents who perceive that they are effective in managing their child's HAs also perceive that the HAs are worn more often and that they are more involved in their child's speech and language development.

Degree of hearing loss was also a predictor of amount of daily HA use (Walker et al., 2013). Children with severe losses wore their HAs more than children with milder losses, although, once again, age was a mitigating factor. Slightly more than half of the parents whose children had mild-to-moderate hearing loss reported HA use in preschool. In contrast, almost all the parents of children with hearing in the moderate-to-severe range reported full-time HA use by that age. By 5 years of age, HA use by the two groups was about the same. Parents of children with mild-to-moderate hearing loss might not be as aware of the importance of consistent HA use for their child during infancy, but by the preschool years deficits in speech and language acquisition can begin to appear, motivating an increase in HA use. This finding highlights the need for information and coaching for families of children with hearing levels in the mild-to-moderate range.

A study by Tomblin, Oleson, Ambrose, Walker, and Moeller (2014) also provides useful information for families. These researchers examined the association between aided threshold levels and length of HA use with speech and language outcomes in 180 children who were 3 and 5 years old and were enrolled in the OCHL study. Measures of the gain in hearing ability modestly but significantly correlated with levels of speech and language development. Higher levels of audibility are attained when the degree of hearing loss is less and HAs are well fitted; thus, children with milder degrees of hearing loss have the best access to their auditory environments when wearing HAs. In addition, the amount of benefit from aided hearing interacted with duration of HA use. Thus, children with the best aided hearing levels who were fitted early and had longer periods of HA use had the best speech and language outcomes. Further evidence supporting the importance of daily HA use for children with mild levels of hearing loss was provided by Walker, Holte, and colleagues (2015), who examined the effects of consistent HA use on speech, language, and speech perception outcomes of 5- and 7-year-old children with mild hearing loss. The children were separated into three groups based on patterns of HA use. After controlling for age at confirmation of hearing loss, level of audibility, and enrollment in early intervention, only daily HA use predicted significant differences in the children's scores on vocabulary and grammar. Together, these findings confirm the importance of providing ongoing support to families as they work to achieve consistent HA use for children with mild hearing loss.

In a more recent study of 296 of the OCHL children, Walker, McCeery, et al. (2015) analyzed whether or not there were trends that predicted HA use. Many of the children across three age groups (infant, preschool, and school age) started out as consistent HA users, defined as 8 or more hours of use per day, and maintained a high level of use. Infants had the lowest percent of consistent users (64%). A subgroup of infants (27%) started out wearing their HAs inconsistently but increased use over time, and 10% of the babies were inconsistent users throughout infancy. Among the preschoolers, 79% were consistent HA users, 11% began the preschool period as inconsistent but increased use over time, and 10% were inconsistent throughout the preschool years. By school age, 84% of the children wore their HAs consistently. Clearly, chronological age is a factor in how much of the time children wore their HAs. Although most of the children in the OCHL study wore their HAs consistently, 10% to 16% of them did not. Even in this group of children whose parents reported high levels of consistent HA use, some children never achieved consistent access to their auditory environments, regardless of age or context.

Be willing to provide encouragement and support to parents in the efforts they make toward the goal of consistent HA use. Take the time to discuss the situations they find the most challenging and to acknowledge the frustration they might be experiencing. Families who are made to feel they have failed at a task are unlikely to reveal that they continue to need help. If a toddler always removes the hearing aids in the car, a temporary solution might be to have the parent remove them prior to entering the car and replace them at the end of the trip. More proactively, if the child is fitted with an FM system, the parent or perhaps a sibling might be able to keep the child engaged by talking about the passing scenery and what they are seeing. This strategy can provide enough distraction, not to mention language-learning opportunities to keep the child engaged. Let parents know it is "OK'" to pick their HA battles. If a tired, hungry, and very grumpy 14-month-old pulls her hearing aids out, it is unlikely that reinserting them will be successful. After lunch and a nap, the child is likely to be much more receptive. Like all of us, families want to be reinforced for what they can do and "not judged for what they are unable to do" (Roush, 2000, p. 164). Acknowledging the challenges and offering to help problem solve those situations with families is a reasonable and proactive tactic.

One of the most powerful strategies to support families who struggle with consistent device use can be to connect them with another family who has struggled but ultimately been successful with HA use or other challenges of childhood hearing loss. When an audiologist knows a family who would be a particularly good partner to that of a newly identified child, and has their permission, it can very helpful to ask permission for the "experienced" family to call the family who is new to the world of HAs and EI services. Parent-to-parent support and coaching is a strategy that is widely acknowledged as effective, but one many of us still fail to employ. Local chapters of Hands and Voices (http://handsandvoices.org) or the Alexander Graham Bell Association for the Deaf and Hard of Hearing (agbell.org) can be sources of support and information for families. Being aware of any parent groups in your area and having contact information available for parents is a component of comprehensive care for children and families. Creating a shared understanding of the importance of device use and a team approach (a team that will eventually include the child) to hearing device management is a cornerstone to successful device use.

Device Management

In addition to daily use, the devices must be kept in good working condition to provide consistent access to audition. Yet many parents experience challenges managing their child's instruments. Elfenbein (1994) reported that although parents were aware of the need to check their child's hearing aids, they lacked the necessary equipment and skills to accomplish the task. Even when they did check the hearing aids, they frequently missed cues that the device was not functioning properly. In a 2001 study of their early experiences with their child's HAs, parents reported their greatest concerns were care and maintenance of the HAs and feeling overwhelmed by the technology provided for their child (Sjoblad, Harrison, Roush, & McWilliam). In their 2009 study, Moeller et al. queried parents of young children regarding their early experiences with hearings aids. One of the findings was that many parents need ongoing support in the management of their child's hearing technologies throughout early childhood. Most manufacturers of hearing aids and cochlear implants provide information about care and maintenance of the device at the time of purchase as well as on their websites. However, as DesJardin and colleagues have repeatedly shown, parental self-efficacy requires involvement and hands-on practice. Information alone is not sufficient for mastery of a skill to occur.

Before sending the family home with new hearing instruments, it is important to demonstrate a listening and maintenance check. As important as this initial demonstration is in developing a parent's sense of comfort and competence, it is only the first of many steps in establishing consistent use of optimally functioning devices. The family's EI professionals, who are likely to interact with the family on a much more frequent basis than the audiologist, can become excellent partners in establishing both consistent device use and monitoring equipment status. Although many EI professionals are likely to require training in these tasks, the payoff in regard to child and family outcomes can be substantial.

After a comprehensive listening and hearing aid check has been demonstrated, ask the parent or EI to practice it with you. It will almost certainly be necessary to provide cues the first time through. Coaching them as they begin to master the task in addition to demonstrating it provides a multidimensional learning experience. Well-illustrated written instructions can also help as they learn to do the check at home. Some clinicians call a few days after the initial HA fitting to ask if there are questions they can help answer. Access to Skype, FaceTime, or similar technologies can provide easy access to visual demonstration, which might be helpful. On the family's first return visit, reinforce the importance of conducting this daily task by asking them to run through the HA check to confirm that they are comfortable with the process. Although this might require more time than the audiologist would like to devote to the task, the time spent assuring that parents are comfortable assessing device function is well worth the investment. Once it is clear that one family member is knowledgeable about and confident in the ability to complete a routine check, that individual should be asked to teach one other person in the household how to conduct a check. Not only is teaching a skill the final step in mastery, it assures that more than one person in the family can complete the task.

In the future, the family and EI professionals will need to learn how to check each device and each combination of devices the child uses. For example, if more than one program/memory is available or an FM system is used, they must listen to each of these to determine that the signal is clear and undistorted. If an FM system is used at home, instruct the family how to set the FM microphone/transmitter close to radio or television and listen to the signal as they move to different areas of the house to check for interference. As the child becomes older and begins to use the telephone, that signal will need to be tested as well. By this point, most children will be old enough to become involved in monitoring their own equipment. Each time a new program or device is added to the child's array, remind the family to include it in the daily listening check.

Most parents will appreciate having their audiologist acknowledge that HAs, FM, or CIs are complex instruments and that learning how to care for and maintain them will be a process rather than a one-time review. Such an acknowledgement is likely to create an atmosphere in which families and others feel comfortable asking questions or for assistance. Finally, assure families and any other professionals working with the child that they should not hesitate to contract you if they have conducted maintenance and listening checks and yet continue to be concerned about the child's rate of progress. For example, if they notice a decrease in the child's previous levels of speech perception, a decrease in speech production abilities, or if the child makes little or no progress over a specified period of time, an appointment with the pediatric audiologist should be scheduled immediately.

Although a daily maintenance check might initially require more time as families are learning to master the task, they should be encouraged that once they are familiar with it, the maintenance check will typically take only a few minutes a day. The daily check is most likely to become part of the family's routine if it is completed at the same time every day. For some families this might be after the child goes to sleep in the evening, for others it might be first thing in the morning or at naptime. When a family has difficulty incorporating the daily maintenance check into their routine, having them listen to the difference between the signal produced by a well versus a poorly functioning instrument might be motivating.

Ling Six Sound Test

In addition to the hearing aid maintenance check, the family should also learn how to conduct a quick listening check using the Ling Six Sound Test (Ling, 1989). The sounds included in the Ling Six Sound Test, /ah/, /ee/, /oo/, /s/, /sh/, and /m/, were selected because they cover the range of speech sounds we hear and say, from the lowest frequencies in /m/ around 500 Hz, to the highest in /s/, which contains frequencies as high as 8400 Hz, depending on the vowel context and the gender of the speaker (Boothroyd & Medwetsky, 1992). Each sound should be presented at a normal conversational level. When the child is an infant, an adult will use a stethoset to conduct a daily listening check. The adult will produce each sound while listening for clarity with no distortion or unwanted noise in the signal as each of the Ling Six Sounds is presented. The Ling Six Sound Test can be used by anyone—audiologists, speech-language pathologists, teachers, and parents—to conduct a listening check. It can also be used for a variety of purposes ranging from simple detection of the presence of sound, to discrimination, and identification, and for a variety of purposes. A broader discussion can be found in the literature; however, the goal here is to establish a practice of a daily listening check by the family.

As soon as the child is old enough to respond reliably, and this will depend on the interplay of degree of hearing loss, cognitive ability, chronological age, and, to some degree, personality, the child should become the listener. Their response can be any of a wide variety of actions including clapping or some other physical activity such as tossing a toy in a box. Then as soon as they are able, the child should be encouraged to imitate the sounds as they are presented. Children who were prescriptively fitted with hearing aids soon after birth and are able to hear sounds across the speech spectrum are likely to imitate some of the sounds by 18 months of age, and some will begin to produce the vowels much earlier.

Families should be reminded that this is an auditory-only task. The child should not be able to see speaker's mouth; however, placing a hand or an object too close to the mouth can distort the signal. Sitting beside the child or producing the sounds when they are not focused on the speaker's face is a more natural approach. Modeling the technique is helpful and requires only a few minutes. Remind families and EI professionals to (a) practice presenting all the sounds at relatively equal degrees of intensity (given the frequency range the word *relatively* is stressed); (b) vary the order of presentation of the sounds so that the child does not learn a specific presentation pattern, (c) wait until the child is not looking directly at your face before presenting a sound or sit beside rather than in front of the child; and (d) present all sounds at the same distance from the child. When parents begin to explore the range of their child's listening abilities, sounds will be presented at varying distances; however, for the purpose of checking the working condition of the equipment, distance should be constant. Presentation of the sounds, one at a time and waiting for the child to imitate provides a check of the overall integrity of the system. Whether the child is fitted with HAs or has CI(s), use of the Ling Six Sound Test is an excellent way to monitor device function and is available on several websites.

The Roles of Distance and Noise in Facilitating Communication Development

Understanding how distance and noise affect audibility is a key element in developing listening and language skills in a child with hearing loss. The role of distance in relation to audibility might be one of the least abstract and therefore most easily understood by parents and the professionals who work with the child's family. The inverse square rule, known to all audiologists, states that the sound pressure of a spherical wave-front radiating from a point source decreases by 50% as the distance is doubled. Measured in decibels (dB), it decreases by 6.02 dB as the distance is doubled. The behavior is actually not inverse-square but is inverse-proportional. However, simply translated, it means that as a sound source becomes more distant, the more difficult it will be for the child to hear and understand the sound. As basic as this concept might seem, it is not immediately evident to most individuals. Many parents and even some professionals do not understand the importance of distance. A simple demonstration using a nonsense word spoken at a normal conversational level and having the adult begin at a distance of 12 to 15 feet away from the sound source can assist in explaining the important role distance plays. One of the strategies employed in auditory-verbal therapy when the child fails to respond to the auditory signal is reducing the distance between the sound source and child. Reducing distance is an easy, low-tech strategy adults interacting with the child should know about and use. The pediatric audiologist might be the only person in the child's sphere who is aware of this information.

Noise is another enemy of listening, especially for young children. Even 15-year-olds performed more poorly than adults in speech identification in the presence of noise or reverberation (Johnson, 2000). Children who are DHH are faced with the added challenge of trying to decode an auditory signal that is degraded by their impaired auditory system. Young children typically live in very noisy environments. Homes are often filled with the sounds of other children, the television, radio, or video games. In child-care centers and preschools, the sounds and noise of childhood activities and mishaps reverberate. Providing children who have hearing loss with as many opportunities as possible to listen in situations in which the auditory signal is accessible is absolutely necessary for successful language development. Recent research at the University of Washington reported that television exposure of young children between 2 and 48 months of age was associated with significantly reduced child vocalizations. In addition, the number of words uttered to them by adults with television on was reduced. Every additional hour of television exposure resulted in further reduction in both child and adult scores. Not only does television increase noise in the environment, Christakis et al. 2009, demonstrated that when television was on, significantly less language was directed to the child by adults in the home. Ambrose, VanDam, and Moeller (2014) studied the quantity of adult words, adult-child conversational turns, and electronic media in the auditory environment on 28 children who were hard-of-hearing to examine whether these variables contributed to the children's language outcomes. The children were all within 6 months of their second birthday when LENA (Language ENvironment Analysis) technology was used to collect full-day acoustic recordings. The authors reported that toddlers who engaged in more conversational turns with adults demonstrated stronger linguistic outcomes than those who engaged in fewer conversational turns. In homes with high rates of electronic media exposure in the auditory environment, frequency of conversational interactions was decreased. Thirty percent of households in the United States report that the television is on all of the time. Young children who are at risk for developing auditory-based language are even more vulnerable to the negative effects of television than children with hearing in the normal range. Encourage families to be aware of the noise level in the child's environments, and whenever possible turn off the television and reduce extraneous noise.

Involving Families in Establishing Access to Audition

When parents are able to identify positive changes in their child's auditory behavior, they might be more likely to persevere in device use (Harrison, 2000). A useful tool to share with parents and EI professionals who are less familiar with the influence noise and distance have on listening is the test of Early Listening Function (ELF) developed by Karen Anderson (2002). The ELF was designed to obtain an estimate of a child's functional use of hearing as it relates to distance and noise. The concept that is presented and reinforced in the ELF is that of the child's "Listening Bubble," which represents the variable area surrounding a child within which sounds with differing degrees of loudness can be heard. The "bubble" is wider for louder sounds and more restricted for those that are quieter. The ELF describes 12 specific, contrived listening activities that can easily be conducted at home. Parents are asked to determine if their child exhibits a behavioral response at specified distances, in quiet and "typically noisy" conditions. As they perform the tasks described in the ELF, parents gain knowledge about how far away their child can hear a variety of sounds under several different listening conditions. The activities can be conducted over a period of days or even weeks. In fact, one strategy that has been successful is to break the ELF into smaller subsets of activities. When the family completes the activities and returns for their next appointment, their observations are shared and discussed with their pediatric audiologist. The next set is then sent home. Engaging the professionals providing EI services in administration of the ELF creates valuable learning opportunities for those who are unfamiliar with the challenges created by hearing loss and can assist in opening communication between the audiologist and the EI providers. The results of the activities provide parents with a clear understanding of exactly how far away from a sound their child can be and what the listening conditions must be for the child to be able to hear.

Results from the ELF guide parents and professionals in discovering the role distance and noise play in a child's specific listening ability. One family might learn that although a sound is audible in quiet conditions at a distance of 9 feet, in noisy conditions the same sound is inaudible at 6 feet. Another might learn that their child's listening bubble is less than 6 feet for a sound in quiet and in noise the child is unable to hear the sound at all. As parents gain expertise in estimating the size of their child's listening bubble, they begin to become knowledgeable about the conditions that must be present in the child's auditory environment for listening and language learning to occur. The ELF is available online at http://home.earthlink.net/~karenlanderson/ELF.html

Families who have been sufficiently supported in learning about their child's listening environment and understand the importance of device use have accomplished two very important tasks. First, they have learned to provide the conditions necessary for consistent auditory access. Perhaps even more importantly, in the process they have acquired knowledge and learned new skills that increase their self-efficacy regarding management of their child's hearing loss. The key elements of "self-efficacy," or belief in our ability to accomplish a goal, are knowledge and confidence. Whether the professional is a teacher of the deaf and hard of hearing, a speech-language pathologist, early childhood special educator, or an audiologist, the essential components to developing parental self-efficacy are to (a) provide parents with knowledge, and then (b) support them in persisting in mastering a goal until they are successful. The importance of both of these elements of self-efficacy as it relates to parent-child relationships was demonstrated by Conrad, Goss, Fogg, and Ruchala (1992) who reported that when mothers saw themselves as being less competent, an increase in knowledge alone failed to change the quality of mother-child interactions. Simply providing parents with information is not always sufficient. Mastery of a goal is essential to achieving self-efficacy, and those parents who do not think of themselves as able to be successful need support to incrementally achieve the goals that will foster their child's development. Partnerships among audiologists, speech pathologists, early intervention specialists, and families are often necessary to accomplish mastery.

The Building Blocks of Language Learning

Most parents who decide to have their child fitted with HAs do so because they envision them as children, and eventually as young adults, who use oral language to communicate. Thus, reinforcing the relationship between early sound awareness, which requires early and consistent device use, and the development of speech and language is a logical place to begin the ongoing conversation how to master that goal. All children require extensive exposure to the elements of language in order to acquire it. Those whose auditory access is diminished or distorted by hearing loss require at least as much exposure, if not significantly more, in order to extract the information from which language is constructed. Recent studies suggest that inconsistent hearing aid use can be a primary source of individual differences in language and speech outcomes of early identified infants (Jones & Feilner, 2013; Moeller et al., 2009; Walker et al., 2015; Walker et al., 2013). Linking early speech perception to later language development can be helpful in explaining the need for early and consistent device use to parents. Indirect evidence of the role speech perception plays in language and reading development can be found in studies of children with normal hearing. Much of this work comes from the area of reading and learning disabilities and is drawn from studies of children who have normal peripheral hearing but appear to be unable to use auditory information in an effective manner. Reed (1989) demonstrated that children with reading disabilities were much poorer at discriminating consonants compared to children the same age with no reading challenges. Links between deficits in speech perception abilities and reduced language skills have been strongly established in children with specific language impairment (Leonard, McGregor, & Allen, 1992). These studies are representative of a large body of work supporting the idea that a child's ability to extract information accurately from an auditory signal is directly related to later language and reading development. Hearing loss obviously creates a barrier to the acquisition of information from an auditory signal. Hearing aids and cochlear implants can, when fitted and used optimally, provide the only means to access the information essential to development of speech and language.

Development of the phonological representations that underlie spoken language production depends on perceptual access to the auditory signal (Kuhl, 2000). The relationship between babies' ability to discriminate between vowels at 6 months of age and their later vocabulary, as measured by the number of words produced, was described Kuhl, Conboy, Padden, Nelson, and Pruitt, (2005). Six-month-old babies who were able to discriminate between two simple vowels /i/ (tea) and /u/ (two) had larger vocabularies when they were 18 and 24 months old as measured by the MacArthur Communicative Development Inventory (Fenson et al., 1993). Furthermore, babies with the highest level of vowel discrimination had the largest vocabularies. Early vocabulary development is vitally important because it remains one of the strongest predictors of overall language ability at school age. Language ability is, in turn, a strong predictor of academic achievement. These findings, in conjunction with a number of supporting studies, led Kuhl and her colleagues to propose a theory of Native Language Neural Commitment (NLNC).

Simply stated, NLNC posits that language acquisition depends on early phonetic learning in a baby's native language. Babies who are most able to capture phonemic contrasts such as those in the words "tea" and "two" are creating neural connections essential for native language development. When infants are born, and for several months afterward, they are responsive to phonemes in their own language as well as those of other, very different languages. By the time they are a year old, their ability to discriminate nonnative phonemes has declined significantly. The notion of neural commitment proposes that early phonetic learning alters perception and, thus, influences future phoneme and language learning ability. This theory hypothesizes that the trajectory of language learning between 7 and 30 months of age is highly dependent on an infant's level of sophistication in learning native language phonemic structure before the age of 12 months. In fact, in a study of 6-month-old infants, Kuhl, Williams, Lacerda, Stevens, and Lindbolm (1991) demonstrated that exposure to a specific language in the first half year of life altered the infants' phonetic perception. The implications for the importance of early and consistent auditory access are clear.

The NLNC theory is supported by recent evidence. By the time English-speaking toddlers with normal hearing are 25 to 29 months old, they are able to produce vowels with 88% accuracy and consonants with 64% accuracy. By their third birthdays, just a few months later, accuracy has risen to 95% for vowels and 73% for consonants (McIntosh & Dodd, 2008). Ambrose et al. (2014) investigated the speech sound production abilities of 70 children who were hard of hearing. Their goals were to compare their productions to those of children with normal hearing, to identify sources of risk for children who were hard of hearing, and finally to determine whether speech sound production skills at age 2 years predict those skills at age 3 years. By age 2 years, children who were hard of hearing had vowel production similar to that of children with normal hearing; however, consonant production was weaker. Similar vowel production is likely a function of the more robust intensity and frequency characteristics of English vowels. The children were divided into two age groups at HA fitting, those with normal hearing or children who were hard of hearing but fitted with hearing aids before 6 months and those who were fitted with hearing aids after 6 months of age. Better outcomes for consonant accuracy were associated with HA fitting before 6 months of age. A follow-up analysis revealed that there was no difference between children with normal hearing and those fitted with HAs by 6 months. There was also a significant effect for degree of hearing loss on consonant production scores, with 2-year-olds whose hearing losses were more than 45 dB HL doing less well. It was also the case that the children's scores at 2 years of age predicted performance a year later on a speech sound production test. For professionals who work with families choosing an oral/auditory approach, this work offers support and motivation for promoting early consistent use of amplification that can provide access to audition. The predictive relationship between performance at 2 and 3 years of age also provides evidence that counters a "wait and see approach" when a child is not making progress in speech sound acquisition. The possibility that the HA is not providing adequate access to audition should be explored.

Even when hearing loss is identified at birth and hearing aids are optimally fitted, children with profound hearing loss are not likely to have access to audition to the degree that children with normal hearing do. Studies conducted by Stelmachowicz and her colleagues (Stelmachowicz et al., 2008; Stelmachowicz, Pittman, Hoover, & Lewis, 2001; Stelmachowicz, Pittman, Hoover, Lewis, & Moeller, 2004) have suggested that reduced audibility in the high frequencies (because of the bandwidth of hearing instruments) restricts access to important phonemes in English and thus plays a role in the delays in phonological development often exhibited by children with hearing impairment. McGowen, Nittrouer, and Chenausky (2008) found that even when profoundly deaf infants were identified at birth and consistently used amplification, at the age of 12 months they had fewer multisyllabic utterances with consonants; produced fewer fricatives (/f/, /s/, and /sh/) and fewer stops with alveolar-velar stop place (/t/, /d/); and had more restricted front-back tongue position for vowels. This was attributed to restricted output of hearing aids.

Most hearing aids are capable of providing audibility only to approximately 3000 Hz. However, according to Boothroyd and Medwetsky (1992), some of the phonemes that carry important information in English require audition in frequencies up to 8300 Hz, depending on age and gender of the speaker and the vowel context. It is reasonable to assume that babies are unlikely to produce phonemic content to which they have never had access. Recent advances in hearing aid technology, specifically frequency compression strategies that provide audibility of important high-frequency phonemes, might provide infants with more of the information they need to hear the high-frequency phonemes necessary for vocabulary and language acquisition (Glista et al., 2009). Later language development appears to depend heavily on acquisition of the phonemic elements of a language prior to 12 months of age. This requires exposure to language for most of a child's waking hours from birth. The consequences of failing to establish a pattern of consistent hearing aid use as early as possible in a child's life can very negatively affect later language outcomes. These effects can be seen as early as 2 years of age.

Language Facilitation Strategies

The First Few Months

Beginning in the first few days of an infant's life, parents and babies engage in mutual, reciprocal gazing. Babies only a few weeks old will attempt, often quite successfully, to imitate facial expressions. A bit later they begin to vocalize in response to an adult's simple vocal model. This interaction, while quite endearing, is also an important communication benchmark indicating the establishment of "conversational turn-taking" and the earliest steps in developing joint attention and gestural communication. At this early point, a communicative relationship has begun to develop between a parent and child. A positive communicative strategy that parents can begin to use with very young babies is *waiting*. Encourage parents to model a face or a sound for their baby and then wait . . . and wait awhile longer, to allow the baby time to organize a response. The strategy of waiting is one that will be useful across the child's language acquisition years, and it is never too early for adults, parents, and professionals to implement. Most adults enjoy this type of interaction with babies, but few are aware of the developmental importance of the activity. Knowledge that establishing mutual gazing and attempts at imitation of facial expressions are early forms of communication and an early developmental step might promote increased interaction between parents and their infant.

Very young infants can easily be positioned so that they are supported and close enough to clearly see the parents' or caregivers' faces. An ideal situation is to have the adult sit on the floor with his or her back against a wall or sturdy furniture with their legs together and knees bent so that they form an inverted V. Place the baby so that the back rests against the parent's thighs and the feet are on the parent's chest. In this position, the baby has a clear view of the adult's face, is secure and comfortable, and the adult is an ideal visual and auditory distance from the child. In addition, both of their hands are free. As the baby grows, an infant seat can be used while maintaining a similar distance, at least initially, for interactions. In the beginning, encourage parents to interact with their babies in the simplest ways. Look at them and smile, tell them they are adorable. If the baby's eyes open widely, encourage the parents to imitate. Have them smile, or open their mouths and then wait for the baby to imitate them. At this stage, the goal is to develop mutual gazing, reciprocity, and early turn taking; thus, it is essential that the baby be able to clearly see the adult's face. Later, it might be more appropriate for the adult to position himself or herself beside the child some of the time.

The Value of Routines

The earliest communication between adults and babies is based on an adult successfully reading the baby's cues and then responding appropriately to those cues. If a baby is fussy and has not been fed for several hours, the mother might interpret the behavior as hunger and feed her. The mother's behavior is a signal to the baby, who might quieten for a few moments when she sees preparations for a feeding underway. The baby has successfully communicated a need and, in turn, the parent has successfully communicated that the need has been understood. The easier a baby's cues are to read, the more successful the parents will feel in responding; and the more predictable the parent's response, the more competent the baby can become in signaling his or her needs or states to the parents. Successful parent-infant communication, which in the earliest weeks is similar regardless of hearing status, contributes to parents' sense of self-efficacy. The fundamental aspect of this earliest communication is reciprocity. The adult reads the baby's cues and then responds with cues or behaviors that the baby can easily understand. These successful interactions provide a perfect platform for early language learning. Every daily activity, whether it is feeding, bathing, burping, or dressing, can become a routine, something that is done in about the same way, with a similar outcome and at roughly the same time every day. Routines promote predictability through repetition, which is important to language learning for all children. Listening and language development depend on providing an environment that provides a wealth of opportunities to interact with competent language users (i.e., parents, siblings, and other caregivers). Predictability, consistency, and repetition are particularly important when barriers or challenges such as hearing loss are present. The earlier a child learns that sound is meaningful and can be predictive (the sounds of food preparation mean eating and feeling satisfied), the more likely the child is to integrate a wide range of sounds, including those of the child's native language, into his or her auditory awareness.

Routines provide an ideal context for the words, phrases, and sentences and other communicative acts to which the baby is exposed every day, day after day, in a predictable manner. Coaching parents to (a) identify their own routines, (b) recognize the language that can be incorporated into those routines, and (c) understand the importance of repetition in the routines, allows them to incorporate language learning activities without increasing either stress or time to their day. In fact, being knowledgeable about strategies that support their child's language learning will likely reduce stress. Understanding how to use everyday routines also reinforces the idea that communication goes on throughout the entire day and is not a special event during a specified period of time that has to be set aside to "work with" the child.

Early Strategies: Birth to Three Months

From birth until the baby is about 3 to 4 months of age, encourage parents to talk about the child's immediate realm of experience; what the child is *feeling* or *experiencing* at that moment. "You are so tired and sleepy. It's time to go to bed." Or, "Oooooh, you're all clean, let's get you nice and dry." If there are any concerns about the parents' understanding of baby talk or "motherese," demonstrate speaking in a sing-song manner typical of the speech that experienced parents use. Many, but certainly not all parents, seem to understand that such a manner of speaking is more engaging to babies. Motherese typically has a slightly higher pitch with clearly spoken words. It is slower with longer pauses between words and phrases, and vowels are slightly elongated. The vowel stretching that is found in motherese ("Ooooooh, you're aaall cleeeean!"), is an example of acoustic highlighting, a technique for focusing the child's attention on a specific piece of auditory information. The acoustic stretching of phonetically relevant information in infant-directed speech focuses the child's attention on acoustic cues and appears to play an important role in speech discrimination. Tsao, Liu, and Kuhl (2004) used vowel stretching, typical in motherese and a recognized measure of speech intelligibility, as a measure of speech clarity. They found that the degree to which mothers engaged in vowel stretching was strongly related to infant speech perception skill at 6 months of age. When they measured the language ability of those babies at 13, 16, and 24 months, there were significant correlations between individual infant's speech perception skills and his or her later language abilities, including word understanding, word production, and phrase understanding as measured by the MacAuthur-Bates Development Communicative Inventory years (Fenson et al., 1993). It is also the case that adults using motherese tend to repeat their utterances. Again, repetition is an important element of early language learning, and for children whose access to spoken language is degraded by hearing loss, repetition should be significantly increased. When children are developing typically, motherese begins to disappear by the time the child is about 2 years of age. However, clearly articulated speech, with some acoustic highlighting, is a technique used for children with hearing loss throughout childhood and beyond. It is one of the important early strategies for developing listening and language abilities.

Early Strategies: Three to Six Months

As babies develop, their head and neck control matures, permitting them to look from left to right as well as up and down. In addition, their visual field becomes wider and deeper providing expanded visual access to their environments. As a baby's world expands, so will the objects and experiences to which they are exposed. Around the time the baby is about 3 months of age, parents should begin to include vocabulary and language related to events or objects the surrounding the child. People or objects that reappear frequently, such as the names of siblings or other family members, pets, toys, or events that occur as part of daily routines, are typical examples. Linking words to objects, people, or activities assists the baby in attaching meaning to words and phrases. Guide parents to tune into what the baby appears to be interested in and comment or describe where they are visually focused. If something interesting is occurring and the baby is unaware of it, hold or turn the baby so he or she can see, draw the baby's attention, and then comment, "There's a bird." or "Look, Mommy's home!" Family routines remain a foundation for language acquisition. If, for example, weekday mornings include taking an older sibling to the school bus stop with the family dog in tow, vocabulary and language might focus on the sibling's name, the dog's name, school bus, stroller, or articles of clothing needed for the weather. Phrases such as "time for the bus" or "let's go" and "bye-bye" can also be part of the language routine. Critical elements in facilitating early language learning are (a) talking about what is in the baby's immediate experience; (b) using language that names or describes someone or something in which the baby is *interested;* and, (c) ideally, providing opportunities to talk about the person, object, or event repeatedly.

Six to Twelve Months

Although people and objects in the child's environments remain the primary topics of conversation for many more months, in the second half of the child's first year, language topics expand to keep pace with the baby's cognitive, social, and motor development. For example, if a fire truck roars past with sirens blazing, a parent might comment, "That was a loud fire truck." Likewise, when an older brother gets on the school bus and rides away, he can no longer be seen. He is not immediately present. However, it is entirely reasonable to talk about him and say, "Bye-bye, Nick, see you later." The objects and events are no longer in the baby's immediate environment; however, because of their saliency, one because it was big, red, and noisy, the other because he is such an important person in the baby's life, they can be referenced and their existence beyond the present moment has begun to be established.

At around this time, parents' vocabulary typically begins to expand to include descriptors of people and objects. Words such as *happy*, *soft*, *clean*, and *dirty* begin to appear more frequently. Other children are described as *big girl* or *crying baby*. The more opportunities a child has to interact with adults who are able to establish responsive, mutual communication focusing on the child's feelings, experiences, and environment in a predictable manner, the more likely they are to acquire new sounds and words. Even as topics, vocabulary, and language expand, it continues to be important to pay attention to how far away from a sound source the child is and the level of noise in the environment. These factors should always be considered unless an FM system is being used. Use of clear speech with characteristics of motherese and waiting for a response should be characteristic of the adults' style of interaction by this time.

Book Sharing

Picture books for babies offer an excellent resource for facilitating vocabulary and language learning. At around 5 to 6 months of age, when the baby is old enough to have developed good head control and sit up with only slight props, parents can begin to use sturdy picture books with bright, interesting pages as a platform for language learning.

The baby should be positioned so that she or he can easily see both the book and the parent's face. Some parents seem to understand intuitively how to share books with infants, while others require guidance. If a relationship with a speech-language pathologist or other early service provider has been established, working with them to develop book sharing skills with the parents can provide reinforcement for what will hopefully become an enjoyable activity for both the parent and the child. With both the baby and the adult in a comfortable position, have the adult point to a picture, or if the child is already attending to the book, point to their focus of attention, and then comment about the object, "It's a cute puppy." Next, the adult should look at the baby and once eye contact has occurred, return the baby's gaze to the picture, point to the same object and comment on the picture again. The act of directing the child's attention through the use of eye gaze and pointing is strategic in developing "joint attention" (Figure 34–1). Joint attention is the process by which one individual alerts another to a person, object, or event through nonverbal means, such as gazing or pointing. Joint attention occurs when two partners share attention to the same subject. Learning to engage in joint attention is critical for a child's language, cognitive, and social development. Book sharing not only creates opportunities for linguistic interaction, it is an activity that perfectly supports development of joint attention.

Some adults believe they need to read all the text in a book in much the same manner an adult might read to a linguistically competent 4-year-old. Babies, particularly those with hearing loss, are unable to manage this level of interaction and will respond negatively.

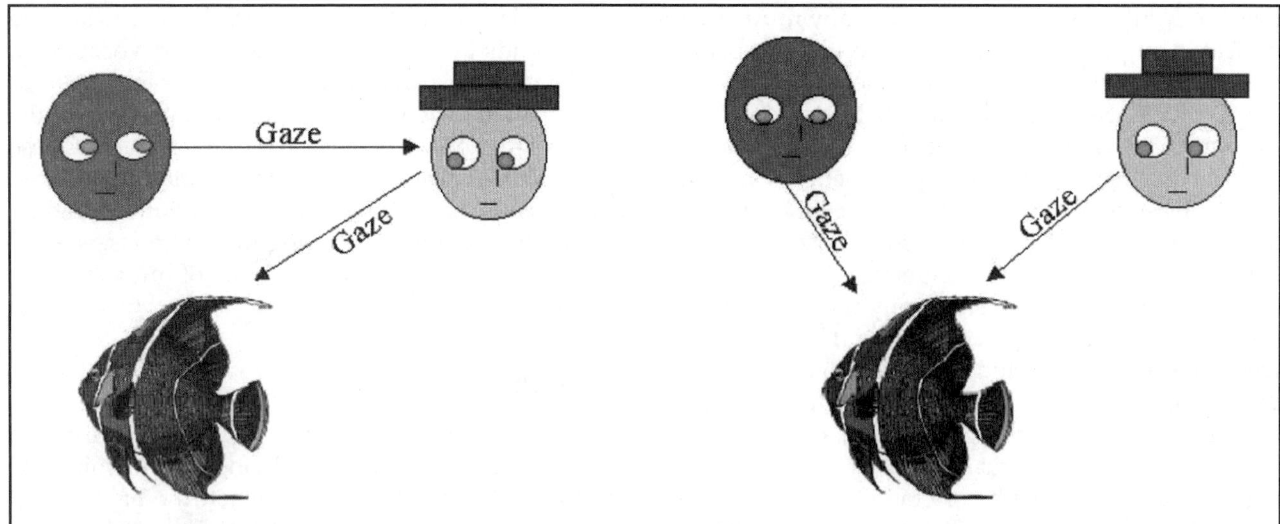

FIGURE 34–1. Joint Attention: Using eye contact or gesture to show or direct the attention of another person. (Reprinted with permission from http://eigsti.psy.uconn.edu/jt_attn.html by Inge-Marie Eigsti.)

Parents who have employed this approach to book sharing often report that their child does not like to read books. Pointing at, describing, and commenting to the child about the pictures constitutes how book sharing is ideally conducted at this age. Adults can also incorporate gestures such as pretending to sniff the picture of a flower, or scratching behind the ear of a picture of a puppy and then actually scratching behind the baby's ear to maintain the baby's attention. Language and vocabulary should be descriptive and responsive to the baby's focus of attention, using an engaging voice with characteristics of motherese in a relatively quiet environment. As the baby's vocabulary and language understanding expand, the complexity of the pictures in books and the language used in book sharing should always match or be slightly beyond that of the child's.

Prelinguistic Communication: The Foundation of Language

Understandably, parents of a child with a hearing loss can become so focused on speech and oral language that they are unaware of the importance of nonverbal prelinguistic foundations of communication upon which later oral language is constructed. Coaching parents to be aware of and responsive to those early communication acts is extremely important in building language competency. Two of the basic prelinguistic constructs are *intent* and *gesture*, which are intricately linked. Behavior that clearly seeks to engage an adult's attention or assistance can be called *intentional communication* and does not appear until the child understands that behavior can have an effect on the world (an adult). Learning cause and effect depends on the cognitive and biological development of the child, as well as the types of experiences the child has had with adults. Iverson and Thal (1998) describe gestures as actions produced with the intent to communicate, typically with fingers, hands, and arms but sometimes including other parts of the body or lips. Gestures can be interpreted only in context and can be involve a variety of objects and events.

More than 30 years ago, Elizabeth Bates demonstrated that infant gesture and nonverbal communicative functions or intentions provide a foundation for later verbal overlay. Prelinguistic communication is the only means of signaling early intentionality that typically developing children, regardless of their hearing status, begin to develop early in of the first year of life. Not only is a child's level of prelinguistic communication an indicator of his or her current linguistic and cognitive development, it can serve as a predictor of later language competence (Crais, Douglass, & Campbell 2004; Mundy et al., 2007; Stoel-Gammon, 1999). Thus, being aware of and appropriately responding to prelinguistic communication reinforces the child's earliest attempts at communicating. For many years, the production of gestures by children with hearing loss was strongly discouraged as being a precursor of sign-language. Some programs went so far as to discourage toddlers from waving "bye-bye." However, more recently, the foundational role of gesture in the emergence of language has resulted in a different perspective regarding this fundamental communicative function.

The earliest gestures emerge between 7 and 9 months of age (Carpenter, Mastergeorge, & Coggins, 1983) and are referred to as *deictic gestures*. Deictic gestures, which account for about 88% of the gesture repertoire in infants and toddlers, are divided into two categories: contact and distal gesture (Thal & Tobias, 1992). Contact gestures generally require physical contact between the child and an object or caregiver. Examples of deictic gestures with an object might be pushing an offered bottle away as if to say, "I don't want that." These often first appear as an open-handed gesture indicating that an object is desired or rejected. Another example of a deictic gesture is turning the head away from an object as an indication of refusal. Distal deictic gestures require no direct contact and typically involve pointing or reaching. One of the most universally recognized is a baby reaching with both arms up, indicating a desire to be picked up. Understanding the communicative value of a deictic gesture provides parents with opportunities to respond to the baby's communicative act and to provide appropriate linguistic input. For example, if a baby turns his head away from a spoonful of food, it might be because he has had enough, or it might be that he does not care for strained peas. The parent's response depends on the knowledge of the context. If the baby has been eating spoonful after spoonful of peas and then turns his head, a logical interpretation of the gesture would be that he is full and the appropriate adult language is something such as, "All done," "No more," or "You're full!" If the baby turns his head at the first spoonful, another interpretation is more probable.

The second major type of gesture, *representational gesture*, appears near the end of the first year, around 12 months of age (Bates, Benigni, Bretherton, Camaioni, & Volterra, 1979) and typically occurs after deictic gestures emerge and are established. Representational gestures establish a reference and also indicate particular semantic or meaningful content. These gestures are used primarily to add information to a communicative exchange or to maintain the "listener's" attention. They can be *conventional* gestures that are used socially, such as blowing a kiss or waving good-bye, or they can be *object-related* gestures that signify some feature of the referent, for example, pretending to give a baby-doll a bottle or sniffing a flower.

Representational gestures often emerge within familiar routines and games such as peek-a-boo that parents and other caregivers use to engage children (Accredolo & Goodwyn, 1988). Representational gestures tend to require the parent's modeling of the gesture, and so, are dependent on parent practices, the amount of parental input, and the family routines. All of these are influenced by culture, beliefs, and tradition. One family might indicate "hungry" by rubbing their tummies, while another might do so by putting their fingers to the mouth. The importance of representational gestures as they relate to facilitating language development among children with hearing loss is that higher levels of gestural production have been associated with higher levels of comprehension among typically developing hearing children (Bates Bretherton, & Snyder, 1988) and that the use of gesture is communicatively functional. Clearly, in order for gestures to provide a framework for later language learning to occur, language must be present in conjunction with gesture. Parents who react to their child's gestures with an action plus appropriate vocabulary and language are providing a rich linguistic environment that will promote language learning in a manner that responding without language cannot. Being aware of the role gesture plays in the development of communication and the opportunities gesture provides for adults to engage in meaningful, responsive, and reciprocal language can be pivotal in developing parent-child linguistic interaction in the early months of life.

Gesture Function

Understanding the function of a gesture is critical to determining an accurate response and the language to use. The function of children's prelinguistic communicative acts was first described by Bruner (1981) who identified three functional categories of prelinguistic communication, including behavior regulation, social interaction, and joint attention. Behavior regulation functions overlap both deictic and representational gestures. Behavior regulation and social interaction emerge prior to joint attention; however, they emerge in an overlapping rather than sequential manner. Crais and her colleagues (2004) and Carpenter et al. (1983) have begun to describe the emergence of gestural communicative functions.

Behavior regulation is a term used to describe a baby's attempts to manage adult behavior. Behavior regulation includes both *protesting* and *requesting* gestures and their age of emergence is the most predictable of all gestures. Protesting is commonly the first to appear at approximately 6 months of age and can be expressed by pushing an object away or turning the head, for example, deictic gestures, which were discussed earlier. Requesting gestures begin at roughly the same time or shortly thereafter. These gestures include the request of either objects or actions. Object requests, which are generally observed first, typically involve the child's arm outstretched in the direction of an object, such a toy or a person, and *might* be accompanied by vocalization. "Oh, you want the red truck" might be the parent's response. Requesting an action, such as playing peek-a-boo, is more sophisticated communication and commonly emerges several months later at 8 to 9 months of age.

Social interaction gestures, Bruner's second functional category, emerge shortly after birth and develop complexity throughout infancy (Bruner, 1981). First, there is an initial period, early in life when the infant attends to social partners. This is seen first as mutual gazing and then might involve other parts of the body. Gestural greetings can be seen in 3-month-olds who smile and coo in response to an attentive adult. A bit later, a social interaction gesture might take the form of a body movement, such as a 6-month-old repeatedly kicking her legs to gain attention.

The next period of development in social interaction is marked by the infant's efforts and growing ability to maintain a shared attentional focus to objects and events with social partners, often involving social games and object sharing. A 10-month-old might pull a blanket on her head as a social gesture to initiate a game of peek-a-boo. A few months later the toddler might blow a kiss or wave bye-bye and might produce a verbal approximation of "bye-bye." These conventional gestures typically promote a reciprocal gesture or utterance from the person to whom they were directed. Thus, conversational turn taking advances to the next level.

In the last 3 months of the first year of life, a prelinguistic milestone occurs when babies begin to intentionally communicate their interests and needs to others. Joint attention, initiated by the *child*, is the final prelinguistic communication function to emerge. It does so in stages, beginning as early as 9 months of age when the baby shows or gives objects directly to an adult. Within the next few months the baby will simply point to a person, object, or event often while vocalizing, in order to draw the adult's attention to the object of interest. Around 15 to18 months of age, toddlers will point in response to an adult's language prompting, "Where's the kitty?" or request information from the adult by pointing at something and then looking at the adult for comment of explanation. Finally, as oral language emerges, the toddler will use gesture to clarify a word approximation when it is not understood. For example, in an attempt to request juice the toddler might repeat "ooz," point to the refrigerator, and then look back at the adult to ascertain that the adult is attending and understands the request.

Transition from Prelinguistic to Linguistic Communication

As children move from the nonverbal prelinguistic stage to the early stages of verbal language, parent strategies for supporting language acquisition must also evolve. The *Division of Early Childhood (DEC) Recommended Practices in Early Intervention* (Sandall, McLean, & Smith, 2000) notes the importance of appropriate parent responsiveness to best support language development in young children. When parents are able to fine-tune their responses to their child's utterance, language development appears to occur at an optimal rate. Not surprisingly, parent response to a child utterance should be governed by the complexity of the utterance. When children are at the one-word level, the types of parent responses recommended by the *DEC Recommended Practices* include both *imitation and expansion*. Imitation is simply responding to a child's utterance with the word the child has said, albeit in the adult rather than child form. If the child holds out stuffed bunny and says, "Bebe," the adult imitation should be "Bunny" or "It's Bunny" unless, of course, the bunny's name is Bebe. Expansion involves the simple addition of elements to the child's utterance to produce a slightly more complex model. For example, in response to "gawgee," the adult model might be, "Brown doggie" or "Yes, that's a brown doggie," or "It's a big doggie!" The adult has expanded the child's one-word utterance to a two-word utterance or a simple sentence with one adjective, modeling the next level of complexity for them.

When the two- to three-word level is attained, adult responses evolve in complexity to include strategies such as *parallel talk, recasting*, and *asking open-ended questions*. Parallel talk occurs most frequently as an adult plays along with a young child in a form of parallel play during which the child and adult play with similar toys but do not engage in coordinated, cooperative play. Children from the age of 2 to 3 years are typically at the two- to three-word level and engage in parallel play with other children as well as adults. Parallel talk is related to the activities around which play is centered. It might involve description of the toys or actions of the toys. It could be suppositional, "I think my baby is hungry. I'm going to feed her." The adult does not necessarily expect the child to respond but is simply modeling appropriate linguistic content for the situation in which they are engaged. Recasting is a more complex language facilitating technique but is contingent on the child's utterance. In recasting, the child's language is restated or "recast" in a changed sentence structure that maintains and refers to the central meaning of the child's production. For example, if the child observes someone fall from a bike and says, "fall down," the adult recast might be, "He was going too fast. That's why he fell down."

Open-ended questions promote the most complex response the child is capable of making and are appropriate for children who are firmly into the two-word utterance stage. Asking a how, what, or why question avoids a simple yes or no response. Thus, asking,"What's Daddy doing?" supports the more elaborate and developmentally appropriate response, "Daddy singing," than if the child had simply been asked, "Is Daddy singing?"

Although the strategies and language adults use to promote a child's language development evolve continually from early infancy through toddlerhood and into early childhood, it continues to be the case that all young children learn language within the context of their daily routines and through daily interactions with their parents. Although the services of a professional with specialization in providing speech and language service to infants and toddlers with hearing loss should be available to every family, the reality is quite different. However, whether or not services with an expert are available, there is a need for proactive management with the involvement of family members and those who provide services to them. Family involvement is the key to child success in all areas of development. The information presented in this chapter should be sufficient to create a solid foundation for a child's communication development in the earliest years of life if parents are supported by a pediatric audiologist who is both knowledgeable and understanding.

References

Acredolo, L., & Goodwyn, S. (1988). Symbolic gesturing in normal infants. *Child Development 59*, 450–466. doi:10.2307/1130324

Ambrose, S. E., Unflat Berry, L. M., Walker, E. A. Harrison, M., Oleson, J., & Moeller, M. P. (2014). Speech sound production in two-year-olds who are hard of hearing. *American Journal of Speech-Language Pathology, 23*(2), 91–104. doi:10.1044/2014_AJSLP-130039

Ambrose, S. E., VanDam, M., & Moeller, M.P. (2014). Linguistic input, electronic media, and communication outcomes of toddlers with hearing loss. *Ear and Hearing, 35*(2), 139–147. doi:10.1097/AUD.0b013e3182a76768

Anderson, K. (2002). Early Listening Function (ELF). Parent involvement: The magic ingredient in successful child outcomes: Improving parent participation using the ELF and the CHILD. *Hearing Review, 9*(11), 24–26.

Bamford, J., Uus, K., & Davis, A. (2005). Screening for hearing loss in childhood: Issues, evidence and current approaches in the UK. *Journal of Medical Screening, 12*(3), 119–124. doi:10.1258/0969141054855256

Bandura, A. (1986). *Social foundations of thought and action: A social cognitive theory.* Englewood Cliffs, NJ: Prentice Hall.

Bates, E., Benigni, L., Bretherton, I., Camaioni, L., & Volterra, V. (1979). *The emergence of symbols: Cognition and communication in infancy.* New York, NY: Academic Press.

Bates, E., Bretherton, I., & Snyder, L. (1988). *From first words to grammar: Individual differences and dissociable mechanisms.* New York, NY: Cambridge University Press.

Boothroyd, A., & Medwetsky, L. (1992). Spectral distribution of /s/ and the frequency response of hearing aids. *Ear and Hearing, 13,* 150–157.

Bruner, J. (1981). The social context of language acquisition. *Language and Communication, 1,* 155–178.

Calderon, R., Bargones, J., & Sidman, S. (1998). Characteristics of hearing families and their young deaf and hard-of-hearing children: Early intervention follow-up. *American Annals of the Deaf, 143,* 347–362.

Calderon, R., & Naidu, S. (2000). Further support for the benefits of early intervention for children with hearing loss. *Volta Review, 100*(5), *Monograph,* 53–84.

Carpenter, M., Mastergeorge, A. M., & Coggins, T. (1983). The acquisition of communicative intentions in infants eight to fifteen months of age. *Language and Speech, 26*(2), 101–116.

Christakis, D., Gilkerson, J., Richards, J., Zimmerman, F., Garrison, M., Xu, D., . . . Yapanel, U. (2009). Audible television and decreased adult words, infant vocalizations, and conversational turns: A population based study. *Archives of Pediatric and Adolescent Medicine, 163*(6), 554–558.

Conrad, B., Goss, D., Fogg, L., & Ruchala, P. (1992). Maternal confidence, knowledge, and quality of mother-child interactions: A preliminary study. *Infant Mental Health Journal, 13,* 353–362.

Crais, E., Douglass, D., & Campbell, C. (2004). The intersection of the development of gestures and intentionality. *Journal of Speech, Language and Hearing Research, 47*(3), 678–694.

DesJardin, J. L. (2003). Assessing parental perceptions of self-efficacy and involvement in families of young children with hearing loss. *Volta Review, 103*(4), 391– 409.

Desjardin, J. L. (2005). Maternal perceptions of self-efficacy and involvement in the auditory development of young children with prelingual deafness. *Journal of Early Intervention, 27*(3), 193–209.

DesJardin, J. L., & Eisenberg, L. S. (2007). Maternal contributions: Supporting language development in young children with cochlear implants. *Ear and Hearing, 28*(4), 456–469. doi:10.1097/AUD.0b013e31806dc1ab

Elfenbein, J. (1994). Monitoring preschooler's hearing aids: Issues in program design and implementation. *American Journal of Audiology, 3*(2), 65–70. doi:10.1044/1059-0889.0302.65

Fenson, L., Dale, P., Resnick, S., Thal, D., Bates, E., Hartung, J., . . . Reilly, J. (1993). *MacArthur Communicative Development Inventories: User's guide and technical manual.* San Diego, CA: Singular.

Glista, D., Scollie, S., Bagatto, M., Seewald, R., Parsa, V., & Johnson, A. (2009). Evaluation of nonlinear frequency compression: Clinical outcomes. *International Journal of Audiology, 48*(9), 632–644. doi:10.1080/14992020902971349

Halpin, K. S., Smith, K. Y., Widen, J. E., & Chertoff, M. E. (2010). Effects of universal newborn hearing screening on an early intervention program for children with hearing loss birth to 3 years of age. *Journal of the American Academy of Audiology, 21*(3), 169–175. doi:10.3766/jaaa.21.3.5

Harrison, M. (2000). How do we know we've got it right? Observing performance with amplification. In R. Seewald (Ed.), *A Sound Foundation Through Early Amplification: Proceedings of an international conference.* pp. 119–140. Chicago, IL: Phonak.

Harrison, M., Page, T. A., Oleson, J., Spratford, M., Unflat-Berry, L., Peterson, A., . . . Moeller, M. P. (2015). Factors affecting early services for children who are hard of hearing. *Language, Speech, and Hearing Services in the School* doi:10.1044/2015_LSHSS-14-0078

Holte, L., Walker, E., Oleson, J., Spratford, M., Moeller, M. P., Roush, P., . . . Tomblin, J. B. (2012). Factors influencing follow-up to newborn hearing screening for infants who are hard-of-hearing. *American Journal of Audiology, 21*,163–174. doi:10.1044/1059-0889(2012/12-0016)

Iverson, J., & Thal, D. (1998). Communication transitions: There's more to the hand than meets the eye. In A. Wetherby, S. Warren, & J. Reichle (Eds.), *Transitions in prelinguistic communication* (pp. 59–86). Baltimore, MD: Brookes.

Johnson, C. E. (2000). Children's phoneme identification in reverberation and noise. *Journal of Speech, Language, and Hearing Research, 43,* 144–157. doi:10.1044/jslhr.4301.144

Jones, C., & Feilner, M. (2013). What do we know about the fitting and daily life usage of hearing instruments in pediatrics? In J. L. Northern (Ed.), *A Sound Foundation Through Early Amplification 2013: Proceedings of the Sixth International Conference* (pp. 97–104). Stäfa, Switzerland: Phonak AG.

Kennedy, C., McCann, D., Campbell, M. J., Kimm, L., & Thornton, R. (2005). Universal newborn screening for permanent childhood hearing impairment: An 8-year follow-up of a controlled trial. *Lancet, 366*(9486), 660–662. doi:10.1016/S0140-6736(05)67138-3

Kuhl, P. K. (2000). A new view of language acquisition. *Proceedings of the National Academy of Sciences, 97*(22), 11850–11857. doi:10.1073/pnas.97.22.11850

Kuhl, P., Conboy, B., Padden, C., Nelson, T., & Pruitt, J. (2005). Early speech perception and later language development: Implications for the critical period. *Language Learning and Development, 1*(3&4), 237–264. doi:0.1080/15475441.2005.9671948

Kuhl, P. Williams, K., Lacerda, F., Stevens, K., & Lindbolm, B. (1991). Linguistic experience alters phonetic perception by 6 months of age. *Science, 255*, 606–608. doi:10.1126/science.1736364

Leonard, L., McGregor, K., & Allen, G. (1992). Grammatical morphology and speech perception in children with specific language impairment. *Journal of Speech and Hearing Research 35,* 1076–1085. doi:10.1044/jshr.3505.1076

Ling, D. (1989). *Foundations of spoken language for the hearing-impaired child.* Washington, DC: Alexander Graham Bell Association for the Deaf.

McGowen, R., Nittrouer, S., & Chenausky, K. (2008). Speech production in 12-month-old children with and without hearing loss. *Journal of Speech, Language, and Hearing Research, 51,* 879–888. doi:10.1044/1092-4388(2008/064)

McIntosh, B., & Dodd, B. J. (2008). Two-year-olds' phonological acquisition: Normative data. *International Journal of Speech-Language Pathology, 10*(6), 460-469. doi:10.1080/17549500802149683

Moeller, M. P. (2000). Early intervention and language development in children who are deaf or hard of hearing. *Pediatrics, 106*(3), 43–50. doi:10.1542/peds.106.3e43

Moeller, M. P., Hoover, B., Peterson, B., & Stelmachowicz, P. (2009). Consistency of hearing aid use with early identified infants. *American Journal of Audiology, 18*, 14–23. doi:10.1044/1059-0889(2008/08-0010)

Morton, C. C., & Nance, W. E. (2006). Newborn hearing screening—A silent revolution. *New England Journal of Medicine, 354*(20), 2151–2164. doi:10.1056/NEJMra050700

Mundy, P., Block, J., Delgado, C., Pomares, Y., Vaughan, A., Van Hecke, A., & Parlade, M. (2007). Individual differences and the development of joint attention in infancy. *Child Development, 78,* 938–954. doi:10.1111/j.1467-8624.2007.01042.x

Reed, M. (1989). Speech perception and the discrimination of brief auditory cues in dyslexic children. *Journal of Experimental Child Psychology, 48,* 270–292. doi:10.1016/0022-0965(89)90006-4

Roush, J. (2000). Implementing parent-infant services: Implementing parent-infant services: Advice from families. In R. Seewald (Ed.), *A sound foundation through early amplification: Proceedings of an international conference* (pp. 159–166). Chicago, IL: Phonak.

Sandall, S., McLean, M. E., & Smith, B. J. (2000). *DEC recommended practices in early intervention/early childhood special education*. Longmont, CO: Sopris West.

Shulman, S., Besculides, M., Saltzman, A., Ireys, H., White, K. R., & Forsman, I. (2010). Evaluation of the universal newborn hearing screening and intervention program. *Pediatrics, 126*(Suppl. 1), S19–S27. doi:10.1542/peds.2010-0354F

Sjoblad, S., Harrison, M., Roush, J., & McWilliam, R. (2001). Parents' reactions and recommendations after diagnosis and hearing aid fitting. *American Journal of Audiology, 10,* 24–31. doi:10.1044/1059-0889(2001/004)

Spencer, P. E. (2004). Individual differences in language performance after cochlear implantation at one to three years of age: Child, family and linguistic factors. *Journal of Deaf Studies and Deaf Education, 9*(4), 395–412. doi:10.1093/deafed/enh033

Stelmachowicz, P., Nishi, K., Sangsook, C., Lewis, D., Hoover, B., Dierking, D., & Lotto, A. (2008). Effects of stimulus bandwidth on the imitation of English fricatives by normal-hearing children. *Journal of Speech, Language and Hearing Research, 51*(5), 1369–1380. doi:10.1044/1092-4388(2008/07-0115)

Stelmachowicz, P., Pittman, A., Hoover, B., & Lewis, D., (2001). Effect of stimulus bandwidth on the perception of /s/ in normal- and hearing-impaired children and adults. *Journal of the Acoustical Society of America, 110*(4), 2183–2190. doi:http://dx.doi.org/10.1121/1.1400757

Stelmachowicz, P. G., Pittman, A. L., Hoover, B. M., Lewis, D. L., & Moeller, M. P. (2004). The importance of high-frequency audibility in the speech and language development of children with hearing loss. *Archives of Otolaryngology, 130*, 556–562. doi:10.1001/archotol.130.5.556

Stika, C. J., Eisenberg, L. S., Johnson, K. C., Henning, S. C., Colson, B. G., Ganguly, D. H., & DesJardin, J. L. (2015). Developmental outcomes of early identified children who are hard of hearing at 12 to 18 months of age. *Early Human Development, 91*(1), 47–56. doi:/10.1016/.earlhumdev.2014.11.005

Stoel-Gammon, C. (1999). Role of babbling and phonology in early linguistic development. In A. Wetherby, S. Warren, & J. Reichle, (Eds.), *Transitions in paralinguistic communication* (pp. 87–111). Baltimore, MD: Brookes.

Swanepoel, D., Störbeck, C., & Friedland, P. (2009). Early hearing detection and intervention in South Africa. *International Journal of Pediatric Otorhinolaryngology, 73*(6), 783–786. doi:http://dx.doi.org/10.1016/j.ijporl. 2009.01.007

Thal, D., & Tobias, S. (1992). Relationships between language and gesture in normally developing and late-talking toddlers. *Journal of Speech, Language, and Hearing Research, 337*, 147–170. doi:10.1044/jshr.3506.1289

Tomblin, J. B., Oleson, J., Ambrose, S. E., Walker, E., & Moeller, M. P. (2014). The influence of hearing aids on the speech and language development of children with hearing loss. *JAMA Otolaryngology-Head and Neck Surgery, 140*(5), 403–409. doi:10.1001/jamaoto.2014267

Tsao, F., Liu, H., & Kuhl, P. (2004). Speech perception in infancy predicts language development in the second year of life: A longitudinal study. *Child Development, 75*(4), 1067–1084.

Walker, E. A., Holte, L., McCreery, R. W., Spratford, M., Page, T., & Moeller, M. P. (2015). The influence of hearing aid use on outcomes of children with mild hearing loss. *Journal of Speech, Language, and Hearing Research, 58*(5), 1611–1625. doi:10.1044/2015_JSLHR-H-15-0043

Walker, E. A., McCeery, R. W., Spratford, M., Oleson, J. J., Van Buren, J., Roush, P., & Moeller, M. P. (2015). Trends and predictors of longitudinal hearing aid use for children who are hard of hearing. *Ear and Hearing, 36*, 38S–47S. doi:10.1097/AUD.0000000000000208

Walker, E. A., Spratford, M., Moeller, M. P., Oleson, J., Hua, O., Roush, P., & Jacobs, S. (2013). Predictors of hearing aid use time in children who are hard of hearing. *Language, Speech, and Hearing Services in the Schools, 44*, 73–88. doi:10.1044/0161-1461(2013/12-005)

Watkin, P., McCann, D., Law, C., Mullee, M., Petrou, S., Stevenson, J., & Kennedy, C. (2007). Language ability in children with permanent hearing impairment: The influence of early management and family participation. *Pediatrics, 120*(3), e694–e701. doi:10.1542/peds.2006-2116

Woods, J., Kashinath, S., & Goldstein, H. (2004). Effects of embedding caregiver-implemented teaching strategies in daily routines on children's communication outcomes. *Journal of Early Intervention, 26*(3), 175–193. doi:10.1177/105381510402600302

Potential Meets Reality in Early Intervention for Children With Hearing Loss

Amy McConkey Robbins

Introduction

This chapter explores issues related to the gaps that currently exist between the technology available to identify babies with hearing loss (HL) at very early ages and the reality of serving those babies and their families in a timely and comprehensive way. I explore these gaps recognizing the monumental progress that has been made in this arena over the last 20 years. It has taken the perseverance, creative use of resources, devoted energies, and the best minds in our field to make universal newborn hearing screening (UNHS) possible in the United States and in many other countries. That UNHS is so widely used is a dream come true for many, including this author. The screening of all infants, though a necessary and momentous first step, was never intended to be the end goal but rather the beginning of a long-term process to ensure communicative competence and, ultimately, improve the quality of life of these children (Bamford, 1998). This is reflected in the term *early hearing detection and intervention* (EHDI), more commonly used than UNHS, and implying a more comprehensive continuum of care.

The challenges clinicians face in serving babies and families after HL has been diagnosed in infancy are formidable. As with any health care movement that involves rapid changes in technology, legislative policies that impact multiple agencies, and urgency for widespread professional education, challenges are inevitable. It is incumbent on those of us working in EHDI to recognize the many ways in which we have succeeded, to acknowledge where we are falling short in our service to babies who are deaf and hard of hearing (D/HH) and their families, and to explore what might be done to manage children and families effectively, even within this gap between the vast potential of early detection of HL and the reality—the gap between "what could be" and "what is."

The Value of Early Screening and Diagnosis of Hearing Loss

The undeniable value of early screening and diagnosis of HL is covered at length elsewhere in this volume and is not repeated here, as this chapter deals primarily with communication intervention after HL is diagnosed. From the standpoint of a speech-language pathologist, I reinforce the importance of EHDI by noting that babies who are identified in the first six months of life and who shortly thereafter receive appropriate early intervention demonstrate substantially better communication outcomes than do later-identified children. (See *Joint Committee on Infant Hearing [JCIH] Year 2007 Position Statement* and *Supplement to the JCIH Statement* [JCIH, 2007, 2013] for extensive references.) Conversely, if HL is not identified and treated early, the consequences to spoken language are detrimental and often irreparable.

The issues in this chapter relate to families who have made an informed choice to value auditory development, who want their children to wear amplification, and who place importance on the development of spoken language, whether through methods of auditory-oral, auditory-verbal, cued speech, or spoken language augmented by manual signs. Issues of families who choose a strictly manual communication approach for their child, or where amplification is not a priority are beyond the scope of this chapter.

Advances in Serving This Population

Considering the tremendous changes over the last decade, we must acknowledge that many improvements have occurred in how babies who are D/HH and their families are served. Such improvements include the fact that hearing screening of newborns is now commonplace, thereby dramatically lowering the average age at which HL is diagnosed:

- many techniques have been designed specifically to assess hearing and fit hearing aids and cochlear implants on infants and toddlers;
- curricula have been published to help early interventionists guide families in developing the baby's communication potential;
- research on brain plasticity provides evidence to families and clinicians of the benefits of early auditory stimulation and the critical time-sensitive windows for auditory cortical development;
- some universities have recognized the need to include early intervention (EI) topics in their students' curricula and practicum;
- the importance of understanding adult learning styles, how they impact EI services, and clinicians' sensitivity to these has been recognized;
- preservice and in-service programs are becoming available so that clinicians who previously served only older children can learn the principles and practices of EI; and
- IDEA, the U.S. federally mandated Individuals with Disabilities Education Improvement Act legislation, stipulates that parents be informed of and offered choices about communication methods, and that they have a voice as full members of the team that writes the Individualized Family Service Plan (IFSP).

All of these actions represent improvement in our efforts to serve very young children with HL and their families.

The Potential of Early Intervention for Babies Who Are D/HH and Families

There is general agreement that the purpose of identifying HL through UNHS is not just to "know early" but to "act early." Extracting key points from the Joint Committee on Infant Hearing (JCIH) Year 2007 Position Statement, we could define "acting early" as diagnosing the hearing loss accurately before age 3 months, fitting appropriate amplification within 1 month of initial confirmation of HL, and providing family-centered early intervention by a clinician knowledgeable and experienced with this population before age 6 months. For purposes of this chapter, the term *early intervention* (EI) is used to mean parent-baby services directed at improving communication skills (i.e., auditory, speech, language and pragmatics). "Parent" also includes grandparents, relatives, guardians, and any caregivers who interact with the child. The term *audiologic management* is used to mean the diagnosis and monitoring of the HL, and the fitting and maintaining of appropriate hearing instruments, recognizing that there can be considerable overlap between the two.

There has been overwhelming success in screening nearly all newborns in the United States, yet the steps that follow this screening in the widely used 1-3-6 month time frame of infant hearing management have a much lower rate of success. This represents one of the first gaps between potential and reality—the technology exists to successfully screen almost all newborns, but at least one third of those who fail the screening do not undergo further evaluation for HL by the recommended 3-month benchmark. In a technical paper (American Speech and Hearing Association [ASHA], 2008c) written by an ASHA working group and commissioned by the Centers for Disease Control and Prevention (CDC), it was noted that various EHDI jurisdictions designate infants and their families who miss the 3-month benchmark for confirmation of HL as "lost to follow-up" or "lost to documentation," without agreement about the definition of those terms. More recently, it has been suggested that these two designations might be combined under the broader heading of "lost to system" (LTS). State EHDI programs are working diligently to reduce the number of LTS infants. Indeed, progress toward this end is being made, with some EHDI jurisdictions reporting impressively low numbers of children who are LTS. Solutions to reducing overall LTS rates are ongoing and described elsewhere in this volume, but it is important to mention the issue here because high LTS rates early in the process create another gap between the potential and the reality of EI, largely due to a cascade effect. Based on national data, at least one third of the children eventually referred for therapy services are behind the recommended schedule (i.e., older than age 6 months) when starting early intervention, in many cases because they did not meet the previous benchmark on time (i.e., confirmation of HL before three months; CDC, 2008).

Early Intervention Begins With the Audiologist

In 1998, as UNHS was just becoming a reality, Bamford (1998) cautioned that

> It is important for us to reestablish in pediatric audiology a wider perspective; there is always a danger that pediatric audiology might be implemented as a narrow health-based discipline in which the outcome measures of importance stop at age of identification and age of HA fitting. (p. 353)

Taking Bamford's broader view of success, not just as the fitting of amplification, the long-term goals of early identification of HL are the child's achievement of communicative competence and enhanced quality of life. Achieving these goals becomes more realistic if pediatric audiologists recognize the important role they play in fostering a baby's communication development during the weeks and months of early confirmation of HL and fitting of amplification. A traditional model of the management of infants with HL would assign this role to early interventionists—speech-language pathologists or deaf educators. However, the foundation that is established by the audiologist during the earliest weeks and months with a family whose baby has an HL often sets the stage for either informed, involved families who have high expectations, or for passive families who struggle with managing their child who is D/HH and with achieving full-time use of amplification in a timely way. If audiologists begin the discussion of communication progress with families, EI can be thought of as overlapping with the fitting of amplification in infants. This is a role some audiologists are willing but unprepared to play, largely because they do not have tools readily available to (a) guide families who are struggling with full-time HA use, and (b) connect such use directly to the development of auditory and spoken language proficiency. Throughout this chapter, suggestions are provided to help audiologists discuss with parents the direct connection between full-time use of amplification and spoken language development.

Features of Early Intervention for Infants With Hearing Loss and Their Families

We have acknowledged that an initial gap exists between the technology available to screen babies at birth and the success rate of confirming HL before age 3 months, and that this creates an additional gap by delaying the age at which a substantial number of infants who are D/HH begin receiving EI. Another gap between potential and reality is covered in detail in the next section: the gap between what have been identified as appropriate EI practices and the actual services many babies who are D/HH and families receive through federally mandated IDEA Part C programs (in the United States, Part C of IDEA governs early intervention services for infants and toddlers with disabilities under age 3 years). Several official documents outline the characteristics of appropriate EI. For example, a position paper from an ASHA Ad Hoc Committee (ASHA, 2008a) addresses recommended practices for speech-language pathologists who conduct EI with infants or toddlers who have disabilities. This document outlines four guiding principles of EI:

1. Services are family centered and culturally and linguistically responsive.
2. Services are developmentally supportive and promote children's participation in their natural environments.
3. Services are comprehensive, coordinated, and team based.
4. Services are based on the highest quality evidence that is available.

As we discover, the EI services many children who are D/HH receive fall short of adhering to one or more of these principles. For some families, there are considerable barriers to receiving EI that approximates the four principles above. Barriers to meeting these four guiding principles are multilayered and differ widely across EHDI jurisdictions. The next section reviews the four principles and provides examples illustrating the barriers some families and clinicians encounter.

Principle 1: Services Are Family Centered and Culturally and Linguistically Responsive

"Family-centered" service has been the term of choice in EI for at least a decade, yet it remains an unattained goal in some cases. An often reported obstacle to family-centered services is that many clinicians were trained in a traditional therapy model and are accustomed to conducting intervention as a "teacher-student" dyad. In a traditional therapy model, interactions are primarily controlled by the clinician, while the parent quietly observes, or in some cases, is not even present in the room. This is in conflict with a family-centered philosophy of EI in which the clinician does not "teach" the baby, but rather models effective communication techniques, coaches, and encourages parents who gradually assume a greater leadership role during sessions. The goal of a family-centered model is that parents naturally incorporate techniques learned in EI to foster good language, speech, auditory, and pragmatic skills with their baby during everyday activities. This shift in philosophy might be difficult for some seasoned clinicians to embrace.

A fundamental feature of "family-centered" EI is that it honors the choice of communication methodology and the goals families have expressed and written in the IFSP. This is also directly related to services being "culturally and linguistically responsive," as culture and language are deeply entwined in the fabric of families. Parents have reported facing multiple barriers to securing EI that are consistent with their communication choice and language. Five common barriers are reviewed herein. First, there might be no clinician in the geographic area who is trained to conduct EI in the communication method chosen by the parents. Second, the family might speak a language other than English, and there are neither clinicians nor interpreters in the geographic area who speak the language, or interpreters are available but the Part C program will not authorize their services. Third, there can be clinicians in the geographic area trained in the chosen communication method, but their caseloads are full and families must wait until a therapy spot becomes available, which might be a matter of 6 months or more. Fourth, highly trained and experienced EI clinicians are available but might not be approved as Part C providers because they conduct primarily center-based EI rather than home-based EI. This will be discussed further as it relates to "natural environment" policies. These four barriers result from the paucity of EI clinicians who are knowledgeable about HL, or fluent in another language, or authorized as Part C providers, relative to the number of babies being diagnosed and referred for EI services.

Communication Bias

The fifth barrier to "family-centered and culturally/linguistically responsive" EI is of a different nature. It relates to the bias toward a particular communication method that might exist among members of the eligibility determination (ED) team that confirms a child's eligibility and authorizes EI services (such teams and their titles vary across states; ED team is used here as a generic term). Professional bias at this level might be overt, with families being told outright that one communication method is superior to others, or it might be insidious, where team members make subtle remarks in verbal or written form that families worry about, find offensive, or begin to internalize. For example, the parents of one deaf toddler receiving Part C services attended her annual IFSP review with their ED team. The parents reported that she had recently received a cochlear implant and was making excellent progress learning to listen with it. An audiologist on the team asked the parents, "Do you realize you have just tethered your child to a fragile technology for the rest of her life?" The mother later reported:

> Clearly this was not a legitimate question but a statement of concern or even opposition about the irreversible choice we had made for our child. My husband and I were not dissuaded by this insensitive and hurtful "question" because we were well-informed when we decided on the cochlear implant, and our decision was reinforced by the amazing changes in our daughter's listening and speech since her initial stimulation. But we were angered to think what effect this insidious question might have had on the confidence level of less secure families attempting to do what they believed was in the best interest of their child.

Communication bias can manifest itself as a failure by professionals to describe the range of options available to families, including support groups or parent advocacy groups consistent with the family's choice. (See Martin, Nicholson, & Hall, 2012, for a review of family decision-making processes and support.) Parents sometimes report that only in hindsight, as they look back at their early experiences with the ED Team and the IFSP, do they realize what they were *not* told. One parent remarked,

> I knew there was a program in the city that taught deaf children using an oral method, but it was never mentioned as an option when the ED team described EI choices to us. Only one option was mentioned and given all-around accolades by the team, so knowing absolutely nothing about deafness, we assumed every child who was D/HH and their parents were taught American Sign Language (ASL) during EI. We enrolled her in ASL EI and followed their recommendation to join an ASL parent-child playgroup at our state school for the deaf. The ED team eventually authorized speech therapy services as well, but recommended a speech language pathologist with no experience or knowledge of HL. Only later, as our daughter was approaching age three and we explored preschool options, did we realize that through Part C, she had been eligible to receive EI from listening and spoken language

(LSLS) certified practitioners, either instead of or in addition to our ASL involvement.

A Therapeutic Alliance on Behalf of the Child

Central to the integrity of a professional who evaluates, authorizes, or conducts EI should be the conviction that parents have a right to know of all the communication options available to children who are D/HH, to make choices for their child, and know that these choices will be honored and supported, even if they are not the same choices the professional would make. For example, a clinician with a strong bias toward listening and spoken language was deeply puzzled by a family's choice to teach sign to their baby and used pressure to dissuade the family from this option, stating erroneously that, "no child who uses sign will ever learn to talk." Such actions clearly violate the spirit of respect for family choice. The ethical, professional code demands that in all of these cases, parent choice must be honored after the family has been informed of all communication options in an unbiased way. A negative and often long-lasting consequence occurs when professionals do not honor parent choice in that the clinician and the family fail to form what has been termed a therapeutic alliance on behalf of the child (ASHA, 2008a; Dinnebeil, Hale, & Rule, 1996). "Therapeutic alliance" (Bordin, 1979), a concept widely used in psychotherapy, is based on collaborative problem solving, accountability, and alignment of purpose. In other words, the parent and clinician know that they are both fully committed to doing everything they can to help a child fulfill his or her potential. Establishing such an alliance with families over time is the platform that makes even difficult conversations civil and productive. Bordin (1979) identified three main elements of a successful therapeutic alliance: agreement on the goals of treatment, agreement on the tasks to achieve those goals, and a personal bond made up of reciprocal positive feelings. The optimal therapeutic alliance is forged when the parent and professional share beliefs with regard to the goals of treatment and view the methods used to achieve these as efficacious and relevant. Such an alliance is required if a child is to benefit from the collaboration between professionals and parents who demonstrate mutual respect and are united in their efforts on behalf of the child.

"Proving" a Child With Hearing Loss Requires Intervention

Another family's experience involved their 2-month-old infant with a moderate-to-severe loss diagnosed after UNHS. During the IFSP process, they expressed their goal that he develop auditory skills, learn to talk, and be mainstreamed in regular school by age 5 years. The EI service offered to the family through Part C was to send a deaf, signing, and nonspeaking adult into their home to conduct EI, accompanied by a reverse oral interpreter. When the family protested that this was not consistent with their communication choice, they were told that although it is known that babies who are D/HH have "language" delays from birth, a "speech" delay cannot be documented until 12 months of age, and therefore the team could not authorize an oral therapist until the child was 1 year old. The team explained that at age 12 months, the baby's speech could be tested and a speech delay possibly "proven." They mentioned that even at that time, there would be a long wait for a provider if the baby did show a speech delay. The family's response was to borrow money from relatives to pay for oral EI for their baby, outside of the Part C program. Although rules for eligibility differ across states, the state in which this family lived considers children immediately eligible for EI services, "if they have a diagnosed medical condition [permanent hearing loss being one of them] that has a high probability of resulting in a delay." The regulations state that children with these medical conditions are eligible for EI even if they are not exhibiting delays at the time of diagnosis. Therefore, a specific "speech" delay should not need to be documented for a child with permanent HL to be eligible for services. The presence of the HL already puts the baby at risk for language, auditory, and speech delays, even in children with mild-to-severe hearing losses (Ambrose, Unflat Berry, Walker, Harrison, Oleson, & Moeller, 2014) much in the same way that clinicians following babies with Down syndrome do not have to "prove" the child will be delayed; the presence of Down syndrome automatically qualifies a child for services.

The JCIH Year 2007 Statement lists as one of the obstacles to successful EHDI implementation the fact that, "Children may not qualify for services before demonstrating language delays (a prevention model versus deficit model)" (p. 23). This document also asserts that, "All families of infants with any degree of bilateral or unilateral permanent hearing loss should be considered eligible for early intervention services" (p. 3). The wait-and-see, failure-based model of intervention has been shown to be ineffective and a disservice to families, going back many decades in the literature. It also is more costly over time, because children who do not begin intervention until a later age make slower progress than those who begin intervention early (Moeller, 2000), take longer to "catch up," require such intervention for a longer period of time, and are more likely to require special education placement rather than typical classroom placement when they begin school.

Principle 2: Services Are Developmentally Supportive and Promote Children's Participation in Their Natural Environments

The first part of this principle, that services be developmentally supportive, faces several obstacles. We have already noted that there is a severe shortage of clinicians who are experienced and knowledgeable about working with babies who are D/HH and their families. The legislation and policies mandating services from birth onward to children with HL were set in place years before an adequate number of clinicians received training and practice in working within an EI context. Because of this severe shortage, some EI services currently are being provided by those with no experience or knowledge of HL, or no experience with children younger than age 3 years. Professionals are hired, despite their lack of experience, because of the mandate to provide EI under Part C. However, doing therapy with a 4- or 5-year-old is very different from working with a 7-month-old and his or her parent(s), regardless of whether the baby has a HL or not. As noted earlier, a shift in intervention philosophy is needed when working with babies. One of the characteristics effective EI clinicians tend to possess is flexibility, given that infants and toddlers have less reliable behavior than older children, will often fluctuate in their compliance, or might spend the entire session sleeping. A creative clinician adequately trained and experienced in EI, recognizes these behaviors as an expected part of working with such young children. A productive session still is entirely possible by abandoning a lesson plan to do something that grabs the baby's attention, or in the case of a sleeping infant, focusing more on parent discussion and information sharing. Robbins (2003) outlines four essential differences between parent-infant EI and traditional therapy and provides suggestions for clinicians who must make adjustments in the way they approach intervention with infants and toddlers with HL.

Natural Environment Policies

The second part of this principle, that services promote children's participation in their natural environments is a well-intentioned goal, given that the purpose of any intervention is to develop skills that carry over into real life. Nonetheless, misguided implementation of the natural environments policy has had negative consequences for many children who are D/HH and families. Increasingly rigid interpretation of "natural environments" has meant that in some EHDI jurisdictions, the location in which EI occurs (i.e., intervention always must take place in the child's home) takes precedence over any other considerations, including a clinician's knowledge and experience, efficient use of the expertise of a limited number of specialists in HL, the conditions within the home environment, and family choice. Some families strongly prefer that EI take place in their home, citing the reduction in stress at having a clinician come to their residence, or the elimination of the hardship of locating transportation to appointments, or the desire to see communication techniques demonstrated in their own home, among others. For these families, no one would argue that home-based EI be available to them (JCIH, 2007). Other families express a preference for center-based services, noting that, as parents, they can give their full attention to their baby and the therapy session when they are not distracted by the frequent interruptions that occur in their home. Some families live in homes that are not conducive to conducting EI for children with HL, such as the case of a multigenerational extended family where the baby who was D/HH and her mother lived with many relatives, including two uncles who worked night shifts and slept during the day, requiring complete silence in the home. A reason cited by some families who prefer center-based EI is the frequent contact available there with other parents who are also raising a child with HL, alleviating a sense of isolation. Some families report that center-based services allow them to observe other children with HL, to see the range of performance and individuality of each child, and to feel optimism at seeing older children who are making good progress. Such contact is also possible for families who received home-based EI, but this involves organizing additional meetings or groups, rather than spontaneous interactions.

No One Solution Fits All Families

Given that there is no research evidence that demonstrates that early intervention with children who are D/HH is more effective if it is conducted in the home rather than in a clinic or other setting (Yoshinaga-Itano, Stredler Brown, & Beams, 2004), it seems logical that different families require different settings for EI, and many families can benefit from a combination of home sessions and clinic sessions. Ultimately, "natural environment" is a *family-centered philosophy* of dealing with parents and their infants, not a definition of the physical space in which intervention takes place. Some have commented that, for an infant in particular, the "natural environment" is wherever the mother [or other caregiver] is.

Another issue that must be considered in relation to "natural environment" policies with children who are D/HH is how we can make the most effective use of the available clinical time of the relatively few trained EI professionals. We have noted repeatedly that there is a severe shortage of EI specialists trained to work with babies who are D/HH. As written in a summary document (Marge & Marge, 2005) from the 2004 Consensus Conference, *Effective Interventions for Infants and Young Children with Hearing Loss*, "In some instances [of early intervention delivery] . . . when the service provider must travel long distances, home visitation may not be practical or financially feasible" (p. 16).

Auditory Conditions in the Child's Home

Experts agree that controlling the auditory environment is critical when a baby is first learning to listen with hearing aids (HAs) or cochlear implant (CIs), but achieving this control might be impossible if a family lives in an apartment complex next to neighbors who play loud rock music during EI sessions, or for a family with four other children who disrupt session, and pull the parent's attention away from the task at hand. The deleterious effects on auditory development of a baby living in a chaotic, noisy environment with constant background auditory "clutter" cannot be overstated. This is an example of a case where a home visit by the EI provider would be critical, to see the characteristics of this family's daily life. By noting the excessive background noise, the clinician could make recommendations about reducing this noise, including educating the family about the negative effects of loud background noise on the baby's communication development, moving the television or video games to another location in the home, engaging one of the other children during EI activities and rotating between sessions so that everyone feels included, or finding quiet, motivating activities for the other children to do on their own during the EI sessions. For long-term productive intervention, this might well be a family that is best served by conducting most sessions at a center where the auditory environment can be controlled and the child's listening skills developed. Just as each family has individual characteristics, so EI solutions should be individualized to meet current best practices and be consistent with parent choice.

It is widely accepted that the goal of intervention is to enable children to participate in their natural environments—that is, in the venues and activities in which nondisabled children participate. However, to say we wish to *promote* learning that will be transferred to the natural environment is very different from saying that intervention must always be *conducted* in the natural environment. An increasing number of formal documents have expressed concern about the overly restrictive interpretation of "natural environment" and have recommended that multiple options be offered to families. For example, under the "Early Intervention section," the JCIH Year 2007 document states that, "the committee recommends that both home-based and center-based intervention options should be offered" (p. 3). In a Fact Sheet approved by the Joint Committee of ASHA and the Council on Education of the Deaf (CED), "Natural Environments for Infants and Toddlers Who Are Deaf or Hard of Hearing and Their Families" (ASHA, 2004), the committee noted that the individual needs of a child should be given considerable weight in the IFSP team's decision about location of services. The document states:

> While the IFSP team is required to justify why services may need to be provided in settings other than a natural environment, ASHA-CED believes the team should not feel compelled to provide an undue burden of justification, *as this would violate the spirit of the requirement that the IFSP be based on the individual needs of the child.* (Sec. 303.340)

Principle 3: Services Are Comprehensive, Coordinated, and Team Based

Providing coordinated rather than fragmented services is often a challenge when children are receiving services from more than one professional or agency, but the problem is compounded in the case of EI with babies who are D/HH. Reasons for this include the ways different states in the United States transition children from the hearing detection program to Part C services, restrictions on agencies sharing information due to the U.S. Family Education Rights and Privacy Act (FERPA) regulations, policies limiting reimbursement for clinical hours spent in team meetings or team conference calls, and the sheer number of children who are D/HH who receive a variety of therapies from different clinicians. The latter reflects the fact that approximately 40% of children with hearing loss also have at least one other disability (Mitchell & Karchmer, 2011; Parrish & Roush, 2004), meaning that almost half of children who are D/HH will require EI services from two or more clinicians. Many clinicians do not have training or experience in working with children who are D/HH with complex needs and must rely on a team of experts from different disciplines for guidance.

Co-Treatment of Children With Complex Needs

Published literature and clinical experience suggest that an excellent way to provide coordinated, team-based services, particularly to children with complex needs, is to co-treat a child. Using this model, two clinicians work together for a few sessions to share with each other techniques and expertise in their respective areas. This author has had the experience of working with a child with both HL and vision impairment (VI), and learned valuable information over a period of three joint sessions from the VI therapist. Her input changed how I positioned the child in therapy and taught me to utilize the limited vision he had to its fullest potential. Conversely, the VI therapist was unaware of the value of full-time HA use or the amount of residual, aidable hearing the child had. In three sessions together, she was amazed at the power of audition to connect this child to his environment, to give him the security of knowing his parents were near by the sound of their voices, and to provide access to musical experiences. As a result of teaming for just three sessions, she became an advocate for this child's full-time use of HAs and incorporated many listening techniques into her EI with him.

Principle 4: Services Based on the Highest Quality Evidence That Is Available

A glaring barrier to meeting this principle within EI is the shortage of clinicians qualified, experienced, and knowledgeable about working with babies who are D/HH and their families. As previously noted, some clinicians providing EI do not have even basic training working with children who are D/HH and do not have familiarity with current literature that would guide evidence-based practices. Because Part C programs cannot locate a sufficient number of clinicians trained to provide EI to babies who are D/HH and families, many of the clinicians serving this population have no experience with issues of communication choice, the impact of hearing loss on language development, how hearing aids or cochlear implants work, or techniques to achieve full-time device use in the home. This is a cause of great concern, considering that the JCIH (2007) statement asserts that, "The key component of providing quality EI service is the expertise of the provider specific to HL" (p. 17). This assertion is borne out by published research studies (Moeller, 2000; Yoshinaga-Itano et al., 1998).

Early Intervention and Qualified Providers

The reality of the shortage of qualified providers became apparent to a family whose baby with identified hearing loss was authorized to receive speech-language EI services. After an exhaustive search, the family discovered that all the trained Part C EI clinicians in their geographic area had caseloads with a 6- to 9-month waiting list. As an alternative, the Part C program authorized a developmental therapist to visit the home on a weekly basis, in spite of the fact that the child had no disabilities except HL. (*Developmental therapist* is a generic term, varying across jurisdictions, which refers to persons providing "general" EI. Persons labeled as developmental therapists span the continuum from clinicians highly knowledgeable about children with developmental disabilities to former second-grade teachers who do not have experience with either special needs children or family-centered EI. Developmental therapists with no EI experience are required to work under the direct supervision of a credentialed developmental therapist for 12 months, although in many cases the supervisor has no expertise or experience with children who are D/HH, hearing aids or other issues relevant to this population.) The family, fully self-educated about the importance of acting early, decided to pay privately for EI from a speech-language pathologist specialized in HL and to receive Part C services from the developmental therapist.

The baby's mother noted that the developmental therapist was kind and nurturing but could offer no guidance on issues specific to HL. The developmental therapist was amazed that the baby wore his HAs full-time within a few weeks after fitting, as a result of sessions with the private SLP. The developmental therapist asked the mother to give her tips on how she might help her other families with babies who were D/HH achieve this. The mother was distressed to learn (a) that this developmental therapist was the primary EI provider for families of babies who were D/HH, given that she admitted having no training or knowledge of this area; and (b) that the babies who were D/HH and being followed by the developmental therapist were all inconsistent users of amplification even after extended periods of time, largely because the developmental therapist was not familiar with the techniques to achieve this goal. Given that this was not her area of expertise, the developmental therapist was unfamiliar with the research literature regarding the powerful influence of early auditory experiences that HAs and CIs provide, how brain development is changed when babies receive consistent auditory input at early ages, and how young an age was meant by "early." All these factors combined to unintentionally deny the babies who were D/HH in this therapist's practice access to services that met even basic standards of care, much less were evidence based.

Families as the Source of Some Barriers

The sources of some of the barriers found in EI service provision are created by the families of children who are D/HH themselves. Even in a perfectly planned program, clinicians report family related challenges that are daunting and discouraging. A few illustrations of such challenges are given not as a comprehensive list but as examples of a much broader set of challenges, and they include the following:

- Families do not show up for scheduled appointments or are not home when clinicians have traveled long distances to conduct EI at a child's residence.
- Personal family conflicts interfere with the delivery of EI, such as when divorced parents cannot agree upon services for their child or when a baby is at the father's home when the clinician arrives at the mother's home for the scheduled EI session.
- Parents fail to follow through with suggestions provided by the EI clinician, causing the child's communication progress to plateau.
- Parents experience prolonged periods of anger or resentment after the diagnosis, treating the EI clinician with hostility in a "blame the messenger" scenario, or become depressed to the point of requiring mental health care.
- Families do not have a predictable schedule for their child who is D/HH, with regular routines for meals, bathing, and bedtime. Without these routines, which are essential for babies to feel secure in their world, there are often concomitant problems with behavior and compliance.
- Families question the presence of an HL in their baby or doubt the benefit provided by the HAs. This has been shown to occur more often in parents whose children have milder degrees of hearing loss (Moeller, Hoover, Peterson, & Stelmachowicz, 2009; Walker, Spratford, Moeller, Oleson, Ou, Roush, & Jacobs, 2013).

Under these conditions, the chances of success in achieving full-time HA use are severely compromised. The clinician will need to reevaluate various supports and information that can be important for the family to have including creative ways to characterize hearing loss for different parents. Studies on variations across adult learning preferences suggest that professionals should be cognizant of these variations and flexible enough to accommodate different parent learning styles (Martin et al., 2012). In addition, terms such as *mild* and *moderate* can cause parents to underestimate the impact of hearing loss on development, whereas simulations of these degrees of loss allow parents to experience the sensory impairment themselves (Haggard & Primus, 1999). Audiologists should be familiar with the most common emotional reactions and challenges of hearing aid use that parents self-report (Munoz, Olson, Twohig, Preston, Blaiser, & White, 2014).

Summary of Barriers Within EI Service Provision

In the sections above, some of the barriers that contribute to the gap between "what could be" and "what actually is" in the provision of EI services for babies who are D/HH and their families were reviewed. Though these barriers differ across jurisdictions and individual families, some common themes reappear. These are

- inadequate number of early interventionists with expertise in hearing loss, relative to the number of babies being identified and referred for EI services;
- regulations within Part C that create roadblocks or prevent clinicians from providing state-of-the-art EI;
- interpretation of certain regulations, particularly those related to "natural environments" that constrain the EI services available and create disincentives for experienced clinicians to become Part C providers and limit parent choice;
- failure of some ED teams or other EI professionals to provide families unbiased information about the range of communication options available to babies with HL; and
- barriers that originate within the child's home or family that limit the child's auditory or language progress. Chief among the latter is the lack of full-time HA use by some babies with HL.

Full-Time Device Use— A Disconnect?

Let us consider the last point mentioned above, that of failure to achieve full-time HA use, even among some early identified infants. Because early interventionists vary so greatly in their knowledge of HAs and their ability to advise families about a baby's acceptance of amplification, audiologists become fundamental partners in this critical aspect of EI: achieving full-time HA use. The reasons for lack of full-time HA use result from a number of different factors that we have already mentioned, and certainly differ widely. However, for some families, there might be a disconnect between our explanation of highly technical, computer-generated test results (i.e., auditory brainstem response [ABR], auditory steady-state response [ASSR], otoacoustic emissions [OAEs], and real-ear hearing aid verification) and the parent's understanding of hearing loss and importance of full-time use of HAs, thereby undermining the potential of EHDI to mitigate the detrimental effects of HL on communication development.

Traditionally, many audiologists included parents as part of the audiologic assessment. Rather than presenting technically complex graphic results obtained with limited parent input, the child was often tested in a sound booth, seated on a parent's lap. During testing the audiologist would periodically query, "Mrs. Jones, do you think Johnny heard that last sound?" The parents became a part of the assessment team and developed ownership and belief in the test results. With newborn infant hearing assessment, a natural shift occurred to a reliance on technology (i.e., ABR, OAE), with the unfortunate consequence of a dramatic reduction in parent involvement in the assessment process. Similarly, digital hearing aid verification procedures, such as on-ear speech mapping and simulated on-ear measurements utilizing real-ear-to-coupler differences (RECDs) and prescriptive targets, are wonderful tools that are technologically superior for predicting speech audibility than traditional pure tone–aided audiograms obtained in the sound booth. These new measurements represent "good science." Unfortunately, these technologies that more accurately assess the appropriateness of the hearing aid's programming do not automatically improve parents' understanding of hearing aid benefit. On the contrary, it is not uncommon in this authors' experience for parents to come away from real-ear verification appointments with several printouts and no understanding of what the testing showed or what the printouts mean. From the standpoint of being user friendly, a traditional audiogram with aided and unaided results made sense to parents; they could clearly see the difference between what their child heard with and without HAs. In addition, most parents sat in the sound booth while their child was tested and actually experienced the intensity levels of the presentation stimuli. This involvement in the testing made their child's hearing loss real to them.

One Parent's Story

A mother of a 4-year-old child with bilateral severe sensorineural hearing loss explained her experience this way:

> Billy's dad and I certainly believed the ABR results that confirmed he had a significant HL at 3 months of age and intellectually understood the importance of aiding him right away. But the reality of HL and the value of his HAs didn't truly sink in for us until a few months later. That's when he sat on my lap in the sound booth, and I watched his responses to sound without his HAs, and then while wearing them. The difference was so dramatic that I re-committed myself to ensuring Billy always had access to sound via his HAs. Over time, I became familiar with audiograms and could explain Billy's HL to others by showing them the difference between his aided and unaided results. This was especially important because early on, his grandparents didn't seem to believe he had a HL; they kept saying he looked so "normal." They certainly didn't grasp the importance of the HAs and didn't insist he keep them in during his frequent visits with them. It was only after I showed and explained the audiogram to them that they became "believers" in the importance of HAs and were firm about the rule that he always wear them. After a few predictable but unsuccessful attempts to test limits about this rule, Billy complied with full-time HA use at his grandparents' home. It has never been an issue since then.

This mother continues,

> Recently, Billy completed real-ear verification testing and in contrast to booth testing, I felt completely removed from the process of whatever they were assessing, which actually was unclear to me. Upon completion, I was given a paper with squiggly lines accompanied by techno-jargon with which I was unfamiliar. As the audiologist pointed to various marks on the graph and pronounced the aids appropriate for Billy, I began to feel the knowledge I thought I had about Billy's hearing sucked right out of me. I sensed I knew less now than I had before! I pondered a question in my mind for a long time after the real-ear speech mapping was performed, "How do I gain access to what those test results really mean for Billy and his listening skills with hearing aids?"

This is a poignant question for a parent to pose and one that deserves a frank answer. Although no one would advocate returning to an inferior technology, such as relying exclusively on aided audiograms, we might wonder how a better balance could be achieved between the use of newer, more accurate assessment technologies and ensuring that parents understand those assessment results as well as they understood aided audiograms. Is there a user-friendly protocol for graphically displaying the results of such tests as real-ear verification that clearly communicates the findings to parents or nonaudiology colleagues? Clearly, no professional intentionally sacrifices a parent's comprehension of test results, yet if parents come away from testing confused and unsure about the value of HAs, we might be setting into motion a chain of events that leads to an undervaluing of HAs by the parents, and more difficulty achieving full-time amplification in early identified babies. This possibility is supported by data from Munoz et al. (2014) and Moeller (2007) showing that an alarmingly high percentage of parents of early identified babies struggle to achieve full-time HA use, even over an extended period of time. In fact, when the children in the Moeller study were 24 to 28 months of age, only five of 14 (36%) early identified children had achieved use of HAs during all waking hours. This finding was replicated in the Munoz et al. (2014) study in which only 35% of parents reported that their toddler (mean age = 22 months) wore hearing aids during all waking hours. As asserted by McCreery, Walker, and Spratford (2015), "The benefits of amplification are only achievable if children wear hearing aids consistently." Although the causes of part-time use in these infants are likely multifaceted, we could hypothesize that the type of assessment used and the way results were shared with families might be contributing factors.

The Two Owners of Test Results

Is it possible that with the advent of newer and more accurate technologies, our profession has thrown the baby out with the bath water? Have we abandoned aided testing in the sound booth completely? Perhaps a combination of assessments is the most pragmatic approach, given that hearing test results have two "owners." The first owner is the audiologist, who interprets the test information to make the most accurate diagnosis and provide the best care on the baby's behalf. This first owner finds real-ear verification measures to be the superior technique. But, there is a second "owner" of test results—the parents—and it might be appropriate to utilize aided audiograms focusing on speech stimuli in the booth, not in place of real-ear measures but in addition to them, to be certain that parents understand the results and the enormous benefits of full-time amplification to their baby's development.

To summarize, the development of more accurate technology to confirm hearing loss does not automatically transfer to better ability to convey the results to parents or to nonaudiology colleagues, such as early interventionists. This represents an additional gap between potential and reality: the difficulty clinicians encounter in translating highly technical test results so that parents can understand and believe the results. If doubt remains in parents' minds about whether their baby really needs to wear HAs full time, the "therapeutic alliance on behalf of the child" might take a long time to develop, or might never be an alliance that has mutual trust and confidence at its core.

The Amplification-Communication Connection: A Three-Phase Program for Audiologists

Audiologists who treat a baby with newly diagnosed HL typically focus on the critical jobs of verifying the degree of HL and fitting HAs as early as possible. The pediatric audiologist is often the professional with whom the parents have the most contact in the early period following diagnosis of HL. (See Smith & Wolfe, 2015, for a review of the most common questions parents pose.) In that capacity, audiologists have the potential to establish with parents a foundation that fosters communication development in their child with HL. If this foundation is established convincingly, progress during the subsequent stages of EI and educational placement can be highly effective. Conversely, if parents do not understand the direct connection between the consistent, full-time use of HAs and the role they, the parents, play in nurturing communication development, the speech and language achievement of even early identified babies can be adversely affected. For more information about the program outlined below, see Robbins (2002, 2007). The Three-Phase program described here encompasses the period immediately following diagnosis of HL in babies. The time frame for this period might be only a few weeks or might last up to 6 months, a point when all babies and their parents should be enrolled in an ongoing EI program with an experienced and knowledgeable therapist. As we have noted, unfortunately, this is one of the goals of EHDI that is not yet a reality for every family. Even after an EI program is established, the audiologist often has more knowledge and experience with HL than the EI provider. Thus, the audiologist remains an integral part of the child and family's support team.

Three Phases and Their Goals

The three phases within the program are as follows: Phase I starts at diagnosis and lasts until the first fitting of HAs (often loaners); Phase II encompasses the early weeks after the initial fitting of amplification; Phase III begins after HA adjustment and tapers, but does not end when the baby and family are enrolled in an EI communication program. The audiologist's role in giving input related to communication development differs at each of the three phases, largely because the emotional status, needs, and processing capabilities of parents change over time. Families respond to the news of deafness in a variety of unique ways, yet there are some common reports parents have given. These reports often tell of a sense of helplessness or despair families felt as they waited for upcoming appointments, after receiving the diagnosis of HL. These parents have reported their desire to *do* something, to take action that would help their child rather than simply waiting for the next audiology appointment. In these cases, it is important to give parents some tasks on which to focus so they feel empowered to have a positive effect on their child's communication. Receiving this news from the audiologist is essential. Some parents later lament that the audiologist handled issues of hearing and the HAs but deferred questions of communication to the speech-language pathologist or other early interventionist whom the parents did not meet until weeks or months later. Importantly, if the audiologist treats the HAs as a domain separate from communication, families might not make the connection that the full-time use of amplification is the foundation of auditory and spoken language progress.

Because parents of newly identified babies are likely to best retain information if it is presented in both oral and written forms (Munoz et al., 2014), audiologists are advised to accompany their verbal discussion of the communication goals with a printed sheet that reviews this information. A handout version of the goals at each of the three stages entitled "Journey with Hearing Loss" appears in the following figures. Hearing health care professionals might assume it is self-evident that HAs and communication development are inextricably linked, though data reviewed in this chapter and clinical experience suggest that parents of babies who are D/HH might not recognize that link unless it is explicitly and repeatedly explained.

Phase I

At Phase I (Figure 35–1), caution is advised in supplying too much technical information, as many parents experience disbelief, grief, and a sense of being overwhelmed at the time of diagnosis. This is a period when parents require time to absorb the news and react emotionally. If professionals are uncomfortable responding to parents' emotional reactions in Phase I, they might inadvertently utilize the counterproductive "technical jargon" or "hit and run" approaches (Hersch & Amon, 1973) with families. Feedback from parents suggests that these approaches often leave families feeling lost and powerless to effect change in their child with HL. At Phase I, audiologists will, of course, review the hearing test results and respond to the many questions parents ask at this stage. A sense of optimism can be conveyed to families if the audiologist also reviews the communication goals on the Phase I, Journey with Hearing Loss, handout (see Figure 35–1).

Phase II

When families come for the initial HA fitting at Phase II, our first communication advice is an equipment issue, where the audiologist gives the family multiple opportunities to become familiar with the HAs. Giving the parents Handout II at this time (Figure 35–2) will serve as a reminder to cover these points, knowing that the audiologist has much to accomplish in the limited appointment time. But, at this appointment, both parents, not just one, should repeatedly practice opening the battery door, inserting the battery, and manipulating other parts of the HA. The majority of parents have never held a HA in their hands, much less tried to insert a tiny earmold in the ear of a 6-week-old baby. Demonstrating putting the aid in, then letting both parents practice at least twice can make the difference at this stage. The author has had initial EI sessions with babies who have already had several audiology appointments, including HA fitting, but whose families do not know how to change the battery, struggle to the point of frustration to insert the earmold, or have one parent who feels incapable and always defers to the other parent to handle the HAs. This point is mentioned, not as a criticism of audiologists, but as a reminder that practice makes perfect. To save time during audiology appointments, families can practice inserting the HAs and changing batteries while the audiologist is engaged in other tasks.

Professional standards dictate that we approach each family about the importance of full-time HA use with sensitivity to their unique situation and coping skills.

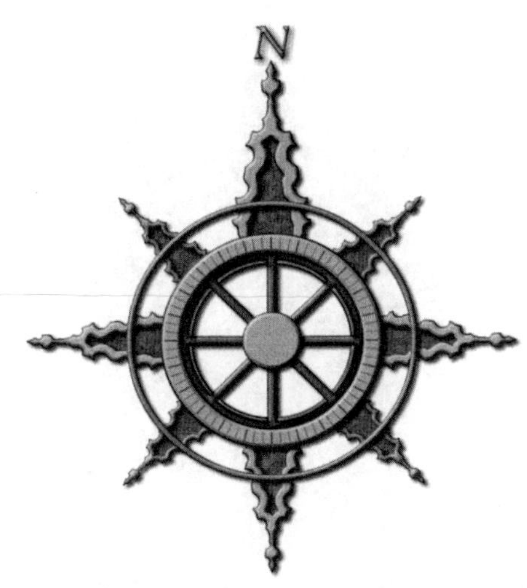

The Journey with Hearing Loss – Phase I

Lifetime Goals

Be confident! You can and will master what you need to know about raising a child with hearing loss.

Have high expectations! Your child can and will achieve much if you expect that he or she can do much.

Develop autonomy and responsibility! Your child can and will grow up to be an independent and responsible person.

Here are three things you can do right now to reach these lifetime goals:

1. **Continue to talk to your child.** Speak close to your child's face and use plenty of facial expression.

2. **Write down your thoughts and feelings in your journal.** You can also write down any questions you might have for the audiologist or teacher so you can remember to ask them.

3. **Sign up for the home correspondence course through the John Tracy Clinic.** (800-522-4582 or www.johntracyclinic.org)

FIGURE 35–1. Handout to use during Phase I with families of newly diagnosed babies. (Adapted from Robbins, A. M. [2002]. Empowering parents to help their newly diagnosed child gain communication skills, *Hearing Journal*, *55*[11], 55–59.)

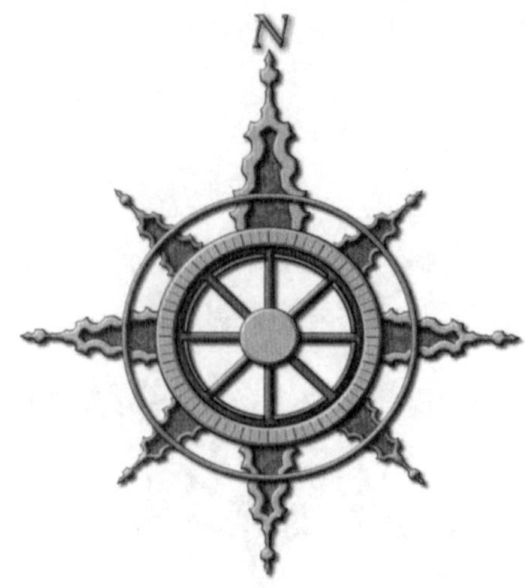

The Journey with Hearing Loss – Phase II

Lifetime Goals

Be confident! You can and will master what you need to know about raising a child with hearing loss.

Have high expectations! Your child can and will achieve much if you expect that he or she can do much.

Develop autonomy and responsibility! Your child can and will grow up to be an independent and responsible person.

Here are four things you can do right now to reach these lifetime goals:

1. **Use a hearing aid calendar to record when your child is wearing the hearing aids.** You can record your child's responses to sound, any equipment problems or questions you have for the audiologist or teacher.

2. **Use your child's name with a purpose.** It's important for your child to know his name. Make sure you are calling your child's name for a *reason*, not just to see her response.

3. **Help your child become aware of important sounds in your home.** Use a hand-to-ear response at home when sounds occur. When you hear something your child should attend to, say "I hear that!" or "Listen" and put your hand to your ear.

4. **Pay attention to the sounds your child makes.** As your child learns to use sound, she will become aware of how to use her voice to get your attention. Your child will learn to recognize sounds in your home. Use your journal to record changes in your child's responses. Writing them down will be helpful for you, your audiologist and your teacher.

FIGURE 35–2. Handout to use during Phase II with families of newly diagnosed babies. (Adapted from Robbins, A. M. [2002]. Empowering parents to help their newly diagnosed child gain communication skills, *Hearing Journal*, *55*[11], 55–59.)

It is also important that we convey how common it is for families to struggle with device use, a struggle that will likely vary as a function of age, situation, and emotional state (Walker et al., 2013). If the data from Munoz et al. (2014) and Moeller (2007) are representative of the larger group of children with HL, this is a discouraging trend. However, it remains unknown whether audiologists are explicitly making the connection for families early and often, as in, "Your baby needs full-time HA use if her brain's auditory centers are to develop fully." Some families can be given this information repeatedly, provided with appropriate support and techniques and still elect not to insist on full-time HA use. But if families have never been told, gently but bluntly, that listening development depends on the baby having consistent and dependable auditory input all day long, how do we expect them to figure this out?

Providing parents with real-life examples creates a mental snapshot that can be worth a stack of pamphlets or research articles. I have shared with parents the importance of consistent auditory input for their baby by relaying stories such as,

> I worked with a 4-year-old boy whose parents did not insist on full-time HA use when he was first fitted as an infant, because he went through phases of pulling them out or whining when they were inserted. When he behaved this way, his family allowed him to leave the HAs out, not recognizing that all babies will pull the aids out and require reinsertion, and most babies will whine at HA insertion until the parents get very adept and swift with the process. The parents hoped the baby's full-time use would happen naturally as he got older. On the contrary, as the baby became a toddler, the harder it was to change the "rule" that had been established. That rule, unintentionally reinforced, was that the child, not his family, was in control of the HAs. A child who fails to achieve full-time device use within 3 months of initial fitting is at high risk for ongoing power struggles over the HAs for years to come, as was this 4-year old boy.

The clinician should express optimism to parents that, with the team's support, their child's full-time HA use is achievable.

Phase III

At Phase III (Figure 35–3), the audiologist should gently but thoroughly query the parents about HA adjustment and hours of daily use. It is particularly important at this interval to remind the family that the earlier a baby accepts HAs and wears them full time, the sooner the benefit and the more consistent the auditory input to the baby's brain. Toward that end, the audiologist can provide assistance only if the family feels secure enough to honestly report HA adjustment problems. If asked, "Katy is wearing her HAs full-time, isn't she?" parents might feel a sense of failure at admitting that Kathy is not wearing the HAS full-time. Techniques for probing families about full-time use must be sensitive to the family's desire to please the professionals or the family's embarrassment at not achieving full-time use. Horton (personal communication, August 30, 2008) suggests some nonthreatening ways to gain an accurate picture of a child's HA use. These suggestions include asking parents the following:

- "When was the last time you changed the battery in Sally's HA?"
- "How comfortable is Dad (or the child-care provider or other significant person) with inserting the HAs?"
- "Tell me about situations when Sophie doesn't wear her HAs." (This gives parents "permission" to provide an honest report.)
- "When do you get the most resistance from Sophie about wearing her HAs?" (This implies that all babies show some resistance.)
- "What problem with Sophie's HA use could I help you most with today?"

Resources for Families Struggling With Full-Time Hearing Aid Use

When parents report challenges or frustrations with their baby's acceptance of HAs, an array of resources is available to support families in working toward the goals of full-time use of amplification. Recall that findings from Walker et al. (2013) and Moeller et al. (2009) suggest that young children of different ages present different kinds of challenges. Suggested resources include the following:

- Printed or video materials are available that discuss HA adjustment issues unique to infants and toddlers. Parent-friendly suggestions are found in the first several lessons of the "Listen Around the Clock" section of Rossi's (2003) parent-infant program. Rossi gives many practical examples of how a baby benefits from full-time device use and emphasizes that a baby's listening development is jeopardized if full-time use is not established.
- Samples of products designed specifically to keep a baby's HAs in place are available, such as special

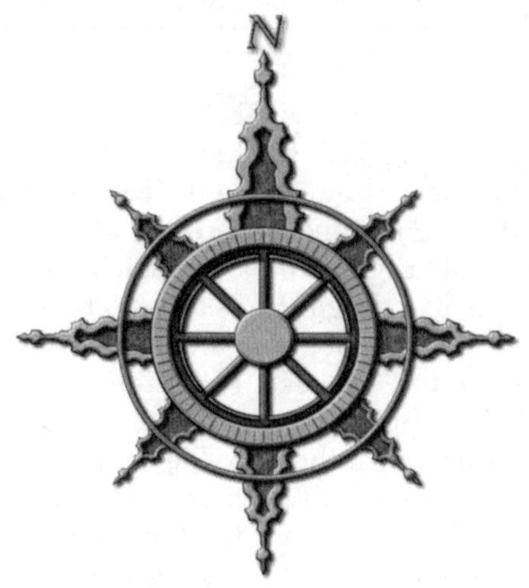

The Journey with Hearing Loss – Phase III

Lifetime Goals

Be confident! You can and will master what you need to know about raising a child with hearing loss.

Have high expectations! Your child can and will achieve much if you expect that he or she can do much.

Develop autonomy and responsibility! Your child can and will grow up to be an independent and responsible person.

Here are three things you can do right now to reach these lifetime goals:

1. **Imitate the sounds your child makes.** Babies and young children enjoy playing with sounds and love to use them to communicate to you.

2. **Help your child put meaning to sound.** For example, if you've been playing "How Big is (your child's name)? SOOOO Big!" with your child face-to-face, try to get the same response from your child when standing behind him.

3. **Choose a few sounds in your home that will help your child learn.** Many children love to hear the telephone ring, the dog bark, a musical instrument playing or someone knowing at the door. When you hear one of those sounds, make a big deal about it with your child.

FIGURE 35–3. Handout to use during Phase III with families of newly diagnosed babies. (Adapted from Robbins, A. M. [2002]. Empowering parents to help their newly diagnosed child gain communication skills, *Hearing Journal*, *55*[11], 55–59.)

clips and some styles of bonnets or caps. The website http://www.babyhearing.org has photos and descriptions of many available products to keep hearing aids on little ears. Information on the website is available in both English and Spanish.

- A dedicated weekly HA calendar is useful, on which parents record the number of hours of HA use each day, as well as pertinent information about equipment problems, baby's resistance to putting HAs on, or problems pulling them out. Parents might also note whenever their child responds to sounds, and the nature of the response, such as a startle, cessation of activity, or eye widening. Some studies suggest that parents consistently overestimate HA use time in their babies when compared to data-logging within the devices themselves. However, there is still value in encouraging parents to be good observers and reporters of all aspects of their child's hearing aid use and auditory behaviors. Families can bring the calendar to audiologic appointments to discuss HA use and problems.
- Baby seats that are conducive to HA use and fully support an infant's trunk and upper body without any padding across the back of the head are available. This contrasts to most infant seats or high chairs where the baby's head rests back on a surface, often causing the HAs to move out of position or to be pulled out by the baby.
- Data logging is a feature built into most current HAs that allows clinicians and families to keep track of actual use time.
- A wealth of resources is available on Karen Anderson's website: http://www.successforkidswithhearingloss.com, including simulations of varying degrees of hearing loss for parents.
- An invaluable source of support can be found in advice from other families who are able to share real-life tips about things that have worked with their babies. Experiences of many parents can be found in the "Parent to Parent" section of the website: http://www.babyhearing.org

To complete the visit at Stage III, the *Journey with Hearing Loss* handout can be reviewed and given to parents, focusing on the child's developing communication skills through listening. Families should be advised that another fundamental reason to establish full-time HA use quickly is to ascertain whether HAs provide adequate access to spoken language. If they do, we expect to see certain positive changes in the baby's speech and listening behaviors. If not, the family should know there are other options, including educational ones, such as visual communication (sign language or cued speech), and medical ones (cochlear implantation).

The Power of Parental Influence

Parents continue to have powerful influence over their child's communication development, long after Stage III when they are enrolled in an ongoing intervention program. Moeller et al. (2007) cite statistics from Dunst (2001) that indicate that 2 hr per week in therapy make up only 2% of a normal-hearing toddler's waking hours, whereas everyday activities such as diapering and feeding occur at least 2,000 times before the first birthday. This statistic is a convincing statement about the power of families to influence, positively or negatively, their child's communication after HA fitting. Parents who take advantage of only 10 interactions each waking hour of a child's day will have provided more than 36,000 teachable moments between ages 1 and 2 years (Moeller et al., 2007). Consider the lost opportunity if the child is not wearing amplification during these interactions. If this is case, are audiologists and other hearing health care professionals emphasizing this fact to parents repeatedly? If families are struggling over time with HA compliance, Horton (personal communication, August 30, 2008) suggests providing additional stories that demonstrate the detrimental effect of inconsistent HA use. She has shared with families in her EI practice this example of a 4-year-old boy with moderate-severe hearing loss who said, "My parents smarter than me. When we makin' microwave popcorn, it ready every time them open the door! But when I open it, popcorn sometimes ready and sometimes not. Them is lucky!" This story makes the point that first, this 4-year-old has delayed syntactic development as a result of inconsistent auditory input via HAs, particularly because grammatical morphemes in English are often at the ends of words and are acoustically subtle. For example, without HAs, the child did not hear the difference between "it ready" and "it's ready." The second point is that children must hear a grammatical form hundreds of times before they begin to use it. Suppose half of this child's exposure to those forms occurred when he was not wearing HAs; his mastery would be slower than that of a child with similar loss who wore HAs full-time, or might never occur. Finally, the story shows parents that, without full-time HA use, the child did not hear the microwave buzzer often enough to associate it with food being ready. He never made the connection that his parents knew the popcorn was ready because they heard a buzzer go off, erroneously interpreting this as luck.

Parents' Most Important Decisions

Audiologists can offer a realistic optimism to families that has a lasting effect on the attitude and coping skills of parents. Moeller and Condon (1998) have noted that most of the decisions parents are required to make after diagnosis relate to communication mode, amplification, and educational choices. But, they suggest that professionals reinforce that the most important decision parents will make are not these technical ones, but rather (1) the decision to have high expectations for their child; (2) the decision to give the child autonomy and responsibility; and (3) the decision to be confident in their ability to parent a child with a hearing loss. These decisions are so fundamental that they are included at the top of each of the handouts in Figures 35–1 through 35–3 to remind families they are capable of handling the difficult but rewarding task of raising their baby who is D/HH.

Cochlear Implants Provide Another Viable Intervention Option

The now common option of providing cochlear implants to profoundly deaf babies has far-reaching implications for EI services and the qualifications of EI providers. Although the topic of early cochlear implantation is too extensive to cover here, the reader is referred to Chapters 29 and 30 in this volume. In almost every instance in which "hearing aids" have been used in this chapter, the words *cochlear implants* could be substituted. That is, issues of full-time device use, knowledge, and experience of the clinician, valuing of family choice, parent understanding of test results, and the need for urgency in treatment to take advantage of sensitive periods of development, are as applicable to babies who receive cochlear implants as to those who wear HAs. Due to the vast body of published literature demonstrating the effectiveness of early cochlear implantation, families should be made aware of this treatment option during discussions of communication and educational choices.

A Review of the Gaps Between Potential and Reality

This chapter has described some of the gaps that currently exist between the potential and the reality of EI services for infants with HL and their families. Readers will recognize that none of these gaps exist in isolation; rather they are interrelated, forming a web of challenges facing our profession:

- Almost all newborns are screened for HL with the primary goals of early diagnosis and HA fitting, EI services, and subsequent competence in communication; yet at least one third of newborns needing further audiological evaluation before age 3 months are lost to the system (LTS).
- Children who are LTS experience a chain reaction of delays—their HL is not confirmed through diagnostic evaluation by age 3 months, causing them to miss the next goal of enrollment in Part C EI before age 6 months.
- A substantial number of infants with confirmed hearing loss are not fitted with HAs within 1 month of diagnosis, as recommended by JCIH (2007).
- Once babies are fitted with HAs and families are enrolled in Part C intervention, the services they receive might not meet professional standards of care.
- Clinicians providing EI encounter system roadblocks and family circumstances that limit the effectiveness of their intervention.
- The technologies used to more accurately assess hearing and to confirm HA benefit in children might not yield results that are easily interpreted by some parents and therapists.
- Though babies are identified at young ages, a substantial number might not wear HAs on a full-time basis; this undermines one of the primary goals of infant hearing screening—providing access to sound to ensure communicative competence.

Finding Solutions and Closing the Gaps

Acknowledging the gaps that exist between what is and what could be brings us to the ongoing work of closing these gaps. Early in this chapter we cited some positive advances toward improving our services to babies who are D/HH and families. Some of these are mentioned again as they directly relate to improving the quality of EI that professionals provide:

1. An urgent need exists to rapidly increase the number of specialists trained to provide EI to babies who are D/HH and their families. Current action to address this need includes the following:
   - University training programs in audiology, speech-language pathology, and deaf education

have begun to include EI coursework or practicum in their curriculum so that students graduate with some basic knowledge in this area. Some programs provide the option of obtaining an "emphasis" in EI.

- For clinicians who have already completed college degrees, a range of continuing education options are available to learn about (a) EI practices and (b) children with HL. Beginning with those that involve short-term commitments, there are 1-hour online courses or multiple hour "virtual conferences" offered through such agencies as ASHA, hearing aid companies, and cochlear implant manufacturers.

2. Clinicians conducting EI require materials specifically designed for babies who are D/HH and their parents. A key ingredient to successful EI with children who are D/HH is the use of developmentally appropriate materials. Fortunately, excellent resources are available for this population.
   - Rossi's "Learn to Talk Around the Clock Toolbox" (2003) has step-by-step lessons that are user friendly, even for early interventionists who lack extensive experience with HL. An accompanying videotape demonstrates the Signature Behaviors that parents learn to use with their child who is D/HH to enhance listening and spoken language.
   - A second program by Rossi (2007) is written specifically for child-care providers. "Learn to Talk Around the Clock at Childcare" addresses a need that has existed for a long time because a considerable number of babies who are D/HH spend most of their waking hours with a child-care provider, not with their parents. Though parent education remains our primary focus, materials written for child-care providers require a different level of complexity and a realistic approach to the amount of time the provider can give any one child. Rossi's child-care lesson kits come with colored bracelets, each of which is a reminder to child-care providers of a skill they should target that day.
   - The John Tracy Correspondence Course free home lessons (http://www.johntracyclinic.org) can be accessed anywhere in the world and give parents a sense of empowerment as they observe their baby's progress.
   - The Cottage Acquisition Scales for Listening, Language and Speech (CASLLS) help clinicians monitor progress in children who are D/HH and select communication goals that are developmentally appropriate (http://www.sunshinecottage.org). Other materials from this website incorporate Learning-to-Listen sounds and the concept of Listening Age.
3. Support from other parents is needed by families of newly identified babies who are D/HH.
   - State chapters in the United States of the Guide-by-Your-Side program (http://www.handsandvoices.com) of Hands and Voices helps families make connections with other families of children who are D/HH and encourages mentoring of families with newly identified babies by experienced parents.
   - The website, http://www.babyhearing.org, and its Spanish version, "La Audicion de mi Bebe," has a vast array of information and resources including quotes from parents who reflect on their experiences with their child who is D/HH.
4. Professionals working with infants who are D/HH require training about presenting unbiased options to families. Day-long workshops and other materials from such groups such as Hands and Voices (http://www.handsandvoices.org) address issues of discussing communication options with parents of children who are D/HH in an unbiased and family centered manner.
5. Government agencies need feedback from clinicians and parents whose lives are directly affected by EHDI and Part C Policies:
   - Grassroots and organizational pressures are needed to influence the ways in which Part C policies are interpreted, particularly those related to natural environments and the qualifications of those who provide EI services for infants with HL.
   - The National Center for Hearing Assessment and Management (NCHAM), Utah State University, has resources and data available on their extensive website (http://www.infanthearing.org) that cover all aspects of EHDI, including legislative mandates and public policies.
6. The development of user-friendly ways to translate highly technical hearing test results for parents should be a priority. The best technology is only as good as the parents' belief in its validity and their subsequent commitment to full-time HA use. Newer, more precise measurements of hearing are questionable leaps forward if families understand less about their child's HL and cannot easily recognize the benefit provided by HAs. Audiologists report a desire for training in how to counsel families, including how to explain test results to parents (Harrison & Roush, 2002), yet most university programs in audiology offer limited coursework on the

principles and techniques of counseling. "Counseling" within the context of managing infants and families should not be viewed as a separate service but as an approach to conveying information, providing support, and listening to families that is infused into ongoing clinical services. An excellent resource about the audiologist's roles in counseling is the Guidelines for Counseling document (ASHA, 2008b).

7. Continued funding for research is imperative to further explore such topics as brain plasticity, sensitive windows for cortical development, and evidence based clinical practices. Results from research studies should inform clinical procedures so that professionals provide intervention consistent with best practices. Conversely, clinical reports and dilemmas help frame the questions that lead investigators in new research directions.

Conclusion

There is a maxim in quantum physics, "When you change the way you look at things, the things you look at change." Change for the better is within our profession's grasp but is not guaranteed. The same level of energy and commitment of resources that brought UNHS into existence against many odds must be mustered if we are to improve EI services as dramatically as UNHS changed early identification of HL. This becomes a requirement that we "change the way we look at things" by taking a different perspective, both individually and collectively, altering the way we look at what we do. This requirement is a call, not just to examine the relatively small realm of our own specialized role in serving babies who are D/HH and their families, but to view the entire EHDI system broadly, and to recommit ourselves to moving "what is" ever closer to "what could be."

Acknowledgment. The author wishes to thank Amy Birath and Julia Renshaw for providing helpful input to the author.

References

Ambrose, S. E., Unflat Berry, L., Walker, E., Harrison, M., Oleson, J., & Moeller, M. P. (2014). Speech sound production in 2-year-olds who are hard of hearing. *American Journal of Speech-Language Pathology, 23*, 91–104.

American Speech Language Hearing Association (ASHA; 2004). *Fact sheet. Natural environments for infants and toddlers who are deaf or hard of hearing and their families. Joint committee of ASHA and CED*. Retrieved August 16, 2010, from http://www.asha.org/policy

American Speech Language Hearing Association (ASHA; 2008a). *Ad hoc committee. Roles and responsibilities of speech-language pathologists in early intervention: Technical report*. Retrieved May 20, 2015, from http://www.asha.org/policy

American Speech Language Hearing Association (ASHA; 2008b). *Guidelines for audiologists providing informational and adjustment counseling to families of infants and young children with hearing loss birth to 5 years of age*. Retrieved from http://www.asha.org/policy

American Speech Language Hearing Association (ASHA; 2008c). *Working group. Loss to follow-up in early hearing detection and intervention programs: Technical report*. Retrieved May 10, 2015, from http://www.asha.org/policy

Bamford, J. (1998). Early identification . . . what then? In F. Bess (Ed.), *Children with hearing impairments: Contemporary trends* (p. 353). Nashville, TN: Vanderbilt Bill Wilkerson Press.

Bordin, E. S. (1979). The generalizability of the psychoanalytic concept of the working alliance. *Psychotherapy, 16*, 252–260.

Centers for Disease Control and Prevention (CDC; 2008). *Summary of 2006 national EHDI data*. Retrieved July 21, 2008, from http://www.cdc.gov/ncbddd/ehdi/data.htm

Consensus Conference. (2004). *Effective interventions for infants and young children with hearing loss*. September 10–12. Washington, DC: Author.

Dinnebeil, L. A., Hale, L. M., & Rule, S. (1996). A qualitative analysis of parents' and service coordinators' descriptions of variables that influence collaborative relationships. *Topics in Early Childhood Special Education, 16*, 322–347.

Dunst, C. J. (2001). *Parent and community assets as sources of young children's learning opportunities*. Asheville, NC: Winterberry Press.

Haggard, R. S., & Primus, M. A. (1999). Parental perceptions of hearing loss classification in children. *American Journal of Audiology, 8*, 83–92.

Harrison, M., & Roush, J. (2002). Information for families with young deaf and hard of hearing children: Reports from parents and pediatric audiologists. In R. C. Seewald & J. S. Gravel (Eds.), *A sound foundation through early amplification: Proceedings of the second international conference* (pp. 233–249). Stäfa, Switzerland: Phonak AG.

Hersch, B., & Amon, C. (1973). An approach to reporting the diagnosis of hearing loss to parents of a hearing-impaired child. In J. Northern & M. Downs (Eds.), *Hearing in children* (pp. 167–170). Baltimore, MD: Williams & Wilkins.

Joint Committee on Infant Hearing (JCIH; 2007). Position statement: Principles and guidelines for early hearing detection and intervention programs. *Pediatrics, 120*, 898–921.

Joint Committee on Infant Hearing of the American Academy of Pediatrics. (2013). Supplement to the JCIH 2007 position statement: Principles and guidelines for early intervention after confirmation that a child is deaf or hard of hearing. *Pediatrics, 131*(4), e1324–e1349. doi:10.1542/peds.2013-0008

Marge, D., & Marge, M. (Eds.). (2005). *Report and recommendations for the 2004 national consensus conference on effective educational and health care interventions for infants and young children with hearing loss.* Syracuse, NY: SUNY Upstate Medical University.

Martin, P., Nicholson, N., & Hall, C. (2012). Family support in early hearing detection and intervention (EHDI) systems. *Perspectives on Hearing and Hearing Disorders in Childhood, 22*(1), 11–21.

McCreery, R. W., Walker, E. A., & Spratford, M. (2015). Understanding limited use of amplification in infants and children who are hard of hearing. *Perspectives on Hearing and Hearing Disorders in Childhood, 25*, 15–23.

Mitchell, R. E., & Karchmer, M. A. (2011). Demographics and achievement characteristics of deaf and hard of hearing students. In M. Marschark & P. Spencer (Eds.), *The Oxford handbook of deaf studies, language and education* (Vol. 1, 2nd ed.). Oxford, UK: Oxford University Press.

Moeller, M. P. (2000). Early intervention and language development in children who are deaf and hard of hearing. *Pediatrics, 106*(3), e43. Retrieved August 16, 2010, from http://www.pediatrics.org/cgi/cntent/full/106/3/e43

Moeller, M. P., & Condon, M. (1998). Family matters: Making sense of complex choices. In F. Bess (Ed.), *Children with hearing impairment, contemporary trends.* Nashville, TN: Vanderbilt Bill Wilkerson Press.

Moeller, M. P., Hoover, B., Peterson, B., & Stelmachowicz, P. (2009). Consistency of hearing aid use. *American Journal of Audiology, 18*(1), 14–23.

Moeller, M. P., Hoover, B., Putman, C., Arbataitis, K., Bohnenkamp, G., Peterson, B., . . . Stelmachowicz, P. G. (2007). Vocalizations of infants with hearing loss compared to infants with normal hearing. Part I: Phonetic development. *Ear and Hearing, 28*(5), 605–627.

Munoz, K., Olson, W. A., Twohig, M. P., Preston, E., Blaiser, K., & White, K. R. (2014). Pediatric hearing aid use: Parent-reported challenges. *Ear and Hearing, 36*, 279–287.

Parrish, R., & Roush, J. (2004). When hearing loss occurs with other disabilities. *Volta Voices, 11*(7), 20–21.

Robbins, A. M. (2002). Empowering parents to help their newly diagnosed child gain communication skills. *Hearing Journal, 55*(11), 55–59.

Robbins, A. M. (2003). Communication intervention for infants and toddlers with cochlear implants. *Topics in Language Disorders, 23*, 16–33.

Robbins, A. M. (2007). Monitoring communication progress in early intervention. In R. Seewald & J. Bamford (Eds.), *A sound foundation through early amplification 2007: Proceedings of the fourth international conference* (pp. 95–105). Stäfa, Switzerland: Phonak AG.

Rossi, K. (2003). *Learn to talk around the clock.* Washington, DC: A. G. Bell.

Rossi, K. (2007). *Learn to talk around the clock at childcare.* Omaha, NE: Learn to Talk Around the Clock Products.

Smith, J., & Wolfe, J. (2015). Anticipate families' most common hearing healthcare questions. *Hearing Journal, 68*(4), 22, 23, 26, 28.

Walker, E. A., Spratford, M., Moeller, M. P., Oleson, J., Ou, H., Roush, R., & Jacobs, S. (2013). Predictors of hearing aid use time in children with mild-to-severe hearing loss. *Language, Speech, and Hearing Services in Schools, 44*, 73–88.

Yoshinaga-Itano, C., Stredler Brown, A., & Beams, D. (2004). *Evidence-based programming for infants and young children with hearing loss.* Paper commissioned for Consensus Conference: Effective interventions for infants and young children with hearing loss, September 10–12. Washington, DC.

36

Support for Adolescents With Hearing Loss

Kris English

Introduction

Developmental experts tend to use the onset of puberty as the starting point for adolescence. The end of adolescence is harder to define and will reflect cultural values but typically is considered to be the end of the teenage years (Blakemore, 2008). As to the experiential nature of adolescence, there is overall agreement with Ginott's (1969) observation of adolescence as a "period of curative madness, in which every teenager has to remake his personality. He has to free himself from childhood ties with parents, establish new identification with peers, and find his own identity" (p. 25).

This period of "curative madness" requires adolescents to manage the stress of change on many fronts: personal and physical, emotional and social. These stressors take a toll on self-confidence, self-efficacy, and self-esteem (Robins & Trzesniewski, 2005; Figure 36–1). When teens also live with the additional challenge of hearing loss, their pediatric audiologists should be part of their support system during the transition to young adulthood.

This chapter will review adolescent development from two perspectives: *psycho-emotional* and *cognitive*. Psycho-emotional concerns are intentionally presented first to emphasize the "gatekeeping" impact of emotions on thinking and problem solving. Simply put, intense emotions prevent us from learning; if a patient is emotionally distraught, information cannot be processed (Goleman, 2005). We waste precious time on patient education when emotions, even if unexpressed, are the primary concern. Our ability to help adolescents express their thoughts and feelings could make all the difference in our overall effectiveness, and therefore must be addressed first.

Summaries of these two perspectives will conclude with recommendations for the audiologist's role, and a set of support strategies. Throughout, the themes of *development* and *counseling* will be integrated; as teens work their way through the developmental milestones of adolescence, we want to be available to support their transitions with supportive counseling expertise.

Psycho-Emotional Development

What's Going On?

Whether it occurred recently or long ago, pediatric audiologists should occasionally revisit our own teen years and the emotions we experienced at that time. Looking back, we can remember difficult moments of mortification, confusion, mood swings, and feeling misunderstood or unaccepted. Because time gives perspective, we might shrug off the memories as "typical teen drama." But rather than distance ourselves from those memories, it is helpful to view them as a necessary set of experiences; by doing so, we enhance our ability to empathize with our patients' experiences.

Like all acquired skills, developing "emotional intelligence" (Goleman, 2005) is a process and includes these stages:

- knowing one's own emotions (self-awareness);
- managing emotions (shaking off bad moods, self-restraint);
- motivating oneself (delaying gratification, controlling impulsivity);
- recognizing emotion in others (empathy); and
- handling relationships (managing emotions in others).

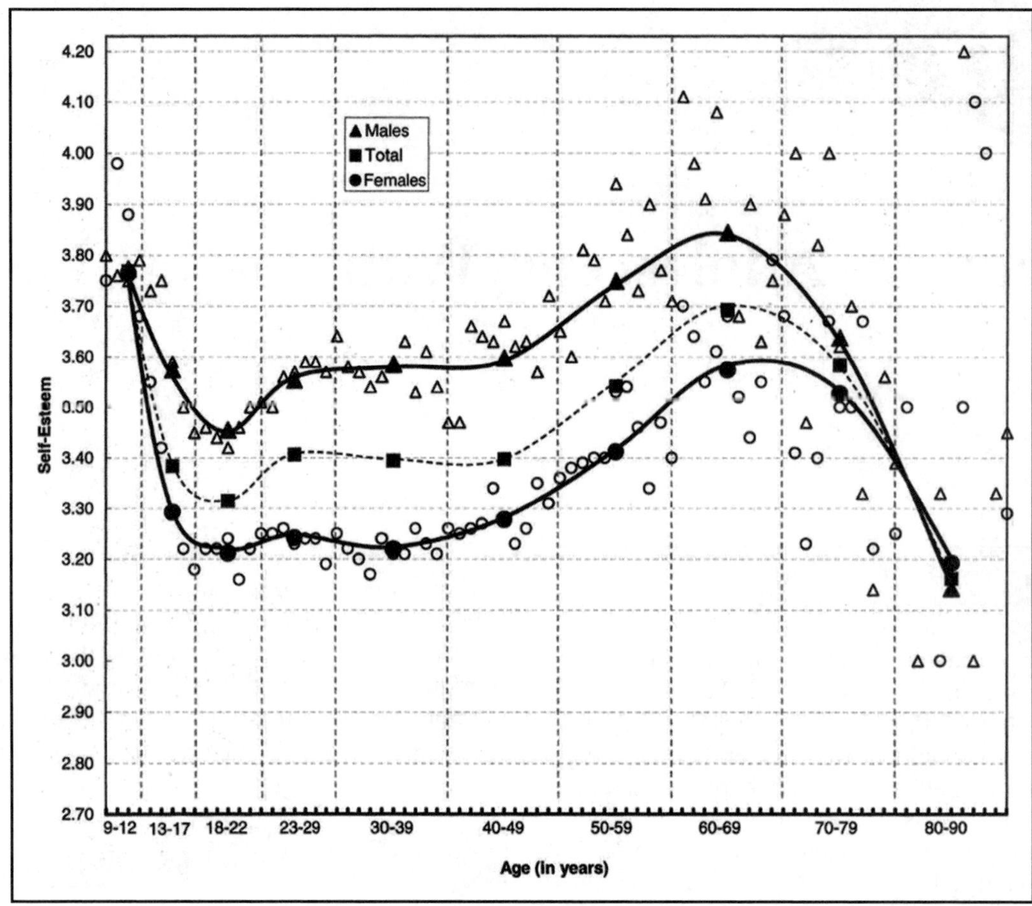

FIGURE 36–1. Mean levels of self-esteem across the life span. When children enter their teen years, their sense of self-esteem is deeply affected, females more than males, according to the Single-Item Self-Esteem Scale: "I see myself as someone who has high self-esteem." (N = 326,641). (From Robins, R.W., Trzesniewski, K. H., Tracy, J. L., Gosling, S. D., & Potter, J. [2002]. Global self-esteem across the lifespan. *Psychology and Aging, 17*, 428. Copyright © 2002 by the American Psychological Association. Reprinted with permission.)

These stages are building blocks, but the process is not strictly linear or time-locked, which is one reason why adolescence can be a turbulent time. Some teen patients struggle with the first-stage skill of self-awareness. (To explore this topic further, see Suggested Learning Activities at the end of the chapter.) Other teens can usually manage their emotions, but temporarily revert because of social pressures. Much depends on temperament and a positive history in handling adversity, of course, so some teens are already "mature for their age" in the areas of empathy and relationships.

How Emotions Affect Cognition

As teens mature as emotional beings, they of course are also developing as thinkers. However, these are not independent processes. Damasio (2005) has summarized several years of neurological research to explain the relationship between emotions and cognition, providing valuable insights regarding effective patient interaction.

It has long been established that reasoning, problem solving, and evaluating/storing new information (i.e., *thinking*) is a function of the brain's frontal cortex. However, before this kind of high-level analysis can occur, all new input is first processed by the amygdala, serving as the "gatekeeper" to the frontal cortex. The amygdala first analyzes the potential of threat: Am I in danger? Is this going to hurt me? Is this something that I don't understand? If threat is perceived, the amygdala triggers a release of adrenaline, which increases respiration rates and blood pressure (i.e., the classic physiological stress response called "flight or fight"). We experience this stress as a range of emotions, including shock, fear, and anger, or milder reactions such as disappointment or uncertainty.

Importantly, during these moments, access to the frontal cortex is effectively blocked. Although we might feel obligated to press on with explanations or recommendations, the information is not reaching our intended destination (the listener's frontal cortex). For the time being, survival (physical or psychological) takes precedence, and our listener functions more as an emotional being and less as a thinker.

The amygdala is still developing during the teen years. Combined with hormonal changes, emotional responses during the teen years can be intense experiences.

Implications: Risk of Communication Mismatch

Goleman (2005) reports that we generally use both our "thinking mind" and "feeling mind" throughout the day; however, depending on circumstances, one will take precedence over the other. To communicate effectively with our teen patients, we are challenged not only to determine which "mind" they are using at any given point, but also to respond appropriately. Simply put, we should strive to *match our response* to a patient's "mind"—that is, provide information to a request for information with information, and provide emotional support to a request for emotional support.

This simple logic apparently is not as easy as it sounds. For instance, Ekberg, Grenness, and Hickson (2014) found that although most patients in their study expressed a range of emotional concerns, their audiologists usually did not address them, resulting in a "communication mismatch." Related studies show that when patients feel unheard, they are less likely to follow our recommendations, resulting in poorer patient outcomes (Adams, Cimino, Arnold, & Anderson, 2012; Grenness, Hickson, Laplante-Levesque, Meyer, & Davidson, 2015). It takes practice and constant monitoring to ensure that we are "on the same page" at any given moment. Communication mismatch can have serious consequences and will described in the next section.

The Audiologist's Role

Teens' emotional development can be supported with adult conversation, especially when the conversation means "teens talk more; adults talk less." However, audiologists anecdotally report frustration and awkwardness when communicating with teen patients, likely because we have not anticipated how to gradually shift our conversation from parent to patient. To that end, we might keep this advice in mind:

> Adolescents will not simply "open up" to adults on demand. Effective communication requires that an emotional bond form, however briefly, between the professional and the adolescent. Professionals must find a way to relate comfortably to adolescents, and be flexible enough to accommodate the wide range of adolescents they are likely to encounter. And, professionals must recognize that developing effective communication with the adolescents with whom they work requires effort on their part. It might take a number of sessions of nonjudgmental listening to establish the trust needed for a particular adolescent to share with an adult what he or she is thinking and feeling. It might take even longer before an adolescent feels comfortable asking an adult for help with an important decision. (American Psychology Association, 2002, p. 3)

The skills described above are directly related to understanding the differences between the "thinking mind" and "feeling mind" discussed earlier. If we are not paying attention, we are likely to "mismatch" our response (Ekberg et al., 2014; English, Rojeski, & Branham, 2000). This mismatch most often occurs when teens describe *how they feel*, whereas our response indicates *what we think*. This mismatch is often a result of training, wherein we are prompted to give information to demonstrate to our supervisor that we indeed know specific information. However, teen patients are not our supervisors; a different audience needs a different approach. Consider the following example.

Dialogue #1

Teen: *I'm going to stop using the FM in school. I hate it and besides, I hear fine without it.*

Audiologist: *I highly doubt that. Your classrooms are bound to be very noisy, and you've mentioned before that you prefer to sit in the back of the classroom.*

In this exchange, the teen expressed *how she feels*, and the audiologist replied with *what he thinks*. We can easily imagine the teen's reaction: resentment, annoyance, and closing down to any further conversation. A "matched" response would have actively addressed the "feeling mind," such as, "You hate it?" Audiologists can learn to avoid communication mismatches by "raising their antenna" to listen at a deeper level to the subtext, and then respond with reflective comments that invite more conversation (Clark & English, 2014).

How do we prevent mismatches? When in doubt, address both possibilities. After providing information, step back and ask the patient about the emotional components of the comment.

Dialogue #2

Teen: *I'm going to stop using the FM in school. I hate it and besides, I hear fine without it.*

Audiologist: *I highly doubt that. Your classrooms are bound to be very noisy, and you've mentioned before that you prefer to sit in the back of the classroom. (Stops, recognizes the mismatch). But . . . more importantly, I didn't know you hate the FM system.*

Teen: *It's a hassle, and people make jokes about the mic.*

Audiologist: (avoiding temptation to problem solve the "hassle"): *They're teasing you?*

Teen: *Not in a mean way, more like they are bored and looking for something to talk about. I just don't want it to be about me.*

Audiologist: [nods head]

Teen: *Kids just do that, you know? But if there was a different a way to manage the mic . . .*

Audiologist: *Have you thought of any possibilities? We could brainstorm . . .*

Dialogue #2 did not take much more time than Dialogue #1 (perhaps 20 s longer), and yet it resulted in a different, more productive outcome. The audiologist recognized the emotion in the comment and invited the teen to expand. The teen perceived that the audiologist accepts whatever she has to say, and we learn that although she wanted to vent a little, she was not especially angry or upset. When the audiologist indicated that he trusts the teen, the teen in turn considered trusting the audiologist. When the teen felt understood and accepted, she signaled a readiness to shift to problem solving.

Caveat: Professional Boundaries

Audiologists must be especially sensitive to their role in this kind of audiologic (nonprofessional) counseling (Kennedy & Charles, 2001). Although it is quite appropriate to provide counseling support for the expected challenges associated with hearing loss, at all times we must be cognizant of our professional boundaries, and also stay alert for "red flags" when a referral to a professional counselor is needed. For instance, living with hearing loss involves many typical challenges, such as the experience of not realizing someone was talking. However, similar experiences can require different responses on our part. Compare these two reports:

- "It's really embarrassing when the teacher calls on me for an answer, but not knowing because she didn't look at me."
- "My stepfather gets really angry when I don't hear him talking from another room. Last week he hit me because he thought I was deliberately ignoring him."

We know instinctively that the second comment requires expertise beyond our scope of practice. Our work settings must have policies to guide us through a referral process whenever we have even a doubt about a patient's safety and well-being (Stone & Olswang, 1989).

Support Strategies

As mentioned earlier, adolescents should not be expected to "open up" to adults on demand. Fortunately, there are several resources available to help the audiologist get the conversational ball rolling. When we employ joint attention on a teen's self-report, for instance, conversations can flow naturally. The teen will likely disclose some challenges on the self-report, and by inviting more details, the audiologist effectively joins the teen's ongoing thought processes.

This approach has many advantages, including (a) giving the audiologist a familiar starting point, (b) giving the teen conversational control, and (c) helping the audiologist understand the teen's life in a meaningful way. Two applications to this approach are described in the following sections.

Self-Assessment of Communication: Adolescents (SAC-A)

A tool specifically designed for this purpose is called the *Self-Assessment of Communication—Adolescents* (SAC-A; Elkayam & English, 2003). This instrument, found in Figure 36–2, was adapted from an adult version (Schow & Nerbonne, 1982) and purposefully stays true to the spirit of the original by addressing more than situational listening challenges (classrooms, etc.).

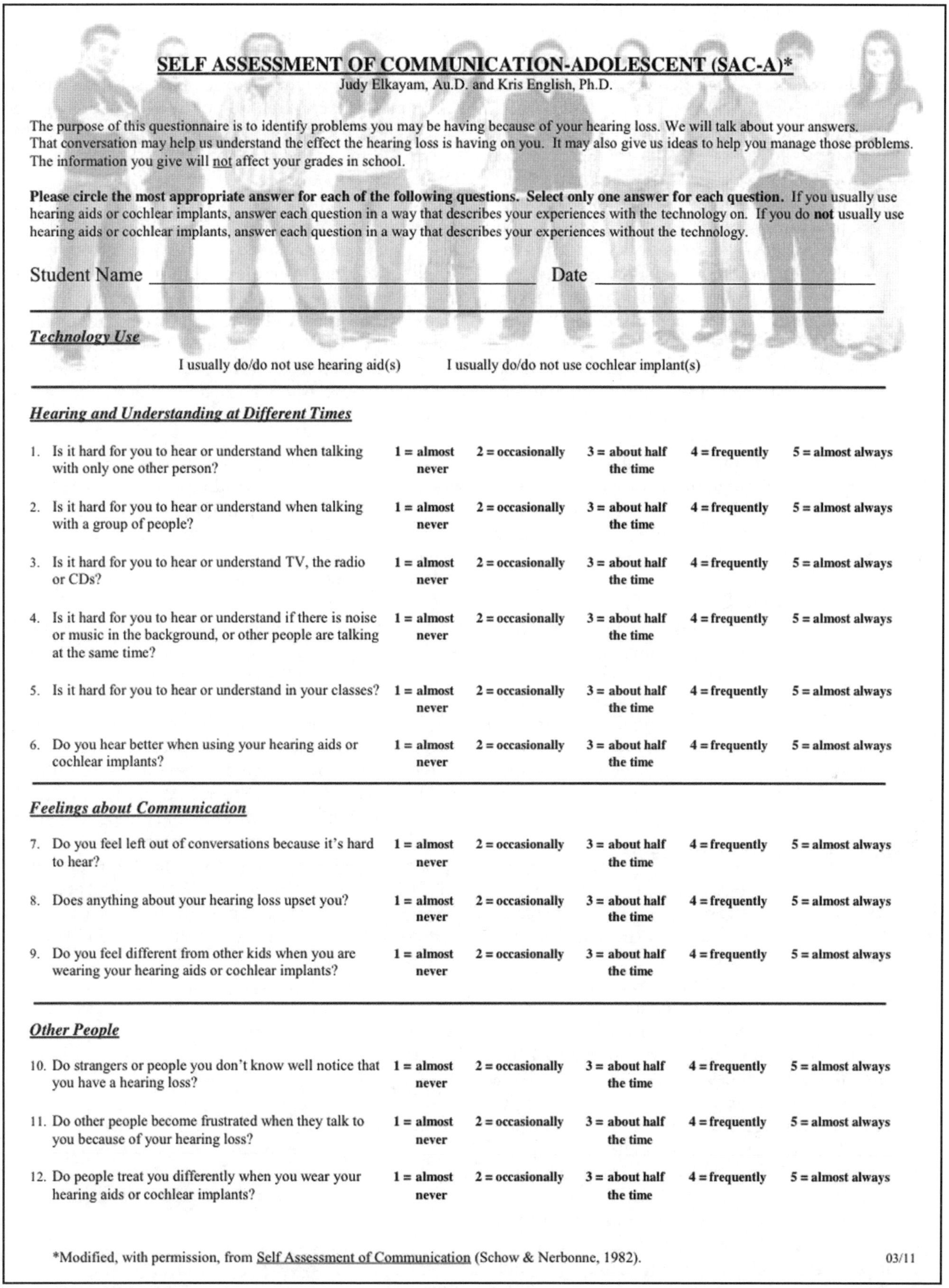

SELF ASSESSMENT OF COMMUNICATION-ADOLESCENT (SAC-A)*

Judy Elkayam, Au.D. and Kris English, Ph.D.

The purpose of this questionnaire is to identify problems you may be having because of your hearing loss. We will talk about your answers. That conversation may help us understand the effect the hearing loss is having on you. It may also give us ideas to help you manage those problems. The information you give will not affect your grades in school.

Please circle the most appropriate answer for each of the following questions. Select only one answer for each question. If you usually use hearing aids or cochlear implants, answer each question in a way that describes your experiences with the technology on. If you do **not** usually use hearing aids or cochlear implants, answer each question in a way that describes your experiences without the technology.

Student Name ______________________________ Date ____________________

Technology Use

I usually do/do not use hearing aid(s) I usually do/do not use cochlear implant(s)

Hearing and Understanding at Different Times

1. Is it hard for you to hear or understand when talking with only one other person?	**1 = almost never**	**2 = occasionally**	**3 = about half the time**	**4 = frequently**	**5 = almost always**
2. Is it hard for you to hear or understand when talking with a group of people?	**1 = almost never**	**2 = occasionally**	**3 = about half the time**	**4 = frequently**	**5 = almost always**
3. Is it hard for you to hear or understand TV, the radio or CDs?	**1 = almost never**	**2 = occasionally**	**3 = about half the time**	**4 = frequently**	**5 = almost always**
4. Is it hard for you to hear or understand if there is noise or music in the background, or other people are talking at the same time?	**1 = almost never**	**2 = occasionally**	**3 = about half the time**	**4 = frequently**	**5 = almost always**
5. Is it hard for you to hear or understand in your classes?	**1 = almost never**	**2 = occasionally**	**3 = about half the time**	**4 = frequently**	**5 = almost always**
6. Do you hear better when using your hearing aids or cochlear implants?	**1 = almost never**	**2 = occasionally**	**3 = about half the time**	**4 = frequently**	**5 = almost always**

Feelings about Communication

7. Do you feel left out of conversations because it's hard to hear?	**1 = almost never**	**2 = occasionally**	**3 = about half the time**	**4 = frequently**	**5 = almost always**
8. Does anything about your hearing loss upset you?	**1 = almost never**	**2 = occasionally**	**3 = about half the time**	**4 = frequently**	**5 = almost always**
9. Do you feel different from other kids when you are wearing your hearing aids or cochlear implants?	**1 = almost never**	**2 = occasionally**	**3 = about half the time**	**4 = frequently**	**5 = almost always**

Other People

10. Do strangers or people you don't know well notice that you have a hearing loss?	**1 = almost never**	**2 = occasionally**	**3 = about half the time**	**4 = frequently**	**5 = almost always**
11. Do other people become frustrated when they talk to you because of your hearing loss?	**1 = almost never**	**2 = occasionally**	**3 = about half the time**	**4 = frequently**	**5 = almost always**
12. Do people treat you differently when you wear your hearing aids or cochlear implants?	**1 = almost never**	**2 = occasionally**	**3 = about half the time**	**4 = frequently**	**5 = almost always**

*Modified, with permission, from Self Assessment of Communication (Schow & Nerbonne, 1982). 03/11

FIGURE 36–2. Self-Assessment of Communication—Adolescents.

Its 12 questions do not take much time to answer, but once shared, the audiologist-teen dyad can approach topics that might not have been brought up otherwise.

For example, Joseph, age 14 years, has been Dr. Beecham's patient for over 10 years. Joseph has experienced a growth spurt and now is taller than Dr. B. The audiologist recognizes a need to shift her conversations from parent to patient but is unsure how. At the next appointment, she asks Joseph to independently complete the SAC-A in the waiting room, and then asks to look at it when all gather in the consult room. She notes the wide range of responses: Questions 1 through 6 do not indicate any concerns, but for Question 8 (Does anything about your hearing loss upset you?), Joseph circled, "almost always." To make sure she does not break any trust, the audiologist waits until Joseph is in the testing booth, and before hearing aids are removed, asks, "Your answer about your hearing loss bothering you . . . is that something we could talk about with your mother present?" Joseph replies, "Yes. I'd like my folks to know how hard things can be. We never talk about it."

Questionnaires and scales such as the SAC-A are by definition closed-set queries, but the responses to those queries can serve as a springboard for open-ended conversations. All the while, the topics themselves are focused on hearing loss, keeping us within our scope of practice. If additional problems are revealed, we know how to refer for professional counseling support. See Resources at the end of the chapter for more suggestions.

Screening for Bullying Problems

Teens face many challenges, but one that can directly impact personal health and safety is the problem of bullying. Although bullying has always been a concern, it is now a topic receiving national attention. The Centers for Disease Control and Prevention indicates that in the United States, one in three children reports being bullied, and that children who have disabilities are up to three to four times more likely to be bullied than children with no disabilities (Banks, Kendall, Banks, & Gover, 2009; Hamburger, Basile, & Vivolo, 2011; Sullivan, 2006). Although bullying occurs throughout childhood, the incidence rate peaks in the early teen years, ages 12 to 15 years (Finkelhor, Turner, Shattuck, & Hamby, 2013).

In 2011, the White House Summit on Bullying stressed in no uncertain terms that bullying is not a "rite of passage," and must be recognized as a public health and safety issue (White House Blog, 2011). However, children often choose not to tell adults when they are being bullied, usually confusing "telling" with "tattling." They might also be embarrassed to acknowledge that other children do not like them or that they cannot stop the bullying themselves, or worry that adults will make the situation worse (Petrosino, 2010; Smith & Shu, 2000).

Keeping in mind our recurring theme that "adolescents will not simply 'open up' to adults on demand," ideally we would have an appropriate screening tool to help us broach this topic. Several screeners are available, but they are designed for large group data collection rather than to guide a personal conversation. Instead, the American Academy of Pediatrics (APA; 2009) recommends a protocol of questions to pose during wellness exams and patient visits, such as the following:

- I'd like to hear about how school is going.
- How many good friends do you have in school?
- Do you ever feel afraid to go to school? Why?
- Do other kids ever bully you at school, in your neighborhood, or online?
- Who bullies you? When and where does it happen?
- What do they say or do?
- What do you do if you see other kids being bullied?
- Who can you go to for help if you or someone you know is being bullied?

When it comes to bullying and teens with hearing loss, what is the role of the pediatric audiologist? Like pediatricians, should we also screen for bullying problems as a standard of care? A survey of over 300 pediatric audiologists indicated that although concern for bullying was high, screening for the problem rarely occurred (Squires, Spangler, DeConde Johnson, & English, 2013). However, these respondents felt it appropriate for audiologists to bring up the topic as a matter of routine, and of course be ready with more information should the need arise.

Using the set of APA questions above as a guide, following is a sample discussion with a teen (Janie) and her mother:

Dialogue #3

Audiologist: *Well, Janie, and Mom too of course, now that we are done with your regular hearing tests, and we've adjusted your hearing aids a bit, do you have any questions about anything?*

Janie/Mom: *No questions, things look great!*

Audiologist: *And Janie, how are things in general? I know you just celebrated your 13th birthday, so that puts you in . . . 7th grade, right? What can you tell me about school these days?*

Janie: *It's good. I am getting good grades. Too much homework but . . . Most of my teachers are good about using the FM.*

Mom: *We are so proud of Janie. She is very independent.*

Audiologist: *I did want to ask you about something kind of serious—it's about bullying. I know your school has some anti-bullying programs; could you tell me about that?*

Janie: *A person in the school is the harassment/ bullying safety officer. She talks to us about this at assemblies and stuff. She's okay.*

Mom: *The school offers flyers, posters and programs and they have a zero tolerance policy about bullying . . . they have it covered.*

Audiologist: *Good to know! The school and your teachers really care. But Janie, even with all that support—do you ever notice any bullying?*

Mom: *Not with a zero tolerance policy! Kids wouldn't do that.*

Janie: *Well, actually, Mom, it does happen. Like my friend Torie—there are a couple kids who are really mean to her all the time.*

Mom: *That's terrible! How can the teachers let that happen?*

Audiologist: *Janie, you were saying it happens all the time—to you, too? Do you get bullied?*

Mom: *Of course not! I would know if that were happening.*

Janie: *No, no problems . . .*

Mom: *Yes, exactly, because I would know.*

Audiologist: *For lots of reasons, we are learning that kids tend not to tell. Does that make sense, Janie, that a kid may not want to tell?*

Janie: *A kid probably wouldn't talk about it . . . it could make things worse.*

Mom: *Janie honey, you would tell me, though, right?*

Janie: (starts to cry). *I'm not sure! Maybe it's not bullying...*

Audiologist: *Now that's a good point. It can be confusing. But let's try to understand it, if you'll answer some questions.* (Janie nods) *So when this happens, does it involve a friend?*

Janie: *This girl? She is definitely not a friend. She is really mean, her and her friend together.*

Audiologist: *Mean, and not just a kidding-around kind of thing?* (Janie nods) *What we are talking about—was it a one-time hassle?*

Janie: *I wish. No it keeps happening . . . I can see on their faces when they are ready to do something, I get really scared sometimes, and it feels like I am going to barf. They come at me from behind and start saying stuff loud so everyone can hear about me being stupid because I can't hear. They have torn up my homework. And more . . .*

Mom: *I can't believe this!*

Audiologist: *Mom, this is becoming pretty clear, even though she's kept it to herself. It's not friendly teasing, and it's not a one-time disagreement or fight—since it keeps happening, and is meant to harm, it qualifies as bullying. A lot of kids don't realize how POWER plays into it, but the situation is not one where Janie has as much power as these girls.*

(To Janie): *This was hard to talk about, huh? But good for you, this is so important. You have a right to feel safe and be safe. Mom and Janie, our clinic has developed a partnership with your school and we have materials for you, too—but what do you want to do now?*

Mom: *Janie, I think we need to talk to the principal and the safety officer. You can come with me or I can talk to them first and then you can talk to them.*

Audiologist: *Make sure Janie knows who to talk to, and make sure that person will follow through. We also have some new material about what can go on an IEP and supplemental services, and info about some good websites . . .*

Although we cannot say whether this discussion will make a difference in Janie's life, we do have strong evidence that a history of being bullied has long-term effects. A study from the United Kingdom (Takizawa, Maughan, & Arseneault, 2014) tracked a cohort of over 7,700 children born in 1958 for 50 years, and in 2014 reported that children with a history of being bullied had higher rates of depression, anxiety disorders, and suicide ideation than their nonvictimized peers. They concluded that "victimization by bullies is increasingly considered along maltreatment and neglect as a form of childhood abuse" (p. 777).

Reporting possible abuse is already within audiology's scope of practice, and although a new challenge, screening for bullying problems is a logical extension of that responsibility (Squires et al., 2013). The responsibility entails much preparation—timely access to referral sources, development of support materials, communication with schools and communities, and so on. See Learning Activity #3 to explore this conversation further.

Up to this point, we have focused on teen patients' psycho-emotional development. The next section will discuss concerns related to our patients as learners and thinkers.

Cognitive Development

Much has been written in the last decade about brain development during the teen years. Parents, teachers, advisors, and others now have the science to confirm what they have long observed: that teens are not yet young adults in the neurocognitive sense. This section will provide a brief overview of adolescent brain development and learning, and how adolescents-as-learners can be effectively engaged in patient education.

What Is Going On

Although their bodies have reached adult proportions, teens' brains are still developing, most importantly in the region of the frontal cortex. As mentioned at the beginning of this chapter, this "executive center" of the brain is involved with judgment, organization, planning, and strategizing. As teens begin to mature, their frontal lobes begin to thicken with gray matter, as depicted in Figure 36–3. This image displays the dynamic sequence of gray matter maturation in a longitudinal magnetic resonance imaging (MRI) study of 13 children, scanned every 2 years for 8 to 10 years (Blakemore, 2008).

As audiologists, our concerns are the functional implications. How do we convey information to this

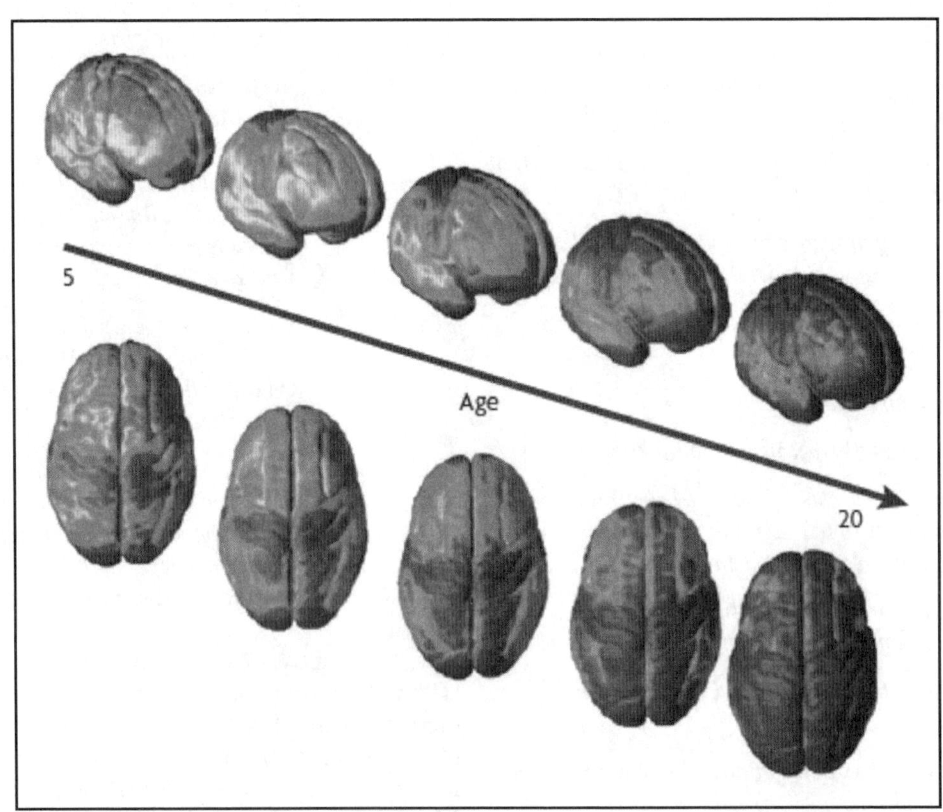

FIGURE 36–3. Dynamic sequence of gray matter maturation in a longitudinal MRI study of 13 children, scanned every 2 years for 8 to 10 years (Blakemore, 2008).

brain? Gilbert (2011) cautions us not to assume too much too soon:

> Ask an adolescent a really straightforward question like, "Swimming with sharks—good idea or bad idea?" and see what happens. This is exactly what researchers did, measuring the time it took for the adolescent to come up with an answer. An adult brain knows immediately the answer is bad idea, without a great deal of thinking. The child's brain would probably want to know what the shark's name was and if they could bring a friend. The teenage brain, on the other hand, hesitates because, well, there are lots of answers to that question and, hey, I want to make sure I'm not missing anything here. The spurt in neural connectivity they are experiencing, especially in their immature pre-frontal cortex (PFC), means that their brains have many, many possible ways to get from A—is swimming with sharks dangerous?—to B. (p. 65)

As our pediatric patients grow into adolescence, we recognize the need to broaden our patient education efforts to include the patient as well as the parent. As time moves on, our goals for all teens should include the ability to describe their hearing loss to others, make their own appointments, explain their hearing and other health problems clearly, and understand hearing and other health care recommendations. This development needs guidance and practice. In this domain, practice opportunities include problem solving, decision making, and self-expression. Sylwester (2007) maintains that the best way to help teens understand their own development is through conversation.

The Audiologist's Role

Viewing our teen patient as learner, we now need to consider our role as educator. Ultimately, any time we convey information, we are teaching. We teach whenever we explain and demonstrate new information to teens' family members, an activity that likely occurs at every appointment. However, audiologists are not always familiar with the science of *teaching effectively*. The fact that information was conveyed does not ensure that the learner understood it. In fact, research shows that explaining alone usually does not result in real understanding.

The act of learning something new involves a fairly well-understood neurologic process. Stimuli that holds the learner's attention long enough, and have sufficient meaning to the learner, will create a permanent change in brain function: synaptic connections become more efficient, allowing the learner to create new connections to previously learned information, making it easier to retrieve and use at a later point (Mason, Reid, & Hagaman, 2012; Suter & Suter, 2008; Zull, 2002).

Our patient education skills do not generate much discussion in the profession and could be taken for granted, but that would be a grave mistake. If not careful, we might apply a range of ineffective practices, such as

- using words our patients cannot process;
- explaining with more detail than patients can remember;
- conveying information unrelated to patients' questions; and
- providing information without helping patients apply it to their lives.

Regarding that last point, information designed to "help patients apply it to their lives" elevates *patient education* to a new level of responsibility. We are not only talking about providing information, but also using information as a vehicle for change.

This concept is relatively new. Falvo (2011) notes that although "many people think of patient education as the transfer of information . . . the real goal is *patient learning*, in which patients are not only provided with information, but helped to incorporate it into their daily lives" (p. 21). We are invited to redefine this process, to evolve from *a monologue of information giving* into *an interactive framework for change*, to include not only knowledge dissemination but also knowledge implementation.

Knowledge Dissemination

We have abundant knowledge to share about test results, anatomy, etiologies, genetics, recommendations, and treatments. However, as part of effective patient education, this knowledge base is just the first of several considerations. Even as we disseminate information, we cannot assume the patient understands us, or will remember what we said accurately. Our two concerns are the following:

- Comprehension: Does our patient understand? The easiest way to find out is to ask:
  - "Would you like a detailed explanation, or a big-picture summary?"
  - "Do you prefer information conveyed verbally, or in writing, or both?"
  - "To be sure we are on the same page, could you share with me your understanding of the situation?"

- Recall: Will our patient remember what we said? Converting working memory traces to long-term memory depends on repetition and review; otherwise, the neural cells that had been temporarily excited will reset itself and act as if nothing happened (Medina, 2008). Solutions include
  - easy-to-read handouts to take home for later review;
  - lists of websites with relevant video demonstrations or patient/parent testimonials; and
  - intentional review of the information in follow-up appointments.

Knowledge Implementation

This second step in effective patient education aims to "help patients help themselves." The following items are interrelated; each item is designed to engage the patient not just as a learner but also as a partner in the change process.

- Readiness: No one does anything until he or she is ready. A simple way to discuss this variable is the classic 1 through 10 scale. If 1 means "no way" and 10 means "ready right now," what will a patient say when we ask, "How ready are you to try hearing aids again, use communication repair strategies, advocate for yourself?"
- Self-efficacy: When confronted with change, teen patients will ask themselves a very reasonable question: "Can I do this?" That is, do I believe in my ability to control my desired outcomes? Self-efficacy does not depend on "being smart," but on knowing one can control one's effort and persistence (Elliot & Dweck, 2007). To help patients answer the question, we can ask them for examples in their past when they successfully dealt with similar challenges. "Small wins" provide concrete evidence that a task is within one's abilities.
- Support system: The value of social support cannot be underestimated (Taylor, 2002). However the teen patient defines it, find a way to include trusted "others" into the learning process.
- Patient-defined goals: When we confirm that a patient is ready to use our information, believes in his or her ability to do so, and has a support system to help with the process, we are ready to focus on goals. Effective patient education requires the patient, not the audiologist, to identify the problems to solve and the goals to accomplish. These goals represent the patient's internal motivation and personal expertise. When the goals are identified, the audiologist's role is to teach appropriate problem-solving skills and help the patient test them out.

Support Strategies

This section presents support strategies designed to improve patient education. The two skill sets addressed here include (a) self-advocacy skills and (b) health literacy.

Self-Advocacy Skills

On a daily basis, pediatric audiologists advocate for patients and families. By definition, an advocate seeks support for the rights and well-being of others, or the advancement of a cause. By application, pediatric audiologists have advocated for universal newborn screening, timely and effective interventions, family support, and more. Beyond our patients' first years, we advocate for appropriate educational settings, extracurricular accommodations, advanced technologies, and continuity of care.

When our patients reach adolescence, we face a new challenge—empowering teen patients to learn the skills needed to advocate for themselves. Learning to be one's own advocate is, of course, another developmental process. For teens with hearing loss, it starts with understanding the rationale for these skills, which include these real-world realities:

- College faculty, career trainers, and employers might not know about the rights of persons with hearing loss.
- The legal protections available through the school years change after high school graduation.
- Adults are generally expected to present their concerns personally, rather than rely on others.

In addition to learning about the changes in law and related implications, teens need practice and feedback as they develop communication and interpersonal skills to effectively explain their rights to others. These rights include acoustic access in classrooms and public places, and nondiscrimination when applying to college, vocational training, or employment positions.

Teen patients with Individual Education Plans (IEPs) usually receive school-based support in developing self-advocacy skills, to include goals such as, (a) assume responsibility for one's technology and educational materials; (b) develop introductory financial management skills (e.g., balancing a checkbook and explaining responsible credit card use); and (c) schedule and attend regular meetings with the career counselor. However, many teens with hearing loss do not have IEPs, so pediatric audiologists will want to share resources with patient and families to provide a self-taught option. A list of sample materials can be found in the Resources section below. Readers are encouraged to review a curriculum (English, 2012) designed to provide this support, with lessons on setting goals, expressing needs, negotiating, resolving conflicts, and transitioning to post–high school settings.

A Specialized Self-Advocacy Skill: Health Literacy

Patient education is not inherently easy. Every audiologist has had those moments when we realize our patient does not understand us. Sometimes the patient is emotionally distraught and cannot concentrate, and sometimes we unintentionally provide more information than the patient-as-learner can process.

Another variable to consider is the patient's *health literacy*. In addition to reading abilities, health literacy as measured by the National Assessment of Adult Literacy (NAAL; 2006) includes the ability to interpret graphs, do basic calculations (numeracy skills), and use a computer. We cannot take any patient's health literacy for granted; in fact, the NAAL reports that more than a third of adults in the United States (77 million) have limited (basic and below basic) health literacy skills (Figure 36–4). Persons at basic/below basic literacy levels are not able to read or fully understand a newspaper article, fill out forms for Social Security, Medicaid, or Medicare, or follow a bus schedule or calendar (Weiss, 2007). Relatedly, low health literacy is linked to more mistakes in medication usage, more emergency room visits and hospitalizations, and a higher risk of death. Relevant to audiology, it could mean misunderstanding instructions for hearing aid use, misinterpreting Internet sites about cochlear implant candidacy or auditory processing problems, or an inability to complete scales/questionnaires or provide a medical history.

Health literacy skills are affected by age, education, income, health insurance status, and first language acquisition. But as Weiss (2007) warns us, "You can't tell by looking" (p. 16).

Health literacy is a topic of high interest these days because health-related information continues to grow in complexity. Zarcadoolas, Pleasant, and Greer (2005) define health literacy as "the wide range of skills, and competencies that people *develop* to seek out, comprehend, evaluate and use health information" (emphasis added; p. 196). Such development can occur independently on the patient's end, but it also can occur as a result of effective communication with health care providers. In other words, if we educate effectively, a patient's health literacy level should increase over time.

Berkman, Davis, and McCormack (2010) define health literacy as "the degree to which individuals can obtain, process, understand, and communicate about health-related information needed to make informed health decisions" (p. 16). They added the phrase "communicate about" to the Institute of Medicine's 2004 definition because they considered oral communication skills (listening and speaking) to be a critical part of health care—as do audiologists and others. For instance, Ishikawa and Yano (2008) point out that in addition to NAAL's consideration of functional skills (reading, interpreting graphs, computation, computer use), a patient's *communication skills* are also essential, including the ability to

- articulate health concerns,
- describe symptoms accurately,
- ask pertinent questions, and
- understand verbal information accurately.

Another dimension to health literacy is *media literacy*, or the ability to critically evaluate media messages in all formats. And although not mentioned in the health literacy literature, audiologists might want to add *understanding and use of technology* (apart from computers) as a health literacy skill.

Each of these skills is directly relevant to teen patients with hearing loss. The differences between pediatric and adult audiology care are extensive, but an easy transition cannot be taken from granted. Compared to pediatric appointments, adult-level audiologic care includes shorter appointments that involve higher levels of language and terminology. Some of the advanced skills expected of adult patients include being able to

- provide accurate and complete information for a case history;
- manage insurance forms and appointments, and prescription dosages and refills; and
- communicate effectively with the health care provider (i.e., explain symptoms clearly, ask relevant questions, understand explanations and instructions).

Teens might not be prepared for this higher level of engagement with the health care system. To support this developmental process, Pajevic and English (2014) adapted a transition model developed by the Royal College of Nursing (2004). Their model (see Figure 36–4) includes three stages, each one fully respecting the goals and values of every family. Following is a "walk-through" depicting health-literacy transition planning.

Transition Planning in Health Care

A Proposed Three-Stage Model

Early Stage (13-14 yrs)

The Audiologist Will:

- Introduce the concept of transition
- Seek parents' thoughts on transition process
- Discuss eventual, gradual withdraw of parents from appointments
- Introduce concept of confidentiality

Sample Goals/The Patient Will:

- Explain degree, history of hearing loss
- Manage hearing technology
- Identify and repair communication challenges
- Identify support systems

Middle Stage (14-15 yrs)

The Audiologist Will:

- Discuss new thoughts/concerns of parents and patient
- Update transition plan
- Suggest 5 minutes one-on-one with patient, family steps out

Sample Goals/The Patient Will:

- Keep appointment calendar
- Become expert in hearing technology
- Know how to contact help in emergencies
- Be able to provide basic info for case history, family history

Late Stage (16-18 yrs)

The Audiologist Will:

- Update transition plan
- Provide relevant materials, info
- Suggest 10 minutes one-on-one with patient, family steps out

Sample Goals/The Patient Will:

- Maintain a personal health file
- Schedule own appointments
- Fill out health history form
- Explain legal rights and accommodations in health care

FIGURE 36–4. Transition planning in health care: a three-stage model.

Stage 1, or the Early Stage, would begin around age 13 to 14 years. During this beginning phase, we introduce the concept of transition, describe the rationale and general goals, and provide written support materials for home reading. We emphasize the collaborative nature of a transition plan, wherein the family and teen take the lead and the audiologist provides support. If the patient and family agree, we draft an initial plan, subject to revision at each appointment.

At this stage, we should determine our patients' knowledge of their hearing loss and their ability to describe it to others. Does the teen need practice, information, or clarification? We can also inquire about the patient's participation in school, friendships, sports, and other activities. Throughout, we listen for any concerns that would warrant a referral to counseling or social work. Finally, we ask families to consider *gradually* withdrawing from future appointments. Our role during this stage is to "plant the transition seed," help the family consider some initial goals, and provide educational materials and other resources.

Stage 2, the Middle Stage, can begin around age 14 to 15 years. During this stage, we address any new concerns and developments (general health, school, friendships, part-time work, etc.). We can start describing how the adult health care system differs from pediatric care, and depending on patient maturity, we might ask the patient to start keeping track of appointments. We should evaluate the patient's level of responsibility in managing hearing aids or implants. When families are willing, they would yield 5 minutes at the end of the appointment for one-on-one conversations with the patient. During these 5 minutes, we can clarify the concept of confidentiality and give the teen an opportunity to ask questions.

Stage 3, the Late Stage, begins around age 16 to 18 years. As before, the plan and goals are adjusted as the patient continues to mature. We can now encourage the patient to demonstrate expertise in addressing communication needs and self-advocacy. Developing a personal health file could be an age-appropriate goal (e.g., family and medical history, inoculation records, emergency and other contacts, insurance information). The topic of health records gives us the opportunity to address the importance of keeping health and personal information secure. The patient might practice conveying case history information, complete intake forms, and scheduling appointments. We continue to provide relevant educational materials, discuss rights and accommodations, and share advanced information on communication strategies and support groups. The one-on-one consultation could be expanded to 10 to 15 minutes, continuing to encourage participation and communication skill development.

Conclusion

Supporting adolescents through their transition from childhood to young adulthood is somewhat underexplored in audiology but is essential nonetheless. In this chapter, we have considered the teen patient's psycho-emotional and cognitive development, and the role of the audiologist in supporting the natural desire to assume more responsibility and independence, and to have more opportunity to express one's needs and practice decision making, all the while within the context of family. Adolescent patient challenges are not unique to audiology (e.g., see Naimi et al., 2009; Taddeo, Edegy, & Frappier, 2008; Weissberg-Benchell et al., 1995), but we know our population best, and therefore must continue to develop patient-centered conversations, transition plans, and relevant support materials for adolescents living with hearing loss.

Suggested Learning Activities

1. This chapter mentioned that "some teen patients struggle with first-stage skills (self-awareness)." Based on your experience with teens and your own teen years, identify two possible reasons and compare thoughts with a classmate or colleague.
2. In teams of two, assign one person to role-play a teen with hearing loss who has completed the SAC-A. The other team member assumes the role of audiologist. Conduct a dialogue that gives the teen ample opportunity to expand on answers, and the audiologist ample opportunity to refrain from solving the teen's problems.
3. Review Dialogue #3, "Screening for Bullying Problems." Note that the audiologist did not ask the direct question, "Are you being bullied?" How would you describe her approach? During the conversation, how did the teen's responses change, and what did the audiologist say to facilitate those changes?
4. How would a pediatric audiologist introduce the topic of health literacy and health transition planning to a teen patient and his or her family?

Resources

Bullying Prevention and Intervention:

- Hands & Voices (handsandvoices.org) is coauthoring information on age-specific development of safety skills with Kidpower: http://deafed-childabuse-neglect-col.wiki.educ.msu.edu/
- PACER's National Bullying Prevention Center: http://www.pacer.org/bullying/resources/students-with-disabilities/
- StopBullying.gov: http://www.stopbullying.gov/prevention/talking-about-it/index.html
- Office for Civil Rights and Prohibited Disability Harassment: http://www2.ed.gov/about/offices/list/ocr/docs/disabharassltr.html

Self-Advocacy Development

- *Knowledge is Power (KIP): A program to help students learn about their hearing loss.* (2009). Educational Audiology Association. This binder of multigrade lessons addresses topics in legislation and transition as well as anatomy, hearing evaluations, etiologies, and technology. Available at http://www.edaud.org
- Guide to Access Planning (GAP): Self-advocacy competency checklist. An online self-evaluation of skills and goal identification. Available at http://www.phonakpro.com/us/b2b/en/pediatric/GAP/teens_youngadults/self_advocacy/self-advocacy_checklist.html

References

Adams, K., Cimino, J., Arnold, R. M., & Anderson, W. (2012). Why should I talk about emotion? Communication patterns associated with physician discussion of patient expressions of negative emotion in hospital admission encounters. *Patient Education and Counseling, 89*, 44–50

American Academy of Pediatrics. (2009). Position statement: Role of the pediatrician in youth violence prevention. *Pediatrics, 124*, 393–402. Retrieved from http://pediatrics.aappublications.org/content/124/1/393

American Psychology Association. (2002). *Developing adolescents: A reference for professionals.* Washington, DC: Author.

Banks, M., Kendall, E., Banks, M. E., & Gover, R. M. S. (Eds.). (2009). *Disabilities: Insights from across fields and around the world.* Westport, CT: Praeger.

Berkman, N. D., Davis, T. C., & McCormack, L. (2010). Health literacy: What is it? *Journal of Health Communication: International Perspectives, 15*(2), 9–19.

Blakemore, S. (2008). The social brain in adolescence. *Neuroscience, 9*, 267–277.

Clark, J. G., & English, K. (2014). *Counseling-infused audiologic care.* Boston, MA: Allyn & Bacon.

Damasio, A. (2005). *Descartes' error: Emotion, reason, and the human brain.* London, UK: Penguin.

Ekberg, K., Grenness, C., & Hickson, L. (2014). Addressing patients' psychosocial concerns regarding hearing aids within audiology appointments for older adults. *American Journal of Audiology, 23*, 337–350.

Elkayam, J., & English, K. (2003). Counseling adolescents with hearing loss with the use of self-assessment/significant other questionnaires. *Journal of the American Academy of Audiology, 14*(9), 485–499. SAC-A Retrieved from http://www.audiology.org/sites/default/files/journal/JAAA_14_09_03.pdf

Elliot, A. J., & Dweck, C. S. (Eds.). (2007). *Handbook of competence and motivation.* NY: Guilford Press.

English, K. (2012). *Self-advocacy for students who are deaf or hard of hearing* (2nd ed.). Retrieved from http://gozips.uakron.edu/~ke3/Self-Advocacy.pdf

English, K., Rojeski, T., & Branham, K. (2000). Acquiring counseling skills in mid-career: Outcomes of a distance education course for practicing audiologists. *Journal of American Academy of Audiology, 11*, 84–90.

Falvo, D. (2011). *Effective patient education: A guide to increased adherence* (4th ed.). Sudbury, MA: Jones & Bartlett.

Finkelhor, D., Turner, H. A., Shattuck, A., & Hamby, S. L. (2013). Violence, crime, and abuse exposure in a national sample of children and youth: An update. *JAMA Pediatrics, 167*(7), 614–621.

Gilbert, I. (2011). *Why do I need a teacher when I've got Google?* London, UK: Routledge.

Ginott, H. (1969). *Between parent and teenager.* New York, NY: Macmillan.

Goleman, D. (2005). *Emotional intelligence: Why it might matter more than IQ.* New York, NY: Bantam Books.

Grenness, C., Hickson, L., Laplante-Levesque, A., Meyer, C., & Davidson, B. (2015). The nature of communication throughout diagnosis and management planning in initial audiologic rehabilitation consultations. *Journal of American Academy of Audiology, 26*, 36–50.

Hamburger, M. E., Basile, K. C., & Vivolo, A. M. (2011). *Measuring bullying victimization, perpetration, and bystander experiences: A compendium of assessment tools.* Atlanta, GA: Centers for Disease Control and Prevention, National Center for Injury Prevention and Control.

Institute of Medicine. (2004). *Health literacy: A prescription to end confusion.* Washington, DC: National Academies Press. Retrieved from http://www.nap.edu/catalog/10883.html

Ishikawa, H., & Yano, E. (2008). Patient health literacy and participation in the health-care process. *Health Expectations, 11*, 113–122.

Kennedy, E., & Charles, S. (2001). *On becoming a counselor: A basic guide for nonprofessional counselors and other helpers* (3rd ed.). New York, NY: Crossroad.

Mason, L., Reid, R., & Hagaman, J. (2012). *Building comprehension in adolescents*. Baltimore, MD: Paul H. Brookes.

Medina, J. (2008). *Brain rules*. Seattle, WA: Pear Press.

Naimi, D. R., Freedman, T. G., Ginsburg, K., Bogen, D., Rand, C. S., & Apter, A. J. (2009). Adolescents and asthma: Why bother with our meds? *Journal of Allergy and Clinical Immunology, 123*(6), 1335–1341.

National Assessment of Adult Literacy. (2006). *The health literacy of America's adults: Results from the 2003 National Assessment of Adult Literacy*. Washington, DC: U.S. Department of Education.

Pajevic, E., & English, K. (2014). Teens as health care consumers: Planned transition and empowerment. *Audiology Today*, *26*(6), 14–18.

Petrosino A. (2010). *What characteristics of bullying, bullying victims, and schools are associated with increased reporting of bullying to school officials?* Washington, DC: National Center for Education Evaluation and Regional Assistance.

Robins, R. W., & Trzesniewski, K. H. (2005). Self-esteem development across the lifespan. *Current Directions in Psychological Science*, *14*(3), 158–162.

Royal College of Nursing. (2004). *Adolescent transition care: Guidance for nursing staff.* Retrieved from https://www.bspar.org.uk/DocStore/FileLibrary/PDFs/RCNGuidanceAdolescentTransitionalCare.pdf

Schow, R., & Nerbonne, M. (1982). Communication Screening Profile: Use with elderly clients. *Ear and Hearing*, *3*(3), 135–147.

Smith, P. K., & Shu, S. (2000). What good schools can do about bullying: Findings from a survey in English schools after a decade of research and action. *Childhood, 7*, 193–212.

Squires, M., Spangler, C., DeConde Johnson, C., & English, K. (2013). Bullying is a safety and health issue: How pediatric audiologists can help. *Audiology Today, 25*(5), 18–26.

Stone, J. R., & Olswang, L. B. (1989). The hidden challenge in counseling. *ASHA, 31*, 27–31.

Sullivan, P. (2006). Children with disabilities exposed to violence: Legal and public policy issues. In M. Feerick & G. Silverman (Eds.), *Children exposed to violence* (pp. 213–237). Baltimore, MD: Paul H. Brookes.

Suter, P. M., & Suter, W. N. (2008). Timeless principles of learning: A solid foundation for enhancing chronic disease self-management. *Home Healthcare Nurse, 26*(2), 82–88.

Sylwester, R. (2007). *The adolescent brain: Reaching for autonomy*. Thousand Oaks, CA: Corwin Press.

Taddeo, D., Edegy, M., & Frappier, J. Y. (2008). Adherence to treatment in adolescents. *Paediatrics & Child Health, 13*(1), 19–24.

Takizawa, R., Maughan, B., & Arseneault, B. (2014). Adult health outcomes of childhood victimization: Evidence from a five-decade longitudinal British birth cohort. *American Journal of Psychiatry, 171*(7), 777–784.

Taylor, S. (2002). *The tending instinct: How nurturing is essential to who we are and how we live.* New York, NY: Henry Holt.

Weiss, B. (2007). *Health literacy and patient safety: Help patients understand. Manual for clinicians* (2nd ed.). Chicago, IL: American Medical Association.

Weissberg-Benchell, J., Glasgow, A. M., Tynan, W. D., Wirtz, P., Turek, J., & Ward, J. (1995). Adolescent diabetes management and mismanagement. *Diabetes Care, 18*, 177–182.

White House Blog. (2011, March). President Obama and the First Lady at the White House Conference on Bullying Prevention. Retrieved from https://www.whitehouse.gov/blog/2011/03/10/president-obama-first-lady-white-house-conference-bullying-prevention

Zarcadoolas, C., Pleasant, A., & Greer, D. (2005). Understanding health literacy: An expanded model. *Health Promotion International, 20*(2), 195–203.

Zull, J. (2002). *The art of changing the brain: Enriching the practice of teaching by exploring the biology of learning*. Sterling, VA: Stylus.

Minimal Hearing Loss in Children

Heather Porter, Fred H. Bess, and Anne Marie Tharpe

Introduction

In the 1-year period between 1964 and 1965, a rubella epidemic resulted in approximately 12.5 million cases of rubella leading to approximately 20,000 children born with a variety of handicapping conditions including hearing loss in the United States (National Communicable Disease Center, 1969; Vernon, Grieve, & Shaver, 1980). As such, the following decade was one in which pediatric audiologists were necessarily focused on the identification and management of children with severe-to-profound degrees of hearing loss. Hence, it is not surprising that the profession of audiology during that time gave only limited consideration to mild degrees of hearing loss. That is, when compared to children with severe-to-profound hearing loss, many of whom had additional handicapping conditions, the potential impact of mild degrees of hearing loss on children seemed inconsequential. However, for the last several decades, children with mild degrees of hearing loss have garnered the interest of audiologists, especially since the 1980s when studies were expanded to include a population of children referred to as having minimal hearing loss (Bess, 1982, 1985; Bess & Tharpe, 1986). A review of definitions of minimal hearing loss appears below.

A time-honored maxim among physicians, educators, and many audiologists has been that children with minimal degrees of hearing loss, including unilateral hearing loss, generally experience few, if any, communicative or psychoeducational difficulties. Historically, the typical management strategy for this population has been relatively complacent. Once the hearing loss has been identified, parents are told that the hearing loss exists, and they are often assured that no problems will occur as a result of the loss. Preferential seating in the classroom is recommended, and occasionally some type of amplification is suggested on a trial basis. Because of the long-standing belief that minimal hearing loss is without significant consequence, many of these children are not always considered educationally handicapped, and in many school districts, they are not eligible for special services. Despite the widespread impression that minimal hearing loss is not a serious problem, there is a lack of experimental evidence to support such an assumption. In fact, numerous studies have appeared over the last few decades to support the notion that the impact of minimal hearing loss is not minimal at all.

In one of the first studies on the topic, Quigley and Thomure (1969) identified school-aged children with hearing loss who were not receiving support services (n = 116). The majority of children identified were children with hearing threshold levels of less than 26 dB HL (82.7%). As a group, the identified children scored below expected levels on subtests of the Sanford Achievement Test (i.e., word meaning, paragraph meaning, and language) and, on average, were one grade behind expected levels based on age. A contemporary review of minimal hearing loss in children leads one to several realities. First, the majority of studies on children with minimal hearing loss have reported a variety of auditory, educational, and psychoeducational complications (e.g., Bess, Dodd-Murphy, & Parker, 1998; Bess & Tharpe, 1984; Bess, Tharpe, & Gibler, 1986; Crandell, 1993; Culbertson & Gilbert, 1986; Jenson, Johansen, & Børre, 1989; Most, 2004, 2006; Oyler, Oyler, & Matkin, 1988). However, a few studies have reported no such difficulties (Hallmo, Moller, Lind, & Tonning, 1986; Tieri, Masi, Ducci, & Marsella,

1988). Second, definitions of normal hearing sensitivity vary, and one consequence of this variation in definition is confusion and indecision regarding intervention (Gravel, Knightly, & McKay, 2008). Third, nomenclature within our profession appears to promote a lack of importance for certain hearing loss categories. The term *minimal hearing loss* carries a connotation of minimal consequence. In fact, a survey of parental impressions of commonly used terms to describe degrees of hearing loss suggested that specific terminology (e.g., slight, minimal, mild) might result in an underestimation of the potential magnitude of the disability (Haggard & Primus, 1999). Finally, but not without significant influence, is the adherence of educators and health care specialists to a failure-based model of intervention that includes "wait-and-see" policies that support monitoring a child's development and intervening only at the point of academic failure.

This chapter presents a contemporary overview of children with minimal hearing loss. To this end, topic areas to be covered include etiology, prevalence, screening and diagnostic challenges, auditory performance, and intervention options. The chapter concludes with a section on future directions and research needs.

Definition of Minimal and Mild Hearing Loss

A starting point in our discussion of minimal hearing loss should reasonably be the definition of minimal and mild hearing loss. Because of the importance of acute hearing for the normal development of speech and language, some investigators have suggested that the definition of hearing sensitivity for children should be more conservative than for adults; specifically, a pure-tone threshold average (PTA) between 10 and 15 dB (Clark, 1981; Diefendorf & Gravel, 1996). Mild hearing loss is typically defined as hearing sensitivity between 26 and 40 dB HL, which suggests that minimal loss is defined as a PTA greater than or equal to 15 and less than or equal to 25 dB HL. However, the category of minimal hearing loss is broad, and both the degree of hearing loss and the configuration of hearing loss are important. The most commonly accepted definitions of minimal and mild hearing loss were proposed by the Centers for Disease Control (CDC) Early Hearing Detection Intervention Program (2005), which adapted the following definitions of minimal hearing loss originally proposed by Bess et al. (1998) with minor modifications:

- unilateral sensory/neural hearing loss—average air-conduction thresholds (.5, 1.0, 2.0 kHz) greater than or equal to 20 dB HL in the impaired ear and an average air-bone gap no greater than 10 dB at 1.0, 2.0, and 4.0 kHz and average air-conduction thresholds in the normal hearing ear less than or equal to 15 dB HL;
- bilateral sensory/neural hearing loss—average air-conduction thresholds between 20 and 40 dB HL bilaterally with average air-bone gaps no greater than 10 dB at frequencies 1.0, 2.0, and 4.0 kHz; and
- high-frequency sensory/neural hearing loss—air-conduction thresholds greater than 25 dB HL at two or more frequencies above 2 kHz (i.e., 3.0, 4.0, 6.0, or 8.0 kHz) in one or both ears with air-bone gaps at 3.0 and 4.0 kHz no greater than 10 dB.

Others have used different definitions (Ross, Visser, Holstrum, & Kenneson, 2005), but regardless of the definition used, an effort should be made for standardized terminology to enable meaningful comparisons of data across studies. Our attempts to evaluate data on the impact of minimal and mild hearing loss on children obtained across studies are compromised when we are not using uniform definitions.

Prevalence

A shift has occurred in the incidence and prevalence of certain causative factors and degrees of hearing loss in the past 40 to 50 years. Disorders that resulted in severe-to-profound sensory/neural hearing loss in the 1950s and 1960s, such as rubella and meningitis, are no longer as prevalent as they once were. As the result of health care improvements, we now have a better understanding of the pathogenesis of disease and have developed new and effective immunizations. In addition, our ability to manage the complications associated with premature delivery has resulted in dramatically improved infant survival rates. Although we are grateful for the lowered limit of viability, these small and fragile babies face high morbidity. Those born weighing less than 750 g are at highest risk of lifelong morbidity, including hearing loss. These hearing losses tend to be milder in degree than what was observed decades ago. Hence, today, pediatric audiologists are being asked to serve a distinctively different group of children than we served in the past.

In 2012, about 97% of infants were screened for hearing loss in the United States (3,820,624 per

3,953,986 live births; CDC, 2014). Of the 46 states and territories offering epidemiological data, hearing loss was diagnosed in approximately 1.6 per 1,000 infants screened. Others have reported similar prevalence rates (Dalzell et al., 2000; Finitzo, Albright, & Neal, 1998; Prieve et al., 2000). Of those infants screened for hearing loss, approximately 0.03% was diagnosed with minimal hearing loss (minimal bilateral = 0.02%; unilateral = 0.006%). Interestingly, studies on the prevalence of unilateral hearing loss in school-aged children suggest a much higher prevalence within the general population relative to infancy. For example, Bess and coworkers (1998) reported unilateral hearing loss in 37/1,218 (3.0%) of children in third, sixth, and ninth grades. Additionally, Niskar et al. (1998) investigated 6,166 children aged 6 to 19 years and noted that 14.2% of these children had low-frequency or high-frequency unilateral hearing loss. More recently, Wake et al. (2006) found slight to mild bilateral sensory/neural hearing loss in 55/6,581 (0.88%) of first- and fifth-grade children surveyed.

The aforementioned data suggest that by the time children reach school age, the prevalence of minimal hearing loss increases from approximately 0.03% to about 1% to 14%—a substantial increase. Why is there such a large discrepancy in prevalence rates of minimal hearing loss from birth to school-aged children? Possible explanations include (1) newborn screening programs that are not designed to detect minimal or mild degrees of hearing loss; (2) progressive or late-onset hearing losses; (3) variability as a result of differing definitions/inclusion criteria; (4) low follow-up rates in newborn screening programs that result in underestimation of true prevalence; and (5) a large percentage of cases missed to follow-up.

Etiology

Information about the etiology of minimal hearing loss has been limited. In fact, whereas the etiology of unilateral hearing loss is unknown for 30% to 60% of cases in children (Brookhouser, Worthington, & Kelly, 1991; English & Church, 1999; Ghogomu, Umansky, & Lieu, 2014), even less is known about the etiology of minimal bilateral hearing loss in children. A summary of major etiologic factors associated with minimal hearing loss is shown in Table 37–1.

Congenital cytomegalovirus (CMV) is the most common cause of nongenetic hearing loss and the leading cause of UHL in children (Nance, 2007). CMV infection occurs in 0.2% to 2.5% of all live births; however, it does not always present with symptoms (Leung, Sauve, & Davies, 2003). By age 6 years, 35% of infants with symptomatic CMV and 11% of infants with nonsymptomatic CMV have hearing loss (Fowler, Dahle, Boppana, & Pass, 1999). Nance, Lim, and Dodson (2006) found congenital CMV and genetic mutations related to connexin[1] to be two major causes of deafness at birth, and enlarged vestibular aqueduct syndrome (EVAS) and congenital CMV as the major causes for late onset prelingual hearing loss.

Other infections can also be responsible for minimal hearing loss. Prior to 1967 when the mumps vaccine was introduced, mumps was the leading cause of acquired UHL. Since that time, there has been a 90% to 95% decrease in the incidence of mumps; however, more recent outbreaks have been noted in the United States and the United Kingdom (Cohen et al., 2007; Dayan et al., 2008). Bacterial and viral meningitis can also cause hearing loss. Although viral meningitis is more common than bacterial meningitis, hearing loss is often associated with the bacterial form of this condition. Hearing loss, ranging from mild unilateral to profound bilateral, is the most common complication of bacterial meningitis among children (Baraff, Lee, & Schriger, 1993). Approximately 30% of cases of hearing loss resulting from bacterial meningitis are unilateral (Kutz, Simon, Chennupati, Giannoni, & Manolidis, 2006).

Enlarged vestibular aqueduct syndrome (EVAS) is the most common form of inner ear malformation associated with sensory/neural hearing loss (Boston et al., 2007). In the majority of cases, hearing loss associated with EVAS is bilateral, but cases of UHL have been reported (Govaerts et al., 1999). Additional malformations shown to cause hearing loss, such as Chiari malformation, might occur unilaterally more often than bilaterally (Simons, Ruscetta, & Chi, 2008).

Other less common causes of minimal hearing loss in children include auditory neuropathy spectrum disorder (ANSD), sudden idiopathic hearing loss, and congenital aural atresia and microtia. Though ANSD is typically bilateral, unilateral cases have been reported (Podwall, Podwall, Gordon, Lamendola, & Gold, 2002). Sudden idiopathic hearing loss typically occurs unilaterally; however, the prevalence is lower in children than adults (Roman, Aladio, Paris, Nicollas,

[1]Connexin is a subunit of connexon, a protein that forms a gap junction between cells. These junctions are essential to the function of the inner ear as they permit intercellular exchange of potassium and calcium.

Table 37–1. Summary of Etiologic Factors Associated With Minimal Hearing Loss

Cause	Frequency of Occurrence	Reference
Congenital cytomegalovirus (CMV)	This occurs in 0.2% to 2.5% of all live births. Hearing loss results in ~7% to 40% of cases. This is the leading cause of unilateral hearing loss in children.	Leung, Sauve, & Davies, 2003; Nance, 2007
Bacterial meningitis	Approximately 10% to 30% of cases result in at least a unilateral hearing loss. Approximately 14% are minimal bilateral, ~4% to 30% are unilateral.	Kutz, Simon, Chennupati, Giannoni, & Manolidis, 2006
Viral/bacterial mumps	Approximately 80% to 95% of cases of hearing loss caused by viral or bacterial mumps are unilateral.	Unal et al., 1998
Enlarged vestibular aqueduct syndrome (EVAS)	Most cases are moderately severe or greater in degree. Approximately 20% of cases of EVAS are unilateral.	Govaerts et al., 1999
Chiari malformation	The majority of cases (~65%) are unilateral.	Simons, Ruscetta, & Chi, 2008
Auditory neuropathy spectrum disorder (ANSD)	Most cases of ANSD are bilateral; ~33% are minimal bilateral. Some cases of unilateral hearing loss have been reported.	Podwall, Podwall, Gordon, Lamendola, & Gold, 2002
Sudden sensory/neural hearing loss (SNHL)	Approximately 85% of cases of sudden SNHL in children are unilateral.	Roman, Aladio, Paris, Nicollas, & Triglia, 2001
Atresia	Congenital atresia or microtia occurs in approximately 1 out of 10,000 live births. Approximately 70% of cases of atresia are unilateral.	Schuknecht, 1989
Gap junction beta-2 (*GJB2*)	Over 80 mutations of *GJB2* are responsible for hearing loss. Some cases of UHL have been reported, but most cases are profound.	Kenna, Wu, Cotanche, Korf, & Rehm, 2001; Wilcox et al., 2000
Prematurity	Approximately 5% of premature infants have minimal bilateral or unilateral hearing loss.	Herrgård, Karjalainen, Martikainen, & Heinonen, 1995

& Triglia, 2001). Only about 3.5% of cases of sudden idiopathic hearing loss occur in patients under 14 years of age (Nakashima & Yanagita, 1993). Congenital aural atresia or microtia occurs in approximately 1 per 10,000 to 20,000 live births as part of syndromic or nonsyndromic disorders (Melnick & Myrianthopoulos, 1979; Schuknecht, 1989). The severity of anomaly can range from mild to more severe symptoms that could include absence of the middle ear structures in combination with anotia. Unilateral aural atresia occurs in approximately 70% of cases of atresia (Schuknecht, 1989). Other possible causes of minimal hearing loss, not referenced in Table 37–1, include noise-induced hearing loss and head trauma (Brookhouser et al., 1991; Niskar et al., 1998).

It is suspected that over 500 genes, with some containing hundreds of mutations, are likely to contribute to hearing loss. For each of the six most frequent causative genes that have been identified to date for autosomal recessive nonsyndromic hearing loss (*GJB2*,

SLC26A4, MYO15A, OTOF, CDH23, TMC1), at least 20 mutations have been reported (Phillips et al., 2013). Mutations involving the gap junction beta-2 (*GJB2*) gene[2] are the most frequent cause of deafness in many populations (Nance & Kearsey, 2004). *GJB2* is a small gene that contains a single coding exon but over 300 different mutations have been reported (Human Gene Mutation Database: http://www.hgmd.org). Most reports of hearing loss related to *GJB2* have been profound, but associations with less severe and unilateral hearing loss have been reported (Kenna, Wu, Cotanche, Korf, & Rehm, 2001; Wilcox et al., 2000).

As we learn more about genetic testing and identify children with hearing loss at an earlier age, we should become better able to identify the causes of minimal hearing loss. Currently, identification of etiology at birth can be accomplished in approximately 60% of late-onset prelingual cases of hearing loss (Nance et al., 2006). Although this is an improvement over past estimates, the need for continued improvement is essential. Morton and Nance (2006) suggest an etiologic focus on newborn hearing screening—a focus that also identifies infants at risk for late-onset hearing loss. By screening for four causes of hearing loss, the majority of children with congenital deafness and late-onset prelingual deafness could be identified shortly after birth: *GJB2* deafness, mitochondrial *A1555G*3 mutations,[3] Pendred's syndrome, and congenital CMV (Nance et al., 2006). Recent studies continue to document etiology for approximately 50% of patients (Declau, Boudewyns, Van den Ende, Peeters, & van den Heyning, 2008). This type of large-scale, early etiologic work not only helps to identify children with, and those at risk for, prelingual hearing loss, but also helps to define the causes of early onset minimal hearing loss in children.

Progression of Minimal Hearing Loss

Although children might initially be identified with minimal hearing loss, progression of hearing loss is possible, and vigilant monitoring of hearing sensitivity is therefore recommended. Changes in hearing sensitivity are expected in about 20% of children (Fitzpatrick, Whittingham, & Durieux-Smith, 2014; Pittman & Stelmachowicz, 2003). For example, Fitzpatrick and coworkers (2014) reported a progression of hearing loss in 22% of a large group of children (*N* = 337) with minimal bilateral or unilateral hearing loss. In a group identified since UNHS was implemented, 33 of 102 (32.4%) experienced an average threshold change of 20 dB or greater—26 of these children had average threshold changes of more than 20 dB.

The progression of unilateral to bilateral hearing loss in some children is also a possibility (e.g., Declau et al., 2008; Edwards, 2008; Fitzpatrick et al., 2014; Neault, 2005). Fitzpatrick and colleagues (2014) reported that approximately 11% of infants confirmed with unilateral hearing loss via diagnostic testing following failed newborn hearing screening were later found to have bilateral hearing loss. Furthermore, Neault (2005) reported 36% of infants who unilaterally failed a hearing screening were diagnosed with bilateral hearing loss, and 64% were confirmed to have unilateral hearing loss. Hence, more than one third of unilateral refers who exhibited hearing loss at the time of the audiologic examination showed bilateral hearing loss rather than unilateral hearing loss. Similarly, Edwards (2008) reported 4.5% of infants who unilaterally failed a hearing screening were eventually diagnosed with bilateral hearing loss, and 26% were confirmed to have unilateral hearing loss. In addition, Declau and colleagues (2008) reported 8.3% of infants with unilateral hearing screening failures were ultimately diagnosed with bilateral hearing loss. Clearly, a need exists for hearing health care professionals to develop a better understanding of the progression of hearing loss in both children with minimal bilateral hearing loss and children with unilateral loss.

Impact of Auditory Deprivation

Early auditory experiences shape the way the brain processes and perceives sound. As such, the potential effects of auditory deprivation are an important consideration with regard to the difficulties experienced by children with hearing loss. In general, auditory deprivation has been described as a systematic decrease over time in performance associated with the reduced availability of acoustic information (Palmer, 1999).

[2]Also known as connexin 26 (*Cx26*), this gene codes for proteins that form gap junctions between cells. Recall that these junctions are essential to the function of the inner ear as they permit intercellular exchange of potassium and calcium. Mutations of *GJB2/Cx26* are responsible for 30% to 40% of genetic deafness (Pandya et al., 2003).

[3]Mutations of *A1555G* are associated with sensitivity to aminoglycosides and account for 10% of hearing loss attributed to ototoxicity in the United States (Nance et al., 2006).

Detrimental effects of auditory deprivation on speech understanding have been shown for adults. Silverman, Silman, Emmer, Schoepflin, and Lutolf (2006) reported that word recognition performance of adults with asymmetric hearing loss declined in the poorer ear of adults who did not utilize amplification compared to a group of adults with asymmetric hearing loss who wore amplification.

Neural changes occur within the anatomic structure of the brain in cases of hearing loss. Although the greatest effects can reasonably be expected for more severe degrees of hearing loss, mild-to-moderate hearing loss is not without consequence in the developing auditory pathway. For example, induced mild-to-moderate conductive hearing loss in developing gerbils results in alterations in the timing of neural synapses and spikes, suggesting a possible contribution to auditory processing difficulties experienced by individuals with minimal hearing loss (Xu, Kotak, & Sanes, 2007).

In addition to differences in the auditory pathway of individuals with bilateral hearing loss compared to those with normal hearing sensitivity, differences in the auditory pathway of individuals with unilateral hearing loss can be expected to differ from those with normal hearing sensitivity as well. For example, adults with congenital unilateral deafness have reduced activation in the left lateral temporal cortex when compared to normal hearing controls during speech-reading tasks (MacSweeney et al., 2001). In cases of monaural stimulation, people with normal hearing display contralateral activation on functional magnetic resonance imaging (fMRI; Jäncke, Wüstenberg, Schulze, & Heinze, 2002); however, people with unilateral hearing loss display bilateral activation patterns (Scheffler, Bilecen, Schmid, Tschopp, & Seelig, 1998; Tschopp et al., 2000). Schmithorst and coworkers (2005) reported children with left unilateral hearing loss and right unilateral hearing loss had some differences in their fMRI responses to random tonal stimuli. Although robust activation was seen in the auditory cortex bilaterally for both groups, children with left unilateral hearing loss displayed increased activation in the superior temporal areas, and those with right unilateral hearing loss showed increased activation in the inferior frontal areas. These results suggest a differing cortical reorganization that is dependent on the laterality of hearing loss.

Structural changes suggested by imaging studies in individuals with unilateral hearing loss have also been demonstrated in animal models. Animal studies have shown reorganization of the auditory brainstem (Illing, Kraus, & Meidinger, 2005) as well as cortical reorganization (Hutson, Durham, Imig, & Tucci, 2007; Popescu & Polley, 2010) following unilateral deafness in rats and gerbils. Unilateral ablations tend to cause reorganization of the auditory pathway resulting in a strengthening of the functional role of the intact ear. Independent of whether unilateral ablation occurs in a developing or adult animal, the pathway from the intact ear to the ipsilateral cortex is strengthened (Syka, 2002).

The anatomic and physiologic asymmetry for speech perception in the brain provides a theoretical framework for poorer outcomes for children with right ear hearing loss versus left ear hearing loss. The evidence for outcome differences between those with right ear and left ear hearing loss is explored later in this chapter.

Screening and Diagnostic Challenges

Screening principles and methods are thoroughly addressed in Chapter 15 and will not be repeated here. However, a brief mention of screening and diagnostic factors relevant to minimal hearing loss is warranted.

Most infants with hearing loss greater than or equal to 35 to 40 dB will be identified through current newborn hearing screening programs (Benito-Orejas, Ramirez, Morais, Almaraz, & Fernandez-Calvo, 2008; Bess & Humes, 2008). But, as noted previously, those with lesser degrees of loss or with progressive or late-onset losses might not be found. Even if newborn hearing screening programs were designed to target these losses, a number of technical barriers to early identification of minimal and mild hearing loss in the newborn period have been suggested (Gravel et al., 2005):

- Current otoacoustic emissions (OAEs) and auditory brainstem response audiometry (ABR) technologies do not reliably distinguish between normal and mild hearing loss (Gravel et al., 2005). Because of the variability in ear canal volume and geometry, the intensity of the stimuli varies somewhat from infant to infant. At this time, screening instruments do not automatically calibrate the stimulus levels for each ear.
- The configuration of loss in some hearing-impaired ears could result in screening ABR and OAE results that are indistinguishable from normal hearing ears (i.e., significant loss at some frequencies but normal hearing over a range of frequencies; Norton et al., 2000);
- Manufacturer provided pass-fail criteria are often insufficient to determine the validity of specific pass-fail criteria and automated screening algorithms.

Therefore, identifying minimal hearing loss in the newborn period is likely to remain problematic for the foreseeable future. Our ability to distinguish permanent minimal hearing loss from temporary conductive loss, such as that resulting from otitis media with effusion, is also a significant challenge and impacts our financial resources dedicated to hearing screening follow-up. Furthermore, beyond the newborn period, there is no systematic hearing-screening program for children prior to school entry. Even pure-tone screening in the schools fails to identify most children with minimal sensory/neural hearing loss. In fact, if a 25 dB HL criterion is used to screen school-age children, as many as 62% of those with minimal hearing loss would be missed; when screening at a more sensitive cutoff level such as 20 dB HL close to 40% of those children with minimal hearing loss could be missed (Dodd-Murphy, Murphy, & Bess, 2014). Given the documented increase in prevalence of minimal and mild hearing loss between the newborn period and school age, and the potential impact of such losses on psychoeducational development, this is a public health need that requires further examination and action.

Clinical Evaluation of Minimal Hearing Loss

Because hearing screening programs do not target minimal and mild degrees of hearing loss, these children are not likely to be referred for diagnostic evaluations. Without the usual indicators pointing to a possible hearing loss, such as obvious speech or language deficits, suspicion of minimal to mild hearing loss in infancy and early childhood based on parental observation is not likely. However, even if hearing loss is suspected, the accuracy of current diagnostic methods used to define minimal to mild hearing loss in infants and young children might be suboptimal (Cone-Wesson, Sininger, & Widen, 2005; Rance & Rickards, 2002). Specifically, the variability in electrophysiologic (i.e., ABR and auditory steady-state response [ASSR]) and behavioral tests (i.e., visual reinforcement audiometry [VRA]) is felt to limit one's ability to differentiate minimal and mild losses from normal hearing sensitivity.

All pediatric hearing evaluations should incorporate a multifaceted test battery approach as opposed to the use of only one test to determine hearing status. As discussed in Chapter 18, the 2007 Joint Committee on Infant Hearing (JCIH) recommends that audiological assessments include a child and family history and a combination of both physiological and behavioral tests appropriate for a child's developmental age. The following discussion focuses on specific testing strategies that can be employed by audiologists to decrease the likelihood of missing or misdiagnosing minimal to mild hearing loss in children.

Behavioral Testing

Starting at approximately 6 months developmental age, behavioral testing can be included as a reliable component in the pediatric test battery. Whenever possible, ear-specific testing, as opposed to sound-field testing, should be employed. Insert earphones are recommended unless contraindicated, and bone conduction should be utilized if air-conduction responses are not within normal range. More detail on methods of pediatric behavioral hearing testing can be found in Chapter 23.

Accuracy in estimating thresholds, whether using electrophysiological or behavioral tests, is directly linked to the stepsize used during a test session. That is, to detect a minimal or mild hearing loss, using a small stepsize and bracketing approach of, for example, down 10 dB and up 5 dB would be more accurate than a larger stepsize and bracketing approach of down 20 dB and up 10 dB. Likewise, use of a predetermined stopping level commensurate with normal hearing sensitivity could result in a less accurate measure of hearing sensitivity than continuing to test until threshold is obtained. Furthermore, a predetermined stopping level that is too high could result in missing some cases of minimal hearing loss. For example, a stopping level of 10 dB would be better to detect a minimal loss than a stopping level of 25 dB. However, utilization of small stepsizes and testing until threshold is obtained requires additional time that might not be available with restless children. Furthermore, young children with normal hearing might be more likely to respond only to suprathreshold signals between 15 and 30 dB, making it difficult to ascertain a minimal or mild hearing loss. It is important to remember that if one uses large stepsizes and high stopping levels, minimal hearing loss will likely be missed.

Physiologic Testing

Frequency-specific testing is recommended when utilizing auditory brainstem responses (ABRs) for purposes of threshold estimation. Unlike click-evoked responses, which contain a wide range of frequencies, frequency-specific stimuli are better predictors of audiometric thresholds and will assist in identifying varying hearing loss configurations, such as high-frequency losses. Clicks, on the other hand, test for responses in the 1- to 4-kHz range. As with behavioral testing, if one is attempting to identify all types and degrees of hearing loss, testing should include high-frequency stimuli (e.g., 3000 or 4000 Hz) in addition to lower frequencies.

Another limitation of using ABR to identify minimal or mild degrees of loss is that we do not know the actual sound pressure level of the stimulus at the eardrum of the baby being tested. That is, even when using a signal of, for example, 35 dB nHL, the sound pressure level at the eardrum will vary from baby to baby depending on the volume of the ear canal and the age of the baby; the smaller the ear canal volume, the larger is the SPL at the eardrum, thus exceeding the presumed 35 dB nHL chosen for use. Therefore, one might obtain normal ABR recordings from a child with minimal to mild hearing loss. Additional discussion of ABR testing can be found in Chapter 21.

Otoacoustic emissions (OAEs) are a useful contribution to our pediatric test battery. Transient-evoked OAEs, or TEOAEs, are typically evoked from all normal hearing ears and are absent if losses exceed approximately 30 to 35 dB HL (Benito-Orejas et al., 2008; Bess & Humes, 2008). Distortion product OAEs, or DPOAEs are also typically present in normal hearing ears but absent if hearing loss exceeds 40 to 50 dB HL (Gorga, Neely, & Dorn, 1999). Therefore, although OAEs are a quick and relatively inexpensive indicator of gross hearing status, they are likely to miss minimal and mild degrees of hearing loss. See Chapter 20 of this volume for discussion of promising approaches to the use of OAEs for detecting mild hearing loss.

Another diagnostic challenge is the presence of otitis media with effusion, which is often accompanied by minimal to mild degrees of conductive hearing loss in the speech frequency range. Distinguishing between a transient loss secondary to otitis media with effusion and a permanent hearing loss requires the convergence of several diagnostic indicators including bone-conduction thresholds, immittance audiometry, and pneumatic otoscopy. The presence of an abnormal tympanogram is an excellent predictor of otitis media with effusion. Acoustic stapedial reflex testing can also supply information about the functional status of the middle ear and cochlea. However, acoustic stapedial reflexes can be present within the normal range even in the presence of minimal or mild hearing loss. (See Chapter 19 for additional information on immittance testing in children.)

Audiologic uncertainty about either the type or degree of hearing loss can delay definitive diagnosis and intervention. As noted previously, we have known for decades that children with milder hearing losses are identified later than children with more severe losses (e.g., Elssman, Matkin, & Sabo, 1987). In a survey of pediatric audiology practices in the United States and the United Kingdom, Bamford and colleagues (2001) shed additional light on why we might be seeing that delay. They queried audiologists about the age at which they thought they would achieve "audiologic certainty" in young children defined as reliable estimates of hearing thresholds for low, mid, and high frequencies, and clarity on whether the loss was sensory/neural, conductive, or mixed, for children with varying degrees of hearing loss with no risk factors and no other obvious disabilities. Eighty percent or more of the respondents indicated that they reached audiologic certainty about 3 months sooner for children with severe or profound hearing loss than for those with mild hearing losses.

Functional Auditory Assessment

If it is the case that audiologists are not as confident in their ability to diagnose minimal to mild losses with our current audiologic test battery as they are with greater degrees of loss, functional auditory measures might provide an enhancement to the battery and, thus, add a degree of confidence to the diagnosis. Furthermore, although some of these assessments are designed to supplement the diagnostic test battery, others are used to determine the degree of handicap that might be associated with the hearing loss and can guide professionals toward appropriate intervention options. Note that *handicap* is defined as the loss or limitation of opportunities to take part in the life of the community on an equal level with others (World Health Organization, 1980). By assessing listening behaviors in real-world settings, outside the confines of the soundproof booth where most formal audiologic testing takes place, functional assessments can contribute information about what a child hears and, perhaps more importantly, how the child uses what is heard in everyday situations. Typically, these assessments consist of parent or teacher questionnaires. Some of these tools are designed specifically to identify the subtle differences in listening behavior by those with minimal and mild degrees of hearing loss. A summary of functional auditory assessments that are designed to identify or assist in managing minimal to mild losses can be found in Table 37–2.

Table 37–2. Functional Auditory Assessment Measures for Use With Children With Minimal to Mild Hearing Losses

ABEL: Auditory Behavior in Everyday Life (Purdy, Farrington, Moran, Chard, & Hodgson, 2002)	
Age range: 2 to 12 years	*Purpose:* Twenty-four item questionnaire with three subscales (Aural-Oral, Auditory Awareness, Social/Conversational skills) that evaluates auditory behavior in everyday life.
CHILD: Children's Home Inventory for Listening Difficulties (Anderson & Smaldino 2000)	
Age range: 3 to 12 years	*Purpose:* Parent and child questionnaire with 15 situations that rate how well the child understood speech.
ELF: Early Listening Function (Anderson, 2000)	
Age range: 5 months to 3 years	*Purpose:* Twelve listening situations in which the parent and audiologist observe the child and record the distance the child responds to the auditory stimuli.
LIFE: Listening Inventory for Education (Anderson & Smaldino, 1996)	
Age range: 6 years and up	*Purpose:* Questionnaire that identifies classroom situations that are challenging for the child. There are two formats of the questionnaire: a teacher questionnaire with 16 items and a child questionnaire with 15 items.
Little Ears (Kühn-Inacker, Weichbold, Tsiakpini, Coninx, & D'Haese, 2003)	
Age range: 0 years and up	*Purpose:* Questionnaire for the parent with 35 age-dependent questions that assesses auditory development.
LSQ: Listening Situations Questionnaire (Grimshaw, 1996)	
Age range: 7 years and up	*Purpose:* Questionnaire for the parent and child with eight situations. Responses focus on help of amplification, difficulty of understanding, and satisfaction of amplification.
PEACH: Parents' Evaluation of Aural/Oral Performance of Children (Ching, Hill, & Psarros, 2000)	
Age range: Preschool to 7 years	*Purpose:* Interview with parent with 15 questions targeting the child's everyday environment. Includes scoring for five subscales (Use, Quiet, Noise, Telephone, Environment).
Preschool SIFTER: Preschool Screening Instrument for Targeting Educational Risk (Anderson & Matkin, 1996)	
Age range: 3 to 6 years	*Purpose:* Questionnaire with 15 items completed by the teacher which identifies children at risk for educational failure with five subscales (academics, attention, communication, participation, behavior).
SIFTER: Screening Instrument for Targeting Educational Risk (Anderson, 1989)	
Age range: 6 years and above	*Purpose:* Questionnaire with 15 items completed by the teacher which identifies children at risk for educational failure with five subscales (academics, attention, communication, participation, behavior).
TEACH: Teachers' Evaluation of Aural/Oral Performance of Children (Ching, Hill, & Psarros, 2000)	
Age range: Preschool to 7 years	*Purpose:* Interview with teacher with 13 questions targeting the child's everyday environment. Includes scoring for five subscales (Use, Quiet, Noise, Telephone, Environment).

Note. Age refers to child's developmental, as opposed to chronological, age level. Adapted with permission from Oticon.

Auditory Performance of Children With Minimal Hearing Loss

Research performed within laboratory environments offers experimental control, allowing for the investigation of specific aspects of hearing that contribute to listening in real-world environments. For example, it is possible to isolate a specific ear, and to use auditory stimuli that have well-defined frequency and temporal characteristics. Some aspects of auditory performance are particularly difficult for children with unilateral hearing loss, such as localization and understanding speech in noise when the speech signal is presented to the ear with hearing loss. Studies examining the auditory performance of children with minimal hearing loss are discussed in detail in the sections below.

Localization Difficulties for Children With Unilateral Hearing Loss

Children with unilateral hearing loss experience greater problems localizing sounds on the horizontal plane than normal hearing listeners. For example, children with unilateral hearing loss have significantly greater errors localizing 500-Hz and 3000-Hz pure tones than children with normal hearing in quiet (Bess et al., 1986; Humes, Allen, & Bess, 1980) and in background cafeteria noise (Humes et al., 1980). Furthermore, localization errors can be expected to increase as the degree of hearing loss in the impaired ear worsens (Bess et al., 1986; Humes et al., 1980). Results from other studies also illustrate the detrimental effect of unilateral hearing loss on localization. For example, infants and children as young as 6 months and adults as old as 80 years with unilateral hearing loss—some temporary and conductive—have all demonstrated localization difficulties (Morrongiello, 1988; Priwin, Jönsson, Hultcrantz, & Granström, 2007).

It is noteworthy that though the negative effects of localization have been documented in research studies, they might go unnoticed by children in real-world situations. In a study of sound localization in children with severe unilateral hearing loss, 57% of the participants were unaware of problems prior to joining in the study (Newton, 1983). This suggests that children might not reliably report their sound localization ability. Such findings have implications for safety considerations.

Speech Understanding in Children With Minimal Hearing Loss

Children with unilateral hearing loss exhibit difficulty understanding speech stimuli, especially under adverse listening conditions (Bess et al., 1986; Rothpletz, Wightman, & Kistler, 2012). The mean syllable recognition scores for a group of children with unilateral hearing loss and their normal hearing counterparts are shown in Figure 37–1.

Children with unilateral hearing loss exhibit poorer speech recognition scores than children with normal hearing in both monaural direct (speech to good ear, noise to impaired ear) and monaural indirect (noise to good ear, speech to impaired ear) conditions (Bess et al., 1986). In addition, the more adverse the listening condition—that is, the lower the signal-to-noise ratio (SNR)—the greater the discrepancy between children with unilateral hearing loss and children with normal hearing. Children with unilateral hearing loss performed significantly poorer than normal hearing children in the monaural indirect condition. Even in situations where the signal of interest is directed to the good ear with noise directed to the hearing impaired ear, children with unilateral hearing loss did not perform as well as their peers with normal hearing. These results are similar to the more recent findings of Rothpletz and colleagues (2012) showing poorer performance for listeners with unilateral hearing loss for conditions in which the target speech and maskers were colocated at 0 degrees azimuth. However, in that study, listeners with unilateral hearing loss did not have poorer performance than listeners with normal hearing in all listening conditions.

The ability to perform well on speech-in-noise tasks is also affected by degree of unilateral impairment. Ruscetta, Arjmand, and Pratt (2005) found that children aged 6 to 14 years with severe-to-profound unilateral hearing loss required a significantly greater SNR to perform as well as children with normal hearing on sentence and syllable recognition tasks. Similarly, Bess et al. (1986) showed poorer speech recognition in noise performance for children with severe-to-profound unilateral hearing loss compared to children with mild-to-moderate unilateral hearing loss. Other research has also demonstrated that some children and adults with unilateral hearing loss have difficulty understanding speech in noise (Priwin et al., 2007; Welsh, Welsh, Rosen, & Dragonette, 2004). These findings could have real-world implications as children with unilateral hearing loss who exhibit poor speech recognition abilities have been shown to be more likely to struggle academically than children with good recognition abilities. Bess and colleagues (1986) examined speech recognition abilities of children with unilateral hearing loss who had failed a grade in school and those who had not failed a grade and found a tendency for children who have poor speech perception ability to experience more difficulty in school.

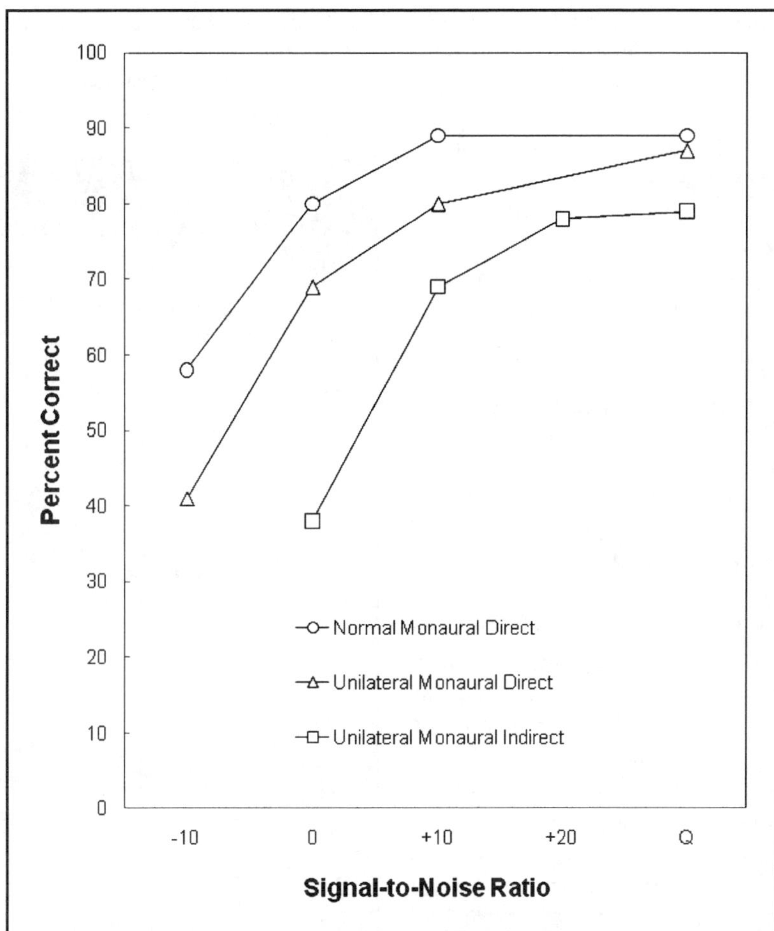

FIGURE 37–1. Mean sound-field composite scores (in percent) on the Nonsense Syllable Test (NST) across several signal-to-noise ratio (SNR) conditions for normal-hearing children and children with UHL. The children were assessed in the monaural direct and monaural indirect conditions. Children with normal hearing were assessed with speech in the right ear and noise in the left ear. (Reprinted with permission from Bess, F., Tharpe, A., & Gibler, A. [1986]. Auditory performance of children with unilateral sensory/neural hearing loss. *Ear and Hearing, 7*[1].)

Although some research has shown an effect of side of impairment on speech-in-noise tasks, the generalizability of the results are often limited by a small sample size and an unequal numbers of participants with right versus left ear impairment. Bess and colleagues (1986) demonstrated that children with right ear unilateral hearing loss performed more poorly than children with normal hearing and children with left ear hearing impairment on speech recognition tasks across various SNR conditions. Jensen, Johansen, and Børre (1989) also showed that children with right ear unilateral hearing loss exhibited poorer performance on speech in noise tests than children with left ear unilateral hearing loss, whereas children with left ear unilateral hearing loss performed similarly to children with normal hearing. They also investigated ear effects on nonverbal intelligence tests and reported that children with right ear unilateral hearing loss performed significantly poorer than children with left ear unilateral hearing loss. Such information could shed some light on findings, such as those by Bess and Tharpe (1986) and Oyler et al. (1988), that suggest children with right ear hearing loss are more likely to have failed a grade in school than children with left ear hearing loss. However, as mentioned above, unequal numbers of children with right versus left ear impairment might have influenced the generalizability of these findings. A greater proportion of children in Bess and Tharpe (1986) and Oyler et al. (1988) had right ear impairment (60% and 64%, respectively). It should also be mentioned that some studies suggest that children with right ear unilateral hearing loss and left ear unilateral hearing loss perform similarly on language performance measures (e.g., Lieu, Tye-Murray, Karzon, & Piccirillo, 2010).

Finally, children with minimal bilateral sensory/neural hearing loss also can experience problems in speech recognition—especially, under adverse listening conditions such as background noise or reverberation. Crandell (1993) examined the effects of commonly reported classroom SNRs (+6 dB, +3 dB, 0 dB, −3 dB, −6 dB) on the speech recognition of children with bilateral minimal hearing loss. Results revealed that children with minimal hearing loss exhibited poorer sentence recognition scores than children with normal hearing for most listening conditions. In addition, Crandell reported that the performance decrement between the two groups increased as the listening condition worsened (Table 37–3.) Others have reported similar results (Blair, 1977; Boney & Bess, 1984). Collectively, these studies provide evidence that children with permanent minimal to mild bilateral hearing loss experience greater difficulty understanding speech than their normal-hearing peers, particularly under acoustic conditions that simulate those typically found in school classrooms. Importantly, Lewis, Valente, and Spalding (2014) recently demonstrated the potential implications of minimal hearing loss on auditory performance in a simulated classroom environment for cognitively demanding tasks. Although children with minimal hearing loss in that study performed near ceiling on a sentence recognition task, they had poorer performance than children with normal hearing when comprehension of a prerecorded spoken story was assessed. This study highlights the potential difficulties children with minimal hearing loss can have acquiring knowledge from auditory information in a classroom setting.

Table 37–3. Means and Standard Deviations (SD), in Percent Correct, of Normal-Hearing and Minimally Hearing-Impaired Children for the Bamford-Kowal-Bench Sentences Across Six Test Conditions

Test Condition	Normal Hearing	Minimal Hearing Loss
Quiet		
Mean	99.7	96.3
SD	(0.7)	(6.9)
+6 dB		
Mean	96.2	83.5
SD	(6.0)	(14.6)
+3 dB		
Mean	94.7	74.9
SD	(5.6)	(21.0)
+0 dB		
Mean	93.2	67.3
SD	(5.2)	(21.1)
−3 dB		
Mean	84.4	53.8
SD	(7.6)	(22.1)
−6 dB		
Mean	70.7	38.1
SD	(15.4)	(25.4)

Note. Reprinted with permission from Crandell, C. (1993). Speech recognition in noise by children with minimal degrees of sensory/neural hearing loss. *Ear and Hearing*, *14*(3).

Real-World Outcomes for Children With Minimal Hearing Loss

Learning and Educational Issues

When compared to children with normal hearing, children with minimal hearing loss appear to be more likely to experience academic difficulties. In general, many children with unilateral hearing loss experience educational, social, emotional, and behavioral problems in school (Bess & Tharpe, 1984; Culbertson & Gilbert, 1986; Lieu, Tye-Murray, & Fu, 2012; Stein, 1983), and degree of hearing loss alone might not be a good predictor of a child's language or educational performance (Davis, Elfenbein, Schum, & Bentler, 1986; Moeller, 2007). A few studies have concluded that there are no adverse academic outcomes associated with minimal hearing loss (Briscoe, Bishop, & Norbury, 2001; Wake et al., 2006), but there is a collective body of evidence to suggest otherwise.

Brookhouser and colleagues (1991) demonstrated that 59% of 172 children with unilateral hearing loss experienced academic or behavioral problems. They found no correlation between degree of impairment and amount of academic difficulty, although more recent evidence suggests that children with profound unilateral hearing loss tend to have worse verbal cognitive and oral language scores than children with less severe unilateral hearing loss (Lieu, Karzon, Ead, & Tye-Murray, 2013). Degree of hearing loss often acts in accord with other variables that contribute to development. Age of identification, family motivation, intervention plans, and the presence of additional disabilities, among other factors contribute to the overall development of children with hearing loss (e.g., Moeller, 2000; Porter, Sladen, Ampah, Rothpletz, & Bess, 2013).

Although not all children with minimal hearing loss experience functional difficulties, some are clearly at risk for problems. Most studies suggest that children with minimal hearing loss (both unilateral and minimal bilateral) are significantly more likely than their normal hearing peers to have to repeat a grade in school or access resource assistance for a variety of academic or cognitive deficits (Bess et al., 1998; Blair, Peterson, & Viehweg, 1985; Davis et al., 1986; Lieu et al., 2012; Most, 2004; Ross et al., 2005; Yoshinaga-Itano, Johnson, Carpenter, & Brown, 2008). Approximately 35% of children with unilateral hearing loss will fail at least one grade, and an additional 15% to 60% will be in need of resource assistance in the schools.

Bess and Tharpe (1984) reported that many children with unilateral hearing loss failed at the first-grade level; however, one-half of the subjects failed grades above the first grade. In another study of 1,218 children with mild sensory/neural hearing loss, two thirds of whom had unilateral hearing loss, 37% failed at least one grade and exhibited significantly greater dysfunction than normal hearing children on subtests of a screening tool for functional status that included behavior, energy, stress, social support, and self-esteem (Bess et al., 1998). Other studies have also noted excessive behavior problems in a significant proportion of children with unilateral hearing loss (Brookhouser et al., 1991; Stein, 1983). Interestingly, Bess and colleagues (1998) noted significant differences between children with minimal bilateral hearing loss and those with unilateral hearing loss. Children with unilateral hearing loss reported poorer communication with family members and greater difficulty getting along well with others than children with minimal bilateral hearing loss. In general, when teacher questionnaires have been utilized to document classroom performance of children with minimal hearing loss, teachers observe higher levels of dysfunction in classroom settings for these children as compared to their peers with normal hearing (Dodd-Murphy & Murphy, 2007; Most, 2004; Tharpe, Ricketts, & Sladen, 2004).

It is informative to examine statistics regarding grade failures in view of the general population. Oyler et al. (1988) collected teacher survey data and found 24% of students with unilateral hearing loss failed at least one grade compared to an overall district rate of 2%. Children with right ear hearing loss were more likely to have failed a grade than children with left ear hearing loss and children with severe-to-profound hearing loss were more likely to have failed a grade than children with lesser degrees of impairment. Overall, 41% of children with unilateral hearing loss had received additional educational services compared to an average district rate of 8.6%. Interestingly, teacher ratings of behavior were similar for children with unilateral hearing loss and children with normal hearing. Although unilateral hearing loss does not always have obvious repercussions on speech and language acquisition, children with unilateral hearing loss should be monitored for subtle speech and language problems. Some screening tests for speech and language problems might not be sensitive to the types of problems the children with unilateral hearing loss experience. Discussions with teachers and parents regarding the child's performance at home and in school can provide valuable information on the child's developmental progress.

Importantly, not everyone has found that children with minimal hearing loss are at risk for educational difficulties. For instance, Keller and Bundy (1980) reported no differences on standardized test scores between children with unilateral hearing loss, siblings used as a control group, and national norms. Lack of statistical power (limited sample size) has been suggested as the possible reason no differences were seen between groups (Lieu, 2004). Tieri and colleagues (1988) found parental report of academic difficulty in the majority of cases of a cohort of 280 children with unilateral hearing loss; they did not, however, identify any specific speech or language problems. Additionally, Hallmo and colleagues (1986) reported no differences in linguistic development or academic progress in children with unilateral hearing loss; however, these inferences were not based on a standardized test measure and they did not include a control group. Finally, Stein (1983) noted that of 19 children with unilateral hearing loss, only one student needed to repeat a grade. Within this group, however, 42% were reported to have excessive behavior problems. Hence, even if educational difficulties are not noted in some children with hearing loss, behavioral problems can exist.

Language and Cognitive Skills

Mixed evidence exists regarding specific implications for language development in children with minimal hearing loss (Borg et al., 2002; Kiese-Himmel, 2002;

Klee & Davis-Dansky, 1986; Peckham & Sheridan, 1976). Some evidence has shown differences in early word usage between children with unilateral hearing loss and children with normal hearing. Kiese-Himmel (2002) reported that children with unilateral hearing loss were delayed in using two-word phrases, but not in acquisition and use of their first words. Borg and colleagues (2002) offered further evidence for an adverse effect of unilateral hearing loss on language development—they reported that children with unilateral hearing loss had significantly delayed language development compared to peers with normal hearing. Recently, Lieu et al. (2010) demonstrated that school-aged children with unilateral hearing loss had worse language skills than their siblings with normal hearing. Persistent negative effects of unilateral hearing loss were seen on language scores after adjustment for confounding variables such as IQ, family income, and maternal level of education. Children with unilateral hearing loss also were more likely to have received speech therapy and have individualized education plans (IEPs) or other educational accommodations suggesting academic difficulty.

Studies have also suggested that children with unilateral hearing loss might not be at high risk for language and cognitive skills. Peckham and Sheridan (1976) reported a higher proportion of speech difficulties in a longitudinal study of 44 children with severe unilateral hearing loss; however, only four children still had poor speech intelligibility at 11 years. In addition, Klee and Davis-Dansky (1986) found no differences between children with unilateral hearing loss and children with normal hearing on six standardized language tests. However, within the group of children studied, it was noted that children with unilateral hearing loss of 60 dB HL or greater had lower full-scale IQ scores as measured by the WISC-R compared to children with less severe losses. Additionally, eight children who failed a grade in elementary school had significantly lower verbal IQ scores than children with unilateral hearing loss who were academically successful. From these data, the authors suggest that children with unilateral hearing loss might have language difficulties, but that the tests they chose to use in this study were not sensitive enough to measure them.

Speech and language assessments of children with minimal degrees of bilateral hearing loss have been lacking. Most studies have examined children with minimal bilateral hearing loss as part of a larger group of children with greater degrees of loss, making conclusions specific to children with minimal losses difficult at best. However, studies of vocabulary, reading comprehension, and language use have shown that children with mild hearing loss perform poorer than children with normal hearing (Blair, Peterson, & Viehweg, 1985). In a more recent population-based study by Wake et al. (2006), no statistically significant differences on tests of language, reading, and behavior were found for a large cohort of children with slight or mild sensory/neural hearing loss when compared to those with normal hearing. However, phonological short-term memory and phonological discrimination were poorer in the children with hearing loss than in those with normal hearing.

Psychosocial Skills

It has been well documented that a percentage of children with minimal hearing loss experience social, emotional, and behavioral problems in school (Bess et al., 1998; Bess & Tharpe, 1984; Brookhouser et al., 1991; Culbertson & Gilbert, 1986; Keller & Bundy, 1980). To illustrate, behavior-rating data by teachers on several behavioral dimensions for both unilaterally hearing-impaired children and normal children are shown in Figure 37–2.

Note that children with unilateral hearing loss had a higher percentage of negative teacher ratings than children with normal hearing. The group of children with unilateral hearing loss received more negative ratings on attention to task, peer relations, dependence/independence, emotional stability, and total negative responses. The only behavioral category in which no differences were found between the two groups was organization skills.

Poor behavior ratings and dysfunction in the areas of self-esteem, energy, and social support have also been documented for some children with minimal hearing loss—both unilateral and bilateral (Bess et al., 1998; Brookhouser et al., 1991; Culbertson & Gilbert, 1986). Children with hearing loss experience difficulty following communication in conversations with multiple talkers, following most conversations in noise, and hearing from a distance. These difficulties can have implications for psychosocial development (Moeller, 2007). In addition, it has been reported that some children with hearing loss experience self-esteem detriment, increased stress, increased energy expenditure, strained peer relations, and decreased social support (Bess et al., 1998; Stinson, Whitmire, & Kluwin, 1996).

Even though some children with minimal hearing loss experience no difficulties, minimal hearing loss must be considered a risk factor given that at least one third of the population experience psychoeducational problems. Recent research supports findings of psy-

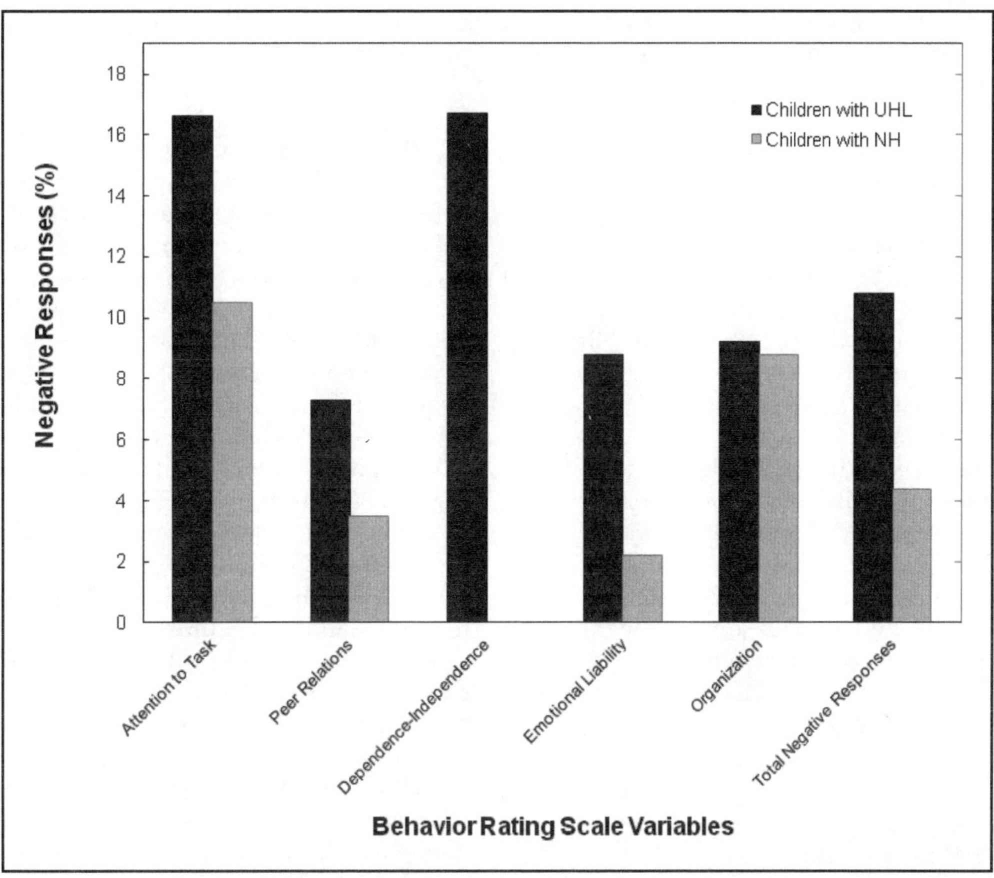

FIGURE 37–2. Behavioral characteristics of children with UHL and children with normal hearing. (Data from Culbertson & Gilbert, 1986.)

chosocial difficulties in those with unilateral hearing loss. Priwin and colleagues (2007) noted a moderate-to-high degree of self-assessed hearing problems in children and adults aged 3 to 80 years. This suggests that although problems might not be noted in observable behaviors, children with unilateral hearing loss can experience problems with socialization and self-perceived quality of life that might not be apparent to their parents.

Teacher expectations of students with unilateral hearing loss might be lower for children with hearing loss compared to peers with normal hearing. Dancer, Burl, and Waters (1995) reported that Screening Tool for Targeting Educational Risk (SIFTER) scores were significantly lower for children with unilateral hearing loss compared to children with normal hearing, suggesting increased risk for academic difficulty; however, no differences were found between groups in terms of teacher ratings of whether students were working to expectations. This might suggest that teachers had lower expectations for children with hearing loss. It is reasonable to consider that lower expectations could affect students' willingness to challenge themselves and the teachers' willingness to challenge these students academically.

Along those lines, there is some evidence to suggest that children with minimal to mild hearing loss might have less energy because of increased listening effort and subsequent fatigue relative to normal hearing children (Hicks & Tharpe, 2002). To the extent that this is true, effort expended to listen in the classroom setting might be a contributing factor to academic difficulties.

Impact on Auditory Skills

For children with hearing loss to understand speech optimally, the signal ideally should be 30 dB more intense than the room noise. Any SNR less than +30 dB has been shown to produce degradation in word recognition among individuals with impaired hearing.

Unfortunately, the ambient noise levels in typical classroom environments are often too high to produce an appropriate SNR. Numerous studies over several decades have documented the poor acoustic conditions of classrooms (see, for example, Cruckley, Scollie, & Parsa, 2011; Knecht, Nelson, Whitelaw, & Feth, 2002; Picard & Bradley, 2001). This situation is compounded by the fact that individuals with hearing loss exhibit greater difficulty in speech recognition than normal listeners under the same noise conditions. Other factors that contribute to the adversity of the listening condition and can possibly produce a synergistic effect include reverberation; speaker-listener distance; the degree, configuration, and type of hearing loss; type of amplification; age of the child; linguistic abilities of the child; the complexity of the message; classroom acoustics properties; and classroom lighting. We have learned earlier in this chapter that the acoustic environment imposes a significant negative effect on speech understanding in children with minimal hearing loss. That is, the poorer the acoustic environment, the more difficult it is to hear and understand clearly, resulting in academic difficulties.

Clinical Management of Minimal Hearing Loss

The appropriate course of action for the clinical management of minimal hearing loss is often not immediately apparent to many pediatric audiologists. The idea that not all children with minimal hearing loss struggle academically or demonstrate speech and language delays can result in hesitation to recommend intervention. Oftentimes, children with minimal hearing loss might not be eligible for intervention services, and amplification can be a prohibitive financial burden for many families. Moreover, it can be difficult for families to accept that a minimal hearing loss is present, let alone a problem (Moeller, Hoover, Peterson, & Stelmachowicz, 2009). Finally, evidence indicates that children with milder hearing losses are less likely to wear hearing aids in school than children with more severe losses (Gustafson, Davis, Hornsby, & Bess, 2015). Despite these barriers to intervention, it is clear that some children with minimal hearing loss struggle, and therefore, the most professionally responsible approach is recommended. That is, all children with hearing loss should be provided with the tools necessary to help them reach their full potential. The following section describes recommendations for the clinical management of minimal hearing loss.

Counseling and Education

Before any management can be initiated, family members of children with minimal hearing loss and the professionals who work with them must all be aware of the value of normal hearing and the risks associated with hearing loss. If not convinced that a risk of developmental or academic problems exists, it is likely that efforts to provide services will be declined.

Keep in mind that depending on the environmental listening conditions, children with minimal hearing loss can often hear much of a speech signal. Therefore, family members and others who observe these children will note that they respond to a variety of environmental sounds. It might be difficult for observers to understand that multiple factors contribute to the way in which children with minimal hearing loss process auditory stimuli (e.g., noise, reverberation, presentation side of signal of interest). One way to educate individuals about the hearing difficulties associated with minimal hearing loss is through the use of hearing loss simulations. Different configurations of minimal hearing loss have been simulated and can be found on the Internet, and recorded versions can be obtained from professional audiology organizations or hearing aid manufacturers. For simulating unilateral hearing loss, one simple option is to provide a single earplug for a family member or school personnel to wear during a counseling session or meeting, which can provide a relatively effective demonstration of what a child experiences.

Etiologic Evaluation

As previously discussed, the etiology of minimal hearing loss in children often remains unknown. The paucity of identified causative factors with this group of children might be related to the later age at which minimal hearing loss is often identified compared to more severe degrees of hearing loss. Recall that minimal bilateral hearing loss is not targeted for newborn hearing screening programs, and that unilateral hearing losses are often lost to follow-up following unilateral failure on newborn hearing screening evaluations. Encouragingly, there is some evidence to suggest that minimal hearing loss is being identified earlier in childhood than has historically been reported (Fitzpatrick et al., 2014). Earlier identification of hearing loss can provide opportunities for determining etiology that are not available for cases of delays in identification of hearing loss until school age. For example, congenital CMV is the primary cause of nongenetic, sensory hearing loss and the leading cause of unilateral prelinguistic hearing loss in children (Nance, 2007). However, to determine the presence of congenital CMV in children, testing must be conducted in the first week of life, prior to other forms of noncongenital exposure to the virus (e.g., from family members, especially young children). Because congenital, not acquired, CMV is associated with hearing loss, a positive test obtained after the newborn period is not effective in determining etiology. In addition, delays in identification of hearing loss might affect parental memory of possible maternal illnesses that can indicate the etiology of the hearing loss.

In addition to the late identification of minimal hearing loss that might be contributing to an inability to define the causative factors, the medical community might not be as aggressive in searching for etiology of these losses as it is for more severe degrees of hearing loss. Etiologic evaluations of *all* degrees of hearing loss should include a careful history and physical exam, and selective use of genetic, radiographic imaging, and laboratory assessment. Determining hearing loss etiology helps to individualize our parent counseling and inform our management decisions.

Intervention Options

The audiologic management of children with minimal hearing loss must be made on a case-by-case basis. Although approximately 25% to 40% of children with minimal hearing loss appear to be at high risk for academic difficulty, it is unclear exactly which of these children will fall into that risk category and require some form of intervention and which children will not. Some evidence exists to suggest that late identification of hearing loss and low levels of maternal education are specific risk factors for psychoeducational difficulties in children with minimal hearing loss (Porter et al., 2013). Intervention options for children with these characteristics should be given careful consideration. It is possible that further research in this area will reveal additional characteristics associated with increased difficulties for children with minimal hearing loss. Therefore, at this point in time, all children with permanent minimal hearing loss must be considered at risk for psychoeducational difficulties and managed accordingly.

Environmental Modifications (Daycare and School Environments)

As noted above, high levels of noise and reverberation can have adverse effects on the speech perception abilities of children with minimal hearing loss. The American National Standard Institute (ANSI) and the American Speech, Hearing, Language Association (ASHA) have recommended standards for classroom acoustics (ANSI, 2010; ASHA, 2005). Several steps should be taken to ensure adherence to these guidelines:

- Measure background noise levels in A-weighted decibels (dBA).
- Measure or estimate reverberation time.
- Measure or estimate SNR.

Following measurement or estimation of these acoustic conditions, a comparison must be made to acceptable standards. ASHA (2005) recommends the following acoustic conditions in educational settings:

- Unoccupied classroom noise levels must not exceed 35 dBA.
- Unoccupied classroom reverberation times must not surpass 0.6 s in smaller classrooms (<10,000 ft^3) or 0.7 s in larger rooms (>10,000 ft^3 and <20,000 ft^3).
- SNR should be at least 15 dB at the level of a child's ear.

In addition, ANSI S12.60-2010 provides acoustic guidelines for learning spaces greater than 20,000 ft^3. There is some evidence to suggest that today's classrooms are not meeting these guidelines for background noise. Reported background noise measurements for typical classrooms range from about 40 to 70 dBA (Crandell & Smaldino, 1995; Cruckley et al., 2011; Knecht et al., 2002).

Of course, there is no guarantee that adequate acoustics will overcome the effects of degraded speech across distance for children with hearing loss. Regardless of the degree of hearing loss or whether the child is using hearing technology, the primary signal should be presented in close proximity of the student, when possible. Hearing technology, especially frequency-modulated (FM) or digital modulation (DM) systems, can overcome many of these adverse acoustic effects. However, many children with minimal hearing loss do not use hearing technology either because it is assumed that such losses are inconsequential, or school systems do not provide the technology except for more severe degrees of hearing loss. Therefore, in the absence of technologic listening enhancements, or in addition to such equipment, low-tech interventions can be employed. Although many acoustic modifications to the listening environment will require the expertise of acoustical engineers, architects, and audiologists, some modifications can be accomplished via simple steps including

- strategic placement of carpet remnants throughout the classroom;
- placement of sound-absorbing materials on the walls to reduce reverberation times (e.g., cork boards, window curtains);
- placement of sound-reducing pads on feet of chairs (e.g., tennis balls, foot covers); and
- installment of acoustic ceiling tiles.

Such modifications to the physical structure of a room improve the SNR, decrease reverberation time, and decrease the overall ambient noise levels.

Types of Hearing Technology

Much like children with other degrees of hearing loss, there are a variety of technology options for children with minimal hearing loss. National organizations in the United States have agreed that hearing technology recommendations for children with minimal hearing loss should be considered on a child-by-child basis (American Academy of Audiology, 2013; CDC, 2005). The reason for this approach, as noted previously, is that although children with minimal hearing loss are at risk for academic difficulty, it is unclear exactly which children will require some form of intervention and which children will not. Also complicating the issue of amplification for children with minimal hearing loss are findings suggesting young children and children with milder hearing loss wear hearing aids less consistently than older children and children with more severe hearing loss (Gustafson et al., 2015; Walker et al., 2013). Therefore, each child's hearing, speech-language, psychosocial, and educational development should be monitored closely. Once the degree, configuration, and type of hearing loss have been determined, it is appropriate to consider the hearing technologies available to help children with minimal hearing loss reach their full potential.

Hearing technologies are described in more detail elsewhere in this handbook. This section focuses specifically on the application of these technologies in children with minimal hearing loss. The type of technology is selected based on the individual needs and activities of each child. For example, there might be a need for a personal FM system for use outside of the school environment if a child participates in activities that impose a distance from a speaker of interest when good communication is critical (e.g., bike riding, horseback riding). Therefore, it is important for audiologists to collect information about a child's activities and interests both inside and outside the home when determining the types of technology that might be valuable. Both those with unilateral hearing loss and those with minimal bilateral hearing loss can be considered for hearing technologies; however, some technologies (e.g., CROS hearing aids) are only appropriate for those with unilateral hearing loss.

Conventional Hearing Aids. Audiologic uncertainty can result in concerns regarding an accurate determination of the degree of hearing loss for some individuals with minimal hearing loss (e.g., infants, young children, and children with significant developmental delays). This uncertainty can give rise to concerns about the possibility of overamplification resulting in a lack of sufficient amplification for these children. However, as with all amplification fittings, the use of real-ear measurements for verification purposes is of particular importance for the safety and efficacy of hearing aid use in children.

Prescriptive methods have been developed for use with infants and young children and incorporate the real-ear-to-coupler difference (RECD) to determine gain and output values for safe and audible sound levels (e.g., Desired Sensation Level Approach [DSL], Seewald & Scollie, 2003). However, the prescribed targets serve as a starting place, not a final goal, for gain and output settings, and adjustments in fittings should be individualized. For children with minimal degrees of hearing loss, it is particularly important to measure RECDs, as opposed to using age averages, because the individual variability can be quite large. Figure 37–3 demonstrates the variability that can be seen in RECD measurements in the infant population. This figure represents a clinical sample of 30 infants (2 months to 6 months of age). See Chapter 25 for more detailed discussion of prescriptive hearing aid fitting for infants and children.

When infants and young children are fitted with conventional hearing aids, the size of their external ear canals influences their RECD, which in turn informs how much hearing aid gain is prescribed. Given the expected large RECDs in infants and young children, it is possible that the prescribed gain at each frequency for those with minimal degrees of loss will be only a few decibels. In such circumstances, one should consider whether the expenditures of cost and effort warrant the purchase of a hearing aid or if, alternatively,

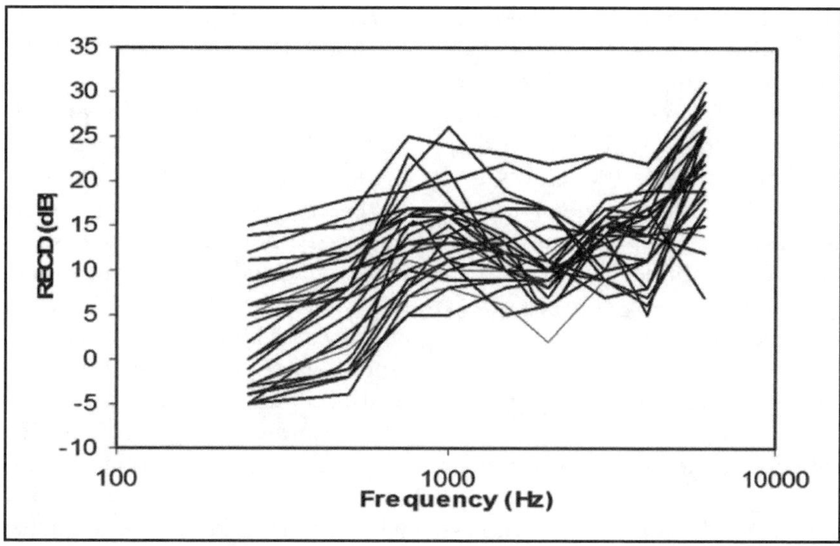

FIGURE 37–3. Real-ear-to-coupler (RECD) values across frequency from infants 2 to 6 months of age. (Republished with permission of American Academy of Audiology, from Bagatto, M. P., Seewald, R. C., Scollie, S. D., & Tharpe, A. M. [2006]. Evaluation of a probe-tube insertion technique for measuring the real-ear-to-coupler difference [RECD] in young infants. *Journal of the American Academy of Audiology*, *17*, 573–581; permission conveyed through Copyright Clearance Center, Inc.)

the goals of improved SNR and audibility could be immediately accomplished by instructing families to use effective communication strategies. For example, families can be counseled to obtain the child's attention prior to initiating communication, maintain close proximity to their infant when speaking, or speak to the better hearing side for those with unilateral hearing loss. In addition, parents can maintain an acoustically friendly environment in the home by reducing extraneous background noise such as televisions and stereos, or managing the play activities of siblings. If amplification is not recommended in infancy, amplification needs and options should be revisited as an infant moves into childhood and gains mobility and independence. That is, when children become ambulatory, the distance from their caregivers is such that they might not be able to receive an adequate level of speech input any longer, thus, a change in recommendations might be needed.

As the category of minimal hearing loss encompasses a range of audiologic configurations, consideration should be given to hearing aid characteristics as they apply specific configurations of hearing loss. For example, for children with minimal to mild bilateral hearing loss, linear processing with compression limiting or low-threshold compression might provide comfortable listening and minimize loudness tolerance problems. Feedback cancellation circuitry might not be necessary because the low amount of recommended gain is unlikely to produce feedback unless coupled to an open earmold. The hearing aid noise floor should be considered when fitting low-gain hearing instruments in children to ensure that the amount of benefit from amplification is not negated by the amount of low-level noise emitted by the hearing aid. Finally, open-ear fittings might be appropriate for older children to avoid occluding the ear from natural, audible signals in the environment. However, in infants and young children, open-ear fittings might not be possible because of the small size of the ear canal.

The audibility of high-frequency phonemes, such as /s/ and /z/, are critical for receptive and expressive language development and are of particular importance to consider for children with high-frequency hearing loss. High-frequency phonemes indicate plurality (e.g., shoe versus shoes), possession (e.g., the girl's sweater), contractions (e.g., that's right), and third-person present tense (e.g., she sits). For perception of these critical phonemes, audibility is required at least through 8000 Hz (Stelmachowicz, Pittman, Hoover, & Lewis, 2002). The use of frequency-lowering technology (nonlinear frequency compression) has been shown to effectively enhance the audibility of high-frequency phonemes in children with mild-to-moderate losses (Glista et al., 2009; Wolfe, Caraway, John, Schafer, & Nyffeler, 2009).

Bagatto and Tharpe (2014) recently proposed a comprehensive guideline to assist with determining the appropriateness of hearing aids for infants and preschool-aged children with minimal bilateral hearing loss (Figure 37–4). In accordance with national guidelines to consider the fitting of amplification on children with minimal hearing loss on a case-by-case basis, they recommended consideration of

- configuration and degree of loss (e.g., high frequency or flat);
- ear canal and earmold acoustics (e.g., possibility for venting);
- hearing aid gain/output and noise floor (e.g., access to speech);
- family factors (e.g., readiness, motivation); and
- child factors (e.g., developmental status).

Recommendations for amplification for children with unilateral hearing loss depend on the severity of the loss, the age of the child, and other factors, such as the child's and family's motivation for using the device. Although the benefits of conventional hearing aid fittings on children with unilateral hearing loss have not been thoroughly documented, it is reasonable to expect that children with unilateral hearing loss would experience some of the advantages of binaural hearing if aided. These advantages include improved speech understanding in noise, binaural summation, and improved localization skills. However, the provision of bilateral hearing does not ensure that a listener will enjoy the binaural benefits that are available from two normal-hearing ears. That is, it is possible that by

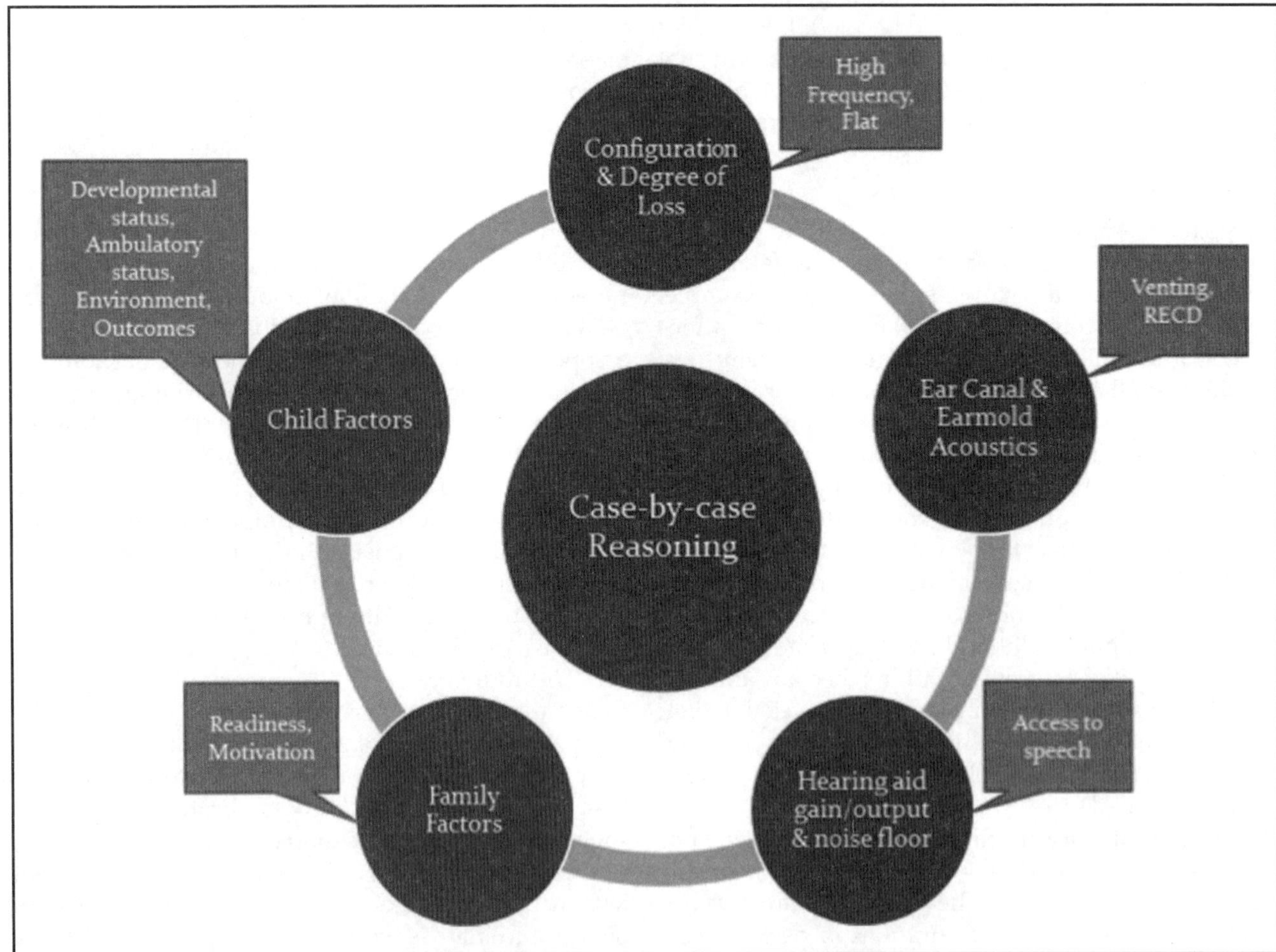

FIGURE 37–4. Factors to consider when determining the appropriateness of a hearing aid for an infant or child with minimal bilateral hearing loss. (From Bagatto & Tharpe, 2014. Reprinted with permission from Phonak, AG.)

aiding one ear, a reduction in speech perception relative to unaided performance can occur. This phenomenon of decreased bilateral performance when an individual receives asymmetric auditory input is referred to as *binaural interference* (Jerger, Silman, Lew, & Chmiel, 1993). In a study of child and adult listeners, Rothpletz, Tharpe, and Grantham (2004) found evidence of bilateral interference in adults but not children, when listening to asymmetrically degraded speech. However, neither children nor adults demonstrated a binaural advantage under the same listening conditions.

Another consideration in fitting amplification to a child with unilateral hearing loss is that of when to fit the amplification relative to possible auditory deprivation effects. As previously noted, unilateral hearing loss is typically not considered of great importance and, thus, hearing technology is often not considered until school age or later, if at all. However, researchers have speculated that binaural hearing is a skill learned early in childhood and cannot be fully recovered later in life (Litovsky, Johnstone, & Godar, 2006). Even instances in which hearing thresholds are improved following corrective surgery for unilateral atresia, improvements in binaural hearing are modest (Byun et al., 2015). It is possible that leaving an impaired ear unaided during infancy and early childhood might limit the benefits (i.e., binaural hearing abilities) a child might receive compared to being fit earlier in life.

Contralateral-Routing-of-Signal (CROS) Hearing Aids. The traditional option for individuals with UHL whose hearing is considered to be "unaidable" with a conventional hearing aid is a contralateral-routing-of-signal (CROS) hearing aid system (often referred to as a *conventional* CROS). The premise of a CROS system is that signals coming to the poorer ear are routed, via a wired or wireless connection, to a receiver coupled to an open earmold on the normal-hearing ear, thus, eliminating head-shadow effects (i.e., diffraction effects of the head) and allowing better perception of sounds originating on the side of the impaired ear.

Although a CROS aid can provide an effective option for children with unilateral hearing loss, one must also consider the possible limitations. For example, in classroom settings, it often is difficult to control the dynamic nature of sound throughout the room. A child might be seated such that the desired signal (usually speech) is routed to the normal-hearing ear one minute, but then background noise might be routed to the normal-hearing ear the next. If a CROS aid is under consideration, one must note whether the child possesses the maturity to monitor the environment and adjust his or her location accordingly. Therefore, young children typically are not considered candidates for CROS devices.

Transcranial CROS. Reported limitations of CROS amplification (i.e., having to wear a device on each ear, poor sound quality) led to the application of transcranial hearing technology. The principle behind the transcranial CROS fitting is that by fitting a high-power in-the-ear, completely-in-the-canal, or behind-the-ear hearing aid deep into the osseous portion of the ear canal of the impaired side, enough output will be produced to stimulate the contralateral cochlea via bone conduction. However, evidence supporting the use of transcranial fittings in children with unilateral hearing loss has been lacking and their use with adults has been received with mixed results.

Bone-Anchored Hearing Aids (BAHA). Although originally intended for use by individuals with conductive or mixed hearing loss, the BAHA has gained popularity for individuals who have profound unilateral hearing loss. At the time of this writing, the BAHA has been approved by the U.S. Food and Drug Administration for implanting children over 5 years of age. The BAHA provides transcranial delivery of the signal via bone conduction from the impaired side to the normal cochlea. Specifically, a BAHA utilizes direct percutaneous coupling of a vibrating transducer to a titanium implant anchored in the temporal bone and is now a CROS option for those with unilateral hearing loss. (See Chapter 31 for a detailed discussion of BAHA devices.)

Most of the efficacy research on this device has been with adults, not children. For children younger than the age of 5 years, conventional transcutaneous coupling of bone-conduction sound is required. This can be achieved by either a traditional bone-conduction hearing aid worn with a rigid headband or the application of the BAHA external sound processor coupled to a soft band worn around the child's head. Proper placement, retention, comfort, and overall ergonomics of use have been reported to be superior with the soft band BAHA compared to the traditional rigid band bone-conduction devices. As the BAHA and the transcranial CROS provide transcranial delivery of the signal in individuals with profound unilateral hearing loss, one could speculate that in adverse listening situations, the introduction of noise to the impaired ear, which is sent to the normal hearing ear, would have similar negative listening effects as those associated with a conventional CROS aid.

Cochlear Implants. Recently, cochlear implants have begun to be considered as an intervention option for adults with moderate-to-profound unilateral hearing loss, and are undergoing clinical trial investigations to determine the efficacy of this treatment option (e.g., Dillon, 2014). Preliminary results suggest improved localization and quality-of-life measures for adult cochlear implant recipients (for review, see vanZon, Peters, Stegeman, Smit, & Grolman, 2015). More research is needed to determine the viability of cochlear implants as an intervention for children with unilateral hearing loss.

Frequency Modulation (FM) Systems. FM systems have many useful applications for children with hearing loss because they incorporate a microphone in close proximity to a talker's mouth, or directly connect to the sound source, and the sound is transferred via FM radio waves to the listener. This arrangement maintains a listening advantage above the level of background noise without reverberation and other effects that degrade the primary signal of interest.

If a child is not wearing personal hearing aids, FM options include use of a low-gain ear-level FM-only device on a normal or near-normal hearing ear; a classroom sound-field FM (or infrared system) with speakers installed in the ceiling or around the periphery of a room; or a desktop style of FM with a speaker placed directly in front of the student. Limited research is available to determine the most preferred configuration, but both ear-level FM systems and desktop FM systems outperform classroom sound-field systems, in terms of improving the SNR, for students with hearing loss. Classroom sound-field systems improve the overall audibility of the teacher's voice for all students in the class and are relatively cost effective. However, in terms of size, portability, and audibility, ear-level FM systems have obvious advantages over larger speaker choices, but usually have an increased cost. Moreover, ear-level FM systems are easily worn in settings outside of the classroom—for example, in the car when parents want to converse with their child in the back seat, when a caregiver wants to talk with a child being pushed in a stroller, or on field trips when considerable distances are expected between the primary speaker and listener. For children who already use ear-level amplification, another FM option becomes available, that of coupling an FM receiver directly to hearing aids or BAHAs. For children with unilateral hearing loss, the decision to route an FM signal to an ear with hearing loss, rather than to the normal hearing ear, will depend on the ability of that ear to process and understand speech. The use of an FM system might not provide any benefit and might even be a detriment if the ear to which the FM signal is routed cannot process the talker's voice adequately.

Tharpe and colleagues (2004) examined various fitting configurations (monaural or bilateral with open or skeleton earmolds) of an ear-level FM system on children with minimal to mild degrees of hearing loss (including some children with UHL). Outcome measures included speech perception ability and configuration preference as reported by the children. The children enrolled in the study demonstrated significantly better speech perception ability in noise (originating from a variety of sources around the child's head) when wearing any of the FM configurations as opposed to the unaided condition. This FM benefit was significantly enhanced when using bilateral FM placement relative to monaural placement in only two of the sound source locations. All but one of the children enrolled in this study reported that they liked wearing the ear-level FM device, and their families chose to purchase the system at the end of the study. Furthermore, all of the children who wanted to keep the FM systems wanted a monaural configuration. It was speculated that monaural usage allowed the students to use the opposite ear for communicating with classmates. Because of the varied amplification and FM coupling options available, FM candidacy should be considered carefully. FM options should be considered for all children with minimal hearing loss in the classroom setting. Current FM options make it possible to choose an FM system for a child to be used as the primary amplification intervention or as an adjunct to the child's primary hearing aid. This makes FM systems a viable option for many individuals with minimal hearing loss. See Chapter 27 in this volume for detailed coverage of remote microphone systems.

Future Research Directions

The overview on minimal hearing loss presented in this chapter raises a number of research questions that are worthy of investigation. For example, although not every child with minimal hearing loss experiences problems with communication or psychoeducational achievement, it is known that many of these children will indeed have difficulties—difficulties that have the potential to compromise social emotional learning and educational progress. The challenge is to identify early the children with minimal hearing loss who are at-risk for problems so that a timely intervention strategy can be implemented. Developmental issues concerned with attention, memory, listening effort, and fatigue are undefined for children with minimal hearing loss. To this end, future research is needed to delineate the specific deficits that underlie the academic and psychosocial adversity seen in this population. Moreover, it is important to establish whether the problems seen in these children will lessen over time. That is, will the children eventually learn to compensate for the adversities imposed by the minimal hearing loss?

Another important area of research includes the social and emotional correlates of minimal hearing loss in children. Psychosocial skills are known to play an important role in an individual's receipt of social, academic and emotional rewards. Emotional-behavioral functioning of children with hearing loss is thought to be a significant predictor of educational performance. In addition, it is well documented that problems in social and emotional development are linked to peer status, school maladjustment, school dropout, and juvenile delinquency. Because social-emotional competence is important to later emotional health and development, it is essential for us to develop a better understanding of the underlying psychosocial factors that contribute to poor social development. Future research should define the peer relationships of children and adolescents with minimal hearing loss and seek to answer the following questions: (a) What factors underlie poor peer relationships for some children with minimal hearing loss? and (b) do children with minimal hearing loss experience transient periods of poor function or are the social/emotional problems present over the long term?

Questions also remain regarding the benefit of intervention for children with minimal hearing loss. Though it is not apparent that all children with minimal hearing loss need intervention to avoid academic and psychosocial problems, it is possible that all children with minimal hearing loss can receive benefit from some type of intervention. Children with minimal hearing loss might not fail a grade or require additional academic assistance, but it is not unreasonable to consider that children who receive intervention have a better chance of reaching their full potential. Outcomes associated with various types of amplification (i.e., traditional air conduction hearing aids, BAHA, and ear-level and sound field FM systems) for children with minimal hearing loss are undefined and merit future study. Future research is also needed to outline evidence-based practices concerning general management, support, and intervention for children with minimal hearing loss and their families. Longitudinal studies are needed as they could begin to delineate the effects of early intervention on academic achievement and psychosocial constructs for older school-aged children.

Efforts should be made to improve early identification of minimal hearing loss, including improvements to technology for early identification and diagnosis. Future research must include systematic etiologic evaluations. By understanding the causes of minimal hearing loss, we might be better able to identify children at risk for progressive loss or other developmental disabilities that can be associated with the etiology of the hearing loss. To this effect, prevalence data in newborns and school-aged children also reflect a need for further investigation. This information will be useful when making policy decisions relative to school-aged children, establishing newborn hearing screening protocols, and justifying funding for intervention and future research.

Afterword

It is generally believed that minimal hearing loss in children does not produce handicapping conditions. An evidence-supported case is made that children with minimal hearing loss experience a variety of auditory, linguistic, and cognitive problems that appear to be compromising, in some unknown way, educational progress. The major conclusion from this chapter is that a growing body of scientific-based research exists to support the premise that school, and ultimately, lifelong consequences result from the presence of minimal hearing loss in childhood. To be sure, a need exists to develop a better understanding of minimal hearing loss in children—research is needed in such areas as identification, diagnosis, prevalence, etiology, educational and social risk factors, and management strategies. Indeed, we cannot afford to do less.

References

American Academy of Audiology. (2013). *Clinical practice guidelines: Pediatric amplification.* Retrieved June 7, 2015, from http://galster.net/wp-content/uploads/2013/07/AAA-2013-Pediatric-Amp-Guidelines.pdf

American National Standards Institute. (2010). *ANSI/ASA S12.60-2010/Part 1 American National Standard Acoustical Performance Criteria, Design Requirements, and Guidelines for Schools, Part 1: Permanent Schools.* Washington, DC: Author.

American Speech-Language-Hearing Association. (2005). *Acoustics in educational settings: position statement* [Position statement]. Retrieved from http://www.asha.org/policy

Bagatto, M. P., Seewald, R. C., Scollie, S. D., & Tharpe, A. M. (2006). Evaluation of a probe-tube insertion technique for measuring the real-ear-to-coupler difference (RECD) in young infants. *Journal of the American Academy of Audiology, 17*, 573–581.

Bagatto, M. P., & Tharpe, A. M. (2014). Decision support guide for hearing aid use in infants and children with minimal/mild bilateral hearing loss. In J. Northern (Ed.), *A sound foundation through early amplification 2013: Proceedings of the sixth international conference*, (pp. 1–8). Stafa, Switzerland: Phonak.

Bamford, J., Beresford, D., Mencher, G., DeVoe, S., Owen, V., & Davis, A. (2001). Provision and fitting of new technology hearing aids: Implications from a survey of some "good practice services" in UK and USA. In R. C. Seewald & J. S. Gravel (Eds.), *A sound foundation through early amplification: Proceedings of the second international conference* (pp. 213–219). Stäfa, Switzerland: Phonak AG.

Baraff, L., Lee, S., & Schriger, D. (1993). Outcomes of bacterial meningitis in children: A meta-analysis. *Pediatric Infectious Disease Journal, 12*(5), 389–394.

Benito-Orejas, J. I., Ramirez, B., Morais, D., Almaraz, A., & Fernandez-Calvo, J. L. (2008). Comparison of two-step transient evoked otoacoustic emissions (TEOAE) and automated auditory brainstem response (AABR) for universal newborn hearing screening programs. *International Journal of Pediatric Otorhinolaryngology, 72*(8), 1193–1201. doi:10.1016/j.ijporl.2008.04.011

Bess, F., Dodd-Murphy, J., & Parker, R. (1998). Children with minimal sensorineural hearing loss: Prevalence, educational performance, and functional status. *Ear and Hearing, 19*(5), 339–354.

Bess, F. H. (1982). Children with unilateral hearing loss. *Journal of the Academy of Rehabilitative Audiology, 15*, 141–144.

Bess, F. H. (1985). The minimally hearing-impaired child. *Ear and Hearing, 6*(1), 43–47.

Bess, F. H., & Humes, L. E. (2008). *Audiology: The fundamentals.* Philadelphia, PA: Lippincott Williams & Wilkins.

Bess, F., & Tharpe, A. (1984). Unilateral hearing impairment in children. *Pediatrics, 74*(2), 206–216.

Bess, F., & Tharpe, A. (1986). Case history data on unilaterally hearing-impaired children. *Ear and Hearing, 7*(1), 14–19.

Bess, F., Tharpe, A., & Gibler, A. (1986). Auditory performance of children with unilateral sensorineural hearing loss. *Ear and Hearing, 7*(1), 20–26.

Blair, J. C. (1977). Effects of amplification, speech reading and classroom environments on reception of speech. *Volta Review, 79*, 443–449.

Blair, J., Peterson, M. E., & Viehweg, S. H. (1985). The effects of mild sensorineural hearing loss on academic performance of young school-age children. *Volta Review, 93*, 87–93.

Boney, S., & Bess, J. H. (1984, November). *Noise and reverberation effects on speech recognition in children with minimal hearing loss.* Paper presented at the American Speech-Language-Hearing Association, San Francisco, CA.

Borg, E., Risberg, A., McAllister, B., Undemar, B., Edquist, G., Reinholdson, A., & Willstedt-Svensson, U. (2002). Language development in hearing-impaired children. Establishment of a reference material for a "Language test for hearing-impaired children," LATHIC. *International Journal of Pediatric Otorhinolaryngology, 65*(1), 15–26.

Boston, M., Halsted, M., Meinzen-Derr, J., Bean, J., Vijayasekaran, S., Arjmand, E., & Greinwald, J. (2007). The large vestibular aqueduct: A new definition based on audiologic and computed tomography correlation. *Otolaryngology-Head and Neck Surgery, 136*(6), 972–977.

Briscoe, J., Bishop, D. V. M., & Norbury, C. F. (2001). Phonological processing, language, and literacy: A comparison of children with mild-to-moderate sensorineural hearing loss and those with specific language impairment. *Journal of Child Psychology and Psychiatry, 42*(3), 329–340.

Brookhouser, P., Worthington, D., & Kelly, W. (1991). Unilateral hearing loss in children. *Laryngoscope, 101*(12), 1264–1272.

Byun, H., Moon, I. J., Woo, S., Jin, S. H., Park, H., Chung, W., . . . Cho, Y. S. (2015). Objective and subjective improvement of hearing in noise after surgical correction of unilateral congenital aural atresia in pediatric patients: A prospective study using the Hearing in Noise Test, the Sound-Spatial-Quality Questionnaire, and the Glasgow Benefit Inventory. *Ear and Hearing,* Advance online publication. doi:10.1097/AUD.0000000000000149

Centers for Disease Control and Prevention (CDC; 2014). *2012 Annual data early hearing detection and intervention (EHDI) program.* Retrieved April 2015, from http://www.cdc.gov/ncbddd/hearingloss/2012-data/2012_type_asha_web.pdf

Centers for Disease and Control and Prevention, Early Hearing Detection and Intervention Program, & The Marion Downs Hearing Center. (2005). *National Workshop of Mild and Unilateral Hearing Loss.* Breckenridge, Colorado.

Ching, T. C., Hill, M., & Psarros, C. (2000, August). *Strategies for evaluation of hearing aid fitting for children.* Paper presented at the International Hearing Aid Research Conference, Lake Tahoe, CA. Retrieved from http://www.nal.gov.au

Clark, J. G. (1981). Uses and abuses of hearing loss classification. *ASHA, 23*, 493–500.

Cohen, C., White, J., Savage, E., Glynn, J., Choi, Y., Andrews, N., & Ramsay, M. E. (2007). Vaccine effectiveness estimates, 2004–2005 mumps outbreak, England. *Emerging Infectious Diseases, 13*(1), 12–17.

Cone-Wesson, B., Sininger, Y., & Widen, J. (2005). *Issues associated with conducting diagnostic audiologic evaluations in children with suspected mild and unilateral hearing loss.* Proceedings from a National Workshop on Mild and Unilateral Hearing Loss. Breckenridge, CO. Retrieved from http://www.cdc.gov/ncbddd/hearingloss/documents/unilateral/mild_uni_2005-workshop_proceedings.pdf

Crandall, C. (1993). Speech recognition in noise by children with minimal degrees of sensorineural hearing loss. *Ear and Hearing, 14*, 210–216.

Crandell, C. C., & Smaldino, J. J. (1995). Classroom acoustics. In R. J. Roeser & M. P. Downs (Eds.), *Auditory disorders in school children: The law, identification, remediation* (3rd ed., pp. 219–234). New York, NY: Thieme Medical.

Cruckley, J., Scollie, S., & Parsa, V. (2011). An exploration of nonquiet listening at school. *Journal of Educational Audiology, 17*, 23–35.

Culbertson, J., & Gilbert, L. (1986). Children with unilateral sensorineural hearing loss: Cognitive, academic, and social development. *Ear and Hearing, 7*(1), 38–42.

Dalzell, L., Orlando, M., MacDonald, M., Berg, A., Bradley, M., Cacace, A., & Prieve, B. (2000). The New York State universal newborn hearing screening demonstration project: Ages of hearing loss identification, hearing aid fitting, and enrollment in early intervention. *Ear and Hearing, 21*(2), 118–130.

Dancer, J., Burl, N., & Waters, S. (1995). Effects of unilateral hearing loss on teacher responses to the SIFTER. Screening Instrument for Targeting Educational Risk. *American Annals of the Deaf, 140*(3), 291–294.

Davis, J., Elfenbein, J., Schum, R., & Bentler, R. (1986). Effects of mild and moderate hearing impairments on language, educational, and psychosocial behavior of children. *Journal of Speech and Hearing Disorders, 51*(1), 53–62.

Dayan, G., Quinlisk, M., Parker, A., Barskey, A., Harris, M., Schwartz, J., & Seward, J. F. (2008). Recent resurgence of mumps in the United States. *New England Journal of Medicine, 358*(15), 1580–1589.

Declau, F., Boudewyns, A., Van den Ende, J., Peeters, A., & van den Heyning, P. (2008). Etiologic and audiologic evaluations after universal neonatal hearing screening: Analysis of 170 referred neonates. *Pediatrics, 121*(6), 1119–1126. doi:10.1542/peds.2007-1479

Diefendorf, A., & Gravel, J. (1996). Behavioral observation and visual reinforcement audiometry. In S. Gerber (Ed.), *The handbook of pediatric audiology* (pp. 55–83). Washington, DC: Gallaudet University Press.

Dillon, M. *Cochlear implantation in cases of single-sided deafness (CI in SSD).* ClinicalTrials.gov. Bethesda, MD: National Library of Medicine. 2000–2015. Retrieved from https://clinicaltrials.gov/ct2/show/NCT02203305; NLM Identifier: NCT02203305

Dodd-Murphy, J., & Murphy, W. (2007, November). *Educational risk and perception of hearing difficulty in school children.* Paper presented at American Speech-Language-Hearing Association National Convention, Boston, MA.

Dodd-Murphy, J., Murphy, W., & Bess, F. H. (2014). Accuracy of school screenings in the identification of minimal sensorineural hearing loss. *American Journal of Audiology, 23*(4), 365–373. doi:10.1044/2014_AJA-14-0014

Edwards, M. (2008). *Follow-up of unilateral failures in a newborn hearing screening program.* Nashville, TN: Vanderbilt.

Elssmann, S. F., Matkin, N. D., & Sabo, M. P. (1987). Early identification and habilitation of hearing impaired chil dren: Fact or fiction. *Proceedings of a symposium in audiology.* Conducted at Rochester Methodist Hospital, Rochester, MN.

English, K., & Church, G. (1999). Unilateral hearing loss in children: An update for the 1990s. *Language, Speech, and Hearing Services in Schools, 30*(1), 26–31.

Finitzo, T., Albright, K., & Neal, J. O. (1998). The newborn with hearing loss: Detection in the nursery. *Pediatrics, 102*(6), 1452–1460.

Fitzpatrick, E. M., Whittingham, J. A., & Durieux-Smith, A. (2014). Mild bilateral and unilateral hearing loss in childhood: A 20-year view of hearing characteristics, and audiologic practices before and after newborn hearing screening. *Ear and Hearing, 35,* 10–18.

Fowler, K. B., Dahle, A. J., Boppana, S. B., & Pass, R. F. (1999). Newborn hearing screening: Will children with hearing loss caused by congenital cytomegalovirus be missed? *Journal of Pediatrics, 135*(1), 60–64.

Ghogomu, N., Umansky, A., & Lieu, J. (2014). Epidemiology of unilateral sensorineural hearing loss with universal newborn hearing screening. *Laryngoscope, 124,* 295–300.

Glista, D., Scollie, S., Bagatto, M., Seewald, R., Parsa, V., & Johnson, A. (2009). Evaluation of nonlinear frequency compression: Clinical outcomes. *International Journal of Audiology, 48*(1), 632–644.

Gorga, M. P., Neely, S. T., & Dorn, P. A. (1999). Distortion product otoacoustic emission test performance for a priori criteria and for multifrequency audiometric standards. *Ear and Hearing, 20,* 345–362.

Govaerts, P. J., Casselman, J., Daemers, K., De Ceulaer, G., Somers, T., & Offeciers, F. E. (1999). Audiological findings in large vestibular aqueduct syndrome. *International Journal of Pediatric Otorhinolaryngology, 51*(3), 157–164.

Gravel, J., Knightly, C., & McKay, S. (2008). *Minimal hearing loss in infants and young children.* Unpublished RO1 grant work; presented by Carol Knightly. The Children's Hospital of Philadelphia, PA.

Gravel, J. S., White, K. R., Johnson, J. L., Widen, J. E., Vohr, B. R., James, M., & Meyer, S. (2005). A multisite study to examine the efficacy of the otoacoustic emission/automated auditory brainstem response newborn hearing screening protocol: Recommendations for policy, practice, and research. *American Journal of Audiology, 14*(2), S217–S228. doi:10.1044/1059-0889(2005/023)

Grimshaw, S. (1996). *The extraction of listening situations which are relevant to young children, and the perception of normal-hearing subjects of the degree of difficulty experienced by the hearing impaired in different types of listening situations.* Nottingham, UK: MRC Institute of Hearing Research.

Gustafson, S., Davis, H., Hornsby, B. W., & Bess, F. (2015). Factors influencing hearing aid use in the classroom. *American Journal of Audiology.* doi:10.1044/2015_AJA-15-0024

Haggard, R. S., & Primus, M. A. (1999). Parental perceptions of hearing loss classification in children. *American Journal of Audiology, 8,* 83–92.

Hallmo, P., Moller, P., Lind, O., & Tonning, F. M. (1986). Unilateral sensorineural hearing loss in children less than 15 years of age. *Scandinavian Audiology, 15*(3), 131–137.

Herrgård, E., Karjalainen, S., Martikainen, A., & Heinonen, K. (1995). Hearing loss at the age of 5 years of children born preterm—A matter of definition. *Acta Paediatrica, 84,* 1160–1164.

Hicks, C. B., & Tharpe, A. M. (2002). Listening effort and fatigue in school-age children with and without hearing loss. *Journal of Speech, Language, and Hearing Research, 45,* 573–584.

Humes, L. E., Allen, S. K., & Bess, F. H. (1980). Horizontal sound localization skills of unilaterally hearing-impaired children. *Audiology, 19,* 508–518.

Hutson, K., Durham, D., Imig, T., & Tucci, D. (2007). Consequences of unilateral hearing loss: Cortical adjustment to unilateral deprivation. *Hearing Research, 237*(1–2), 19–31.

Illing, R., Kraus, K., & Meidinger, M. (2005). Reconnecting neuronal networks in the auditory brainstem following unilateral deafening. *Hearing Research, 206*(1–2), 185–199.

Jäncke, L., Wüstenberg, T., Schulze, K., & Heinze, H. (2002). Asymmetric hemodynamic responses of the human auditory cortex to monaural and binaural stimulation. *Hearing Research, 170*(1–2), 166–178.

Jensen, J., Johansen, P., & Børre, S. (1989). Unilateral sensorineural hearing loss in children and auditory performance with respect to right/left ear differences. *British Journal of Audiology, 23*(3), 207–213.

Jerger, J., Silman, S., Lew, H., L., & Chmiel, R. (1993). Case studies in binaural interference: Converging evidence from behavioral and electrophysiologic measures. *Journal of the American Academy of Audiology, 4*, 122–131.

Joint Committee on Infant Hearing (JCIH; 2007). Year 2007 position statement: Principles and guidelines for early hearing detection and intervention programs. *Pediatrics, 120*(4), 898–921.

Keller, W., & Bundy, R. (1980). Effects of unilateral hearing loss upon educational achievement. *Child: Care Health Development, 6*, 93–100.

Kenna, M. A., Wu, B.-L., Cotanche, D. A., Korf, B. R., & Rehm, H. L. (2001). Connexin 26 studies in patients with sensorineural hearing loss. *Archives of Otolaryngology-Head and Neck Surgery, 127*(9), 1037–1042. doi:10.1001/archotol.127.9.1037

Kiese-Himmel, C. (2002). Problemas auditivos sensorineurales unilaterales en niños: Análisis de 31 casos consecutivos [Unilateral sensorineural hearing impairment in childhood: Analysis of 31 consecutive cases]. *International Journal of Audiology, 41*(1), 57–63.

Klee, T., & Davis-Dansky, E. (1986). A comparison of unilaterally hearing-impaired children and normal-hearing children on a battery of standardized language tests. *Ear and Hearing, 7*(1), 27–37.

Knecht, H., Nelson, P., Whitelaw, G., & Feth, L. (2002). Background noise levels and reverberation times in unoccupied classrooms: Predictions and measurements. *American Journal of Audiology, 11*, 65–71.

Kühn-Inacker, H., Weichbold, V., Tsiakpini, L., Coninx, S., & D'Haese, P. (2003). *Little Ears: Auditory questionnaire*. Innsbruck, Austria: MED-EL.

Kutz, J., Simon, L., Chennupati, S., Giannoni, C., & Manolidis, S. (2006). Clinical predictors for hearing loss in children with bacterial meningitis. *Archives of Otolaryngology-Head and Neck Surgery, 132*(9), 941–945.

Leung, A., Sauve, R., & Davies, H. (2003). Congenital cytomegalovirus infection. *Journal of the National Medical Association, 95*(3), 213–218.

Lewis, D. E., Valente, D. L., & Spalding, J. L. (2014). Effect of minimal/mild hearing loss on children's speech understanding in a simulated classroom. *Ear and Hearing, 36*(1), 136–144.

Lieu, J. (2004). Speech-language and educational consequences of unilateral hearing loss in children. *Archives of Otolaryngology-Head and Neck Surgery, 130*(5), 524–530.

Lieu, J., Karzon, R., Ead, B., & Tye-Murray, N. (2013). Do audiologic characteristics predict outcomes in children with unilateral hearing loss. *Otology and Neurotology, 34*(9), 1703–1710.

Lieu, J., Tye-Murray, N., & Fu, Q. (2012). Longitudinal study of children with unilateral hearing loss. *Laryngoscope, 122*, 2088–2095.

Lieu, J., Tye-Murray, N., Karzon, R., & Piccirillo, J. (2010). Unilateral hearing loss is associated with worse speech language scores in children. *Pediatrics, 125*(6), e1348–e1355.

Litovsky, R. Y., Johnstone, P. M., & Godar, S. P. (2006). Benefits of bilateral cochlear implants and/or hearing aids in children. *International Journal of Audiology, 45*(Suppl.), S78–S91.

MacSweeney, M., Campbell, R., Calvert, G., McGuire, P., David, A., Suckling, J., . . . Brammer, M. J. (2001). Dispersed activation in the left temporal cortex for speech-reading in congenitally deaf people. *Proceedings of the Royal Society of London, 268*(1466), 451–457.

Melnick, M., & Myrianthopoulos, N. (1979). External ear malformations: Epidemiology, genetics and natural history. *Birth defects: Original article series* (Vol. XV, pp. 1–140). New York, NY: Alan R. Liss.

Moeller, M. P. (2000). Early intervention and language development in children who are deaf and hard of hearing. *Pediatrics, 106*(3), e43.

Moeller, M. (2007). Current state of knowledge: Psychosocial development in children with hearing impairment. *Ear and Hearing, 28*(6), 729–739.

Moeller, M. P., Hoover, B., Peterson, B., & Stelmachowicz, P. (2009). Consistency of hearing aid use. *American Journal of Audiology, 18*(1), 14–23.

Morrongiello, B. (1988). Infants' localization of sounds along the horizontal axis: Estimates of minimum audible angle. *Developmental Psychology, 24*(1), 8–13.

Morton, C., & Nance, W. (2006). Newborn hearing screening—A silent revolution. *New England Journal of Medicine, 354*(20), 2151–2164.

Most, T. (2004). The effects of degree and type of hearing loss on children's performance in class. *Deafness and Education International, 6*(3), 154–166.

Most, T. (2006). Assessment of school functioning among Israeli Arab children with hearing loss in the primary grades. *American Annals of the Deaf, 151(3)*, 327–335.

Nakashima, T., & Yanagita, N. (1993). Outcome of sudden deafness with and without vertigo. *Laryngoscope, 103*, 1145–1149.

Nance, W. E. (2007). Marion Downs lecture: How can newborn hearing screening be improved? *Audiology Now*. Denver, CO.

Nance, W. E., & Kearsey, M. J. (2004). Relevance of connexin deafness (DFNB1) to human evolution. *American Journal of Human Genetics, 74*, 1081–1087.

Nance, W. E., Lim, B., & Dodson, K. (2006). Importance of congenital cytomegalovirus infections as a cause for prelingual hearing loss. *Journal of Clinical Virology, 35*(2), 221–225.

National Communicable Disease Center. (1969). *Rubella surveillance.* Bethesda, MD: U.S. Department of Health, Education, and Welfare.

Neault, M. (2005). Progression from unilateral to bilateral loss. In *National Workshop on Mild and Unilateral Hearing Loss: Workshop Proceedings.* Breckenridge, CO: Centers for Disease Control and Prevention.

Newton, V. (1983). Sound localization in children with a severe unilateral hearing loss. *International Journal of Audiology, 22*(2), 189–198.

Niskar, A., Kieszak, S., Holmes, A., Esteban, E., Rubin, C., & Brody, D. (1998). Prevalence of hearing loss among children 6 to 19 years of age. The third national health and nutrition examination survey. *American Medical Association, 279,* 1071–1075.

Norton, S. J., Gorga, M. P., Widen, J. E., Folsom, R. C., Sininger, Y., Cone-Wesson, B., . . . Fletcher, K. (2000). Identification of neonatal hearing impairment: Evaluation of transient evoked otoacoustic emission, distortion product otoacoustic emission, and auditory brain stem response test performance. *Ear and Hearing, 21*(5), 508–528.

Oyler, R., Oyler, Anne, L., & Matkin, N. (1988). Unilateral hearing loss: Demographics and educational impact. *Language, Speech, and Hearing Services in the Schools, 19*(2), 201–210.

Palmer, C. (1999). Deprivation and acclimatization in the human auditory system: Do they happen? Do they matter? *Hearing Journal, 52,* 23–25.

Pandya, A., Arnos, K., Xia, X., Welch, K., Blanton, S., Friedman, T., & Nance, W. E. (2003). Frequency and distribution of *GJB2* (connexin 26) and *GJB6* (connexin 30) mutations in a large North American repository of deaf probands. *Genetics in Medicine, 5*(4), 295–303.

Peckham, C., & Sheridan, M. (1976). Follow-up at 11 years of 46 children with severe unilateral hearing loss at 7 years. *Child: Care, Health and Development, 2*(2), 107–111.

Phillips, L. L., Bitner-Glindzicz, M., Lench, N., Steel, K. P., Langford, C., Dawson, S. J., Davis, A., Simpson, S., & Packer, C. (2013). The future role of genetic screening to detect newborns at risk of childhood-onset hearing loss, *International Journal Audiology, 52,* 124–133.

Picard, M., & Bradley, J. (2001). Revisiting speech interference in classrooms. *Audiology, 40,* 221–244.

Pittman, A. L., & Stelmachowicz, P. G. (2003). Hearing loss in children and adults: Audiometric configuration, asymmetry, and progression, *Ear and Hearing, 24*(3), 198–205.

Podwall, A., Podwall, D., Gordon, T., Lamendola, P., & Gold, A. (2002). Unilateral auditory neuropathy: Case study. *Journal of Child Neurology, 17*(4), 306–309.

Popescu, M. V. & Polley, D. B. (2010). Monaural deprivation disrupts development of binaural selectivity in auditory midbrain and cortex. *Neuron, 65*(5), 718–731.

Porter, H., Sladen, D. P., Ampah, S. B., Rothpletz, A., & Bess, F. H. (2013). Developmental outcomes in early school-age children with minimal hearing loss. *American Journal of Audiology, 22,* 263–270.

Prieve, B., Dalzell, L., Berg, A., Bradley, M., Cacace, A., Campbell, D., & Stevens, F. (2000). The New York State universal newborn hearing screening demonstration project: Outpatient outcome measures. *Ear and Hearing, 21*(2), 104–117.

Priwin, C., Jönsson, R., Hultcrantz, M., & Granström, G. (2007). BAHA in children and adolescents with unilateral or bilateral conductive hearing loss: A study of outcome. *International Journal of Pediatric Otorhinolaryngology, 71*(1), 135–145.

Purdy, S., Farrington, D. R., Moran, C. A., Chard, L. L., & Hodgson, S. A. (2002). ABEL: Auditory Behaviour in Everyday Life. *American Journal of Audiology, 11,* 72–82.

Quigley, S., & Thomure, F. (1969). *Some effects of hearing impairment upon school performance.* Retrieved June 18, 2010, from http://files.eric.ed.gov/fulltext/ED044869.pdf

Rance, G., & Rickards, F. (2002). Prediction of hearing threshold in infants using auditory steady-state evoked potentials. *Journal of the American Academy of Audiology, 13*(5), 236–245.

Roman, S., Aladio, P., Paris, J., Nicollas, R., & Triglia, J. (2001). Prognostic factors of sudden hearing loss in children. *International Journal of Pediatric Otorhinolaryngology, 61*(1), 17–21.

Ross, D. S., Visser, S., Holstrum, J., & Kenneson, A. (2005). Minimal hearing loss and cognitive performance in children: Brief update. *Proceedings from a National Workshop on Mild and Unilateral Hearing Loss,* Breckenridge, CO. Retrieved from http://www.cdc.gov/ncbddd/hearingloss/documents/unilateral/mild_uni_2005-workshop_proceedings.pdf

Rothpletz, A. M., Tharpe, A. M., & Grantham, D. W. (2004). The effect of asymmetrical signal degradation on binaural speech recognition in children and adults. *Journal of Speech, Language and Hearing Research, 47,* 269–280.

Rothpletz, A. M., Wightman, F. L., & Kistler, D. J. (2012). Informational masking and spatial hearing in listeners with and without unilateral hearing loss. *Journal of Speech, Language, and Hearing Research, 55*(2), 511–531.

Ruscetta, M., Arjmand, E., & Pratt, S. (2005). Speech recognition abilities in noise for children with severe-to-profound unilateral hearing impairment. *International Journal of Pediatric Otorhinolaryngology, 69*(6), 771–779.

Scheffler, K., Bilecen, D., Schmid, N., Tschopp, K., & Seelig, J. (1998). Auditory cortical responses in hearing subjects and unilateral deaf patients as detected by functional magnetic resonance imaging. *Cerebral Cortex, 8*(2), 156–163.

Schmithorst, V., Holland, S., Ret, J., Duggins, A., Arjmand, E., & Greinwald, J. (2005). Cortical reorganization in children with unilateral sensorineural hearing loss. *NeuroReport, 16*(5), 463–467.

Schuknecht, H. (1989). Congenital aural atresia. *Laryngoscope, 99*(9), 908–917.

Seewald, R. C., & Scollie, S. D. (2003). An approach for ensuring accuracy in pediatric hearing instrument fitting. *Trends in Amplification, 7,* 29–40.

Silverman, C., Silman, S., Emmer, M., Schoepflin, J., & Lutolf, J. (2006). Auditory deprivation in adults with asymmetric, sensorineural hearing impairment. *Journal of the American Academy of Audiology, 17*(10), 747–762.

Simons, J. P., Ruscetta, M. N., & Chi, D. H. (2008). Sensorineural hearing impairment in children with Chiari I malformation. *Annals of Otology, Rhinology, and Laryngology, 117*(6), 443–447.

Stein, D. M. (1983). Psychosocial characteristics of school-aged children with unilateral hearing loss. *Journal of the Academy of Rehabilitative Audiology, 16*, 12–22.

Stelmachowicz, P., Pittman, A., Hoover, B., & Lewis, A. (2002). Aided perception of /s/ and /z/ by hearing-impaired children. *Ear and Hearing, 23*, 316–324.

Stinson, M. S., Whitmire, K., & Kluwin, T. N. (1996). Self perceptions of social relationships in hearing-impaired adolescents. *Journal of Educational Psychology, 88*(1), 132–143.

Syka, J. (2002). Plastic changes in the central auditory system after hearing loss, restoration of function, and during learning. *Physiological Reviews, 82*(3), 601–636.

Tharpe, A. M., Ricketts, T., & Sladen, D. P. (2004). FM systems for children with minimal to mild hearing loss. In D. Fabry, & C. D. Johnson (Eds.), *Access conference proceedings* (pp. 191–197). Chicago, IL: Phonak AG.

Tieri, L., Masi, R., Ducci, M., & Marsella, P. (1988). Unilateral sensorineural hearing loss in children. *Scandinavian Audiology Suppl., 30*, 33–36.

Tschopp, K., Schillinger, C., Schmid, N., Rausch, M., Bilecen, D., & Scheffler, K. (2000). Detection of central auditory compensation in unilateral deafness with functional magnetic resonance tomography. *Laryngo-rhino-otologie, 79*(12), 753–757.

Unal, M., Katircioglu, S., Can Karatay, M., Suoglu, Y., Erdamar, B., & Aslan, I. (1998). Sudden total bilateral deafness due to asymptomatic mumps infection. *International Journal of Pediatric Otorhinolaryngology, 45*(2), 167–169.

vanZon, A., Peters, J., Stegeman, I., Smit, A. L., & Grolman, W. (2015). Cochlear implantation for patients with single-sided deafness or asymmetrical hearing loss: A systematic review of the evidence. *Otology and Neurotology, 36*(2), 209–219.

Vernon, M., Grieve, B., & Shaver, K. (1980, November). Handicapping conditions associated with the congenital rubella syndrome. *American Annals of the Deaf, 125*(8), 993–997.

Wake, M., Tobin, S., Cone-Wesson, B., Dahl, H., Gillam, L., McCormick, L., . . . Williams, J. (2006). Slight/mild sensorineural hearing loss in children. *Pediatrics, 118*(5), 1842–1851. doi:10.1542/peds.2005-3168

Walker, E. A., Spratford, M., Moeller, M. P., Oleson, J., Ou, H., Roush, P., & Jacobs, S. (2013). Predictors of hearing aid use time in children with mild-to-severe hearing loss. *Journal of Language, Speech, and Hearing Services in Schools, 44*, 73–88. doi:10.1044/0161-1461(2012/12-0005)

Welsh, L., Welsh, J., Rosen, L., & Dragonette, J. (2004). Functional impairments due to unilateral deafness. *Annals of Otology, Rhinology, and Laryngology, 113*(12), 987–993.

Wilcox, S. A., Saunders, K., Osborn, A. H., Arnold, A., Wunderlich, J., Kelly, T., & Dahl, E. E. (2000). High frequency hearing loss correlated with mutations in the *GJB2* gene. *Human Genetics, 106*(4), 399–405.

Wolfe, J., Caraway, T., John, A., Schafer, E. C., & Nyffeler, M. (2009). Studies suggest that non-linear frequency compression helps children with moderate loss. *Hearing Journal, 62*(9), 32–37.

World Health Organization (WHO; 1980). *A manual of classification relating to the consequences of disease.* Published in accordance with resolution WHA29.35 of the Twenty-ninth World Health Assembly, May 1976, Geneva, Switzerland.

Xu, H., Kotak, V. C., & Sanes, D. H. (2007). Conductive hearing loss disrupts synaptic and spike adaptation in developing auditory cortex. *Journal of Neuroscience, 27*(35), 9417–9426.

Yoshinaga-Itano, C., Johnson, C. D., Carpenter, K., & Brown, A. S. (2008). Outcomes of children with mild bilateral hearing loss and unilateral hearing loss. *Seminars in Hearing, 29*, 196–211.

Moderate to Profound Sensory/Neural Hearing Loss in Children

Karen C. Johnson, Amy S. Martinez, Laurie S. Eisenberg, and Dianne M. Hammes Ganguly

Introduction

In this chapter, we discuss the impact of moderate to profound bilateral hearing loss on auditory abilities in young children, specifically those related to speech perception and production. In considering the two, which are intrinsically linked in development, we are dealing with moving and complex targets. Until relatively recently, much of what has been reported in the literature was based on outcomes in older children, often identified at ages well beyond 1 year. With the widespread implementation of early hearing detection and intervention (EHDI) programs a decade ago, many more children with hearing loss are now being diagnosed well under 1 year of age. Consequently, studies regarding the development of speech perception and production skills in very young children who are deaf and hard of hearing are beginning to emerge.

Early identification of children with hearing loss has also generated interest in evaluating the impact of early intervention on speech perception and production, including the fitting of sensory devices at younger ages. To this end, research tools that were developed to examine speech feature perception in normal hearing infants and children with profound hearing loss in the era prior to pediatric cochlear implantation are being adapted for use with a new generation of infants and toddlers who are deaf and hard of hearing. In adapting such tools, the goal is to examine basic auditory-perceptual abilities while minimizing the influence of cognitive, linguistic, and task demands.

We have organized this chapter around a conceptual framework of perceptual development of speech perception and production in young children with hearing loss. We also discuss more recent outcomes for children with severe and profound hearing losses in the context of the changing criteria for cochlear implantation, the advent of pediatric auditory brainstem implantation, and the contribution of multimodal processing.

Classification of Hearing Loss

For the purpose of this chapter, we will be considering children whose auditory detection thresholds in both ears average 40 dB HL (i.e., three-frequency pure-tone average; at 500, 1000, and 2000 Hz) or greater. In the absence of a universally adopted classification scheme for hearing loss,[1] we are using the following ranges to categorize hearing loss by degree: moderate, 40 to 55 dB HL; moderately severe, 56 to 69 dB HL; severe, 70 to 89 dB HL; profound, 90 dB HL and greater.

Because much of the literature concerning auditory abilities in children with hearing loss does not distinguish among clinical subtypes (e.g., conductive

[1]See Centers for Disease Control (CDC), 2015; National Institute on Deafness and Other Communication Disorders (NIDCD), 2006; World Health Organization (WHO), 2015.

versus sensory/neural), our discussion will include children with permanent conductive and mixed losses, as well as those with primarily sensory (cochlear) disorders. Nevertheless, it is assumed that the majority of children with permanent loss described herein exhibit some degree of cochlear involvement and the perceptual consequences that typically accompany sensory loss.

Prevalence of Moderate to Profound Hearing Loss

Large-scale population studies in the United States (Kancherla, Van Naarden Braun, & Yeargin-Allsopp, 2013; Van Naarden Braun et al., 2015) and the United Kingdom (Kennedy, McCann, Campbell, Kimm, & Thornton, 2005) put the estimated annual prevalence of permanent childhood hearing loss greater than or equal to 40 dB between 1.2 to 1.4 cases per 1,000. In these studies, degree of hearing loss is almost equally divided between those categorized as "moderate" and "moderately severe" (approximately 40 to 70 dB HL) versus those categorized as "severe" or "profound" (approximately 71 dB HL or greater). Late-onset, progressive, and acquired losses are estimated to account for approximately 25% of permanent hearing loss in children 9 to 10 years of age (Kennedy et al., 2005; Weichbold, Nekahm-Heis, & Welzl-Mueller, 2006). Thus, the impact of hearing loss on child development will depend not only on its degree, but also on its age of onset and progression (along with other numerous child, family, and intervention-related factors).

Conceptual Framework

A framework that we have found useful in considering the effects of early childhood hearing loss is Aslin and Smith's (1988) model of perceptual development. This model is organized around three levels assumed to underlie development in all perceptual systems including sensory primitives, perceptual representation, and cognitive/linguistic processing. These levels reflect not only the stages in perceptual processing from sensory reception at the periphery to assignment of relevance and meaning at higher cortical centers, but also the transition from less to more complex processing of sensory stimuli made possible with neuromaturation and auditory/linguistic experience.

Moeller and Carney (Carney, 1996; Moeller & Carney, 1993) adopted and extended Aslin and Smith's three-tiered model to describe the development of both speech perception and production, which typically emerge in parallel in normal hearing infants and young children. Level I, sensory/production primitives, corresponds to the most basic stage of auditory perception (sound detection) and production (primitive vocalizations). Level II, perceptual/production representation, involves the coding at higher levels within the neural system that underlies phonetic discrimination and complex vocal utterances at the pre-word stage. Level III involves the cognitive/linguistic processing that allows for word recognition and phonemic-syllabic representation. Table 38–1 summarizes these three levels of auditory perception and speech production for typically hearing children, along with the likely impact of hearing loss.

Sensory Primitives (Level 1)

Typically Hearing Children

Speech Perception. At the most basic level of auditory perception, sound is transformed into a pattern of neural stimulation, reflecting the frequency, intensity, and temporal characteristics of the auditory stimulus. The structures responsible for encoding these parameters (cochlea, auditory nerve, and brainstem) are morphologically mature by the end of the second trimester of gestation (Moore & Linthicum, 2007), and the onset of auditory function is evident by 26 to 28 weeks of gestation (Birnholtz & Benacerraf, 1983; Starr, Amlie, Martin, & Sanders, 1977). Studies examining the intrauterine acoustic environment in animal models (summarized by Gerhardt & Abrams, 2000) suggest that the prosodic features of speech (i.e., pitch contours, rhythm, and stress) are all available to the fetus, as are cues underlying the perception of voicing (Griffiths, Brown, Gerhardt, Abrams, & Morris, 1994). There is also evidence of rudimentary frequency discrimination on the part of the fetus during the third trimester of gestation (Shahidullah & Hepper, 1994), and newborns have been shown to demonstrate preferences for acoustic stimuli to which they have been repeatedly exposed during the fetal period (DeCasper & Fifer, 1980; Lecanuet & Schaal, 1996). Thus, by the time he or she is born, the typically hearing and developing infant has been detecting and responding to sound in utero for 2 to 3 months. It has been suggested that this early experience not only assists infants in attending to specific sounds or speech features shortly following birth, but also forms the basis for transnatal learning (Granier-Deferre, Bassereau, Ribeiro, Jacquet, & DeCasper, 2011;

Table 38–1. Impact of Hearing Loss (HL) on Speech Perception and Production

Level of Perception	*Speech Perception*	*Speech Production*
Level I. Sensory Primitives	Encoding of physical characteristics of auditory input (frequency, intensity, duration, and temporal pattern) by the cochlea, auditory nerve, and brainstem into pattern of neural activity. Sound detection occurs at this level. Impact of HL*:* Reduces or eliminates the sensory primitive, depending on degree and extent of auditory damage. The fitting and programming of sensory devices targets this stage, attempting to provide as much access to the auditory input (e.g., speech spectrum) as possible.	Cries, "vegetative sounds," undifferentiated vocalizations, and vocal play; developmental progression toward adult-like speech in duration, formant transitions, and vowel space secondary to anatomical maturation and auditory experience. Impact of HL*:* Similar repertoire of early vocalization types to typically hearing peers. Emergence of later production primitives may be prolonged, depending on degree of loss, timing, or effectiveness of sensory device use.
Level II. Perceptual Representations	Complex encoding at higher, more neural levels; discrimination and categorization based on complex acoustic features. Impact of HL*:* The ability to differentiate speech pattern contrasts decreases as HL increases. Vowel contrasts are perceived with greater accuracy than consonant contrasts; consonant voicing and front place of articulation are perceived with greater accuracy than manner and rear place of articulation.	Production of more complex vocal sequences resembling adult speech patterns in timing, syllabic structure, and phonetic content—"canonical babbling." Impact of HL*:* Delayed onset of babbling, restricted consonant repertoire, and smaller proportion of multisyllabic consonant-vowel (CV) utterances compared to hearing peers. Greater degrees of HL are associated with longer delays and greater restrictions in vocal output.
Level III. Cognitive/Linguistic Processing	Complex neural code transformed into meaningful words; listeners are able to break down words into component phonemes, but processing primarily at whole word level. Further development with maturation of the higher auditory/cortical centers, accumulating experience with the ambient language, and the expansion of receptive and expressive language skills. Impact of HL*:* Children with HL in moderate to severe range typically achieve open-set recognition for speech that is made audible; however, word and sentence recognition decrease systematically as degree of HL increases. Children with profound hearing loss exhibit a range of speech perception abilities, depending on the degree and quality of auditory access provided by sensory devices (HAs, CIs, or ABIs).	Clear phonemes and syllabic patterns from the parent language can be identified in vocal repertoire of infants and toddlers. Phonemes in speech strings begin to be used meaningfully in real words. Orderly progression in speech sound acquisition occurs throughout childhood. The majority of typically hearing and developing children are intelligible to unfamiliar listeners by approximately 4 years of age. Impact of HL*:* Most children with moderate and severe HL develop intelligible speech; many children with profound HL using CI(s) also develop intelligible speech. Phonologic development follows typical progression but may be delayed depending on degree of HL, the age of sensory intervention, and the quality of auditory access provided by sensory devices. Fricative and affricates are particularly vulnerable to omission and substitution by children with all degrees of HL.

Note. ABI = auditory brainstem implant; *CI* = cochlear implant; *HA* = hearing aid; *HL* = hearing loss. Based on Aslin and Smith's (1988) model of perceptual development and Moeller and Carney's (1993) application of the model to describe auditory and vocal development.

Mampe, Friederici, Christophe, & Wermke, 2009; Moon & Fifer, 2000; Partanen et al., 2013). Nevertheless, it is only after birth that infants are exposed to the full range of sound in their environment (Werner, 2007).

In the newborn, the abilities to detect, discriminate, and locate sounds are immature compared to adults (Olsho, Koch, Carter, Halpin, & Spetner, 1988; Schneider, Trehub, & Thorpe, 1991; Tharpe & Ashmead, 2001; Trehub, Schneider, & Endman, 1980). Auditory sensitivity, frequency and temporal resolution, and sound source localization continue to mature throughout the course of infancy and childhood and are dependent on further auditory experience.[2]

Speech Production. The most basic level of speech output is represented by the cries, vegetative sounds (associated with feeding and protection of the airway), undifferentiated vocalizations, and vocal play characteristic of infants during the first half year of life. Due to anatomic and neuromuscular immaturities of the vocal tract, these early sound productions are, for the most part, qualitatively distinct from those characteristic of adults in terms of frequency, resonance, and duration (Kent & Murray, 1982; Oller, 1980; Stark, 1980). Nevertheless, it appears that babies only a few days old are able to exert sufficient respiratory-laryngeal control to produce cries reflective of the prosody of the ambient language (Mampe et al., 2009).

With maturation, the vocal tract develops toward one that more closely resembles that of the adult human, enabling the articulatory capacity that underlies speech. Beginning around 3 months of age, infants are able to produce vocalizations that perceptually match the vowels produced by an adult speaker (Kuhl & Meltzoff, 1996). This is considered to reflect not only the infant's emerging laryngeal and articulatory motor control, but vocal learning via imitation as well. Around 4 months of age, the infant begins to combine vowel-like and consonant-like productions, during what has been referred to as "marginal babbling" by (Oller, 1980) and "vocal play" by (Stark, 1980). Although the consonant and vocalic elements in these utterances do not yet match those of adult speech in duration, formant transitions, or vowel space, the developmental progression toward adult-like targets over the first six months provides evidence that the infant's early auditory experience with the ambient language, combined with maturation and the propensity to imitate, converge to shape subsequent vocal and speech production.

Impact of Hearing Loss

Speech Perception. The primary impact of hearing loss is to reduce or eliminate the sensory primitive, and it is at this level that sensory intervention is targeted (Carney, 1996; Moeller & Carney, 1993). Without sensory assistance, children with hearing losses of moderate or greater severity will have inconsistent, incomplete, or possibly no access to speech produced by themselves or others.[3] For most of these children, appropriately fitted hearing aids (HAs) might bring much of the speech spectrum into the audible range. Still, depending on the configuration of the hearing loss and bandwidth of the sensory device, some components of speech (e.g., low amplitude, high frequency) might continue to be inaudible (Boothroyd & Medwetsky, 1992; Glista et al., 2009; Stelmachowicz, Pittman, Hoover, & Lewis, 2002; Stelmachowicz, Pittman, Hoover, Lewis, & Moeller, 2004).

For some children with profound loss, it might not be possible to provide sufficient gain to access much beyond the temporal envelope of speech signals, available in the lower frequencies. As hearing loss increases beyond 110 dB HL, any response to sound using acoustic amplification is likely to be based more on vibration than actual audition (Boothroyd & Cawkwell, 1970). For children with severe and profound hearing losses, cochlear implants (CIs) might provide better access to acoustic signals across a broader frequency range than HAs.

Beyond the issue of audibility, the broadened frequency tuning and poorer temporal resolution that often accompany cochlear dysfunction will alter the pattern of neural activation sent forward to the next stage of perception processing. In addition, the necessity for listening to signals processed through acoustic amplification is likely to further impact speech perception, given the intrastimulus masking (i.e., upward spread of masking, backward masking) that might occur at high intensity levels (Boothroyd, 1978; Moore, 1996). Any or all of these factors might play a role in the reduced speech perception abilities demonstrated by individuals with cochlear involvement.[4]

Speech Production. Studies comparing the vocal characteristics of infants with hearing loss to those of normal hearing infants over the first few months of life have highlighted differences in fundamental frequency (F0), utterance duration, and proportion of unvoiced

---

[2]For a comprehensive review of developmental aspects of human hearing, the reader is referred to Werner, Fay, and Popper (2012).
[3]Re: average speech spectra (Cornelisse, Gagne, & Seewald, 1991; Pittman, Stelmachowicz, Lewis, & Hoover, 2003).
[4]For excellent summaries about cochlear processing and the perceptual consequences of cochlear impairment, see Moore (1996, 2008).

elements in total utterances between the two groups (Clement, Koopmans-van Beinum, & Pols, 1996; van den Dikkenberg-Pot, Koopmans-van Beinum, & Clement, 1998). Overall, compared to typically hearing infants, those with profound hearing loss tend to produce longer utterances, with a greater proportion of voiceless to voiced productions. Fundamental frequency also tends to be higher in deaf infants. These differences become significant by 8.5 to 10.5 months of age. Such findings suggest that vocal development is shaped not only by physical maturation of the vocal and articulatory mechanism, but by speech auditory perception and feedback as well.

Perceptual Representation (Level II)

Typically Hearing Children

Speech Perception. Although sensory primitives are necessary for perception, an intermediate stage of processing is required to encode the neural stimulation patterns generated at the sensory periphery into perceptual units that are directly relevant to the real world (Aslin & Smith, 1988; Clement et al., 1996). In auditory perception, this stage corresponds to the prelinguistic encoding of complex acoustic features that underlies discrimination at the phonemic level. Nearly a half-century of research has demonstrated that humans are born with an astonishing array of abilities for differentiating and categorizing the sounds of speech.[5] Newborns are able to recognize and show preference for their mother's voice (DeCasper & Fifer, 1980). Electrophysiologic evidence suggests that the mother's voice elicits language-relevant pre-attentional processing in newborns, whereas the voice of a stranger elicits more voice-specific processing (Beauchemin et al., 2010). Furthermore, infants a few days old have been shown to distinguish between their mother's native language and another language (Moon, Cooper, & Fifer, 1993) even when spoken by the same (bilingual) woman (Mehler et al., 1988). Prenatal exposure to the ambient language also appears to alter perception of specific speech features underlying vowel discrimination in newborns (Moon, Lagercrantz, & Kuhl, 2013).

The studies cited above build on classic experiments conducted in the 1970s and 1980s demonstrating that, within the first six months of life, infants are able to discriminate the majority of phonetic contrasts required to perceive most segmental features underlying speech perception. These include voicing (Eimas, Siqueland, Jusczyk, & Vigorito, 1971), place and manner of articulation (Eimas, 1974; Eimas & Miller, 1980b), and vowel identity (Kuhl & Miller, 1982). In addition, infants demonstrate the ability to manage the variability introduced into speech by different talkers (Juszyck, Pisoni, & Mullennix, 1992; Kuhl, 1983), and speaking rates (Eimas & Miller, 1980a; Miller & Eimas, 1983).

Speech Production. Around six months of age, infants with normal hearing begin to demonstrate the coordinated phonation and articulatory gestures required to produce well-formed consonant-vowel (CV) syllables (Oller, 1980). The combining of CV syllables in repeated or alternating sequence, referred to as *canonical babbling*, typically emerges between the ages of 5 to 10 months of age (Nathani, Ertmer, & Stark, 2006; Oller, 2000). Its onset is quite sudden and, in terms of its quality, timing, and frequency transitions, canonical babbling sounds noticeably like adult "speech" (Oller & Eilers, 1988). Because the syllable is considered to be the "phonetic building block" of adult speech (Oller & Eilers, 1988), canonical babbling marks an important boundary between prelexical and lexical stages of phonological development and is a necessary precursor for the first spoken words (Oller, Wieman, Doyle, & Ross, 1976; Vihman, Ferguson, & Elbert, 1986).

Impact of Hearing Loss

Speech Perception. In contrast to the vast literature regarding discriminative abilities in normal hearing infants and children, this intermediate stage of perceptual processing has received comparatively limited attention in children with hearing loss. Until relatively recently, much of what we know about this level of representation in deaf and hard of hearing children came from seminal studies conducted in older children by pioneering investigators in the 1970s and 1980s (Boothroyd, 1984; Erber, 1972, 1979; Erber & Alencewicz, 1976; Hack & Erber, 1982; Smith, 1975). The aim of this research was to determine which speech features were available to children with different degrees of loss, in order to identify the acoustic and prosodic cues that might be made more accessible through focused auditory training. A second goal was to investigate the contribution of nonauditory sources of information (e.g., visual, tactile) for children who had little or no access to acoustic information with amplification, for the purpose of suggesting supplementary or alternative approaches to sensory intervention (e.g., lipreading, vibrotactile devices).

[5]For reviews summarizing development of speech perception in typically developing infants, see Jusczyk and Luce (2002), Houston (Chapter 3 in this volume), and Kuhl (2004).

In a series of investigations in school aged children, Erber and colleagues determined that, in general, those with hearing loss in the severe range (approximately 70 to 95 dB HL) were able to discriminate between consonants on the basis of voicing and manner (e.g., plosive versus nasal; Erber, 1972, 1979; Erber & Alencewicz, 1976). Place of articulation (e.g., bilabial, alveolar, velar) was discriminated with less consistency (Erber, 1972). Importantly, the ability to perceive most consonants meant that children with severe hearing loss typically were able to identify the number of syllables within words, although words containing voiced continuant consonants (e.g., /m/, /n/) at syllable boundaries were more difficult to segment than those marked by stops or plosives (Erber, 1971, 1979). In contrast, children with hearing losses greater than 95 dB HL tended to have access only to the gross temporal and intensity cues (waveform envelope) available in the lower frequency regions and through vibrotactile reception (Cramer & Erber, 1974; Zeiser & Erber, 1977). The inability to access the spectral information underlying consonant perception meant that these children also had difficulty identifying syllabic boundaries and thus the pattern of speech (Erber, 1971).

Boothroyd (1984) used pairs of consonant-vowel-consonants (CVCs) to examine contrast perception in 120 orally educated children with hearing losses ranging from moderate to profound (55 to 130 dB HL). Employing a four-alternative forced-choice paradigm (Speech Pattern Contrast test; SPAC), eight contrasts were assessed, including vowel height, vowel place, consonant voicing, consonant continuance (manner), consonant place, temporal (syllabic) pattern, pitch variation, and talker gender. Performance decreased with increasing hearing loss. Children with hearing losses averaging 55 to 74 dB HL were able to perceive all contrasts with 66% or greater accuracy. Children with hearing losses in the 75 to 89 dB HL range scored above chance on all contrasts except consonant place. Children with hearing losses greater than or equal to 90 dB HL showed systematic decreases in the ability to discriminate segmental contrasts as hearing loss increased from 90 to 130 dB HL. In this group of subjects, temporal pattern (number of syllables) and vowel height were the contrasts that remained most perceivable with increasing degrees of hearing loss.

With the advent of pediatric cochlear implantation, there was renewed interest in the acoustic-phonemic level of perceptual representation. Drawing largely on the work of Erber and Boothroyd, a number of tools were compiled to assess a hierarchy of discrimination skills below the level of word recognition in children with profound hearing loss and limited verbal skills. These tools included the Discrimination After Training (DAT) test (Thielemeir, Brimacombe, & Eisenberg, 1982), the Minimal Pairs test (Robbins, Renshaw, Miyamoto, Osberger, & Pope, 1988), the Early Speech Perception test (ESP; Moog & Geers, 1990), and the Change-No Change procedure (Carney et al., 1993; Robbins, Osberger, Miyamoto, Renshaw, & Carney, 1988). Researchers used such measures to examine outcomes in profoundly deaf children using early generations of CI devices and to compare rate of change in speech perception abilities across children using different types of sensory devices (single-channel versus multichannel CIs; CIs versus HAs versus tactile aids).

In general, it was demonstrated that the single-channel implant (3M/House) primarily provided enhanced suprasegmental information (timing, intensity, stress, duration) compared to that provided by the power-gain HAs being used at the time, with some limited encoding of low-frequency segmental (speech feature) cues (Eisenberg, Berliner, Thielemeir, Kirk, & Tiber, 1983). Nevertheless, a small subset of children (primarily those with acquired hearing loss) obtained enough segmental information to discriminate between spondees in closed-sets and obtain "nonzero" open-set recognition (Thielemeir, Tonokawa, Petersen, & Eisenberg, 1985). Children using the multichannel Nucleus-22 demonstrated, on average, better vowel and consonant perception than those using either the single-channel implant (Chute, Hellman, Parisier, & Selesnick, 1990; Miyamoto et al., 1992) or tactile aids (Carney et al., 1993; Robbins, Osberger, et al., 1988). Furthermore, speech feature discrimination for children using multichannel devices tended to be comparable to that demonstrated by children with pure-tone averages (PTAs) in the 90 to 100 dB HL range using HAs (Geers & Brenner, 1994; Osberger et al., 1991). The significance of this comparison was that, at the time, children with PTAs in the range of 90 to 100 or 105 dB HL were still generally considered to have functional hearing for the purpose of developing spoken communication.

The children who participated in the early CI studies described above were generally school aged. With the implementation of early hearing detection and intervention (EHDI) programs during the past decade, attention again turned toward assessing speech pattern contrast perception for the purpose of evaluating the impact of sensory intervention in very young children (i.e., HAs, CIs, and auditory brainstem implants [ABIs]) on developing speech perception abilities in early identified deaf and hard of hearing children (Kosky & Boothroyd, 2003; Mahshie, Core, & Larsen, 2015; Martinez, Eisenberg, Boothroyd, & Visser-Dumont, 2008; Uhler, Yoshinaga-Itano, Gabbard, Rothpletz, &

Jenkins, 2011). Most of the measures derive from the speech pattern contrast test (SPAC; Boothroyd, 1984). To this end, Boothroyd and colleagues have extended the SPAC concept to young children by developing a test battery for the purpose of assessing speech pattern contrast perception in children as they mature (i.e., ages 6 months to 5 years; Eisenberg, Martinez, & Boothroyd, 2007). This progressive test battery consists of four measures: Visual Reinforcement Assessment of the Perception of Speech Pattern Contrast (VRASPAC), Play Assessment of Speech Pattern Contrasts (PLAYSPAC), Online Imitative Test of Speech Feature Contrast Perception (OLIMSPAC), and Video Speech Pattern Contrast Test (VIDSPAC). All of the measures examine the same six phonetic contrasts: vowel height (e.g., "aa" versus "oo"), vowel place (e.g., "ee" versus "oo"), consonant voicing (e.g., "d" versus "t"), consonant continuance or manner (e.g., "t" versus "s"), consonant place in the front (alveolar versus bilabial position, e.g., "d" versus "b"), and consonant place in the rear position (alveolar versus velar, e.g., "d" versus "g"). However, each measure employs a different behavioral response task, based on the child's age and developmental abilities, to determine whether phonetic change has been perceived.

The test developed specifically for infants, VRASPAC (Martinez et al., 2008) uses a visually reinforced head turn to indicate that a child has detected a phonetic change in a series of replicated syllables. For each phonetic contrast, results are plotted according to the confidence level that the child's head turn responses are not random. Figure 38–1 shows VRASPAC results obtained over a 9-month period from a child with profound hearing loss. Diagnosed at 1 month of age, this child was fitted with amplification by the age of 2 months. He was implanted bilaterally (Nucleus 24) in sequential surgeries at 12 months (right ear) and 14 months (left ear) of age, with device activation at 13 and 15 months of age, respectively. The top graph shows results obtained from this child at 10 months of age, prior to implantation. With amplification, this child was able to detect a change in vowel height with greater than 90% confidence, but could not be conditioned to respond to a change in vowel place. The more difficult consonant contrasts were not attempted. The middle graph shows this child's results at the age of 16 months, 1 and 3 months following activation of his first and second implants, respectively. With just 3 months of experience using his first cochlear implant, this child demonstrated the ability to detect consonant continuance in addition to vowel height, at a confidence level of over 90%. Again, he could not be conditioned to respond consistently to vowel place or to consonant place in the frontal position. Consonant voicing and consonant place in the rear position were not tested. The bottom graph shows results obtained 3 months later, 6 months following activation of his first CI and 4 months following the second CI. At this interval, he met or exceeded the 90% confidence level for detection for five of the six contrasts.

Employing the VRASPAC algorithm described above, Uhler and colleagues (2011) tracked phoneme discrimination in three infant/toddlers with severe to profound hearing loss who received cochlear implants between the ages of 12 and 16 months. Seven normal hearing age-matched controls were tested over the same time period. Discrimination was assessed for the following contrasts: /sa-ma/ (contrast in all acoustic aspects); /a-u/, /a-i/, /u-i/ (vowel place); /ta-da/ (consonant voicing); and /pa-ka/ (consonant place). Testing was conducted pre-CI activation, on the second day following CI activation, then at 1, 2, and 3 months postactivation. By the 3-month postactivation time point, all three toddlers were able to discriminate at least three out of the five phoneme contrasts with 90% confidence or greater. Furthermore, after 3 months of CI experience, there was no difference in discrimination performance between two of the CI recipients and their normal hearing age-matched peers.

VRASPAC and PLAYSPAC also were used to track emerging speech contrast detection in two English-speaking children who had been implanted with ABIs in Europe, prior to the initiation of the pediatric ABI clinical trials in the United States. For PLAYSPAC, the child is conditioned to perform a motor activity (e.g., putting a peg on a board, dropping a block in a bucket) in response to perceiving a speech feature change. Figure 38–2 shows postactivation results obtained for "ABI 1" and "ABI 2," who were implanted at ages 2 years 2 months and 2 years 6 months, respectively. ABI 1 was diagnosed with profound hearing loss at the age of 5 months. Imaging studies conducted at the age of 10 months revealed hypoplasia of right cochlea and aplasia of the left cochlea. ABI 2 was diagnosed with bilateral agenesis of the auditory nerves at the age of 24 months. After an initial period of medical follow-up at their European ABI center, both children traveled to our center for further consultation and audiologic follow-up. The top half of the figure shows results for both children within the first two years following device activation. At 24 months post, ABI 1 was able to detect a change in vowel place but not vowel height. At 16 months postactivation, ABI 2 was able to detect a change in vowel height but not vowel place. Neither child could be conditioned to respond to a change in consonant continuance; in addition, ABI 2 could not be conditioned to respond to consonant

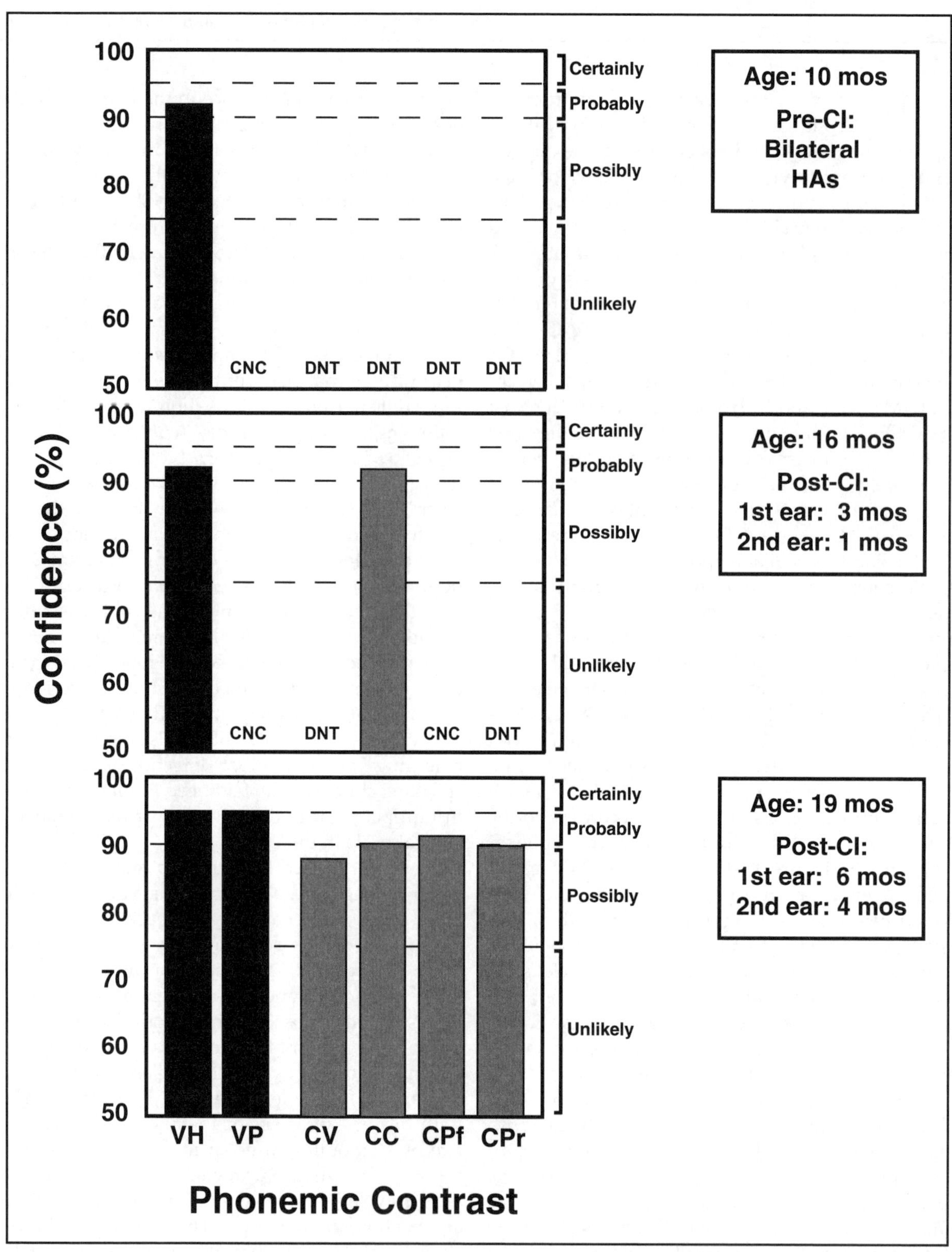

FIGURE 38–1. VRASPAC results for a young child with profound hearing loss at three test intervals: prior to sequential bilateral cochlear implantation (*top*), and at 3 months (*middle*) and 6 months (*bottom*) following activation of the first implanted ear. Trials to which the child could not be conditioned are indicated by "CNC." Contrast conditions that were not tested are indicated by "DNT." The six speech pattern contrasts tested were vowel height (VH), vowel place (VP), consonant voicing (CV), consonant continuance/manner (CC), consonant place in the front position (CPf), and consonant place in the rear position (CPr). (CI = cochlear implant; HA = hearing aid.)

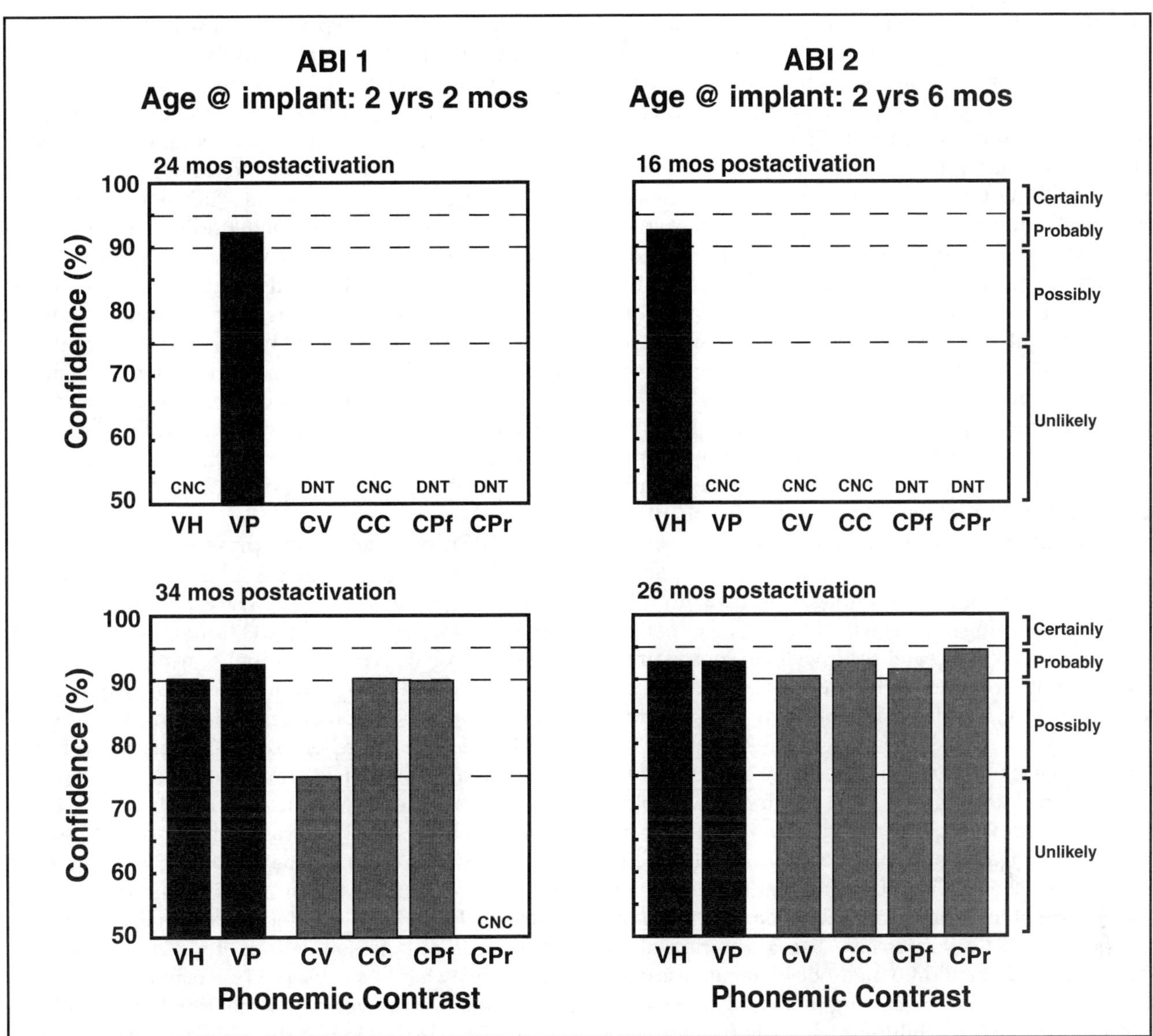

FIGURE 38–2. VRASPAC/PLAYSPAC results for two children, ABI 1 (*left*) and ABI 2 (*right*), at two test intervals following activation of their auditory brainstem implants (ABI). ABI 1 was tested using VRASPAC at 24 months postactivation (*top*) and PLAYSPAC at 34 months postactivation (*bottom*). ABI 2 was tested using PLAYSPAC at both the 16-month (*top*) and 26-month (*bottom*) postactivation intervals. The six speech pattern contrasts tested were vowel height (VH), vowel place (VP), consonant voicing (CV), consonant continuance/manner (CC), consonant place in the front position (CPf), and consonant place in the rear position (CPr). Trials to which the children could not be conditioned are indicated by "CNC." Contrast conditions that were not tested are indicated by "DNT."

voicing. The remaining consonant contrasts were not tested. The bottom half of Figure 38–2 shows results obtained for both children 10 months later. At 36 months postactivation, ABI 1 demonstrated the ability to detect four out of the six contrasts with 90% confidence or greater. At 26 months postactivation, ABI 2 was able to detect changes in all six contrasts. As these cases illustrate, the period over which the ability to detect speech pattern contrasts emerges in children with ABIs tends to be protracted compared to the relatively rapid skill acquisition for young children receiving CIs.

The OLIMSPAC (Boothroyd, Eisenberg, & Martinez, 2010) differs from the VRASPAC and PLAYSPAC in that it requires the child to imitate the syllable heard. "On-line" refers to the fact that the child's responses are scored by an examiner while the test is in progress, as opposed to off-line by a panel of judges in the earlier IMSPAC version (Boothroyd, 1985; Kosky & Boothroyd, 2003). Mahshie and colleagues (2015) used a modification of the OLIMSPAC to examine relationships between auditory perception and production of speech contrasts in 15 children who had been implanted by 3 years of age. In this study, the OLIMSPAC was used to assess speech perception for six contrast features (vowel height, vowel place, consonant voicing, consonant continuance, and consonant place of articulation—front and back), whereas a picture-naming task was used to examine speech production. Speech perception and production were scored in terms of percent correct. Vowel contrasts were perceived with more accuracy than consonant contrasts. Among the consonant contrasts, children's scores on average were lower for continuance and back place of articulation as compared to consonant voicing and front place of articulation. This pattern of findings, in which the two vowel features are perceived with greater accuracy than consonants, is consistent with earlier studies involving children using CIs (Eisenberg, Martinez, & Boothroyd, 2003; Martinez et al., 2008) and HAs (Boothroyd, 1984; Erber, 1972). Median speech production scores were 100% for all features, demonstrating that most children were able to produce them with consistency and accuracy. For five out of the six features, accuracy of production exceeded accuracy of perception, indicating that these young CI users were able to produce articulatory contrasts that they did not always perceive using audition alone. This finding that children might be better at producing speech features than perceiving them is also consistent with past reports in children using CIs (Boothroyd & Boothroyd-Turner, 2002) and HAs (Boothroyd, Eran, & Hanin, 1996).

The ability of infants and young children with cochlear implants to discriminate speech contrasts also has been examined by using visual habituation. Houston, Pisoni, Iler Kirk, Ying, and Miyamoto (2003) used a modified visual habituation procedure to compare attention to speech and speech pattern discrimination in a group of 16 deaf infants implanted at less than 2 years of age with those of 48 normal hearing infants, ages 6 and 9 months. Normal hearing infants and those with CIs alike spent significantly longer periods of time looking at a visual display paired with a novel sound stimulus ("ahhh") compared to the one to which they had previous habituated ("hop, hop, hop"). However, during the habituation phase of the experiment, the infants with CIs spent less time looking at the visual display paired with sound ("hop, hop, hop") overall than did normal hearing infants. Taken together, these investigators interpreted their findings as providing evidence that following cochlear implantation, deaf infants are able to detect and discriminate some sound patterns, although their attention to sound might be weaker than that displayed by normal hearing infants. The visual habitual technique with variants is gaining traction as a means to assess different aspects of speech perception in young children (Core, Brown, Larsen, & Mahshie, 2014; Houston, Horn, Qi, Ting, & Gao, 2007; Warner-Czyz, Houston, & Hynan, 2014).

Speech Production. In the presence of hearing loss of moderate or greater degree, the onset of canonical babbling typically is delayed. The extent of the delay is variable, with reports of some children (usually, but not always, those with more residual hearing) demonstrating canonical babbling within the age range of normal-hearing peers (Koopmans-van Beinum, Clement, & Van Den Dikkenberg-Pot, 2001; Moeller, Hoover, Putman, Arbataitis, Bohnenkamp, Peterson, Wood, et al., 2007). Most children with hearing loss do not start babbling, however, until well after their normal hearing age-mates, and the delay tends to lengthen as degree of hearing loss increases from moderate to profound (Carney, 1996; Moeller, Hoover, Putman, Arbataitis, Bohnenkamp, Peterson, Wood, et al., 2007). This pattern of delay has been observed even among the majority of infants who were early identified and amplified (Davis, Morrison, von Hapsburg, & Warner Czyz, 2005; Moeller, Hoover, Putman, Arbataitis, Bohnenkamp, Peterson, Wood, et al., 2007). Furthermore, some children with severe and profound hearing losses do not produce enough canonical syllables within their ongoing vocalizations to be considered "consistent"[6] (Davis et al., 2005; Oller & Eilers, 1988; Oller, Eilers, Bull, & Carney, 1985; von Hapsburg & Davis, 2006).

Notable exceptions to these trends have been described for infants with profound hearing loss who have received cochlear implants. In 2000, the FDA lowered the approved age for cochlear implantation of infants with profound hearing loss from 24 months to

[6]Re: canonical babbling ratio (CBR), or proportion of canonical syllables produced versus overall vocalizations. A CBR of 0.20 is typically used as the minimum criterion for the canonical babbling stage (Oller & Eilers, 1988; Schauwers, Gillis, Daemers, De Beukelaer, & Govaerts, 2004; von Hapsburg & Davis, 2006).

12 months. Soon thereafter, reports began to appear in the literature of young children with CIs beginning to babble 1 to 6 months after device activation (e.g., Ertmer & Mellon, 2001; Moore & Bass-Ringdahl, 2002; Schauwers et al., 2004). Further advancement in vocal behavior and expansion of phonetic inventories following cochlear implantation also was reported, with some CI children attaining vocal and verbal milestones with fewer months of auditory experience than typically hearing children (Ertmer & Mellon, 2001; Ertmer & Jung, 2012; Ertmer, Young, & Nathani, 2007; Moore & Bass-Ringdahl, 2002; Schauwers et al., 2004).

Cognitive/Linguistic Processing (Level III)

Typically Hearing Children

Speech Perception. Beginning at about 6 months, the normally hearing infant shows an increasing ability to recognize those sounds (Werker & Tees, 1984), sound sequences (Juscyzk, Friederici, Wessles, Svenkerud, & Juscyzk, 1993), and rhythmic/stress patterns (Juscyzk, Cutler, & Redanz, 1993) that are likely to appear in the words of the ambient language. This knowledge underlies the infant's developing ability to segment words from fluent speech, which in turn provides the basis for the building of a lexicon. Processing begins to take place at the level of the whole word rather than the phonemes that compose it (Carney, 1996).

Speech perception skills continue to develop throughout childhood and adolescence with further maturation of the auditory pathways and other cortical centers, accumulating exposure to and experience with the ambient language, and expansion of the child's own receptive and expressive language skills. In addition, a number of more generalized cognitive factors and information processing skills are likely to play an important role in the child's developing abilities to comprehend spoken language. These include, but might not be limited to, selective attention, lexical access, working memory, verbal rehearsal speed, and multimodal processing (e.g., Kirk et al., 2012; Pisoni, 2000; Pisoni et al., 2008; Pisoni, Kronenberger, Roman, & Geers, 2011).

Speech Production. Around nine months of age, an infant's vocalizations and syllabic patterns begin to shift from universal forms that are easiest to produce toward those that are used in the ambient language (Werker & Tees, 1999). These advanced forms include syllables of increasing complexity and jargon (Nathani et al., 2006). By 12 to 15 months of age, normal hearing infants and toddlers begin to produce their first recognizable words (Kent & Bauer, 1985; Stoel-Gammon, 1985; Vihman et al., 1986).

Normal hearing children continue to develop and master their phonological skills over the course of childhood. Ages 1 to 4 years are characterized by an orderly progression in speech sound acquisition that includes vowels, diphthongs, stops, nasals, and glides (Kent, 2004; Stoel-Gammon, 1985). Among vowels, central, low-mid-front and low-front vowels precede high vowels in order of acquisition (Kent & Bauer, 1985). Among consonants, voiced stop consonants precede voiceless stops and stop consonants produced in the frontal position precede those produced in the rear position (Stoel-Gammon, 1988). Fricatives, liquids, and initial consonant clusters are finally mastered during ages 5 to 9 years (Kent, 2004; Smit, Hand, Freilinger, Bernthal, & Bird, 1990). Despite the fact that not all speech sounds have yet been acquired, 3-year-old children typically are judged to be 50% to 80% intelligible by unfamiliar listeners (Vihman, 1988), and 4-year-olds are judged to be roughly 70% to 100% intelligible (Gordon-Brannan, 1994).

Impact of Hearing Loss

Speech Perception. In the presence of hearing loss, the output at the perceptual representation stage is reduced, incomplete, or absent. This inconsistent or lack of access to the sound patterns of the ambient language is likely to delay the development of lexical representation underlying word recognition (Moeller, Hoover, Putman, Arbataitis, Bohnenkamp, Peterson, Lewis, et al., 2007; Nott, Cowan, Brown, & Wigglesworth, 2009). Delays in language development further restrict a child's ability to "fill in the blanks" in complex or difficult listening situations.

Despite the number of cognitive, linguistic, and other nonauditory influences on word and sentence recognition, it is at this level that speech perception is typically assessed for clinical purposes. In many instances, an attempt is made to control for such influences by restricting the response set to a fixed number of alternatives (i.e., "closed-set"). This approach is often used to assess young children or other individuals who might have limited vocabularies and/or verbal abilities (e.g., Elliot & Katz, 1980; Jerger, Lewis, Hawkins, & Jerger, 1980; Moog & Geers, 1990; Ross & Lerman, 1970). In other instances, no attempt is made to limit responses to a set of predetermined alternatives (i.e., "open-set"), so as to better reflect the demands of "real-world" listening (Kirk, French, & Choi, 2009). In doing so, open-set measures also tap into the listener's linguistic and cognitive processing skills as well as auditory-perceptual capabilities.[7]

In general, children with hearing losses in the moderate and severe range achieve open-set recognition for speech that is made audible (Blamey, Sarant, et al., 2001; Eisenberg, Kirk, Martinez, Ying, & Miyamoto, 2004; Hicks & Tharpe, 2002). Nevertheless, word and sentence recognition tend to decrease systematically as degree of hearing loss increases. As part of a larger study comparing speech perception, speech production, and language outcomes in children using HAs versus CIs, Blamey, Sarant, and colleagues (2001) conducted a series of regression analyses on open-set word recognition scores as a function of child age and degree of loss. For the 40 children using HAs with hearing losses ranging from moderate to profound, consonant-nucleus-consonant (CNC) word scores (Peterson & Lehiste, 1962) decreased by approximately 5% for every 10 dB of threshold change across a range of 40 to 103 dB HL, after accounting for child age. The rate of change was slightly steeper for BKB sentences scored for key words (Bamford-Kowal-Bench Sentence Test; Bench, Doyle, & Greenwood, 1987), which decreased by approximately 6% for every decibel of loss.

Children with profound hearing loss also exhibit a range of speech perception abilities (Boothroyd, Geers, & Moog, 1991; Erber & Alencewicz, 1976). Early evidence regarding the range of speech perception abilities in this population was provided by Erber and Alencewicz (1976) using a newly developed speech perception battery that subsequently became known as the Monosyllable-Trochee-Spondee (MTS) test. Using a closed-set format with picture card depictions of the word items, the test is scored in two ways: correct identification of syllabic stress pattern and correct identification of the word itself. Presenting data obtained on 126 ears (67 children), these investigators showed that children with average hearing thresholds less than 110 dB HL achieved a wide range of scores for closed-set word identification. Analyzing these same word scores further, Boothroyd et al. (1991) showed that most subjects with hearing losses less than 90 dB HL identified words within syllable categories with 70% to 100% accuracy. Those with hearing losses greater than 110 dB HL tended to score at chance (25%) or below.

Children with profound hearing loss who use CIs are likely to achieve open-set word recognition similar to that exhibited by children with severe hearing loss who use HAs (Blamey, Sarant, et al., 2001; Boothroyd & Eran, 1994; Eisenberg et al., 2004). Children with severe to profound loss who use a CI are likely to achieve open-set speech recognition similar to that demonstrated by children with moderate to severe hearing loss who use HAs (Fitzpatrick et al., 2012). Although the majority of growth in speech recognition abilities tends to occur within the first three to five years following implantation, continued improvement has been observed beyond 5 years (Beadle et al., 2005; Davidson, Geers, Blamey, Tobey, & Brenner, 2011; Tyler et al., 2000; Uziel et al., 2007).

Open-set speech recognition is strongly associated with speech production and language skills; growth in the former can be accounted for by further development in the latter (Blamey, Sarant, et al., 2001; Davidson et al., 2011; Eisenberg, Martinez, Holowecky, & Pogorelsky, 2002; Eisenberg et al., in press). In particular, the recognition of complex speech materials such sentences in quiet and noise is positively associated with vocabulary and syntax skills (Eisenberg et al., 2002; Eisenberg et al., in press). The relationship between speech perception and language skill appears to asymptote once an equivalent language age of 10 to 11 years old is achieved (Davidson et al., 2011).

Nevertheless, a small subset of children does not develop functional open-set speech recognition, even after 5 years or more of CI use for a variety of reasons (Barnard et al., 2015; Tyler et al., 2000; Uziel et al., 2007). In a recent investigation examining poorer speech recognition outcomes in a large, longitudinal cohort of pediatric CI recipients (Barnard et al., 2015), the characteristics associated with an inability to progress to open-set testing after 5 years of implant experience included older age at initial fitting of amplification prior to CI, poorer aided detection thresholds pre-CI, complicated perinatal history (prematurity/admission to the NICU), and lower maternal sensitivity to communication needs. All but one in the subset of children who failed to achieve open-set recognition (94%) relied on some level of sign support to communicate, whereas 84% of the group with open-set skills communicated exclusively by spoken language (i.e., no sign support).

Speech Production. During the transition from prelexical vocalization to first words, infants and toddlers with hearing loss exhibit a more restricted range of phonetic elements compared to normal hearing children the same age (Kent, Osberger, Netsell, & Hus-

[7]One limitation of open-set testing is that the child is asked to repeat each item heard. For children with hearing loss, who might not have intelligible speech or display specific articulation deficits, scoring the words or sentences correct presents a challenge. Some clinicians might ask the child to write, sign, or describe the meaning of the word.

tedde, 1987; Moeller, Hoover, Putman, Arbataitis, Bohnenkamp, Peterson, Wood, et al., 2007; Stoel-Gammon, 1988). They also tend to be slower in moving from production of simpler to more complex syllabic forms (Koopmans-van Beinum et al., 2001; Moeller, Hoover, Putman, Arbataitis, Bohnenkamp, Peterson, Lewis, et al., 2007; Moeller, Hoover, Putman, Arbataitis, Bohnenkamp, Peterson, Wood, et al., 2007; Stoel-Gammon, 1988). The extent of hearing loss plays a significant role in early speech sound acquisition; children with milder degrees of hearing loss tend to demonstrate larger phonetic and syllabic repertoires than children with more severe losses (Davis et al., 2005; Moeller, Hoover, Putman, Arbataitis, Bohnenkamp, Peterson, Wood, et al., 2007). Nevertheless, acquisition of first true words is likely to be delayed even among infants who were early identified and fitted with sensory devices within the first year of life (Moeller, Hoover, Putman, Arbataitis, Bohnenkamp, Peterson, Lewis, et al., 2007; Nott et al., 2009).

In general, the overall pattern of phonologic development in most children with hearing loss follows that demonstrated by normal hearing children, albeit somewhat delayed (Moeller, Hoover, Putman, Arbataitis, Bohnenkamp, Peterson, Lewis, et al., 2007; Stoel-Gammon, 1983). Furthermore, many of the production errors observed in older children with hearing loss are characteristic of younger children with normal hearing (McDermott & Jones, 1984; Oller et al., 1985; Stoel-Gammon, 1983). The pattern of production errors appears to be similar across children, with the number and types of errors increasing as degree of loss increases (Markides, 1970; McDermott & Jones, 1984; Smith, 1975; Stoel-Gammon, 1983).

Fricatives and affricates appear to be particularly vulnerable to omission and substitution across children with all degrees of hearing loss (Elfenbein, Hardin-Jones, & Davis, 1994). In a longitudinal study of phonetic development, Moeller, Hoover, Putman, Arbataitis, Bohnenkamp, Peterson, Wood, and colleagues (2007) observed different developmental trajectories for fricatives/affricates versus nonaffricates between children with early identified hearing loss and normal-hearing controls. Not only did the group with hearing loss produce fewer fricative/affricates than the group with normal hearing at a comparable age, but the gap in usage between the two also widened with age. Relevant to these findings are previous studies from the same laboratory showing the peak energy of /s/ to be outside the bandwidth of current hearing aids (Stelmachowicz et al., 2002; Stelmachowicz et al., 2004). In addition, fricatives tend to be low in amplitude, particularly in connected speech and in the final position in words. Thus, children with hearing loss, even of milder degrees, might not have consistent access to phonemes within this class in the course of daily listening across a number of environments.

Exceptions to the patterns of phonologic development described above have been noted for some young CI recipients, in whom the order of vowel and consonant acquisition might diverge from that typically observed in normal hearing children (Ertmer, 2001; Ertmer et al., 2007). In addition, different patterns in the accuracy of production have been noted between the two groups (Ertmer & Goffman, 2011; Warner-Czyz & Davis, 2008; Warner-Czyz, Davis, & MacNeilage, 2010). At the level of the individual child, these differences likely reflect a combination of age at implantation, the manner in which acoustic information is encoded via the CI, and the child's prelexical/lexical stage of development at the time of implantation.

Most children with moderate and severe hearing losses develop intelligible speech (Boothroyd, 1984; Elfenbein et al., 1994; Monsen, 1978). Children with profound loss vary widely in their production skills (Boothroyd, 1984; Monsen, 1978; Smith, 1975; Svirsky, Chin, & Miyamoto, 2000). The amount of residual hearing appears to be the key factor in development of intelligible speech (Boothroyd, 1984; Svirsky et al., 2000).

Many children with profound loss using CIs are able to develop intelligible speech (e.g., Blamey, Barry, et al., 2001; Tobey, Geers, Brenner, Altuna, & Gabbert, 2003; Tomblin, Peng, Spencer, & Lu, 2008). Although speech skill development in children with CIs tends to lag behind that of normal hearing children, as a group they tend to perform within one standard deviation of their normal hearing peers (Blamey, Barry, et al., 2001). The most rapid progress typically is observed over the first six years of device use (Blamey, Barry, et al., 2001; Tomblin et al., 2008), with children implanted at younger ages (<2.5 years) showing steeper rates of growth than children implanted at older ages (Connor, Craig, Raudenbush, Heavner, & Zwolan, 2006). Nevertheless, continued skill growth with continued CI use has been observed beyond 10 years and well into adolescence (Tobey, Geers, Sundarrajan, & Shin, 2011).

Improved speech intelligibility with increased auditory experience using a CI reflects, in part, positive changes in a number of the elements of connected speech, including increased accuracy in vowel and consonant production (Chin, 2003, 2007; Serry & Blamey, 1999; Tobey et al., 2003), and shortening in overall sentence duration to that approaching more normal values (Tobey et al., 2003; Uchanski & Geers, 2003). Improved speech intelligibility is also associated with advances in CI technology (Tobey et al., 2000).

However, not all children using CIs develop intelligible speech, even after many years of implant use (Beadle et al., 2005; Uziel et al., 2007). One factor observed to correlate with communication outcomes in children with profound hearing loss is mode of communication. Specifically, children whose educational settings emphasize an oral-aural approach consistently have shown better speech perception and production outcomes than children from settings using total communication, whether using CIs (Chin, 2003; Geers, Strube, Tobey, Pisoni, & Moog, 2011; Tobey et al., 2003; Tobey et al., 2011; Uchanski & Geers, 2003) or HAs (Boothroyd, 1984; Svirsky et al., 2000).

Impact of Adverse Listening Conditions

Speech perception scores obtained in quiet, under the controlled conditions of the laboratory or clinic, belie the amount of difficulty that children, with or without hearing loss, might experience. For children, the ability to detect and understand speech under adverse or degraded conditions is not equivalent to that demonstrated by adults (Eisenberg, Shannon, Martinez, Wygonski, & Boothroyd, 2000; Fallon, Trehub, & Schneider, 2000; Hall, Grose, Buss, & Dev, 2002; Johnson, 2000; Neuman, Wroblewski, Hajicek, & Rubinstein, 2010). These are skills that continue to develop throughout childhood, not reaching adult-like performance until well into adolescence (Eisenberg et al., 2000; Elliott, 1979; Fallon et al., 2000; Johnson, 2000).

Children with hearing loss experience greater difficulty understanding speech under degraded or complex listening conditions than their normal hearing peers (Crandell, 1993; Finitzo-Hieber & Tillman, 1978; Hicks & Tharpe, 2002). In general, when tested under the same noise conditions, younger children demonstrate poorer speech recognition than older children (Gravel, Fausel, Liskow, & Chobot, 1999) and children with greater degrees of hearing loss (Erber, 1971). Still, children with minimal hearing loss can demonstrate significant decrements in performance compared to normal hearing children, as listening conditions become increasingly adverse (Crandell, 1993). Furthermore, even when relatively high levels of performance can be maintained in noise, it is likely to require more effort on the part of children with hearing loss compared to their normally hearing peers (Hicks & Tharpe, 2002).

Figure 38–3 illustrates the impact of listening in competition on two groups of 3- to 4-year-old children (K. C. Johnson and L. V. Dumont, unpublished data, 2007). Shown are mean percent correct identification scores obtained on a closed-set sentence identification test for 10 children with normal hearing and 10 children with hearing loss. For the children in the hearing loss group, PTAs ranged from 30.0 to 78.3 dB HL; all were fitted with bilateral amplification. Stimuli were sentences from the Pediatric Speech Identification (PSI) test (Jerger et al., 1980), presented at 70 dB(A) from a loudspeaker located in front of the child (0° azimuth). The child's task was to point to the picture depicting the sentence heard from a set of five alternatives. In the competing conditions, single-talker competition was introduced from a speaker located behind the child (180° azimuth) and varied in 10-dB steps relative to the target to generate a range of message-to-competition ratios (MCRs), from relatively easy (+10 MCR) to difficult (−10 MCR). At +10 MCR, the easiest condition, both groups of children scored at or near ceiling. As the listening difficulty increased, performance decreased for both groups. However, the rate of decline was more pronounced for the hearing loss group. At 0 MCR, mean performance for the hearing loss group (85%) was slightly below that of the normal hearing group (95%). At −10 MCR, the most difficult listening condition, sentence identification for the children with hearing loss was markedly poorer (10%) than that shown by the majority of children with normal hearing (57%).

Sensory Device Use in Children With Severe to Profound Hearing Loss

For children with severe and profound losses, cochlear implantation has become the standard of care. Over half of the children diagnosed with severe to profound hearing loss in the United States currently undergo cochlear implantation (Bradham & Jones, 2008). Studies conducted with early generations of multichannel cochlear implants suggested that children with profound losses in excess of 100 dB HL derived greater benefit from CIs than from HAs (Geers & Brenner, 1994; Meyer, Svirsky, Kirk, & Miyamoto, 1998; Osberger et al., 1996). Studies involving successive generations of CIs, suggest that a cochlear implant enables the child with severe to profound hearing loss to function more like a child with severe (Blamey, Sarant, et al., 2001; Eisenberg et al., 2004; Mahshie et al., 2015) or moderately severe (Fitzpatrick et al., 2012) hearing loss.

In children with symmetrical severe to profound losses, bilateral cochlear implantation has become com-

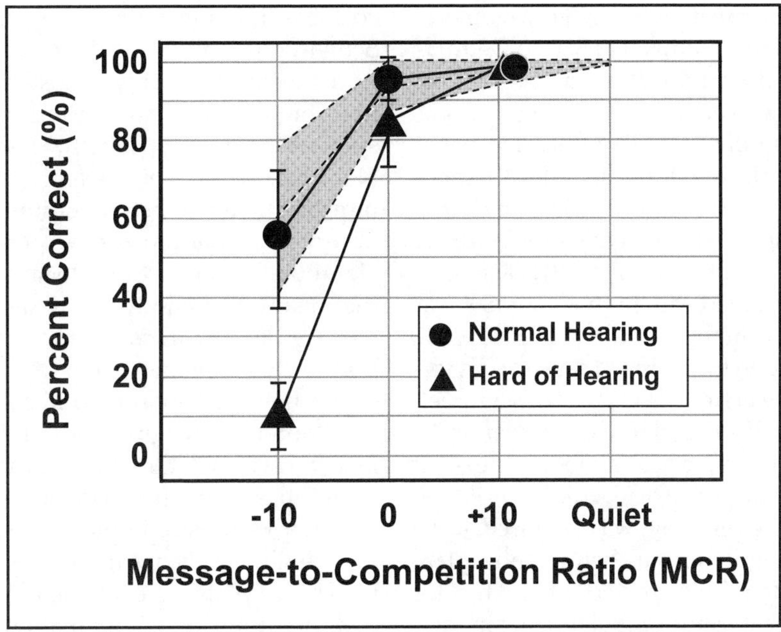

FIGURE 38–3. Performance on the Pediatric Speech Intelligibility Test (PSI sentences) at three message-to-competition ratios (MCRs; −10, 0, +10) for 10 children with normal hearing (filled circles) and 10 children with hearing loss (filled triangles). The shaded area represents the mean and ± 2 standard errors for a reference group of eight children with normal hearing (mean age: 4.75 years; range: 3.41 to 6.25 years).

monplace. Children are either implanted sequentially (requiring two different surgeries) or simultaneously (two devices implanted during the same surgery). The goal of bilateral implantation is the same as for the fitting of two HAs—to provide binaural hearing for enhanced sound localization and improved speech recognition in noise. A host of studies conducted in children over the past decade point to a general advantage in the use of two implants versus one, although improvements under the bilateral condition were not universal.[8]

In most of these studies, participants were children who had been implanted sequentially, with various periods of delay between the first and second CIs. Improved performance tended to be associated with reduced periods of auditory deprivation in the second implanted ear (e.g., Litovsky, Johnstone, & Godar, 2006; Peters, Litovsky, Parkinson, & Lake, 2007). In studies in which a binaural advantage was not observed, study participants tended to be those with relatively brief periods of experience using the second implant (e.g., Grieco-Calub, Litovsky, & Werner, 2008; Litovsky et al., 2004) or with a protracted period of auditory deprivation in the second implanted ear (e.g., Galvin, Mok, & Dowell, 2007; Peters, Litovsky, Lake, & Parkinson, 2004).

In cases in which only one ear is implanted, CI users are often encouraged to continue use of a HA in the ear opposite to the implant (bimodal fitting), so that they might benefit from low-frequency acoustic cues. Research on bimodal device configurations in children has shown, in general, improved speech recognition compared to use of a CI alone, particularly in the presence of noise (Dettman et al., 2004; Holt, Kirk, Eisenberg, Martinez, & Campbell, 2005). There is also evidence of emerging localization ability over time (Ching, Psarros, Hill, Dillon, & Incerti, 2001; Litovsky et al., 2006). However, some children show no difference

[8]For summaries of studies examining bilateral CI and bimodal fittings, the reader is referred to reviews by Ching, van Wanrooy, and Dillon (2007); Johnston, Durieux-Smith, Angus, O'Connor, and Fitzpatrick (2009); and Schafer, Amlani, Seibold, and Shattuck (2007).

or even poorer performance in noise using two devices compared to one CI alone (Ching et al., 2001; Dettman et al., 2004; Holt et al., 2005; Litovsky et al., 2006; Schafer & Thibodeau, 2006). Factors influencing bimodal benefit can include amount of residual hearing in the aided ear (Morera et al., 2005), the length of experience with the hearing aid (Holt et al., 2005), and optimization of the hearing aid fitting to balance loudness between the two devices (Ching et al., 2001). The hearing loss in the nonimplanted ears in these studies was generally reported to be in the severe range.

An emerging trend in the fitting of sensory devices in children has been the use of CIs in cases of asymmetric hearing loss, with a profound loss in one ear and a moderate or moderately severe hearing loss in the other ear. In the early years of pediatric cochlear implantation, even the better hearing ear was required to be in the profound hearing loss range before an implant would be recommended. This created a hardship for some children with significant residual hearing in their better hearing ear, but who were not progressing with the use of amplification to the extent typically demonstrated by children with bilateral profound loss using CI(s). Today, many centers implant children with this type of audiometric profile in the poorer ear, thereby enabling the pairing acoustic amplification in the better hearing ear and electrical stimulation in the poorer hearing ear. Investigators point to the complementary information resulting from combining low-frequency acoustic input from the better ear with the mid-to-high frequency electrical input from the cochlear implant in the poorer ear (Kong, Stickney, & Zeng, 2005; Ching et al., 2007).

A significant development in sensory device use among children with profound loss has been the ABI (Eisenberg et al., 2008; Shannon et al., 2009). Developed for use in adults with neurofibromatosis type 2 (NF2; Edgerton, House, & Hitselberger, 1981; Eisenberg, Maltan, Portillo, Mobley, & House, 1987; Hitselberger, House, Edgerton, & Whitaker, 1984), the ABI provides stimulation to the cochlear nucleus in the brainstem (Brackmann et al., 1993; Shannon et al., 1993). In 2000, two multichannel versions of the device were approved by the U.S. Food and Drug Administration for sole use in patients with NF2, 12 years and older, undergoing surgical resection of their auditory nerve.

Over the next 10 years, surgeons in Europe began implanting ABIs in non-NF2 adults, as well as children as young as 14 months old (Colletti et al., 2002; Colletti et al., 2005; Nevison et al., 2002). Pediatric candidates for ABI include children with absent or abnormal cochleae or cochlear nerves, injuries to the auditory nerve, extensive ossification in the cochlea, and use of cochlear implants with no benefit (Kaplan et al., 2015; Sennaroglu et al., 2011). Reported outcomes in children have indicated an array of post-ABI performance, ranging from detection and pattern perception to open-set speech recognition (Colletti, Shannon, & Colletti, 2014; Noij et al., 2015). Not unexpectedly, more rapid rates of improvement and better auditory outcomes have been observed in children with acquired hearing loss due to eighth nerve injury or cochlear ossification. However, the majority of children who are implanted with the ABI are those with cochlear or cochlear nerve aplasia. Within this etiologic group, the poorest auditory outcomes have been observed in children with additional developmental/cognitive disabilities, which is prevalent in this population. Among those without additional disabilities, better performance was achieved for those children who were implanted earlier. As of this writing, clinical trials are underway at four CI centers in the United States to evaluate the safety and efficacy of auditory brainstem implantation in young children.

A word of caution is in order when comparing auditory access through acoustic amplification versus electric stimulation. Whereas real-ear measures can be used to determine the spectral information available to the child through the HA, no corresponding measure exists for CIs, let alone ABIs. Thus, access to sound across the frequency region important for speech perception is frequently (and crudely) estimated through a sound field detection audiogram. It is important to note that although detection levels using the implant might be brought to within what generally is considered the "mild hearing loss" range, electrical stimulation is not equivalent to acoustic stimulation and the child will still be required to map meaning onto these sensations. Thus, a child with profound hearing loss who demonstrates sound-field thresholds of 15 dB HL using a CI or ABI cannot be expected to have comparable suprathreshold performance as a child with similar aided or unaided thresholds. It can be assumed only that the implant processor has been adjusted in such a way that the child is able to detect soft sounds at different frequencies.

Multimodal Perception

Speech communication is multimodal in that auditory and visual cues provide complementary information to the listener. With greater degrees of hearing loss, the visual modality is likely to play an increasingly important role in providing access to the sensory primitives and perceptual representations upon which speech perception develops at the cognitive/linguistic level.

In early infancy, children are sensitive to the associations between auditory and visual speech sounds. In their seminal study of bimodal speech perception in infants, Kuhl and Meltzoff (1982) demonstrated that infants ages 18 to 20 weeks are able to match vowel sounds to facial displays of articulation, spending more time looking at the matching than the nonmatching face. Follow-up studies have shown that infants as young as 2 months of age are able to match auditory information and visual information on the face (Patterson & Werker, 1999, 2003). It has been suggested that auditory-visual integration plays a role in the development of articulation (Kuhl & Meltzoff, 1982; Patterson & Werker, 1999) and the learning of phonemic boundaries (Teinonen, Aslin, Alku, & Csibra, 2008).

Deaf toddlers who receive CIs also begin to show evidence of matching phonetic information within 9 months of device activation (Barker & Tomblin, 2004). Furthermore, deaf children who use CIs begin to integrate the audiovisual information in words following activation gradually, whereas deaf children using HAs might not (Bergeson, Houston, & Miyamoto, 2010). Children with mild to moderate hearing loss using HAs are able to match audio and visual information in much the same way as children with normal hearing (Bergeson et al., 2010). Thus, children with early auditory deprivation secondary to hearing loss are able to begin to use audition in support of audiovisual processing, although the process might take several months of experience to unfold.

Children with hearing loss rely on the combination of auditory and visual cues to maximize comprehension of spoken language. With assistance from their sensory devices, many children with hearing loss learn to perceive and produce vowels and consonants (Eisenberg et al., 2003). Much of the acoustic information that enables differentiation among vowels or processing of consonant voicing and manner features is found in the time/intensity domain, cues that are generally accessible across a wide range of frequencies. Place of articulation is restricted to the frequency/time domain, and listeners with hearing loss often experience difficulty differentiating between speech sounds that are most reliant on the higher-frequency spectral cues (e.g., /i/ versus /u/, or /b/ versus /d/). The addition of the visual modality can resolve perceptual ambiguities in the acoustic signal, particularly in adverse listening conditions (Erber, 1971; Sumby & Pollack, 1954).

A number of investigators have compared auditory-visual versus auditory-only and visual-only perception of speech in children with hearing loss. Early studies were aimed at assessing children with severe to profound hearing loss (Erber, 1971, 1972; Hack & Erber, 1982), although more recent investigators have evaluated children with a broad range of hearing losses (Eisenberg et al., 2003; Seewald, Ross, Giolas, & Yonovitz, 1985; Tillberg, Ronnberg, Svard, & Ahlner, 1996). After CIs became commercially available for children with profound hearing loss, studies were conducted to evaluate the multimodal benefits with this sensory device (Bergeson, Pisoni, & Davis, 2003, 2005; Bergeson et al., 2010; Geers & Brenner, 1994; Kirk et al., 2007; Lachs, Pisoni, & Kirk, 2001; Schorr, Fox, van Wassenhove, & Knudsen, 2005). Despite the use of different speech materials with children of different ages, degrees of hearing loss, and sensory device types, results across studies have been generally consistent; speech recognition is more accurate when assessed via the auditory-visual modality relative to auditory-only or visual-only modalities. In addition, children with greater amounts of residual hearing have been shown to benefit more from both auditory-visual and auditory-only delivery of speech than children with little residual hearing (Erber, 1972; Seewald et al., 1985). Children with CIs who demonstrate higher language skills also perform more accurately on measures of speech recognition presented in auditory-visual and auditory-only formats than those with poorer language skills (Kirk et al., 2007). Moreover, children with CIs who derive greater benefit from visual enhancement of the auditory speech signal have more intelligible speech than children who receive little or no benefit from the addition of visual speech cues (Lachs et al., 2001). Finally, children implanted at earlier ages (2.5 years and younger) have been shown to develop better auditory-visual integrative skills than children implanted at later ages (Schorr et al., 2005).

In view of the fact that auditory-visual processing of speech is reflective of real-world communication and demonstrates underlying perceptual skills, it is interesting that standard audiologic practice focuses almost exclusively on the administration of speech recognition tests in the auditory-only modality. Audiologic assessment of speech recognition in auditory-visual, auditory-only, and visual-only modalities would provide a more complete glimpse of how a child with hearing loss is performing with his or her sensory device. Thus, it is quite promising that new directions in test development are beginning to emphasize multimodal speech processing and that such tests might be available for future clinical use (see Kirk et al., 2009; Kirk et al., 2012).

Conclusions

In this chapter we have attempted to highlight important research findings relating to the speech perception and production abilities of children with moderate to profound hearing loss. In reviewing the early literature, one can point to a general trend for performance to decrease with increasing severity of hearing loss. However, confounding variables that have impacted outcome data in the past include the duration and degree of auditory deprivation experienced by the child and the quality of the sensory assistance available at the time.

More recent evidence suggests that differences among groups categorized by hearing loss are becoming obscured as the result of a number of factors, including technologic innovations in cochlear implants and digital hearing aids, improved assessment and device fitting protocols, and widespread implementation of EHDI programs. Thus, the children we describe today might not be representative of children with hearing loss a few years hence, as the influence of these factors become more fully realized. Future reports based on longitudinal studies currently tracking early identified infants fitted with contemporary sensory devices might provide further insight regarding the impact of hearing loss, per se, versus the confounding effects of long-term auditory deprivation that have clouded our picture in the past.

Acknowledgments. This work was supported, in part, by grants R01 DC004797, R01 DC009561, and U01 DC013031 from the National Institutes on Deafness and Other Communication Disorders (NIDCD) of the National Institutes of Health (NIH).

References

Aslin, R. N., & Smith, L. B. (1988). Perceptual development. *Annual Reviews of Psychology, 39*, 435–473.

Barker, B. A., & Tomblin, B. J. (2004). Bimodal speech perception in infant hearing aid and cochlear implant users. *Archives of Otolaryngology-Head and Neck Surgery, 130*(5), 582–586.

Barnard, J. M., Fisher, L. M., Johnson, K. C., Eisenberg, L. S., Wang, N.-Y., Quittner, A. L., . . . The CDaCI Investigative Team. (2015). A prospective longitudinal study of U.S. children unable to achieve open-set speech recognition 5 years after cochlear implantation. *Otology and Neurotology, 36*(6), 985–992.

Beadle, E. A. R., McKinley, D. J., Nikolopoulos, T. P., Brough, J., O'Donoghue, G. M., & Archbold, S. M. (2005). Long-term functional outcomes and academic-occupational status in implanted children after 10 to 14 years of cochlear implant use. *Otology and Neurotology, 26*, 1152–1160.

Beauchemin, M., González-Frankenberger, B., Tremblay, J., Vannasing, P., Martínez-Montes, E., Belin, P., . . . Lassonde, M. (2010). Mother and stranger: An electrophysiological study of voice processing in newborns. *Cerebral Cortex, 21*(8), 1705–1711.

Bench, J., Doyle, J., & Greenwood, K. M. (1987). A standardization of the BKB/A Sentence Test for children in comparison with the NAL-CID Sentence Test and CAL-PBM Word Test. *Australian Journal of Audiology, 9*, 39–48.

Bergeson, T. R., Houston, D. M., & Miyamoto, R. T. (2010). Effects of congenital hearing loss and cochlear implantation on audiovisual speech perception in infants and children. *Restorative Neurology and Neuroscience, 28*(2), 157–165.

Bergeson, T. R., Pisoni, D. B., & Davis, R. A. O. (2003). A longitudinal study of audiovisual speech perception by children with hearing loss who have cochlear implants. *Volta Review, 103*(4 Monograph), 347–370.

Bergeson, T. R., Pisoni, D. B., & Davis, R. A. O. (2005). Development of audiovisual comprehension skills in prelingually deaf children with cochlear implants. *Ear and Hearing, 26*(2), 149–164.

Birnholtz, J., & Benacerraf, B. (1983). The development of human fetal hearing. *Science, 222*, 516–518.

Blamey, P. J., Barry, J., Bow, C., Sarant, J., Paatsch, L., & Wales, R. (2001). The development of speech production following cochlear implantation. *Clinical Linguistics and Phonetics, 15*, 363–382.

Blamey, P. J., Sarant, J. Z., Paatsch, L. E., Barry, J. G., Bow, C. P., Wales, R. J., . . . Toohrt, R. (2001). Relationships among speech perception, production, language, hearing loss, and age in children with impaired hearing. *Journal of Speech, Language, and Hearing Research, 44*(2), 264–285.

Boothroyd, A. (1978). Speech perception and sensorineural hearing loss. In M. Ross & T. G. Giolas (Eds.), *Auditory management of hearing-impaired children: Principles and prerequisites for intervention* (pp. 117–144). Baltimore, MD: University Park Press.

Boothroyd, A. (1984). Auditory perception of speech contrasts by subjects with sensorineural hearing loss. *Journal of Speech and Hearing Research, 27*(1), 134–144.

Boothroyd, A. (1985). Evaluation of speech production of the hearing impaired: Some benefits of forced-choice testing. *Journal of Speech, Language, and Hearing Research, 28*(2), 185–196.

Boothroyd, A., & Boothroyd-Turner, D. (2002). Postimplantation audition and educational attainment in children with prelingually acquired profound deafness. *Annals of Otology, Rhinology, and Laryngology, supplement, 189*, 79–84.

Boothroyd, A., & Cawkwell, S. (1970). Vibrotactile thresholds in pure tone audiometry. *Acta Otolaryngologica, 69*(6), 381–387.

Boothroyd, A., Eisenberg, L. S., & Martinez, A. S. (2010). An On-Line Imitative Test of Speech-Pattern Contrast Perception (OLIMSPAC): Developmental effects in normally hearing children. *Journal of Speech, Language, and Hearing Research, 53*(3), 531–542.

Boothroyd, A., & Eran, O. (1994). Auditory speech perception capacity of child implant users expressed as equivalent hearing loss. *Volta Review, 96*, 151–167.

Boothroyd, A., Eran, O., & Hanin, L. (1996). Speech perception and production inchildren with hearing impairment. In F. Bess, J. S. Gravel, & A. M. Tharpe (Eds.), *Amplification for children with auditory deficits* (pp. 55–74). Nashville, TN: Bill Wilkerson Center Press.

Boothroyd, A., Geers, A. E., & Moog, J. S. (1991). Practical implications of cochlear implants in children. *Ear and Hearing, 12*(4 Suppl.), 81S–89S.

Boothroyd, A., & Medwetsky, L. (1992). Spectral distribution of /s/ and the frequency response of hearing aids. *Ear and Hearing, 13*(3), 150–157.

Brackmann, D. E., Hitselberger, W. E., Nelson, R. A., Moore, J., Waring, M. D., Portillo, F., . . . Telischi, F. F. (1993). Auditory brainstem implant: I. Issues in surgical implantation. *Otolaryngology-Head and Neck Surgery, 108*(6), 624–633.

Bradham, T., & Jones, J. (2008). Cochlear implant candidacy in the United States: Prevalence in children 12 months to 6 years of age. *International Journal of Pediatric Otorhinolaryngology, 72*(7), 1023–1028.

Carney, A. E. (1996). Audition and the development of oral communication competency. In F. E. Bess, J. S. Gravel, & A. M. Tharpe (Eds.), *Amplification for children with auditory deficits* (pp. 29–53). Nashville, TN: Bill Wilkerson Press.

Carney, A. E., Osberger, M. J., Carney, E., Robbins, A. M., Renshaw, J. J., & Miyamoto, R. T. (1993). A comparison of speech discrimination with cochlear implants and tactile aids. *Journal of the Acoustical Society of America, 94*(4), 2036–2049.

Centers for Disease Control and Prevention (CDC; 2015). *Metropolitan Atlanta Developmental Disabilities Surveillance Program (MADDSP) Case definitions: Hearing loss.* National Center on Birth Defects and Developmental Disabilities. Retrieved August 18, 2015, from http://www.cdc.gov/ncbddd/developmentaldisabilities/casedefinitions.html

Chin, S. B. (2003). Children's consonant inventories after extended cochlear implant use. *Journal of Speech, Language, and Hearing Research, 46*(4), 849–862.

Chin, S. B. (2007). Variation in consonant cluster production by pediatric cochlear implant users. *Ear and Hearing, 28*(2 suppl.), 7S–10S.

Ching, T. Y. C., Psarros, C., Hill, M., Dillon, H., & Incerti, P. (2001). Should children who use cochlear implants wear hearing aids in the opposite ear? *Ear and Hearing, 22*(5), 365–380.

Ching, T. Y. C., van Wanrooy, E., & Dillon, H. (2007). Binaural-bimodal fitting or bilateral implantation for managing severe to profound deafness: A review. *Trends in Amplification, 11*(3), 161–192.

Chute, P. M., Hellman, S. A., Parisier, S. C., & Selesnick, S. H. M. D. (1990). A matched-pairs comparison of single and multichannel cochlear implants in children. *Laryngoscope, 100*(1), 25–28.

Clement, C. J., Koopmans-van Beinum, F. J., & Pols, L. C. W. (1996). Acoustical characteristics of sound production of deaf and normally hearing infants. *Proceedings of the Fourth International Conference on Spoken Language Processing* (Vol. 3, pp. 1549–1552). Philadelphia, PA.

Colletti, L., Shannon, R. V., & Colletti, V. (2014). The development of auditory perception in children after auditory brainstem implantation. *Audiology and Neuro-otology, 19*(6), 386–394.

Colletti, V., Carner, M., Fiorino, F., Sacchetto, L., Miorelli, V., Orsi, A., . . . Pacini, L. (2002). Hearing restoration with auditory brainstem implant in three children with cochlear nerve aplasia. *Otology and Neurotology, 23*(5), 682–693.

Colletti, V., Carner, M., Miorelli, V., Guida, M., Colletti, L., & Fiorino, F. (2005). Auditory brainstem implant (ABI): New frontiers in adults and children. *Otolaryngology-Head and Neck Surgery, 133*(1), 126–138.

Connor, C. M., Craig, H. K., Raudenbush, S. W., Heavner, K., & Zwolan, T. A. (2006). The age at which young deaf children receive cochlear implants and their vocabulary and speech-production growth: Is there an added value for early implantation? *Ear and Hearing, 27*(6), 628–644.

Core, C., Brown, J. W., Larsen, M. D., & Mahshie, J. (2014). Assessing speech perception in children with cochlear implants using a modified hybrid visual habituation procedure. *Ear and Hearing, 35*(5), 555–564.

Cornelisse, L. E., Gagne, J.-P., & Seewald, R. C. (1991). Ear level recordings of the long-term average spectrum of speech. *Ear and Hearing, 12*(1), 47–54.

Cramer, K. D., & Erber, N. P. (1974). A spondee recognition test for young hearing-impaired children. *Journal of Speech and Hearing Disorders, 39*(3), 304–311.

Crandell, C. C. (1993). Speech recognition in noise by children with minimal degrees of sensorineural hearing loss. *Ear and Hearing, 14*(3), 210–216.

Davidson, L. S., Geers, A. E., Blamey, P. J., Tobey, E. A., & Brenner, C. A. (2011). Factors contributing to speech perception scores in long-term pediatric cochlear implant users. *Ear and Hearing, 32*(1 Suppl.), 19S–26S.

Davis, B. L., Morrison, H. M., von Hapsburg, D., & Warner Czyz, A. D. (2005). Early vocal patterns in infants with varied hearing levels. *Volta Review, 105*(1), 7–27.

DeCasper, A. J., & Fifer, W. P. (1980). Of human bonding: Newborns prefer their mothers' voices. *Science, 208*, 1174–1176.

Dettman, S. J., D'Costa, W. A., Dowell, R. C., Winton, E. J., Hill, K. L., & Williams, S. S. (2004). Cochlear implants for children with significant residual hearing. *Archives of Otolaryngology-Head and Neck Surgery, 130*(5), 612–618.

Edgerton, B., House, W., & Hitselberger, W. (1981). Hearing by cochlear nucleus stimulation in humans. *Annals of Otology, Rhinology, and Laryngology Supplement, 91*(2 Pt. 3), 117–124.

Eimas, P. D. (1974). Auditory and linguistic processing of cues for place of articulation by infants. *Perception and Psychophysics, 16*(3), 513–521.

Eimas, P. D., & Miller, J. L. (1980a). Contextual effects in infant speech perception. *Science, 209*(4461), 1140–1141.

Eimas, P. D., & Miller, J. L. (1980b). Discrimination of information for manner of articulation. *Infant Behavior and Development, 3*, 367–375.

Eimas, P. D., Siqueland, E. R., Jusczyk, P., & Vigorito, J. (1971). Speech perception in infants. *Science, 171*(3968), 303–306.

Eisenberg, L. S., Berliner, K. I., Thielemeir, M. A., Kirk, K. I., & Tiber, N. (1983). Cochlear implants in children. *Ear and Hearing, 4*(1), 41–50.

Eisenberg, L. S., Fisher, L. M., Johnson, K. C., Ganguly, D. H., Grace, T., Niparko, J. K., . . . the CDaCI Investigative Team. (In press). Sentence recognition in quiet and noise by pediatric cochlear implant users: Relationships to spoken language. *Otology and Neurotology*.

Eisenberg, L. S., Johnson, K. C., Martinez, A. S., DesJardin, J. L., Stika, C. J., Dzubak, D., . . . Rector, E. P. (2008). Comprehensive evaluation of a child with an auditory brainstem implant. *Otology and Neurotology, 29*(2), 251–257.

Eisenberg, L. S., Kirk, K. I., Martinez, A. S., Ying, E. A., & Miyamoto, R. T. (2004). Communication abilities of children with aided residual hearing: Comparison with cochlear implant users. *Archives of Otolaryngology-Head and Neck Surgery, 130*(5), 563–569.

Eisenberg, L. S., Maltan, A. A., Portillo, F., Mobley, J. P., & House, W. F. (1987). Electrical stimulation of the auditory brain stem structure in deafened adults. *Journal of Rehabilitation and Research Development, 24*(3), 9–22.

Eisenberg, L. S., Martinez, A. S., & Boothroyd, A. (2003). Auditory-visual and auditory-only perception of phonetic contrasts in children. *Volta Review, 103*(4 Monograph), 327–346.

Eisenberg, L. S., Martinez, A. S., & Boothroyd, A. (2007). Assessing auditory capabilities in young children. *International Journal of Pediatric Otorhinolaryngology, 71*(9), 1339–1350.

Eisenberg, L. S., Martinez, A. S., Holowecky, S. R., & Pogorelsky, S. (2002). Recognition of lexically controlled words and sentences by children with normal hearing and children with cochlear implants. *Ear and Hearing, 23*(5), 450–462.

Eisenberg, L. S., Shannon, R. V., Martinez, A. S., Wygonski, J., & Boothroyd, A. (2000). Speech recognition with reduced spectral cues as a function of age. *Journal of the Acoustical Society of America, 107*(5), 2704–2710.

Elfenbein, J. L., Hardin-Jones, M. A., & Davis, J. M. (1994). Oral communication skills of children who are hard of hearing. *Journal of Speech, Language, and Hearing Research, 37*(1), 216–226.

Elliott, L. L. (1979). Performance of children aged 9 to 17 years on a test of speech intelligibility in noise using sentence material with controlled word predictability. *Journal of the Acoustical Society of America, 66*(3), 651–653.

Elliot, L. L., & Katz, D. R. (1980). *Northwestern University Children's Perception of Speech (NU-CHIPS): Technical manual*. St. Louis, MO: Auditec of St. Louis.

Erber, N. P. (1971). Auditory and audiovisual reception of words in low-frequency noise by children with normal hearing and by children with impaired hearing. *Journal of Speech, Language, and Hearing Research, 14*(3), 496–512.

Erber, N. P. (1972). Auditory, visual, and auditory-visual recognition of consonants by children with normal and impaired hearing. *Journal of Speech and Hearing Research, 15*(2), 413–422.

Erber, N. P. (1979). Speech perception by profoundly hearing-impaired children. *Journal of Speech and Hearing Disorders, 44*(3), 255–270.

Erber, N. P., & Alencewicz, C. M. (1976). Audiologic evaluation of deaf children. *Journal of Speech and Hearing Disorders, 41*(2), 256–267.

Ertmer, D. J. (2001). Emergence of a vowel system in a young cochlear implant recipient. *Journal of Speech, Language, and Hearing Research, 44*(4), 803–813.

Ertmer, D. J., & Goffman, L. (2011). Speech production accuracy and variability in young cochlear implant recipients: Comparisons with typically developing age-peers. *Journal of Speech, Language, and Hearing Research, 54*(1), 177–189.

Ertmer, D. J., & Jung, J. (2012). Prelinguistic vocal development in young cochlear implant recipients and typically developing infants: Year 1 of robust hearing experience. *Journal of Deaf Studies and Deaf Education, 17*(1), 116–132.

Ertmer, D. J., & Mellon, J. A. (2001). Beginning to talk at 20 months: Early vocal development in a young cochlear implant recipient. *Journal of Speech, Language, and Hearing Research, 44*(1), 192–206.

Ertmer, D. J., Young, N. M., & Nathani, S. (2007). Profiles of vocal development in young cochlear implant recipients. *Journal of Speech, Language, and Hearing Research, 50*(2), 393–407.

Fallon, M., Trehub, S. E., & Schneider, B. A. (2000). Children's perception of speech in multitalker babble. *Journal of the Acoustical Society of America, 108*(6), 3023–3029.

Finitzo-Hieber, T., & Tillman, T. W. (1978). Room acoustics effects on monosyllabic word discrimination ability for normal and hearing-impaired children. *Journal of Speech, Language, and Hearing Research, 21*(3), 440–458.

Fitzpatrick, E. M., Olds, J., Gaboury, I., McCrae, R., Schramm, D., & Durieux-Smith, A. (2012). Comparison of outcomes in children with hearing aids and cochlear implants. *Cochlear Implants International, 13*(1), 5–15.

Galvin, K. L., Mok, M., & Dowell, R. C. (2007). Perceptual benefit and functional outcomes for children using sequential bilateral cochlear implants. *Ear and Hearing, 28*(4), 470–482.

Geers, A. E., & Brenner, C. (1994). Speech perception results: Audition and lipreading enhancement. *Volta Review, 96*, 97–108.

Geers, A. E., Strube, M. J., Tobey, E. A., Pisoni, D. B., & Moog, J. S. (2011). Epilogue: Factors contributing to long-term outcomes of cochlear implantation in early childhood. *Ear and Hearing, 32*(1 Suppl.), 84S–92S.

Gerhardt, K. J., & Abrams, R. M. (2000). Fetal exposures to sound and vibroacoustic stimulation. *Journal of Perinatology, 20*(8 Pt. 2), S20–S29.

Glista, D., Scollie, S., Bagatto, M., Seewald, R., Parsa, V., & Johnson, A. (2009). Evaluation of nonlinear frequency compression: Clinical outcomes. *International Journal of Audiology, 48*(9), 632–644.

Gordon-Brannan, M. P. (1994). Assessing intelligibility: Children's expressive phonologies. *Topics in Language Disorders, 14*(2), 17–25.

Granier-Deferre, C., Bassereau, S., Ribeiro, A., Jacquet, A.-Y., & DeCasper, A. J. (2011). A melodic contour repeatedly experienced by human near-term fetuses elicits a profound cardiac reaction one month after birth. *PLoS One, 6*(2), e17304.

Gravel, J. S., Fausel, N., Liskow, C., & Chobot, J. (1999). Children's speech recognition in noise using omni-directional and dual-microphone hearing aid technology. *Ear and Hearing, 20*(1), 1–11.

Grieco-Calub, T. M., Litovsky, R. Y., & Werner, L. A. (2008). Using the observer-based psychophysical procedure to assess localization acuity in toddlers who use bilateral cochlear implants. *Otology and Neurotology, 29*(2), 235–239.

Griffiths, S. K., Brown, W. S., Gerhardt, K. J., Abrams, R. M., & Morris, R. J. (1994). The perception of speech sounds recorded within the uterus of a pregnant sheep. *Journal of the Acoustical Society of America, 96*(4), 2055–2063.

Hack, Z. C., & Erber, N. P. (1982). Auditory, visual, and auditory visual perception of vowels by hearing-impaired children. *Journal of Speech and Hearing Research, 25*, 100–107.

Hall, J. W., III, Grose, J. H., Buss, E., & Dev, M. B. (2002). Spondee recognition in a two-talker masker and a speech-shaped noise masker in adults and children. *Ear and Hearing, 23*(2), 159–165.

Hicks, C. B., & Tharpe, A. M. (2002). Listening effort and fatigue in school-age children with and without hearing loss. *Journal of Speech, Language, and Hearing Research, 45*(3), 573–584.

Hitselberger, W., House, W., Edgerton, B., & Whitaker, S. (1984). Cochlear nucleus implants. *Otolaryngology-Head and Neck Surgery, 92*(1), 52–54.

Holt, R. F., Kirk, K. I., Eisenberg, L. S., Martinez, A. S., & Campbell, W. (2005). Spoken word recognition development in children with residual hearing using cochlear implants and hearing aids in opposite ears. *Ear and Hearing, 26*(4 Suppl.), 82S–91S.

Houston, D. M., Horn, D. L., Qi, R., Ting, J. Y., & Gao, S. (2007). Assessing speech discrimination in individual infants. *Infancy, 12*(2), 119–145.

Houston, D. M., Pisoni, D. B., Iler Kirk, K., Ying, E. A., & Miyamoto, R. T. (2003). Speech perception skills of deaf infants following cochlear implantation: A first report. *International Journal of Pediatric Otorhinolaryngology, 67*(5), 479–495.

Jerger, S., Lewis, S., Hawkins, J., & Jerger, J. (1980). Pediatric Speech Intelligibility Test. I. Generation of test materials. *International Journal of Pediatric Otorhinolaryngology, 2*, 217–230.

Johnson, C. E. (2000). Children's phoneme identification in reverberation and noise. *Journal of Speech, Language, and Hearing Research, 43*(1), 144–157.

Johnson, K.C., & Dumont, L.V. (2007). *[Identification scores for normal hearing children and children with hearing loss]*. Unpublished raw data.

Johnston, J. C., Durieux-Smith, A., Angus, D., O'Connor, A., & Fitzpatrick, E. (2009). Bilateral paediatric cochlear implants: A critical review. *International Journal of Audiology, 48*(9), 601–617.

Juscyzk, P. W., Cutler, A., & Redanz, N. (1993). Infant preference for the predominant stress patterns of English words. *Child Development, 64*, 675–687.

Juscyzk, P. W., Friederici, A. D., Wessles, J., Svenkerud, V. Y., & Juscyzk, A. M. (1993). Infants' sensitivity to the sound patterns of native language words. *Journal of Memory and Language, 32*, 402–420.

Jusczyk, P. W., & Luce, P. A. (2002). Speech perception and spoken word recognition: Past and present. *Ear and Hearing, 23*(1), 2–40.

Juszyck, P. W., Pisoni, D. B., & Mullennix, J. (1992). Some consequences of stimulus variability on speech processing by 2–month old infants. *Cognition, 43*, 253–291.

Kancherla, V., Van Naarden Braun, K., & Yeargin-Allsopp, M. (2013). Childhood vision impairment, hearing loss and co-occurring autism spectrum disorder. *Disability and Health Journal, 6*(4), 333–342.

Kaplan, A. B., Kozin, E. D., Puram, S. V., Owoc, M. S., Shah, P. V., Hight, A. E., . . . Lee, D. J. (2015). Auditory brainstem implant candidacy in the United States in children 0–17 years old. *International Journal of Pediatric Otorhinolaryngology, 79*(3), 310–315.

Kennedy, C., McCann, D., Campbell, M. J., Kimm, L., & Thornton, R. (2005). Universal newborn screening for permanent childhood hearing impairment: An 8-year follow-up of a controlled trial. *Lancet, 366*(9486), 660–662.

Kent, R. D. (2004). Development, pathology and remediation of speech. In J. Slifka, S. Manuel, & M. Matthies (Eds.), *From sound to sense: 50+ years of discoveries in speech* (pp. 148–163). Cambridge, MA: Massachusetts Institute of Technology.

Kent, R. D., & Bauer, H. R. (1985). Vocalizations of one-year-olds. *Journal of Child Language, 12*(03), 491–526.

Kent, R. D., & Murray, A. D. (1982). Acoustic features of infant vocalic utterances at 3, 6, and 9 months. *Journal of the Acoustical Society of America, 72*(2), 353–365.

Kent, R. D., Osberger, M. J., Netsell, R., & Hustedde, C. G. (1987). Phonetic development in identical twins differing in auditory function. *Journal of Speech and Hearing Disorders, 52*(1), 64–75.

Kirk, K. I., French, B. F., & Choi, S. (2009). Assessing spoken word recognition in children with cochlear implants. In L. S. Eisenberg (Ed.), *Clinical management of children with cochlear implants* (pp. 217–250). San Diego, CA: Plural.

Kirk, K. I., Hay-McCutcheon, M. J., Holt, R. F., Gao, S., Qi, R., & Gerlain, B. L. (2007). Audiovisual spoken word recognition by children with cochlear implants. *Audiological Medicine, 5*(4), 250–261.

Kirk, K. I., Lindsay, P., French, B., Gotch, C., Eisenberg, L. S., & Young, N. (2012). Assessing spoken word recognition in children who are deaf or hard of hearing: A translational approach. *Journal of the American Academy of Audiology, 23*(6), 464–475.

Kong, Y. Y., Stickney, G. S., & Zeng, F. G. (2005). Speech and melody recognition in binaurally combined acoustic and electric hearing. *Journal of the Acoustic Society of America, 117*, 1351–1361.

Koopmans-van Beinum, F. J., Clement, C. J., & Van Den Dikkenberg-Pot, I. (2001). Babbling and the lack of auditory speech perception: A matter of coordination? *Developmental Science, 4*(1), 61–70.

Kosky, C., & Boothroyd, A. (2003). Validation of an on-line implementation of the Imitative Test of Speech Pattern Contrast Perception (IMSPAC). *Journal of the American Academy of Audiology, 14*(2), 72–83.

Kuhl, P. K. (1983). Perception of auditory equivalence classes for speech in early infancy. *Infant Behavior and Development, 6*, 263–285.

Kuhl, P. K. (2004). Early language acquisition: Cracking the speech code. *Nature Reviews Neuroscience, 5*(11), 831–843.

Kuhl, P. K., & Meltzoff, A. N. (1982). The bimodal perception of speech in infancy. *Science, 218*(4577), 1138–1141.

Kuhl, P. K., & Meltzoff, A. N. (1996). Infant vocalizations in response to speech: Vocal imitation and developmental change. *Journal of the Acoustical Society of America, 100*(4 Pt. 1), 2425–2438.

Kuhl, P. K., & Miller, J. D. (1982). Discrimination of auditory target dimensions in the presence or absence of variation in a second dimension by infants. *Perception and Psychophysics, 31*(3), 279–292.

Lachs, L., Pisoni, D. B., & Kirk, K. I. (2001). Use of audiovisual information in speech perception by prelingually deaf children with cochlear implants: A first report. *Ear and Hearing, 22*(3), 236–251.

Lecanuet, J.-P., & Schaal, B. (1996). Fetal sensory competencies. *European Journal of Obstetrics and Gynecology and Reproductive Biology, 68*(1–2), 1–23.

Litovsky, R. Y., Johnstone, P. M., & Godar, S. P. (2006). Benefits of bilateral cochlear implants and/or hearing aids in children. *International Journal of Audiology, 45*(Suppl. 1), S78–S91.

Litovsky, R. Y., Parkinson, A., Arcaroli, J., Peters, R., Lake, J., Johnstone, P., & Yu, G. (2004). Bilateral cochlear implants in adults and children. *Archives of Otolaryngology-Head and Neck Surgery, 130*(5), 648–655.

Mahshie, J., Core, C., & Larsen, M. D. (2015). Auditory perception and production of speech feature contrasts by pediatric implant users. *Ear and Hearing, 36*(6), 653–663.

Mampe, B., Friederici, A. D., Christophe, A., & Wermke, K. (2009). Newborns' cry melody is shaped by their native language. *Current Biology, 19*(23), 1994–1997.

Markides, A. (1970). The speech of deaf and partially-hearing children with special reference to factors affecting intelligibility. *British Journal of Disorders of Communication, 5*(2), 126–140.

Martinez, A., Eisenberg, L., Boothroyd, A., & Visser-Dumont, L. (2008). Assessing speech pattern contrast perception in infants: Early results on VRASPAC. *Otology and Neurotology, 29*(2), 183–188.

McDermott, R. P., & Jones, T. A. (1984). Articulation characteristics and listeners' judgments of the speech of children with severe hearing loss. *Language, Speech, and Hearing Services in Schools, 15*(2), 110–126.

Mehler, J., Jusczyk, P., Lambertz, G., Halsted, N., Bertoncini, J., & Amiel-Tison, C. (1988). A precursor of language acquisition in young infants. *Cognition, 29*(2), 143–178.

Meyer, T. A., Svirsky, M. A., Kirk, K. I., & Miyamoto, R. T. (1998). Improvements in speech perception by children with profound prelingual hearing loss: Effects of device, communication mode, and chronological age. *Journal of Speech, Language, and Hearing Research, 41*(4), 846–858.

Miller, J. L., & Eimas, P. D. (1983). Studies on the categorization of speech by infants. *Cognition, 13*(2), 135–165.

Miyamoto, R. T., Osberger, M. J., Robbins, A. M., Myers, W. A., Kessler, K., & Pope, M. L. (1992). Longitudinal evalutation of communication skills of children with single- or multichannel implants. *American Journal of Otology, 13*(3), 215–222.

Moeller, M. P., & Carney, A. E. (1993). Assessment and intervention with preschool hearing-impaired children. In J. Alpiner & P. McCarthy (Eds.), *Rehabilitative audiology in children and adults* (2nd ed., pp. 106–135). Baltimore, MD: Williams & Wilkins.

Moeller, M. P., Hoover, B., Putman, C., Arbataitis, K., Bohnenkamp, G., Peterson, B., Lewis, D., Estee, S., Pittmanm, A., & Stelmachowicz, P. (2007). Vocalizations of infants with hearing loss compared with infants with normal hearing: Part II—Transition to words. *Ear and Hearing, 28*(5), 628–642.

Moeller, M. P., Hoover, B., Putman, C., Arbataitis, K., Bohnenkamp, G., Peterson, B., Wood, S., Lewis, D., Pittman, A., & Stelmachowicz, P. (2007). Vocalizations of infants with hearing loss compared with infants with normal hearing: Part I—Phonetic development. *Ear and Hearing, 28*(5), 605–627.

Monsen, R. B. (1978). Toward measuring how well hearing-impaired children speak. *Journal of Speech, Language, and Hearing Research, 21*(2), 197–219.

Moog, J. S., & Geers, A. E. (1990). *Early speech perception test for profoundly hearing-impaired children.* St. Louis, MO: Central Institute for the Deaf.

Moon, C., Cooper, R. P., & Fifer, W. P. (1993). Two-day-olds prefer their native language. *Infant Behavior and Development, 16*(4), 495–500.

Moon, C. M., & Fifer, W. P. (2000). Evidence of transnatal auditory learning. *Journal of Perinatology, 20*(8 Pt. 2), S37–S44.

Moon, C., Lagercrantz, H., & Kuhl, P. K. (2013). Language experienced in utero affects vowel perception after birth: A two-country study. *Acta Paediatrica, 102*(2), 156–160.

Moore, B. C. J. (1996). Perceptual consequences of cochlear hearing loss and their implications for the design of hearing aids. *Ear and Hearing, 17*(2), 133–161.

Moore, B. C. J. (2008). Basic auditory processes involved in the analysis of speech sounds. *Philosophical Transactions of the Royal Society of London B: Biological Sciences, 363*(1493), 947–963.

Moore, J. A., & Bass-Ringdahl, S. (2002). Role of infant vocal development in candidacy for and efficacy of cochlear implantation. *Annals of Otology, Rhinology, and Laryngology, supplement, 189*, 52–55.

Moore, J. K., & Linthicum, F. H., Jr. (2007). The human auditory system: A timeline of development. *International Journal of Audiology, 46*(9), 460–478.

Morera, C., Manrique, M., Ramos, A., Garcia-Ibanez, L., Cavalle, L., Huarte, A., . . . Estrada, E. (2005). Advantages of binaural hearing provided through bimodal stimulation via a cochlear implant and a conventional hearing aid: A 6-month comparative study. *Acta Oto-laryngologica, 125*(6), 596–606.

Nathani, S., Ertmer, D. J., & Stark, R. E. (2006). Assessing vocal development in infants and toddlers. *Clinical Linguistics and Phonetics, 20*(5), 351–369.

National Institute on Deafness and Other Communication Disorders (NIDCD; 2006). *NIDCD outcomes research in children with hearing loss. Statistical report: Prevalence of hearing loss in U.S. children, 2005.* Retrieved August 18, 2015, from http://www.nidcd.nih.gov/funding/programs/hb/outcomes/Pages/report.aspx

Neuman, A. C., Wroblewski, M., Hajicek, J., & Rubinstein, A. (2010). Combined effects of noise and reverberation on speech recognition performance of normal-hearing children and adults. *Ear and Hearing, 31*(3), 336–344.

Nevison, B., Laszig, R., Sollmann, W.-P., Lenarz, T., Sterkers, O., Ramsden, R., . . . Wallenberg, E. (2002). Results from a European clinical investigation of the Nucleus® Multichannel Auditory Brainstem Implant. *Ear and Hearing, 23*(3), 170–183.

Noij, K. S., Kozin, E. D., Sethi, R., Shah, P. V., Kaplan, A. B., Herrmann, B., . . . Lee, D. J. (2015). Systematic review of nontumor pediatric auditory brainstem implant outcomes. *Otolaryngology-Head and Neck Surgery, 153*(5), 739–750.

Nott, P., Cowan, R., Brown, M., & Wigglesworth, G. (2009). Early language development in children with profound hearing loss fitted with a device at a young age. Part I—The time period taken to acquire first words and first word combinations. *Ear and Hearing, 30*(5), 526–540.

Oller, D. K. (1980). The emergence of the sounds of speech in infancy. In G. H. Yeni-Kromshian, J. F. Kavanaugh, & C. A. Ferguson (Eds.), *Child phonology, Vol. 1: Production* (pp. 93–112). New York, NY: Academic Press.: Academic Press.

Oller, D. K. (2000). *The emergence of the speech capacity.* Hove, UK: Psychology Press.

Oller, D. K., & Eilers, R. E. (1988). The role of audition in infant babbling. *Child Development, 59*(2), 441–449.

Oller, D. K., Eilers, R. E., Bull, D. H., & Carney, A. E. (1985). Prespeech vocalizations of a deaf infant: Comparison with normal metaphonological development. *Journal of Speech, Language, and Hearing Research, 28*(1), 47–63.

Oller, D. K., Wieman, L. A., Doyle, W. J., & Ross, C. (1976). Infant babbling and speech. *Journal of Child Language, 3*(1), 1–11.

Olsho, L. W., Koch, E. G., Carter, E. A., Halpin, C. F., & Spetner, N. B. (1988). Pure-tone sensitivity of human infants. *Journal of the Acoustical Society of America, 84*(4), 1316–1324.

Osberger, M. J., Robbins, A. M., Miyamoto, R. T., Berry, S. W., Myres, W. A., Kessler, K., & Pope, M. L. (1991). Speech perception abilities of children with cochlear implants, tactile aids, or hearing aids. *American Journal of Otology, 12*(Suppl.), 105–115.

Osberger, M. J., Robbins, A. M., Todd, S. L., Riley, A. I., Kirk, K. I., & Carney, A. E. (1996). Cochlear implants and tactile aids for children with profound hearing impairment. In F. E. Bess, J. S. Gravel, & A. M. Tharpe (Eds.), *Amplification for children with auditory deficits* (pp. 283–308). Nashville, TN: Bill Wilkerson Press.

Partanen, E., Kujala, T., Näätänen, R., Liitola, A., Sambeth, A., & Huotilainen, M. (2013). Learning-induced neural plasticity of speech processing before birth. *Proceedings of the National Academy of Sciences, 110*(37), 15145–15150.

Patterson, M. L., & Werker, J. F. (1999). Matching phonetic information in lips and voice is robust in 4.5-month-old infants. *Infant Behavior and Development, 22*(2), 237–247.

Patterson, M. L., & Werker, J. F. (2003). Two-month-old infants match phonetic information in lips and voice. *Developmental Science, 6*(2), 191–196.

Peters, B., Litovsky, R., Lake, J., & Parkinson, A. J. (2004). Sequential bilateral cochlear implantation in children. *International Congress Series, 1273*, 462–465.

Peters, B. R., Litovsky, R., Parkinson, A., & Lake, J. (2007). Importance of age and postimplantation experience on speech perception measures in children with sequential bilateral cochlear implants. *Otology and Neurotology, 28*(5), 649–657.

Peterson, G. E., & Lehiste, I. (1962). Revised CNC lists for auditory tests. *Journal of Speech and Hearing Disorders, 27*(1), 62–70.

Pisoni, D. B. (2000). Cognitive factors and cochlear implants: Some thoughts on perception, learning, and memory in speech perception. *Ear and Hearing, 21*(1), 70–78.

Pisoni, D. B., Conway, C. M., Kronenberger, W. G., Horn, D. L., Karpicke, J., & Henning, S. (2008). Effcacy and effectiveness of cochlear implants in deaf children. In M. Marscharck & P. C. Hauser (Eds.), *Deaf cognition: Foundations and outcomes* (pp. 52–101). Oxford, UK: Oxford University Press.

Pisoni, D. B., Kronenberger, W. G., Roman, A. S., & Geers, A. E. (2011). Measures of digit span and verbal rehearsal speed in deaf children after more than 10 years of cochlear implantation. *Ear and Hearing, 32*(1 Suppl.), 60S–74S.

Pittman, A. L., Stelmachowicz, P. G., Lewis, D. E., & Hoover, B. M. (2003). Spectral characteristics of speech at the ear: Implications for amplification in children. *Journal of Speech, Language, and Hearing Research, 46*(3), 649–657.

Robbins, A. M., Osberger, M. J., Miyamoto, R. T., Renshaw, J. J., & Carney, A. E. (1988). Longitudinal study of speech perception by children with cochlear implants and tactile aids: Progress report. *Journal of the Academy of Rehabilitative Audiology, 21*, 11–28.

Robbins, A. M., Renshaw, J. J., Miyamoto, R. T., Osberger, M. J., & Pope, M. L. (1988). *Minimal Pairs Test.* Indianapolis, IN: Indiana University School of Medicine.

Ross, M., & Lerman, J. (1970). A picture identification test for hearing-impaired children. *Journal of Speech, Language, and Hearing Research, 13*(1), 44–53.

Schafer, E. C., Amlani, A. M., Seibold, A., & Shattuck, P. L. (2007). A meta-analytic comparison of binaural benefits between bilateral cochlear implants and bimodal stimulation. *Journal of the American Academy of Audiology, 18*(9), 760–776.

Schafer, E. C., & Thibodeau, L. M. (2006). Speech recognition in noise in children with cochlear implants while listening in bilateral, bimodal, and FM-system arrangements. *American Journal of Audiology, 15*(2), 114–126.

Schauwers, K., Gillis, S., Daemers, K., De Beukelaer, C., & Govaerts, P. J. (2004). Cochlear implantation between 5 and 20 months of age: The onset of babbling and the audiologic outcome. *Otology and Neurotology, 25*(3), 263–270.

Schneider, B. A., Trehub, S. E., & Thorpe, L. (1991). Developmental perspectives on the localization and detection of auditory signals. *Perception and Psychophysics, 49*(1), 10–20.

Schorr, E. A., Fox, N. A., van Wassenhove, V., & Knudsen, E. I. (2005). Auditory-visual fusion in speech perception in children with cochlear implants. *Proceedings of the National Academy of Sciences, 102*(51), 18748–18750.

Seewald, R. C., Ross, M., Giolas, T. G., & Yonovitz, A. (1985). Primary modality for speech perception in children with normal and impaired hearing. *Journal of Speech, Language, and Hearing Research, 28*(1), 36–46.

Sennaroglu, L., Colletti, V., Manrique, M., Laszig, R., Offeciers, E., Saeed, S. R., . . . Konradsson, K. (2011). Auditory brainstem implantation in children and non-neurofibromatosis type 2 patients: A consensus statement. *Otology and Neurotology, 32*, 187–191.

Serry, T. A., & Blamey, P. J. (1999). A 4-year investigation into phonetic inventory development in young cochlear implant users. *Journal of Speech, Language, and Hearing Research, 42*(1), 141–154.

Shahidullah, S., & Hepper, P. G. (1994). Frequency discrimination by the fetus. *Early Human Development, 36*(1), 13–26.

Shannon, R. V., Colletti, L., Eisenberg, L. S., Johnson, K. C., Carner, M., & Colletti, V. (2009). Auditory branstem implants in children. In L. S. Eisenberg (Ed.), *Clinical management of children with cochlear implants* (pp. 655–662). San Diego, CA: Plural.

Shannon, R. V., Fayad, J., Moore, J., Lo, W. W., Otto, S., Nelson, R. A., & O'Leary, M. (1993). Auditory brainstem implant: II. Postsurgical issues and performance. *Otolaryngology-Head and Neck Surgery, 108*(6), 634–642.

Smit, A. B., Hand, L., Freilinger, J. J., Bernthal, J. E., & Bird, A. (1990). The Iowa Articulation Norms Project and its Nebraska replication. *Journal of Speech and Hearing Disorders, 55*(4), 779–798.

Smith, C. R. (1975). Residual hearing and speech production in deaf children. *Journal of Speech, Language, and Hearing Research, 18*(4), 795–811.

Stark, R. E. (1980). Stages of speech development in the first year of life. In G. H. Yeni-Kromshian, J. F. Kavanaugh, & C. A. Ferguson (Eds.), *Child phonology. Vol. 1: Production* (pp. 73–92). New York, NY: Academic Press.

Starr, A., Amlie, R., Martin, W., & Sanders, S. (1977). Development of auditory function in newborn infants revealed by auditory brainstem potentials. *Pediatrics, 60*, 831–839.

Stelmachowicz, P. G., Pittman, A. L., Hoover, B. M., & Lewis, D. E. (2002). Aided perception of /s/ and /z/ by hearing-impaired children. *Ear and Hearing, 23*(4), 316–324.

Stelmachowicz, P. G., Pittman, A. L., Hoover, B. M., Lewis, D. E., & Moeller, M. P. (2004). The importance of high-frequency audibility in the speech and language development of children with hearing loss. *Archives of Otolaryngology-Head and Neck Surgery, 130*(5), 556–562.

Stoel-Gammon, C. (1983). The acquisition of segmental phonology by normal and hearing-impaired children. In I. Hochberg, H. Levitt, & M. J. Osberger (Eds.), *Speech of the hearing impaired: Research, training, and personnel preparation* (pp. 267–280). Baltimore, MD: University Park Press.

Stoel-Gammon, C. (1985). Phonetic inventories, 15–24 months: A longitudinal study. *Journal of Speech, Language, and Hearing Research, 28*(4), 505–512.

Stoel-Gammon, C. (1988). Prelinguistic vocalizations of hearing-impaired and normally hearing subjects: A comparison of consonantal inventories. *Journal of Speech and Hearing Disorders, 53*(3), 302–315.

Sumby, W. H., & Pollack, I. (1954). Visual contribution to speech intelligibility in noise. *Journal of the Acoustical Society of America, 26*(2), 212–215.

Svirsky, M. A., Chin, S. B., & Miyamoto, R. T. (2000). Speech intelligibility of profoundly deaf pediatric hearing aid users. *Volta Review, 102*(4), 175–198.

Teinonen, T., Aslin, R. N., Alku, P., & Csibra, G. (2008). Visual speech contributes to phonetic learning in 6-month-old infants. *Cognition, 108*(3), 850–855.

Tharpe, A. M., & Ashmead, D. H. (2001). A longitudinal investigation of infant auditory sensitivity. *American Journal of Audiology, 10*(2), 104–112.

Thielemeir, M. A., Brimacombe, J. A., & Eisenberg, L. S. (1982). Audiological results with the cochlear implant. *Annals of Otology, Rhinology, and Laryngology Supplement, 91*(2 Pt 3), 27–34.

Thielemeir, M. A., Tonokawa, L. L., Petersen, B., & Eisenberg, L. S. (1985). Audiological results in children with a cochlear implant. *Ear and Hearing, 6*(3 Suppl.), 27S–35S.

Tillberg, I., Ronnberg, J., Svard, I., & Ahlner, B. (1996). Audiovisual speech reading in a group of hearing aid users: The effects of onset age, handicap age and degree of hearing loss. *Scandinavian Audiology, 25*, 267–272.

Tobey, E. A., Geers, A. E., Brenner, C., Altuna, D., & Gabbert, G. (2003). Factors associated with development of speech production skills in children implanted by age five. *Ear and Hearing, 24*(1 Suppl.), 36S–45S.

Tobey, E. A., Geers, A. E., Douek, B. M., Perrin, J., Skellet, R., Brenner, C., & Toretta, G. (2000). Factors associated with speech intelligibility in children with cochlear implants. *Annals of Otology, Rhinology, and Laryngology Supplement, 185*, 28–30.

Tobey, E. A., Geers, A. E., Sundarrajan, M., & Shin, S. (2011). Factors influencing speech production in elementary and high school-aged cochlear implant users. *Ear and Hearing, 32*(1 Suppl.), 27S–38S.

Tomblin, J. B., Peng, S.-C., Spencer, L. J., & Lu, N. (2008). Long-term trajectories of the development of speech sound production in pediatric cochlear implant recipients. *Journal of Speech, Language, and Hearing Research, 51*(5), 1353–1368.

Trehub, S. E., Schneider, B. A., & Endman, M. (1980). Developmental changes in infants' sensitivity to octave-band noises. *Journal of Experimental Child Psychology, 29*(2), 282–293.

Tyler, R. S., Kelsay, D. M. R., Teagle, H. F. B., Rubenstein, J. T., Gantz, B. J., & Christ, A. M. (2000). 7-year speech perception results and the effects of age, residual hearing, and pre-implant speech perception in prelingually deaf children using the Nucleus and Clarion Cochlear Implants. *Advances in Otorhinolaryngology, 57*, 305–310.

Uchanski, R. M., & Geers, A. E. (2003). Acoustic characteristics of the speech of young cochlear implant users: A comparison with normal-hearing age-mates. *Ear and Hearing, 24*(1 Suppl.), 90S–105S.

Uhler, K., Yoshinaga-Itano, C., Gabbard, S. A., Rothpletz, A. M., & Jenkins, H. (2011). Longitudinal infant speech perception in young cochlear implant users. *Journal of the American Academy of Audiology, 22*(3), 129–142.

Uziel, A. S., Sillon, M., Vieu, A., Artieres, F., Piron, J.-P., Daures, J.-P., & Mondain, M. (2007). Ten-year follow-up of a consecutive series of children with multichannel cochlear implants. *Otology and Neurotology, 28*(5), 615–628.

van den Dikkenberg-Pot, I., Koopmans-van Beinum, F. J., & Clement, C. J. (1998). Influence of lack of auditory speech perception on sound productions of deaf infants. *Proceedings of the Institute of Phonetic Sciences* (Vol. 22, pp. 47–60). Amsterdam, the Netherlands: University of Amsterdam.

Van Naarden Braun, K., Christensen, D., Doernberg, N., Schieve, L., Rice, C., Wiggins, L., . . . Yeargin-Allsopp, M. (2015). Trends in the prevalence of autism spectrum disorder, cerebral palsy, hearing loss, intellectual disability, and vision impairment, metropolitan Atlanta, 1991–2010. *PLoS One, 10*(4), e0124120.

Vihman, M. M. (1988). Early phonological development. In J. Bernthal & N. Bankson (Eds.), *Articulation and phonological disorders* (2nd ed., pp. 60–109). Baltimore, MD: Williams & Wilkins.

Vihman, M., Ferguson, C. A., & Elbert, M. (1986). Phonological development from babbling to speech: Common tendencies and individual difference. *Applied Psycholinguistics, 7*, 3–40.

von Hapsburg, D., & Davis, B. L. (2006). Auditory sensitivity and the prelinguistic vocalizations of early-amplified infants. *Journal of Speech, Language, and Hearing Research, 49*(4), 809–822.

Warner-Czyz, A. D., & Davis, B. L. (2008). The emergence of segmental accuracy in young cochlear implant recipients. *Cochlear Implants International, 9*(3), 143–166.

Warner-Czyz, A. D., Davis, B. L., & MacNeilage, P. F. (2010). Accuracy of consonant–vowel syllables in young cochlear implant recipients and hearing children in the single-word period. *Journal of Speech, Language, and Hearing Research, 53*(1), 2–17.

Warner-Czyz, A. D., Houston, D. M., & Hynan, L. S. (2014). Vowel discrimination by hearing infants as a function of number of spectral channels. *Journal of the Acoustical Society of America, 135*(5), 3017–3024.

Weichbold, V., Nekahm-Heis, D., & Welzl-Mueller, K. (2006). Universal newborn hearing screening and postnatal hearing loss. *Pediatrics, 117*(4), e631–e636.

Werker, J. F., & Tees, R. C. (1984). Cross-language speech perception: Evidence for perceptual reorganization during the first year of life. *Infant Behavior and Development, 7*(1), 49–63.

Werker, J. F., & Tees, R. C. (1999). Influences on infant speech processing: Toward a new synthesis. *Annual Review of Psychology, 50*, 509–535.

Werner, L. A. (2007). Issues in human auditory development. *Journal of Communication Disorders, 40*(4), 275–283.

Werner, L., Fay, R. R., & Popper, A. N. (Eds.). (2012). *Human auditory development*. New York, NY: Springer.

World Health Organization (WHO; 2015). *Grades of hearing impairment.* Retrieved August 18, 2015, from http://www.who.int/pbd/deafness/hearing_impairment_grades/en/

Zeiser, M. L., & Erber, N. P. (1977). Auditory/vibratory perception of syllabic structure in words by profoundly hearing-impaired children. *Journal of Speech, Language, and Hearing Research, 20*(3), 430–436.

School-Age Children

Carolyne Edwards

Introduction

When children reach school age, the focus of our audiologic attention changes in response to the different players involved. Assessment and management of school-aged children demand a comprehensive view of their educational setting and the people who now enter their school life. On the professional side, those people include the classroom teacher, special education teacher, principal, teacher of the deaf and hard of hearing, educational audiologist, speech-language pathologist, and other support personnel as needed. On the personal side, children now must interact with a large group of other children, who might or might not have hearing loss depending on the school setting. Family members are the one constant throughout and therefore carry the history of where their child began and the direction for the future.

Audiologists must now focus on how to create the most optimal integration of children with hearing loss into the elementary school setting. Although educational audiologists are best known for their direct mandate in children's auditory needs in the school system, it behooves all audiologists to see themselves as vital contributors to children's educational progress and to ensure that the necessary steps are taken to provide for the learning needs of all children with hearing loss.

Creating Optimal Integration for Children With Hearing Loss

Audiologists contribute to children's successful integration into the school setting in the following ways:

- assessment of children under a variety of listening conditions to provide:
  - an ongoing picture of the growth in children's listening abilities and
  - the communication strategies necessary for optimal understanding of speech in the classroom;
- description of children's auditory functioning in layperson terms so that all personnel who work with children who have hearing loss develop appropriate expectations of their auditory capabilities;
- description of the social-emotional impact of hearing loss so that personnel working with children with hearing loss can incorporate that knowledge into their strategies;
- evaluation of amplification needs on an ongoing basis in order to respond to the changing auditory demands of the classroom;
- communication with the team of key support personnel at the school level to ascertain concerns and issues that need to be addressed by the audiologist; and
- provision of the counseling needs of children and their families as the school demands change.

Assessment of Listening Skills

Audiologic assessment has moved well beyond diagnosis and monitoring of hearing levels in the last 30 years. In the early years, the only audiological information requested at school case conferences was the pure-tone audiogram and the degree of hearing loss. In recent years, educational and clinical audiologists alike have forwarded information to school personnel to describe

- the type and degree of hearing loss;
- auditory potential based on degree of hearing loss;
- current auditory capacity to understand speech;
- predictors of the child's listening difficulty;
- the effects of middle ear function on the child's hearing levels and everyday functioning; and
- the effect of the child's hearing loss on functioning within current school setting.

Although traditional testing protocols consisted of the pure-tone audiogram, middle ear measurement, speech awareness or reception thresholds, and a word discrimination score, there is a wide variety of speech tests now available to measure understanding of speech under varying conditions. The audiologist is able to provide a comprehensive description of a child's listening skills and then measure changes over time. This information is critical to the school staff's understanding of the child's current and future needs in the classroom.

Degree of Hearing Loss

Degree of hearing loss is the most well-reported and understood characteristic of audiologic testing. Anderson's *Relationship of Hearing Loss to Listening and Learning Needs* (2007) continues to provide valuable descriptors of auditory functioning in layperson language for hearing levels ranging from unilateral hearing loss to bilateral minimal to profound sensorineural hearing loss (Appendix 39–A). Audiologists would be wise to include these descriptors in their reports to schools.

Children with minimal hearing loss, unilateral hearing loss, precipitously sloping hearing loss, and progressive hearing loss require special mention in audiological reports due to their unique characteristics. Because we are unable to predict which children with minimal hearing loss will show difficulties, it is wise to describe a child with minimal hearing loss as "at risk for academic, linguistic and/or social emotional delays" so that their needs can be monitored. For children with unilateral hearing loss, it is important to emphasize the impact of the hearing loss in the impaired ear versus the normal hearing ear. The effect of the hearing loss for children with precipitously sloping hearing loss will often be underestimated due to their better low-frequency hearing levels, so it is important to acknowledge the discrepancy between their presentation and performance. Educators can also be alerted to the importance of close monitoring of children with progressive hearing loss to determine the need for any changes in communication strategies or counseling for those children and their families.

Type of Hearing Loss

Often the type of hearing loss is no longer prominent in audiologic reporting as the child enters the school years. However, at the time of school entry it is useful to differentiate the functional differences between the child with conductive hearing loss and the child with sensorineural hearing loss so that educators know what to expect with regard to speech perception and speech intelligibility.

Middle Ear Function

The presence of abnormal middle ear function for children with sensorineural hearing loss is significant to educators for one or more reasons and can be reported as such:

- The pure-tone thresholds obtained on the audiogram do not reflect the child's optimal hearing levels.
- The child might perform more poorly than usual and need a higher volume setting or a different program on the hearing aid.
- The child might need more support and communication strategies in the classroom.
- The child might be more fatigued than usual if hearing levels are significantly poorer than typical levels.

Normal middle ear function indicates that the pure-tone thresholds reflect the child's optimum potential for understanding of speech.

Speech Perception Ability

The original purpose of speech testing was to obtain a validation of pure-tone thresholds and a measure of understanding of speech using a single word discrimination test. Unlike the adult population where the results are given directly to the individual with hearing loss, results of testing for children are sent to school settings so that educators can understand the impact of hearing loss. Although formal word discrimination testing continues to be the most common speech perception test used in clinics, it gives only a cursory representation of the child's ability to function in the classroom, given the variety of listening conditions encountered in the school. Therefore, additional tests are useful and round out the audiologic results to increase relevance of speech testing in the educational environment.

Testing Different Modalities

The impact of hearing loss is well known to audiologists, but school personnel often have little background knowledge in the area of audition. Therefore, when an audiologist can present speech perception scores that demonstrate a child's capacity to understand speech by listening only and by listening and speechreading (as seen in Table 39–1), teachers have a better idea of the impact of various listening conditions.

Although speechreading cues enhance comprehension of speech, Child #1 will not be affected by the loss of speechreading cues to the same degree as the other three children in the examples in Table 39–1. When the teacher looks away or turns to the blackboard to write, Child #2, Child #3, and Child #4 will lose critical information. Notice the difference between Child #3 and Child #4. Optimal performance for Child #3 is reliance on a combined listening and speechreading input, whereas Child #4 is functioning primarily through visual information only. By testing auditory only, visual only, and auditory-visual, audiologists can provide this information.

Testing Different Intensity Levels and Speech-to-Noise Ratios

Classroom listening conditions vary considerably depending on the grade level, the classroom activity, the number of students in the class, the location of the student in the classroom and proximity to the teacher, and the acoustical conditions of the classroom. Testing at speech-to- noise ratios of +5 dB or 0 dB will best replicate challenging acoustic conditions in most classrooms without the use of classroom amplification systems (Crandell & Smaldino, 2002; Hetu, Truchon-Gagnon, & Bilodeau, 1990).

Table 39–2 presents sample scenarios. Notice that Child #2 will have considerably more difficulty than Child #1 when the teacher is at a distance (quiet conversational speech levels) or in the presence of background noise when the teacher is within close proximity.

Test results such as the scenarios presented above can highlight for audiologists the importance of recommending additional amplification technologies such

Table 39–1. Sample Speech Perception Scores

Child #1		
	By listening only	92%
Child #2		
	By listening only	48%
	By listening and speechreading	92%
Child #3		
	By listening only	16%
	By listening and speechreading	76%
	By speechreading only	48%
Child #4		
	By listening only	0%
	By listening and speechreading	56%
	By speechreading only	60%

Table 39-2. Sample Scenarios

Child #1		
	Word recognition at normal conversational speech	92%
	Word recognition at quiet conversational speech	56%
	Word recognition at normal conversational speech in background noise (S/N = + 5 dB)	68%
Child #2		
	Word recognition at normal conversational speech	56%
	Word recognition at quiet conversational speech	12%
	Word recognition at normal conversational speech in background noise (S/N = + 5 dB)	16%

as personal FM system versus a sound-field system, a boom microphone versus a lapel microphone, and strategies such as seating locations away from noise sources in the classroom. The quantitative data offered by speech perception scores are useful in describing the child's auditory difficulties in the classroom, potential problems, and recommended solutions to educators. See Chapter 27 in this volume for more information on FM systems.

Testing Different Speech Materials

One of the easiest modifications for word recognition testing is to record a child's responses and then score the number of phonemes correct in addition to the number of words correct. This is useful when discrimination scores are low, in order to obtain more information on a child's auditory perceptual ability.

Although the word recognition scores for both children in Table 39–3 are the same, the phoneme scores are significantly different, suggesting far more auditory perceptual errors for the second child. These difficulties will be apparent on spelling tasks and often will be reflected in the child's speech intelligibility.

For children with high-frequency hearing loss, Gardner's high frequency monosyllabic word list (Berger, 1977) continues to be useful to demonstrate to the child, teacher, or parents the listening challenges that are not clearly seen with administration of a conventional word list that has no special emphasis on high-frequency phonemes.

Although word recognition testing is a more reliable and valid indicator of auditory perception, it does not represent the nature of the speech that a child faces in the classroom. The child is faced with sentence material, and often a series of sentences presented without pause in the classroom. It is difficult to standardize norms for children's performance on phrase or sentence material as it is highly language dependent. Therefore, testing that goes beyond word recognition is not used as a precise comparative measure of performance from year to year, but rather as an indication of the degree of enhancement in understanding speech when moving from word to sentence materials using materials such as BKB sentences (Bamford, Koval, & Bench, 1979), or the Speech–in-Noise Test (SPIN; Kalikow, Stevens, & Elliott, 1977).

In some cases such as precipitous hearing loss, the difference between word recognition and sentence recognition is great, often showing very low scores on word recognition of 30% or less and high scores on sentence materials ranging from 76% to 100% with the addition of the acoustic and contextual clues provided by connected speech. The child's functioning in the classroom can be better described by including both word and sentence measures than either measure alone.

There are a variety of other speech materials using phrase or sentence recognition or comprehension tasks that can be used to gain a broader understanding of a child's auditory abilities (DeConde Johnson, Benson, & Seaton, 1997a; Edwards 1991, 1999). The reader is referred to these references for further elaboration of pediatric speech test batteries for school-aged children.

Table 39–3. Word Versus Phoneme Scoring

Child #1		
	Word recognition at 50 dB HL	32%
	Phoneme recognition at 50 dB HL	66%
Child #2		
	Word recognition at 50 dB HL	32%
	Phoneme recognition at 50 dB HL	36%

Description of Auditory Functioning

Many educators have little familiarity with the nature of audiologic testing. Therefore, audiologic assessment and reporting that can translate clinical findings into meaningful descriptions of classroom functioning are essential to produce changes in educators' understanding of the auditory needs of the child.

Audiologists can describe the nature of the hearing loss in terms of implications for the classroom, specifically the challenges that the child will have in the classroom. The questions below can be used as a guide to the type of information valuable to educators.

- What is the child's capacity to understand speech?
  - by listening only?
  - by listening and watching the teacher's face?
  - How much does the child rely on hearing alone?
  - Will the child be able to understand the teacher when they are not facing each other?
  - Is the child reliant on watching the teacher's face to understand speech?
- Which speech sounds are difficult to hear?
  - Does the child have difficulty hearing high-frequency speech sounds such as /s/, /f/, voiceless "th" or "ch" or /t/?

The /s/ sound is a grammatically loaded sound in the English language that signifies plurals, possessives, and change in verb tense. If a child is unable to hear the /s/, it is useful for the teacher to know so the child can be provided with other grammatical clues instead.

- How will distance affect the child's understanding of speech?
  - without amplification?
  - with hearing aid(s) or cochlear implants?
  - with classroom hearing technology?

School situations such as classroom discussion, listening in the gymnasium during sports activities, gatherings of the whole school for assemblies, the playground and class trips involve distance listening. The degree of difficulty children experience for softer levels of speech will affect their ability to respond in these situations. Identifying the child's degree of difficulty in these situations will be helpful to a child's teachers. Furthermore, educators will need to know how much change to expect when a child uses classroom hearing technology.

- How will noise affect a child's understanding of speech?
  - without amplification?
  - with hearing aid/s?
  - with classroom hearing technology?

School situations such as small group work, seminar groups, and listening in the gymnasium during sports activities involve listening in noise. The degree of difficulty children experience in noise will affect their ability to respond and learn in these situations. Again, educators need to know how much improvement will occur when classroom hearing technology is used.

- What modifications will assist the child in hearing better?
  - proximity to the teacher?
  - use of classroom amplification system?
  - repetition and buddy systems?
  - visual supports—speechreading and written supplements?

For children not using FM systems who have difficulty listening at a distance, sitting close to the teacher during circle time for primary levels or row seating near the teacher for higher grades will be beneficial. Most children with hearing loss will benefit from the use of classroom hearing technology of some kind *if* there are large group teaching situations in which they are involved. Evaluation of candidacy for an FM system is best done at the school level where the educational audiologist and the teacher of the deaf and hard of hearing, and occasionally the speech language pathologist, are in direct contact with the classroom teacher and can assess the nature of the classroom structure and its suitability for the use of such systems. The clinical audiologist can raise the issue of FM use for consideration with the parents and child as soon as the child enters school. Furthermore, the audiologist needs to ensure that hearing aid settings are compatible with FM use. See Chapter 26 for detailed discussion of FM system use.

When a child has difficulty in quiet listening situations by listening only, it is wise to ensure that there are other strategies put into place to support comprehension, such as repetition of instructions by the teacher, or a buddy system where a classmate is selected to provide repetition of instructions as required by the child. Similarly, when a child is dependent on speechreading for accurate listening, the importance of speechreading needs to be underlined. Educators need to be aware that when they turn their backs to write on the blackboard or to address another child, the understanding by the child with hearing loss will be compromised. Writing key words or instructions on the blackboard, the overhead projector, or on interactive white boards will assist the child by supplementing the loss of speechreading information. In summary, audiologists must ensure that the implications of audiologic testing are translated into concrete actions for those working with children in the classroom setting.

Social-Emotional Impact of Hearing Loss

Children's sense of difference from their family and friends starts to develop between ages 7 and 9 years (Rall, 2007). Even with the best technology available, we cannot change the fact that children with hearing loss will have more difficulty hearing under degraded listening conditions (such as noise and distance) than their hearing peers. However, what we can impact is children's attitudes toward their differences.

Accurate perspective comes from acceptance of both the similarities *and* the differences from others. Some children will imagine their difference as greater than they appear to others, and some children might imagine their differences as less than they appear to others. Without adequate input and feedback from others in their environment, either viewpoint can lead to inappropriate use of communication strategies due to an inaccurate perspective of auditory needs.

Children with hearing loss often identify their own listening difficulties but do not know that normal-hearing peers also have difficulty listening in noise, with the resulting feeling that others will never understand their experience. That feeling of separation from others must be bridged in order to bring a greater sense of self-worth.

Audiologists can encourage classroom teachers to support sharing of listening difficulties by all students in the class so that children with hearing loss begin to understand that everyone, normal hearing or hearing impaired, has difficulty hearing in noise to varying degrees. When children with hearing loss understand that they are not alone in their experience of auditory challenges, it gives them more confidence to ask for help and implement strategies to enhance communication. If teachers can make all children in the class part of the solution, communication strategies become inclusive rather than isolating (Edwards, 1996, 2005).

Simulation of hearing loss using earplugs (Appendix 39–B) is an effective way to educate individuals about hearing loss (Edwards, 2005). Whether we give earplugs to a child's classmates, teachers, or to a child's parents for a personal experience of mild loss, the experience of simulated hearing loss is powerful and memorable for most people and can elicit a surprising empathy for the person with hearing loss.

Children need an opportunity to share their thoughts and feelings about hearing loss for acknowledgement and validation of their experiences. Sharing can reveal what is working and what is not working in the classroom, what strategies to continue, what strategies need to be discarded, and what new strategies need to be implemented. Audiologists can use such tools such as the Listening Inventory for Education–Revised (L.I.F.E.-R; Anderson, Smaldino, & Spangler, 2011), Child Home Inventory for Home Listening Difficulties (C.H.I.L.D.; Anderson & Smaldino, 2000), or scales such as the Children's Peer Relationship Scale (English, 2002), Secondary School Survey (Lambert & Goforth 2001), and the Self Assessment of Communication-Adolescent (Wright, English, & Elkayam, 2010) to elicit comments on listening ease or lack thereof for a child. Alternately, audiologists can use open-ended questions and discussion starters such as the following:

- How do you feel about your FM system?
- What do your classmates understand about your hearing loss?
- What is difficult to explain to your classmates?
- What is frustrating about school right now?
- What is working in the classroom and what is not?

Such information can then lead to discussion of strategies that might assist students in the classroom and with their peers.

Audiologists can support the development of children's self-advocacy skills in the clinical setting and the educational setting. Children need to understand their own audiogram, and be knowledgeable about the cause of their hearing loss, the implications of their hearing loss, and any progression of hearing loss through the years. They must have an increasing understanding of their hearing technology and how best to use it, and the types of hearing concerns that they should report to their audiologist. Audiologists can be effective teachers in these subject areas.

Educational audiologists in the school system can engage the child in decisions about the type of education to be provided to their classmates and teacher about hearing loss and the degree of involvement of the child in such programming. Often the student knows more about their hearing devices than their classroom teachers; it is important to encourage the classroom teacher to draw on the student's expertise when possible.

Having children teach others about their hearing loss builds confidence and empowers students to learn how to manage their hearing impairment. The ways in which we support children will change with their age. For younger children, they can show their classmates how their hearing aid works with support personnel such as the educational audiologist or the teacher of the deaf and hard of hearing present as support. Older students can teach others about their hearing loss through science projects, class presentations, lessons on sound, or being part of a hearing awareness day in the school where various booths are created to teach others about hearing loss and hearing aids. Giving children experiences in managing their own hearing needs teaches them what works and what does not, increases their awareness of options, and improves their decision-making ability and their ability to negotiate solutions.

Audiologists also need to be aware of a child's educational placement in order to intuit the challenges that might be confronted. Children in the mainstream can feel the pressure to be the same as their peers and therefore might minimize any interventions that demonstrate their differences from others. Children in self-contained classes in the mainstream often feel more secure in their class with other hearing impaired peers but might need more support for their visits to the general education classes. Children in schools for the deaf often are secure in their school setting with their deaf peers but face their greatest challenges in their social community at home, either as day students who by the time they arrive home on the bus have little energy to interact with people other than their family, or as residential students whose weekend visits with their families leave only brief opportunities to interact with the hearing world.

Ongoing Evaluation of Hearing Technology Needs

Most children with hearing loss are candidates for some form of classroom amplification. As described in detail in Chapter 27 of this volume, there are a myriad of FM system configuration options now available for children with varying degrees of hearing loss as well as for children with normal hearing. Table 39–4 shows many of the possible choices facing audiologists when making a recommendation for an FM system for a school child.

As the reader can see, audiologists must gather information on the child's hearing aids, the type of classroom setting, the structure and scheduling of the classroom setting, the type of instruction, the teacher's use of the system, and the child's willingness to accept a device, to select the optimal FM system for a child. Then these choices must be reviewed annually to ensure the equipment can be modified to include any additional amplification needs arising from changing classroom structure or demands.

Table 39–4. Selection of Amplification System

Type of Classroom Amplification System	
1. Personal FM System	***2. Sound-Field System***
FM Receiver Options	**Nature of Signal Transmission**
Ear-level hearing aid with FM receiver attached	FM system
Universal FM receiver attached to audio shoe	Infrared system
Dedicated/integrated FM receiver	**Speaker Type**
Ear-level hearing aid and neckloop FM receiver	Totable
FM receiver only in ear level case	Portable
FM body worn receiver	Stationary
With earphones	Single speaker
Cochlear implant	Multiple speakers
FM receiver with ear-level processor	Wall mounted
FM receiver with body worn processor	Ceiling mounted
Neckloop FM receiver	**Sound-Field Transmitter Options**
FM Transmitter Options	Transmitter type
Transmitter type	Single-channel transmitter
Single-channel transmitter	Dual-channel transmitter
Dual-channel transmitter	Multichannel transmitter
Multichannel transmitter	Pass-around microphone
Pass-around microphone	Coupling
Coupling	Over-the-ear boom microphone
Lapel microphone	Collar microphone
Boom microphone	Lapel microphone
Collar microphone	

The important questions that audiologists must ask to ascertain the need for change are the following:

➤ *What has changed, if anything, in the classroom structure?*

If there is team teaching in the classroom, the FM system will have to provide multiple transmitters working within the same classroom without interference. Different manufacturers have different ways of addressing this. If the child has an educational assistant who does the primary work with the child, one must consider a second transmitter on a different frequency and determine who will wear the "primary" transmitter. If there is small group work in the classroom, a pass-around microphone might be necessary. The child might prefer a different type of microphone (boom versus lapel) depending on the vocal characteristics of the teacher's voice.

➤ *Has the child changed from a single classroom to rotary classes?*

For children with sound-field systems, this is the time to discuss a change to a personal FM system. If the student is averse to a personal FM system, a totable or portable system, rather than stationary loudspeaker system, can be considered.

➤ *Are there any interference problems reported this year?*

Transmission frequency might need to be changed if the student reports interference. With a change in classrooms, the frequency that the child was previously using might no longer be suitable. Interference can occur in one area of the school and not in another.

And, of course, any time that the child's hearing aids change, the FM system must be evaluated with the new amplification to ensure compatibility and transparency. The other outstanding issue that occurs with the use of FM systems is the monitoring and maintenance of such systems.

With sound-field systems, it is immediately obvious to everyone when the system is not working. However, with personal FM systems, we are dependent on the child reporting a problem or one of the school staff checking the system to ensure adequate functioning. The historical data on adequate functioning of hearing aids are quite discouraging, so it is critical to ensure that a staff member has been trained to check the personal FM system in combination with the hearing aid(s) and does so on a routine basis.

Despite the enhanced speech-to-noise ratio when the FM transmitter is in use by the teacher, children with hearing loss are still acoustically challenged during small group work. Overhearing is an important part of language development for normal hearing children and children with hearing loss (Moeller, 2008), and yet children with hearing loss do not have many technological or acoustic options to assist with overhearing. The FM system is not a viable option for the rapid communication that occurs in small groups and so enhancement of classroom acoustical conditions is the only option available. Unfortunately, there has been less emphasis on improving classroom acoustics in recent years.

Carpeting classrooms is still the most effective way to reduce the noise of classroom chairs scraping on the floor and provide some absorption of children's voices, particularly if carpet underpadding is added (Crandell & Smaldino, 2005). Tennis balls placed on the bottom of chair legs will reduce the noise of chairs scraping against the hard floor surfaces but will not provide any absorption of the overall classroom noise. Precut tennis balls are commercially available through several companies in Canada and the United States. For acoustical design modifications to classrooms, readers are referred to Melancon, Truchon-Gagnon, and Hodgson (1990) for a comprehensive guide.

Working With Other Professionals

The audiologist's mandate within the educational setting is to ensure that every aspect of audition is addressed for the child with hearing loss. Depending on the extent of involvement, audiologists can be seen on a continuum from a peripheral consultant to an integral part of the team of professionals working with the child with hearing loss.

What is unique about the audiologist's role in providing information regarding auditory perception? Audiologists can

- provide the school staff with a clear sense of expectations for the child's understanding of speech in the classroom;
- identify the communication challenges that a child will have in the classroom;
- determine the contribution of hearing loss to the child's reported academic, social, or behavioral difficulties, especially for children with multiple learning challenges;
- provide the information necessary for working with the child's hearing aids;
- provide recommendations for classroom hearing technology;

- educate the class regarding hearing loss and amplification devices;
- meet with the child as needed regarding any hearing related concerns;
- meet with parents regarding any hearing-related concerns;
- support interactions between the child with hearing loss and other classmates; and
- meet with hearing resource staff regarding auditory programming.

It is important that audiologists anticipate the areas of difficulty that might arise with school personnel to manage proactively. For example, for children with subtle hearing loss such as those with minimal, mild, or unilateral hearing losses, school personnel often do not notice any obvious hearing difficulties with the child. Rather than beginning with an explanation of the potential effects of subtle hearing loss, it might be more useful to get feedback from the staff about *any* areas of concern first, prior to sharing information. That will allow the audiologist to build on staff information and align with them rather than create resistance at the beginning by assuming that others have also seen the problem.

When other personnel report speech, language, emotional, and learning concerns for a child, audiologists must be prepared to state which of those issues are likely associated with hearing loss and which are not associated with hearing loss. This is particularly helpful for teachers, parents, speech language pathologists, and school psychologists when too much or too little attention is focused on the effects of the hearing loss.

Counseling Needs of Children and Families

It is essential that children and parents have an opportunity to express their feelings related to the hearing loss as feelings arise. What feelings can emerge? Isolation can occur when the child feels different from his or her peers. Frustration and anger can occur when children cannot change the environment, and the differences from their peers become evident. Denial of hearing loss or increased dependency can emerge as default strategies to cope with hearing loss. Children can feel lost or want to give up when there is not enough support available in the environment to cope.

Parents can experience similar feelings when they are unable to change their child's reality and make it better for their child and when they do not have other parents with whom to share. Luterman and Kurtzer-White (1999) found that when parents of preschool hearing-impaired children were asked what the most important factor was in their adjustment to the diagnosis of their child's hearing loss, they indicated that it was meeting other parents, specifically other parents of children with hearing loss.

Often parents are not aware of the many areas of support that are available to them. The Family Needs Survey (DeConde Johnson, Benson, & Seaton, 1997b) can empower parents to ask for the support they need. By having the family fill out the survey before meeting with the audiologist, parents learn more about the questions they can ask relating to general information, specific information about hearing and hearing loss, communication, educational resources, family and social support, child care, and community services, and financial support. By the time they see an audiologist, they are better informed as to the support services that could be useful to them at that time and are equipped to ask questions about those services.

Acceptance of a child's hearing loss is often presented as a one-time experience, but in reality, each time there is a new demand in a child's environment that is constrained by hearing loss, parents are faced with a new demand for acceptance of the hearing loss. There are natural transitions within the educational environment that have corresponding changes in listening, communication, and social emotional demands. Transitions occur for a child and family at elementary school entry, movement from primary to junior grades, from senior grades to secondary level, and final years of preparation for higher education at the secondary level. Audiologists need to be aware of those changing demands as children grow older and offer technological, strategy, and counseling support as needed.

Parents hold the balance and perspective between the child's current reality and the dream of who their child can be. Audiologists must be sensitive to these demands and be able to acknowledge and discuss both the reality of the current situation and a child's auditory potential in the context of a child's school performance.

Although much attention is given to the tutoring and academic support that parents provide, we must not forget their role in modeling an attitude and approach to hearing loss that will support the child through the school years. Through counseling at different stages of the child's development, audiologists can help parents to model principles essential for acceptance and growth of the child's individuality.

Perspective is key in facilitating a child's understanding of oneself both as a person and as a child with hearing loss. Parents can model perspective by acknowledging and naming difficult communicative situations for the child. When the child recognizes those situations, parents can then teach the child *choice* by discussing and modeling a variety of communication strategies to explore under acoustically challenging situations. When parents reinforce the child's use of strategies to improve listening, they support the development of the child's *decision-making* skills. The child learns that decision-making is an ongoing process in response to a communicative situation, and that there are no mistakes, but rather simply more opportunities to learn. Finally, parents can stand behind their children when their children begin to advocate for their own communicative needs—providing *independence with support*. That is a critical step prior to children having to advocate independently. Audiologists can show parents how to model each of these steps for their child in order to co-empower both the child and family.

Summary

The audiologic management of the child with hearing loss through the school years is broad-ranging and multifaceted, and is directed by the child's clinical and educational audiologists. Audiologists must work with the child, the family, the educators, and other school personnel in order to ensure that audiologic information is meaningful and relevant to the child's progress. The information from the school staff is essential to shape the audiologic recommendations for further assessment, changes in amplification, implications of hearing loss, and directions for counseling for the child and family. Ease of communication among all of the personnel involved with a child can ensure that all of a child's auditory needs are being addressed. When the young adults graduating from secondary school can successfully implement those auditory, communication, and technological strategies and know where to access resources and services as needed, our job is done.

References

Anderson, K. (2007). *Relationship of hearing loss to listening and learning needs*. Retrieved from Karen Anderson Audiology Consulting website http://www.kandersonaudconsulting.com/

Anderson, K. L., & Smaldino, J. J. (2000). Children's Home Inventory for Listening Difficulties (C.H.I.L.D). *Educational Audiology Review, 17*(3 Suppl.).

Anderson, K. L., Smaldino, J. J., & Spangler, C. (2011). *Listening Inventory for Education- Revised (L.I.F.E.-R)*. Retrieved from http://successforkidswithhearingloss.com/tests/

Bamford, J., Koval, A., & Bench, J. (1979). *Speech hearing tests and the spoken language of partially hearing children*. New York, NY: Academic Press.

Berger, K. (1977). *Speech audiometry materials*. Kent, OH: Herald.

Bess, F. (1982). Children with unilateral hearing loss. *Journal of Rehabilitative Audiology, 15*, 131–144.

Bess, F., Dodd-Murphy, J., & Parker, R. (1998). Children with minimal sensorineural hearing loss: Prevalence, educational performance and functional status. *Ear and Hearing, 19*(5), 339–355.

Crandell, C., & Smaldino, J. (2002). *Classroom acoustics*. Paper presented at the American Academy of Audiology National Convention, Philadelphia, PA.

Crandell, C., & Smaldino, J. (2005). Acoustical modifications in classrooms. In C. Crandell, J. Smaldino, & C. Flexer (Eds.), *Sound field FM amplification: Applications to speech perception and classroom acoustics* (2nd ed., pp. 132–141). New York, NY: Thomson Delmar Learning.

DeConde Johnson, C., Benson, P., & Seaton, J. (1997a). Assessment practices. In C. DeConde Johnson & J. Seaton (Eds.), *Educational audiology handbook* (pp. 478–488). San Diego, CA: Singular.

DeConde Johnson, C., Benson, P., & Seaton, J. (1997b). Family needs survey—Appendix 10-B. In C. DeConde Johnson & J. Seaton (Eds.), *Educational audiology handbook* (pp. 443–444). San Diego, CA: Singular.

Edwards, C. (1991). Assessment and management of listening skills in school-aged children. *Seminars in Hearing 12*(4), 389–401.

Edwards, C. (1996). Auditory intervention for children with mild auditory deficits. In F. Bess, J. Gravel, & A. M. Tharpe (Eds.), *Amplification for children with auditory deficits* (pp. 383–398). Nashville, TN: Bill Wilkerson Center Press.

Edwards, C. (1999). Current directions in educational audiology. In J. Katz & L. Medwetsky (Eds.), *Handbook of clinical audiology* (4th ed.). Baltimore, MD: Williams & Wilkins.

Edwards, C. (2005). From system selection to enhancement of listening skills: Considerations for the classroom. In C. Crandell, J. Smaldino, & C. Flexer (Eds.), *Sound field FM amplification: Applications to speech perception and classroom acoustics* (2nd ed., pp. 166–191). New York, NY: Thomson Delmar Learning.

English, K. (2002). *Counseling children with hearing impairment and their families*. Boston, MA: Allyn & Bacon.

Hetu, R., Truchon-Gagnon, C., & Bilodeau, S. (1990). Problems of noise in school settings: A review of the literature and the results of an exploratory study. *Journal of Speech Language Pathology and Audiology, 14*(3), 31–39.

Kalikow, D., Stevens, K., & Elliott, L. (1977). Development of a test of speech intelligibility in noise using sentence materials with controlled word predictability. *Journal of the Acoustical Society of America, 61*, 1337–1351.

Lambert, D., & Goforth, D. (2001). Middle school hard of hearing survey. *Educational Audiology Review, 18*, 13–19.

Lieu, J. E. (2004). Speech-language and educational consequences of unilateral hearing loss in children. *Archives of Otolaryngology-Head and Neck Surgery, 130*, 524–530.

Luterman, D., & Kurtzer-White, E. (1999). Identifying hearing loss: Parents' needs. *American Journal of Audiology, 8*(1), 13–18.

Melancon, L., Truchon-Gagnon, C., & Hodgson, M. (1990). *Architectural strategies to avoid noise problems in child care centres*. Montreal, Canada: Groupe d'acoustique de l'Universite de Montreal.

Moeller, M. P. (2008). Building sound foundations: What's in a word? In R. Seewald & J. Bamford (Eds.), *A Sound Foundation Through Early Amplification 2007: Proceedings of the fourth international conference* (pp. 19–31). Stäfa, Switzerland: Phonak AG.

Rall, E. (2007). *Supporting psychosocial development of children with hearing loss*. Poster session presentation at the Sound Foundation through Early Amplification. Fourth International Conference, Chicago, IL.

Wright, K., English, K., & Elkayam, J. (2010). Reliability of the Self-Assessment of Communication-Adolescent (SAC-A). *Journal of Educational Audiology, 16*, 4–10.

APPENDIX 39–A

Relationship of Hearing Loss to Listening and Learning Needs

16-25 dB HEARING LOSS		
Possible Impact on the Understanding of Language and Speech	**Possible Social Impact**	**Potential Educational Accommodations and Services**
Impact of a hearing loss that is approximately 20 dB can be compared to ability to hear when index fingers are placed in your ears. Child may have difficulty hearing faint or distant speech. At 16 dB student can miss up to 10% of speech signal when teacher is at a distance greater than 3 feet. A 20 dB or greater hearing loss in the better ear can result in absent, inconsistent or distorted parts of speech, especially word endings (s, ed) and unemphasized sounds. Percent of speech signal missed will be greater whenever there is background noise in the classroom, especially in the elementary grades when instruction is primarily verbal and younger children have greater difficulty listening in noise. Young children have the tendency to watch and copy the movements of other students rather than attending to auditorily fragmented teacher directions.	May be unaware of subtle conversational cues that could cause child to be viewed as inappropriate or awkward. May miss portions of fast-paced peer interactions that could begin to have an impact on socialization and self concept. Behavior may be confused for immaturity or inattention. May be more fatigued due to extra effort needed for understanding speech.	Noise in typical classroom environments impede child from having full access to teacher instruction. Will benefit from improved acoustic treatment of classroom and sound-field amplification. Favorable seating necessary. May often have difficulty with sound/letter associations and subtle auditory discrimination skills necessary for reading. May need attention to vocabulary or speech, especially when there has been a long history of middle ear fluid. Depending on loss configuration, may benefit from low power hearing aid with personal FM system. Appropriate medical management necessary for conductive losses. Inservice on impact of "minimal" 15 – 25 dB hearing loss on language development, listening in noise and learning, required for teacher.

26-40 dB HEARING LOSS		
Possible Impact on the Understanding of Language and Speech	**Possible Social Impact**	**Potential Educational Accommodations and Services**
Effect of a hearing loss of approximately 20 dB can be compared to ability to hear when index fingers are placed in ears therefore a 26 – 40 dB hearing loss causes greater listening difficulties than a "plugged ear" loss. Child can "hear" but misses fragments of speech leading to misunderstanding. Degree of difficulty experienced in school will depend upon noise level in the classroom, distance from the teacher, and configuration of the hearing loss, even with hearing aids. At 30 dB can miss 25-40% of the speech signal; at 40 dB may miss 50% of class discussions, especially when voices are faint or speaker is not in line of vision. Will miss unemphasized words and consonants, especially when a high frequency hearing loss is present. Often experiences difficulty learning early reading skills such as letter/sound associations. Child's ability to understand and succeed in the classroom will be substantially diminished by speaker distance and background noise, especially in the elementary grades.	Barriers begin to build with negative impact on self-esteem as child is accused of "hearing when he/she wants to," "daydreaming," or "not paying attention." May believe he/she is less capable due to difficulties understanding in class. Child begins to lose ability for selective listening, and has increasing difficulty suppressing background noise causing the learning environment to be more stressful. Child is more fatigued due to effort needed to listen.	Noise in typical class will impede child from full access to teacher instruction. Will benefit from hearing aid(s) and use of a desk top or ear level FM system in the classroom. Needs favorable acoustics, seating and lighting. May need attention to auditory skills, speech, language development, speechreading and/or support in reading and self-esteem. Amount of attention needed typically related to the degree of success of intervention prior to 6 months of age to prevent language and early learning delays. Teacher inservice on impact of so called "mild" hearing loss on listening and learning to convey that it is often greater than expected.

Please Consider Indicated Items in the Child's Educational Program:

_____Teacher inservice and seating close to teacher _____Hearing monitoring at school every ____mos. _____Amplification monitoring

_____Contact your school district's audiologist _____Protect ears from noise to prevent more loss _____Educational support services/evaluation

_____Screening/evaluation of speech and language _____Note-taking, closed captioned films, visuals _____FM system trial period

_____Educational consultation/ program supervision by specialist(s) in hearing loss _____Regular contact with other children who are deaf or hard of hearing

_____Periodic educational monitoring such as October and April teacher/student completion of SIFTER, LIFE

NOTE: All children require full access to teacher instruction and educationally relevant peer communication to receive an appropriate education. Distance, noise in classroom and fragmentation caused by hearing loss prevent full access to spoken instruction. Appropriate acoustics, use of visuals, FM amplification, sign language, notetakers, communication partners, etc. increase access to instruction. Needs periodic hearing evaluation, rigorous amplification checks, and regular monitoring of access to instruction and classroom function (monitoring tools at www.hear2learn.com or www.SIFTERanderson.com).

Relationship of Hearing Loss to Listening and Learning Needs

41-55 dB HEARING LOSS

Possible Impact on the Understanding of Language and Speech	Possible Social Impact	Potential Educational Accommodations and Services
Consistent use of amplification and language intervention prior to age 6 months increases the probability that the child's speech, language and learning will develop at a normal rate. Without amplification, understands conversation at a distance of 3-5 feet, if sentence structure and vocabulary are known. The amount of speech signal missed can be 50% or more with 40 dB loss and 80% or more with 50 dB loss. Without early amplification the child is likely to have delayed or disordered syntax, limited vocabulary, imperfect speech production and flat voice quality. Addition of a visual communication system to supplement audition may be indicated, especially if language delays and/or additional disabilities are present. Even with hearing aids, child can "hear" but may miss much of what is said if classroom is noisy or reverberant. With personal hearing aids alone, ability to perceive speech and learn effectively in the classroom is at high risk. A personal FM system to overcome classroom noise and distance is typically necessary.	Barriers build with negative impact on self esteem as child is accused of "hearing when he/she wants to," "daydreaming," or "not paying attention." Communication will be significantly compromised with this degree of hearing loss if hearing aids nor worn. Socialization with peers can be difficult, especially in noisy settings such as cooperative learning situations, lunch or recess. May be more fatigued than classmates due to effort needed to listen.	Consistent use of amplification (hearing aids + FM) is essential. Needs favorable classroom acoustics, seating and lighting. Consultation/program supervision by a specialist in childhood hearing impairment to coordinate services is important. Depending on intervention success in preventing language delays, special academic support necessary if language and academic delays are present. Attention to growth of oral communication, reading, written language skills, auditory skill development, speech therapy, self esteem likely. Teacher inservice required with attention to communication access and peer acceptance.

56-70 dB HEARING LOSS

Possible Impact on the Understanding of Language and Speech	Possible Social Impact	Potential Educational Accommodations and Services
Even with hearing aids, child will typically be aware of people talking around him/her, but will miss parts of words said resulting in difficulty in situations requiring verbal communication (both one-to-one and in groups). Without amplification, conversation must be very loud to be understood; a 55 dB loss can cause a child to miss up to 100% of speech information without functioning amplification. If hearing loss is not identified before age one year and appropriately managed, delayed spoken language, syntax, reduced speech intelligibility and flat voice quality is likely. Age when first amplified, consistency of hearing aid use and success of early language intervention strongly tied to speech, language and learning development. Addition of visual communication system often indicated if language delays and/or additional disabilities are present. Use of a personal FM system will reduce the effects of noise and distance and allow increased auditory access to verbal instruction. With hearing aids alone, ability to understand in the classroom is greatly reduced by distance and noise.	If hearing loss was late-identified and language delay was not prevented, communication interaction with peers will be significantly affected. Children will have greater difficulty socializing, especially in noisy settings such as lunch cooperative learning situations, or recess. Tendency for poorer self-concept and social immaturity may contribute to a sense of rejection; peer inservice helpful.	Full time, consistent use of amplification (hearing aids + FM system) essential. May benefit from frequency transposition (frequency compression) hearing aids depending upon loss configuration. May require intense support in development of auditory, language, speech, reading and writing skills. Consultation/supervision by a specialist in childhood hearing impairment to coordinate services is important. Use of sign language or a visual communication system by children with substantial language delays or additional learning needs, may be useful to access linguistically complex instruction. Note-taking, captioned films, etc. accommodations often needed. Requires teacher inservice.

Please Consider Indicated Items in the Child's Educational Program:

_____Teacher inservice and seating close to teacher _____Hearing monitoring at school every ____mos. _____Amplification monitoring

_____Contact your school district's audiologist _____Protect ears from noise to prevent more loss _____Educational support services/evaluation

_____Screening/evaluation of speech and language _____Note-taking, closed captioned films, visuals _____FM system trial period

_____Educational consultation/ program supervision by specialist(s) in hearing loss _____Regular contact with other children who are deaf or hard of hearing

_____Periodic educational monitoring such as October and April teacher/student completion of SIFTER, LIFE

NOTE: All children require full access to teacher instruction and educationally relevant peer communication to receive an appropriate education. Distance, noise in classroom and fragmentation caused by hearing loss prevent full access to spoken instruction. Appropriate acoustics, use of visuals, FM amplification, sign language, notetakers, communication partners, etc. increase access to instruction. Needs periodic hearing evaluation, rigorous amplification checks, and regular monitoring of access to instruction and classroom function (monitoring tools at www.hear2learn.com or www.SIFTERanderson.com).

Relationship of Hearing Loss to Listening and Learning Needs

71-90 dB & 91+ dB		
Possible Impact on the Understanding of Language and Speech	**Possible Social Impact**	**Potential Educational Accommodations and Services**
The earlier the child wears amplification consistently with concentrated efforts by parents and caregivers to provide rich language opportunities throughout everyday activities and/or provision of intensive language intervention (sign or verbal), the greater the probability that speech, language and learning will develop at a relatively normal rate. Without amplification, children with 71-90 dB hearing loss may only hear loud noises about one foot from ear. When amplified optimally, children with hearing ability of 90 dB or better should detect many sounds of speech if presented from close distance or via FM. Individual ability and intensive intervention prior to 6 months of age will determine the degree that sounds detected will be discriminated and understood by the brain into meaningful input. Even with hearing aids children with 71-90 dB loss are typically unable to perceive all high pitch speech sounds sufficiently to discriminate them or benefit from incidental listening, especially without the use of FM. The child with hearing loss greater than 70 dB may be a candidate for cochlear implant(s) and the child with hearing loss greater than 90 dB will not be able to perceive most speech sounds with traditional hearing aids. For full access to language to be available visually through sign language or cued speech, family members must be involved in child's communication mode from a very young age.	Depending on success of intervention in infancy to address language development, the child's communication may be minimally or significantly affected. Socialization with hearing peers may be difficult. Children in general education classrooms may develop greater dependence on adults due to difficulty perceiving or comprehending oral communication. Children may be more comfortable interacting with peers who are deaf or hard of hearing due to ease of communication. Relationships with peers and adults who have hearing loss can make positive contributions toward the development of a healthy self-concept and a sense of cultural identity.	There is no one communication system that is right for all hard of hearing or deaf children and their families. Whether a visual communication approach or auditory/oral approach is used, extensive language intervention, full-time consistent amplification use and constant integration of the communication practices into the family by 6 months of age will highly increase the probability that the child will become a successful learner. Children with late-identified hearing loss (i.e., after 6 months of age) will have delayed language. This language gap is difficult to overcome and the educational program of a child with hearing loss, especially those with language and learning delays secondary to hearing loss, requires the involvement of a consultant or teacher with expertise in teaching children with hearing loss. Depending on the configuration of the hearing loss and individual speech perception ability, frequency transposition (frequency compression) aids or cochlear implantation may be options for better access to speech. If an auditory/oral approach is used, early training is needed on auditory skills, spoken language, concept development and speech. If culturally deaf emphasis is selected, frequent exposure to Deaf, ASL users is important. Educational placement with other signing deaf or hard of hearing students (special school or classes) may be a more appropriate option to access a language-rich environment and free-flowing communication. Support services and continual appraisal of access to communication and verbal instruction is required. Note-taking, captioning, captioned films and other visual enhancement strategies necessary. Training in pragmatic language use and communication repair strategies helpful. Inservice of general education teachers is essential.

Please Consider Indicated Items in the Child's Educational Program:

_____Teacher inservice and seating close to teacher _____Hearing monitoring at school every ____mos. _____Amplification monitoring
_____Contact your school district's audiologist _____Protect ears from noise to prevent more loss _____Educational support services/evaluation
_____Screening/evaluation of speech and language _____Note-taking, closed captioned films, visuals _____FM system trial period
_____Educational consultation/ program supervision by specialist(s) in hearing loss _____Regular contact with other children who are deaf or hard of hearing
_____Periodic educational monitoring such as October and April teacher/student completion of SIFTER, LIFE

NOTE: All children require full access to teacher instruction and educationally relevant peer communication to receive an appropriate education. Distance, noise in classroom and fragmentation caused by hearing loss prevent full access to spoken instruction. Appropriate acoustics, use of visuals, FM amplification, sign language, notetakers, communication partners, etc. increase access to instruction. Needs periodic hearing evaluation, rigorous amplification checks, and regular monitoring of access to instruction and classroom function (monitoring tools at www.hear2learn.com or www.SIFTERanderson.com).

Relationship of Hearing Loss to Listening and Learning Needs

UNILATERAL HEARING LOSS

Possible Impact on the Understanding of Language and Speech	Possible Social Impact	Potential Educational Accommodations and Services
Child can "hear" but can have difficulty understanding in certain situations, such as hearing faint or distant speech, especially if poor ear is aimed toward the person speaking. Will typically have difficulty localizing sounds and voices using hearing alone. The unilateral listener will have greater difficulty understanding speech when environment is noisy and/or reverberant, especially when normal ear towards the overhead projector or other competing sound source and poor hearing ear towards the teacher. Exhibits difficulty detecting or understanding soft speech from the side of the poor hearing ear, especially in a group discussion.	Child may be accused of selective hearing due to discrepancies in speech understanding in quiet versus noise. Social problems may arise as child experiences difficulty understanding in noisy cooperative learning, or recess situations. May misconstrue peer conversations and feel rejected or ridiculed. Child may be more fatigued in classroom due to greater effort needed to listen, if class is noisy or has poor acoustics. May appear inattentive, distractible or frustrated, with behavior or social problems sometimes evident.	Allow child to change seat locations to direct the normal hearing ear toward the primary speaker. Student is at 10 times the risk for educational difficulties as children with 2 normal hearing ears and 1/3 to 1/2 of students with unilateral hearing loss experience significant learning problems. Children often have difficulty learning sound/letter associations in typically noisy kindergarten and grade 1 settings. Educational and audiological monitoring is warranted. Teacher inservice is beneficial. Typically will benefit from a personal FM system with low gain/power or a sound-field FM system in the classroom, especially in the lower grades. Depending on the hearing loss, may benefit from a hearing aid in the impaired ear.

MID-FREQUENCY HEARING LOSS or REVERSE SLOPE HEARING LOSS

MID-FREQUENCY HEARING LOSS or REVERSE SLOPE

Possible Impact on the Understanding of Language and Speech	Possible Social Impact	Potential Educational Accommodations and Services
Child can "hear" whenever speech is present but will have difficulty understanding in certain situations. May have difficulty understanding faint or distant speech, such as a student with a quiet voice speaking from across the classroom. The "cookie bite" or reverse slope listener will have greater difficulty understanding speech when environment is noisy and/or reverberant, such as a typical classroom setting. A 25 – 40 dB degree of loss in the low to mid-frequency range may cause the child to miss approximately 30% of speech information, if unamplified; some consonant and vowel sounds may be heard inconsistently, especially when background noise is present. Speech production of these sounds may be affected.	Child may be accused of selective hearing or "hearing when he wants to" due to discrepancies in speech understanding in quiet versus noise. Social problems may arise as child experiences difficulty understanding in noisy cooperative learning situations, lunch or recess. May misconstrue peer conver-sations, believing that other children are talking about him or her. Child may be more fatigued in classroom setting due to greater effort needed to listen. May appear inattentive, distractible or frus-trated.	Personal hearing aids important but must be precisely fit to hearing loss. Child likely to benefit from a sound-field FM system, a personal FM system or assistive listening device in the classroom. Student is at risk for educational difficulties. Can experience some difficulty learning sound/letter associations in kindergarten and 1st grade classes. Depending upon degree and configuration of loss, child may experience delayed language development and articulation problems. Educational monitoring and teacher inservice warranted. Annual hearing evaluation to monitor for hearing loss progression is important.

Please Consider Indicated Items in the Child's Educational Program:

_____Teacher inservice and seating close to teacher _____Hearing monitoring at school every ____mos. _____Amplification monitoring

_____Contact your school district's audiologist _____Protect ears from noise to prevent more loss _____Educational support services/evaluation

_____Screening/evaluation of speech and language _____Note-taking, closed captioned films, visuals _____FM system trial period

_____Educational consultation/ program supervision by specialist(s) in hearing loss _____Regular contact with other children who are deaf or hard of hearing

_____Periodic educational monitoring such as October and April teacher/student completion of SIFTER, LIFE

NOTE: All children require full access to teacher instruction and educationally relevant peer communication to receive an appropriate education. Distance, noise in classroom and fragmentation caused by hearing loss prevent full access to spoken instruction. Appropriate acoustics, use of visuals, FM amplification, sign language, notetakers, communication partners, etc. increase access to instruction. Needs periodic hearing evaluation, rigorous amplification checks, and regular monitoring of access to instruction and classroom function (monitoring tools at www.hear2learn.com or www.SIFTERanderson.com).

Relationship of Hearing Loss to Listening and Learning Needs

HIGH FREQUENCY HEARING LOSS		
Possible Impact on the Understanding of Language and Speech	**Possible Social Impact**	**Potential Educational Accommodations and Services**
Child can "hear" but can miss important fragments of speech. Even a 25-40 dB loss in high frequency hearing may cause the child to miss 20%-30% of vital speech information if unamplified. Consonant sounds t, s, f, th, k, sh, ch likely heard inconsistently, especially in noise. May have difficulty understanding faint or distant speech, such as a student with a quiet voice speaking from across the classroom and will have much greater difficulty understanding speech when in low background noise and/or reverberation is present. Many of the critical sounds for understanding speech are high pitched, quiet sounds, making them difficult to perceive; the words: cat, cap, calf, cast could be perceived as "ca," word endings, possessives, plurals and unstressed brief words are difficult to perceive and understand. Speech production may be affected. Use of amplification often indicated to learn language at a typical rate and ease learning.	May be accused of selective hearing due to discrepancies in speech understanding in quiet versus noise. Social problems may arise as child experiences difficulty understanding in noisy cooperative learning situations, lunch or recess. May misinterpret peer conver-sations. Child may be fatigued in classroom due to greater listening effort. May appear inattentive, distractible or frustrated. Could affect self concept.	Student is at risk for educational difficulties. Depending upon onset, degree and configuration of loss, child may experience delayed language and syntax development and articulation problems. Possible difficulty learning some sound/letter associations in kindergarten and 1st grade classes. Early evaluation of speech and language skills is suggested. Educational monitoring and teacher inservice is warranted. Will typically benefit from personal hearing aids and use of a sound-field or a personal FM system in the classroom. Use of ear protection in noisy situations is imperative to prevent damage to inner ear structures and resulting progression of the hearing loss.

FLUCTUATING HEARING LOSS		
Possible Impact on the Understanding of Language and Speech	**Possible Social Impact**	**Potential Educational Accommodations and Services**
Of greatest concern are children who have experienced hearing fluctuations over many months in early childhood (multiple episodes with fluid lasting three months or longer). Listening with a hearing loss that is approximately 20 dB can be compared to hearing when index fingers are placed in ears. This loss or worse is typical of listening with fluid or infection behind the eardrums. Child can "hear" but misses fragments of what is said. Degree of difficulty experienced in school will depend upon the classroom noise level, the distance from the teacher and the current degree of hearing loss. At 30 dB can miss 25-40% of the speech signal; child with a 40 dB loss associated with "glue ear" may miss 50% of class discussions, especially when voices are faint or speaker is not in line of vision. Will frequently miss unstressed words, consonants and word endings.	Barriers begin to build with negative impact on self esteem as the child is accused of "hearing when he/she wants to," "daydreaming," or "not paying attention." Child may believe he/she is less capable due to understanding difficulties in class. Typically poor at identifying changes in own hearing ability. With inconsistent hearing, the child learns to "tune out" the speech signal. Children are judged to have greater attention problems, insecurity, distractibility and lack self esteem. Tend to be non-participative and distract themselves from classroom tasks; often socially immature.	Impact is primarily on acquisition of early reading skills and attention in class. Screening for language delays is suggested from a young age. Ongoing monitoring for hearing loss in school, communication between parent and teacher about listening difficulties and aggressive medical management is needed. Will benefit from sound-field FM or an assistive listening device in class. May need attention to development of speech, reading, self esteem, or listening skills. Teacher inservice is beneficial.

Please Consider Indicated Items in the Child's Educational Program:

_____Teacher inservice and seating close to teacher _____Hearing monitoring at school every ____mos. _____Amplification monitoring

_____Contact your school district's audiologist _____Protect ears from noise to prevent more loss _____Educational support services/evaluation

_____Screening/evaluation of speech and language _____Note-taking, closed captioned films, visuals _____FM system trial period

_____Educational consultation/ program supervision by specialist(s) in hearing loss _____Regular contact with other children who are deaf or hard of hearing

_____Periodic educational monitoring such as October and April teacher/student completion of SIFTER, LIFE

NOTE: All children require full access to teacher instruction and educationally relevant peer communication to receive an appropriate education. Distance, noise in classroom and fragmentation caused by hearing loss prevent full access to spoken instruction. Appropriate acoustics, use of visuals, FM amplification, sign language, notetakers, communication partners, etc. increase access to instruction. Needs periodic hearing evaluation, rigorous amplification checks, and regular monitoring of access to instruction and classroom function (monitoring tools at www.hear2learn.com or www.SIFTERanderson.com).

Source: Reprinted with permission from Karen L. Anderson, Audiology Consulting website: http://www.kandersonaudconsulting.com/

APPENDIX 39–B

Simulation of Hearing Loss Handout (Edwards, 2005)

Direct experience often produces optimum learning. Most teachers who are faced with the prospect of a child with hearing loss in their classroom for the first time, express concern about their ability to address the child's needs in their class. By giving the teacher some direct experience with hearing loss, you can provide them with

- an empathetic understanding of the communication demands on a child with hearing loss in the classroom;
- an understanding of the teaching strategies that are detrimental to communication in the classroom;
- an understanding of the teaching strategies that are beneficial to a child with hearing loss in the classroom.

Use of foam earplugs can simulate a mild conductive hearing loss of approximately 25 to 35 dB. The following points are important to emphasize to school staff.

- The simulation only creates a mild hearing loss, and so students with moderate, severe, or profound hearing loss will experience greater difficulty than that experienced with the earplugs.
- The simulation reflects what children with mild hearing loss might hear without a hearing aid, or what children with moderate or moderately severe hearing loss might hear with the hearing aid on.
- Use of the earplugs simulates a conductive rather than a sensorineural hearing loss, because the earplugs are simply impeding the passage of sound through the external ear. This is an important distinction, as the staff must realize that the distortion of speech sounds and the susceptibility to noise seen with children with sensorineural hearing loss cannot be simulated through the use of earplugs alone.
- The simulation produces an accurate perception of the hearing loss often seen with children with recurrent otitis media. Although many teachers might not have experiences with children with sensorineural hearing loss, all primary teachers will have a number of children in their classes each year with histories of recurrent otitis media. (Otitis media is the single most common reason for a child to visit the family physician, and the most common cause of hearing loss in children.)

Suggested Procedure

After explaining the purpose of the exercise, hand out a pair of foam earplugs to each group member. Ask the participants to hold the plugs by the rounded edge and roll them between their fingers to compress them to approximately 1/3 to 1/4 of their original size.

Then have everyone insert the compressed plugs into their ear canals so that the canals are completely occluded. If the participants do not hear a clear difference in the loudness of the sound after inserting the plugs, the plugs have not been inserted correctly. Have the individuals remove and reinsert the earplugs. Then ask the participants to get out a sheet of paper and pencil to write down what you say. There are a number of concepts that you want to demonstrate during the simulation.

- The farther away the speaker is from the listener, the more difficult the listening task.
- Restricting speechreading cues makes the listening task more difficult.
- Presence of background noise increases the difficulty of the listening task.
- The type of material presented will vary the difficulty of the task. Single words are much more difficult to identify than sentences, where contextual clues can provide a great deal of information.
- The intensity of vowels is greater than that of consonants, thus increasing the ease of vowel recognition.
- High frequency consonants such as /s/, /f/, /ch /, /k/, /t/, and the voiceless /th/ are usually the most difficult sounds to hear, particularly the /f/ and voiceless /th/, as they are the softest of all of the consonants.
- Listening under difficult conditions is fatiguing, resulting in a tendency to tune out or daydream.
- Listening can be very frustrating when speakers are far away, are covering their mouths, or when background noise is present. The listener can experience anger or frustration towards the speaker or towards the sources of background noise.
- Additional visual supplements such as writing on the blackboard or the overhead projector can be of great assistance in following the conversation, and reduce the strain of listening.

Ask participants to write numbers 1 to 15 on the side of the page. In order to demonstrate the aforementioned concepts, present words and sentences in the following way:

<table>
<tr><th colspan="2">Write the word . . .</th></tr>
<tr><td>1. please</td><td rowspan="5">By hearing alone (mouth covered); quiet conversational level; move around while you are talking</td></tr>
<tr><td>2. great</td></tr>
<tr><td>3. sled</td></tr>
<tr><td>4. pants</td></tr>
<tr><td>5. rat</td></tr>
<tr><th colspan="2">Write the word . . .</th></tr>
<tr><td>6. bad</td><td rowspan="5">By hearing alone (mouth covered); create background noise (papers rustling, keys jingling, book dropping on floor . . .); quiet conversational level; move around while you are talking</td></tr>
<tr><td>7. pinch</td></tr>
<tr><td>8. such</td></tr>
<tr><td>9. bus</td></tr>
<tr><td>10. need</td></tr>
</table>

Write the word . . .	
11. ways	By hearing and speechreading (mouth uncovered); quiet conversational level; background noise sporadic
12. five	
13. mouth	
14. rag	
15. put	

Now ask the participants to number their page from 1 to 10 and tell them that you will now say some sentences.

1. Walking is my favorite exercise.	by hearing alone (mouth covered); background noise sporadic
2. Here's a nice quiet place to rest.	
3. Somebody cleans the floors every night.	
4. It would be much easier if everyone would help.	
5. Open your window before you go to bed.	
6. Do you think that she should stay out so late?	by hearing and speechreading (mouth uncovered); background noise sporadic
7. How do you feel about beginning work at a different time every day?	
8. Move out of the way.	
9. The water is too cold for swimming.	
10. Why should I get up so early in the morning?	

- *It is important to use a quiet conversational voice level rather than a normal conversational level for maximum effect.*
- *Because sentences are considerably easier to identify than are single words, they are presented through hearing alone in noise, rather than in quiet.*
- *The background noise can be sporadic or continuous; the listeners will experience the frustration in either situation.*
- *When moving around, ensure that you rotate around the entire room so that everyone can experience both optimal and least desirable listening conditions.*

Then, have the participants take up their answers WITH THE EARPLUGS STILL INSERTED. When a person gives his or her answer, ensure that the rest of the group has heard it. If not, ask the person to change the way that he or she has presented the answer so that others will understand better (such as repeating the response, saying the word or sentence louder, facing the group, spelling the word, or adding an accompanying gesture). Write down the various answers on a board or overhead projector to provide a visual supplement. Underline the correct answer from all of the choices provided by the participants.

Once all of the words and sentences have been reviewed, HAVE THE GROUP TAKE OUT THE EAR-PLUGS. Initiate a group discussion of the following issues:

- their emotional reactions to the overall experience;
- the causes of specific frustrations experienced;
- insights about the experiences of children with hearing loss in the classroom;
- ways in which they could change their teaching strategies to address the needs of children with hearing loss.

The discussion deepens the experience of the simulation of hearing loss and allows participants themselves to determine the necessary changes in teaching strategies.

Source: Reprinted with permission from Edwards, C. (2005). From system selection to enhancement of listening skills: Considerations for the classroom. In C. Crandell, J. Smaldino, & C. Flexer (Eds.), *Sound field FM amplification: Applications to speech perception and classroom acoustics* (2nd ed.). New York, NY: Thomson Delmar Learning.

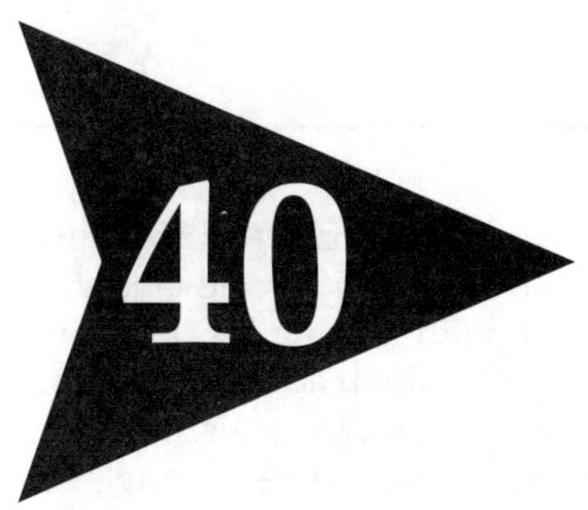

Providing Services in Educational Contexts: Defining the Role of the Educational Audiologist

Patricia M. Chute and Mary Ellen Nevins

Introduction

With an undeniable societal emphasis on early learning, it could be posited that an increasing number of pediatric clinical audiologists also take on the role as educational audiologists. For school districts that have limited numbers of these professionals or none at all, it behooves pediatric clinicians to expand their roles beyond the traditional ones of identifying hearing loss and fitting sensory devices. Auditory access is foundational for a child's learning about the world using the sense of hearing. Those audiologists who identify hearing loss and ameliorate its effects unlock the potential of auditory learning to make a substantive contribution to the child's development across domains. But, their contribution goes beyond the numbers on the audiogram or the percentage of speech recognition obtained with a hearing aid or cochlear implant. It requires an ongoing relationship with the professionals who will utilize those "numbers" to support the development of spoken language skills. More importantly, the relationship of listening to spoken language and spoken language to literacy is becoming clearer as more research is being conducted in this area. It has been suggested that successful reading is intimately connected with what one has learned from listening. Given this relationship, the pediatric audiologist is the "first responder" to the learning emergency that hearing loss poses. Actions taken by pediatric audiologists launch the literacy journey through early detection and subsequent fitting of listening technologies that provide optimal audibility. More than ever, it is clear that education does not begin with formal school enrollment but commences with input from families and caregivers to build spoken language and early literacy skills.

That said, audiologists who commit to providing specialized, school-based services, will need an additional knowledge base and an expert skill set that is subject, of course, to larger trends, reforms, initiatives, and policy changes to meet the needs of students in educational environments. Education in the United States has reached a pivotal time in which the evolution of technology has transformed the manner in which children learn and the way they demonstrate that learning in assessment tasks in our schools (Spangler, 2015). The national agenda to improve outcomes to make an American education more competitive with other countries has resulted in the adoption of a Common Core along with a stringent teacher evaluation system. This has fashioned a perfect storm that, in many cases, has created an environment that is at best conciliatory and at worst contentious. For the child with special needs, educators and support personnel feel caught in a tug of war between trying to teach while adhering to new mandates. For children who are deaf and hard of hearing, residual debate that pertains to modality of language acquisition persists. Yet, state-of-the-art listening technologies support the education of the large majority of children for learning through auditory-based instruction. This most often occurs in mainstream environments where other technologies and teaching paradigms have been incorporated in the daily lesson plan. Pedagogy now involves flipped classrooms in which "in-and out-of-school learning" is encouraged. At home, students have a first pass at learning through Web-based materials. In the classroom, they work on application of new content in engaging learning experiences facilitated by a teacher as opposed to listening to instruction. The use of tablets with downloadable applications creates exciting conditions to support learning with unlimited access to topics ranging from science to art. Interfacing listening technologies with learning technologies has become a primary responsibility of today's educational audiologist. Ensuring that the best technologies are in use is as important as the initial diagnosis and the initial fitting of hearing devices, which for many children now occurs in the first few weeks of life.

Changes that have also occurred in the political climate of the late 20th and early 21st centuries have set the stage for early identification and treatment of hearing loss for greater numbers of children. It is against this backdrop that educational considerations for children with any degree of hearing loss must be viewed with the expectation for improved outcomes that reflect contemporary and future possibilities. Today, it is by parental choice (or limited intervention services) that a child, whose sole challenge is hearing loss, uses manual communication through sign language or a sign system. Auditory access provided by any one of a number of sensory devices offers the potential for spoken language learning through the auditory channel. In most cases, the clinical pediatric audiologist serves as a portal through which children identified with hearing loss access the intervention system. This professional requires knowledge of the law, evidenced-based practices, and communication choices. The influence of the pediatric audiologist cannot be overstated as the need for positive exchanges with the child's parents at the time of identification is crucial for timely follow-up.

A clinical pediatric audiologist is the professional with the most knowledge regarding the level of hearing loss and the sensory device best suited to achieve communication goals set by the parents. As the degree of hearing loss increases, the complexity of the decision-making process for communication choice and educational opportunities increases commensurately. Offering cautious optimism for the potential of spoken language outcomes through utilization of available technologies gives hearing parents (who number more than 90% of parents of children with severe-to-profound hearing loss) a sense of hope at an extraordinarily difficult time. These parents become the primary advocates and standard bearers for the child with hearing loss and often require concentrated and expedient access to information and communication with professionals.

Unfortunately, there appears to be a correlation between socioeconomic status (SES) and communication opportunity; children from homes with a higher SES tend to have greater access to listening and spoken language educational options than do their less affluent peers (Geers & Brenner, 2003; Hoff & Tian, 2005; Hyde & Power, 2006; Kirkham, Baroody, Siddique, Nevins, & Suskind, 2009; Sorkin & Zwolan, 2008). This correlation of outcomes with income crosses all aspects of health care, not just those with hearing loss. Although there is increasing attention to the needs of families of children who are deaf or hard of hearing who are living in poverty (Voss & Lenihan, 2010) as well as promising interventions specifically for families of low socioeconomic status (Sachs et al., 2014), the issues facing children from lower incomes prevail. Auditory access and auditory-based intervention could be considered a basic right of every child with hearing loss for families who consider listening and spoken language a desired outcome. It is with technology and education provided by expert professionals that the effects of childhood hearing loss can be ameliorated and allow a child the opportunity to develop spoken communication skills. The pediatric audiologist is often the gatekeeper to this process.

Whether counseling parents of newly identified infants and toddlers or working with school-aged children, the pediatric audiologist is considered the foremost professional charged with assessing and monitoring the auditory abilities of a child with hearing loss. Professionals who further identify as *educational* audiologists also play an important role in the early hearing detection and intervention (EHDI) process. Macione and Johnson (2015) suggested that educational audiologists have a responsibility to support families through the development of the Individual Family Service Plan (IFSP) under IDEA Part C. Thus, it is critical for educational audiologists to be articulate about the communication opportunities and the educational placement options that are available to children who are deaf or hard of hearing from which parents can choose. Regrettably, the number of available educational audiologists in any one school district is far outnumbered by the number of children requiring services. This places a stress on the system that requires parents to be the lead advocates as advised by their clinical pediatric audiologist for their child in the school setting.

Educational Placement Options

Each placement option has certain features that might make it more or less attractive and suitable for any individual child. Population density and geographic locale can preclude the possibility that parents will have access to a continuum of options from which to select. Furthermore, family goals for the child who is deaf or hard of hearing, as well as whole-family priorities, create a filter that can constrain the field of appropriate options. Although not all placements fit neatly into one category, the following basic descriptions might provide a starting point from which to consider the child-program match that is best for any family. In some states, early intervention programming is managed by the Department of Education; when this is the case, consideration of "educational placement" begins soon after identification of hearing loss. In cases in which early identification is managed by the Department of Health or other agency, additional considerations regarding providers might be in effect (e.g., licensed provider locations or identification of certified individual providers). Regardless, it is unequivocal that locating appropriate service providers for family's choice of communication, amplification, and education options is among the highest priority tasks of the audiologist working with families of newly identified infants and toddlers. That said, there are a number of established and categorical educational options that have characteristics that can be identified and defined. The following discussion acknowledges the features of each of the named placement options. Keep in mind that it is not unlikely that a child will attend a number of different program types throughout an educational career as instructional needs change over time. It is important for all health professionals, from the pediatrician to the clinical pediatric audiologist or speech-language pathologist, to understand the different options and how they might impact learning.

General Education/Mainstream Placement

Most children who are deaf or hard of hearing will be educated in the general education environment, most often referred to as the *mainstream*. Degree of hearing loss seems to be the key aspect of the profile of the child in general educational settings. Simply stated, the lesser the degree of hearing loss, the more likely it is that a child will be placed in a general education program. As the degree of educationally significant hearing loss increases, so does the importance of the placement recommendation. Children with the cognitive, academic, and linguistic capacity to learn alongside their typically developing peers can attend school in their local neighborhoods. In its truest sense, mainstream education works best for children with sufficient skills to learn in this environment through the instruction of a classroom teacher. In-class accommodations, such as frequency modulation or digital modulation (FM/DM) systems, Communication Access Real-time Translation (CART), or other commercially available voice-to-text technologies might be required to assure access. However, once access is provided, children in the mainstream are expected to "keep pace" with their peers. Supported as needed by a team of professionals that can include an educational audiologist, a speech-language pathologist, and oftentimes a teacher of children who are deaf or hard of hearing, mainstreamed children are academically and socially integrated in a public or private general education school. (If a child presents with additional learning needs, services might be required of an occupational therapist, a physical therapist, a reading specialist, and/or school psychologist.) In many circumstances, children in the mainstream are "singletons" and might represent the first child with educationally significant hearing loss enrolled in a particular school program.

General Education/Inclusion

The term *inclusion* is often used synonymously with mainstream education; however, here it represents a different classroom configuration and a different staffing model from that of the mainstream. For the most part, children in included classrooms have good linguistic and academic potential, but benefit from instruction that is co-delivered by a general education teacher and a certified teacher of children who are deaf or hard of hearing. Oftentimes, inclusion is manifested by a small group of children with hearing loss clustered within a general education classroom (that is, reduced in class size to provide accommodations for instructional needs of the children who are deaf or hard of hearing). The unique staffing of two teachers in a single classroom affords children with hearing loss the best of both worlds—grade-level academic content with the instructional vigilance of a certified teacher of children who are deaf or hard of hearing. When well executed, inclusion models create instructional teams that have equal status in the classroom, while at the same time assigning equal status to all students regardless of hearing acuity. There are a number of co-teaching models that have been used successfully in inclusion classrooms but require administrative support, and teams that are well suited for collaboration are essential. Often, this model can be found in densely populated, urban areas where there is a critical mass of children with hearing loss such that this is one option on the continuum of service delivery models. Alarmingly, the term *inclusion* is often overextended and is used when a child with hearing loss is placed, regardless of educational ability, in a class of typically developing children.

Regional Cooperatives/Urban Programs

Metropolitan areas with a large number of children with hearing loss can often support a "program" for children that has many classrooms, different communication tracks, and instruction across the age span. Similarly, suburban counties or intermediate unit/districts form cooperatives to pool resources to serve children with all special needs, including hearing loss. Small instruction or self-contained classrooms might be more numerous at the younger ages as children with hearing loss receive the language foundation that can allow them to move on to other instructional environments with their typically developing peers. Regardless, regional/urban programs provide, at the very least, opportunities for social mainstreaming. Although content instruction takes place in classrooms with other students with hearing loss, activities such as physical education, art, and music, as well as lunch and recess are scheduled so that all participate. Partial academic mainstreaming might be offered, subject by subject, as a student's individual achievement warrants. It generally is the case that programs within this designation have the critical mass (and the administrative vision) to provide a full continuum of placement options.

Private (OPTION) Schools for Children With Hearing Loss

There is a long-standing history of private schools as a placement choice for students with hearing loss that offer listening and spoken language instruction (previously referred to as auditory/oral). Ever-increasing auditory access has created demand for more of this instructional emphasis, and in a number of major cities, private school programs meet this need. Often considered model programs, many OPTION schools (http://www.optionschools.org) specialize in the infant to preschool-aged child and often employ "reverse mainstreaming" in which typically developing hearing children are invited to enroll and participate in classrooms with a small teacher-to-student ratio and language-rich instruction. An increasing number of OPTION schools have added after-school speech and language therapy for primary- and elementary-aged students as well as teletherapy for early intervention to the comprehensive services that they offer.

State Schools for Deaf Children

Although not every state in the United States has a school designated as a state school for the deaf (and a few have more than one state school), these campuses and the staff and community that surround them have become centers for the majority of individuals who identify with Deaf Culture. These schools' long-standing presence in the state education systems has made them a natural place to turn for the management of early intervention in many states. However, strong ties to the community of Deaf individuals might make it difficult for professionals there to offer parents a world view that reflects a hearing culture. Respect for and a desire to provide auditory access through hearing aids and cochlear implants might not be a priority at some state schools. However, at other state schools, sweeping legal and technological changes in the last 30+ years have created the dissonance that has resulted in a more egalitarian approach to the audiologic management of hearing loss in young children of both deaf and hearing parents.

Regardless of the educational setting, educational audiologists become key members of interprofessional teams that will effectively monitor a child's auditory needs throughout the child's school career. Using an age-based organizational template, three major roles of the educational audiologist will now be considered—that of assessor/evaluator, habilitation oversight manager, and advocate. The relative weight of each of these components will change over time as the child moves through early intervention and the educational system. Embedded within these discussions is an acknowledgement of the pervasive skills of the educational audiologist in counseling, in communicating, and in collaborating.

Early Intervention

For children to reach their fullest potential, early detection and intervention are key. In the United States, the Individuals with Disabilities Education Act (IDEA), stipulates that parents be informed and offered choices about communication methods, and that they have a voice as full members of the team that writes the Individualized Family Service Plan (IFSP). Part C of IDEA governs all early intervention services for infants and toddlers with disabilities under 3 years of age. It is an unfortunate reality that the path of a deaf or hard-of-hearing child's entry into the Part C, birth to 3 years, educational system, is often controlled by the least specialized and underprepared professional in the chain of referral—the service coordinator. This individual might come from a field such as psychology, social work, or nursing and might not have any formal education concerning children who are deaf or hard of hearing. In fact, in the recent Supplement to the JCIH 2007 Position Statement: Principles and Guidelines for Early Intervention after Confirmation that a Child is Deaf or Hard of Hearing (AMA, 2013), the Joint Committee on Infant Hearing asserted:

> Unfortunately, most EI systems currently provide limited access to professionals with expertise in listening and spoken language and do not collect system-wide outcome data on children's development of listening and spoken language skills. Such data are essential to ensure that families and children have received high-quality intervention with targeted outcomes. Many EI systems do not offer professional development opportunities to ensure continuous improvement for the EI providers, nor do they offer consultation/mentorship and/or direct observation to guarantee fidelity of the intervention implementation. These are critical areas of need if best practices in listening and spoken language are to be established. In order to assist the service coordinator, the pediatric audiologist should be knowledgeable of the vast store of information that exists for early hearing detection and intervention services. . . . Since the pediatric audiologist is the lead professional that parents encounter when the hearing loss is confirmed, it is critical for this professional to have knowledge of the resources available to assist parents in making subsequent decisions. (p. 1331)

If parents are relying on audiologic input to make decisions about listening devices and communication choices (i.e., should a cochlear implant be considered? should the hearing aid be changed? should sign language be introduced?), then hearing data cannot exist in a vacuum that only measures performance under carefully controlled conditions. It is vital that the clinical pediatric clinical audiologist collaborate with other key professionals (including the school-based educational audiologist if one is available) to provide the context in which services are linked to the parents' desired outcome for their child. Collaboration encompasses communication, coordination, and cooperation and is more than any one of these entities.

Communication is not synonymous with report dissemination. This relegates communication to a product-oriented outcome. True communication requires interaction between and among the parties of interest. When parents become the messengers and are asked to assume the responsibility for distributing reports among agencies, the result is often a disjointed collection of information with no substantive integration. For communication to be truly effective, there must be coordination that facilitates the communicative *exchange* that takes place in response to agency reports.

Coordinating appointments and activities and collating results is a role that is assigned to the various health and education professionals providing services to the family of the child who is deaf or hard of hearing. Although every professional has an individual role, coordination requires that *one* individual accepts the responsibility of managing the information that is being generated across disciplines. The coordination of this effort requires cooperation among professionals to ensure that all relevant data are considered, thus encouraging the best possible outcome for the child and family. The nature of a collaborative relationship is dependent on a cooperative spirit among professionals. It must be respectful and have as its goal a genuine concern for the child without bias or prejudice for one particular outcome; it allows for individual expertise to be considered fully within the context of mutual esteem. Thus, communication, coordination, and cooperation represent the foundation of a true collaborative effort. When previous experiences with collaboration have been positive, it is more likely that there will be expectations for a positive outcome; unfortunately, the reverse is often true. Negative experiences with collaborative groups might color the outcomes of future efforts. Furthermore, if collaboration is imposed by administration and not viewed as a best practice approach to service delivery, the quality of the interactions can be compromised. In order to be a productive member of a collaborative group, one must project a sincere belief in the value of the professional expertise of the other members of the group. There should be no sense of competition among service providers; the needs of the child transcend each individual's area of expertise. It is the collective construction of a comprehensive plan to meet the family's needs that becomes the desired outcome of this effort. Clear and unambiguous conversations about the implications of hearing loss and its effect on the development of communication is imperative to this process that starts at the pediatric audiologist's point of intersection with other professionals: the initial evaluation.

Assessment

Clinical pediatric audiologists evaluate children for many purposes: initial diagnosis, sensory device fitting, or monitoring progress with auditory skill development. The initial identification of hearing loss may occur as a result of the referral process of universal newborn hearing screening, physician recommendation, or parental concern. The diagnosis is often a culmination of data gathered over multiple visits. A comprehensive battery of tests provides a cohesive picture of the status of the auditory system. It is at this point that the pediatric audiologist as counselor is most critical. As parents learn the news of their child's hearing loss, there is often a tendency for them to pass through the various stages of grief that have been documented in the psychological literature. These stages take into account denial, anger, bargaining, depression, and acceptance (Kubler-Ross, 1969). Professionals must respect parents' actions during this challenging time. Although there is an urgency to begin habilitation through the dispensing of a sensory aid, some parents might disengage from the process as a mechanism for coping and appear to be nonadherent.

For clinical pediatric audiologists, there is a need to offer both information and support at this juncture. All audiologists (regardless of the population they service) are trained to provide informational counseling concerning the degree, type, and severity of hearing loss along with the sensory aid recommendation for ameliorating the loss. However, parents are often in the early stages of grief when a large amount of this information is being imparted. For this reason, a great deal of the subject matter is poorly received and often misunderstood. Research indicates that patients forget 40% to 80% of the information provided at any medical appointment (Kessels, 2003). Half of the information that is remembered is incorrect. Furthermore, pediatric audiologists who address only the informational aspects of hearing loss and not the emotional effects of that information can thwart the development of the important relationship necessary to assist families in moving past the initial stage of grief. As families enter subsequent stages, they might "shop around" to identify another professional who will provide a diagnosis they find more acceptable or one who will be more sensitive to their needs. Seeking second and third opinions often causes delays in the ultimate fitting of amplification and in accessing early intervention services. Professionals walk a fine line in providing necessary support as families adjust to the diagnosis, yet encouraging intervention in a timely manner. Families who have been given the news that they have a child with a disability must first learn to make room in their life for the disability but not make the disability their life. This concept is not one that can be grasped in a single session, and as assessment progresses it requires continual attention.

The assessment process that begins in early intervention persists throughout childhood to monitor changes that might occur in functional auditory capacity. The introduction of new technologies might be required to remediate hearing loss that changes over time. Assessment should be viewed as an activity that is dynamic and is constructed to ensure the best outcome for the child. Families who embrace this concept will contribute to their child's progress; those who withdraw will increase the likelihood that additional roadblocks might impede positive growth. Assessment is seen as a shared responsibility of the managing pediatric audiologist, the family, and the early intervention system. Once habilitation is initiated, the early intervention period creates a productive intermingling of evaluation, response, and reevaluation and may be the point of entry of the traditional school-based, educational audiologist (Macione & Johnson, 2015) as part of the collaborative team.

Habilitation

If assessment answers the question, "What is the level of hearing loss?" then habilitation must answer the question, "How can the hearing loss be treated in the most effective manner?" The habilitation process begins with the selection of the proper sensory device or devices (see Chapters 25 through 32) coupled with appropriate intervention. Monitoring performance with hearing aids or cochlear implants is necessary to ensure development of age-appropriate auditory, speech, and language skills. It is incumbent on the clinical pediatric audiologist and educational audiologist to stay current with technology that can affect the outcomes of the early intervention plan.

A primary factor in determining the appropriateness of a prescribed sensory aid is to benchmark a child's performance against other children with hearing loss of the same magnitude. A pediatric audiologist cannot merely check the sensory device for proper function but must evaluate it relative to the child's outcomes in the areas of spoken language, auditory perception, and educational progress. The view from the sound-treated audiometric test suite should not be simply one of measuring functional gain or even word recognition scores; an all-encompassing measurement of child performance in light of the age at identification, duration of sensory aid use, and communication development is also required. To make a truly informed decision about the successful use of the selected sensory device, mode of communication, or educational environment, pediatric audiologists should gather information from a variety of sources to consider the role audition is playing in the child's overall development. Anything less would be ineffective.

It is never more critical to be part of an interprofessional collaborative team than in evaluating the effectiveness of the sensory device and the habilitation plan during the EI period. There has been a long-standing association between pediatric audiologists and speech-language pathologists. Communication with teachers of children who are deaf or hard of hearing is customary, but the early intervention system has created an even wider circle of professional colleagues with whom pediatric audiologists must interact. With a mandate for considering all the child's needs during the period of greatest development, pediatric audiologists are challenged to make the implications of hearing loss clear to nonspeech and hearing professionals as they deliver services within their scope of practice.

Thus, the role of the pediatric audiologist does not begin and end with the fitting of a sensory device. The overall benefits of amplification and its contribution to the development of spoken language skills must be monitored. In addition, this professional should, in fact, provide oversight of the use of amplification, the amount and type of services that a child receives, and the venue in which these services are available. The hallmark of the early intervention period is the provision of family centered services in the natural environment. To date, this generally has been interpreted as home-based interventions in which parents are counseled and guided in learning to facilitate their child's language development.

Advocacy

Advocacy can take many forms. It can include negotiating for services, ensuring device function, or educating others about the implications of hearing loss in daily living. Some components of advocacy are legal and others are personal. Those that are legal require families to be knowledgeable about rights and privileges within their local education communities. As most families have no legal background or knowledge of special education law, becoming an advocate might seem overwhelming. This task is compounded by the fact that they might still be struggling with the identification of hearing loss. There are multiple resources that families can access both locally and nationally to assist them in the process. One advocacy organization that can provide good assistance is Hands and Voices, a national, nonprofit parent-driven group (http://www.handsandvoices.org). As its name implies, all families of children with hearing loss, as well as concerned professionals, are welcome as members in this group. Their local, state, and national activities, as well as publications, are especially valuable to families in the area of legal advocacy. Personal advocacy issues focus on the day-to-day usage of the sensory device in conjunction with the development of an identity as an individual with hearing loss. Self-awareness of auditory access should be targeted as an early intervention goal. Even young children can learn personal advocacy skills by informing interventionists when there are problems with their sensory aids. By developing responsibility at a young age, the early intervention professional is supporting the acquisition of the more complex advocacy skills that will be required in the future.

Pediatric audiologists might assume the role of chief advocate for the child and family during the birth-to-3-years period. For computer savvy and Internet-secure families, the Internet can provide a wealth of information and resources to assist in the development of advocacy skills (see, for example, The Parent Advocacy Training course, http://www.listeningandspokenlanguage.org/PAT/). For families with less computer access or those who live in remote areas, learning about hearing loss and its implications for education might require more time. Modeling the types of questions that should be addressed during the Individual Family Service Plan (IFSP) process can be one method of assisting parents in the development of advocacy skills. Part of the pediatric audiologist's role is to transition the parent to become the key individual advocating for the child during the period of early intervention. Regardless of who performs advocacy activities during the early intervention period, plans should be considered for transferring this role to the child over time.

Preschool- and School-Aged Children

Although hearing loss is identified early for many children, there remain a number of youngsters for whom identification is delayed until academic pressures raise questions about hearing acuity. In addition, there are other children who are born with normal hearing that later diminishes over time. Regardless of when diagnosis occurs, audiologic management within the educational system is required to ensure that a child has every advantage to access curriculum. As indicated earlier, pediatric audiologists who work solely within a school district are known as educational audiologists. Educational audiologists are certified and licensed individuals who identify their primary place of employment as a local school or educational agency. The Educational Audiology Association (EAA) is an international organization of pediatric audiologists and related professionals who deliver hearing services to children in educational settings. Often working in conjunction with clinical pediatric audiologists, educational audiologists are specialists in the fitting of assistive devices that augment personal listening technologies in the learning environment. The EAA website (http://www.edaud.org) has numerous publications and position statements to assist professionals working in schools.

Emphasis on audiologic services for children with confirmed hearing loss does not negate the need for additional programs that focus on identification of auditory processing problems and the promotion of hearing conservation education. The responsibilities of an educational audiologist also can be captured in assessment, (re)habilitation, and advocacy.

Assessment

Most often, the primary role of the educational audiologist is to monitor those children within the school district who have already been identified with hearing loss so that changes in performance are documented over time. It is important that the school-based educational audiologist remain in constant communication with the clinical pediatric audiologist to ensure appropriate sensory device function. In addition to this role, educational audiologists will screen typically developing children based on local mandates or referrals by teachers. Children with normal hearing acuity but poor auditory perception might be screened for auditory processing disorders by the educational audiologist to determine whether additional referral or technology is required.

In addition to assessing individual children, it is the responsibility of educational audiologists to assess the acoustic environment of learning spaces within the school. Evaluation of classroom ambient noise and reverberation and identification of strategies to reduce noise are within the purview of this professional. Measuring the functionality of any sensory device and personal or classroom FM/DM system should also be part of educational audiologists' scope of practice. (For more detailed information on Classroom Acoustics and FM/DM systems, see Chapter 27 in this volume.) Educational audiologists can assess a child's listening capabilities within any learning space through a number of questionnaires as rated by the classroom teacher or other professionals. These instruments include the Functional Listening Evaluation (FLE; Johnson & VonAlmen, 1997), Screening Identification for Targeting Educational Risk (SIFTER; Anderson, 2004), Listening Inventories for Education (LIFE; Anderson & Smaldino, 1999), Early Listening Function (ELF; Anderson, 2002), and Children's Home Inventory for Listening Difficulty (CHILD; Anderson & Smaldino, 2000).

(Re)habilitation

Stated job responsibilities or personal preference can determine whether or not the educational audiologist takes an active role in providing (re)habilitation services to children with hearing loss. This is well within recognized scope of practice but often is dependent on the needs of an individual school district. The educational audiologist's primary (re)habilitative responsibility is to participate in a collaborative team to ensure that the child is receiving the most appropriate services.

Educational audiologists collaborate with clinical pediatric audiologists, classroom teachers, teachers of children who are deaf or hard of hearing, and speech-language pathologists in a partnership to emphasize the interrelationships of hearing acuity, auditory skill development, spoken language acquisition, and academic success. Within this collaborative team, educational audiologists communicate the potential and limitations of a child's sensory device while the teacher and speech-language pathologist share information regarding the child's language and academic development. The complex relationship between listening and language is explored through the dialogue that occurs during these professional exchanges (Garber & Nevins, 2012). As audiology is the platform on which subsequent skills are developed, no discussion of a child's performance can take place without an audiologist to contextualize it as a function of access to sound. When access is the issue, pediatric audiologists assume responsibility to explore the appropriate options so that learning can commence. When access issues have been ruled out, attention should be placed on provision of services. Specifically, professionals providing services and the quality of those services should be examined. Finally, once access and service provision have been verified, the team can turn its attention to the possibility that learning challenges are limiting performance.

Even when children in the mainstream are operating at their "personal best" in listening, spoken language, and academics, there continue to be linguistic issues that might not be obvious to a general education teacher. The acquisition of Tier Two vocabulary (Beck, McKeown, & Kucan, 2002), which is a challenge that many children face, is even more pronounced in children with hearing loss, as acoustic access is not precise. With deficits in vocabulary, reading comprehension at increasingly more complex levels is at risk. Educational audiologists should be knowledgeable about the potential hurdles that obstruct a child's continued success by raising awareness of vocabulary development issues with the classroom teacher. Similarly, difficulty in understanding colloquial or figurative language can preclude a child from being able to understand narratives written with a rich use of idiomatic language. These "linguistic hazards" (Nevins, 2009) are not only associated with children who have hearing loss and might be equally problematic for the child with auditory processing problems.

Children with learning issues related to auditory processing require the attention of educational audiologists to make available and monitor technology that enhances signal reception. It is not enough to simply provide technology; educational audiologists must educate school personnel in its proper use and maintenance. Finally, educational audiologists are also responsible for hearing conservation education. With the growing number of young children using MP3 players, there is increasing concern regarding the potential for noise-induced hearing loss at earlier ages (Vogel, Brug, Hosli, van der Ploeq, & Raat, 2008).

Advocacy

During the school-aged period, the child requiring audiologic services should begin to assume the responsibilities for self-advocacy. Clearly, younger children can be limited in this task by their cognitive and linguistic abilities. It should not be presumed, however, that children are unable to communicate their auditory needs and wants. As they grow physically, linguistically, and emotionally, children might be ready to assume more responsibility for management of both their sensory aids and acoustic environment. It is likely that these skills will not develop without coaching. Conscious and intentional facilitation of the development of self-advocacy should be a part of children's Individualized Educational Programs (IEPs).

A self-advocacy curriculum often includes components of identity, self-image, technology, legal rights, and community resources for children who are deaf or hard of hearing. These should be guided by professionals with expertise in each of these areas and engage parents and children in the process. Discussions regarding identity and self-image might emphasize how hearing loss affects relationships. Strategies that teach children how to negotiate communication outside the academic setting likely will assist them into their teenage years. Comprehensive resources that might drive curriculum development in this area include *Educational Advocacy* (Johnson, DesGeorge, & Seaver, 2013) and *Building Skills for Success in the Fast-Paced Classroom* (Anderson & Arnoldi, 2011). In addition, the website Supporting Success for Children with Hearing Loss (http://successforkidswithhearingloss.com) provides resources that can be shared with parents and children of all ages for those who wish to explore the learning and social issues of children with hearing loss.

Adolescents and Young Adults

Generally speaking, the child who enters high school will often emerge as a very different young adult. Each child's journey is individual and will be influenced by personality, learning style, talent, and motivation. Fitting in with peers is sometimes a function of the use of colloquial expressions, slang, and, in some cases, even sarcasm. Children who are deaf or hard of hearing might have more challenges in this area as the subtleties of the language get lost. The use of technologies that provide the child with auditory access might be the very reason that the child feels disconnected. Strategic counseling by educational audiologists can help the child to accept the trade-off between auditory access and peer pressure to conform.

Assessment

Adolescents often will bring years of sensory device use and therapy experience with them to the high school. The role of educational audiologists is to ensure that technology is the most advanced and appropriate for the student. In addition, educational audiologists should guide the selection of other electronics that interface with listening devices to ensure proper use. Like the majority of their peers, teens with hearing loss wish to utilize smartphones that are Internet accessible and also act as a source of entertainment. Educational audiologists can guide students to the best technology that will yield the greatest advantage given the constraints of any particular hearing loss.

The various assistive technologies that are available for independent living should be reviewed at this juncture. As teenagers begin to consider life outside the cocoon of the home environment, it is important for them to be able to respond to the myriad sounds that are used for signaling or alerting. Exploring the wide range of devices that are available to support independence is an important part of the role of educational audiologists in the high school years.

(Re)habilitation

It is not unexpected that during the adolescent years, students will reject previously prescribed technology that sets them apart from their age-mates. Research indicates that the largest number of nonusers of hearing aids, cochlear implants, and FM systems is in the adolescent population (Tyler et al., 1997). To circumvent limited use, a good relationship with an educational audiologist, clinical pediatric audiologist, and other educational team members is necessary. Contrasting performance outcomes with and without sensory aids is often a mechanism for demonstrating benefit for this age group. In addition, the use of "contracts" to shape behavior has been successfully implemented by professionals who work with the adolescent population.

Traditional one-on-one therapy paradigms should not be the only service offered to this age group. Self-study that is accessible at any hour of the day might better fit adolescents' learning and lifestyle. With more information available through the Internet, students with hearing loss can now access listening exercises that are online and always available. Many sites designed for English as Second Language (ESL) users provide excellent resources that can be accessed for guided practice at home. Music videos can also serve as therapy material that engages the adolescent in a manner that can enhance listening and speaking. Pragmatics and functional communication in group settings with peers can be emphasized at this age rather than specific listening targets or speech production.

Functional communication takes place in listening environments that are often degraded by competing noise. For the student with hearing loss, strategies to reduce the effects of background noise rely heavily on speech reading. The use of Continuous Discourse Tracking (CDT; DeFilipo & Scott, 1978) encourages the development of speech-reading skills and diminishes the deleterious effects of communicating in less than optimal listening conditions.

(Re)habilitation strategies for the adolescent include functional practice and continued counseling. A broader view of the lifelong implications of hearing loss and acceptance of the strengths and limitations that it brings to the student is required. This creates a seamless transition from rehabilitation to self-awareness and self-advocacy.

Advocacy

The current information-driven society has made advocacy more important than ever. New technology has made communication easier; new technology has made it more difficult. The adolescent or young adult who is deaf or hard of hearing can now exchange information more easily with the advent of text messaging on a local or global scale. Texting has removed the isolation of the individual with hearing loss but has simultaneously placed communication skills on display to a larger audience. Social networking through sites such as Facebook, Twitter, and Snapchat provide opportunities for individuals to exchange information in a forum that is not face-to-face. However, such forums can create a false sense of communicative competence. In the virtual world, communication is only limited by the ability to create comprehensible text messages. In the nonvirtual world, communication challenges are real and include background noise, insufficient lighting, and poor acoustics. Once individuals with hearing loss step into the real world, they must advocate for support systems to allow equal access. These systems might include closed-captioning, infrared technology in theaters, and accommodations in travel and public buildings. At no time is this more important than for the student who is deaf or hard of hearing than when entering college.

The technology of the cochlear implant has enabled children to attend regular district schools and progress through the educational system to enter colleges alongside their hearing age-mates. In the past, most students with severe-to-profound hearing loss attended colleges specifically designed for deaf students. Services were provided without question; there was no need for the student to practice advocacy skills. Today, public and private institutions of higher education are now among the choices available to students with hearing loss with sufficient skills to compete for admission. It is imperative that students know their legal rights and the systems that must be in place to accommodate their needs. Once in college, student success will be dependent on a variety of factors—one of which is student engagement.

Data from the U.S. National Survey of Student Engagement indicate that students who are engaged in curricular and extracurricular activities are more likely to be successful and graduate within 4 years of entering college (Wasley, 2006). When a student is fully integrated both in and out of class, there is a greater need for self-advocacy skills that transcend the academic environment. Some students find the advocacy role more challenging due to limited opportunities in their youth. Parents who diligently assumed the role of advocate without training their children for a future as independent students were unwittingly shortsighted. Although the "helicopter parent" is a familiar sociological phenomenon for many millennial children, the overall effect often is counterproductive for students who are striving for independence. An autonomous student is one who presents with the typical skills of registering for classes, paying bills, and managing a class schedule. In addition, the student who is deaf or hard of hearing must secure services that will support learning. Educational audiologists and clinical audiologists can be part of the transition team that provides information to the student and parent to help prepare for postsecondary culture.

Similarly, students who enter directly into the workforce should ensure that the work environment is conducive to communicative success. As transition plans are developed within the educational setting, consideration of the acoustics of the workplace and the assistive technology that can aid the individual in the proper performance of work responsibilities might be offered by educational audiologists. Whether in the workplace or the college setting, the greatest obstacle to success occurs when the individual fails to self-identify. Recognizing hearing loss as part of the fabric that makes each individual unique removes its stigma and strengthens the personal adjustment that opens the door to lifelong success.

Summary

Never has it been a more exciting time to be an educational audiologist than today. The quantity and quality of technologies available to school-based audiologists make their role as advocate and educational liaison increasingly relevant in support of a child's learning. More so than any other professional who touches a child, the educational audiologist has a vantage point that allows a holistic view of development and learning. From assessment to advocacy, educational audiologists have influence over the educational lifetime of children who are deaf or hard of hearing and play a dynamic role in ameliorating the effects of hearing loss, be it unilateral, minimal, or profound. Their continued presence and commitment to the field elevates the potential outcomes for the children with whom they work. Tomorrow's promise of medical and technological advances for children with hearing loss coupled with the blurring of the societal view of differences between and among its citizens creates an unprecedented potential for educational parity for all. Knowledgeable professionals with the skills and dispositions to support access, both auditory and educational, are an important part of any child's journey to productive citizenship. Those who choose educational audiology are poised to make an incalculable contribution to this end.

References

American Academy of Pediatrics, Joint Committee on Infant Hearing. (2013). Supplement to the JCIH 2007 position statement: Principles and guidelines for early intervention after confirmation that a child is deaf or hard of hearing. *Pediatrics*, *131*(4), 1324–1349.

Anderson, K. (2002). Early Listening Function (ELF). Parent involvement: The magic ingredient in successful child outcomes: Improving parent participation using the ELF and the CHILD. *Hearing Review*, *9*(11), 24–27, 56.

Anderson, K. (2004). *Secondary Screening Instrument for Targeting Educational Risk (SIFTER).* Retrieved November 24, 2009, from http://www.hear2learn.com

Anderson, K. L., & Arnoldi, K. A. (2011). *Building skills for success in the fast-paced classroom Optimizing achievement for students with hearing loss*. Hillsboro, OR: Butte.

Anderson, K., & Smaldino, J. (1999) Listening inventories for education: A classroom measurement tool. *Hearing Journal*, *52*(10), 74–76.

Anderson, K., & Smaldino, J. (2000). Children's Home Inventory of Listening Difficulties (CHILD). *Educational Audiology Review*, *17*, 3.

Beck, I. L., McKeown, M. G., & Kucan, L. (2002). *Bringing words to life.* New York, NY: Guilford Press.

DeFilipo, C., & Scott, B. (1978). A method for training and evaluating the reception on ongoing speech. *Journal of the Acoustical Society of America*, *63*, 1186–1192.

Educational Audiology Association. (2009). *Recommended professional practices for educational audiology.* Retrieved April 22, 2015, from http://c.ymcdn.com/sites/www.edaud

.org/resource/resmgr/imported/Professional%20Practices_pos09_REVISED.pdf

Garber, A. S., & Nevins, M. E. (2012). Child-centered collaborative conversations that maximize listening and spoken language development for children with hearing loss. *Seminars in Speech and Language*, *33*, 264–272.

Geers, A., & Brenner, C. (2003). Background and educational characteristics of prelingually deaf children implanted by five years of age. *Ear and Hearing*, *24*(1 Suppl.), 2S–14S.

Hoff, E., & Tian, C. (2005). Socioeconomic status and cultural influences on language. *Journal of Communication Disorders*, *38*(4), 271–278.

Hyde, M., & Power, D. (2006). Some ethical dimensions of cochlear implantation for deaf children and their families. *Journal of Deaf Studies and Deaf Education*, *11*(1), 102–111.

Johnson, C. D., DesGeorges, J., & Seaver, L. (2013). *Educational advocacy for students who are deaf or hard of hearing: The hands and voices guidebook.* Boulder, CO: Hands & Voices.

Johnson, C. D., & Von Almen, P. (1997). The Functional Listening Evaluation. In C. D. Johnson, P. V. Benson, & J. B. Seaton (Eds.), *Educational audiology handbook* (pp. 336–339). San Diego, CA: Singular.

Kessels, R. (2003). Patient's memory for medical information. *Journal of the Royal Society of Medicine*, *96*(5), 219–222.

Kirkham, E. S. C., Baroody, F., Siddique, J., Nevins, M. E., & Suskind, D. (2009). Health disparities in pediatric cochlear implantation: An audiologic perspective. *Ear and Hearing*, *5*, 515–525.

Kubler-Ross, E. (1969). *On death and dying*. New York, NY: MacMillan.

Macione, M., & Johnson, C. D. (2015). The role of educational audiologists in the EHDI process. In L. Schmeltz (Ed.). *The EHDI eBook.* Retrieved from http://www.infanthearing.org/ehdi-ebook/2015_ebook/1a-CoverPgAcknowledgeTOC2015.pdf

Nevins, M. E. (2009). *Skating on thin academic ice: Idiosyncratic gaps that threaten even our most successful children in the mainstream.* 21st Annual Mainstream Conference, Clarke School for the Deaf, Northampton, MA, Parent Advocacy Training course. Retrieved from http://www.listeningandspokenlanguage.org/PAT/

Sachs, C., Shay, S., Repplinger, L., Leffel, K., Sapolich, S., Suskind, E., . . . Suskind, D. (2014). Pilot testing of a parent-directed intervention (Project ASPIRE) for underserved children who are deaf or hard of hearing. *Child Language, Teaching and Therapy*, *30*(1), 91–102.

Sorkin, D. L., & Zwolan, T. A. (2008). Parental perspectives regarding early intervention and its role in cochlear implantation in children. *Otology and Neurotology*, *29*(2), 137–141.

Spangler, C. (2015). *Positive "disruptions" for a new school year: Accessing educational technology to maximize auditory access and learning for all.* Retrieved April 22, 2015, from http://www.listeningandspokenlanguage.org/EdTechAccess/

Tyler, R. S., Fryauf-Bertschy, H., Kelsay, D. M., Gantz, B. J., Woodworth, G. P., & Parkinson, A. (1997). Speech perception by prelingually deaf children using cochlear implants. *Archives of Otolaryngology-Head and Neck Surgery*, *117*(3 Pt. 1), 180–187.

Vogel, I., Burg, J., Hosli, E. J., van der Ploeq, C. P., & Raat, H. (2008). MP3 players and hearing loss: Adolescents' perceptions of loud music and hearing conservation. *Journal of Pediatrics*, *152*(3), 400–404.

Voss, J., & Lenihan, S. (2010). Improving outcomes for children living in poverty. *Volta Voices*, *18*(1), 16–19.

Wasley, P. (2006). Underrepresented students benefit most from "engagement." *Chronicle of Higher Education*, *53*(13), A39–A40. Retrieved November 30, 2009, from Education Module (Document ID: 1191531481).

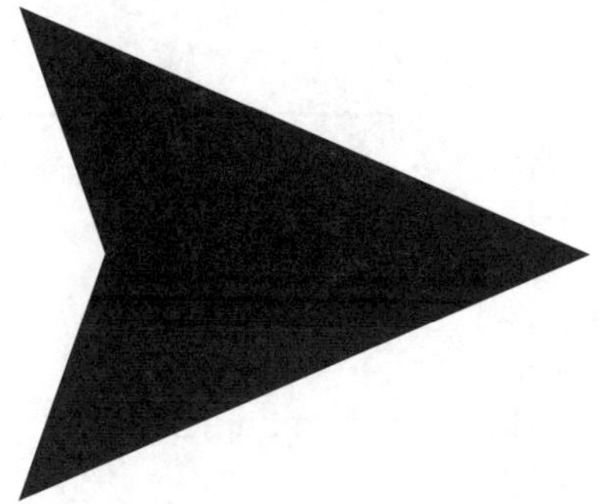

Index

360-degree effect review, 358
3M/House single-channel implant, 821
4P (deletion problem), 610
5P (Cri-du-chat syndrome), 610

A

AAA (American Academy of Audiology), 285
AABR (automated auditory brainstem response), 185
  false positives, 345
  refer rate variation, 342
  screening device parameter options, 343–346
    frequencies targeted, 343–344
    severities targeted, 343–344
  signal detection algorithms, 345
AAP (American Academy of Pediatrics), 393, 414, 818, 876
ABI (Auditory brainstem implants), 173, 175, 793
  future of, 795
Abnormalities
  environmental, 17
  external ear, 17–18
  genetic, 17
  inner ear, 18–19
  middle ear, 18
ABR (Auditory brainstem response), 143, 164, 228
  ANSD (Auditory neuropathy spectrum disorder) and, 227, 247
  auditory steady-stage response, 525–539
    air-conduction stimuli, 531–536
    analysis techniques, 525–527
    artificial, 530–531
    bone-conduction stimuli and, 536–539
    calibration of stimuli for brainstem, 529
    frequency specificity of brainstem, 529
    multiple, 528–529
    problem of new technology/methodology, 529–530
  behavioral threshold using, 507–508
  bone-conduction, 207, 516–517
    assessment, 514–516
  brainstem integrity and, 282
  central auditory processing disorders and, 570
  click, 479–480, 486–487, 517, 532, 542
    diagnostic tests, 494
    middle ear assessment and, 209
    phase-versus-frequency function, 477
    physiologic testing and, 390–391, 893
    recording recommendation, 493
    tympanometry and, 457
  cochlear hearing loss and, 228, 391
  conductive loss assessment and, 511–514
  couple bone oscillator to infant's head, 524
  defined, 228
  Down syndrome and, 617
  establishing normative data, 524–525
  frequency-specific threshold analysis, 539–540
  frequency-specificity of tone, 522
  gentamicin and, 184
  historical perspective on, 551
  implementation of new clinical techniques, 506–507, 507
  infant threshold analysis and, 505–542
  intrinsic sensitivity limitations of, 334–335
  limitations of, 339–340, 894
  maximum stimulus intensities for, 523
  newborns and, 450
  OAEs (Otoacoustic emissions) and, 485
  prenatal heroin exposure, 184
  protocols and sequence testing, 540–542
  required information, 506
  response
    could not assess, 506–507
    not present, 506–507
    presence/absence, 520–522
    present, 506–507
  screening specificity, 338–339

ABR (Auditory brainstem response) *(continued)*
stimulus onset polarity, 522–523
tone
interpretation of, 517–520
technical details, 517
tonepip, 819
transient tone-evoked, 510–511
transient vs. steady-state responses, 505–506
waveform noisiness, 520
Absolute auditory sensitivity, 67–68
thresholds, 68
ACEMg, 192
Acadian patients, 140, 141
Acetaminophen, 157, 229
Acoustic impedance measures, 615–616
Acoustic neuromas, 182
bilateral, 170
Acoustic reflex, 467
test limitations of, 468
threshold, pseudohypacusis and, 301–302
Acoustics
auditory processing disorder (APD) and, 680
children
with hearing loss and, 679
with normal hearing, 679–680
ear canal, 634–641
clinical measurements of external, 635–637
ACPT (Auditory Continuous Performance Test), 280, 287
Activity analysis vs. coverage analysis, 370
Acute otitis media, 156–157
effect of genes on, 218
risk factors for, 218–219
with effusion, 216–217
Adaptive Test of Temporal Resolution, 276
Adenoidectomy, 190, 219, 455
ADHD (Attention deficit hyperactivity disorder), 680
auditory late responses, 578–579
auditory neuropathy spectrum disorder (ANSD), 580
autism spectrum disorder, 579–580
Adolescents
bullying problems and, 876–878
cognitive development, 878–883
communication difficulties with, 873–874
audiologist's role, 873
self-assessment, 874–876
psycho-emotional development and, 871–878
responding to, 873
Adult-directed speech (ADS), rhythm/intonation effects on, 51–52
Adults, with hearing loss, 531–534
AEPs (Auditory evoked potentials), 617, 618
brainstem, 414
estimating behavioral thresholds using, 507–508
AER (Auditory evoked responses)
audio steady-state response (ASSR) and, 617
central auditory processing disorders and, 570
cochlear implants and, 766
early hearing detection and, 818
frequency specific testing and, 893
screening challenges, 892
Age-appropriate tests, 622
Age, prevalence of hearing impairment and, 94–95
Agency for Healthcare Research and Quality, 155, 156
Air-conduction hearing devices, 783
Air-conduction pure-tone average (PTA), 212
Air-conduction stimuli, 531–536
Alcohol
hearing loss and, 184–185
prenatal exposure to, 184
Alexander Graham Bell Association for the Deaf and Hard of Hearing, 415, 427, 834
Algorithms
comparison of NSL and DSL, 645–646
desired sensational level multistage input/output, 644
generic vs. proprietary, 642–643
National Acoustics Laboratories (NAL), 644–645
signal detection, 29
Allophones, 54
Alpha-lipoic acid, 192
Alport syndrome, 111, 137–138, 152, 610
hearing loss and, 438
ALR (Auditory late response)
acoustic change complex, 580–581
AMRL and, 563
anatomical changes in, 576–577
anatomic/physiologic correlates maturation, 569–570
attention deficit hyperactivity disorder, 578–579
audiologic intervention effects, 577–578
brain lesions/injury, 575–576
central auditory processing disorder (CAPD), 570–572
central auditory processing index, 572–573
changes in scalp distribution, 567–568
clinical applications of, 570
developmental changes in, 565–567
morphology/refractoriness, 568–569
electrophysiological assessment of, 551–582
future directions for clinical research, 581–582
introduction to, 562–563
language/learning difficulties, 573–575
measurement and analysis, 563
nonpathologic factors, 565

normal hearing and, 565
in pediatric populations, 565
Alternating polarity, 522–523
American Academy of Audiology (AAA), 285, 415
American Academy of Audiology (AAA) Pediatric Amplification Clinical Practice Guideline, 680
American Academy of Family Medicine, 155
American Academy of Family Physicians, 393
American Academy of Ophthalmology and Otolaryngology, 414, 818
American Academy of Otolaryngology-Head and Neck Surgery, 155, 393, 415
American Academy of Pediatrics (AAP), 393, 414, 818, 876
American Asylum for the Education and Instruction of the Deaf and Dumb, 816
American National Standard Institute (ANSI), 599, 903
American School for the Deaf, 816
American Speech and Hearing Association, 818
American Speech-Language-Hearing Association (ASHA), 269, 414, 903
Amifostine, 192
Amikacin, hearing loss and, 185–186
Aminoglycosides, 191
hearing loss and, 185–187
induced deafness, 141–142
AMLR (Auditory middle latency response), 551–562, 565, 575
brain injury and, 561
in children with normal hearing, 557
developmental changes in
anatomic correlates, 557–558
recording parameters, 558–559
state of arousal and, 559
electrophysiological assessment of, 551–582
as index of depth of anesthesia, 560
measurement and analysis, 552, 554–555
nonpathologic factors, 555
in pediatric populations, 555, 557
clinical applications of, 559–562
rationale for application in children, 551–552
vs. ALR, 563
Amoxicillin, 157
Amplification, 819–821
goals of, pediatric, 680–681
recommendations for, 906
signal audibility and, 719
speech recognition and, 715
Amplification-communication-connection, 859–866
Amplitude spectrum plots, age-related changes, 71–73
Amygdala, 872–873
AN (Auditory neuropathy), 170–173
otoacoustic emissions (OAEs), and, 492
AN/AD (Auditory neuropathy/dys-synchrony), 142
Analgesics, 176
Analysis timing, 366
Animal models
abnormal neural connections and, 28
auditory system development and, 24
classification and, 4
cochlear implants and, 739
cross-model remapping and, 576
hair cell neural transmission and, 11
hearing loss structural changes and, 892
importance of, 3
intrauterine acoustic environment in, 916
temporal bone studies and, 229
Anomalies, craniofacial anomalies, 152, 208
assessment of children with, 209–216
aural atresia, 212
cleft lip/palate and, 215–216
congenital aural atresia, 210–211
congenital CHL, 212
Down syndrome and, 215
microtia, 210–211
Anotia, 17, 890
ANSD (Auditory neuropathy spectrum disorder), 170–173, 254–264, 492, 890
amplification and, 714–715
audiologic clinical profile, 233–238
auditory
brainstem response and, 247
late responses, 580
system pathways integrity, 280–285
behavioral audiometry, 250–251
binaural processing, 276–278
brainstem responses and, 508
case studies, 241–243
cochlear implants and, 253
counseling families, 253–254
decisions guide, 251–252
diagnosis/management of, 231–233
diagnostic criteria, 248–249
hearing aids/FM systems, 251–252
identification of, 227–228
listening as active process, 278–280
management of, 247–265
mechanisms producing patterns of, 228–229
medical aspects of, 229–230
medical assessment, 251
MEMRs (Middle ear muscle reflexes), 467
physiologic measures, 249–250
prevalence of, 230–231
professional practice, 285–287
screening for, 230

ANSI (American National Standard Institute), 599, 903
Anterior cardinal vein, 5
Anteroventral cochlear nucleus (AVCN), 25
AOAEs (automated otoacoustic emissions)
  false positives, 345
  refer rate variation, 342
  screening device parameter options, 343–346
    frequencies targeted, 343–344
    severities targeted, 343–344
  signal detection algorithms, 345
APDs (Auditory processing disorders), acoustics and, 678
Apramycin, 192
Area variations, refer rates, 371
Arnold Chiari malformation, 251
Articulation Index theory, 719–721
ASHA (American Speech-Language-Hearing Association), 269, 414, 903
Ashkenazi Jews, 136, 141
Assessment information, importance of accurate, 641
Associative learning, infants, 55
ASSR (Auditory steady-state response), 143, 525–539, 819
  air-conduction stimuli, 531–536
  analysis techniques, 525–527
  artificial, 530–531
  auditory-evoked potentials (AEP) and, 617
  bone-conduction stimuli and, 536–539
  calibration of stimuli for brainstem, 529
  frequency specificity of brainstem, 529
  historical perspective on, 551
  infant threshold analysis and, 505–542
  multiple, 528–529
  problem of new technology/methodology, 529–530
  stimulus paradigms, 527–528
Asymmetric hearing, 753
Atresia, 890
  congenital aural, 213
Atresiaplasty, 177, 212, 214
Attention deficit hyperactivity disorder (ADHD), 680
  auditory late responses, 578–579
  auditory neuropathy spectrum disorder (ANSD), 580
  autism spectrum disorder, 579–580
Attention disorders, behavioral indicators, 280
Attention, increasing, 621
Audibility, 719–721
Audiologic assessment
  attendance for, 374–377
  basic approach, 374–375
Audiologists
  Early Hearing Detection and Intervention (EHDI) Guidelines and, 419–420
  educational
    adolescents/young adults and, 969–971
    advocacy by, 967
    assessment and, 966
    children and, 967–969
    defining role of, 961–971
    early intervention and, 965–966
    habilitation and, 966–967
    placement options, 963–964
  geneticists and, 133
  working with other professionals, 948–949
Audiology
  describing functioning, 944–945
  profession of, 816–817
Audiology diagnostic test
  management of, child who fails audiology diagnostic test, 154–155
  medical home and, 158
Audiometric test sessions, comparing different, 639–641
Audiometry
  behavioral, acoustic and environmental factors, 602–603
  control trials in, 602
  conventional/conditioned, 598–602, 623–624
  effects of external ear on, 637–641
  play, 598–602
    conditioned, 600–602
    speech perception and, 602–605
  pure-tone, 143, 390, 522, 599
    behavioral audiometric measures and, 594
    pseudohypacusis and, 298, 299, 300
Audition
  development access to, 831–837
    device management and, 834–835
    distance and noise in, 835–836
    involving families, 836–837
    Ling Six Sound Test, 835
Auditory assessment, optimizing, 618–624
Auditory brainstem implants (ABI), 173, 175, 793
  future of, 795
Auditory brainstem response (ABR), 143, 175, 228, 506–507
  ANSD (Auditory neuropathy spectrum disorder and, 227, 247
  auditory steady-state response, 525–539
    air-conduction stimuli, 531–536
    analysis techniques, 525–527
    artificial, 530–531
    bone-conduction stimuli and, 536–539
    calibration of stimuli for brainstem, 529
    frequency specificity of brainstem, 529

multiple, 528–529
problem of new technology/methodology, 529–530
stimulus paradigms, 527–528
behavioral thresholds using, 507–508
bone-conduction, 207
bone-conductive assessment, 514–516
brainstem integrity and, 282
central auditory processing disorders and, 570
cochlear hearing loss and, 228, 391
conductive loss assessment and, 511–514
couple bone oscillator to infant's head, 524
defined, 228
Down syndrome and, 617
establishing normative data, 524–525
frequency-specific threshold analysis, 539–540
frequency specificity of tone, 522
gentamicin and, 185
historical perspective on, 551
infant threshold analysis and, 505–542
intrinsic sensitivity limitations of, 334–335
limitations of, 339–340, 894
maximum stimulus intensities for, 523
newborns and, 450
OAEs (Otoacoustic emissions) and, 485
prenatal heroin exposure, 184
protocols and sequence testing, 540–542
required information, 506
response
could not assess, 506–507
not present, 506–507
presence/absence, 520–522
present, 506–507
screening specificity, 338–339
stimulus onset polarity, 522–523
testing, 164
tone
interpretation of, 517–520
technical details, 517
tonepip, 819
transient tone-evoked, 508, 510–511
transient vs. steady-state responses, 505–506
waveform noisiness, 520
Auditory Continuous Performance Test (ACPT), 280, 287
Auditory development
age related changes, 67–69
sources of, 68–69
cochlear implants and, 752–754
in a growing child, 753–754
normal children, 67–82
reasons to study, 67
stimulating with cochlear implant, 749–752
Auditory evoked potentials (AEPs), 302, 617, 618
brainstem, 414
estimating behavioral thresholds using, 507–508
Auditory evoked responses (AER)
audio steady-state response (ASSR) and, 617
central auditory processing disorders and, 570
cochlear implants and, 766
early hearing detection and, 818
frequency specific testing and, 893
screening challenges, 892
Auditory Fusion Test–Revised, 276
Auditory implants
cognitive status and, 799–800
future of, 793–804
listening effort/fatigue and, 800–802
SSD (Social Security Disability) and, 799
Auditory late response (ALR)
acoustic change complex, 580–581
AMRL and, 563
anatomical changes in, 576–577
anatomic/physiologic correlates maturation, 569–570
attention deficit hyperactivity disorder, 578–579
audiologic intervention effects, 577–578
brain lesions/injury, 575–576
central auditory processing disorder (CAPD), 570–572
central auditory processing index, 572–573
changes in scalp distribution, 567–568
clinical applications of, 570
developmental changes in, 565–567
morphology/refractoriness, 568–569
electrophysiological assessment of, 551–582
future directions for clinical research, 581–582
introduction to, 562–563
language/learning difficulties, 573–575
measurement and analysis, 563
nonpathologic factors, 565
normal hearing and, 565
in pediatric populations, 565
Auditory meatus, 15
external, 17
Auditory middle latency response (AMLR), 551–562, 565, 575
brain injury and, 560–561
in children with normal hearing, 557
developmental changes in, 559
anatomic correlates, 557–558
recording parameters, 558–559
electrophysiological assessment of, 551–582
as index of depth of anesthesia, 560
measurement and analysis, 552, 554–555

Auditory middle latency response (AMLR) *(continued)*
nonpathologic factors, 555
in pediatric populations, 555, 557
clinical applications of, 559–562
rationale for application in children, 551–562
vs. ALR, 563
Auditory nerve
from cochlear implant, electrophysiologic responses, 743
electrical stimulation of, 740, 742
Auditory neuropathy (AN), 170–173
otoacoustic emissions (OAEs), and, 492
Auditory neuropathy spectrum disorder (ANSD), 170–173, 227–243, 492, 890
amplification and, 714–715
audiologic clinical profile, 233–238
auditory late responses, 580
auditory system pathways integrity, 280–285
behavioral audiometry, 250–251
binaural processing, 276–278
brainstem responses and, 508
case studies, 241–243, 254–264
cochlear implants and, 253
counseling families, 253–254
decisions guide, 251–252
diagnosis/management of, 231–233
diagnostic criteria, 248–249
hearing aids/FM systems, 252–253
identification of, 227–228
listening as active process, 278–280
management of, 247–265
mechanisms producing patterns of, 228–229
medical
aspects of, 229–230
assessment, 251
MEMRs (Middle ear muscle reflexes), 467
otoacoustic emissions (OAEs), 746
physiologic measures, 249–250
prevalence of, 230–231
professional practice, 285–287
screening for, 230
Auditory neuropathy/dys-synchrony (AN/AD), 142
Auditory ossicles, middle ear, 13
Auditory pathways, childhood deafness and, 746–747
Auditory performance, of children with minimal hearing loss, 896–898
Auditory plasticity, limitations of, with cochlear implants, 754
Auditory processing
deficits, 280
described, 269–271
disorders in children, 269–289
auditory attention, 278–280
binaural processing, 276–278
current practice patterns, 286–287
neural integrity, 280–285
professional practice, 285–287
rehabilitation, 288–289
screening, 286
stimulus encoding, 271–276
Auditory processing disorders (APDs)
acoustics and, 680
position papers, 285
Auditory skills, hearing loss and, 901–902
Auditory steady-state response (ASSR), 143, 525–539, 819
air-conduction stimuli, 531–536
analysis techniques, 525–527
artificial, 530–531
auditory-evoked potentials (AEP) and, 617
bone-conduction stimuli and, 536–539
calibration of stimuli for brainstem, 529
frequency specificity of brainstem, 529
historical perspective on, 551
infant threshold analysis and, 505–542
multiple, 528–529
problem of new technology/methodology, 529–530
stimulus paradigms, 527–528
Auditory stimulation, fetus response to, 49–50
Auditory system, 5
animal models and, 24
awakening the, 740, 742–749
biologic development of, 23–45
early growth of periphery, 24–27
changes in childhood bilateral deafness, 745
evoked potential measures, 30–35
plasticity, 42–45
abnormal, 42–43
Auditory training, 288–289
Auditory tube, middle ear, 14–15
Auditory verbal therapy (AVT), 165
Auditory, thresholds, 165, 172
Audits, device, 374
Aural atresia, 17
congenital, 210–211, 364, 387, 889–890
treatment for, 212, 214, 216
Auricle, 15
Auricular fistulas, 18
Auriculocondylar syndrome, 18
Austen-Lynch model, 296
Autism spectrum disorder (ASD), 680
auditory late responses, 579–580
Automated auditory brainstem response (AABR), 185
false positives, 345
refer rate variation, 342

screening device parameter options, severities targeted, 343–344
signal detection algorithms, 345
Automated otoacoustic emissions (AOAEs)
false positives, 345
refer rate variation, 342
screening device parameter options, 343–346
frequencies targeted, 343–344
severities targeted, 343–344
signal detection algorithms, 345
AVCN (Anteroventral cochlear nucleus), 25

B

Bacterial meningitis, 890
Bacterial mumps, 890
BAHA hearing devices, 175, 176, 212, 783, 791, 907
congenital aural atresia and, 212
reconstructive surgery and, 175
Baseline cohort, 365
Basic discrimination ability, 271
Battery operated, hearing aids, 819
Battery, ingestion of, 664
BC (Bone conduction), 143
described, 781
thresholds, 143
BCDs (Bone conduction devices), 782
indications for, 781–783
vs. skin-drive devices, 783–788
BCEHP (British Columbia Early Hearing Program), 505
Beckwith-Wiedemann syndrome, 18
Behavior
operant, 592
respondent, 592–594
Behavioral audiometry, 173, 581–582
acoustic and environmental factors, 602–603
behavioral responses and, 593
measurements, 594–602
measures, pure-tone audiometry and, 594
obtaining ear-specific thresholds in, 634
optimizing audiologic assessment and, 618–624
respondent behavior, 592–594
Behavioral hearing screening, 389–390
Behavioral observation, 594
Behavioral observation audiometry (BOA), 594, 619–620
visual reinforcement audiometry (VRA) and, 619–620
Behavioral pure-tone screening, 390
Behavioral remote microphone system verification, 707
Behavioral responses
acceptable in conventional audiometry, 598
in visual reinforcement audiometry (VRA), 595–596
Behavioral testing, 893
Behavioral thresholds
estimating, 507–508
high-frequency, 69
Behavioral pure tone-screening, 390
Behind-the-ear (BTE) hearing aids, 649,727
amplification, 820
care and maintenance of, 664
CROS amplification and, 907
ear hook and, 666
earmolds and, 662
Bell, Alexander Graham, 816, 819
Bell Laboratories, 359
Benchmarks, described, 361
BiCHIP (Bilateral Children's Hearing Implant Profile), 772
Bilateral acoustic neuromas, 170
Bilateral Children's Hearing Implant Profile (BiCHIP), 772
Bilateral cochlear implants, 754–755
candidacy, 803–804
Bilateral deafness, childhood changes in, 745
Binary cutoffs, 365–366
Binaural
hearing system
developmental plasticity of, 28–29
intrinsic vs. extrinsic influences during development, 29–30
integration, 276, 277, 753
interference, 907
processing, 276–278
Birth cohort, 365
Bluetooth digital radio transmission, 683–684, 684–685
BOA (Behavioral observation audiometry), 619–620
visual reinforcement audiometry (VRA) and, 619–620
Body hearing aid, amplification, 820
Bone-anchored hearing aids (BAHA), 175, 783, 791, 793, 907
Bone-anchored implants, 793
Bone-conduction auditory brainstem response, 207
Bone-conduction stimuli, 539
brainstem ASSRs to, 536–539
Bone conduction ABR, responding cochlea isolation, 516–517
Bone conduction (BC), 781–791
described, 781
thresholds, 143
Bone conduction devices (BCDs), 173, 212, 781–791, 783
categories, 782
indications for, 781–783
implantable, 175
screenings and, 213

Bone conduction devices (BCDs) *(continued)*
semi-implantable, 214
vs. skin-drive devices, 783–788
Bone-conductive tone, ABR (Auditory brainstem response), 514–516
Bone oscillator, couple to infant's head, 524
congenital aural atresia and, 212
reconstructive surgery and, 176, 177
Bonet, Jaun Pablo, 815
Book sharing, 841
Branchiootorenal syndrome (BOR), 134, 138, 169, 213
visual inspection and, 614
Brain
cognitive development, 878–883
connecting cochlea to, 25, 27
plasticity, 42
Brain injury
auditory late responses, 575–576
auditory middle latency response (AMLR) and, 560–561
Brain lesions, auditory late responses, 575–576
Brainstem auditory-evoked potentials (AEPs), 414
Brainstem, cochlear implant, electrophysiologic responses to, 743
Branchiooculofacial syndrome, 18
Branchio-otic syndrome, 138
Branchiootorenal (BOR) syndrome, 134, 169, 213
screenings and, 213
Branchiootorenal syndrome, 18, 610
Brånemark, Per-Ingvar, 783
British Columbia Early Hearing Program (BCEHP), 505
British Society for Audiology (BSA), 269
Bronchopulmonary dysplasia (BPD), 610
BSA (British Society for Audiology), 269, 285
BTE (Behind the ear) hearing aids, 649,727
amplification, 820
care and maintenance of, 664
CROS amplification and, 907
ear hook and, 666
earmolds and, 662
Bullying, screening for, 876–878

C

CAA (Canadian Academy of Audiology), 269
CAD (Classroom audio distribution), 689
advantages/limitations of, 695–697
CAEPs (Cortical auditory-evoked potentials), 715, 721
Canadian Academy of Audiology (CAA), 269
Canadian Paediatric Society (CPA), 445
CAPD (Central auditory processing disorder)
auditory late responses, 570–572
language/language disabilities and, 560–561
Carboplatin, 191
Cardinal vein, anterior, 5
Care coordination, 153
Carhart three frequency range, 298
Carnegie stages, of embryonic period, 4, 6
CART (Communication Access Real-time Translation), 963
CASLLS (Cottage Acquisition Scales for Listening, Language and Speech), 867
CDC (Centers for Disease Control and Prevention, 145
Framework for Program Evaluation, 357
program evaluation/quality, 356–358
CEA (Cost-effectiveness analysis), 353, 377
example, 378
Centers for Disease Control and Prevention, 145
Framework for Program Evaluation, 357
program evaluation/quality, 356–358
Central auditory
brain, 36, 42, 43
development, cochlear implants and, 45
neurons, 43
development of, 28–30
plasticity, 43
processing disorder (CAPD)
ABR (Auditory brainstem response) and, 570
auditory late responses, 570–572
in children, 269–289
language/language disabilities and, 560–561
Central Institute for the Deaf, 816
CEOAE (Click evoked otoacoustic emission), 479–480, 486–487, 517, 532, 542
diagnostic tests, 494
middle ear assessment and, 209
phase-versus-frequency function, 477
physiologic testing and, 390–391, 893
recording recommendation, 493
tympanometry and, 457
Change-No Change procedure, 920
CHAPS (Children's Auditory Performance Scale), 285, 287, 571
Charcot-Marie-Tooth disease/syndrome, 142, 150, 152, 235, 262, 398, 438, 492, 746
CHARGE Syndrome, 138, 610
Chiari malformation, 610, 889, 890
Chicken model, 3
CHILD (Children's Home Inventory for Listening Difficulties), 673, 895, 946
Childhood hearing impairment
defined, 89–90
prevalence of, 91–92
variations in, 94–104
severity of, 92–93
site of, 93–94

Childhood Hearing Screening Clinical Practice Guidelines, 394
Children
auditory development in a growing, 753–754
central auditory processing disorders in, 269–289
changes in bilateral deafness, 745
cochlear implants and, 739–755
auditory plasticity limitations, 754
electrophysiological responses evoked by initial, 743–745
complex developmental conditions, audiologic assessment of, 615–618
counseling needs of, 949–950
craniofacial anomalies assessment, 209–216
cytomegalovirus (CVM) and, 182
deafness, auditory pathways and, 746–747
education hearing loss, 661–662
hearing assessment, 632–634
historical perspective on deaf, 815–816
listening effort, 800
listening needs of, 643–644
management of
who fails audiology diagnostic test, 154–155
who fails the rescreen, 154
who fails the screen, 153
who passes the screen, 154
minimal hearing loss and, 887–909
auditory skills and, 901–902
behavioral testing, 893
clinical evaluation of, 893–894
clinical management of, 902–908
etiology of, 889–892
language/cognitive skills, 899–900
learning/educational issues, 898–899
outcomes, 898–902
physiologic testing and, 893–894
prevalence of, 888–889
psychosocial skills and, 899–900
research directions, 908–909
screening/diagnostic challenges, 892–893
speech understanding, 896–898
moderate to profound hearing loss, 915–932
conceptual framework, 928
impact of listening conditions, 928
multimodal perception, 930–931
prevalence of, 916
sensory device used with, 928–930
with normal hearing, auditory late responses and, 565
otoacoustic emissions (OAEs) and, 475–498
screening, 392–393
pure-tone average and deaf, 817
school-age, 941–960
hearing loss, 942
integrating children with hearing-loss, 941
listening skills assessment, 942–944
speech perception ability, 942–943
special needs, 714–715
testing
different modalities, 943–944
intensity levels, 943
speech materials, 944
speech-to-noise ratios, 943–944
unilateral hearing loss and, localization difficulties, 896
with hearing loss
auditory brainstem implants, 175
auditory performance, 896–898
auditory neuropathy (AN), 170–173
background and protocol, 163–165
cochlear implants and, 173–175
communication abilities and, 679
congenital conductive hearing loss, 176–177
ear disease management, 175
functional auditory assessment of, 894
inner ear malformations, 177
intervention for, 821–825
laboratory assessment, 170
management of, 815–825
measuring outcomes of, 713–731
medical diagnostic evaluation, 165–167
medical management of, 173–177
otitis externa, 176
otitis media, 176
radiographic imaging, 167–170
social-emotional impact of, 944–945
state schools for, 964
Children's Auditory Performance Scale (CHAPS), 285, 287, 571
Children's Home Inventory for Listening Difficulties (CHILD), 673, 895
Children's Implant Profile (ChIP), 768, 772
Children's Outcome Worksheets (COW), 673
Children's Peer Relationship Scale, 946
ChIP (Children's Implant Profile), 768, 772
CHL. *See* Conductive hearing loss
Chomsky, Noam, 49
Chromosomal syndromes, hearing impairment and, 111
Chromosomes, described, 133
Cisplatin, 191
Classical conditioning, 592
Classroom audio distribution (CAD), 689
Classroom, induction loop systems, 820
Cleft lip and palate (CLP), 166, 215–216
eustachian tube and, 215

Click evoked otoacoustic emission (CEOAE), 390, 479, 480, 486–487, 517, 532, 542
diagnostic tests, 494
middle ear assessment and, 209
phase-versus-frequency function, 477
physiologic testing and, 390–391
recording recommendation, 493
threshold determination, 506
tympanometry and, 457
Clinical management
of minimal hearing loss, 902–908
counseling/education and, 902
daycare/school environments, 903–904
ethologic evaluation, 902–903
intervention options, 903–908
CLP (Cleft lip and palate), 166, 215–216
conductive hearing loss and, 215–216
CMV (cytomegalovirus), 113, 166, 182–183, 890
hearing loss and, 151, 437
permanent childhood hearing impairment (PCHI) and, 113
screenings and, 213
Cocaine, hearing loss and, 183–184
Cochlea
connecting brain to, 25, 27
development, 8–12
duct, 5
dysplasias, 167
ganglion, 6, 8
hearing loss, 209, 227, 318
auditory brainstem response and, 228, 391
MEMR and, 464
NICU and, 396, 404
OAE screening and, 395–396, 405
Cochlear hypoplasia, 168
postnatal maturation of, 72
sensory epithelium of, 26
tonotopic maps after chronic local excitation, 41–42
Cochlear implants, 173–175, 680, 793–794, 907–908
age and, 752
animal models and, 739
auditory neuropathy spectrum disorder (ANSD) and, 253
bilateral, 754–755
care of, 761–778
central auditory development and, 45
children and, 739–755
auditory development limitations, 752–754
electrophysiological responses evoked by initial, 743–745
described, 739
development of cranial, 821
documentation of performance, 560
evoked potential measures, 32–35
future of, 794–795
limitations of, 752–753
related to deafness, 753
related to unilateral stimulation, 753
medical home and, 157
multichannel, 821
remote microphone technology and, 702–703
stimulating auditory development with, 749–752
stimulating central auditory development, 45
structure/function of, 740
Cochlear inner hair cells, auditory neuropathy spectrum disorder (ANSD) and, 227
Cochlear lesions, tonotopic maps after, 36–39
Cochlear morphology of OAEs, 480
Cochlear nerve deficiency, 171
Cochleotopic projections. *See* Tonotopic projections
Cochleovestibular neuron, 5
Cognition, emotions and, 872–873
Cognitive development, adolescents, 878–883
Cognitive skills
hearing loss and, 899–900
minimal hearing loss and, 899–900
Cognitive status, auditory implants and, 799–800
Communication abilities, 881
difficulties of children with hearing loss and, 679
unilateral hearing loss and, 679, 887
Communication Access Real-time Translation (CART), 963
Communication bias, 852–853
Communication difficulties
adolescents, 873–874
audiologist's role, 873
self-assessment, 874–876
children
with hearing loss, 679
with normal hearing, 679–680
Communities, hearing impairment and, 99–100
Compensatory strategies, 289
Complex developmental conditions, children with, audiologic assessment of, 615–618
Compression, low-threshold, 905
Conditioned play audiometry (CPA), 594, 598–602, 622–623
control trials in, 602
speech perception and, 602–605
Conditioned play procedure, 600–602
conditioning process, 600–601
conventional play audiometry, 600–602
threshold exploration, 601
Conditioning
instrumental, 592–593

Pavlovian, 592
Conduction block, 227
Conduction, thresholds, 175
Conductive hearing loss, 207–222
assessment with ABR, 511–514
case studies, 221–222
Conference on the Deaf Child [1964], 818
Congenital
aural atresia, 213
conductive hearing loss, 176–177
cytomegalovirus (CMV), 890
hearing loss, 133, 387
Connexin-Deafness Homepage, 145
Consanguinity, as hearing impairment risk factor, 105–106
Conscious-unconscious dichotomy, 296
Continuous quality improvement (CQI), 358, 359
basic tools of, 359–361
Control trials, in visual reinforcement audiometry, 598
Conventional
audiometry, 623–624
hearing aids, 904–907
play audiometry, 598–602
acceptable behavioral responses in, 599
conditioned play procedure, 600–602
Cornelisse, Leonard, 644
Cortex
auditory connections development, 30
from cochlear implant, electrophysiologic responses, 743, 745
Cortical auditory-evoked potentials (CAEPs), 715, 721
Cost-effectiveness analysis (CEA), 353, 377
example, 378
Cottage Acquisition Scales for Listening, Language and Speech (CASLLS), 867
Council of Education of the Deaf, 415
Counseling
children/family needs, 949–950
hearing loss and, 902
Countries, hearing impairment and, 96–98
Coverage
equity of, 368
stratification in analysis, 369–370
Coverage analysis, vs. activity analysis, 370
COW (Children's Outcome Worksheets), 673
CPA (Canadian Paediatric Society), 445
CPA (Conditioned play audiometry), 594, 622–623
acceptable behavioral responses in, 599
conditioned play procedure, 600–602
control trials in, 602
reinforcement when using, 599–600
speech perception and, 602–605
CQI (Continuous quality improvement), 358, 359
basic tools of, 359–361
Cranial nerve, development, 15–16
Craniofacial anomalies, 152, 208
assessment of children with, 209–216
aural atresia, 212
cleft lip/palate and, 215–216
congenital aural atresia, 210–211
congenital CHL, 212
Down syndrome and, 215
microtia, 210–211
Crib-O-Gram, 414, 818
Cri-du-chat syndrome, 610
CROS (Contralateral-routing-of-signal) hearing aids, 907
Cross-model
changes in deafness, 745
plasticity, 30, 745
remapping, animal models and, 576
reorganization, 746, 803
Crouzon syndrome, 610
craniofacial anomalies and, 208
Cultural competency, 614
Cytomegalovirus (CMV), 113, 166, 182–183, 890
hearing loss and, 151, 437
delayed-onset hearing loss and, 182
permanent childhood hearing impairment (PCHI) and, 113

D

de Leon, Pedro Ponce, 815
DAI (Direct audio input)
receivers, directly coupled, 702
hearing aids, 649
Dandy-Walker
malformation, 251
syndrome, 169
DAT (Discrimination After Testing), 920
Daycare, 903–904
de Lange syndrome, 610
de l'Epee, Abbe, 816
Deaf and dumb, 815
"The Deaf Child," 817
Deaf children. *See* Children
Deaf mute, 815
Deaf or hard of hearing (DHH)
hearing aids
developmental outcomes, 730
fitting, 715
usage and discomfort, 723

Deafness
auditory pathways and, 746–747
defined, 89
early detection of, 817–819
DEC Recommended Practices, 844
Delayed-onset hearing loss, 154, 181, 314, 388, 398, 403
cytomegalovirus (CMV) and, 182
Deletion problem (4P), 610
Deming, W.E., 359
Deming wheel/cycle/cycle, 359
Desired Sensation Level Approach (DSL), 904
Desired sensation level input/output algorithm, 644
compared to NAL-NL1, 645–646
Desjardin, Jean, 830
Developmental Index of Auditory and Listening (DIAL), 725
Developmentally appropriate tests, 622
Device audits, 374
Diagnostic and Statistical Manual of Mental Diseases (DSM-IV), 580
DIAL (Developmental Index of Auditory and Listening), 725
DIDMOAD, 141
DiGeorge syndrome, 215, 610
Digital radio frequency transmission, 685–688, 687
Digital versus analog systems, remote microphone technology, 694–695
Direct audio input (DAI), hearing aids, 649
Direct-drive bone conduction, 783
advantages of, 784
Directors of Speech and Hearing Programs in State Health and Welfare Agencies, 415
Discrimination After Testing (DAT), 920
Disease, hearing loss and, 190
Diagnostic tests, CEOAE (Click evoked otoacoustic emission), 494
Distance, communication development and, 390, 487–489 834–835
Distortion, otoacoustic emissions (OAEs) and, 476–477, 480
recording recommendation, 493
using higher stimulus levels, 493–494
Distortion product otoacoustic emissions (DPOAEs), 320–322
Divided attention, 279–280
Division of Early Childhood (DEC) Recommended Practices in Early Intervention, 844
D-methionine, 192
Donabedian, Avedis, 351–352
Down syndrome, 135, 610
auditory brainstem response (ABR) and, 617
craniofacial anomalies and, 208
assessment, 215
eustachian tube and, 215
hearing impairment and, 111
inner ear and, 18–19
middle ear and, 18
pass-fail criteria, 395
visual inspection and, 614
Down-slanting eyes, 166
DPOAEs (Distortion product otoacoustic emissions), 320–322, 487–489
recording recommendation, 493
using higher stimulus levels, 493–494
Drugs
hearing loss and, 183–187, 191–192
prescribed, 185–186
maternal exposure to, 113
DSHPSHWA (Hearing Programs in State Health and Welfare Agencies), 432
DSL (Desired Sensation Level Approach), 644, 904
DSM-IV (Diagnostic and Statistical Manual of Mental Diseases), 580
Dual source theory
otoacoustic emissions (OAEs), 475–480
distortion, 476–477
reflection, 476
signatures/sensitivities, 477–479
Duration Pattern Sequencing Test, 286
Dysmorphic evaluation, 143

E

EABRS (Electrically evoked auditory brainstem response), 747
Ear
abnormalities, 18
cochlear development, embryology of, 8–12
disease management, 175
embryology of, 3–19
origins, 3
vestibular development, 12–13
external
abnormalities, 17–18
symptoms associated with, 231
effects of audiometry, 637–641
inner
early, 5
embryology of, 5
malformations, 212
middle
assessment of newborn, 209
auditory ossicles, 13
auditory tube, 14–15
AOM/OME and, 218

cleft lip/palate and, 215
disease and, 184
Down syndrome and, 215
prenatal alcohol exposure and, 184
characteristics of, 449–451
chronic disease, 220
disease, prevalence of, 393
disorders, OAE screening and, 395
early, 13
embryology of, 13
function, 942
hearing loss and, auditory brainstem response and, 228
immittance instrumentation, 451
implants, 793
muscle reflexes, 463–468, 617
auditory neuropathy spectrum disorder (ANSD), 467
normative studies, 464, 466–467
otitis media, 467
muscles, 13–14
postnatal development, 449–451
recommendations on, 208–209
screening, 383–405
for disorders, 393–397
purpose of, 383–387
universal newborn hearing screening (UNHS) and, 456
otic vesicle development, embryology of, 5–8
outer, inspection of, 614
Ear canal, 15
acoustics, 634–641
clinical measurements of external, 635–637
Early Hearing Detection and Intervention (EHDI)
benchmarks, 418
best practice principles, 418–419
data tracking/reporting, 431–434
described, 413
federal legislation and, 429–430
follow-up procedures, 425–427
funding/budgets for, 430–431
future directions, 439–440
goals of, 417–418
guidance for programs, 417–434
guidelines, 150, 309
history of, 413–417
later onset hearing loss, 437–439
lost to follow-up/to documentation, 434–437
principles for, 417–418
public health and, 427–429
role of audiologists, 419–420
screening protocols, 420–424
stakeholders, 427
Ear hook, pediatric, 649
"Early Identification of Hearing Impairment in Infants and Young Children," 818
Ear-specific thresholds, obtaining, 634
Early intervention (EI) programs, 829
features of, 851–857
potential of, 850–851
serving the population, 850
value of, 849–850
Early Listening Function (ELF), 836–837
Early Speech Perception Test (ESP), 252, 920
Earmolds, 662–663
care and maintenance, 663–664
material, 662
tubing, 662–663
venting, 663
Ebselen, 192
ECAP (Electrically evoked compound action potential), 172, 743, 745, 747, 751
Economic conditions, hearing loss and, 99
Ectoderm, 4
Education, hearing loss and, 902
Educational audiologists
adolescents/young adults and, 969–971
advocacy by, 967
assessment and, 966
children and, 967–969
defining role of, 961–971
early intervention and, 965–966
habilitation and, 966–967
placement options, 963–964
Edwards syndrome, 19, 610
Effectiveness, program evaluation and quality, 362–374
Efficacy, of tympanometric screening, 404
Efficiency, evaluation of, 377–380
EHDI (Early Hearing Detection and Intervention)
benchmarks, 418
best practice principles, 418–419
data tracking/reporting, 431–434
described, 413
federal legislation and, 429–430
follow-up procedures, 425–427
funding/budgets for, 430–431
future directions, 439–440
goals of, 417–418
guidance for programs, 413–417
history of, 413–417
later onset hearing loss, 437–439
lost to follow-up/to documentation, 434–437
principles for, 417–418
public health and, 427–429
role of audiologists, 419–420

EHDI (Early Hearing Detection and Intervention) *(continued)*
screening protocols, 420–424
stakeholders, 427
EHDI (Early Hearing Detection and Intervention) Guidelines, 150, 309
goals of, 417–434
EI (Early intervention) programs, 829
Electrically evoked auditory brainstem response (EABRS), 745, 747
Electrically evoked compound action potential (ECAP), 172, 743, 745, 747, 751
Electrically evoked middle latency response (EMLR), 560, 743, 745, 751
Electroacoustic
characteristics, hearing aids, 646–648
performance, verification of, 650–653
remote microphone system verification, 704–705
Electromagnetic induction, 682–683
systems, 689
Electrophysiologic threshold estimates, hearing aid fitting and, 633
Electrophysiological assessment
of AMLR (Auditory middle latency response), 551–582
of auditory late response (ALR), 551–582
Electrophysiological responses
clinical use of initial, 747, 749
evoked by cochlear implant, stimulating auditory development with, 749–752
evoked by initial cochlear implant, 743–745
from auditory nerve, 743
from brainstem, 743
from cortex, 743
from Thalamus, 743
ELF (Early Listening Function), 836–837
Embryology
of the ear, 3–19
cochlear development, 8–12
embryology of, 13
inner, 5
origins, 3
otic vesicle development, 5–8
vestibular development, 12–13
human, 3–5
Embryonic development, 4–5
Carnegie stages of, 4
EMLR (Electrically evoked middle latency response), 560, 743, 745, 751
Emotional intelligence, 871
Emotions, cognition and, 872–873
Encoding, evidence of early, 50
Endoderm, 4
Enlarged vestibular aqueduct syndrome (EVAS), 745, 890
Environmental
abnormalities, 17
toxins, 187–188
EOAE (Evoked otoacoustic emissions), 228, 301
Epidemiology, influences on services, 89
Epithelium, 5
Equity, of coverage, 368
Equivalent ear canal volume (Veq), 454–455
ESP (Early Speech Perception Test), 920
Etiology
evaluation, 902–903
factors, 106–117
changes over time, 111
genetics, 111
syndromic, 111–112
hearing loss and, 11, 889–891
evaluation, 902–903
European Consensus Development Conference on Neonatal Hearing Screening, 415
Eustachi, Bartolomeo, 14
Eustachian tube, 14–15
AOM/OME and, 218
cleft lip/palate and, 215
disease and, 190
Down syndrome and, 184
prenatal alcohol exposure and, 184
EVAS (Enlarged vestibular aqueduct syndrome), 890
Evidence-based, 392
answers, 319
approach, evaluating outcomes with hearing aids, 653
care revolutions, 350
clinical practices, 219
health care, 314
practices, 312, 356, 380, 426, 570, 856, 868, 909
prescriptions, 643
protocols, 404, 615
hearing and fitting hearing aids, 252
review, 383
revision, 771
studies, 212
techniques, 631
Evoked cortical responses, 721
Evoked otoacoustic emissions (EOAE), 228
pseudohypacusis and, 301
Evoked potential
cochlear implants in children and, 32–35
human auditory system development, 30–35
Ewing, Alexander William Gordon, 591
Excellence, need for, 349–350
External auditory meatus, 15, 17

External ear
abnormalities, 17–18
symptoms associated with, 213
development, 15
effects on audiometry, 637–641

F

FAE (Fetal alcohol effect), 18
False and exaggerated hearing loss (FEHL), 296–297
False negative, 384
OAE and ABR, 339–340, 373
False positive, 384
OAE and ABR, 343
errors, 345
OAE and ABR, 339–340
response, 594
decreasing, 621–622
Families, counseling needs of, 949–950
Family
education, hearing loss and, 659–661
experience surveys (FESs), 375–377
information, hearing loss and, 143
involving, 836–837
FAS (Fetal alcohol syndrome), 18, 610
FASDs (Fetal alcohol spectrum disorders), 18
Feeling mind, 873
FEHL (False and exaggerated hearing loss), 296–297
FESs (Family experience surveys), 375–377
Fetal alcohol effect (FAE), 18
Fetal alcohol spectrum disorders (FASDs), 18
Fetal alcohol syndrome (FAS), 18, 610
Fetuses, response to auditory stimulation, 49–50
Fifth rhombomere, 5
Fisher Auditory Problems Checklist, 285
Fixed-gain versus adaptive systems, remote microphone technology, 692–694
Flag levels, refer rates, 372
Flat panel/forced resonance transducers, 691–692
Fletcher average, 298
FM (Frequency modulation) systems, 908
FM (Frequency modulation) radio technology, 684–685
FM (Frequency modulation) systems, 251–252
Focused attention, 69, 278–280, 579, 925
immature, 78
Food and Drug Administration (FDA)
auditory implants and, 799
number of cochlear implants, 157
Forensic analysis, 367
Forensic audit, group selection, 375
Framework for Program Evaluation, 357
Frequency-specific threshold analysis, in infants and children, 539–540
Frequency specificity of the brainstem, auditory steady-stage response and, 529
Friedreich's ataxia, 152, 438, 492, 746
Frontal cortex, 878
FS (Stimulus-frequency) OAEs, 477
F-test using single-point variance, 520
Functional auditory assessment, 894
Functional, defined, 295

G

Gallaudet, Thomas Hopkins, 816
Ganglion fibers, 7
Gap junction beta, 890
Gaussian frequency shift keying (GFSK), 685–688
Gender, prevalence of hearing impairment and, 96
GeneReviews, 145
Genes, effect on AOM/OME, 218
GeneTests, 145
Genetic
abnormalities, 17
hearing loss, 133
screening, molecular, 143–144
testing for disorders, 112
Geneticists, audiologists and, 133
Genetics
hearing impairment and, 111
patterns of inheritance, 133–135
Genotype-phenotype relationships, 136–137
Gentamicin
auditory brainstem response (ABR) and, 185
hearing loss and, 185–186
Germ layers, 4
GFSK (Gaussian frequency shift keying), 685–688
Glial cells, 7
Goal statement, 356
Goldenhar syndrome, 213
craniofacial anomalies and, 208
Goldstein, Max, 816
Gray matter, 878
Great Orchestra of Christmas Charity, 430
Guide to Clinical Preventive Services, 415
Guidelines for Audiologic Screening, 394
Guillain-Barré, 262

H

Hallway conversation, 611
Handicap, defined, 894
Hard-of-hearing child, 817
HAS (High-amplitude sucking paradigm), 52
HCBDD (National Center for Birth Defects and Disabilities), 430

Head trauma, hearing loss and, 117, 152, 438
Health information, hearing loss and, 143
Health Insurance Portability and Accountability Act (HIPAA), 611
Health literacy, 881–882
  transition planning, 881–883
Health Resources and Services Administration (HRSA), 415
Healthy People 2000, 415, 428
Hearing
  asymmetric, 753
  binaural, development plasticity of, 28–29
  in complex sound environments, 79–81
    age related changes, 80–82
  development of cranial, 23–24
  restorative medical interventions, 173
  thresholds, 188
Hearing aids, 251–252, 680
  battery ingestion, 664
  battery operated, 819
  behind the ear, 649,727
    amplification, 820
    care and maintenance of, 664
    CROS amplification and, 907
    ear hook and, 666
    earmolds and, 662
  body, 820
  bone-anchored hearing aids, 175, 783, 791, 793, 907
  care and maintenance, 663–664
  case studies, 726–730
  contralateral-routing-of-signal, 907
  conventional, 904–907
  developmental outcomes, 730–731
  direct audio input (DAI), 649
  documentation of performance, 560
  effectiveness of, for individuals, 713–714
  electroacoustic characteristics, 646–648
  establishing use of, 831–834
  evaluation of, 726
  fitting, 715
  follow-up and monitoring, 668
  management of, 834–835
  over amplification, 664
  physical characteristics, 648–649
  proper placement of, 664–665
  rear-ear measurements, 650
  retention and use, 665–667
  selecting, 641–646, 649
  usage and discomfort, 723
  usage and wear, 667
  using electrophysiologic threshold estimates for fitting, 633
  validation of performance, 667–668
  variables affecting, 632
  wide dynamic range compression (WDRC) circuitry, 644
Hearing assessment
  children, 632–634
  infants, 632–634
Hearing impairment
  childhood, 89–90
  communities and, 99–100
  country and, 96–98
  genetics and, 111
    nonsyndromic, 112
  prevalence of, variations in, 94–104
  risk factors, 104–106
  severity of, 92–93
  sex ratio and, 96
  site of, 93–94
Hearing instrument. *See* Hearing aids
Hearing loss, 303
  adults, 531–534
  behavioral screening procedures, 389–390
  categories, 317–318
  children
    auditory performance and, 896–898
    auditory skills and, 901–902
    children with, auditory brainstem implants, 175
    auditory neuropathy (AN), 170–173
    background and protocol, 163–165
    clinical management of, 902–908
    cochlear implants and, 173–175
    communication abilities and, 679
    congenital conductive hearing loss, 176–177
    ear disease management, 175
    functional auditory assessment, 894
    inner ear malformations, 177
    intervention for, 821–825
    laboratory assessment, 170
    management of, 815–825
    measuring outcomes of, 713–734
    medical diagnostic evaluation, 165–167
    medical management of, 173–177
    otitis externa, 176
    otitis media, 176
    psychosocial skills and, 899–900
    radiographic imaging, 167–170
    social-emotional impact of, 944–945
  classification of, 915–916
  cochlear, 209, 227, 318
    auditory brainstem responses and, 228, 391
    MEMR and, 464
    NICU and, 396, 404
    OAE screening and, 395–396, 408

conceptual framework, 916–928
  cognitive/linguistic processing, 925–928
  perceptual representation, 919–925
  sensory primitives, 916–919
conductive, 207–222
  assessment with ABR, 511–514
congenital, 133, 387
  conductive, 176–177
counseling and education for, 659–662
cytomegalovirus (CMV) and, 182–183
delayed onset, 154, 181, 314, 388, 398, 403
  cytomegalovirus (CMV) and, 182
detection, 43–45
drugs and, 183–187
early intervention programs
  features of, 851–857
  potential of, 850–851
  serving the population, 850
  value of, 849–850
economic, conditions and, 99
etiologic factors of, 890
etiology of, 889–891
false/exaggerated. *See* Pseudohypacusis
genetic, 133
hereditary, evaluation of, 142–143
impact of, speech perception and, 918
infants, 534–536
listening needs and, 643–644
minimal
  auditory performance and, 896–898
  behavioral testing, 893
  clinical evaluation of, 893–894
  etiology of, 889–892
  functional auditory assessment of, 894
  learning/educational issues, 898–899
  outcomes, 898–902
  physiologic testing and, 893–894
  prevalence of, 888–889
  research directions, 908–909
  screening/diagnostic challenges, 892–893
  speech understanding, 896–898
moderate to profound hearing loss, 915–932
  impact of listening conditions, 928
  multimodal perception, 930–931
newborn screening. *See* Newborn hearing screening
noise and, 117, 188–189
nonoccupational, 193–194
nonsyndromic, 135–136
occupational noise, 193
ototoxic treatments and, 116–117
personal listening devices and, 193
postnatal, 189–195
prevalence of permanent, 387–388
preventable, 181–195
prevention of, 194–195
psycho-emotional development and, 871–878
rubella and, 181–182
screening and, 383–405
  methods of, 389
social-emotional impact of, 945–947
structural changes, animal models and, 892
syndromes associated with, 136–141
trauma and, 117
unilateral, 91, 119, 318–319
  academic problems, 898–899
  amplification recommendations, 906
  auditory deprivation and, 892
  auditory performance and, 896–899
  bone-conduction stimuli and, 538
  communication abilities and, 679, 887
  counseling/education and, 902
  cytomegalovirus (CMV) and, 113
  degrees of, 942
  etiology of, 889
    evaluation, 902–903
  hearing technology and, 904–908
  language and cognitive skills and, 899–900
  listening/learning need and, 954
  localization difficulties, 896
  lost to follow-up (LTF), 436
  prevalence of, 889
  psychosocial skills and, 900–901
  public health and, 429
  reorganization, 803
  screenings and, 96, 388
  structural changes, animal models and, 892
  tinnitus and, 798
  universal newborn hearing screening and, 91
  visual reinforcement audiometry, 597
  working with professionals and, 949
Hearing technology
  ongoing needs, 947–948
  types of, 904–908
Heart rate variability (HRV), listening effort and, 801
Hebbian processes, 42, 43
Hemifacial microsomia, 18, 211, 610
Hereditary Hearing Loss and Its Syndromes, 137
Hereditary hearing loss, evaluation of, 142–143
Hereditary Hearing Loss Homepage, 135, 145, 746
Heroin, hearing loss and, 183–184
Herpes, as factor in hearing loss, 151
Heteroplasmy, 135
High-amplitude sucking (HAS) paradigm, 52
High-frequency, behavioral thresholds, 69
HIPAA (Health Insurance Portability and Accountability Act), 611

HL-to-SPL transforms, 638–639
Homoplasmy, 135
HRSA (Health Resources and Services Administration), 415
HRV (Heart rate variability), listening effort and, 801
Hughson-Westlake procedure, 596, 597
Human embryology, 3–5
Human Genome Project, 144
Hunter syndrome, 152
  hearing loss and, 438
Hyperbilirubinemia, 610
Hypoplasia
  auditory nerve, 227, 233
  cochlear, 167, 168, 746, 921
  maxillary, 166
  Stickler syndrome and, 140

I

Identification and Diagnosis of Hearing Loss and Middle-Ear Dysfunction in Preschool and School-Age Children, 394
Idiopathic, defined, 295
IDS (Infant directed speech), rhythm/intonation effects on, 51–52
IEPs (Individual Education Plans), 880–881
Imaging, radiographic, children/infants with hearing loss, 167–170
Immature selective attention, 78
Immittance instrumentation, middle ear, 451
Immunocompromise, 219
Impedance measures, acoustic, 615–616
Implants, 173–175, 680, 793–794, 907–908
  age and, 752
  animal models and, 739
  auditory
    brainstem, 173
    neuropathy spectrum disorder (ANSD) and, 253
  bilateral, 754–755
  central auditory development and, 45
  children and, 739–755, 761–778
    auditory development limitations, 752–754
    electrophysiological responses evoked by initial, 743–745
  development of cranial, 821
  documentation of performance, 560
  evoked potential measures, 32–35
  future of, 793–804
  limitations of, 752–753
    related to deafness, 753
    related to unilateral stimulation, 753
  medical home and, 157
  multichannel, 821
  remote microphone technology and, 702–703
  stimulating auditory development with, 749–752
  stimulating central auditory development, 45
  structure/function of, 740
Incidence, defined, 384
Individual Education Plans (IEPs), 880–881
Induction loop systems, 682, 689
  classroom, 820
Inequity, of coverage, 368
Infant speech perception, 49–61
  birth to six months, 49–54
  six months to one year, 54–61
Infant-directed speech (IDS), rhythm/intonation effects on, 51–52
Infants
  associative learning, 55
  auditory late responses population, 565
  couple bone oscillator to head of, 524
  hearing aid fitting and, electrophysiologic threshold estimates, 633
  hearing assessment, 632–634
  with hearing loss, 534–536
    auditory neuropathy (AN), 170–173
    background and protocol, 163–165
    congenital conductive hearing loss, 176–177
    facilitating communication in, 829–845
    inner ear malformations, 177
    laboratory assessment, 170
    medical diagnostic evaluation, 165–167
    medical management of, 173–177
    otitis externa, 176
    otitis media, 176
    radiographic imaging, 167–170
  hearing loss and, measuring outcomes of, 713–731
  infant threshold analysis and, 505–542
  learning mechanisms in, 54
  listening needs of, 643–644
  mechanisms of learning by, 54–55
  with normal hearing, 534
  otoacoustic emissions (OAEs) and, 475–498
  recognition memory, 55
  sensitivity to rhythm/intonation, 50–51
  social interaction/motivation for, 56
  statistical learning, 55–56
  threshold analysis in, 505–542
  tympanometry of, 456–459
Infant-Toddler Meaningful Auditory Integration Scale (IT-MAIS), 252
Infections
  childhood, PCHI and, 118
  hearing loss and, 152, 190, 191–192
  postnatal, 114
  systemic, 115–116
Information, sources of, 144

Infrared transmission, 688
Inheritance, patterns of, 133–135
Injury, brain,
auditory late responses, 575–576
auditory middle latency response (AMLR) and, 560–561
Inner ear
abnormalities, 18–19
aplasia, 19, 167, 168
early, 5
malformations, 177
Insert receivers, 820
Instrumental conditioning, 592–593
Interference, binaural, 907
International Classification of Functioning, Disability and Health, 316
International Standards Organization (ISO), 524
Intervention options, minimal hearing loss and, 903–908
Interview, patient history, 612–613
Intonation
early speech processing and, 51–52
infants sensitivity to, 50–51
Intrinsic sensitivity limitations
of auditory brainstem response, 335–338
of otoacoustic emissions, 335–338
ISO (International Standards Organization), 524
IQWiG (Institute for Quality and Efficiency in Health Care), 416
IT-MAIS (Infant-Toddler Meaningful Auditory Integration Scale), 252

J

JCIH (Joint Committee on Infant Hearing), 104, 181, 248, 364–365, 414, 818, 824
middle ear recommendations, 108–109, 208–209
screenings and, 364–365
JCNS (National Joint Committee on Newborn Screening), 818
Jervell and Lange-Nielsen syndrome (JLNS), 138–139, 143, 152
hearing loss and, 438
Joint Committee on Infant Hearing (JCIH), 104, 181, 248, 364–365, 414, 818, 824
middle ear recommendations, 208–209
screenings and, 364–365

K

Kanamycin, hearing loss and, 185–186
Kemp, David, 475
Key performance indicators (KPIs), 360–361
KIP (Knowledge is Power Curriculum), 661–662
Klippel Feil syndrome, craniofacial anomalies and, 208
Knowledge
dissemination, 879–880
implementation, 880
Knowledge is Power Curriculum (KIP), 661–662
KPIs (Key performance indicators), 360–361

L

Landau Kleffner syndrome (LKS), 575
Language, central auditory processing disorder (CAPD), 560–561
Language disabilities, central auditory processing disorder (CAPD), 560–561
Language experience effects, on speech discrimination, 53–54
Language facilitation strategies, 839–842
Language learning
building blocks of, 837–845
strategies, 839
Language skills
hearing loss and, 899–900
minimal hearing loss and, 899–900
Language training, 289
Late-onset hearing loss, risk factors for, 151–152
Learning, mechanisms of, in infancy, 54–55
Lexical access, 925
Line array systems, 692
Ling Six Sound Test, 835
Linguistic communication, transition from prelinguistic, 844–845
Listen skills, assessment of, 942–944
Listening bubble, 836
Listening effort, 801
children, 800
heart rate variability, 801
objective estimates of, 800–802
physiologic biomarkers of stress and, 800
pupillometry and, 800–801
skin conductance and, 801–802
subjective estimates of, 802
Listening, impact of adverse conditions, 928
Listening Inventory for Education—Revised, 946
Listening needs, infants and children, 643–644
Literacy, health, 881–882
LKS (Landau Kleffner syndrome), 575
Localization difficulties, unilateral hearing loss and, 896
Logic model, defined, 355
Long-term potentiation (LTP), 42, 43, 859–866
Lost to documentation (LTD), 363
Early Hearing Detection and Intervention (EHDI), 432–437

Lost to follow-up (LTF), 363, 436
  Early Hearing Detection and Intervention (EHDI), 432–437
Low-frequency, thresholds, 27, 68
Low refer rates, 372
Low-threshold
  compression, 905
  signal detection, 24
LTD (Lost to documentation), 363
  Early Hearing Detection and Intervention (EHDI), 432–437
LTF (Lost to follow-up), 363, 436
  Early Hearing Detection and Intervention (EHDI), 432–437
LTP (Long-term potentiation), 42, 43

M

Malingering, defined, 295
Masking level difference (MLD), 247, 276
Massachusetts Department of Public Health, 436
Maternal and Child Health Bureau, 415
Maternal and Child Health Programs, 430
Maximum stimulus intensities for ABR, 523
Measuring outcomes, 713–731
  evaluation of, 715–726
Measurements
  behavioral audiometric, 594–602
  rear-ear, 650
Media literacy, 881
Medicaid, 430
Medical home, 149
  acute otitis media, 156–157
  audiology diagnostic fail, 158
  care coordination, 153
  cochlear implants and, 157
  continued surveillance, 152–153
  hearing screening, 157–158
  medical workup, 153
  middle ear disease and, 155–157
  newborn hearing screening and, 149
  risk factors for hearing loss, 151–152
  surveillance, 155
Medical interventions, hearing, 173
Medical workup, 153
MEE (Middle ear effusion), 393
MELAS, 139
MEMRs (Middle ear muscle reflexes), 463–468
    normative studies, 464
  auditory neuropathy spectrum disorder (ANSD), 467
  muscle reflexes, 466–467
    otitis media, 467
Meningitis
  bacterial, 890
  screenings and, 213
MERRF, 139
Mesoderm, 4
Metacognitive strategies, 289
Methadone, hearing loss and, 183–184
Michel aplasia, 19, 167, 168
Microphone technology, 681
  advantages/limitations of, 695–697
  cochlear implants and, 702–703
  digital versus analog systems, 694–695
  design and operation considerations, 702–703
  electromagnetic induction, 682–683
  fixed-gain versus adaptive systems, 692–694
  near-field magnetic induction, 683–684
  orientation/outcome measurement, 707–708
  performance influencing characteristics, 692–695
  signal delivery methods, 681–688
  sound-field microphone, 689–692
  technology present in
    receivers, 701
    transmitters, 697–701
  types of microphone systems, 688–692
  verification of, 703–707
Microtia, 17–19, 170, 210–211, 889–890
  surgery, 177
Middle ear
  abnormalities, 18
  assessment of newborn, 209
  auditory ossicles, 13
  auditory tube, 14–15
    AOM/OME and, 218
    cleft lip/palate and, 215
    disease and, 184
    Down syndrome and, 215
    prenatal alcohol exposure and, 184
  characteristics of, 449–451
  chronic disease, 220
  disease, prevalence of, 393
  disorders, OAE screening and, 395
  early, 13
  function, 942
  hearing loss and, auditory brainstem response and, 228
  immittance instrumentation, 451
  implants, 793
  muscle reflexes, 463–468, 617
    auditory neuropathy spectrum disorder (ANSD), 467
    normative studies, 464, 466–467
    otitis media, 467
  muscles, 13–14
  postnatal development, 449–451

recommendations on, 208–209
screening, 383–405
for disorders, 393–397
purpose of, 383–387
universal newborn hearing screening (UNHS) and, 456
Middle ear disease (OME), medical home and, 155–156
Middle ear effusion (MEE), 393
Middle latency response (MLR), 555
Minimal hearing loss, in children, 887–909
auditory performance and, 896–898
auditory skills and, 901–902
behavioral testing, 893
clinical evaluation of, 893–894
clinical management of, 902–908
etiology of, 889–892
functional auditory assessment of, 894
language/cognitive skills, 899–900
learning/educational issues, 898–899
outcomes, 898–902
physiologic testing and, 893–894
prevalence of, 888–889
psychosocial skills and, 899–900
research directions, 908–909
screening/diagnostic challenges, 892–893
speech understanding, 896–898
Minimal Pairs test, 920
Mitochondria, described, 135
Mitochondrial
disorders, 610
nuclear genes and, 112
hearing impairment and, 111
MLD (Masking level difference), 247, 276–278, 287
MLNT (Multisyllabic Lexical Neighborhood Test), 252
MLR (Middle latency response), 555
Moderate hearing loss
in children, 915–932
impact of listening conditions, 928
multimodal perception, 930–931
prevalence of, 916
sensory device used with, 928–930
Moderate to profound hearing loss, 915–932
cochlear implants and, 908
homozygous and, 136
impact of listening conditions, 928
multimodal perception, 930–32
lifetime cost of, 388
prevalence of, 94, 387
Molecular genetic screening, 143–144
Motivation, increasing, 621
mtDNA mutation, 135
Multichannel cochlear implants, 821
Multichannel devices, PTA (Pure-tone average) and, 920
Multicultural considerations, 613–614
Multifactorial inheritance, 135
Multifrequency tympanometry, 459
Multimodal perception, moderate/profound hearing loss, 930–931
Multimodal processing, 925
Multiple-comparisons problem, screening, 371–372
Multiple rescreens, 373–374
Multipoint-to-point system, 700
Multisensory communication, 802–803
Multisyllabic Lexical Neighborhood Test (MLNT), 252
Mumps, 890
Muscles, middle ear, 13–14
Myelin, 749
influence of, 568
temporal bone analysis and, 229
Myelination
age and, 31
of Schwann cells, 7
Myingoplasty, defined, 220

N

NAAL (National Assessment of Adult Literacy), 881
N-acetylcysteine, 192
NAL (National Acoustics Laboratories), 644–645
National Acoustics Laboratories (NAL) algorithm, 644–645
compared to DSL, 645–646
National Assessment of Adult Literacy (NAAL), 881
National Center for Birth Defects and Disabilities (HCBDD), 430
National Center for Evidence-Based Practice in Communication Disorders (N-CEP), 436
National Institute for Occupational Safety and Health (NIOSH), 188
National Institute of Deafness and Other Communication Disorders, 818
National Institutes of Health (NIH), 415
National Joint Committee on Newborn Screening (JCNS), 818
National Research Council, 816
Native Language Neural Commitment (NLNC), 838
NBHS (Newborn Hearing Screening Program), 350
effectiveness, 352–353
efficiency, 353–354
equity, 353
N-CEP (National Center for Evidence-Based Practice in Communication Disorders), 436
Near-field magnetic induction (NFMI), 683–684

Neckloop systems
directly coupled, 702
personal induction, 689
Neonatal intensive care unit (NICU)
cochlear hearing loss and, 396, 404
as factor in hearing loss, 151
Neonatal Screening for Early Detection of Hearing Impairment:, 416
Neonatal sepsis, 610
Neonatal, risk factors for hearing loss, 151–152
Neoplastic drugs, 191
Nerve fibres, demyelination of, 227
Nerve, development of cranial, 15–16
Neural
connections, animal models and, 28
dys-synchrony, 227
plasticity, 42
transmission, hair cell, 11
tube, 5
Neurofibromatosis, 152, 438, 793, 795
bilateral acoustic neuromas, 170
cochlear nerve deficiency and, 175
hearing loss and, 438
middle ear muscle reflexes and, 617
type II, 610
Neutral stimulus (NS), 592
Newborn
assessment of middle ear, 209
EHDI (Early Hearing Detection and Intervention)
future directions, 439–440
guidance for programs, 417–434
history of, 413–417
later onset hearing loss, 437–439
lost to follow-up/to documentation, 434–437
hearing screening, 93, 143–144
tympanometry of, 456–459
Newborn and Infant Hearing Screening: Current Issues and Guiding Principles for Action, 416
Newborn and Infant Screening and Intervention Act, 429–430
Newborn hearing screening
conceptual model, 309–312
effectiveness, 352–353
efficiency, 353–354
equity, 353
need for excellence, 349–350
population screening, 314–315
program evaluation/quality, 349–381
quality, 350–352
rules for, 312–314
Newborn Hearing Screening Program (NBHS), 350
NFMI (Near-field magnetic induction), 683–684
NHANES III, 99
NICHQ (National Initiative for Child Healthcare Quality), 437
NICU (Neonatal intensive care unit)
cochlear hearing loss and, 396, 404
as factor in hearing loss, 151
NIH (National Institutes of Health), 415
NIH-NIDCD (National Institutes on Deafness and Other Communication Disorders), 415
NIOSH (National Institute for Occupational Safety and Health), 188
NLNC (Native Language Neural Commitment), 838
NNS (Number needed to screen), 332
Noise
communication development and, 835
hearing loss and, 117, 188–189, 192–193
induced hearing loss, 117
signal detection in, 29
Nonauditory responses, 530–531
Nonoccupational noise, hearing loss and, 193–194
Nonorganic, defined, 295
Nonsyndromic
genetic PCHI, 112
hearing loss, 135–136
Normal hearing, infants with, 534
NS (Neutral stimulus), 592
Nuclear genes, mitochondrial genes and, 112
Nucleus Baha hearing system, 793
Number needed to screen (NNS), 332

O

OAEs (Otoacoustic emissions), 69, 93, 142, 164, 185, 207
abnormal, 490–491
absent, 489–490
acoustic impedance measures and, 616
applying in audiology clinic, 485–491
auditory
brainstem response and, 485
neuropathy and, 492
case studies, 495–497
click evoked, 390, 479, 480, 486–487, 517, 532, 542
diagnostic tests, 494
middle ear assessment and, 209
phase-versus-frequency function, 477
physiologic testing and, 390–391
recording recommendation, 493
threshold determination, 506
tympanometry and, 457
clinical applications of, 414
cochlear hearing loss and, 405
defined, 228

development of, 480–484
cochlear morphology, 480
diagnostic criteria, 248
dual source theory, 475–480
hearing screening sensitivity and, 334–335
in infants and children, 480–484, 632
interpretation of, 489–491
intrinsic sensitivity limitations of, 335–338
limitations of, 339–340
limited effectiveness, 302
middle ear disorder screening, 393
newborns and, 420
screening, 471
normal, 490
otitis media and, 484
otoacoustic emissions (OAEs), 746
ototoxic monitoring and, 492–493
physiologic screening procedures, 390
physiologic testing and, 894
recordings, 207
refer rate variation, 340–342
screening, 320–322
preschool/school-age, 392–393
specificity, 338–339
selection of, 420
TPP measurement, 454
updated approach, 493–495
Observation period censoring, 366
Observation, behavioral, 594
Occupational Safety and Health Administration (OSHA), 188
Occupational noise, hearing loss and, 193
OM (Otitis media)
medical home and, 155–156
with effusion, 216–217
genes effects on, 218
risk factors for, 218–219
treatment for, 219–220
tympanometric screening for, 393
OMIM (Online Mendelian Inheritance in Man), 137, 144
Online Mendelian Inheritance in Man (OMIM), 137, 144
Open-ended questions, 845
Operant
behavior, 592
conditioning, 592–593
Opportunity costs, 314, 350, 352
Organogenesis, 4
OSHA (Occupational Safety and Health Administration), 188
Osseointegration, 175, 783, 799
Osteogenesis imperfecta spectrum, 610
Osteopetrosis, hearing loss and, 438
Otic
placodes, 5
vesicle, development, 5–8
Oticon Medical bone-anchored hearing system, 793
Otitis externa, 176
Otitis media, 176
with effusion, 216–217
genes effects on, 218
risk factors for, 218–219
treatment for, 219–220
tympanometric screening for, 393
MEMR and, 467
otoacoustic emissions (OAEs), and, 484
treatment for, 219–220
with effusion, MEMR and, 467
Otoacoustic emissions (OAEs), 68–69, 93, 142, 164, 207
abnormal, 490–491
absent, 489–490
acoustic impedance measures and, 616
applying in audiology clinic, 485–491
auditory brainstem response and, 485
auditory neuropathy and, 492
auditory neuropathy spectrum disorder (ANSD), 746
case studies, 495–497
click evoked, 390, 479, 480, 486–487, 517, 532, 542
diagnostic tests, 494
middle ear assessment and, 209
phase-versus-frequency function, 477
physiologic testing and, 390–391
recording recommendation, 493
threshold determination, 506
tympanometry and, 457
clinical applications of, 414
cochlear hearing loss and, 405
defined, 228
development of, 480–484
cochlear morphology, 477
diagnostic criteria, 248
dual source theory, 475–480
hearing screening sensitivity and, 334–335
in infants and children, 480–484, 632
interpretation of, 489–491
intrinsic sensitivity limitations of, 334–335
limitations of, 339–340
limited effectiveness, 352
middle ear disorder screening, 393
newborn screening, 491
newborns and, 450
normal, 490
otitis media and, 484
ototoxic monitoring and, 492–493
physiologic screening procedures, 390

Otoacoustic emissions (OAEs) *(continued)*
physiologic testing and, 894
recordings, 227
refer rate variation, 340–342
screening specificity, 338–339
screenings and, 185, 320–322, 892
selection of, 420
TPP measurement, 454
updated approach, 493–495
Otocyst, 5
Otoscopy, visual inspection, 614–615
Ototoxic monitoring, otoacoustic emissions (OAEs) and, 492–493
Ototoxic treatments, hearing loss and, 116–117
Outer ear, visual inspection, 614–615
Overall refer rates, 371
Over amplification, hearing aids, 664
Oversight, program evaluation and quality, 380
Over-the-ear hearing aid, 820
Oxidative phosphorylation (OXPHOS), 135
OXPHOS (Oxidative phosphorylation), 135

P

Paired-comparison tests, 717
Parallel talk, 844
Parent support groups, 427
Parents' Evaluation of Aural/oral performance of Children (PEACH), 718–719
Parent's Guide to Genetics and Hearing Loss, 145
Parent-to-parent support, 427
Pass-fail criteria, 323–326
Patau syndrome, 19, 610
Patient-centeredness, 352
Patent ductus arteriosus, 610
Patient history, 610–614
interpreter use, 614
interview, 612–613
observation/interaction, 610–612
Patients, management of, 144
Pavlovian conditioning, 592
PBK (Phonetically Balanced Kindergarten) words, 252
Polychlorinated biphenyls (PCBs), 187
PCHI (Permanent childhood hearing impairment),burden of, 117–119
PDCA (Plan-do-check-act), 359
PDSA (Plan-do-study-act), 359
PEACH (Parents' Evaluation of Aural/oral performance of Children), 715, 718–719
Peak compensated static admittance (Ytm), 452
Pediatric
amplification, goals of, 680–681
ear hook, 649
prescriptive method, characteristics of, 643
Pendred syndrome, 19, 111, 139, 610
hearing impairment and, 111–112
hearing loss and, 438
Perception, categorical, 52
Perceptual representation, 919–925
hearing loss and
speech perception and, 919–924
speech production and, 924–925
speech perception and, 919
Performance measures, 348
Peri-/intraventricular hemorrhage, 610
Perinatal
asphyxia, 610
risk factors, 105, 113
Permanent childhood hearing impairment (PCHI), 117–119
Permanent childhood hearing loss (PCHL), 90–92, 109, 110, 414–415, 432–434, 437–439
Permanent hearing loss, prevalence of, 387–388
changes over time, 111
communities and, 99–100
by country, 96–98
cytomegalovirus (CMV) and, 113
diseases and, 116
genetics and, 111
global burden of, 117–119
nonsyndromic, 112
prenatal factors, 113–114
prevalence of, 94–96
risk factors for, 104–105
consanguinity as, 105–106
prenatal heroin exposure, 105
rubella and, 112–113
sex ratio and, 96
syndromic, 111–112
systemic, 116
Persistent stapedial artery, 18
Personal induction neckloop systems, 689
Personal listening devices, hearing loss and, 193
Personal remote microphone systems, 688
advantages/limitations of, 702
Personal sound-field (desktop) systems, 692
Phase-versus-frequency function—click-evoked OAEs, 477
Phoneme inventory, sensitivity to, 53
Phonemes, 53–54
Phonetically Balanced Kindergarten (PBK) words, 252
Physiologic biomarkers of stress, listening effort and, 800
Physiologic screening procedures, 390–391
audiologic assessment of, 615–618
minimal hearing loss and, 893–894

Picture books, 841
Pierre Robin sequence, 610
Pinna, 15
Pitch, defined, 73
Pitch Pattern Sequencing Test, 286
Pitch perception
  age related changes, 73–74
    sources of, 75–76
Placodes, 5
Plan-do-check-act (PDCA), 359
Plan-do-study-act (PDSA), 359
Plasticity
  auditory system, 42–45
    abnormal, 42–43
  brain, 42
  defined, 36
  limitations of using implants, 754
Platinum neoplastics, 191
Play audiometry, 598–602
  conditioned, 600–602
  control trials in, 602
  speech perception and, 602–605
Point-to-multipoint system, 700
Polychlorinated biphenyls (PCBs), 187
Polymerase chain reaction (PCR), 152,170
Posteroventral-cochlear nucleus (PVCN), 25
Postnatal
  hearing loss, 189–195
  infections, 114–115
  middle ear development, 449–451
Prelinguistic communication, 842–845
  transition to linguistic communication, 844–845
Prematurity, 890
Prenatal
  alcohol/tobacco use, hearing loss and, 184–185
  infections, 112
Preneural status of auditory system, 390
Preschool, OAEs (Otoacoustic emissions) screening, 392–393
Prescriptive algorithms, 646
  generic vs. proprietary, 642–643
Prescriptive targets, deriving, 646
Private schools, 965
Probe blockage, 340
Profound hearing loss
  in children, 915–932
    prevalence of, 916
  impact of listening conditions, 928
  sensory device used with, 928–930
Program evaluation and quality, 349–381
  attribution, 358
  basic tools of, 359–361
  CDC approach, 356–357
  continuous quality improvement, 358–362
  effectiveness, 362–374
  implementation, 357–358
  oversight and control, 380
  refer rates, 362–374
  reporting proportions, 361–362
Programmable audio input, designated, 702
Proportions, reporting of, 361–362
Prosody
  utterance-level, 56–57
  word-level, 57–59
Pseudohypacusis, 295–304
  case studies, 303
  causes/maintaining factors, 296–297
  demographics of, 296
  interviewing/counseling/referring, 303
  psychosocial considerations, 302–303
  pure-tone audiometry and, 298, 299, 300
  signs/risk factors, 297–298
  speech audiometry and, 298
Psycho-emotional development, 871–878
Psychogenic, defined, 295
Psychosocial considerations, pseudohypacusis, 302–303
Psychosocial skills
  minimal hearing loss and, 899–900
  unilateral hearing loss and, 900–901
PTA (Pure-tone average), 99, 192, 298, 794, 915
  air conduction, 212
  deaf children and, 817
  multichannel devices and, 920
  speech audiometry and, 298
  threshold shift, 784, 788
Public Health England, 416
Public health, Early Hearing Detection and Intervention (EHDI) and, 427–429
PubMed, 3
Pupillometry, listening effort and, 800–801
Pure-tone audiometry, 143, 390, 522, 599
  behavioral, 390
  behavioral audiometric measures and, 594
  pseudohypacusis and, 298, 299, 300
Pure-tone average (PTA), 99, 192, 298, 784, 794, 817, 915
  air conduction, 212
  deaf children and, 817
  multichannel devices and, 920
  speech audiometry and, 298
  threshold shift, 784, 788
Pure-tone probe acoustic reflex test, limitations of, 468
Pure-tone, thresholds, 143, 170, 172, 172–173
PVCN (Posteroventral-cochlear nucleus), 25

Q

QA (Quality assurance), 358
QC (Quality control), 358
QI (Quality improvement), 358, 359
QM (Quality management), 358
Quality assurance (QA), 358
Quality control (QC), 358
Quality improvement (QI), 358
Quality management (QM), 358
Quality, described, 350
Question mark ear, 18

R

Radio frequency microphone systems, 688–689
Radiographic imaging, children/infants with hearing loss, 167–170
Random Gap Detection Test, 276
Real-ear aided response (REAR), 650
Real-ear measurements, simulated, 650–652
Real-ear remote microphone system verification, 705–706
Real-ear unaided responses (REURs), 650
Real-ear unguided gain (REUG), 635–637
Real-ear verification protocols, 650
Real-ear-to-coupler differences (RECD), 252, 635–637, 820, 904
  normative, 640–641
Real-ear-to-dial difference (REDD), 635–637
REAR (Rear-ear aided response), 650
Rear-ear measurements, 650
Recasting, 844
RECD (Real-ear-to-coupler) difference, 252, 635–637, 820, 904
  normative, 640–641
Recognition memory, infants, 55
Recreational drugs, hearing loss and, 183
REDD (Real-ear-to-dial difference), 635–637
Refer rate variation, otoacoustic emissions (OAEs), 340–342
Refer rates
  flag levels, 372
  low, 372
  monitoring over time, 374
  overall, 371
  program evaluation and quality, 362–374
  risk-stratified, 371
  screening, 370–374
Reference equivalent threshold sound pressure levels (RETSPLs), 524, 638
Reflection, otoacoustic emissions (OAEs) and, 476, 480
Reflex measures, wideband acoustic, 468
REIG (Real-ear insertion gain), 650
Reinforcement, interval between response and, 594
Relationship of Hearing Loss to Listening and Learning Needs, 942
Relative operating characteristic (ROC), 326–328
Remote microphone technology, 681
  advantages/limitations of, 695–697
  cochlear implants and, 702–703
  digital versus analog systems, 694–695
  design and operation considerations, 702–703
  electromagnetic induction, 682–683
  fixed-gain versus adaptive systems, 692–694
  near-field magnetic induction, 683–684
  orientation/outcome measurement, 707–708
  performance influencing characteristics, 692–695
  signal delivery methods, 681–688
  sound-field microphone, 689–692
  technology present in
    receivers, 701
    transmitters, 697–701
  types of microphone systems, 688–692
  verification of, 703–707
Rescreens, multiple, 373–374
Residual noise, 520
Respiratory distress syndrome, 610
Respondent behavior, 592–594
Responses
  behavioral
    acceptable in conventional audiometry, 598
    in Visual reinforcement audiometry (VRA), 595–596
  decreasing false, 621–622
  false, 594
  interval between reinforcement and, 594
  judging, 620–621
  thresholds, 187
  transient vs. steady-state, 505–506
Restorative medical interventions, hearing, 173
RETFLs (Reference equivalent threshold force levels), 524
Retinitis pigmentosa (RP), 140–141
Retrocochlear hearing loss, 405
RETSPLs (Reference equivalent threshold sound pressure levels), 524, 638
REUG (Real-ear unguided gain), 635–637
REURs (Real-ear unaided responses), 650
Rhombomere, 5
Rhythm
  early speech processing and, 51–52
  infants sensitivity to, 50–51
Risk factors
  for hearing impairment, 104–106, 151–152
    consanguinity as, 105–106
    perinatal, 105
Risk-stratified refer rates, 371

Routines, value of, 839–840
RP (Retinitis pigmentosa), 140–141
Rubella, 19, 112–113, 181–183
as factor in hearing loss, 151
permanent childhood hearing impairment (PCHI) and, 112–113

S

SAC-A (Self-assessment of communication: adolescents), 874–876
Salicylate, 192
School-age children, 941–960
hearing loss, 942
integrating children with hearing-loss, 941
listening skills assessment, 942–944
OAEs (Otoacoustic emissions) screening, 392–393
speech perception ability, 942–943
testing
different modalities, 943–944
intensity levels, 943
speech materials, 944
speech-to-noise ratios, 943–944
School environment, 903–904
Schools
for deaf children
private, 965
state, 965
Schwann cell myelination, 7
Screened, described, 364
Screening, 286
activity analysis vs. coverage analysis, 370
beyond newborn period, 388–389
characteristics of, 383–387
coverage
equity of, 368–369
stratification in analysis, 369–370
date cohorts, 370–371
device audits, 374
devices, parameter options, 343–346
forensic analysis, 367
goal of, 362–363
for hearing loss, 383–405, 387–393
behavioral procedures, 389–390
methods of, 389
measurement of coverage, 363–367
age distributions, 365–366
analysis timing, 366
binary counts/ratings, 364–365
cohort definition, 365
observation period censoring, 366
target population, 363–364
multiple-comparisons problem, 371–372
multiple rescreens, 373–374
physiologic, 615–618
purpose of, 383–387
refer rates, 370–374
area variations, 371
flag levels, 372
low, 372
subgroup analyses, 371
screening
date cohorts, 370–371
overall and risk-stratified, 371
tympanometric, 393–395, 405, 456
efficacy of, 404
tympanometry, 456
unsuccessful, 370
variations analysis, 369
Screening Identification for Targeting Educational Risk, 285
Screening programs
core values, 356
described, 354–356
EHDI (Early hearing detection and intervention)
described, 413
future directions, 439–440
guidance for programs, 413–417
later onset hearing loss, 437–439
lost to follow-up/to documentation, 434–437
goals, 356
logic models, 355
objectives and evaluation, 356
structure-process-outcome model, 354–355
Screening tests
acceptable, 320–322
challenges, 332–343
efficacy of, 322–332
accuracy, 332
impact of fail/pass results, 329–331
likelihood ratios, 331–332
operating characteristic, 326–328
pass-fail criteria, 323–326
selecting full criteria, 328
sensitivity/specificity, 323
reporting, 329
target disorder definition and, 329
limitations of, OAE and ABR, 339–340
measures of, 322–332
SDT/SAT (Speech detection/awareness thresholds), 624–625
Secondary School Survey, 946
Seewald, Richard, 644
Segmental information, described, 51–52
Segmentation, speech, 50, 57–58
allophones and, 54
nonphonetically based clues, 60–61
subphonemic clues/information, 60

Self-advocacy, 289
  skills, 880–881
    health literacy, 881–882
Self-assessment of communication: adolescents (SAC-A), 874–876, 946
Self-efficacy, elements of, 837
Semicircular canals, 5
Sensitivities, otoacoustic emissions (OAEs) and, 477–479
Sensitivity
  defined, 384
  tympanometry, 455–456
Sensory
  placodes, 5
  primitives, 916–919
Sequencing, time to present next signal, 594
Sex, prevalence of hearing impairment and, 96
Shewhart wheel/cycle/cycle, 359
Signal detection
  algorithms, 29
  in noise, 29
Signal quality, improving, 288
Signal-to-noise ratio, 520–521
Signatures, otoacoustic emissions (OAEs) and, 477–479
SII (Speech Intelligibility Index) model, 719–721
Simulated real-ear measurements, 650–652
Single-frequency
  tympanometry, 459–460
  gene syndrome, hearing impairment and, 111
  point variance, 520
  polarity, 522–523
Skin conductance, listening effort and, 801–802
Skin-drive bone conduction, 783–788
SNHL (Sudden sensory/neural hearing loss), 890
Social drugs, hearing loss and, 183
Sodium thiosulfate, 192
Sound
  hearing in complex environments, 79–82
  representations of, 69
    spectral, 69–73
  temporal representation development, 73–78
Sound-field
  (desktop) systems, 692
    advantages/limitations of, 695–697
  remote microphone systems, 689–692
Spatial hearing
  age related changes, 78–79
    sources of, 79
Specificity
  defined, 384
  tympanometry, 455–456
Spectral resolution, 272
Speech audiometry, 300–301, 614
  optimizing audiologic assessment and, 624–626
  pseudohypacusis and, 298
Speech, best practices for assessment of, 802–803
Speech discrimination, language experience effects on, 53–54
Speech Intelligibility Index (SII) model, 719–721
Speech perception, 625–626, 916–918
  cochlear implants and, 749–750
  conditioned play audiometry and, 602–605
  described, 49
  hearing loss and, 918
  infant
    birth to six months, 49–54
  perceptual representation and, 919–925
  skills, 925
Speech processing
  intonation and, 51–52
  rhythm and, 51–52
Speech production, 918
  hearing loss and, 918–919
Speech recognition, amplification and, 715
Speech recognition threshold (SRT), 298, 625–626
Speech segmentation, 50, 57–58
  allophones and, 54
  nonphonetically based clues, 60–61
  subphonemic clues/information, 60
Speech-to-noise ratios, testing, 943–944
Speech training, 289
SPO (Structure-process-outcome model), 354–355
Spontaneous OAEs (SOAEs), 480
SRT (Speech recognition threshold), 298, 625–626
SSD (Social Security Disability), auditory implants and, 799
St. Joseph's School for the Deaf, 816
Staggered Spondaic Word Test, 279
Standard deviation ratio, 520–521
Standards, described, 361
State schools, for deaf children, 965
Static admittance, 452
Statistical learning, infants, 55–56
Steady-state responses
  auditory brainstem response (ABR), 525–539
  vs. transient, 505–506
Stenger test, 301
Step size, 597–598
Steven's Power Law, 644
Stickler syndrome, 139–140, 610
Stimulus-frequency (FS) OAEs, 477
Stimulus onset polarity, 522–523
Stimulus rate, 558
Strength-Weakness-Opportunity-Threat (SWOT), 431, 437

Streptomycin, hearing loss and, 185–186
Structure-process-outcome model (SPO), 354–355
Subgroup analyses, refer rates, 371
Subjective report measures, 717–719
Subphonemic
  clues, speech segmentation, 60
  information, speech segmentation and, 60
Sudden sensory/neural hearing loss (SNHL), 890
Suprasegmental information, 50
  organizing, 56–59
Sustained attention, 280
Sustained errors, OAE and ABR, 339
SWOT (Strength-Weakness-Opportunity-Threat), 431, 437
Symptomatic cytomegalovirus (CMV), screenings and, 213
Syphilis, as factor in hearing loss, 151
Systemic infections, 115–116

T

Targets, described, 361
Tectorial membrane
  development of, 26
  maturation of, 24
Teenagers
  bullying problems and, 876–878
  cognitive development, 878–883
  communication difficulties with, 873–874
    audiologist's role, 873
    self-assessment, 874–876
  psycho-emotional development and, 871–878
  responding to, 873
Temporal bone studies
  animal models and, 229
  myelin and, 229
Temporal resolution, 76–78, 234, 237, 238, 275–276, 918
  age related changes, 76–77
    sources of, 77–78
  defined, 76
TEOAE (Transient-evoked otoacoustic emissions). 479–480, 486–487, 517, 532, 542
  diagnostic tests, 494
  middle ear assessment and, 209
  phase-versus-frequency function, 477
  physiologic testing and, 390–391, 893
  recording recommendation, 493
  tympanometry and, 457
Teratogens, 17
Test of Everyday Attention for Children (TEA-Ch), 280
Test outcomes, 348
Thalamocortical pathways, 743, 745
Thalamus, from cochlear implant, electrophysiologic responses, 743, 745
"The Deaf Child," 817–819
Thinking mind, 873
Third National Health and Safety Examination Survey, 99
Threat-Opportunity-Weakness-Strength (TOWS), 431, 437
Threshold analysis, in infants, 505–542
Threshold determination, click evoked otoacoustic emissions, 506
Threshold estimation
  AMLR (Auditory middle latency response) and, 559
  electrophysiologic, infant hearing aid fitting and, 633
Threshold, described, 598
Thresholds
  absolute, 68–69
    auditory, 68
  auditory, 165, 172
  behavioral, 69
  bone conduction, 143
  conduction, 175
  ear-specific, obtaining, 634
  estimating behavioral, 507–508
  low-frequency, 27, 68
  pure-tone, 143, 170, 172–173
  response, 187
Time-averaged CEOAE waveform, 486
Tinnitus, 42–43
  suppression, 798–799
Tobacco, hearing loss and, 184–185
Toddlers. *See* Infants
Tone-ABR waveforms, 517
  frequency specificity of, 522
  interpretation of, 517–520
Tonepip ABRs, 819
Tonotopic map
  reorganization
    after chronic local excitation of neonatal cochlea, 41–42
    after cochlear lesions, 36–39
    at subcortical levels, 39–41
Tonotopic projections, plasticity of, 36
TORCH, 181
Total quality management (TQM), 358, 359
Townes and Brocks syndrome, 18
TOWS (Threat-Opportunity-Weakness-Strength), 431, 437
Toxins, environmental, 187–188
Toxoplasmosis, as factor in hearing loss, 151
TPP (Tympanometric peak pressure), 454
TQM (Total quality management), 358, 359

Transcranial CROS, 907
Transcription factors, 5
Transforms, HL-to-SPL, 638–639
Transient errors, OAE and ABR, 339
Transient-evoked otoacoustic emissions. 390, 479, 480, 486–487, 517, 532, 542
Transient responses, vs. steady-state, 505–506
Transient tone-evoked ABR, 508, 510–511
  diagnostic tests, 494
  middle ear assessment and, 209
  phase-versus-frequency function, 477
  physiologic testing and, 390–391
  recording recommendation, 493
  threshold determination, 506
  tympanometry and, 457
Transmitters, remote microphone technology, 697–701
Trauma
  head, hearing loss and, 152, 438
  hearing loss and, 117, 190–191
Treacher Collins syndrome, 17, 134, 213, 610
  visual inspection and, 614
Trisomy 13, 610
  inner ear and, 19
Trisomy 18, 19, 610
Trisomy 21, 135, 610
  craniofacial anomalies assessment, 215
  inner ear and, 18–19
  middle ear and, 18
True negative, 384
True positive, 384
Turner syndrome, 135
  hearing impairment and, 111
TW (Tympanometric width), 452
Tympanic
  cavity, 14–15
  membrane, 15
    reconstruction of, 220–221
Tympanogram, 615
  quantified, 394
Tympanometric
  peak compensated static admittance (Ytm), 452
  peak pressure, 454
  shapes, 451–452
  width, 452
Tympanometry, 394–395
  0.226-kHz, 456–457
  0.66- and 1kHz, 457–459
  multi-frequency, 459
  newborns and infants, 456–459
  screening, 393–395, 405, 456
    efficacy of, 404
  sensitivity/specificity reporting, 455–456
  single-frequency, 459–460
    measurements, 451–455
  wideband acoustic immittance, 459–463
Tympanostomy, 155
  tubes, 156, 165, 176, 190, 255, 454, 455

U

Unconditional stimulus (UCS), 592
"Understanding the Genetics of Deafness: A Guide for Patients and Families," 145
UNHS (Universal newborn hearing screening), 91–92
  English data, 91–92, 94–95
  middle ear and, 456
  prevalence by, 100–104
Unilateral hearing loss, 91, 119, 318–319
  academic problems, 898–899
  amplification recommendations, 906
  auditory
    deprivation and, 892
    performance and, 896–899
  bone-conduction stimuli and, 538
  communication abilities and, 679, 887
  counseling/education and, 902
  cytomegalovirus (CMV) and, 113
  degrees of, 942
  etiology of, 889
    evaluation, 902–903
  hearing technology and, 904–908
  language and cognitive skills and, 899–900
  listening/learning need and, 954
  localization difficulties, 896
  lost to follow-up (LTF), 436
  prevalence of, 889
  psychosocial skills and, 900–901
  public health and, 429
  reorganization, 803
  screenings and, 96, 388
  structural changes, animal models and, 892
  tinnitus and, 798
  universal newborn hearing screening and, 91
  visual reinforcement audiometry, 597
  working with professionals and, 949
Universal newborn hearing screening (UNHS), 91–92
  English data, 91–92, 94–95
  middle ear and, 456
  prevalence by, 100–104
  Position Statement from the Canadian Pediatric Society, 416
U.S. Preventive Services Task Force (USPSTF), 415
Usher syndrome, 140–141, 610
  confirmation of, 140
  genes associated with, 141

hearing impairment and, 111
hearing loss and, 438
USPSTF (U.S. Preventive Services Task Force), 415
Utterance-level prosody, 56–57
Utterances, 56

V

Van Camp, Guy, 145
Variations analysis, screening, 369
Velocardiofacial syndrome, 18
Veq (Equivalent ear canal volume), 454–455
Verbal rehearsal speed, 925
Verification
behavioral remote microphone system verification, 707
electroacoustic remote microphone system verification, 704–705
real-ear remote microphone system verification, 705–706
Vestibular
ganglion, 6
system, 5
Vestibulocochlear ganglion, 16
Viral mumps, 890
Visual inspection, outer ear/otoscopy, 614–615
Visual reinforced operant conditioning audiometry (VROCA), 390
Visual reinforcement audiometry (VRA), 390, 595–598
acceptable behavioral responses in, 595–596
behavioral observation audiometry and, 620–622
control trials in, 598
conventional audiometry, reinforcement when using, 599–600
Hughson-Westlake procedure, 596
reinforcement operations in, 596
starting level, 597
step size, 597–598
training the response for, 596–597
trial duration, 597–598
VOICE for Hearing Impaired Children, 427
Voice onset time (VOT), 52
Volta Bureau, 816
VOT (Voice onset time), 52
VRA (Visual reinforcement audiometry), 390, 595–598
acceptable behavioral responses in, 595–596
behavioral observation audiometry and, 620–622
control trials in, 598
conventional audiometry, reinforcement when using, 599–600
Hughson-Westlake procedure, 596
reinforcement operations in, 596
starting level, 597
step size, 597–598
training the response for, 596–597
trial duration, 597–598
VROCA (Visual reinforced operant conditioning audiometry), 390

W

Waardenburg syndrome, 134, 140, 141, 152, 610
hearing loss and, 438
WAI (Wideband acoustic immittance), 459–463
Walsh, James T., 415, 429–430
Walsh Act, 415, 429–430
Waveform
noisiness, 520
presence/absences, 520–522
WBA (Wideband absorbance), 461–463
WDRC (Wide dynamic range compression) circuitry, hearing aid, 644
White House Summit on Bullying, 876
WHO (World Health Organization), 312, 362, 416
hearing impairment and, 97
International Classification of Functioning, Disability and Health, 316
Wide dynamic range compression (WDRC) circuitry, hearing aid, 644
Wideband absorbance (WBA), 461–463
Wideband
acoustic immittance (WAI), 459–463
acoustic reflex measures, 468
Wolfram syndrome, 141
Word-level prosody, 57–59
Working memory, 925
World Health Organization (WHO), 312, 362, 416
hearing impairment and, 97
International Classification of Functioning, Disability and Health, 316

X

X-linked
deafness, 18
syndromes, hearing impairment and, 111

Y

Y_{tm} (Peak compensated static admittance), 452

Z

Zebrafish model, 5